Bruno Lunenfeld, M.D.

Patricia Payne Mahlstedt, Ed.D.

Alejandro Manzur, M.D.

Dan C. Martin, M.D.

Paul G. McDonough, M.D.

Kathryn F. McGonigle, M.D.

Susan R. Miller, Sc.D.

Daniel R. Mishell, Jr., M.D.

Kamran S. Moghissi, M.D.

Mahmood Morshedi, Ph.D., CTBS, MT (CA)

Ana A. Murphy, M.D.

Robert S. Neuwirth, M.D.

Alan S. Penzias, M.D.

Roger J. Pepperell, M.D.

James S. Prihoda, M.D.

Jaron Rabinovici, M.D.

Valerie S. Ratts, M.D.

Robert W. Rebar, M.D.

Daniel H. Riddick, M.D., Ph.D.

John A. Rock, M.D.

Allen W. Root, M.D.

Zev Rosenwaks, M.D.

Timothy C. Rowe, M.D., F.R.C.S.(C)

Roger C. Sanders, M.D.

Joseph G. Schenker, M.D.

William D. Schlaff, M.D.

Sheldon J. Segal, Ph.D., D.Sc.

Jillian Shaw, Ph.D.

Alvin M. Siegler, M.D.

Yolanda R. Smith, M.D.

Susan J. Spencer, M.D.

Robert J. Stillman, M.D.

Dale Stovall, M.D.

Thomas L. Toth, M.D.

Alan Trounson, Ph.D.

John E. Tyson, M.D.

Lucinda L. Veeck, MLT, D.Sc. (hon)

Kenneth K. Vu, M.D.

Edward E. Wallach, M.D.

Don P. Wolf, Ph.D.

Susan Macduff Wood, M.A.

Samuel S. C. Yen, M.D., D.Sc.

Howard A. Zacur, M.D., Ph.D.

Peter K. Zucker, M.D.

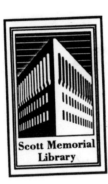

REPRODUCTIVE
Medicine and Surgery

Edward E. Wallach, M.D.

J. Donald Woodruff Professor and Chairman
Department of Gynecology and Obstetrics
The Johns Hopkins University School of Medicine
Baltimore, Maryland

Howard A. Zacur, M.D., Ph.D.

Associate Professor and Director
Division of Reproductive Endocrinology
Department of Gynecology and Obstetrics
The Johns Hopkins University School of Medicine
Baltimore, Maryland

with 616 illustrations

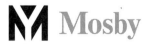

St. Louis Baltimore Boston Carlsbad Chicago Naples New York Philadelphia Portland
London Madrid Mexico City Singapore Sydney Tokyo Toronto Wiesbaden

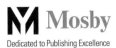

Mosby
Dedicated to Publishing Excellence

A Times Mirror Company

Editor: Stephanie Manning
Developmental Editor: Carolyn Malik
Project Manager: John Rogers
Production Editor: Chuck Furgason
Designer: Renée Duenow
Manufacturing Manager: Theresa Fuchs
Cover design: Carolyn Duffy

Printed in the United States of America
Composition by Carlisle Communications, Ltd.
Printing/binding by Maple Vail Book Mfg

Mosby–Year Book, Inc.
11830 Westline Industrial Drive
St. Louis, Missouri 63146

Library of Congress Cataloging in Publication Data

Reproductive medicine and surgery / [edited by] Edward E. Wallach,
    Howard A. Zacur.— 1st ed.
        p. cm.
    Includes bibliographical references and index.
    ISBN 0-8016-7504-9
        1. Generative organs—Diseases. 2. Generative organs—Surgery.
    3. Infertility. 4. Human reproduction. 5. Human reproductive
    technology. I. Wallach, Edward E., II. Zacur, Howard A.
        [DNLM: 1. Infertility—therapy. 2. Infertility—diagnosis.
    3. Reproduction Techniques. 4. Genital Diseases, Female. WP 570
    R4255 1994]
    RC875.R47 1994
    616.6'5—dc20
    DNLM/DLC
    for Library of Congress   94-29456
                                                                          CIP

95 96 97 98 99 / 9 8 7 6 5 4 3 2 1

CONTRIBUTORS

Anibal A. Acosta, M.D.
The Jones Institute
Eastern Virginia Medical School
Norfolk, Virginia

Eli Y. Adashi, M.D.
Professor and Director
Division of Reproductive Endocrinology
Departments of Obstetrics/Gynecology and Physiology
University of Maryland School of Medicine
Baltimore, Maryland

Barry D. Albertson, Ph.D.
Associate Professor
Department of Medicine
Division of Endocrinology, Diabetes and Clinical Nutrition
Oregon Health Sciences University
Portland, Oregon

Deborah I. Arbit, M.D.
Developmental Endocrinology Branch
National Institute of Child Health and Human Development
National Institutes of Health
Bethesda, Maryland

Ricardo H. Asch, M.D.
Professor
Department of Obstetrics and Gynecology
Assistant Dean of Outreach
College of Medicine
University of California, Irvine
University of California, Irvine Medical Center
Orange, California

Ricardo Azziz, M.D.
Associate Professor
The University of Alabama at Birmingham
Department of Obstetrics and Gynecology
Division of Reproductive Biology and Endocrinology
Birmingham, Alabama

Jose P. Balmaceda, M.D.
Professor, Director
Division of Reproductive Endocrinology and Infertility
Department of Obstetrics and Gynecology
University of California, Irvine
University of California, Irvine Medical Center
Orange, California

Robert L. Barbieri, M.D.
Kate Macy Ladd Professor of Obstetrics, Gynecology
    and Reproductive Biology
Harvard Medical School
Chairman, Department of Obstetrics and Gynecology
Brigham and Women's Hospital
Boston, Massachusetts

John R. Brumsted, M.D.
Associate Professor
Director, Division of Reproductive Endocrinology and Infertility
Head, Section of Gynecology
University of Vermont College of Medicine
Burlington, Vermont

Trudy L. Bush, Ph.D., M.H.S.
Professor
Departments of Epidemiology and Preventative Medicine
University of Maryland
Department of Epidemiology
Johns Hopkins School of Hygiene and Public Health
Baltimore, Maryland

Sue Ellen Carpenter, M.D.
Associate Professor
Director, Pediatric and Adolescent Gynecology
Department of Gynecology and Obstetrics
Emory University School of Medicine
Atlanta, Georgia

Abraham T. K. Cockett, M.D.
Professor and Chairman
Department of Urology,
The University of Rochester Medical Center
Rochester, New York

David S. Cooper, M.D.

Director, Division of Endocrinology
Sinai Hospital of Baltimore
Associate Professor of Medicine
Johns Hopkins School of Medicine
Baltimore, Maryland

Randle S. Corfman, M.D., Ph.D.

The Midwest Center for Reproductive Health
St. Louis Park, Minnesota

Glenn R. Cunningham, M.D.

Professor of Medicine
Baylor College of Medicine
Veterans Affairs Medical Center
Houston, Texas

Marian D. Damewood, M.D.

Associate Director
Women's Hospital Fertility Center and IVF Program
Greater Baltimore Medical Center
Associate Professor
Department of Gynecology and Obstetrics
Johns Hopkins University School of Medicine
Baltimore, Maryland

Owen K. Davis, M.D.

Assistant Professor of Obstetrics/Gynecology
Department of Obstetrics/Gynecology
Cornell University of Medical College
New York, New York

Alan H. DeCherney, M.D.

Louis E. Phaneuf Professor and Chairman
Department of Obstetrics and Gynecology
Tufts University School of Medicine
New England Medical Center Hospitals
Boston, Massachusetts

Michael P. Diamond, M.D.

Director
Division of Reproductive Endocrinology
Associate Professor
Departments of Obstetrics and Gynecology, Surgery
    and Molecular Physiology and Biophysics
Vanderbilt University
Nashville, Tennessee

Patrica K. Donahoe, M.D.

Professor of Surgery
Harvard Medical School
Cambridge, Massachusetts

Gustavo F. Doncel, M.D., Ph.D.

Head, Sperm Biology and Contraceptive Research Laboratory
The Jones Institute for Reproductive Medicine
Norfolk, Virginia

Nicole Fournet, M.D.

Fellow
Division of Reproductive Endocrinology
Department of Obstetrics and Gynecology
UCLA School of Medicine
Los Angeles, California

Victor Gomel, M.D., F.R.C.S. (C)

Professor
Department of Obstetrics and Gynecology
Faculty of Medicine
University of British Columbia
Vancouver Hospital and Health Sciences Centre
British Columbia's Women's Hospital
    and Health Centre
Vancouver, British Columbia
Canada

Sandra B. Goodman, M.D.

Instructor
Division of Reproductive Endocrinology
Department of Gynecology and Obstetrics
The Johns Hopkins Medical Institutions
Baltimore, Maryland

Michael L. Gustafson, M.D.

Division of Pediatric Surgery
Massachusetts General Hospital
Boston, Massachusetts

Jacqueline N. Gutmann, M.D.

Clinical Assistant Professor
University of Pennsylvania
School of Medicine
Philadelphia Fertility Institute
Philadelphia, Pennsylvania

Gilbert G. Haas, Jr., M.D.

Professor and Chief
Section of Reproductive Endocrinology and Infertility
Department of Obstetrics and Gynecology
University of Oklahoma Health Sciences Center
Oklahoma City, Oklahoma

Jouko Halme, M.D., Ph.D.

Director
North Carolina Center for Reproductive Medicine
Cary, North Carolina

John S. Hesla, M.D.

Associate Professor
Department of Obstetrics and Gynecology
Director, Assisted Reproductive Technologies
Emory University School of Medicine
Atlanta, Georgia

Gary D. Hodgen, Ph.D

President, The Jones Institute of Reproductive Medicine
Professor, Department of Obstetrics and Gynecology
Eastern Virginia Medical School
Norfolk, Virginia

George R. Huggins, M.D.

Associate Professor
Department of Obstetrics and Gynecology
The Johns Hopkins Bayview Medical Center
Johns Hopkins University
Baltimore, Maryland

Scot M. Hutchison, M.D.

Assistant Professor
Division of Reproductive Endocrinology
Department of Gynecology and Obstetrics
The Johns Hopkins Medical Institutions
Baltimore, Maryland

Vaclav Insler, M.D., F.R.C.O.G.

Professor of Obstetrics and Gynecology,
Hebrew University and Hadassah Medical School,
    Jerusalem
Director, Department of Obstetrics and Gynecology,
Kaplan Hospital
Rehovot, Israel

Robert B. Jaffe, M.D.

Director
Reproductive Endocrinology Center
Professor and Chairman
Department of Obstetrics and Gynecology
    and Reproductive Sciences
University of California, San Francisco
San Francisco, California

Raphael Jewelewicz, M.D.

Chairman, Department of Obstetrics and Gynecology
Maimonides Medical Center
Professor of Obstetrics and Gynecology
State University of New York
Health Science Center at Brooklyn
Brooklyn, New York

Howard W. Jones, Jr., M.D.

Professor of Obstetrics and Gynecology
Eastern Virginia Medical School
Norfolk, Virginia
Professor Emeritus of Gynecology and Obstetrics
Johns Hopkins University School of Medicine
Baltimore, Maryland

Warren R. Jones, M.D., Ph.D.

Department of Obstetrics and Gynecology
Flinders Medical Center
Bedford Park
South Australia

Howard L. Judd, M.D.

Division of Reproductive Endocrinology
Department of Obstetrics and Gynecology
UCLA School of Medicine
Los Angeles, California

L. Michael Kettel, M.D.

Assistant Professor
Director, Infertility Services
Department of Reproductive Medicine
University of California, San Diego
UCSD Medical Center
San Diego, California

Oscar A. Kletzky, M.D.

Department of Obstetrics and Gynecology
Harbor UCLA Medical Center
Torrance, California

Lawrence C. Layman, M.D.

Assistant Professor
Division of Reproductive Endocrinology
Department of Obstetrics and Gynecology
New England Medical Center
Tufts University School of Medicine
Boston, Massachusetts

Paul W. Ladenson, M.D.

Associate Professor
Department of Internal Medicine
Director, Division of Endocrinology and Metabolism
Johns Hopkins University School of Medicine
The Johns Hopkins Hospital
Baltimore, Maryland

Robert Lindsay, M.B.Ch.B., Ph.D., F.R.C.P.

Chief, Internal Medicine
Helen Hayes Hospital
West Haverstraw, New York
Professor of Clinical Medicine
Columbia University
College of Physicians and Surgeons
New York, New York

D. Lynn Loriaux, M.D., Ph.D.

Professor, Chairman
Department of Medicine
Oregon Health Sciences University
Portland, Oregon

Bruno Lunenfeld, M.D.

Professor
Institute of Endocrinology
Bar-Ilan University
Chaim Sheba Medical Center
Tel-Hashomer, Israel

Patricia Payne Mahlstedt, Ed.D.
Clinical Instructor
Department of Obstetrics and Gynecology
Baylor College of Medicine
Houston, Texas

Alejandro Manzur, M.D.
Clinical Research Fellow
Division of Reproductive Endocrinology and Infertility
Department of Obstetrics and Gynecology
University of California, Irvine
University of California, Irvine Medical Center
Orange, California

Dan C. Martin, M.D.
Reproductive Surgeon
Baptist Memorial Hospital
Clinical Associate Professor
University of Tennessee
Memphis, Tennessee

Paul G. McDonough, M.D.
Professor
Department of Obstetrics and Gynecology
Medical College of Georgia
Augusta, Georgia

Kathryn F. McGonigle, M.D.
Staff Surgeon
Department of Gynecology
City of Hope National Medical Center
Assistant Professor
UCI School of Medicine
Duarte, California

Susan R. Miller, Sc.D.
Senior Research Program Coordinator
Johns Hopkins University
Women's Research Core
Lutherville, Maryland

Daniel R. Mishell, Jr., M.D.
Lyle G. McNiele Professor and Chairman
Department of Obstetrics and Gynecology
University of Southern California
USC School of Medicine
Los Angeles, California

Kamran S. Moghissi, M.D.
Director, Division of Reproductive Endocrinology and Infertility
Department of Obstetrics and Gynecology
Hutzel Hospital
Detroit, Michigan

Mahmood Morshedi, Ph.D., CTBS, MT (CA)
The Jones Institute for Reproductive Medicine
Department of Obstetrics and Gynecology
Eastern Virginia Medical School
Norfolk, Virginia

Ana A. Murphy, M.D.
Associate Professor
Department of Obstetrics and Gynecology
Director, Division of Reproductive Endocrinology
Emory University School of Medicine
Atlanta, Georgia

Robert S. Neuwirth, M.D.
Director of Hysteroscopic Surgery
St. Lukes Roosevelt Hospital Center
College of Physicians and Surgeons
    of Columbia University
New York, New York

Alan S. Penzias, M.D.
Assistant Professor
Division of Reproductive Endocrinology
Department of Obstetrics and Gynecology
Tufts University School of Medicine
Boston, Massachusetts

Roger J. Pepperell, M.D.
Professor and Chairman
Department of Obstetrics and Gynecology
University of Melbourne
Royal Women's Hospital
Carlton, Victoria
Australia

James S. Prihoda, M.D.
Instructor of Molecular Genetics and Internal Medicine
    Center for Human Nutrition
The University of Texas
Southwestern Medical Center
Dallas, Texas

Jaron Rabinovici, M.D.
Department of Obstetrics and Gynecology
Sheba Medical Center
Tel-Hashomer, Israel

Valerie S. Ratts, M.D.
Assistant Professor
Division of Reproductive Endocrinology
Department of Gynecology and Obstetrics
The Johns Hopkins University School of Medicine
Baltimore, Maryland

Robert W. Rebar, M.D.
Professor and Chairman
Department of Obstetrics and Gynecology
University of Cincinnati College of Medicine
Cincinnati, Ohio

Daniel H. Riddick, M.D., Ph.D.
Professor and Chairperson
Department of Obstetrics and Gynecology
University of Vermont College of Medicine
Burlington, Vermont

John A. Rock, M.D.

Professor and Chairman
Department of Obstetrics and Gynecology
Emory University School of Medicine
Atlanta, Georgia

Allen W. Root, M.D.

Professor of Pediatrics
Professor of Biochemistry and Molecular Biology
University of South Florida College of Medicine
Tampa, Florida

Zev Rosenwaks, M.D.

Professor
Director, Reproductive Medicine
Department of Obstetrics and Gynecology
Cornell University Medical College
New York, New York

Timothy C. Rowe, M.D., F.R.C.S. (C)

Associate Professor
Department of Obstetrics and Gynecology
Faculty of Medicine
The University of British Columbia
Vancouver Hospital and Health Science Centre
Vancouver, British Columbia
Canada

Roger C. Sanders, M.D.

Clinical Professor of Radiology and Obstetrics/Gynecology
University of Maryland
Medical Director
Ultrasound Institute of Baltimore
Greenspring Station, Falls Concourse
Baltimore, Maryland

Joseph G. Schenker, M.D.

Professor
Chairman, Department of Obstetrics and Gynecology
Hadassah Medical Organization
Jerusalem, Israel

William D. Schlaff, M.D.

Chief, Section of Reproductive Endocrinology
Associate Professor, Department of Obstetrics and Gynecology
University of Colorado Health Science Center
Denver, Colorado

Sheldon J. Segal, Ph.D., D.Sc.

Distinguished Scientist
The Population Council
New York, New York

Jillian Shaw, Ph.D.

Senior Research Officer
Centre for Early Human Development
Monash Medical Centre
Clayton, Victoria
Australia

Alvin M. Siegler, M.D., D.Sc.

Professor
Department of Obstetrics and Gynecology
State University of New York
Health Sciences Center
Brooklyn, New York

Yolanda R. Smith, M.D.

Instructor
Fellow, Division of Reproductive Endocrinology
Department of Gynecology and Obstetrics
The Johns Hopkins Medical Institutions
Baltimore, Maryland

Susan J. Spencer, M.D.

Postdoctoral Fellow
Reproductive Endocrinology Center
Department of Obstetrics and Gynecology and Reproductive Sciences
University of California, San Francisco
San Francisco, California

Robert J. Stillman, M.D.

Professor
Director, Division of Reproductive Endocrinology
Department of Obstetrics and Gynecology
George Washington University Medical Center
The H.B. Burns Medical Center
Washington, D.C.

Dale Stovall, M.D.

Associate Professor
Obstetrics, Gynecology and Reproductive Services
McGee Women's Hospital
University of Pittsburgh
Pittsburgh, Pennsylvania

Thomas L. Toth, M.D.

Director InVitro Fertilization Program
Division of Reproductive Endocrinology/Infertility
Vincent Memorial Gynecology Service
Harvard Medical School
Massachusetts General Hospital
Boston, Massachusetts

Alan Trounson, Ph.D.

Senior Research Officer
Centre for Early Human Development
Monash Medical Centre
Clayton, Victoria
Australia

John E. Tyson, M.D.

Professor, University of Toronto
Active Staff, Department of Obstetrics and Gynaecology
The Toronto Hospital
Toronto, Ontario
Medical Director, C.A.R.E. Health Resources
Mississauga, Ontario
Canada

Lucinda L. Veeck, MLT, D.Sc. (hon)

The Jones Institute for Reproductive Medicine
Eastern Virginia Medical School
Norfolk, Virginia

Kenneth K. Vu, M.D.

Instructor
Fellow, Division of Reproductive Endocrinology
Department of Gynecology and Obstetrics
The Johns Hopkins Medical Institutions
Baltimore, Maryland

Edward E. Wallach, M.D.

J. Donald Woodruff Professor and Chairman
Department of Gynecology and Obstetrics
The Johns Hopkins University School of Medicine
Baltimore, Maryland

Don P. Wolf, Ph.D.

Professor
Department of Obstetrics and Gynecology
Oregon Health Sciences University
Portland, Oregon

Susan Macduff Wood, M.A.

Research Management Consultant
Research Administration Services
Walnut Creek, California

Samuel S.C. Yen, M.D., D.Sc.

Wallace R. Persons Professor of Reproductive Medicine
Director, Division of Reproductive Endocrinology
University of California, San Diego
La Jolla, California

Howard A. Zacur, M.D., Ph.D.

Associate Professor and Director
Division of Reproductive Endocrinology
Department of Gynecology and Obstetrics
The Johns Hopkins University School of Medicine
Baltimore, Maryland

Peter K. Zucker, M.D.

Assistant Professor
The Johns Hopkins University School of Medicine
Chief of Gynecology
Church Hospital
Baltimore, Maryland

PREFACE

Half a century ago, a small gathering of 21 physicians/scientists with a common purpose met at the Morrison Hotel in Chicago to establish a new organization. Their goal was to develop a professional society dedicated to the investigation and treatment of the infertile couple. The organization founded by 30 visionaries in 1944, calling itself The American Society for the Study of Human Sterility, made a commitment to the investigation of both fundamental and practical aspects of human reproduction with an ultimate goal of meeting the needs of infertile couples. Once firmly established, the organization took on the additional responsibility of producing a scientific journal. The publication, *Fertility and Sterility,* made its debut in 1950. Over the ensuing four decades, *Fertility and Sterility* has come to be recognized as a leading scientific periodical and has subsequently been joined by many other journals throughout the world that focus on human reproduction. Its content reflects the philosophy of its parent organization, namely that reproductive health encompasses not only the amelioration of infertility, but also the appropriate timing and spacing of children within the family. Two name changes transformed The American Society for the Study of Human Sterility first into The American Society for the Study of Sterility (1946) and ultimately into what is now The American Fertility Society (1965).

Egon Diczfalusy recently addressed the question of what constitutes "reproductive health" by restating the World Health Organization's definition of health as "a state of complete physical, mental, and social well-being and not merely the absence of disease or infirmity." Reproductive health can be better identified by supplementing this broad definition with a number of elements: including "the *ability* to procreate, regulate fertility, and enjoy sex; *success* in the outcome of pregnancy, in infant and child survival, growth, and development; and *safety* in pregnancy, childbirth, fertility regulation, and sex" (Diczfalusy E: *Obstet Gynecol Surv* 48:321, 1993).

Much has been accomplished over the past 5 decades to advance the level of reproductive health. Among these achievements have been a detailed understanding of the intricacies of the neuroendocrine regulation of reproductive processes; insights into factors governing folliculogenesis, spermatogenesis, ovulation, fertilization, and implantation; effective modalities to enhance ovarian function for women with ovulatory defects; and the identification and implementation of varied means to suppress ovulation both for contraceptive purposes and for managing estrogen/androgen-dependent conditions that impair fertility. Endocrine assay methodology has progressed to such a degree that we now employ precise, accurate, swift, and practical means for evaluating an individual's hormonal status. Reproductive tract surgical techniques and approaches not only have become refined but also have been re-refined in this short span of time. Today we are able to use delicate instruments and suture material with the aid of magnification to minimize tissue trauma in an attempt to restore normal reproductive tract anatomy. At this point in the evolution of care of the infertile couple, we even employ endoscopic approaches to accomplish objectives that once had been realized through more extensive open abdominal surgery. The incorporation of the video camera and screen into this approach is revolutionizing these techniques, capitalizing on the hand-eye coordination and magnification mastered earlier through experience gained in electron microscopy and microsurgical procedures. Advanced imaging, particularly ultrasonography, has also become a mainstay in the day-to-day management of infertile couples.

The methodology recently developed for identifying chromosomes paved the way for today's genome project. The contributions of Watson and Crick in unraveling the structure of the gene, together with the technology that permits the sequencing of individual genes as well as the identification of their presence, absence, location, or structural integrity, place us on the forefront of a new diagnostic and therapeutic era. The successful birth of a child from in vitro fertilization in 1978 represents the single most dramatic clinical breakthrough in reproductive technology over the past 50 years. This achievement, which has now been duplicated many thousands of times the world over, has become state of the art for care of infertile couples. Combining principles of ultrasonography, endocrine assay, ovarian stimulation, cryopreservation, hormonal manipulation, and microscopic procedures on gametes and embryos, the original in vitro fertilization and embryo transfer process, pioneered by Steptoe and Edwards, has undergone a metamorphosis in its relatively short life span. The incorporation of in vitro fertilization and related techniques into infertility management currently enables many couples previously relegated to a barren existence to benefit from the gift of fertility.

Reproductive Medicine and Surgery was itself conceived based on the creation of a reference text that unifies both medical and surgical aspects of infertility while applying basic and fundamental principles to clinical situations. In planning this text, the editors felt that the full range of reproductive endocrinology and infertility should span from puberty through menopause, from preconception through implantation, and from nidation through early pregnancy. The three elements of reproductive health alluded to by Diczfalusy—*ability, success,* and *safety*—are emphasized throughout this text. Sixty-two chapters, divided into nine parts, draw upon leaders in reproductive medicine and surgery throughout the world who were selected both for their wisdom and for their communication skills. We, as editors, have assumed the responsibility for preparing a significant proportion of the text. We have also attempted to standardize the illustrative material, drawing upon the Department of Art as Applied to Medicine at Johns Hopkins to create attractive and readily coherent figures.

In his play *The Tempest* Shakespeare proposed that "what's past is prologue." During the last half-century, reproductive medicine and surgery can be viewed with Shakespeare's perspective in mind. Viewing the prologue critically, the empiricism that is inherent today in the widespread adaptation of assisted reproductive technology for multiple indications, often with minimum preliminary investigation, itself raises concerns about the future. Improved understanding of the physiological processes that culminate in normal fertility and an appreciation of the molecular and cellular basis for disorders that impair fertility are vital prerequisites for guiding us into the future. Avoidance of empiricism will nourish new advances that can develop only if we create them through a desire to provide answers for unanswered questions. The reader, in a quest for a composite view of reproductive medicine and surgery, can read this text from cover to cover or, seeking specific information on an individual subject or technique, may refer to *Reproductive Medicine and Surgery* as a friendly resource. As the naturalist William Beebe articulated so succinctly, "The isness of things is well worth studying, but it is their whyness that makes life worth living."

ACKNOWLEDGMENTS

The authors wish to acknowledge with gratitude the invaluable role of Ms. Betty Blevins for her extensive editorial input. We also gratefully acknowledge Ms. Belle Fahey and Ms. Kathy Zulty for providing technical assistance in manuscript preparation and in the expeditious ebb and flow of galley and page proofs. The Department of Medical Illustration at Johns Hopkins, specifically Mr. Tim Phelps, were extraordinary in rendering the bulk of the illustrations for our text.

Edward E. Wallach, M.D.
Howard A. Zacur, M.D., Ph.D.

CONTENTS

REPRODUCTIVE
Medicine and Surgery

Part I

REPRODUCTIVE PHYSIOLOGY

Chapter 1

MOLECULAR GENETICS IN REPRODUCTIVE ENDOCRINOLOGY

Lawrence C. Layman, MD
and Paul G. McDonough, MD

Molecular genetics has been one of the most significant developments in science in the past two decades. Recombinant deoxyribonucleic acid (DNA) technology has allowed the study of biochemical disorders at a level hardly conceivable before its inception. In clinical medicine the main impact of molecular biology has been the development and use of DNA probes to study and diagnose human disease. Classically a genetic disorder was assessed by making observations, constructing pedigrees, and determining recurrence risks empirically according to the natural history of the disease. Although this information is integral to the study of human disease, molecular techniques have opened new possibilities for the study of human disease. As more biochemical disorders are studied with recombinant DNA technology, it is now being appreciated that many entities seemingly due to environmental factors contain a strong genetic component. By using molecular techniques such as the Southern blot analysis and polymerase chain reaction, the DNA of an individual with a genetic disorder may be assessed directly for possible causative mutations or for benign mutations that segregate with a disorder facilitating its diagnosis (restriction fragment length polymorphisms). Unique-sequence DNA probes and probes for these restriction fragment length polymorphisms are being generated at an exponential rate. The continued development of molecular techniques to analyze and sequence the human genome ultimately will result in automated DNA diagnosis.

In the field of reproductive biology, a large number of critical genes have been isolated and, in many cases, molecular mutations have been described. At the current pace it is highly likely that in the next decade all monogenic disorders related to reproductive endocrinology will have molecular determinants. As these techniques become automated, the approach to clinical diagnosis will undergo radical changes. DNA analysis provides a very special contribution to clinical medicine—the potential for preclinical diagnosis. Since DNA is present in every nucleated cell and is unaffected by therapy, analysis of any cell in the organism at any time will reveal the altered genotype. A clear understanding of the DNA alterations causing disease will provide for directed approaches to modify or limit the expression of these mutant nucleotides. This chapter focuses on the basic concepts of DNA and ribonucleic acid (RNA);[11,19,35,42,68] a discussion of the various molecular techniques used in genetic diagnosis; and an overview of many of the genes involved in reproduction and, when relevant, their clinical applications.

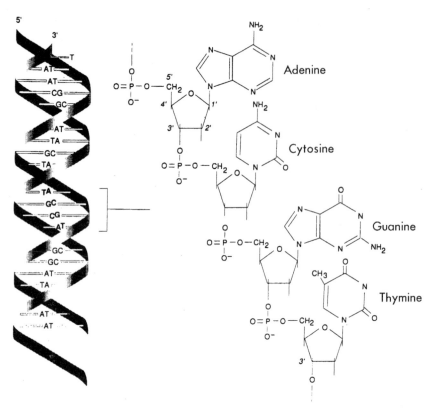

Fig. 1-1. Structure of DNA. (From Gelehrter TD, Collins FS, editors: *Principles of medical genetics,* Baltimore, 1990, Williams & Wilkins.)

BASIC SCIENCE ASPECTS OF MOLECULAR BIOLOGY

DNA structure

The entire foundation on which recombinant DNA techniques reside is the structure of DNA, described by Watson and Crick in 1953. DNA exists as a double-helix molecule composed of two nucleotide chains, each with an outwardly positioned sugar-phosphate backbone and an inwardly directed nitrogenous base (Fig. 1-1).[11,19,35,42,68] Each phosphate is connected by phosphodiester bonds to the five-carbon-atom sugar deoxyribose at the 5' and 3' hydroxyl groups. Note that the carbon atoms of the sugar are designated 1' to 5'. The nitrogenous bases consist of the purines adenine (A) and guanine (G) and the pyrimidines cytosine (C) and thymine (T). These bases are attached at the 1' carbon atom and appear to line up flat, like rungs on a ladder, in the interior of the molecule (Fig. 1-1). The molecule is held together by hydrogen bonds joining two specific nitrogenous bases. G is linked to C by three hydrogen bonds, whereas A is joined to T by two hydrogen bonds. Recombinant DNA technology is based on the observation that complementary bases join specifically (or hybridize) by hydrogen bonds (only C with G and T with A). Each complementary joining of the nitrogenous bases is termed a base pair (bp). A nucleotide is defined as a unit composed of the phosphate, sugar, and nitrogenous base.

The primary structure of DNA with complementary base pairing facilitates transcription of the message and translation into the appropriate protein. The secondary structure (helical configuration) protects DNA from injury, facilitates DNA repair, and may permit or allow binding of certain transcription factors. DNA is further compacted into a tertiary structure so that it can fit into the nucleus of the cell (Fig. 1-2). The nucleotide chains wind about a core of proteins known as histones to form a nucleosome (each nucleosome contains 146 bp of DNA). As demonstrated in Fig. 1-2, the nucleosomes become condensed into fibers that ultimately form bands that can be recognized by chromosomal analysis (karyotype). By standard metaphase staining with Giemsa stain, about 350 to 550 G-bands are seen on a karyotype. With more recent prometaphase extended banding, usually more than 850 bands can be visualized. Since there are about 3×10^6 kilobases (kb) of nucleotides per haploid genome in humans, each band by standard metaphase analysis is about 6000 kb and on extended banding is roughly 3000 kb.

Mitochondrial DNA is also present in the cytoplasm of human cells and is composed of a circular double-stranded genome of about 16,000 bp. Interestingly, messenger RNA (mRNA) is transcribed from both strands. Disorders of mitochondrial DNA theoretically should be present in both males and females; but they are transmitted only by fe-

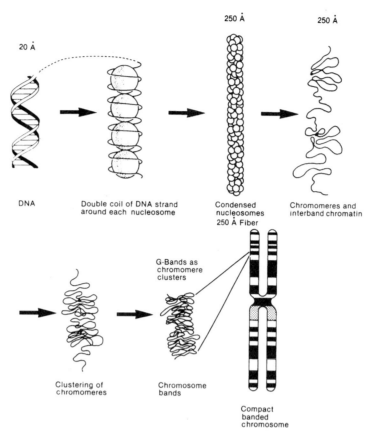

Fig. 1-2. DNA coiling about histones to form nucleosomes and ultimately chromosomal bands. (From Gelehrter TD, Collins FS, editors: *Principles of medical genetics,* Baltimore, 1990, Williams & Wilkins.)

males, since mitochondrial DNA is contained only in maternal cytoplasm.

Gene structure

A gene is a sequence of DNA that is transcribed into RNA and translated into a protein. Genes usually demonstrate independent assortment during meiosis, meaning that they segregate autonomously (i.e., not with other genes). The location of a gene on a chromosome is called its locus, and different forms of the gene on homologous chromosomes are termed alleles. About two thirds of human DNA is single copy, but less than 5% of these sequences actually encode for the estimated 10,000 to 100,000 genes.[19,35] The remaining 30% of DNA is composed of repetitive sequences whose function is unclear, but it has applications in clinical medicine (see DNA fingerprinting) and in gene mapping.[19,35]

Genes, with their regulatory sequences, ensure that their products are synthesized in cells in precisely the right amounts in the appropriate tissues and at the correct time during development. Each cell contains the genetic information necessary to make an entire human being. Certain genes that encode proteins that are vital to every cell, such as enzymes involved in intermediary metabolism, are called "housekeeping genes." Other genes encode proteins that have tissue-specific and often temporal-specific patterns of expression. This is important to the cell; otherwise, a particular specialized cell might make many unnecessary proteins.

Eukaryotic genes are composed of exons, which are the coding regions, and introns, which are the noncoding or intervening sequences between the exons. Prokaryotes such as bacteria do not have introns. If there are three exons, for example, then there are two introns between them (Fig. 1-3). This particular mammalian gene encodes a protein of 100 amino acids, so the coding region is 300 bp (3 bp/codon). Even though only 300 bp are necessary to encode the protein, this theoretical gene may be 1000 bp (1 kb) because of the introns and the regulatory regions. Note that the orientation of the gene is based on the numbering of deoxyribose carbon atoms. By convention, the 5' end of the gene is written on the left, and the 3' end is written on the right. The region of the gene 5' (or upstream) to the initiation of translation is the 5' untranslated region, whereas the area 3' (or downstream) to the stop codon is the 3' untranslated region (Fig. 1-3). These regions are

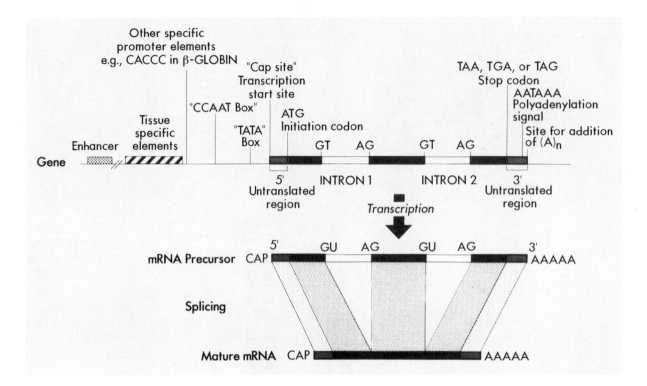

Fig. 1-3. Gene structure displaying three exons (*shaded regions*) and two introns (*nonshaded regions*). Note the consensus sequences. See text for explanation. (From Gelehrter TD, Collins FS, editors: *Principles of medical genetics,* Baltimore, 1990, Williams & Wilkins.)

transcribed into RNA but are not translated into protein. Both regions possess sequences important in gene regulation.

Contained within the 5′ untranslated region is the promoter, a sequence of nucleotides often within 300 to 400 bp upstream to the start of transcription (Fig. 1-3). The promoter functions to localize the exact start site for transcription; controls the quantity of RNA; and, in some cases, regulates tissue-specific expression. Within the promoter there are usually certain sequences that appear in most eukaryotic genes and are termed consensus sequences. The consensus sequence TATA or "TATA box" is present in most eukaryotic genes about 25 to 30 bp upstream to the start of transcription and specifically appears to determine this start site (Fig. 1-3). Less often a "CCAAT box" resides 75 to 80 bp 5′ to this start site and appears to regulate expression quantitatively (Fig. 1-3). Enhancers of expression are often present in the 5′ untranslated region, although they may be located within the gene or long distances from the gene in either direction (3′ or 5′). An enhancer is a short sequence of bases that is able to augment expression regardless of its position in the gene and irrespective of its orientation (5′ to 3′ or reversed 3′ to 5′). There are many examples of enhancers in reproductive biology. The cyclic adenosine monophosphate (cAMP)-responsive element in the alpha subunit of human chorionic gonadotropin (α-hCG) gene allows cAMP to bind to the DNA and increase expression.[33]

Although the DNA content is the same in all cells of the body for a particular individual, only certain tissues express certain genes. This may be related to which regions of the DNA are exposed to RNA polymerase, perhaps by the way in which DNA is folded in the cell. In the 5′ untranslated region some areas termed tissue-specific elements provide this specificity. The site of transcription initiation set by the TATA box is often termed the cap site, since a modified nucleotide (7-methyl guanosine) is added to "cap" the 5′ end of the RNA (Fig. 1-3).

Other consensus sequences in the gene determine the site at which the intron will begin and end. An intron usually starts with a GT sequence (splice donor site) and ends with an AT sequence (splice acceptor site). A short run of other sequences often follows the splice donor site and precedes the splice acceptor site. The introns are spliced out of the RNA before translation (Fig. 1-3). At the 3′ untranslated region of the gene is the consensus sequence AATAAA, which provides a signal for polyadenylation of the RNA (Fig. 1-3). RNA must have a series of As added, the polyadenylate (polyA) tail, to the 3′ end to direct its exit from the nucleus for translation. Elements that regulate genes may be on the same chromosome (called *cis*-acting elements) or on a different chromosome (*trans*-acting factors).

Transcription

RNA consists of three basic types: mRNA, ribosomal RNA (rRNA), and transfer RNA (tRNA). rRNA comprises

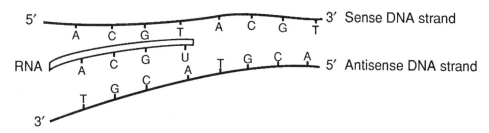

Fig. 1-4. RNA is copied from the antisense DNA strand. Note that the RNA sequence is identical with the top (sense) strand of DNA except that U replaces T.

about 80% to 85% of the cellular RNA in a typical mammalian cell, whereas mRNA is only 1% to 5% of total RNA.[57] RNA is very similar to DNA except that the sugar is ribose, it is single stranded, and uracil (U) replaces thymine. U is complementary to A. In the nucleus, the enzyme RNA polymerase II moves to the promoter and initiates transcription of DNA into mRNA, synthesizing in a 5′ to 3′ direction. The mRNA transcript is synthesized from the "antisense" strand, so it has the same sequence as the "sense" strand of double-stranded DNA (Fig. 1-4). This sense strand is the strand that codes for the protein and is by convention the nucleotide sequence written left to right in the 5′ to 3′ direction. Usually DNA sequences and mRNA sequences are written as the sense strand.

For expression to occur, the promoter must be activated, probably by interaction between certain *trans*-acting and *cis*-acting factors. After RNA polymerase has synthesized the mRNA strand from DNA, the mRNA precursor (often termed heterologous nuclear RNA) initially contains all of the sequences present in the DNA template. Soon, however, the introns are spliced out at the splice donor and acceptor consensus sequences listed above (Fig. 1-3). The AATAAA sequence signals the addition of a series of As, so now the mRNA has no introns and contains the polyA tail.

One consequence of the existence of introns is that different products can be produced from the same gene by a process of differential mRNA splicing. One of the clearest demonstrations of alternative splicing is the calcitonin gene.[12] The two different products, calcitonin and calcitonin gene-related peptide factor (CGRF) are produced in different tissues.[12] Both peptides are coded for by the same gene, but, by using different exons, two distinct and physiologically significant products are produced.[12] Calcitonin is important in the regulation of calcium metabolism, and CGRF is a potent vasodilator. An alternative way in which a gene may encode for more than one protein product involves transcription from both DNA strands. This has been known to occur in prokaryotes for some time but has only recently been recognized in eukaryotes. The only known example of this process in mammals involves the gonadotropin-releasing hormone gene,[2] although it probably also occurs in other eukaryotic genes.

Translation

The translation of mRNA into protein utilizes the "genetic code," whereby an amino acid is specified by a particular triplet of bases termed a codon. Since there are four nitrogenous bases and three possible orders for these bases, 4^3, or 64, possible codons are contained in proteins; thus it was apparent that each of the 20 amino acids (AA) could be encoded by more than one codon (Table 1-1).[19] This has been termed the "degeneracy" of the genetic code.

Certain consensus sequences are important for initiation and termination of translation (Fig. 1-3). The first ATG triplet in the gene sequence (AUG for RNA) indicates the start of translation, and three codons (TAA, TAG, and TGA) specify the stopping point of translation as the ribosome moves along the mRNA (see below). For these sequences to be operative they must be able to be read as a specific triplet codon "in frame." A reading frame is one of the possible ways of reading or translating codons, and an open reading frame refers to a series of codons without a stop codon (TAA, TAG, TGA) so that translation into protein is possible. When identifying candidate genes, there must be evidence of an open reading frame (no stop codon until the appropriate time) if this gene is to be translated. If a stop codon occurs too early as the result of a mutation, a truncated and usually defective protein results. Likewise, mutation may alter the reading frame, which could also result in a dysfunctional protein (see later discussion).

Translation is a complex process occurring on the ribosomes, containing rRNA (Fig. 1-5).[11,19,35,42,68] The mRNA moves out of the nucleus, presumably directed by the polyA tail to the ribosomes, where it becomes the template for translation. The initiation site (AUG) is identified and translation begins. A tRNA contains a codon (termed an anticodon) complementary to an mRNA codon for the specific AA that the tRNA carries (Fig. 1-5). When the tRNA finds a complementary codon on the mRNA, the particular AA is added to the growing peptide chain. The ribosome then moves to the next codon in a 5′ to 3′ direction, adding AAs until a stop codon is reached (Fig. 1-5). The first ATG (AUG) encodes a methionine, which is cleaved from the precursor protein, so the AA following

Table 1-1. The genetic code*

First position (5′ end)	Second position				Third position (3′ end)
	U	**C**	**A**	**G**	
U	Phe	Ser	Tyr	Cys	U
	Phe	Ser	Tyr	Cys	C
	Leu	Ser	STOP	STOP	A
	Leu	Ser	STOP	Trp	G
C	Leu	Pro	His	Arg	U
	Leu	Pro	His	Arg	C
	Leu	Pro	Gln	Arg	A
	Leu	Pro	Gln	Arg	G
A	Ile	Thr	Asn	Ser	U
	Ile	Thr	Asn	Ser	C
	Ile	Thr	Lys	Arg	A
	Met	Thr	Lys	Arg	G
G	Val	Ala	Asp	Gly	U
	Val	Ala	Asp	Gly	C
	Val	Ala	Glu	Gly	A
	Val	Ala	Glu	Gly	G

From Gelehrter TD, Collins FS, editors, *Principles of medical genetics,* Baltimore, 1990, Williams & Wilkins, p. 15.
*Note the three stop codons UAA, UAG, and UGA. Ala, Arg, Asn, Asp, Cys, Glu, Gln, Gly, His, Ile, Leu, Lys, Met, Phe, Pro, Ser, Thr, Trp, Tyr, and Val are the amino acids alanine, arginine, asparagine, aspartic acid, cysteine, glutamic acid, glutamine, glycine, histidine, isoleucine, leucine, lysine, methionine, phenylalanine, proline, serine, threonine, tryptophan, tyrosine, and valine, respectively.

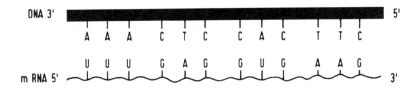

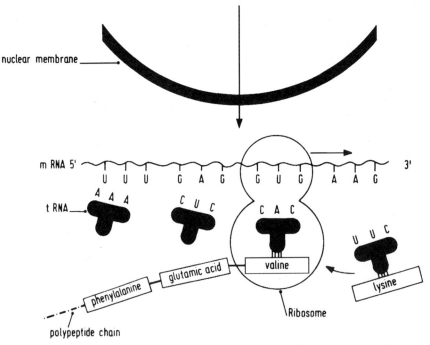

Fig. 1-5. Process of transcription from the antisense DNA strand with subsequent translation in the ribosomes. (From Emery AEH: *An introduction to recombinant DNA,* Chichester, U.K., 1983, John Wiley & Sons.)

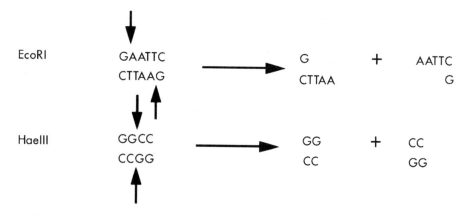

Fig. 1-6. Restriction enzymes. The recognition sequence and the production of staggered ends (with *Eco*RI) and blunt ends (with *Hae* III) are illustrated. (From Layman LC: *Obstet Gynecol Clin North Am* 19:1, 1992.)

this initiation of translation becomes the first AA in the protein. The protein then is released from the ribosome and is utilized by the cell or further modified in the Golgi complex. This is true of the gonadotropin subunits that are glycosylated in the Golgi complex after translation, then joined in an α-β heterodimer.[33] Synthesis occurs such that the 5′ end of the mRNA corresponds to the amino terminus of the protein and the 3′ end to the carboxy terminus. Proteins are usually in a pre-pro or precursor form and are processed to yield the mature peptide.

RECOMBINANT DNA TECHNOLOGY
Restriction enzymes

A key discovery in molecular biology was the identification of enzymes in bacteria that could cut DNA.[11,19,35,42,68] These enzymes recognize specific sequences and cleave DNA into smaller fragments. The enzymes are known as restriction enzymes or restriction endonucleases because they cut within nucleotide sequences rather than at the ends, and they "restrict" their cutting to foreign DNA (i.e., DNA foreign to the bacteria in which they are found). Restriction enzyme recognition sequences generally comprise four to six bases. Restriction enzymes are named for the organism and strain from which they were derived and the order of discovery. For example, *Eco*RI is derived from *Escherichia coli,* strain R, and was the first of this particular strain to be identified. *Eco*RI recognizes the sequence GAATTC and cuts between the G and A. As can be seen in Fig. 1-6, overlapping or "sticky" ends are produced, which tend to facilitate joining with other sequences in cloning. *Hae* III, derived from *Haemophilus aegyptius,* recognizes the sequence GGCC and produces blunt ends, which—as might be expected—do not form as stable recombinants as enzymes producing overlapping ends. Some enzymes, such as *Not* I, are infrequent cutters and they may be useful for certain techniques such as pulsed-field gel electrophoresis.[57]

Cloning

Cloning DNA fragments into vehicles called vectors facilitates the isolation and study of genes. Vectors used in cloning include plasmids, bacteriophages, and cosmids, which are artificial constructs with properties of both bacteriophages and plasmids. Plasmids are circular pieces of double-stranded DNA found in bacteria that confer resistance to certain antibiotics. In general, small fragments of DNA (up to several kilobases) are placed into plasmids and larger ones are placed into bacteriophages. Cosmids can accommodate much larger fragments of DNA. The β-hCG gene cluster (about 60 kb) has been cloned into a cosmid for study of structure and orientation.[33] More recently, yeast artificial chromosomes have been used in cloning because they can accommodate fragments hundreds to thousands of kilobases in size, which is considerably more than cosmids can accommodate.[57]

Vectors containing a gene of interest are placed into bacterial cells, which are then grown in culture so that bacteria and vector will increase in copy number. The gene first must be inserted into the vector. Both the vector and the DNA to be cloned are digested with a certain restriction enzyme (commonly one that cuts sticky ends, such as *Eco*RI or *Hin*dIII). The sticky ends of DNA created by digestion with *Eco*RI can join in a number of ways to form different recombinant molecules, some of which will contain the sequence of interest but others that will not (Fig. 1-7). The variety of plasmid vectors is then inserted into *E. coli* (the *E. coli* are transformed) so that multiple copies or clones of the recombinant plasmid can be generated.

Some method must exist to determine which cells take up the gene chosen to be cloned. The plasmid in the example given has an ampicillin resistance gene, so transformed *E. coli* are grown in culture medium in the presence of ampicillin. Only colonies that have taken up the plasmid will be able to survive and grow in the medium. This eliminates some of the recombinants consisting of only pieces of DNA but without plasmid. Additional steps are

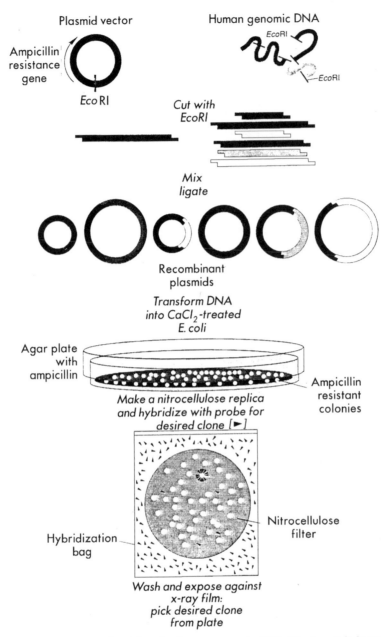

Fig. 1-7. An overview of cloning. Note that human genomic DNA *(the insert)* is inserted into a plasmid with an ampicillin-resistant gene at the *Eco*RI cut site. The plasmid is then placed into bacteria, grown on a plate, blotted onto a membrane (creating a replica of the plate), and hybridized with a labeled DNA probe. Positive clones can be identified and studied further. (From Gelehrter TD, Collins FS, editors: *Principles of medical genetics,* Baltimore, 1990, Williams & Wilkins.)

required to identify the clone of interest. A membrane composed of nitrocellulose or nylon may be blotted onto the colonies in the Petri dish, creating a replica of the colonies (clones) on the plate (Fig. 1-7). This membrane can be denatured to render the DNA single stranded and then hybridized to a labeled single-stranded DNA probe to assess which clones possess the desired gene. By comparing the areas that hybridize to the probe on the membrane

and going back to the plate, the positive clones can be identified, purified, and studied further.[19]

DNA analysis

Southern blot analysis. Genomic DNA from persons suspected of having a genetic disease can be studied for mutations. A piece of single-stranded DNA (i.e., a DNA probe) representing the gene of interest can be hybridized to single-stranded genomic DNA to determine whether that sequence is present and whether mutations exist. Genomic DNA can be permanently immobilized (the Southern blot) on a nitrocellulose or nylon membrane; the analysis was named for E.M. Southern. Similar techniques are available for the study of RNA (northern blot) and proteins (western blot).

To construct a Southern blot, a series of steps is necessary (Fig. 1-8).[11,19,35,42,68] First, double-stranded genomic DNA is extracted from nucleated cells, such as peripheral white blood cells, collected in a heparin or ethylenediaminetetraacetic acid. Red blood cells contain no nuclei and therefore no DNA. Platelets contain mitochondrial DNA but do not possess a nuclear genome for study. DNA can also be extracted from tissue, amniocytes, spermatozoa, oocytes, and even mummified, ancient tissue samples. DNA extraction may be automated in some settings, taking as little as 2 to 4 hours for completion. The cells usually are washed and lysed, and the nuclei are pelleted. The nuclei are lysed, and proteins are digested by proteases. Phenol and chloroform are used to extract proteins, and ethanol is used to precipitate the DNA. The DNA is then placed into solution in a dilute buffer.[57]

Genomic DNA is then cut with a restriction enzyme into many pieces. Agarose gel electrophoresis is performed next, which separates pieces of DNA according to size. Small fragments migrate faster (and farther) from the wells than do larger fragments (Fig. 1-8). The gel is stained with ethidium bromide to assess the adequacy of digestion. This compound intercalates between the base pairs so that DNA fragments can be visualized with ultraviolet light. Although the DNA appears as a smear on the gel, it is really composed of innumerable discrete fragments. Digested genomic DNA is not easily resolved on the agarose gel because of the large number of variably sized fragments and the very large size of the human genome. The DNA is rendered single stranded (denatured) with alkali and then transferred to a nitrocellulose or nylon membrane (Southern blot) by capillary action. The buffer solution travels upward through a filter paper or sponge to the gel, and causes the single-stranded DNA to migrate from the gel to the membrane. Baking at 80°C in a vacuum oven permanently immobilizes the DNA.

A DNA probe is then labeled by nick translation or random primer labeling, usually with [32]P.[57] Nick translation depends on the right combination of two enzymes, deoxyribonuclease I, which nicks double-stranded DNA, and DNA polymerase I, which allows repair of the injured strand.[57] Typically three of the deoxynucleotide triphosphates (deoxyadenosine, -guanosine, and -thymidine [dATP, dGTP, and dTTP]) added are unlabeled; deoxycytidine triphosphate (dCTP) is radioactively labeled. When the polymerase repairs the strand, "hot" phosphorous atoms are added, resulting in a probe with high specific activity. Another technique, random primer labeling, uses unlabeled

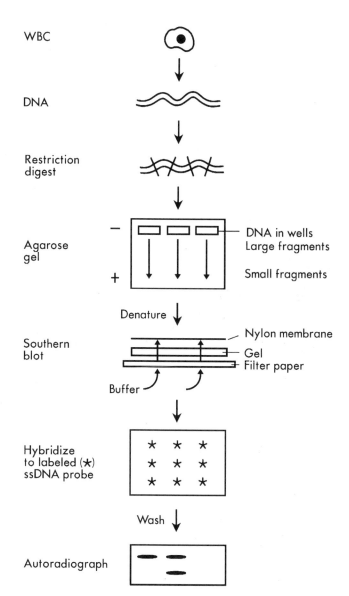

Fig. 1-8. The steps necessary to perform a Southern blot analysis and hybridization. WBC, White blood cell; ssDNA, single-strand DNA. (From Layman LC: *Obstet Gynecol Clin North Am* 19:1, 1992.)

random hexamers to provide a starting point for the polymerase to repair the DNA strand, and one of the deoxynucleotide triphosphates (dNTPs) is radioactive, similar to nick translation.[57] Nonradioactive methods such as biotinylation may also be used. After labeling, the probe is denatured and placed in a solution along with the membrane for hybridization. Hybridization efficiency depends directly on salt concentration and inversely on temperature. The lower the temperature the greater the hybridization, including nonspecific hybridization. The membrane is then washed under controlled conditions of temperature and salt (stringency) to rid it of excess nonspecific hybridization. High-stringency conditions refer to washing the membrane in low salt concentration and at high temperature. In this

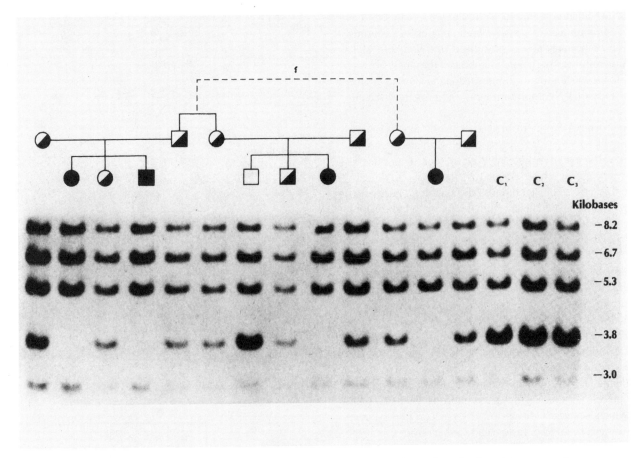

Fig. 1-9. A deletion in the active growth hormone gene is shown in a family with autosomal recessive familial isolated growth hormone deficiency. Note the absence of the 3.8-kb bands in the affected individuals (*shaded symbols*) of the pedigree, a decreased intensity of this band in heterozygotes (*half-shaded symbols*), and normal intensity in those unaffected. (From Phillips JA III et al: *Proc Natl Acad Sci U S A* 76:6372, 1981.)

manner only the fragments of DNA exactly complementary to the probe will join, and background (nonspecific hybridization) will be reduced. The membrane is then exposed to film by a process termed autoradiography, and the film is developed. A band or a pattern of bands is present on the radiograph. Since the sequences of the probe hybridize to complementary sequences on the membrane, the presence or absence of a particular gene can be determined. If the gene is present, the numbers and sizes of the bands on the radiograph are readily ascertained. Typically, fragments from several hundred bases up to 23 kb can be resolved by this technique. If special types of agarose are used, the fragment sizes may be extended to more than 40 kb in the upper range and shortened to less than 50 bp in the lower range. Larger fragments typically require pulsed-field gel electrophoresis; smaller fragments may be assessed by polyacrylamide gel electrophoresis.

The use of Southern blot analysis has greatly aided the diagnosis of a number of genetic disorders. For example, in the rare autosomal recessive disorder of isolated familial growth hormone (GH) deficiency type IA, infants are born with low birth weight and length, have undetectable levels of serum GH, and respond to GH therapy.[51] Phillips et al.[51]

studied these patients at the DNA level by using a DNA probe for the GH gene. The GH gene exists in a cluster of genes on chromosome 17 with human placental lactogen (hPL).[51] There are two genes for GH, two genes for hPL, and one GH-like gene. Only one of the two GH genes is active; the other is a pseudogene and does not appear to be functional in humans.[51] These investigators studied a family with this disorder by Southern blotting with hybridization to a GH DNA probe.[51] As can be seen in Fig. 1-9, all patients demonstrated bands on the autoradiograph corresponding to the gene cluster, since these sequences have greater than 90% homology. However, affected patients lacked the 3.8-kb band containing the active GH gene.[51] Deletions have been identified in other endocrine disorders, including congenital adrenal hyperplasia due to a deficiency in 21-hydroxylase (21-OHase)[56] and 17α-hydroxylase (17α-OHase)[76] and complete androgen insensitivity syndrome.[17] This is an example of a gene deletion causing an endocrine disorder. A deletion is possible in any genetic disorder with very low or undetectable levels of a particular protein. For the deletion or insertion to be picked up by Southern blotting, it usually has to be at least 50 to 100 bp in size. Smaller deletions may

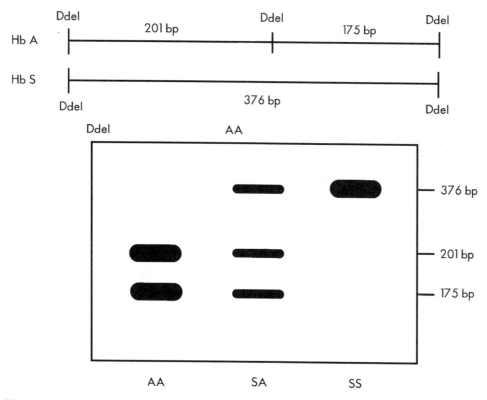

Fig. 1-10. *Dde*I digestion of genomic DNA and subsequent hybridization to a DNA probe for the β-globin gene for sickle cell anemia. Note that affected individuals (hemoglobin [Hb]) (*SS*), heterozygotes (*SA*), and unaffected (*AA*) individuals can be differentiated. See text.

be assessed by other methods such as denaturing gradient gel electrophoresis or DNA sequencing.

Deletions may occur in genes as the result of asymmetric pairing of homologous nucleotide sequences at meiosis. When crossing over occurs at these points, one chromosomal homologue may be duplicated for these sequences and the other will be deleted for these sequences.[42] If the deleted chromosome segregates into a gamete, the resultant individual will be heterozygous for the deletion. Two individuals heterozygous for the same deletion have a one in four risk of producing a conceptus with a homozygous deletion for the particular gene.

Occasionally, a biologically significant mutation can occur precisely at the recognition site of a restriction enzyme. The prototype of this infrequent event is the mutation that occurs in the β-globin gene that causes sickle cell anemia (SS).[18] A point mutation of GAG to GTG results in a single AA substitution of glutamine to valine at position 6 of the β-globin gene. This creates an abnormal β-globin protein that causes red blood cells to sickle under low oxygen tension and causes significant disease. DNA diagnosis of this mutation has been available for well over a decade. The normal human β-globin gene has been isolated, cloned, sequenced, and mapped to the short arm of chromosome 11 (11p). The restriction enzyme *Dde*I possesses the recognition sequence CTNAG, where N is any base.[18] If DNA from an individual with a normal β-globin

gene is digested with *Dde*I, two DNA fragments are consistently produced, one of 175 bp and the other of 201 bp (Fig. 1-10).[18] With the point mutation of the abnormal "sickle gene," the restriction enzyme *Dde*I does not recognize the GTG sequence, fails to cut, and generates the larger 376-bp DNA fragment.[18] The restriction fragments of the normal and abnormal β-globin gene are identified by using a radiolabeled β-globin probe and allowing it to hybridize to the digested β-globin gene DNA fragments.[18] Individuals with two normal β-globin genes (*AA*) show only the normal 175-bp and 201-bp fragments, and they possess two copies of each fragment, corresponding to fragments from both chromosomes 11 (Fig. 1-10). Persons with two mutated β-globin genes (*SS*) demonstrate two copies of the large 376-bp fragment. Individuals who are SA carriers, with one mutated sickle gene and one normal β-globin gene, demonstrate one copy of all three fragments (175 bp, 201 bp, and 376 bp), representing one copy of the normal gene and one copy of the abnormal gene, respectively (Fig. 1-10).[18] The enzyme *Mst*II also recognizes a cut site (CCTNAGG), which can be used similarly for diagnosis.[19] Sickle cell anemia is unique in that the specific base pair substitution is consistently present, and therefore causative of the disorder. This is not to be confused with a restriction fragment length polymorphism, discussed later. In sickle cell anemia, the mutation resulting in loss of the restriction site *is* the causative mutation. With restriction

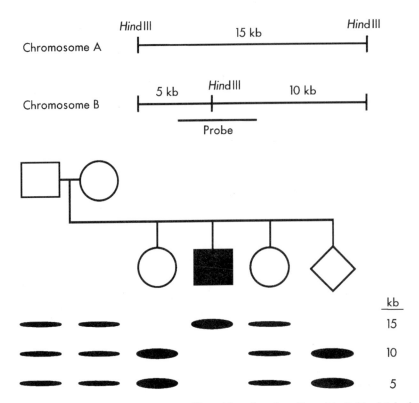

Fig. 1-11. Restriction fragment length polymorphism. Note that the affected individual (*shaded symbol*) is homozygous for the 15-kb fragment, and that no one unaffected (normal or heterozygote) has the genetic disorder. See text for full explanation. (From Layman LC: *Obstet Gynecol Clin North Am* 19:1, 1992.)

fragment length polymorphisms the loss or gain of a restriction site segregates only with the mutation; it is not the causative mutation.

Dot blot analysis. The use of standard Southern blotting for gene analysis is specific, but Southern blotting requires digestion of DNA with a restriction enzyme, electrophoresis transfer, and hybridization. A more rapid method used especially in microbiology is a technique called "slot" or "dot" blotting of DNA or RNA. This technique is used to detect the presence, absence, or amount of a genetic element. In this technique, undigested DNA or RNA is denatured, spotted onto nylon filters in a vacuum apparatus, baked, and hybridized to a labeled probe. This technique is rapid and may be used to screen multiple samples. With radiolabeled probes of high specific activity the resulting sensitivity (i.e., the smallest detectable amount) is about 0.2 to 0.5 pg of DNA.[42] Although the technique is highly sensitive, it may not be as specific as the Southern blot. The signal generated from the hybridization in a slot blot may be nonspecific because appropriate band size is not determined. Dot blotting must be standardized and controlled for each probe and appropriate stringency conditions determined. Nevertheless, it is a valuable technique for the detection of specific DNA or RNA sequences in a sample with microgram quantities of template.

Restriction fragment length polymorphisms. If bands

are present on the radiograph of the Southern blot, then at least part of the gene sequence is present. If a difference between an affected individual and a control subject exists in the pattern of bands on the Southern blot, the two possibilities are true mutations affecting the gene or benign polymorphisms. The study of family members becomes necessary to provide insight into the etiology of the variant bands (Fig. 1-11). For example, consider that fragments produced by digestion of DNA with the restriction enzyme *Hind*III yield 5-, 10-, and 15-kb fragments when hybridized to a DNA probe for a certain genetic disorder (Fig. 1-11). On one chromosome a 15-kb band is present, but on the other there is an additional *Hind*III site so the original 15-kb fragment is cut into 10- and 5-kb fragments. Patients may be homozygous or heterozygous for these alleles. This variation in DNA sequences may be useful for the diagnosis of a genetic disorder if one or several of these fragments are found in affected persons, but not in unaffected persons. In Fig. 1-11, both parents possess one copy each of the 5-, 10-, and 15-kb fragments (they are heterozygous for this mutation of DNA). Each unaffected offspring is either homozygous for allele B (with two copies of 5- and 10-kb bands) or is heterozygous like the parents. An individual with the genetic disorder has two copies of allele A (homozygous for the 15-kb fragment), but no unaffected individual has this pattern. In this family the 15-kb fragment segregates with the disease, so it is a "marker" for this disorder. The technique described is that of restriction fragment length polymorphisms. Even though this 15-kb band may not be the cause of the genetic defect, it appears to segregate with the disease and so may be used for diagnosis.[35]

The benign mutation, or *polymorphism,* is transmitted in a mendelian fashion, as can be seen in Fig. 1-11. It is identified through family studies by Southern blot analysis as a *restriction fragment* (a band on the radiograph), created usually by a loss or gain of a restriction site that is not deleterious to the individual. The *length* refers to the size of the fragment or band. Thus a restriction fragment length polymorphism (RFLP) pertains to a benign mutation in DNA sequences that alters a restriction enzyme cut site. The resulting DNA fragment segregates with a genetic disorder. Several features are important when discussing RFLPs. The band on the radiograph is not the causative mutation; it is merely close physically (or linked) to the causative mutation, so it segregates with the disease-producing mutation. "Close" may mean several thousand kilobases away from the causative gene.

These restriction fragments follow mendelian patterns of inheritance, as is demonstrated in Fig. 1-11. Since this fragment is not the cause of the disease, study of family members is necessary. The RFLP is useful only if there is heterozygosity in the family. In this example the 15-kb fragment segregates with the disease and is said to be "informative." It is possible to predict whether an individual will be affected or unaffected by using the RFLP analysis. The closer the RFLP is to the causative gene, the greater the chance that it will be informative. If every patient in this family had only 15-kb bands, the RFLP would not be informative with the DNA probe used; or if recombination occurred between the marker (RFLP) and the disease-producing gene, the RFLP would not be informative. A recombination frequency of 1% is termed 1 centiMorgan (cM), which corresponds roughly to a physical distance of 1000 kb. Often a group of several markers is used to diagnose genetic disorders by linkage analysis. If the marker is 3000 kb (3 cM) away from the disease-producing gene, the marker should be 97% informative.

There are many examples in the literature of RFLPs. Since the gene for 21-OHase is closely linked to regions of the human leukocyte antigen (HLA) histocompatibility complexes *HLA-DR* and *HLA-B,* RFLPs may be useful for prenatal diagnosis by using probes either from 21-OHase itself or from nearby *HLA-B* or *HLA-DR* regions.[56] Many genetic disorders are capable of being diagnosed by RFLP analysis, and the more informative the RFLPs are, the closer to the causative gene they are likely to be. Once the gene is identified and studied in patients with a genetic disease, a more direct approach may be possible in many cases.

It is important to point out that RFLPs can also be used to determine the parental origin of the extra chromosome in

aneuploidic situations such as trisomy 21. As more and more of these polymorphisms are recognized and RFLPs are identified to cover the entire human genome, every monogenic disorder potentially is diagnosable by this linkage technique.[42] The overall advantage of the technique of RFLPs is that a gene can be linked with one of its flanking DNA polymorphisms. In humans with about 3×10^6 kb of nucleotides per haploid genome, calculations indicate that there would be several million detectable differences in the DNA of any two individuals.[42] This would provide more than sufficient DNA variation to be used to establish linkage of any defective gene to an RFLP. By following an RFLP that segregates with a mutant phenotype it should be possible to recognize recessive carriers, nonpenetrant dominant carriers, and delayed-onset mutant phenotypes such as idiopathic hypogonadotropic hypogonadism (Kallmann syndrome), which generally do not express themselves until adolescence. The ultimate goal is to map the human genome with a series of overlapping RFLPs or at the least no greater distance apart than 1 cM. It has been estimated that 2500 markers would be needed to construct a 1-cM RFLP map.[42] At that point every gene of interest in the genome would be linked to one of these polymorphic loci.[42]

Minisatellites and variable number of tandem repeats. Most RFLPS result from a loss or gain of a restriction site, but there is another kind of RFLP that has been useful for DNA analysis. As mentioned before, there are areas of noncoding repetitive DNA spread throughout the genome. These may vary from a few to several hundred copies of so-called tandem repeats.[5] If a restriction enzyme cuts near, but not within, these tandem repeats many different fragment sizes (bands) may be generated on a Southern blot (Fig. 1-12).[5] Note that, because of the variable number of tandem repeats (VNTRs), it is much more likely for individuals to be heterozygous (Fig. 1-12).[5] Strictly speaking, tandem repeats at one locus on a particular chromosome are termed VNTRs; but if they are located at multiple loci of many different chromosomes, they are termed minisatellites.[5] Often in the literature these terms are used interchangeably.[5]

If a DNA probe is generated from the common core sequences of these VNTR regions, it can hybridize to homologous regions on other chromosomes and generate multiple bands on a Southern blot (Fig. 1-12). This type of pattern has been termed a DNA fingerprint because the bands are unique to different individuals even if they are related (with the exception of identical twins).[28] The odds that two individuals carry exactly the same-sized fragments among these multiple fragments is extremely small.[28] Because of their tremendous variability in the size and number of bands, minisatellites and VNTRs are useful in paternity testing and forensic medicine cases such as child abuse, rape, and murder. As is shown in Fig. 1-13, semen (*S*) taken from the vagina of a murdered woman has bands identical with those of the semen from one of the three

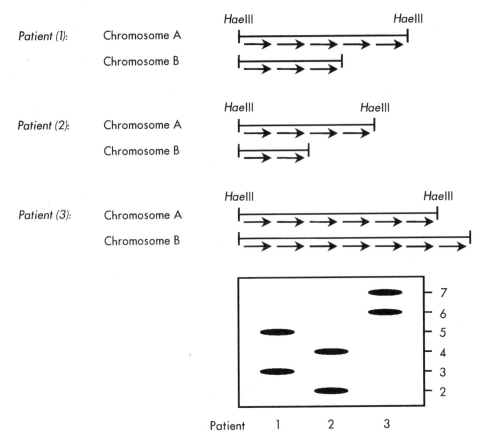

Fig. 1-12. The concept of the variable number of tandem repeats. Note that the fragment sizes reflect the number of tandem repeats each patient possesses, since the restriction enzyme cuts outside the hypervariable region. (From Layman LC: *Obstet Gynecol Clin North Am* 19:1, 1992.)

suspects (*X*).[24] Standardization of methodology with rigorous controls must be implemented for accurate diagnosis.[5]

In situ hybridization. In situ hybridization may be used to localize genes (DNA) on chromosomes and transcripts (RNA) in histologic sections.[37,49] It is similar to blot methods in that a probe is placed directly onto a specimen containing a nucleic acid immobilized on a solid substrate. In situ hybridization for DNA analysis can be performed on chromosomal preparations, frozen sections, cytologic specimens, or formalin-fixed, paraffin-embedded sections.[42] Tissue is affixed to a glass slide and treated with a protease so the probe can gain access to nuclear DNA, which is denatured by heating. A single-stranded probe is added in an overlying hybridization buffer, and hybridization occurs if target DNA complementary to the probe is present. Extensive washing after hybridization removes unbound labeled probe and mismatched sequences. The probe may be detected by using any of a variety of reporting systems, including avidin–biotin enzyme reactions, fluorescence, or autoradiography. Once the hybridization is completed, the nucleic acid duplex can be visualized and quantitated.

The utility of in situ hybridization results from its ability to localize relevant DNA sequences within larger structures, thereby linking biochemistry with cytogenetics or histochemistry. Genes can be localized to specific chromosomes by radioactive probes and the results made visible by autoradiography of the chromosomes. DNA probes complementary to alphoid-repeated sequences located in the centromeres may differentiate chromosomes, facilitating the diagnosis of trisomies.[49] Chromosome-specific DNA probes currently are available that can allow diagnosis of trisomies on chromosomal spreads. Unfortunately, the chromosome 13 probe cross-hybridizes to chromosome 21, and chromosome 14 cross-hybridizes to chromosome 22.[49] Chromosomes 1, 5, and 19 also may be difficult to distinguish.[49] Since trisomies may not be identified in 100% of interphase cells, the clinical use of this technique requires further study. Important information about gene expression can be obtained in relation to the development of specific tissues by identifying the presence of mRNA in histologic sections by autoradiography or fluorescence microscopy. Also, viral genomes can be localized specifically within tissues with this technique.[42]

Polymerase chain reaction. The polymerase chain re-

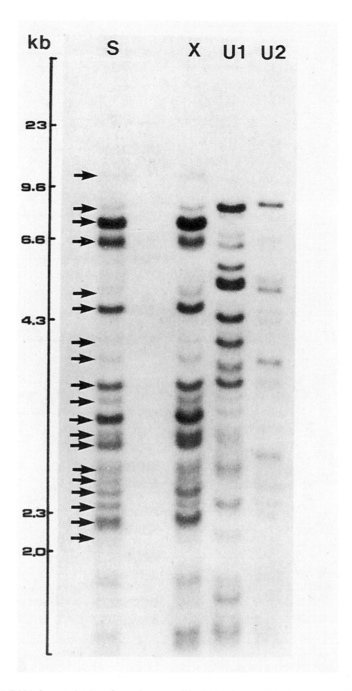

Fig. 1-13. A DNA fingerprint in a forensics case. The DNA fingerprint of semen (*S*) taken from the vagina of a murdered woman is compared with those of the semen from three suspects (*X, U1, U2*). Note that bands match identically with suspect *X,* providing evidence that he is the perpetrator. (From Honma M et al: *J Forensic Sci* 34:222, 1989. Copyright American Society for Testing and Materials, Philadelphia. By permission.)

action (PCR) has revolutionized recombinant DNA technology because of its decreased time commitment, reduced cost, and requirement of a much smaller sample of DNA template. Instead of requiring 5 to 7 μg of DNA and often 1 week of time for a Southern blot, PCR can use nanogram amounts of DNA (or as little as a single cell) and yield results the same day.[13,47] To perform PCR, the sequence of

the gene or at least the boundaries of the region of DNA to be amplified must be known. The procedure consists of three basic steps (Fig. 1-14). In the first step DNA is heated to 94°C to render it single stranded. The temperature is then lowered to 37°C to 55°C, which results in DNA renaturing. Primers, which have been added to the tube, are short pieces of single-stranded DNA (usually about 20 to 30 bp

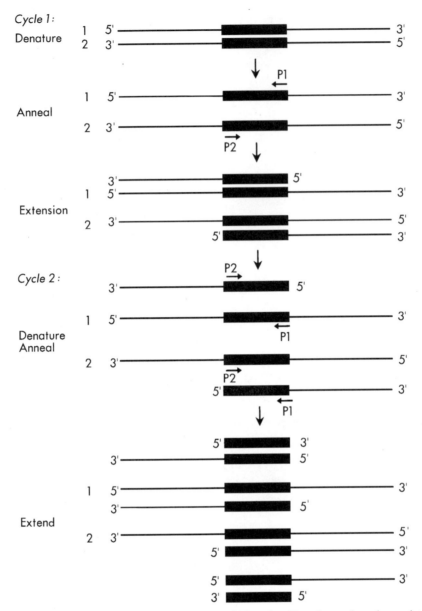

Fig. 1-14. Polymerase chain reaction is shown for 2 of 30 cycles. Note that each cycle consists of denaturation, annealing, and extension. *P1* and *P2* are the primers. Not shown is the presence of enzyme, buffer, and dNTPs. Note that by the end of cycle 2, some of the fragments are of the desired length; they are defined by the primers. (From Layman LC: *Obstet Gynecol Clin North Am* 19:1, 1992.)

long) that are exactly complementary to the 3′ ends of each piece of the double-stranded DNA to be amplified. When the temperature is lowered, these primers will stick or anneal to their complementary regions of the DNA (Fig. 1-14). This is the reason the sequence of part of the DNA template must be known. The time for the annealing step is short, so it selectively allows the short primers to "stick" to their complementary sequences rather than to the whole DNA molecule renaturing. The third step involves increasing the temperature to about 72°C; then, in the presence of an enzyme (usually a thermostable DNA polymerase such as *Taq* polymerase) and deoxynucleotide triphosphates (dATP, dCTP, dGTP, dTTP), synthesis of the second complementary strand of DNA will be completed. Primers provide the necessary starting point to enable the polymerase to extend the molecule. In actuality, the primers, buffer, dNTPs, and enzyme are all added together along with the DNA and placed in an incubator (the thermal cycler) that changes temperature rapidly.

After one cycle of denaturation, annealing, and primer extension the DNA content is doubled so that two double-stranded pieces of DNA result from one piece of double-

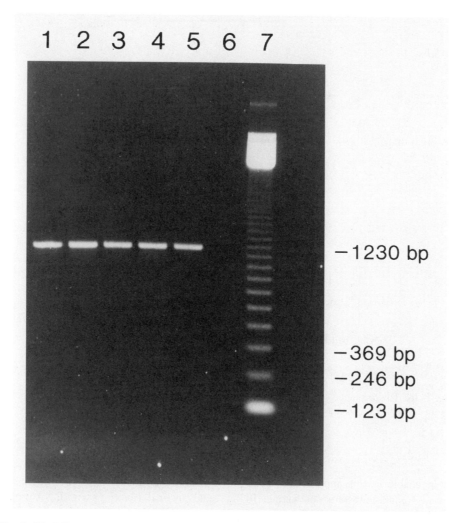

Fig. 1-15. PCR amplification of 1.2-kb fragment containing exon I, intron I, and exon II of the gonadotropin-releasing hormone gene in idiopathic hypogonadotropic hypogonadism (IHH). Lanes *1* to *4* contain DNA from four patients with IHH, lane *5* is a positive control, lane *6* is a negative control, and lane *7* contains the molecular-weight marker. (From Layman LC et al: *Fertil Steril* 57:42, 1992.)

stranded DNA (Fig. 1-14). After two cycles there are four copies; after three cycles there are eight, and so on.[13] In the early stages of the PCR reaction, some of the fragments are longer than the desired product (Fig. 1-14).[13] But since the termini of the amplified regions are defined by the primers (they are physically incorporated into one strand), as the number of cycles increases, successively more of the fragments become the desired length (Fig. 1-14). The amount of DNA being amplified increases exponentially with each cycle, so that the final amount of amplified DNA will be 2^n. After 30 to 35 cycles, which is the typical number of cycles used, the gene of interest may be amplified over 2^{30} or over 1 million-fold, such that it may now be visualized as a band on an agarose gel with ethidium bromide, without the need for DNA probes (Fig. 1-15).[36] However, exponential amplification does not continue indefinitely; in later cycles the product increases linearly, producing the so-called plateau effect.[13,47] Frag-

ments of several kilobases can be amplified reproducibly, but sequences of up to 10 kb have been amplified successfully.

Applications of polymerase chain reaction. Applications of PCR for both research and clinical settings are numerous.[29] Clinically, PCR is used routinely for the diagnosis of genetic diseases.[29] PCR may be used to identify RFLPs, which may allow diagnosis of genetic diseases.[29] For diseases with point mutations or several base deletions or insertions, both normal and mutated oligonucleotide probes (allele-specific oligonucleotide [ASO] probes) may be synthesized and hybridized to PCR products used to construct dot blots (Fig. 1-16). For example, in an autosomal recessive disease, an affected individual would have only the mutated allele, a carrier would have both the normal and mutated alleles, and an unaffected individual would have only the normal sequence (Fig. 1-16). Disorders known to have many different gene

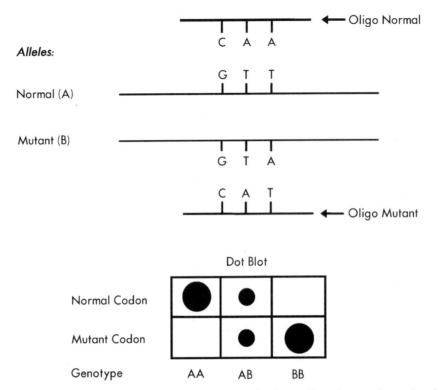

Fig. 1-16. The technique of allele-specific oligonucleotide probing. See text for explanation. (From Layman LC: *Obstet Gynecol Clin North Am* 19:1, 1992.)

mutations are not so amenable to this approach. In such situations the spectrum of mutations must be known in order to develop ASO probes for each of them. Fortunately, certain mutations tend to be more prevalent in specific ethnic groups or geographic areas, which can simplify the process. Hybridization conditions under which labeled ASO probing is used must be carefully controlled and are usually quite stringent. This is particularly true when Southern blots of digested DNA are hybridized to ASOs. If PCR products are transferred to membranes and hybridized to ASO probes, the target sequence is much more enriched, so hybridization conditions are usually not quite as critical. The use of membranes hybridized to ASO probes remains an important approach to DNA diagnosis.

In other diseases such as Duchenne muscular dystrophy, the most common mutations can be assessed by PCR.[6,14] If different fragment sizes are generated for several areas of the gene being evaluated, simultaneous amplification of seven to nine fragments may be performed in one reaction (multiplex PCR).[6,14] This rapid and simple technique permits the detection of deletions over megabase regions of a gene. Multiplex PCR requires considerable sequence data over the gene of interest, or at least in the areas where mutations occur, in order to synthesize oligonucleotide primers. Lack of a band for any of these PCR products could indicate a deletion.

Infectious disease may be diagnosed by Southern blot analysis or dot blotting with DNA probes isolated from the genomes of the particular organism, but recently infections involving human immunodeficiency virus, Lyme disease, human papillomavirus, and other agents have been studied by PCR.[14] PCR has been successfully used in cloning genes, amplifying RNA and DNA from a single cell, gene mapping, genetic engineering, and DNA sequencing, among many other research uses that ultimately may become clinically relevant.[14] PCR has also been used in denaturing gradient gel electrophoresis, which can detect small mutations resulting from differences in the DNA melting temperatures.[14] (See Denaturing Gradient Gel Electrophoresis.)

DNA sequencing by polymerase chain reaction. DNA sequencing by PCR has greatly simplified and shortened the technique, which traditionally involved cloning of the DNA templates. The typical PCR reaction as outlined previously uses similar concentrations of primers and is termed symmetric PCR. DNA sequencing is usually performed using single-stranded DNA, so a variation called asymmetric PCR may be used to amplify selectively a single strand of DNA rather than both strands (Fig. 1-17).[21,22] In asymmetric PCR, one primer is used in excess (for example, in a 100:1 or 50:1 ratio to the second primer).[21,22] Early in the reaction, some of each primer is present to provide enough

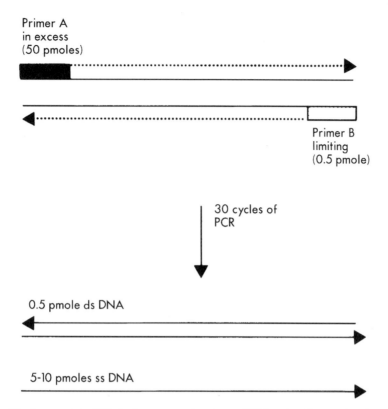

Fig. 1-17. Asymmetric PCR is demonstrated, using a 100:1 ratio of one primer to another. ds DNA, Double-stranded DNA; ss DNA, single-stranded DNA. (From Gyllensten U: In Erlich HA, editor: *PCR technology: principles and applications for DNA amplification,* New York, 1989, Stockton Press.)

template for the remainder of the amplification, which is driven by a single primer. The result is the production of an excess of single-stranded DNA over double-stranded DNA that can be purified and sequenced.[21,22]

Direct sequencing of the PCR product may then be performed. Normally when nucleotides are added to the 3′ end of a synthesized nucleic acid, they are placed onto the 3′ hydroxyl (Fig. 1-1). If a dideoxynucleotide triphosphate (ddNTP) is added to the 3′ hydroxyl, no more nucleotides can be added to the growing chain, so the reaction is terminated. The chain termination method of Sanger et al.[58] is based on the use of ddNTPs. A primer complementary to the strand to be sequenced is labeled, usually with [35S]dATP in the presence of a polymerase (Fig. 1-18).[19] This labeled primer is then divided and placed into four tubes; all four tubes contain dNTPs, but only one of the tubes each contains ddATP, ddCTP, ddGTP, or ddTTP (Fig. 1-18). The G tube, for example, contains all dNTPs in addition to ddGTP; thus incorporation of the ddGTP can occur immediately in some of the templates and later in the reaction in others, since normal dGTP may also be incorporated. The result is that different-sized labeled fragments ending with the same ddNTP will be present in each tube. For each sample being sequenced, four reaction tubes (A, C, G, T) are subsequently loaded into adjacent lanes on a

polyacrylamide gel followed by autoradiography. The sequence can be read from the bottom upward as indicated in Fig. 1-18.

Although the time involved has been reduced greatly, DNA sequencing is not often used in clinical genetic diagnosis unless mutations are confined to a certain region of the gene. If a mutation is too small to be detected by PCR, DNA sequencing may be performed. For example, if a normal 300-bp fragment has a 1-bp deletion, 299 bp may not be easily distinguished from 300 bp on a gel. Many disorders of reproductive endocrinology have 1-bp (point) mutations as demonstrated by DNA sequencing, including androgen insensitivity syndrome,[17] congenital adrenal hyperplasia,[56,76] severe forms of insulin resistance and hyperinsulinism (insulin receptor gene),[67] non–insulin-dependent diabetes mellitus (insulin receptor gene),[67] generalized thyroid hormone resistance (thyroid hormone receptor gene),[70] and some autosomal recessive forms of congenital hypothyroidism (beta subunit of thyroid-stimulating hormone gene).[7,23] If a point mutation occurs, it may or may not affect the protein. If it changes, for example, a TAT to a TAA in the reading frame, a premature stop codon will be produced (Fig. 1-3), and the protein will be truncated and probably not functional. This nonsense mutation, as it is called, has been described in one family with congenital

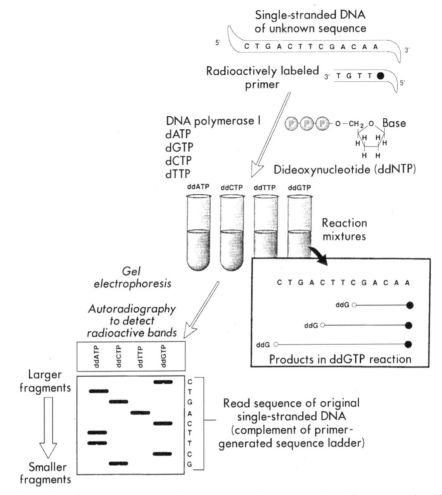

Fig. 1-18. DNA sequencing. See text. (From Gelehrter TD, Collins FS, editors: *Principles of medical genetics,* Baltimore, 1990, Williams & Wilkins.)

hypothyroidism[7] and in the androgen insensitivity syndrome.[17] If the point mutation changes an AA from one to another (a missense mutation), the protein may or may not be affected. This depends on whether the particular AA affects the conformation of the protein. Frameshift mutations, such as a 1-bp deletion, may allow a gene to continue beyond the stop codon or bring a stop codon into frame. A frameshift mutation has evolved in the human ancestral beta subunit of luteinizing hormone (β-LH) gene that allows β-LH to incorporate an additional 24 AAs, producing a new protein subunit, β-hCG.[66]

Pulsed-field electrophoresis. Pulsed-field electrophoresis (PFGE) is a technique capable of resolving fragments of DNA too large to be resolved by conventional agarose gel electrophoresis.[32] Fragments ranging from 50 kb to several megabases may be identified by use of this technique. DNA cannot be extracted by traditional methods. Instead, cells must be cultured, placed in a plug of agarose, and extracted in this medium so that large fragments of DNA will not be sheared. Restriction enzyme digestion, often with an infrequent cutting enzyme such as *Not*I to generate large fragments, follows while the DNA remains in the plug. The

plug is then loaded into the gel and current is applied in several different directions. There are many different types of PFGE depending on the direction of current, including field-inversion gel electrophoresis, orthogonal-field agarose gel electrophoresis, and transverse alternating-field gel electrophoresis, among several others.[32] Recently, the contour-clamped homogeneous electric field has been introduced, which contains 24 electrodes providing current at 120-degree alternating pulses. DNA migrates through the pores of the gel in a zigzag fashion, but the end result is that it runs essentially straight. Large genes such as dystrophin gene in Duchenne and Becker muscular dystrophy and the factor VIII gene are about 1 megabase and 200 kb, respectively, and may be studied with this technique.[19] Yeast and bacterial chromosomes as well as localization of genes may be studied with PFGE.

Denaturing gradient gel electrophoresis. Denaturing gradient gel electrophoresis (DGGE) allows the separation of small DNA fragments because of differences in the melting temperatures of certain regions of the DNA.[48] DNA molecules partially melt when they are exposed to increasing denaturing conditions (heat or denaturant solutions with

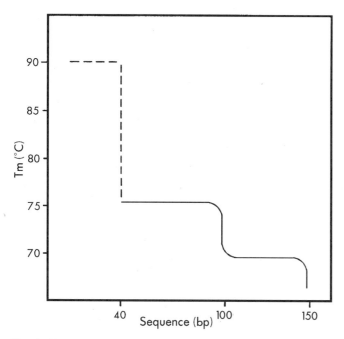

Fig. 1-19. Denaturing gradient gel electrophoresis. The melting domain is shown for a portion of the mouse β-globin promoter. The X axis shows the size of the fragment, and the Y axis demonstrates the melting temperature (*Tm*). DNA will melt at temperatures above the horizontal line, and remain helical when temperatures are below the line. Note that this strand of DNA (*solid line*) melts in two domains, one at 70°C and one at 75°C. If a 40-bp G-C clamp (*broken line*) is added to the fragment, an additional melting domain is created. (From Myers RM et al: In Erlich HA, editor: *PCR technology: principles and applications for DNA amplification,* New York, 1989, Stockton Press.)

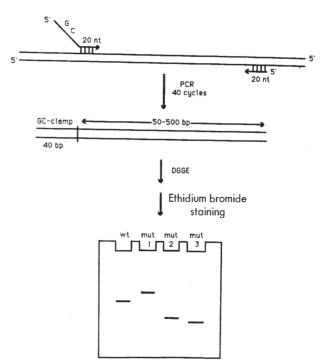

Fig. 1-20. Schematic diagram of PCR with a primer containing a G-C clamp placed at the 5′ end of a 20-nucleotide (*nt*) primer. After PCR, a gel electrophoresis demonstrates the wild-type (*wt*) sequence with three mutated (*mut*) sequences. Note different migration patterns with as little as 1-bp discrepancy. (From Myers RM et al: In Erlich HA, editor: *PCR technology: principles and applications for DNA amplification,* New York, 1989, Stockton Press.)

urea and formamide). Instead of melting as one large molecule, DNA melts in distinct regions called melting domains (Fig. 1-19).[48] These melting domains are dependent on the nucleotide sequence, and temperature differences of several degrees may be obtained with as little as 1-bp difference in sequence. Partially melted DNA migrates more slowly in the gel than does nonmelted DNA. If a fragment with a 1-bp mutation melts in a way that is different from that of the wild type, and both fragments are run on DGGE simultaneously, the 1-bp difference may be resolved. This technique may be applied to Southern blot analysis with digestion of DNA with restriction enzymes, electrophoresis in a polyacrylamide gel with increasing concentrations of denaturant, transfer to a nylon membrane, and hybridization to a DNA probe. Alternatively, a PCR product may be run on DGGE and visualized directly with ethidium bromide without the need for a radiolabeled probe. If the fragment to be amplified does not contain different melting domains, 20 to 40 bp of Gs and Cs (called a G-C clamp) may be added to the 5′ region of one of the primers to create different melting domains (Fig. 1-20). Since G joins C by three hydrogen bonds, the melting temperature is higher, and a higher melting domain may be

created artificially. Since it is at the 5′ region of the primer, additional G-Cs should not affect specificity of the primer annealing to the template. The 3′ end is much more important for exact complementarity, so the polymerase may extend the fragment.

DGGE may detect more than 50% of all single-base changes. The power of this technique may be illustrated by an example: Fragments run under standard conditions on an agarose gel may not demonstrate a difference if even 20 to 50 bp are different, yet the same fragments run under denaturing conditions may be differentiated if there is only a 1-bp change. The potential uses for DGGE are many and include RFLPs (often termed restriction fragment melting polymorphisms [RFMPs]) and the detection of single-base mutations. DGGE is one of many methods to screen top 1-bp changes. Ultimately, DNA sequencing is necessary to identify the particular single-base mutation.

RNA analysis

Northern blot analysis. RNA molecules are analyzed either to assess the quantitative level of expression of certain genes or to identify structural mutations. If a particular disorder results in decreased production of a protein or a defective protein, studies of expression are warranted. For this approach to be a realistic option, tissue from which the gene is expressed must be available. For example, the study of factors regulating transcription for the beta subunit of follicle-stimulating hormone (β-FSH) gene and GnRH gene requires the presence of pituitary tissue and hypothalamus or placenta (or similar tissue) in order to isolate total RNA and ultimately mRNA for study. Northern blot analysis is the method most commonly used to analyze whether a gene is being expressed (whether the DNA template is being transcribed into mRNA), whether an mRNA transcript has the appropriate size, whether a gene is expressed at an appropriate level compared with the control, and whether mRNA is intact or degraded.

In the northern blot technique total RNA is isolated from cells or tissue samples. Commonly, RNA is obtained from tissue by methods that disrupt cells and inactivate ribonucleases simultaneously, such as with guanidine hydrochloride or guanidium thiocyanate.[57] Since mRNA is usually the species to be retrieved and is located within the cytoplasm, the nuclei are pelleted and removed prior to isolation. If the nuclei remain, heterologous nuclear RNA (the mRNA precursor; see Fig. 1-3) would also be extracted, incorrectly reflecting cytoplasmic mRNA. Centrifugation in a cesium chloride gradient will pellet RNA at the base of the tube, whereas DNA often appears as a white band higher up the tube with ethidium bromide staining.[57] The RNA is further purified by ethanol precipitation, but it occasionally requires phenol/chloroform extraction, similar to the method for DNA.[57] Particular care must be taken when extracting RNA because of the abundance of ribonucleases that degrade RNA. Remember that at least 80% to 85% of RNA in a typical mammalian cell is ribosomal (28S, 18S, 5S), and most of the remaining species are composed of low-molecular-weight RNAs such as tRNA or small nuclear RNAs. RNA makes up only 1% to 5% of total RNA.[57] Because mRNA has a 3' polyA tail, this species may be isolated specifically by passing total RNA through an oligo(dT)-cellulose column containing a series of complementary Ts. PolyA mRNA usually yields better results than does total RNA for northern analysis.[57]

Once extracted, the RNA is subjected to electrophoresis through agarose gels under denaturing conditions. Although mRNA is naturally single stranded, the mRNA molecule may fold back on itself and self-anneal over short segments of complementary nucleotides, creating an extensive secondary structure within the molecule. Therefore the mRNA must be denatured with gentle heating and electrophoresis in the presence of a denaturant such as formaldehyde, methyl mercury, or glyoxal so that it migrates through the gel according to its true linear size. Agarose denaturant gels may be stained with ethidium bromide after electrophoresis and visualized in a manner similar to that for Southern blot DNA gels. Transfer to nitrocellulose or nylon membranes and hybridization to a probe (DNA or RNA) are similar to those methods for DNA.

Other analyses. As discussed previously, in situ hybridization may identify and localize RNA molecules in tissue sections. Immunocytochemistry and immunohistochemistry may demonstrate the presence of a protein in certain tissues. This does not determine whether the particular protein is produced there or simply travels there after synthesis and release elsewhere. In situ hybridization allows the determination of whether transcription occurs in a particular tissue. The GnRH gene, for example, has been localized to the medial basal hypothalamus by this technique,[33] as have countless other genes involved in reproduction.

Tissue and cell localization of mRNA transcripts is a rapidly evolving technology and now includes techniques to amplify the target DNA or RNA. The presence of specific mRNAs has been examined in preimplantation mouse embryos by first converting mRNA to complementary DNA (cDNA) by the enzyme reverse transcriptase, followed by DNA amplification with PCR. DNA and RNA from a single cell may be amplified.[54] This level of sensitivity will further understanding of gene expression during embryogenesis.

If a gene is demonstrated to be present by Southern blot analysis, and the exons with their splice sites are normal by DNA sequencing, the promoter may be examined next. A mutation in the promoter could result in low or absent expression despite the presence of a normal structural gene. The mutant promoter may be amplified by PCR, using primers with restriction sites built onto the 5' ends, and then cloned into a plasmid that drives the expression of a so-called reporter gene. Reporter genes are genes that enable assessment of the effects of a promoter from another gene (a heterologous promoter) on the expression of a gene that produces a product that can be quantified.[57] Two examples are chloramphenicol acetyltransferase (CAT) and firefly luciferase.[57] If a heterologous promoter is placed into a plasmid containing the coding regions of either of these genes (and the reporter gene promoter is removed), the amount of chloramphenicol labeled with radioactive carbon (^{14}C) (CAT assay) or the amount of luciferase produced may be quantitated directly.[57] In this way a point mutation in the promoter may be compared with a normal sequence promoter to determine whether the point mutation significantly affects transcription.

Isolation of new genes and gene mapping

Normally a gene is isolated first by assessing the protein product. Typically a cDNA "library" is constructed from all of the mRNA produced in the organ in which the gene is expressed. RNA is isolated and copied into cDNA by the enzyme reverse transcriptase. This process involves the digestion of RNA and the addition of a DNA polymerase and dNTPs so that the cDNA is a double-stranded piece of DNA, that is, a cDNA probe. This cDNA is then cloned into a vector (usually bacteriophage). The bacteriophages are inserted into bacteria by transduction, grown in culture, and isolated from plaques on the plate (representing bacteria lysed by the bacteriophages). The clones can then be blotted onto a membrane (creating a replica of the plate) and screened to determine whether the gene of interest is present.

If the gene has been isolated in another species, a DNA probe cloned from that particular animal can be hybridized to these human clones, since homology often approaches 60% to 80%. Positive clones can be sequenced and the predicted AA sequence determined from the nucleotide sequence. If a DNA probe is not available, a series of oligonucleotide probes covering all possible combinations of a short, conserved AA sequence may be synthesized and hybridized to clones from the cDNA library. Screening a cDNA library in this manner will identify nucleotides for only the transcribed regions of the gene (the mRNA), since introns are not present. If an antibody for the protein is available, the cDNA could be placed in an expression vector, and the protein product could be assessed by western blotting with a labeled antibody.

Once the cDNA has been identified, it can be used to isolate the gene. Generally a genomic library is constructed, which consists of total genomic DNA incompletely cut with a restriction enzyme to generate a variety of different-sized fragments. These fragments of DNA are then cloned into a bacteriophage vector as mentioned previously. The DNA from the plate (each plaque represents a clone) is blotted onto a membrane and screened by hybridization to the cDNA probe. Positive clones are placed back into bacteria and grown (amplified) for confirmation of the gene of interest. DNA is extracted from the clones and digested with a variety of restriction enzymes. Southern blots are then constructed and hybridized to the cDNA. The size of the fragment may be ascertained easily. DNA sequencing follows for definitive confirmation of the gene. Because the clones contain partial digests, the entire gene may not be present on each clone. The nucleotide sequence is examined for consensus sequences (shown in Fig. 1-3) and an open reading frame, providing evidence that the sequence has been transcribed and translated into a protein with the appropriate AA sequence.

This order of protein to RNA to gene is the usual method for characterization of genes. However, if the biochemical basis of the disorder is unknown, a technique referred to as positional cloning or "reverse genetics" is employed. The dystrophin gene for Duchenne muscular dystrophy (DMD) has been identified by using reverse genetics.[19,45] In DMD the protein had not been isolated, so the biochemical abnormality was unknown. The first step in the reverse genetics approach was to identify the chromosome on which the gene resides. This first clue may involve cytogenetics, such as a translocation involving two different chromosomes (in DMD it was a translocation of 21p and Xp).[19,45] Since DMD is known to be X-linked (so the gene should be on the X chromosome), the break point of the translocation revealed valuable information concerning the

localization of the gene, namely Xp.[19,45] A different patient with DMD had a deletion of this region of Xp, so this also was contributory.[19,45] By linkage (RFLP) analysis of many families with DMD, the gene was eventually identified and partially sequenced.[45]

Other techniques for localization of genes also may be used. The creation of combinations of human cells fused with another species, termed somatic cell (nongerm cell) hybrids, is of tremendous value in identifying the chromosomal location of a gene.[19] Usually human cells and mouse cells are grown together in culture under conditions of nutrient deprivation, so that only human/mouse hybrid cells survive. The human cells fuse to mouse cells randomly, and, for unclear reasons, only some of the human chromosomes survive; therefore different sets of chromosomes will be present in each particular hybrid. Cytogenetics techniques can be used to differentiate rodent and human chromosomes and then further to determine which particular human chromosomes are present in a particular hybrid. Southern blots are constructed from DNA taken from a variety of cell panels and hybridized to the particular gene. Mapping can then be performed. For example, sequences for the β-FSH gene hybridize to all panels that contain chromosome 11, indicating that it is localized to chromosome 11.[73] As mentioned previously, in situ hybridization of chromosomes with probes specific for each chromosome also may be used to identify the chromosome on which the gene is located.

Once a gene is located and cloned, the locations of the 5′ and 3′ ends and the sites of the introns are usually determined.[57] Several methods may be used for this purpose, including S1 nuclease mapping, primer extension, and mapping with ribonuclease and radiolabeled RNA probes.[57] S1 nuclease mapping utilizes the ability of RNA to form hybrids with DNA. When DNA is denatured and hybridized to RNA, only DNA transcribed into RNA (the exons) hybridizes to RNA. The introns of the DNA strand will not hybridize with RNA and will form loops, which are digested by the enzyme S1 nuclease. If these RNA/DNA hybrids are then run on a denaturing gel, fragments will be separated on the basis of size. For example, the three exons of different size in Fig. 1-3 could be identified by gel electrophoresis under denaturing conditions. They would appear as one large fragment if nondenaturing conditions were used. These gels can be transferred to nylon membranes and hybridized to fragments of DNA from the gene of interest, which makes it possible to map the 5′ and 3′ regions of the gene. Other methods rely on having the RNA placed into an expression vector and extended in the presence of radiolabeled rNTPs so that radioactive RNA/RNA hybrids are formed. Ribonuclease I digests single-stranded RNA, so the RNA hybrids can now be quantitated by electrophoresis under denaturing conditions and autoradiography. Primer extension analysis depends on the use of a DNA primer radiolabeled at its 5′ terminus, followed by extension by the enzyme reverse transcriptase, which copies the mRNA into cDNA. This labeled cDNA is then analyzed by electrophoresis and autoradiography. Other techniques, including PCR, also have been used to map gene structure.[57]

Gene transfer and gene therapy

The ability to diagnose genetic disorders and replace mutated genes with normal genes is the long-range goal of recombinant DNA. For this to become a reality, a series of events must take place[8,10,19,57]: The gene defect must be known. The normal gene must be cloned and placed into the proper target cell that expresses the gene. The gene must become integrated into the host cell genome without altering normal genes and must be expressed. For somatic cell (nongerm cell) therapy, the transformed cell must have a half-life long enough so that it does not need to be replaced often. For germ line therapy, the gene must insert in a position such that it is transcribed but does not disrupt other existing genes; if it does, these mutations will be transferred from generation to generation (this is the major reason that germ line therapy is less likely for gene therapy than somatic cell therapy). There also must be some method to ensure adequate replacement of the excess defective cells with normal cells. Broadly speaking, the placement of foreign genomes into host cells is termed gene transfer.

Genes may be placed into cells by a process termed transfection. If the DNA becomes integrated into the host genome, transformation is said to occur. Sometimes terminology is confusing, since the term *transformation* has also referred to placing genes into bacteria rendered "competent." The first definition is used in this section. The term *transduction* is usually reserved for insertion of viruses into cells. Commonly the transformation of cells occurs transiently (10% to 40%), but, unfortunately, stable (or permanent) transformation occurs in usually less than 1%.[8,10,19,57] There are many different ways to transfect cloned genes into cells, although the most important ones are calcium phosphate precipitation, electroporation, microinjection (as in the transgenic mouse), and use of retroviruses. When cells are exposed to precipitates of DNA and calcium phosphate, the DNA enters the cell, perhaps by endocytosis.[57] Electroporation involves using a brief period of high-voltage electric shock that creates holes in cells, which permits DNA to enter.[57]

Two techniques have special importance to gene transfer: microinjection of fertilized mouse embryos creating transgenic mice, and the use of retroviruses. Currently microinjection is the only method available for the introduction of genes into mammalian oocytes and preimplantation embryos.[8] With a very finely tipped pipette, DNA is injected directly into the nucleus of fertilized mouse oocytes (Fig. 1-21). The embryos are then transferred to an appropriate female for gestation. Often 10% to 30% of the mouse progeny will integrate the gene and pass it to their offspring. As can be seen in Fig. 1-21, the gene may or

may not be present (by Southern blotting); if present, it may or may not be expressed (by northern blotting). The use of transgenic mice is valuable for the study of gene regulation, tissue-specific gene expression, and mutational analysis, among many other possible uses.[8] As an example, consider the deletion of the GnRH gene in the hypogonadal mouse.[40] (See Gonadotropin-Releasing Hormone Gene.) These mice have hypogonadotropic hypogonadism and are infertile. If the normal gene is microinjected into a fertilized oocyte and incorporated into the mouse genome, some of the first generation will be heterozygotes.[41] If the heterozygotes are bred, one fourth of their progeny should be homozygous for the normal gene. In fact, this gene therapy has reversed the hypogonadism in these mice.[41]

Perhaps the most promising of the techniques for gene therapy in humans is the use of retroviral vectors.[10,19,72] Microinjection is less practical because, although the injection of a fertilized oocyte can lead to incorporation of the desired gene, it can also disrupt some normal genes, the effect of which might not be evident for many years. Moral and ethical considerations are also of major concern. For somatic cell gene therapy, retroviral vectors offer many advantages. Retroviruses are single-stranded RNA viruses that are capable of injecting their RNA into host cells, thereby converting their genomes to DNA by the enzyme reverse transcriptase.[8,72] If the genome is transcribed and packaged, it may lead to additional infected cells. By genetically engineering recombinant retroviruses, the gene to be inserted may be introduced into host cells but lose the capability to reinfect. In this way the gene can be incorporated into host somatic cells without the risk of further infectivity. (For details concerning the life cycles of these viruses and the actual constructs used for transfection, consult references 8 and 72.) This type of therapy often allows stable transformation in 1% to 50% of cells, which makes this modality suitable for gene therapy.[10,57] In fact, retroviruses have been used clinically to introduce normal adenosine deaminase genes into hosts deficient in this enzyme, which if deficient renders the patient extremely susceptible to infection (severe combined immunodeficiency disease). In general, electroporation and recombinant retroviruses increase the proportion of stable transformants (1% for electroporation and 1% to 50% for retroviruses) beyond the capabilities of chemical methods, which are usually less than 1%.[8,10,19,57,72]

For the production of recombinant proteins, the gene is usually cloned into a plasmid containing promoter elements for the particular gene.[38,55] This plasmid is then placed into bacteria, which can provide all of the necessary *trans*-acting factors for expression and translation. For example, recombinant insulin and GH can be produced by this method, since essentially they are not modified posttranslationally.[38] For more complex proteins, such as the glycoproteins FSH and LH, some cell must be used that has the ability to glycosylate.[38,55] These genes are cloned into

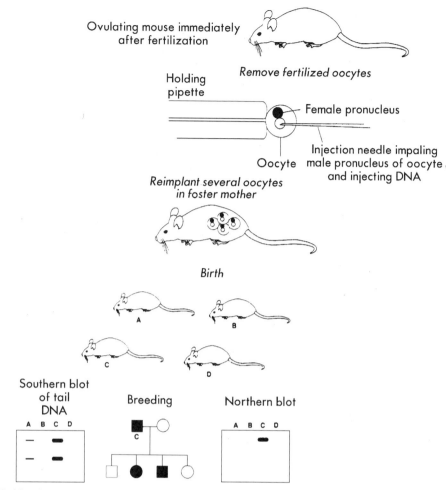

Fig. 1-21. The generation of transgenic mice. See text. (From Gelehrter TD, Collins FS, editors: *Principles of medical genetics,* Baltimore, 1990, Williams & Wilkins.)

expression vectors and transfected into Chinese hamster ovary cells or monkey cells.[55] The gene is transcribed and translated, and, because the animal cell can glycosylate proteins, glycosylated gonadotropins may be produced. These recombinant glycoproteins have been used successfully in primates and rodents, and certainly will become available clinically within the next decade. Many other proteins also will be produced, which will change the practice of medicine markedly by the year 2000.

REPRODUCTIVE GENES AND CLINICAL RELEVANCE

Now that the basic approaches for molecular analysis have been addressed, some of the genes relevant to reproductive endocrinology are discussed. Many of the genes that have been mapped are shown in Fig. 1-22, with the corresponding chromosome location. Note that receptor genes for many proteins are lacking, but these will certainly be cloned in the near future. It is beyond the scope of this chapter to discuss in detail all of the genes important to reproduction. Genes that are better characterized and those relevant to clinical endocrinology are described in the following sections. These include the genes for tropic hormones and their receptors, GnRH, steroid enzymes, steroid hormone receptors, sexual differentiation, and growth factors.

Tropic hormone genes

Gonadotropin-releasing hormone gene. The cDNA and gene for human GnRH have been characterized and localized to 8p.[1,59] The 7.2-kb single-copy gene contains four exons that encode for a 92-AA precursor protein (Fig. 1-23).[1] Exon I encodes for the 5′ untranslated region; exon II codes for a 23-AA signal peptide, the GnRH decapeptide, three AA involved in processing, and the first 11 AA of GnRH-associated peptide (GAP).[1] Exon III encodes for AA 12 to 43 of GAP, and exon IV codes for AA 44 to 56 of GAP and the 3′ untranslated region.[1] The gene is expressed in different areas of the central nervous system (CNS), including the hypothalamus, and in the placenta.[1,59] Inter-

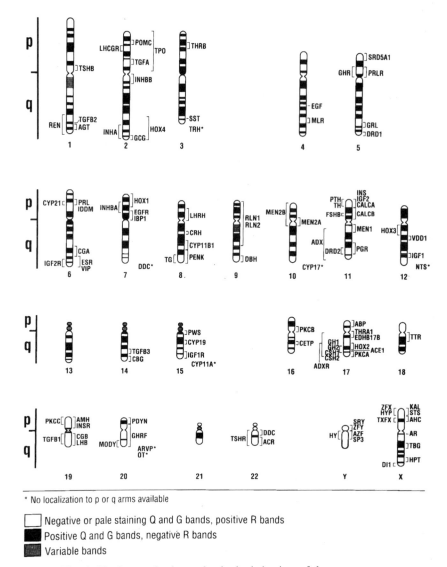

* No localization to p or q arms available

☐ Negative or pale staining Q and G bands, positive R bands
■ Positive Q and G bands, negative R bands
▨ Variable bands

Fig. 1-22. A reproductive endocrinologist's view of the gene map.

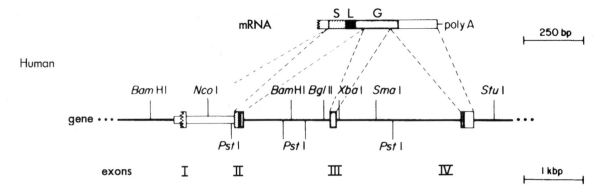

Fig. 1-23. The human GnRH gene is shown. The mRNA is shown at the top of the figure and the gene is shown at the bottom. Exons are displayed as boxes. Dotted lines demonstrate the contribution of the exons to the mRNA. Restriction enzyme cut sites are shown. (From Adelman JP et al: *Proc Natl Acad Sci U S A* 83:179, 1986.)

estingly, the 500-bp mRNA transcribed in the hypothalamus is about 1 kb longer in the placenta, since intron I is not spliced out during transcription. By PCR it has been determined that the hypothalamus and placenta utilize different promoters, with the placental promoter being located more upstream to the hypothalamic promoter.[53] One very unusual characteristic of the GnRH gene is that its opposite (antisense) strand is transcribed from intron I in cardiac muscle and hypothalamus.[2] There is speculation that the transcript termed the SH RNA somehow may be involved in GnRH regulation in the hypothalamus, but its function is unclear in cardiac muscle.[2]

Studies of GnRH deficiency have been performed in a mouse with hypogonadotropic hypogonadism—the hypogonadal mouse.[59] These mice have decreased GnRH, LH, and FSH content in the CNS and transmit this hypogonadism in an autosomal recessive fashion.[59] A large (at least 33 kb) deletion involving exons III and IV of the GnRH gene has been demonstrated to be responsible for the hypogonadal state,[38] which may be restored by GnRH administration, brain grafts containing GnRH neurons, or gene therapy.[41,59] In humans the gene for GnRH has been demonstrated to be present in both men and women with idiopathic hypogonadotropic hypogonadism (IHH) by Southern blotting and by PCR of the exons encoding the structural protein.[33,34,36] Although IHH genetically and clinically is quite heterogeneous, smaller mutations in the gene for GnRH are possible. Additional study of the GnRH gene for point mutations in exons with intron/exon junctions and for promoter, receptor, or postreceptor events may reveal possible factors in IHH.[34]

In the X-linked form of Kallmann syndrome with IHH, anosmia, colorblindness, and associated ichthyosis, a deletion in the gene for steroid sulfatase has been identified.[33] More recently the putative gene for Kallmann syndrome, termed KALIG-1, has been identified on Xp with homologous sequences on Y, and appears to escape X inactivation.[16] Deletions of this gene appear to be present in patients with Kallmann syndrome, suggesting that this gene may be responsible for X-linked Kallmann syndrome.[16] Interestingly, this protein is predicted to have properties that suggest that it might be involved in neural migration.[16] Since GnRH neurons appear to migrate from their origin in the olfactory placode to the position in the hypothalamus,

perhaps a defect in this gene could explain both anosmia and hypogonadotropic hypogonadism.[16] This is in contrast to the hypogonadal mouse, which has a deletion in the GnRH gene, in which the transcripts for exon II (which is not deleted) are in the normal anatomic location.[59]

Gonadotropin genes. The gonadotropins are glycoproteins composed of heterodimers of a common α-subunit and a specific β-subunit.[33] The products of the α- and β-subunits are glycosylated posttranslationally and then assembled. Usually additional modifications of the glycoproteins are made after dimer assembly. Therefore FSH, LH, thyroid-stimulating hormone (TSH), and hCG share in common an α-subunit encoded by a single 9.4-kb gene with four exons located on chromosome 6q.[33] The genes for the β-subunits reside on different chromosomes, with β-TSH localized to 1p, β-FSH localized to 11p, and β-LH and β-hCG clustered on chromosome 19q.[33] All of the β-subunit genes are composed of three exons and two introns.[33] Each of the four human glycoprotein genes contains a CAGY AA sequence (Cys-Ala-Gly-Tyr) region in exon II, which may be important in α–β-subunit assembly.[23]

β-LH–β-hCG gene complex. Originally it was postulated that there were eight β-hCG-like genes,[65] but now there is general agreement that there are six genes for β-hCG and one gene for β-LH oriented on chromosome 19q, as shown in Fig. 1-24.[52] Note that β-hCG-6 is not listed since this was in fact demonstrated to be an artifact of cloning.[52] β-hCG-4 turned out to represent the single gene for β-LH. Some of these genes for β-hCG appear to be pseudogenes and so are not expressed. (See discussion of expression in the following paragraph.) Amino acid similarities between β-hCG and β-LH subunits are approximately 80%, but nucleotide homology surpasses 90%.[66] Each gene is about 1.65 kb, and there are only three restriction sites that differ between β-LH and β-hCG genes.[65] Talmadge et al.[66] proposed that β-hCG arose from a common ancestral β-LH-like gene and, during evolution, acquired a new function. With DNA sequencing of the β-hCG genes, these investigators identified a 1-bp deletion and a 2-bp insertion that allowed β-hCG to extend beyond the stop codon (TAA) and acquire 24 additional AAs at the carboxy terminus.[66] Interestingly, β-CG genes have been isolated only in horses and primates, not in murine species.[33,66] Likewise the α-subunit gene is not expressed in

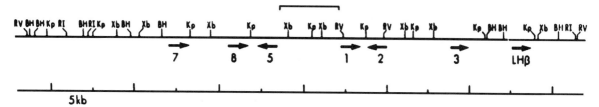

Fig. 1-24. The currently accepted orientation of the β-LH–β-hCG gene complex. Note that β-hCG-4 is actually β-LH. (From Policastro PF et al: *J Biol Chem* 261:5907, 1986.)

the placentas of animals lacking β-CG genes.[33]

Expression of the β-subunit genes appears to be tissue specific.[26,63] The α-subunit is expressed in both the normal pituitary and the normal placenta, in some pituitary adenomas, and in trophoblastic and nontrophoblastic malignancies.[26] β-hCG is expressed only in the placenta, whereas β-LH is expressed in the anterior pituitary and in some pituitary adenomas, but not in the placenta.[26] During early pregnancy, α-subunit expression is double that of β-subunit expression; by the third trimester, the α:β ratio is 12:1.[33] Of the β-hCG genes, β-hCG-5 is the major transcript, with a ratio of 20:1 of β-hCG-5 to β-hCG-3.[33] There is less agreement about which of the other β-hCG genes are transcribed, although β-hCG-1 and β-hC-8 have been reported to be expressed.[33]

Although consensus promoter sequences are located in the same regions of β-hCG and β-LH, these genes appear to utilize different promoters.[33,63] The promoter for β-hCG is more than 300 bp upstream from that of β-LH, so that β-hCG has a longer 5′ untranslated region and that of β-LH is relatively short. Both of the subunit genes of hCG are activated by cAMP.[33,63] An enhancer sequence has been identified within the regulatory region of the α-subunit gene that is composed of two *cis*-acting elements; one sequence contains two repeats of a palindromic cAMP-responsive element (CRE) and a trophoblast-specific element (TSE).[63] Interestingly, only one copy of the palindromic CRE is present in the murine and bovine α-gene promoters, which do not express the α-subunit in the placenta.[63] A point mutation exists within the bovine CRE that renders the homologue nonfunctional, so the α-subunit gene is not expressed in the placenta.[63] In the β-subunit gene, a different CRE has been identified, with at least three protein-binding sites.[63] As opposed to the α-subunit CRE, which binds a transcription factor termed CREB, the β-subunit appears to interact with a different *trans*-acting factor.[63] Thus, although the α- and β-subunit genes are induced by cAMP, their mechanisms of activation are markedly different.[63]

β-FSH and β-TSH genes. The gene for β-FSH was the most recently isolated of the glycoprotein hormone genes. This gene spans over 10 kb[27] and is closely linked to the so-called WAGR locus.[73] Deletions of the WAGR locus may involve β-FSH and result in Wilms' tumor, aniridia, genitourinary abnormalities, and mental retardation.[33] Transcription of β-FSH in the anterior pituitary yields four different species of mRNA resulting from alternate splicing of exon I, and several AATAAA sites for polyadenylation, but the predominant species is a 1.8-kb transcript. In other words, there are two copies of the splice donor site (GT; see Fig. 1-3) that are in the reading frame of exon I. If the first one is read as the splice donor site, the exon is shorter; if the second one is read, the exon length is increased.[27] Two different sites for polyadenylation are present that could result in transcripts with differing lengths of the polyA tail.

Thus an mRNA with an unusually long 3′ untranslated region may be formed.[27] These two mechanisms give rise to four possible mRNAs, although the different mRNAs result in the production of the appropriately sized protein.[27] The gene for β-TSH is a 4.3-kb single copy with a structure similar to the structures of other glycoprotein β-subunit genes.[20] Thyroid-responsive elements have been identified in the 5′ untranslated region, similar to other genes.[20]

Clinical relevance of tropic hormone genes. No mutations have been identified for the gene for the common α-subunit, although two polymorphisms have been identified.[33] The clinical relevance of these RFLPs currently is unknown. Mutations in the α-subunit gene are likely to be more deleterious, since they would involve decreases in all four of the glycoprotein hormones. Two mutations have been described involving β-TSH, both of which are etiologic in congenital forms of hypothyroidism.[7,23] One is a nonsense mutation in exon II, which creates a premature stop codon at AA 11 (of 118AA), so the protein is markedly truncated and dysfunctional.[7] Another mutation is a point mutation in the CAGY region of exon II.[23] When the mutated protein is expressed, the protein is not able to join to the α-subunit, which provides evidence that this conserved region of exon II of the glycoprotein β-subunit genes may be important in dimer assembly.[23] No other mutations have been identified in the β-subunit genes, although polymorphisms have been described for β-FSH and β-LH–β-hCG.[33] The genes for β-FSH and β-LH are present in hypogonadotropic hypogonadism,[36] and the gene for β-FSH is present in IHH even in three patients with undetectable FSH levels basally and after GnRH stimulation.[36] It is unclear whether other mutations in the gonadotropin genes are present in other endocrine disorders.

Tropic hormone receptor genes

The glycoprotein hormone receptors (R), FSHR, LH/hCGR, and TSHR have recently been purified and the cDNAs isolated and sequenced in pig, rat, and human.[31,43,60] In each case, a single gene encodes a large glycoprotein approximately 650 to 750 AA with the NH_2 terminus and COOH terminus being roughly equal in size.[31,43,60] The amino terminus contains four to six potential sites for glycosylation and an area of 14 repeats, which resemble the family of leucine-rich glycoproteins (LRG).[43,60] The carboxy terminus contains seven conserved transmembrane domains, which share sequence homology to G protein receptors.[43,60] These findings suggest that glycoprotein hormone receptor genes evolved by recombination of G protein receptor and *LRG* genes.[31,43,60] The carboxy terminus also possesses potential phosphorylation and proteolytic cleavage sites, characteristic of G proteins.[31,43,60] The large extracellular domain (often over 300 AA) of the receptor contributes to the binding of the glycoprotein hormone (Fig. 1-25).[31,43,60] This is in contradistinction to the other G protein receptors, which generally

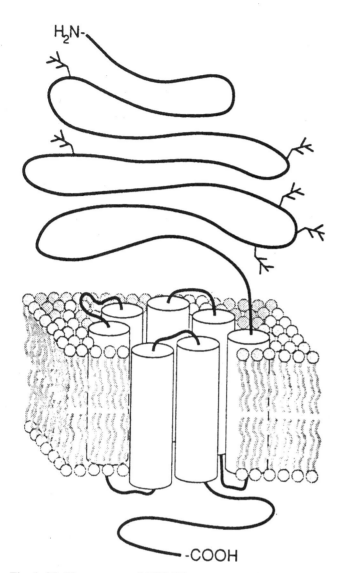

Fig. 1-25. The structure of LH/hCG receptor protein. Above the cell membrane is the extracellular space. Note that most of the amino terminus (H₂N) is extracellular, and the carboxy terminus (COOH) is intracellular. There are seven repeated motifs in the transmembrane domain. (From McFarland KC et al: *Science* 245:494, 1989.)

have smaller extracellular domains and bind small ligands such as dopamine, epinephrine, and norepinephrine.[43,60]

The transcripts of the glycoprotein hormone receptor genes are generally about 2 kb in size.[31,43,60] The porcine and murine mRNAs are of variable sizes, probably secondary to alternate splicing of the gene.[43,60] Recently the genes have been isolated and partially sequenced for the rat LHR/hCGR, FSHR, and TSHR.[31,43,60] The genes for humans are currently being characterized, but it appears that all have similar structures.[31,43,60] In contrast to many G protein receptor genes, which are intronless, the glycoprotein hormone receptor genes contain 11 exons separated by large introns.[31] The rat gene for the LHR/hCGR is over 60 kb in the coding region, which consists of 11 exons and 10

introns.[31] The first 10 exons contain repetitive sequence motifs and encode the NH₂-terminal half of the molecule, whereas exon 11 codes for the COOH-terminal half of the protein.[60] Of particular interest is the finding that exon 11 and the accompanying intron 10 correspond highly to the intronless G protein receptor genes.[31] This finding suggests that gonadotropin receptor genes may be assembled by adding 10 exons to an intronless gene of the other G protein receptors.[31]

Gonadotropin receptor genes may provide useful information about the molecular mechanisms of gonadotropin receptor binding. Their clinical relevance lies in the possibility that gene mutations could contribute to syndromes of hormone resistance. When glycoprotein hormone levels are elevated, mutations of the receptor genes could be contributory. In premature ovarian failure and testicular failure, absence of the receptor gene or mutations in the gene could be the cause of the disorder. Initial work suggests that the genes for the FSHR are present in chromosomally competent ovarian failure, but further characterization of defects will be required. At this time another important tropic hormone receptor gene, the gene for the GnRH receptor, has not been isolated. The gene for the GH receptor has been isolated, and a point mutation in this gene is responsible for Laron dwarfism.[3]

Steroid enzyme genes

Congenital adrenal hyperplasia (CAH) due to 21-OHase deficiency was the first molecular defect described in steroid enzyme genes, but all of the other enzymes in the steroid pathway now have their genes isolated and mapped. Many of the steroid enzymes belong to a class of heme-containing oxidative enzymes that accept electrons from the reduced form of nicotinamide-adenine dinucleotide phosphate (NADPH), termed cytochrome P-450 enzymes.[44] These include P-450c21 (21-OHase), P-450c17 (17α-hydroxylase), P-450c11 (11β-hydroxylase), P-450scc (side chain cleavage), and P-450aro (aromatase).[44] All of these genes have been isolated and mapped (Fig. 1-22), as have other non–cytochrome P-450 steroid enzymes such as 3β-ol-dehydrogenase/Δ⁴⁻⁵-isomerase, 17-ketosteroid reductase, 5α-reductase, and steroid sulfatase (Fig. 1-22). Genes for the proteins adrenodoxin and adrenodoxin reductase, which transfer electrons to the P-450 enzymes, have also been identified.[44]

The cytochrome P-450 genes share some homology in structure, particularly with respect to their heme-binding region in the 3' region of the gene (carboxy terminus of the protein).[44] The sizes and exon/intron organization differ greatly among these genes, which is compatible with the fact that they are distantly related through evolution.[44] The first steroid gene identified was the gene for 21-OHase P-450c21 which has been named P450XIA. The 21-OHase genes exist in tandem with the complement gene C4 in the HLA class III region on the short arm of chromosome 6

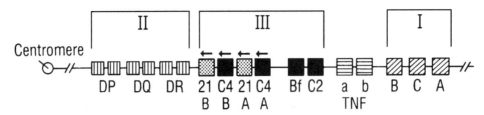

Fig. 1-26. The orientation of the 21-OHase gene with HLA class II region on chromosome 6p. Also shown are HLA classes I and II. (From Speiser PW et al: *N Engl J Med* 319:19, 1988. By permission of the *New England Journal of Medicine.*)

(Fig. 1-26).[44,56,62] The duplication of the 21-OHase and complement genes are shown in Fig. 1-26. Both the P-450c21 and C4 genes are duplicated, with the actively transcribed gene for P-450c21 being the B gene, while the noncoding A gene is a pseudogene. This organization probably arose from a duplication in this HLA region on chromosome 6p, which is a "hot spot" for mutation.[44,56,62] The active B gene and inactive A gene share more than 95% homology, each being about 3.2 kb, with 10 exons, differing only in 10 bases in their coding regions.[44,56]

Mutations in the B gene for 21-OHase are responsible for diverse clinical phenotypes of CAH, which include classic and nonclassic varieties.[44,56] CAH from 21-OHase deficiency, as in the remainder of the steroid enzyme defects, is transmitted in an autosomal recessive mode of inheritance. Several types of mutations have been identified in classic CAH due to 21-OHase deficiency.[44,56] Deletions of the P-450c21 B gene probably constitute about 10% to 20% of the mutations.[56] A variety of point mutations constitute at least 75% of the abnormalities in the gene.[44,56] Interestingly, most of the point mutations convert the active gene into the inactive A gene, a process termed gene conversion.[56] A phenomenon described in yeast, gene conversion differs from unequal crossing over during meiosis, which is the usual mechanism in producing deletions.[44,56] In unequal crossover, pairing occurs between two very similar but nonhomologous genes (for example, the 21-OHase A gene on one chromosome, the B gene on another). When they line up, the resulting gamete either gets a deletion of one gene on one chromosome or a duplication on the other chromosome. With gene conversion, there is no reciprocal product, and the number of genes stays the same.[44] Thus the gamete contains one A gene and one B gene, not like unequal crossover, where one chromosome has two of one gene and one of the other.[44] Interestingly, about half or more of the initially described deletions of the B gene may well represent gene conversions.[56] The absence of a band on a Southern blot with one particular enzyme (often a *Taq* I fragment) is not always associated with no band upon digestion with other enzymes.[56] If a true deletion is present, no bands should be identified with a number of restriction enzymes on Southern blots hybridized to P-450c21 probes.[56] Also, about 25% of patients with CAH demonstrate RFLPs when the cDNA for P-450c21 is used; this observation may be useful in prenatal diagnosis.[56] Probes for the *HLA-B* and *HLA-DR* regions are more polymorphic and may increase the informativeness of diagnosis.[56] Because many of the point mutations occur in certain regions of the gene, CAH may become amenable to diagnosis by multiplex PCR, provided these mutations occur in the population being studied.[46] Point mutations have also been described in nonclassic CAH, but the exact frequency is unclear.[69]

Mutations for P-450c17 have also been identified in humans.[76] Interestingly, both 17α-hydroxylation and 17,20-lyase (desmolase) activity are performed by the P-450c17 protein, encoded by a single gene, with less than 30% homology to P-450c21 gene. A variety of mutations have been described in the P-450c17 gene (named P450XVIIA1).[76] A large (518-bp) deletion and 469-bp insertion have been described, but usually Southern blot analysis is normal for patients with 17α-OHase deficiency.[76] On PCR analysis and DNA sequencing, nonsense mutations, duplications, and frameshift mutations have been described.[76] Results of Southern blot analysis have been normal in studies of several individuals with P-450scc deficiency, which suggests that probably point mutations or small deletions or insertions may be etiologic in this often-fatal disorder.[44] Mutations in other steroid enzyme gene defects have not yet been described but certainly will be in the future.

Steroid hormone receptor genes

When the gene for the glucocorticoid receptor (GR) was identified, the isolation and cloning of similar genes led to the realization that there existed a whole superfamily of genes with properties similar to those of the viral oncogene *erb* A.[15] (An oncogene, as the name suggests, is a gene encoding a protein that produces malignant changes.) Many oncogenes arise from mutations of protooncogenes, which are genes that direct normal cellular growth. These oncogenes permit uncontrolled cellular growth and malignant transformation. Included in this group are receptors that might be expected to be related, including the following:

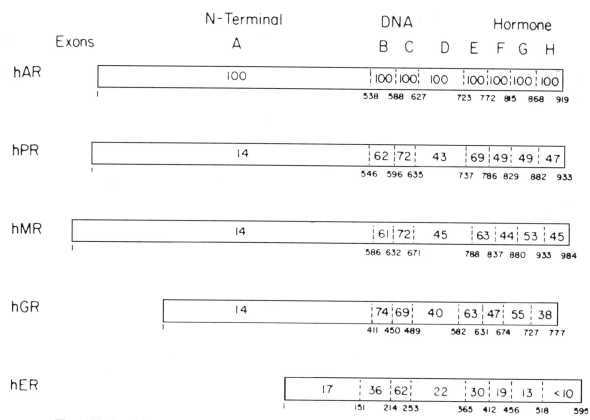

Fig. 1-27. Steroid receptor gene homology for each exon with respect to the hAR gene. See text for details. (From French FS et al: *Recent Prog Horm Res* 46:1, 1990.)

mineralocorticoid receptor (MR), progesterone receptor (PR), estrogen receptor (ER), c-*erb* A β-receptor, vitamin D receptor, and the human androgen receptor (hAR).[15] Interestingly, the product of the protooncogene c-*erb* A β-receptor is the thyroid hormone receptor.[15] Other related receptor genes include the retanoic acid receptor; a second thyroid hormone receptor; the estrogen-related receptor; and hepatic-associated receptor, which has been implicated in hepatic carcinoma. Others with undetermined ligands have also been identified (orphan receptors).[15]

All of these proteins comprise three regions: the amino terminus, a central DNA-binding domain, and a steroid-binding domain at the carboxy terminus (Fig. 1-27). The amino terminus, which is the hypervariable region, shares less homology among receptors than does the DNA-binding domain, which may exhibit anywhere from 40% to 90% homology among receptor genes.[15,17] The function of the amino terminus is probably related to transcription activation or DNA binding (or both), because if this region is deleted, receptor activity is decreased 10- to 20-fold.[15] The DNA-binding domain contains a high proportion of basic residues and two putative zinc fingers, which probably act at hormone-responsive elements (HREs) of the genes they activate.[15,17] In general, each zinc finger is encoded by a separate exon. The function of the steroid-binding domain

is self-explanatory. The proposed mechanisms of action for all of these receptors are similar and involve binding of the ligand (hormone) to the steroid-binding domain.[75] This process, often termed activation, allows the dissociation of a heat shock protein normally "covering" the DNA-binding domain, so that the DNA-binding domain is exposed and able to interact with HREs of other genes (Fig. 1-28).[75] For example, the c-*erb* A β-receptor activates an HRE on the β-TSH gene to regulate transcription. The products of these genes appear to be transcription factors. These interactions provide a link between steroid function and oncogenesis. For example, it is possible that activation of ER and PR in breast and prostate, respectively, plays a role in the development of carcinoma in these organs.[15]

Mutations have been identified in three of these steroid receptor genes. The c-*erb* A β-receptor (thyroid hormone receptor) has been reported to contain point mutations in the triiodothyronine (T_3)-binding domain that have been associated with generalized thyroid hormone resistance (GTHR).[70] An interesting 3-bp deletion has also been described in GTHR. If patients are heterozygous for the deletion, they exhibit typical signs of thyroid resistance— increased free thyroxine (T_4), resistant T_4 action, and inappropriately normal or elevated TSH levels.[71] Patients homozygous for the deletion display markedly elevated

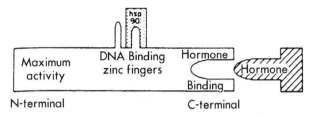

A. DNA molecule with acceptor sites for hormone receptor.

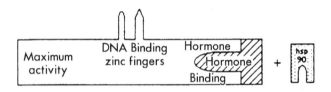

B. Steroid hormone receptor: N-terminal domain required for maximum activity, central DNA-binding domain with 2 zinc fingers, C-terminal zinc finger bound to hsp 90, C-terminal hormone-binding domain.

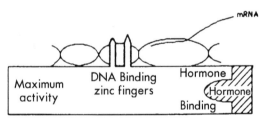

C. Binding of hormone results in a conformational change in the receptor causing dissociation of hsp90, revealing the DNA binding site on the receptor.

D. Binding of the receptor to DNA leads to transcription.

Fig. 1-28. The proposed mechanism of steroid action. Binding of the hormone to the hormone-binding domain allows the dissociation of a heat shock protein from the DNA-binding domain. Now the DNA-binding domain is free to bind to other genes and regulate their expression. (From Witt BR, Thorneycroft IH: *Clin Obstet Gynecol* 33:563, 1990.)

TSH and free T_4 levels and have profound aberrations in brain development and growth.[71] When this mutant receptor was transfected, expressed, and translated, the resultant protein did not bind to the TRE of the β-TSH gene, as does the wild type.[71] This mutant receptor belongs to a class of proteins called dominant negative inhibitors, meaning that the coexistence of a mutant and a wild type interferes with normal activity.[71]

The hAR gene has considerable clinical relevance to reproductive endocrinology. For quite some time, androgen

insensitivity syndrome (AIS), formerly called testicular feminization, was known to be X-linked, and recently the gene was localized to Xq11-q12.[17] The gene consists of eight exons and contains more than 75 kb of DNA. Exon A encodes for the hypervariable amino terminus region, whereas exons B and C encode for the two zinc fingers contained within the DNA-binding domain. Exon D encodes part of the DNA-binding domain and part of the steroid-binding domain. Exons D to G encode for the steroid-binding domain.[17] In the complete form of AIS, in which no receptor has been identified in androgen-sensitive skin, deletions of the entire hAR gene or of varying degrees of the steroid-binding domain have been identified.[17] No RNA is detected by northern blot hybridization in these cases. In complete AIS in which the receptor is present but dysfunctional, no gene deletions are detectable by Southern blotting, but various point mutations principally involving the steroid-binding domain have been identified.[17] Some are nonsense mutations and others are missense mutations. Genetic heterogeneity appears to be present in this disorder, as are the phenotypic effects of the androgen receptor mutations. Point mutations have also been described in the zinc finger region of the DNA-binding domain in the vitamin D receptor gene; these mutations cause autosomal recessive vitamin D rickets.[25]

Sexual differentiation

Since the Y chromosome was presumed to contain sequences responsible for testicular differentiation, search began for the elusive testicular-determining factor (TDF) in humans and Tdy (testis-determining Y chromosome) in mice. Of historic interest only is the identification of the H-Y antigen, a cell surface protein, which was thought to be TDF at one time. That H-Y antigen is not TDF has been proven conclusively.[61] By gene mapping techniques, TDF was determined to be on Yp, and H-Y antigen was localized to Yq.[61] Three maps of the Y chromosome have assisted in the analysis of Y-specific sequences: (1) deletion maps from phenotypic males with a 46,XX karyotype (sex-reversed males) and 46,XY females (Swyer syndrome), (2) meiotic maps from the pseudoautosomal region (regions shared by both the X and Y chromosomes), and (3) long-range restriction maps, linking data gathered from each of the first two maps.[61] Most 46,XX males inherit Y DNA (and TDF) by terminal exchange between the X and Y at meiosis. Homologous pairing of autosomes pair side by side, but X and Y pair end to end. Theoretically, then, 46,XX males must contain a minute amount of Y material (including TDF) because they are phenotypic males. Likewise, 46,XY females contain most of the Y sequences, but they should lack the part of the Y with TDF.

The map of the distal p arm of the Y chromosome is given in Fig. 1-29.[61] Note that the most distal aspect of Yp is the pseudoautosomal region, the region in which interchange of Y and X material occurs. The boundary region is

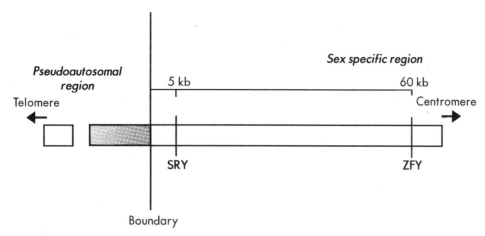

Fig. 1-29. A map of the short (p) arm of the Y chromosome. The pseudoautosomal region is separated from the sex-specific region of Y chromosome by the boundary (*vertical line*). Everything to the right is the sex-specific region (the rest of the p and q arms). The putative TDF sequence termed SRY is located about 5 kb proximal to the pseudoautosomal region. Note that ZFY is further proximal to SRY. (From Sinclair AH et al: *Nature* 346:240, 1990.)

the region between the pseudoautosomal region and the sex-specific region.[61] Originally TDF was thought to reside on a 140-kb fragment just proximal to the boundary region.[50] It encodes a protein rich in cysteine residues with zinc fingers, which are believed to interact with DNA.[50] This sequence became known as ZFY, for zinc finger Y.[50] ZFY was present in a 46,XX male and absent in a 46,XY female, and "Noah's ark blots" demonstrated the presence and absence of the putative Y-specific band in males and females, respectively, from a variety of eutherian mammals.[50] This protein was expressed in testes, was found on the Y chromosome of all eutherian animals tested, was present in the sex-determining region of the mouse Y chromosome, had features common to all transcription factors, and was presumed to be the putative TDF.[50,61] However, ZFY was demonstrated not to be TDF for several reasons: (1) related sequences on X, termed ZFX, were identified and found not to be subject to X inactivation; (2) ZFY sequences are located on autosomes in mettherian mammals (marsupials); (3) Zfy-1- and Zfy-2-related sequences in mice are located on autosomes; and (4) Wᵉ/Wᵉ mutant mice have normal testicular development, but lack Zfy-1 and Zfy-2. Taken together, these data provided strong evidence against ZFY's being TDF.[61]

The strongest candidate currently for TDF was reported by Sinclair et al.[61] They identified a 2.1-kb sequence more distal on Yp than ZFY, located approximately 35 kb proximal to the boundary region (ZFY was 60 kb proximal to the boundary), which was present in four 46,XX males who were negative for ZFY. This sequence was named SRY, for sex-determining region Y, and was identified from overlapping clones (chromosomal walking) 35 kb proximal to the boundary.[61] In this region, only one single-copy clone (pY53.3) hybridized exclusively to male DNA by analysis

of Noah's ark blots.[61] This gene is expressed in testes, has zinc finger domains, and could act as a "switch" to turn on male differentiation.[61] There is the possibility that SRY may act to turn on müllerian-inhibiting substance (MIS) gene expression, thereby causing regression of the müllerian duct structures in genetic males. SRY has been identified in most 46,XX males to date, but it is also present in most 46,XY females with Swyer syndrome.[4] Interestingly, SRY has not been demonstrated in 46,XX true hermaphrodites. Although most true hermaphrodites exhibit sexual ambiguity, one would expect that these patients would have SRY. Perhaps these patients have mutations in the gene. Because SRY has not been identified unequivocally in all 46,XX males, is present in 46,XY females, and is not present in true hermaphrodites, some question still remains as to whether SRY is the true TDF.[4,50,61]

Oncogenes and growth factors

Studies of RNA frequently provide confirmatory and new insights into reproductive biology. The isolation of a large number of human protooncogenes permitted a study of their patterns of expression during human development. The protooncogene N-*myc* studied in human trophoblast is seen on northern blot analysis to have a temporal-specific pattern of expression during early pregnancy.[64] Similarly, the isolation and cloning of the gene for bovine and human MIS provided the opportunity to study the expression of this important gene.[9] Northern blot analysis revealed transcripts for MIS in newborn calf testis, as anticipated; but, surprisingly, transcripts are clearly seen in mature human granulosa cells.[9] Recently these MIS transcripts have been localized in humans by in situ hybridization to testes and ovarian follicles, particularly primordial follicles.[74] These findings have raised interesting biologic questions as to the

Table 1-2. Some genes relevant to reproductive endocrinology

Symbol	Gene	Chromosome	Symbol	Gene	Chromosome
ABP	Sex hormone–binding globulin	17	ACE1	Angiotensin I–converting enzyme	17
ACR	Acrosin	22	ADX	Adrenodoxin	11
ADXR	Adrenodoxin receptor	17	AGT	Angiotensinogen	1
AHC	Congenital adrenal hypoplasia	X	AMH	Antimüllerian hormone (müllerian-inhibiting substance)	19
AR	Androgen receptor	X	ARVP	Arginine vasopressin	20
AZF	Azoospermia	Y	CALCA	Calcitonin (CALC)/ CALC-related peptide, α-subunit	11
CALCB	Calcitonin (CALC)/ CALC-related peptide, β-subunit	11	CBG	Corticosteroid-binding globulin	14
CETP	Cholesterol ester transfer protein	16	CGA	Chorionic gonadotropin, α-subunit	6
CGB	Chorionic gonadotropin, β-subunit	19	CRH	Corticotropin-releasing hormone	8
CSH1,2	Chorionic somatomammotropin 1,2	17	CYP11A	P-450 side chain cleavage	15
CYP11B1	P-450c11 (11β-hydroxylase)	8	CYP17	P-450c17 (17α-hydroxylase)	10
CYP19	P-450 Aromatase	15	CYP21	21-hydroxylase (P-450c21)	6
DDC	Dopa-decarboxylase	7	DBH	Dopamine β-hydroxylase	9
DI1	Nephrogenic diabetes insipidus	X	DRD1	Dopamine receptor D1	5
DRD2	Dopamine receptor D2	11	EDHB17B	17-ketosteroid reductase	17
EGF	Epidermal growth factor (EGF)	4	EGFR	EGF receptor	7
ESR	Estrogen receptor	6	FSHB	Follicle-stimulating hormone, β-subunit	11
GCG	Glucagon	2	GH1,2	Growth hormone 1,2	17
GHR	Growth hormone receptor	5	GHRF	Growth hormone-releasing factor	20
GRL	Glucocorticoid receptor	5	HOX1	Homeobox 1	7
HOX2	Homeobox 2	17	HOX3	Homeobox 3	12
HOX4	Homeobox 4	2	HPT	Hypoparathyroidism	X
HY	H-Y antigen	Y	HYP	Hypophosphatemic, vitamin D–resistant rickets	X
IBP1	Insulin-like growth factor (IGH) 1–binding protein	7	IDDM	Insulin-dependent diabetes mellitus	6
IGF1	IGF 1 [11]	11	IGF1R	IGF 1 receptor	15
IGF2	IGF 2	11	IGF2R	IGF 2 receptor	6
INHA	Inhibin α	2	INHBA	Inhibin βA	7
INHBB	Inhibin βB	2	INS	Insulin	11
INSR	Insulin receptor	19	KAL	Kallmann syndrome	X
LHB	Luteinizing hormone, β-subunit	19	LHCGR	Luteinizing hormone/chorionic gonadotropin receptor	2
LHRH	Gonadotropin-releasing hormone	8	MEN1	Multiple endocrine neoplasia (MEN) 1	11
MEN2A	MEN 2A	10	MEN2B	MEN 2B	10
MLR	Mineralocorticoid receptor	4	MODY	Maturity onset diabetes of the young	20
NTS	Neurotensin	12	OT	Oxytocin	20
PDYN	Prodynorphin	20	PENK	Proenkephalin	8
PGR	Progesterone receptor	11	PKCA	Protein kinase C, α-polypeptide	17
PKCB	Protein kinase C, β-polypeptide	16	PKCC	Protein kinase C, γ-polypeptide	19
POMC	POMC	2	PRL	Prolactin	6
PRLR	Prolactin receptor	5	PTH	Parathyroid hormone	11
PWS	Prader-Willi syndrome	15	REN	Renin	1
RLN 1,2	Relaxin 1,2	9	SP3	Azoospermia factor 3	Y
SRD5A1	5α-Reductase	5	SRY	Sex-determining region Y (SRY)	Y
SST	Somatostatin	3	STS	Steroid sulfatase [X]	X
TBG	Thyroxine binding globulin	X	TG	Thyroglobulin	8
TGFA	Transforming growth factor (TGF), α-subunit	2	TGFB1	TGF, β1-subunit	19
TGFB2	TGF, β2-subunit	1	TGFB3	TGF, β3-subunit	14
TH	Tyrosine hydroxylase	11	THRA1	Thyroid hormone receptor α	17
TPO	Thyroid peroxidase	2	TRH	Thyrotropin-releasing hormone	3
TRHB	Thyroid hormone receptor, β-subunit	3	TSHB	Thyroid-stimulating hormone (TSH) β-subunit	1
TSHR	TSH receptor	14	TTR	Thyroxine-binding prealbumin	18
TXFX	Gonadal dysgenesis, 46,XY	X	VDD1	Vitamin D receptor 1	12
VIP	Vasoactive intestinal polypeptide	6	ZFX	Zinc finger X	X
ZFY	Zinc finger Y	Y			

possible function of the mRNA transcripts for MIS.[74] One might speculate that MIS may play some role in initiating or suppressing the process of meiosis. The homology between the β-subunit of transforming growth factor (β-TGF) and MIS is of particular interest because both are capable of inhibiting the cell cycle and normal cellular growth.[39] Structural comparison of the MIS and β-TGF genes may provide insight into the regions of these proteins responsible for their antitumor activity and improve our understanding of the regulation of cell growth. The homologies among β-TGF, MIS, and the β-subunits of inhibin have led to speculation that the three proteins may be members of a single gene family.[39] A nonsense mutation in the MIS gene has been described in normally virilized males possessing müllerian structures.[30]

SUMMARY

The study of molecular biology is continuing at such a rapid pace that it may be possible in the future to perform DNA testing for many different genetic disorders and infections in the office with simple automated hybridization procedures. Some of the many techniques used in molecular genetics have been described, but it is beyond the scope of this chapter to be all-inclusive. New techniques are being developed continually. Likewise, new genes are being identified with relevance to reproductive endocrinology. There are so many that it is impossible to discuss all of them within the confines of this chapter, but some relevant genes are listed in Table 1-2. It is hoped that a better understanding of molecular biology will enable reproductive biologists to integrate some of these procedures into their armamentaria, which will contribute to significant findings in the future.

REFERENCES

1. Adelman JP et al: Isolation of the gene and hypothalamic cDNA for the common precursor of gonadotropin-releasing hormone and prolactin release-inhibiting factor in human and rat, *Proc Natl Acad Sci USA* 83:179, 1986.
2. Adelman JP et al: Two mammalian genes transcribed from opposite strands of the same DNA locus, *Science* 235:1514, 1987.
3. Amselem S et al: Laron dwarfism and mutations of the growth hormone-receptor gene, *N Engl J Med* 321:989, 1989.
4. Behzadian MA, Tho SPT, McDonough PG: The presence of the testicular determining sequence, SRY, in 46,XY females with gonadal dysgenesis (Swyer syndrome), *Am J Obstet Gynecol* 165:1887, 1991.
5. Butler WJ: Minisatellite probes, *Semin Reprod Endocrinol* 9:56, 1991.
6. Chamberlain JS et al: Deletion screening of the Duchenne muscular dystrophy locus via multiplex DNA Amplification, *Nucleic Acids Res* 16:11141, 1988.
7. Dacou-Voutetakis C et al: Familial hypothyroidism caused by a nonsense mutation in the thyroid-stimulating hormone β-subunit gene, *Am J Hum Genet* 46:988, 1990.
8. DePamphilis ML et al: Microinjecting DNA into mouse ova to study DNA replication and gene expression and to produce transgenic animals, *Biotechniques* 6:662, 1988.
9. Donahoe PK et al: Mullerian inhibiting substance: gene structure and mechanism of action of a fetal regressor, *Recent Prog Horm Res* 43:431, 1987.
10. Eglitis MA, Anderson WF: Retroviral vectors for introduction of genes into mammalian cells, *Biotechniques* 6:608, 1988.
11. Emery AEH: *An introduction to recombinant DNA,* Chichester, UK, 1983, John Wiley & Sons.
12. Emeson RB et al: Alternative production of calcitonin and CGRP mRNA is regulated at the calcitonin-specific splice acceptor, *Nature* 341:76, 1989.
13. Erlich A, Gelfand DH, Saiki RK: Specific DNA amplification, *Nature* 331:461, 1988.
14. Erlich HA, editor: *PCR technology: principles and applications for DNA amplification,* New York, 1989, Stockton Press.
15. Evans RM: The steroid and thyroid hormone receptor superfamily, *Science* 240:889, 1988.
16. Franco B et al: A gene deleted in Kallmann's syndrome shares homology with neural cell adhesion and axonal path-finding molecules, *Nature* 353:529, 1991.
17. French FS et al: Molecular basis of androgen insensitivity, *Recent Prog Horm Res* 46:1, 1990.
18. Geever RF et al: Direct identification of sickle cell anemia by blot hybridization, *Proc Natl Acad Sci U S A* 78:5081, 1981.
19. Gelehrter TD, Collins FS, editors: *Principles of medical genetics,* Baltimore, 1990, Williams & Wilkins.
20. Guidon PT et al: The human thyrotropin β-subunit gene differs in 5′ structure from murine TSH-β genes, *DNA* 7:691, 1988.
21. Gyllensten U: Direct sequencing of in vitro amplified DNA. In Erlich HA, editor: *PCR technology: principles and applications for DNA amplification,* New York, 1989, Stockton Press.
22. Gyllensten UB: PCR and DNA sequencing, *Biotechniques* 7:700, 1989.
23. Hayashizaki Y et al: Thyroid stimulating hormone (TSH) deficiency caused by single base substitution in the CAGYC region of the β-subunit, *EMBO J* 8:2291, 1989.
24. Honma M et al: Individual identification from semen by the deoxyribonucleic acid (DNA) fingerprint technique, *J Forensic Sci* 34:222, 1989.
25. Hughs MR et al: Point mutations in the human vitamin D receptor gene associated with hypocalcemic rickets, *Science* 242:1702, 1988.
26. Jameson JL, Lindell CM, Habener JF: Gonadotropin and thyrotropin α- and β-subunit gene expression in normal and neoplastic tissues characterized using specific messenger ribonucleic acid hybridization probes, *J Clin Endocrinol Metab* 64:319, 1986.
27. Jameson JL et al: Human follicle-stimulating hormone β-subunit gene encodes multiple messenger ribonucleic acids, *Mol Endocrinol* 2:806, 1988.
28. Jeffreys AJ, Wilson V, Thein SL: Individual-specific 'fingerprints' of human DNA, *Nature* 316:76, 1985.
29. Kazazian HH Jr: Use of PCR in the diagnosis of monogenic disease. In Erlich HA, editor: *PCR technology: principles and applications for DNA amplification,* New York, 1989, Stockton Press.
30. Knebelmann B et al: Anti-mullerian hormone bruxelles: a nonsense mutation associated with the persistent mullerian duct syndrome, *Proc Natl Acad Sci U S A* 88:3767, 1991.
31. Koo YB et al: Structure of the luteinizing hormone receptor gene and multiple exons of the coding sequence, *Endocrinology* 128:2297, 1991.
32. Lai E et al: Pulsed field gel electrophoresis, *Biotechniques* 7:34, 1989.
33. Layman LC: Genetics of gonadotropin genes and the GnRH/GAP gene, *Semin Reprod Endocrinol* 9:22, 1991.
34. Layman LC: Idiopathic hypogonadotropic hypogonadism: diagnosis, pathogenesis, genetics, and treatment, *Adolesc Pediatr Gynecol* 4:111, 1991.
35. Layman LC: Basic concepts of molecular biology as applied to pediatric and adolescent gynecology, *Obstet Gynecol Clin North Am* 19:1, 1992.
36. Layman LC et al: Gonadotropin-releasing hormone, follicle-stimulating hormone beta, and luteinizing hormone beta gene structure

in idiopathic hypogonadotropic hypogonadism, *Fertil Steril* 57:42, 1992.

37. Lichter P, Ward DC: Is non-isotopic in situ hybridization finally coming of age?, *Nature* 345:93, 1990.

38. Mange AP, Mange EJ: New genetic technologies. In *Genetics: human aspects,* Sunderland, Mass, 1990, Sinauer Associates.

39. Mason AJ et al: Complementary DNA sequences of ovarian follicular fluid inhibin show precursor structure and homology with transforming growth factor-β, *Nature* 318:659, 1985.

40. Mason AJ et al: A deletion truncating the gonadotropin-releasing hormone gene is responsible for hypogonadism in the hpg mouse, *Science* 234:1366, 1986.

41. Mason AJ et al: The hypogonadal mouse: reproductive functions restored by gene therapy, *Science* 234:1372, 1986.

42. McDonough PG: Molecular biology in reproductive endocrinology. In Yen SSC, Jaffe RB, editors: *Reproductive endocrinology,* Philadelphia, 1991, WB Saunders.

43. McFarland KC et al: Lutropin-choriogonadotropin receptor: an unusual member of the G protein-coupled receptor family, *Science* 245:494, 1989.

44. Miller WL: Molecular biology of steroid hormone synthesis, *Endocr Rev* 9:295, 1988.

45. Monaco AP, Kunkel LM: Cloning of the Duchenne/Becker muscular dystrophy locus, *Adv Hum Genet* 17:61, 1988.

46. Mornet E et al: Distribution of deletions and seven point mutations on CYP21B genes in three clinical forms of steroid 21-hydroxylase deficiency, *Am J Hum Genet* 48:79, 1991.

47. Mullis KB, Faloona FA: Specific synthesis of DNA in vitro via a polymerase-catalyzed chain reaction, *Methods Enzymol* 155:335, 1987.

48. Myers RM, Sheffield VC, Cox DR: Mutation detection by PCR, GC-clamps, and denaturing gradient gel electrophoresis. In Erlich HA, editor: *PCR technology: principles and applications for DNA amplification,* New York, 1989, Stockton Press.

49. Oncor Corporation: *Oncor molecular cytogenetics bibliography,* Gaithersburg, Md, 1991, Oncor.

50. Page DC et al: The sex determining region of the human Y chromosome encodes a finger protein, *Cell* 51:1091, 1987.

51. Phillips JA III et al: Molecular basis for familial isolated growth hormone deficiency, *Proc Natl Acad Sci U S A* 78:6372, 1981.

52. Policastro PF et al: A map of the hCGβ-LHβ gene cluster, *J Biol Chem* 261:5907, 1986.

53. Radovick S et al: Isolation and characterization of the human gonadotropin-releasing hormone gene in the hypothalamus and placenta, *Mol Endocrinol* 4:476, 1990.

54. Rapoli DA et al: Novel method for studying mRNA phenotypes in single or small numbers of cells, *J Cell Biochem* 39:1, 1989.

55. Reddy VA et al: Expression of human chorionic gonadotropin in monkey cells using a single simian virus 40 vector, *Proc Natl Acad Sci U S A* 82:3644, 1985.

56. Reindollar RH, Gray MR: The molecular basis of 21-hydroxylase deficiency, *Semin Reprod Endocrinol* 9:34, 1991.

57. Sambrook J, Fritsch EF, Maniatis T: *Molecular cloning: a laboratory manual,* ed 2, Cold Spring Harbor, NY, 1989, Cold Spring Harbor Laboratory Press.

58. Sanger F, Nicklen S, Coulson AR: DNA sequencing with chain-terminating inhibitors, *Proc Natl Acad Sci U S A* 74:5463, 1977.

59. Seeburg PH et al: The mammalian GnRH gene and its pivotal role in reproduction, *Recent Prog Horm Res* 43:69, 1987.

60. Segaloff DL et al: Structure of the lutropin/choriogonadotropin receptor, *Recent Prog Horm Res* 46:261, 1990.

61. Sinclair AH et al: A gene encodes a protein from the human sex-determining region with homology to a conserved DNA-binding motif, *Nature* 346:240, 1990.

62. Speiser PW, New MI, White PC: Molecular genetic analysis of nonclassic steroid 21-hydroxylase deficiency associated with HLA-B14,DR1, *N Engl J Med* 319:19, 1988.

63. Steger DJ et al: Evolution of placenta-aspecific gene expression: comparison of the equine and human gonadotropin a-subunit genes, *Mol Endocrinol* 5:243, 1991.

64. Su BC et al: Temporal and constitutive expression of homeobox-2 gene (Hu-2), human heat shock gene (hsp-70) and oncogenes C-sis and N-myc in early human trophoblast, *Am J Obstet Gynecol* 159:1195, 1988.

65. Talmadge K, Boorstein WR, Fiddes JC: The human genome contains seven genes for the β-subunit of chorionic gonadotropin but only one gene for the β-subunit of luteinizing hormone, *DNA* 2:281, 1983.

66. Talmadge K, Vamvakopoulos NC, Fiddes JC: Evolution of the genes for the β subunits of human chorionic gonadotropin and luteinizing hormone, *Nature* 307:37, 1984.

67. Taylor SI et al: Mutations in the insulin receptor gene in genetic forms of insulin resistance, *Recent Prog Horm Res* 46:185, 1990.

68. Thompson JS, Thompson MW: The molecular structure and function of chromosomes and genes. In Thompson JS, Thompson MW, editors: *Genetics in medicine,* ed 4, Philadelphia, 1986, WB Saunders.

69. Tusie-Luna M et al: A mutation (Pro-30 to Leu) in CYP21 represents a potential nonclassic steroid 21-hydroxylase deficiency allele, *Mol Endocrinol* 5:685, 1991.

70. Usala SJ et al: A base mutation of the c-erbAβ thyroid hormone receptor in a kindred with generalized thyroid hormone resistance, *J Clin Invest* 85:93, 1990.

71. Usala SJ et al: A homozygous deletion in the c-erbAβ thyroid hormone receptor gene in a patient with generalized thyroid hormone resistance: isolation and characterization of the mutant receptor, *Mol Endocrinol* 5:327, 1991.

72. Verma IM: Gene therapy, *Sci Am,* p 68, Nov 1990.

73. Watkins PC et al: DNA sequence and regional assignment of the human follicle-stimulating hormone β-subunit gene to the short arm of human chromosome 11, *DNA* 6:205, 1987.

74. Whitman GF, Pantazis CG: Cellular localization of mullerian inhibiting substance messenger RNA during human ovarian follicular development, *Am J Obstet Gynecol* 165:1881, 1991.

75. Witt BR, Thorneycroft IH: Reproductive steroid hormones: generation, degradation, reception, and action, *Clin Obstet Gynecol* 33:563, 1990.

76. Yanase T, Simpson ER, Waterman MR: 17α-Hydroxylase/17,20-lyase deficiency: from clinical investigation to molecular definition, *Endocr Rev* 12:91, 1991.

Chapter 2

REPRODUCTIVE EMBRYOLOGY AND SEXUAL DIFFERENTIATION

Michael L. Gustafson, MD
and Patricia K. Donahoe, MD

If an infant is to develop as a phenotypically complete male or female, a cascade of interdependent events must occur in the proper sequence and at the appropriate times in ontogeny. The embryo must have the correct chromosomal constituents. The germ cells must migrate from the endoderm of the yolk sac to the urogenital ridge in the retroperitoneum, where invasion of the developing gonads then occurs. The gonads, in turn, must produce hormones, and the urogenital ridge and external genitalia must have functional receptors to respond normally. These stages of sexual development define the infant's genetic, gonadal, and phenotypic sex, respectively. Should any of these events fail, or occur too late, an infant with abnormal sexual development or incongruent genetic, gonadal, and phenotypic sex may result. Clinically, such patients with ambiguous genitalia present challenges for gender assignment, timely surgical intervention, and appropriate hormonal replacement.

Recent advances in both reproductive endocrinology and molecular biology have improved understanding of the complex processes involved in sexual differentiation and embryologic development of the reproductive tract. For example, the pulsatile nature of hypothalamic gonadotropin-releasing factors and the three-dimensional structure of the gonadotropins have been well characterized. In addition, a factor involved in the migration of gonadotropin-releasing hormone (GnRH)-releasing neurons from the olfactory placode to the hypothalamus recently has been cloned and implicated in the etiology of Kallmann's syndrome. Genes encoding the receptors for luteinizing hormone chorionic gonadotropin (LH-CG), follicle-stimulating hormone (FSH), estrogen, progesterone, and androgen; the steroid enzyme testosterone 5α-reductase; and the hormones müllerian inhibiting substance (MIS), inhibin, and activin recently have all been cloned. Therefore, the structure/function, interactions, and second messengers of these protein molecules and their roles in sexual differentiation are being explored. Other factors responsible for the earliest stages of testis determination have also been identified. How the sex-determining region of the Y chromosome (SRY) gene and the testis-determining factor (TDF) regulate expression of related hormones and receptors, and therefore sexual differentiation, currently is being determined. The availability of many of the above proteins and molecular probes for research purposes, including study of their effects on the central nervous system, makes the area of sexual development an exciting scientific frontier.

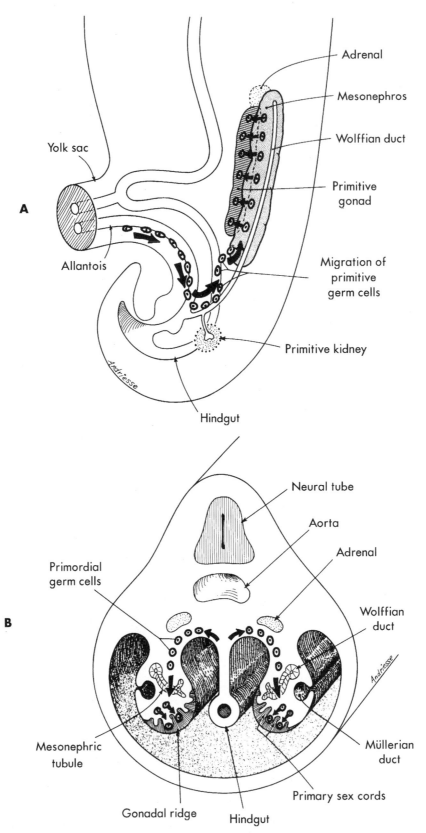

Fig. 2-1. Primordial germ cell migration. **A,** Germ cell migration is depicted during early embryonic development (lateral view). Primordial germ cells first appear in the wall of the yolk sac by 24 days of gestation, and then migrate along the nearby allantois to the hindgut. They subsequently travel via the retroperitoneum to arrive in the undifferentiated gonad. **B,** Completion of germ cell migration, as depicted in transverse section. Germ cells arriving from the hindgut and dorsal mesentery enter the primitive gonadal ridge by the sixth week of gestation. Note the primitive sex cords formed by invaginating coelomic epithelium. (From Donahoe PK, Crawford JD: In Welch KJ et al, editors: *Pediatric surgery,* ed 4, vol 2, Chicago, 1986, Year Book Medical Publishers.)

REPRODUCTIVE EMBRYOLOGY
Gonadal differentiation

Although the presence or absence of a sex-determining gene at the time of fertilization may determine the eventual gonadal sex of the embryo, morphologic development of the gonad as either a testis or an ovary does not occur until much later. A primitive urogenital ridge first forms from mesoderm of the posterior wall of the abdominal cavity and retroperitoneum at approximately 28 days of gestation in the human. The gonadal portion of this ridge results from rapid proliferation of coelomic epithelium and condensation of adjacent mesenchyme.[86] Epithelial strands are seen to extend into the underlying mesenchyme at this "indifferent" stage, giving rise to primitive sex cords that remain attached to the gonadal surface. Human primordial germ cells, meanwhile, first appear among endoderm cells in the wall of the yolk sac at 24 days of gestation.[111] These germ cells migrate along the nearby allantois, the wall of the hindgut, and the dorsal mesentery to enter the primitive gonadal ridge by the sixth week of development[12] (Fig. 2-1). Germ cell migration occurs actively through pseudopod formation, combined with growth and folding of the caudal end of the embryo. According to experimental studies in mice, the arrival of germ cells in the gonad does not appear to be necessary for testicular differentiation.[7] In contrast, the presence of oogonia seems to be essential for normal ovarian differentiation to occur.[65]

In the presence of a TDF a thick layer of fibrous connective tissue—later known as the tunica albuginea—forms around the early gonad, separating the primitive sex cords from the surface epithelium. The formation of the "testes cords" as early as day 42 is the first of many differences between male and female gonadal differentiation. The solid medullary cords, which consist of primordial germ cells and sustentacular cells of Sertoli, acquire lumina shortly before puberty and are then known as the seminiferous tubules of the adult testis.

Sertoli cells are thought to play the major role in support, maturation, and protection of the testicular germ cells and spermatogonia. Accordingly, germ cells that remain outside of the testes cords do not survive. Another primary function of Sertoli cells is to secrete MIS, the glycoprotein hormone responsible for regression of the müllerian ducts in normal males. As detailed later, MIS secretion begins between the seventh and eighth weeks of fetal life, but it continues at low levels throughout adulthood. Other functions of Sertoli cells include synthesis of androgen-binding protein, phagocytosis of degenerating germ cells, secretion of inhibin, and production of a host of other growth factors.

Interstitial cells of Leydig, meanwhile, begin to appear between the medullary testes cords by the seventh to eighth week of fetal development; they are thought to be of mesenchymal origin. These cells initiate testosterone synthesis and secretion by 8 weeks, which is necessary for maintainence and growth of the wolffian duct structures. The number of Leydig cells within the testis increases dramatically between the seventh and fourteenth embryonic weeks, when they account for 50% of the relative testis area.[70] Their number then decreases dramatically (probably by dedifferentiation), such that only relatively few remain in the newborn testis.

In the "female" urogenital ridge (lacking a TDF), on the other hand, the medullary sex cords eventually disappear and are replaced by vascular stroma. The surface epithelium of the resulting primitive ovary then forms a second set of cortical cords around primordial germ cells in the outer mesenchyme during the seventh week. These cell cords ultimately disperse to form the primordial ovarian follicles.

Byskov[7] believes that the mesonephros (the second of the three primitive kidneys) also contributes significantly to the somatic cell population of the gonad. This investigator hypothesizes that a "gonadal blastema" is formed in the gonad medulla by invasion of solid cell cords, with contributions from the adjacent mesonephros, the mesenchymal cells of the urogenital ridge, and the primordial germ cells. Primitive sex cords would then arise from this admixture of gonadal cells, rather than originating solely from coelomic epithelium. According to both theories of gonadal development, however, granulosa cells of the ovary and Sertoli cells of the testis arise from the same primitive bipotential sex cord cell.

Germ cell division

The fate of primordial germ cells in human embryos follows two distinct paths, which are distinguished primarily by the timing of germ cell entry into meiosis. This phenomenon is another of the earliest differences between male and female sexual development. In the developing fetal ovary, germ cells undergo multiple mitotic divisions between the third and seventh months and differentiate into oogonia. These oogonia also undergo multiple mitoses and then differentiate into primary oocytes, which immediately enter prophase of the first meiotic division. Primary oocytes subsequently form clusters of cells in the ovarian cortex that become surrounded by flattened epithelial cells, which ultimately give rise to the follicular or granulosa cells of maturing follicles.

The number of oogonia peaks during the fifth month of development at approximately 7 million.[86] Between the fifth and seventh months, however, most of the oogonia and primary oocytes degenerate. By the time of birth, only primary oocytes individually surrounded by a layer of future granulosa cells remain. The formation of such primordial follicles seems to be regulated by fetal pituitary FSH, which peaks in serum at 20 to 25 weeks.[30] The number of these primordial follicles at birth has been estimated to be 700,000 to 2,000,000.[86] All of the primary oocytes have entered the resting or dictyotene stage of the first meiotic division by this time, where they remain until puberty. At this point, several oocytes resume meiosis with the start of each ovarian cycle, with one or a few completing the first division to form a secondary oocyte and a diploid polar body. Ovulation then occurs when the secondary oocyte is in metaphase of the second division; this meiotic stage is completed only if fertilization occurs. Most of the primordial follicles become atretic during childhood, with approximately 400,000 surviving until puberty.[86]

In sharp contrast, primordial germ cells in the male persist in the primitive sex cords as prespermatogonia until shortly before puberty. A prepubescent burst in mitotic activity of these cells then results in formation of spermatogonia and primary spermatocytes within the seminiferous tubules. Each primary spermatocyte then undergoes first and second meiotic divisions to form two secondary spermatocytes and four haploid spermatids, respectively; spermatids then undergo extensive structural changes, such as acrosome formation and tail development, to form mature spermatozoa. Such cycles of spermatogenesis, which take approximately 74 ± 5 days from spermatogonia to spermatozoa,[37] are initiated continuously within the seminiferous tubules to maintain the sperm cell pool.

The timing of meiosis and pattern of germ cell differentiation are affected by the "gonadal context," or nature of the surrounding gonadal somatic cells. Upadhyay and Zamboni,[102] for example, observed that ectopically located primordial germ cells within the adrenal glands of male mice differentiated as otherwise normal-appearing oocytes. They concluded that germ cells enter meiosis during fetal life and then differentiate as oocytes autonomously unless present in a testicular environment. Interestingly, the timing of germ cell meiosis also seems to be regulated by the sex chromosomes of the surrounding gonadal somatic cells, rather than by those of the invading germ cells themselves.[62]

Genital duct differentiation

Two pairs of genital ducts develop within the urogenital ridge in both male and female embryos. The mesonephric kidney and its excretory duct develop in this region at 4 weeks in the human embryo.[74] The mesonephric, or wolffian, duct lies in the posteromedial aspect of the ridge, drains the mesonephric kidney along its lateral border, and then enters the urogenital sinus caudally (Fig. 2-1). Although the mesonephric kidney degenerates, its duct persists in the presence of testosterone to give rise to the epididymis, vas deferens, and seminal vesicle in fetal males. Proximal remnants of the mesonephric ducts in females are the epoöphoron and paroöphoron (vestigial structures near the ovary), whereas distally Gartner's ducts persist within the vaginal wall.

During the sixth week of gestation, the paramesonephric, or müllerian, ducts develop as paired longitudinal invaginations of coelomic epithelium along the anterolateral aspect of the urogenital ridge, in close proximity to the wolffian duct[86] (Fig. 2-1). In the absence of MIS, these ducts separate further from the wolffian ducts and ultimately give rise to the fallopian tubes, uterus, and upper portion of the vagina. Each duct opens cranially into the coelomic cavity, and then runs lateral and ventral to the wolffian duct until meeting the contralateral müllerian duct in the midline; the dividing uterine septum then disappears by day 66.[92] The caudal tip of the fused ducts abuts the posterior wall of the urogenital sinus to form the müllerian tubercle at about 9 weeks of development.[92] Sinovaginal bulbs, two solid evaginations from the urogenital sinus, then fuse with the müllerian tubercle to form the vaginal plate by the eleventh week. The urogenital sinus is greatly foreshortened and the urethra is pulled toward the perineum as this vaginal plate enlarges. Canalization of the vaginal plate is then completed by 17 weeks of development.[73] The proximal remnant of the müllerian duct in males is the appendix testis; the distal remnant is the prostatic utricle, a small outpouching from the male urethra at the level of the prostate.

The exact line of demarcation between the lower vagina of urogenital sinus origin and the upper vagina of müllerian duct origin is not clear. It is thought that the müllerian duct fusion site at the vaginal plate descends to the level of the hymen, with squamous cells from the urogenital sinus migrating upward and epithelializing an indeterminate portion of the müllerian vagina.[101] It is also possible that direct transformation of columnar müllerian epithelium to stratified squamous epithelium occurs in the vaginal canal.[92]

Fetal inducers, probably of mesenchymal origin, may play important roles in the normal development of the urogenital ridge and hindgut structures. The association of vaginal atresia, caudal regression anomalies, vertebral anomalies, and pelvic kidneys or renal agenesis in many patients suggests a common mesenchymal defect. It has been proposed that the mesonephros and its ducts are obligate inducers for metanephros development and ascent, as well as müllerian duct development.[16] The metanephric duct forms as an outpouching of the lower mesonephric duct and then ascends to meet the metanephric blastema, just posterior and lateral to the urogenital sinus. An ectopically located pelvic kidney may be perceived as failing to undergo normal embryonic ascent from this early position along the mesonephric "scaffolding." The mesonephros is equally critical to development of the müllerian ducts, whose formation seems to be guided by the wolffian duct. Gruenwald[29] has shown, for example, that experimental interruption of the wolffian duct results in failure of müllerian duct development.

If mesonephric resorption occurs prematurely in the fetus, an absent kidney may be associated with an absent or abnormal vas deferens and epididymis in the male, or absent or abnormal müllerian duct formation in the female (Fig. 2-2). If mesonephric resorption occurs after the metanephric blastema and ureteric bud have appeared, a

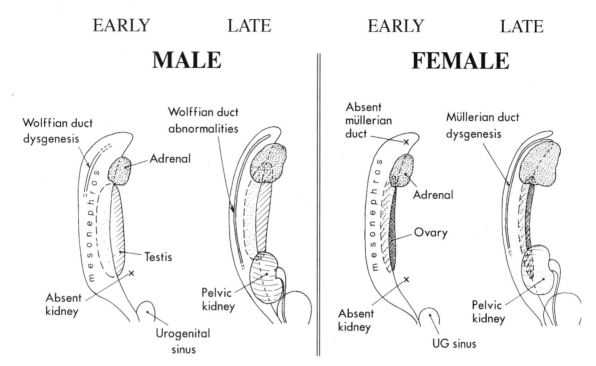

Fig. 2-2. Differentiation of genital ducts: abnormal mesonephric induction. The mesonephros is a posterior structure that provides a retroperitoneal backing for the adrenal superiorly, gonad and the müllerian and wolffian ducts laterally, and the kidney inferiorly. Its extent is seen in the 14-day rat embryo, two thirds of the way through gestation, before renal ascent accelerates. The mesonephros resorbs as the kidney ascends and differentiates. The mesonephros serves as an obligate inducer (1) to renal differentiation and ascent and (2) to the müllerian duct, either through or in conjunction with the mesonephric duct. If, in the male, mesonephric resorption occurs earlier than normal, renal agenesis and wolffian duct agenesis will occur. Later resorption can lead to pelvic kidney with less severe wolffian duct anomalies. Early resorption in the female leads to renal agenesis and müllerian duct atresia. Later resorption in the female can cause pelvic kidney and vaginal atresia. (Modified from Donahoe PK, Hendren WH: *J Pediatr Surg* 15:486, 1980.)

kidney in the pelvic position may result. In the male, this may be associated with anomalies of the vas deferens and epididymis; in the female, if the resorption occurs before müllerian duct development is completed, the pelvic kidney may be associated with distal müllerian duct agenesis, that is, vaginal atresia.

External genitalia differentiation

During the first 6 weeks of fetal development, the primordial external genitalia of male and female embryos are identical. As shown in Fig. 2-3, these bipotential structures include urogenital folds on either side of the cloacal or urogenital membrane, the labioscrotal swellings lateral to the urogenital folds, and the genital tubercle, which is formed by fusion of the urogenital folds cranially. Differentiation then begins at 7 to 8 weeks of development, corresponding to initiation of hormone synthesis by the primitive gonad.

In the presence of testosterone secretion by the fetal testis, the urogenital folds are pulled forward by rapid growth of the genital tubercle to form a urethral groove along the dorsal aspect of the elongating phallus. These folds then fuse in the midline to form the penile urethra. The distal urethra, however, is formed by a cord of ectodermal cells that migrates inward from the glans penis and then canalizes to form the urethral meatus.[86] The labioscrotal swellings migrate caudally from the inguinal region and fuse in the midline to form the scrotum and scrotal septum. Labioscrotal fusion is complete by the twelfth week of gestation; if fusion has not occurred by this stage, subsequent androgen exposure will cause phallic growth but not fusion.

In the female, in the absence of androgenic stimulation, the unfused urogenital folds give rise to the labia minora, and the lateral labioscrotal swellings develop into the labia majora. The midline urogenital groove, meanwhile, remains open as the vestibule. Finally, the clitoris develops from slight enlargement of the genital tubercle.

Gonadal descent

Testicular descent from the posterior abdominal wall to the internal inguinal ring is completed by 12 weeks of development. Between the seventh fetal month and the time of birth, the testis then completes its descent through the

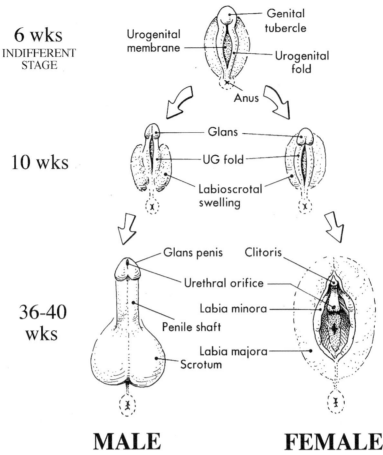

Fig. 2-3. Differentiation and development of external genitalia: differentiation of male and female external genitalia from early indifferent structures in the fetus. (Modified from Sadler TW: *Langman's medical embryology*, Baltimore, 1990, The Williams & Wilkins Co.)

inguinal canal into the scrotum. Ovarian descent, on the other hand, occurs to a level just above the pelvic rim during the twelfth fetal week; the ovary does not descend further in the absence of MIS and testosterone.

The gubernaculum is thought to be a target structure for the hormones involved in testicular descent, particularly during early abdominal migration. It extends from the caudal end of the testis through the inguinal canal eventually to insert on the wall of the scrotal swelling[82] and is at some stages as large as the testis itself. In the female, the gubernaculum equivalent is the round ligament of the uterus, a rudimentary structure that passes through the inguinal canal into the labia majora.

Intersex gonads

It is constructive to compare normal sexual differentiation with that observed in dysgenetic gonad syndromes and true hermaphroditism. Patients with dysgenetic gonads, particularly those with mixed gonadal dysgenesis, have disordered formation, early senescence, and neoplastic transformation of their gonadal tissue.[15,23] Many of these 45,X/46,XY or 46,XY patients have a dysgenetic testis on one side and a streak ovary on the other, although considerable gonadal variability can occur, such as unilateral gonadal agenesis, bilateral streak gonads, and unilateral gonadal tumors.[15,85]

In the absence of appropriate testicular "induction," differentiation of seminiferous tubules does not occur normally and MIS is produced only poorly or too late, leading to retention of müllerian duct structures. Leydig cell differentiation may also be deficient or delayed, leading to subnormal or late production of testosterone and incomplete masculinization. The ovary is also poorly differentiated in these patients, probably because of the absence of a second X chromosome (as discussed later). The streak ovaries are characterized by increased connective tissue elements and diminution of the primary follicles, which worsen and accelerate with time.

Such dysgenetic gonads are prone to neoplastic transformation.[15] Gonadoblastomas, which are often microscopic and bilateral, are an in situ form of malignancy that is most common in the dysgenetic testis; further dedifferentiation can occur in these gonads in the form of more malignant germ cell tumors, such as seminomas/dysgerminomas.[85]

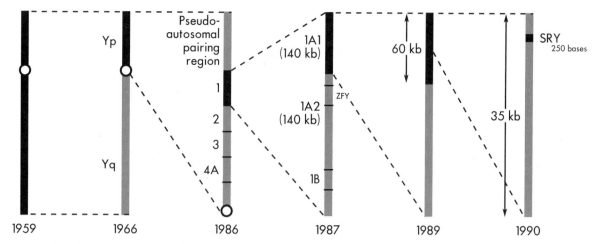

Fig. 2-4. Hunting the testis-determining factor. The chromosomal region thought to include the elusive TDF factor is shown in black. The search has narrowed from 30 to 40 million bases (1959) to the 250 bases encoding the consensus HMG 80-amino acid motif of SRY (1990). 1959, the Y chromosome was shown for the first time to be male-determining; 1966, search narrowed to the short arm; 1986, deletion analysis identified TDF in interval 1; 1987, further analysis limited search to 1A1; 1989, men were found who lacked ZFY; 1990, SRY identified. (From McLaren A.[63] Reprinted by permission from *Nature* 346:216. Copyright © 1990 Macmillan Magazines Ltd.)

Development of the latter group of germ cell malignancies is also common within streak gonads. Tumor expectancy in dysgenetic gonads with a Y chromosome has been calculated at 3% by 10 years, 10% by 13 years, 20% by 15 years, and 75% by 26 years.[58] Muller et al.[68] have reported carcinoma in situ changes in the germ cells of 45,X/46,XY dysgenetic gonads that precede development of clinically detectable tumors. These changes are similar to those observed in carcinoma in situ germ cells of cryptorchid testes and usually warrant gonadectomy. Both persistently elevated gonadotropin levels and the presence of primordial germ cells outside protective seminiferous tubules or ovarian follicles have been postulated to play a role in the neoplastic transformation.

True hermaphrodites, on the other hand, have both testicular and ovarian tissue that is well developed and nondysgenetic.[14] Such patients usually have a 46,XX karyotype, although more complex mosaicisms have been reported. The two gonadal tissue types may be present in a wide variety of combinations; often they occur together to form ovotestes or appear separately as a testis on one side and an ovary on the other. In ovotestes, testicular differentiation is almost always central, with ovarian differentiation at the gonadal poles; therefore, surgical biopsies should always be taken longitudinally through both the poles and the central portion of the gonad.[71] Müllerian duct structures are often present on the side of the ovary but regress on the side of the testicular gonad.

Asymmetry of the internal and external genitalia is frequently noted in the two groups of intersex patients just described. Gonadal symmetry refers to the position of one gonad relative to the other above or below the external inguinal ring. If symmetric, both gonads are located either above or below the inguinal ring, implying that a diffuse biochemical defect is present that is affecting each gonad equally. Such symmetry is observed in patients with male or female pseudohermaphroditism. However, if testicular tissue predominates on one side and ovarian tissue on the other, as is seen with mixed gonadal dysgenesis or true hermaphroditism, then gonadal asymmetry results. The predominantly ovarian gonad remains intraabdominal or inguinal, above the external ring, while the predominantly testicular gonad descends more normally.

REGULATION OF SEXUAL DIFFERENTIATION

The endocrine, paracrine, and autocrine factors required for proper phenotypic expression of sexual development are myriad and complex. A symphonic interaction is essential to ensure appropriate regulation of differentiation.

Testis-determining factor

The central event in fetal sexual differentiation is development of the indifferent gonadal ridge into a testis or an ovary. The critical role of the Y chromosome in this testicular, and thus male, differentiation was first appreciated in the late 1950s[63] (Fig. 2-4). For the first time, Ford et al.[26] and Jacobs and Strong[45] were able to demonstrate that the Y chromosome was associated with testicular differentiation in human intersex gonads. Subsequently, the search for the *TDF* gene was narrowed to the short arm of the Y. A male-specific histocompatibility antigen H-Y was next proposed as the primary testis determinant.[106] However, both men and mice[64] were found who did not fit this paradigm; that is, they possessed testes but lacked H-Y antigen. Therefore, a search was begun for other factors.

By analysis of chromosomal translocations in XX phenotypic males and deletion analysis of XY phenotypic females, Page et al.[75] were able to define a critical region for testis determination that was just proximal to the pseudoautosomal X-Y pairing region on the short arm of the Y chromosome (Fig. 2-4). Within this region they identified a 140-kilobase (kb) segment that was present in one XX male and absent in another XY female patient. A highly conserved gene in this portion of the Y chromosome (called zinc finger Y, or ZFY) encodes a zinc finger containing deoxyribonucleic acid (DNA)-binding protein that was initially thought to be the TDF.[75] However, this region was subsequently shown to be absent in several XX men, [76] and therefore the expression of ZFY, although likely important, was inconsistent with a role as the primary sex-determining gene.

All of the XX men studied, however, had markers positive for segment 1A1 of the Y chromosome, located between the above ZFY gene and the pseudoautosomal X-Y pairing region. In this sex-specific region of the Y, Sinclair et al.[90] recently delimited the search to a region of 35 kb. A single-copy gene that encodes a protein with homology to the phylogenetically distant mating type protein of yeast and to a mammalian high-mobility-group (HMG) protein nuclear transcription factor was identified from this region. This gene, called SRY for sex-determining region of the Y chromosome, is specific to the Y chromosome of all mammals studied and is highly conserved. It remains the best plausible candidate for the TDF gene.

The SRY protein has a strongly conserved 80-amino acid DNA-binding motif (the HMG box). Tissue- and time-specific SRY expression has been demonstrated during early development in male mice, immediately prior to gonadal differentiation, that is, in the somatic cells of the 10.5- to 12.5-day postcoitum urogenital ridge.[31,50] In addition, SRY expression in the fetal testis was shown to be independent of the presence of primordial germ cells. Expression of SRY returns in the mouse and human testis during adulthood and seems to be germ cell-dependent at this stage, since northern blot analyses of sex-reversed testes without spermatogonia were negative. The SRY messenger ribonucleic acid (mRNA) is approximately 1.3 kb in length in the adult testis.[50]

Several animal and human studies support the role of SRY as the primary testis determinant. In a line of XY sex-reversed female mice, the SRY gene was shown to be deleted from the Y chromosome.[31] In similar analyses of two XY human females, de novo mutations resulting in a conservative amino acid change within the DNA-binding motif of SRY in one patient, and a four-nucleotide deletion, frame-shift mutation in this same region in another patient were identified.[5,46] Finally, a number of chromosomally female mice, transgenic for a 14-kb fragment of the mouse Y chromosome containing the SRY gene and its adjacent regulatory sequences, displayed normal fetal testicular development.[51] The adult transgenic testes, however, showed absence of maturing spermatogonia (most likely secondary to the presence of two X chromosomes.)

Thus SRY plays an essential primary role in testis differentiation, most likely by activating a cascade of molecular events that lead to normal gonadal development (Table 2-1). For example, we have recently discovered an element in the promoter region of the MIS gene (designated SRYe) to which the HMG region of SRY binds with high affinity.[34] The specificity of this binding is attested to by its competition with SRY antibody. Similar elements are found in promoter regions of the aromatase gene. Therefore, expression of such sex-specific gene products, which are essential for proper sexual function, is likely to be regulated by SRY.

It should be stressed that many other factors exist that are potentially involved in human sexual differentiation and development but that have not been listed in Table 2-1. Such growth and regulatory factors include the inhibins,[60] activin,[54,103] small-molecular-weight oocyte maturation inhibitor,[98] and such proteins as epidermal growth factor and insulin-like growth factors I and II. All of these proteins have been detected in developing gonads, but their precise roles in gonadogenesis are still under investigation.

X Chromosome and X inactivation

The relatively large X chromosome, to which numerous genetic disorders have been linked, comprises 6% of the genomic DNA. The transcription of X-linked genes in males (with one X chromosome) and females (with two X chromosomes) is equal, secondary to "X inactivation." This phenomenon of "heterochromatinization," which results in transcriptional inactivation of all but one X chromosome in all somatic cells, occurs between the twelfth and eighteenth days in the human embryo.[30] However, several genes on the distal short arm of the X chromosome are known to escape this inactivation, including those in the pseudoautosomal region and the more proximal Xg blood group, steroid sulfatase enzyme, and zinc finger X (ZFX) loci.[87] The ZFX gene has striking homology to the ZFY gene on the Y chromosome described earlier, and both encode transcriptional activators with zinc finger domains that likely bind to identical DNA sequences. Page et al.[75] believe that ZFX and ZFY derived from a common gene on the ancestral autosomal chromosome pair that eventually gave rise to the mammalian X and Y. Classic Turner syndrome (45,X) has been related to monosomy of a gene on the long arm of the X chromosome that encodes an isoform of ribosomal protein S4 (RPS4X), which is known to escape X inactivation.[25] This gene has a Y chromosome homologue encoding another S4 isoform (RPS4Y) that maps to interval 1A1B on the distal short arm of the Y

Table 2-1. Factors involved in sexual determination and differentiation

Factor	Site Expression	Action	Ontogeny
Testis-determining factor	Fetal testis (somatic tubule cells)	Testicular differentiation	Immediately before gonadal differentiation
Second X chromosome	Ovarian oocytes (escape X inactivation)	Ovarian maturation	Somatic cell X inactivation, 2nd-3rd fetal week
Müllerian inhibiting substance	Sertoli cells	Müllerian duct regression; testicular descent; inhibition of germ cell meiosis; gonadal differentiation	By 7th-8th fetal week; decreases by puberty to low adult levels
	Granulosa cells	Inhibition of oocyte meiosis	Puberty and adulthood at low levels
Kallmann syndrome gene	Central nervous system	Production of neural cell adhesion/axonal pathfinding molecule; migration of GnRH-releasing neurons	Early fetal life
Luteinizing hormone (LH)-releasing hormones	Hypothalamus	Regulation of LH secretion	After 10th fetal week
Human chorionic gonadotropin (hCG)	Placenta	Regulation of androgen synthesis; Leydig cell differentiation?	By 6th-8th fetal week
LH	Anterior pituitary	Regulation of androgen synthesis	After 10th fetal week
hCG/LH receptor	Leydig cells	hCG/LH binding; regulation of androgen synthesis	By 6th-8th fetal week
FSH	Anterior pituitary	Formation of primordial ovarian follicles	By mid-fetal life
FSH receptor	Ovarian follicles	Folliculogenesis	By mid-fetal life
Testosterone	Leydig cells	Maintenance of wolffian duct; testicular descent	By 8th fetal week
Testosterone 5-α-reductase	Urogenital sinus, tubercle, folds, swellings; prostate	Conversion of testosterone to dihydrotestosterone (DHT)	By 8th fetal week
DHT	Same as above	Differentiation of male external genitalia; prostatic development; male-pattern hair growth	By 8th fetal week
Androgen receptor	All androgen-responsive cells	Testosterone/DHT-binding; androgen transport to nucleus; transcriptional regulation	Throughout life
Calcitonin gene-related peptide	Genitofemoral nerve	Testicular descent; gubernacular contraction; regulation of gubernacular differentiation	During testicular descent

chromosome, the region implicated by deletional analysis to be involved in 46,XY Turner syndrome. It has therefore been hypothesized that RPS4 "haploinsufficiency" may play a role in the development of the characteristic Turner syndrome phenotype.[25]

It is important to note that female germ cells require two active X chromosomes for normal oocyte formation, whereas male germ cells require X inactivation for normal spermatogenesis.[30] The second X chromosome in the female karyotype is presumed to be responsible for ovarian maturation, since in its absence the ovary undergoes premature degeneration. In patients with Turner syndrome, who have normal germ cell migration, oocytes disappear from the ovary prior to puberty and ovarian failure occurs

prematurely. Likewise, a family with premature ovarian failure was identified that had an interstitial deletion of the long arm of the X chromosome.[52] A Xq26-27 site in this region, which is also thought to escape X inactivation, likely contains one or several genes required for normal ovarian development.

Although two X chromosomes are required for completion of oocyte maturation in the ovary, the presence of two X chromosomes in a "testicular" environment is incompatible with fertility. For example, in XX sex-reversed male mice, germ cells do not survive in normal-appearing seminiferous tubules. Similarly, XXY human males with Klinefelter syndrome are sterile secondary to a germ cell maturational defect.

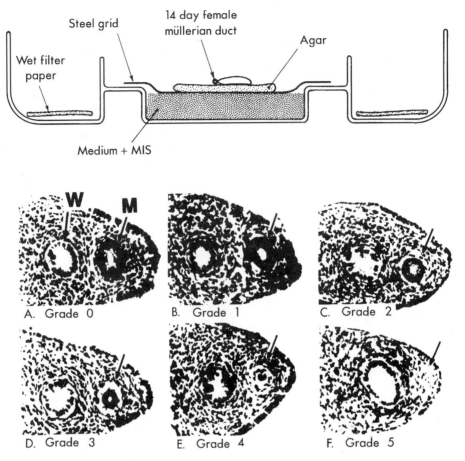

Fig. 2-5. Müllerian inhibiting substance bioassay. The schematic diagram (*top*) depicts the standard organ culture assay for MIS activity, which utilizes 14-day female fetal rat urogenital ridges. **A,** Section of a control ridge in the absence of MIS, demonstrating normal architecture of the müllerian (*M*) and wolffian (*W*) ducts. **B to D,** Intermediate grade 1 to grade 3 regression of the müllerian duct after 72 hours of incubation with recombinant human MIS. Mesenchymal condensation around the duct, basement membrane breakdown, and loss of epithelial cells are characteristic. **E and F,** Further grade 4 to grade 5 regression of the cultured müllerian duct. Some of the tubular epithelial cells have migrated into the surrounding mesenchyme. Note that the adjacent wolffian duct is unaffected. Magnification 100%. (Modified from Donahoe PK et al: *J Surg Res* 23:141, 1977.)

Müllerian inhibiting substance

In the male, Sertoli cells in the seminiferous tubules begin secreting MIS during the seventh to eighth fetal weeks. Taguchi et al.[92] concluded in a study of human embryonic müllerian duct tissue that MIS secretion begins by at least day 51 of gestation. This glycoprotein hormone, composed of two identical 70-kDa subunits, causes regression of the müllerian duct by approximately 64 days of fetal development. According to rat organ culture studies, there appears to be a critical window of müllerian duct responsiveness to MIS, before or after which MIS exposure does not induce full regression. In addition, duct regression is irreversible following appropriate MIS exposure.[18]

In the presence of MIS, condensation of mesenchyme occurs around the epithelial structures of the müllerian duct, followed by basement membrane breakdown. These events are associated with increased hyaluronidase activity and a decrease in hyaluronic acid, laminin, heparan sulfate, fibronectin, and type IV collagen within the basement membrane and mesenchymal matrix.[21,35] Some of the epithelial cells die an apoptotic death,[81] with autophagy of adjacent cells, while others migrate into the surrounding mesenchyme.[35,97] Fig. 2-5 demonstrates such müllerian duct regression in an experimental organ culture assay for MIS activity.[19] A 14.5-day female fetal rat urogenital ridge that has been cocultured with recombinant human MIS for 72 hours shows partial regression (Fig. 2-5, **B** to **D**) and nearly complete regression (Fig. 2-5, **E** and **F**), compared with no regression (Fig. 2-5, **A**) in the absence of MIS; the adjacent wolffian duct is unaffected.

The *MIS* gene, which was cloned in 1986[8] and subsequently mapped to the short arm of chromosome 19,[11]

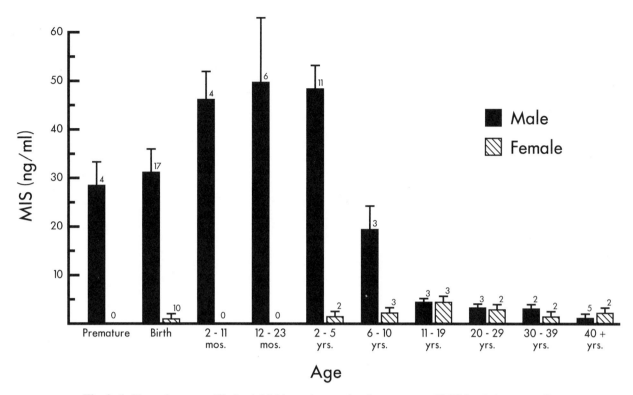

Fig. 2-6. Normal serum müllerian inhibiting substance levels: ontogeny of MIS levels in serum of human male and female subjects. Blood samples were obtained from patients at the age ranges indicated. MIS levels were quantitated by enzyme-linked immunosorbent assay (ELISA). Numbers indicate the numbers of samples per group, and the brackets denote the standard error of the mean. (Modified from Hudson PL et al: An immunoassay to detect human müllerian inhibiting substance in males and females during normal development, *J Clin Endocrinol Metab* 70:16, 1990; © The Endocrine Society.)

belongs to a supergene family of proteins and growth factors that are important in cell growth, differentiation, and regulation. This family includes the beta subunit of transforming growth factor, inhibin, activin, decapentaplegia complex, and bone morphogenesis factors. Members of this family share 20% to 40% amino acid homology at their carboxy-terminal ends, and several are known to undergo cleavage to form biologically active carboxy-terminal dimers. MIS is likewise thought to undergo activation by cleavage at amino acid 427, which produces 55- and 12-kDa fragments; the larger fragment is then believed to undergo secondary cleavage to form 34- and 22-kd peptides. It was not certain until recently which of these protein species was responsible for each biologic activity, but purified carboxy-terminal MIS is now known to be active in both müllerian duct regression and tumor inhibition assays.[57]

Murine monoclonal and rabbit polyclonal antibodies generated against human MIS were used to develop a highly sensitive enzyme-linked immunosorbent assay (ELISA) for the measurement of serum MIS.[39] Normal MIS values were then established for males and females at various ages throughout life (Fig. 2-6). As shown, MIS is present at high levels in normal males for several years postnatally; secretion then falls to a low baseline level by puberty (1 to 5 ng/mL), where it remains throughout adulthood. In contrast, serum MIS is undetectable in newborn females. MIS then becomes detectable at similarly low serum concentrations (1 to 5 ng/mL) between puberty and the onset of menopause, when it again falls below measurable levels. This ELISA has been useful for studying patients with various intersex anomalies, suspected anorchia, retained müllerian ducts, and ovarian sex cord tumors—particularly granulosa cell tumors and sex cord tumors with annular tubules.[32,33] MIS has become a valuable marker for both the presence of functioning testicular tissue and metastatic sex cord tumor, particularly when testosterone and estradiol levels are inconclusive.

MIS is thought to have several functions in addition to its primary role in genital tract development. For example, MIS may be a factor in the higher incidence of respiratory distress syndrome observed in premature males, since it can inhibit fetal rat lung surfactant accumulation and lung

Table 2-2. Correlation of müllerian inhibiting substance in the developing rat gonad with the timing of sex cord and germ cell mitotic/meiotic activities

| Stage of development* | Male (+ SRY) | | Female (autonomous) | |
	Sertoli cells	Germ cells	Granulosa cells	Germ cells
E_{10-11}		Mitosis (prespermatogonia)		Mitosis (oogonia)
$E_{13.5-14}$	(+) MIS			
E_{16}-P_2	(+) MIS; cell division	No meiotic division; cessation of mitosis		First meiotic division (oocytes); cessation of mitosis
P_{3-8}	(↓) MIS; cessation of cell division	Mitosis (spermatogonia)	(+) MIS; cell division in preantral/antral follicles	Meiotic arrest (dictyate stage)
P_{8-15}		(Spermatocytes)		
P_{15}-adult	(−) MIS	Two meiotic divisions (spermatids)	(+) MIS in preantral/antral follicles; (−) MIS in large preovulatory follicles	Resumption of meiosis with ovulation

*E, Embryonic day; P, postnatal day.

maturation in vivo.[9] It is also thought to play a role in testicular descent in the fetus, as described later. MIS contributes to the "freemartin effect" in genetic females who have placental anastomoses to their male twins. In addition to the anticipated regression of their müllerian ducts, these XX females have ovaries with markedly reduced volume, germ cell depletion, and primitive seminiferous tubule formation.[47] By treatment of fetal ovaries with recombinant MIS in vitro, Vigier et al.[104] were able to reproduce these characteristic features, which were subsequently demonstrated to be associated with inhibition of aromatase biosynthesis[105] and the release of testosterone instead of estradiol from MIS-treated ovaries. This phenomenon was therefore termed "endocrine sex reversal."

Such morphologic and endocrine effects have suggested a potential role for MIS in primary gonadal differentiation. When transgenic mice chronically expressing MIS were created, the female animals had blind vaginas, no uteri or fallopian tubes, and fewer germ cells than normal within their newborn ovaries.[4] By 2 weeks of age, germ cells were completely lost and somatic cells were organizing into seminiferous tubulelike structures. By adulthood, these ovaries had degenerated and were no longer detectable. These results suggest that MIS has direct effects on both germ cells and somatic cells during gonadogenesis.

Table 2-2 illustrates several of these possible relationships in the rat model. In both male and female rats, MIS is secreted in the largest amounts at times when meiotic activity of the germ cells is inhibited, with subsequent decreases in MIS secretion accompanied by initiation or resumption of meiosis. The ontogeny of MIS in bovine[94] and rat[99] granulosa cells and the variation in MIS production by these cells during the rat estrous cycle[100] supports

such a critical role for MIS in the regulation of oocyte maturation. In addition, germinal vesicle breakdown of rat oocytes has been shown to be inhibited by MIS in vitro.[93] Similarly, in the B6.YDOM mouse ovotestes, Taketo et al.[95] have noted that MIS-producing seminiferous tubules contain germ cells in meiotic arrest, whereas germ cells in tubules lacking MIS undergo progressive maturation. It is also of note that the periods of greatest mitotic activity of sex cord cells correspond to the times of peak MIS production, both in rapidly growing fetal testes cords and in enlarging pubertal and adult ovarian follicles.

Study of patients with persistent müllerian duct syndrome has provided additional insight into the actions of MIS. These patients are characterized by uterus inguinale (retained uterus and fallopian tubes in an inguinal hernia sac) and unilateral or bilateral cryptorchidism, but they have normal external genitalia and virilization. A point mutation in the *MIS* gene of such a patient, in whom no immunoreactive or bioactive MIS could be detected, was recently identified.[49] This "nonsense" mutation produced a premature stop codon in the fifth exon of the *MIS* gene, resulting in an abnormal protein lacking 178 carboxy-terminal amino acids. The patient with retained müllerian duct had normal testicular differentiation and morphology, which may argue for a role for the NH_2-terminal portion of MIS in male gonadogenesis. Other MIS-positive patients are thought to have MIS receptor defects or to express MIS only after the period of receptor sensitivity has passed.

The ontogeny and tissue specificity of SRY and MIS expression suggest that the *MIS* gene may be induced by SRY and that MIS may then act later to support continued testicular differentiation. In the mouse, SRY is expressed in the urogenital ridge between fetal days 10.5 and 12.5[50]

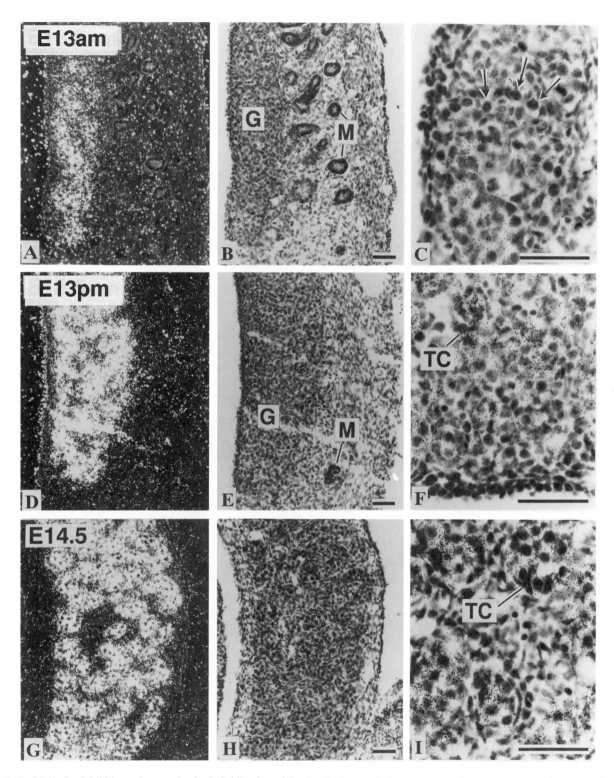

Fig. 2-7. Müllerian inhibiting substance in situ hybridization of the developing testis. The ontogeny of MIS gene expression in relationship to sex cord formation and gonadal differentiation is demonstrated by this study of the fetal rat testis. Left lanes are dark-field views, in which MIS hybridization signals are seen as white grains; middle lanes are bright-field views of the same sections; right lanes are higher magnification, with MIS signals seen as black grains. On the morning of fetal day 13 (*E13am;* **A, B, C**), germ cells with large round nuclei are scattered throughout the gonad (*G*), while somatic cells with ovoid nuclei are not yet organized; MIS signals are seen diffusely over the gonad (*M,* mesonephros). Later that day (*E13pm;* **D, E, F**), some somatic cells are seen organizing around germ cells as early testis cords (*TC*); MIS expression is increased, but in a patchy distribution. By fetal day 14.5 (*E14.5*) (**G, H, I**), testis cord formation is observed throughout the gonad, with intense MIS signal localized to the testis cord Sertoli cells. Magnification 200%. (From Hirobe S et al: *Endocrinology* 131:854, 1992.)

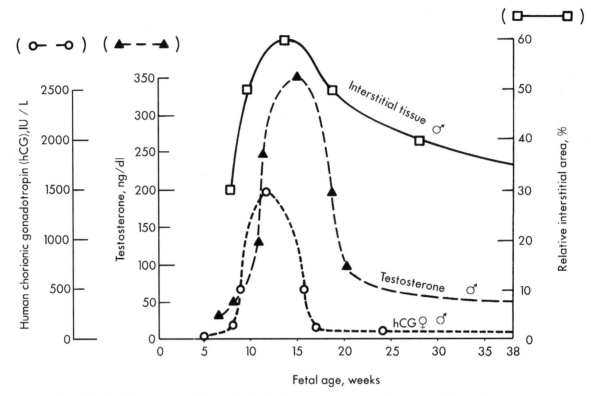

Fig. 2-8. Fetal hormone profile and testicular development: schematic representation of human chorionic gonadotropin (hCG) and testosterone in male fetal serum throughout gestation, correlated with testicular interstitial tissue area. hCG and testosterone values are given on the left ordinate; relative interstitial tissue area is given as a percentage of total tissue area on the right ordinate. (Modified from Pelliniemi LJ, Dym M: In Tulchinsky D, Ryan KJ, editors: *Maternal-fetal endocrinology,* Philadelphia, 1980, WB Saunders.)

(which correlates with fetal days 11.5 to 13.5 in the rat), immediately prior to the onset of testicular differentiation and the expression of MIS mRNA and protein.[69] In the rat, SRY expression has not been fully characterized, but sex cord formation occurs between fetal day 13.5, when in situ studies show that MIS mRNA is first expressed,[38] and fetal day 14.5, when discrete seminiferous tubule formation can first be observed (Fig. 2-7). In addition, we have also recently observed that 12.5-day fetal rat urogenital ridge nuclear extracts bind with high affinity to a regulatory sequence (designated *SRYe*) in the promoter region of the *MIS* gene, and can compete with excess SRY antibody. Therefore, MIS secretion may be an important early event in the cascade of molecular events controlling gonadal differentiation.

Gonadotropins and their releasing factors

Leydig cells appear in the interstitium of the testis during the seventh to eighth fetal weeks and begin testosterone biosynthesis almost immediately. The androgen concentration subsequently increases in testicular tissue, fetal blood, and amniotic fluid over the next several weeks,

peaking at 300 ng/dL in fetal serum at 15 to 18 weeks of development.[79] This surge of androgen synthesis and secretion corresponds with a dramatic increase in the number of Leydig cells in the interstitium and is preceded by an increase in placental human chorionic gonadotropin (hCG) concentration in the fetus, as shown in Fig. 2-8. This rise in placental hCG occurs simultaneously with the appearance of the first Leydig cells. A rapid fall in placental hCG is followed first by a decrease in the relative area of interstitial tissue in the testis and then by a return of serum testosterone to low baseline levels (approximately 75 ng/dL at birth).[79]

The demonstration of hCG in fetal testes,[42] the presence of hCG receptors in fetal Leydig cells,[41] and the correlations between hCG levels and testicular interstitial volume all suggest that hCG may stimulate mesenchymal cell differentiation into Leydig cells. In addition, testosterone synthesis by the interstitial cells seems to be regulated initially by hCG.[40] This seems likely, since hCG and LH have very similar B-subunits, bind to the same receptor, and have the same biologic effects. Neither of the fetal pituitary gonadotropins (luteinizing hormone [LH] and FSH) is detectable in serum before the tenth week of development[48]; they appear to be important in testosterone regulation only late in gestation. It thus makes sense that placental insufficiency may be associated with deficient masculinization of the newborn child or male pseudohermaphroditism. Placental insufficiency, which may be more common than previously appreciated, is suggested by low levels of hCG in pregnancy tests and may explain the deficient genitalia found in the "twin-B syndrome."[13] Children of such pregnancies usually have an excellent response to postnatal testosterone therapy, which can be used prior to genital reconstruction.

Kallmann syndrome and panhypopituitarism, on the other hand, are associated with micropenis, but not such earlier developmental defects as hypospadias or failure of scrotal fusion. Kallmann syndrome is characterized by hypogonadotropic hypogonadism secondary to GnRH deficiency and anosmia (the inability to smell). A gene deletion recently has been identified on the X chromosome in several such patients; this proposed gene encodes a protein with homology to neural cell adhesion and axonal pathfinding molecules, as well as protein kinases and phosphatases.[27] Lack of this protein could therefore result in abnormal migration of both olfactory neurons and GnRH-producing hypothalamic neurons that originate in the olfactory placode. In patients with either of these causes of hypogonadotropic hypogonadism, pulsatile GnRH therapy is currently being used to achieve pubertal maturation.[108] GnRH is administered subcutaneously by a pump at short pulse intervals, which simulates its normal physiologic release and results in appropriate testosterone or estrogen secretion. (See Chapter 34.)

The LH-CG and FSH receptors, both of which have been cloned within the last few years, are related to the G protein-coupled receptor "superfamily."[61,91] Both possess seven membrane-spanning domains, which are characteristic of this family, but each also has a large extracellular domain that presumably is important for ligand binding. (See Fig. 1-25.) There is 50% sequence homology between these extracellular domains and 80% between the transmembrane domains. In response to hCG, LH, and FSH, cells expressing these receptors show an increase in adenylate cyclase activity and an increase in the intracellular second-messenger cyclic adenosine monophosphate.

Despite normal placental hCG, fetal pituitary LH, and normal Leydig cell receptors, deficient masculinization in the newborn male still may occur. Any one of three etiologies, addressed in the following sections, may lead to male pseudohermaphroditism, including inadequate testosterone biosynthesis, an inability to convert testosterone to its more active form of dihydrotestosterone (DHT), and absent or defective androgen receptors.

Sex steroid synthesis

The pathway for normal steroid metabolism and androgen biosynthesis is represented in Fig. 2-9. Most of the synthetic enzymes shown are cytochrome P-450-related oxygenases. Deficiencies in several different enzymes, which are inherited as autosomal recessive traits, can result in deficient biosynthesis of testosterone. 20,22-Desmolase (also known as P-450scc, for side chain cleavage), 3β-hydroxysteroid dehydrogenase, and 17d-hydroxylase deficiencies also interfere with normal cortisol production; therefore, such male infants present with adrenal insufficiency as well as insufficient masculinization. 17,20-Desmolase and the more common 17-ketosteroid reductase defects, on the other hand, result in isolated testosterone deficiency. Barbiturates and hydantoins can inhibit testosterone secretion by inhibiting the P-450scc enzyme and thereby cause male pseudohermaphroditism. After stimulation with hCG in all of these patients, serum testosterone does not increase as expected. Intermediary substrate-product ratios can then provide information to localize further the defect in the steroid biosynthetic pathway.

If a 21-hydroxylase or 11-hydroxylase defect occurs in the adrenal steroidogenic pathway shown in Fig. 2-9, congenital adrenal hyperplasia can result.[66] In the female fetus, this will result in masculinization or female pseudohermaphroditism. Decreased synthesis of cortisol stimulates overproduction of adrenocorticotropic hormone from the pituitary, which in turn stimulates P-450scc activity and increased adrenal androgen secretion. Virilization of the female fetus results from this in utero androgen exposure. The uterus, fallopian tubes, and ovary develop normally, but the distal vagina often fails to reach the perineum, resulting in a urogenital sinus deformity. The more severely masculinized the patient, the more proximal will be the conjoining of the vagina to the urethra. Masculinization of the external genitalia also can be severe, with profound clitoral enlargement and labioscrotal fusion. In contrast, male infants with this enzyme defect usually have a normal phenotype,[17] but they can be detected by genital and areolar hyperpigmentation.

The role of estrogen in early sexual differentiation may be constitutive, because both male and female embryos exist in a sea of maternal estrogen. Rabbit and human fetal ovaries are capable of synthesizing estradiol from cholesterol, although the 3β-hydroxysteroid dehydrogenase activity is only a fraction of that observed in the fetal testis. It is of interest and extreme biologic importance that no congenital anomalies manifesting abnormalities of the estrogen receptor have been found.

Testosterone 5α-reductase

In the male, differentiation of the external genitalia requires reduction of testosterone to DHT by the microsomal enzyme steroid 5α-reductase. This enzyme activity appears in the urogenital sinus and urogenital tubercle, folds, and swellings before the onset of sexual differentiation.[89,110] Under the influence of the resulting DHT, the tubercle lengthens considerably, the urogenital folds fuse to form the penile urethra, the labioscrotal swellings form the

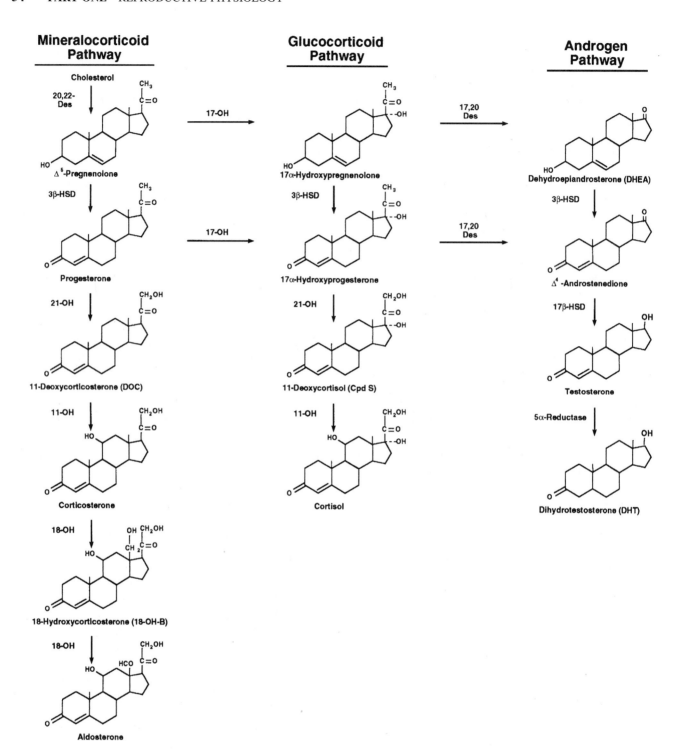

Fig. 2-9. Normal pathways of steroid metabolism and androgen biosynthesis: normal pathways for steroid metabolism, demonstrating the related mineralocorticoid, glucocorticoid, and androgen synthetic enzymes. A single enzyme deficiency therefore affects more than one pathway (*Des,* desmolase; *OH,* hydroxylase; *HSD,* hydroxysteroid dehydrogenase). (Modified from Donahoe PK, Crawford JD: In Welch KJ et al, editors: *Pediatric surgery,* ed 4, vol 2, Chicago, 1986, Year Book Medical Publishers.)

scrotum, and the prostate develops as an outpouching of the urogenital sinus. In contrast, wolffian duct derivatives do not develop the capacity for DHT formation until late in development.[89,110] Therefore, the conversion of testosterone to DHT does not seem to be required for normal differentiation of the epididymis, vas deferens, and seminal vesicle. Both testosterone and DHT exert their effects through androgen receptor binding, although DHT has been shown to have somewhat higher affinity than testosterone.[109]

The inability to convert testosterone to DHT because of a steroid 5α-reductase deficiency results in a rare form of male pseudohermaphroditism, originally referred to as pseudovaginal perineoscrotal hypospadias.[72,80,107] This autosomal recessive defect results in deficiency of the external genitalia, with a clitoral-like phallus, severe perineoscrotal hypospadias, an undifferentiated prostatic utricle into which drain normal genital ducts, and normally differentiated testes. The genes for two human 5α-reductase isozymes recently have been cloned from prostatic tissue.[2,3] The first of these appears to be of only minor significance in genital structures and is normal in affected patients. The second isozyme, on the other hand, has much greater expression in genital and prostatic tissue and has been found to be deleted in two related patients with 5α-reductase deficiency.

Such patients undergo significant masculinization at puberty; therefore, it seems appropriate that they should be raised as males. Dramatic growth of the phallus and external genitalia occurs, accompanied by an increase in muscle mass and deepening of the voice.[80] The characteristic poor response to endogenous androgen in the newborn period and this vigorous response at puberty are not fully understood, but they are a distinct clinical entity. It is of interest that these postpubertal patients report normal erections, ejaculations, and libido, but lack normal body and facial hair growth, acne formation, and temporal hairline recession. The prostate also remains small, being barely palpable in patients over 30 years of age. This observation has potential clinical applications, because blockade of 5α-reductase activity could be useful in the treatment of benign prostatic hypertrophy or prostatic carcinoma.

The testosterone-DHT ratio is increased in the serum of postpubertal males with this enzyme defect. Prepubertally, when the basal level of androgen is low, such an abnormality may not be appreciated until hCG stimulation is performed. The diagnosis has also been confirmed by assaying 5α-reductase activity in cultured skin fibroblasts.

The period of maximal responsiveness of the phallus to testosterone stimulation remains somewhat controversial. Traditionally, it was thought that the phallus was more responsive to androgen immediately after birth and that a normal newborn infant may have higher 5α-reductase activity,[83] more abundant androgen receptors,[30,83] and more hyperplastic tissue.[1] Therefore, improved growth of the phallus would be possible with early treatment. However,

other investigators now believe that the phallus should respond appropriately regardless of the time treatment is initiated.[67] The natural histories of patients with 5α-reductase deficiency support this latter hypothesis, since these patients masculinize sufficiently at puberty for gender-appropriate function.

Androgen receptor

The effects of both testosterone and DHT on sexual differentiation and virilization are mediated through binding to a high-affinity nuclear receptor. This receptor, which is a 100 kDa monomeric protein encoded by a gene on the X chromosome, belongs to the supergene family of steroid hormone receptors[22] (Fig. 2-10). All of these proteins are characterized by a hypervariable amino-terminal region, a cysteine-rich DNA-binding domain, and a hydrophobic steroid-binding domain. Binding of steroid ligand to receptor is thought to result in transcriptional activation (or inactivation). Consensus oligonucleotide probes complementary to the highly conserved DNA-binding domains of the other steroid receptors were used to clone the androgen receptor gene.[10,55,96] In the DNA-binding domain, the glucocortoid and progesterone receptors are more than 90% homologous to the androgen receptor, whereas the steroid ligand-binding regions are only about 50% homologous. The amino-terminal domain, which is the most dissimilar to other steroid hormone receptors, is postulated to have a role in transcriptional activation or modulation of DNA binding.

The syndrome of complete androgen insensitivity, or testicular feminization, is now known to be secondary to a variety of genetic defects in the androgen receptor. A point mutation[56] and a large deletion[6] in the androgen-binding domain of the receptor gene have been described, as well as aberrant splicing[84] and a premature termination codon in the messenger RNA.[59] In addition, a point mutation in the steroid-binding domain and a single base pair deletion resulting in a frame-shift mutation have been described in the experimental testicular-feminized rat[113] and mouse[36] androgen receptors, respectively. Most recently, X-linked spinal and bulbar muscular atrophy was found to be associated with an androgen receptor gene mutation; these patients have many more tandem cytosine-adenine-guanine (CAG) repeats in the NH_2 terminus of the gene, resulting in larger polyglutamine tracts in the receptor protein and altered transcriptional regulation.[53] These defects result in either reduced androgen receptor mRNA and/or protein, or in a protein with functional impairment in binding or transcriptional activation. Androgen-binding assays of cultured skin fibroblasts obtained by biopsy can be performed in the evaluation of this type of male pseudohermaphroditism.

Testicular descent

Normal gonadal descent in the male fetus is thought to occur as a two-step process. The first stage involves

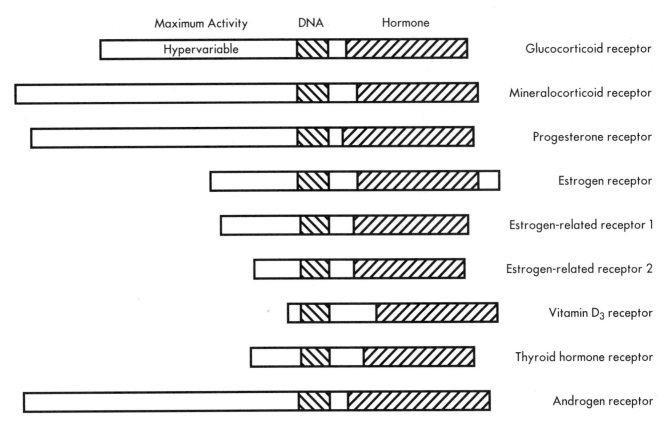

Fig. 2-10. Steroid receptor homology. Steroid receptor family members all display a level of homology for a zinc finger DNA-binding region, a hormone-binding region, and a region required for maximal activity that probably regulates DNA binding. (Modified from Evans RM: *Science* 240:889. Copyright 1988 by the American Association for the Advancement of Science.)

transabdominal movement of the gonad, followed by a second stage of inguinal and transscrotal descent.[44] The abdominal migration of the testis occurs while MIS is still markedly elevated and may be regulated by this hormone. The second stage of descent, on the other hand, is thought to be a neuronally mediated, testosterone-driven event.

Consistent with this two-stage hypothesis, patients with the persistent müllerian duct syndrome and an MIS or MIS receptor defect have abdominal testes, whereas females with congenital adrenal hyperplasia and markedly elevated testosterone levels have normally located ovaries.[88] Two studies have likewise suggested that cryptorchid testes secrete less MIS than age-matched controls, although whether this is cause or effect remains unclear.[20,112] Human patients and experimental mice with complete androgen insensitivity, meanwhile, have arrested descent of the gonad just past the level of the internal inguinal ring.[43]

It is likely that the gubernaculum plays a central role in testicular descent and is acted upon by MIS, testosterone, and other regulatory factors. The early abdominal phase of migration is associated with rapid growth of the distal gubernacular "bulb," with marked cellular proliferation and deposition of hyaluronic acid, sulfated glycosaminogly-

cans, and collagen within this structure.[24] A 1988 in vitro study of fetal porcine gubernacular fibroblasts obtained during this stage measured growth in response to MIS, androgens, inhibin, and several other fetal growth factors. None of these factors increased DNA synthesis significantly, but a low-molecular-weight factor—tentatively named descendin—present in same-stage fetal testicular extracts did so.[24]

The later inguinal phase of descent is associated with cessation of cellular proliferation, regression of the extraabdominal "bulb," and gubernacular differentiation. In animal studies, the gubernacular mesenchymal tissue has been shown to possess both androgen receptors and age-specific 5α-reductase activity, supporting a role for testosterone in differentiation and function during this stage.[28] Park and Hutson,[78] however, have proposed that androgens act indirectly upon this structure via the genitofemoral nerve. Early studies in which division of this nerve prevented second-stage testicular descent, as well as gubernacular differentiation, prompted their current work. They have recently shown that the 37-amino acid peptide neurotransmitter, calcitonin gene-related peptide (CGRP), is present in motor neurons of the genitofemoral nerve and their nerve cell bodies.[78] In addition, there is marked sexual dimorphism between the size and number of these cell bodies within the lumbar spinal cord, with larger and more numerous cells observed in male rodents than in female rodents. Moreover, newborn male rat gubernacula excised and placed in organ culture demonstrated continuous rhythmic contractions in response to added CGRP (40 to 230 beats per minute). The gubernaculum therefore appears to be a highly active structure, with regulation during this stage by CGRP, the genitofemoral nerve, and testosterone.

FUTURE DIRECTIONS

With increased understanding of reproductive embryology, the normal stages of sexual development, and the molecular mechanisms underlying sexual differentiation, a greater appreciation of abnormalities of sexual ambiguity will be possible. As the next step, this knowledge may make rational and timely fetal intervention for such genetic defects a viable option in the future, as is now being done for congenital adrenal hyperplasia.[77] Earlier treatment may produce a more "normal" newborn and preclude the long delays in medical or surgical therapy that often occur today. With such intervention, the complexity of the genital abnormality, as well as its clinical management and surgical reconstruction, may decrease significantly. In addition, the use of drugs designed from improved understanding of nonsteroidal molecular defects may augment steroid replacement therapy to provide these children with a more normal existence.

REFERENCES

1. Allen TD: Microphallus: clinical and endocrinological characteristics, *J Urol* 119:750, 1978.
2. Andersson S, Russell DW: Structural and biochemical properties of cloned and expressed human and rat steroid 5-alpha-reductases, *Proc Natl Acad Sci U S A* 87:3640, 1990.
3. Andersson S et al: Deletion of steroid 5-alpha-reductase 2 gene in male pseudohermaphroditism, *Nature* 354:159, 1991.
4. Behringer RR et al: Abnormal sexual development in transgenic mice chronically expressing mullerian inhibiting substance, *Nature* 345:167, 1990.
5. Berta P et al: Genetic evidence equating SRY and the testis-determining factor, *Nature* 348:448, 1990.
6. Brown TR et al: Deletion of the steroid-binding domain of the human androgen receptor gene in one family with complete androgen insensitivity syndrome: evidence for further genetic heterogeneity in this syndrome, *Proc Natl Acad Sci U S A* 85:8151, 1988.
7. Byskov AG: Differentiation of mammalian embryologic gonad. *Physiol Rev* 66:71, 1986.
8. Cate RL et al: Isolation of the bovine and human genes for mullerian inhibiting substance and expression of the human gene in animal cells, *Cell* 45:685, 1986.
9. Catlin EA et al: Sex specific fetal lung development and MIS, *Am Rev Respir Dis* 141:466, 1990.
10. Chang C, Kokontis J, Liao S: Molecular cloning of human and rat complementary DNA encoding androgen receptors, *Science* 240:324, 1988.
11. Cohen-Hagenauer O et al: Mapping of the gene for anti-mullerian hormone to the short arm of the human chromosome 19, *Cytogenet Cell Genet* 44:2, 1987.

12. Donahoe PK, Crawford JD: Ambiguous genitalia in the newborn. In Welch KJ et al, editors: *Pediatric surgery,* ed 4, vol 2, Chicago, 1986, Year Book.
13. Donahoe PK, Crawford JD, Hendren WH: Management of neonates and children with male pseudohermaphroditism, *J Pediatr Surg* 12:1045, 1977.
14. Donahoe PK, Crawford JD, Hendren WH: True hermaphroditism: a clinical description and a proposed function for the long arm of the Y chromosome, *J Pediatr Surg* 13:293, 1978.
15. Donahoe PK, Crawford JD, Hendren WH: Mixed gonadal dysgenesis, pathogenesis and management, *J Pediatr Surg* 14:287, 1979.
16. Donahoe PK, Hendren WH: Pelvic kidney in infants and children: experience with 16 cases, *Pediatr Surg* 15:486, 1980.
17. Donahoe PK, Powell DM, Lee MM: Clinical management of intersex abnormalities. In Wells SA et al, editors: *Current problems in surgery,* vol 28, St Louis, 1991, Mosby-Year Book.
18. Donahoe PK et al: The production of mullerian inhibiting substance by the fetal, neonatal, and adult rat, *Biol Reprod* 15:329, 1976.
19. Donahoe PK et al: A graded organ culture assay for the detection of mullerian inhibiting substance, *J Surg Res* 23:141, 1977.
20. Donahoe PK et al: Mullerian inhibiting substance in human testes after birth, *J Pediatr Surg* 12:323, 1977.
21. Donahoe PK et al: Molecular dissection of mullerian duct regression. In Trelstad RL, editor: *The role of extracellular matrix in development,* New York, 1984, Alan R Liss.
22. Evans RM: The steroid and thyroid hormone receptor superfamily, *Science* 240:889, 1988.
23. Federman DD: *Abnormal sexual development: a genetic and endocrine approach to differential diagnosis,* Philadelphia, 1967, WB Saunders.
24. Fentener van Vlissingen JM et al: In vitro model of the first phase of testicular descent: identification of a low molecular weight factor from fetal testis involved in proliferation of gubernaculum testis cells and distinct from specified polypeptide growth factors and fetal gonadal hormones, *Endocrinology* 123:2868, 1988.
25. Fisher EMC et al: Homologous ribosomal protein genes on the human X and Y chromosomes: escape from X inactivation and possible implications for Turner syndrome. *Cell* 63:1205, 1990.
26. Ford CE et al: A sex-chromosome anomaly in a case of gonadal dysgenesis (Turner's syndrome), *Lancet* 1:711, 1959.
27. Franco B et al: A gene deleted in Kallmann's syndrome shares homology with neural cell adhesion and axonal path-finding molecules, *Nature* 353:529, 1991.
28. George FW: Developmental pattern of 5-alpha-reductase activity in the rat gubernaculum, *Endocrinology* 124:727, 1989.
29. Gruenwald P: The relation of the growing mullerian duct to the wolffian duct and its importance for the genesis of malformations, *Anat Rec* 81:1, 1941.
30. Grumbach MM, Conte FA: Disorders of sex differentiation. In Wilson JD, Foster DW, editors: *Williams textbook of endocrinology,* Philadelphia, 1992, WB Saunders.
31. Gubbay J et al: A gene mapping to the sex-determining region of the mouse Y chromosome is a member of a novel family of embryonically expressed genes, *Nature 346:245, 1990.*
32. Gustafson ML et al: Mullerian inhibiting substance: a novel tumor marker for ovarian sex cord tumor with annular tubules, *N Engl J Med* 326:466, 1992.
33. Gustafson ML et al: Mullerian inhibiting substance in the diagnosis and management of intersex and gonadal abnormalities, *J Pediatr Surg,* 28:439, 1993.
34. Haqq CM et al: SRY recognizes conserved DNA sites in sex specific promoters, *Proc Natl Acad Sci U S A* 90:1097, 1993.
35. Hayashi A et al: Periductal and matrix glycosaminoglycans in rat mullerian duct development and regression, *Dev Biol* 92:16, 1982.
36. He WW, Kumar MV, Tindall DJ: A frame-shift mutation in the androgen receptor gene causes complete androgen insensitivity in the testicular-feminized mouse, *Nucleic Acids Res,* 19:2373, 1991.

37. Heller CG, Clermont Y: Kinetics of the germinal epithelium in man, *Recent Prog Horm Res* 20:545, 1964.

38. Hirobe S et al: Mullerian inhibiting substance messenger ribonucleic acid expression in granulosa and Sertoli cells coincides with their mitotic activity, *Endocrinology,* 131:854, 1992.

39. Hudson PL et al: An immunoassay to detect human mullerian inhibiting substance in males and females during normal development, *J Clin Endocrinol Metab* 70:16, 1990.

40. Huhtaniemi IT: Studies on steroidogenesis and its regulation in human fetal adrenal and testis, *J Steroid Biochem* 8:491, 1977.

41. Huhtaniemi IT, Korenbrot CC, Jaffe RB: hCG binding and stimulation of testosterone biosynthesis in the human fetal testis, *J Clin Endocrinol Metab* 44:963, 1977.

42. Huhtaniemi IT, Korenbrot CC, Jaffe RB: Content of chorionic gonadotropin in human fetal tissues, *J Clin Endocrinol Metab* 46:994, 1978.

43. Hutson JM: Testicular feminization: a model for testicular descent in mice and men, *J Pediatr Surg* 21:195, 1986.

44. Hutson JM, Donahoe PK: The hormonal control of testicular decent, *Endocr Rev* 7:270, 1986.

45. Jacobs PA, Strong JA: A case of human intersexuality having a possible XXY sex-determining mechanism, *Nature* 183:302, 1959.

46. Jager RJ et al: A human XY female with a frame shift mutation in the candidate testis-determining gene SRY, *Nature* 348:452, 1990.

47. Jost A, Vigier B, Prepin J: Freemartins in cattle: the first steps of sexual organogenesis, *J Reprod Fertil* 29:349, 1972.

48. Kaplan SL, Grumbach MM, Aubert ML: The ontogenesis of pituitary hormones and hypothalamic factors in the human fetus: maturation of central nervous system regulation of anterior pituitary function, *Recent Prog Horm Res* 32:161, 1976.

49. Knebelmann B et al: Anti-mullerian hormone bruxelles: a nonsense mutation associated with the persistent mullerian duct syndrome, *Proc Natl Acad Sci U S A* 88:3767, 1991.

50. Koopman P et al: Expression of a candidate sex-determining gene during mouse testis differentiation, *Nature* 348:450, 1990.

51. Koopman P et al: Male development of chromosomally female mice transgenic for SRY, *Nature* 351:117, 1991.

52. Krauss CM et al: Familial premature ovarian failure due to an interstitial deletion of the long arm of the X chromosome, *N Engl J Med* 317:125, 1987.

53. LaSpada AR et al: Androgen receptor gene mutations in X-linked spinal and bulbar muscular atrophy, *Nature* 352:77, 1991.

54. Ling N et al: Pituitary FSH is released by a heterodimer of the beta-subunits from the two forms of inhibin, *Nature* 321:779, 1986.

55. Lubahn DB et al: Cloning of human androgen receptor complementary DNA and localization to the X chromosome, *Science* 240:327, 1988.

56. Lubahn DB et al: Sequence of the intron/exon junctions of the coding region of the human androgen receptor gene and identification of a point mutation in a family with complete androgen insensitivity, *Proc Natl Acad Sci U S A* 86:9534, 1989.

57. MacLaughlin DT et al: Mullerian duct regression and antiproliferative bioactivities of mullerian inhibiting substance reside in its carboxy-terminal domain, Endocrinology 131:291, 1992.

58. Manuel M, Katayama KP, Jones HW: The age of occurrence of gonadal tumors in intersex patients with a Y chromosome, *Am J Obstet Gynecol* 124:205, 1976.

59. Marcelli M et al: Definition of the human androgen receptor gene structure permits the identification of mutations that cause androgen resistance: premature termination of the receptor protein at amino acid residue 588 causes complete androgen resistance, *Mol Endocrinol* 4:1105, 1990.

60. Mason et al: Complementary DNA sequences of ovarian follicular fluid inhibin show precursor structure and homology with transforming growth factor-beta, *Nature* 318:659, 1985.

61. McFarland KC et al: Lutropin-choriogonadotropin receptor: an un-usual member of the G protein-coupled receptor family, *Science* 245:494, 1989.

62. McLaren A: Meiosis and differentiation of mouse germ cells, *Symp Soc Exp Biol* 38:7, 1984.

63. McLaren A: What makes a man a man?, *Nature* 346:216, 1990.

64. McLaren A et al: Male sexual differentiation in mice lacking H-Y antigen, *Nature* 312:552, 1984.

65. Merchant H: Rat gonadal and ovarian organogenesis with and without germ cells: an ultrastructural study, *Dev Biol* 44:1, 1975.

66. Miller WT, Levine LS: Molecular and clinical advances in congenital adrenal hyperplasia, *J Pediatr* 111:1, 1987.

67. Money J, Lehne GK, Pierre JF: Micropenis: adult follow-up and comparison of size against new norms, *J Sex Marital Ther* 10:105, 1984.

68. Muller J et al: Carcinoma in situ of the testis in children with 45X/46XY gonadal dysgenesis, *J Pediatr* 106:431, 1985.

69. Munsterberg A, Lovell-Badge R: Expression of the mouse antimullerian hormone gene suggests a role in both male and female sexual differentiation, *Development* 13:613, 1991.

70. Niemi M, Ikonen M, Hervonen A: Histochemistry and fine structure of the interstitial tissue in the human foetal testis. In Wolstenholme GEW, O'Connor M, editors: *Ciba Foundation colloquia on endocrinology, vol 16, Endocrinology of the testis,* London, 1967, J & A Churchill.

71. Nihoul-Fekete C et al: Preservation of gonadal function in true hermaphroditism, *J Pediatr Surg* 19:50, 1984.

72. Opitz JM et al: Pseudovaginal perineoscrotal hypospadias, *Clin Genet* 3:1, 1972.

73. O'Rahilly R: The embryology and anatomy of the uterus. In *The uterus,* Baltimore, 1973, Wilkins & Wilkins.

74. O'Rahilly R: Prenatal human development. In Wynn RM, editor: *Biology of the uterus,* New York, 1977, Plenum Press.

75. Page DC et al: The sex-determining region of the human Y chromosome encodes a finger protein, *Cell* 51:1091, 1987.

76. Palmer MS et al: Genetic evidence that ZFY is not the testis-determining factor, *Nature* 342:931, 1990.

77. Pang S et al: Prenatal treatment of congenital adrenal hyperplasia due to 21-hydroxylase deficiency, *N Engl J Med* 322:111, 1990.

78. Park WH, Hutson JM: The gubernaculum shows rhythmic contractility and active movement during testicular descent, *J Pediatr Surg* 26:615, 1991.

79. Pelliniemi LJ, Dym M: The fetal gonad and sexual differentiation. In Tulchinsky D, Ryan KJ, editors: *Maternal-fetal endocrinology,* Philadelphia, 1980, WB Saunders.

80. Peterson RE et al: Male pseudohermaphroditism due to steroid 5-alpha-reductase deficiency, *Am J Med* 62:170, 1977.

81. Price JM, Donahoe PK, Ito Y: Involution of the female mullerian duct of the fetal rat in the organ-culture assay for the detection of mullerian inhibiting substance, *Am J Anat* 156:265, 1979.

82. Radhakrishnan J et al: Observations on the gubernaculum during descent of the testis, *Invest Urol* 16:365, 1979.

83. Rajfer J, Namkung PC, Petra PH: Ontogeny of 5-alpha-reductase and the androgen receptor in the penis, *Clin Androl* 7:53, 1981.

84. Ris-Stalpers C et al: Aberrant splicing of androgen receptor mRNA results in synthesis of a nonfunctional receptor protein in a patient with androgen insensitivity, *Proc Natl Acad Sci U S A* 87:7866, 1990.

85. Robboy SJ et al: Dysgenesis of testicular and streak gonads in the syndrome of mixed gonadal dysgenesis, *Hum Pathol* 13:700, 1982.

86. Sadler TW: *Langman's medical embryology,* Baltimore, 1990, Williams & Wilkins.

87. Schneider-Gadicke A et al: ZFX has a gene structure similar to ZFY, the putative human sex determinant, and escapes X inactivation, *Cell* 57:1247, 1989.

88. Scott JES: The Hutson hypothesis: a clinical study, *Br J Urol* 60:74, 1987.

89. Siiteri PK, Wilson JD: Testosterone formation and metabolism

during male sexual differentiation in the human embryo, *J Clin Endocrinol Metab* 38:113, 1974.

90. Sinclair AH et al: A gene from the human sex-determining region encodes a protein with homology to a conserved DNA-binding motif, *Nature* 346:240, 1990.

91. Sprengel R et al: The testicular receptor for follicle stimulating hormone: structure and functional expression of cloned cDNA, *Mol Endocrinol* 4:525, 1990.

92. Taguchi O et al: Timing and irreversibility of mullerian duct inhibition in the embryonic reproductive tract of the human male, *Dev Biol* 106:394, 1984.

93. Takahashi M, Koide SS, Donahoe PK: Mullerian inhibiting substance as oocyte meiosis inhibitor, *Mol Cell Endocrinol* 47:225, 1986.

94. Takahashi M et al: The ontogeny of mullerian inhibiting substance in granulosa cells of the bovine ovarian follicle, *Biol Reprod* 35:447, 1986.

95. Taketo T et al: Delay of testicular differentiation in the B6.YDOM ovotestis demonstrated by immunocytochemical staining for mullerian inhibiting substance, *Dev Biol* 146:386, 1991.

96. Tilley WD et al: Characterization and expression of a cDNA encoding the human androgen receptor, *Proc Natl Acad Sci U S A* 86:327, 1989.

97. Trelstad RL et al: The epithelial-mesenchymal interface of the male rat mullerian duct: loss of basement membrane integrity and ductal regression, *Dev Biol* 92:27, 1982.

98. Tsafriri A, Pomerantz SH: Oocyte maturation inhibitor, *Clin Endocrinol Metab* 15:157, 1986.

99. Ueno S et al: Cellular localization of mullerian inhibiting substance in the developing rat ovary, *Endocrinology* 124:1000, 1989.

100. Ueno S et al: Mullerian inhibiting substance in the adult rat ovary during various stages of the estrous cycle, *Endocrinology* 125:1060, 1989.

101. Ulfefder H, Robboy SJ: The embyological development of the human vagina, *Am J Obstet Gynecol* 126:769, 1976.

102. Upadhyay S, Zamboni L: Ectopic germ cells: natural model for the study of germ cell sexual differentiation, *Proc Natl Acad Sci U S A* 79:6584, 1982.

103. Vale et al: Purification and characterization of an FSH releasing protein from porcine ovarian follicular fluid, *Nature* 321:776, 1986.

104. Vigier B et al: Purified bovine AMH induces a characteristic freemartin effect in fetal rat prospective ovaries exposed to it in vitro, *Development* 100:43, 1987.

105. Vigier B et al: Anti-mullerian hormone produces endocrine sex reversal of fetal ovaries, *Proc Natl Acad Sci U S A* 86:3684, 1989.

106. Wachtel SS et al: Possible role for H-Y antigen in the primary determination of sex, *Nature* 257:235, 1975.

107. Walsh PC et al: Familial incomplete male pseudohermaphroditism, type 2: decreased dihydrotestosterone formation in pseudovaginal perineoscrotal hypospadias, *N Engl J Med* 291:944, 1974.

108. Whitcomb RW, Crowley WF: Clinical review 4: diagnosis and treatment of isolated gonadotropin-releasing hormone deficiency in men, *J Clin Endocrinol Metab* 70:3, 1990.

109. Wilbert DM, Griffin JE, Wilson JD: Characterization of the cytosol androgen receptor of the human prostate, *J Clin Endocrinol Metab* 56:113, 1983.

110. Wilson JD, Lasnitzki I: Dihydrotestosterone formation in fetal tissues of the rabbit and rat, *Endocrinology* 89:659, 1971.

111. Witschi E: Migration of the germ cells of the human embryos from the yolk sac to the primitive gonadal folds, *Contrib Embryol* 32:67, 1948.

112. Yamanaka J et al: Serum levels of mullerian inhibiting substance in boys with cryptorchidism, *J Pediatr Surg* 26:621, 1991.

113. Yarbrough WG et al: A single base mutation in the androgen receptor gene causes androgen insensitivity in the testicular feminized rat, *J Biol Chem* 265:8893, 1990.

Chapter 3

THE HYPOTHALAMUS AND REPRODUCTIVE DISORDERS

Samuel S. C. Yen, MD, DSc

To be fully versed in reproductive disorders, an understanding of the hypothalamic control of reproductive hormones (follicle-stimulating hormone [FSH], luteinizing hormone [LH], and prolactin) and metabolic hormones (thyroid-stimulating hormone [TSH], adrenocorticotropic hormone [ACTH], and growth hormone [GH]) as well as neurohypophysial hormones is required. For example, reproductive dysfunction may be associated with GH excess (acromegaly), with ACTH excess (Cushing syndrome), and with thyroid deficiency and excess. In fact, patients with amenorrhea due to hypothalamic lesions may have abnormal hormonal secretion by both adenohypophysial and neurohypophysial systems. Furthermore, neuroendocrine regulation of reproductive homeostasis has been recognized to involve circadian rhythmicity and sleep-wake cycles within the 24-hour biologic clock. These dynamic processes are properties of a hypothalamic pacemaker (the suprachiasmatic nucleus) and they invoke cyclic changes of almost all clinically discernible physiologic variables such as body temperature, blood pressure, and pituitary hormone release.[5] Frequent sequential measurement of plasma hormones has led to the recognition that most hormones are secreted episodically (ultradian rhythm); several have prominent circadian rhythmicity, some are linked to the sleep-wake cycle, and others are synchronized with food ingestion and a dark-light cycle.[5,47,76,123] These entrained neuroendocrine rhythms have emerged as critical indexes of "glandular" function of the brain, and with growing appreciation that desynchronization of these rhythms may underlie a number of important reproductive disorders.[1,76]

To date, five hypophysiotropic hormones have been isolated: thyrotropin-releasing hormone (TRH), gonadotropin-releasing hormone (GnRH), somatostatin (SS), corticotropin-releasing factor (CRF), and GH-releasing hormone (GHRH). The amino acid sequence of each of these neuropeptides is shown in Fig. 3-1. These peptidergic neuronal systems, originally thought to be unique to the hypothalamus, are now found in many regions of the brain, the brainstem, and spinal cord. Furthermore, they are present in the peripheral and central autonomic nervous system; the exocrine and endocrine glands; the diffuse endocrine tissues of the gastrointestinal, respiratory, and reproductive tracts; and the placenta.

This chapter deals with the control of adenohypophysial function by all of the established hypothalamic hormones. Clinical manifestation, diagnosis, and management of menstrual disorders of hypothalamic origin are presented.

HYPOTHALAMIC-ADENOHYPOPHYSIAL SYSTEM

Median eminence

The median eminence is the final common pathway for neurohumoral control of the anterior pituitary. It receives peptidergic neurons of the tuberohypophysial tract and their neuropeptides, the releasing and release-inhibiting hormones. From the substance of the median eminence, these

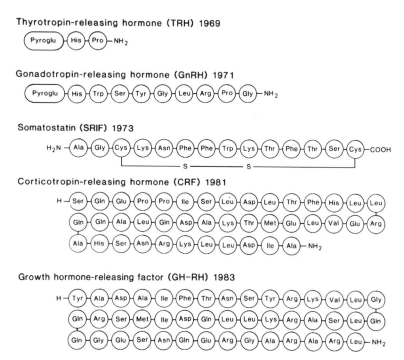

Fig. 3-1. Amino acid sequences of the hypophysiotropic peptides of hypothalamic origin that have been isolated, characterized, and synthesized since 1969.

hypophysiotropic hormones are delivered to the portal capillaries, where they act on target cells with specific receptors. The endothelium of these capillary loops is fenestrated, thus permitting macromolecules to enter without a functional blood-brain barrier. Axons of the neurohypophysial neurons also pass through this region with terminals abutting on portal vessels, where high concentrations of vasopressin, oxytocin, and neurophysin are delivered to the portal blood. For this reason and because the dorsomedial zone of the adenohypophysis receives a part of its blood supply from the adjacent neural lobe, there exists a potential for interaction between the two lobes of the pituitary.[79]

Portal system

The portal system connecting the median eminence and the adenohypophysis serves to deliver hypothalamic hormones to target cells in the anterior pituitary in the regulation of biosynthesis and secretion. Retrograde flow from the pituitary to the hypothalamus also appears to occur, and constitutes the mode of "short loop" feedback whereby pituitary hormones may have direct effects on hypothalamic function.[56,79]

In the portal blood, all of the known hypothalamic neuropeptides are present in high concentration. In addition, catecholamines, dopamine, norepinephrine, and epinephrine also are secreted into the portal blood in concentrations severalfold higher than in peripheral blood.[80] Biogenic amines, in addition to serving as neurotransmitters, may have a direct neurohormonal role in the regulation of hypothalamic-hypophysial function.

HYPOTHALAMIC GONADOTROPIN-RELEASING HORMONE–GONADOTROPE SYSTEM

The elucidation of the structure of the 10-amino acid hypothalamic GnRH in 1971,[73] followed by its total synthesis, led to a rapid advance in the understanding of central regulation of reproductive function. The pulsatile nature of hypothalamic GnRH release is now known to determine episodic pituitary gonadotropin secretion. The periodicity and amplitude of the pulsatile rhythm of GnRH–gonadotropin secretion are critical in determining gonadal activation specifically and reproductive function generally. The attribute of the self-priming effect of GnRH on its own action is expressed only at the physiologic periodicity (60 to 90 minutes) by way of up-regulation of GnRH receptors on the gonadotrope; slower frequency causes anovulation and amenorrhea, and higher frequency or constant exposure of GnRH induces refractory gonadotropin responses resulting in a state of down-regulation. At the molecular level, the activation of gene expression for alpha and beta subunits (α-gonadotropin; β-LH, β-FSH), dimerization of α, β- subunits, and glycosylation is also governed by intermittency of GnRH inputs to the gonadotrope.

Gonadotropin-releasing hormone neuronal system

Distribution. The GnRH neuronal system has been mapped in detail by using immunocytochemical methods. GnRH neurons are not grouped into distinct nuclei, but appear as loose networks spread through several anatomic divisions. There are considerable differences in the distribution of GnRH neurons among various mammalian species: primates, including humans, have GnRH neurons located mainly in the arcuate nucleus of the medial basal hypothalamus (MBH) and the preoptic area of the anterior hypothalamus, whereas in rodents very few GnRH neurons have been detected in the arcuate nucleus. The most prominent network in the rodent is composed of neurons forming a loose continuum of the septo-preoptico-infundibular pathway.[6,107,111]

Axons from GnRH neurons project to many sites within the brain. One of the most distinct projections is from the MBH to the median eminence, terminating in an extensive plexus of boutons on the primary portal vessel that delivers GnRH to its target cells—the gonadotropes. Axons of GnRH neurons also project to the limbic system and circumventricular organs other than the median eminence, such as the organum vasculosum of the lamina terminalis and neurohypophysis in humans and other mammals.[3] The neuroendocrine role of these projections is unclear at the present time.

Ontogeny

Origin. During early development, neurons expressing GnRH immunoreactivity are found in the epithelia of the olfactory placode, and GnRH cells course across the nasal septum and traverse the nervus terminalis into the forebrain. Thereafter, most GnRH cells form an arch through the developing forebrain into the anlagen of the septum and hypothalamus, extending into the preoptic area by embryonic day 14. This migratory route of GnRH neurons, studied in mice, supports the notion of an olfactory pit origin, since increasing numbers of GnRH cells are found in the septal-preoptic-hypothalamic area, with a concomitant decrease in the numbers of GnRH cells in the olfactory pit and nasal septum as gestation advances.[103] Immunocytochemistry and in situ hybridization reveal a similar migratory pattern of GnRH neurons from the nasal region to the basal hypothalamus in fetal rhesus monkeys.[95] An olfactory epithelial origin for GnRH neurons and the absence of olfactory bulbs account for the anosmia associated with hypogonadotropic hypogonadism in patients with Kallmann syndrome.[32,102] The Kallmann gene locus on the X chromosome—Xp22.3—has been identified; the syndrome develops when deletion or translocation of this gene occurs.[32] As a consequence, GnRH neurons fail to migrate into the brain. They appear to have been hooked up with numerous GnRH cells along the early migration route, but they are totally or partially absent in the brain beyond the meninges.[102]

During fetal life. LH-containing cells develop in the human fetal anterior pituitary as early as 9 weeks of gestation,[51] and GnRH immunoactivity has been found in the human hypothalamus at 11 weeks.[12] Furthermore, isolated MBH from the midgestational (20 to 23 weeks) human fetus releases GnRH in a pulsatile manner in vitro.[90] The fetal gonadotrope has the capacity to respond in vivo and in vitro to GnRH stimulation with the release of LH.[99] Thus, long before midgestation in the human fetus, the hypothalamic GnRH pulse generator and the pituitary gonadotrope constitute a functional unit for maintaining LH and FSH secretion.

Concentrations of immunoreactive LH in serum and the pituitary are significantly greater in the human female fetus than in the human male fetus at midgestation.[93] Since GnRH secretion at this time is quantitatively similar in male and female MBHs,[88,89] this sex-associated difference in LH secretion may reflect a negative feedback action by factors from the fetal testis that attenuate the pituitary sensitivity to GnRH stimulation. Indeed, during repetitive GnRH pulse administrations, pituitary LH responses are sixfold greater in female fetuses than in male fetuses.[99]

During sexual maturation. The onset of puberty is brain-driven by way of an increase in pulsatile release of hypothalamic GnRH. It is initiated in the absence of gonads, as has been observed in patients with gonadal dysgenesis[98]; and in the infantile monkey, puberty can be activated prematurely by exogenous pulses of GnRH.[127]

The ontogeny of pulsatile GnRH-gonadotropin secretion appears to conform to a U-shaped curve (Fig. 3-2); the elevated gonadotropin levels found during the first year of life are followed by a progressive decline, reaching a quiescent hypogonadotropic state at age 6 to 8 years with a parallel decrease in pituitary responsiveness to exogenous GnRH. Since the gonadotropin nadir occurs in the absence of ovarian function,[98] this prepubertal restraint on gonadotropin secretion can be attributed entirely to the central inhibition of hypothalamic GnRH secretion. Although endogenous opioids are a most attractive candidate as a central inhibitor of GnRH neuronal activities, studies in monkeys[74] and humans[81] have failed to support this hypothesis. Instead, evidence suggests that the onset of puberty, but not the prepubertal gonadotropin nadir, is associated with an increased opioidergic tone[81] and enhanced proopiomelanocortin gene expression in the arcuate nucleus.[125] The role of the putative excitatory neurotransmitter, aspartate, in the activation of GnRH neuronal secretion during puberty should be considered; prolonged, intermittent, intravenous injection of an analogue of aspartate, *N*-methyl-D-asparate, results in onset of precocious puberty in immature monkeys.[84]

The pubertal activation of the GnRH secretory program (the upswing of the U-shaped curve; see Fig. 3-2) implies a decline in hypothalamic inhibitors or an increase in stimulators, either mechanism permitting a progressive increase in GnRH-LH pulse amplitude without changing

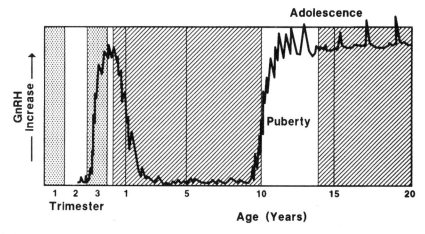

Fig. 3-2. Diagrammatic representation of the ontogeny of GnRH secretion from fetal life to adolescence. GnRH neuronal activity is well established during the second half of gestation. The relatively active GnRH pulsatility appears to be sustained in early neonatal life, followed by a progressive decline during the first year of life. Note the prepubertal nadir and the upswing of GnRH secretory activity at the onset of puberty, which is followed by irregular LH surges during adolescence in girls—the U-shaped curve. (Redrawn from Yen SSC: In Roland R, editor: *Neuroendocrinology of reproduction,* Amsterdam, 1988, Excerpta Medica.)

frequency.[98] In addition, the sleep-entrained amplification of GnRH-LH pulsatility is critical to activation of pituitary-ovarian function.[50] Before the hypothalamic-pituitary-ovarian axis is synchronized, luteal phase defects and anovulatory cycles are common occurrences in adolescent girls.[4]

Gonadotropin-releasing hormone gene and its expression

GnRH gene sequences were first isolated in 1984 from a human genomic deoxyribonucleic acid (DNA) library.[105] Analysis of the nucleotide sequence of messenger ribonucleic acid (mRNA) reveals that the GnRH decapeptide is derived from the posttranslational processing of a large precursor molecule, prepro-GnRH. The prepro-GnRH molecule consists of 92 amino acids with a tripartite structure: the decapeptide is preceded by a signal peptide of 23 amino acids and followed by a glycine-lysine-arginine sequence (position 11 to 13) essential for proteolytic processing and carboxy-terminal amidation of GnRH molecules. The last 56 amino acid residues are designated as GnRH-associated peptide (GAP), which may have prolactin-inhibiting properties.[106] It is a single gene located on the short arm of chromosome 8. The human gene contains four exons: exon 2 encodes pro-GnRH, exon 3 and parts of exons 2 and 4 encode the GAP protein, and a long 3' untranslated region is also encoded in exon 4. Placental pro-GnRH mRNA is longer than hypothalamic pro-GnRH mRNA because of an encoded 900-base pair intron that may modify or be regulated by tissue-specific promoters.[106]

By using nucleic acid probes for in situ hybridization of prepro-GnRH mRNA as well as precursor-specific and GAP-specific antisera, the molecular processing within the GnRH neurons is found to occur primarily in the cell body (soma). The cleavage products, GnRH and GAP, are then transported to the nerve terminals and secreted in tandem into the portal circulation.[1,52,96,106] In the basal hypothalamus of proestrous rats, GnRH decapeptide and pro-GnRH mRNA are found in the same cell with a high degree of correlation ($r = .9$), whereas the correlation in male rats is relatively low ($r = .56$), suggesting that molecular components of the GnRH system are regulated by reproductive states.[97] Within the brain, GAP is invariably co-localized with GnRH, but the functional significance of this tight association is unclear.[1]

Gonadotropin-releasing hormone pulse generator

In a series of elegant experiments conducted in the rhesus monkey by Knobil and associates, it was firmly established that the GnRH neuronal system within the MBH exhibits a rhythmic behavior with acute and short-lasting volleys of electrical multiunit activity. These volleys occur at approximately hourly intervals, have their origin in the vicinity of the arcuate nucleus within the MBH, and show a remarkable synchronism between pulses of GnRH in the portal blood and LH pulses in the peripheral blood.[16,17,55] Thus a short-term rhythm at hourly intervals within the MBH that governs the pulsatile discharge of GnRH from the nerve terminals at the median eminence represents the key controller of pituitary gonadotropin secretion and hence the entire reproductive process.

In humans, hypothalamic pulsatile GnRH secretion and the site of the putative GnRH pulse generator have been largely extrapolated from studies in nonhuman primates. In humans, this functional-anatomic relationship of the pulse generator has been confirmed in isolated human MBHs. Discrete pulsatile GnRH release from the MBH of the human fetus (20 to 23 weeks of gestation) and adult can be observed in an in vitro perfusion system. The periodicity of GnRH pulses is approximately 60 minutes for the fetal MBH and 60 to 100 minutes for the adult MBH.[90] Thus in humans, as in monkeys, the hypothalamic GnRH pulse-generating system is located entirely within the MBH.

GnRH pulse generator activities and associated LH pulses are subject to neuromodulation. Blockade of α-adrenergic inputs by phentolamine and dopaminergic activity by metoclopramide inhibit the frequency of pulse generators or arrest it altogether, suggesting that the central catecholaminergic systems exert modulating inputs. Morphine and endogenous opioids have an inhibitory effect that can be reversed abruptly by the administration of the opiate antagonist naloxone. CRF administered peripherally promptly suppresses the GnRH pulse generator activity. This inhibitory effect of CRF is mediated through the activation of endogenous opiate.[55] γ-Aminobutyric acid represents another potent GnRH inhibitor as observed in experimental animals; in humans demonstration of this inhibitory role has not been performed.

Neuropeptide Y and aspartate are putative excitatory neuromodulators of GnRH release. Although aspartate appears to exert its effect directly by increasing the activity of the GnRH pulse generator, neuropeptide Y requires gonadal steroids for its action.

Action of gonadotropin-releasing hormone

Receptors: up-regulation and down-regulation. The first step in GnRH action is its recognition by specific receptors localized exclusively in the plasma membrane of the gonadotrope. GnRH receptors initially are distributed evenly on the cell surface, but coupling with GnRH induces dimerization of receptors and formation of clusters, which then become internalized. Subsequent to their internalization, there is a substantial degradation of hormone-receptor complex in the lysosomes. A significant fraction of GnRH receptors is rapidly shuttled back to the cell surface. This recycling process is causally related, in part, to the up-regulation of GnRH receptors by GnRH.[43]

The GnRH receptor is a 60-kd glycoprotein that contains sialic acid residues; the oligosaccharide portion is essential for the functional expression of the receptor on the cell surface of the gonadotropes. A negatively charged domain interacts predominantly with arginine at position 8 of the GnRH molecule. GnRH induces and maintains a state of receptor cross-linking (microaggregation), thereby triggering subsequent events of the hormone action. Prolonged or continuous exposure to GnRH or its agonists results in profound suppression of gonadotropin release, known as down-regulation. A GnRH antagonist, on the other hand, is capable of binding to the receptor but is unable to induce dimerization of receptors, and thus it reduces gonadotropin secretion by occupying the receptor without triggering the hormone action.[43]

Gonadotropin synthesis and release. GnRH is a humoral link between the neural and endocrine components of reproductive function. As such, after binding to its receptor, GnRH induces a complex series of cellular responses resulting in hormone secretion and in biosynthesis of α- and β-subunits of LH and FSH, dimerization of α, β-subunits, and glycosylation processes.

Physiologic regulation of LH and FSH biosynthesis and secretion by GnRH involves the integration of hormonal influences by ovarian steroids (estradiol and progesterone), inhibin, activin and folliculostatin. These ovarian factors, all of which are targeted on the gonadotrope, induce changes in gene expression of the common α-subunit and specific β-subunits of LH and FSH and account for the differential secretion of FSH and LH by the same gonadotrope.[40]

HYPOTHALAMIC DYSFUNCTION AND REPRODUCTIVE DISORDERS

Congenital and destructive lesions

Isolated gonadotropin deficiency (Kallmann syndrome). A syndrome involving hypogonadotropic hypogonadism associated with anosmia or hyposmia was described by Kallmann and associates[49] in 1944. Included in the original observations were families in which members were afflicted with additional disorders, such as colorblindness, synkinesis, mental retardation, and a series of congenital midline defects. The syndrome commonly refers to an isolated gonadotropin deficiency (IGD) that occurs more frequently in males than in females. Review of autopsy materials disclosed anatomic evidence of partial or complete agenesis of the olfactory apparatus in association with secondary hypogonadism.[23]

The pathogenesis of the hypogonadotropinism in IGD syndrome recently has been discovered. As mentioned earlier, the ontogeny of GnRH-expressing cells involves migration from the olfactory placode into the hypothalamus. This remarkable observation, originally made in mice,[103] has been confirmed in several species, including the human fetus.[32,102] A gene has now been isolated from the critical region on Xp22.3 to which the syndrome locus has been assigned; partial or complete deletion and translocation of this gene locus are responsible for development of the syndrome.[32] The predicted protein has significant similarities to proteins involved in neural cell adhesion and axonal pathfinding. Thus the developmental defect in GnRH neurons in a fetus with Kallmann syndrome is their failure, along with the olfactory and terminalis nerves, to migrate into the hypothalamus. It should be noted that earlier studies have detected several modes of inheritance, including three different genetic defects in this syndrome.[44]

Clinical features. The salient feature of IGD or Kallmann syndrome is gonadotropin deficiency resulting in hypogonadism, which includes failure of both gametogenic function and sex steroid production. Because the appearance of secondary sex characteristics is dependent on sex steroids, sexual infantilism is the prominent manifestation of this syndrome. The degree of hypogonadism in male patients with IGD varies over a wide range from complete testicular immaturity and Leydig cell atrophy (aleydigism) to a mild syndrome of hypoleydigism, with testicular size approaching normal and with spermatid formation. In the latter clinical situation, the disparity between the development of gametogenic function and deficient testosterone production was considered to be a consequence of isolated LH deficiency. Faiman and colleagues[27] later demonstrated that these patients exhibited very low LH secretion in the face of normal circulating quantities of FSH. Thus normal spermatogenesis with androgen insufficiency owing to isolated LH deficiency was confirmed and the term *fertile eunuch syndrome* was introduced. It is likely that this syndrome represents an incomplete form of GnRH deficiency.

In women, the clinical features of IGD also vary widely, with secondary sex characteristics ranging from classic eunuchoidal features to moderate breast development.[110] Primary amenorrhea is common. The ovaries of patients with IGD rarely contain follicles past the primordial stage, suggesting that early stages of follicular maturation require amounts of gonadotropin beyond those secreted by these patients.[42] Thus, in both males and females, this syndrome has a high degree of clinical, biochemical, developmental, and genetic heterogeneity.

Pathophysiology. In IGD syndrome, circulating levels of LH and FSH are usually undetectable, although low-normal values occasionally are found. Most patients exhibit subnormal LH and FSH release in response to GnRH stimulation. Complete unresponsiveness to GnRH is relatively uncommon.[124,130,134] The varying degrees of gonadotrope responsiveness to GnRH in these patients include failure of both LH and FSH levels to increase, appropriate increases in levels of both LH and FSH, and an increase in FSH only or in LH only.[124,130] These findings are consistent with those observed in patients with isolated monohormonal deficiency of LH or FSH.[87]

Heterogeneity of hypothalamic GnRH secretory episodes in these patients also has been observed[124]; it varies from complete absence of pulsatile LH activity to low-frequency and low-amplitude pulses to nearly normal patterns of pulsatile LH secretory episodes. In the latter group, the defect appears to be the secretion of biologically inactive LH molecules, the majority of which are α-subunit. The heterogeneous basis for the IGD syndrome may reflect the degree of migration failure of GnRH neurons from the olfactory placode to the arcuate nucleus in the hypothalamus during development.

Management. The diagnosis of IGD can be made only when mass lesion of the hypothalamic-pituitary site is excluded by either magnetic resonance imaging or computed tomography scanning and by the presence of otherwise normal pituitary function.[124] Careful assessment of the presence or absence of anosmia and hyposmia, the stage of pubertal development, and the clinical manifestation of sexual infantism and eunuchoid features is of paramount importance.

In female patients, induction of ovulation and resulting pregnancy can be accomplished readily by the use of pulsatile modes of GnRH delivery. An average dose of 5 μg per pulse has been remarkably successful in the activation of gonadotropin secretion and ovarian cyclicity. Ovulation with attainment of normal pregnancies has occurred in a high percentage of patients.[19,62,75] Thus, for women, the defective GnRH secretory activity can be replaced effectively by the use of an automatic portable-pump GnRH delivery system with a delivery interval of 1 hour. Slower or faster frequency tends to induce abnormal follicular development and luteal phase defects. Higher doses of GnRH (i.e., 10 μg per pulse) can override the negative feedback control system, as evidenced by an increased amplitude of LH pulses resulting in development of multiple follicles and ovulation.[64] Use of GnRH to induce ovulation is discussed in detail in Chapter 34. In men, long-term subcutaneous delivery of GnRH at 2-hour intervals has been successful in inducing puberty and stimulating sustained testosterone secretion and spermatogenesis, with the ability to impregnate for some patients.[31,46]

Hypothalamic hypopituitarism. In this section, the features that distinguish the failure of pituitary cells (primary hypopituitarism) from a lack of appropriate hypothalamic-releasing factors (secondary or hypothalamic hypopituitarism) in patients with pituitary hypofunction are discussed. Both types of hypopituitarism may involve a single pituitary hormone (monotropic deficiency) or several and even all pituitary hormones (panhypopituitarism).

Although the incidence of hypopituitarism secondary to hypothalamic dysfunction is unknown, increasing recognition of this type of pituitary hypofunction has emerged in recent years. The anatomic and neuroendocrine relationships in hypopituitarism secondary to hypothalamic dysfunction depend on the size and location of the lesion(s). The cause can be secondary to compression, infiltration, and destruction depending on the nature of the lesion. The clinical clues for hypothalamic causes of hypopituitarism are as follows:

1. Hyperprolactinemia (loss of hypothalamic prolactin-inhibiting factors)
2. Clinical and laboratory evidence of pituitary hormone deficiencies
3. Visual impairment (optic chiasma compression)
4. Diabetes insipidus (interrupting nerve tract from hypothalamus to neurohypothesis)

Craniopharyngioma. Craniopharyngioma of the suprasellar region is a common cause of hypopituitarism. Retardation of growth and calcification of the sella region on X-ray examination are frequent findings in children.[45] Headache, visual disturbance, and varying degrees of pituitary hormone deficiency are common features.[48]

Germinoma. Germinoma, previously known as ectopic pinealoma or atypical teratoma of the pineal gland, is another relatively common lesion. The histologic features of this tumor are the same as those in seminoma of the testis and dysgerminoma of the ovary. Thus the term *germinoma* has been adopted to emphasize identity with its gonadal counterparts.

Endodermal sinus tumor. Endodermal sinus tumor, a rare but highly malignant tumor of the hypothalamus, requires some emphasis; it is a germ cell tumor and is also found in the ovaries and testes, as well as the cervix and vagina, of infants and children. To date, a few such tumors also have been identified in the region of the pineal gland.[10,13] This tumor has a typical honeycomb pattern and is believed to be derived from antecedents of the yolk sac ("yolk-sac carcinoma"). It is a highly vascular tumor capable of producing alpha-fetoprotein and it metastasizes early to various regions of the brain, including the hypothalamus.

Hand-Schüller-Christian disease. Hand-Schüller-Christian disease (histiocytosis X), a condition with multifocal eosinophilic granulomas, is a rare cause of a hypothalamic destructive lesion in children; it produces hypopituitarism with delayed puberty, growth retardation, and diabetes insipidus (40%).[14,26]

It has been 40 years since Lichtenstein's concept linked eosinophilic granuloma of bone, Letterer-Siwe disease, and Hand-Schüller-Christian syndrome under the term *histiocytosis X,*[63] now more correctly called Langerhans cell histiocytosis. Reassessment of these and other distinctive histiocytosis syndromes in children has revealed mononuclear phagocytes (histiocytes) and their interactions with other cells; the Langerhans cell, a unique histiocyte, has been clearly associated with Lichtenstein histiocytosis X.[77]

Clinically, three classic features suggest a hypothalamic basis for hypopituitarism: (1) the presence of diabetes insipidus, (2) the modest elevation of prolactin levels along with reduced levels of other pituitary hormones, and (3) visual disturbances.[113] Other symptoms suggesting hypothalamic involvement are obesity, psychiatric disturbances, and hypersomnolence. Growth retardation in children may be the first presenting complaint in those seeking medical evaluation.[113] A definitive diagnosis by biopsy is essential. Once the diagnosis is established, radiation therapy can be effective. GH deficiency in children has serious consequences, and therapy with either recombinant GH or frequent injections of GHRH is indicated. Restoration of GH secretion is accompanied by a prompt increase in serum levels of insulin-like growth factor.[39]

Head injuries. Head injuries, especially those sustained in head-on automobile collisions, can cause hypothalamic damage resulting in hypopituitarism with elevated prolactin levels that may or may not respond to TRH stimulation. The presence of hyperprolactinemia provides critical evidence of the hypothalamic site of damage and serves to discriminate it from pituitary panhypopituitarism. It is believed that automobile accidents resulting in whiplash injury may cause transection of the pituitary stalk during the acute forward motion of the head. Patients with such injuries may have permanent diabetes insipidus, a feature consistent with stalk transection. Prolonged hypotension, hypovolemia, and unconsciousness may precipitate either hypothalamic ischemia or portal vein thrombosis, which represents another mechanism for the development of hypopituitarism that sometimes follows head injury.

Irradiation. External irradiation for pituitary tumors can cause damage to the hypothalamus and impair its function. Pituitary cells are relatively radioresistant, whereas the brain and its nerves are more radiosensitive. Thus changes in pituitary function after radiation therapy for pituitary tumor may be attributable to an indirect effect of hypothalamic damage. Under this circumstance, hypopituitarism develops slowly and is frequently associated with modest elevation of prolactin levels. Irradiation of the head and neck for the treatment of cancer of the nasopharynx frequently results in hypopituitarism. In two prospective studies in which the time course and relative deficiency of hypothalamic-pituitary function following cranial irradiation (1200 to 6000 Gy) were evaluated. The progressive impairment of the hypothalamic-pituitary function becomes evident as early as 1 year after radiotherapy, and further impairments of GH, FSH/LH, TSH, and ACTH have occurred in relation to time and dose.[58,65]

Functional hypothalamic amenorrhea

Cessation of menstrual cycles in young women without clinically demonstrable abnormalities of the pituitary-ovarian axis represents one of the most common types of amenorrhea. The term *functional hypothalamic amenorrhea* refers to the nonorganic nature of the amenorrhea; it is a reversible disorder. Functional hypothalamic amenorrhea includes a variety of physiologic and pathophysiologic conditions and is thus nonspecific.

Psychogenic amenorrhea. With the increasing recognition that psychogenic stress causes hypothalamic dysfunction, it is appropriate to regard amenorrhea accompanied by psychologic stress in the absence of organic disease as functional hypothalamic amenorrhea of the psychogenic type. It should be recognized that psychogenic variables and the subsequent development of dysfunction or dysfunction overcome by adaptation are important concepts in the assessments of these patients. Recent studies have revealed a multitude of neuroendocrine-metabolic aberrations in this syndrome.

Pathophysiology. Half a century ago, Albright and Hal-

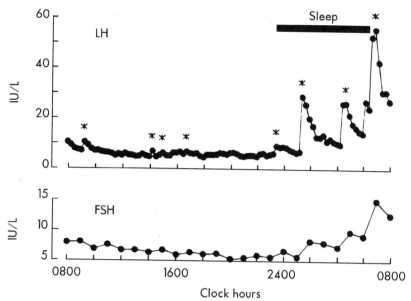

Fig. 3-3. Pulsatile LH pattern and serum FSH concentrations in a patient with functional hypothalamic amenorrhea. Note the sleep-associated pubertal pattern of augmentation of LH pulse amplitude. (From Berga S et al: *Clin Endocrinol* 72:151, 1991.)

stead,[2] Klinefelter et al.,[54] and Reifenstein[92] collectively offered indirect evidence for a hypothalamic mechanism by which psychogenic stress impairs ovarian function via reduced pituitary gonadotropin secretion. With the discovery of GnRH, it became clear that the pituitary-ovarian function is intact in such patients[57,133] and that the disorder is a consequence of reduced pulsatile GnRH secretion.[8,19,91] Identification and characterization of pulsatile patterns of LH secretion, which reflect episodic secretory activity of hypothalamic GnRH, have revealed a variety of abnormalities. The degree of impairment of GnRH secretion varies widely, as evidenced by the diversity of pulsatile LH activity. In general, the frequency and amplitude of the pulses are diminished and, in some cases, a pubertal pattern with amplification of pulsatile LH activity in association with sleep is evident (Fig. 3-3).[8,19,91] The spectrum of abnormalities most likely reflects a pathophysiologic continuum with changing hypothalamic GnRH activity with time and status of stress/adaptation.[53,131] In severe cases, when few quasipulses of LH are present, the ovarian activity virtually ceases, as reflected by markedly reduced levels of estradiol, androstenedione, and testosterone. Thus the entire hypothalamic-pituitary-ovarian system is functionally regressed to the prepubertal state, and subsequent recovery resembles that seen in neuroendocrine activation by the GnRH pulse generator (Fig. 3-4). In contrast, patients with modest LH pulse amplitudes but significantly reduced numbers of LH pulses have a substantial degree of ovarian secretion of estradiol and normal levels of androgens. Under this setting, spontaneous menses may occur in some cases. The continuum of hypothalamic-pituitary-ovarian dysfunc-

tion in psychogenic amenorrhea accounts for the lack of a consistent pattern or erratic GnRH pulse generator activity as well as the gonadotropin responses to exogenous GnRH stimulation; low, normal, or exaggerated GnRH responses have been observed.

The presence of identifiable psychogenic factors in some cases and the spontaneous reversal of the amenorrhea following appropriate counseling in others suggest a suprahypothalamic site as a primary cause of hypothalamic GnRH secretory malfunction. Ovulation and pregnancy can be achieved readily by pulsatile administration of GnRH with appropriate frequency and dose,[19,62,75] indicating that the random or irregular GnRH secretory program is the immediate underlying cause of amenorrhea in this syndrome.

Defective gonadotropin-releasing hormone secretion. Since substantial evidence suggests that hypothalamic β-endorphin and dopamine function as modulators of the secretory activity of GnRH neurons, reduced pulsatile frequency or amplitude (or both) may be causally related to inappropriate elevations of hypothalamic opioidergic and dopaminergic neuronal activities in patients with psychogenic amenorrhea. Studies using the opioid receptor antagonist naloxone and the dopamine (D_2) receptor antagonist metoclopramide (MCP) have demonstrated increments of LH secretion after the blockade of both receptors.[9,53,86] These findings are extended by showing the reversal of LH pulse frequency and amplitude toward a normal range in response to a 24-hour infusion of D_2 receptor blockade (MCP)[9] and induction of ovulatory cycles by administration of the long-acting opioid receptor

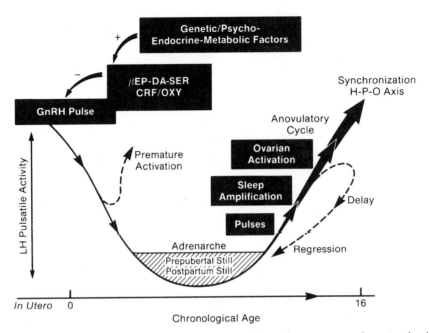

Fig. 3-4. Diagrammatic display of the U-shaped curve relating a time-compressed neuroendocrine event of puberty. The prepubertal restraint of GnRH-LH pulses due to the expression of hypothalamic inhibitors or modulators such as β-endorphin (*β-EP*), dopamine (*DA*), serotonin (*SER*), CRF, and oxytocin (*OXY*) is depicted. The final synchronization of the hypothalamic-pituitary-ovarian (*H-P-O*) axis in generating ovulatory cycles follows a sequence of decline of inhibitory mechanisms, initiation of GnRH-LH pulsatile activity, and the sleep-entrained amplifications. The time course of these events is determined by genetic, nutritional, psychologic, and social-environmental factors. Interruptions of this sequence of events occur in several clinical abnormalities, as exemplified by premature activation in central precocious puberty and a delay or regression to the prepubertal state in patients with anorexia nervosa.

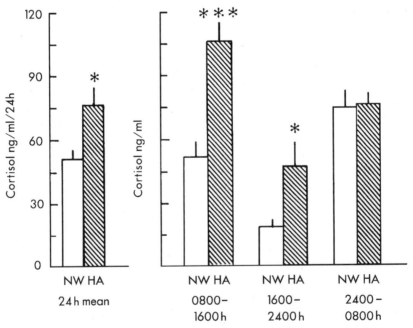

Fig. 3-5. Integrated cortisol levels for 24-hour mean (±SE) values and for 8-hour segments of the day and evening are elevated in patients with hypothalamic amenorrhea (*HA*) compared with those of matched controls (*NW*). Note: The night cortisol levels are in the normal range.

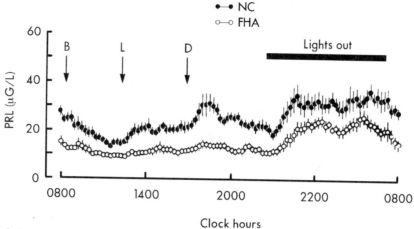

Fig. 3-6. Mean (± SE) 24-hour serum PRL levels measured at 15-minute intervals in 10 normal control women in the early follicular phase (*NC*) and 10 women with functional hypothalamic amenorrhea (*FHA*). *B,* Breakfast; *L* lunch; *D,* dinner. (From Berga SL et al: *J Clin Endocrinol Metab* 68:301, 1989.)

antagonist naltrexone.[126] These responses are by no means uniform; patients with prepubertal levels of LH showed no response, and the defect is unrelated to pituitary sensitivity to GnRH.[86]

Hypercortisolism. It is well known that emotional stress and depression are associated with activation of the pituitary-adrenal axis and blunting of the circadian rhythm of cortisol secretion.[41,100] Not unexpectedly, patients with functional hypothalamic amenorrhea are found to have hypersecretion of cortisol with a selective increase in the amplitude of secretory episodes during the day and evening hours (Fig. 3-5). The 24-hour mean cortisol level is increased without alteration in the circadian rhythm of cortisol. The ACTH response to CRF stimulation is blunted, reflecting the negative feedback effect of hypercortisolism. These findings suggest that an increased CRF drive centrally is involved in this syndrome.[8,11,114] That CRF can inhibit the GnRH-gonadotropin axis has been well demonstrated in a variety of in vivo and in vitro experiments in both rodents and primates. This effect of CRF appears to be mediated by endogenous opioids, since naloxone administration can reverse this CRF effect.[38,78,82,128] It is conceivable that an increased CRF drive at the hypothalamic or suprahypothalamic level may link hypercortisolism to emotional stresses, since a similar relationship has been shown in experimentally imposed psychologic stresses in humans.[116]

Hypoprolactinemia. The 24-hour serum prolactin (PRL) levels of patients with functional hypothalamic amenorrhea at all time points were lower than those of normally cycling women during the early follicular phase (Fig. 3-6). The 24-hour integrated PRL value was reduced by 39%. However, the sleep-associated increments were greater in patients with functional hypothalamic amenorrhea.[8] The neuroendocrine mechanisms to account for the decreased PRL secretion are not clear, but the link of an elevated inhibitory action of endogenous hypothalamic dopaminergic activity may be considered. It is unrelated to estrogen levels, since both estradiol and estrone concentrations are not different from those of controls.

Changes in growth hormone and thyroid hormones. The 24-hour secretory pattern of GH is selectively increased during the nocturnal hours (Fig. 3-7). Despite a normal 24-hour TSH secretory profile, serum triiodothyronine (T_3) and thyroxine (T_4) levels are significantly reduced in patients with functional hypothalamic amenorrhea.[8] Neuroendocrine mechanisms to account for these changes are unclear. These findings may be related to the compensatory response to relative nutritional deficits in these patients. (See later discussion of malnutrition.) Collectively, multihormonal aberrations appear to occur in this syndrome.

Amplification of nocturnal melatonin secretion. Aberrations of nocturnal melatonin secretion in women with functional hypothalamic amenorrhea are found. Although daytime melatonin concentrations are similar, the integrated nocturnal melatonin secretion is threefold greater in these patients when compared with the season and with secretion by age-matched cycling women in the early follicular phase. This increase in melatonin is due to an elevated peak amplitude and extended duration with a delay in the offset time.[7] The underlying mechanisms of the amplified nocturnal melatonin secretion in women with functional hypothalamic amenorrhea are unknown. It is not related to body weight, LH pulses, or the ovarian steroid influence and cannot be explained by seasonal differences, because both patients and control subjects are exposed to the same light-dark environment. This amplification of nocturnal melatonin secretion may reflect an increased central adrenergic activity and probably has no effect on gonadotropin secretion.[30,122]

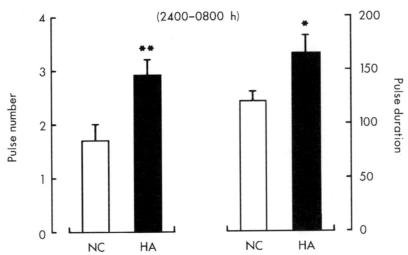

Fig. 3-7. Significant increases in nocturnal GH secretory activities, in both pulse amplitude and duration, are present in patients with hypothalamic amenorrhea (*HA*), compared with normal controls (*NC*).

Management of functional hypothalamic amenorrhea. The underlying cause of psychogenic amenorrhea appears to be intimately related to social-environmental stress of sufficient intensity and duration. The degree of vulnerability is determined by the predisposing factors and adaptability of the individual. Failure of coping results in decompensation and subclinical depression with accompanying changes in neuroendocrine-metabolic systems. The cessation of menses represents nature's device to prevent exposure of the young to an unfavorable environment when the potential mother is preoccupied with constant adjustment for her own survival.

The multiple hormonal aberrations and the variation of their expressions represent a continuum of neuroendocrine disorders with a time course construct that resembles the U-shaped curve described for the onset of puberty (Fig. 3-4).

1. Activation of hypothalamic-pituitary-cortisol secretory activity occurs selectively during the daylight hours.
2. Reduced pulsatile frequency or amplitude (or both) of GnRH-gonadotropin release results in progressive ovarian functional impairment from luteal phase defect to complete arrest (amenorrhea).
3. There is indirect evidence of an increased hypothalamic inhibitor on GnRH secretion, that is, CRF and opioid peptides.
4. Hypoprolactinemia and amplification of nocturnal melatonin secretion may represent additional expressions of reproductive curtailment.
5. Increased nocturnal GH secretion and low T_3 and T_4 levels may reflect an adaptive response to nutritional deficits.
6. Recovery is associated with a progressive increase in frequency of pulsatile GnRH-gonadotropin release, and its sleep-associated amplification resembles that seen at the initiation of puberty.

Successful management requires an established rapport between physician and patient. A careful and detailed history concerning parental, sexual, social, environmental, and interpersonal relationships, and the availability of support during childhood and adolescence, is imperative. Careful exclusion of organic disease, reassurance, and appropriate and timely positive reinforcement are potent modes of management. When spontaneous recovery does not ensue within 6 to 8 months after psychologic guidance, additional measures may be required, such as estrogen-progestin replacement and clomiphene citrate induction of ovulation. If pregnancy is desired and clomiphene fails, induction of ovulation by pulsatile administration of GnRH has a high degree of success.

Exercise-related menstrual dysfunction

The rapid increase in popularity of physical exercise during the past decade has led to the recognition of deleterious effects of strenuous exercise on reproductive function.[67] The cause-effect relationship of this association is difficult to quantitate because physiologic responses to various forms of exercise and athleticism have not been fully characterized and because of the presence of individual lifestyle variables, which also influence reproductive function.[71] Thus the type, duration, and intensity of exercise and the body composition, psychologic background, and stress factors of individuals participating in exercise programs are confounding factors to be considered in assessing exercise-related neuroendocrine-metabolic consequences.[66]

Clinical features. Menstrual abnormalities have been reported in connection with a wide variety of sports, including middle-distance and long-distance running, swimming, ballet dancing, and field events. Varying degrees of menstrual disorders are related to the length and intensity of the activity. They are greater at the end of the athletic season, and there is a positive correlation between weekly training mileage and incidence of amenorrhea. Even joggers ("slow and easy," 5 to 30 miles/wk) have significantly fewer menses per year than their less energetic counterparts.[22]

It is important to distinguish among the different physical activities and the age at which they were started. When training starts before the menarche, as in gymnastics and ballet dancing, menarche is delayed by about 3 years, and the incidence of secondary amenorrhea or chronic anovulation in later life is also higher.[20] This age-related effect was also found in a group of college swimmers and runners; each year of training prior to menarche delayed it by an average of 5 months.[20]

Exercise amenorrhea may be sport specific. The incidence is much greater in high-intensity runners and ballet dancers (40% to 50%), whereas it is lower in swimmers independent of training intensity (approximately 12%).[101] This difference may be attributable to the relatively high percentage of body fat among swimmers (approximately 20%), compared with runners (15%) and ballet dancers (about 15%).[34] In addition, runners with amenorrhea have significantly less daily protein intake and greater weight loss than have runners without amenorrhea.[104] These observations support the hypothesis elaborated by Frisch and McArthur[35] that the integrity of menstrual function depends on critical levels of body weight, specifically the lean-fat ratio, with at least a level of 22% body fat being required for normal menses.[35] The proposed body composition mechanism for the development of amenorrhea should be viewed as a general principle, because there are obvious exceptions: (1) Athletic amenorrhea can occur with or without weight loss. (2) If training is interrupted in ballet dancers (e.g., through injury), menses return without changes in body weight or the lean-fat ratio. (3) Although a 10% to 15% loss of body weight (reflecting a 30% loss of body fat) can produce amenorrhea, the underlying mechanism is likely multifactorial rather than a reduced extraglandular formation of estrogen from androgen by the fat compartment. The lean body mass, mainly the muscle, must be taken into account as an important site for aromatization of androgen to estrogen.[66]

Pathophysiology. Vigorous exercise and its associated variables appear to induce a progressive dysfunction of ovarian cyclicity that includes (1) luteal phase defects, (2) anovulatory cycles and amenorrhea, and (3) delayed menarche in prepubertal girls.

Defective gonadotropin-releasing hormone secretion. Abnormalities of hypothalamic GnRH secretion, as reflected by pulsatile LH frequency and amplitude, have been observed in patients with exercise amenorrhea. Pituitary gonadotropin responses to GnRH are increased for both LH and FSH as compared with normal controls.[69,119] A spectrum of reduced frequency and/or amplitude of LH pulses resembling those described in patients with psychogenic amenorrhea is found.[21,69,119] Furthermore, randomly occurring pulsatile LH activity varied from month to month, as illustrated by repeated studies in the same individuals. Defects in pulsatile LH release have also been observed in "normally menstruating" runners in whom pulsatile LH frequency was reduced and amplitude was increased above those of sedentary controls.[21,69,119] Although these runners had regular menstrual bleeding, the integrity of ovarian function was impaired, as reflected by luteal phase defects.[69] Thus altered pulsatile patterns of gonadotropin secretion may lead to impaired folliculogenesis as an initiating cause of a continuum of luteal phase defects, anovulatory cycles, and amenorrhea.

This formulation is supported by a well-controlled prospective study of 28 untrained college women with documented normal ovulatory cycles. Bullen and associates[15] demonstrated that progressive increases in the intensity of exercise (from running 4 miles/d to running 10 miles/d during a 4-week span), particularly if compounded by weight loss, induced a remarkable increase over time in the incidence of luteal phase defects (63%) and anovulation (81%). These findings represent a transition from initial to long-term impacts of vigorous exercise, which, with time, can lead to functional arrest of the hypothalamic-pituitary-ovarian axis, resulting in hypoestrogenic amenorrhea.

Thus high-intensity endurance exercise exerts a central inhibitory effect on the hypothalamic GnRH secretory function that is discernible even before clinical evidence of altered menstrual cyclicity. The recovery likely follows a progressive and time-related increase in GnRH pulsatile activity.

Hypercortisolism. The neuroendocrine link between exercise-induced menstrual disorders and inhibition of GnRH secretion is unclear. However, recent studies indicate that the hypothalamic-pituitary-adrenal axis is altered in athletic women.[69] The 24-hour urinary cortisol levels and serum cortisol concentrations are elevated.[24,69,121] With equal exercise intensity, women athletes with amenorrhea have elevated serum cortisol levels throughout the 24-hour circadian rhythm, whereas women athletes with cyclic menses exhibit hypercortisolism only during the early morning hours.[69] This relative hypersecretion of cortisol is accompanied by a normal circadian rhythm of ACTH and blunted responses to CRF in both groups of athletic women. The adrenal sensitivity to ACTH appears to be increased as judged by the ratio of cortisol-ACTH in response to exogenous CRF.[69] Thus the maintenance of normal ACTH secretion in the face of elevated cortisol levels and increased endogenous CRF drive may be implicated. If proven, the well-known inhibitory effect of CRF on GnRH pulse generator activity may be accountable, at least in part,

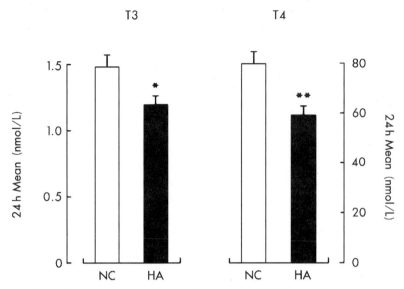

Fig. 3-8. Significant decreases in serum T_4 and T_3 with normal TSH levels (not shown) are found in patients with hypothalamic amenorrhea (*HA*), compared with matched controls (*NC*).

for the erratic pattern of LH pulses in these patients.

Fuel expenditure. The fundamental physiologic requirement in response to any mode of exercise is, of course, energy expenditure. Utilization of metabolic fuels is measured by oxygen consumption ($\dot{V}o_2$), which is estimated to be 3.5 mL/min per kilogram at rest.

At the beginning of exercise, the energy demands are met by the anaerobic fuel metabolism (i.e., the production of lactate). The initial oxygen deficit (anaerobic metabolism) will be shifted, within seconds or minutes, to an aerobic metabolic pathway. Circulating glucose provided by glycogenolysis in liver and muscle is the major source of fuel.[28] With sustained exercise, plasma glucose levels are maintained by gluconeogenesis in the liver from substrates derived from muscle alanine. When exercise is extended beyond 60 minutes, the contribution of fat becomes progressively important, with more than 50% of the metabolic fuel being derived from plasma and muscle triglycerides and free fatty acids. The metabolic contribution by protein is a late event, and mobilization of amino acids (via protein breakdown in the muscle) occurs. The relative contribution of amino acids to the pool of metabolic fuel is small (5% to 10%), and they serve to provide gluconeogenesis via the alanine-glucose cycle.[37] This sequence of metabolic events in response to energy demands of exercise is, of course, dependent on body composition and dietary patterns. The lean body composition and relatively low caloric intake frequently encountered in individuals pursuing strenuous exercise result in fuel deficits. In this regard, the recently observed global hypothyroidemia (T_3, T_4, fT_4, fT_3) (Fig. 3-8) with normal TSH levels and increased levels of insulin-like growth factor (IGF) BP-1 (binding protein) with reduced bioavailability of free IGF-I[18] may represent a protective mechanism for conservation of metabolic fuels.

Activation of neuroendocrine systems. Acute bouts of exercise induce, within minutes, a multitude of hormonal changes as well as activation of the sympathetic nervous system after the onset of controlled exercise experiments. It is apparent that the release of ACTH, cortisol, β-endorphin, GH, PRL, melatonin, epinephrine, and norepinephrine is activated within minutes of exercise.[70,109,112,117] These rapid discharges of stress hormones undoubtedly exert cellular actions and interactions in the modulation of metabolic demands and blood flow. The neuroendocrine mechanisms that account for the multihormonal responses and the sympathetic nervous system activation are unclear. The rapidity of responses and the concomitant release of the proopiomelanocortin family of peptides implicate CRF-mediated events, which may also be responsible for the activation of norepinephrine and epinephrine release.

Hypermelatoninemia. An acute increase in melatonin levels occurs in response to acute exercise.[112,117] The daytime resting melatonin levels are elevated in women athletes but there is a striking increase in melatonin secretion at nighttime that occurs only in amenorrheic women athletes (Fig. 3-9).[60] This elevated nocturnal melatonin secretion is characterized by a 2-hour delay in offset, and it is independent of opioidergic and dopaminergic systems. The proposition that elevated melatonin may serve as a timekeeper for reproduction is consistent with the observation of seasonal variation in gonadotropin and ovarian function in women participating in exercise training programs; the short photoperiod in autumn (increased melatonin secretion) is associated with low FSH and follicular and luteal defects, whereas the long photoperiod in the spring (decreased melatonin secretion) seems partly overcome by

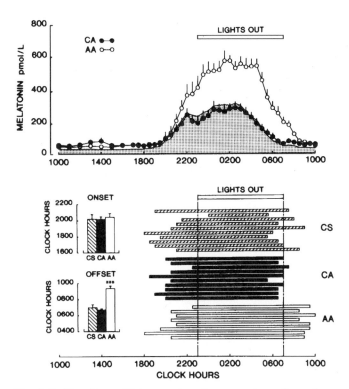

Fig. 3-9. *Top,* Serum 24-hour melatonin pattern in cycling athletes (*CA*) and amenorrheic athletes (*AA*) with comparable degrees of exercise training, psychometric tests, body compositions and dietary consumption. The data (mean ± SE) are plotted against values for regularly cyclic, sedentary women (*shaded area*). *Bottom,* The onset, offset, and duration of nocturnal melatonin rise are displayed in reference to clock hours and compared among groups (*insets*). CS, Control subjects. (From Laughlin G, Loucks AB, Yen SSC: *J Clin Endocrinol Metab* 73:1321, 1991.)

the suppressive effects of physical training on ovarian function.[94]

Risks and benefits of exercise. In recent years, various exercise regimens have been promoted for increasing health and longevity. The beneficial effects of exercise have been identified, especially its role in retarding an age-related increase in serum lipids and insulin resistance, cardiovascular diseases, and bone mineral loss,[85] and its association with a lower lifetime occurrence of breast cancer.[36]

Osteopenia. Modest exercise programs are reported to increase total body calcium and lumbar vertebral density in postmenopausal women. On the other hand, bone mineral content has been found to be significantly reduced in athletes with amenorrhea compared with matched, normally cycling peers.[25] This manifestation may be related to the lower serum estradiol and estrone levels and altered metabolic pathways of estrogens in amenorrheic athletes; 2-hydroxylation with the formation of biologically inactive catecholestrogens is increased, compared with that in cycling athletes performing similar exercise, and the extent of 2-hydroxylation of estradiol is positively correlated with the degree of body leanness.[108] Thus, low body fat and

ovarian inactivity contribute to chronic estrogen deficiency, which may explain the decrease in bone density. In another study, mineral density of the lumbar spine in amenorrheic runners was lower than that in normal cycling women and age-matched controls but higher than that in less intense runners with secondary amenorrhea.[72] These observations indicate that strenuous exercise may reduce the impact of amenorrhea on bone loss, but amenorrheic runners remain at high risk for osteopenia and fracture.

Status of lipoproteins. Regular physical activity, both occupational and recreational, is associated with increases in plasma high-density lipoprotein (HDL) and decreases in low-density lipoprotein (LDL).[59,115,129] Apolipoproteins (APO) A-I and B are major proteins of HDL and LDL, respectively, and are better predictors of coronary heart disease. Lower levels of plasma APO B are found in both amenorrheic and eumenorrheic female athletes. However, amenorrheic athletes have lower APO A-I levels and a lower APO A-I: APO B ratio and thus reverse the beneficial effect of physical exercise.[59]

Management of exercise-related menstrual dysfunction. The approaches to counseling and management of patients with exercise-associated amenorrhea and infertility must take into account the fact that many women include regular exercise as an important part of their lifestyles. Appropriate care for these patients should include imparting up-to-date information concerning the beneficial and deleterious effects of strenuous exercise on the reproductive and skeletal systems.

Physiologic responses to exercise mainly involve the activation of cellular and compartmental fuel mobilization, redistribution, and utilization. This is accomplished by a multitude of changes in neuroendocrine signals from the brain. Although the mechanisms by which these complex activational processes act are unclear, the integrity of neuroendocrine-metabolic homeostasis is influenced by the mode, frequency, duration, and intensity of exercise regimens. Perhaps even more important is quantity and quality of food intake, which determines the body composition. Thus an understanding of balanced inputs and expenditures is of obvious importance.

Guidance and information exchange with the patient may result in moderation of exercise and establishment of optimal nutritional needs. The fact that exercise-associated amenorrhea is reversible adds further incentive for the patient to make rational decisions with respect to major problems of amenorrhea—infertility and osteoporosis.

Supplementation with estrogen-progestin, multivitamins, and calcium is an important consideration, but the primary aim in management is to provide guidance in terms of exercise moderation and fuel economy.

Malnutrition-related amenorrhea

In affluent sections of Western societies, the availability of food usually is not a factor in determining nutritional states of an individual. In recent years, however, a number of reproductive disorders have emerged that appear to be related to dieting and a desire for leanness. Weight loss, whether occurring in the setting of food restriction or exercise, may cause delayed puberty, delayed menarche, and amenorrhea.

Given the demands of reproduction—to provide nutrients to the fetus and to nurse the newborn infant—female body composition is crucial to the extent that reproduction is curtailed when the fat depots and lean body mass are reduced to suboptimal levels. Because of these special constraints, women in comparison to men are endowed with a significant amount of fat beginning at the time of puberty, an endowment that is maintained throughout adult life.[33] This sex difference in body composition is biologically relevant to ensure sufficient energy storage as a reproductive strategy. Thus modification of body composition by food restriction, either voluntary or involuntary, is appropriately accompanied by anovulation and amenorrhea, an important device for endogenous contraception in the face of inability to meet a large caloric demand.

The importance of body weight and neuroendocrine control of ovarian function is conspicuously displayed by primitive desert-dwelling hunter-gatherers of the !Kung San (bushman) population of Botswana in the Kalahari Desert, South Africa. In this ecologic environment, seasonal changes in nutrition, body weight, and activity exist, and the women have a peak time of giving birth—exactly 9 months after attainment of maximal weight, when conceptions occur.[118] Thus a seasonal suppression of ovulation and an increased prevalence of luteal phase defects, as documented by hormonal studies, occur in these women at a time when they are most active and have lowest body weight. This corresponds to the winter months, when food availability is most limited, the search for food is most intense, and endurance physical efforts are made (bushwomen often carry children 30 or more miles per day).[61]

The precise causal relationship between food deprivation and cessation of cyclic menstrual function is not entirely clear. Several findings implicate hypothalamic dysfunction as the basis for the onset of amenorrhea: altered temperature regulation and a reduced pulsatile LH activity with a reversion to a peripubertal sleep-entrained episodic LH secretory program.[83,120] Moderate dietary restriction and weight loss in normal, cycling women have been associated with a reduction of estradiol levels and anovulation in the face of normal LH levels,[83] and severe starvation of healthy women for 2½ weeks induced a reversal of the LH pulse to prepubertal patterns.[29]

REFERENCES

1. Ackland JF et al: Molecular forms of gonadotropin-releasing hormone associated peptide (GAP): changes within the rat hypothalamus and release from hypothalamic cells in vitro, *Neuroendocrinology* 48:376, 1988.

2. Albright F, Halsted J: Studies on ovarian dysfunction, II: the application of the "hormonal measuring sticks" to the sorting out and to the treatment of the various types of amenorrhea, *N Engl J Med* 212:250, 1935.

3. Anthony ELP, King JC, Stopa EG: Immunocytochemical neurohypothesis: evidence for multiple sites of releasing hormone secretion in humans and other mammals, *Cell Tissue Res* 236:5, 1984.

4. Apter D, Viinikka L, Vihko R: Hormonal pattern of adolescent menstrual cycles, *J Clin Endocrinol Metab* 47:944, 1978.

5. Aschoff J: The circadian system in man. In Krieger DT, Hughes JC, editors: *Neuroendocrinology,* Sunderland, Mass, 1980, Sinauer Associates.

6. Barry J, Barette B: Immunofluorescence study of LRF neurons in primates, *Cell Tissue Res* 164:163, 1975.

7. Berga SL, Mortola JF, Yen SSC: Amplification of nocturnal melatonin secretion in women with functional hypothalamic amenorrhea, *J Clin Endocrinol Metab* 66:242, 1988.

8. Berga SL et al: Neuroendocrine aberrations in women with functional hypothalamic amenorrhea, *J Clin Endocrinol Metab* 68:301, 1989.

9. Berga SL et al: Acceleration of LH pulse frequency in functional hypothalamic amenorrhea by dopaminergic blockade, *J Clin Endocrinol Metab,* 72:151, 1991.

10. Bestle J: Extragonadal endodermal sinus tumors originating in the region of the pineal gland, *Acta Pathol Microbiol Scand* 74:214, 1968.

11. Biller BMK et al: Abnormal cortisol secretion and response to corticotropin-releasing hormone in women with hypothalamic amenorrhea, *J Clin Endocrinol Metab* 70:311, 1990.

12. Bloch B et al: Immunohistochemical detection of proluteinizing hormone-releasing hormone peptides in neurons in the human hypothalamus, *J Clin Endocrinol Metab* 74:135, 1992.

13. Borit A: Embryonal carcinoma of the pineal region, *J Pathol* 97:165, 1969.

14. Braunstein GD, Kohler PO: Pituitary function in Hand-Schüller-Christian disease: evidence for deficient growth hormone release in patients with short stature, *N Engl J Med* 286:1225, 1972.

15. Bullen BA et al: Induction of menstrual disorders in untrained women by strenuous exercise, *N Engl J Med* 312:1349, 1985.

16. Carmel PW, Araki S, Ferin M: Pituitary stalk portal blood collection in rhesus monkeys: evidence for pulsatile release of GnRH, *Endocrinology* 99:243, 1976.

17. Clarke IJ, Cummins JT: The temporal relationship between gonadotropin releasing hormone (GnRH) and luteinizing hormone (LH) secretion in ovariectomized ewes, *Endocrinology* 111:1737, 1982.

18. Crist DM, Hill JM: Diet and insulinlike growth factor I in relation to body composition in women with exercise-induced hypothalamic amenorrhea, *J Am Coll Nutr* 9:200, 1990.

19. Crowley WF Jr et al: The physiology of gonadotropin-releasing hormone (GnRH) secretion in men and women, *Recent Prog Horm Res* 41:473, 1985.

20. Cumming DC, Wheeler GD: Exercise-associated changes in reproduction: a problem common to women and men. In Reisch RE, editor: *Adipose tissue and reproduction,* Basel, 1990, Karger.

21. Cumming DC et al: Defects in pulsatile LH release in normally menstruating runners, *J Clin Endocrinol Metab* 60:810, 1985.

22. Dale E, Gerlach DH, Wilhite AL: Menstrual dysfunction in distance runners, *Obstet Gynecol* 54:47, 1979.

23. De Morsier G: Etudes sur les dysraphies cranioencephaliques, *Schweiz Arch Neurol Neurochir Psychiatr* 74:309, 1954.

24. Ding JH et al: High serum cortisol levels in exercise-associated amenorrhea, *Ann Intern Med* 108:530, 1988.

25. Drinkwater BL et al: Bone mineral content of amenorrheic and eumenorrheic athletes, *N Engl J Med* 311:277, 1984.

26. Dunger DB et al: The frequency and natural history of diabetes insipidus in children with Langerhans-cell histiocytosis, *N Engl J Med* 321:1157, 1989.

27. Faiman C et al: The "fertile eunuch" syndrome: demonstration of isolated luteinizing hormone deficiency by radioimmunoassay technique, *Mayo Clin Proc* 43:661, 1968.

28. Felig P, Wahren J: Fuel homeostasis in exercise, *N Engl J Med* 293:1078, 1975.

29. Fichter MM, Pirke KM: Hypothalamic pituitary function in starving healthy subjects. In Pirke KM, Ploog D, editors: *The psychobiology of anorexia nervosa.* Berlin, 1984, Springer-Verlag.

30. Fideleff H et al: Effect of melatonin on the basal and stimulated gonadotropin levels in normal men and postmenopausal women, *J Clin Endocrinol Metab* 42:1014, 1976.

31. Finkelstein JS et al: Pulsatile gonadotropin secretion after discontinuation of long term gonadotropin-releasing hormone (GnRH) administration in a subset of GnRH-deficient men, *J Clin Endocrinol Metab* 69:377, 1989.

32. Franco B et al: A gene deleted in Kallmann's syndrome shares homology with neural cell adhesion and axonal path-finding molecules, *Nature* 353:529, 1991.

33. Friis-Hansen B: Hydrometry of growth and aging. In Brozek J, editor: *Human body composition: approaches and applications,* Symposia of the Society for the Study of Human Biology, vol 7, Oxford, UK 1965, Pergamon Press.

34. Frisch RE: Body fat, menarche, fitness and fertility. In Reisch RE, editor: *Adipose tissue and reproduction,* Basel, 1990, Karger.

35. Frisch RE, McArthur JW: Menstrual cycles: fatness as a determinant of minimum weight for height necessary for their maintenance or onset, *Science* 185:949, 1974.

36. Frisch RE et al: Lower prevalence of breast cancer and cancers of the reproductive system among former college athletes compared to non-athletes, *Br J Cancer* 52:885, 1985.

37. Galbo H et al: The effect of fasting on the hormonal response to graded exercise, *J Clin Endocrinol Metab* 52:1106, 1981.

38. Gambacciani M, Yen SSC, Rasmussen DD: GnRH release from the medial basal hypothalamus: in vitro inhibition by corticotropin-releasing factor, *Neuroendocrinology* 43:533, 1986.

39. Gelato MC, Loriaux DL, Merriam GR: Growth hormone responses to growth hormone-releasing hormone in Hand-Schüller-Christian disease, *Neuroendocrinology* 50:259, 1989.

40. Gharib SD et al: Molecular biology of the pituitary gonadotropins, *Endocr Rev* 11:177, 1990.

41. Gold PW et al: Responses to corticotropin-releasing hormone in the hypercortisolism of depression and Cushing's disease, *N Engl J Med* 314:1329, 1986.

42. Goldenberg RL et al: Ovarian morphology in women with anosmia and hypogonadotropic hypogonadism, *Am J Obstet Gynecol* 126:91, 1976.

43. Hazum E, Conn PM: Molecular mechanism of gonadotropin releasing hormone (GnRH) action, I: the GnRH receptor, *Endocr Rev* 9:379, 1988.

44. Hermanussen M, Sippell WG: Heterogeneity of Kallmann's syndrome, *Clin Genet* 28:106, 1985.

45. Hoff JT, Patterson RH Jr: Craniopharyngiomas in children and adults, *J Neurosurg* 36:299, 1972.

46. Hoffman AR, Crowley WF Jr: Induction of puberty in men by long-term pulsatile administration of low-dose gonadotropin-releasing hormone, *N Engl J Med* 307:1237, 1982.

47. Ishizuka B, Quigley ME, Yen SSC Yen: Pituitary hormone release in response to food ingestion: evidence for neuroendocrine signals from gut to brain, *J Clin Endocrinol Metab* 57:1111, 1983.

48. Jenkins JS, Gilbert J, Ang V: Hypothalamic-pituitary function in patients with craniopharyngiomas, *J Clin Endocrinol Metab* 43:394, 1976.

49. Kallmann FJ, Schoenfeld WA, Barrera SE: The genetic aspects of primary eunuchoidism, *Am J Ment Defic* 48:203, 1944.

50. Kapen S et al: Effect of sleep-wake cycle reversal on luteinizing hormone secretory pattern in puberty, *J Clin Endocrinol Metab* 39:293, 1974.

51. Kaplan SL, Grumbach MM, Aubert ML: The ontogenesis of pituitary hormones and hypothalamic factors in the human fetus: maturation of central nervous system regulation of anterior pituitary function, *Recent Prog Horm Res* 32:161, 1976.

52. Kelly MJ et al: Effects of ovariectomy on GnRH mRNA, pro-GnRH and GnRH levels in the preoptic hypothalamus of the female rat, *Neuroendocrinology* 49:88, 1989.

53. Khoury SA et al: Diurnal patterns of pulsatile luteinizing hormone secretion in hypothalamic amenorrhea: reproducibility and responses to opiate blockade and an α_2-adrenergic agonist, *J Clin Endocrinol Metab* 64:755, 1987.

54. Klinefelter HF Jr, Albright F, Griswold GC: Experience with a quantitative test for normal or decreased amounts of follicle-stimulating hormone in the urine in endocrinological diagnosis, *J Clin Endocrinol Metab* 3:529, 1943.

55. Knobil E: The electrophysiology of the GnRH pulse generator, *J Steroid Biochem* 33:669, 1989.

56. Kreiger DT, Liotta AS: Pituitary hormones in brain: where, how, and why?, *Science* 205:366, 1979.

57. Lachelin GCL, Yen SSC: Hypothalamic chronic anovulation, *Am J Obstet Gynecol* 130:825, 1978.

58. Lam KSL et al: Early effects of cranial irradiation on hypothalamic-pituitary function, *J Clin Endocrinol Metab* 64:418, 1987.

59. Lamon-Fava S et al: Effect of exercise and menstrual cycle status on plasma lipids, low density lipoprotein particle size, and apolipoproteins, *J Clin Endocrinol Metab* 68:17, 1989.

60. Laughlin G, Loucks A, Yen SSC: Marked augmentation of nocturnal melatonin secretion in amenorrheic athletes but not in eumenorrheic athletes, *J Clin Endocrinol Metab* 73:1321, 1991.

61. Lee RB: *!Kung San: men, women and work in a foraging society,* New York, 1978, Cambridge University Press.

62. Leyendecker G, Wildt L, Hansmann M: Pregnancies following chronic intermittent (pulsatile) administration of GnRH by means of a portable pump (Zyklomat): a new approach in the treatment of infertility in hypothalamic amenorrhea, *J Clin Endocrinol Metab* 51:1214, 1980.

63. Lichtenstein L: Histiocytosis X, integration of eosinophilic granuloma of bone, Letterer-Siwe disease and Schüller-Christian disease as related manifestations of a single nosologic entity, *Arch Pathol* 56:84, 1953.

64. Liu JH et al: Induction of multiple ovulation by pulsatile administration of gonadotropin releasing hormone (GnRH), *Fertil Steril* 40:18, 1983.

65. Littley MD et al: Radiation-induced hypopituitarism is dose-dependent, *Clin Endocrinol* 31:363, 1989.

66. Longcope C et al: Aromatization of androgens by muscle and adipose tissue in vivo, *J Clin Endocrinol Metab* 46:16, 1978.

67. Loucks AB, Horvath SM: Athletic amenorrhea: a review, *Med Sci Sports Exerc* 17:56, 1985.

68. Loucks AB, Laughlin G, Yen SSC: Thyroid hormone deficiency in women athletes, *J Clin Endocrinol Metab* 75:514, 1992.

69. Loucks AB et al: Alterations in the hypothalamic-pituitary-ovarian and the hypothalamic-pituitary-adrenal axes in athletic women, *J Clin Endocrinol Metab* 68:402, 1989.

70. Luger A et al: Acute hypothalamic-pituitary-adrenal responses to the stress of treadmill exercise, *N Engl J Med* 316:1309, 1987.

71. Malina RM et al: Age at menarche and selected menstrual characteristics in athletes at different competitive levels and in different sports, *Med Sci Sports* 10:218, 1978.

72. Marcus R et al: Menstrual function and bone mass in elite women distance runners, *Ann Intern Med* 102:158, 1985.

73. Matsuo H et al: Structure of the porcine LH- and FSH-releasing hormone, I: the proposed amino acid sequence, *Biochem Biophys Res Commun* 43:1334, 1971.

74. Medhamurthy R, Gay VL, Plant TM: The prepubertal hiatus in gonadotropin secretion in the male rhesus monkey (Macaca mulatta) does not appear to involve endogenous opioid peptide restraint of hypothalamic gonadotropin-releasing hormone release, *Endocrinology* 126:1036, 1990.

75. Miller DS et al: Pulsatile administration of low dose gonadotropin-releasing hormone (GnRH) for the induction of ovulation and pregnancy in patients with hypothalamic amenorrhea, *JAMA* 250:2937, 1983.

76. Moore-Ede MC, Czeisler CA, Richardson GS: Circadian timekeeping in health and disease, *N Engl J Med* 309:530, 1983.

77. Nezelof C, Basset F, Rousseau MF: Histiocytosis X: histogenetic arguments for a Langerhans cell origin, *Biomedicine* 18:365, 1973.

78. Olster DH, Ferin M: Corticotropin-releasing hormone inhibits gonadotropin secretion in the ovariectomized rhesus monkey, *J Clin Endocrinol Metab* 65:262, 1987.

79. Page RB: Directional pituitary blood flow: a microcine-photographic study, *Endocrinology* 112:157, 1983.

80. Paradisi R et al: High concentrations of catecholamines in human hypothalamic-hypophysial blood, *J Clin Invest* 83:2079, 1989.

81. Petraglia F et al: Naloxone-induced luteinizing hormone secretion in normal, precocious, and delayed puberty, *J Clin Endocrinol Metab* 63:1112, 1986.

82. Petraglia F et al: Corticotropin-releasing factor decreases plasma luteinizing hormone levels in female rats by inhibiting gonadotropin-releasing hormone release into hypophyseal portal circulation, *Endocrinology* 120:1083, 1987.

83. Pirke KM et al: The influence of dieting on the menstrual cycle of healthy young women, *J Clin Endocrinol Metab* 60:1174, 1985.

84. Plant TM et al: Puberty in monkeys is triggered by chemical stimulation of the hypothalamus, *Proc Natl Acad Sci USA* 86:2506, 1989.

85. Powell KE et al: Physical activity and the incidence of coronary heart disease, *Annu Rev Public Health* 8:253, 1987.

86. Quigley ME et al: Evidence for an increased dopaminergic and opioid activity in patients with hypothalamic hypogonadotropic amenorrhea, *J Clin Endocrinol Metab* 50:949, 1980.

87. Rabin D et al: Isolated deficiency of follicle-stimulating hormones: clinical and laboratory features, *N Engl J Med* 287:1313, 1972.

88. Rasmussen DD et al: Endogenous opioid regulation of gonadotropin-releasing hormone release from the human fetal hypothalamus in vitro, *J Clin Endocrinol Metab* 57:881, 1983.

89. Rasmussen DD et al: Human fetal hypothalamic GnRH neurosecretion: dopaminergic regulation in vitro, *Clin Endocrinol* 25:127, 1986.

90. Rasmussen DD et al: Pulsatile gonadotropin-releasing hormone release from the human mediobasal hypothalamus in vitro: opiate receptor-mediated suppression, *Neuroendocrinology* 49:150, 1989.

91. Reame NE et al: Pulsatile gonadotropin secretion in women with hypothalamic amenorrhea: evidence that reduced frequency of gonadotropin-releasing hormone secretion is the mechanism of persistent anovulation, *J Clin Endocrinol Metab* 61:851, 1985.

92. Reifenstein EC Jr: Psychogenic or "hypothalamic" amenorrhea, *Med Clin North Am* 30:1103, 1946.

93. Reyes RI et al: Studies on human sexual development, II: fetal and maternal serum gonadotropin and sex steroid concentrations, *J Clin Endocrinol Metab* 38:612, 1974.

94. Ronkainen H et al: Physical exercise-induced changes and season-associated differences in the pituitary-ovarian function of runners and joggers, *J Clin Endocrinol Metab* 60:416, 1985.

95. Ronnekleiv OK, Resko JA: Ontogeny of gonadotropin-releasing hormone-containing neurons in early fetal development of rhesus macaques, *Endocrinology* 126:498, 1990.

96. Ronnekleiv OK et al: Immunohistochemical demonstration of pro-GnRH and GnRH in the preoptic-basal hypothalamus of the primate, *Neuroendocrinology* 45:518, 1987.

97. Ronnekleiv OK et al: Combined immunohistochemistry for gonadotropin-releasing hormone (GnRH) and pro-GnRH, and in situ hybridization for GnRH messenger ribonucleic acid in rat brain, *Mol Endocrinol* 3:363, 1989.

98. Ross JL, Loriaux DL, Cutler GB: Developmental changes in neuroendocrine regulation of gonadotropin secretion in gonadal dysgenesis, *J Clin Endocrinol Metab* 57:288, 1983.

99. Rossmanith WG et al: Pulsatile GnRH-stimulated LH release from the human fetal pituitary in vitro: sex-associated differences, *Clin Endocrinol* 33:719, 1990.

100. Rupprecht R et al: Blunted adrenocorticotropin but normal β-endorphin release after human corticotropin-releasing hormone administration in depression, *J Clin Endocrinol Metab* 69:600, 1989.

101. Sanborn CF, Martin BJ, Wagner WW: Is athletic amenorrhea specific to runners? *Am J Obstet Gynecol* 143:859, 1982.

102. Schwanzel-Fukuda M, Bick D, Pfaff DW: Luteinizing hormone-releasing hormone (LHRH)-expressing cells do not migrate normally in an inherited hypogonadal (Kallmann syndrome), *Mol Brain Res* 6:311, 1989.

103. Schwanzel-Fukuda M, Pfaff DW: Origin of luteinizing hormone-releasing hormone neurons, *Nature* 338:161, 1989.

104. Schwartz B et al: Exercise-associated amenorrhea: a distinct entity?, *Am J Obstet Gynecol* 141:662, 1981.

105. Seeburg PH, Adelman JP: Characterization of cDNA for precursor of human luteinizing hormone releasing hormone, *Nature* 311:666, 1984.

106. Seeburg PH et al: The mammalian GnRH gene and its pivotal role in reproduction, *Recent Prog Horm Res* 43:69, 1987.

107. Silverman A-J, Jhamandas J, Renaud LP: Localization of luteinizing hormone-releasing hormone (LHRH) neurons that project to the median eminence, *J Neurosci* 7:2312, 1987.

108. Snow RC, Barbieri RL, Frisch RE: Estrogen 2-hydroxylase oxidation and menstrual function among elite oarswomen, *J Clin Endocrinol Metab* 69:369, 1989.

109. Sotsky MJ, Shilo S, Shamoon H: Regulation of counterregulatory hormone secretion in man during exercise and hypoglycemia, *J Clin Endocrinol Metab* 68:9, 1989.

110. Spitz IM et al: Isolated gonadotropin deficiency: a heterogenous syndrome, *N Engl J Med* 290:10, 1974.

111. Standish LJ et al: Neuroanatomical localization of cells containing gonadotropin-releasing hormone messenger ribonucleic acid in the primate brain by in situ hybridization histochemistry, *Mol Endocrinol* 1:371, 1987.

112. Strassman RJ et al: Increase in plasma melatonin, β-endorphin, and cortisol after 128.5-mile mountain race: relationship to performance and lack of effect of naltrexone, *J Clin Endocrinol Metab* 69:540, 1989.

113. Strauss JH et al: Hypothalamic hypopituitarism in an adolescent girl: assessment by a direct functional test of the adenohypophysis, *J Clin Endocrinol Metab* 39:639, 1974.

114. Suh BY et al: Hypercortisolism in patients with functional hypothalamic-amenorrhea, *J Clin Endocrinol Metab* 66:733, 1988.

115. Sutherland WHF, Woodhouse SP: Physical activity and plasma lipoprotein lipid concentrations in men, *Atherosclerosis* 37:285, 1980.

116. Symington T, Duguid WP, Davidson JN: Effect of exogenous corticotropin on histochemical pattern of human adrenal cortex and comparison with changes during stress, *J Clin Endocrinol Metab* 16:580, 1956.

117. Theron JJ, Oosthuizen JMC, Routenbach MM: Effect of physical exercise on plasma melatonin levels in normal volunteers, *S Afr Med J* 66:838, 1984.

118. Van der Walt LA, Wilmsen EN, Jenkins T: Unusual sex hormone patterns among desert-dwelling hunter-gatherers, *J Clin Endocrinol Metab* 46:658, 1978.

119. Veldhuis JD et al: Altered neuroendocrine regulation of gonadotropin secretion in women distance runners, *J Clin Endocrinol Metab* 61:557, 1985.

120. Vigersky RA et al: Hypothalamic dysfunction in secondary amenorrhea associated with simple weight loss, *N Engl J Med* 297:1141, 1977.

121. Villanueva AL et al: Increased cortisol production in women runners, *J Clin Endocrinol Metab* 63:133, 1986.

122. Weinberg U et al: Melatonin does not suppress the pituitary luteinizing hormone response to LH-RH in man, *J Clin Endocrinol Metab* 51:161, 1980.

123. Weitzman ED: Biologic rhythms and hormone secretion patterns. In Krieger DT, Hughes JC, editors: *Neuroendocrinology,* Sunderland, Mass, 1980, Sinauer Associates.

124. Whitcomb RW, Crowley WF Jr: Clinical review, 4: diagnosis and treatment of isolated gonadotropin-releasing hormone deficiency in men, *J Clin Endocrinol Metab* 70:3, 1990.

125. Wiemann JN, Clifton DK, Steiner RA: Pubertal changes in gonadotropin-releasing hormone and proopiomelanocortin gene expression in the brain of the male rat, *Endocrinology* 124:1760, 1989.

126. Wildt L, Leyendecker G: Induction of ovulation by the chronic administration of naltrexone in hypothalamic amenorrhea, *J Clin Endocrinol Metab* 64:1334, 1987.

127. Wildt L, Marshall GR, Knobil E: Experimental induction of puberty in the infantile female rhesus monkey, *Science* 207:1373, 1980.

128. Williams CL et al: Corticotropin-releasing factor and gonadotropin-releasing hormone pulse generator activity in the rhesus monkey, *Neuroendocrinology* 52:133, 1990.

129. Williams PT et al: Lipoprotein subfractions of runners and sedentary men, *Metabolism* 35:45, 1986.

130. Yeh J et al: Pituitary function in isolated gonadotrophin deficiency, *Clin Endocrinol* 31:375, 1989.

131. Yen SSC: Reproductive strategy in women: neuroendocrine basis of endogenous contraception. In Roland R, editor: *Neuroendocrinology of reproduction,* Amsterdam, 1988, Excerpta Medica.

132. Yen SSC, Rebar RW: Endocrine rhythms in gonadotropins and ovarian steroids with reference to reproductive processes. In Krieger DT, editor, *Endocrine rhythms,* vol 1, New York, 1979, Raven Press.

133. Yen SSC et al: Hypothalamic amenorrhea and hypogonadotropism: responses to synthetic LRF, *J Clin Endocrinol Metab* 36:811, 1973.

134. Yen SSC et al: Pituitary gonadotrophin responsiveness to synthetic LRF in subjects with normal and abnormal hypothalamic-pituitary-gonadal axis, *J Reprod Fertil* 20:137, 1973.

Chapter 4

PUBERTY IN THE FEMALE
Normal and Aberrant

Allen W. Root, MD

Puberty* in the female is the period of development during which the reproductive endocrine system matures, the secondary physical characteristics (growth, thelarche, pubarche) of adolescence appear, and the individual becomes capable of conceiving and bearing offspring.

PHYSICAL CHANGES OF PUBERTY
Growth

Increase in the rate of linear growth is the earliest manifestation of puberty in the majority of females. Approximately 20% of the adolescent increase in height is achieved before the onset of breast budding.[54] The rate of linear growth accelerates between 8 and 10 years of age; the peak height velocity (PHV) is achieved at 11 to 12 years, approximately 6 to 12 months before menarche. The average girl gains about 25 cm in height during the adolescent period, 11 cm of which can be directly attributed to the effects of ovarian sex hormones.[120] The mean PHV of 8.3 cm/y (range 6.1 to 10.4) is reached at an average age of 11.4 years (range 9.6 to 13.3) in North American girls. Growth rate decelerates thereafter, and adult height is reached at 15.2 years. In early-maturing American girls, the mean PHV of 10.4 cm/y is achieved at 9.6 years and is substantially greater than the mean PHV of 6.2 cm/y reached at 13.3 years in late-maturing American girls.[255] In normal American girls, the tempo of growth and sexual maturation has no effect on final stature in the majority of subjects, because the longer growing period of the late-maturing girl compensates for the more rapid, but less prolonged, growth spurt of the early-maturing subject.[255] However, LaFranchi et al.[129] report that girls with marked constitutional delay in growth and sexual maturation achieve adult stature somewhat below average (−1.3 SD). In Japanese girls there is a direct correlation between the age of PHV and adult stature; late-maturing girls are taller than early maturers.[253]

---

*In this discussion the terms *puberty* and *adolescence* are employed synonymously.

Growth is determined by the genetic background of the individual, superimposed on which are socioeconomic, nutritional, psychophysiologic, and disease factors. Pituitary growth hormone (GH) and the thyroid hormones regulate growth of the infant and prepubertal child, whereas the sex steroid hormones are of fundamental importance in the rapid growth of puberty.[20] Thyroid hormone is essential for pubertal growth to occur, but it is not the primary stimulus to the pubertal growth spurt. Adrenal androgens may also influence linear growth. In children with central precocious puberty receiving gonadotropin-suppressing doses of a gonadotropin-releasing hormone (GnRH) agonist, linear growth rates correlate directly with the serum concentrations of dehydroepiandrosterone sulfate (DHAS).[273]

The adolescent growth spurt is the result of the pubertal increase in the secretion of both gonadal sex hormones and pituitary GH and is superimposed on the basal growth rate of childhood.[120] In girls, estrogen appears to be the primary hormonal factor stimulating pubertal growth. Low levels of estrogens stimulate growth, but high doses of estrogens inhibit growth by accelerating the rate of skeletal maturation and the closure of the epiphyseal cartilage growth plates.[54] In boys, both androgens and GH are clearly necessary to achieve maximal adolescent growth.[20] The contribution of GH to pubertal growth in the female is less clear; in girls with central precocious puberty and GH deficiency, the rate of linear growth may be as rapid as in girls with intact GH secretion, but the duration of adolescent growth is briefer and final attained height is compromised.[7]

In girls, the secretion of GH as assessed by measurement of serum GH concentrations every 20 to 30 minutes for 24 hours (or for 12 hours overnight) begins to increase in the late prepubertal period.[47, 207] The nocturnal mean GH concentration is significantly increased over prepubertal values in normal girls by Tanner stages II to III of pubic hair growth and breast development, and maximal GH levels coincide with the age of PHV. The mean nocturnal concentration of GH determined by frequent sampling increases from 4.2 ± 1.0 (mean $\pm$ SEM) to 10.0 ± 0.8 ng/mL between pubertal stages I and IV, declining to 3.9 ± 0.7 ng/mL in pubertal stage V.[47] The increase in mean GH concentrations in adolescence is the result of increase in the amplitude of the GH secretory pulse, not in the frequency of GH secretory episodes, which average 7 per 24 hours. The daily GH production rate is inversely proportional to body mass in males,[155] whereas the nocturnal mean GH concentration correlates inversely with body mass in girls.[207]

The pubertal increase in GH secretion is thought to be due to the effects of sex hormones (specifically estrogens, although androgens may also have an effect), which amplify the GH secretory pulse. In girls with delayed adolescence, pulsatile administration of GnRH leads to increased nocturnal secretion of GH, which is significantly elevated by Tanner stage III breast development.[244, 246] The mechanism(s) by which sex hormones amplify GH secretion are incompletely understood, but they probably alter the secretory relationships of the GH-regulating hypothalamic neurohormones, GH-releasing hormone (GHRH), and somatostatin (SRIH).[201] The secretion of GH in response to provocative stimuli is increased in prepubertal children and adult males after only 2 to 3 days of pretreatment with estrogens, indicating the rapidity with which this effect can occur.[164] In both young and old adult females endogenous secretion of GH is greater than that in adult males.[100] In both sexes the mean 24-hour GH concentration is directly related to the serum concentration of free estradiol, but not to the total or free testosterone level.[100] Estrogen might suppress SRIH or enhance GHRH release from the hypothalamus or alter the response of the pituitary somatotroph to either or both neurohormones. Studies of the direct effects of estrogens on the rat somatotroph have been inconsistent. Fukata and Martin[81] recorded no effect of estradiol on basal or stimulated secretion of GH, whereas Simard et al.[235] reported opposite findings. Whether there is a direct effect of estrogens on the neurons that produce the GH-regulating neuropeptides or an indirect effect on a neurotransmitter(s) is unknown. In normal young adult women in the luteal phase of the cycle, administration of the cholinergic agonist pyridostigmine has no effect on GHRH-induced GH secretion.[10] Since cholinergic stimulation impairs SRIH release from hypothalamic neurons, this observation suggests that at this stage of the menstrual cycle, SRIH secretion is low. Thus estrogens may stimulate GHRH release rather than inhibit SRIH secretion. In the *castrated male rat*, testosterone and dihydrotestosterone, but not estradiol, increase hypothalamic GHRH messenger ribonucleic acid (mRNA) expression,[284] while both androgens and estrogens increase expression of hypothalamic SRIH mRNA.[40, 269] Stanhope et al.[244] suggest that the early pubertal rise in GH secretion may not be sex hormone–mediated but due to other hypothalamic and/or gonadal factors. Activin (vide infra) is a peptide found in the gonad and pituitary that might be involved in the regulation of pituitary GH secretion during adolescence.[146]

In serum, approximately 50% of circulating GH is bound to a high-affinity GH-binding protein (GHBP) that is the extracellular domain of the plasma cell membrane receptor for GH.[138] The percentage of GH bound to GHBP increases progressively through childhood and adolescence to adult values[234]; GHBP values correlate negatively with mean 24-hour GH concentrations in males.[154] The metabolic activity of GH is influenced by GHBP; thus GHBP inhibits the binding of GH to cell membrane receptors, GH-induced production of insulin-like growth factor I (IGF-I) and GH-mediated conversion of preadipocytes.[142, 151] The role of GHBP in the regulation of the adolescent growth spurt requires further study.

The pubertal increase in GH secretion is accompanied by an increase in serum concentrations of IGF-I, which has direct mitogenic and differentiating effects on chondrocytes of the epiphyseal growth plate. [43, 114, 136, 207] The maximal level of this GH-dependent growth factor coincides with the age of the PHV and likely contributes to the pubertal acceleration of growth. The pubertal increase in production of IGF-I reflects the interaction of both growth and sex hormones. [67] Serum concentrations of IGF-I decline in late adolescence until adult values are reached. The level of the GH-induced IGF–binding protein 3 (IGFBP-3) also increases during puberty in boys and is correlated positively with total daily GH production, plasma IGF-I, and serum testosterone concentrations. [68, 155] In addition to its transport function, IGFBP-3 may have direct and indirect effects on cartilage growth and sexual maturation. [43, 136] Serum concentrations of IGFBP-1, which has inhibitory effects on IGF action, decline during puberty, perhaps under the influence of insulin. [102, 103]

Physiologic concentrations (1 and 10 ng/mL) of human (h) GH alone increase the secretion of estradiol from cultured luteinized granulosa cells of healthy adult women in vitro and augment in an *additive* manner the estrogen secretory response to human follicle-stimulating hormone (FSH). Neither FSH nor the combination of hGH and FSH increases the secretion of IGF-I, which remains undetectable in this system. [156] The GHBP has been demonstrated in follicular fluid, suggesting the presence of GH receptors in the human ovary. [87] Since exposure to hGH does not increase mRNA for IGF-I in mature, luteinized human granulosa cells [263] and hGH does not act synergistically with FSH, the data suggest that hGH has a direct stimulating effect on the granulosa cell that is independent of both IGF-I and FSH.

Nevertheless, the IGFs (IGF-I, particularly) play a major role in ovarian function. This IGF is synthesized by granulosa cells under the regulation of GH, FSH, and estrogen. [2] It is thought to act in a paracrine/autocrine manner on adjacent cells or its cell of origin to influence differentiation and/or function. Both FSH and luteinizing hormone (LH), augmented by GH, up-regulate (rat) granulosa cell receptors for IGF-I. Adashi et al. [2] suggest that IGF-I (1) amplifies gonadotropin action on the ovary; (2) integrates and coordinates granulosa-theca cell function and follicular maturation; (3) is involved in the selection of a "dominant" follicle for ovulation; and (4) participates in the development of follicles in the fetal, neonatal, and adolescent periods. In addition, the GHBP, mRNA for IGF-II, and the peptide itself are detectable in mature, luteinized granulosa cells, and both IGF-I and IGF-II have been identified in human follicular fluid. [87, 91] In these cells the synthesis of IGF-II is under the control of gonadotropins, not GH.

IGF-I stimulates aromatase activity in human granulosa cells and granulosa-luteal cells and may be produced by developing human granulosa cells, as it is by rat and porcine granulosa cells of developing follicles. [172] Receptors and expression of mRNA for the IGF receptors have been found in human luteinized granulosa cells and in rat granulosa cells. [91] IGFBPs are also synthesized by human and animal granulosa cells and may play facilitatory or inhibitory roles through their effects on the IGFs. In experimental animals IGF-I stimulates adenyl cyclase and aromatase activities; synthesis of LH receptor protein and protoglycan; secretion of progesterone, inhibin, and androstenedione; and expression of mRNA for the P-450 side-chain cleavage enzyme. In human mature granulosa cells IGF-I stimulates aromatase activity and progesterone secretion, whereas in human thecal cells IGF-I stimulates androstenedione and testosterone secretion. [91] IGF-I acts synergistically with LH and FSH to affect ovarian function. IGF-II and insulin itself also act on the ovary, primarily through the IGF-I receptor, however. [87] It has been hypothesized that in hyperandrogenic females, IGF-I may be of pathogenetic significance by causing excessive ovarian androgen synthesis and secretion. [87, 212] These observations indicate that IGF-I, either synthesized by the human ovarian granulosa cell and acting in a paracrine/autocrine manner or produced elsewhere and transported to the ovary, is important in ovarian development and function. Other growth factors may be important in this process as well. This subject is discussed in detail in Chapter 10.

GH accelerates the rate of pubertal maturation in the female rhesus monkey and in humans. [55, 276] In intact female rhesus monkeys, administration of GH advances the age of the initial increase in serum concentrations of LH and the age of first ovulation (in 60% of treated animals) but not the age of menarche. [276] In humans, GH administration may lower the age at which adolescence begins. In untreated subjects with isolated GH deficiency, puberty begins at approximately 16 years of age, but at an appropriate bone age (10 to 10.5 years). In 37 girls with isolated deficiency of GH treated with somatotropin, the age of pubertal onset was younger but still significantly delayed (12.1 vs. 11.2 years [control subjects] for Tanner stage II breast development). [55] However, in GH-treated subjects the rate of progression from Tanner breast stage II to breast stage IV was more rapid (1.5 years) than in control subjects (2.0 years). Thus in this series GH lowered the age of pubertal onset in GH-deficient girls and accelerated the rate of pubertal progression. In hypogonadotropic, hypogonadal women concomitant administration of hGH lowers the amount of gonadotropin necessary for induction of ovulation. [104] These effects of somatotropin reflect the influence of GH and IGF-I on the ovary and their augmentation of gonadotropin-mediated ovarian function. [91] GH also acts directly in mammary tissue to enhance mammary gland development and function. GH binds to the prolactin receptor, a process mediated by zinc. [52] In transgenic mice expressing hGH, mammary gland development and secretion of milk protein occur at younger ages than in control animals.[11] In women with isolated deficiency of GH, administration of GH improves breast development,[232] presumably by direct effect and perhaps through a synergistic effect with estrogen.

Serum concentrations of insulin increase during puberty as a result of insensitivity to its peripheral metabolic effects.[4] The enhanced postreceptor resistance to insulin has been attributed to rising GH and IGF-I values during puberty rather than to sex hormones.[34, 99] The elevated insulin concentrations of adolescence correlate with increasing IGF-I values and favor the growth-promoting effects of this hormone.[238, 249] Insulin lowers serum levels of IGFBP-1 (an IGFBP that inhibits the effect of IGF-I on cellular anabolism) and of sex hormone–binding globulin (SHBG), thus increasing serum levels of free sex hormones); it also increases amino acid transport, which enhances cell growth and replication, and fat deposition, which alters body composition.[62, 102, 103] Insulin also has gonadotropin-like activity; it stimulates steroidogenesis by acting on steroidogenic enzymes through ovarian theca or granulosa cell receptors for insulin or IGF-I and functions synergistically with LH and FSH by altering ovarian receptor number/affinity for the gonadotropins.[185] The hyperinsulinemia of puberty has effects on ovarian maturation and function as well as on linear growth and body composition. Thus there is a coordinated metabolic milieu that enhances the adolescent growth spurt involving the sex hormones, SHBG, insulin, GH, GHBPs, IGF-I and the IGFBPs (Fig. 4-1).

In addition to effects on GH secretion, estrogens act directly on epiphyseal cartilage to increase the synthesis of proteoglycans, collagen, and IGF-I and to enhance osteoblast proliferation.[7, 49, 56, 67] Patients with primary or secondary hypogonadism (except those with gonadal dysgenesis) achieve normal adult heights, indicating that sex hormones are not essential for linear growth, but they have no defined adolescent growth spurt and their body proportions are eunuchoid.[20] Truncal growth during the adolescent growth spurt is stimulated by sex hormones, whereas the increase in leg length is primarily influenced by GH. Further evidence for the importance of estrogen in the adolescent growth spurt in girls is the observation that in patients with 46,XY testicular feminization (complete androgen insensitivity), the mean age at spontaneous PHV and the PHV at adolescence are similar to those of normal girls; although the adult height of the 46,XY female is closer to that of adult males than to adult females, the latter observation reflects other height-regulating genes on the Y

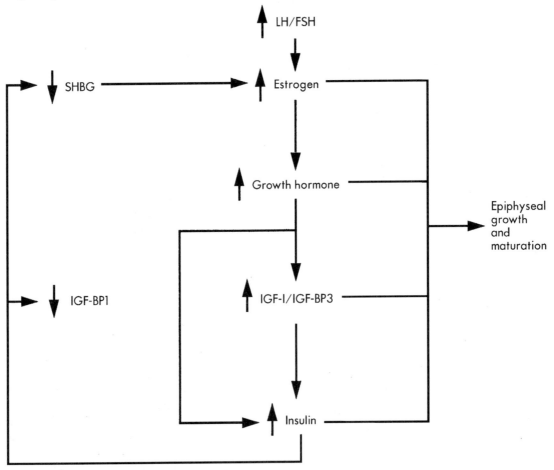

Fig. 4-1. Factors that regulate the adolescent growth spurt.

chromosome.[239,283] In GH-deficient children receiving a fixed dose of GH, sex hormones accelerate growth[20] (Fig. 4-2). Nevertheless, there is an attenuated sex hormone-mediated growth spurt in pubertal patients with deletion of the genes for GH or its receptor.[7] Estrogens increase endogenous serum concentrations of IGF-I in the absence of GH; IGF-I levels in GH-deficient subjects with central precocious puberty are lower than those in eusomatotropic patients with central precocious puberty but are higher than those in prepubertal GH-deficient children.[7, 36] These observations indicate that the acceleration of linear growth during adolescence requires both GH and the sex hormones.

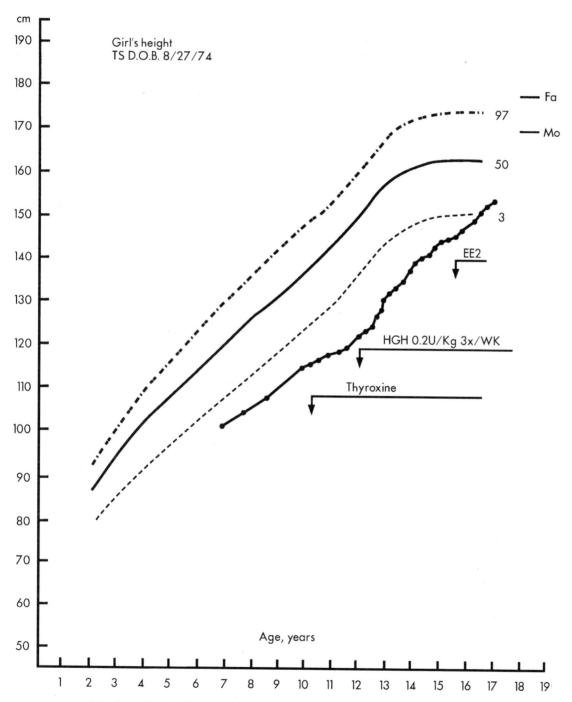

Fig. 4-2. Growth of a girl with idiopathic anterior panhypopituitarism. While she was receiving a constant dose of growth hormone, addition of estrogen at 15 years of age resulted in acceleration of linear growth rate. *EE2,* Ethinyl estradiol.

Body composition

During puberty in the female there is a 120% increase in body fat content and a 44% increase in lean body mass, with consequent decline in the ratio of lean body mass to fat from 5:1 at the beginning of the adolescent growth spurt to 3:1 at menarche.[79] Body mass index (BMI) ($BMI = weight/height^2 = kg/m^2$) increases with age and is greater in postmenarcheal than in premenarcheal girls of the same age.[93, 94] Body fat content is approximately 24% of body weight at menarche. The contribution of body fat to the regulation of pubertal development in the female is a matter of controversy.[78] The age of menarche is weakly related to the percentage of body fat, but there is wide variability.[247] Frisch [78,79] initially suggested that at menarche a "critical" weight of 47 kg was achieved. From her data Frisch[79] concluded that for menarche to occur, at least 17% of body weight had to be fat. These data were dependent on the measurement of total body water and subsequent calculations of lean body mass, assuming that water accounts for 72% of lean body mass. The validity of the "critical weight" concept of menarche has been criticized by a number of investigators on the basis of unreliable estimates of body composition and statistical analyses, the wide variations in weights at menarche in girls of similar heights, and the presence of confounding factors to explain such variability.[230] Stark et al.[247] determined weight and height at menarche in 4,427 English girls and found that weight accounted for no more than 18% of the variability in age of menarche, although heavier girls tended to have earlier menarche, a well-known association. Furthermore, relative weight (weight for height) was unimportant in the timing of menarche. Parra et al.[175] observed a closer relationship between the pubertal increase in gonadotropin secretion and lean body mass than that with total body fat. deRidder et al.[57] could find no relationship between gonadotropin or total plasma sex steroid levels and body fat mass in early pubertal (Tanner breast stage II) girls.

Garn et al.[83] report that "maturational timing has a greater long-term effect on the level of fatness than the level of fatness [has] on maturational timing." Early-maturing white women (menarche <11 years) tend to be 1 cm shorter and 5 kg heavier than late-maturing (menarche>14 years) women. The increase in weight in earlier-maturing females is attributed to fat rather than to a large skeletal frame size. With advancing puberty there are changes in fat distribution. There is a significant increase in hip circumference due to increased fat deposition and a decline in the waist-hip ratio in white and Hispanic females.[92] Early pubertal girls with fat distributed predominantly about the hips have higher gonadotropin and sex hormone values than do slimmer girls, suggesting a relationship between ovarian activity and body fat distribution.[57]

Body fat content continues to increase as the female matures; in the average adult woman, 28% of body weight is fat.[79] When weight loss leads to secondary amenorrhea in adult women, menses resume when the threshold weight for menarche is exceeded by at least 10% because of the higher body fat content of the mature female.

That energy metabolism influences the reproductive endocrine system is reflected by the menstrual dysfunction observed after weight loss and the delayed adolescence of highly trained women athletes with a paucity of body fat.[78,262] The mechanism(s) by which metabolic signals control the reproductive endocrine system is unclear but may involve an effect of metabolic substrates (glucose, amino or fatty acids, glycerol, or other metabolites), hormones (such as insulin or sex or thyroid hormones), or even body temperature on neurotransmitters that regulate the frequency and amplitude of GnRH secretion from the hypothalamus. Processes within the pituitary or gonads themselves may also be targets of metabolic influence. Fat is a metabolically active tissue that converts androgens to estrogens; weight loss may alter this function. Furthermore, levels of SHBG are increased (and concentrations of free sex hormone are reduced) in malnourished subjects. Thus a variety of signals may "inform" higher central nervous system (CNS) centers of the nutritional and energy states of the body.

Short stature and delayed puberty are common in girl gymnasts, but this reflects heritable factors rather than the sport itself. Parents of competitive gymnasts are shorter and lighter in weight (and menarche has occurred later in mothers of these girls) than are parents of competitive female swimmers or sedentary girls.[256] Thus girls with these familial traits apparently select gymnastics as a sport, rather than that the sport and its training requirements lead to these growth and developmental characteristics. Normal growth but delayed pubertal development is common in highly trained adolescent females engaged in long-distance running, swimming, and ballet.[196] Although total body weight may be normal or increased, the percentage of body fat is often low (<10%). Thelarche and menarche may be delayed 1 to 3 years in ballet dancers, whereas pubarche (adrenarche) is usually normal. When injured and forced to a sedentary state, adolescent development may progress rapidly in these girls despite little or no change in body weight or composition, suggesting that calories initially used for exercise are now diverted to reproductive maturation. Stager et al.[242] argue that in female athletes the age of menarche is "later" rather than "delayed," because ages of onset of athletic training and menarche may determine the choice to be an athlete rather than be a consequence of the athletic activity itself. Hormonal changes that accompany delayed puberty or secondary amenorrhea of the female athlete include decrease in frequency and amplitude of LH (i.e., GnRH) pulsatile secretion, a normal or increased gonadotropin secretory response to GnRH, and normal or low-normal prolactin levels and low sex steroid levels.

Table 4-1. Tanner stages of breast development and pubic hair growth in American females*

Tanner stage	Characteristics	Mean age	Age range (y)
Breast			
I	Prepubertal; elevation of papilla only		
II	Breast bud; mound of subareolar tissue less than or equal to diameter of enlarging areola		
III	Enlargement with diameter greater than that of the areola	10.9	8.9-12.9
IV	Projection of areola and papilla and formation of a secondary mound above the plane of the breast	11.9	9.9-13.9
V	Adult; projection of papilla only; areolar border in plane of breast	12.9	10.4-15.3
		14.5	11.3-17.8
Pubic hair			
I	Prepubertal; no sexual hair		
II	Sparse growth of long, straight, or slightly curled hair on the pubis or labia		
III	Rim of coarse, dark, curled hair confined to the lower pubis	11.2	9.0-13.4
IV	Adult-type sexual hair confined to the inverted triangular suprapubic region	11.9	9.7-14.1
V	Adult distribution of sexual hair with spread to the medial aspects of the thighs	12.6	10.4-14.8
		14.6	12.4-16.8

*Data are from references 212 and 270.

Thelarche

Thelarche (breast budding or Tanner stage II breast development) is the earliest physical sign of adolescence in approximately 84% of girls. Paralleling the increase in breast size are increases in the widths of the areola and nipple and the appearance of Montgomery's tubercles.[197] Tanner breast staging describes the contours of the breast, not breast volume, which is extremely variable. At thelarche 87.2% of final adult height has been reached.[133] Early in adolescence thelarche may be unilateral, and it may transiently regress, apparently a reflection of the irregular secretion of estrogen at this time. In North American girls thelarche occurs at a mean age of 10.9 years (±2 SD 8.9 to 12.9 years) (Table 4-1), approximately 1.7 to 2.1 years before menarche.[211, 212, 270] Ordinarily the adolescent female progresses through each stage of breast development, but in some girls breast development may cease at Tanner stage IV, whereas others progress from Tanner stage III directly to stage V.[48] A mature breast (Tanner stage V) is usually achieved 3 to 4 years after thelarche.[270] In some girls adult breast development may not be achieved until 18 years. Breast development occurs earlier and adult breast formation is often reached at a younger age in black females than in white females.[94, 97] In a North Carolina study 6% of normal white girls and 29% of normal black girls had breast development by 6 years of age.[97] One hundred percent of 10-year-old white females and 85% of black girls had thelarche in this survey. Adult breast development is present in 30% of 12-year-old black girls but in only 14% of white 12-year-old girls.[94]

Pubarche

Pubic hair growth (pubarche) begins at an average age of 11.2 years and is the initial manifestation of adolescence in 16% of North American girls. Approximately 3 years elapse before adult pubic hair distribution is reached (Table 4-1).

At pubarche 85.1% of adult stature has been achieved.[133] Pubic hair growth begins at a younger age and reaches the adult stage at an earlier age in black females than in white females. In a North Carolina study 25% of black girls and 9% of white girls had pubic hair by 6 years of age.[97] Kaplowitz et al.[118] have also noted a high incidence of pubic hair growth among black females. Seventy-five percent of 10-year-old black females and 25% of white females had pubic hair growth in this report. Nineteen percent of 12-year-old black girls but only 5% of white girls have Tanner stage V pubic hair.[94]

An adult axillary odor often precedes pubic hair growth. Axillary hair appears 2 years after pubic hair is visible. Breast and pubic hair stages usually correlate well.[94] In Swiss girls pubarche precedes thelarche by 0.5 year, and a male pattern of pubic hair growth (Tanner stage VI: spreading of pubic hair up the linea alba) occurs in 16% of 18-year-old females.[133] Acne occurs in many girls between 11 and 15 years of age; among Swiss females 81% have acne of variable degree during the second decade of life.[133]

The androgens responsible for pubic hair growth are of both adrenal and ovarian origin, but primarily from the latter source. Thus girls with gonadal dysgenesis develop pubic hair, but it is often sparse and appears at older ages and with higher DHAS concentrations than in normal females. On the other hand, girls with primary hypoadrenocorticism develop and maintain normal pubic and axillary hair growth in the absence of adrenal androgens (personal observation).

Menarche

Menarche, the first menstrual period, occurs approximately 2 years after thelarche and pubarche at an average age of 12.7 years for white girls and 12.4 years for black girls in North America.[212, 254] It coincides with Tanner stages III to IV breast development and occurs after the

PHV has been achieved. Only rarely (<1%) is menarche the very first sign of puberty. If more than 4 years elapse without menarche after thelarche, an explanation for this delay needs to be sought. At menarche 95.3% of final height has been reached.[133] Although initially irregular and anovulatory, menstrual periods tend to regularize and to become ovulatory approximately 2 years after menarche. There is great variability in the length of the menstrual cycle and in the duration of menses in normal adolescent females.[48] In the first postmenarcheal year 70% of cycles are 21 to 35 days in duration; 23% are shorter and 7% are longer than this interval. By the fifth postmenarcheal year 88% of cycles are 21 to 35 days in length; 3% are shorter and 9% are longer. Fourteen percent of menstrual cycles are ovulatory in the first postmenarcheal year, 50% by the end of the second year, and 87% in the fifth postmenarcheal year.[133]

Other physical changes of adolescence

During puberty, thyroid volume increases twofold to threefold (from 2 to 5 mL) and is related to body weight; it enlarges more rapidly in girls than in boys.[252] The increase in thyroid volume during adolescence may reflect an increased need for iodine during this period. There is also an increase in thyroid function early in adolescence.

Skeletal maturation advances during adolescence under the influence of sex hormones, thyroid hormone, and GH. Bone mineral density increases during childhood and adolescence (Table 4-2). By single-photon absorptiometry, cortical radial bone mineral content is greater in boys than in girls and in black children than in white children 1 to 6 years of age and increases with age and weight.[139] By using dual-photon absorptiometry of trabecular spinal bone, bone mineral content is found to correlate with weight, height, BMI, and age in children 5 to 12 years of age.[183] During adolescence, trabecular spinal bone mineral density increases in the later pubertal stage in response to rising levels of sex hormones and vitamin D metabolites.[88, 158] Bone mineral density is greater in black adolescents than in white or Hispanic adolescents. In females after age 7 years bone mineral density is equal to or slightly greater than that in males.[86, 88, 158] In adolescent females bone mineral density correlates with weight, estrogen secretion, and testosterone concentrations.[58] In mature young women (20 years of age) with low estrogen output, bone mineral density is lower than in peers with greater estrogen exposure. Interestingly, increased intake of dietary fiber adversely affects bone mineralization by decreasing estrogen levels due to decreased enterohepatic circulation.[58]

By pelvic ultrasound ovarian size increases during puberty and its morphology changes. In the infant female the mean ovarian volume is 0.7 mL, and the ovary is homogeneous.[219] Between ages 2 and 8 years ovarian weight increases as a result of increases in medullary stroma and ovarian follicle number and size.[13] Between 7 and 10 years

Table 4-2. Bone mineral content in female children and adolescents

Chronologic age (y)	Race*	Bone mineral content (g/cm²)	Reference
<3	B	0.19	139
3-5	B	0.31	
5-7	B	0.41	
<3	W	0.16	
3-5	W	0.24	
5-7	W	0.34	
5	Mixed	0.64	183
6	Mixed	0.64	
7	Mixed	0.72	
8	Mixed	0.69	
9	Mixed	0.73	
10	Mixed	0.78	
11	Mixed	0.84	
12	W	0.95	88
13	W	0.80	
14	W	0.96	
15	W	0.90	

*B, Black; W, white.

of age mean ovarian volume increases twofold while the girl is still prepubertal (i.e., absence of thelarche); it increases another threefold between 10 and 17 years of age (Fig. 4-3).[33] Uterine weight increases between 2 and 8 years, whereas uterine volume (2.5 mL) remains constant between 7 and 10 years of age and increases fourfold in the next year and sixfold between 11 and 17 years of age (Fig. 4-3). Growth of the uterine corpus accounts for the bulk of pubertal uterine growth. Rising LH, FSH, and estradiol concentrations parallel and correlate with the increases in uterine and ovarian volumes. By 4 to 5 years of age ovarian follicular cysts less than 9 mm in diameter are present in 10% to 20% of girls. The number, size, and frequency of ultrasonographically visualized ovarian cysts gradually increases between 6 and 12 years; by the latter age, cysts are present in 80% of ovaries and cysts greater than 10 mm are present in 20% of girls. Even in postmenarcheal girls, however, a homogeneous ovarian appearance is seen in 20% of normal subjects. Ovarian cyst number and size increase markedly between 8 and 10 years of age (even before onset of thelarche), when 5- to 10-mm follicular cysts appear. Cysts greater than 10 mm in diameter are observed after 10 years of age. Between 10 and 12.5 years of age, ovaries have a "multi (follicular) cystic" ultrasonographic appearance with more than six follicular cysts 4 mm or more in diameter.[33, 278] The ultrasonographic pattern of multicystic ovaries of the adolescent girl differs from that of polycystic ovaries; in the latter ovarian stroma is increased and the small cysts are subcapsular; in multicystic ovaries, medullary stroma is scant and the follicular cysts "fill" the ovary.[33] The increase in number and size of

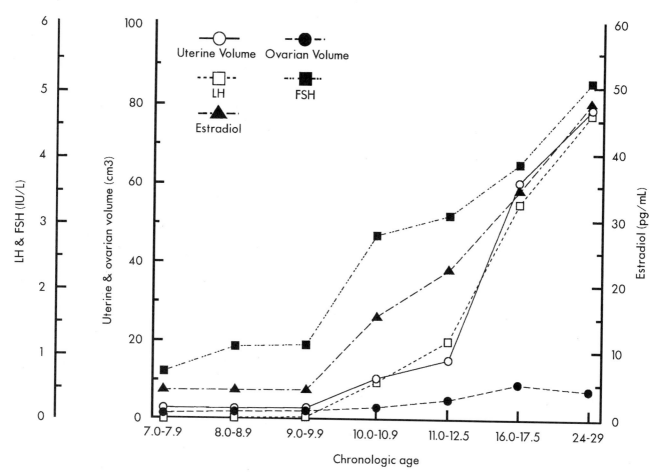

Fig. 4-3. Relationship of serum concentrations of LH, FSH, and estradiol to ovarian and uterine volumes and chronologic age. (Drawn from data in reference 33.)

follicles in pubertal girls is the response to increased gonadotropin (and GnRH) secretion.

Vaginal length increases prepubertally, and enlarges still further to menarche and beyond. Vaginal epithelium becomes cornified, and the clitoris and labia enlarge with estrogen exposure.[270]

MATURATION OF THE REPRODUCTIVE ENDOCRINE SYSTEM IN FEMALES

The female reproductive endocrine system involves the hypothalamus, anterior pituitary, and ovaries (Fig. 4-4). Ovaries develop from the bipotential gonadal ridge in the absence of a functioning testicular determining factor (TDF)[61] present on the short arm of the Y chromosome. The rete ovarii is derived from the mesonephric tubules. A second X chromosome is *not* required for ovarian differentiation. Thus in the 45,X fetus ovarian morphology at 3 months of gestation is indistinguishable from that of the 46,XX

fetus. However, the rate of oocyte degeneration is much more rapid in the 45,X than in the 46,XX fetus, indicating the necessity of the second X chromosome for oocyte "maintenance."[96] The rapid degeneration of oocytes in the 45,X ovary leads to the characteristic fibrous streak gonad of the girl with gonadal dysgenesis. Germ cells migrate into the gonad from the yolk sac entoderm early in the first trimester. After migration oogonia undergo mitotic division, which is concluded by the seventh month of gestation.[211] After completion of mitotic division oogenesis begins; the oogonia enter the prophase of meiosis and become oocytes, which peak in number (6 to 7 million) in the fifth gestational month.[250] Oocytes (or primordial follicles) either become atretic or, under the influence of fetal gonadotropins, are encircled by granulosa cells to become primary follicles, which first appear in the fourth month of gestation and are maximum between the fifth and ninth months.

In late gestation primary follicles progress to preantral

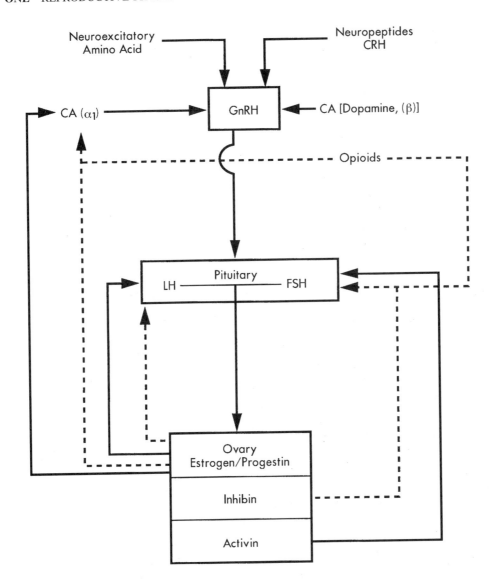

Fig. 4-4. Regulation of hypothalamic-pituitary-ovarian function. CA, Chronologic age.

follicles (several hundred granulosa cells surrounding an enlarging oocyte enclosed within a layer of theca cells, ranging in diameter from 0.05 to 0.2 mm). By term, one or two antral follicles (fluid-filled antrum, mature oocyte, well-developed theca, diameter of 1 to 2 mm) are present. More than 6 million germ cells are present in midgestation; by term the number has fallen to 2 million and declines exponentially thereafter. During infancy and early childhood, primary follicles develop and some become antral follicles in response to episodic gonadotropin secretion.[211] By 7 years of age, several antral follicles (>5 mm in diameter) are present in both ovaries, most of which become atretic. The number of antral follicles (>1 mm) increases to a peak between 15 and 20 years of age.[211] Small antral follicles become large antral follicles (>10 mm in diameter) and either are recruited for ovulation or undergo atresia.

Hypothalamic-pituitary development and the pituitary-portal vascular system are complete by the end of the first trimester.[190] Pituitary size increases with somatic development. During adolescence there is a marked increase in pituitary volume as determined by magnetic resonance imaging.[66]

Gonadotropins and estrogens

GnRH is the primary regulator of pituitary-gonadal function by stimulating gonadotropin secretion. This decapeptide is secreted episodically, and the frequency and amplitude of the GnRH pulse determines the pattern of gonadotropin secretion. Pulsatile secretion of GnRH is essential for its action, as continuous exposure of the gonadotrope to GnRH results in its desensitization and inhibition of function. The secretory pattern of GnRH varies with the stage of development; GnRH secretion is increased in utero and in the neonate and young infant; the amplitude of GnRH pulsation is dampened during childhood, only to increase in frequency and amplitude with the onset of puberty. These developmental changes in GnRH release are reflected in the pattern of gonadotropin secretion throughout life.[42, 45]

The arcuate nucleus is the site of GnRH production; GnRH is a decapeptide synthesized as part of a large prohormone containing 91 amino acids.[205] Neurons that synthesize GnRH develop from the medial olfactory placode early in gestation (which accounts for the association of abnormalities of smell and gonadotropin deficiency states, i.e., Kallmann syndrome), cross the nasal septum, and eventually locate in the preoptic area and arcuate nucleus of the medial basal hypothalamus, in which is also located the "GnRH pulse generator."[224] GnRH is secreted from nerve terminals in the median eminence into the pituitary portal vasculature and transported to the anterior pituitary. Luteinizing hormone and FSH are synthesized by pituitary gonadotropes, under stimulation by GnRH.[13] The gonadotropins are families of related heterogeneous forms of glycoproteins of molecular weights of 28 to 30 kd with identical alpha subunits (92–amino acid peptide coded on chromosome 6q12-q21) and distinct beta subunits that confer biologic activity on the intact molecule. (β-LH is a 112–amino acid protein encoded on chromosome 19; β-FSH is a 111–amino acid peptide encoded on chromosome 11p13.[13]) The gonadotropins contain varying amounts of carbohydrates and sialic acid that confer differing physicochemical (size, charge, clearance) and biologic properties on LH and FSH. In general, isoforms of the gonadotropins that do not have sialic acid residues (i.e., are more basic) are cleared rapidly from serum, whereas sialylated molecules have longer half-lives. Alterations in carbohydrate composition do not inhibit binding of the gonadotropins to their cell membrane receptors; however, deglycosylation and removal of galactose leaves an LH molecule that binds to its receptor with higher affinity than intact hormone, but has decreased biologic activity.[13] Some isoforms of LH (FSH) bind to its receptor but inhibit its function. Overall biologic activity of serum LH and FSH depends on the relative proportions of their various isoforms in the circulation.[13]

Immunoreactive GnRH is present in the human fetal brain by 32 days of gestation, and pituitary immunoreactive LH and FSH are identifiable by 9 weeks of gestation.[215] Whether the fetal ovary is capable of secreting estrogens is uncertain, as the placenta is the major source of estrogens in utero. The importance of fetal pituitary gonadotropin secretion to ovarian and oocyte maturation is indicated by the poorly developed antral follicles of the anencephalic 46,XX fetus[250] and by the adverse effect of hypophysectomy on ovarian germ cell and oocyte number in the fetal rhesus monkey.[211]

Fetal hypothalamic levels of GnRH and pituitary and serum concentrations of LH and FSH are maximal between the 17th and 24th weeks of gestation.[12, 211] Serum and pituitary levels of immunoreactive (I) LH and FSH are substantially higher in female fetuses than in male fetuses.[12] Serum values of the gonadotropins decline in the third trimester, presumably the consequence of the acquisition of sensitivity to the negative feedback effects of sex hormones and possibly to the onset of inhibitory control of hypothalamic function by higher CNS centers and the early establishment of "central restraint" of GnRH secretion (Fig. 4-5). Fetal serum concentrations of bioassayable (B) FSH are often greater than values recorded in agonadal subjects; they are higher than I-FSH values, peak at 23 to 24 weeks of gestation, are higher in female fetuses than in male fetuses, and decline by 35 to 40 weeks of gestation when B-FSH levels are similar in the two sexes.[12, 13] That the female fetus synthesizes and secretes more gonadotropins in midgestation than does the male fetus may be due to greater sensitivity of the male fetal hypothalamic-pituitary unit to the inhibitory effects of testosterone, or to the synthesis by the male fetal pituitary of short-lived isoforms of the gonadotropins.[13] Fetal serum concentrations of estrogen are high but are derived primarily from the fetoplacental unit (fetal adrenals provide androgenic precursors of estrogens to the placenta, which has aromatase activity). Plasma concentrations of "free" testosterone reportedly are low in the female fetus, but values increase in the last month of gestation to levels similar to those in the male fetus.[12] The source and significance of the late gestational rise in plasma free testosterone concentrations are unknown.

At birth serum gonadotropin concentrations are relatively low but then increase.[211] The rise in serum LH and FSH concentrations in the female neonate is related to the fall in serum estrogen levels that follows birth. Estrogen concentrations range up to 50 pg/mL in female infants, with maximal values between 2 and 6 months of age.[211] The higher gonadotropin (particularly FSH) concentrations found in female infants than in male infants possibly also reflect, in part, a lesser ovarian secretion of the gonadal peptide inhibin, compared with that of the testes.[31] In addition, the high gonadotropin concentration in the female infants may be due to relative lack of CNS inhibitory input to the hypothalamus. The posterior hypothalamus is the site through which central inhibitory input is delivered to the GnRH-secreting neurons, although the mechanism by which restraint is exercised is unknown.[223] During the first 2 years of life the dominant inhibitory influence on gonadotropin secretion is sex steroid–negative feedback. This is evidenced by the substantially higher LH and FSH values present in agonadal infants as compared with intact infants during this interval.[46, 148, 215]

Between 2 and 4 years of age, serum gonadotropin levels decline in girls to nadir values between 4 and 10 years of age.[46] The midchildhood decline in gonadotropin secretion is relatively independent of gonadal function, as a similar pattern is recorded in agonadal children and ova-

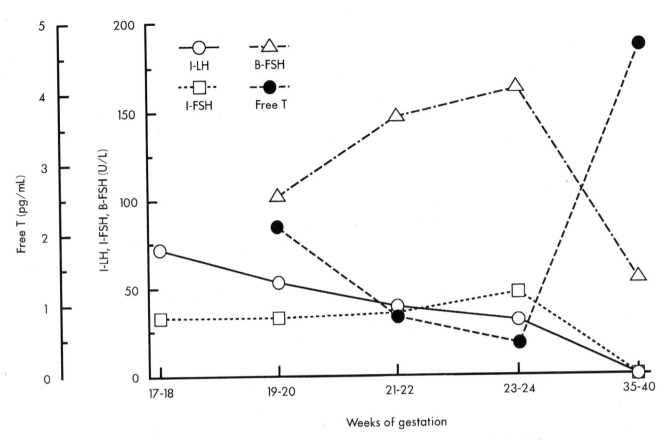

Fig. 4-5. Plasma concentrations of I-LH, I-FSH, B-FSH, and free testosterone in the female fetus. (Drawn from data in reference 12.)

riectomized rhesus monkeys, although some effects of the negative feedback of sex hormone are still identifiable at this period; thus basal LH and FSH levels are a bit higher in agonadal children than in intact children of comparable age.[46,215] Thus at this point the "central restraint" or inhibition of hypothalamic GnRH and pituitary gonadotropin secretion is maximal. The earliest hormonal indicator of puberty is an increase in the amplitude and frequency of the nocturnal secretion of I LH (and thus of GnRH) recorded in late prepubertal subjects (Fig. 4-6). This is followed by an increase in daytime LH concentrations and rising I-FSH and estradiol levels as puberty progresses (see Fig. 4-3).

Newly developed time-resolved immunofluorometric assays (IFA) and immunoradiometric assays (IRMA) of LH and FSH have provided further insight into gonadotropin secretion in childhood because of their greatly increased sensitivity and greater similarity to biologic assays.[112] Early measurements of bioassayable urinary LH and FSH had indicated that the prepubertal child secreted gonadotropins, findings confirmed by radioimmunoassay of urinary and serum gonadotropin specimens. Such studies suggested that even in prepubertal children LH and FSH are secreted episodically and in the female child cyclically.[113] However, serum gonadotropin values (particularly LH) are often below the range of detection by conventional radioimmu-

noassays. Utilizing IFAs for LH and FSH, Apter et al.[5] report that in prepubertal girls sampled at 1200 to 1400 hours the mean LH concentration is 0.04 mIU/mL (World Health Organization International Reference Preparation [WHO IRP] 68/40), and increases tenfold with thelarche (see Fig. 4-3). Significantly, LH and estradiol concentrations double even before the onset of thelarche. Serum LH concentrations are 116 times higher in young adult women in the early follicular phase of the menstrual cycle than in prepubertal girls. Serum FSH concentrations approximate 1 mIU/mL (second IRP pituitary FSH/LH 78/549) in prepubertal girls, increase twofold before thelarche and approximately threefold in Tanner breast stage II, and are 6.7 times higher in adult women than in prepubertal girls. In the study by Apter et al.[5] estradiol concentrations triple with thelarche, paralleling the rising LH and FSH concentrations; they are approximately fifteenfold higher in the early follicular phase of the cycle in young adult women than in prepubertal girls.

These investigators also report that in prepubertal 6-year-old girls there is episodic nocturnal secretion of LH at values below the sensitivities of most IRMAs and radioimmunoassays.[279] The mean number of LH pulses in girls is 1.8 per 12 hours (boys 2.2, range 1 to 6) and the mean pulse amplitude is 0.35 mIU/mL (boys 0.16). The

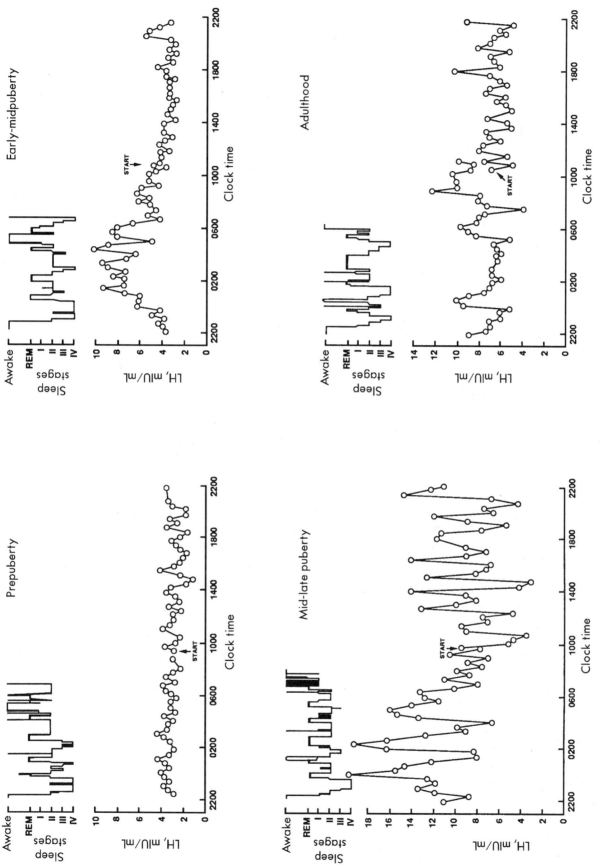

Fig. 4-6. Ontogeny of the diurnal variation in the secretion of LH in females. (Redrawn from Katz JT et al: Toward an elucidation of the psychoendocrinology of anorexia nervosa. In Sachar EJ, editor: *Hormones, behavior and psychopathology*, New York, 1976, Raven Press, p 265.)

mean nocturnal pulse interval in prepubertal girls is 111 minutes (boys 169 minutes). The mean nocturnal LH concentration in girls is 0.19 mIU/mL (boys 0.10) and the minimal level is 0.12 mIU/mL (boys 0.09). There are no sex differences in nocturnal LH secretory patterns. In prepubertal girls the mean nocturnal FSH concentration is 1.95 mIU/mL (boys 0.46), the pulse amplitude is 1.62 mIU/mL (boys 0.19), the pulse nadir is 1.30 mIU/mL (boys 0.45), the number of pulses is 1.67 per 12 hours (boys 2.13), and the mean pulse interval is 160 minutes (boys 209). The mean FSH concentration, pulse amplitude, and pulse nadir are higher in girls than in boys. Approximately 50% of LH and FSH pulses are concordant.

The nocturnal pulses of LH and FSH recorded in prepubertal girls (and boys) cluster about the point of sleep onset and wane with increasing duration of sleep.[279] There is also a significant increase (+71%) in post–sleep-onset concentrations of LH and FSH as compared with presleep values in prepubertal girls (+75% in boys). Fujieda et al.[80] measured LH concentrations by IFA over a 24-hour period in 16 prepubertal children (11 males, 4 females) and found pulsatile secretion of LH with 6 to 15 LH peaks per 24 hours and a day-night difference, with LH secretion being greater at night. Similar (but less sensitive) data have been provided by IRMAs of LH and FSH. For instance, Garibaldi et al.[82] report serum LH concentrations in early prepubertal children to be less than 0.25 mIU/mL (WHO IRP 68/40); LH levels increase to 1.0 mIU/mL in late prepubertal subjects and to 1.5 mIU/mL in Tanner stage II breast development, rising still further to 9.9 mIU/mL by Tanner breast stage V. In this study serum LH concentrations remained undetectable in 60% of late prepubertal and 40% of early pubertal subjects, indicating the continuum of LH secretion as the child gradually enters puberty. Since the secretion of LH (and FSH) is entrained on the release of GnRH, the pulsatility of LH secretion in prepubertal subjects implies that GnRH is also released episodically by the hypothalamus and that night-day differences in LH secretion are present in the prepubertal child; thus the GnRH pulse generator is functional in the preadolescent child.

Prepubertally, the serum gonadotropin secretory response to GnRH is maximal in the female infant, with substantially more FSH than LH released in response to this decapeptide (a pattern distinct from that of the male infant). The gonadotropin response to GnRH declines during childhood (sometimes to undetectable levels), although generally basal and GnRH-provoked FSH concentrations remain higher in girls than in boys throughout childhood.[190] With the onset of adolescence, the LH secretory response to GnRH increases, whereas the FSH response declines (Fig. 4-7). GnRH administered at proper time intervals (once every 60 to 90 minutes) has a "self-priming" effect; that is, each successive pulse of GnRH stimulates a greater secretory pulse of LH; more frequent (every 10 minutes or continuous infusion) administration of GnRH inhibits LH

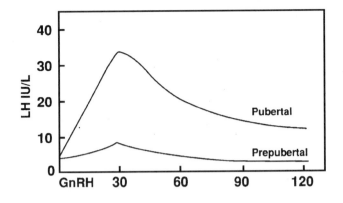

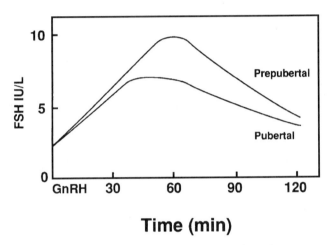

Time (min)

Fig. 4-7. Maturity-related change in the gonadotropin secretory response to GnRH in females from an FSH-predominant to an LH-predominant pattern. (Redrawn with permission from Schwartz ID, Root AW: Puberty in girls: early, incomplete, or precocious? *Contemp Pediatr* 7 [1]:147, 1990. Copyright 1990 by *Contemporary Pediatrics.*)

secretion, whereas less frequent administration (every 3 hours) favors FSH rather than LH release. The gonadotrope membrane receptors for GnRH are up-regulated by GnRH when administered hourly but down-regulated when administered more frequently. The proper timing of exposure of the gonadotrope to exogenous (or endogenous) pulsatile GnRH results in the sequential changes in pituitary secretion of gonadotropins, ovarian follicular development, ovulation, and sex hormone production characteristic of the fertile woman. Alterations in GnRH pulse frequency have pathologic effects.[153]

By using conventional but sensitive radioimmunoassays (reference second IRP of human menopausal gonadotropins [hMG]; relative to WHO IRP 68/40, second IRP-hMG LH values are approximately 1.5 to 2 times higher), Oerter et al.[171] characterized spontaneous 24-hour patterns of LH and FSH secretion (in samples obtained at 20-minute

Table 4-3. Criteria for pubertal gonadotropin secretion*

Criterion†	Females		Males	
Peak LH:FSH (GnRH)	>0.66	(96%)†	>3.6	(65%)†
Peak [LH] (GnRH)	>15	(96%)	>30	(78%)
Maximal nocturnal [LH]	>10	(92%)	>12	(90%)
Maximal increment [LH] (GnRH)	>12	(88%)	>25	(83%)
Mean increment nocturnal [LH]	>6.7	(88%)	>9	(86%)
Mean nocturnal [LH]	>5	(80%)	>7	(81%)

*Data are from reference 171.
†Sensitivity with 100% specificity. LH values are expressed in international units per liter, second IRP-hMG.

intervals) and GnRH-induced gonadotropin secretion in prepubertal and adolescent female subjects. Pulsatile secretion of LH and FSH was observed in all subjects. Although the LH secretory peak frequency increased from 9 to 12 per 24 hours and the FSH secretory peak frequency increased from 6 to 9 per 24 hours between the prepubertal female and the Tanner breast stage V female, the changes were not significant. The most rapid LH pulse frequencies were recorded between 2200 and 0200 hours, immediately after onset of sleep. Mean nocturnal (2000 to 0800 hours) LH and FSH concentrations were higher than daytime values in both prepubertal and pubertal subjects, the levels increasing with advancing puberty primarily because of an increase in secretory pulse amplitudes. In females with Tanner stage V breast development the day-night difference in LH and FSH secretion disappeared. (Prolactin values were also measured in this study and did not change with advancing adolescence.) In females in response to GnRH, peak LH concentrations increased and peak FSH concentrations decreased with progression of puberty. A maximal nocturnal LH concentration greater than 10 mIU/mL, a peak LH secretory response to GnRH of greater than 15 mIU/mL, and a post–GnRH peak LH:FSH ratio greater than 0.66 defined the pubertal state with more than 90% sensitivity and 100% specificity (Table 4-3).

Although day-night differences in LH concentrations ordinarily are not present in the adult subject, there is marked suppression of LH (and GnRH) secretion in the early follicular and early luteal phases of the menstrual cycle of the adult woman.[72, 130] The nocturnal LH pulse frequency is increased in the mid- and late follicular phases of the menstrual cycle.[72] Despite similar serum estradiol values, the nocturnal LH secretory patterns of normal, early pubertal girls and girls with central precocious puberty differ markedly from those of young adult women in the early follicular phase of the cycle.[130] This observation suggests that there is a different mechanism(s) of nocturnal regulation of GnRH-LH secretion in these two groups. In the young adult woman, inhibition of endogenous opioid action by naloxone increases nocturnal GnRH-mediated LH release in the early follicular phase.[216] However, opioid blockade has no effect on daytime or nighttime secretion of

LH in prepubertal or early pubertal subjects. The neurotransmitter regulatory control of nocturnal LH secretion in the early puberty subject is unknown.[85]

The bioactivity of circulating LH may be measured by the rat or mouse interstitial cell testosterone secretion (RICT) assay, in which the end point is the amount of testosterone secreted by interstitial cells in vitro in response to the bioactivity of LH (or human chorionic gonadotropin [hCG]) in the test sample. With the RICT it has been shown that bioactive LH and hCG concentrations are higher than I-LH and hCG values in cord serum samples from female infants and decline during the first week after birth as hCG is cleared from plasma; B-LH remains measurable in serum from females through infancy and childhood at values near assay sensitivity with B:I ratios greater than 1. Bioactive LH values increase significantly with each pubertal stage in girls and boys and to a greater extent than do levels of I-LH, resulting in progressively higher B:I ratios with advancing adolescence.[13]

An increase in the B:I ratio reflects a change in the structure of the LH molecule that confers upon it greater bioactive potency per unit of immunoreactive mass. The amount, type, and site of oligosaccharide incorporated into the LH molecule during post-translational processing results in the formation of isohormones of LH with differing charge, half-lives, receptor-activating affinity, and in vivo and in vitro bioactivity.[39] The change to a more bioactive isoform of LH secreted during puberty is the result of GnRH-stimulated LH secretion and of sex hormones that modify post-translational processing of LH.[259, 261] Some of the variability of the B:I ratio and its changes with stimulation by GnRH, suppression by GnRH agonists, and during the menstrual cycle are attributable to the radioimmunoassay of LH, which spuriously overestimates low levels of LH, perhaps lowering B:I ratios inappropriately. Nevertheless, data indicate that the species of LH changes during adolescence and that these isoforms are more biologically active. Bioassayable LH concentrations increase eightfold between Tanner breast stages I and V, whereas I-LH levels increase only threefold.[13, 192] The B:I ratio increases progressively with advancing development (from 1.1 in Tanner breast stage I to 4.1 in breast stage V). Reiter et al.[193] used a sensitive RICT bioassay and report that 70% of serum samples from prepubertal girls have detectable B-LH values, and that pulsatile B-LH as well as I-LH patterns of secretion are identifiable.

Bioactive FSH (B-FSH), assayed by the rat Sertoli cell aromatase induction assay, is measurable in prepubertal girls and does not change during adolescence.[14] Beitins et al.[14] report that mean B-FSH concentrations range from 8.4 mIU/mL (National Hormone and Pituitary Program [NHPP] hFSH-3, 3100 U/mg) in prepubertal girls to 12.1 mIU/mL in the female with adult breast development and are similar in adult women in the follicular and luteal phases of the menstrual cycle (6.2 and 4.3 mIU/mL, respectively). Serum I-FSH concentrations increased insignificantly from 2.0 to 3.6 mIU/mL between Tanner breast stages I and V, and the FSH B:I ratio fluctuated between 0.8 and 1.5 in this study; the similarity of B-FSH and I-FSH in girls during adolescence suggests that the bulk of the FSH secreted by females is bioactive. In adult women in midcycle, the serum levels of B-FSH increase threefold whereas I-FSH values barely change, resulting in a B:I of 4.4 at this point in the cycle. (In boys during puberty B-FSH concentrations are similar to those of girls, but I-FSH levels are generally lower, resulting in higher B:I FSH ratios than in girls.) Since I-FSH concentrations as measured by IFA[5] increase during female adolescence and B-FSH concentrations apparently do not change, further studies of bioactive and immunoreactive FSH and their relationships utilizing similar standards are required to clarify the changes in the secretion of the mass of FSH that occurs during puberty.

Endogenous GnRH and exogenous GnRH preferentially increase the release of more bioactive LH isoforms with a consequent increase in the LH B:I ratio.[13, 59] Administration of testosterone, dihydrotestosterone, or estradiol decreases secretion of bioactive (and immunoreactive) LH and depresses LH B:I ratios. However, in postmenopausal women, estrogen increases the secretory rate and mass of B-LH induced by GnRH, perhaps by increasing the expression of GnRH receptors on the gonadotrope plasma cell membrane.[259] In peripubertal boys B-FSH is secreted episodically before and after the onset of sleep; pulses of B-FSH do not correlate well with meager pulsatile secretion of I-FSH in such subjects.[13] Intravenous pulses of GnRH (25 ng/kg every 1 to 2 hours) administered to boys with idiopathic hypogonadotropism initially increase B-FSH concentrations whereas release of I-FSH and I-LH is meager, implying preferential secretion of bioactive isoforms of FSH by GnRH in this situation.[13]

In adult women FSH B:I ratios increase at midcycle, suggesting that estradiol alters endogenous GnRH-induced secretion of FSH, preferentially increasing the release of isoforms of FSH with increased bioactivity; LH B:I ratios change only slightly during the midcycle surge of gonadotropin secretion.[13] In girls with gonadal dysgenesis, estrogens decrease the LH B:I ratio but increase the FSH B:I ratio.[13] Estrogens increase preferentially the secretion of basic (rather than acidic) isoforms of FSH, which are more rapidly cleared from serum. During puberty in the female it is likely that the predominant isoforms of FSH are more basic and short-lived and less biopotent than those in the male.[13] This may have important implications for the development of normal cyclic hypothalamic-pituitary-ovarian function in the female (vide infra).

Other hormonal changes of puberty

Androgens. In females androgens are secreted by the adrenal cortex (androstenedione [A], dehydroepiandrosterone [DHEA] and its sulfate [DHAS]) and ovaries (A, DHEA) under the stimulatory regulation of adrenocorticotropin (ACTH) and LH, respectively. Adrenal androgen secretion by the fetal adrenal cortex begins at 8 to 10 weeks of gestation under the control of ACTH.[202] In the neonate, high levels of DHEA, DHAS, and A fall quickly over the first 3 months and more slowly over the next 9 months as the fetal adrenal zone degenerates. Between 3 and 7 years of age the zona reticularis of the adrenal cortex, the site of androgen synthesis, appears and enlarges. Between 6 and 8 years serum concentrations of DHEA and DHAS increase and the "adrenarche" ensues (Table 4-4). Serum concentrations of A increase between 8 and 10 years of age. Adrenal androgens stimulate pubic and axillary hair growth in girls with gonadal dysgenesis, but in normal subjects ovarian androgens are primarily involved, as sexual hair develops normally in patients with primary adrenal insufficiency.

The mechanism of the adrenarche is unknown, but it may be the result of growth of the adrenal with increasing concentrations of steroid intermediary metabolites, which suppress adrenal 3β-hydroxysteroid dehydrogenase activity and increase 17,20-lyase activity, thus increasing adrenal production of DHEA and DHAS. A number of other explanations for the adrenarche have been suggested, none of which has been substantiated.[202, 210]

During adolescence serum concentrations of DHEA, DHAS, A, and testosterone (the latter primarily the result of peripheral conversion of androstenedione) increase with advancing breast and pubic hair stages. In the adult female 90% of circulating DHAS, 50% of DHEA and A, and 25% of testosterone are of adrenal origin; 20% of DHEA, 50% of A, and 25% of testosterone are of ovarian origin. The remainder of the circulating androgens are derived from peripheral conversion of precursors.

SHBG concentrations are high in the infant, decline during childhood, and fall slightly during adolescent development in the female (whereas in the male SHBG levels decline significantly during late childhood and adolescence).

Gonadal peptides. In addition to sex steroid hormones, the ovary produces a number of peptides involved in the regulation of hypothalamic-pituitary function as endocrine

Table 4-4. Mean serum androgen concentrations in females: birth to adulthood*

Stage of development	DHEA (ng/dL)	DHAS (µg/dL)	Androstenedione (ng/dL)	Testosterone (ng/dL)
Age				
Birth (cord)	593	134	74	
1-3 d	325	160	13	<10
1 mo	34	25		<10
6 mo	52	<10	<10	<10
1 y	91	<10	13	<10
2-6 y	<50	<10	14	<10
8 y	100	35	29	<10
10 y	125	50	49	15
12 y	400	75	68	26
14 y	400	100	133	25
Breast				
I	145	41	34	13
II	190	41	57	15
III	267	99	102	22
IV	274	87	126	21
V	325	86	118	26
Pubic hair				
I	50	30	20	<10
II	250	110	60	21
III	250	125	75	29
IV-V	600	210	120	38

*Data are from reference 202.

hormones and, in all likelihood, as paracrine (possibly even autocrine) regulatory elements of gonadal activity.[281] The inhibins are glycoprotein heterodimers of an α-subunit (molecular weight [MW] 18 kd) and two β-subunits (β-A and β-B, MW 14 kd).[260] The genes for the α-, β-A, and β-B subunits of inhibin are located on chromosomes 2q, 7, and 2p, respectively (Fig. 4-8). A primary function of inhibin is to depress the synthesis and secretion of pituitary FSH acting in concert with estrogens, although it also has inhibitory effects on GnRH-induced LH release under some circumstances and inhibitory and stimulatory effects on gonadal function as well as on extrareproductive activities (Table 4-5). In the female, inhibin is synthesized by granulosa cells and is partially under the control of FSH, which stimulates its secretion.[160] (Luteinizing hormone and hCG are also able to stimulate inhibin secretion in males, suggesting that it may be synthesized by Leydig cells as well as Sertoli cells in males.[30])

Serum immunoreactive inhibin concentrations are measurable in female infants and comparable to values recorded in the follicular phase of the menstrual cycle (but only one quarter the levels recorded in male infants) and decline to undetectable values by 1 year of age.[31] By 6 years of age serum inhibin concentrations are again measurable and increase as adolescent sexual maturation progresses (Fig. 4-9).[29] At each pubertal stage, serum levels of inhibin in males are twice those in females. There is a weak but positive correlation among serum concentrations of FSH, LH, estradiol and inhibin, and between age and inhibin

Table 4-5. Comparison of actions of inhibin and activin

Site	$\alpha\beta$-Inhibin*	Action	$\beta\beta$-Activin*
Pituitary	–	Basal FSH	+
Pituitary	–	GnRH→FSH/LH	+
Pituitary	+	GHRH→GH	–
Pituitary		Basal ACTH	–
Gonad	+	LH→Androgen	–
Gonad	–	FSH→Estrogen	+
Placenta	–	hCG→Progesterone	+
Bone marrow	–	Erythropoiesis	+
Brain		Oxytocin	+

From Vale W et al: In Sporn MB, Roberts AB, editors: *Peptide growth factors and their receptors II*, Berlin, 1990, Springer-Verlag, p 235.
*–, Inhibitory; +, stimulatory.

levels. During the menstrual cycle serum inhibin concentrations increase in the late follicular phase, peak coincident with the midcycle surge of LH and FSH, decline, and then rise still further to maximal values in the mid- to late luteal phase.[159] In adult women inhibin values correlate inversely with FSH and positively with serum estradiol and progesterone levels. Inhibin is present in the human placenta, and maternal serum concentrations of inhibin are high.[160] These observations suggest that inhibin is an important regulatory hormone for FSH (and possibly LH), as well as for gonadal steroidogenesis, but there are no data linking inhibin to the alteration in GnRH pulse frequency or amplitude involved in the onset of puberty.

Activin is a heterodimer glycoprotein composed of the

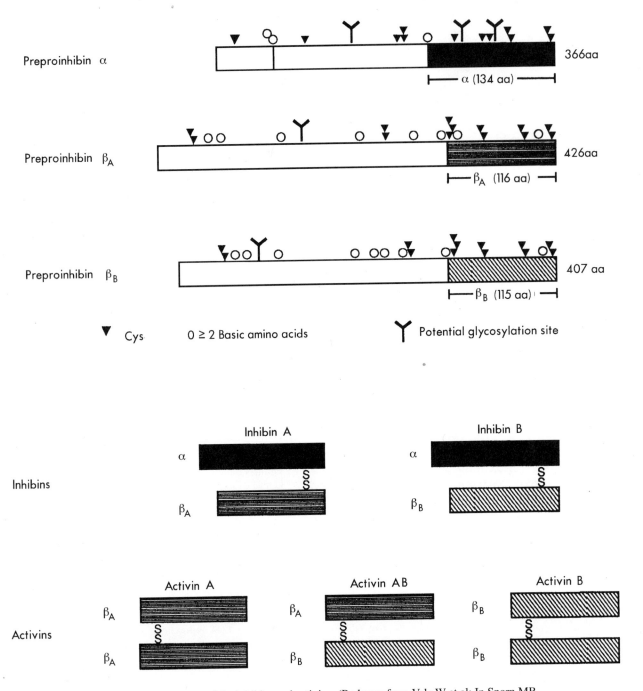

Fig. 4-8. Subunit structure of the inhibins and activins. (Redrawn from Vale W et al: In Sporn MB, Roberts AB, editors: *Peptide growth factors and their receptors II,* Heidelberg, 1990, Springer-Verlag.)

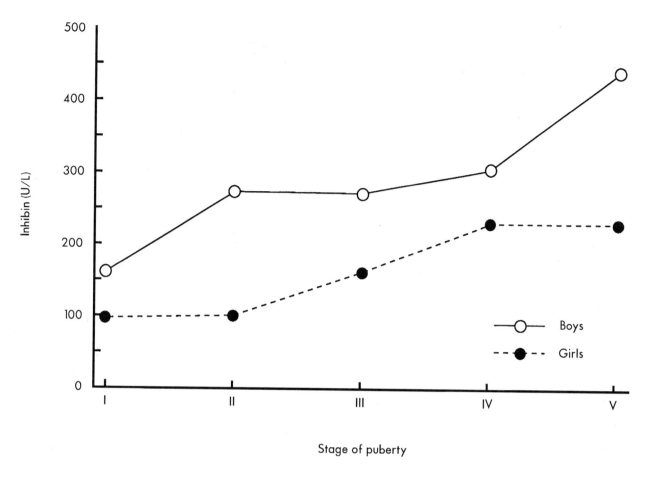

Fig. 4-9. Changes in serum concentrations of inhibin with advancing puberty in females and males. (Drawn from data in reference 28.)

same subunits as inhibin in differing combination (Fig. 4-8), but it has physiologic effects exactly opposite to those of inhibin (Table 4-5). Serum concentrations of activin have not been measured, and its role (if any) in the onset and regulation of puberty is unknown.

Inhibin and activin are structurally similar to transforming growth factor-β (TGF-β). This growth factor synergistically increases FSH-mediated aromatase activity and increases LH receptor number and thymidine incorporation; it stimulates FSH secretion from pituitary cells in culture.[160] Inhibin antagonizes these effects of TGF-β.

Müllerian inhibiting substance (MIS) is a glycoprotein that inhibits differentiation of the müllerian ducts and is secreted primarily by Sertoli cells.[162] It is also synthesized by luteinized graulosa cells, primarily under the regulation of LH/hCG. MIS is another member of the TGF-β family of growth factors. It is a homodimer of subunits of MW 57 kd. MIS inhibits oocyte meiosis, but its role in ovarian development and function is unknown at present.[38] Serum concentrations of MIS are extremely low or undetectable in infants and young girls (whereas MIS values in boys are

quite high) and increase slightly between 11 and 19 years, when male levels have fallen to female values; levels remain measurable but extremely low thereafter.[107, 115] In the female MIS is primarily important as a paracrine regulator of ovarian function. Its role in the gonadal mechanisms that lead to increased ovarian sensitivity to gonadotropin stimulation is unknown. Additional information is available in Chapter 2.

Human follistatin is a single-chain, glycosylated, 317–amino acid polypeptide found in follicular fluid that inhibits FSH release and FSH-mediated secretion of estradiol.[281] The role of this peptide in pubertal growth and development is unknown.

Melatonin. Melatonin (*N*-acetyl-5-methoxytryptamine) is an indoleamine synthesized primarily in the pineal gland from tryptophan.[194] Its secretion is entrained to the photoperiod through the retina and optic nerves; there is increased secretion during darkness, when signals from the suprachiasmatic nucleus via the superior cervical ganglion release norepinephrine in the pineal. This adrenergic neurotransmitter increases serotonin-*N*-acetyltransferase activ-

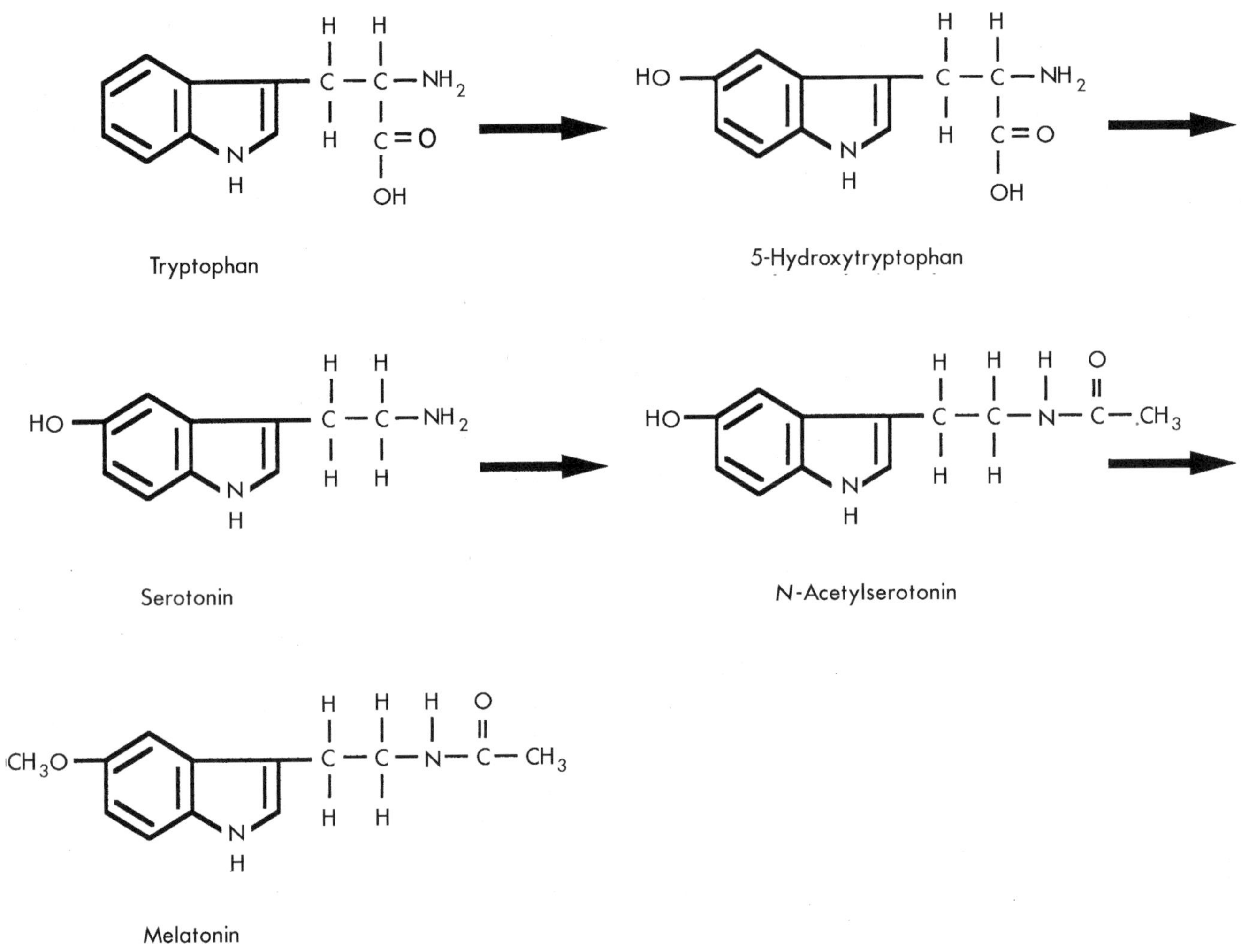

Fig. 4-10. Biosynthesis of melatonin from tryptophan in the pineal gland. (Redrawn with permission from Wurtman RJ, Axelrod J, Kelly DE: *The pineal,* New York, 1968, Academic Press, p 60.)

ity and *N*-acetyl-serotonin values. Following methylation (hydroxyindole-*O*-methyltransferase) *N*-acetyl-serotonin is converted to melatonin (Fig. 4-10). This indoleamine inhibits gonadotropin secretion by altering the frequency of pulsatile GnRH release in experimental animals and delaying maturation of the hypothalamic GnRH pulse generator; its physiologic role in humans is uncertain. Melatonin concentrations in serum and cerebrospinal fluid increase at night in prepubertal and adult subjects. Morning values of serum melatonin (<20 pg/mL) do not change with maturation. Nocturnal serum melatonin concentrations are low in infancy, increase to a peak at 1 to 3 years and then decline steadily to adult values.[265] Nocturnal concentrations fall with advancing development (prepubertal <7 years, 195 pg/mL; young adults, 49 pg/mL), and there is a negative correlation between nocturnal melatonin and LH concentrations throughout puberty.[264] The decrease in nocturnal serum concentrations of melatonin between 1 and 20 years

is inversely correlated to the increase in body weight and surface area, suggesting that increase in body size and volume of distribution may explain the change in nocturnal serum levels of melatonin. In support of this concept is the finding that 24-hour urine melatonin (6-hydroxymelatonin sulfate) excretion is similar in children, adolescents, and adults.[282] However, nocturnal urinary melatonin excretion is greater in children and adolescents than in adults, as is melatonin excretion expressed in terms of body weight, surface area, or creatinine excretion.

Although the hypothesis that declining melatonin values increase pulsatile GnRH secretion at puberty is attractive, there are no data to support this concept in humans. Pinealectomy of the infantile gonadectomized male rhesus monkey does not alter gonadotropin secretion or prevent the prepubertal fall in gonadotropin levels characteristic of this species.[182]

Other hormones. The developmental changes in the

secretion of GH, IGF-I, and insulin have been described. Fasting and posthyperglycemia serum concentrations of insulin increase twofold during adolescence, while fasting glucose levels and glucose tolerance remain normal. In young adults basal and stimulated insulin values decline but not to prepubertal values.[34, 99] The pubertal increase in insulin resistance coincides with Tanner stage II or III breast development, the peak height velocity, and the point of rising endogenous GH secretion.[99] The insulin resistance of puberty is restricted to peripheral glucose metabolism, since suppression of hepatic glucose production and substrate (branched-chain amino acids, free fatty acids, β-hydroxybutyrate) responses to insulin are not affected by adolescence.[4] Only peripheral glucose uptake is impaired during puberty. It has been suggested that the increased concentrations of insulin during puberty relate to its growth-promoting anabolic effects.[62]

There is a steady decline in serum concentrations of thyroxine (T_4) and triiodothyronine (T_3) from infancy to adulthood.[73] No change in basal thyrotropin (TSH) levels has been recorded after the neonatal period. However, Michaud et al.[161] report that there is a (prepubertal) peak in serum TSH concentrations at 9 years of age and maximal T_4 and T_3 concentrations between 10 and 11 years in iodine-sufficient Chilean boys and girls coinciding with the onset of clinical signs of puberty. There may also be increased conversion of T_4 to T_3 at this point. Whether there is any physiologic relevance of these observations in regard to the onset of pubertal development is uncertain. During puberty there is a transient increase in thyroid gland size.

Urinary free cortisol excretion increases a bit with advancing adolescence, but there is considerable individual variability.[89] When normalized for body surface area, however, there is little variability in urinary free cortisol excretion with age or pubertal development.

There is an increase in the serum concentrations of 1,25-dihydroxyvitamin D_3 (1,25$(OH)_2D_3$) during adolescence. The peak serum concentration of 1,25$(OH)_2D_3$ is achieved at 12 years in girls and coincides with PHV and endogenous secretion of GH. Growth hormone and estradiol are reported to enhance renal 25-hydroxyvitamin D-1α-hydroxylase activity, and may contribute to the rise in 1,25$(OH)_2D_3$ values, but the importance of this vitamin D metabolite to adolescent growth and maturation is unknown.[199]

Regulation of the onset of puberty

The hypothalamic-pituitary-ovarian axis begins to function in utero and remains functional thereafter at varying levels of activity. In midchildhood, "central restraint" is imposed on hypothalamic secretion of GnRH, which wanes during adolescence (Fig. 4-11). In addition, there is increased inhibitory "sensitivity" to the gonadotropin-suppressive effects of sex steroid hormone during later

infancy and childhood (Fig. 4-12). The cellular mechanisms through which central restraint of gonadotropin secretion is mediated, how it is regulated, and how it is removed are unknown. The primary consequence of central restraint is to decrease the amplitude and the frequency of endogenous GnRH pulsatile secretion in late infancy through neurotransmitter control of the GnRH–synthesizing/secreting arcuate neurons. The inhibitory neurotransmitters involved are unknown. Although opioids and dopaminergic neurotransmitters inhibit the secretion of LH in mature subjects, neither opioid or dopamine antagonists lower LH concentrations in prepubertal children.[85, 215]

As central restraint wanes, the amplitude and frequency of GnRH pulses increase, initially immediately after the onset of sleep. No brain monoamines, pineal gland secretory products, or other neurotransmitters have been identified that are definitively related to the midchildhood central restraint of GnRH secretion mediated through the posterior hypothalamus.[215] In the infantile female rhesus monkey, Wildt et al.[275] demonstrated that administration of pulses of exogenous GnRH (6 µg every hour) leads to full sexual maturation, including cyclic gonadotropin, estrogen, and progestin secretion, ovulation, and menstruation, all of which regress to the prepubertal state when the GnRH pulse is discontinued. Thus sexual development in the female primate requires the establishment of a regular pattern of GnRH secretion of sufficient magnitude and frequency to permit stimulation of gonadotropin secretion in the intact subject. This process is reversible and reproducible as evidenced by data from amenorrheic adult women with anorexia nervosa. In these subjects the 24-hour profile of LH secretion has reverted to the prepubertal pattern of low LH concentrations with little change during the 24-hour pattern; as the patient gains weight and improves psychologically, there is initially a nocturnal increase in LH secretion that progresses sequentially to the adult pattern of gonadotropin secretion. In the anorectic female before improvement, pulsatile administration of exogenous GnRH leads to increased LH secretion and patterns of LH release similar to those of the pubertal girl.[152]

The frequency of GnRH pulsation is regulated by catecholamines, opioids, and glutamate.[24, 153] α-Adrenergic input increases the frequency of GnRH release.[153] Endorphins and enkephalins (endogenous opioids) depress the amplitude and frequency of GnRH release and may be the peptide neurotransmitters through which sex steroid hormones (estrogens, androgens, progestins) exert inhibitory effects on gonadotropin secretion.[153] The major endogenous opioid-regulating LH secretion in humans is probably β-endorphin acting through µ-opiate receptors on GnRH release.[85] However, the opiate antagonists naloxone and naltrexone do not increase LH concentrations or pulse frequency during the day or night in prepubertal or early pubertal subjects, implying that central restraint and inhibiting sensitivity to sex hormones are not exercised through

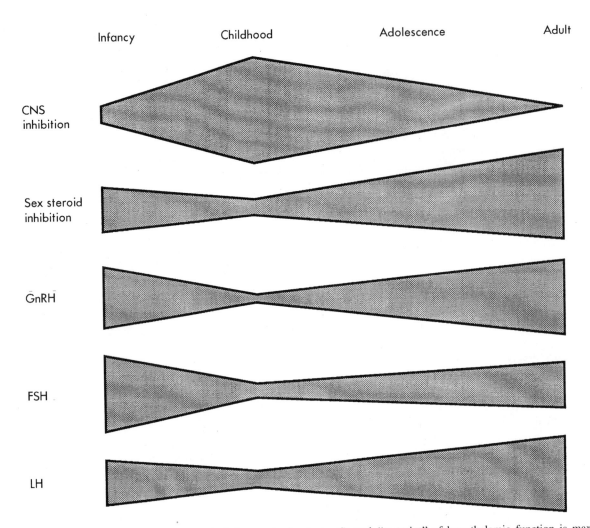

Fig. 4-11. Schematic mechanism for the control of the onset of puberty. Central "restraint" of hypothalamic function is maximal in midchildhood. Sex steroid inhibitory regulation of GnRH is present in infancy, early childhood, and adulthood. Pulsatile secretion of GnRH is depressed in midchildhood, increasing with the onset of puberty. FSH secretion is high in the infant female, declines, and increases again at puberty. LH secretion is modest in infancy, minimal in childhood, and increases significantly during adolescence.

increased release of central endogenous opioids in the prepubertal or early puberty subject. Adrenergic, Y-aminobutyric acid (GABA)ergic, and serotoninergic neurotransmitters also modulate the secretion of GnRH and LH in experimental animals, but their role in determining the onset of puberty in humans is as yet unestablished.

Agonists of the neuroexcitatory amino acids glutamate and aspartate stimulate LH release in rats and monkeys in vivo.[21,84,277] These agents act through the N-methyl-D,L-aspartate (NMDA) receptor to stimulate release of GnRH from hypothalamic neurons.[21] In male rats NMDA receptors controlling the pulsatile release of GnRH are transiently activated in the prepubertal period.[24] The ultrashort loop inhibitory feedback effect (see also Chapter 30) exerted by GnRH on its own secretion is mediated through the NMDA receptor in this species; the sensitivity of this autoinhibitory effect of GnRH is reduced in the late prepubertal period of the male rat.[22] Thus the increased frequency of GnRH pulsatility at puberty may be related, in part, to decreased ultrashort loop inhibitory feedback of GnRH mediated through the neuroexcitatory amino acids. However, the mechanism by which the change might be achieved remains enigmatic. Furthermore, the interrelationship of the neuroexcitatory amino acids and the NMDA receptor to the onset of puberty is even more complex, because inhibition of GnRH release through the NMDA receptor can also be demonstrated in the prepubertal male rat.[25] Thus the peripubertal change in this system implies yet a higher level of control. The applicability of this system to females and to puberty in the primate requires further evaluation.

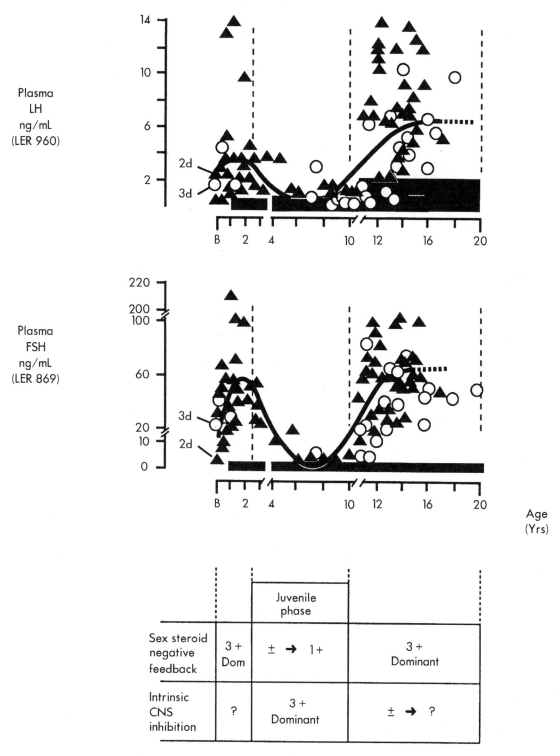

Fig. 4-12. Biphasic changes in serum concentrations of LH and FSH in girls with gonadal dysgenesis in relationship to factors regulating GnRH release during infancy, childhood, and adolescence. (Redrawn with permission from Rosenthal SM, Grumbach MM: The neuroendocrinology of puberty: recent advances. In Adashi EY, Mancuso S, editors: *Major advances in human female reproduction,* New York, 1990, Raven Press, p 27.)

Although pulsatile nocturnal secretion of LH (and GnRH) is present in prepubertal subjects, the marked increase in frequency and amplitude of GnRH/LH secretion at night shortly after the onset of sleep in the late prepubertal and early to midpubertal adolescent is noteworthy. This nocturnal increase implies that central restraint is first diminished by sleep and that whatever the mechanism of this early pubertal change in GnRH secretory pattern, it may be progressively expressed throughout the 24-hour period. The nocturnal increase in GnRH/LH secretion at this early pubertal stage might suggest transient increase in refractoriness to sex hormone–negative feedback at this point in the 24-hour period. However, since girls without ovaries (gonadal dysgenesis) demonstrate a temporal pattern of LH secretion similar to that of intact females, the role of estrogen in this nocturnal phenomenon is also questionable. The nocturnal increase in GnRH/LH release is not mediated by endogenous opioids, since naloxone is without effect on nocturnal LH secretion at this developmental stage. Another nocturnal event perhaps related to increased nocturnal GnRH/LH secretion might involve GH, whose release also increases shortly after sleep onset. As previously recorded, GH decreases the age of onset of pubertal development and accelerates the rate of sexual maturation in girls with isolated GH deficiency. However, the fact that puberty occurs in girls with isolated GH deficiency argues against somatotropin as a primary influence on GnRH secretion. Neither prolactin nor melatonin, both of which are secreted during sleep, seems to be of primary importance in maturation of the reproductive endocrine system in man. The pituitary adrenocortical axis is functional at night; corticotropin-releasing hormone (CRH) inhibits GnRH release, and cortisol suppresses GnRH-stimulated gonadotropin secretion.[212] However, no pubertal changes in the activity of this unit have been documented. A delta sleep–inducing peptide stimulates LH secretion in rodents.[111] Its role in human maturation is unknown.

Once initiated, the increase in amplitude and frequency of GnRH release stimulates the secretion of both LH and FSH. In addition to stimulating gonadotropin secretion, GnRH also enhances the synthesis of LH by increasing transcription of the genes for both of its subunits and by increasing release of isoforms with enhanced biologic activity.[13,153] In females, in addition to momentary episodic and circadian fluctuation, gonadotropin secretion also varies monthly even in prepubertal girls, suggesting inherent, primary rhythmicity in the GnRH-gonadotropin system.

Sex hormones exert inhibitory and stimulatory effects on LH and FSH secretion; the inhibitory effect of sex hormones on GnRH release begins to develop in the latter half of the midtrimester of gestation and matures during infancy and childhood, when maximal inhibitory sensitivity is present[190]; with onset of puberty, inhibitory sensitivity to sex hormones declines. Waning sensitivity to sex hormone–induced suppression of GnRH/LH release is probably a phenomenon secondary to a basic higher CNS mechanism that regulates GnRH synthesis and release. In late adolescence, females develop a positive gonadotropin-releasing feedback response to estrogen, an important trigger for the midcycle surge of LH and FSH release. Positive feedback of estrogen requires increasing levels of estradiol to values above 200 pg/mL, increased pituitary sensitivity to GnRH (i.e., increase in GnRH receptor number or intracellular response mechanisms), and sufficient GnRH and LH stores to enhance LH release.[190]

The effects of GnRH on gonadotropin synthesis and secretion are modified by the sex hormone milieu; estradiol can both inhibit the secretion of GnRH and LH and enhance the LH secretory response to GnRH, as well as trigger the positive feedback effect. Progesterone increases the LH secretory response to GnRH after preexposure to estrogen, but decreases GnRH pulse frequency. Estrogens inhibit FSH secretion, perhaps in association with gonadal inhibin. Activin has been identified in the pituitary gland and may exert a paracrine stimulatory effect on FSH secretion.[149] In the prepubertal period, FSH induces its own receptors and those of LH and stimulates the growth of ovarian stroma and follicular development by enhancing division of granulosa cells.[13] Nevertheless, FSH increases ovarian aromatase activity only slightly in the prepubertal ovary, thus leading to follicular atresia and loss of oocyte number, but this gonadotropin is essential for maintenance of the prepubertal ovary, and by induction of LH receptors "prepares" the ovary for pubertal stimulation by LH.[13]

With greater frequency and amplitude of GnRH/LH pulsations, increased ovarian androgen production leads to greater estrogen secretion, resulting in breast and uterine growth and feedback inhibition of gonadotropin secretion, perhaps in concert with inhibin and activin. The increasing sensitivity of the ovary to the actions of the gonadotropins that occurs during puberty may be mediated not only by the gonadotropins themselves, but also in part by the IGF-I axis, which amplifies the effects of LH and FSH.[2] As puberty progresses, ovarian size increases; there is increased follicular growth and coordinated, sequential secretion of androgens and estrogens and ultimately cyclic pituitary-ovarian function, ovulation, and corpus luteum formation and progestin secretion. The intense, short-lived midcycle increase in biopotency of both LH and FSH induces changes in a dominant ovarian follicle leading to ovulation. Beitins and Padmanabhan[13] suggest that the various gonadotropin isoforms secreted during adolescence and the menstrual cycle have differing physiologic functions: the acidic, longer half-lived, less biopotent isoforms of FSH stimulate growth and maintain ovarian function, while the more basic, shorter half-lived, more biopotent isoforms of FSH are necessary for rapidly occurring events such as ovulation.

To summarize, in girls puberty is characterized by the following:

1. Increase in GnRH pulse frequency and amplitude, leading to
2. A self-priming effect of GnRH on the gonadotrope, and
3. Increase in LH pulse frequency, amplitude, and biopotency, and to
4. Modest increase in I-FSH secretion but no change in FSH biopotency, resulting in
5. Enhanced ovarian "sensitivity" to gonadotropins (perhaps aided by GH/IGF-I), to increased secretion of endogenous estrogen, and to
6. Ovarian follicle development, leading to ovulation and corpus luteum formation,
7. Progesterone secretion, which decreases GnRH pulse frequency, and
8. Reinforcement of the inherent, feminine, cyclic pattern of gonadotropin secretion.

This sequence is accompanied by a decline in the inhibitory sensitivity of the hypothalamic-pituitary unit to sex hormones and by development of a positive feedback effect of estradiol, which triggers the midcycle surge of gonadotropin secretion.

DELAYED ADOLESCENCE

Adolescence is delayed in the female if (1) no signs of secondary sexual development have appeared by 13 years of age (+2 SD [1 SD $\cong$ 1 year] above the mean ages of thelarche and pubarche) or (2) if menarche has not occurred within 4 years after thelarche.[233] Since pubarche and thelarche can be dissociated (as in girls with gonadal dysgenesis or hypogonadotropism), absence of thelarche (evidence of gonadarche) by 13 years or its failure to occur within 6 to 12 months after pubarche (except in girls with premature adrenarche) should also prompt inquiry. Causes of delayed adolescence in the female are listed in the box. In a series of 326 females evaluated between 11 and 27 years of age for delayed adolescence in a reproductive

---

Causes of delayed adolescence

I. Constitutional delay in growth and sexual development

II. Nutritional disorders

  A. Deprivation
    1. Anorexia nervosa
    2. Refusal to thrive
    3. Fear of obesity
    4. Zinc deficiency
    5. Hypothalamic tumor

  B. Obesity

III. Hypogonadotropic hypogonadism

  A. Hypothalamic dysfunction
    1. Idiopathic deficiency of GnRH
      a. Isolated
      b. Familial
        (1) with anosmia (Kallmann syndrome)
      c. With other pituitary deficits
    2. Insult to CNS
      a. Congenital anomaly
        (1) Prader-Willi syndrome
      b. Trauma
      c. Irradiation
      d. Infections
      e. Neoplasm
    3. Functional
      a. Systemic disease
      b. Stress
        (1) psychogenic
      c. Athletics

  B. Pituitary dysfunction
    1. Congenital anomaly
      a. Empty sella turcica
    2. Deficiency of gonadotropes

    3. Trauma
    4. Vascular insult
    5. Neoplasm
      a. Prolactinoma

IV. Hypergonadotropic hypogonadism
  A. Gonadal dysgenesis
    1. Chromosomal anomaly
    2. Normal chromosomes
  B. Trauma/surgery
  C. Autoimmune oophoritis
  D. Infections
  E. Irradiation
  F. Chemotherapy
  G. Galactosemia
  H. Gonadotropin resistance
  I. 17α-Hydroxylase deficiency

V. Hyperandrogenism
  A. Polycystic ovary syndrome
    1. Primary
    2. Secondary
      a. Nonclassic congenital adrenal hyperplasia
      b. 17-Ketoreductase deficiency
      c. Cushing's syndrome
      d. Hyperprolactinemia
      e. Hypersomatotropism
      f. Insulin resistance disorders

VI. Other disorders
  A. Müllerian duct agenesis (Mayer-Rokitansky-Küster-Hauser syndrome)
  B. Complete androgen insensitivity syndrome
  C. Transverse vaginal septum
  D. Imperforate hymen

Table 4-6. Causes of delayed adolescence in 326 females evaluated in a reproductive endocrinology clinic*

Cause	No.	%
Constitutional delay in growth and sexual development	32	10
Nutritional disorders	9	3
Hypogonadotropic hypogonadism	37	13
Hypothalamic ($n = 35$)		
Pituitary ($n = 2$)		
Systemic disease	16	5
Hyperprolactinemia	5	<2
Hypergonadotropic hypogonadism	141	43
Gonadal dysgenesis	(136)	(42)
Abnormal chromosomes ($n = 84$)		
Normal chromosomes ($n = 52$)		
Irradiation to ovaries ($n = 3$)		
Infection ($n = 2$)		
Anatomic malformation	58	18
Müllerian duct agenesis ($n = 45$)		
Other ($n = 13$)		
Hyperandrogenism	22	7
Androgen insensitivity	4	<2
Other	2	<2

*Data are from reference 188.

Table 4-7. Causes of delayed adolescence in 53 females evaluated in a pediatric endocrinology clinic*

Cause	No.	%
Constitutional delay in growth and sexual development	14	26
Nutritional disorders	2	4
Hypogonadotropic hypogonadism	19	36
Hypothalamic ($n = 18$)		
Pituitary ($n = 1$)		
Systemic disease	6	6
Hypergonadotropic hypogonadism	10	19
Gonadal dysgenesis ($n = 8$)		(15)
Other ($n = 2$)		
Anatomic malformation	2	4

*Data are from reference 126.

endocrinology clinic, 43% of patients were found to have ovarian failure, most commonly due to a chromosome anomaly (Table 4-6).[188] Ten percent of girls had constitutional delay in growth and sexual development (vide infra). In a subset of 290 females with pubertal amenorrhea, 265 had primary amenorrhea and 25 had secondary amenorrhea.[189] Forty-nine percent of girls with primary amenorrhea had primary ovarian failure (gonadal dysgenesis), 28% of patients with primary amenorrhea were hypogonadotropic, 16% had müllerian duct aplasia, and 6% were hyperandrogenic; 48% of subjects with secondary amenorrhea were hypergonadotropic, 32% hyperandrogenic and 12% hypogonadotropic. Of 53 girls with delayed adolescence evaluated by Krainz et al.[126] in a pediatric endocrine clinic, 14 (26%) had constitutional delay in growth and sexual development, 19 (36%) were hypogonadotropic, and 8 (15%) had gonadal dysgenesis (Table 4-7). In general, in pediatric endocrine clinics, females account for 15% to 25% of children found to have constitutional delay in growth and sexual development.[129]

Constitutional delay in growth and sexual development

Constitutional delay in growth and sexual development (CDGD) is an alteration in the timing and tempo of growth and sexual maturation and does not represent a significant pathologic disorder. In 30% of girls with CDGD this pattern of growth and development is familial.[129] Although it is brought to the physician's attention more frequently in boys, CDGD occurs with probably equal frequency in girls as well, but is better tolerated because of somewhat fewer psychosocial stresses in girls unless the pattern becomes extreme. A typical course of such a girl is depicted in Fig. 4-13.

CDGD in the female is characterized by the following[129, 209]:

1. Birth length and weight are normal.
2. Deceleration of linear growth rate occurs between 6 and 24 months of age, such that length falls to or below the 3rd percentile.[105]
3. Thereafter a normal linear growth velocity maintains height in a channel that is parallel to or slightly below the 3rd percentile (but seldom more than -3 SD below mean height for age) until onset of adolescent development.
4. Onset of puberty occurs before 16 years of age.
5. Bone age for height and onset of pubertal development (10 to 11 years) are appropriate.
6. Deceleration of linear growth rate occurs before initiation of the pubertal growth spurt.
7. Normal sequential pubertal development occurs once the process is initiated.
8. Prepubertal followed by normal pubertal hormonal secretion occurs once adolescence begins. (In patients with CDGD pubarche is delayed as well as gonadarche, and DHAS concentrations are appropriate for bone age.)
9. Function of the reproductive endocrine system is normal as an adult.
10. There is absence of any serious chronic systemic, genetic, or endocrinologic nutritional or psychologic disorder.

LaFranchi et al.[129] followed 13 females with CDGD to adult stature (20.5 years) and recorded a mean adult height of 156 cm (-1.3 SD below the mean adult height for females) and 5.3 cm below the estimated target height calculated from midparental heights; achieved heights approximated the predicted heights (Bayley-Pinneau method). In another series of 32 girls with CDGD, mean adult height was 157.8 cm, also within the lower half of the adult height range but much closer to the target height (-0.65 SD).[27] These observations suggest that girls with CDGD do not

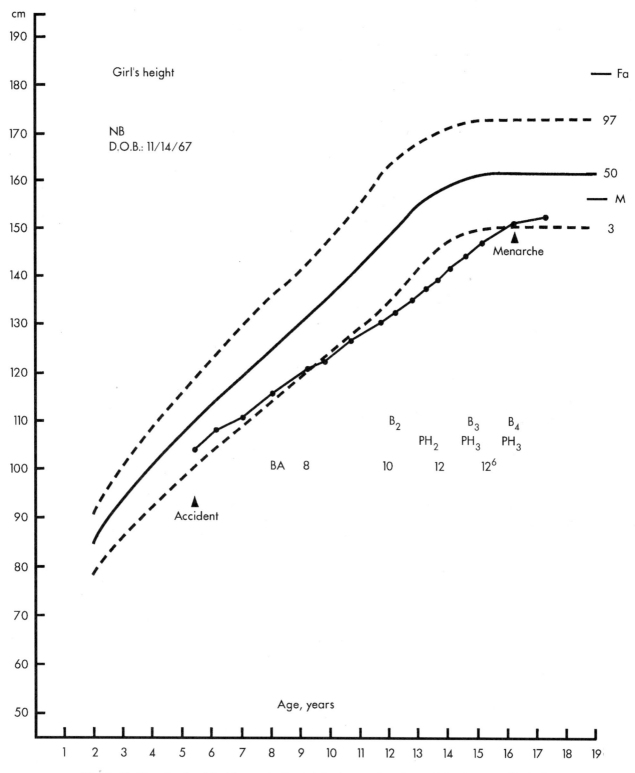

Fig. 4-13. Growth of a girl with constitutional delay in growth and sexual development. She had sustained a mild head injury in an automobile accident as a child, which had no influence on her patterns of growth and sexual maturation. *B*, Tanner breast stage; *PH*, Tanner pubic hair stage; *BA*, bone age.

achieve an average adult height but may also reflect the severity of the growth retardation of these subjects that prompted referral to pediatric endocrine centers. It has been suggested that children with CDGD may have subnormal secretion of GH, and there may be a small subset of children who do, but in the majority of subjects with CDGD who reach their predicted heights, a significant GH-deficient state is unlikely.[129]

Nutritional disorders

In the prepubertal child with anorexia nervosa (AN), absence of weight gain and deceleration of linear growth are the primary manifestations. In the peripubertal girl AN may also present with arrest of linear growth and weight gain and failure of initiation or progression of adolescent development. In the pubertal girl, AN is manifested by weight loss, slowing of linear growth, and arrest of or regression of sexual development; in the postmenarcheal female with AN, secondary amenorrhea may precede weight loss and persist after recovery of weight.[198] In the early pubertal girl who develops AN, estrogen secretion may cause advancement of epiphyseal maturation in the absence of cartilage proliferation, resulting in severe compromise of adult stature.[204]

In patients with AN the primary reproductive abnormality is at the hypothalamic level with decreased endogenous GnRH release and consequent hypogonadotropism. Administration of pulsatile doses of GnRH stimulates LH secretion, and improvement in the disorder leads to sequential restoration of hypothalamic-pituitary-ovarian function in a pattern ontogenously similar to that of normal puberty.[153] The primary hypothalamic abnormality in females with AN is unknown but may relate to aberrations of (opiatergic, adrenergic) neurotransmitter control of the GnRH-secreting neuron. In patients with AN there is altered activity of the hypothalamic-pituitary-adrenal axis with increased serum cortisol concentrations. This is due in part to the decreased catabolism of cortisol secondary to the functional hypometabolic state of malnutrition (decreased T_3 concentrations) and to stress-induced release of hypothalamic CRH.[212] This hypothalamic peptide stimulates increased secretion of ACTH and β-endorphin (from proopiomelanocortin). Both β-endorphin and cortisol, as well as CRH itself, contribute to the hypogonadotropic state. Endogenous opioids and CRH depress GnRH release, whereas cortisol inhibits the LH secretory response to GnRH.[212] The pathophysiology of AN is distinct from that of simple weight loss, in which the menstrual pattern follows closely the pattern of weight loss or gain.[262]

Many children and adolescents with CDGD are a bit underweight (usually <15% below ideal body weight for size), and increase in caloric intake and weight gain improves their rates of linear growth and sexual maturation. In some subjects with "primary" anorexia noted since early childhood, weight has been substantially decreased (>20% below ideal body weight for size) since late infancy, and this is accompanied by slow rates of growth and delayed sexual maturation. Children with "refusal to thrive" (Fig. 4-14) are characterized by (1) decreased caloric intake since early childhood or even infancy; (2) generally good health with no identifiable systemic or endocrinologic disorder, specific nutritional deficiency, "fear of obesity," or psychopathology consistent with anorexia nervosa; and (3) continued linear growth, normal but delayed adolescence, and an adult height consistent with their genetic potential.

Delayed adolescence is also recorded in subjects who diet voluntarily because of "fear of obesity" and in those with severe zinc deficiency.[140, 220] Zinc deficiency of this magnitude is unusual in the experience of this writer, but it can be encountered in patients with chronic inflammatory bowel disease (due to malabsorption of zinc) and in patients with sickle cell disease (due to hyperzincuria).

Women athletes may have delayed puberty or secondary amenorrhea due to or associated with decreased body fat content as discussed earlier under "Body Composition." In these athletes elevated β-endorphin and cortisol secretion perhaps contributes to the hypogonadotropic state.[212]

Obesity in females is usually associated with early adolescence and somewhat earlier menarche (approximately 12.4 years) than in girls of average weight, but when morbid obesity is present amenorrhea may occur. This may be due to increased production of estrone from adrenal androstenedione by fat (which has aromatase activity) and inhibition of GnRH secretion and/or of GnRH action on the gonadotrope. In other females obesity accompanies the hyperandrogenic state.

Hypogonadotropic hypogonadism

Hypothalamic or pituitary lesions may cause decrease in secretion of gonadotropins (Table 4-6). Congenital isolated deficiency of GnRH may occur as a sporadic or familial disorder; when familial, it may be transmitted as an autosomal dominant or autosomal recessive characteristic[188]; isolated GnRH deficiency has been found in association with progressive cerebellar ataxia and/or cerebellar hypoplasia.[1] The structure of the gene for GnRH has been normal in patients with isolated GnRH deficiency studied to date.[169,268] In the majority of subjects with the Prader-Willi syndrome of hypotonia, hypomentia, hypogonadism, and obesity, deletion of the (paternal) 15q11-13 segment is present.[63] These patients have isolated deficiency of GnRH and a form of hypothalamic obesity presumably associated with dysfunction of the ventromedial nucleus.[1] Because of the embryologic origin of GnRH-secreting neurons from the olfactory cortex,[224] deficiency of GnRH and disorders of olfaction (hyposmia, anosmia) are often associated (Kallmann syndrome) as a sporadic or familial (autosomal recessive) disorder.

Congenital deficiency of GnRH may be idiopathic or

Patient 13 D.O.B 10/ 6/ 68

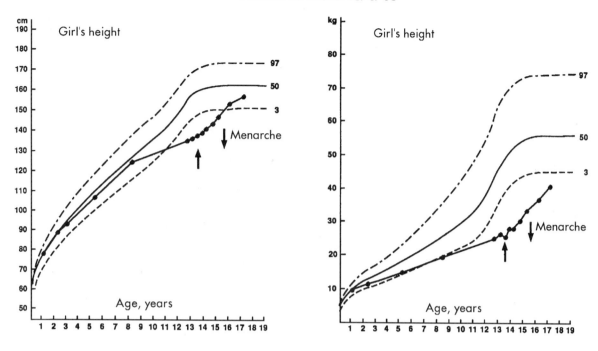

Patient 14 D.O.B. 1/ 24/ 69

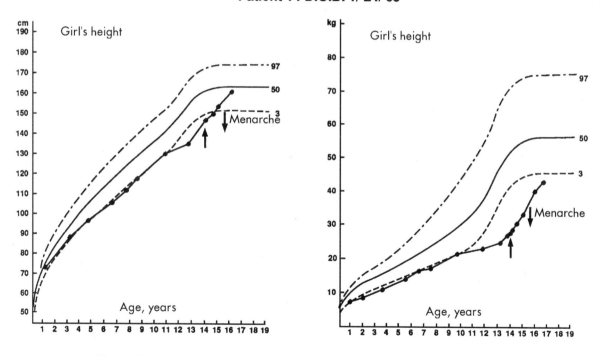

Fig. 4-14. Growth and maturational patterns of two girls with "refusal to thrive."

may occur in patients with congenital malformations of the CNS, particularly those involving midline cranial structure (holoprosencephaly, absence of the corpus callosum, septooptic dysplasia, anophthalmia, transection of the pituitary stalk with hypoplasia of the anterior pituitary, and an "ectopic" neurohypophysis). Hypothalamic hypopituitarism may be secondary to birth trauma, particularly in breech deliveries, or may be acquired as a result of trauma; irradiation; inflammatory or infiltrative disorders; or neoplasms involving the hypothalamus, pituitary stalk (craniopharyngioma), or contiguous structures (optic nerves or chiasm). Isolated deficiency of GnRH was present in 23 of 326 patients (7%) with delayed adolescence evaluated in a reproductive endocrine unit[188] and in 2 of 53 females (4%) investigated in a pediatric endocrine clinic,[126] and is thus rather uncommon. More frequently GnRH deficiency is one of a complex of hypothalamic neurohormonal defects often involving GHRH, CRH, and thyrotropin-releasing hormone (TRH) in a variety of combinations leading to the hypopituitary state with variable anterior pituitary hypofunction. Primary congenital or acquired abnormalities of the pituitary may be associated with defective gonadotropin secretion as an isolated occurrence (aplasia of the gonadotropes) or as part of a multihormonal deficiency state. Isolated deficiency of GH or peripheral insensitivity to somatotropin due to a receptor defect (Laron syndrome) is associated with delayed adolescence; in these patients puberty begins at an appropriate bone age and progresses normally to full reproductive capability. Secondary sexual characteristics such as breast development may be less prominent, since GH appears to synergize with sex steroid hormone action on peripheral tissues.[232]

Pituitary adenomas, particularly GH-secreting neoplasms, may destroy the gonadotropes, whereas pituitary ACTH and prolactin-secreting adenomas impair pituitary gonadotropin secretion. Hypercortisolemia of Cushing syndrome inhibits GnRH-stimulated secretion of LH, whereas β-endorphin depresses GnRH release in a manner analogous to that which occurs in states of high stress (malnutrition, athletic activity, depression, anxiety, other forms of psychogenic hypothalamic amenorrhea). The abnormality is reversible with neurosurgical removal of the ACTH-secreting adenoma (or successful irradiation or chemotherapy).

Hyperprolactinemia may be associated with functional hypogonadotropism in the presence of a microadenoma (<10 mm in diameter) or in subjects with a functional defect due to ingestion of a psychoactive drug (such as chlorpromazine or a similar agent). Hyperprolactinemia inhibits GnRH release, perhaps due to a compensatory increase in dopamine turnover. Administration of GnRH to hyperprolactinemic subjects stimulates normal or exaggerated LH secretory responses.[9,106] Prolactin-secreting macroadenomas may lead to direct interference with gonadotrope function. Howlett et al.[106] reported 10 females (16 to 25 years of age) with hyperprolactinemia, all of whom had

normal onset of breast and pubic hair growth but had either primary ($n = 8$) or secondary ($n = 2$) amenorrhea 4 to 9 years after pubertal onset; the latter subjects each had one menstrual period at 20 and 22 years, respectively. Eight patients had galactorrhea of variable degree (trace to spontaneous); two had microadenomas and eight had macroadenomas with suprasellar or lateral extension in seven subjects. Badawy et al.[9] studied nine hyperprolactinemic females (18 to 27 years of age), all of whom had normal thelarche and pubarche; four had primary amenorrhea and five had oligomenorrhea. One of the latter had galactorrhea. There was no relationship between size of the adenoma and amenorrhea, although patients with primary amenorrhea had eightfold higher prolactin values than did those with oligomenorrhea (995 vs. 128 ng/mL, respectively). Thus in adolescent females with hyperprolactinemia, the onset of puberty is usually normal, but development fails to progress normally or to be sustained; galactorrhea may not be prominent. In the majority of subjects (80%) treated with a dopamine agonist, prolactin concentrations fall (often to the normal range), tumor size decreases, menses occur or resume, and fertility is achieved if desired.

Chronic systemic disease can impede adolescent development. Severe anemia (sickle cell disease, thalassemia); heart disease; respiratory insufficiency (cystic fibrosis); compromise of renal, hepatobiliary, or gastrointestinal (chronic inflammatory bowel disease, gluten-sensitive enteropathy) function; and metabolic (diabetes mellitus) and hormonal disorders (hypothyroidism, hyposomatotropism) are often associated with delayed adolescence.[95,126] In such patients irregular or depressed hypothalamic secretion of GnRH is the primary cause of the hypogonadal state.[191] In pubertal aged patients with chronic renal disease, gonadal steroid levels are low; gonadotropin values may be normal, slightly elevated, or low, but the response to GnRH is blunted or delayed.[221] The mechanism(s) by which pulsatile GnRH release is altered or depressed in these girls is unknown, but may be related to nutritional deprivation; altered metabolic substrates or metabolites; abnormal acid-base balance; hypoxemia; or stress-induced secretion of CRH, cortisol, and β-endorphin, which inhibit gonadotropin secretion. Cure or successful treatment of these diseases leads to restoration of pubertal development; in the majority of disorders adolescent sexual maturation will ensue even in the continued presence of the underlying disease, albeit at an older age. Although sexual maturation occurs in these patients, the adolescent growth spurt often is attenuated, and adult stature frequently is compromised. Psychogenic factors acting through stress-related mechanisms may also be associated with delayed or arrested adolescent development and amenorrhea.

Hypergonadotropic hypogonadism

Primary ovarian failure may be due to congenital or acquired abnormalities of gonadal function. Gonadal dysgenesis (Turner syndrome) associated with an abnormality

Table 4-8. Clinical characteristics of girls with gonadal dysgenesis and an abnormality of the X chromosomes*

Characteristic	%
Growth retardation	100
Face	
Epicanthal folds	
Posteriorly rotated ears	
Micrognathia	60
Highly arched palate	35
Strabismus	17
Ptosis	10
Neck	
Short	40
Low posterior hairline	40
Pterygium coli (webbed)	23
Trunk	
Abnormal upper-lower ratio	90
Shield chest	
Pectus excavatum	
Scoliosis	12
Extremities	
Cubitus valgus	45
Brachymetacarpals/tarsals	35
Genu valgum	30
Edema of hands/feet	21
Dysplastic nails	12
Madelung's deformity	7
Cardiovascular disorders	
Bicuspid aortic valve	33
Coarctation of aorta	10
Mitral valve prolapse	9
Hypertension without coarctation	7
Aortic dissection	
Renal disorders	
Duplication of collecting system	33
Horseshoe kidney	
Ectopic kidney	
Renal agenesis	
Renal vascular anomaly	
Gastrointestinal disorders	
Telangiectasia	
Lymphangiectasia	
Inflammatory bowel disease	
Cognition/personality	
Deficiency in	
Spatiotemporal processing	
Perceptual stability	
Visual-motor coordination	
Motor learning	
Feminine personality	
Social immaturity	
Associated disorders	
Hypergonadotropic hypogonadism	94
Autoimmune thyroid disease	43
Carbohydrate intolerance	40
Diabetes mellitus	
Hyposomatotropism	
Gonadoblastoma (with Y)	
Multiple skin nevi	25

*Data are from references 96 and 145.

of X chromosome number or structure (isochromosome, deletion of all or part of the long or short arm) is the most common form of primary ovarian failure encountered in the pediatric endocrine clinic (Table 4-8). Many of these girls are identified before the adolescent period when referred for growth retardation or somatic characteristics typical of such children (Table 4-8). Among 53 girls evaluated for delayed adolescence by Krainz et al.,[126] only 8 (15%) had gonadal dysgenesis; since this pediatric endocrine unit cares for 70 girls with this disorder, the majority (89%) presented other chief complaints. In another pediatric endocrine unit, 35% of 165 subjects with gonadal dysgenesis were referred for evaluation of delayed puberty.[145] In the report by Reindollar et al.,[188] 84 of 326 girls (26%) with delayed puberty evaluated in their reproductive endocrine unit had gonadal dysgenesis associated with an abnormality of the X chromosome: 33% had the sex chromosome karyotype 45,X and 10% were 45,X/46,XX; in 26% an X isochromosome was present; 19% had a Y chromosome in the karyotype (and thus were at risk for development of gonadoblastoma); sex chromosome mosaicism was found in 56% of these patients (Table 4-9). Among 165 patients with gonadal dysgenesis followed by Lippe[145] in a pediatric endocrine clinic, 50% had 45,X, 16% had an X isochromosome, 6% had a Y chromosome or fragment, and 28% had sex chromosome mosaicism. Gonadal dysgenesis also occurs in patients with the 46,XX and 46,XY karyotypes; these karyotypes were present in 48 of 326 (15%) and 9 of 326 (3%) females, respectively, with delayed adolescence reported by Reindollar et al.[188] In this series 40% (57 of 141) of patients with gonadal dysgenesis had a normal karyotype and 60% had an anomaly of the X chromosome. No such patients were observed by Lippe.[145]

Gonadal dysgenesis occurs in 1 in 2000 to 1 in 5000 liveborn girls; an abnormality of the X chromosome is the most common chromosome defect in spontaneously aborted fetuses, and more than 90% of conceptuses with such an anomaly are aborted.[96] In the newborn period peripheral edema and webbing of the neck suggest the presence of gonadal dysgenesis but can also be seen in

Table 4-9. Chromosomal anomalies in patients with gonadal dysgenesis*

Karyotype†	Ref 188 (N = 141)		Ref 145 (N = 165)	
45,X	28	(19.9%)	95	(57.6%)
46,XXqi	11	(15.6%)	27	(16.4%)
45,X/46,XX	8	(5.7%)	15	(9.1%)
45,X/46,XY	16	(11.3%)	10	(6.0%)
46,XXr	3	(2.1%)	8	(4.8%)
46,XXq− or p−	5	(3.5%)	8	(4.8%)
45,X/47,XXX	1	(0.7%)	2	(1.2%)
46,XX	48	(34.0%)	None	
46,XY	9	(6.4%)	None	

*Data are from references 145 and 188.
†q, Long arm; p, short arm; i, isochromosome; r, ring; −, deletion.

infants with the pseudo–Turner syndrome of Noonan, as well as in other disorders; in childhood, growth retardation and somatic characteristics (Table 4-8) focus attention on the diagnosis, and failure of adolescent development may occasionally bring this child to medical attention in the second decade of life. It should be appreciated that the somatic characteristics of gonadal dysgenesis are expressed variably, even in girls with the 45,X karyotype, and often far less so in patients with X chromosome mosaicism or structural abnormalities. Fisher et al.[74] have isolated X- and Y-associated genes that encode isoforms of ribosomal protein S4. On the X chromosome this gene is located near the X-inactivation site. The authors suggest that insufficiency of gene product may be involved in the development of the physical characteristics of Turner syndrome. Because the rates of oocyte degeneration and the failure of ovarian function are variable, many girls with (45,X) gonadal dysgenesis will develop thelarche, and some (6%)[145] experience menarche but usually then develop secondary amenorrhea. In the series of girls with pubertal amenorrhea reported by Reindollar et al.,[189] 5 of 84 subjects (6%) with an X chromosome anomaly and 7 of 41 patients (17%) with 46,XX gonadal dysgenesis had secondary amenorrhea. Indeed, 14 patients with the 45,X karyotype have conceived 22 times and delivered 14 liveborn offspring.[96] Forty-nine women with mosaic Turner syndrome have conceived 117 times and delivered 69 live infants. Serum concentrations of LH and FSH (particularly) are greatly increased in the neonate and infant with gonadal dysgenesis, as is the gonadotropin secretory response to GnRH. Serum levels of LH and FSH decline in midchildhood, as does GnRH-provoked secretion of the gonadotropins (see Fig. 4-12). At 10 to 12 years gonadotropin concentrations increase (FSH before LH) into the castrate range.[46]

The cause of the short stature in patients with gonadal dysgenesis is unknown. Although there are some data that suggest that such children may have a subtle primary osteodystrophy, Rimoin and co-workers state that "The skeletal defects [are] not ... sufficiently severe ... to account for their short stature."[147] These workers believe that:

Growth retardation in Turner syndrome is of multifactorial causation involving the nonspecific growth retardation of aneuploidy, ovarian dysgenesis with lack of gonadal steroid stimulation of childhood and pubertal growth, the lack of gonadal steroid-induced hGH and somatomedin during puberty, and a variety of lymphatic and vascular malformations in utero....[147]

Pelvic irradiation and chemotherapy are becoming increasingly more common causes of primary ovarian failure as the number of children surviving neoplasia and its treatment expands. Irradiation of the pelvis directly injures the ovary. Chemotherapy has adverse effects on ovarian morphology, diminishing primordial follicles and decreasing follicular growth in prepubertal girls and increasing

stromal hyalinization and follicular destruction in older subjects.[8] Nevertheless, in the majority of girls less than 17 years of age receiving chemotherapy for neoplasia or nephrosis, ovarian function is not impaired, at least in the short term. Long-term consequences of such therapy in childhood and puberty are unknown.[8]

Bilateral gonadectomy of prepubertal girls is uncommon but has occurred as a consequence of trauma or bilateral ovarian torsion, sometimes associated with ovarian cysts that may occur in hypothyroid prepubertal girls.[143] Gonadectomy of the male pseudohemaphrodite reared as a female in childhood leads to hypergonadotropic hypogonadism, which requires treatment. In the girl with galactosemia, ovarian failure may occur because galactose is toxic to the ovary.[122] Antibodies to ovarian steroid cells may result in ovarian dysfunction and failure, usually as part of a complex of autoimmune polyendocrinopathies.[3] Rarely, viral oophoritis will lead to bilateral ovarian dysfunction. Resistance to gonadotropin action may occur primarily or sometimes in association with antibodies to the FSH receptor, or in patients with pseudohypoparathyroidism type IA.[37]

Hyperandrogenism

Hyperandrogenism—whether of adrenal, ovarian, or exogenous origin—leads to ovarian follicular atresia and disruption of the normal feedback interrelationships of the hypothalamic-pituitary-ovarian unit.[210] Testosterone, after conversion to dihydrotestosterone by 5α-reductase at target sites, causes the prepubertal pilosebaceous vellus follicle to differentiate into a terminal sexual hair follicle or into a sebaceous gland.[210] Hyperandrogenism is frequently associated with hirsutism and acne; hirsutism is an excessive male pattern of hair growth.

In the polycystic ovary (PCO) syndrome there are frequently multiple small subcapsular ovarian cysts with increased medullary stroma, but the ovary may also be histologically and ultrasonographically normal with all intermediate gradations of architectural abnormalities. Clinically, the PCO syndrome is characterized by obesity, hirsutism, and amenorrhea, but many hyperandrogenic adolescent females do not have this phenotype. Rosenfield[210] suggests that PCO syndrome is a gonadotropin-dependent disorder arising as the result of intrinsic dysregulation of the P-450c17α enzyme (with both 17α-hydroxylase and 17,20-lyase activities), leading to increased ovarian androgen production and disruption of normal ovarian androgen-estrogen relationships.

The PCO syndrome is often associated with insulin resistance and significant hyperinsulinism. Since insulin acts synergistically with FSH to stimulate granulosa cell growth and function, inhibition of insulin activity may depress granulosa cell function. Secondarily, insulin, perhaps acting through normal or hybrid receptors for IGF-I, may also lead to increased theca cell synthesis of androgens through enhanced sensitivity to LH and up-regulation of LH receptors.[64,184,212] Insulin also decreases SHBG synthesis, leading to an increase in free (bioactive) androgen levels. However, PCO syndrome is the final common pathway that also follows functional abnormalities in other components of the reproductive system; thus, a primary increase in LH secretion due to dysfunction of the hypothalamus with increased frequency of GnRH release may lead to increased LH and decreased FSH production, favoring ovarian androgen production. Increased androgen production by the adrenal gland or increased androgen ingestion may result in the PCO syndrome, as well as may the excessive production of prolactin or of IGF-I that occurs in the hypersomatotropic subject. This disorder begins in the late prepubertal–early pubertal subject; it may be associated with primary or secondary amenorrhea or menstrual irregularity, although pubarche and thelarche are usually normal.[243] The PCO syndrome may also evolve in the girl who presents initially with isosexual precocity.[203] The characteristic laboratory findings in these patients are increased serum concentrations of free testosterone and decreased SHBG concentrations. Serum concentrations of LH may be modestly elevated, but not to castrate values (type I), but may also be normal (type II); FSH concentrations are normal.

Rosenfield[210] also describes a syndrome of "exaggerated adrenarche," which in his experience occurs as frequently as and often in association with ovarian hyperandrogenism. These subjects have increased ACTH-stimulated secretion of Δ^5-17-hydroxypregnenolone and DHEA but normal GnRH-provoked gonadotropin secretory responses, suggesting that they do not have deficiency of 3β-hydroxysteroid dehydrogenase activity.

Hyperandrogenism may also occur in patients with nonclassic congenital adrenal hyperplasia, Cushing syndrome, adrenal tumor, and insulin-resistant syndromes.[210] Partial deficiency of ovarian 17-ketosteroid reductase activity leads to impaired conversion of androgens to estrogens; to compensatory increases in serum concentrations of androstenedione, testosterone, and estrone; and clinically to hirsutism, secondary amenorrhea, and PCO syndrome.[174]

Other causes of delayed adolescence in the female

Deficiency of ovarian (and adrenal) 17α-hydroxylase (P-450c17α) activity prevents synthesis of estrogens (and androgens) and the development of secondary sexual characteristics.[280] The enzyme P-450C17α is found in the endoplasmic reticulum of the adrenal cortex, ovary, and testis. It is a 508–amino acid peptide whose gene is encoded on chromosome 10. Females with deficiency of 17α-hydroxylase are sexually immature but phenotypically normal, with normal but infantile internal genitalia, tall stature, a eunuchoid habitus, and low-renin hypertension (due to increased synthesis of adrenal steroids with mineralocorticoid activity [deoxycorticosterone]), hypokalemia,

metabolic alkalosis, and increased serum LH and FSH values.

A defect in the synthesis, ligand-binding capacity, or DNA-activating activity of the androgen receptor leads to syndromes of complete and partial androgen insensitivity (CAIS, PAIS). Males with CAIS are phenotypic, relatively hairless, females with normal breast development but a blind shallow vaginal pouch and hence primary amenorrhea (testicular feminization syndrome). In infancy these girls often have inguinal hernias with gonads in the vaginal canals or labia majora. Patients with PAIS vary in phenotype and include individuals with ambiguity of the external genitalia, minor anomalies of the male external genitalia, infertility, or only decreased muscle bulk.[258]

Phenotypically normal 46,XX girls with agenesis of müllerian duct structures (fallopian tubes, uterus, and upper third of vagina) have normal thelarche and pubarche but primary amenorrhea (Mayer-Rokitansky-Küster-Hauser syndrome). The pathogenesis of this disorder is unknown, but it might be due to inappropriate in utero production of MIS by the ovaries or other fetal source. Müllerian duct aplasia can also be seen in patients with a variety of congenital anomalies (such as cryptophthalmos in the Frazier syndrome and other eponymic syndromes). Reindollar et al.[188] found müllerian aplasia in 45 of 326 girls (14%) with delayed adolescence. Primary amenorrhea but normal secondary sexual characteristics occurs in girls with cervical atresia, transverse vaginal septum, or imperforate hymen.

Evaluation of the female with delayed sexual development

Evaluation of the reproductive system should be considered (1) in a sexually immature girl of 13 years or older; (2) if there has been arrest of pubertal maturation once initiated, particularly if more than 5 years have passed after thelarche without menarche; (3) if secondary amenorrhea is longer than 6 months in duration (excluding pregnancy, of course); or (4) if there is a striking dissociation between development of androgen- and estrogen-mediated signs of sexual development.

The evaluation should begin with careful historical review and thorough physical examination (Fig. 4-15). Details of the patterns of linear growth, weight gain or loss, and sexual development (if any) should be recorded; the history of any known illness (diabetes mellitus, systemic disease) should be reviewed and symptoms or signs suggestive of ongoing chronic disease (headaches, visual disturbances) sought. Attention to the nutritional and psychosocial history is important, as is information concerning drug, radiation, or chemotherapy exposure. The family history should be reviewed to identify members with similar patterns of delayed puberty. Plotting of past measurements of height and weight is essential, because these patterns may provide important diagnostic clues to the

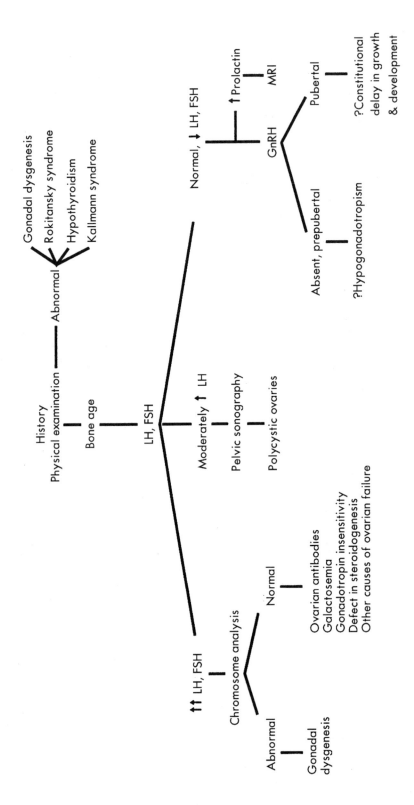

Fig. 4-15. Evaluation of the girl with delayed adolescence. (Redrawn with permission from Schwartz ID, Root AW: Puberty in girls: early, incomplete, or precocious? *Contemp Pediatr* 7[1]:147, 1990. Copyright 1990 by *Contemporary Pediatrics*.)

presence of disordered pituitary function, nutritional deprivation, and systemic disease.

During the physical examination, height, weight, limb and trunk lengths, blood pressure, and pulse should be recorded (and height and weight plotted). Hypertension in the eunuchoid, sexually immature teenager may suggest 17α-hydroxylase deficiency. Significantly short stature would be consistent with defective pituitary function, chronic systemic disease, or nutritional deprivation. Initial visual examination may reveal facial and somatic findings consistent with gonadal dysgenesis (Table 4-9), hyposomatotropism (immature face, peritruncal fat), hypothyroidism, glucocorticoid excess, pseudohypoparathyroidism type I, or other recognizable disorder. The degree of hirsutism and acne formation should be estimated. Visual fields, pupillary responsivity, extraocular eye movement, and fundi should be carefully inspected; midline cranial defects (cleft lip or cleft palate, optic nerve hypoplasia) may be associated with hypothalamic dysfunction. Dental age, which correlates modestly well with skeletal maturity (bone age), should be recorded. Olfactory sensation should be tested. Configuration of the neck, position of the posterior hairline, chest configuration, heart murmur(s), peripheral pulsations, and the presence of cubitus valgus or brachymetacarpals/brachymetatarsals should be noted. The stages of breast and pubic hair development should be recorded, the anatomy and degree of estrogenization of the external genitalia estimated, and the presence of a uterus confirmed by rectal examination. Occasionally direct vaginal examination is necessary to define müllerian duct–derived structures or intravaginal anatomic anomalies. (See Chapter 7, Primary Amenorrhea, for a complete discussion.)

If the history and physical examination do not give specific direction for further evaluation, a general survey to exclude systemic disease is indicated, which should include estimation of bone age, complete blood count (for anemia), urinalysis, erythrocyte sedimentation rate (for inflammatory bowel disease, collagen-vascular disease), automated chemistry profile, and T_4 measurement. Measurement of IGF-I is indicated if the patient is short but not malnourished; IGF-I values in subjects with CDGD tend to be appropriate for bone age and low for chronologic age.[209] It is next most appropriate to measure serum concentrations of immunoreactive LH and FSH; usually a random sample is satisfactory, but for more exact (but still preliminary) assessment, sampling at 20-minute intervals for 40 minutes (three samples) and pooling aliquots of each specimen for one integrated LH measurement gives a more accurate picture of endogenous LH secretion. Subsequently, patients may be separated into those with greatly elevated LH/FSH values (hypergonadotropic), those with modestly elevated LH values (PCO syndrome type I, androgen deficiency or resistance syndromes), and those with normal/low serum LH/FSH values (Fig. 4-15). It is not possible to distinguish between normal and low basal gonadotropin concentrations by utilizing conventional radioimmunoassays because of assay insensitivity; with IRMAS and IFAs it may be possible to distinguish between normal and low LH/FSH values as related to the degree of skeletal maturation.[82,279] Measurement of serum concentrations of bioassayable LH and FSH have not proven helpful in distinguishing between prepubertal children with CDGD and those with hypogonadotropic hypogonadism until signs of sexual maturation have appeared, when B-LH values rise in the former and do not change in the latter subjects.[13]

In females with hypergonadotropism, determination of the karyotype is essential to identify patients with gonadal dysgenesis and its variants. Other causes of primary ovarian failure may be evident from the history (irradiation, chemotherapy, oophorectony, trauma, galactosemia). The presence of anti-ovarian hormones, particularly in association with other autoimmune disorders (autoimmune polyglandular disease type I: hypoadrenalism, hypoparathyroidism, vitiligo), is consistent with autoimmune oophoritis.

Defects in steroidogenesis may be identified by measuring steroid levels in basal and stimulated states. In patients with 17α-hydroxylase deficiency, basal and ACTH-stimulated concentrations of progesterone, desoxycorticosterone (DOC), 18-hydroxyDOC, corticosterone, and 18-hydroxycorticosterone are increased.[280] In subjects with deficiency of 17-ketoreductase, basal and hCG-stimulated concentrations of androstenedione, testosterone, and estrone are increased.[174] In patients with deficiencies of 3β-hydroxysteroid dehydrogenase, 21-hydroxylase, and 11β-hydroxylase, the characteristically elevated steroid metabolites are 17α-hydroxypregnenolone and DHEA, 17α-hydroxyprogesterone and androstenedione, and desoxycortisol, respectively. Patients with end-organ insensitivity to gonadotropin action may be suspected by their clinical phenotype (pseudohypoparathyroidism type I: short stature, developmental delay, brachymetacarpals, hypocalcemia) or by an ovarian biopsy specimen that reveals a pattern of primary ovarian follicles in various stages of development.[37]

Hypogonadotropism associated with chronic systemic disease or nutritional disorders is suggested primarily by the history, physical examination, and chemical screens and/or by evaluation of the pattern of weight loss (or lack of weight gain) and the psychologic profile. The finding of hyperprolactinemia should prompt a search for a pituitary adenoma. In subjects with known malformations or other insults to the hypothalamus or pituitary or identified by magnetic resonance or computed tomographic scanning, particularly in association with further defects in anterior pituitary function, anosmia, or an eponymic syndrome with hypogonadism (Prader-Willi syndrome), the diagnosis of hypogonadotropic hypogonadism may be relatively clear. However, the differentiation between idiopathic hypogonadotropic hypogonadism and CDGD is difficult, particularly in the young subject. Basal gonadotropin levels are similar in the two entities; sampling of nocturnal LH concentrations does not distinguish between the two entities because patients with hypogonadotropism occasionally may have increased nocturnal LH values, as do normal late prepubertal and early pubertal subjects[236]; bone age is delayed and similar to height age in patients with CDGD, whereas height and bone age are usually normal for chronologic age (until 13 years) in patients with hypogonadotropism, after which the rate of skeletal maturation declines. The presence of multicystic ovaries determined by pelvic ultrasound suggests pulsatile LH secretion, whereas cysts are usually not found in the hypogonadotropic female. Adrenal androgen concentrations are appropriate for bone age in girls with CDGD and for chronologic age in subjects with hypogonadotropism. In prepubertal girls a significant FSH secretory response to GnRH may identify the subject with intact gonadotropin secretion,[23] but the absolute reliability of this finding in distinguishing the subject with CDGD from the hypogonadotropic patient is uncertain. Clearly the LH secretory response to GnRH does not distinguish between the two entities.[236] However, the combined criteria of Oerter et al.,[171] which include gonadotropin secretion at night and in response to GnRH (Table 4-3) may be used to identify the girl who has entered early puberty. In patients with hypogonadotropism the incremental LH secretory

response to GnRH may be normal for a pubertal individual, but the peak value is often reached later than in the subject with intact hypothalamic-pituitary function (Fig. 4-16). This pattern of LH secretion resembles that of TSH to TRH seen in patients with hypothalamic-pituitary dysfunction, which reflects anterior pituitary mass and the secretion of β-TSH rather than intact TSH.[28,69]

Rosenfield and co-workers[65,213,214] studied the effects of the long-acting GnRH agonist nafarelin ([6-[3-(2-naphthyl)-D-alanine]] GnRH acetate) on secretion of LH, FSH, estradiol, and sex steroid hormone intermediates in adult, pubertal, and prepubertal females. In response to nafarelin (1.0 µ/kg subcutaneously) with sampling sequentially for 24 hours, there is a marked increase in FSH secretion, with peak concentrations (20 to 110 mIU/mL) reached 4 hours after nafarelin administration in prepubertal girls (0.2 to 6.0 years of age); LH peak concentrations range from approximately 15 to 80 mIU/mL at +4 hours, and estradiol values are maximal (12 to 92 pg/mL) between +16 and +20 hours after GnRH agonist injection. Peak LH, FSH, and estradiol values after nafarelin are high in children younger than 2 years, decline in midchildhood, and increase again with the onset of puberty. The biphasic responsivity of the pituitary-ovarian unit documented with GnRH agonist stimulation is similar to that observed when

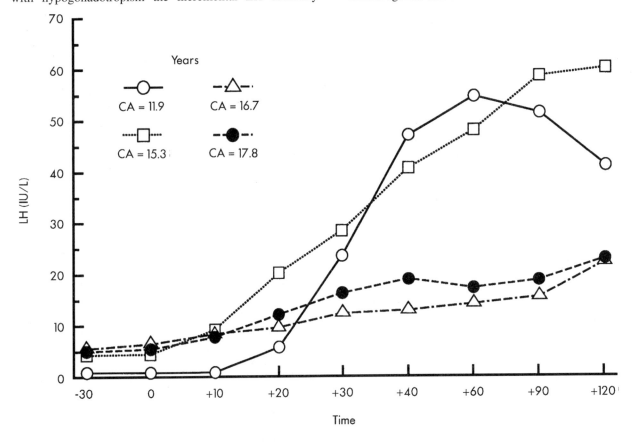

Fig. 4-16. Changing LH secretory responses to GnRH in a girl with an "empty" sella turcica and evolving hypogonadotropism. *CA,* Chronologic age.

measuring basal gonadotropin values and the peak gonadotropin secretory responses to native GnRH; however, the estradiol secretory response to GnRH agonist is greater than that to native GnRH, in all likelihood due to the more intense and prolonged gonadotropin response to the longer-acting analogue of GnRH. In children (3.5 to 8.8 years) with primary ovarian dysfunction (Turner syndrome), there is a rapid increase in FSH concentrations within 1 hour after nafarelin administration (30 to 60 mIU/mL) that is greater than that in normal adult women in the midfollicular phase (<22 mIU/mL), but there is no increase in estradiol concentrations in those children. In females with (proven) hypogonadotropism the response to nafarelin is variable. In patients with multiple anterior pituitary hormone deficiencies, LH, FSH, and estradiol secretory responses to GnRH agonist are absent, but in girls with idiopathic, isolated hypogonadotropism, the secretory response is variable and sometimes even normal for a pubertal subject. The heterogeneity of response to nafarelin reflects the variability of this disorder itself. The higher prolactin secretory response to TRH and/or metoclopramide in males with CDGD, compared with hypogonadotropic subjects, has been advocated as a distinguishing feature between these two disorders; however, these observations are not consistent.[51] The applicability of such studies in females is uncertain. Chlorpromazine also stimulates prolactin secretion, but because of its sedative property has not been extensively evaluated in this situation.

Thus the diagnosis of idiopathic, isolated hypogonadotropism remains difficult. Rosenfield[212] suggests that:

In the delayed prepubertal teenage girl with bone age greater than 11 years . . ., gonadotropin deficiency is *possible* if there is a midline facial defect, CNS dysfunction or abnormal CT or MRI brain scan, *probable* if the bone age is greater than 13 years without puberty, there is anosmia or panhypopituitarism, the sleep-associated increase in LH is lacking, the GnRH agonist test yields a flat response, and *diagnostic* if the bone age is greater than 16 years.

The presence of hyperandrogenism is suggested by the clinical findings of acne and hirsutism (often in association with obesity) and documented by the presence of an elevated free testosterone concentration. The total testosterone concentration may be normal or high (but not in the virilizing range), and the SHBG concentration is decreased. Pelvic ultrasound may reveal a polycystic pattern or may be normal. The differential diagnosis of hyperandrogenism can be approached by the scheme of Rosenfield[212]: dexamethasone suppressibility (1 mg/m² for 5 to 7 days) of androgens and cortisol secretion differentiates between glucocorticoid-suppressible and -nonsuppressible forms of hyperandrogenism; testing with ACTH identifies functional adrenal abnormalities of 3β-hydroxysteroid dehydrogenase and 21β- and 11β-hydroxylase activities. Administration of nafarelin to women with PCO syndrome, a gonadotropin-

dependent process,[64,65] leads to exaggerated early LH, 17-hydroxyprogesterone, and androstenedione secretion and decreased FSH release when compared with normal women in the early follicular phase of the menstrual cycle. Since the clinical and biochemical manifestations of hyperandrogenism may be subtle, serial measurements of serum androgen values is recommended when the cause of delayed or arrested adolescence is obscure.

Therapeutic management of the female with delayed adolescence

Appropriate treatment of the female with delayed adolescence is dependent on a thorough understanding of its etiology and pathophysiology in the individual patient. In girls with CDGD, reassurance and observation are the mainstays of therapy. Although girls with CDGD may be concerned about their immature sexual appearance, severe personality disturbances are uncommon.[157] The use of GH in such patients is experimental; in all likelihood GH ultimately will prove useful and practical *only* if a functional deficit in the secretion of endogenous GH can be documented. Very rarely, androgens (oxandrolone, 0.1 mg/kg per day, or testosterone depot, 20 mg intramuscularly monthly) may be administered to such girls for no more than 6 months to increase the linear growth rate[209]; occasionally the administration of estrogen (estradiol cypionate, intramuscularly 0.5 mg monthly; ethinyl estradiol, 5 μg orally daily; or micronized estradiol, 0.5 to 1.0 mg orally daily or cyclically with a progestin) may be indicated for the girl with extreme CDGD who is quite concerned about her immature appearance.[209,226] Pulsatile nocturnal administration of GnRH (1 to 2 μg per pulse for four or five pulses at 90-minute intervals) for 12 months will induce complete and sustained pubertal development, including menses, in girls with CDGD; whether shorter periods of such therapy will trigger ongoing adolescent development is unknown.[245]

In girls with nutritional disorders, athletic amenorrhea, or psychogenic or stress-related amenorrhea, resolution of the underlying conflict, improved nutrition, weight gain, and increase in body fat content will result in progression or resumption of adolescent development. In girls with secondary amenorrhea associated with anorexia nervosa, weight often must be restored to a value 10% greater than the weight at menarche in order for menses to resume.[212] In subjects with hyperprolactinemia, prolactin secretion may be suppressed and tumor size decreased with dopamine agonists such as bromocriptine.[9,106] Occasionally, neurosurgical removal of a prolactinoma is required if medical therapy fails to alleviate visual impairment or increased intracranial pressure.

Females with hypogonadotropic hypogonadism can be feminized with cyclic estrogen-progestin (micronized estradiol, 0.5 to 1.0 mg, between days 1 and 21 and medroxyprogesterone acetate, 10 mg, between days 12 and 21 of each month) or pulsatile GnRH administration.[226,245] When pulsatile GnRH was administered intravenously every 1.5 to 2 hours to one adult and four teenaged hypogonadotropic females (chronologic age 16 to 26 years, bone age 12 to 13.25 years) with hypothalamic dysfunction, Schoemaker et al.[222] observed both anovulatory and ovulatory cycles and normal and deficient corpus luteum function as normal ovulatory cycles were established, recapitulating normal pubertal development and maturation of pituitary and ovarian function. Fertility can be realized in hypogonadotropic women by the administration of GnRH or gonadotropins.[45,108] (See also Chapter 30.)

In the girl with primary ovarian dysfunction, estrogen and progestin administration (vide supra) will induce secondary sexual characteristics and menses (if a uterus and patent vagina are present). In patients with gonadal dysgenesis, administration of hGH is followed by acceleration of linear growth rate and increased adult height prediction.[208] When a Y chromosome or fragment (identified by probes for Y-associated DNA) is present in the karyotype of a girl with gonadal dysgenesis, removal of the streak gonads is recommended because of the high incidence of gonadoblastoma in such patients.[96,145] Adult women with primary ovarian dysfunction may become pregnant and deliver liveborn children with donated ova and in vitro fertilization.[231]

Hyperandrogenic females have normal pubertal development if androgen values return to normal with appropriate therapy. In subjects with PCO syndrome, cyclic progestin administration or ovarian suppression with estrogen-progestin or GnRH analogues, may be required.[45] Glucocorticoid suppression of ACTH secretion depresses androgen concentrations in patients with nonclassic forms of congenital adrenal hyperplasia and permits reasonable pituitary-ovarian function; in patients with deficiency of P-450c17α, ACTH suppression and replacement of sex hormones will alleviate hypertension and bring about secondary sexual development.[280] In one woman with P-450c17α deficiency, ovarian follicular development has been induced by GnRH analogue therapy, with recovery of an ovum and successful in vitro fertilization.[187] Correction of surgically amenable lesions (imperforate hymen, transverse vaginal septum) permits menstruation. Hormonal therapy is not required for 46,XX girls with müllerian agenesis, since ovarian function is normal. Surgical or mechanical therapy ultimately may be necessary to facilitate coital function in women with attenuation of the vagina. Surrogate motherhood may be considered in the appropriate situation, since these women ovulate normally.[124] In patients with testicular feminization, gonadectomy and replacement estrogen administration is recommended.

SEXUAL PRECOCITY

In the female, sexual precocity is defined by Rosenfield[212] as the appearance of thelarche before age 7.5 years,

pubarche before age 8.5 years, and menarche before age 9.5 years. In other texts any sign of sexual development before age 8 years is considered premature sexual development.[206] However, it must be recalled that a substantial number of girls, particularly black girls, develop pubarche and thelarche before this age[98] and progress thereafter into early but nevertheless normal adolescence. These children represent early-maturing girls who are the counterparts to late-maturing children with CDGD. As with the latter subjects, the majority of such children when identified require only reassurance and observation. Causes of isosexual precocity are listed in the box on p. 39. True and complete, central isosexual precocity (TC/CIP) occurs more frequently in girls than in boys, suggesting that the factor(s) "restraining" amplified GnRH secretion are more "fragile" in girls; whether this reflects an intrinsic genetic influence or the sex hormone milieu is unknown. Among 95 girls with isosexual precocity evaluated at the National Institutes of Health (NIH) over a 5-year period, 60 (63%) had idiopathic TC/CIP; 14 (15%) had hypothalamic hamartomas, 13 (14%) had other CNS lesions, and 2 (2%) had TC/CIP evolving from adrenal virilizing disorders.[180] Six girls (6%) had the Albright-McCune-Sternberg syndrome.

True and complete central isosexual precocity

In girls with TC/CIP, normally regulated, mature hypothalamic-pituitary-ovarian function occurs at a prematurely young age. This designation is preferred to the term *central precocious puberty* because the latter does not distinguish between patients with intact central pubertal mechanisms and those with CNS neoplasms that may cause either TC/CIP or may secrete gonadotropins (germinomas secrete hCG), which rarely may cause sexual maturation in the female independently of hypothalamic regulatory control; the latter are best considered under the category of pseudoprecocious puberty in which sexual development is not under hypothalamic GnRH influence (refer to the box on p. 117).

Precocious increase in the frequency and amplitude of GnRH secretion in the female is most frequently idiopathic; it may also be the result of congenital anomalies (septooptic dysplasia, hydrocephalus, arachnoid cysts) or acquired insults to the CNS (empty sella, trauma, inflammatory disorders, neoplasms, cranial irradiation). Familial forms of TC/CIP have occurred in both sexes in the same family.[169] In such families results of analysis of the gene structure of GnRH have been normal.[169,268] With the presently available precise imaging procedures, 20% to 40% of children with "idiopathic" TC/CIP are found to have CNS lesions, the majority of which are hypothalamic hamartomas sited in the posterior hypothalamus.[233] Cacciare et al.[32] report that hamartomas were present in 33% of girls with TC/CIP, an incidence twice that of the NIH experience.[180] Hamartomas are congenital, non-neoplastic heterotopic malformations composed of neurons, fiber bundles, and glial cells.[195]

Causes of isosexual precocity in females

I. *True and complete, central isosexual precocity*

  A. IDIOPATHIC
    1. After exposure to sex hormones
      a. Congenital adrenal hyperplasia
      b. Adrenal/ovarian tumor
      c. Albright-McCune-Sternberg syndrome
  B. CONGENITAL ANOMALY OF THE CNS
    1. Hamartoma
    2. Hydrocephalus
    3. Septooptic dysplasia
    4. Arachnoid cyst
  C. ACQUIRED INSULT TO THE CNS
    1. Inflammation
      a. Meningitis
      b. Encephalitis
      c. Abscess
    2. Trauma
    3. Irradiation
    4. Neoplasm
      a. Optic glioma (neurofibromatosis)
      b. Astrocytoma
      c. Ependymoma
      d. Craniopharyngioma

II. *Pseudoisosexual precocity*

  A. hCG-SECRETING NEOPLASM
    1. Germinoma
    2. Hepatoblastoma
  B. OVARIAN
    1. Follicular/luteal cysts
    2. Granulosa cell tumor
    3. Neurocutaneous syndromes
      a. Albright-McCune-Sternberg syndrome
      b. Tuberous sclerosis
  C. NONCLASSIC CONGENITAL ADRENAL HYPERPLASIA
  D. EXOGENOUS INGESTION

III. *Incomplete isosexual precocity*

  A. PREMATURE THELARCHE
  B. PREMATURE MENARCHE
  C. PREMATURE PUBARCHE/ADRENARCHE

IV. *Causes of vaginal bleeding*

  A. FOREIGN BODY
  B. VAGINITIS
  C. URETHRAL PROLAPSE
  D. SEXUAL ABUSE
  E. NEOPLASM

the medial basal hypothalamic site of GnRH synthesis and the "pulse generator."[223] Children with TC/CIP manifesting before age 3 years are most likely to have hamartomas.[233]

Sockalosky et al.[240] describe precocious sexual development in 5 of 10 prepubertal girls between ages 4 and 8 years admitted to a regional trauma center and rehabilitation center with severe cranial injuries (coma for >14 days) in whom sexual development began 2 to 17 months after head injury, bone age advanced rapidly, and hormonal data were consistent with a central form of isosexual precocity. Imaging of the CNS revealed dilatation of the third ventricle in the majority of affected children. Sexual precocity may also occur in children experiencing peripartum insults to the CNS. There is an association between sexual precocity in girls and sexual abuse, but cause and effect are uncertain in this situation.[98]

Precocious or early adolescent sexual development is being recognized with increasing frequency in children who have survived chemotherapy and cranial irradiation (18 to 24 Gy) therapy for leukemia and solid brain tumors. Many of these children tend to have deficiency of spontaneous GH secretion but have normal stimulated GH release (and are primary examples of "GH neurosecretory dysfunction"[16]). Leiper et al.[135] reported that 20% ($N = 24$) of 121 girls who survived chemotherapy and cranial irradiation (at mean age 3.9 years) began sexual development before 8 years and another 12% ($N = 12$) before 9.8 years; in 58% ($N = 21$) of these subjects the expected increase in linear growth rate was attenuated, suggesting concomitant deficiency of GH secretion.

Dissociation of pubertal sexual development from acceleration of linear growth in girls is often indicative of an endocrine abnormality such as hyposomatotropism, hypothyroidism, or hypercortisolism. In the study by Quigley et al.,[186] among 20 girls who survived therapy for acute lymphoblastic leukemia, thelarche and menarche occurred at significantly younger ages, and the interval between thelarche and menarche was significantly shorter than that in control subjects; 90% had decreased GH secretion. Further study of this population revealed elevated (tenfold) basal concentrations of FSH, an increase threefold in GnRH-mediated secretion of FSH and LH, and decreased serum concentrations of inhibin, suggestive of ovarian injury secondary to chemotherapy with compensatory increase in gonadotropin secretion suggestive of a "failing ovary." The long-term fertility of these females is as yet unknown. At higher doses of cranial irradiation, gonadotropin deficiency may develop as well.

TC/CIP may follow successful therapy of states of pseudoisosexual precocity that have resulted in advanced bone age and presumably hypothalamic "maturation" to the point of increased GnRH secretion. This may occur after treatment of the hyperandrogenic state of congenital adrenal hyperplasia in females or evolve spontaneously

Many of the hamartomas found in patients with TC/CIP contain GnRH, but it is uncertain whether these lesions are the site of an "ectopic GnRH pulse generator" or lead to hypothalamic maturation because of their location in the posterior hypothalamus, which interrupts inhibitory input to

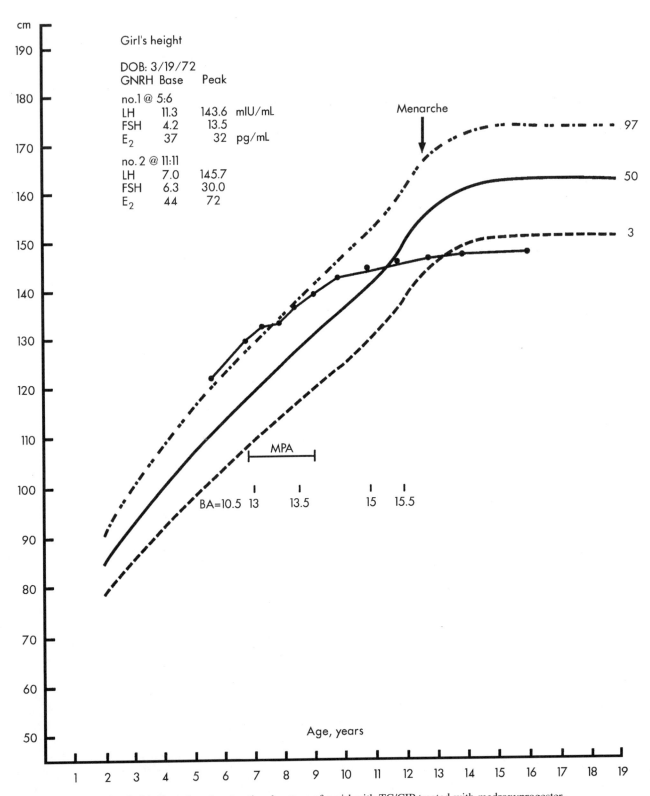

Fig. 4-17. Growth and maturational pattern of a girl with TC/CIP treated with medroxyprogesterone acetate (*MPA*). Note the rapid early growth and compromised adult stature.

from the hyperestrogenic state of the Albright-McCune-Sternberg syndrome of fibrous dysplasia (vide infra). Young girls with primary hypothyroidism have large, cystic ovaries on ultrasound examination and often develop thelarche; galactorrhea and vaginal bleeding can also occur in these patients.[143] The pathophysiology of this disorder is unclear; although measurable, the gonadotropin secretory response to GnRH is usually prepubertal.[228] The hyperestrogenic state may be the result of decreased catabolism of normally secreted gonadotropins and/or of estrogens by the prepubertal subject with consequent prolonged biologic activity, the secretion of biologically distinct isoforms of FSH and LH as a consequence of hypothyroidism, or an effect of both the gonadotropins and the increased secretion of prolactin characteristic of primary hypothyroidism. Sexual precocity regresses completely with restoration of the euthyroid state.

In girls with TC/CIP, thelarche is usually the first clinical manifestation; pubic hair growth occurs as a consequence of ovarian androgen production. (Adrenarche occurs at the usual chronologic age in girls with TC/CIP; usually the levels of the adrenal androgens DHEA and DHAS are low and in the preadrenarcheal range.) The rates of linear growth and sexual maturation accelerate, but the rate of increase in bone age exceeds that of the height increment, resulting in ultimate short stature (Fig. 4-17). Puberty advances, and menarche ensues. (Fertility is normal in these patients, and menopause does not occur prematurely[168]). The vaginal mucosa is estrogenized clinically and by vaginal cytology. By ultrasonography girls with TC/CIP have uterine and ovarian volumes and architecture appropriate for the stage of sexual development and in advance of girls of similar chronologic age.[219] Basal endogenous diurnal and nocturnal and GnRH-stimulated gonadotropin and estrogen concentrations are appropriate for the stage of sexual maturation.[206] Random serum estradiol concentrations are within the prepubertal range in many girls with TC/CIP, but often increase into the pubertal range after administration of native GnRH. Markedly elevated pubertal serum concentrations of estradiol are observed 12 and 24 hours after the administration of the GnRH agonist nafarelin to such patients.[213] There is increased secretion of GH in girls with TC/CIP and high IGF-I values in accord with the stage of pubertal development.

As classically described, TC/CIP—once initiated—is a progressive maturational phenomenon. However, there are many patients in whom the pattern of growth and development proceeds at a more relaxed pace; it starts, arrests, or regresses or is even transient.[177,229] First, it is important to recognize the girl with normal early adolescence in whom thelarche or pubarche may occur at 6 to 8 years, with slow progression to a somewhat earlier-than-average age of menarche, but still one that is greater than 9.5 to 10 years of age. Kreiter et al.[127] describe seven girls with TC/CIP presenting at a mean age of 5.8 years with thelarche and pubarche, comparable bone and height ages, and similar

predicted and target heights in whom there was little or no progression in sexual development or discordant increase in bone or height age over the next 2 years, during which interval the predicted adult height increased slightly. A similar group of 17 girls with idiopathic TC/CIP in whom bone age was less than 2 years in advance of chronologic age had a mild, nonprogressive, and even transient form of precocious puberty with no compromise of predicted adult height.[75]

Pescovitz et al.[181] studied GnRH-stimulated immunoreactive gonadotropin secretion in 58 girls with thelarche and no underlying structural abnormality of the CNS. They identified six clinically distinguishable groups varying from those with isolated breast development (premature thelarche) to those with TC/CIP. Basal FSH and LH concentrations were similar in all groups except the group with TC/CIP, in which LH values were twofold higher than in other groups. The peak LH secretory response to GnRH increased and the peak FSH release decreased with advancing development (Fig. 4-18). Thus the gonadotropin secretory response to GnRH varied from a prepubertal (FSH predominant) to a pubertal (LH predominant) pattern with advancing signs of sexual development. However, there was considerable overlap in LH and FSH secretory responses to GnRH and of peak LH:FSH ratios among the girls with intermediary forms of sexual development. Nocturnal LH secretion appropriately increased in girls with TC/CIP, but was occasionally increased in subjects with typical premature thelarche as well. This range of clinical and laboratory findings across a spectrum of sexually precocious girls implies a continuum of hypothalamic GnRH secretory patterns leading to variable manifestations of precocious sexual development. The fact that this variability in sexual development is described perhaps exclusively in girls is further evidence of the intrinsic instability of the factor(s) restraining GnRH secretion in females.

Pseudoisosexual precocity

Isosexual precocity not under regulation of hypothalamic GnRH is defined as pseudoprecocious puberty, which may be the result of exposure to gonadotropins or sex hormones of endogenous or exogenous origin; estrogens may be secreted by the ovary or adrenal or may be ingested from exogenous sources (please refer to the box on p. 117). Secretion of hCG by germinomas arising from the pineal gland or other CNS sites, hepatoblastomas, or retroperitoneal or thoracic tumors is a rare paraneoplastic cause of pseudoisosexual precocity in girls, because this gonadotropin has primarily LH-like bioactivity; thus estrogen secretion is only occasionally enhanced in the female with these tumors.[206] Depending on the intracranial site, however, a germinoma may interfere with hypothalamic-pituitary function (as may any CNS tumor) and lead to TC/CIP, either primarily or after successful radiotherapy. The presence of high circulating levels of the β-subunit of hCG (β-hCG) is

(a)

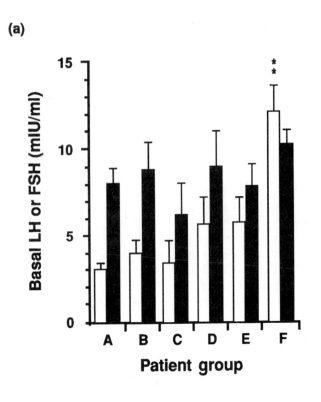

(b)

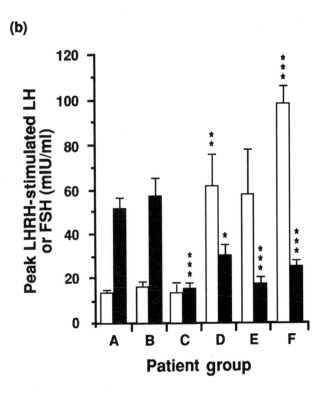

Group	Breast	Pubic hair	Rapid growth	BA > 2SD CA
A	+	−	−	−
B	+	−	−	+
C	+	+	−	−
D	+	−	+	+
E	+	+	+ or	+
F	+	+	+	+

A, premature thelarche; F, TC/CIP.

(Redrawn with permission from Pescovitz OH et al: Premature thelarche and central precocious puberty: the relationship between clinical presentation and the gonadotropin response to luteinizing hormone-releasing hormone, *J Clin Endocrinol Metab* 67:474-479, 1988; © The Endocrine Society.)

Fig. 4-18. Patterns of basal LH (*open bars*) and FSH (*closed bars*) concentrations **(a)** and of the gonadotropin secretory responses to GnRH **(b)** in girls with varying forms of isosexual precocity ($*P < 0.05$; $**P < 0.01$; $***P < 0.001$ compared with group A).

the biochemical hallmark of hCG-secreting neoplasms. Although unlikely, administration of exogenous gonadotropins to a prepubertal girl could conceivably produce sexual precocity.

Autonomous secretion of estrogens by ovarian follicular or lutein cysts is an unusual cause of pseudoisosexual precocity (Fig. 4-19). In children with ovarian cysts the onset of estrogen secretion (thelarche) is abrupt, and estradiol concentrations are extremely high. Serum gonadotro-pin concentrations are low and do not change after GnRH administration. Skeletal maturation is often normal, and pelvic ultrasound usually reveals a single ovarian cyst more than 3 cm in diameter. The cause of these cysts is uncertain. They may reflect the normal waxing and waning of small follicular cysts under gonadotropin (FSH) regulation typical of the prepubertal female, one of which grows to disproportionate size and becomes autonomous. The interesting question of whether some children with recurrent

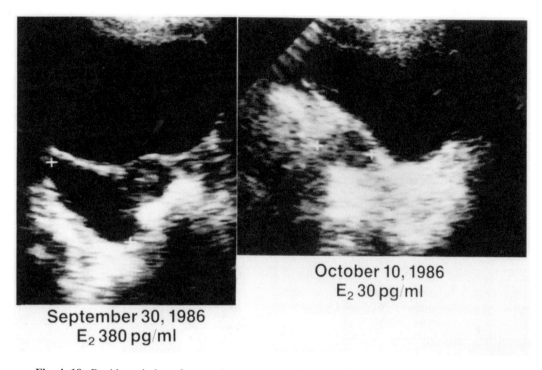

September 30, 1986
E₂ 380 pg/ml

October 10, 1986
E₂ 30 pg/ml

Fig. 4-19. Rapid resolution of an ovarian cyst in an 18-month-old infant girl who presented with a 3-week history of thelarche.

estrogen-secreting ovarian cysts may have an autoimmune process with development of an immunoglobulin with FSH-like activity has been raised but requires more evaluation.[248] Many of these cysts regress spontaneously, and surgical intervention is not required unless torsion occurs or the abnormality persists for more than 6 to 8 weeks.[70] Serial ultrasonograms and serum estradiol measurements are necessary to be certain the process resolves. A multicystic ovary found by ultrasonography mandates evaluation of thyroid function and treatment with thyroxine, if the child is hypothyroid. Occasionally a very large ovarian cyst may be associated with pubertal gonadotropin secretion.

Arisaka et al.[6] describe a girl who underwent unilateral oophorectomy at 3 years of age for an immature teratoma. At 7 years she developed thelarche. Shortly thereafter she was found to have a 5-cm follicular cyst and an exaggerated LH secretory response to GnRH. The large ovarian cyst in this patient might reflect prolonged exposure to increased gonadotropin secretion in a unilateral gonadectomized subject. Perilongo et al.[179] studied a 2-year-old girl with thelarche of 8 months' duration and recent onset of vaginal bleeding who had a 5-cm luteinized ovarian cyst; further evaluation revealed a hypothalamic hamartoma and an exaggerated LH secretory response to GnRH. These observations document the necessity to follow closely all girls with ovarian cysts to be certain that these represent isolated lesions and are not secondary manifestations of primary CNS mechanisms of precocious sexual development requiring alternative therapy.

Solid functional granulosa cell, theca cell, mixed granulosa-theca cell, or mixed germ cell–sex cord–stromal ovarian tumors causing pseudoisosexual precocity may be malignant.[128,179] Thus an aggressive surgical approach to such patients with unilateral salpingo-oophorectomy is justified.

The Albright-McCune-Sternberg triad of polyostotic fibrous dysplasia, irregularly edged café au lait pigmentation of the skin, and a variety of functional endocrine abnormalities (the most common of which in girls is isosexual precocity) is associated with rhythmic ovarian cyst formation, autonomous ovarian function, and episodic secretion of estradiol, which correlates with cyst formation, leading to thelarche and occasionally to vaginal bleeding.[76] Initially, serum gonadotropin values are low and rise little or not at all during sleep or after GnRH administration. With advancing age and skeletal maturation, the regulation of ovarian function changes and becomes gonadotropin mediated.[76,176,206] The child thus evolves from one with pseudoisosexual precocity to one with TC/CIP. Other endocrinopathies associated with the Albright-McCune-Sternberg syndrome include hyperthyroidism, hyperadrenocorticism, and hypersomatotropism. Hypophosphatemia and hyperphosphaturia are also seen in some patients.[134] These abnormalities represent disordered endocrine/paracrine regulation of cellular function, probably mediated through errors in the signaling mechanism that regulates the generation of cyclic AMP. Activating mutations of the α-subunit of membrane-associated G-stimulating protein have been detected in four patients with the Albright-McCune-Sternberg syndrome. In two subjects histidine was substituted for arginine at position 201; in two other patients cysteine was substituted at the same site. Both mutations led to increased activity of the G-stimulatory protein and consequently to increased cyclic AMP activity and (presumably) cellular function.[267] Studies of immunoglobulins with FSH-mimicking bioactivity in such subjects (although probably not involved) would be of interest.[248] A circulating primate-specific Leydig cell–stimulating factor has been identified in the serum of boys with Leydig cell hyperplasia[150]; similar studies would be of interest in patients with the Albright-McCune-Sternberg syndrome as well. Although the course of the fibrous dysplastic process is not predictable (and may be associated with fractures or deformities), the prognosis for linear growth and mature reproductive function is good, with apparently normal fertility and a normal (or prolonged) reproductive period.[134] However, breast carcinoma has been observed in two young (11 and 35 years old) affected females, necessitating close follow-up of such patients.[134]

Pseudoisosexual precocity (thelarche and pubarche) has been observed in a girl with nonclassic, 21-hydroxylase–deficient congenital adrenal hyperplasia; it was suggested that the thelarche of this child was the result either of increased adrenal secretion of estrogen or of peripheral aromatization of adrenal androgens.[116] Ingestion of exogenous estrogens either by prescription[231] or by accident in unexpected forms in foodstuffs may also induce thelarche. Ling et al.[144] observed 23 girls with thelarche and vaginal bleeding ($N = 14$), which they attributed to ingestion of estrogen-containing agents ($N = 20$) or to breastfeeding while their mothers were pregnant or receiving estrogens. An estrogen-secreting adrenal tumor is a rare cause of pseudoisosexual precocity in the female.[44]

Incomplete isosexual precocity

The term *incomplete isosexual precocity* implies isolated, transient, nonprogressive signs of sexual development without systemic manifestations that are of little or no clinical consequences to the child. As discussed earlier, however, there is significant overlap between these limited forms of isosexual precocity and those of greater import.[181]

Premature thelarche. Premature thelarche is the isolated development of unilateral (44%) or bilateral (56%) breast tissue with no other signs of sexual maturation at the initial examination and during follow-up.[41,137] It occurs most commonly between 1 and 3 years of age. These girls have normal linear growth, bone age appropriate for chronologic age, and no sexual hair. Serum concentrations of estrogens are low, but the vaginal maturation index may transiently reveal some cornified cells; basal and GnRH-stimulated gonadotropin values are appropriate for the chronologic age of the child. The breast thermographic pattern for girls with premature thelarche is similar to that in prepubertal girls.[77] They do not progress further into adolescent development; breast tissue may remain stationary in size or may regress.[206] Most neonates have palpable breast buds (unless delivered before 36 weeks of gestation), which may increase in size for the first 2 months of life (probably in response to the elevated secretion of FSH typical in the female neonate) and then regress slowly to disappear by 10 to 12 months of age. Therefore, when evaluating a young infant with thelarche, it is important to know whether breast development has been present since birth or had regressed only to recur.

The frequency with which thelarche is observed in female infants and the data of Pescovitz et al.[181] suggest that premature thelarche is the result of pituitary-ovarian function and ovarian estrogen secretion during this interval. In some instances precocious breast development may be the result of ingestion of estrogen-like substances contained in food or other environmental agents. Wilcox et al.[274] demonstrated that soya flour and linseed contain estrogen-like substances (phytoestrogens, isoflavones, coumestans, lignans, resorcyclic acid lactones) that can estrogenize the vaginal mucosa of postmenopausal women. There are no data concerning the relationship between soy formula and premature thelarche, but since thelarche is distinctly uncommon in male infants and children who also receive this nutrient, it is probably not of major pathogenetic significance. "Epidemics" of thelarche have occurred in girls and boys in Puerto Rico and Italy, thought to be related to estrogen contamination of foodstuffs.[217] Immunoglobulin G antibodies to the estrogen receptors have been found in human serum, with high levels present in serum from young females.[166] These anti–estrogen receptor immunoglobulins are reported to have estrogen-like activity.[19] The anti–estrogen receptor antibody is thought to be a naturally occurring response to environmental estrogens with development of an idiotype antibody that recognizes the estrogen receptors. Further studies of this immunoglobulin in relation to the pathogenesis of premature thelarche seem warranted. Thelarche is also the initial sign of TC/CIP, and therefore a period of observation is necessary before the diagnosis of premature thelarche is made.

The natural history of the girl with premature thelarche is variable. Breast development regresses in 32%, persists unchanged in 57%, increases in size in 11%, or regresses and periodically reappears.[163] Among 68 Israeli girls with premature thelarche, 85% had had breast tissue since birth or had developed breast tissue before 2 years of age.[110] In 91% of these infants, breast tissue regressed or persisted without increase in size. In 4 of 10 children in whom breast development began after 2 years, progressive breast enlargement was observed. Of 59 Thai girls with premature thelarche, breast development regressed over 3 to 66 months in 27%, persisted in 46%, and continued to enlarge in 27%.[41] In this series and that of Ilicki et al.[110] there was a bimodal distribution of age of onset of thelarche, with the majority of patients presenting before 2 years of age or after 5 to 6 years of age. Very few children presented with thelarche between 2 and 6 years of age. Those girls with persistent or enlarging breasts primarily were in the older age group, suggesting that these subjects may be those with early adolescence.[97] As adolescents and adults, girls with premature thelarche are thought to have a normal and intact reproductive endocrine system.

Premature menarche. Premature menarche is the isolated appearance of uterine (vaginal) bleeding in otherwise prepubertal girls with no evidence of a pathologic cause (vide infra) for such bleeding. It has much the same significance and pathogenesis as premature thelarche, although premature menarche is far less common. Nevertheless, vaginal bleeding in an infant or child (except the estrogen withdrawal vaginal bleeding of the newborn infant female) is a matter of concern to parent and physician and merits evaluation. Approximately 38 girls with premature menarche have been reported.[206,218] These patients ranged in age from 3 months to 9 years; vaginal bleeding may occur only once, but is more likely to be recurrent. Eventually vaginal bleeding ceases, and later sexual development commences and progresses normally with normal adult fertility.[167] The gonadotropin secretory pattern in response to GnRH is usually prepubertal and FSH predominant. Estrogen levels are often slightly elevated; nocturnal secretion of LH is pulsatile when vaginal bleeding has occurred in the previous 3-week period, but regresses to a prepubertal pattern after vaginal bleeding has ceased for several months.[218] Pelvic ultrasound examination reveals ovaries and uterus of prepubertal size and architecture.[218]

Premature pubarche. Premature pubarche is the isolated appearance of pubic hair, but in general the term refers to manifestations of androgenic activity (apocrine axillary odor, pubic and/or axillary hair) occurring at an inordinately young age.[206] Linear growth rate is usually normal; bone age is appropriate for or slightly in advance (<2 years) of chronologic age; there is no virilization; a few microcomedones may be visible.[210] As the child is followed, the amount of pubic hair may increase slowly; but other signs of sexual maturation do not appear until the appropriate age, and then maturation progresses normally.[109] The long-term course of females with premature

adrenarche is not clearly documented, and whether some of these subjects develop hyperandrogenism as adults is a consideration. Most commonly, premature pubarche is accompanied by a measurable increase in adrenal androgen secretion, hence the term *premature adrenarche.* As we have seen, the normal age of pubarche/adrenarche is variable, particularly among black females, 25% of whom may have pubic hair by age 6 years.[97] Black females are referred to the author's pediatric endocrine unit for evaluation of an adult axillary odor or pubic hair growth with great frequency.[202] In a 15-year period, 82 girls were evaluated for premature pubarche, of whom 29 (36%) were black (a considerably higher proportion than the 8% of black patients in our total pediatric endocrinology population). Of 10 girls less than 4 years of age with premature pubarche, 7 (70%) were black. Nevertheless, in white girls the appearance of pubic hair growth or other androgenic manifestation may be considered premature if it occurs before age 8 years.

Premature pubarche due to premature adrenarche is accompanied by increased serum concentrations of DHEA and DHAS and a steroidogenic secretory response to ACTH comparable to that of a normal adolescent at that stage of pubic hair growth. Adrenarche is characterized by an increase in synthesis and secretion of 3β-hydroxysteroids (Δ^5-17α-hydroxypregnenolone, Δ^5-androstene-3β, 17β-diol sulfate, DHEA, DHAS) and in androstenedione, suggesting decreased activity of 3β-hydroxysteroid dehydrogenase and increased activity of 17,20-lyase (P-450c17α) perhaps due to changes in the adrenal steroid microenvironment that influences the kinetics of the enzyme synthesizing these hormones.[165,202,210,257] In addition, serum concentrations of SHBG are reported to be lower in girls with premature adrenarche than in age-appropriate, prepubertal girls, suggesting that free androgen levels are higher than total values would indicate.[165]

The proportion of children with premature pubarche who have a subtle defect in adrenal steroidogenesis is low. Some patients with premature pubarche clearly have a nonclassic form of 21-hydroxylase–deficient congenital adrenal hyperplasia that can be identified only by measuring the 17α-hydroxyprogesterone secretory response to ACTH or by measuring serum concentrations of 17α-hydroxyprogesterone serially over a 24-hour period, because there may be marked diurnal variability in the secretion of this metabolite.[210] The reported incidence of 21-hydroxylase deficiency among series of female children with premature pubarche has varied from none to 32%, and the reported incidence of deficiency of 3β-hydroxysteroid dehydrogenase activity has varied from none to 20%.[170] No children with premature pubarche associated with 11β-hydroxylase deficiency have been identified in two studies (Table 4-10).[170] The variability in the incidence of nonclassic congenital adrenal hyperpasia reflects, in part, different populations studied and, in part, the criteria employed for

Table 4-10. Incidence of nonclassic congenital adrenal hyperplasia in girls with premature pubarche*

No.	P-450c21	3-bHSD†	P-450c11
175	11 (6%)		
125		15 (12%)	
65			None

*Data are from reference 170.
†3β-HSD, 3β-hydroxysteroid dehydrogenase.

this diagnosis. Rosenfield[210] suggests that a diagnosis of nonclassic 3β-hydroxysteroid dehydrogenase deficiency as a cause of premature pubarche be made only if the secretory responses to ACTH of Δ^5-17α-hydroxypregnenolone and DHEA exceed those of normal adults by twofold, there are subnormal secretory responses of 17α-hydroxyprogesterone and androstenedione, *and* bone age is more than 2 years in advance of chronologic age.

Premature growth of pubic hair may also be seen in girls with age-appropriate or even low serum concentrations of DHAS; often DHEA values are increased in these girls and serial measurements demonstrate rising adrenal androgen levels over time. Premature pubarche may be a presenting manifestation of a virilizing tumor or cyst of the ovary, a virilizing neoplasm of the adrenal, Cushing disease, cortisol resistance, or cortisone reductase deficiency, the latter due to a compensatory increase in adrenal androgen secretion.[210]

Nonhormonal causes of vaginal bleeding

Vaginal discharge or vaginal bleeding in the prepubertal girl may be due to chemical or infectious vulvovaginitis; an intravaginal foreign body; urethral prolapse; sexual abuse; accidental genital trauma; or vaginal or uterine neoplasm such as sarcoma botryoides or endodermal, clear-cell, or mesonephric carcinoma.[50] Sexual precocity is present in 7% of girls who have been sexually abused; whether precocious sexual development is causally related to the abuse or is the response of the abuser to a sexually precocious child is unknown.[98]

In adolescent girls irregular vaginal bleeding is most frequently due to dysregulation of hypothalamic-pituitary-ovarian function; many of the causes of genital bleeding or vaginal discharge listed for prepubertal girls may also occur in this age group.

Evaluation of the female with isosexual precocity

Careful historical review and physical examination initiate the evaluation of the sexually precocious child (Fig. 4-20). Medical history may reveal the presence of an intracranial insult (peripartum trauma; infectious disease; trauma; tumor; irradiation; congenital anomalies; or symptoms suggestive of CNS disease such as visual disturbances, seizures, headaches, and personality changes) or exposure to exogenous sex hormones or other drugs with estrogenic properties. The patterns of linear growth, onset and progression of sexual characteristics, and the family pattern of sexual maturation should be documented. Physical examination should record height, weight, stage(s) of sexual maturation, the presence of diagnostic skin lesions (irregularly bordered "coast of Maine" café au lait spots characteristic of the Albright-McCune-Sternberg syndrome; smooth-bordered "coast of California" café au lait spots and axillary freckling observed in patients with neurofibromatosis, which can be associated with an optic or hypothalamic glioma; or ash-leaf spots typical of tuberous sclerosis), ocular or other signs of CNS dysfunction, findings suggestive of hypothyroidism, palpable adnexal or intravaginal masses, and uterine size.

Skeletal maturation is then assessed: if bone age is appropriate for chronologic age and linear growth rate has been normal, incomplete forms of sexual precocity should be considered. If bone age is significantly delayed (>1 year) behind chronologic age, particularly if linear growth rate is slow, evaluation of thyroid function is important to exclude hypothyroidism. In the girl with premature thelarche, serum estradiol concentrations and gonadotropin secretory dynamics are characteristically prepubertal, although nocturnal gonadotropin secretion may be pulsatile (but is not routinely evaluated). Practically, if the child with suspected premature thelarche has a characteristic history, unremarkable findings on physical examination (including rectal examination) other than for thelarche, normal bone age, and low estrogen level, further hormonal evaluation is not necessary, but follow-up to document the clinical course is mandatory, since thelarche in some of these children evolves into TC/CIP. In the child with suspected premature menarche, however, more complete evaluation including pelvic ultrasound examination and testing with GnRH, as well as prolonged follow-up, are necessary since isolated menses in a prepubertal child is a rather unusual problem.

In the girl with premature pubarche, virilizing signs of hyperandrogenism (acne, clitorimegaly, hirsutism, rapid growth rate, extremely tall stature, and bone age >2 years in advance of chronologic age) are absent; serum DHEA, DHAS, and testosterone concentrations are within the adrenarchal range. Search for an ovarian or adrenal source of androgen secretion is necessary if virilization is present, the bone age is advanced, the growth rate is rapid, and/or serum levels of testosterone and/or DHAS are markedly elevated. Studies of ACTH-stimulated adrenal biosynthetic pathways, GnRH agonist-stimulated ovarian steroidogenesis, and ovarian and adrenal imaging should be undertaken when clinically appropriate. In the protocol proposed by Rosenfield,[210] if initial measurement reveals an elevated free testosterone concentration in a subject with excessive acne, hirsutism, menstrual irregularity, clitorimegaly, and so forth, dexamethasone suppression is followed by testing with ACTH to distinguish among patients with PCO syn-

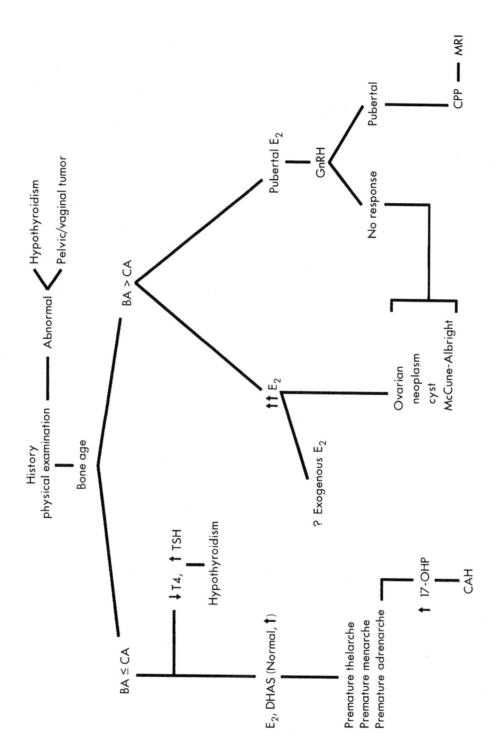

Fig. 4-20. Evaluation of the girl with isosexual precocity. (Redrawn with permission from Schwartz ID, Root AW: Puberty in girls: early, incomplete, or precocious? *Contemp Pediatr* 7[1]:147, 1990. Copyright 1990 by *Contemporary Pediatrics*.)

drome, Cushing disease, congenital adrenal hyperplasia, and other causes of hyperandrogenemia. Serum DHAS concentrations greater than 600 μg/dL are found in subjects with adrenal neoplasms; testosterone values greater than 150 ng/dL suggest a virilizing ovarian or adrenal tumor, although such values may also be found in patients with hyperthecosis.[60]

Girls with thelarche due to an ovarian cyst often do not have rapid growth rate or advanced height or bone ages, because of the acuteness of this disorder. Estradiol concentrations are markedly elevated (200 to 300 pg/mL), gonadotropin secretion is suppressed, and a large (>3 cm), unilateral ovarian cyst is visualized by ultrasonography. Because such cysts occasionally may be due to a central process, careful follow-up and further evaluation is undertaken as indicated. Ovarian sex hormone–secreting neoplasms are often solid, although a cystic component may be present also. Estrogen levels are high in the patient with a granulosa cell tumor; inhibin values may also be increased.[132] The Albright-McCune-Sternberg syndrome is identified by its characteristic triad, although all three characteristics are not present in all patients: 60% of girls with this syndrome have all three characteristics, 30% have café au lait spots and sexual precocity but not fibrous dysplasia, and 10% do not have café au lait spots.[134] Serum estradiol concentrations fluctuate in relation to ovarian cyst size and number; gonadotropin secretion is blunted or prepubertal until there has been sufficient hypothalamic maturation to initiate increased GnRH secretion leading to secondary TC/CIP.

Girls with TC/CIP are characterized by rapid linear growth rate; tall stature; progressive sexual development with thelarche, pubarche, and menarche; advanced skeletal maturation; and pubertal nocturnal and GnRH-provoked gonadotropin secretion (LH predominant).[171,181] Bioactive LH but not bioactive FSH concentrations are higher in girls with TC/CIP than in normal prepubertal subjects or patients with pseudoisosexual or incomplete isosexual precocity (except in rare instances of hCG-secreting neoplasms).[13,266] Adrenal androgen levels are low initially in the majority of girls with TC/CIP, increasing at an appropriate chronologic age.[273] Pelvic ultrasound helps to distinguish between girls with premature thelarche (in whom uterine and ovarian volume are appropriate for age-matched control girls) and those with TC/CIP (in whom uterine and ovarian volumes are greater than, and ovarian architecture is similar to, these features in pubertally matched controls).[219] In girls with premature pubarche, ovarian structure and uterine and ovarian volumes are age appropriate. Magnetic resonance and/or computed tomographic imaging of the CNS is necessary in all girls with TC/CIP to identify a surgically remediable cause of this disorder, such as an arachnoid cyst.[251] Among 73 girls with TC/CIP, Rieth et al.[195] found 8 patients (11%) with hypothalamic masses, 7 of which were hamartomas and 1 a teratoma; 2 girls (3%) had

gliomas of the optic nerve or anterior hypothalamus (1 with neurofibromatosis); 6 girls (8%) had hydrocephalus; and 1 (1%) had a suprasellar subarachnoid cyst; overall, 17 of 73 girls (23%) with TC/CIP had demonstrable CNS lesions, emphasizing the utility of the imaging techniques.

Therapeutic management of the female with isosexual precocity

Appropriate therapy of the sexually precocious girl requires correct diagnostic categorization; long-term follow-up with repetitive clinical and laboratory evaluation are often necessary before the diagnosis and optimal therapeutic management of the individual child can be determined. The parents of children with premature thelarche need to be reassured and the child observed to document her course; since there is a spectrum of clinical and laboratory states between premature thelarche and TC/CIP,[181] it is important to assess periodically the growth rate, skeletal maturation, and hormonal status of girls in whom breast development persists or increases. In girls with isolated premature menarche periodic reevaluation is essential.

In girls with premature pubarche initial reassurance and observation are appropriate. No medical therapy is necessary for girls with premature adrenarche. If a diagnosis of nonclassic congenital adrenal hyperplasia can be established, adrenal-suppressive therapy with glucocorticoids is necessary. However, in girls with premature pubarche and minor abnormalities in cortisol biosynthesis (some of whom perhaps are "carriers" of an abnormal gene for 21-hydroxylase) or in girls with "exaggerated adrenarche," the utility of adrenal suppression is uncertain.[210] In children with virilizing tumors of the ovary or adrenal, surgical removal of the tumor is essential. The adolescent girl with hyperandrogenism due to PCO syndrome should be encouraged to lose weight if obese; cyclic administration of a progestin (medroxyprogesterone acetate, 10 mg nightly for 5 days every 1 to 2 months) may be useful in some girls with irregular menstrual patterns. When dysfunctional uterine bleeding is resistant to cyclic progestin therapy, an oral estrogen/progestin (ethinyl estradiol, 35 μg/ethynodiol diacetate, 1 mg [Demulen 1/35]) may be indicated.[210] Treatment of hirsutism due to ovarian hyperandrogenism in the older adolescent may require ovarian suppression, sometimes in combination with an androgen antagonist.[210]

Estrogen- or androgen-secreting neoplasms of the ovary or adrenal require surgical removal. Postoperatively, long-term follow-up is necessary because some children will enter puberty prematurely if the exposure to high sex hormone concentration has been of sufficient duration to induce hypothalamic maturation. Prospective assessment of GnRH-mediated gonadotropin secretion may permit early diagnosis of evolving TC/CIP more readily than clinical observation alone. If TC/CIP develops, therapy with a GnRH agonist is warranted (vide infra). Management of the girl with an ovarian cyst (not due to hypothyroidism) is a matter of controversy. Some investigators advocate immediate surgical removal.[125] This writer recommends serial clinical, ultrasonographic, and hormonal evaluation for 6 to 8 weeks before surgery, since many of these cysts will regress spontaneously.[141] Grumbach and Kaplan[90] report that administration of medroxyprogesterone, by inhibiting FSH secretion or interfering with steroidogenesis, accelerates regression and prevents recurrence of autonomously functioning ovarian follicular cysts. Careful follow-up of these children is necessary, and search for a primary cause is indicated if clinically or hormonally appropriate.[179]

In the young girl with Albright-McCune-Sternberg syndrome at the stage of functional ovarian autonomy, suppression of estrogen synthesis with the aromatase inhibitor testolactone has been clinically effective. Feuillan et al.[71] administered testolactone (20 mg/kg increasing to 40 mg/kg daily in four divided doses) to five girls with this disorder who responded with decreased serum estradiol concentrations and ovarian volumes, decline in the rates of linear growth and skeletal maturation, and cessation of menses. During testolactone administration, the gonadotropin secretory response to GnRH increased as estrogen-mediated inhibition of GnRH release was alleviated. Since the natural history of this disorder is the evolution of TC/CIP from gonadotropin-independent isosexual precocity,[176] the addition of a GnRH agonist to testolactone is necessary when central stimulation of gonadotropin secretion occurs.[101]

Treatment of the girl with TC/CIP has been dramatically altered with the introduction of agonists of GnRH which, after initial stimulation of pituitary-ovarian function, inhibit gonadotropin secretion by down-regulating GnRH receptor number on the gonadotropin plasma membrane and by altering the synthesis of the gonadotropins leading to primary secretion of the α-subunit.[15,131] It is necessary to emphasize that all girls with TC/CIP do not require therapy with GnRH agonist (GnRHa), particularly those whose sexual maturation begins after 6 to 7 years of age and progresses slowly and whose bone age and height age are comparable, with little expected compromise in adult stature. These latter patients are identified by a bone age-height age ratio of 1.0 and predicted adult height (method of Bayley/Pinneau) similar to target height ([height of mother + height of father ± 13 cm]/2) (2 SD = ± 9.0 cm). Since the course of a child with TC/CIP is variable (it may be transient or advance quite slowly), a period of observation of 6 to 12 months should follow the initial diagnostic studies, particularly in girls with idiopathic TC/CIP. Children with a known insult to the CNS as a cause of TC/CIP are more likely to have progressive sexual maturation. Surgically remediable lesions (arachnoid cyst, hydrocephalus, neoplasm, or abscess) should be corrected primarily and the child's progress reassessed serially after successful surgery before initiating GnRHa. Neurosurgical removal of a hypothalamic hamartoma is not usually recommended

since the TC/CIP caused by this disorder is responsive to gonadotropin suppression and the clinical course is benign, unless the lesion is so large as to cause obstructive hydrocephalus and/or seizures.[26,195] Irradiation and/or chemotherapy for an intracranial neoplasm should be completed and the child reevaluated serially, especially for development of GH deficiency, before GnRH therapy of the sexual development is initiated.

The objectives of the management of children with TC/CIP as outlined by Grumbach and Kaplan[90] are as follows:

1. Identification and treatment of an identifiable, correctable CNS lesion
2. Regression of sexual characteristics and arrest of pubertal progression
3. Suppression of the rapid rates of linear growth and skeletal maturation to preserve and increase (if possible) final adult stature
4. Management of any psychosocial, behavioral, or educational problems that may accompany precocious puberty
5. Prevention of sexual abuse and pregnancy
6. Reinitiation of pubertal development at an appropriate point, and preservation of fertility

Criteria for treatment of a girl with documented TC/CIP with GnRHa are as follows[117,127]:

1. Rapidly advancing progressive thelarche and pubarche over 6 to 12 months of observation
2. Cyclic menses before age 7
3. Rapid linear growth rate and progression of skeletal maturation
4. Decrease in predicted height of 5 cm by sequential estimation over 6 months or more
5. Predicted adult height less than 152.5 cm unless comparable to target height

It should be emphasized that these criteria are flexible and should be considered in relationship to the clinical/hormonal/psychosocial status of the individual child. As a group, children with precocious puberty tend to have more behavioral problems and less social competence than do prepubertal girls of the same age, although clearly there are many individual exceptions to these observations.[157] Children with lower intellectual competence may be more vulnerable to behavioral disturbances, but the majority of girls with idiopathic TC/CIP are of average to high-average intelligence. As adolescents, girls who had TC/CIP as children are generally well adjusted and psychosexually appropriate for chronologic age. (Since young girls with TC/CIP are fertile, even closer parental supervision than usual is necessary.)

In the majority of girls with TC/CIP, except for short stature and whatever psychosocial problems may attend early sexual development, the process is usually benign.[206]

Table 4-11. Agonists of GnRH employed in the treatment of central isosexual precocity*

GnRH†	1 PyroGlu	2 His	3 Trp	4 Ser	5 Tyr	6 Gly	7 Leu	8 Arg	9 Pro	10 Gly-NH₂
Tryptorelin (Decapeptyl)		. . . .				D-Trp	. . . .			
Leuprolide		. . . .				D-Leu	. . . .			EthNH₂
Buserelin		. . . .				D-Ser(tBU)	. . . .			EthNH₂
Nafarelin		. . . .				D-Nal(2)	. . . .			EthNH₂
Deslorelin		. . . .				D-Trp	. . . .			EthNH₂
Histrelin		. . . .				D-His(ImB21)	. . . .			EthNH₂

*Data are from references 45 and 271. EthNH₂, Ethylamide; tBU, t-butyl-D-serine; D-Nal(2), D-naphthylalanine.
†Dosages: Tryptorelin, 20-40 μg/kg/d subcutaneously (sc); 50-100 μg/kg/mo intramuscularly (im). Leuprolide, 20-40 μg/kg/d sc; 140-300 μg/kg/mo im. Buserelin, 20-40 μg/kg/d sc; 1200-1800 μg/d intranasally. Nafarelin, 4-8 μg/kg/d sc; 800-1600 μg/d intranasally. Deslorelin, 4-8 μg/kg/d sc.

Therefore, selection of the girl with TC/CIP for GnRHa treatment using the guidelines listed is important. A number of GnRHa have been used in the successful therapy of children with TC/CIP (Table 4-11). In general, native GnRH has been modified to decrease its rate of degradation and thus increase its effective biologic half-life. These modifications have included removal of the amino-terminal glycine amide and replacement by an alkylamine ethylamide and substitution of a D-amino acid at position 6 (glycine by D-tryptophan, D-serine, D-leucine) or hydrophobic alteration at the same position (D-Nal [2]⁶). Even with these chemical modifications, daily (and sometimes twice and thrice daily) injections of GnRHa are required to achieve complete gonadotropin secretion.²³⁷ Intranasal administration of these analogues four times daily (but at much higher doses) also suppresses pituitary gonadotropin secretion in most, but not all, recipients. Suspension of GnRHa in biodegradable microcapsules of lactide-glycolide copolymer yields depot forms of GnRHa that are effective for 21 to 28 days, thus decreasing substantially the frequency of injections and increasing effective gonadotropin suppression.²⁷¹

Administration of a GnRHa to a child with TC/CIP leads to suppression of spontaneous secretion of gonadotropins and gonadal sex hormones over the 24-hour period, inhibition of GnRH-stimulated gonadotropin release, and decline in spontaneous secretion of GH and in IGF-I concentrations. Clinically, this is accompanied by cessation of menses (if present; one episode of vaginal bleeding often occurs 10 to 14 days after initiation of GnRHa therapy and reflects the initial surge in gonadotropin and sex hormone secretion due to the agonist property of these compounds), arrest or regression of thelarche and pubarche, decline in linear growth rate, and decline in the rate of skeletal maturation.⁴⁵

Boepple et al.¹⁷ report that in 40 girls with TC/CIP treated with [D-Trp⁶, Pro⁹ ethylamide] GnRH (4 to 8 μg/g

per day subcutaneously) for 3 years, secretion of spontaneous and stimulated gonadotropins was suppressed and serum estradiol levels and vaginal cytologic maturation index declined to prepubertal values. In this series growth velocity declined from 10.1 cm/y (+3.3 SD for chronologic age) before treatment to 5.8, 4.6, and 3.2 cm/y during the first through third years of GnRHa administration, respectively. The change in the bone age–chronologic age ratio was less than 1.0 during therapy and the predicted adult height increased by 6.7 cm after 3 years of treatment. Grumbach and Kaplan,⁹⁰ using the same GnRHa, treated 12 girls with TC/CIP for 3 years; they recorded essentially similar laboratory and clinical observations; three girls experienced recurrent hot flushes as a consequence of estrogen withdrawal. These investigators also administered nafarelin intranasally to 17 girls with TC/CIP with comparable findings to the response to [D-Trp⁶, Pro⁹ ethylamide] GnRH, although the period before gonadotropin suppression was longer after nasal administration (12 weeks) than after subcutaneous administration (2 weeks). Kreiter et al.¹²⁷ treated 14 girls with TC/CIP with intranasal nafarelin and reported arrest of sexual development, suppression of gonadotropin and estrogen secretion within 6 months, decreased rates of linear growth and skeletal maturation, and slightly improved height prediction (+2 cm) after 2 years of therapy. However, these investigators point out that in a group of untreated girls with TC/CIP but similar height and bone ages, predicted height increased 2.7 cm over a 2-year period. They conclude that GnRHa therapy can *preserve* height potential in such patients.

Oostdijk et al.¹⁷³ treated 74 girls with a depot form of D-Trp⁶ GnRH (Decapeptyl) (50 to 100 μg/kg at 4-week intervals). Menses ceased promptly in each of the 12 postmenarcheal girls, breast growth arrested and perhaps regressed slightly, gonadotropin and sex hormone secretion decreased promptly, growth rate declined to one-half the pretreatment growth velocity, skeletal maturation slowed,

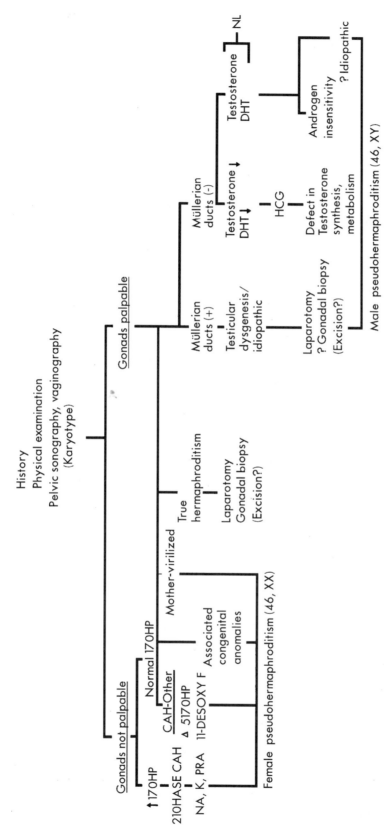

Fig. 4-21. Evaluation of the neonate with ambiguous genitalia. 17OHP, 17-Hydroxyprogesterone; 21OHASE, 21-hydroxylase; CAH, congenital adrenal hyperplasia; DHT, dihydrotestosterone; NL, normal; 11-DESOXY F, 11-desoxy cortisol; PRA, plasma renin activity. (Redrawn from Root AW: Abnormalities of sexual differentiation and maturation. In Kaye R, Oski FA, Barness LA, editors: *Core textbook of pediatrics*, Philadelphia, 1989, JB Lippincott.)

and predicted height increased (+2.2 cm) after 18 months of therapy. Similar observations have been made after administration of depot-leuprolide.[119]

Once treatment with a GnRHa is initiated and effective suppression of gonadotropin and sex hormone secretion is achieved, 3-month clinical and hormonal evaluation is recommended. Periodic assessment of skeletal maturation and pelvic ultrasonography are important also.

After termination of GnRHa therapy between 11 and 13 years of age, pituitary-ovarian function reactivates promptly and cyclic menses occur within 12 months in the majority of subjects. In 60% of girls, menses resume within 2 years after cessation of GnRHa therapy.[90,149,178] Kauli et al.[123] reported that seven of eight girls with TC/CIP treated with D-Trp[6]-GnRH after 8 years of age for 15 to 41 months achieved heights that exceeded pretreatment-predicted heights by 1.0 to 16.3 cm. In three subjects adult-achieved height exceeded pretreatment-predicted height by 6.4, 11.8, and 16.3 cm. On the other hand, Boepple et al.[18] report that in 27 girls with TC/CIP treated with GnRHa the average increase in final height was only 2.4 cm over predicted height, within the expected change suggested by Kreiter et al.[127] Paul et al.[178] report that in 15 children (11 females) with TC/CIP treated with GnRHa, final height was at target height in 7 of 15 and within 2 SD of target height in 6 of 15. Thus current data do not as yet permit definitive assessment of the effect of GnRHa therapy on achieved final height. Successful therapy depends on selection of an effective dose of GnRHa administered to a compliant patient. It is possible—perhaps even probable—that as selection criteria for treatment are more rigidly defined, younger children are treated for longer periods, and long-acting preparations of GnRHa are employed (thus enhancing gonadotropin suppression and lessening the chance for noncompliance) significantly increased final heights will be attained. In patients with GH deficiency and TC/CIP (due to CNS irradiation primarily) combined GH and GnRHa are required to optimize growth.[35,36]

Side effects of GnRHa are few; occasionally local erythema at the injection site is seen; anaphylaxis is rare.[90] Antibodies to the GnRHa may occasionally develop, but the clinical significance of these immunoglobulins is uncertain. This writer has observed one patient who developed recurrent sterile abscesses at the site of injection of a depot form of GnRHa. Development of GnRH analogues with antagonist activity is progressing rapidly; these agents, which block GnRH action and have immediate onset of prolonged action, will prove useful in the treatment of children with TC/CIP.[45]

Appropriate psychologic support for children with sexual precocity and their families is important.[157] Such support consists primarily of informing the patients of the situation and calm reassurance as to eventual outcome as appropriate.

Heterosexual precocious puberty

Heterosexual precocity in the genetic female may be congenital, resulting in female pseudohermaphroditism, or acquired, leading to virilization (please see the box below).

The most common cause of female pseudohermaphroditism is classic 21-hydroxylase–deficient congenital adrenal hyperplasia due to an abnormality in the gene structure for P450c21. Two *CYP21* genes are present on the short arm of the sixth chromosome; one is a shortened pseudogene (*CYP21A*) and the other (*CYP21B*) the active gene. Deletions, base substitutions, gene conversions, and other errors have been described in the *CYP21B* structure, leading to deficiency of enzyme activity, impairment of cortisol and aldosterone biosynthesis, and compensatory increase in fetal adrenal androgen synthesis resulting in masculinization of the external genitalia (fusion of labial-scrotal and urethral folds and clitoral hypertrophy, occasionally with complete incorporation of the urethra into the enlarged phallus, but more commonly with a residual urogenital sinus) with normal development of the ovaries and müllerian duct derivatives. An elevated serum concentration of 17α-hydroxyprogesterone suppressed by administration of glucocorticoids is the biochemical hallmark of this disorder.[53,272] Virilization of the external genitalia of the female fetus may be due to the 11β-hydroxylase–deficient and 3β-hydroxysteroid dehydrogenase–deficient forms of congenital adrenal hyperplasia, to a maternal source of andro-

---

Causes of heterosexual precocious puberty in females

I. Prenatal virilization

A. CONGENITAL ADRENAL HYPERPLASIA
   1. Deficiency of P450c21
   2. Deficiency of P450c11

B. MATERNAL ANDROGENS
   1. Congenital adrenal hyperplasia
   2. Luteoma
   3. Ingestion

C. IDIOPATHIC CAUSES
   1. Associated with other anomalies

II. Acquired virilization

A. NONCLASSIC CONGENITAL ADRENAL HYPERPLASIA
   1. Deficiency of P 450c21
   2. Deficiency of P 450c11
   3. Deficiency of 3 β-hydroxysteroid dehydrogenase

B. ADRENAL CAUSES
   1. Virilizing neoplasm
   2. Cushing syndrome

C. OVARIAN CAUSES
   1. Arrhenoblastoma
   2. Hyperthecosis
   3. Deficiency of 17-ketoreductase

D. ANDROGEN INGESTION (COMPETITIVE ATHLETICS)

gen, or to association with congenital anomalies of the genitourinary tract and a variety of eponymic syndromes. A scheme for the evaluation of a newborn with ambiguous genitalia is presented in Fig. 4-21. Acquired sources of virilization in the female are discussed earlier in this chapter.

ACKNOWLEDGMENT

The author thanks Ms. Sandy Tyo and Ms. Lucille Curtin for exceptional secretarial assistance.

REFERENCES

1. Abrams GM, Valiquette G: Neuroendocrinology: clinical and experimental, *Curr Opin Neurol Neurosurg* 4:466, 1991.
2. Adashi EY et al: Growth factors and follicle function. In Adashi EY, Mancuso S, editors: *Major advances in human female reproduction,* New York, 1990, Raven Press.
3. Ahonen P et al: Clinical variation of autoimmune polyendocrinopathy-candidiasis-ectodermal dystrophy (APECED) in a series of 68 patients, *N Engl J Med* 322:1829, 1990.
4. Amiel SA et al: Insulin resistance of puberty: a defect restricted to peripheral glucose metabolism, *J Clin Endocrinol Metab* 72:277, 1991.
5. Apter D et al: Serum luteinizing hormone concentrations increase 100-fold in females from 7 years of age to adulthood, as measured by time-resolved immunofluorometric assay, *J Clin Endocrinol Metab* 68:53, 1989.
6. Arisaka O et al: Ovarian cysts in precocious puberty, *Clin Pediatr* 28:44, 1989.
7. Attie KM et al: The pubertal growth spurt in eight patients with true precocious puberty and growth hormone deficiency: evidence for a direct role of sex steroids, *J Clin Endocrinol Metab* 71:975, 1990.
8. Averette HE, Boike GM, Jarell MA: Effects of cancer chemotherapy on gonadal function and reproductive capacity, *CA* 40:199, 1990.
9. Badawy SZA, Marshall L, Refaie A: Primary amenorrhea-oligomenorrhea due to prolactinomas in adolescent and adult girls, *Adolesc Pediatr Gynecol* 4:27, 1991.
10. Barbarino A et al: Sexual dimorphism of pyridostigmine potentiation of growth hormone (GH)-releasing hormone-induced GH release in humans, *J Clin Endocrinol Metab* 73:75, 1991.
11. Bchini O et al: Precocious mammary gland development and milk protein synthesis in transgenic mice ubiquitously expressing human growth hormone, *Endocrinology* 128:539, 1991.
12. Beck-Peccoz P et al: Maturation of hypothalamic-pituitary-gonadal function in normal human fetuses: circulating levels of gonadotropins, their common α-subunit and free testosterone, and discrepancy between immunological and biological activities of circulating follicle-stimulating hormone, *J Clin Endocrinol Metab* 73:525, 1991.
13. Beitins IZ, Padmanabhan V: Bioactivity of gonadotropins, *Endocrinol Metab Clin North Am* 20:85, 1991.
14. Beitins IZ et al: Serum bioactive follicle stimulating hormone concentrations from prepuberty to adulthood: a cross-sectional study: *J Clin Endocrinol Metab* 71:1022, 1990.
15. Bhasin S, Swerdloff RS: Mechanisms of gonadotropin-releasing hormone agonist action in the human male, *Endocr Rev* 7:106, 1986.
16. Blatt J, Bercu BB, Gillin JC: Reduced pulsatile growth hormone secretion in children after therapy for acute lymphoblastic leukemia, *J Pediatr* 104:182, 1984.
17. Boepple PA et al: Impact of sex steroids and their suppression on skeletal growth and maturation, *Am J Physiol* 255(*Endocrinol Metab* 18):E559, 1988.
18. Boepple PA et al: Final heights in girls with central precocious puberty (CPP) following GnRH agonist (GnRHa)-induced pituitary-gonadal suppression, *Pediatr Res* 29:74A, 1991.
19. Borkowski A et al: Estrogen-like activity of a subpopulation of natural antiestrogen receptor autoantibodies in man, *Endocrinology* 128:3283, 1991.
20. Bourguignon JP: Linear growth as a function of age at onset of puberty and sex steroid dosage: therapeutic implications, *Endocr Rev* 9:467, 1988.
21. Bourguignon JP, Gerard A, Franchimont P: Direct activation of gonadotropin-releasing hormone secretion through different receptors to neuroexcitatory amino acids, *Neuroenocrinology* 49:402, 1989.
22. Bourguignon JP, Gerard A, Franchimont P: Maturation of the hypothalamic control of pulsatile gonadotropin-releasing hormone secretion at onset of puberty, II: reduced potency of an inhibitory autofeedback, *Endocrinology* 127:2884, 1990.
23. Bourguignon JP et al: Hypopituitarism and idiopathic delayed puberty: a longitudinal study in an attempt to diagnose gonadotropin deficiency before puberty, *J Clin Endocrinol Metab* 54:733, 1982.
24. Bourguignon JP et al: Maturation of the hypothalamic control of pulsatile gonadotropin-releasing hormone secretion at onset of puberty, I: Increased activation of *N*-methyl-D-aspartate receptors, *Endocrinology* 127:873, 1990.
25. Bourguignon JP et al: ANMDA-receptor mediated restraint of pulsatile GnRH secretion is removed at onset of puberty, *Endocrinology* 128:306A, 1991.
26. Boyko OB et al: Hamartomas of the tuber cinerium: CT, MR, and pathologic findings, *AJNR* 12:309, 1991.
27. Bramswig JH et al: Adult height in boys and girls with untreated short stature and constitutional delay of growth and puberty: accuracy of five different methods of height prediction, *J Pediatr* 117:886, 1990.
28. Brown RS, Bhatia V, Hayes E: An apparent cluster of congenital hypopituitarism in central Massachusetts: magnetic resonance imaging and hormonal studies, *J Clin Endocrinol Metab* 72:12, 1991.
29. Burger HG et al: Serum inhibin concentrations rise throughout normal male and female puberty, *J Clin Endocrinol Metab* 67:689, 1988.
30. Burger HG et al: Human chorionic gonadotropin raises serum immunoreactive inhibin levels in men with hypogonadotropic hypogonadism, *Reprod Fertil Dev* 2:137, 1990.
31. Burger HG et al: Serum gonadotropin, sex steroid and immunoreactive inhibin levels in the first two years of life, *J Clin Endocrinol Metab* 72:682, 1991.
32. Cacciari E et al: How many cases of true precocious puberty in girls are idiopathic?, *J Pediatr* 102:357, 1983.
33. Cacciatore B et al: Ultrasonic characteristic of the uterus and ovaries in relation to pubertal development and serum LH, FSH and estradiol concentrations, *Adolesc Pediatr Gynecol* 4:15, 1991.
34. Caprio S et al: Increased insulin secretion in puberty: a compensatory response to reduction in insulin sensitivity, *J Pediatr* 114:963, 1989.
35. Cara JF, Kreiter M, Rosenfield RL: Height prognosis of children with coexistent growth hormone deficiency and true precocious puberty: effect of combined treatment with gonadotropin releasing hormone agonist, *Pediatr Res* 29:75A, 1991.
36. Cara JF et al: Growth hormone deficiency impedes the rise in plasma insulin-like growth factor-I levels associated with precocious puberty, *J Pediatr* 115:64, 1989.
37. Case records of the Massachusetts General Hospital: Resistant ovary syndrome, *N Engl J Med* 315:1336, 1986.
38. Cate RL, Donahoe PK, MacLaughlin DT: Müllerian-inhibiting substance. In Sporn MB, Roberts AB, editors: *Peptide growth factors and their receptors,* vol 2, Berlin, 1990, Springer-Verlag.
39. Chappel S: Biological to immunological ratios: reevaluation of a concept, *J Clin Endocrinol Metab* 70:1494, 1990 (editorial).
40. Chowen-Breed JA, Steiner RA, Clifton DK: Sexual dimorphism and testosterone-dependent regulation of somatostatin gene expression in

the periventricular nucleus of the rat brain, *Endocrinology* 125:357, 1989.

41. Churesigaew S: Natural history of premature thelarche, *J Med Assoc Thai* 72:198, 1989.

42. Clayton RN, Catt KJ: Gonadotropin-releasing hormone receptors: characterization, physiological regulation and relationship to reproductive function, *Endocr Rev* 2:186, 1981.

43. Clemmons DR: Insulin-like growth factor binding proteins, *Trends Endocrinol Metab* 1:412, 1990.

44. Comite F et al: Isosexual precocious pseudopuberty secondary to a feminizing adrenal tumor, *J Clin Endocrinol Metab* 58:435, 1984.

45. Conn PM, Crowley WF Jr: Gonadotropin-releasing hormone and its analogues, *N Engl J Med* 324:93, 1991.

46. Conte F, Grumbach MM, Kaplan SL: A diphasic pattern of gonadotropin secretion in patients with gonadal dysgenesis, *J Clin Endocrinol Metab* 40:670, 1975.

47. Cook JS et al: Growth hormone secretion during puberty in normal children, *Pediatr Res* 29:76A, 1991.

48. Copeland KC: Variations in normal sexual development, *Pediatr Rev* 8:47, 1986.

49. Corvol MT et al: Evidence for a direct *in vitro* action of sex steroids on rabbit cartilage cells during skeletal growth: influence of age and sex, *Endocrinology* 120:1422, 1987.

50. Cowan BD, Morrison JC: Management of abnormal genital bleeding in girls and women, *N Engl J Med* 324:1710, 1991.

51. Cristiano AM et al: Prolactin response to metoclopramide does not distinguish patients with hypogonadotrophic hypogonadism from delayed puberty, *Clin Endocrinol* 28:75, 1988.

52. Cunningham BC et al: Zinc mediation of the binding of human growth hormone to the human prolactin receptor, *Science* 250:1709, 1990.

53. Cutler GB Jr, Laue L: Congenital adrenal hyperplasia due to 21-hydroxylase deficiency, *N Engl J Med* 323:1806, 1990.

54. Cutler GB Jr et al: Pubertal growth: physiology and pathophysiology, *Recent Prog Horm Res* 42:443, 1986.

55. Darendeliler F et al: Growth hormone increases rate of pubertal maturation, *Acta Endocrinol* 122:414, 1990.

56. Dayani N et al: Estrogen receptors in cultured rabbit articular chondrocytes: influence of age, *J Steroid Biochem* 31:351, 1988.

57. deRidder CM et al: Body fat mass, body fat distribution and plasma hormones in early puberty in females, *J Clin Endocrinol Metab* 70:888, 1990.

58. Dhuper S et al: Effects of hormonal status on bone density in adolescent girls, *J Clin Endocrinol Metab* 71:1083, 1990.

59. Dufau ML et al: Effect of luteinizing hormone releasing hormone (LHRH) upon bioactive and immunoreactive serum LH levels in normal subjects, *J Clin Endocrinol Metab* 43:658, 1976.

60. Dunaif A: Case records of the Massachusetts General Hospital, *N Engl J Med* 318:1449, 1988.

61. Editorial: The secret of sex?, *Lancet* 2:348, 1990.

62. Editorial: Insulin resistance in puberty, *Lancet* 337:1259, 1991.

63. Editorial: Imprinting makes an impression, *Lancet* 338:413, 1991.

64. Ehrmann DA, Rosenfield RL: An endocrinologic approach to hirsutism, *J Clin Endocrinol Metab* 71:1, 1990.

65. Ehrmann DA, Rosenfield RL: Gonadotropin-releasing hormone agonist testing of pituitary-gonadal function, *Trends Endocrinol Metab* 2:86, 1991.

66. Elster AD et al: Pituitary gland: MR imaging of physiologic hypertrophy in adolescence, *Radiology* 174:681, 1990.

67. Ernst M, Heath JK, Rodan GA: Estradiol effects on proliferation, messenger ribonucleic acid for collagen and insulin-like growth factor-I, and parathyroid hormone-stimulated adenylate cyclase activity in osteoblastic cells from calvariae and long bones, *Endocrinology* 125:825, 1989.

68. Ernst M, Rodan GA: Increased activity of insulin-like growth factor (IGF) in osteoblastic cells in the presence of growth hormone (GH):

positive correlation with the presence of the GH-induced IGF-binding protein BP-3, *Endocrinology* 127:807, 1990.

69. Faglia G et al: Excess of β-subunit of thyrotropin (TSH) in patients with idiopathic central hypothyroidism due to secretion of TSH with reduced biological activity, *J Clin Endocrinol Metab* 56:908, 1983.

70. Fakhry J et al: Sonography of autonomous follicular ovarian cysts in precocious pseudopuberty, *J Ultrasound Med* 7:597, 1988.

71. Feuillan PP et al: Treatment of precocious puberty in the McCune-Albright syndrome with the aromatase inhibitor testolactone, *N Engl J Med* 315:1115, 1986.

72. Filicori M et al: Characterization of the physiologic pattern of episodic gonadotropin secretion throughout the human menstrual cycle, *J Clin Endocrinol Metab* 62:1136, 1986.

73. Fisher DA et al: Serum T4, TBG, T3 uptake, T3, reverse T3 and TSH concentrations in children 1-15 years old, *J Clin Endocrinol Metab* 45:191, 1977.

74. Fisher EM et al: Homologous ribosomal protein genes on the human X and Y chromosomes: escape from X inactivation and possible implications for Turner syndrome, *Cell* 63:1205, 1990.

75. Fontoura M et al: Precocious puberty in girls: early diagnosis of a slowly progressive variant, *Arch Dis Child* 64:1170, 1989.

76. Foster CM et al: Ovarian function in girls with McCune-Albright syndrome, *Pediatr Res* 20:859, 1986.

77. Frejaville E et al: Breast contact thermography for differentiation between premature thelarche and true precocious puberty, *Eur J Pediatr* 147:389, 1988.

78. Frisch RE: Body fat, puberty and fertility, *Biol Rev* 59:161, 1984.

79. Frisch RE: Fatness and fertility, *Sci Am* 258:88, 1988.

80. Fujieda K, Hosoda A, Matsuura N: Day-night rhythm and pulsatile gonadotropin secretion in prepubertal children, *Endocrinology* 128:1105A, 1991.

81. Fukata J, Martin JB: Influence of sex steroid hormones on rat growth hormone-releasing factor and somatostatin in dispersed pituitary cells, *Endocrinology* 119:2256, 1986.

82. Garibaldi LR et al: Serum luteinizing hormone concentrations as measured by a sensitive immunoradiometric assay in children with normal, precocious or delayed pubertal development, *J Clin Endocrinol Metab* 72:888, 1991.

83. Garn SM et al: Maturational timing as a factor in female fatness and obesity, *Am J Clin Nutr* 43:879, 1986.

84. Gay VL, Plant TM: N-Methyl-D-L aspartate elicits hypothalamic gonadotropin-releasing hormone release in prepubertal male rhesus monkeys (Macaca mulatta), *Endocrinology* 120:2289, 1987.

85. Genazzani AR, Petraglia F: Opioid control of luteinizing hormone in humans, *J Steroid Biochem* 33:751, 1989.

86. Gilsanz V et al: Vertebrae bone density in children: effect of puberty, *Radiology* 166:847, 1988.

87. Giordano G, Barreca A, Minuto F: Growth factors and puberty. In Adashi EY, Mancuso S, editors: *Major advances in human female reproduction,* New York, 1990, Raven Press.

88. Glastre C et al: Measurement of bone mineral content of the lumbar spine by dual energy X-ray absorptiometry in normal children: correlations with growth parameters, *J Clin Endocrinol Metab* 70:1330, 1990.

89. Gomez MT et al: Urinary free cortisol values in normal children and adolescents, *J Pediatr* 118:256, 1991.

90. Grumbach MM, Kaplan SL: Recent advances in the diagnosis and management of sexual precocity, *Acta Paediatr Jpn Overseas Ed* 30(suppl):155, 1988.

91. Guidice LC: The insulin-like growth factor autocrine-paracrine system and its role in ovarian folliculogenesis. Syllabus: *Frontiers in reproductive endocrinology,* Washington, DC, April 22-26, 1991, pp 95-108.

92. Hammer LD et al: Impact of pubertal development on body fat distribution among white, Hispanic and Asian female adolescents, *J Pediatr* 118:975, 1981.

93. Hammer LD et al: Standardized percentile curves of body-mass index for children and adolescents, *Am J Dis Child* 145:259, 1991.

94. Harlan WR, Harlan EA, Grillo GP: Secondary characteristics of girls 12 to 17 years of age: the US health examination survey, *J Pediatr* 96:1074, 1980.

95. Hein K: The interface of chronic illness and the hormonal regulation of puberty, *J Adolesc Health Care* 8:530, 1987.

96. Heinze HJ, Root AW: The Turner syndrome of gonadal dysgenesis, *Clin Pract Gynecol* 3:125, 1992.

97. Herman-Giddens MF, MacMillan JP: Prevalence of secondary sexual characteristics in a population of North Carolina girls 3 to 10, *Adolesc Pediatr Gynecol* 4:21, 1991.

98. Herman-Giddens ME, Sandler AD, Friedman NE: Sexual precocity in girls: an association with sexual abuse?, *Am J Dis Child* 142:431, 1988.

99. Hindmarsh P et al: Changes in serum insulin concentrations during puberty and their relationship to growth hormone, *Clin Endocrinol* 28:381, 1988.

100. Ho Ky et al: Effects of sex and age on the 24 hour profile of growth hormone secretion in man: importance of endogenous oestradiol concentrations, *J Clin Endocrinol Metab* 64:51, 1987.

101. Holland FJ: Gonadotropin-independent precocious puberty, *Endocrinol Metab Clin North Am* 20:191, 1991.

102. Holly JMP et al: Levels of the small insulin-like growth factor-binding protein are strongly related to those of insulin in prepubertal and pubertal children but only weakly so after puberty, *J Endocrinol* 121:383, 1989.

103. Holly JMP et al: Relationship between the pubertal fall in sex hormone binding globulin and insulin-like growth factor binding protein-I: a synchronized approach to pubertal development?, *Clin Endocrinol* 31:277, 1989.

104. Homberg R et al: Cotreatment with human growth hormone and gonadotropins for induction of ovulation: a controlled clinical trial, *Fertil Steril* 53:254, 1990.

105. Horner JM, Thorsson AV, Hintz RL: Growth deceleration patterns in children with constitutional short stature, *Pediatrics* 62:529, 1978.

106. Howlett TA et al: Prolactinomas presenting as primary amenorrhea and delayed or arrested puberty: response to medical therapy, *Clin Endocrinol* 30:131, 1989.

107. Hudson PL et al: An immunoassay to detect human müllerian inhibiting substance in males and females during normal development, *J Clin Endocrinol Metab* 70:16, 1990.

108. Hurley DM et al: Induction of ovulation and fertility in amenorrheic women by pulsatile low-dose gonadotropin-releasing hormone, *N Engl J Med* 310:1069, 1984.

109. Ibanez L et al: Growth, maturation and final height in premature pubarche, *Acta Paediatr Scand Suppl* 366:129A, 1990.

110. Ilicki A et al: Premature thelarche: natural history and sex hormone secretion in 68 girls, *Acta Paediatr Scand* 73:756, 1984.

111. Iyer KS, McCann SM: Delta sleep inducing peptide (DSIP) stimulates the release of LH, but not FSH via a hypothalamic site of action in the rat, *Brain Res Bull* 19:535, 1987.

112. Jaakkola T et al: The ratios of serum bioactive/immunoreactive luteinizing hormone and follicle stimulating hormone in various clinical conditions with increased and decreased gonadotropin secretion: reevaluation by a highly sensitive immunometric assay, *J Clin Endocrinol Metab* 70:1496, 1990.

113. Jakacki RI et al: Pulsatile secretion of luteinizing hormone in children, *J Clin Endocrinol Metab* 55:453, 1982.

114. Jorgensen JOL et al: Short-term changes in serum insulin-like growth factors (IGF) and IGF binding protein 3 after different modes of intravenous growth hormone (GH) exposure in GH-deficient patients, *J Clin Endocrinol Metab* 72:582, 1991.

115. Josso N et al: An enzyme linked immunoassay for anti-müllerian hormone: a new tool for the evaluation of testicular function in infants and children, *J Clin Endocrinol Metab* 70:23, 1990.

116. Kalter-Leibovici O et al: Late onset 21-hydroxylase deficiency in a girl mimicking true sexual precocity, *J Pediatr Endocrinol* 3:121, 1989.

117. Kaplan SL, Grumbach MM: Pathophysiology and treatment of sexual precocity, *J Clin Endocrinol Metab* 71:785, 1990.

118. Kaplowitz PB, Cockrell JL, Young RB: Premature adrenarche: clinical and diagnostic features, *Clin Pediatr* 29:28, 1986.

119. Kappy M et al: Suppression of gonadotropin secretion by a long-acting gonadotropin-releasing hormone analog (leuprolide acetate, Lupron depot) in children with precocious puberty, *J Clin Endocrinol Metab* 69:1087, 1989.

120. Karlberg J: On the construction of the infancy-childhood-puberty growth standard, *Acta Paediatr Scand Suppl* 356:26, 1989.

121. Katz JT et al: Toward an elucidation of the psychoendocrinology of anorexia nervosa. In Sachar EJ, editor: *Hormones, behavior and psychopathology*, New York, 1976, Raven Press.

122. Kaufman FR, Donnell GN, Lobo RA: Ovarian androgen secretion in patients with galactosemia and premature ovarian failure, *Fertil Steril* 47:1033, 1987.

123. Kauli R, Kornreich L, Laron Z: Pubertal development, growth and final height in girls with sexual precocity after therapy with the GnRH analogue D-Trp[6]-LHRH, *Horm Res* 33:11, 1990.

124. Kolata G: When grandmother is the mother, until birth, *New York Times* CXL:48,683, Aug 5, 1991, p A1, A11.

125. Kosloske AM et al: Treatment of precocious pseudopuberty associated with follicular cysts of the ovary, *Am J Dis Child* 138:147, 1984.

126. Krainz PL, Hanna CE, LaFranchi SH: Etiology of delayed puberty in 146 children evaluated over a 10 year period, *J Pediatr Endocrinol* 2:165, 1987.

127. Kreiter M et al: Preserving adult height potential in girls with idiopathic true precocious puberty, *J Pediatr* 117:364, 1990.

128. Lacson AG, Gillis DA, Shawwa A: Malignant mixed germ cell-sex cord-stromal tumors of the ovary associated with isosexual precocious puberty, *Cancer* 61:2122, 1988.

129. LaFranchi S, Hanna CE, Mandel SH: Constitutional delay of growth: expected versus final adult height, *Pediatrics* 87:82, 1991.

130. Landy H et al: Sleep modulation of neuroendocrine function: developmental changes in gonadotropin-releasing hormone secretion during sexual maturation, *Pediatr Res* 28:213, 1990.

131. Landy H et al: Altered patterns of pituitary secretion and renal excretion of free α-subunit during gonadotropin-releasing hormone agonist-induced pituitary desensitization, *J Clin Endocrinol Metab* 72:711, 1991.

132. Lappohn RE et al: Inhibin as a marker for granulosa-cell tumors, *N Engl J Med* 321:790, 1989.

133. Largo RH, Prader A: Pubertal development in girls: variability and interrelationships, *Pediatrician* 14:212, 1987.

134. Lee PA, Van Dop C, Migeon CJ: McCune-Albright syndrome long-term follow-up, *JAMA* 256:2980, 1986.

135. Leiper AD et al: Precocious or early puberty and growth failure in girls treated for acute lymphoblastic leukemia, *Horm Res* 30:72, 1988.

136. LeRoith D et al: Insulin-like growth factors and their receptors in normal physiology and pathologic states, *Trends Endocrinol Metab* 2:134, 1991.

137. Leung AKC: Premature thelarche, *J Singapore Paediatr Soc* 31:64, 1989.

138. Leung DW et al: Growth hormone receptor and serum binding protein: purification, cloning and expression, *Nature* 330:537, 1987.

139. Li JY et al: Bone mineral content in black and white children 1 to 6 years of age: early appearance of race and sex differences, *Am J Dis Child* 143:1346, 1989.

140. Lifshitz F: Nutritional dwarfing in adolescents, *Growth Genet Horm* 3(4):1, 1987.

141. Lightner ES, Kelch RP: Treatment of precocious pseudopuberty associated with ovarian cysts, *Am J Dis Child* 138:126, 1984.

142. Lim L et al: Regulation of growth hormone (GH) bioactivity by a recombinant human GH-binding protein, *Endocrinology* 127:1287, 1990.

143. Lindsay AN, Voorhess ML, MacGillivray MH: Multicystic ovaries detected by sonography, *Am J Dis Child* 134:588, 1980.

144. Ling X et al: Isosexual precocious puberty: clinical analysis of 109 patients, *Chin Med J [Engl]* 100:865, 1987.

145. Lippe B: Turner syndrome, *Endocrinol Metab Clin North Am* 20:121, 1991.

146. Logan A: Headlines for hormones, *Lancet* 338:376, 1991.

147. Lubin MB, Gruber HE, Lachman RS: Skeletal abnormalities in the Turner syndrome. In Rosenfeld RG, Grumbach MM, editors: *Turner syndrome*, New York, 1990, Marcel Dekker.

148. Lustig RH et al: Ontogeny of gonadotropin secretion in congenital anorchidism: sexual dimorphism versus syndrome of gonadal dysgenesis and diagnostic considerations, *J Urol* 138:587, 1987.

149. Manasco PK et al: Resumption of puberty after long term luteinizing hormone-releasing hormone agonist treatment of central precocious puberty, *J Clin Endocrinol Metab* 67:368, 1988.

150. Manasco PK et al: A novel testis-stimulating factor in familial male precocious puberty, *N Engl J Med* 324:227, 1991.

151. Mannor DA et al: Plasma growth hormone (GH)-binding proteins: effect on GH binding to receptors and GH action, *J Clin Endocrinol Metab* 78:30, 1991.

152. Marshall JC, Kelch RP: Low dose pulsatile gonadotropin-releasing hormone in anorexia nervosa: a model of human pubertal development, *J Clin Endocrinol Metab* 49:712, 1979.

153. Marshall JC, Kelch RP: Gonadotropin-releasing hormone: role of pulsatile secretion in the regulation of reproduction, *N Engl J Med* 315:1459, 1986.

154. Martha PM Jr et al: Growth hormone-binding protein activity is inversely related to 24-hour growth hormone release in normal boys, *J Clin Endocrinol Metab* 73:175, 1991.

155. Martha PM Jr et al: The maturity related rise of IGF-BP-3 concentration: a reflection of endogenous growth hormone production, *Pediatr Res* 29:81A, 1991.

156. Mason HD et al: Direct gonadotropic effect of growth hormone on estradiol production by human granulosa cells *in vitro*, *J Endocrinol* 126:R1, 1990.

157. Mazur T, Clopper RR: Pubertal disorders, psychology and clinical management, *Endocrinol Metab Clin North Am* 20:211, 1991.

158. McCormick DP et al: Spinal bone mineral density in 335 normal and obese children and adolescents: evidence for ethnic and sex differences, *J Bone Miner Res* 6:507, 1991.

159. McLachlan RI et al: Circulating immunoreactive inhibin levels during the normal human menstrual cycle, *J Clin Endocrinol Metab* 65:954, 1987.

160. McLachlan RI et al: Advances in the physiology of inhibin and inhibin related peptides, *Clin Endocrinol* 29:77, 1988.

161. Michaud P et al: A prepubertal surge of thyrotropin precedes an increase in thyroxine and 3,5,3'-triiodothyronine in normal children, *J Clin Endocrinol Metab* 72:976, 1991.

162. Miller WL: Immunoassays for human müllerian inhibitory factor (MIF): new insights into the physiology of MIF, *J Clin Endocrinol Metab* 70:8, 1990.

163. Mills LJ et al: Premature thelarche: natural history and etiologic investigation, *Am J Dis Child* 135:743, 1981.

164. Moll GW Jr, Rosenfeld RL, Fang VS: Administration of low dose estrogen rapidly and directly stimulates growth hormone production, *Am J Dis Child* 140:124, 1986.

165. Montalto J et al: Serum 5-androstenedione-3β,17β-diol sulphate, sex hormone binding globulin and free androgen index in girls with premature adrenarche, *J Steroid Biochem* 33:1149, 1989.

166. Mudarris A, Peck EJ Jr: Human anti-estrogen receptor antibodies: assay, characterization, and age and sex-related differences, *J Clin Endocrinol Metab* 64:246, 1987.

167. Murram D, Dewhurst J, Grant DB: Premature menarche: a follow-up study, *Arch Dis Child* 58:142, 1983.

168. Murram D, Dewhurst J, Grant DB: Precocious puberty: a follow up study, *Arch Dis Child* 59:77, 1984.

169. Nakayama Y et al: Analysis of gonadotropin-releasing hormone gene structure in families with familial central precocious puberty and idiopathic hypogonadism, *J Clin Endocrinol Metab* 70:1233, 1990.

170. Oberfield SE, Mayes DM, Levine LS: Adrenal steroidogenic function in a black and Hispanic population with precocious pubarche, *J Clin Endocrinol Metab* 70:76, 1990.

171. Oerter KE et al: Gonadotropin secretory dynamics during puberty in normal girls and boys, *J Clin Endocrinol Metab* 71:1251, 1990.

172. Oliver JE et al: Insulin-like growth factor I gene expression in rat ovaries is confined to the granulosa cells of developing follicles, *Endocrinology* 124:2671, 1989.

173. Oostdijk KW et al: Treatment of children with central precocious puberty by a slow-release gonadotropin-releasing hormone agonist, *Eur J Pediatr* 149:308, 1990.

174. Pang S et al: Hirsutism, polycystic ovarian disease, and ovarian 17-ketosteroid reductase deficiency, *N Engl J Med* 316:1295, 1987.

175. Parra A et al: The relationship of plasma gonadotrophins and steroid concentrations to body growth in girls, *Acta Endocrinol* 98:161, 1981.

176. Pasquino AM et al: Precocious puberty in the McCune-Albright syndrome: progression from gonadotropin-independent to gonadotropin-dependent puberty in a girl, *Acta Paediatr Scand* 76:841, 1987.

177. Pasquino AM et al: Transient true precocious puberty, *Eur J Pediatr* 148:735, 1989.

178. Paul DL et al: Long-term effects of GnRH agonists on heights and gonadotropin-gonadal function in children with true precocious puberty, *Pediatr Res* 29:83A, 1991.

179. Perilongo G, Ross A, Hale D: Isosexual precocious puberty associated with an ovarian mass, *Med Pediatr Oncol* 16:273, 1988.

180. Pescovitz OH et al: The NIH experience with precocious puberty: diagnostic subgroups and response to short-term luteinizing hormone releasing hormone analogue therapy, *J Pediatr* 108:47, 1986.

181. Pescovitz OH et al: Premature thelarche and central precocious puberty: the relationship between clinical presentation and the gonadotropin response to luteinizing hormone-releasing hormone, *J Clin Endocrinol Metab* 67:474, 1988.

182. Plant TM, Zorub DS: Pinealectomy in agonadal infantile male rhesus monkeys (*Macaca mulatta*) does not interrupt initiation of the prepubertal hiatus in gonadotropin secretion, *Endocrinology* 118:227, 1986.

183. Ponder SW et al: Spinal bone mineral density in children aged 5.00 through 11.99 years, *Am J Dis Child* 144:1346, 1990.

184. Poretsky L: On the paradox of insulin-induced hyperandrogenism in insulin-resistant states, *Endocr Rev* 12:3, 1991.

185. Poretsky L, Kalin M: The gonadotropic function of insulin, *Endocr Rev* 8:132, 1987.

186. Quigley C et al: Normal or early development of puberty despite gonadal damage in children treated for acute lymphoblastic leukemia, *N Engl J Med* 321:143, 1989.

187. Rabinovici J et al: *In vitro* fertilization and primary embryonic cleavage are possible in 17α-hydroxylase deficiency despite extremely low intrafollicular 17β-estradiol, *J Clin Endocrinol Metab* 68:693, 1989.

188. Reindollar RH, Tho SPT, McDonough PG: Delayed puberty: an updated study of 326 patients, *Adolesc Pediatr Gynecol*, 1993 (in press).

189. Reindollar RH, Tho SPT, McDonough PG: Pubertal amenorrhea: a subset of 290 patients, *Adolesc Pediatr Gynecol*, 1993 (in press).

190. Reiter EO: Neuroendocrine control processes: pubertal onset and progression, *J Adolesc Health Care* 8:479, 1987.

191. Reiter EO, Stern RC, Root AW: The reproductive endocrine system

in cystic fibrosis, I: basal gonadotropin and sex steroid levels, *Am J Dis Child* 135:422, 1981.

192. Reiter EO et al: Bioassayable luteinizing hormone during childhood and adolescence and in patients with delayed pubertal development, *J Clin Endocrinol Metab* 54:155, 1982.

193. Reiter EO et al: Pulsatile release of bioactive luteinizing hormone in prepubertal girls: discordance with immunoreactive luteinizing hormone pulses, *Pediatr Res* 21:409, 1987.

194. Reiter RJ: Pineal gland: interface between the photoperiodic environment and the endocrine system, *Trends Endocrinol Metab* 2:13, 1991.

195. Rieth KG et al: CT of cerebral abnormalities in precocious puberty, *AJR* 148:1231, 1987.

196. Rogol AD: Pubertal development in endurance-trained female athletes, *Growth Genet Horm* 2(1):5, 1986.

197. Rohn RD: Nipple (papilla) development in puberty: longitudinal observations in girls, *Pediatrics* 79:745, 1987.

198. Root AW: Biologic aspects of eating behaviors. In Powers PS, Fernandez RC, editors: *Current treatment of anorexia nervosa and bulemia,* Basel, 1984, S Karger.

199. Root AW: Calcium phosphate, and magnesium disorders. In Colon AR, Ziai M, editors: *Pediatric pathophysiology,* Boston, 1985, Little, Brown.

200. Root AW: Abnormalities of sexual differentiation and maturation. In Kaye R, Oski FA, Barness LA, editors: *Core textbook of pediatrics,* Philadelphia, 1989, JB Lippincott.

201. Root AW: Neurophysiological regulation of the secretion of growth hormone, *J Endocrinol Invest* 12(suppl 3):3, 1989.

202. Root AW, Diamond FB Jr: Androgens in the pediatric patient. In Frajese G et al, editors: *Reproductive medicine: medical therapy,* Amsterdam, 1989, Excerpta Medica.

203. Root AW, Moshang TJ: Evolution of the hyperandrogenism-polycystic ovarian syndrome from isosexual precocious puberty: report of two cases, *Am J Obstet Gynecol* 149:763, 1984.

204. Root AW, Powers PS: Anorexia nervosa presenting as growth retardation in adolescents, *J Adolesc Health Care* 4:25, 1983.

205. Root AW, Rogol AD: Regulation of the endocrine system. In Kappy M, Blizzard R, Migeon C, editors: *Wilkins' endocrinology of childhood and adolescence,* ed 4, Springfield, Ill, Charles C Thomas (in press).

206. Root AW, Shulman DI: Isosexual precocity: current concepts and recent advances, *Fertil Steril* 45:749, 1986.

207. Rose SR et al: Spontaneous growth hormone secretion increases during puberty in normal girls and boys, *J Clin Endocrinol Metab* 73:428, 1991.

208. Rosenfeld RG et al: Three year results of a randomized prospective trial of methionyl human growth hormone and oxandrolone in Turner syndrome, *J Pediatr* 113:393, 1988.

209. Rosenfield RL: Diagnosis and managment of delayed puberty, *J Clin Endocrinol Metab* 70:559, 1990.

210. Rosenfield RL: Hyperandrogenism in peripubertal girls, *Pediatr Clin North Am* 37:1333, 1990.

211. Rosenfield RL: The ovary and female sexual maturation. In Kaplan SA, editor: *Clinical pediatric endocrinology,* ed 2, Philadelphia, 1990, WB Saunders Co.

212. Rosenfield RL: Puberty and its disorders in girls, *Endocrinol Metab Clin North Am* 20:15, 1991.

213. Rosenfield RL et al: The rapid ovarian secretory response to pituitary stimulation by the gonadotropin-releasing hormone agonist nafarelin in sexual precocity, *J Clin Endocrinol Metab* 63:1386, 1986.

214. Rosenfield RL et al: Use of nafarelin for testing pituitary-ovarian function, *J Reprod Med* 34:1044, 1989.

215. Rosenthal SM, Grumbach MM: The neuroendocrinology of puberty: recent advances. In Adashi EY, Mancuso S, editors: *Major advances in human female reproduction,* New York, 1990, Raven Press.

216. Rossmanith WG, Yen SSC: Sleep associated decrease in luteinizing hormone pulse frequency during the early follicular phase of the menstrual cycle: evidence for an opioidergic mechanism, *J Clin Endocrinol Metab* 65:715, 1987.

217. Saenz de Rodriquez CA, Bongiovanni AM, Conde de Borrego L: An epidemic of precocious development in Puerto Rican children, *J Pediatr* 107:393, 1985.

218. Saggese G et al: Gonadotropin pulsatile secretion in girls with premature menarche, *Horm Res* 33:5, 1990.

219. Salardi S et al: Pelvic ultrasonography in girls with precocious puberty, congenital adrenal hyperplasia, obesity or hirsutism, *J Pediatr* 112:880, 1988.

220. Sandstead HH: Zinc deficiency: a public health problem?, *Am J Dis Child* 145:853, 1991.

221. Schaefer F et al: Pulsatile gonadotropin secretion in pubertal children with chronic renal failure, *Acta Endocrinol* 120:14, 1989.

222. Schoemaker J et al: Induction of first cycles in primary hypothalamic amenorrhea with pulsatile luteinizing hormone-releasing hormone: a mirror of female pubertal development, *Fertil Steril* 48:204, 1987.

223. Schultz N, Terasawa E: Posterior hypothalamic lesions advance the time of the pubertal changes in luteinizing hormone release in ovariectomized female rhesus monkeys, *Endocrinology* 123:445, 1988.

224. Schwandel-Fukuda M, Pfaff DW: Origin of luteinizing hormone-releasing hormone neurons, *Nature* 338:161, 1989.

225. Schwartz ID, Root AW: Puberty in girls: normal or delayed?, *Contemp Pediatr* 6(11):83, 1989.

226. Schwartz ID, Root AW: When adolescence is delayed, *Contemp Ob/Gyn* 34(5):95, 1989.

227. Schwartz ID, Root AW: Puberty in girls: early, incomplete, or precocious?, *Contemp Pediatr* 7(1):147, 1990.

228. Schwarz HP, Duck SC, Johnson DA: Isolated precocious menstruation in primary hypothyroidism, *Adolesc Pediatr Gynecol* 4:33, 1991.

229. Schwarz HP, Tschaeppeler H, Zuppinger K: Case report: unsustained central sexual precocity in four girls, *Am J Med Sci* 299:260, 1990.

230. Scott EC, Johnston FE: Critical fat, menarche, and the maintenance of menstrual cycles: a critical review, *J Adolesc Health Care* 2:249, 1982.

231. Serhal PF, Craft IL: Oocyte donation in 61 patients, *Lancet* 2:1185, 1989.

232. Sheikholislam BM, Stempfel RS Jr: Hereditary isolated somatotropin deficiency: effects of human growth hormone administration, *Pediatrics* 49:362, 1972.

233. Shulman DI: Isosexual precocious puberty, *Pediatrician* 14:261, 1987.

234. Silbergeld A et al: Serum growth hormone binding protein activity in healthy neonates, children and young adults: correlation with age, height and weight, *Clin Endocrinol* 31:295, 1989.

235. Simard J et al: Stimulation of growth hormone release and synthesis by estrogens in rat anterior pituitary cells in culture, *Endocrinology* 119:2004, 1986.

236. Sizonenko PC: Delayed sexual maturation, *Pediatrician* 14:202, 1987.

237. Sizonenko PC, Reznik Y, Aubert ML: Urinary excretion of [D-Ser(t-Bu)6, Des-Gly 10] GnRH ethylamide (buserelin) during therapy of central precocious puberty: a multicenter study, *Acta Endocrinol* 122:553, 1990.

238. Smith CP et al: Relationship between insulin, insulin-like growth factor-I, and dehydroepiandrosterone sulfate concentrations during childhood, puberty and adult life, *J Clin Endocrinol Metab* 68:932, 1989.

239. Smith DW, Marokus R, Graham JM Jr: Tentative evidence of Y-linked statural gene(s): growth in the testicular feminization syndrome, *Clin Pediatr* 24:189, 1985.

240. Sockalosky J et al: Precocious puberty after traumatic brain injury, *J Pediatr* 110:373, 1987.

241. Southwood TR et al: Unconventional remedies used for patients with juvenile arthritis, *Pediatrics* 85:150, 1990.

242. Stager JM, Wigglesworth JK, Hatler LK: Interpreting the relationship between age of menarche and prepubertal training, *Med Sci Sports Exerc* 22:54, 1990.

243. Stanhope R, Adams J, Brook CGD: Evolution of polycystic ovaries in a girl with delayed menarche: a case report, *J Reprod Med* 33:482, 1988.

244. Stanhope R, Pringle PJ, Brook CGD: The mechanism of the adolescent growth spurt induced by low dose pulsatile GnRH treatment, *Clin Endocrinol* 28:83, 1988.

245. Stanhope R et al: Induction of puberty by pulsatile gonadotropin-releasing hormone, *Lancet* 2:552, 1987.

246. Stanhope R et al: New concepts of the growth spurt of puberty, *Acta Paediatr Scand Suppl* 47:30, 1988.

247. Stark O, Peckham CS, Moynihan C: Weight and age at menarche, *Arch Dis Child* 64:383, 1989.

248. Stokvis-Brantsma WH et al: Sexual precocity induced by ovarian follicular cysts: is autoimmunity involved?, *Clin Endocrinol* 32:603, 1990.

249. Strauss DS: Growth-stimulatory actions of insulin *in vitro* and *in vivo*, *Endocr Rev* 5:356, 1984.

250. Styne DM: The testes: disorders of sexual differentiation and puberty. In Kaplan SA, editor: *Clinical pediatric endocrinology*, ed 2, Philadelphia, 1990, WB Saunders.

251. Sweasey TA et al: Stereotactic decompression of a prepontine arachnoid cyst with resolution of precocious puberty, *Pediatr Neurosurg* 15:44, 1989.

252. Tajtakova M et al: Thyroid volume by ultrasound in boys and girls 6-16 years of age under marginal iodine deficiency as related to the age of puberty, *Klin Wochenschr* 68:503, 1990.

253. Tanaka T et al: Analysis of linear growth during puberty, *Acta Paediatr Scand Suppl* 347:25, 1988.

254. Tanner JM: Issues and advances in adolescent growth and development, *J Adolesc Health Care* 8:470, 1987.

255. Tanner JM, Davies PSW: Clinical longitudinal standards for height and height velocity for North American children, *J Pediatr* 107:317, 1985.

256. Theintz GE et al: Growth and pubertal development of young female gymnasts and swimmers: a correlation with parental data, *Int J Sports Med* 10:87, 1989.

257. Toscano V et al: Changes in steroid pattern following acute and chronic adrenocorticotropin administration in premature adrenarche, *J Steroid Biochem* 32:321, 1989.

258. Trifiro M et al: Androgen insensitivity: basic mechanisms and clinical relevance. In Root AW, editor: *Proceedings of the seventh Lilly international symposium on endocrine disorders*, Tampa, Fla, May 1, 1991, Bugamor Pharma.

259. Urban RJ, Veldhuis JD, Dufau ML: Estrogen regulates the gonadotropin-releasing hormone-stimulated secretion of biologically active luteinizing hormone, *J Clin Endocrinol Metab* 72:660, 1991.

260. Vale W et al: The inhibin/activin family of hormones and growth factors. In Sporn MB, Roberts AB, editors: *Peptide growth factors and their receptors II*, Heidelberg, 1990, Springer-Verlag.

261. Veldhuis JD, Johnson ML, Dufau ML: Preferential release of bioactive luteinizing hormone in response to endogenous and low dose exogenous gonadotropin-releasing hormone in man, *J Clin Endocrinol Metab* 64:1275, 1987.

262. Vigersky RA et al: Hypothalamic dysfunction in secondary amenorrhea associated with simple weight loss, *N Engl J Med* 297:1141, 1977.

263. Voutilainen R, Miller WL: Coordinate trophic hormone regulation of mRNAs for insulin-like growth factor II and the cholesterol side-chain cleavage enzyme, P450 SSC, in human steroidogenic tissues, *Proc Natl Acad Sci U S A* 84:1590, 1987.

264. Waldhauser F et al: Fall in nocturnal serum melatonin during prepuberty and pubescence, *Lancet* 1:362, 1984.

265. Waldhauser F et al: Alterations in nocturnal serum melatonin levels in humans with growth and aging, *J Clin Endocrinol Metab* 66:648, 1988.

266. Wang C et al: Serum bioactive follicle-stimulating hormone levels in girls with precocious sexual development, *J Clin Endocrinol Metab* 70:615, 1990.

267. Weinstein LS et al: Activating mutations of the stimulatory G protein in the McCune-Albright syndrome, *N Engl J Med* 325:1688, 1991.

268. Weis J, Crowley WF Jr, Jameson JL: Normal structure of the gonadotropin-releasing hormone (GnRH) gene in patients with GnRH deficiency and idiopathic hypogonadotropic hypogonadism, *J Clin Endocrinol Metab* 69:299, 1989.

269. Werner H et al: Steroid regulation of somatostatin mRNA in the rat hypothalamus, *J Biol Chem* 263:7666, 1988.

270. Wheeler MD: Physical changes of puberty, *Endocrinol Metab Clin North Am* 20:1, 1991.

271. Wheeler MD, Styne, DM: The treatment of precocious puberty, *Endocrinol Metab Clin North Am* 20:183, 1991.

272. White PC, New MI, Dupont B: Congenital adrenal hyperplasia, *N Engl J Med* 316:1519;1580, 1987.

273. Wierman ME et al: Adrenarche and skeletal maturation during luteinizing hormone releasing hormone analogue suppression of gonadarche, *J Clin Invest* 77:121, 1986.

274. Wilcox G et al: Oestrogenic effects of plant food in postmenopausal women, *Br Med J* 301:905, 1990.

275. Wildt L, Marshall G, Knobil E: Experimental induction of puberty in the infantile female rhesus monkey, *Science* 207:1373, 1980.

276. Wilson ME et al: Effects of growth hormone on the tempo of sexual maturation in female rhesus monkeys, *J Clin Endocrinol Metab* 68:29, 1989.

277. Wilson RC, Knobil E: Acute effects of *N*-methyl-D,L-aspartate on the release of pituitary gonadotropins and prolactin in the adult female rhesus monkey, *Brain Res* 248:177, 1982.

278. Wood DF, Franks S: Delayed puberty, *Br J Hosp Med* 41:223, 1989.

279. Wu FCW et al: Patterns of pulsatile luteinizing hormone and follicle stimulating hormone secretion in prepubertal (midchildhood) boys and girls and patients with idiopathic hypogonadotropic hypogonadism (Kallmann's syndrome): a study using an ultrasensitive time-resolved immunofluorometric assay, *J Clin Endocrinol Metab* 72:1229, 1991.

280. Yanase T, Simpson ER, Waterman MR: 17α-Hydroxylase/17,20 lyase deficiency: from clinical investigation to molecular definition, *Endocr Rev* 12:91, 1991.

281. Ying S-Y: Inhibins, activins and follistatins: gonadal proteins modulating the secretion of follicle-stimulating hormone, *Endocr Rev* 9:267, 1988.

282. Young IM et al: Constant pineal output and increasing body mass account for declining melatonin levels during human growth and sexual maturation, *J Pineal Res* 5:71, 1988.

283. Zachmann M et al: Pubertal growth in patients with androgen insensitivity: indirect evidence for the importance of estrogens in pubertal growth of girls, *J Pediatr* 108:694, 1986.

284. Zeitler P et al: Growth hormone-releasing hormone messenger ribonucleic acid in the hypothalamus of the adult male rat is increased by testosterone, *Endocrinology* 127:1362, 1990.

Chapter 5

OVARIAN FOLLICULAR GROWTH AND MATURATION

Thomas L. Toth, MD
and Gary D. Hodgen, PhD

Ovarian function is, of course, a principal component of female reproductive physiology from intrauterine development to the postmenopausal status. In this chapter an attempt is made to set the stage for a broader number of issues in reproductive medicine that either derive from or impinge on the fundamental processes of ovarian follicular growth and maturation. After discussion of crucial basic issues in follicular formation, central hormonal feedback, and events of the mature ovarian/menstrual cycle, specific clinical correlates are addressed in which intervention in certain pathophysiologic states can be successful in managing ovarian follicular growth and maturation therapeutically. It is hoped that these tenets of reproductive medicine prove useful to practitioners, investigators, and students alike.

FOLLICULAR FORMATION

Germ cells arise in the yolk sac on approximately day 24 of fetal life and migrate to the gonadal ridge during the fifth week of development to form the indifferent gonad. In the female, these germ cells initially reside within nests without intervening stroma, which are known as the cell syncytium. The migration of stroma cells between the oocytes marks the development of the primordial follicles.[73] Nuclear maturation of the oocyte arrests in the diplotene stage of the first meiotic division, where it remains until ready to resume meiosis and potentially develop into a mature oocyte. (See Chapter 50.) It appears that hormonal input is necessary for embryologic development of ovarian follicles, as indicated by failure of gonadal development in the anencephalic human fetus[48] and by decreased numbers of oocytes after fetal hypophysectomy in monkeys.[39] The duration of this resting state, in which no further development occurs, may last for as little as a few days or as long as 50 years. Nonetheless, germ cell depletion occurs, reducing the number of oocytes from 5 million to 7 million during fetal life to only approximately 400,000 at menarche.

HYPOTHALAMIC-PITUITARY-OVARIAN INTERACTIONS

Ovarian function cannot be explained without consideration of the other endocrine organ systems that communicate stimulatory or inhibitory signals to the ovary and to which the ovary feeds back. Functionally, the hypothalamus, pituitary, and ovary are linked; this relationship is the hypothalamic-pituitary-ovarian axis. The mediators of communication among them are blood-borne hormones.

Anatomically the hypothalamus is composed of nuclei; in turn, discrete hypothalamic areas control specific responses recognized by changes in hormone secretion from the pituitary. As concerns reproduction, the principal releasing hormone that allows gonadotropin secretion from the pituitary is gonadotropin-releasing hormone (GnRH). GnRH from the arcuate nucleus is transported to the median eminence, where it is released into the pituitary portal vascular bed. The intimate connection between these structures allows high concentrations of the hypothalamic releasing hormones to have an impact on the pituitary without systemic passage.

The pituitary gonadotropin follicle-stimulating hormone (FSH) primarily functions to produce proliferation of the granulosa cells and to stimulate aromatase enzyme for estrogen synthesis. Luteinizing hormone (LH) stimulates the transformation of estrogen-secreting ovarian stromal cells to progesterone-secreting cells. In addition, LH is crucial to promoting final oocyte maturation and ovulation in the periovulatory interval.

The predominant ovarian hormones exerting peripheral, central, and intraovarian effects are the steroids estradiol (E_2) and progesterone (P), although other steroids play active roles in ovarian and hypothalamic-pituitary events. The synchronous actions of these substances are now known to be necessary and sufficient for preparation of a fertile endometrium. Also, by means of feedback on the hypothalamus and pituitary, E_2 and P modulate the ovarian cycle.

Not all ovarian effects on hypothalamic-pituitary function can be explained on the basis of steroid hormone action. Similarly, not all intraovarian phenomena, such as selective follicular development and oocyte maturation, can be accounted for by local actions of E_2 and P. Therefore another class of reproductive hormones, known as nonsteroidal ovarian factors (inhibin, oocyte maturation inhibitor, gonadotropin surge-inhibiting factor, and growth factors), seems to be involved in the regulation of pituitary and gonadal function through paracrine and autocrine regulation.

GONADOTROPIN-INDEPENDENT DEVELOPMENT

The earliest development and changes that occur as the primordial follicles leave their resting state and resume development are independent of gonadotropin stimulation. A primary follicle is derived from a primordial follicle; this progression is characterized by oocyte enlargement from approximately 15 to 100 μm, development of a zona pellucida, and the presence of at least two layers of granulosa cells.[20] Specialized gap junctions between granulosa cells and oocytes appear at this time and are thought to be important in cell-to-cell communication and transport[20] (Fig. 5-1). This gonadotropin-independent development occurs during the juvenile, prepubertal, and reproductive years through the climacteric and is unaffected by changes in circulating gonadotropin or sex steroid dynamics. It is demonstrated clinically in patients with olfactogenital dysplasia (Kallmann syndrome) who have a congenital defi-

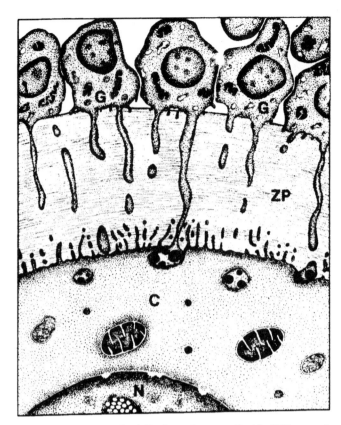

Fig. 5-1. Structure of a fully formed zona pellucida (*ZP*) around an oocyte in a graafian (secondary) follicle. Microvilli arising from the oocyte interdigitate with processes from granulosa cells (*G*). These processes penetrate into the cytoplasm of the oocyte (*C*) and may provide nutrients and maternal protein. *N*, Oocyte nucleus. (From Baker TG: In Austin CR, Short RV, editors: *Germ cells and fertilization,* Cambridge, UK, 1972, Cambridge University Press.)

ciency of gonadotropin secretion and also in patients who are status posthypophysectomy.[28] In both circumstances, the normal process of primary follicular development appears to be unaltered.

In addition, the absence of gonadotropin stimulation will not prolong the total life span of the oocytes, excessive gonadotropin stimulation will not prematurely exhaust the oocyte supply, and contraceptive steroids will not affect the departure of follicles from their resting state.[73] Moreover, oocytes and follicular maturation can be arrested at this stage until eventually undergoing atresia or maturation. It is clear, therefore, that this process continues independent of the circulating gonadotropin and sex steroid milieu.

GONADOTROPIN-DEPENDENT DEVELOPMENT

The morphologic distinguishing feature of the development of secondary follicles and the beginning of gonadotropin sensitivity is the development of a fluid-filled cavity, or antrum. This accumulation of fluids is both the result of the secretion of mucopolysaccharides by granulosa

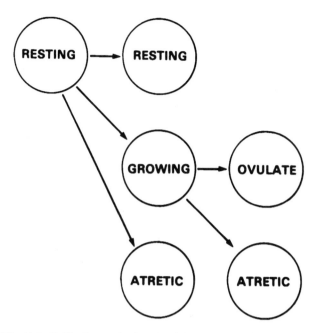

Fig. 5-2. Folliculogenesis. Ovarian follicles may be found in four basic conditions: resting, growing, atretic, or ready to ovulate. (From Goodman AL, Hodgen GD: In Greep RO, editor: *Recent progress in hormone research,* New York, 1983, Academic Press.)

cells and the transudation of plasma proteins from the newly acquired theca layer with its vasculature around the lamina basalis. Overt connection of this follicular apparatus to the peripheral blood stream is coincident with the onset of gonadotropin-dependent follicular growth. This stage of follicular development has only two possible consequences, ovulation or atresia, with the latter occurring in more than 99% of cases (Fig. 5-2).

The gonadotropin-sensitive interval of folliculogenesis has been studied more extensively and is better understood than the gonadotropin-insensitive intervals. In the gonadotropin-sensitive interval, the classic morphologic and endocrine dynamics of folliculogenesis are well defined, and thus an understanding of these dynamics can lead to meaningful clinical intervention.

It is well established that women produce a single fertilizable oocyte approximately every 4 weeks. This is true despite the fact that follicles leave their resting state with the potential to develop to maturity in a continuous process. Therefore, there must be a means of stimulating adequate development of the follicle destined to ovulate while allowing all of the others to undergo atresia. The dynamics of this process have been characterized and separated into the intervals of recruitment, selection, dominance, and ovulation (Fig. 5-3).

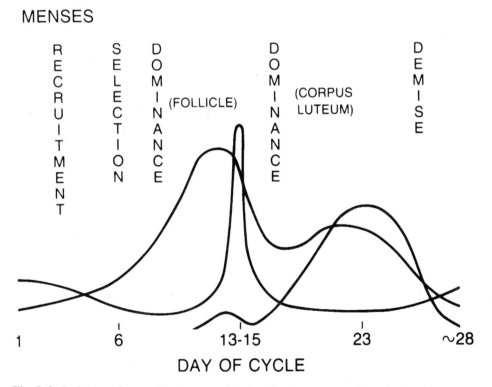

Fig. 5-3. Definition of terms. The terms used to describe the sequence of principal ovarian events during follicular maturation and corpus luteum function are temporally defined in the menstrual cycle. The curves depict idealized (stereotypic) patterns of E_2, pituitary gonadotropins, and P in peripheral circulation. (From Hodgen GD: *Fertil Steril* 38:281, 1983.)

Recruitment

The term *recruitment* indicates that a follicle has entered a gonadotropin-dependent, rapid growth phase. Recruitment includes the entry of primordial follicles and the reentry of slightly more advanced follicles that may have been transiently at rest. This group of quasi-synchronous follicles, referred to as a cohort,[14] must achieve ovulation or become atretic within a single cycle (Fig. 5-4). This unalterable state is supported by Pederson's study[69] in mice suggesting that once a follicle leaves the resting stage, it must continue to mature or succumb to atresia.

Although recruitment of primordial follicles may not be exclusively dependent on gonadotropins (as evidenced by follicles at various preantral stages of development in the ovaries of hypophysectomized subjects and patients with hypogonadotropic hypogonadism [Kallmann syndrome]), inadequate gonadotropin stimulation during this critical period will lead to atresia.[14,58] In normal menstrual cycles, circulating gonadotropin levels are too low throughout most of the cycle to stimulate progression of follicular development beyond this early stage. However, as the corpus luteum function fails at the end of a nonconception cycle, E_2 and P levels decline and their suppression of the hypothalamic-pituitary axis decreases. This results in a narrow window during each monthly menstrual cycle in which the circulating milieu is favorable for the rescue of these follicles, so that further development might occur.

In women this threshold level of gonadotropin concentration must occur at the correct time in order for follicular development to occur at all, as evidenced by the progressive decline in the ability of gonadotropins to stimulate new follicular growth (from less-developed antral follicles) from the midfollicular phase to ovulation during a spontaneous menstrual cycle.[37] Use of the term *rescue* is not to suggest that once a follicle begins to degenerate in vivo it will be able to return to the ovulatory pathway.[42] Rather, this term refers to the recruitment of multiple follicles that have gained gonadotropin sensitivity and possess the ability to proceed to ovulation.[31] These follicles are morphologically indistinguishable, and ablation of any of these recruited follicles does not result in a delay of ovulation. As folliculogenesis progresses, the developing granulosa cells secrete more E_2. The concomitant decline in FSH concentration induced by the rising E_2 levels does not, however, adversely affect the most mature follicles. In the process of developing, the more mature follicle has increased its number of FSH receptors and is capable of sustained growth even in the presence of lower FSH concentrations.[66] This concept that FSH controls folliculogenesis, but not the growth of the dominant follicle exclusively, is supported by others.[65] Other hormones probably are involved in this process, including nonsteroidal gonadal factors such as inhibin and possibly paracrine-autocrine hormones and also including a number of growth factors. This complex inter-

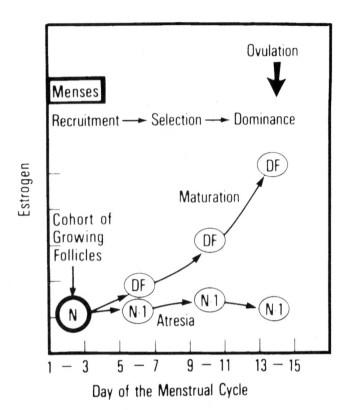

Fig. 5-4. Time course for recruitment, selection, and ovulation of the dominant ovarian follicle, with onset of atresia among other follicles of the cohort. (From Hodgen GD: *Fertil Steril* 38:281, 1983.)

action of pituitary hormones, gonadal steroids, and purported nonsteroidal gonadal factors is required to coordinate the reproductive axis in ovarian follicular development.

Inhibin has been recognized as a key factor for the appropriate regulation of pituitary FSH secretion. Characterization of inhibin proteins and their genes in animals and women has led to a proposed regulation of inhibin secretion in vivo and in vitro as a classic endocrine closed-loop feedback system in which ovarian inhibin is an important negative regulator of pituitary FSH secretion, and ovarian inhibin secretion is in turn under FSH control (Fig. 5-5). Specifically in women it is proposed that the dominant follicle secretes increasing amounts of inhibin to limit further FSH secretion, thus controlling its own rate of development and preventing the development of new asynchronous follicles (Fig. 5-6). Furthermore, on the basis of a significant inverse relationship observed during the luteal phase of both spontaneous and ovulation-induced cycles, inhibin secretion by the corpus luteum may be important in suppressing FSH, thereby preventing the development of new follicles before regression of the corpus luteum.[7,61]

Growth factors are implicated in important roles in intragonadal regulation of growth and differentiation of

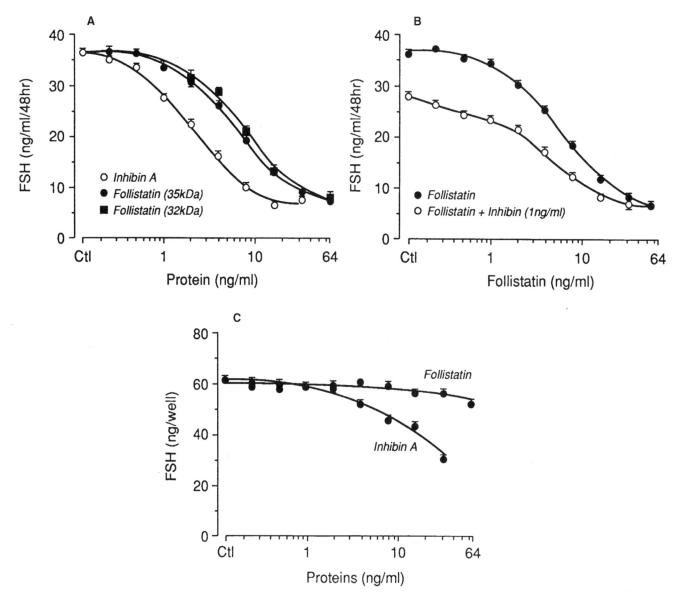

Fig. 5-5. The effects of follistatin and inhibin on FSH secretion and synthesis in rat anterior pituitary cells. **A,** Dose-response curves of inhibin A and of 35-kd and 32-kd follistatin on the suppression of spontaneous FSH release. **B,** Additive effect of follistatin and inhibin on the suppression of FSH release. Multiple doses of 35-kd follistatin alone and in the presence of a constant dose of inhibin were added to the cells. The open circles show additivity at the lower doses of follistatin plus inhibin, but identical E_{max} for follistatin alone or in combination with inhibin in the high doses. **C,** The effects of inhibin and follistatin on pituitary FSH content. Inhibin clearly suppresses the intracellular content of FSH, whereas follistatin is much less effective. (Redrawn from Ling N et al: In Hodgen GD, Rosenwaks Z, Spieler J, editors: *Physiological roles and possibilities in contraceptive development,* Proceedings from the CONRAD International Workshop on Non-Steroidal Gonadal Factors, Norfolk, Va, Jan 6–8, 1988, The Jones Institute Press.)

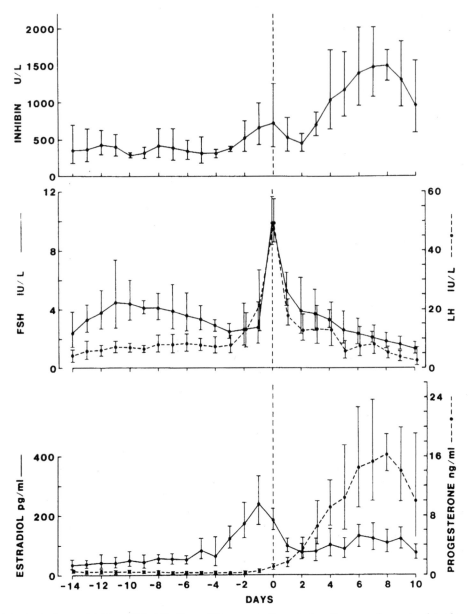

Fig. 5-6. Serum inhibin, FSH, LH, E$_2$, and P concentrations during the normal menstrual cycle. Data from six subjects are normalized around the end of the day of the LH surge (*broken line*). The data are expressed as a geometric mean (67% confidence intervals, four to six observations per point). (From McLachlan RI et al: In Hodgen GD, Rosenwaks Z, Spieler J, editors: *Physiological roles and possibilities in contraceptive development,* Proceedings from the CONRAD International Workshop on Non-Steroidal Gonadal Factors, Norfolk, Va, Jan 6–8, 1988, The Jones Institute Press.)

Table 5-1. Growth factor gene expression or growth factor production by cells of the reproductive system

Growth factor or oncogene*	Cell or tissue of origin†
IGF-I	Ovary, uterus, Sertoli cell, placenta
IGF-II	Granulosa cell, placenta
TGF-α	Theca, decidua, pituitary, mammary
TGF-β type 1	Ovary, bone
TGF-β type 2	MCF-7 cells, prostatic adenocarcinoma
EGF	Ovarian follicle, uterus
FGF	Granulosa cells
PDGF	Cytotrophoblast
HER-2/neu	Breast
IGF-like	Breast, granulosa cell
EGF-like	Breast
TGF-β-like	Sertoli cell
TGF-β-like	Sertoli cell
Seminiferous growth factor	Sertoli cell

From Schomberg DW: In Hodgen GD, Rosenwaks Z, Spieler J, editors: *Physiological roles and possibilities in contraceptive development,* Proceedings from the CONRAD International Workshop on Non-Steroidal Gonadal Factors, Norfolk, Va, Jan 6-8, 1988, The Jones Institute Press, p. 330.
*IGF-I and IGF-II, Insulin-like growth factors I and II; TGF-α and TGF-β, transforming growth factors alpha and beta; EGF, epidermal growth factor; FGF, fibroblast growth factor; PDGF, platelet-derived growth factor; HER-2/neu, Epididymal growth factor receptor.
†MCF-7, Macrophage chemotactic factor 7.

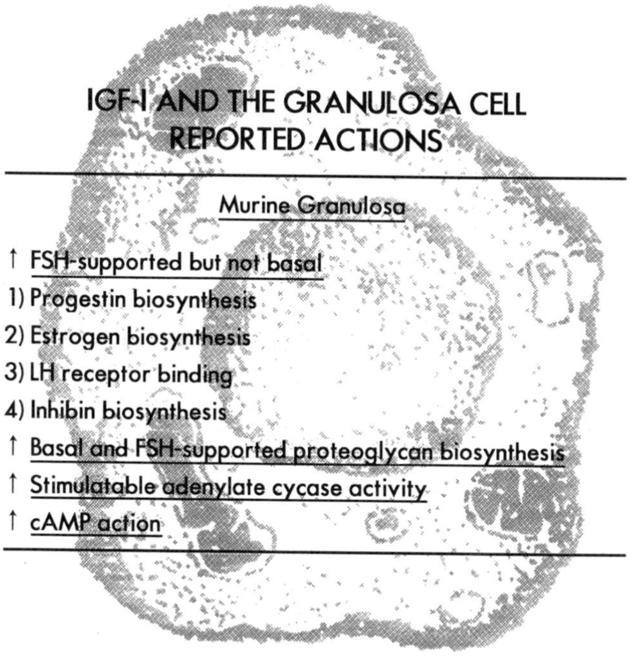

IGF-I AND THE GRANULOSA CELL REPORTED ACTIONS

Murine Granulosa

↑ FSH-supported but not basal
1) Progestin biosynthesis
2) Estrogen biosynthesis
3) LH receptor binding
4) Inhibin biosynthesis
↑ Basal and FSH-supported proteoglycan biosynthesis
↑ Stimulatable adenylate cycase activity
↑ cAMP action

Fig. 5-7. Reported actions of Sm-C/IGF-I in reference to the rat granulosa cell. (From Adashi EY et al: In Hodgen GD, Rosenwaks Z, Spieler J, editors: *Physiological roles and possibilities in contraceptive development,* Proceedings from the CONRAD International Workshop on Non-Steroidal Gonadal Factors, Norfolk, Va, Jan 6-8, 1988, The Jones Institute Press.)

follicular development, although the mechanisms of regulation have not been completely defined (Table 5-1). Among potential regulators, somatomedin C/insulin-like growth factor I (Sm-C/IGF-I) may serve as a central signal, with the granulosa cell its site of production, reception, and action in an autocrine control mechanism. Thus Sm-C/IGF-I may promote replication and differentiation of the developing granulosa cell by amplifying gonadotropin action. Additionally, it may also provide paracrine input to the adjacent theca-interstitial cell compartment through enhancement of ovarian androgen production and therefore of the aromatizing capabilities of the granulosa cell in estrogen production of the developing follicle; thus Sm-C/IGF-I is implicated in coordinating follicular development by coupling the androgen to estrogen biosynthesis[2,80] (Fig. 5-7).

The process of recruitment begins at the end of the luteal phase of the previous cycle, from the onset of menses to approximately day 5 to day 7 of the current cycle.[14] The mechanism involved in the initiation of recruitment is poorly understood, but it may depend on ovarian paracrine mechanisms.[74] It has been hypothesized that the primary follicle/oocyte initiates gonadotropin sensitivity, although

the theca, through an LH receptor response, is perhaps the progenitor cell of the follicle. LH induces an "angiogenesis factor" from the theca, increasing the blood supply and subsequent E_2 synthesis from these specific follicles. This factor may determine which follicles ultimately become dominant or atretic.[46] Angiogenesis factor has been suggested to be angiotensin II.[21,82] Thus, through vascular stimulation and subsequent E_2 production, the theca may initiate the FSH response of the granulosa cells, which in turn may begin the maturation of the oocyte cytoplasm.[46] Eventually, only a single follicle will be able to utilize its hormonal milieu efficiently enough to sustain development, and the interval of recruitment will be completed.

Selection

The term *selection* is used to indicate the final reduction of the cohort size down to the species-characteristic ovulatory quota. Selection is the culmination of the process of recruitment and marks the time when the influence of a single follicle creates an environment in which only it can adequately mature and reach ovulation (Fig. 5-8). In women, spontaneous multiple ovulation is atypical, although not a rarity. The process of selection operates with great precision. This has been demonstrated physiologically by experiments in which the largest follicle was ablated. If the ovaries were in the stage of recruitment (prior to

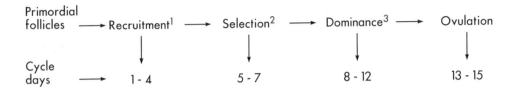

Definitions:

1 = Cohort may be: N = 1 or N =>1

2 = A single follicle is destined to ovulate;
    no surrogate follicles

3 = Dominance may be:

Active = Dominant follicle supresses
         maturation of other follicles

Passive = Dominant follicle thrives uniquely,
          despite the suppressive milieu

Fig. 5-8. Folliculogenesis in the primate ovarian cycle. The cohort of follicles from which the ovulatory follicle is derived begins to grow (gonadotropin dependent) about day 1 of the menstrual cycle. The number of follicles in a cohort is unknown but typically is reduced to the ovulatory quota (unity in women and in these monkeys) by the midfollicular phase. (Redrawn from Hodgen GD: *Fertil Steril* 38:281, 1983.)

selection of the dominant follicle), ablation of the most advanced follicle had little impact; another follicle became dominant, and a normal follicular phase was completed without delay.[33,67] However, if ablation of the largest follicle destroyed the follicle destined to ovulate, the expected surge of E_2 and gonadotropin secretion did not occur at midcycle but was delayed by about 2 weeks. Since this delay approximated the length of a typical follicular phase, it appeared that no other follicle was capable of substituting for the cauterized follicle to accommodate a timely ovulation. Instead, the delay suggested that the follicle destined to ovulate already had been selected by the day of cautery, that is, by the midfollicular phase, and that the next follicle to ovulate was the product of a new cohort of one or more follicles that developed after cautery. With use of this technique in a serial fashion, it was determined that a single follicle becomes destined to ovulate and form the corpus luteum sometime between day 5 and day 7 of the normal 28-day cycle.[33]

The evidence for selection of a dominant follicle also may be defined endocrinologically. Despite perfusion of both ovaries with the same peripheral blood (and therefore similar exposure to pituitary gonadotropins), typically only one of two ovaries sponsors recruitment and selection of the single dominant follicle destined for ovulation. Random comparisons of sex steroid hormone levels in venous effluent from the two ovaries and peripheral venous blood during ovulatory cycles have shown that both ovaries produce estrogens, androgens, and progestogens throughout the cycle; however, once a dominant follicle has become

overtly identifiable, levels of estrogens, androgens and progestogens are dramatically elevated in the venous effluent from the ovary containing that follicle.[14] Indeed, results of earlier studies showed that when the dominant ovarian follicle was present, the opposite ovary could be removed without effect, meaning that there was unambiguous ovarian asymmetry when the dominant structure was recognizable.[31,32] Accordingly, by sequentially sampling ovarian venous effluents after the spontaneous onset of menses, secreted steroid hormones could identify ovarian asymmetry and indicate dominant follicle selection.[15] In fact, there was a uniform, clear-cut disparity of E_2 secretion by cycle days 5 to 7.[15] There are also differences in the intraovarian milieu. It has been shown that follicles destined to become atretic contain decreased levels of E_2 and P and increased levels of androgens relative to those of the dominant follicle.[63]

Furthermore, observations made in the primate ovarian cycle with the use of fluorescein-labeled human chorionic gonadotropin (hCG) to localize in vivo binding around the dominant follicle demonstrated the identification of the dominant follicle on or before day 7 of the menstrual cycle, even though its size (antral diameter) was often not yet a distinguishing factor.[16] Accordingly the follicular pool (total ovarian mass) has been conceptualized to be intermixed before selection of the dominant ovarian follicle, so that symmetric (unigonadal) conditions exist initially. In contrast, after emergence of ovarian asymmetry (bigonadal), such as occurs on selection of the dominant ovarian follicle, the destiny of each ovary is distinctly separate for the

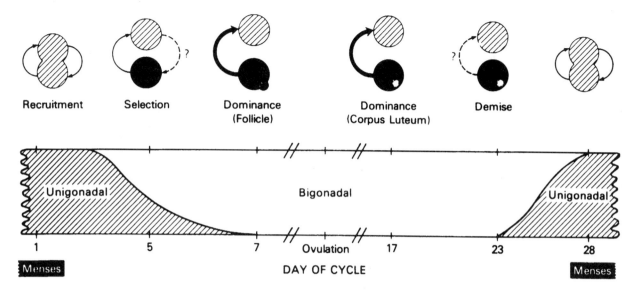

Fig. 5-9. Transient nature of asymmetric ovarian function in the primate menstrual/ovarian cycle. The terms *unigonadal* and *bigonadal* may be used interchangeably with the terms *symmetric* and *asymmetric,* respectively. (From diZerega GS, Hodgen GD: *Endocr Rev* 2:27, 1981.)

duration of the cycle. That is, one ovary supports the dominant ovarian follicle and then the corpus luteum, whereas the other ovary is gametogenically quiescent in that cycle[34] (Fig. 5-9).

Dominance

The interval of growth preceding ovulation but following selection is called *dominance* and is achieved between days 5 and 7 of an idealized 28-day ovarian menstrual cycle. The dominant ovarian follicle is the sole follicle destined to ovulate, and somehow it continues to thrive in a milieu it has helped to make inhospitable to others. It is unknown whether this capacity to thrive results from a unique, newly acquired ability of the dominant follicle or from a preexisting ability originally shared by the entire cohort but retained only by the dominant follicle. The progressive abolition of the ability of human menopausal gonadotropin (hMG) to stimulate follicular growth as ovulation approaches supports the existence of an inhibitory activity (possibly ovarian) designed to suppress the selection and maturation of less-developed antral follicles from the midfollicular phase of the human spontaneous menstrual cycle.[37] However, it appears that the follicle that most rapidly acquires aromatase activity and LH receptors probably becomes the dominant ovarian follicle.[41] This follicle controls the endocrine milieu as it prepares itself, the reproductive tract, and the hypothalamic-pituitary axis for ovulation.

Follicular growth continues during dominance with enlargement of the antrum and proliferation of the granulosa and thecal layers. LH and FSH receptors are up-regulated by the combined effects of E_2 and FSH as the follicle prepares itself for the LH/FSH surge and eventual ovula-

tion. This growth appears to be relatively independent of FSH support as ovulation approaches[76] and therefore may be dependent on intrinsic factors.[65]

The increasing quantities of estrone and E_2 secreted by the granulosa cells play a critical role in coordinating the development of the different portions of the reproductive tract. The hypothalamic-pituitary axis requires estrogen priming of approximately 200 pg/mL for at least 36 hours to develop the ability to discharge an LH surge sufficient for ovulation.[53] Although the specific degree of priming necessary is unknown, the endometrium also requires estrogen priming in order to be able to respond appropriately to the secretion of P during the luteal phase. Similarly, estrogen stimulation of the endocervix and fallopian tube is required for normal gamete and embryo transport.[45] Therefore, the secretory products of the developing follicle prepare and synchronize the entire reproductive system for ovulation, fertilization, and implantation.

Midcycle dynamics

Once the growth of the dominant follicle has achieved the necessary level and the systemic hormonal effects are adequate, cascading physiologic processes occur that stimulate the final maturational changes within the follicle and induce ovulation. The precise means by which the oocyte communicates that it is ready for ovulation (if it does) is poorly understood.

The most prominent marker for impending ovulation is the midcycle LH surge (Fig. 5-10), which is preceded by an accelerated increase in serum E_2 levels. Ovulation often occurs within 10 to 12 hours after the peak and 36 hours after the onset of the LH surge.[27,68] As described later, LH has specific effects on the oocyte and the follicle and is

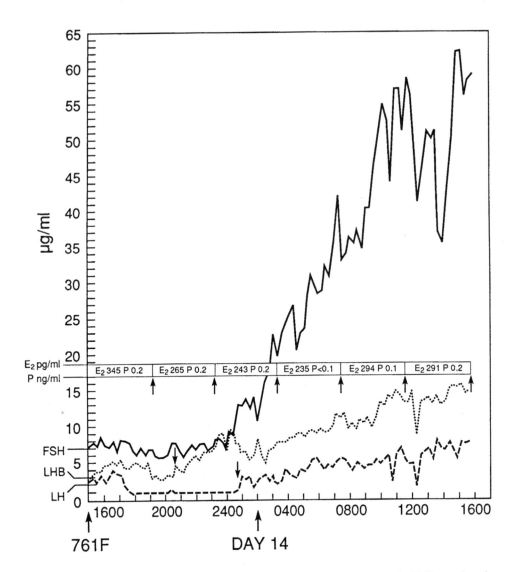

Fig. 5-10. Plasma concentrations of FSH determined by radioimmunoassay and of LH quantitated by radioimmunoassay and in vitro bioassay on day 14 of the menstrual cycle, when E_2 concentrations were approximately 300 pg/ml (periovulatory). E_2 and P concentrations for samples pooled over 4 hours are presented in the center. (Redrawn from Marut EL et al: *Endocrinology* 109:227, 1981.)

under the control of an ovarian pacemaker that dictates the timing of these periovulatory events.

Several specific biochemical and biophysical phenomena occur at the time of ovulation, most of which are associated with the LH surge and its metabolic effects. The oocyte remains in the diplotene stage of meiosis I until the LH surge. At this time, the resumption of meiosis occurs, the first polar body is extruded, and the oocyte becomes ready for fertilization. This process probably is not a stimulatory event but rather a release from prior inhibition. The most suggestive evidence for this is the well-documented phenomenon that, when oocytes are removed from follicles, they can undergo nuclear maturation in vitro.[75] An ovarian peptide, oocyte maturation inhibitor, has been postulated as the agent responsible for preventing premature maturation of the oocyte.[85] Oocyte maturation

inhibitor has not been isolated or characterized in humans or primates, but teleologically it makes sense that the limited supply of female gametes would be protected from premature changes that would render them unsuitable for future cycles.

At the time of the LH surge, the granulosa cells surrounding the follicle begin to become transformed or luteinized. These cells enlarge and, along with a decrease in rough endoplasmic reticulum and increased lipid content, become more specialized toward synthesis and secretion of P and estrogen instead of the predominantly estrogenic and peptidergic products of the follicular phase. This rapid increase in P levels is responsible for inducing and coordinating several of the physiologic changes seen elsewhere in the reproductive system. The concept of regulators of follicular maturation is appealing in explaining the differ-

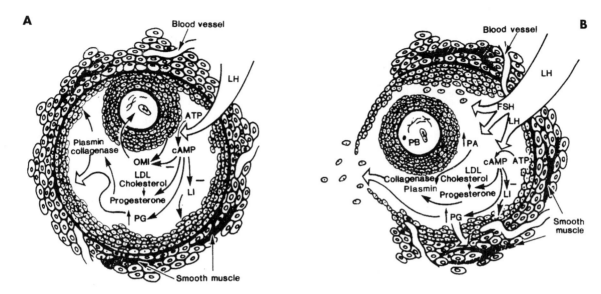

Fig. 5-11. Mechanism of ovulation. (1) Rising LH levels stimulate an increase in cyclic adenosine monophosphate (*cAMP*). (2) cAMP mediates luteinization and resumption of meiosis, overcoming the action of local inhibitor, luteinization inhibitor (*LI*), and oocyte maturation inhibitor (*OMI*). (3) As luteinization proceeds, progesterone levels rise, enhancing the activity of proteolytic enzymes and increasing follicle wall distensibility. (4) Prostaglandin (*PG*) levels increase and, together with plasmin and collagenase, may serve to digest the follicle wall. (5) The midcycle LH surge brings about completion of reduction division and formation of the first polar body (*PB*). (6) Midcycle FSH stimulates expansion of the cumulus and production of plasminogen activator (*PA*). (7) Continued enzymatic digestion results in follicle wall rupture. (8) PGs may stimulate contraction of smooth muscle in the theca externa, causing oocyte expulsion. (9) Branching vessels penetrate the luteinized granulosa. *LDL*, low-density lipoprotein; *ATP*, adenosine triphophate. (From Fritz MA, Speroff L: *Fertil Steril* 38:509, 1982.)

ential behavior of neighboring follicles from cycle to cycle.[9]

Mechanism of ovulation

At present, there are five proposed mechanisms of oocyte extrusion: proteolysis, prostaglandin synthesis, mucification, smooth muscle activity, and angiogenesis factor (Fig. 5-11).

Proteolysis. Large amounts of plasminogen activator are produced from periovulatory granulosa and theca cells.[77] The increase in tissue plasminogen activator produces a parallel increase in intrafollicular plasmin content (and other serine proteases), which weakens the follicular wall and probably produces activation of latent collagenase.[89] The activity of these enzymes is regulated by collagenase inhibitors, which have been found in different species, including humans.[12] These inhibitors, in concert, control the site and extent of tissue remodeling that occurs during ovulation.[3]

Prostaglandin synthesis. Throughout the follicular phase, the dominant follicle accumulates prostaglandins of the E and F series. This process is enhanced by the occurrence of the LH surge.[55] Although the exact mecha-

nism by which prostaglandins have an impact on ovulation is unknown, it has been demonstrated in animal models that indomethacin in vivo can inhibit ovulation and result in the formation of luteinized unruptured follicles.[50] This inhibition can be reversed by exogenous administration of prostaglandins.[87] In addition, histamine and bradykinin probably modulate ovulation.[5,54]

Mucification. FSH and LH stimulate the production and deposition of hyaluronic acid, a nonsulfated glycosaminoglycan, around the oocyte within the corona radiata, which disperses the cumulus and separates the oocyte-cumulus complex from the granulosa membrane. This action facilitates the extrusion of the oocyte at the time of follicular rupture.[18] Follicular fluid also contains sulfated glycosaminoglycans, which inhibit hyaluronic acid–synthesizing activity by cumulus cells.[19] It is hypothesized that the function of these sulfated glycosaminoglycans may be to inhibit precocious cumulus expansion and prevent early demise of the oocyte after ovulation.[78]

Smooth muscle activity. Smooth muscle, which is found in the follicle wall, may facilitate extrusion of the oocyte by maintaining tension on the follicular wall. The ovary is an innervated structure and LH is associated with prostaglandin synthesis, which has been demonstrated to stimulate ovarian smooth muscle activity.[88]

Angiogenesis factor. Before follicular rupture, the antrum remains avascular; however, during and after release of the ovum, transient hemorrhage and neovascular development occur and are preludes to corpus luteum formation. This is important for the delivery of lipoproteins and other substrates to the luteal cells. In fact, studies have demonstrated angiogenic activity in follicular fluid of humans.[24] Renin, angiotensin II, transforming growth factor beta, cytokines, and interleukin-1 have been demonstrated to modulate angiogenesis in follicular fluid.[6,21,57,60,71] It seems likely that these substances might promote follicular rupture.

Function of corpus luteum

Luteal function is dependent both qualitatively and quantitatively on normal development of the granulosa and theca cells during the preceding follicular phase. Inadequate proliferation of these gonadal stroma cells during the follicular phase or incomplete luteinization during the early luteal phase results in decreased secretion of E_2 and P. This, in turn, may result in altered function of the fallopian tube and endometrium, possibly resulting in abnormal gamete or embryo transport and decreased opportunities for implantation. Indeed, deficiencies in either the duration of the P secretion or the amount secreted during the postovulatory phase of the menstrual cycle have been widely correlated with reproductive failure. (See Chapter 24.)

Studies of human follicular and antral fluid have suggested that at least three criteria need to be fulfilled before the rupturing follicle can be transformed into an appropriately functional corpus luteum: (1) there must be sufficient numbers of granulosa cells in the follicle before ovulation, because thereafter granulosa luteal cells cease proliferation; (2) the follicle must contain granulosa cells with the capacity to secrete sufficient P after ovulation; and (3) the granulosa cells, as well as the theca cells, must be responsive to trophic stimuli, especially LH and hCG.[62]

The corpus luteum is not an autonomously functioning unit but is dependent on continued LH support.[44] Experiments have demonstrated that removal of LH support through medical or surgical hypophysectomy or neutralizing antibodies to LH results in decreased P production and shortened luteal phases.[38,86] Maintenance of corpus luteum function is not necessarily dependent on a pulsatile gonadotropin stimulation, but it has been demonstrated with the tonic stimulation provided by an intramuscular injection of hCG. Typically, however, P release from the corpus luteum is pulsatile and corresponds to the endogenous gonadotropin pulses.[23,40]

The corpus luteum undergoes luteolysis with its declining capacity to produce P and E_2 if adequate LH (in the

nonfertile cycle) or hCG (in the fertile cycle) stimulation is not provided. Alternatively, luteolysis may be an active process; rising E_2 levels in the midluteal phase may suppress LH secretion or its action, or increased intraovarian production of prostaglandin $F_{2\alpha}$ in the late luteal phase may inhibit P synthesis.[25]

Finally, the corpus luteum is necessary to maintain gestation in humans until the placental unit becomes competent to secrete adequate P. This interval is known as the luteal-placental shift. Classic studies examining pregnancy maintenance after luteectomy or oophorectomy in women have shown that this interval occurs approximately 8 weeks after the last menses.[11]

CLINICAL CORRELATES
Ovulation induction for anovulatory states

The objective of ovulation induction in anovulatory conditions is to modify pathophysiologic conditions so as to replicate the temporal, quantitative, and qualitative events of the natural fertile menstrual cycle. Defects of the ovarian cycle are the primary cause of infertility in 15% to 20% of infertile couples; therefore, a full understanding of the origin and mechanisms of the ovarian pathophysiology is important to the clinician. This pretreatment evaluation is critical in determining the opportunity for success with ovulation induction. (See Chapter 30.)

Whatever the method used for ovulation induction, conditions of the follicular phase must allow progressive maturation of one or more ovarian follicles with concurrent proliferation of the uterine endometrium. Not uncommonly, the iatrogenic effects of the therapeutic course contribute to failure in treatment. Forcing an oocyte out of the ovary is not enough to achieve a pregnancy. Indeed, both the gametogenic and hormonogenic factors must act in concert during ovulation induction, as they do in the spontaneous fertile menstrual cycle. (See Chapter 31.)

Ovarian wedge resection. Even before medical therapies for ovulation induction were available, elimination of one third to one half of the ovarian mass from patients with polycystic ovary disease often induced ovulation and ovarian cyclicity lasting a few months or years. The means by which this disease prevents ovulation is not fully understood; however, it is clear that often the wedge resection accommodates a disinhibition involving a relative FSH deficiency and an LH excess. Liabilities of the wedge resection include adhesive disease, limited efficacy, and operative risks.[47] Newer methods of ovarian laser cortical ablation are yet to be established in terms of efficacy and possible long-term sequelae.

Bromocriptine. Central defects that result in hyperprolactinemia can cause an associated deficiency of gonadotropin secretion. Administration of the ergot alkaloid bromocriptine, a dopamine agonist, or other related compounds can inhibit pituitary prolactin release concur-

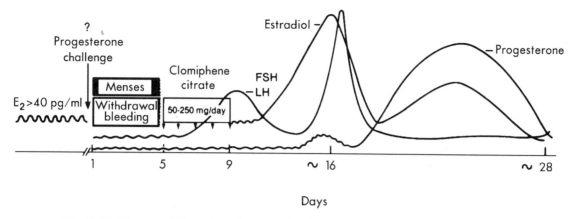

Fig. 5-12. Conceptual illustration of a conventional regimen of clomiphene citrate for induction of ovulation. Note that circulating E₂ levels (best results at or above 40 pg/mL) must be high enough to augment the transient elevation of serum FSH and LH derived from clomiphene treatment. Spontaneous menses or P withdrawal bleeding indicates sufficient estrogen for endometrial proliferation and ovulation induction. (From Hodgen GD: *Fertil Steril* 38:281, 1983).

rently with resumption of the ovarian cycle and ovulation in patients with overt hyperprolactinemia.[72] (See Chapter 9.)

Clomiphene citrate. The indications favoring use of clomiphene citrate, a nonsteroidal weak estrogen, are paradoxical, yet convincing. (See Chapter 32.) Best results occur in patients already near the threshold for spontaneous ovulation. Indeed, intact pituitary and ovarian function is essential. Patients with sufficient endogenous estrogen, to a level allowing withdrawal bleeding after a P challenge, are appropriate candidates for this form of ovulation induction therapy. The actual mechanisms by which clomiphene citrate promotes ovulation are only partially understood. In part, administration of clomiphene citrate in the midfollicular phase causes transient small elevations of gonadotropin secretion that contribute to the promotion of fertile ovulations (Fig. 5-12). The previously discussed mechanism for selection of one dominant follicle can be overcome, and it is not uncommon to mature up to three follicles during a cycle of therapy. Hyperstimulation syndrome is observed infrequently with this agent. It has been demonstrated that high-dose clomiphene citrate treatment with its attenuating (antiestrogen) effects on normal follicular maturation may cause ovarian refractoriness and latent luteal irregularities that may impair fecundity, despite augmentation of pituitary gonadotropin section.[59]

Exogenous gonadotropins. Anovulatory patients who are most deficient in pituitary gonadotropin and estrogen secretion, that is, hypopituitary-hypogonadal women, are often appropriate candidates for exogenous gonadotropins. (See Chapter 33.) This is particularly true when the pituitary response to GnRH is diminished or the pituitary gland is absent. Ovulation induction by administration (direct injection) of a gonadotropin preparation results in a high rate of ovarian response to the supraphysiologic levels of FSH or LH (or both) provided. Usually several follicles mature quasi-synchronously, and spontaneous LH surges often are absent. Accordingly, injections of hCG as the "surrogate" LH surge frequently lead to multiple ovulations and a significant rate of multiple pregnancies if the stimulation is excessive. Hyperstimulation syndrome, resulting in a massive third-space fluid shift into the peritoneal cavity and even ovarian rupture, is a potential complication. (See Chapter 35.) The use of daily rapid estrogen assays, along with ovarian ultrasound monitoring, greatly diminishes this risk.[4,29,81]

It is clear that the supraphysiologic milieu attained during gonadotropin administration will prevent the process of selection of a single dominant follicle as in the natural cycle (Fig. 5-13). The elevated gonadotropin concentrations tend to accelerate development: follicular maturity adequate to produce mature oocytes is present by approximately cycle day 7 to cycle day 10 with this treatment regimen, compared with about cycle day 14 in the normal menstrual cycle.[52]

Pulsatile gonadotropin-releasing hormone. Since appreciation of the physiology of the essential pulsatile GnRH secretion, the use of a "mechanical hypothalamus" has brought a solution to ovulation induction when the causative factor is dysfunction of the hypothalamus. (See Chapter 34.) Interestingly, even with an unvarying intermittent pulse schedule and a wide dose schedule, both subcutaneously and intravenously, the temporal and endocrine characteristics of cycles induced by GnRH pulse therapy are similar to those of the spontaneous menstrual cycle (Fig. 5-14). There is normally a spontaneous LH surge when there is maturation of one dominant follicle. The

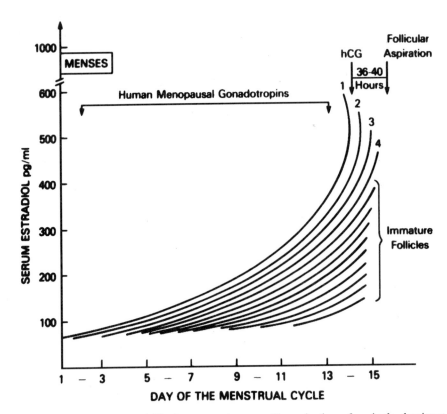

Fig. 5-13. hMG/hCG-stimulated follicular maturation overrides selection of a single dominant follicle in the natural cycle. Note that only a few follicles can be regarded to be developing quasi-synchronously. If hCG is given too late, the most advanced follicles may yield postmature eggs of low potential viability. (From Hodgen GD: In Jones HW Jr et al, editors: *In vitro fertilization—Norfolk,* Baltimore, 1986, Williams & Wilkins.)

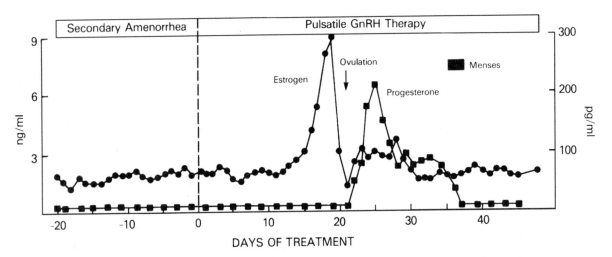

Fig. 5-14. Ovulation induced by pulsatile administration of GnRH for treatment of secondary amenorrhea and anovulatory infertility in primates. A mechanical pump delivered the GnRH pulse intravenously (6 µg per pulse) once every 90 minutes. Note elevation of circulating estrogen levels emanating from the dominant follicle before ovulation, followed by normal serum progesterone levels in the luteal phase with continued GnRH therapy. In these monkeys with secondary amenorrhea (>8 months), only 3 weeks of GnRH therapy was required to induce ovulation. (From Sopelak VM et al: *JAMA* 251:1477, 1984.)

corpus luteum is dependent on continued GnRH pulse therapy throughout the luteal phase; alternatively, hCG can be substituted for corpus luteum support. Although the risk of multiple pregnancies and hyperstimulation has been demonstrated with ovulatory induction by pulsatile GnRH therapy, this risk is greatly lessened.[10,56]

Ovulation induction for normal endocrine states

Before the era of in vitro fertilization, much of the information on the human menstrual cycle was based on peripheral blood hormone measurements and focused on ovarian hormonogenesis and its interactions with the hypothalamic-pituitary axis. With the ability to examine follicular fluids and oocytes obtained during the natural cycle or after a stimulation protocol, ovarian hormonogenesis can now be correlated with gametogenesis, fertilizability of the oocyte, and even viability of the early conceptus. (See Chapter 45.)

The first birth by in vitro fertilization was accomplished in the natural cycle without ovarian stimulation. However, methods to promote multiple follicular development, improve oocyte yield, and control ovarian stimulation have resulted in increased pregnancy rates. (See Chapter 46.) Stimulation of endocrinologically normal menstruating women with exogenous gonadotropins that override the natural cycle has increased understanding of gonadotropin–granulosa cell–oocyte interaction.

A number of treatment methods have been used to obtain multiple follicle development and increased oocyte retrieval. Typically, gonadotropin therapy begins on menstrual cycle day 2 or day 3, when a greater number of follicles are still available for recruitment. This timing, along with the increased concentrations of gonadotropins, results in an ongoing development of multiple follicles. Initiation of gonadotropin therapy later in the cycle reduces the number of quasi-synchronous follicles available for recruitment because of the declining number of follicles remaining in the cohort that have not begun the process of atresia. However, if the gonadotropin levels are maintained sufficiently high so as to recruit other small follicles that may have entered the stage of gonadotropin sensitivity, these smaller follicles will lag behind the follicles that were recruited earlier and are unlikely to produce fertilizable oocytes, and in fact may increase the risk of hyperstimulation. A comparison in monkeys of a "step-up" protocol and a "step-down" protocol of dosages of hMG/hCG demonstrated better synchronization of follicular rupture and reduced susceptibility to delayed ovulations with the step-down protocol.[1]

Most endocrinologically normal ovulating women undergoing exogenous gonadotropin therapy do not have timely spontaneous LH surges.[22] It has been suggested that this inhibition of positive estrogen feedback is due to an inhibitory substance, termed gonadotropin surge-inhibiting factor (GnSIF), produced by supraphysiologic ovarian stimulation.[79] Although GnSIF has not yet been isolated, data strongly suggest that primate ovaries secrete a nonsteroidal factor (GnSIF), distinct from inhibin, that inhibits the spontaneous estrogen-induced LH/FSH surge. It has been hypothesized that the physiologic role of GnSIF is maintenance of the ovulatory quota through prevention of ovulation at an inappropriate time. A decrease in GnSIF to an appropriate level during the late follicular phase may be one factor involved in timely ovulation. Inhibin levels in follicular fluid containing mature granulosa cells were significantly higher than those in fluid containing immature granulosa cells, whereas GnSIF activity was evident in both, suggesting that GnSIF is more selective in suppressing GnRH-stimulated LH secretion and does not affect basal (FSH) gonadotropin production, as does inhibin.[13]

GnRH agonists have further enhanced multiple follicular development for assisted reproductive techniques. GnRH agonists have been applied successfully in two fashions, long and short agonist-gonadotropin regimens[43] (Fig. 5-15). Reduction in treatment cancellation rates (fewer premature LH surges) and enhancement of synchrony of the follicular cohort have been observed with protocols utilizing GnRH agonists because of their suppressive effect on endogenous gonadotropins.[84] In addition, increases in both the average number of oocytes collected and the percentage of oocytes that are meiotically mature are reported with use of GnRH agonists.[17]

It is debatable whether occasional reactivation of the antecedent corpus luteum in demise through re-elevation of P levels during initial treatment can potentially impair oocytes or endometrial quality. GnRH agonists have been demonstrated to have direct effects on ovarian and follicular physiology independent of their influence on the gonadotropin milieu;[70] however, the clinical consequences of this possibility are apparently very limited. Whether the long or short agonist-gonadotropin protocol is more favorable depends on many variables, including the stimulation regimen, monitoring systems, patient population, clinician's expertise, and the techniques of the embryology laboratory.[49,64]

FUTURE CONSIDERATIONS

Recombinant human FSH, which recently has been engineered by several groups,[26] may improve oocyte recovery rates by providing a more individualized treatment regimen using any ratio between FSH and LH doses desired, according to the individual's endocrinologic status. Also, recombinant gonadotropins may diminish the interlot biopotency variability of extracts from urine, which can complicate current dosing regimens.[83]

GnRH antagonists offer some potential advantages over GnRH agonists. The lack of an initial flare-up effect of endogenous gonadotropin secretion results in a virtually

GnRH agonist plus gonadotropins

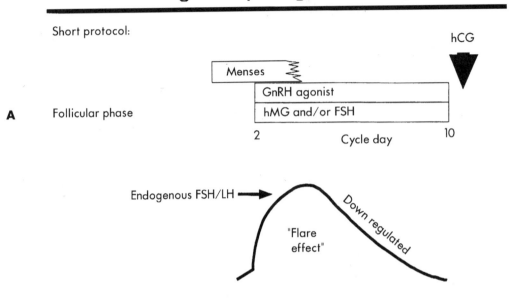

GnRH agonist plus gonadotropins

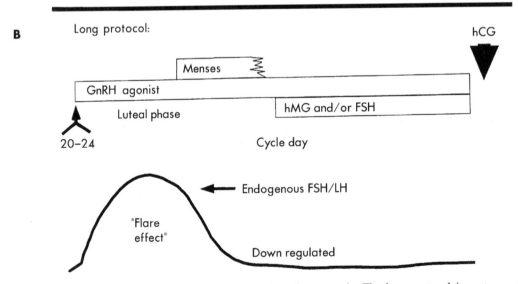

Fig. 5-15. Short (**A**) and long (**B**) agonist-gonadotropin protocols. The long protocol is more versatile overall, whereas the short protocol can save money, provided treatment is effective. (From Hodgen GD: *Contemp Obstet Gynecol* 35:10, 1990.)

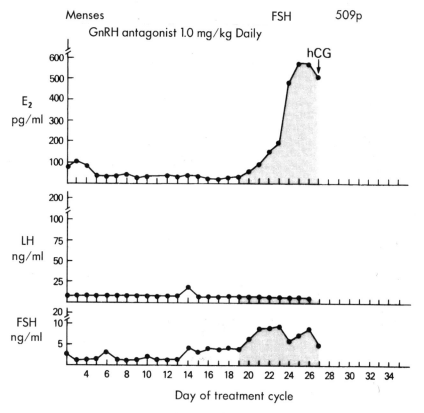

Fig. 5-16. GnRH antagonist (Ac-PClPhe[1], PClPhe[2], DTryp[3], DArg[6], DAla[10])-GnRH HCl, followed by FSH therapy in intact cycling monkeys. Note suppression of endogenous gonadotropin secretion and ovarian responsiveness to FSH treatments as indicated by elevations of E_2 in serum. (From Hodgen GD: In Jones HW Jr et al, editors: *In vitro fertilization—Norfolk,* Baltimore, 1986, Williams & Wilkins.)

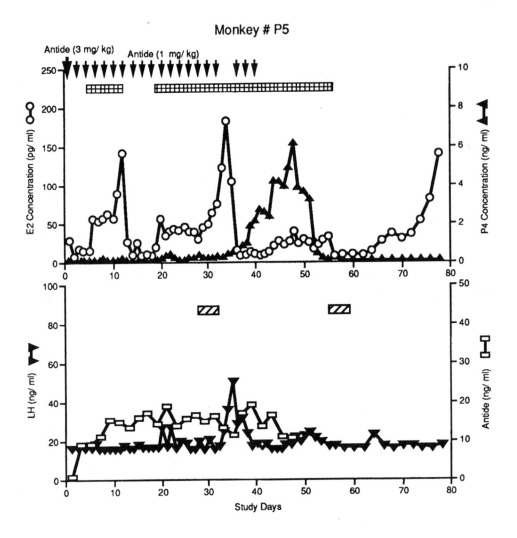

Fig. 5-17. Circulating concentrations of P (m), E₂ (○), Antide (□), and LH (.) in a representative intact monkey treated with Antide plus pulsatile GnRH in a sustaining dose regimen comprising an initial 3-mg/kg dose of Antide (.) with subsequent 1-mg/kg doses administered on alternate days to achieve sustained levels of Antide. Pulsatile GnRH (■) was given at a dose of 5 μg per pulse (one 1-minute pulse per hour) from study day 5 until study day 26. Thereafter, pulsatile GnRH was given at a dose of 10 μg per pulse.

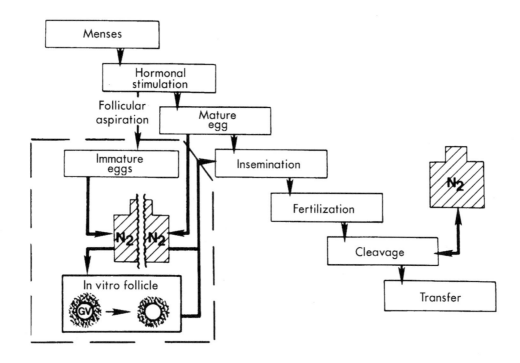

Fig. 5-18. Illustration of the ongoing effort to develop techniques that will permit maturation of oocytes in an in vitro follicle germinal vesicle (*GV*). (From Hodgen GD: In Jones HW Jr et al, editors: *In vitro fertilization—Norfolk,* Baltimore, 1986, Williams & Wilkins.)

immediate "medical hypophysectomy," thus allowing a simultaneous start of the GnRH antagonist and exogenous gonadotropins[36,51] (Fig. 5-16). Also, the antagonists do not down-regulate pituitary GnRH receptor functions; therefore the pituitary remains responsive to exogenous GnRH. This combination of GnRH antagonist and pulsatile GnRH delivered via a pump may offer a new treatment regimen for patients who manifest chronic hyperandrogenemia and the sequelae of endocrinopathy and ovulatory dysfunction[35] (Fig. 5-17).

Among the most important developments in the future will be the ability to mature oocytes in vitro, that is, to harvest dictyate stage oocytes from the ovary for storage and subsequent maturation in an "in vitro follicle" (Fig. 5-18). This would enable patients in need of pelvic irradiation or chemotherapy to preserve their entire pool of oocytes before treatment. It would also avert numerous ethical and legal dilemmas presented by the storage of human embryos. Although significant advances are needed, including the ability to separate reliably all oocytes from their stroma, to cryopreserve oocytes, and to mature immature oocytes in vitro, some preliminary experiments have provided the impetus for future therapy.[8,30]

REFERENCES

1. Abbasi R et al: Cumulative ovulation rate in human menopausal/human chorionic gonadotropin-treatment monkeys: "step-up" versus "step-down" dose regimens, *Fertil Steril* 47:1019, 1987.
2. Adashi EY et al: Insulin-like growth factor 1: a paradigm for putative intraovarian regulators. In Hodgen GD, Rosenwaks Z, Spieler J, editors: *Physiological roles and possibilities in contraceptive development,* Proceedings from the CONRAD International Workshop on Non-Steroidal Gonadal Factors, Norfolk, Va, Jan 6–8, 1988, The Jones Institute Press.
3. Beers WH: Follicular plasminogen and plasminogen activator and the effect of plasmin on ovarian follicular wall, *Cell* 6:379, 1975.
4. Ben-Rafael Z et al: Abortion rate in pregnancies following ovulation induced by human menopausal gonadotropin/human chorionic gonadotropin, *Fertil Steril* 39:157, 1983.
5. Brännström M, Hellberg P: Bradykinin potentiates LH-induced follicular rupture in the rat ovary perfused *in vitro, Hum Reprod* 4:475, 1989.
6. Brown MR et al: Endothelin releasing activity in calf serum and porcine follicular fluid, *Biochem Biophys Res Commun* 173:807, 1990.
7. Burger H et al: Inhibin-regulation and mechanism of action, In Hodgen GD, Rosenwaks, Z, Spieler J, editors: *Physiological roles and possibilities in contraceptive development,* Proceedings from the CONRAD International Workshop on Non-Steroidal Gonadal Factors, Norfolk, Va, Jan 6–8, 1988, The Jones Institute Press.
8. Cha KY et al: Pregnancy after *in vitro* fertilization of human follicular oocytes collected from nonstimulated cycle, their culture *in vitro* and their transfer in a donor oocyte program, *Fertil Steril* 55:109, 1991.
9. Channing CP et al: Ovarian follicular and luteal physiology. In Greep RO, editor: *Reproductive physiology III,* vol 22, *International Review of Physiology,* Baltimore, 1980, University Park Press.
10. Crowley WF, MacArthur JW: Simulation of the normal menstrual cycle in Kallmann's syndrome by pulsatile administration of luteinizing hormone-releasing hormone (LHRH), *J Clin Endocrinol* 51:173, 1980.
11. Csapo AI et al: The significance of the human corpus luteum in pregnancy maintenance, *Am J Obstet Gynecol* 112:1061, 1972.
12. Curry TE Jr et al: Identification and characterization of metalloproteinase inhibitor activity in human ovarian follicular fluid, *Endocrinology* 123:1611, 1988.

13. Danforth DR, Hodgen GD: The regulation of pituitary gonadotropin secretion by GnSIF gonadotropin surge-inhibiting factor and inhibin. In Hodgen GD, Rosenwaks Z, Spieler J, editors: *Physiological roles and possibilities in contraceptive development,* Proceedings from the CONRAD International Workshop on Non-Steroidal Gonadal Factors, Norfolk, Va, Jan 6–8, 1988, The Jones Institute Press.

14. diZerega GS, Hodgen GD: Folliculogenesis in the primate ovarian cycle, *Endocr Rev* 2:27, 1981.

15. diZerega GS et al: Asymmetrical ovarian estradiol secretion during the follicular phase of the primate menstrual cycle, *J Clin Endocrinol* 51:689, 1980.

16. diZerega GS et al: Fluorescence localization of LH/hCG uptake in the primate ovary: characterization of the preovulatory ovary, *Fertil Steril* 34:379, 1980.

17. Droesch K et al: Value of suppression with a gonadotropin-releasing hormone agonist prior to gonadotropin stimulation for *in vitro* fertilization, *Fertil Steril* 51:292, 1989.

18. Eppig JJ: Regulation of cumulus oophorous expansion by gonadotropins *in vivo* and *in vitro, Biol Reprod* 23:545, 1980.

19. Eppig JJ, Ward-Bailey PF: Sulfated glycosaminoglycans inhibit hyaluronic acid synthesizing activity in mouse cumuli oophori, *Exp Cell Res* 150:459, 1984.

20. Erickson GF: Normal ovarian function, *Clin Obstet Gynecol* 21:31, 1978.

21. Fernandez LA et al: Renin-like activity in ovarian follicular fluid, *Fertil Steril* 44:219, 1985.

22. Ferraretti AP et al: Serum luteinizing hormone during ovulation induction with human menopausal gonadotropin for *in vitro* fertilization in normally menstruating women, *Fertil Steril* 40:742, 1983.

23. Filicori M, Butler JT, Crowley WF: Neuroendocrine regulation of the corpus luteum in the human: evidence for pulsatile progesterone secretion, *J Clin Invest* 73:1638, 1984.

24. Frederick JL, Shimanuki T, diZerega GS: Initiation of angiogenesis by human follicular fluid, *Science* 224:389, 1984.

25. Fritz MA, Speroff L: The endocrinology of the menstrual cycle: the interaction of folliculogenesis and neuroendocrine mechanisms, *Fertil Steril* 38:509, 1982.

26. Galaway AB et al: *In vitro* and *in vivo* bioactivity of recombinant human follicular-stimulating hormone and partially deglycosylated variants secreted by transfected eukaryotic cell lives, *Endocrinology* 127:93, 1990.

27. Garcia JE, Jones GS, Wright GL: Prediction of the time of ovulation, *Fertil Steril* 36:308, 1981.

28. Gauthier G: Olfactogenital dysplasia at puberty, *Acta Neuroveg* 21:345, 1960.

29. Gemzell C: Induction of ovulation with human gonadotropins, *Recent Prog Horm Res* 21:179, 1965.

30. Godsen RG: Restitution of fertility in sterilized mice by transferring primordial ovarian follicles, *Hum Reprod* 5:117, 1990.

31. Goodman AL, Hodgen GD: Between-ovary interaction in the regulation of follicle growth, corpus luteum function and gonadotropin secretion in the primate ovarian cycle, I: effects of follicle cautery and hemiovariectomy during the follicular phase in cynomolgus monkeys, *Endocrinology* 104:1304, 1979.

32. Goodman AL, Hodgen GD: Between-ovary interaction in the regulation of follicle growth, corpus luteum function and gonadotropin secretion in the primate ovarian cycle, II: effects of luteectomy and hemiovariectomy during the luteal phase in cynomolgus monkeys, *Endocrinology* 104:1310, 1979.

33. Goodman AL et al: Regulation of folliculogenesis in the rhesus monkey: selection of the dominant follicle, *Endocrinology* 100:155, 1977.

34. Goodman AL, Hodgen GD: The ovarian triad. In Greep RO, editor: *Recent progress in hormone research,* New York, 1983, Academic Press.

35. Gordon K et al: A novel regimen of gonadotropin-releasing hormone (GnRH) antagonist plus pulsatile GnRH: controlled restoration of gonadotropin secretion and ovulation induction, *Fertil Steril* 54:1140, 1990.

36. Gordon K et al: The use of a GnRH antagonist (Antide) as adjunctive therapy with gonadotropins for ovulation induction in cynomolgus monkeys. Paper presented at the Annual Meeting of the Canadian Fertility and Andrology Society, Quebec, Oct 3–6, 1990 (abstract 42).

37. Gougeon A, Testart J: Influence of human menopausal gonadotropin on the recruitment of human follicles, *Fertil Steril* 54:848, 1990.

38. Groff TR et al: Effects of neutralization of luteinizing hormone on corpus luteum function and cyclicity in *Macaca fasicularis, J Clin Endocrinol Metab* 59:1054, 1984.

39. Gulyas BJ et al: Effects of fetal or maternal hypophysectomy on endocrine organs and body weight in infant rhesus monkeys (*Macaca fasicularis*): with particular emphasis on oogenesis, *Biol Reprod* 16:216, 1977.

40. Healy DL et al: Pulsatile progesterone secretion: its relevance to clinical evaluation of corpus luteum function, *Fertil Steril* 41:114, 1984.

41. Hillier SG et al: Superovulation strategy before *in vitro* fertilization, *Clin Obstet Gynecol* 12:687, 1985.

42. Hirshfield AN: Rescue of atretic follicles *in vitro* and *in vivo, Biol Reprod* 40:181, 1989.

43. Hodgen GD: Uses of GnRH analogs in IVF-ET, *Contemp Obstet Gynecol* 35:10, 1990.

44. Hutchinson JS, Zeleznik AJ: The rhesus monkey corpus luteum is dependent on pituitary gonadotropin secretion throughout the luteal phase of the menstrual cycle, *Endocrinology* 115:1780, 1984.

45. Jansen RP: Endocrine response of the fallopian tube, *Endocr Rev* 5:525, 1984.

46. Jones GS: Corpus luteum: composition and function, *Fertil Steril* 54:21, 1990.

47. Jones HW Jr: Polycystic ovarian syndrome: a retrospective study on the therapeutic effect of ovarian wedge resection after unsuccessful treatment with clomiphene citrate (editorial), *Obstet Gynecol Surv* 38:483, 1983.

48. Kaplan SL, Grumbach MM, Aubert ML: The ontogenesis of pituitary hormones and hypothalamic factors in the human fetus: maturation of the central nervous system regulation of anterior pituitary function, *Recent Prog Horm Res* 32:161, 1976.

49. Katayma KP et al: Short-term use of gonadotropin-releasing hormone agonist (Leuprolide) for *in vitro* fertilization, *J In Vitro Fert Embryo Transfer* 5:332, 1988.

50. Katz E et al: Effects of systemic administration of indomethacin on ovulation, luteinization, and steroidogenesis in the rabbit ovary, *Am J Obstet Gynecol* 161:1361, 1989.

51. Kenigsberg D, Hodgen GD: Ovulation inhibition by administration of weekly gonadotropin-releasing hormone antagonist, *J Clin Endocrinol Metab* 62:734, 1986.

52. Kenigsberg D et al: Medical hypophysectomy, II: variability of ovarian response to gonadotropin therapy, *Fertil Steril* 42:116, 1984.

53. Knobil E: The neuroendocrine control of the menstrual cycle, *Recent Prog Horm Res* 36:53, 1980.

54. Krishna A, Terranova PF: Alterations in mass cell degranulation and ovarian histamine in the proestrus hamster, *Biol Reprod* 32:1211, 1985.

55. LeMaire WJ, Leidner R, Marsh JM: Pre- and post-ovulatory changes in the concentration of prostaglandins in rat graafian follicles, *Prostaglandins* 9:221, 1975.

56. Leyendecker G, Wildt L, Hansmann M: Pregnancies following intermittent (pulsatile) administration of GnRH by means of a portable pump ("Zyklomat"): a new approach to the treatment of infertility in hypothalamic amenorrhea, *J Clin Endocrinol Metab* 51:1214, 1980.

57. Loukides JA et al: Human follicular fluids contain tissue macrophages, *J Clin Endocrinol Metab* 71:1363, 1990.

58. Lunenfeld B, Kraiem Z, Echkol A: Structure and function of the growing follicle, *Clin Obstet Gynecol* 3:27, 1976.

59. Marut EL, Hodgen GD: Antiestrogenic action of high-dose clomiphene in primates: pituitary augmentation but with ovarian attenuation, *Fertil Steril* 38:100, 1982.

60. Masure S, Opdenakker G: Cytokine-mediated proteolysis in tissue remodeling, *Experientia* 45:542, 1989.

61. McLachlan RI et al: The physiology of inhibin in women. In Hodgen GD, Rosenwaks Z, Spieler J, editors: *Physiological roles and possibilities in contraceptive development,* Proceedings from the CONRAD International Workshop on Non-Steroidal Gonadal Factors, Norfolk, Va, Jan 6–8, 1988, The Jones Institute Press.

62. McNatty KP, Sawyers RS: Relationship between the endocrine environment within the graafian follicle and the subsequent rate of progesterone secretion by human granulosa cells *in vitro, J Endocrinol* 66:391, 1975.

63. McNatty KP et al: The microenvironment of the human antral follicle: intrarelationships among the steroid levels in antral fluid, the population of granulosa cells, and the status of the oocyte *in vivo* and *in vitro, J Clin Endocrinol Metab* 49:851, 1979.

64. Meldrum DR et al: Timing of initiation and dose schedule of leuprolide influence the time course of ovarian suppression, *Fertil Steril* 50:400, 1988.

65. Messinis IE, Templeton AA: The importance of follicle-stimulating hormone increase for folliculogenesis, *Hum Reprod* 5:153, 1990.

66. Moon YS, Tsang BK, Simpson C, Armstrong DT: 17-β-estradiol biosynthesis in culture granulosa and theca cells of human ovarian follicles: stimulation by follicle-stimulating hormone, *J Clin Endocrinol Metab* 47:263, 1978.

67. Nilsson L, Wikland M, Hamberger L: Recruitment of an ovulatory follicle in the human following follicle-ectomy and luteectomy, *Fertil Steril* 37:30, 1982.

68. Pauerstein CJ et al: Temporal relationships of estrogen, progesterone, and luteinizing hormone levels to ovulation in women and infrahuman primates, *Am J Obstet Gynecol* 130:876, 1978.

69. Pederson T: Follicle kenetics in the ovary of cyclic mouse, *Acta Endocrinol* 64:304, 1970.

70. Pellicer A, Miro F: Steroidogenesis *in vitro* of human granulosa-luteal cells pretreated *in vivo* with gonadotropin-releasing hormone analogs, *Fertil Steril* 54:590, 1990.

71. Pepper MS et al: Transforming growth factor-beta 1 modulates basic fibroblast growth factor-induced proteolytic and angiogenic properties of endothelial cells *in vitro, J Cell Biol* 111:743, 1990.

72. Pepperell RJ, McBain JC, Healy DL: Ovulation induction with bromocriptine in patients with hyperprolactinemia, *Aust N Z J Obstet Gynaecol* 17:181, 1977.

73. Peters H, Himelstein-Braw R, Faber M: The normal development of the ovary in childhood, *Acta Endocrinol* 82:617, 1976.

74. Peters H et al: The effect of gonadotropin on follicle growth initiation in the neonatal mouse ovary, *J Reprod Fertil* 35:139, 1973.

75. Pincus G, Enzmann EV: Comparative behaviors of mammalian eggs *in vivo* and *in vitro:* activation of ovarian eggs, *J Exp Med* 62:655, 1935.

76. Ravindranath N et al: Effect of FSH deprivation at specific times on follicular maturation in the bonnet monkey (*Macaca radiata*), *J Reprod Fertil* 87:231, 1989.

77. Reich R, Miskin R, Tsafriri A: Follicular plasminogen activator: involvement in ovulation, *Endocrinology* 116:516, 1985.

78. Sato E, Miyamoto H, Koide SS: Glycosaminoglycans in porcine follicular fluid promoting viability of oocytes in culture, *Mol Reprod Dev* 26:391, 1990.

79. Schenken RS, Hodgen GD: Follicle-stimulating hormone induced ovarian hyperstimulation in monkeys: blockade of the LH surge, *J Clin Endocrinol Metab* 57:50, 1983.

80. Schomberg DW: Growth factors and reproduction. In Hodgen GD, Rosenwaks Z, Spieler J editors: *Physiological roles and possibilities in contraceptive development,* Proceedings from the CONRAD International Workshop on Non-Steroidal Gonadal Factors, Norfolk, Va, Jan 6–8, 1988, The Jones Institute Press.

81. Schwartz M, Jewelewicz R: The use of gonadotropins for induction of ovulation, *Fertil Steril* 35:3, 1981.

82. Speth RC, Jusain A: Distribution of angiotensin-converting enzyme and angiotensin II-receptor binding sites in the rat ovary, *Biol Reprod* 38:695, 1988.

83. Stone BA et al: Responses of patients to different lots of human menopausal gonadotropins during controlled ovarian hyperstimulation, *Fertil Steril* 52:745, 1989.

84. Thanki KH, Schmidt CL: Follicular development and oocyte maturation after stimulation with gonadotropins versus leuprolide acetate/gonadotropins during *in vitro* fertilization, *Fertil Steril* 54:656, 1990.

85. Tsafriri A, Dekel N, Bar-Ami S: The role of oocyte maturation inhibitor in follicular regulation of oocyte maturation, *J Reprod Fertil* 64:541, 1982.

86. VandeWiele RL et al: Mechanism regulating the menstrual cycle in women, *Recent Prog Horm Res* 26:63, 1970.

87. Wallach EE et al: Effectiveness of prostaglandin $F_{2\alpha}$ in restoration of hMG-hCG induced ovulation in indomethacin-treated rhesus monkeys, *Prostaglandins* 10:129, 1975.

88. Wright KH et al: Studies of rabbit ovarian contractility using chronically implanted transducers, *Fertil Steril* 27:310, 1976.

89. Yoshimura Y, Wallach EE: Studies of the mechanism(s) of mammalian ovulation, *Fertil Steril* 47:22, 1987.

Chapter 6

IMPLANTATION

Sue Ellen Carpenter, MD

Endometrial development
 Epidermal growth factor
 Insulinlike growth factors I and II
 Colony-stimulating factor #1
 Leucocyte inhibiting factor
Adhesion
Trophoblast invasion
 Plasminogen activator
 Type 4 collagenase
Immunoregulation of implantation
 Human leucocyte antigen = G
 TLX antigen
 Immunosuppressive mechanisms
Summary

Implantation involves a complex set of interactions between the developing blastocyst and the uterine epithelium. Apposition of the blastocyst and uterus, cellular adhesion, trophoblast invasion, and endometrial decidualization are required for the successful formation of the mature placenta (Fig. 6-1). The processes involved, because they are complex, time dependent, and species specific, have been difficult to study. Due to technical and ethical constraints, our understanding of human implantation must often be extrapolated from animal models. However, understanding the early cellular events of implantation is invaluable to the treatment of patients with recurrent abortion, and in the advancement of the assisted reproductive technologies.

After fertilization, the human embryo takes 5.5-6 days to traverse the oviduct. Successful implantation requires a receptive endometrium with synchronously developed elements, including glandular and surface endometrium, fibroblasts, stromal cells, smooth myocytes, vascular endothe-

lium macrophages, and monocytes. The first phase of the menstrual cycle is estradiol dominant. Estrogen stimulation of the endometrium results in mitosis of the glandular epithelium, stroma, and vascular epithelium. The second half, or secretory phase, of the menstrual cycle is progesterone dominant, and results in the differentiation of these elements.[41]

Various growth factors present in the endometrium are considered to be the mediators of steroid hormone action in the endometrium. Decidualization of the endometrium is characterized by transformation of the fibroblastic stromal cells into large epithelial cells. In humans, the decidual reaction is progesterone driven, and begins in the late luteal phase of the menstrual cycle. The role of decidual cells is uncertain. The presence of lymphoid-like cells in the decidua has led to the speculation that decidual cells regulate the invasiveness of the trophoblast and participate in immunoprotection of the embryo. It is recognized that inadequate decidualization at the time of implantation is associated with infertility and pregnancy loss.

ENDOMETRIAL DEVELOPMENT
Epidermal growth factor

Epidermal growth factor (EGF) is a proposed polypeptide mediator of estradiol action in the uterus.[40] EGF is a potent mitogen that interacts with a specific cell surface receptor. Using immunohistochemical techniques, Slowey et al. recently reported EGF and EGF-Receptor expression in the glandular epithelium of cycling baboons.[52] No difference in expression was found between the late follicular and mid-luteal phase endometrium. However, there was a shift from glandular to stromal expression of EGF and EGF-R in the decidua during the first trimester of pregnancy. The authors propose that EGF and EGF-R may play a role in implantation and decidualization.

In humans, EGF and EGF messenger ribonucleic acid (mRNA) have been demonstrated in the glandular epithelium and in stromal cells. In general, no cycle dependence is noted.[18,7,19,39] Hofman et al., working with human

158

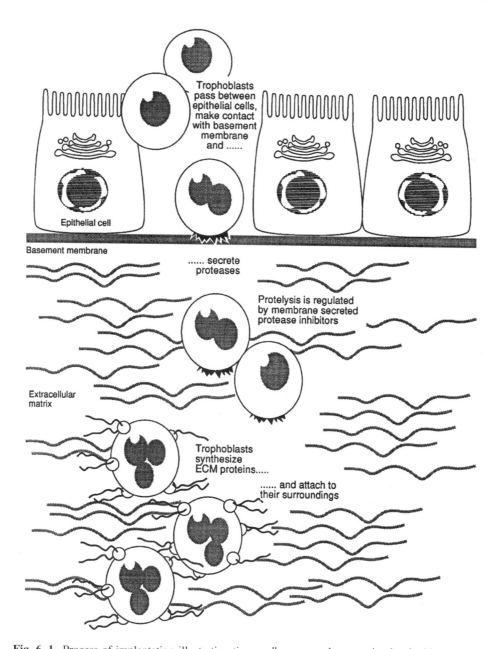

Fig. 6-1. Process of implantation illustrating tissue adherence and penetration by the blastocyst.

decidua, found that EGF staining of the surface epithelium was intense with only light staining of stromal cells.[24] Most immunohistochemical studies of EGF-receptor numbers show staining in both epithelium and stromal cells without cycle dependence.[15] Binding studies are more sensitive to receptor number than immunocytochemistry. Using the more sensitive technique, studies have reported increased numbers of binding sites and increased kD in proliferative endometrium as compared with secretory endometrium.[4,55,56] In situ hybridization techniques applied to endometrial biopsies taken from cycling women have shown an increase in EGF-R mRNA in the periovulatory phase in both the glandular and stromal cells.[32] This effect appears to be a response to increasing estradiol levels, and has also been shown in the preimplantation phase in rabbits.

Regulation of EGF-receptor expression has been studied in vitro. Estrogen, progesterone, and EGF have been shown to have an effect, although the in vivo effect of each has not been clearly determined.[55,47,54]

The presence of EGF and EGF-R in the endometrium, and their interactions with estrogen and progesterone, suggest that they play a role in cellular proliferation and differentiation. Successful decidualization and implantation are dependent on this preparation. EGF and EGF-R may still be shown to play a role in syncytiotrophoblast interaction as well.

Insulin-like growth factors I and II

Insulin-like growth factors (IGF-I and IGF-II) are low molecular weight peptides that promote cellular mitosis and differentiation. They bind to specific receptors on target cell surfaces, and circulate, bound to specific binding proteins that regulate IGF action. In humans, the IGF-I gene is expressed primarily in the proliferative and early secretory endometrium, suggesting that IGF-I is an estromedin in this tissue.[3,16] The IGF-II gene is expressed abundantly in mid to late secretory endometrium and early pregnancy decidua, suggesting a role for IGF-II in differential functions of the endometrium.[16] IGF receptors are present in human endometrium, and total IGF binding capacity (IGF receptors and IGF binding proteins) are cycle and steroid dependent.[49]

Insulin-like growth factor binding protein-1 (IGFBP-1) is produced by endometrial stromal cells in the late secretory phase and in early pregnancy decidua.[30] IGFBP-1 mRNA production is modulated by progesterone. IGFBP-1 inhibits IGF binding to its receptor in human secretory endometrium.[49] During early pregnancy, IGFBPs may limit IGF-mediated trophoblast growth.[48,27]

Colony-stimulating factor 1

Cytokines are proteins that modulate a variety of cellular functions, including cellular proliferation and differentiation, and induction of new antigenic epitopes and cell adhesion molecules. Colony-stimulating factor 1 (CSF-1) is a cytokine that was initially described as a growth factor required for the survival, proliferation, and differentiation of monocytes. It has been reported that a 1000-fold increase in uterine CSF-1 occurs in pregnant mice. This finding has led to investigation of the role of CSF-1 in placentation.[53] Homozygous mutant crosses of mice without CSF-1 are consistently infertile.[2] CSF-1 receptor is expressed on macrophages, decidual cells, and trophoblasts in pregnant mice. In humans, CSF-R protein and mRNA are expressed in the decidual glandular epithelium and in the placenta, and increases during gestation.[26,45] CSF-1 production by placental villous core mesenchymal cells is stimulated by interleukin-1β (IL-1β). It has been suggested that decidual IL-1β may regulate placental CSF-1 production.[37] CSF-1 also regulates the synthesis of human placental lactogen and chorionic gonadotropin.[11] Thus, in addition to its role as a modulator of uterine macrophage number, CSF-1 seems to play a crucial role in placental growth and function.

Leucocyte-inhibiting factor

Leucocyte-inhibiting factor (LIF) is another cytokine that is pleiomorphic in its function. Originally described as a regulator of hematopoietic cell line function, LIF now has been shown to be essential to implantation in mice.[53] Females lacking the LIF gene are fertile, but their blastocysts fail to implant and do not develop. The site of the most abundant LIF expression is the uterine endometrial glands, specifically on day 4 of murine pregnancy.[2] Analysis of LIF expression in pseudopregnant mice, and in females undergoing delayed implantation, showed that it is under maternal control, that its expression coincides with blastocyst formation, and that it always precedes implantation. These results suggest that a principal function of LIF in vivo may be to regulate the growth and to initiate the implantation of blastocysts.

ADHESION

Adhesion of the developing preembryo to the uterine lining is recognized as the important early step in successful implantation. Histological studies of the embryonic uterine interface, taken during the process of implantation in various animal models, show increasing distortion of the two surfaces and the formation of primitive junctional complexes. Characterization of the interaction of cells, with each other and with the components of the extracellular matrix, is essential to understanding a large number of physiological and pathological phenomena, such as organogenesis, cell differentiation, tumor metastasis, and inflammation. In all of these processes, a wide array of cell surface molecules, classified as *adhesion receptors,* have been implicated. Four major families have been identified: integrins, immunoglobulins, selectins, and leucocyte homing receptors.

Integrins are a family of cell surface molecules comprising at least 23 heterodimers of 15 different α chains and nine different β chains.(Fig. 6-2) The term *integrin* reflects the capacity of these molecules to integrate the extracellular and intracellular medium by transferring information in

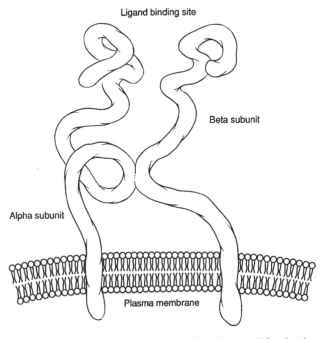

Fig. 6-2. An integrin molecule illustrating the α and β subunits.

both directions.[26] The interaction of integrins with their ligands can evoke intracellular signals that induce changes in cellular morphology, gene expression, and cellular proliferation. On the other hand, the state of cellular activation and intracellular signals regulates the functional activity of integrins in terms of their affinity for their ligands.[45]

The role of integrins and other adhesion molecules in human implantation is being investigated. Lessey et al. have used immunoperoxidase staining to describe the distribution of nine different α and β integrin subunits in human endometrial tissue at different stages of the normal and abnormal human menstrual cycle.[37] Glandular epithelial cells expressed mainly collagen/laminin receptors; stromal cells expressed mainly fibronectin receptors. Expression of α_1 on glandular epithelium was found only in the secretory phase. Expression of both subunits of the vitronectin receptor $\alpha_v\beta_3$ also was cycle specific. The β_3 subunit appeared abruptly on cycle day 20. Discordant luteal-phase biopsies (more than three days "out of phase") from infertility patients showed delayed epithelial β_3 staining. The authors conclude that integrin moieties are regulated in cycling endometrium, and propose that disruption of integrin expression may be associated with decreased uterine receptivity and infertility.

Damsky et al. have investigated distribution patterns of extracellular matrix components and adhesion receptors along the invasive pathway during cytotrophoblast development.[11] Morphologically, this process begins when polarized chorionic villus cytotrophoblasts form multilayered columns of nonpolarized cells and invade the uterus. Damsky et al. compared adhesion molecule expression by cytotrophoblasts in villi, cell columns, and the uterine wall, and found striking changes in distribution between the fetal and maternal compartments of first-trimester placenta. The polarized cytotrophoblasts of chorionic villi are anchored to the trophoblast basement membrane, which contains laminin, fibronectin, and collagen type IV. The integrin $\alpha_6\beta_4$ appears to be the most important receptor complex mediating this interaction. Tenascin, a high molecular weight extracellular matrix component, was expressed exclusively adjacent to column formation regions of the anchoring villi, and may play a role in the induction of invasion. Distally, along the invasive cell columns, $\alpha_5\beta_1$ was seen to interact with fibronectin of cytotrophoblast origin. In the placental bed, where the column structure is lost and cytotrophoblasts are present as clusters of irregularly shaped cells interspersed among the decidual cells of the endometrium, no cell-associated extracellular matrix was identified. Subsequent investigation into this transition may lead to a better understanding of inadequate trophoblast invasion that causes pregnancy loss or excessive trophoblast invasion, as in choriocarcinoma.

In animal models, additional molecular features of blastocyst adhesion have been described. In the rabbit, rat, and mouse, there is a decrease in the thickness of the glycocalyx of the endometrial surface, as well as a decrease in the number of anionic sites. In some species, these changes are embryo specific, occurring only when the embryo is present or only at the site of embryo-uterus contact. The implication of the thinning of the glycocalyx is unknown. It is probable that the process leads to the unmasking of specific binding sites for trophoblasts.[6]

Cell surface changes on the mouse blastocyst at implantation have also been explored. Sialic acid containing glycoproteins contributes a significant negative charge to the blastocyst surface. At implantation, these membrane components decrease.[29] These changes occur both in vivo and in vitro, indicating that they occur independent of maternal/uterine influence. Additional evidence suggests that histocompatibility antigens (of which H-2 is a glycoprotein) also decrease their expression upon activation.[51] Decreased sialic acid content and surface negative charge have been associated with increased membrane deformability and loss of contact inhibition by transformed cells in vitro.[58,42,43] The acquisition of similar properties by the trophectoderm may correlate with the ability to penetrate and invade maternal tissues.

TROPHOBLAST INVASION
Plasminogen activator

Invasion and remodeling of uterine endometrium and vasculature by trophoblasts is a complex process dependent on several proteases. In order to ensure adequate blood supply to the fetus, marked changes in the spiral arterioles must occur. These changes include a disruption of the endothelium, a loss of musculoelastic tissue, and an increase in vessel diameter, all of which facilitate a 10-fold increase in the delivery of maternal blood to the placenta.[13] Because secretion and autocrine binding of urokinase-type plasminogen activator (uPA) is a common mechanism used by cells to facilitate plasmin-dependent tissue invasion, several investigators have explored the expression and regulation of plasminogen activators at implantation. As with all activities having to do with placentation, these mechanisms must be temporally regulated.

Expression of urokinase-type plasminogen activator in mouse embryos has been found in invasive and migratory trophoblast cells at 5.5 and 6.5 days gestation.[59] At 7.5 days, uPA mRNA was localized to trophoblast cells that had reached the deep layers of the uterine wall. At 10.5 days, uPA was undetectable.

Urokinase receptors are present on the cell membranes of first-trimester human cytotrophoblasts. They are also present on term cells, but in diminished numbers. In culture, uPA receptor sites are saturated with endogenous ligand.[50] Cell surface receptors have been hypothesized to localize uPA activity to focal sites on the cell membrane, thereby imparting a direction to the migration of trophoblasts through the basement membrane. Persistence of the receptor on term trophoblasts may prevent fibrin accretion in the placental intervillous spaces. Prourokinase is secreted by and binds to trophoblast with high affinity. All prourokinase on the cell surface is rapidly converted to the active two chain enzyme. Trophoblast in both the first trimester and term converts plasminogen to plasmin. Trophoblasts also produce plasminogen activator inhibitor-1 and -2 (PAI-1 and -2). No plasminogen activator activity is detected in a trophoblast-conditioned medium. This suggests that cell-associated plasminogen activation is more effective than in the extracellular matrix.

To investigate the potential role of prostaglandins in regulation of plasminogen activator activity in mice, Cedars et al. inhibited prostaglandin synthesis just prior to implantation.[5] In treated versus control animals, the degree of vascularity and number of implantation sites was reduced. The embryos tended to remain in the lumen with minimal evidence of invasion. Cultured implantation sites had significantly decreased protein synthesis, plasminogen activation, and PAI activity. The authors suggest that prostaglandin of endometrial origin may be a signal to the embryo to release PA and initiate implantation.

The α_2-macroglobulin receptor/low-density lipoprotein receptor-related protein (α_2MR/LRP) is responsible for binding and internalization of the protease scavenger, α_2-macroglobulin, and very low-density lipoprotein (VLDL) enriched lipoprotein E. It has been shown that α_2MR/LRP binds to the uPA/PAI-1 complex and may be responsible for clearing inactivated UPA from cell surfaces. The expression of α_2MR/LRP and its modulator, receptor-associated protein (RAP), in implantation sites has also been reported. Human cytotrophoblasts and syncytiotrophoblasts from first-trimester chorionic villi, and syncitiotrophoblasts from third-trimester chorionic villi, express α_2MR/LRP and RAP. These proteins may regulate lipoprotein uptake and hence, steroidogenesis. In addition, α_2MR/LRP and RAP have been identified in the first trimester invading trophoblasts deep in the maternal decidua, suggesting a role for these proteins in protease regulation and modulation of trophoblast invasion. In mice, LDL receptor-related protein has been shown to be essential for implantation.[23]

Type IV collagenase

Cytotrophoblast invasion requires degradation of basement membrane collagen type IV. Both enzyme activity and immunoreactive protein studies have confirmed the synthesis specifically of type IV collagenase by invading cytotrophoblasts.[14,36] This activity is markedly decreased in term cells as opposed to first-trimester cytotrophoblasts. Among a variety of metalloproteinases investigated 92-kD type IV collagenase, which was unique to cytotrophoblast, was most critical for invasion. Control of type IV collagenase production is uncertain. Steroid hormone, EGF, I1-1, CSF-1, and TGFα are all possibly direct or indirect regulatory substances. Trophoblast invasion may also be regulated by factors controlling metalloproteinase activation. The control mechanism may be of maternal or embryonic origin.

Isolated first-trimester cytotrophoblasts, placed on a laminin-rich extracellular matrix substrate and evaluated by scanning electron microscopy, have a remarkable morphology of their multicellular aggregates. Elaborate cell processes extend from the surfaces of cells at the periphery of the aggregate.[36] Further observations of the migrating cells have led investigators to suggest that the formation of these cell processes is important to invasion, and that modulation of the repertoire of cytokeratins in cytotrophoblasts might be similar to observed behavior of invading tumor cells. By contrast, cytotrophoblasts isolated from term placenta form smaller aggregates, lack invadopodia, and do not penetrate the surface of an experimental extracellular matrix.

IMMUNOREGULATION OF IMPLANTATION
Human leucocyte antigen-(HLA-G)

How the semiallogenic embryo escapes immunorejection is one of the most important questions in the study of implantation. The placental cytotrophoblast is the only fetal cell type that is exposed to maternal uterine decidua and blood. Because of their position at the maternal fetal interface, the trophoblasts are thought to shield the fetus by serving as a barrier to maternal effector cells. Several mechanisms may be involved: 1) eliciting local production of maternal suppressor cells, 2) protective blocking antibodies, or 3) being nonrecognizable.[33] Mice that undergo experimental delay of implantation express paternal H-2 antigens that disappear after the onset of implantation.[20] The inability to type HLA human cytotrophoblasts with standard typing allosera has suggested the absence of class I antigens as a possible explanation for maternal tolerance toward placenta of a different HLA type.[8] However, some trophoblasts bind reagents that recognize monomorphic determinants on class I antigens. A new cell-associated and soluble major histocompatibility complex (MHC) antigen, called *HLA-G*, has been identified on first-trimester cytotrophoblasts and in the surrounding cellular environment.[33] This molecule differs from other known HLA by its size, its immunological characteristics, and its absence of polymorphism. Expression of HLA-G in third-trimester cytotrophoblasts is greatly reduced, suggesting that HLA-G is developmentally regulated. It has been proposed that HLA-G may act as an immunological shield for the placenta. A nonpolymorphic class I molecule would not stimulate MHC-restricted rejection by maternal effector cells. HLA-G might activate maternal suppressor cells, or soluble HLA-G might directly suppress maternal cytotrophic response, by binding to receptors of the cytotoxic cells and blocking recognition of non-MHC target structures on trophoblasts.

TLX antigen

TLX, the trophoblast-lymphocyte cross-reactive antigen, is so named for the ability of rabbit antisera, raised against human trophoblast membranes, to recognize an antigen common to trophoblasts and peripheral lymphocytes.[38] Anti-TLX antisera have immunosuppressive properties. Based on the observation that the serum of women with recurrent abortion lacks immunosuppressive action, it was proposed that anti-TLX blocking antibodies could be important to maintaining normal early pregnancy. Binding of antibodies to the antigen on lymphocytes in the decidua would prevent the lymphocytes from interacting with other potentially harmful molecules. One report suggests that TLX may be a membrane cofactor protein of the complement system.[46]

Immunosuppressive mechanisms

The placenta acts as a mechanical immunological barrier by filtering maternal lymphocytes. In addition, trophoblasts are known to be unusually resistant to lysis by maternal effector cells. Two lymphoid suppressor cells have been described in human endometrium: a large, nonspecific progesterone-induced cell, and a small, granulated lymphoid cell that is seen in the first-trimester decidua.[12] Activation of these suppressor cells is thought to be trophoblast dependent. The cells produce a soluble factor that interferes with the action of IL-2. IL-2 is known to play a crucial role in graft-rejection mechanisms. In mice, a similar molecule, closely related to TGF-β_2, has also been identified.[9] TGF-β molecules are known to be potent immunosuppressors. Lala has also shown that human decidual cells and decidual macrophages inhibit IL-2 production and induce down regulation of IL-2 receptors. The effect of decidua on IL-2 is mediated through the secretion of PGE$_2$.[34]

The production of complement components by human endometrium has recently been demonstrated.[28] Immunocytochemical methods have been used to localize the complement component, C3.[22] C3 plays a controlling role in the classic and alternative pathways of complement activation, and participates in phagocytic and immunoregulatory processes.[35] Activation of the alternative pathway requires factor B, factor D, and properdin. Cell surface complement regulation is achieved by membrane cofactor proteins and decay-accelerating factor. Complement receptors 1, 2, and 3 mediate the biological function of C3.

C3 has been localized to the glandular epithelium in the luteal phase. Factor B and decay-accelerating factor have a similar pattern of expression. Membrane cofactor protein is formed throughout the menstrual cycle, suggesting it is not hormonally regulated. Complement receptor 1 is found in the stromal compartment of luteal tissue.[22] A direct action of progesterone on C3 gene expression has been suggested by the presence of a progesterone-response element on the gene.[57] Other inflammatory mediators of complement synthesis, such as IL-1, have also been implicated in being regulated by progesterone.

The presence of various complement cofactors within the same cells of the endometrium suggests a functional complement system. However, the exact function of the system in reproduction is uncertain. Functions may vary, depending upon the specific factors expressed in different cells. For example, membrane cofactor protein is present on acrosome reacted sperm and may play a role in fusion. In trophoblast, expression of decay-accelerating factor, which dissociates the alternative pathway convertase, may play an important role in protecting the semiallogenic fetus from maternal complement-mediated attack.[25]

SUMMARY

Successful mammalian implantation is the summation of a series of complex, morphologically described events: decidualization, apposition, adhesion, invasion, and growth. Recent research has focused on the molecular events that govern these processes. Many of the humoral agents discussed in this chapter are pleiomorphic in their function. The study of their role in implantation may expand the understanding of their roles in other physiological and pathological processes. Moreover, better knowledge of the molecular basis of implantation will improve the ability to treat patients with recurrent pregnancy loss, unexplained infertility, and those with the need for advanced reproductive technologies.

REFERENCES

1. Bartocci A, Pollard JW, Stanley ER: Regulation of CSF-1 during pregnancy, *J Exp Med* 164:956, 1986.
2. Bhatt H, Burnet L, Stewart C: Uterine expression of leukemia inhibitory factor coincides with the onset of blastocyst implantation, *Proc Natl Acad Sci U S A* 88:11408, 1991.
3. Boehm KD, Daimon M, Gorodeski IG et al: Expression of the insulin-like anul platelet-derived growth factor genes in human uterine tissues, *Mol Reprod Devel* 27:93, 1990.
4. Bonaccorsi G, Pansini F, Segala V et al: Modification of number and of affinity of endometrial EGF receptors during the menstrual cycle, *Eur J Obstet Gynecol Reprod Biol* 33:177, 1989.
5. Cedars MI, Wei C, Pennington E et al: Effect of inhibition of prostaglandin synthesis on plasminogen activator (PA) activity and embryo implantation, Presented at the 40th meeting of the *Society for Gynecologic Investigation,* March, 1993.
6. Chavez DJ, Andeson TL: The glycocalyx of the mouse uterine luminal epithelium during estrus, early pregnancy, the peri-implantation period and delayed implantation, *Biol Reprod* 32:1135, 1985.
7. Chegini N, Rossi MJ, Masterson BJ: Platelet-derived growth factor (PDGF), epidermal growth factor (EGF), and EGF and PDGF β receptors in human endometrial tissue: localization and in vitro action, *Endocrinology* 130:2373, 1992.
8. Clark DA, Slapsys R, Chaput A et al: Immunoregulatory molecules of trophoblast and decidual suppressor cell origin at the maternofetal interface, *Am J Reprod Immunol Microbiol* 10:100, 1986.
9. Clark DA, Flanders KC, Banwatt D et al: Murine pregnant decidua produces a unique immunosuppressive molecule to TGF β-2, *J Immunol* 144:3008, 1990.

10. Coukos G, Gafvels M, Wisel S et al: Expression of the α2-macroglobulin receptor/low-density lipoprotein receptor-related protein (α_2MR/LRP) in human trophoblasts, *Am J Pathol* 144:383, 1994.

11. Damsky CH, Fitzgerald ML, Fisher SJ: Distribution patterns of extracellular matrix components and adhesion receptors are intricately modulated during first-trimester cytotrophoblast differentiation along the invasive pathway, in vivo, *J Clin Invest* 89:210, 1990.

12. Daya S, Rosenthal KL, Clark DA: Immunosuppressor factors produced by decidua-associated suppressor cells: a proposed mechanism for fetal allograft survival, *Am J Obstet Gynecol* 156:344, 1987.

13. DeWolf F, DeWolf-Peters C, Brosens I et al: The human placental bed: electron microscopic study of trophoblastic invasion of spiral arteries, *Am J Obstet Gynecol* 137:58, 1980.

14. Fisher SV, Aui TY, Zhang L et al: Adhesive and degradative properties of human placental cytotrophoblast cells in vitro, 109:891, 1989.

15. Guidice L: Growth factors and growth modulators in human uterus endometrium: their potential relevance to reproductive medicine, *Fertil Steril* 61:1, 1994.

16. Guidice LC, Dsupin BA, Jin IH et al: Differential expression of mRNAs encoding insulin-like growth factors and their receptors in human uterine endometrium and decidua, *J Clin Endocrinol Metab* 76:1115, 1993.

17. Guilbert LJ, Athanassakis I, Branch DR et al: The placenta as an immune endocrine interface: placental cells as targets for lymphohematopoietic cytokine stimulation. In Wegmann TG, Gill TJ, Nisbet-Brown E, editors: *Molecular and cellular immunology of the maternal-fetal interface*, New York. 1991, Oxford University.

18. Haining RE, Cameron IT, van Papendorp C et al: Epidermal growth factor in human endometrium: proliferative effects in culture and immunocytochemical localization in normal and endometriotic tissues, *Hum Reprod* 6:1200, 1991.

19. Haining RE, Schofield JP, Jones DS et al: Identification of mRNA for epidermal growth factor and transforming growth factor-α present in low copy number in human endometrium using reverse transcriptase-polymerase chain reaction, *J Mol Endocrinol* 6:207, 1991.

20. Hakansson S, Heyner S, Sundquist K et al: The presence of paternal H-2 antigens in hybrid mouse blastocysts during experimental delay of implantation and the disappearance of these antigens after onset of implantation, *Int J Fertil* 20:137, 1975.

21. Harty JR, Kauma SW: Interleukin-1β stimulates colony-stimulating factor-1 production in placental villous core mesenchymal cells, *J Clin Endocrinol Metab* 75:947, 1992.

22. Hasty LA, Lambris JD, Lessey BA et al: Hormonal regulation of complement components and receptors throughout the menstrual cycle, *Am J Obstet Gynecol* 170:158, 1994.

23. Herz J, Clouthier DE, Hammer RE: LDL receptor-related protein internalizes and degrades UPA-PAI-1 complexes and is essential for embryo implantation, *Cell* 71:411, 1992.

24. Hofmann GE, Scott Jr RT, Bergh PA et al: Immunohistochemical localization of epidermal growth factor in human endometrium, decidua, and placenta, *J Clin Endocrinol Metab* 73:882, 1991.

25. Holmes CH, Simpson KL, Wainwright SD et al: Preferential expression of the complement regulatory protein decay accelerating factor at the fetomaternal interface during human pregnancy, *J Immunol* 144:3099, 1990.

26. Hynes RO: Integrins: versatility, modulation, and signalling in cell adhesion, *Cell* 69:11, 1992.

27. Irwin JC, de las Fuentes LA, Dsupin BA et al: Insulin-like growth factor regulation of human endometrial stromal cell function: coordinate effects on insulin-like growth factor binding protein-1, cell proliferation and prolactin secretion, *Regul Pept* 48:165, 1993.

28. Isaacson KB, Galman M, Coutifaris C et al: Endometrial synthesis and secretion of complement component-3 by patients with and without endometriosis, *Fertil Steril* 33:836, 1990.

29. Jenkinson EV, Searle RF: Cell surface changes on the mouse blastocyst at implantation, *Exp Cell Res* 106:386, 1977.

30. Julkunen M, Koistinen R, Suikkari A-M et al: Identification by hybridization histochemistry of human endometrial cells expressing mRNAs encoding a uterine β-lactoglobulin homologue and insulin-like growth factor-binding protein-1, *Mol Endocrinol* 4:700, 1990.

31. Kauma SW, Aukerman SL, Eierman D et al: Colony-stimulating factor-1 and c-fms expression in human endometrial tissues and placenta during the menstrual cycle and early pregnancy, *J Clin Endocrinol Metab* 73:746, 1991.

32. Kleinstein J, Westermann W, Gustmann C et al: Estrogen induces expression of endometrial EGF-receptor before implantation, *Am J Reprod Immunol* 30:58, 1993.

33. Kovats S, Main EK, Litnach C et al: A class I antigen, HLA-G, expressed in human trophoblasts, *Science* 48:220, 1990.

34. Lala PK: Similarities between immunoregulation in pregnancy and in malignancy: the role of PGE$_2$, *Am J Reprod Immunol* 20:147, 1989.

35. Lambris JD: The multifunctional role of C3, the third component of complement, *Immunol Today* 9:387, 1988.

36. Lebeach CL, Werb Z, Fitzgerald ML, et al: 92kD type IV collagenase mediates invasion of human cytotrophoblasts, *J Cell Biol* 113:437, 1991.

37. Lessey BA, et al: Integrin adhesion molecules in the human endometrium, *J Clin Invest* 90:188, 1992.

38. McIntyre JA: In search of trophoblast-lymphocyte crossreactive (TLX) antigens, *Am J Reprod Immunol Microbiol* 17:100, 1988.

39. Murphy LJ, Gong Y, Murphy LC: Growth factors in normal and malignant uterine tissue, *Ann N Y Acad Sci* 622:383, 1991.

40. Nelson KG, Takahashi T, Bossert NL et al: Epidermal growth factor replaces estrogen in the stimulation of female genital-tract growth and differentiation, *Proc Natl Acad Sci U S A* 88:21, 1991.

41. Noyes RW, Hertig AT, Rock J: Dating the endometrial biopsy, *Fertil Steril* 1:3, 1950.

42. Ohta N, Pardee AB, McAuslan BR et al: Sialic acid contents and controls of normal and malignant cells, *Biochem Biophys ACTA* 158:98, 1968.

43. Perdue JF, Kletzien R, Wray VL: The isolation and characterization of plasma membrane from cultured cells, *Biochem Biophys ACTA* 266:505, 1972.

44. Pollard JW, Hunt JS, Wiktov-Jedizeczak W et al: A pregnancy defect in osteopetrotic (op/op) mouse demonstrates the requirement for CSF-1 in female fertility, *Dev Biol* 148:273, 1991.

45. Postigo AA Sanchez Madrid F: Adhesion and homing molecules, *Transplant Proc* 25(1):65, 1993.

46. Purcell DFJ, McKenzie IFC, Johnson M et al: CD46 (Huly-M5) antigen of humans includes the TLX antigen and the MCP of complement, *J Reprod Immunol (suppl)*16:207, 1989.

47. Reynolds RK, Talavera F, Roberts JA et al: Regulation of epidermal growth factor and insulin-like growth factor-I receptors by estradiol and progesterone in normal and neoplastic endometrial cell cultures, *Gynecol Oncol* 38:396, 1990.

48. Ritvos O, Ranta T, Jalkanen J et al: Insulin-like growth factor (IGF) binding protein from human decidua inhibits the binding and biological action of IGF-I in cultured choriocarcinoma cells, *Endocrinology* 122:150, 1989.

49. Rutanen E-M, Pekonen F, Makinen T et al: Soluble 34K binding protein inhibits the binding of insulin-like growth factor I to its receptors in human secretory phase endometrium: evidence for autocrine/paracrine regulation of growth factor action, *J Clin Endocrinol Metab* 66:173, 1988.

50. Sappino AP, Huarte J, Belin D et al: Plasminogen activators in tissue remodeling and invasion: mRNA localization in mouse ovaries and implanting embryos, *J Cell Biol* 109:2471, 1989.

51. Searle RF, Selens MH, Elson V et al: Detection of alloantigens during preimplantation development and early trophoblast differentiation in the mouse by immunoperoxidase labeling, *J Exp Med* 143:348, 1976.

52. Slowey MJ, Verhage HG, Fazleabas AT: Epidermal growth factor (EGF) and EGF-receptor (R) localization in the baboon (*Papio*

anubis) uterus during the menstrual cycle and early pregnancy, Presented at the 40th meeting of the *Society for Gynecologic Investigation,* March, 1993.

53. Stewart CL, Kaspar P, Burnet L et al: Blastocyst implantation depends on natural expression of leukemia inhibitory factor, *Nature* 359:76, 1992.

54. Strowitzki T, Wiedemann R, Hepp H: Influence of growth factors EGF, IGF-1 and human growth hormone on human endometrial cells in vitro, *Ann N Y Acad Sci* 626:308, 1991.

55. Taketani Y, Mizuno M: Evidence of direct regulation of epidermal growth factor receptors by steroid hormones in human endometrial cells, *Hum Reprod* 6:1365, 1991.

56. Troche V, O'Connor DM, Schaudies RP: Measurement of human epidermal growth factor receptor in the endometrium the menstrual cycle, *Am J Obstet Gynecol* 165:1499, 1991.

57. Vik DP, Amiquet P, Moffat GJ et al: Structural features of the human C3-gene: intron/exon organization, transcriptional start site, and promoter region sequence, *Biochemistry* 30:1080, 1991.

58. Weiss L: *J Cell Biology* 26:735, 1965.

59. Zini JM, Munay SC, Graham CH et al: Characterization of urokinase receptor expression by human placental trophoblasts, *Blood* 79:2917, 1992.

Part II

REPRODUCTIVE CYCLE DISORDERS

Chapter 7

PRIMARY AMENORRHEA

Oscar A. Kletzky, MD

No breast development and uterus present
Breast development and uterus absent
No breast development and uterus absent
Breast development and uterus present

The transition from prepuberty to puberty is accompanied by changes in the concentrations and patterns of both serum luteinizing hormone (LH) and follicle-stimulating hormone (FSH) associated with follicular growth and ovum maturation, resulting in the adult state of normal menstrual and ovulatory cycles. Failure to complete this complex sequence of gonadotropic-gonadal maturation during puberty may result in the disorder of primary amenorrhea. Karyotype aberrations, genetic abnormalities, developmental defects of the müllerian ducts, and a variety of central nervous system disorders may be associated with primary amenorrhea. The understanding of the processes leading to normal puberty, as well as the clinical presentation of primary amenorrhea and its correlation with possible errors in gonadal development, müllerian duct anomalies, genital differentiation, and hypothalamic-pituitary function, will increase the physician's ability to correctly diagnose and treat patients with primary amenorrhea.

Early in fetal development the gonad is indifferent, having the potential to develop into either sex. Normally these gonads differentiate into ovaries in genetic females with XX sex chromosomes and into testes in genetic males with XY sex chromosomes. Both the wolffian and müllerian ducts are present early in the fetal life of both male and female fetuses, and on completion of the genetic sex differentiation of these ducts, they will develop into female or male organs. In females the upper one third of the vagina, the uterus, and the fallopian tubes will derive from the müllerian ducts; in males the epididymides, seminal vesicles, and vasa deferentia will develop from the wolffian ducts.[21] In genetic males differentiation of these organs depends on the secretion of testosterone and the presence of a müllerian-inhibiting factor (MIF). In the target tissues, the enzyme 5α-reductase converts testosterone to dehydrotestosterone, which then stimulates the differentiation of the glans penis. Independent of testosterone actions, MIF induces the regression of the müllerian ducts. In contradistinction, differentiation of the female genital tract is independent of fetal gonadal function. Therefore, irrespective of whether or not ovaries are formed, the internal genital organs and external genitalia will differentiate along normal female lines. These embryonic changes are discussed in detail in Chapter 2.

As puberty approaches, nocturnal LH pulses are detected, FSH levels rise, and the ovaries are stimulated. The secretion of ovarian sex steroid hormones induces the development of secondary sexual characteristics. In this chapter women with ambiguous external genitalia, imperforate hymen, or transverse vaginal septum are not discussed (please refer to the box on p. 170). Although these conditions need to be considered in the differential diagnosis, they are not discussed here because these patients have cryptomenorrhea and not primary amenorrhea. Cryptomenorrhea (from the Greek *kryptos* [hidden] and *menorhoia* [menses]) is a condition generated from an imperforate hymen. Usually the diagnosis is made postpubertally, at which time menstrual blood begins to accumulate and results in cyclic pain. Depending on the organ in which the blood collects there may be hematocolpos (vagina), hematometra (uterus), or hematosalpinx (fallopian tube). The treatment is a simple incision of the hymen with excision of a small portion to prevent its closure.

As one of the initial changes at puberty, girls begin to develop breasts and the appearance of axillary and pubic hair. Although the age and rate at which these changes occur are variable, they usually occur in an orderly and synchronous manner that culminates with the first menstrual period at a mean (± SD) age of 12.9 ± 1.2 years. The absence of a spontaneous episode of uterine bleeding by age 16½ (mean + 3 SD) makes the diagnosis of primary amenorrhea.[11] Since breast development initiates at a mean age of 10.8 ± 1.10 (SD) years and pubic hair at a mean age

---

Classification of disorders in patients with primary amenorrhea with normal external genitalia

Primary amenorrhea without breast development; uterus present

1. Hypothalamic failure secondary to
   a. Inadequate gonadotropin releasing hormone synthesis
   b. Inadequate gonadotropin releasing hormone release
   c. Neurotransmitter defect
   d. Congenital anatomic defect
2. Pituitary failure due to
   a. Isolated gonadotropic insufficiency
   b. Chromophobe adenoma
   c. Craniopharyngioma
3. Gonadal failure due to
   a. 45,X (Turner syndrome)
   b. 46,X abnormal X (e.g., short or long arm deletion)
   c. Mosaicism (e.g., X/XX, X/XX/XXX)
   d. 46,XX or 46,XY pure gonadal dysgenesis
   e. 17∝-Hydroxylase deficiency with 46,XX karyotype

Primary amenorrhea with breast development; uterus absent

1. Androgen insensitivity (testicular feminization)
2. Congenital absence of uterus

Primary amenorrhea without breast development; uterus absent

1. 17,20-Desmolase deficiency
2. Agonadism
3. 17α-Hydroxylase deficiency

Primary amenorrhea with breast development; uterus present

1. Hypothalamic causes
2. Pituitary causes
3. Ovarian causes
4. Uterine causes

Modified from Mashchak CA et al: *Obstet Gynecol* 57:715, 1981.

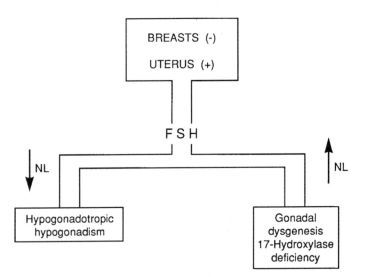

Fig. 7-1. Diagnostic evaluation of patients with primary amenorrhea with absence of breast development and uterus present. *NL,* Normal level. Arrow pointing up indicates level above normal; arrow pointing down indicates level below normal. (Redrawn from Mashchak et al: *Obstet Gynecol* 57:715, 1981, with permission of The American College of Obstetricians and Gynecologists.)

of 11 ± 1.21 years, an earlier diagnostic work-up is justified when there is not breast development by age 15 or the patient has failed to menstruate within 3 to 4 years after the onset of breast development and the appearance of pubic hair. It is recommended that after taking a careful history and conducting a complete physical examination attention be directed toward the presence or absence of breast development and a uterus. The presence of breast tissue will indicate that the hypothalamic-pituitary-ovarian axis did function and resulted in estrogen secretion. The presence of a uterus will be indicative of structurally correct development. By using these two parameters (breast and uterus), patients with primary amenorrhea and normal female external genitalia can be subdivided into four different diagnostic categories[30]:

1. No breast development and uterus present
2. Breast development and uterus absent
3. No breast development and uterus absent
4. Breast development and uterus present

NO BREAST DEVELOPMENT AND UTERUS PRESENT

The differential diagnosis of patients with no breast development and uterus present includes hypogonadotropic hypogonadism due to either hypothalamic or pituitary failure and gonadal dysgenesis. The measurement of the FSH level in a single serum sample is helpful in making the differentiation (Fig. 7-1). Patients with hypogonadotropic hypogonadism have low or low normal serum FSH levels, whereas patients with gonadal dysgenesis have elevated FSH levels (in the menopausal range). The measurement of serum LH and estradiol levels are of no additional diagnostic value (Fig. 7-2). Hypogonadotropic hypogonadism is one of the most common causes of primary amenorrhea. It may occur as a result of an intrinsic hypothalamic derangement or the presence of abnormalities of the neural regulatory mechanism that controls the qualitative or quantitative adequacy of gonadotropin-releasing hormone (GnRH) synthesis and release.[25,34] Some patients with an autosomal

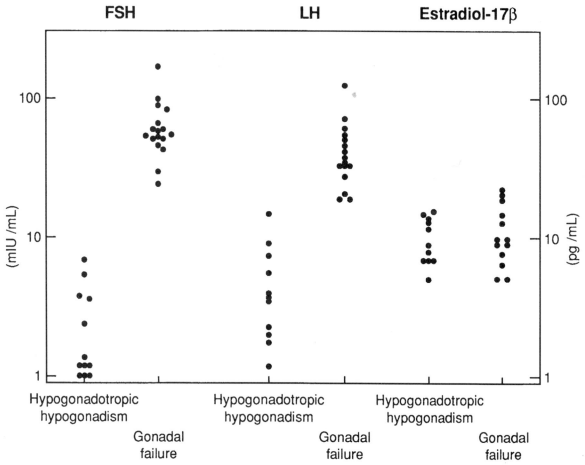

Fig. 7-2. Serum levels of FSH, LH, and estradiol in patients with hypogonadotropic hypogonadism and gonadal failure. (Redrawn from Mashchak et al: *Obstet Gynecol* 57:715, 1981, with permission of The American College of Obstetricians and Gynecologists.)

dominant trait and less frequently with a recessive trait also have anosmia (Kallmann syndrome). Therefore it is recommended that all patients in this group at least be tested with such substances as coffee, tobacco, orange peel, and cocoa to determine the integrity of the olfactory system. Strenuous physical activities beginning before the onset of menstruation may delay maturation of the hypothalamic-pituitary-ovarian axis, resulting in no breast development and primary amenorrhea. In fact, about 6 months' delay in age at menarche has been reported to occur for each previous year of strenuous physical training.[12,13]

Although uncommon, a craniopharyngioma or a prolactinoma occasionally may be present; therefore it is recommended that these patients have a computed tomography scan or magnetic resonance imaging (MRI) of the hypothalamic-pituitary area.[34]

The differentiation between a hypothalamic origin and a pituitary origin in patients with hypogonadotropic hypogonadism can be established by performing a GnRH test. If there is an appropriate LH response (>20 mIU/mL) 30 minutes after the intravenous administration of 100 μg of GnRH, the diagnosis is hypothalamic failure due to failure to produce or secrete adequate levels of GnRH. However, if the pituitary has not been previously primed with endogenous or exogenous GnRH, a lack of an adequate response to a single bolus of GnRH may not indicate primary pituitary gonadotropin deficiency. Therefore patients with an inadequate LH response to GnRH should be retested after being treated with daily doses of GnRH for up to 10 days (Fig. 7-3).[25] Absence of a serum LH response to a subsequent GnRH test usually indicates pituitary failure. Thalassemia major (Fig. 7-4) and retinitis pigmentosa are examples of pituitary diseases in which the patient presents with primary amenorrhea due to primary deficiency in gonadotropin production.[4,26] Patients with hypogonadotropic hypogonadism can be induced to ovulate with the pulsatile administration of GnRH[27] or alternatively with human menopausal gonadotropins.

Patients with gonadal dysgenesis have hypogonadotropic hypogonadism due to either a genetic or an enzymatic abnormality that resulted in the failure of gonadal development or abnormal functioning of the ovaries.[38] Genetic abnormalities are seen in about 30% of patients with primary amenorrhea.[36] The most common chromosomal abnormality is the complete absence of a sex chromosome, 45,X, or Turner syndrome.[39]

The incidence of Turner syndrome has been reported to be between 1/2000 and 1/7000 live births.[36] These patients usually present with short stature (almost always less than 60 inches or 150 cm), streak gonads, and sexual infantilism. Many of these patients have also some type of somatic abnormalities such as webbed neck, short fourth metacarpal, cubitus valgus, and shieldlike chest with wide-set nipples, coarctation of the aorta, and renal anomalies.[39] Also, there is an increased incidence of Hashimoto's thy-

roiditis and diabetes mellitus in these patients.[10, 16] It is of interest to note that the majority of fetuses with gonadal dysgenesis are aborted, making this (45,X) the most common chromosomal abnormality found in spontaneous abortions.[3] Frequently, infants born with Turner syndrome have lymphedema and are of low birth weight. The gonads of those fetuses surviving are devoid of primary follicles and consequently cannot synthesize ovarian steroids. The lack of estrogen secretion and the absence of central negative feedback allows the gonadotropin levels to be elevated into the menopausal range. With the exception of patients who have a Y chromosome or patients with clinical evidence of androgen excess, the streak gonads should not be surgically removed.

Less common genetic causes of primary amenorrhea are a structurally abnormal X chromosome, mosaicism, pure gonadal dysgenesis (46,XX and 46,XY) and 17α-hydroxylase deficiency with a 46,XX karyotype.[9,15,29,35] Patients with structurally abnormal X chromosomes may have a deletion of the long or short arm of one X chromosome. Usually patients with deletion of the long arm have normal stature and no somatic abnormalities, but they have streak ovaries and sexual infantilism.[2,19] Some of these patients have delayed epiphyseal closure and are eunuchoid in appearance. Usually patients with short arm deletion are short. Patients with an isochromosome of the long arm of the X chromosome have the same features as those patients with Turner syndrome. Other chromosomal aberrations include a ring X and a minute fragmentation of the X chromosome.[8,9,18] The most common form of mosaicism in these patients is 4,X/46,XX.[8] About 80% of these patients are shorter than their peers but taller than patients with Turner's syndrome, and more than 60% have evidence of some type of somatic anomaly. About 20% of these patients have been reported to have spontaneous menses.

Patients with pure gonadal dysgenesis (46,XX, 46,XY with bilateral gonadal streaks) usually do not have the physical stigmata of those with Turner syndrome. They are difficult to diagnose prepubertally because they have a female phenotype. Postpubertally, they present with infantilism, eunuchoid features, and elevated serum levels of gonadotropins. The label *pure gonadal dysgenesis* was introduced by Harnden and Stewart[17] in 1959, and it has been suggested to restrict this label to patients with an XX or XY karotype and the physical characteristics just described. It is probably a genetic disorder, since it has been reported among siblings. Some of these patients may present with a history of a few episodes of spontaneous uterine bleeding at the time of puberty, indicating a brief period of estrogen secretion. In that situation the patient may have developed breasts. Patients with 17α-hydroxylase deficiency and a 46,XX karyotype present with hypertension, hypokalemia, high serum progesterone levels, and elevated levels of serum FSH and LH.[15,29]

Because of the absence of the enzyme 17α-hydroxylase,

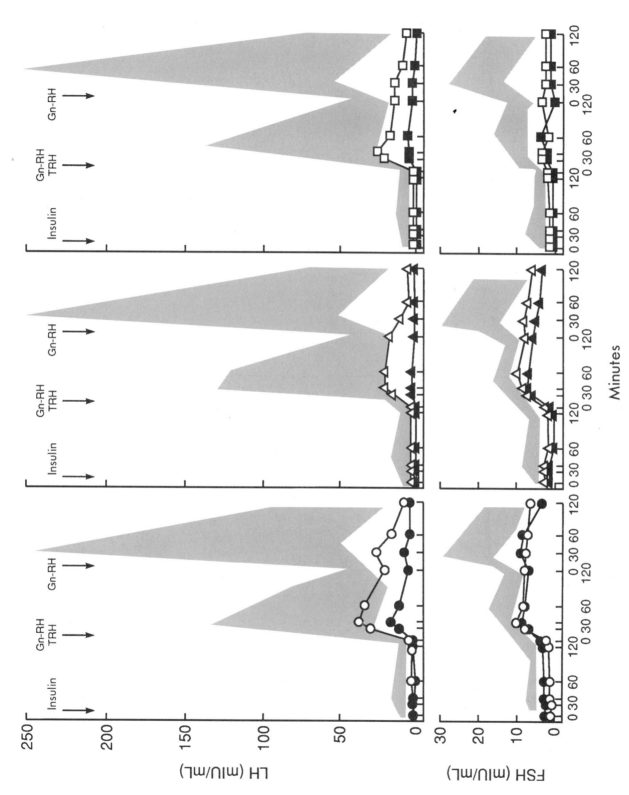

Fig. 7-3. Serum LH and FSH responses to GnRH stimulation in three patients with hypothalamic-hypogonadotropic hypogonadism before (*solid symbols*) and after (*open symbols*) priming with GnRH for 4 consecutive days. Shaded areas represent the 95% confidence limits of ovulatory women studied in the early follicular phase. (Redrawn from Kletzky OA et al: Idiopathic hypogonadotropic hypogonadal primary amenorrhea, *J Clin Endocrinol Metab* 46:808, 1978; © The Endocrine Society.)

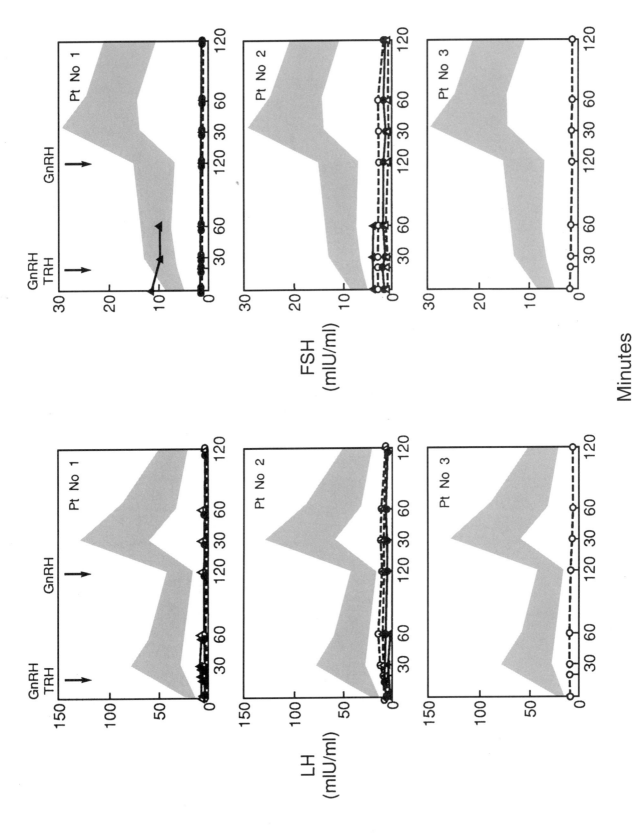

Fig. 7-4. Serum LH and FSH responses in three female patients with thalassemia major to GnRH stimulation test before any treatment (*open circles*; patient 1 was on estrogen replacement and was studied only once), after priming with GnRH for 7 days (*solid circles*), with estradiol for 7 days (*open triangles*), and after human menopausal gonadotropin treatment (*solid triangles*). (Redrawn from Kletzky OA et al: Gonadotropin insufficiency in patients with thalassemia major, *J Clin Endocrinol Metab* 48:901, 1979; © The Endocrine Society.)

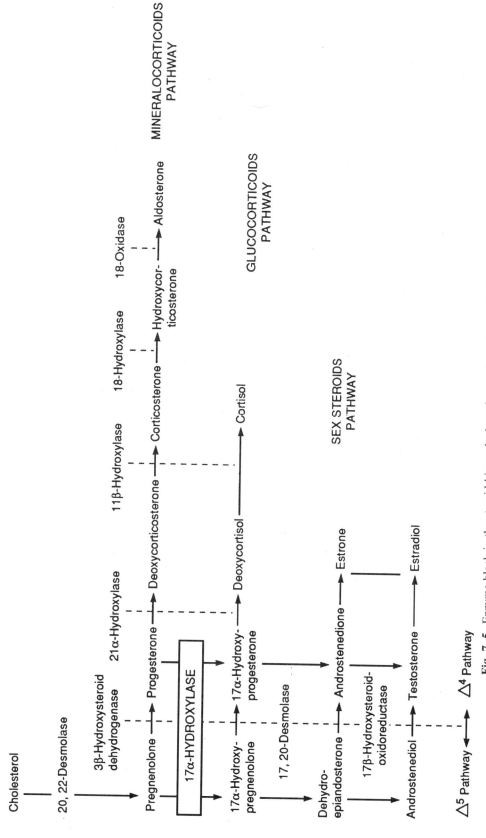

Fig. 7-5. Enzyme block in the steroid biosynthetic pathway of a patient with 17-hydroxylase deficiency.

progesterone is not converted to hydroxyprogesterone, which in turn is not converted to deoxycortisol and finally to cortisol (Fig. 7-5). Thus serum progesterone levels are elevated and cortisol levels are diminished. The absence of a negative feedback effect of cortisol results in additional increases in corticotropin (ACTH) secretion, which further stimulates the steroid pathway. Since ACTH also stimulates the mineralocorticoid pathway, which is not blocked (pregnenolone → progesterone → deoxycorticosterone → corticosterone → hydroxycorticosterone → aldosterone), there is sodium retention with hypertension and hypokalemia.[17] The ACTH test confirms the diagnosis of 17-hydroxylase deficiency because these patients demonstrate a marked increase in serum progesterone levels with no change in the levels of 17-hydroxyprogesterone. These patients respond very well to the treatment with glucocorticoids. ACTH secretion is suppressed, normalizing the concentration of all mineralocorticoids, and consequently serum potassium levels increase and blood pressure decreases. Because of the enzymatic block, these patients do not produce sex steroids and therefore appropriate treatment should include estrogen. If the diagnosis is made during childhood, estrogen should be prescribed at puberty.

Patients with gonadal dysgenesis are sterile and can carry a pregnancy only if a donor egg is fertilized in vitro and transferred into the uterus. Although most of these patients show no signs of secondary sex characteristics, occasionally an individual with mosaicism or Turner syndrome may synthesize enough estrogen to produce some degree of breast development, have a sporadic menstrual period, and even ovulate and become pregnant. Estrogen-

progesterone replacement should be prescribed to all these patients in order to induce breast development and cyclic menstrual bleeding and to prevent osteoporosis.

Breast tissue is extremely sensitive to the administration of estrogen, and therefore only small doses of estrogen should be prescribed initially. It is recommended to start with 0.3 mg of conjugated estrogen daily or 10 μg of ethinyl estradiol for several months before increasing the dose. The general idea is to mimic the slow normal process of breast growth that occurs at puberty. The use of larger doses of estrogen will not necessarily induce larger breasts, and the final breast size will be the same. The degree of breast development is best ascertained by palpating and measuring the diameter of the breastplate. However, it may not be easy to determine its exact limits; thus the distance between the anterior axillary line and the midsternum line at the level of the nipple should be measured. As the breast develops and grows, the distance between these two stationary lines will increase, representing the growth of breast tissue. Usually progestin therapy is added to estrogen therapy to prevent hyperplasia of the endometrium and also to induce regular menstrual bleeding. In our experience, progestin therapy does not modify the estrogen effect of breast development.

A karyotype analysis is necessary only in patients in whom serum FSH levels are elevated. The gonads or streak ovaries do not need to be surgically removed unless the karyotype demonstrates the presence of a Y chromosome or there is clinical evidence of excess androgen production, such as hirsutism or acne.[37]

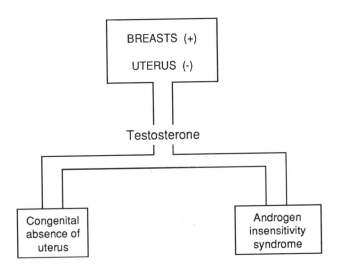

Fig. 7-6. Diagnostic evaluation of patients with primary amenorrhea with normally developed breasts and absent uterus. (Redrawn from Mashchak CA et al: *Obstet Gynecol* 57:715, 1981, with permission of The American College of Obstetricians and Gynecologists.)

BREAST DEVELOPMENT AND UTERUS ABSENT

The differential diagnosis of patients with breast development and uterus absent includes the androgen insensitivity syndrome (testicular feminization) and congenital absence of the uterus (Fig. 7-6). Patients with androgen insensitivity syndrome have testicles; patients with absence of the uterus have ovaries. Therefore, any method designed to detect ovulation, such as a biphasic basal body temperature curve or an elevated serum progesterone level, should be sufficient to establish the differential diagnosis. In addition, patients with androgen insensitivity syndrome have serum testosterone levels in the normal male range (300 ng/dL to 800 ng/dL), and patients with congenital absence of the uterus have serum testosterone levels in the normal female range (20 ng/dL to 80 ng/dL) (Fig. 7-7).[30] Only those patients with serum testosterone levels in the male range should have a karyotype analysis to confirm the diagnosis.

Thus an individual with this syndrome has a female phenotype with normal breasts, short vagina, testicles, and a 46,XY karyotype.[32] Patients with the complete form of the disease also have complete absence of axillary and pubic hair.

Because the testes secrete MIF in utero, the müllerian ducts regress and the upper third of the vagina, the uterus, and the fallopian tubes do not develop. Prepubertally the testes are of normal size and configuration, and they are usually located intraabdominally, in the inguinal canal or in the labia majora. Postpubertally the testes reveal Leydig cell hyperplasia, and small seminiferous tubules with few spermatogonia and no spermatozoa.[7] Serum estrogen levels deriving from peripheral conversion of testosterone and androstenedione and from direct testicular secretion induce complete breast development.[22] In addition, serum LH levels can be moderately elevated, which in turn maintain steroid secretion.

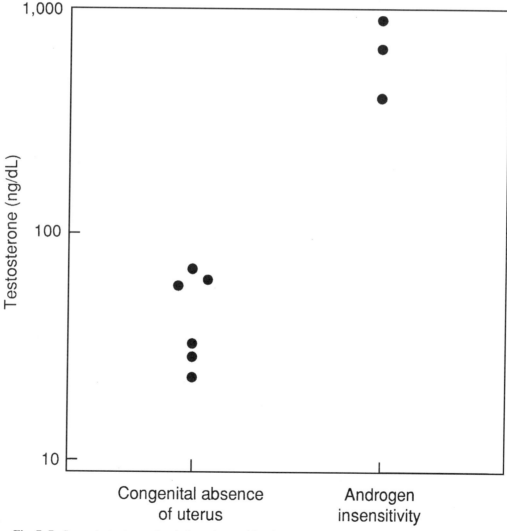

Fig. 7-7. Serum testosterone levels in patients with primary amenorrhea, breast development, and no uterus. (Redrawn from Mashchak CA et al: *Obstet Gynecol* 57:715, 1981, with permission of The American College of Obstetricians and Gynecologists.)

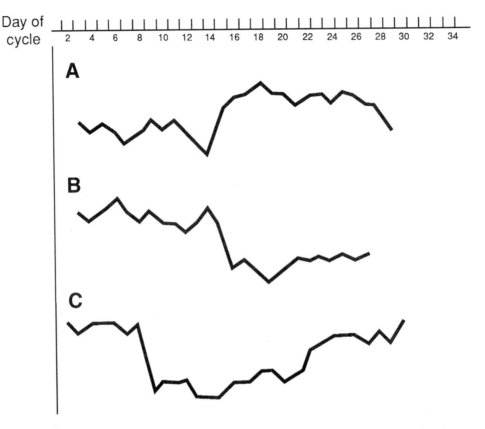

Fig. 7-8. Basal body temperature (BBT) graphs illustrating various possible patterns of ovulatory cycles in patients with congenital absence of the uterus. Pattern *A* represents the usual biphasic curve; pattern *B* is the biphasic graph of a patient starting to record her BBT in the early luteal phase; pattern *C* is the biphasic graph of a patient starting her record in the middle of the luteal phase.

After gonadectomy steroid levels decrease into the hypogonadal range and gonadotropins increase into hypergonadotropic levels. Dysgerminomas or gonadoblastomas have been reported in 22% of patients with androgen insensitivity. It is usually recommended to postpone the surgical removal of these gonads until the patient undergoes spontaneous and complete natural breast development. Afterward, estrogen replacement therapy is prescribed to prevent osteoporosis. The vaginal pouch can be enlarged by utilizing appropriate vaginal dilators. If dilators cannot give acceptable results, a skin graft can be used to create a neovagina. These procedures should be initiated when the patient is prepared to have regular sexual intercourse. In counseling these patients, we recommend that the word *gonad* be used and not *testicle* because it is very difficult for these phenotypical female patients to accept the notion of having testicles instead of normal ovaries. Also we recommend avoiding the specific mention of a Y chromosome because it is commonly known that only male individuals carry an XY karyotype. Instead they should be told that they have an abnormal sex chromosome.

When one testicle is demonstrated during the course of a routine inguinal hernia repair, it may be appropriate to remove both testicles during the same surgical procedure instead of delaying it for a later date. These patients may adopt a child if they wish to become parents.

Patients with congenital absence of the uterus have normally functioning ovaries and therefore they have normal secondary sexual characteristics. They often experience cyclic breast and mood alterations compatible with ovulation. If the basal body temperature is used to detect ovulation the physician should be aware of possible unusual biphasic temperature curves. Because the beginning of the cycle is unknown the patient may start taking her temperature at any time of the cycle (i.e., during the luteal phase), and therefore the elevation will be seen at the beginning and not at the end of the cycle (Fig. 7-8). Alternatively, measurement of the serum testosterone level clearly establishes the differential diagnosis. Those with congenital absence of the uterus will have serum testosterone levels in the normal female range. Since anomalies of the kidneys or urinary collecting system have been reported in up to 40% of these patients, an intravenous pyelogram should be ordered.[20,34] Congenital fusion of the cervical vertebrae has been reported in 5% of these patients, which adds rigidity to the neck.

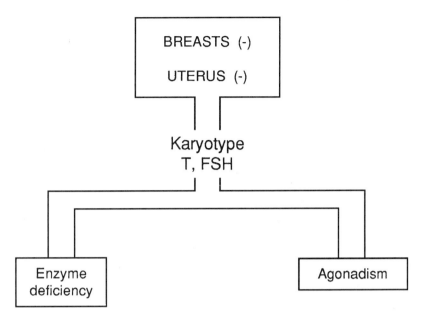

Fig. 7-9. Diagnostic evaluation of patients with primary amenorrhea, no breast development, and absent uterus. (Redrawn from Mashchak CA et al: *Obstet Gynecol* 57:715, 1981, with permission of The American College of Obstetricians and Gynecologists.)

These patients do not require hormone replacement because their endocrine axis is intact. Because they have normally functioning ovaries they could have their own genetic children by transferring a fertilized egg into the uterus of a surrogate mother.

NO BREAST DEVELOPMENT AND UTERUS ABSENT

Patients with no breast development and uterus absent are extremely rare. All reported cases have a male karyotype, elevated gonadotropin levels, and serum testosterone values within or below the normal female range (Fig. 7-9). Some patients have hypertension and hypokalemia. These patients are different from those with gonadal failure because they do not have a uterus; they are different from patients with androgen insensitivity syndrome because they do not have breast development, and their serum testosterone levels are in the female range. Some patients have been reported to have 17,20-desmolase deficiency, another had agonadism and others had 17α-hydroxylase deficiency and a 46,XY karyotype. The diagnosis of 17,20-desmolase deficiency can be made only by studying the steroid pathways in incubated gonadal tissue (Fig. 7-10). These studies will reveal that 17-hydroxypregnenolone is not converted to dehydroepiandrosterone and that 17-hydroxyprogesterone is not converted to androstenedione.[14] Consequently patients are unable to synthesize testosterone and estradiol, whereas they maintain their capacity to synthesize cortisol and deoxycorticosterone.

The diagnosis of agonadism may be suggested by the lack of testosterone response to the daily intramuscular administration of 5000 IU of human chorionic gonadotropin for 5 days. Confirmation can be obtained by demonstrating the absence of testes at laparoscopy.[6] Irrespective of the etiologic diagnosis of patients with no breast development and absent uterus, if gonadal tissue is present it should be removed to prevent a malignant transformation (46,XY). These patients should receive estrogen replacement therapy to induce breast development and to prevent osteoporosis and cardiovascular disease.

The diagnosis of 17α-hydroxylase deficiency can be suspected in patients with hypertension, primary amenorrhea with no breasts, and absent uterus.[1,33] Since these patients have a 46,XY karyotype they can be distinguished from patients with the androgen insensitivity syndrome by the lack of breasts and the presence of hypertension. Management of these patients is similar to that for patients with 17α-hydroxylase deficiency and a 46,XX karyotype.

BREAST DEVELOPMENT AND UTERUS PRESENT

Approximately one third of all patients with primary amenorrhea have normal breasts and a palpable uterus.[30] They are subdivided into four etiologic subgroups: (1) polycystic ovary syndrome (PCO), (2) hypothalamic dysfunction, (3) hypothalamic-pituitary failure, and (4) ovarian failure. All patients with primary amenorrhea are approached diagnostically in a manner similar to that for patients with secondary amenorrhea.[23,24]

Because 25% of these patients are found to have hyperprolactinemia and radiographic evidence of a prolactinoma

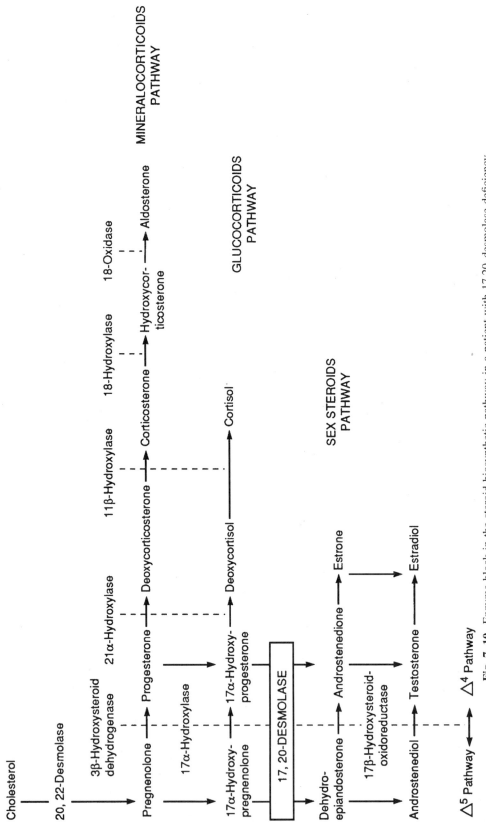

Fig. 7-10. Enzyme block in the steroid biosynthetic pathway in a patient with 17,20-desmolase deficiency.

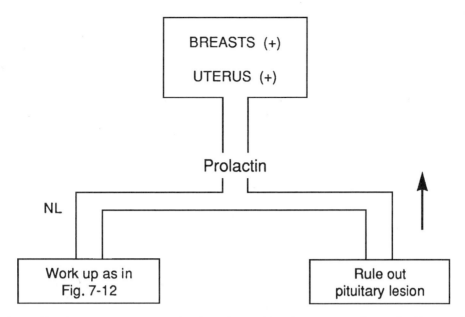

Fig. 7-11. Initial diagnostic evaluation in patients with primary amenorrhea and with normal breasts and uterus present.

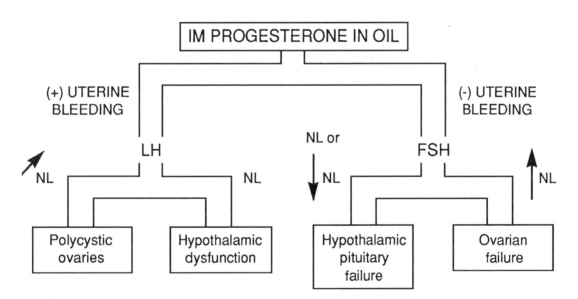

Fig. 7-12. Diagnostic evaluation in patients with primary amenorrhea and with normal breasts and uterus present. *NL,* Normal level. Arrow pointing up indicates level above normal, arrow pointing down indicates level below normal, slanted arrow indicates moderate elevation.

it is recommended that the work-up begin with the measurement of serum prolactin [30] (Fig. 7-11). In patients with normal serum prolactin levels it is important initially to determine the estrogen status by giving a single injection of 100 mg of progesterone in oil intramuscularly or 20 mg of oral progestin for 5 days. Patients with low levels of estrogen (<40 pg/mL) do not have uterine bleeding in response to the progesterone challenge, whereas patients with normal estrogen levels (>40 pg/mL) will have uterine bleeding response after the administration of progesterone.

Even a minimal amount of bleeding 2 to 14 days later is sufficient to consider this a positive response.

The differential diagnosis for patients who have uterine bleeding after the administration of progesterone is PCO or hypothalamic dysfunction (Fig. 7-12). This differential diagnosis can be obtained with the measurement of a single serum LH level. In our laboratory a serum LH value of 25 mIU/mL or greater is diagnostic in about 70% of patients with PCO. The determination of the LH:FSH ratio does not have additional diagnostic value above that given by serum

LH alone. If clinically indicated, patients with PCO should also have androgen studies performed. Those patients with normal serum LH levels are diagnosed as having hypothalamic dysfunction. This diagnosis includes patients with amenorrhea induced by medications, stress, or weight loss and those with amenorrhea of idiopathic etiology.

Both groups of patients (those with PCO and those with hypothalamic dysfunction who have uterine bleeding after progesterone challenge) respond very well to the administration of clomiphene citrate for the induction of ovulation. For patients not desiring to conceive we recommend the monthly administration of 5 mg daily of an oral progestin to induce periodic bleeding and sloughing of the endometrium. Because of the low probability of ovulation in these patients, a barrier method of contraception is appropriate. The use of an oral steroid contraceptive is not necessary because sufficient levels of endogenous estrogen are secreted by the patient's ovaries. However, it may be indicated in patients with PCO and a significant degree of hirsutism or acne in whom it is more important to reduce the levels of serum testosterone. If the amenorrhea is associated with the use of medications or is secondary to stress and weight loss, the treatment should be directed toward the elimination of the etiologic factor.

The differential diagnosis of patients with amenorrhea who do not bleed after the administration of progesterone is between hypothalamic-pituitary failure and premature ovarian failure.[23,24] This differential diagnosis can be accomplished with the measurement of a single FSH level, which clearly identifies the two different diagnoses (Fig. 7-12). Patients with low serum FSH levels have the diagnosis of hypothalamic-pituitary failure, and patients with elevated serum FSH levels carry the diagnosis of premature ovarian failure. The hypothalamic-pituitary failure group includes patients with severe weight loss, associated or not with anorexia nervosa, hypothalamic lesions, Sheehan's syndrome, or nonsecreting pituitary adenomas. The majority of patients with hypothalamic failure do not require further testing of the hypothalamic-pituitary axis. Patients with Sheehan syndrome should have an insulin-induced hypoglycemia test for a more complete and thorough evaluation of hypothalamic-pituitary function.[31] Patients with hypothalamic failure who wish to conceive do not respond to the administration of clomiphene citrate and therefore need to be treated with human menopausal gonadotropins. Patients who do not wish to conceive should be given estrogen-progestin replacement therapy to prevent osteoporosis and cardiovascular disease. Long-term follow-up of patients with hypothalamic-pituitary failure indicates that a large proportion of them show evidence of partial or complete recovery.[5] Patients with a non-secreting pituitary adenoma may require adenomectomy, depending on size of the adenoma.

Patients with the diagnosis of premature ovarian failure should have a karyotype performed if they are younger than age 25 years to rule out a mosaicism with a Y chromosome. In such cases a gonadectomy is indicated before the occurrence of the malignant transformation of the gonads. An autoimmune disorder is probably the most common cause of premature ovarian failure.[28] Significant levels of antibodies produced against the ovaries, oocytes, or gonadotropin receptors, as well as other endocrine glands (adrenal, thyroid, parathyroid) have been reported. Because measurements of antithyroid antibodies and antimicrosomal antibodies are the only tests available to the clinician, these tests should be ordered for all these patients who are younger than age 35 years. Many of these patients with elevated antithyroid and antimicrosomal antibodies may have normal thyroid function. As long as thyroid function is normal these patients should not receive thyroid replacement therapy; however, they should be followed yearly to detect any thyroid hypofunction. A patient with premature ovarian failure can benefit from advanced reproductive technologies by receiving a donor egg fertilized in vitro and transferred into her uterus. Otherwise these patients should be treated with estrogen-progestogen to prevent osteoporosis and cardiovascular disease.

REFERENCES

1. Abad L et al: Male pseudohermaphroditism with 17-alpha-hydroxylase deficiency: a case report, *Br J Obstet Gynaecol* 87:1162, 1980.
2. Baughman FA et al: Two cases of primary amenorrhea with deletion of the long arm of X chromosome (46,XXq−), *Am J Obstet Gynecol* 102:1065, 1968.
3. Carr DH: Chromosome studies in selective spontaneous abortions and early pregnancy loss, *Obstet Gynecol* 37:570, 1971.
4. Chang RJ et al: Hypogonadotropic hypogonadism associated with retinitis pigmentosa in a female sibling: evidence for gonadotropin deficiency, *J Clin Endocrinol Metab* 53:1179, 1981.
5. Davajan V et al: 10 Year follow up of patients with secondary amenorrhea and normal prolactin, *Am J Obstet Gynecol* 164:1666, 1991.
6. Federman DD: *Abnormal sexual development: a genetic and endocrine approach to differential diagnosis,* Philadelphia, 1967, WB Saunders.
7. Ferenczy A, Richart RM: The fine structures of the gonads in the complete form of testicular feminization, *Am J Obstet Gynecol* 113:399, 1972.
8. Ferguson-Smith MA: Karyotype-phenotype correlations in gonadal dysgenesis and their bearing on the pathogenesis of malformation, *J Med Genet* 2:1432, 1965.
9. Ferguson-Smith MA: Phenotypic aspects of sex chromosome aberrations, *Birth Defects* 5:3, 1969.
10. Forbes AP, Engel E: The high incidence of diabetes mellitus in 41 patients with gonadal dysgenesis and their close relatives, *Metab Clin Exp* 12:428, 1963.
11. Frisch RE, Revel R: Height and weight at menarche and a hypothesis of menarche, *Arch Dis Child* 46:695, 1971.
12. Frisch RE, Wyshak G, Vincent LE: Delayed menarche and amenorrhea in ballet dancers, *N Engl J Med* 143:859, 1982.
13. Frisch RE et al: Delayed menarche and amenorrhea of college athletes in relation to age of onset of training, *JAMA* 246:1559, 1981.
14. Goebelsmann U et al: Male pseudohermaphroditism consistent with 17,20 desmolase deficiency, *Gynecol Invest* 7:138, 1976.
15. Goldsmith O, Soloman DH, Horton R: Hypogonadism and mineralo-

corticoid excess: the 17-hydroxylase deficiency syndrome, *N Engl J Med* 277:673, 1967.

16. Hamilton CR, Modawer M, Rosenberg HS: Hashimoto's thyroiditis and Turner's syndrome, *Arch Intern Med* 122:69, 1968.

17. Harnden DG, Stewart JSS: The chromosomes in a case of pure gonadal dysgenesis, *Br Med J* 2:1285, 1959.

18. Hecht F, MacFarlane JC: Mosaicism in Turner's syndrome reflects the lethality of XO, *Lancet* 2:1197, 1969.

19. Hsu LYV, Hirschhorn K: Genetic and clinical consideration of long arm deletion of the X chromosome, *Pediatrics* 45:656, 1970.

20. Jones HW, Rock JA: *Reparative and constructive surgery of the female generative tract,* Baltimore, 1983, Williams & Wilkins.

21. Jost A, Vigier B, Prepin J: Studies on sex differentiation in mammals, *Recent Prog Horm Res* 29:1, 1973.

22. Kelch RP et al: Estradiol and testosterone secretion by human, simian and canine testes in males with hypogonadism and in male pseudohermaphrodites with the feminizing testes syndromes, *J Clin Invest* 51:824, 1972.

23. Kletzky OA et al: Classification of secondary amenorrhea based on distinct hormonal patterns, *J Clin Endocrinol Metab* 41:660, 1975.

24. Kletzky OA et al: Clinical categorization of patients with secondary amenorrhea using progesterone induced uterine bleeding and measurement of serum gonadotropin levels, *Am J Obstet Gynecol* 121:695, 1975.

25. Kletzky OA et al: Idiopathic hypogonadotropic hypogonadal primary amenorrhea, *J Clin Endocrinol Metab* 46:808, 1978.

26. Kletzky OA et al: Gonadotropin insufficiency in patients with thalassemia major, *J Clin Endocrinol Metab* 48:901, 1979.

27. Knobil E: The neuroendocrine control of ovulation, *Hum Reprod* 3:469, 1988.

28. Luborsky JL et al: Ovarian antibodies detected by immobilized antigen immunoassay in patients with premature ovarian failure, *J Clin Endocrinol Metab* 70:69, 1990.

29. Mallin SR: Congenital adrenal hyperplasia secondary to 17-hydroxylase deficiency, *Ann Intern Med* 70:69, 1969.

30. Mashchak CA et al: Clinical and laboratory evaluation of patients with primary amenorrhea, *Obstet Gynecol* 57:715, 1981.

31. Morente C, Kletzky OA: Pituitary response to insulin-induced hypoglycemia in patients with amenorrhea of different etiologies, *Am J Obstet Gynecol* 148:375, 1984.

32. Morris JM, Mahesh VB: Further observations on the syndrome "testicular feminization," *Am J Obstet Gynecol* 87:731, 1963.

33. New MI: Male pseudohermaphroditism due to 17 alpha-hydroxylase deficiency, *J Clin Invest* 459:1930, 1970.

34. Reindollar RH, Byrd JR, McDonough PG: Delayed sexual development: a study of 252 patients, *Am J Obstet Gynecol* 140:371, 1981.

35. Rimoin DL, Schimke NR: *Genetic disorders of the endocrine glands,* St Louis, 1971, CV Mosby.

36. Rosen GF, Kaplan B, Lobo RA: Menstrual function and hirsutism in patients with gonadal dysgenesis, *Obstet Gynecol* 17:677, 1988.

37. Rosen GF et al: The endocrinologic evaluation of a 45,X true hermaphrodite, *Am J Obstet Gynecol* 157:1272, 1987.

38. Santen RJ, Paulsen CA: Hypogonadotropic eunuchoidism: clinical study of the mode of inheritance, *J Clin Endocrinol Metab* 36:47, 1988.

39. Turner HH: A syndrome of infantilism, congenital webbed neck and cubitus-valgus, *Endocrinology* 23:566, 1938.

Chapter 8

ABNORMAL UTERINE BLEEDING

Howard A. Zacur, M.D., Ph.D.
and Kenneth K. Vu, M.D.

MENSTRUAL DISORDERS

Evaluation of the patient with a menstrual-cycle disturbance requires an understanding of the integrative physiological events involving the hypothalamus, pituitary gland, ovaries, and uterus. (See Chapter 5 on ovarian follicular growth and maturation.) In this chapter, the effect of ovarian secretion of 17-beta estradiol and progesterone on uterine endometrial growth and differentiation is reviewed and the physiological mechanisms involved in menstruation are discussed. Different patterns of menstrual-cycle disturbances are then mentioned, followed by an account of the methods used to evaluate and treat these disturbances.

Physiological review

The first half of the human menstrual cycle, known as the *follicular* or *proliferative* phase, involves the recruitment and selection of a dominant ovarian follicle. During this time, the ovarian secretion of 17-beta estradiol produces changes within the lining, or endometrium, of the uterus. The outer surface of this lining is composed of secretory and ciliated cells.[62] An increase in height of these lining cells as they change in shape from cuboidal to tall columnar cells may be observed as ovulation approaches, but much more marked changes are observed in tissues deep in the endometrial lining. Beneath the endometrial lining are the straight necks of endometrial glands that are surrounded by packed stromal cells. During the luteal phase of the cycle, this outermost of the three endometrial layers is known as the *compacta* or *compact layer.* Beneath this is a middle layer with tortuous glands surrounded by less dense stroma, called the *spongiosa* or *spongy layer.* This layers rests on the *basalis* or *basal layer,* containing the blind ends of the glands (Fig. 8-1).

These endometrial layers or zones were elegantly described by Bartelmez in 1957. During the follicular phase of the menstrual cycle, endometrial proliferation is characterized histologically by stromal and glandular cell mitoses, a process that ultimately results in increased thickening of the entire endometrium. Under the influence of estradiol, the number of receptors for estradiol and progesterone within the endometrial glands and stroma increase during the follicular phase of the cycle. After ovulation, a decline in the numbers of estradiol and progesterone endometrial receptors is observed, an effect thought to be mediated by progesterone itself (Fig. 8-2). However, progesterone receptors do remain within the endometrium after ovulation and their presence allows progesterone to cause differentiation of the endometrium. Tortuosity and complexity of the

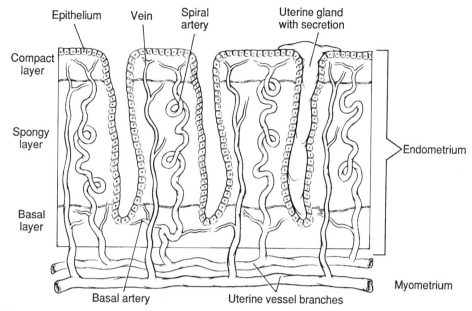

Fig. 8-1. The endometrium depicted as an outer lining beneath which three histologically identifiable layers may be found resting upon the myometrium.

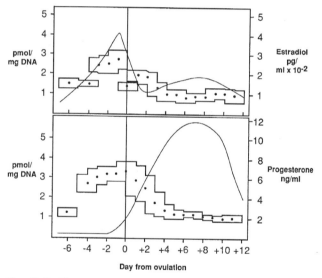

Fig. 8-2. Changes in number of estrogen and progesterone receptors during the human menstrual cycle. Each point represents a mean value enclosed in a rectangle whose abscissa represents the preceding to following day, and whose ordinate is equal to twice the standard error of the mean. Mean steroid concentrations are depicted as solid lines. (Modified from Levy et al: Estradiol and progesterone receptors in human endometrium: normal and abnormal menstrual cycles and early pregnancy, *Am J Obstet Gynecol* 136:646, 1980.)

endometrial glands, coupled with spiraling of the spiral arteries and decidualization of stromal cells, are some of the histological changes that are observed during the luteal phase of menstrual cycle that result, in part, from progesterone stimulation. Synthesis and secretion of a variety of cell proteins, such as prolactin from decidualized stromal cells, occur at this time in response to stimulation by progesterone.

The first day of menstrual-blood flow is defined as the first day of the menstrual cycle and ends on the day of bleeding of the next cycle. From cycle-day one until ovulation is defined as the follicular phase (because of ovarian follicular development during this time) or the proliferative phase (because of endometrial histological changes occurring during this time). The time period from ovulation until menstruation is referred to as the luteal phase (reflecting coexisting ovarian changes) or the secretory phase (reflecting endometrial changes). The entire time period from cycle-day one until the first day of bleeding for the next cycle is termed the *menstrual-cycle interval* (Fig. 8-3).

Length of the follicular phase of the menstrual cycle may vary from seven to 21 days, but the length of the luteal phase is relatively constant at 14 ± 2 days, if pregnancy does not occur, due to the fixed life span of the corpus luteum. Mechanisms responsible for the fixed life span of the corpus luteum remain undetermined. If pregnancy does not occur, the corpus luteum undergoes luteolysis, resulting in a decline in the concentration of progesterone and estradiol, which precedes menstruation. If pregnancy occurs, the corpus luteum is maintained by human chorionic gonadotropin (HCG) stimulation and the corpus luteum provides the necessary progesterone for pregnancy during the first 6 to 8 weeks of gestation. One consequence of the fixed luteal phase interval is that variation of the menstrual-cycle length results from delayed or accelerated follicle growth, which in turn affects the proliferative-phase length. On rare occasions, a short luteal phase (less than 10 days)

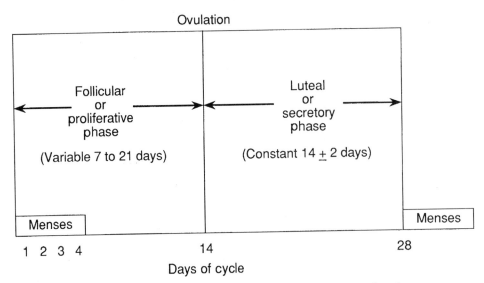

Fig. 8-3. Depiction of different phases of the human menstrual cycle.

due to an abbreviated corpus-luteum life span may be detected, or persistence of the corpus luteum, in the absence of pregnancy, may be noted.

Changes occurring in the uterus prior to menstruation were described by Markee over 50 years ago from a series of classic experiments (which have never been repeated) using human endometrial tissue that had been transplanted into the anterior eye chamber of the monkey.[38] Observations from this study resulted in the realization that the onset of menstruation begins with compression of the endometrium, followed by increased coiling and spasm of the spiral arteries, ultimately resulting in tissue necrosis and vessel rupture with leakage of blood. Initial compression of the endometrium is now thought to result from the loss of fluid from endometrial stroma precipitated by the release of digestive enzymes from lysosomes. Lysosomes are small, intracellular vacuoles containing a variety of enzymes (over 60 are known) that participate in digestion. Lysosomes are found within epithelial, stromal, and glandular cells of the endometrium and much evidence suggests that enzyme accumulation in lysosomes increases between the proliferative and luteal phases of the menstrual cycle. However, prior to menses, the uterine stroma is infiltrated by migratory leukocytes that also contain large numbers of lysosomes. It is believed, but still unproven, that the release of lysosomes from endometrial cells and/or leukocytes is responsible for the initiation of the menstrual period. An excellent review of this subject was written recently by Wang and Fraser.[60] The collapse in the endometrial stroma has traditionally been suggested as either a cause or a consequence of spiral artery spasm and rupture, but an alternative explanation for these vascular changes was offered recently. Endothelin-1 is a protein produced in human endometrial tissue that can cause vasoconstriction.[16] Its activity is regulated in part by the presence of a

membrane metalloendopeptidase that degrades the endothelin-1 peptide.[49,58] The activity of metalloendopeptidase is increased by progesterone.[6] Thus, it is possible that the vascular spasm observed prior to menstruation may be triggered by increased endothelin-1 activity resulting from the falling progesterone levels prior to menses.

Endometrial shedding begins at multiple sites within the uterine cavity at the onset of menses and then spreads throughout the uterine cavity so that complete shedding of the endometrial lining takes place within 24 hours. As tissue is shed, damaged blood vessels are exposed, the tips of which are initially plugged by platelets that are later replaced by a fibrin clot. Menstrual blood itself does not clot due to the presence of the activated fibrin degradation enzyme, plasmin, which is also released by the endometrium during menses. Release of the peptidases, urokinase and trypsin, from shed endometrial tissue converts the precursor plasminogen, which is also released by stromal cells, to plasmin. Endometrial tissue, fluid, and blood are eventually expelled into the vagina by the uterus, which has been induced to begin contracting during this process, presumably by the release of prostaglandins $F_2\alpha$ and E_2 from disrupted endometrial and myometrial tissues.

In a large prospective study of 476 normal women, Hallberg et al. attempted to determine the normal volume of blood loss during menses and the normal duration of menses.[27] Volunteers were provided with sanitary pads to collect menstrual blood; these were returned and then treated with 5% sodium hydroxide (NaOH) to create alkaline hematin, which could be measured spectrophotometrically to provide an estimate of hemoglobin lost during menses. This was then converted to milliliters of blood using volunteers' own venous hemoglobin concentrations as a reference. In this study involving women from age 15 to 50 years, it was determined that the average total

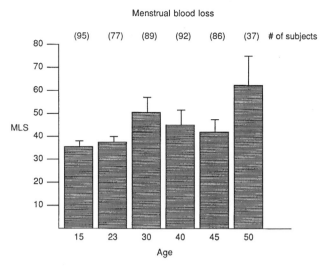

Fig. 8-4. Average measured blood loss (with standard error of mean) in volunteers from ages 15 to 50. (From Hallberg et al: *Acta Obstet Gynecol Scand* 45:320, 1966.)

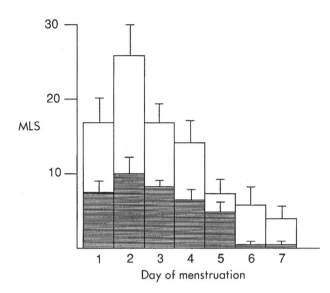

Fig. 8-5. Total fluid loss and blood loss during each day of menses in 28 women. Blood loss is signified by hatched bars. (From Fraser et al: *Obstet Gynecol* 65:194, 1985.)

menstrual-blood loss for an individual is approximately 40 ml, a value not significantly altered by age (Fig. 8-4). However, if this study had been limited to women who possessed a venous hemoglobin concentration of greater than 12 g/100 ml (a transformation presumably excluding women who are anemic as a consequence of menorrhagia) the 95th percentile for this subgroup would have been 76.4 ml. Using this information, the authors conclude that menorrhagia, or excessive menstrual bleeding, can be defined as menstrual-blood loss exceeding 80 ml. Using similar techniques in another country and with a different group of women, Fraser et al. confirmed the findings of Hallberg et al. and noted that, for most women, the second day of menses represented the day of maximal blood loss.[21] Surprisingly, this study observed that only about half of the total menstrual fluid lost during menses was blood, and that desquamated cells and uterine fluid transudate were responsible for the additional volume (Fig. 8-5).

Interpreting disturbances in the menstrual cycle requires a knowledge of the normal menstrual-cycle interval and its variations. Treloar et al. recorded the menstrual-cycle patterns of 2700 women, some of whom were followed from menarche to menopause, and the results showed that variations in the menstrual-cycle interval are quite common.[54] In fact, only one of their subjects consistently had a menstrual-cycle interval of 28 days. The average menstrual-cycle interval for an individual is most commonly 28 days, but the cycle length may frequently be as short as 21 days or as long as 35 days. Surprisingly, very few of the women in this study ever "skipped a month." In fact, only 1% of the subjects were classified as having abnormal menstrual cycles. The greatest variations in the menstrual-cycle interval occurred within seven years of the onset of menarche

and seven years prior to the onset of menopause. Changes within the hypothalamic pituitary ovarian axis were thought to be responsible for these variations (Fig. 8-6).

ABNORMAL BLEEDING

A variety of terms have been used to describe menstrual-cycle disturbances. These terms and brief definitions are presented in the box below. Menstrual-cycle disturbances commonly complained of by patients and not described in this box include midcycle spotting, breakthrough bleeding, and premenstrual spotting or staining. All of these disturbances can be classified as *polymenorrheas*, but the volume and timing of blood loss within what could otherwise be described as a normal menstrual interval are not adequately presented under the general polymenorrhea term.

Ovulatory disturbances, rather than müllerian tract anomalies (e.g., cervical stenosis and uterine synechiae), are usually responsible for menstrual-cycle intervals exceeding 35 days; whereas both structural anomalies (e.g., leiomyo-

Menstrual-cycle disturbances	
Dysfunctional uterine bleeding	Vaginal bleeding without apparent organic cause
Oligomenorrhea	Menses occurring at intervals greater than 35 days
Polymenorrhea	Menses occurring at intervals less than 21 days
Menorrhagia or hypermenorrhea	Menstrual blood loss exceeding 80 ml

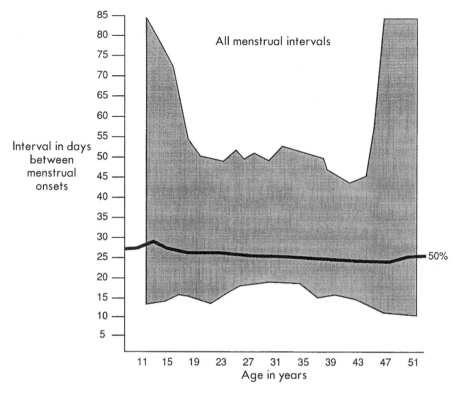

Fig. 8-6. Menstrual cycle intervals in 2,700 women (From Treloar et al: *Int J Fertil* Vol 12, No 1, Part 2:77, 1967).

mata) and ovulatory disturbances may result in irregular or excessive vaginal bleeding. The magnitude of blood loss is of special concern because excessive bleeding may be life-threatening in the acute setting. Excessive bleeding over a prolonged interval may cause anemia, resulting in fatigue and illness. Because of these responses to menorrhagia, it is not unexpected that menorrhagia is frequently listed as the reason for performing the half million hysterectomies performed each year in North America.

A woman's age at the onset of a menstrual-cycle disturbance is an important physiological variable that must be accounted for in evaluating a patient with a menstrual-cycle complaint. While large variations in menstrual-cycle intervals are expected seven years following menarche and seven years prior to menopause, the risk of cervical and uterine malignancies increases with age. Consequently, the possibility of malignancy causing abnormal uterine bleeding should be considered in women who are over the age of 35. For these women, endometrial sampling to exclude a malignant or premalignant condition has been recommended by the American College of Obstetricians and Gynecologists as an initial step of evaluation.[59] The risk of malignancy is less in women between 13 and 20 years of age. Women presenting with menstrual-cycle disturbances between the ages of 20 and 35 are most commonly affected by structural anomalies, as well as disturbances of pregnancy (e.g., ectopic pregnancy, threatened abortion).

Anovulatory dysfunctional uterine bleeding

Most causes of irregular menstrual-cycle bleeding are attributable to anovulation (please see the box below). Production of ovarian estradiol in the absence of postovulation progesterone may stimulate endometrial proliferation until bleeding results. The actual cause of uterine bleeding in this setting remains unknown, although the proliferating endometrium is vascular and lacking in stromal support,

---

Anovulatory menstrual-cycle disturbances

Dysfunctional uterine bleeding

Chronic anovulation condition (e.g., polycystic ovarian disease syndrome, PCOS)

Oligomenorrhea

Chronic anovulatory condition (e.g., hypothalamic amenorrhea)
Perimenarchal
Perimenopausal

Polymenorrhea

Chronic anovulation (e.g., PCOS)
Perimenopausal

Menorrhagia

Chronic anovulation (e.g., PCOS)

causing it to be sensitive to any decline in estrogen level. Sensitivity of this type may also account for the midcycle spotting seen in some ovulating women when a fall in the estradiol level occurs prior to ovulation. In some anovulatory women, the uterine endometrium may be so stimulated by unopposed estrogen that any transient decline in the level of estrogen may provoke significant bleeding from multiple foci. This type of uterine bleeding does not result from an identifiable cause and is called *dysfunctional uterine bleeding* (DUB).

Ovulatory dysfunctional uterine bleeding

Abnormal menstrual-cycle bleeding without an apparent cause may also occur in women who ovulate (please refer to the box below). Disturbances in corpus-luteum function are usually responsible for this. Defective or inadequate luteal phases are caused by insufficient corpus-luteum progesterone production, or deficient endometrial progesterone-receptor number or function. Premenstrual spotting or early onset of menses may be seen in women with luteal-phase disturbances. Short luteal phases are those with a time interval between luteinizing-hormone (LH) surge and menstrual onset of less than 10 days. Conversely, the luteal phase, in the absence of pregnancy, may be prolonged, a condition known as *Halban disease*. The cause of this disorder remains unknown.

In most cases, menstrual-cycle disturbances that occur during ovulatory cycles are explainable. Organic factors such as polyps, leiomyomata, pregnancy, or defects in coagulation are frequently found in these patients.

Ovulatory versus anovulatory state

From the preceding discussion, it follows that there are practical implications for classifying a patient with a menstrual-cycle disturbance as having an anovulatory or ovulatory problem. Diagnosis of anovulation in a person with a menstrual-cycle disturbance usually identifies a patient with DUB. Diagnosis of ovulation occurring in the presence of a menstrual-cycle disturbance usually suggests the presence of coexisting organic pathology.

Ovulation may be documented by measuring the serum progesterone level, taking the basal body temperature, monitoring the level of urinary LH excreted daily, or taking a timed biopsy from the endometrial cavity. A serum progesterone concentration exceeding 3 ng/ml (300 ng/dl), detected during the luteal phase of the cycle, is indicative of ovulation. Serum progesterone levels less than 3 ng/ml are found during the follicular phase. A sustained upward shift in the oral basal body temperature of 0.3° to 1° F is indicative of ovulation due to the temperature-altering effect of progesterone on brain-stem function. Recording the oral temperature with a simple device, such as a digital thermometer, at approximately the same time each day, is all that is required of the patient. For example, a biphasic temperature shift is observed in the ovulatory individual who takes her temperature at around the same time each day in the afternoon. Another simple method is detection of the midcycle, urinary LH surge, using a "dipstick" that changes color in the presence of elevated LH, in daily urine samples taken first thing in the morning. This method is much more expensive, however, due to the reagents used. Likewise, biopsy of the endometrium to detect secretory changes resulting from corpus-luteum progesterone secretion may also be used to document an ovulatory state, but this is an invasive and costly method. In spite of this, when vaginal bleeding occurs and the use of exogenous hormonal agents is contemplated, performance of an endometrial biopsy may help to diagnose the bleeding disorder and thus, be efficient by avoiding alternative diagnostic procedures.

Changes in the echogenicity of the endometrial cavity during the menstrual cycle have been reported using sonographic techniques.[47] Thus, ultrasonography can be used to reveal evidence of ovulation, though the cost-effectiveness of this technique remains an issue. However, determination of the endometrial thickness by transvaginal ultrasonography may have clinical utility in evaluating patients with postmenopausal bleeding because endometrial stripe thickness less than 5 mm is associated with "tissue insufficient for diagnosis" when an endometrial biopsy has been attempted.[26]

Anovulatory menstrual-cycle bleeding disorders

Determining that a menstrual-cycle derangement is occurring in an anovulatory patient should prompt a careful investigation to determine if a hormonal cause is responsible. Causes of anovulatory vaginal bleeding include hyperandrogenemic chronic anovulation syndrome, also known as *polycystic ovary syndrome* or *disease;* hypothalamic-pituitary-ovarian axis dysfunction as com-

---

Ovulatory menstrual-cycle disturbances

Dysfunctional uterine bleeding

Midcycle withdrawal bleeding: etiology uncertain; midcycle decline in estradiol

Oligomenorrhea

Usual cause, but some patients with Asherman syndrome may exhibit this
Pregnancy

Polymenorrhea

Uterine leiomyomata or polyps
Cervical, uterine neoplasia
Pregnancy; ectopic pregnancy

Menorrhagia

Uterine leiomyomata
Blood-clotting disorders

monly seen in the perimenarchal interval; and gonadal failure observed during the perimenopausal period. Anovulation due to stress, weight loss or gain, systemic disease, drug use, or hyperprolactinemia may also be seen.[51]

Ovulatory menstrual-cycle bleeding disorders

Determination that abnormal vaginal bleeding is occurring in an ovulatory individual should strongly suggest that the bleeding results from structural changes within the uterus due to polyps, leiomyomata, or from pregnancy such as implantation, missed abortion, or ectopic gestation. Coagulation disorders, infection, endometriosis, vascular anomalies, and neoplasms are frequently found in ovulatory women with abnormal menstrual-cycle bleeding. These topics are discussed in greater detail below.

Coagulation disorders

In women older than 35 years of age, the possibility of malignancy must be considered and excluded as a routine part of the evaluation, despite the fact that the explanation for most menstrual-cycle disturbances at this age are benign. In adolescent girls, most menstrual-cycle disturbances are caused by anovulation resulting from the maturation of the hypothalamic-pituitary-ovarian axis. However, Claessens and Cowell reported that 19% of adolescents who presented to them with acute menorrhagia were found to have a primary coagulation disorder.[8] During menstruation, the normal physiological mechanisms involved in blood-clot formation and lysis must operate harmoniously to allow normal menstrual-blood volume loss.[7] Coagulation disorders may be primary, such as idiopathic thrombocytopenic purpura, or hereditary, as in the autosomal-dominant von Willebrand disease that may result in life-threatening menorrhagia. Other coagulation disorders may also be acquired. The ingestion of various foods and spices (e.g., Szechwan purpura, onion and garlic, cumin or turmeric) may inhibit platelet aggregation and cause mild hemorrhagic diatheses.[28,37,50] As might be expected, the use of anticoagulants for treatment of thrombosis is associated with increased menstrual-blood loss.[55] Lower platelet counts following chemotherapy treatment may cause bleeding in some patients.

Thyroid disorders

Significant menstrual-blood loss has been reported in women with clinical hypothyroidism.[44] The cause of excessive bleeding in these patients remains unclear, although altered hormonal metabolism and anovulation have been suggested as possible explanations. Recently, 15 out of 67 apparently euthyroid women presenting with menorrhagia were found to have mild hypothyroidism on the basis of an upper normal to mildly elevated fasting thyroid stimulating hormone (TSH) level, as well as an exaggerated TSH response (exceeding 30 mU/L) to 200 µg of thyrotropin releasing hormone (TRH) administered intravenously. In eight patients who were available for follow-up, menorrhagia disappeared following institution of L-thyroxine treatment.[63]

Infections

Irritation or infection of the genital tract, such as vaginitis, cervicitis, or endometritis, may result in abnormal bleeding during the menstrual cycle. Chlamydial and gonorrheal infections may be identified by cultures taken from the endocervical canal. Endometritis may also be detected with the use of cultures, but is more commonly identified histologically after an endometrial biopsy sample has been obtained. *Trichomonas* and fungal infections may be identified by mixing the vaginal discharge with saline or potassium hydroxide on a slide and examining it under a microscope. Recently, *Mobiluncus* species (motile rods exhibiting wavelike, rapid motion in a straight line or arched direction) were identified in wet smears of 14 women with vaginal bleeding or spotting. Treatment with metronidazole 500 mg tid for 10 days resulted in the disappearance of *Mobiluncus* and absence of bleeding.[31]

Endometriosis

Pelvic endometriosis is frequently found during the course of an infertility evaluation, and it also may be present in women complaining of polymenorrhea, menorrhagia, or premenstrual spotting.[52,61] Causes for the bleeding seen in patients with endometriosis include direct tissue injury by the endometrial implants (e.g., cervical endometriosis) or hormonal dysfunction resulting from the presence of pelvic endometriosis. Alternatively, the presence of endometriosis in women with menstrual-cycle disturbances may be coincidental and not causal. Menorrhagia, menstrual irregularity, and premenstrual spotting were found to occur with equal frequency in women with endometriosis compared to those with pelvic adhesions or normal pelvis.[36]

Contraceptive practices

Intrauterine device (IUD). Insertion of a foreign body, such as an IUD, into the uterine cavity, has long been known as a cause of increased menstrual-blood loss. This is due presumably to interference with the normal contractile mechanisms of the uterine musculature regulating blood loss. Inert devices, such as the Lippes Loop, have been reported to cause the greatest blood-volume losses; devices that contain copper or progesterone cause the least.[1]

Sterilization. Anecdotal reports have suggested in the past that tubal ligation could cause menstrual-cycle disturbances. These reports were given some support from the analysis of DeStefano et al., who reviewed the menstrual characteristics of 719 women who had undergone tubal sterilization. Menstrual cycles were defined as exhibiting adverse bleeding if two or more of the following were identified: (1) menstrual-flow duration exceeding six days, (2) average use of more than 12 full pads or tampons per period, (3) moderate or severe large clots with menstrual flow, and (4) moderate or severe spotting, or intermenstrual bleeding. This study showed an increasing trend of adverse bleeding as time passed following tubal ligation.[13] Rulin et al. also reported that slightly more cramping with an increase in menstrual flow was seen following tubal ligation in women with natural cycles, but this was not statistically significant.[45] The cause for such bleeding disturbances remains unidentified, although alterations in ovarian-blood flow resulting in altered steroid production have been suggested.

An increase in menstrual-cycle disturbances following tubal sterilization was suggested in 1951 by Williams et al.[65] Although a physiological effect from tubal sterilization can be postulated to occur as a result of interference with the blood supply between the ovary and uterus, convincing evidence of such an effect on the menstrual cycle has been difficult to obtain. For example, Rulin et al., in a prospective longitudinal study, failed to demonstrate a change in menstrual-cycle parameters following tubal sterilization. They did note, however, that women using oral contraceptives prior to undergoing tubal sterilization experienced an increase in menstrual-cycle flow following the tubal ligation[46] when oral-contraceptive usage ceased. More recently, DeStefano et al. reported on a two-year follow-up of women who participated in a study with the Centers for Disease Control. This follow-up study, known as the Collaborative Review of Sterilization (CREST study), failed to demonstrate an increase in the prevalence of altered menstrual function following tubal sterilization.[14] However, when these same patients were questioned five years after tubal sterilization, an increase in menstrual abnormalities was reported, suggesting again that menstrual-cycle changes may take time to develop following tubal sterilization.[64]

Oral contraceptives. Episodes of irregular and unpredictable spotting are frequent occurrences during initial use of the oral-contraceptive pill. This may reflect differences in dosages of estrogens and progestins contained with the pill preparation to affect endometrial proliferation and decidualization, as well as differences in individual absorption and metabolism of pill steroids. Development of abnormal vaginal bleeding in an individual taking an oral contraceptive who had previously experienced regular withdrawal bleeding with an oral contraceptive signals the need to search for an organic explanation of the bleeding. It could be due to the presence of an endometrial or endocervical polyp, submucous leiomyoma, or undiagnosed pregnancy. Alternatively, the risk of infection should be considered since 19 of 65 women (29.2%) who experienced intermenstrual spotting while taking an oral contraceptive

were found to have positive immunological testing for *C. trachomatis.*[30]

Vascular anomalies

An unusual cause of menorrhagia is that of a uterine vascular anomaly. Although arteriovenous malformation of the uterus is uncommon, six cases were reported recently by Fleming et al.[19] Vascular anomalies are rarely detected before hysterectomy, but this problem should be considered in difficult cases. Arteriography may be required to identify these vascular anomalies.

Malignancy

Heightened concern about the presence of reproductive-tract malignancy is customary when evaluating menstrual-cycle disturbances in women older than 35 years of age.

Neoplastic causes of abnormal menstrual-cycle bleeding patterns may also, unfortunately, be seen in women younger than 35 years of age. Postcoital bleeding or spotting should prompt a gynecological evaluation that includes a careful inspection of the vagina and cervix, as well as a pap smear and colposcopy. Cervical adenocarcinoma may be found in the patient with postcoital spotting who has a negative pap smear.

Existence of intrauterine malignancy may only come to light when younger women with persistent menstrual-cycle disturbances are evaluated hysteroscopically. Endometrial biopsies or curettages are blind procedures that may miss the abnormal endometrial focus in some patients.

Pipelle endometrial biopsy and sonographic endometrial strip-thickness measurement are becoming recognized as effective methods to screen for malignancy.[25] When malignancy is not detected in the older woman, diagnostic and operative hysteroscopy may be effective in identifying and treating the cause of abnormal bleeding. In one series of 110 women with persistent postmenopausal bleeding, 90% were identified as having either polyps or submucous fibroids.[53] Some recent studies have suggested that the prevalence of endometrial cancer in postmenopausal women presenting with vaginal bleeding is less than 10%. As a consequence, it has even been proposed that delaying endometrial sampling for low-risk patients until bleeding recurs may warrant consideration as a "cost-effective" strategy.[17]

Documentation of menstrual-blood loss

A major difficulty in clinical studies that assess changes in menstrual-blood loss is the technique used to determine blood loss. Duration of menses and the number of pads or tampons used have proven to be unreliable indicators. In 69 women who presented with a convincing complaint of menorrhagia in a recent study, only 38% were found to have a measured menstrual loss exceeding 80 ml. No significant correlation was found between the number of pads or tampons used and measured blood loss.[20] Possible explanations for the discrepancy between perceived and actual blood loss depend upon the duration of menses and the accurate impression of tampon use, which correlates with blood loss. Variations in tampon use may also reflect age, race, education, physical activity, availability of toilet facilities, and differences in tampon absorbency. Another source of confusion is that 60% of the menstruum is accounted for by fluid and only 40% is accounted for as whole blood.[21] For practical purposes, a change in duration of menstrual flow (i.e., from four to seven days) should be considered abnormal even though the patient does not have menorrhagia by definition.

Evaluation

Evaluation of the anovulatory patient must include an investigation for hormonal causes. Details of such an investigation are beyond the scope of this chapter and may be found in other chapters of this textbook dealing with such topics as hyperandrogenemic chronic anovulation syndrome (PCO), puberty, menopause, and amenorrhea. Whether the bleeding disturbances occur in a woman who is ovulatory or anovulatory, evaluation of the endometrium by biopsy, dilatation and curettage, or hysteroscopy should be considered. Histological examination detects prolonged anovulatory status by revealing the presence of endometrial hyperplasia, atypia, or carcinoma. Hysteroscopy can reveal the presence of an endocervical or endometrial polyp, as well as a submucous leiomyoma. Foreign bodies and retained pregnancy tissues may also be identified hysteroscopically. A detailed discussion of hysteroscopic findings and their causes may be found in Chapter 58.

Failure to detect a structural cause for a bleeding abnormality in a patient who is ovulatory should prompt investigation for uncommon causes. Coagulation disorders may be detected by obtaining a platelet count, prothrombin time (PT) and partial thromboplastin time (PTT), or bleeding time. Thyroid disorders may be detected by obtaining a sensitive TSH measurement and performing a TRH stimulation test. In rare cases, a uterovascular anomaly may be suspected and a pelvic angiogram obtained.

Some protocols for the evaluation of the patient with menstrual-cycle disturbances have recommended the use of exogenously administered progesterone as part of the evaluation. Demonstration of withdrawal bleeding to this exogenously administered hormone suggests an underlying hormonal disturbance. This approach is entirely satisfactory for many patients who receive continual medical care from physicians knowledgeable about their patients' past gynecological and medical histories. In the absence of such knowledge, progesterone use in the acute setting without first determining if the bleeding is ovulatory or anovulatory may inadvertently prolong the time required to make a proper diagnosis.

THERAPY

Treatment of the menstrual-cycle disturbance in large part depends on the diagnosis rendered. In young women with isolated anovulatory cycles resulting in abnormal bleeding patterns, reassurance is usually best. In perimenopausal women with cycle irregularity resulting from anovulation, reassurance may be given after malignancy has been excluded by inspection, pap smear, and endometrial sampling.

Combination oral-contraceptive pill therapy is very effective in producing regular episodes of uterine withdrawal bleeding in women with chronic anovulation syndrome or in perimenopausal patients. Progesterone or progestin therapy alone may also be tried in individuals not wishing to use contraceptive pills. Two drugs have been used for this purpose. Medroxyprogesterone acetate given in 5 mg or 10 mg amounts for 10 to 13 days each month, every other month, or even every third month has been prescribed. Norethindrone acetate has also been given as a 5 mg tablet for five to 10 days each month as an alternative. Monitoring of the endometrium by periodic biopsy may be individualized depending on the underlying cause of anovulation and frequency of progestin administration. Side effects from use of either progestin are generally mild with depressive mood changes being particularly troublesome.

Identification of uterine anomalies such as polyps or leiomyomata has frequently resulted in surgical treatments such as uterine curettage, myomectomy, or hysterectomy. An alternative method of managing patients with leiomyomata and menorrhagia has been to administer analogues of gonadotropin releasing hormone (GnRH), which cause marked reduction in fibroid size after three to five months of use.[9,18] Unfortunately, the effect of this therapy usually lasts only as long as the treatment continues, with regrowth following cessation of drug use. Reduced growth-factor binding, decreased number of receptors for estradiol and progesterone[2,34], and reduced uterine-blood flow[39] have all been suggested as possible mechanisms of action for gonadotropin-releasing hormone agonists. Side effects of therapy include irregular spotting and symptoms of estrogen withdrawal, such as hot flushes. On rare occasions, vaginal hemorrhage from degenerating submucous leiomyomata may be encountered.[22]

One possible solution, at the present time, to the problem of fibroid regrowth and resumption of menorrhagia in a perimenopausal patient following cessation of GnRH agonist therapy, is to provide continual gonadotropin-releasing hormone agonist therapy coupled with hormone replacement; for example 0.625 mg of conjugated estrogens given daily with 10 mg of medroxyprogesterone acetate given for 10 to 13 days each month. This has been termed *addback* therapy.[23]

Worthy of further investigation are the observations of Murphy et al. who reported 20% decreases in myoma volume in women treated with the antiprogesterone RU486 (mifepristone). Side effects appeared to be less severe than those observed by others with GnRH analogue therapy but larger clinical studies are needed to validate this.[40] Information on the rate of regrowth of leiomyomata following cessation of RU486 treatment is not currently available.

Destruction or "ablation" of the endometrium by means of electrocautery, diathermy, or laser have been advocated for some patients with menstrual-cycle disturbances.[12,24,33,43,57] Follow-up of these patients has been limited due to the recent introduction of these procedures. Amenorrhea is reported in 27% to 74% of women treated by ablation with approximately 10% of patients reporting an unsatisfactory outcome.[29,35]

Hysteroscopic examination following endometrial ablation has revealed the existence of a narrow tubular cavity[5] without obliteration of the cavity as observed in some women diagnosed with Asherman syndrome. Nevertheless, the concern remains that ablative procedures may bury functional endometrial tissue, leading to future difficulty in detecting endometrial dysplasia. These fears have recently been realized with the report of an endometrial cancer detected five years after endometrial ablation. In this single case, bleeding occurred after five years of amenorrhea resulting from endometrial ablation. The patient was evaluated by an endometrial biopsy that detected the malignancy, reported after hysterectomy as a moderately differentiated, superficially invasive adenocarcinoma arising in an endometrial polyp FIGO stage II/III, nuclear grade II.[10] It is unclear whether the ablation procedure advanced or delayed the diagnosis of disease in this case. The effectiveness of endometrial ablation as a therapeutic procedure may also depend upon the preoperative method of endometrial hormonal suppression[4], as well as the wattage used with the lasers[11] or electrode.[48]

Use of modulated (coagulating) and unmodulated (cutting) wave forms have been employed to accomplish electrocautery endometrial ablation. Above 90 watts of power, it appears that using either cutting or coagulating wave forms results in thermal damage (in vitro) to a depth of 3 mm into the myometrium when a single pass with a 2.5 mm roller bar electrode is used.[42] However, when wattages of 40 or less are used, thermal damage does not exceed a depth of 3 mm into the myometrium. Surprisingly, even at power settings exceeding 100 watts, using either a wire loop or roller ball, histologically normal endometrial glands (implying glandular survival) are visible following human uterine ablation in vitro.[32]

Occasionally menorrhagia may be diagnosed in ovulatory women who are otherwise without abnormal findings. Reduction in blood loss in these patients may be obtained by using oral-contraceptive pills to produce endometrial atrophy. If there are objections to contraceptive pill use, prostaglandin synthesis inhibitors may be prescribed to reduce blood loss with mefenamic acid begun immediately prior to and through menses (500 mg po tid). The mechanism responsible for the ability of mefenamic acid to reduce blood loss remains unclear, although recent data suggest improved platelet aggregation and increased vasoconstriction may be responsible.[56]

Use of other agents

Inhibition of fibrinolysis with epsilon-aminocaproic acid (EACA) or tranexamic acid has been used successfully to reduce blood loss for menorrhagic individuals[41], but side effects such as nausea, dizziness, and diarrhea limit the use of these agents.

Infrequently, the need may arise to administer medications to control bleeding prior to providing additional treatment. Intravenous conjugated estrogens at a dosage of 25 mg every four hours has been used for this purpose.[15] For individuals without organic pathology, 72% of those receiving two doses of estrogen stopped bleeding within 10 hours, compared to 38% of subjects who received placebos. Following cessation of bleeding, oral administration of conjugated estrogens for three weeks may be given followed by progestin-induced withdrawal bleeding. Alternatively, administration of combination oral contraceptive with two to four pills per day, tapering to one pill per day over a period of 21 days may be tried.

CONCLUSION

Evaluation of menstrual-cycle disturbances may be organized by age and whether the bleeding disturbance is occurring in an ovulatory or anovulatory individual. Diagnostic use of endometrial biopsies, hysteroscopy, and transvaginal ultrasound are procedures that are becoming increasingly valued and will presumably result in decreased numbers of perfunctory dilation and curettage procedures being performed. Present and future medical therapies include oral-contraceptive pills, prostaglandin synthesis inhibitors, GnRH analogues, and RU486. Use of these treatments ultimately may lead to a reduction in the number of hysterectomies performed for menstrual-cycle disturbances. The success of endometrial ablation as an alternative to hysterectomy is currently being evaluated.

REFERENCES

1. Andrade ATL, Pizarro E, Shaw ST et al: Consequences of uterine blood loss caused by various intrauterine contraceptive devices in South American women, *Contraception* 38:1, 1988.
2. Baird DT, West CP: Medical management of fibroids, *Br Med J* 296:1684, 1988.
3. Bartelmez GW: The phases of the menstrual cycle and their interpretation in terms of the pregnancy cycle, *Am J Obstet Gynecol* 74:931, 1957.
4. Brooks PG, Serden SP, Davos I: Hormonal inhibition of the endometrium for resectoscopic endometrial ablation, *Am J Obstet Gynecol* 164:1601, 1991.
5. Brooks PG, Serden SP: Endometrial ablation in women with abnormal uterine bleeding age fifty and over, *J Reprod Med* 37:682, 1992.

6. Casey ML, Smith JW, Naga K et al: Progesterone-regulated cyclic modulation of membrane metalloendopeptidase (enkephalinase) in human endometrium, *J Biol Chem* 266(34):23041, 1991.

7. Christiaens GCML, Sixma JJ, Haspels AA: Hemostasis in menstrual endometrium: a review, *Obstet Gynecol Surv* 37:281, 1982.

8. Claessens EA, Cowell CA: Acute adolescent menorrhagia, *Am J Obstet Gynecol* 139:277, 1981.

9. Coddington CC, Collins RL, Shawker TH et al: Long-acting gonadotropin hormone-releasing hormone analog used to treat uteri, *Fertil Steril* 45:624, 1986.

10. Copperman AB, DeCherney AH, Olive DL: A case of endometrial cancer following endometrial ablation for dysfunctional uterine bleeding, *Obstet Gynecol* 82:640, 1993.

11. Davis JA: Hysteroscopic endometrial ablation with the neodymium-YAG laser, *Br J Obstet Gynecol* 96:928, 1989.

12. DeCherney AH, Diamond MP, Lavy G et al: Endometrial ablation for intractable uterine bleeding: hysteroscopic resection, *Obstet Gynecol* 70:668, 1987.

13. DeStefano F, Perlman JA, Peterson HB et al: Long-term risk of menstrual disturbances after tubal sterilization, *Am J Obstet Gynecol* 152:835, 1985.

14. DeStefano F, Huezo CM, Peterson HB et al: Menstrual changes after tubal sterilization, *Obstet Gynecol* 62:673, 1983.

15. Devore GR, Owens O, Kase N: Use of intravenous Premarin in the treatment of dysfunctional uterine bleeding—a double-blind randomized control study, *Obstet Gynecol* 59:285, 1982.

16. Economos K, MacDonald PC, Casey ML: Endothelin-1 gene expression and protein biosynthesis in human endometrium: potential modulator of endometrial blood flow, *J Clin Endocrinol Metab* 74:14, 1992.

17. Feldman S, Berkowitz RS, Tosteson AN: Cost-effectiveness of strategies to evaluate postmenopausal bleeding, *Obstet Gynecol* 81:968, 1993.

18. Filicori M, Hall DA, Loughlin JS et al: A conservative approach to the management of uterine leiomyoma; pituitary desensitization by a luteinizing hormone-releasing hormone analogue, *Am J Obstet Gynecol* 147:726, 1983.

19. Fleming H, Oster AG, Pickel H et al: Arteriovenous malformations of the uterus, *Obstet Gynecol* 73:209, 1989.

20. Fraser IS, McCarron G, Markham R: A preliminary study of factors influencing perception of menstrual blood loss volume, *Am J Obstet Gynecol* 149:788, 1984.

21. Fraser IS, McCarron G, Markham R et al: Blood and total fluid content of menstrual discharge, *Obstet Gynecol* 65:194, 1985.

22. Friedman AJ: Vaginal hemorrhage associated with degenerating submucous leiomyomata during leuprolide acetate treatment, *Fertil Steril* 52:152, 1989.

23. Friedman AJ: Treatment of leiomyomata uteri with short-term leuprolide followed by leuprolide plus estrogen-progestin hormonal replacement therapy for 2 years: a pilot study, *Fertil Steril* 51:526, 1989.

24. Goldrath MH, Fuller TA, Segal S: Laser photovaporization of endometrium for the treatment of menorrhagia, *Am J Obstet Gynecol* 140:14, 1981.

25. Goldschmit R, Katz Z, Blickstein I et al: The accuracy of endometrial pipelle sampling with and without sonographic measurement of endometrial thickness, *Obstet Gynecol* 82:727, 1993.

26. Goldstein SR, Nachtigall M, Snyder JR et al: Endometrial assessment by vaginal ultrasonography before endometrial sampling in patients with post-menopausal bleeding, *Am J Obstet Gynecol* 163:119, 1990.

27. Hallberg L, Hogdahl Am, Nilsson L et al: Menstrual blood loss: a population study, *Acta Obstet Gynecol Scand* 45:320, 1966.

28. Hammerschmidt DE: Szechwan purpura, *N Engl J Med* 302:1191, 1980.

29. Ke RW, Taylor PJ: Endometrial ablation to control excessive bleeding, *Hum Reprod* 6:574, 1991.

30. Krettek JE, Arkin SI, Chaisilwattana P et al: *Chlamydia trachomatis* in patients who used oral contraceptives and had intramenstrual spotting, *Obstet Gynecol* 81:728, 1993.

31. Larsson PG, Bergman BB: Is there a causal connection between motile curved rods, *Mobiluncus* species, and bleeding complications? *Am J Obstet Gynecol* 154:107, 1986.

32. Letterie GS, Hibbert ML, Britton BA: Endometrial histology after electrocoagulation using different pressure settings, *Fertil Steril* 60:647, 1993.

33. Lomano JM: Dragging technique versus blanching technique for endometrial ablation with the Nd:YAG laser in the treatment of chronic menorrhagia, *Am J Obstet Gynecol* 159:152, 1988.

34. Lumsden MA, West CP, Bramley T et al: The binding of EGF to the human uterus and leiomyomata in women rendered hypo-estrogenic by continuous administration of an LHRH agonist, *Br J Obstet Gynecol* 12:1299, 1988.

35. Magos AI, Baumann R, Lockwood GM et al: Experience with the first 250 endometrial resections for menorrhagia, *Lancet* 337:1074, 1991.

36. Mahmood TA, Templeton AA, Thompson L et al: Menstrual symptoms in women with pelvic endometriosis, *Br J Obstet Gynecol* 98:558, 1991.

37. Makheja AN, Vanderhock JY, Bryant RW et al: Altered arachidonic acid metabolism in platelets by onion or garlic extracts, *Adv Prostaglandin Thromboxane Leukotriene Res* 6:309, 1980.

38. Markee JE: Menstruation in intraocular endometrial implants in the rhesus monkey, *Contrib Embryol Carnegie Inst,* Washington, DC 28:219, 1940.

39. Matta WHM, Stabile I, Shaw RW et al: Doppler assessment of uterine blood flow changes in patients with fibroids receiving gonadotropin-releasing hormone agonist Buserelin, *Fertil Steril* 49:1083, 1988.

40. Murphy AA, Kettel LM, Morales AJ et al: Regression of leiomyomata in response to the antiprogesterone RU486, *J Clin Endocrinol Metab* 76:513, 1993.

41. Nilsson L, Rybo G: Treatment of menorrhagia, *Am J Obstet Gynecol* 110:713, 1971.

42. Onbargi LC, Hayden R, Valle RF et al: Effects of power and electrical current density variations on an in vitro endometrial ablation model, *Obstet Gynecol* 82:912, 1993.

43. Phipps JH, Lewis BV, Roberts T et al: Treatment of functional menorrhagia by radiofrequency-induced thermal endometrial ablation, *Lancet* 335:374, 1990.

44. Rogers J: Medical progress: menstruation and systemic disease, thyroid disorders, *N Engl J Med* 259:271, 1958.

45. Rulin MC, Davidson AR, Philliber SG et al: Changes in menstrual symptoms among sterilized and comparison women: a prospective study, *Obstet Gynecol* 74:149, 1989.

46. Rulin MC, Turner JH, Dunworth R et al: Post-tubal sterilization syndrome—a misnomer, *Am J Obstet Gynecol* 151:13, 1985.

47. Sakamoto C, Nakano H: The echogenic endometrium and alteration during the menstrual cycle, *Int J Gynaecol Obstet* 20:255, 1982.

48. Soderstrom RM: Electricity inside the uterus, *Clin Obstet Gynecol* 35:262, 1992.

49. Sokolovsky M, Galron R, Kloog Y et al: Endothelins are more sensitive than sarafotoxins to neutral endopeptidase: possible physiological significance, *Proc Natl Acad Sci USA* 87:4702, 1990.

50. Srivastava KC: Extracts from two frequently consumed spices, cumin and turmeric, inhibit platelet aggregation and alter eicosanoid biosynthesis in human blood platelets, *Prostaglandins Leukot Essent Fatty Acids* 37:57, 1989.

51. Steinkampf MP: Systemic illness and menstrual dysfunction, *Obstet Gynecol Clin North Am* 17:311, 1990.

52. Stevenson CS, Campbell CG: The symptoms, physical findings and clinical diagnosis of pelvic endometriosis, *Clin Obstet Gynecol* 3:441, 1960.

53. Townsend DE, Fields G, McCausland A et al: Diagnostic and operative hysteroscopy in the management of persistent post-menopausal bleeding, *Obstet Gynecol* 82:419, 1993.

54. Treloar AE, Boynton RE, Behn BG et al: Variation of the human menstrual cycle through reproductive life, *Int J Fertil* Vol 12, No 1, Part 2:77, 1967.

55. van Eijkeren MA, Christiaens GCML, Haspels AA et al: Measured menstrual blood loss in women with a bleeding disorder or using oral anticoagulant therapy, *Am J Obstet Gynecol* 162:1261, 1990.

56. van Eijkeren MA, Christiaens GCML, Geuze HJ et al: Effects of mefenamic acid on menstrual hemostasis in essential menorrhagia, *Am J Obstet Gynecol* 166:1419, 1992.

57. Vancaille TG: Electrocoagulation of the endometrium with the ball-end resectoscope, *Obstet Gynecol* 74:425, 1989.

58. Vijayaraghavan J, Scili AG, Carretero OA et al: The hydrolysis of endothelins by neutral endopeptidase (enkephalinase), *J Biol Chem* 265:14150, 1990.

59. Visscher HC, editor: *Precis IV: update in obstetrics and gynecology,* Washington, DC, 1990, American College of Obstetricians and Gynecologists.

60. Wang IYS, Fraser IS: Lysosomes: an important mediator in the female reproductive tract, *Obstet Gynecol Surv* 45:18, 1989.

61. Wentz AC: Premenstrual spotting: its association with endometriosis with no luteal-phase inadequacy, *Fertil Steril* 33:605, 1980.

62. White AJ, Buchsbaum HJ: Scanning electron microscopy of the human endometrium, *Gynecol Oncol* 1:330, 1973.

63. Wilansky DL, Greisman B: Early hypothyroidism in patients with menorrhagia, *Am J Obstet Gynecol* 160:673, 1989.

64. Wilcox LS, Martinez-Schnell B, Peterson HB et al: Menstrual function after tubal sterilization, *Am J Epidemiol* 135:1368, 1992.

65. Williams EL, Jones HE, Merrill RE: The subsequent course of patients sterilized by tubal ligation, *Am J Obstet Gynecol* 61:423, 1951.

Chapter 9

EVALUATION AND THERAPY OF HYPERPROLACTINEMIA

Howard A. Zacur, M.D., Ph.D.
and Scot M. Hutchison, M.D.

EVALUATION AND THERAPY OF HYPERPROLACTINEMIA

A human pituitary prolactin hormone was identified in 1971 through the efforts of Friesen et al., using affinity column chromatographic techniques.[52] Prior to this time, the existence of a human prolactin molecule was doubted by the scientific community, which believed that lactogenic activities in human and subhuman primates were mediated by human growth hormone. Once its existence was confirmed, sensitive radioimmunoassays to measure prolactin were developed, and this rapidly led to an understanding of the normal changes in the concentration of this hormone under different physiological conditions. Abnormal elevations in prolactin soon became detectable and hyperprolactinemia was established as the etiology for many previously unexplained cases of impotence and amenorrhea.

Mild, chronic elevations in serum prolactin may result in altered reproductive biologic function, but mild, acute elevations in serum prolactin may be seen in response to normal physiologic stimuli and have no sustained adverse effect on reproductive function. Knowledge of the factors regulating serum prolactin is important in understanding both *physiologic* and *pathophysiologic* hyperprolactinemia. Once understood, the physician can then proceed with evaluation and treatment of the affected patient.

PHYSIOLOGY OF PROLACTIN SECRETION

Secretion of this 199 amino acid protein of approximately 23,000 molecular weight (MW)[100] occurs almost exclusively from lactotropes (or mammotrophs) located in the lateral wings of the anterior pituitary gland.[6] These cells may also be found within the dura mater of the brain, which may explain the peculiar observation that measurable prolactin levels are detectable in individuals who have been hypophysectomized. Prolactin is also secreted by decidual cells of the uterus during the late luteal phase of the menstrual cycle or during pregnancy,[114] as well as from cells of the myometrium itself.[160] Very little, if any, decidual or myometrial prolactin is believed to enter the general circulation under usual circumstances. It is thought that under rare circumstances, prolactin may be secreted by neoplastic cells (e.g., bronchogenic carcinoma),[151] although this concept has been disputed.[91]

The gene for human prolactin has been located on chromosome 6.[106] Although early ribonucleic acid (RNA) blot hybridization studies suggested that the genes for prolactin in the lactotrope and decidual cell were identical, recent investigations have indicated that the human decidual prolactin mRNA is elongated relative to the pituitary transcript at its 5′ end.[33] As a consequence, it has been suspected that promoter activities may be different for the two prolactin genes. Thus, while the protein product of the prolactin gene would be identical from the two different tissues, differences may exist in the regulation of hormone secretion in these tissues. Failure of dopamine added in vitro (to inhibit) or thyrotropin releasing hormone (TRH) (to stimulate) decidual cell prolactin release, in contrast to the responses observed with pituitary cell prolactin release, may be examples of this difference.

REGULATION OF PITUITARY PROLACTIN SECRETION

Prolactin release from the anterior pituitary gland is regulated, in part, by release of stimulating or inhibiting agents from the hypothalamus. In contrast to other pituitary hormones, prolactin secretion is chronically inhibited because transection of the pituitary stalk results in elevation of peripheral prolactin levels with reduced concentrations of other pituitary hormones.[35,36] Dopamine, which is released from axons terminating on pituitary portal vessels, is currently believed to be the agent most responsible for inhibiting prolactin secretion.[82] This conclusion is inferred from studies that have measured dopamine concentrations in pituitary portal blood;[8] from documentation of dopamine binding to receptors on lactotropes;[29] and from observation of diminished prolactin synthesis and release, in vitro and in vivo, following exogenous dopamine administration.

Dopamine receptors exist in several forms. Two of the better known receptors are referred to as D_1 and D_2. Stimulation of the D_1 receptor results in stimulation of adenylate cyclase activity; stimulation of the D_2 receptor results in lowered cellular levels of adenosine 3′ :5′ = cyclic phosphate (cyclic AMP).[134] The dopamine receptor responsible for inhibiting prolactin release is D_2.[29] Not all lactogenic cells possess equally functional dopamine receptors[103] and differences among lactotropes in their responsiveness to dopamine have been described as evidence of lactotrope heterogeneity.[81] This is an important biological concept that may be expressed clinically as hyperprolactinemia that is resistant to dopamine therapy.[141]

Regulation of prolactin secretion is complex due to multifactorial control[167] (Fig. 9-1). Prolactin may inhibit its own secretion directly at the level of the pituitary gland,[169] or indirectly by increasing hypothalamic dopamine turnover.[42,51] Gamma-aminobutyric acid (GABA) can inhibit pituitary prolactin secretion,[124] as can the 56 amino acid peptide encoded before gonadotropin-releasing hormone (GnRH), which has been called gonadotropin hormone–releasing hormone associated peptide (GAP).[101] Depending upon dosage, with lower concentrations being inhibitory

and higher ones stimulatory, endothelin-3, a small 21 amino acid peptide present in the hypothalamus, has also been shown to affect prolactin release.[121]

Stimulatory agents of pituitary prolactin secretion also exist. Estrogens can stimulate prolactin secretion by stimulating prolactin gene transcription[133] or by diminishing hypothalamic dopamine release.[27] TRH and vasoactive intestinal peptide (VIP) can directly stimulate pituitary prolactin release.[119,147] GnRH has also been shown to have prolactin-releasing effects.[101] Table 9-1 summarizes these activities.

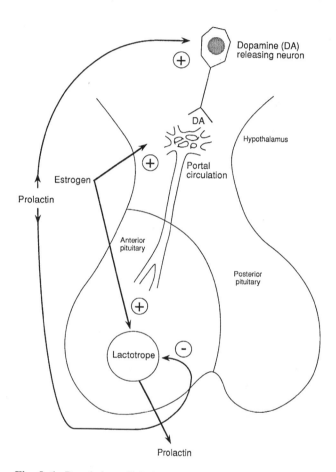

Fig. 9-1. Regulation of pituitary prolactin secretion is complex. Normally under continuous inhibition by hypothalamic dopamine, prolactin release may be stimulated by diminishing the amount of dopamine or blocking its site of action. Prolactin secretion may be stimulated directly by estrogen, which may act at the gland or hypothalamus.

Table 9-1. Regulation of prolactin secretion

Inhibitory agents	Stimulatory agents
Prolactin[169,42]	Estrogen[133]
GABA[124]	TRH[147]
GAP[101]	VIP[119]
Endothelin-3[121]	GnRH[11]

PROLACTIN MEASUREMENT

One of the most common methods of measuring the concentration of prolactin in human serum is through the use of an immunoassay system. Reagents for performing a prolactin assay may be obtained from commercial or institutional sources. It should be remembered that each assay system may be different in terms of its reference material, labeled hormone tag, use of unlabelled or labelled antiserum, and method used to separate bound hormone from free hormone. Details for different standard assay procedures may be found in Chapter 62.

Establishment of a "normal" prolactin concentration is the responsibility of every clinical laboratory that performs a human prolactin assay; however, the range of "normal" from each laboratory may be different. Therefore, it is not surprising to learn that the same serum sample given to different laboratories for prolactin measurement may be reported as having different values.[43] For most laboratories, a normal range of 0-20 ng/ml for serum prolactin concentrations in women has been established, with slightly lower values (0-15 ng/ml) reported for men.

In the past, bioassays depended upon the well-known biologic action of prolactin to stimulate milk production from mammary-gland tissues. Bioassays utilizing the pigeon crop sac[115] or mouse mammary gland[63] have been developed, but these are tedious to perform and lack sensitivity. A radioreceptor assay also has been developed to measure prolactin, but it is less sensitive than current radioimmunoassay methods.[132] Recently, Tanaka et al. described a new bioassay system using Nb2 rat lymphoma cells that has a sensitivity rivaling that of immunoassay.[146] This new bioassay for prolactin depends upon the use of tumorigenic lymphoma cells taken from a transplantable lymphoma of estrogenized male rats of the Noble (Nb) strain. These cells may be continuously grown in culture supplemented with fetal calf serum. Cell division ceases in the absence of serum supplement but resumes upon addition of prolactin. The ability of prolactin to affect ornithine decarboxylase activity and thymidine incorporation into Nb2 lymphoma cells exposed to this hormone implies that an interrelationship may exist between prolactin and the immune system.[44]

An understanding of the differences between immunoassays and bioassays has important clinical consequences. For example, prolactin is a heterogenous molecule as it circulates in different forms.[117] *Little prolactin* (23,000 MW); *big prolactin* (48,000-56,000 MW); and *big, big prolactin* (100,000 MW) have all been described and found in varying concentrations in human serum. Biologic activity varies, with the bigger forms of the molecule being less biologically active[54,162] than the smaller forms. Big prolactin and big, big prolactin are believed to reflect dimers and tetramers of the native prolactin molecule. These molecules are different from prolactin isohormones, which have different biological and immunological activities.[104] Differ-

ences in glycosylation of the usual prolactin molecule may account for isohormones.

It is important to realize that a rise and fall in prolactin concentration may reflect assay variability and not clinical circumstances. For example, in a prolactin assay with a 10-15% interassay variation, a prolactin value of 100 ng/ml could also be read as 85 or 115 ng/ml. It is useful to remember that immunological measurement of a biologically *inactive* prolactin molecule is possible as well, which may be the explanation for the hyperprolactinemic patient who has regular menses and no difficulty conceiving.

Prolactin measurement in body fluids

In addition to its measurement in serum and plasma, prolactin may be measured in other body fluids. These fluids include cerebral spinal fluid,[57] amniotic fluid,[153] cervical mucus,[131] milk,[45] and semen.[130] Prolactin has also been reported to have been measured in urine;[136] however, fragments of the prolactin molecule may exist in urine,[169] as well as other substances, and these may interfere with the prolactin assay.[45] All of these factors may cause erroneous measurements resulting in the absence of a reliable method for measurement of urinary prolactin.

Biologic variation

Physical and emotional stresses are well-known causes of transient hyperprolactinemia in humans.[102] Therefore, an accurate prolactin measurement may not be obtained when blood is drawn following a stressful event. Interestingly, to provoke a response, the stressful event must be acute; neither prolonged emotional[85] nor physical stress[1] is associated with elevated prolactin concentrations.

Prolactin levels rise during sleep[122] whether sleep occurs at night or during the day (Fig. 9–2). When sleep occurs at night, prolactin levels rise, steadily drop as morning nears, and then gradually increase again as afternoon approaches.[5] The biological significance of a sleep-associated rise in prolactin remains unclear, but a relationship between this rise and the function of the human immune system has been suggested.[44]

Food ingestion during the day results in a transient rise in the serum prolactin concentration after lunch or dinner, but not after breakfast.[53,109] High-protein meals cause a release of both prolactin and cortisol,[16] while high-fat meals cause a selective increase in serum prolactin.

Controversial evidence exists to support relative hyperprolactinemia occurring during the periovulatory interval of the human menstrual cycle.[168] This prolactin rise may be a consequence of lactotrope stimulation from the midcycle estradiol surge, or from an increase in frequency or amplitude of GnRH, a polypeptide known to stimulate prolactin release.[84]

Stimulation of the anterior chest wall by suckling,[103] breast implants,[120] chest-wall surgery,[96] or herpes zoster may result in elevated prolactin levels. This presumably

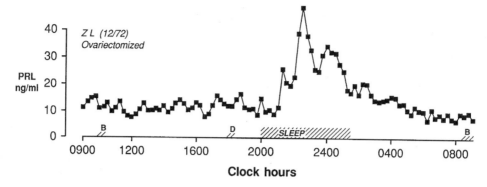

Fig. 9-2. Changes in prolactin concentrations over 24 hours in an ovariectomized woman. A rise in the prolactin concentration is observed with onset of sleep. From Yen SSC and Jaffe RB (eds): *Reproductive Endocrinology*, Philadelphia, 1978, W. B. Saunders.

results from altered hypothalamic-dopamine release induced by messages from afferent sensory nerve fibers located in the anterior chest wall.

Prolactin concentrations rise during gestation[153] and are believed to result from the corresponding increase in serum estrogen levels stimulating the hypothalamus and pituitary. If breastfeeding does not occur following delivery, prolactin levels rapidly fall to normal levels at the end of the first postpartum week. If breastfeeding occurs, prolactin concentrations may remain elevated for a prolonged time period depending upon the frequency, duration, and intensity of the suckling stimulus.[48]

PHARMACOLOGIC EFFECTS

Pituitary prolactin secretion is predominately under inhibitory regulation of the hypothalamus, which is believed to exert its influence via the release of dopamine into pituitary portal blood. Drugs or medications that diminish dopamine of hypothalamic origin or block its action at the level of the lactotroph within the pituitary gland are expected to increase serum prolactin levels.

Tranquilizing drugs such as phenothiazenes e.g., chlorpromazine,[64] fluphenazine,[74] butyrophenones (e.g., pimozide,[21] haloperidol,[74]) substituted benzamides (e.g., sulpiride[94]), or metoclopramide[142]) block dopamine receptors and produce elevated concentrations of serum prolactin. Opiates, whether endogenous or exogenously administered, cause a rise in prolactin levels, which is mediated by two mechanisms: direct stimulation of GnRH release, which in turn stimulates prolactin release;[118] and a reduction in hypothalamic-dopamine activity, again causing prolactin release.[159] Effects of benzodiazepines are controversial, some reports claim no change in prolactin levels following their use[31,163] and others claim an increase.[32] Tricyclic antidepressants and monoamine oxidase inhibitors may also cause prolactin elevations[138,152] by affecting dopamine or serotonin activity, although there is some disagreement on this point.[90]

Increased prolactin levels have also been reported in women using oral-contraceptive pills.[170] This increase may reflect hypothalamic or pituitary regulation of prolactin secretion by estrogens contained within the pill, possibly via upregulation of prolactin receptors. Less is known about the ability of the progestins, norethindrone or norgestrel, to affect prolactin secretion. Medroxyprogesterone acetate may[108] or may not[144] cause a prolactin rise.

Hyperprolactinemia has been noted in some women taking lithium for manic-depressive illness.[60] This effect presumably results from the hypothyroid state induced by this drug, which is capable of inhibiting thyroxine release from the thyroid gland.[143] During states of hypothyroidism, hypothalamic TRH may stimulate additional pituitary prolactin release.

HYPERPROLACTINEMIA AND AMENORRHEA

In nonpregnant women, prolactin elevations are associated with anovulation and amenorrhea. Prolactin, acting on the hypothalamus and/or ovary, is believed responsible for this response. Prolactin has been shown *in vitro* to modulate progesterone secretion from incubating luteinized granulosa cells.[89] In McNatty's study, either low or high prolactin concentrations diminished granulosa cell steroid production. It was therefore suspected that this could occur *in vivo*, resulting in reduced ovarian steroid production and, in turn, adversely affecting hypothalamic regulation of gonadotropin release.

Pituitary secretion of luteinizing hormone (LH) reflects hypothalamic release of GnRH into the portal bloodstream, and norepinephrine and opioids are some of the neurotransmitters that may affect GnRH release. Dopamine is a neurotransmitter that is of particular importance because it is inhibitory for GnRH release.[76] When prolactin is secreted by lactotropes into the circulation, some of this hormone is released into pituitary portal blood, and flows in a retrograde fashion into the hypothalamus. When this happens, hypothalamic neurons release dopamine in response to prolactin.[42] Under conditions of elevated prolactin, it is assumed that GnRH release, as well as LH release, and future prolactin release would be inhibited by this autoregulatory loop.

In women who breastfeed postpartum, prolactin levels may remain elevated for days or months, depending upon the frequency or intensity of nursing. For example, a recent study showed that the average time for return of the first ovulation for women who were breastfeeding was 27 weeks in the United States and 38 weeks in Manila.[48] Although the rise in the prolactin level may account in part for this postpartum delay in resumption of ovulation, nipple stimulation itself can decrease GnRH release directly through afferent impulses to the hypothalamus. For example, in a study involving rhesus monkeys, nipple stimulation by suckling suppressed gonadotropin secretion, while prolactin levels in the same animal were suppressed by bromocriptine treatment.[123]

DIAGNOSIS OF HYPERPROLACTINEMIA

The diagnosis of hyperprolactinemia should be made only when all known causes of hyperprolactinemia have been excluded. To accomplish this, blood samples for prolactin measurement should be taken, if possible, from individuals who are awake, nonstressed, fasted, taking no medications, and in the follicular phase of a menstrual cycle, if menses occur. More than one blood sample should be obtained to verify the diagnosis if an elevated value is initially obtained. When it has been clearly demonstrated that hyperprolactinemia exists, an evaluation of the hyperprolactinemic patient may begin.

Evaluation

Obtaining a comprehensive history is extremely helpful to exclude drug use, as well as to exclude coexisting medical conditions known to cause hyperprolactinemia. For example, primary hypothyroidism is a well-known cause of hyperprolactinemia,[62] presumably due to increased hypothalamic TRH activity that results in increased pituitary prolactin secretion. Laboratory studies indicate that TRH is also a potent stimulator of prolactin release.[55,77] Thyroxine therapy can normalize prolactin levels and even diminish the size of a prolactin-secreting pituitary adenoma when found.

Chronic renal disease may cause prolactin elevation in 20-30% of patients with some degree of renal insufficiency, and in 80% of those requiring dialysis. This hyperprolactinemia was thought to be due to an increased production rate and a decreased metabolic clearance of prolactin.[78] Retention of a pituitary prolactin-stimulating factor as a result of impaired renal function, rather than a reduction in prolactin clearance, is believed to account for this phenomenon.[135]

In patients with cirrhosis, prolactin levels may be elevated regardless of alcohol use.[93] This may result from hypothalamic dopamine alteration[25] rather than hepatic injury per se.

Hyperprolactinemia has also been reported to occur in 3.2-66.7% of women diagnosed with polycystic ovarian syndrome (PCOS).[4,97] An increased estrogenic milieu in patients with PCOS is frequently used to explain this condition. However, in a recent review of the literature on this topic, it was noted that the true frequency of hyperprolactinemia in PCOS patients may not exceed that observed in the general population.[171] This suggests that hyperprolactinemia and PCOS are induced by separate mechanisms. Higher estimates of hyperprolactinemia in women with PCOS may have been reported in earlier studies that were not rigorously controlled to account for all of the factors known to physiologically increase prolactin levels.

When taking the patient's history, previous head trauma should be noted, as well as a history of seizure disorders. Regulatory neural pathways within the central nervous system (CNS) could be disrupted as a result of trauma or seizures. This could account for the hyperprolactinemia by affecting hypothalamic release of inhibitors or stimulators of pituitary prolactin secretion.

Physical examination of the hyperprolactinemic patient should place emphasis on examination of the thyroid gland and breasts. Demonstration of thyroid enlargement, with or without pretibial edema, could point toward hypothyroidism as a contributing factor for hyperprolactinemia. On breast examination, the presence of galactorrhea should be sought. Fluid expressed from the nipple after compression of breast tissue may be microscopically checked to reveal the presence of lipid-laden droplets diagnostic of galactorrhea.

Conversely, existence of galactorrhea is not synonymous with hyperprolactinemia. Hyperprolactinemia may be found in only 20-30% of women with galactorrhea.[65] An explanation for breast-milk discharge in women with normal prolactin levels remains unclear. However, increased breast-receptor sensitivity to normal levels of circulating prolactin has been suggested. During the breast examination, the presence of previous chest-wall injury or irritation should be sought, as well as breast augmentation. All of these changes to the anterior chest wall may result in stimulating afferent nerve impulses to the CNS, ultimately causing pituitary prolactin release.

Laboratory and radiologic evaluation

Initial laboratory testing of the patient with suspected hyperprolactinemia includes repeated measurement of the serum prolactin concentration under controlled conditions to confirm a hyperprolactinemic state. Measurement of the plasma thyrotropin-stimulating hormone (TSH), using a sensitive radioimmunoassay, is also frequently performed to exclude primary hypothyroidism.

Radiologic studies of the pituitary gland are obtained because approximately 40% of patients with elevated prolactin also have a detectable radiographic abnormality.[13] Suggested radiographic imaging techniques include magnetic resonance imaging (MRI) with gadolinium enhancement of the pituitary gland, or computerized tomography (CT scanning) of the pituitary with contrast enhancement. MRI can exquisitely display the anatomic relationships of the pituitary and what is contained within it, as well as the structures adjacent to the pituitary, including the brain stem,

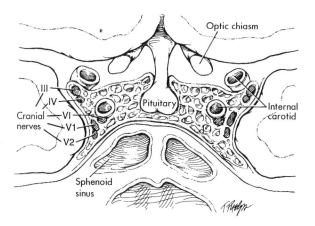

Fig. 9-3. Diagram of the anatomy imaged by an MRI, which was performed to localize a pituitary lesion.

the floor of the sella turcica, the internal carotid arteries, and the optic chiasm (Fig. 9-3). Lesions within the pituitary gland are suspected if the pituitary is enlarged, abnormally shaped, has deviation of the infundibulum, or exhibits irregularities in the density of the contrast material within the gland itself. If the lesion within the pituitary gland is less than 1 cm in maximum width, it is referred to as a *microadenoma*. If it is greater than 1 cm in maximum diameter, it is called a *macroadenoma* (Fig. 9-4).

Normal size of the pituitary gland is determined by measuring its vertical height using a coronal section of the gland at right angles to the diaphragm of the sella. A 7-9 mm height of the gland is considered normal for women; 5-7 mm is considered normal for men.[164] The normal superior shape of the pituitary gland is flat or concave. When a convex shape is noted, a pituitary adenoma is often suspected.[14,17]

Many types of nonneoplastic, low-density areas on MRI imaging with contrast may be found within the otherwise normal pituitary gland. These include neuroepithelial cysts, Rathke's cleft cysts, and arachnoid cysts. Low-density intrapituitary areas have also been found coincidentally in subjects undergoing radiographic imaging, for reasons

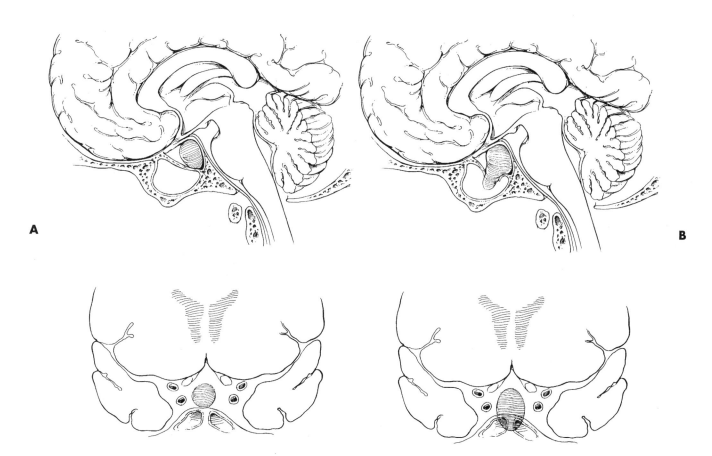

A

B

Fig. 9-4. MRI image of a pituitary macroadenoma followed over time, **A.** Erosion through the sella floor and into the sphenoid sinus is observed in the follow-up study, **B.**

other than hyperprolactinemia. The term *incidentaloma* has been used to describe these images.[92]

Nomenclature

When a pituitary lesion is detected by radiographic imaging of a person with hyperprolactinemia, the commonest terms used to describe this lesion are *pituitary tumor* or *pituitary adenoma*. It is impossible to correctly diagnose the abnormality as a tumor or adenoma without obtaining a specimen of the lesion for histologic examination. True neoplastic lesions of the pituitary gland are extremely rare. When a neoplasm is present, it exhibits the cytologic changes expected of a malignancy; that is, nuclear and/or cytoplasmic atypicalities, as well as mitoses and invasion of adjacent structures. A pituitary adenoma is also rare, but when present, it is defined by encapsulation of a distinct cellular growth.

The pituitary abnormality most commonly observed in women with hyperprolactinemia is nodular hyperplasia of the lactotropes. These prolactin-secreting cells are not encapsulated, do not exhibit cystological or nuclear atypia, and respond to physiological stimuli. Therefore, use of the terms *tumor* or *adenoma* to describe these lesions is incorrect. Perhaps a better term to use is *prolactinoma,* since when a patient hears the terms *tumor* or *adenoma,* the thought of a malignant brain tumor is frequently brought to mind.

The most common type of radiographically identified lesion within the pituitary is a prolactinoma that is directly responsible for hyperprolactinemia. Nonsecreting pituitary lesions are the next most commonly identified pituitary lesion that may cause indirect hyperprolactinemia. This is attributable to disruption of the inhibitory influence of the hypothalamus on prolactin secretion by lactotrope cells adjacent to the lesion. Together, lactotrope and nonhormone-producing tumors account for 30% to 40% of all pituitary lesions.[71] Gonadotropic cell adenomas are responsible for 10-20%,[140] and adrenocorticotropic-secreting tumors and growth hormone-producing tumors are each responsible for 10-20% of the total.[71,92] The frequency with which pituitary adenomas may be found at autopsy in individuals not suspected of having pituitary disease prior to death range from 1.5-26.7% in 13 studies reviewed by Molitch and Russell.[92]

Additional evaluation

Once a pituitary lesion has been identified, its ability to affect vision by compressing the optic chiasm should be assessed. If the adenoma is confined within a normal-sized pituitary gland, or the pituitary and its mass are not adjacent to the optic chiasm, visual-field testing is usually normal and it is not necessary to request this test. If doubt or concern exists, or the lesion is large and adjacent to the optic chiasm, ophthalmologic examination with perimetry studies to exclude field defects are required. Hyperprolactinemic patients with identifiable pituitary lesions are also more likely to complain of headaches, whether the lesion is confined to the gland or exceeds its borders.[145] An explanation for this latter phenomenon is lacking.

Although most pituitary lesions involve lactotropes as previously mentioned, other hormone-producing adenomas may be present and their existence should be sought. Gonadotrope or thyrotrope adenomas may be excluded in the premenopausal hyperprolactinemic patient by measuring basal levels of LH, follicle-stimulating hormone (FSH), and TSH respectively. Growth hormone-producing adenomas may be excluded by measuring the serum level of insulin-like growth factor 1 (IGF-1; formerly called somatomedin C).[20] If this value is normal, a growth hormone-producing adenoma may be excluded. If the value is elevated, oral administration of 75-100 gm of glucose may be given. Failure to suppress growth hormone levels to less than 2 mg/L 60 minutes after glucose is ingested is suggestive of the presence of a growth hormone adenoma.[18]

Adrenocorticotropic hormone (ACTH)-producing adenomas are unlikely to be present if cortisol secretion is normal. This is verified by demonstrating that the free cortisol in a 24-hour urine collection is not elevated.[28] Alternatively, if a sensitive and accurate assay is available, the ACTH concentration may be measured to detect an elevation in hormone concentration.

Use of so-called challenge tests of the pituitary, with GnRH, TRH, L-dopa, and insulin, does not distinguish between a hypothalamic or pituitary disorder responsible for the pituitary lesion and these tests are not routinely used.[155] These tests may be of use in assessing pituitary hormone reserve prior to and following medical or surgical therapy as part of a clinical research protocol.

PROLACTIN AND BONE DENSITY

Osteopenia has been noted in women with hyperprolactinemia and secondary amenorrhea.[68,125] Diminished bone density in these women may result from the hypoestrogenism commonly found in amenorrheic, hyperprolactinemic women, rather than as a direct result of prolactin on bone turnover. Progressive bone loss in untreated hyperprolactinemic women has been noted after 2 years of follow-up,[9] but not after 5 years.[127] Increased radial bone density in hyperprolactinemic women has been observed following implementation of oral dopaminergic therapy with bromocriptine,[69] but not to values comparable with normal controls.

Exogenous estrogen therapy is effective in preventing postmenopausal bone loss in endocrinologically normal women.[79] Administration of estrogens to amenorrheic, hyperprolactinemic women who cannot tolerate dopamine-agonist therapy has not been routinely advocated due to the concern that pituitary adenoma growth is stimulated. In a recent study of 38 women with hyperprolactinemia and amenorrhea, no adverse changes in CT-scan measurements of the pituitary gland were reported when these women were given estrogen hormone replacement or oral-contraceptive pills.[26] Until additional corroborative data is available, caution must be advised before providing estrogen therapy to hyperprolactinemic patients.

MANAGEMENT

Existence of a pituitary lesion, desire to conceive, extent of bone loss, and pregnancy are factors affecting the management of the hyperprolactinemic patient. It is useful to categorize therapy plans based on these factors as is done below, categorizing patients into groups according to the presence or absence of radiographically detectable pituitary lesions, and the patient's desire for childbearing.

Hyperprolactinemia without a pituitary lesion: pregnancy not currently desired

Patients with elevated prolactin levels who do not have evidence of a pituitary lesion on baseline evaluation are at minimal risk for future development of an adenoma. These patients are likely to demonstrate no change or even a decline in prolactin concentrations when followed over time without treatment.[87,139] Yearly prolactin measurement is appropriate for these patients, as are periodic bone-density measurements for patients who are also amenorrheic. Repeated CT or MRI imaging of the sella turcica is unlikely to reveal evidence of rapid growth of a pituitary lesion. Consequently, repeated radiographic imaging over short intervals of time is rarely indicated.

Indications for therapy include declining bone density, desire to conceive, or desire to resume cyclic menstruation. Standard therapy involves administration of the long-acting dopamine agonist, bromocriptine (see below). It has been reported that long-term therapy (5-6 years) with this drug does not result in cumulative problems.[24] Long-term cardiovascular effects of hypoestrogenism secondary to hyperprolactinemia must also be considered if prolactin-lowering drugs are not given. Use of hormone replacement may be considered in view of results from recent studies indicating a lack of effect in increasing prolactin levels in hyperprolactinemic patients receiving such therapy.[26] Future studies may prove that hormone-replacement therapy does not increase serum prolactin in these patients, and therefore may be safe and efficacious in preventing bone loss.

Hyperprolactinemia without a pituitary abnormality: pregnancy desired

Bromocriptine mesylate was approved for clinical use for the treatment of female infertility in 1978.[154] It is an ergot alkaloid-derived, dopamine-receptor agonist. Following oral administration, peak plasma levels are obtained within 1-3 hours. A suppressive effect on prolactin levels may be observed for 14 hours.[107,154] Side effects are numerous and common, and include orthostatic hypotension, nausea, nasal stuffiness, and fatigue. No evidence

exists to demonstrate an increased teratogenic risk to fetuses conceived while maternal bromocriptine is being taken.[34] Increased spontaneous abortion rates or multiple pregnancy rates have not been observed.[150] Other ergot alkaloid dopamine agonists that have been developed include pergolide,[40] metergoline,[11] cabergoline,[39] and terguride.[19] Comparable responses to therapy have been reported with all ergot-derived dopamine agonists,[30] but only bromocriptine has received FDA approval for infertility treatment. Pergolide may be prescribed in the United States for treatment of Parkinson's disease, and it has also been used successfully to treat hyperprolactinemia in Europe.[72]

The lowest dose of bromocriptine should be prescribed initially, with dosage titrated to response.[141] To reduce the severity of adverse reactions, the medication should be taken with food and begun at bedtime with half of a 2.5 mg tablet. After several days, the dose may be increased to a 2.5 mg tablet at bedtime, if indicated by follow-up prolactin levels. Additional 2.5 mg tablets can be taken in the morning and afternoon if required to normalize the prolactin level. Following each dosage escalation, a serum prolactin level should be measured. Prolactin levels are normalized in 90% of patients receiving medication, and ovulation results in most cases.

For some patients, side effects from drug use may be severe enough to discontinue treatment. Vaginal administration of bromocriptine has been reported to be effective for some of these individuals,[61,66] with lack of a first-pass hepatic effect thought to be responsible for the diminished side effects.

Many of the bothersome side effects from bromocriptine administration result from the stimulation of both D_1 and D_2 dopamine receptors by this drug. For example, nasal stuffiness and nausea are side effects that may result from D_1 dopamine-receptor stimulation. Another nonergot-derived dopamine agonist has been developed that is a potent D_2 dopamine-receptor agonist with weak D_1-receptor activity. It is an octahydrobenzol[g]quinoline, currently known as CV 205-502, that has a prolonged suppressive effect on serum prolactin and comparatively few side effects.[156] Unfortunately, CV 205-502 is available only for clinical research studies at the present time in the United States.

Hyperprolactinemic patients who are unable to tolerate dopamine agonists, but who desire to conceive, may be given other ovulation-inducing drugs. Clomiphene citrate given alone is unlikely to induce ovulation in hyperprolactinemic patients, but when given with human chorionic gonadotropin (hCG), a 90% ovulation rate has been reported.[110] Menotropin therapy may also be used successfully to induce ovulation in hyperprolactinemic patients.[38]

After instituting treatment with bromocriptine, resumption of ovulation followed by menses usually occurs within 8 weeks. Contraception is advised until the first menses is observed in order to minimize the prolonged use of bromocriptine during pregnancy. Bromocriptine therapy should be stopped once pregnancy is diagnosed. Reassuringly and somewhat surprisingly, neither the low prolactin concentrations induced by bromocriptine,[166] nor the rebound in prolactin following cessation of bromocriptine postconception,[10] results in pregnancy loss as might be expected by possible alteration in corpus-luteum function due to elevated prolactin levels.

Pregnancy appears to proceed uneventfully in hyperprolactinemic women treated with bromocriptine in order to conceive,[111] and breastfeeding for these patients postpartum is not contraindicated.[67] Monitoring the serum prolactin level during pregnancy is not informative because prolactin concentrations are normally elevated during pregnancy and fluctuate widely.[165] Adverse remote consequences to the patient's pituitary function as a result of a bromocriptine-induced pregnancy have not been reported, and a reduction in prolactin levels with return of menstruation has been reported in some hyperprolactinemic women postpartum.[112] A decline in postpartum prolactin levels has also been reported for euprolactinemic individuals postpartum.[98]

Hyperprolactinemia with a pituitary lesion: pregnancy not currently desired

For hyperprolactinemic patients with a microadenoma of the pituitary gland that has been identified radiographically, current data reveal that adenoma size remains unchanged over time for most untreated women.[86,126,137,161] A change in the prolactin concentration may not be correlated with changes in tumor growth[86] and many patients may experience a spontaneous decline in prolactin levels with resumption of menses[137] when no treatment is provided. If the patient is amenorrheic and does not desire treatment, the risks of osteoporosis and possible cardiovascular disease should be explained. Individuals who ovulate, menstruate, and have an identifiable pituitary lesion may also be followed expectantly. In a recent report summarizing findings in an autopsy series involving 486 subjects, undiagnosed pituitary adenomas were identified in 78 glands. Over half of these women had a case history available for review that demonstrated previous fertility.[2] Thus, the mere existence of a pituitary lesion seen on MRI or CT scan may not warrant a recommendation for medical or surgical therapy to protect future health or fertility.

When treatment is required, medical or surgical therapy may be offered. Since these modalities are quite successful, radiation treatment is no longer recommended because remote hypopituitarism is a significant side effect,[58] and a return to the euprolactinemic state following such therapy is lengthy.[49,58]

Surgical therapy for microadenomas, consisting of partial transsphenoidal hypophysectomy, is also declining in frequency due to the risk of complications[75] and a 16–17% chance of postoperative return of hyperprolactinemia.[116,128]

A persistent beneficial effect of surgery would be expected if the etiologic factor for pituitary microadenoma formation existed within the pituitary gland. Resumption of hyperprolactinemia would be predicted if a suprasellar cause for the hyperprolactinemic state were responsible. Unfortunately, data are not yet available on the risk of microadenoma recurrence following partial transsphenoidal hypophysectomy.

Medical therapy with bromocriptine for hyperprolactinemic patients with a pituitary adenoma remains the treatment of choice.[22,88] Administered as previously described, bromocriptine in dosages up to 2.5 mg tid results in normalization of prolactin levels, shrinkage of the microadenoma,[12] and resumption of ovulation in most subjects.[154] Cessation of bromocriptine therapy after short-term use usually results in a return to the hyperprolactinemic state with regrowth of the prolactinoma.[148] However, long-term administration of bromocriptine (one year or more) has been reported to result in prolactin concentrations lower than observed prior to treatment, with persistent pituitary adenoma size reduction for up to 1 year following withdrawal of bromocriptine treatment.[59,95,113,157] A reduction of lactotrope-cell volume, rather than necrosis, has been noted in pituitary adenomas in one study after 4 to 6 weeks of bromocriptine therapy.[149] In another study, prolonged therapy for over 8 months resulted in actual adenoma cell necrosis.[47] Institution of a protocol for dopamine-agonist therapy that progressively increases the amount of medication needed to suppress prolactin levels so that a minimum dose is used has been recommended.[80] Cessation of dopamine-agonist therapy after long-term use with close followup has also been suggested as a possible treatment protocol.[37] Macroprolactinomas also have been successfully treated using the new dopamine agonist, CV 205-502[129,158] (currently available only for investigational use), which has also been used to treat prolactinomas resistant to bromocriptine.[15] Recommendations as discussed for microadenomas may also apply to the well-informed patient with a macroadenoma. Joint management of patients with macroadenomas by neuroophthalmologists and neurosurgeons is frequently helpful.

Hyperprolactinemia with a pituitary lesion: pregnancy desired

Hyperprolactinemic women with either a micro- or macroadenoma of the pituitary gland who desire to conceive have been able to do so following prolactin suppression with bromocriptine or surgery. In the past, many patients with microadenomas were treated surgically prior to attempting pregnancy, but more recently bromocriptine treatment has proved successful[23,34,46,50,56,83] as pregnancy has proceeded uneventfully in most instances. Cesarean sections, when done, are performed for obstetrical indications and breastfeeding is allowed. Headaches and visual-field defects occur in some patients, but spontaneous resolution of the field defects postpartum is usually observed.[73] On rare occasions, a significant hemorrhage within the pituitary occurs.[41] Most patients may be followed expectantly during pregnancy with visual-field testing at each trimester. Should symptomatic adenoma enlargement occur, bromocriptine therapy may be instituted.

Management recommendations for patients who have pituitary macroadenomas and who desire to conceive have consisted of three approaches. First, prophylactic partial transsphenoidal hypophysectomy prior to attempting to conceive has been advised. If surgery is performed, a risk remains for massive pituitary expansion in pregnancy as a recent case report illustrates.[7] Second, continuous bromocriptine throughout pregnancy, once pregnancy has been diagnosed, has been recommended,[70] but data exist from only a small series of patients and the remote consequences of prolonged bromocriptine therapy on fetal growth and future mental development of the child remains to be determined. Third, cessation of bromocriptine use, which is the protocol for patients with microadenomas, may be followed for patients with macroadenomas. Although concern remains that rapid and substantial growth of the macroadenoma may occur during pregnancy following cessation of bromocriptine use, early reports have indicated few adverse effects when treatment was stopped during eight pregnancies in four women with pituitary macroadenomas who also had suprasellar extension.[3]

If pregnancy is not desired and the size of the macroadenoma remains stable, indications for treatment include diminished libido, unmanageable galactorrhea, and osteoporosis. Adverse consequences of the hypoestrogenic state on cardiovascular disease should be discussed, and benefits of hormone replacement should be mentioned.[99] In untreated hyperprolactinemic hypogonadal men, elevated serum lipids have been reported.[105] If these untoward effects on lipids are confirmed in women, treatment may be recommended in the future.

SUMMARY

Changes in serum prolactin levels occurring as a consequence of normal, as well as pathophysiologic, events have been discussed. A plan for the evaluation of the symptomatic or infertile hyperprolactinemic patient has been presented. Options for therapy influenced by the desire to conceive have been reviewed. With the passage of time, a greater understanding of prolactin physiology and pathology has been achieved allowing physicians to be of greater help in diagnosing and treating patients with hyperprolactinemia.

REFERENCES

1. Aakvaag A, Sand T, Opstad PK et al: Hormonal changes in serum in young men during prolonged physical strain, *Eur J Appl Physiol* 39:283, 1978.
2. Abd El-Hamid MW, Joplin GF, Lewis PD: Incidentally found small pituitary adenomas may have no effect on fertility, *Acta Endocrinol* 117:361, 1988.
3. Ahmed M, Al-Dossary E, Woodhouse NJY: Macroprolactinomas with suprasellar extension: effect of bromocriptine withdrawal during one or more pregnancies, *Fertil Steril* 58:492, 1992.
4. Alger M, Vazquez-Matute L, Mason M et al: Polycystic ovarian disease associated with hyperprolactinemia and defective metaclopromide response, *Fertil Steril* 34:70, 1980.
5. Armeanu ML, Frolich M, Lequin RM: Circadian rhythm of prolactin during the menstrual cycle, *Fertil Steril* 46:315, 1986.
6. Asa SL, Penz G, Kovacs K et al: Prolactin cells in the human pituitary: a quantitative immunocytochemical analysis, *Arch Pathol Lab Med* 106:360, 1982.
7. Belchetz PE, Carty A, Clearkin LG et al: Failure of prophylactic surgery to avert massive pituitary expansion in pregnancy, *Clin Endocrinol* 25:325, 1986.
8. Ben-Jonathan N, Oliver C, Weiner HJ et al: Dopamine in hypophysial portal plasma of the rat during the estrous cycle and throughout pregnancy, *Endocrinology* 100:452, 1977.
9. Biller BMK, Baum HB, Rosenthal DI et al: Progressive trabecular osteopenia in women with hyperprolactinemic amenorrhea. *J Clin Endocrinol Metab* 75:692, 1992.
10. Bennink HJ: Intermittent bromocriptine treatment for the induction of ovulation in hyperprolactinemic patients, *Fertil Steril* 31:267, 1979.
11. Bohnet HG, Kato K, Wolf AS: Treatment of hyperprolactinemic amenorrhea with metergoline, *Obstet Gynecol* 67:249, 1986.
12. Bonneville JF, Poulignot D, Cattin F et al: Computed tomographic demonstration of the effects of bromocriptine on pituitary microadenoma size, *Radiology* 143:451, 1982.
13. Brenner SH, Lessing JB, Quagliarello J et al: Hyperprolactinemia and associated pituitary prolactinomas, *Obstet Gynecol* 65:661, 1985.
14. Brown SB, Irwin KM, Enzman DR: CT characteristics of the normal pituitary gland, *Neuroradiology* 24:259, 1983.
15. Brue T, Pellegrini I, Gunz G et al: Effects of the dopamine agonist CV 205-502 in human prolactinomas resistant to bromocriptine, *J Clin Endocrinol Metab* 74:577, 1992.
16. Carlson HE, Wasser HL, Levin SR et al: Prolactin stimulation by meals is related to protein content, *J Clin Endocrinol Metab* 57:334, 1983.
17. Chambers EF, Turksi PA, LaMasters D et al: Regions of low density in the contrast-enhanced pituitary gland: normal and pathologic processes, *Radiology* 144:109, 1982.
18. Chang-DeMoranville BM: Diagnosis and endocrine testing in acromegaly, *Endocrinol Metab Clin North Am* 21:649, 1992.
19. Ciccarelli E, Touzel R, Besser M et al: Terguride—a new dopamine agonist drug: a comparison of its neuroendocrine and side effect profile with bromocriptine, *Fertil Steril* 49:589, 1988.
20. Clemmons DR, Van Wyk JJ, Ridgeway EC et al: Evaluation of acromegaly by radioimmunoassay of somatomedin-C, *N Engl J Med* 301:1138, 1979.
21. Collu R, Jequiever JC, Leboeuf G et al: Endocrine effects of pimozide, specific dopaminergic blocker, *J Clin Endocrinol Metab* 41:981, 1975.
22. Corenblum B: Successful outcome of ergocryptine-induced pregnancies in twenty-one women with prolactin-secreting pituitary adenomas, *Fertil Steril* 32:183, 1979.
23. Corenblum B, Hanley DA: Bromocriptine reduction of prolactinoma size, *Fertil Steril* 36:716, 1981.
24. Corenblum B, Taylor PJ: Long-term follow-up of hyperprolactinemic women treated with bromocriptine, *Fertil Steril* 40:596, 1983.
25. Corenblum B, Shaffer EA: Hyperprolactinemia in hepatic encephalopathy may result from impaired central dopaminergic transmission, *Hum Metab Res* 21:675, 1989.
26. Corenblum B, Donovan L: The safety of physiological estrogen plus progestin replacement therapy and with oral contraceptive therapy in women with pathological hyperprolactinemia, *Fertil Steril* 59:671, 1993.

27. Cramer OM, Parker CR, Porter JC: Estrogen inhibition of dopamine release into hypophysial portal blood, *Endocrinology* 104:419, 1979.

28. Crapo L: Cushing's syndrome: a review of diagnostic tests, *Metabolism* 28:955, 1979.

29. Creese I, Sibley DR, Leff SE: Agonist interactions with dopamine receptors: focus on radioligand-binding studies, *Fed Proc* 43:2779, 1984.

30. Crosignani PG, Ferrari C, Liuzzi A et al: Treatment of hyperprolactinemic states with different drugs: a study with bromocriptine, metergoline, and lisuride, *Fertil Steril* 37:61, 1982.

31. D'Armiento M, Bisignani G, Reda G: Effect of bromazepam on growth hormone and prolactin secretion in normal subjects, *Horm Res* 15:224, 1981.

32. DeMarinis L, Mancini A, Calabro F et al: Plasma prolactin response to gonadotropin-releasing hormone during benzodiazepine treatment, *Psychoneuroendocrinology* 13:325, 1988.

33. DiMattia GE, Gellerson B, Duckworth ML et al: Human prolactin gene expression: the use of alternative non-coding exon in decidual and the IM-9-P₃ lymphoblast cell line, *J Biol Chem* 25616412-21 265:16412, 1990.

34. Divers WA, Yen SSC: Prolactin-producing microadenomas in pregnancy, *Obstet Gynecol* 62:425, 1983.

35. Everett JW: Luteotropic function of autografts of the rat hypophysis, *Endocrinology* 54:685, 1954.

36. Everett JW: Functional corpora lutea maintained for months by autografts of rat hypophysis, *Endocrinology* 58:786, 1956.

37. Faglia G: Should dopamine agonist treatment for prolactinomas be life-long? (Commentary), *Clin Endocrinol* 34:173, 1991.

38. Farine D, Dor J, Lupovici N et al: Conception rate after gonadotropin therapy in hyperprolactinemia and normoprolactinemia, *Obstet Gynecol* 65:658, 1985.

39. Ferrari C, Barbieri C, Caldara R et al: Long-lasting prolactin-lowering effect of cabergoline, a new dopamine agonist, in hyperprolactinemic patients, *J Clin Endocrinol Metab* 63:941, 1986.

40. Franks S, Horrocks PM, Lynch SS et al: Treatment of hyperprolactinemia with pergolide mesylate: acute effects and preliminary evaluation of long-term treatment, *Lancet* 2:659, 1981.

41. Freeman R, Wezenter B, Silverstein M et al: Pregnancy-associated subacute hemorrhage into a prolactinoma resulting in diabetes insipidus, *Fertil Steril* 58:427, 1992.

42. Fuxe Y, Hokflet T, Nilsson O: Factors involved in the control of the activity of the tuberoinfundibular neurons during pregnancy and lactation, *Neuroendocrinology* 5:257, 1969.

43. Gaines Das RE, Lotes MP: International reference preparation of human prolactin for immunoassay: definition of the international unit. Report of a collaborative study and comparison of estimates of human prolactin made in various laboratories, *J Endocrinol* 80:157, 1979.

44. Gala RR: Prolactin and growth hormone in the regulation of the immune system, *Proc Soc Exp Biol Med* 198:513, 1991.

45. Gala RR, Singhakowinta A, Brennan MJ: Studies on prolactin in human serum, urine and milk, *Horm Res* 6:310, 1975.

46. Gemzell C, Wang CF: Outcome of pregnancy in women with pituitary adenoma, *Fertil Steril* 31: 363, 1979.

47. Gen M, Uozumi T, Ohta M et al: Necrotic changes in prolactinomas after long-term administration of bromocriptine, *J Clin Endocrinol Metab* 59:463, 1984.

48. Gray RH, Campbell OM, Apelo R et al: Risk of ovulation during lactation, *Lancet* 353:25, 1990.

49. Grossman A, Cohen BL, Charlesworth M et al: Treatment of prolactinomas with megavoltage radiotherapy, *Br Med J* 288:1105, 1984.

50. Hammond CB, Haney AF, Land MR et al: The outcome of pregnancy in patients with treated and untreated prolactin-secreting pituitary tumors, *Am J Obstet Gynecol* 147:148, 1983.

51. Hökflet T, Fuxe K: Effects of prolactin and ergot alkaloids on the tubero-infundibular dopamine (DA) neurons, *Neuroendocrinology* 9:100, 1972.

52. Hwang P, Guyda H, Friesen H: A radioimmunoassay for human prolactin, *Proc Natl Acad Sci USA* 68:1902, 1971.

53. Ishizuka B, Quigley ME, Yen SCC: Pituitary hormone release in response to food ingestion: evidence for neuro-endocrine signals from gut to brain, *JCEM* 57:1111, 1983.

54. Jackson JC, Wortsman J, Malarkey WB: Characterization of a large molecular weight prolactin in women with idiopathic hyperprolactinemia and normal menses, *J Clin Endocrinol Metab* 61:258, 1985.

55. Jacobs LS, Snyder PJ, Wilbur JF et al: Increased serum prolactin after administration of synthetic thyrotropin-releasing hormone (TRH) in man, *JCEM* 33:996, 1977.

56. Jewelewicz R, Vande Wiele RL: Clinical course and outcome of pregnancy in twenty-five patients with pituitary microadenomas, *Am J Obstet Gynecol* 136:339, 1980.

57. Jimerson DC, Post RM, Skyler J et al: Prolactin in cerebral spinal fluid and dopamine function in man, *J Pharm Pharmacol* 28:845, 1976.

58. Johnston DG, Hall K, Kendall-Taylor P et al: The long-term effects of megavoltage radiotherapy as sole or combined therapy for large prolactinomas: studies with high-definition computerized tomography, *Clin Endocrinol* 24:675, 1986.

59. Johnston DG, Prescott RWG, Kendall-Taylor P et al: Hyperprolactinemia—long-term effects of bromocriptine, *Am J Med* 75:868, 1983.

60. Kable WT: Drug-induced primary hypothyroidism and hyperprolactinemia, *Fertil Steril* 35:483, 1981.

61. Katz E, Schran H, Adashi EY: Successful treatment of a prolactin-producing pituitary adenoma with intravaginal bromocriptine mesylate: a novel approach to intolerance to oral therapy, *Obstet Gynecol* 73:517, 1989.

62. Keye WR, HoYuen B, Knopf RF et al: Amenorrhea, hyperprolactinemia and pituitary enlargement secondary to primary hypothyroidism: successful treatment with thyroid replacement, *Obstet Gynecol* 48:697, 1976.

63. Kleinberg DL, Frantz AG: Human prolactin: measurement in plasma by in vitro bioassay, *J Clin Invest* 50:1557, 1970.

64. Kleinberg DL, Noll GL, Frantz AG: Chlorpromazine stimulation and L-dopa suppression of plasma prolactin in man, *J Clin Endocrinol Metab* 33:873, 1971.

65. Kleinberg DL, Noel GL, Franz AL: Galactorrhea: a study of 235 cases, including 48 with pituitary tumors, *N Engl J Med* 296:589, 1977.

66. Kletzky OA, Vermesh M: Effectiveness of vaginal bromocriptine in treating women with hyperprolactinemia, *Fertil Steril* 51:269, 1989.

67. Kletzky OA, Marrs RP, Davajan V: Management of patients with hyperprolactinemia and normal or abnormal tomograms, *Am J Obstet Gynecol* 147:528, 1983.

68. Klibanski A, Neer R, Beitins IZ et al: Decreased bone density in hyperprolactinemic women, *N Engl J Med* 303:1511, 1980.

69. Klibanski A, Greenspan SL: Increase in bone mass after treatment of hyperprolactinemic amenorrhea, *N Engl J Med* 315:542, 1986.

70. Konopka P, Raymond JP, Merceron RE et al: Continuous administration of bromocriptine in the prevention of neurological complications in pregnant women with prolactinomas, *Am J Obstet Gynecol* 146:935, 1983.

71. Kovacs K: Pathology of pituitary tumors, *Endocrinol Metab Clin North Am* 16:529, 1987.

72. Lamberts SWJ, Quik RFP: A comparison of the efficacy and safety of pergolide and bromocriptine in the treatment of hyperprolactinemia, *J Clin Endocrinol Metab* 72:635, 1991.

73. Lamberts SWJ, Seldenrath HJ, Kwa HG et al: Transient bitemporal hemianopsia during pregnancy after treatment of galactorrhea-amenorrhea syndrome with bromocriptine, *J Clin Endocrinol Metab* 44:180, 1977.

74. Langer G, Sachan EJ, Gruen PH et al: Human prolactin responses to neuroleptic drugs correlate with antischizophrenic potency, *Nature* 266:639, 1977.

75. Laws ER: Pituitary surgery, *Endocrinol Metab Clin North Am* 16:647, 1987.

76. Leblanc H, Lachelin GCL, Abu-Fadil S et al: Effects of dopamine infusion on pituitary hormone secretion in humans, *J Clin Endocrinol Metab* 43:668, 1976.

77. LeDafniet M, Brand AM, Bression D et al: Evidence of receptors for thyrotropin-releasing hormone in human prolactin-secreting adenomas, *JCEM* 57:425, 1983.

78. Lim VS, Kathpalia S, Frohman LA: Hyperprolactinemia and impaired pituitary response to suppression and stimulation in chronic renal failure: reversal after transplantation, *JCEM* 48:101, 1979.

79. Lindsay R, Hart DM: The minimum effective dose of estrogen for prevention of postmenopausal bone loss, *Obstet Gynecol* 63:759, 1984.

80. Luizzi A, Dallabonzana D, Oppizzi G et al: Low doses of dopamine agonists in the long-term treatment of macroprolactinomas, *N Eng J Med* 313:656, 1985.

81. Lyque EH, Munoz de Toro M, Smith PI et al: Subpopulations of lactotropes detected with the reverse hemolytic plaque assay show differential responsiveness to dopamine, *Endocrinology* 118:2120, 1986.

82. MacLeod RM, Fontham EH, Lehmeyer JE: Prolactin and growth hormone production as influenced by catecholamines and agents that affect brain catecholamines, *Neuroendocrinology* 6:283, 1970.

83. Magyar DM, Marshall JR: Pituitary tumors and pregnancy, *Am J Obstet Gynecol* 132:739, 1978.

84. Mais V, Yen SSC: Prolactin-releasing action of gonadotropin-releasing hormone in hypogonadal women, *J Clin Endocrinol Metab* 62:1089, 1986.

85. Malarkey WB, Hall JC, Pearl DK et al: The influence of academic stress and season on 24-hour concentration of growth hormone and prolactin, *J Clin Endocrinol Metab* 73:1089, 1991.

86. March CM, Kletzky OA, Davajan V et al: Longitudinal evaluation of patients with untreated prolactin-secreting pituitary adenomas, *Am J Obstet Gynecol* 139:835, 1981.

87. Martin T, Kim M, Malarkey W: The natural history of idiopathic hyperprolactinemia, *J Clin Endocrinol Metab* 60:855, 1985.

88. McGregor AM, Scanlon MF, Hall K et al: Reduction in size of a pituitary tumor by bromocriptine therapy, *N Engl J Med* 300:291, 1979.

89. McNatty KP, Sawers RS, McNeilly AS: A possible role for prolactin in control of steroid secretion by the human Graafian follicle, *Nature* 250:653, 1974.

90. Meltzer HY, Fang VS, Tricou BJ et al: Effect of antidepressants on neuroendocrine actions in humans. In Costa E, Racagri G, editors: *Typical and atypical antidepressants: clinical practice,* New York, 1982, Raven.

91. Molitch ME, Schwartz S, Mukherji B: Is prolactin secreted ectopically? *Am J Med* 70:803, 1981.

92. Molitch ME, Russell EJ: The pituitary incidentaloma, *Ann Intern Med* 112:925, 1990.

93. Morgan MY, Jakobovits AW, Gore MB et al: Serum prolactin in liver disease and its relationship to gynecomastia, *Gut* 19:170, 1978.

94. Mori M, Kobayachi I, Shimoyama S et al: Effect of sulpiride on serum growth hormone and prolactin concentrations following L-dopa administration in man, *Endocrinol Jpn* 24:149, 1977.

95. Moriondo P, Travaglini P, Nissim M et al: Bromocriptine treatment of microprolactinomas: evidence of stable prolactin decrease after drug withdrawal, *J Clin Endocrinol Metab* 60:764, 1985.

96. Morley JE, Dawson M, Hodgkinson H et al: Galactorrhea and hyperprolactinemia associated with chest wall injury, *J Clin Endocrinol Metab* 45:931, 1977.

97. Murdoch AP, Dunlop W, Kendall-Taylor P: Studies of prolactin secretion in polycystic ovarian syndrome, *Clin Endocrinol* 24:165, 1986.

98. Musey VC, Collins DC, Musey PI et al: Long-term effect of a first pregnancy on the secretion of prolactin, *N Engl J Med* 316:229, 1987.

99. Nabulsi AA, Folsom AR, White A et al: Association of hormone replacement therapy with various cardiovascular risk factors in postmenopausal women, *N Engl J Med* 328:1069, 1993.

100. Nicoll CS, Mayer GL, Russel SM: Structural features of prolactins and growth hormones that can be related to their biological properties, *Endocr Rev* 7:169, 1986.

101. Nikolics K, Mason AJ, Szonyi E et al: A prolactin-inhibiting factor within the precursor for human gonadotropin-releasing hormone, *Nature* 316:511, 1985.

102. Noel GL, Suh HK, Stone JG et al: Human prolactin and growth-hormone release during surgery and other conditions of stress, *J Clin Endocrinol Metab* 35:840, 1972.

103. Nold GC, Suh HK, Franz AG: Prolactin release during nursing and breast stimulation in postpartum and non-postpartum subjects, *J Clin Endocrinol Metab* 38:413, 1974.

104. Nyberg F, Roos P, Wide L: Human pituitary prolactin: isolation and characterization of three isohormones with different bioassay and radioimmunoassay activities, *Biochem Biophys Acta* 625:255, 1980.

105. Oppenheim DS, Greenspan SL, Zervas NT et al: Elevated serum lipids in hypogonadal men with and without hyperprolactinemia, *Am Int Med* 111:288, 1989.

106. Owerbach D, Rutter WJ, Cooke NE et al: The prolactin gene is located on chromosome 6 in humans, *Science* 212:815, 1981.

107. Parkes D: Bromocriptine, *N Engl J Med* 301:873, 1979.

108. Perez-Lopez FR, Roncero MC: Induced prolactin release in women under long-term medroxyprogesterone acetate treatment, *Obstet Gynecol* 45:267, 1975.

109. Quigley ME, Ropert JF, Yen SSC: Acute prolactin release triggered by feeding, *J Clin Endocrinol Metab* 52:1043, 1981.

110. Radwanska E, McGarrigle HH, Little V et al: Induction of ovulation in women with hyperprolactinemic amenorrhea using clomiphene and human chorionic gonadotropin or bromocriptine, *Fertil Steril* 32:187, 1979.

111. Randall S, Laing I, Chapman AJ et al: Pregnancies in women with hyperprolactinemia: obstetric and endocrinological management of 50 pregnancies in 37 women, *Br J Obstet Gynaecol* 89:20, 1982.

112. Rasmussen C, Bergh T, Nillus SJ et al: Return of menstruation and normalization of prolactin in hyperprolactinemic women with bromocriptine-induced pregnancy, *Fertil Steril* 44:31, 1985.

113. Rasmussen C, Bergh T, Wide L: Prolactin secretion and menstrual function after long-term bromocriptine treatment, *Fertil Steril* 48:550, 1987.

114. Riddick DH, Luciano AA, Kusmik WF et al: De novo synthesis of prolactin by human decidua, *Life Sci* 23:1213, 1978.

115. Riddle O, Bates RW, Dykshorn S: The preparation, identification and assay of prolactin—a hormone of the anterior pituitary, *Am J Physiol* 105:191, 1933.

116. Rodman EF, Molitch ME, Post KD et al: Long-term follow-up of transsphenoidal selective adenomectomy for prolactinoma, *JAMA* 252:921, 1984.

117. Rogoe AD, Rosen SW: Prolactin of apparent large molecular size: the major immunoreactive prolactin component in plasma of a patient with pituitary tumor, *J Clin Endocrinol Metab* 38:714, 1974.

118. Ropert JF, Quigley ME, Yen SSC: Endogenous opiates modulate pulsatile luteinizing-hormone release in humans, *J Clin Endocrinol Metab* 52:583: 1981.

119. Ruberg M, Rotsztein WH, Arancibia S et al: Stimulation of prolactin release by vasoactive intestinal peptide (VIP), *Eur J Pharmacol* 51:319, 1978.

120. Ruiz-Velasco V: Hyperprolactinemia and mammary prostheses: a report of eight cases, *J Reprod Med* 31:267, 1986.

121. Samson WK, Skala KD, Alexander B et al: Possible neuroendocrine actions of endothelin-3, *Endocrinology* 128:1465, 1991.

122. Sassin JF, Frantz AG, Weitzman ED et al: Human prolactin: 24-hour pattern with increased release during sleep, *Science* 77:1205, 1972.

123. Schallengerger E, Richardson DW, Knobil E: Role of prolactin in the lactational amenorrhea of the rhesus monkey (Macaca Mulatta), *Biol Reprod* 25:370, 1981.

124. Schally AV, Redding TW, Arimua A et al: Isolation of gamma-amino butyric acid from pig hypothalami and demonstration of its prolactin release-inhibiting (PIF) activity in vivo and in vitro, *Endocrinology* 100:681, 1977.

125. Schlechte JA, Sherman B, Martin R: Bone density in amenorrheic women with and without hyperprolactinemia, *J Clin Endocrinol Metab* 56:1120, 1983.

126. Schlechte J, Dolan K, Sherman B et al: The natural history of untreated hyperprolactinemia: a prospective analysis, *J Clin Endocrinol Metab* 68:412, 1989.

127. Schlechte J, Walkner L, Kathol M: A longitudinal analysis of premenopausal bone loss in healthy women and women with hyperprolactinemia, *J Clin Endocrinol Metab* 75:698, 1992.

128. Serri O, Rasio E, Beauregard H et al: Recurrence of hyperprolactinemia after selective transsphenoidal adenomectomy in women with prolactinoma, *N Engl J Med* 309:280, 1983.

129. Serri O, Beauregard H, Lesage J et al: Long-term treatment with CV 205-502 in patients with prolactin-secreting pituitary macroadenomas, *J Clin Endocrinol Metab* 71:682, 1990.

130. Sheth AR, Mugatwala PP, Shah G et al: Occurrence of human prolactin in semen, *Fertil Steril* 26:905, 1975.

131. Sheth AR, Vaidya RA, Raiker RS: Presence of prolactin in human cervical mucus, *Fertil Steril* 27:397, 1976.

132. Shiu RPG, Kelly PA, Friesen HG: Radioreceptor assay for prolactin and other lactogenic hormones, *Science* 180:968, 1973.

133. Shull JD, Gorski J: Estrogen regulates the transcription of the rat prolactin gene through the least two independent mechanisms, *Endocrinology* 116:2456, 1985.

134. Sibley DR, Monsma FJ: Molecular biology of dopamine receptors, *Trends Pharmacol Sci* 13:61, 1992.

135. Sievertsen GD, Lim VS, Makawatase C et al: Metabolic clearance and secretion rates of human prolactin in normal subjects and inpatients with chronic renal failure, *J Clin Endocrinol Metab* 50:846, 1980.

136. Sinha Y, Selby FW, Vander Laan WP: Radioimmunoassay of prolactin in the urine of mouse and man, *J Clin Endocrinol Metab* 36:1039, 1973.

137. Sisam DA, Sheenhan JP, Sheeler LR: The natural history of untreated microprolactinomas, *Fertil Steril* 48:67, 1987.

138. Slater SL, Lipper S, Shiling DJ et al: Elevation of plasma-prolactin by monoamine oxidase inhibitors, *Lancet* 2:275, 1977.

139. Sluijmer AV, Lappöhn RE: Clinical history and outcome of 59 patients with idiopathic hyperprolactinemia, *Fertil Steril* 58:72, 1992.

140. Snyder PJ: Gonadotroph cell pituitary adenoma, *Endocrinol Metab Clin North Am* 16:755, 1987.

141. Soto-Albors CE, Randolph JF, Ying YK et al: Medical management of hyperprolactinemia: a lower dose of bromocriptine may be effective, *Fertil Steril* 48:213, 1987.

142. Sowers JR, McCallum RW, Hershman JM et al: Comparison of metoclopramide with other dynamic tests of prolactin secretion, *J Clin Endocrinol Metab* 43:679, 1976.

143. Spaulding SW, Burron GW, Bermudez F et al: The inhibitory effect of lithium on thyroid hormone release in both euthyroid and thyrotoxic patients, *J Clin Endocrinol Metab* 35:905, 1972.

144. Spellacy WN, Buhi WC, Burk SA: Stimulated plasma prolactin levels in women using medroxyprogesterone acetate or an intrauterine device for contraception, *Fertil Steril* 26:970, 1975.

145. Strebel PM, Zacur HA, Gold EM: Headache hyperprolactinemia and prolactinomas, *Obstet Gynecol* 68:195, 1986.

146. Tanaka T, Shiu RP, Gout PW et al: A new sensitive and specific bioassay for lactogenic hormones: measurement of prolactin and growth hormone in human serum, *J Clin Endocrinol Metab* 51:1058, 1980.

147. Tashjian AH, Barowsky NJ, Jensen DK: Thyrotropin-releasing hormone: direct evidence for stimulation of prolactin production by pituitary cells in culture, *Biochem Biophys Res Commun* 43:516, 1979.

148. Thorner MD, Perryman RL, Rogol AD et al: Rapid changes of prolactinoma volume after withdrawal and reinstitution of bromocriptine, *J Clin Endocrinol Metab* 53:480, 1981.

149. Tindall GT, Kovacs K, Horrath E et al: Human prolactin-producing adenomas and bromocriptine: a histological, immunocytochemical, ultrastructural, and morphometric study, *J Clin Endocrinol Metab* 55:1178, 1982.

150. Turkalj I, Bran P, Krupp P: Surveillance of bromocriptine in pregnancy, *JAMA* 247:1589, 1982.

151. Turkington RW: Ectopic production of prolactin, *N Engl J Med* 285:1455, 1971.

152. Turkington RW: Prolactin secretion in patients treated with various drugs, *Arch Intern Med* 130:349, 1972.

153. Tyson JE, Hwant P, Guyda H et al: Studies of prolactin secretion in human pregnancy, *Am J Obstet Gynecol* 113:14, 1972.

154. Vance ML, Evans WS, Thorner MO: Bromocriptine, *Ann Intern Med* 10:78, 1984.

155. Vance ML, Throner MD: Prolactinomas, *Endocrinol Metab Clin North Am* 16:731, 1987.

156. Vance ML, Cragun JR, Reimnitz C et al: CV 205-502 treatment of hyperprolactinemia, *J Clin Endocrinol Metab* 68:336, 1989.

157. Van't Verlaat JW, Croughs RJM: Withdrawal of bromocriptine after long-term therapy for macroprolactinomas; effect on plasma prolactin and tumor size, *Clin Endocrinol* 34:175, 1991.

158. Van't Verlaat JW, Croughs RJM et al: Treatment of macroprolactinomas with a new non-ergot, long-acting, dopaminergic drug, CV 205-502. *Clin Endocrinol* 33:619, 1990.

159. Wardlaw SL, Wehrenberg WB, Ferin M et al: Failure of beta-endorphin to stimulate prolactin release in the pituitary stalk sectioned monkey, *Endocrinology* 107:1663, 1980.

160. Waters CA, Daly DC, Chapitis J et al: Human myometrium: a new potential source of prolactin, *Am J Obstet Gynecol* 147:639, 1983.

161. Weiss MH, Teal J, Gott P et al: Natural history of microprolactinomas: six-year follow-up, *Neurosurgery* 12:180, 1983.

162. Whitaker MD, Klee GG, Kao PC et al: Demonstration of biological activity of prolactin molecular weight variants in human sera, *J Clin Endocrinol Metab* 58:826, 1984.

163. Wilson JD, King DJ, Sheridan B: Tranquilizers and plasma prolactin, *Br Med J* 1:123, 1979.

164. Wolpert SM: The radiology of pituitary adenomas. *Endocrin Metab Clinics* 16:553, 1987.

165. Woodhouse NJY, Niles N, McDonald D et al: Prolactin levels in pregnancy: comparison of normal subjects with patients having micro- or macroadenomas after early bromocriptine withdrawal, *Horm Res* 21:1, 1985.

166. Ylikorkala O, Huhttaniemi I, Tuimala R et al: Subnormal postconceptional levels of prolactin do not interfere with the early events of pregnancy, *Fertil Steril* 32:286, 1979.

167. Zacur HA, Foster GV, Tyson JE: Multifactorial regulation of prolactin secretion, *Lancet* 1:410, 1976.

168. Zacur HA, Lake CR, Zeigler M et al: Plasma dopamine hydroxylase activity and norepinephrine levels during the human menstrual cycle, *Am J Obstet Gynecol* 130:148, 1978.

169. Zacur HA, Mitch WE, Tyson JE et al: Autoregulation of rat pituitary prolactin secretion demonstrated by a new perfusion method, *Am J Physiol* 242: E226, 1982.

170. Zacur HA: Oral contraceptive pills and prolactin, *Semin Reprod Endocrinol* 7:239, 1989.

171. Zacur HA, Foster GV: Hyperprolactinemia and polycystic ovarian sydrome, *Semin Reprod Endocrinol* 10:236, 1992.

Chapter 10

HYPERANDROGENISM

Robert L. Barbieri, MD

BACKGROUND AND PHYSIOLOGY

Androgens have long been described as those steroids capable of stimulating growth of the male secondary sex glands, such as the prostate. A modern definition of androgens would be those steroids able to bind to the androgen receptor and alter the transcription of specific genes. In humans, testosterone (T) and dihydrotestosterone (DHT) are the major androgens. Androstenedione (A) and dehydroepiandrosterone sulfate (DHEAS) are important androgen precursors.[26]

Hyperandrogenism is the state of increased androgen production and action. Hyperandrogenism is a common endocrinopathy in women of reproductive age. In most cases of hyperandrogenism, the ovary, the adrenal, and the pilosebaceous unit contribute to the androgen overproduction.[55] Androgen overproduction in women is associated with hirsutism, acne, oligoovulation or anovulation, infertility, endometrial hyperplasia, and metabolic abnormalities such as hypertriglyceridemia, decreased high-density lipoprotein (HDL) cholesterol, hypertension, and non–insulin-dependent diabetes mellitus. The diseases and syndromes that cause hyperandrogenism are reviewed in this chapter.

Androgen biosynthesis

Androgen biosynthesis is discussed in two parts. First, the biosynthetic steps involved in the production of A and T are reviewed (Fig. 10-1). A discussion of the metabolism of A and T to 3α- and 5α- reduced metabolites follows (Fig. 10-2).

In women, two organs, the adrenal and the ovary, are capable of synthesizing A and T from cholesterol. In the adrenal and corpus luteum, the cholesterol used for steroid synthesis is derived from circulating low-density lipoprotein (LDL) cholesterol. The circulating LDL cholesterol binds to LDL receptors on the cell membrane, and the receptor complexes enter the cells by a process of receptor aggregation (capping) and endocytosis. The cholesterol in the LDL particle is released by the action of lysosomal enzymes. In ovarian theca, granulosa cells, and stroma, cholesterol for steroid biosynthesis is obtained from two sources: circulating LDL cholesterol and de novo synthesis of cholesterol from acetate.[80,88]

Cholesterol metabolism begins with the transport of cholesterol to the mitochondria, where it binds to the cholesterol side-chain cleavage (CSCC) enzyme and is metabolized to pregnenolone (Fig. 10-1). The conversion of cholesterol to pregnenolone is the rate-limiting step in steroid biosynthesis. In the adrenal gland, adrenocorticotropin (ACTH) stimulates CSCC activity. In ovarian stroma and theca, luteinizing hormone (LH) stimulates CSCC activity. Pregnenolone is transported out of the mitochondria and metabolized to the core Δ^5 steroids (17-hydroxypregnenolone and dehydroepiandrosterone [DHEA] and the core Δ^4 steroids (progesterone, 17-hydroxyprogesterone, and A) by two enzyme systems[78] (17-hydroxylase, 17,20-lyase and 3β-hydroxysteroid dehydrogenase-isomerase) (Fig. 10-1). Androstenedione is metabolized to testosterone by the 17-ketosteroid oxi-

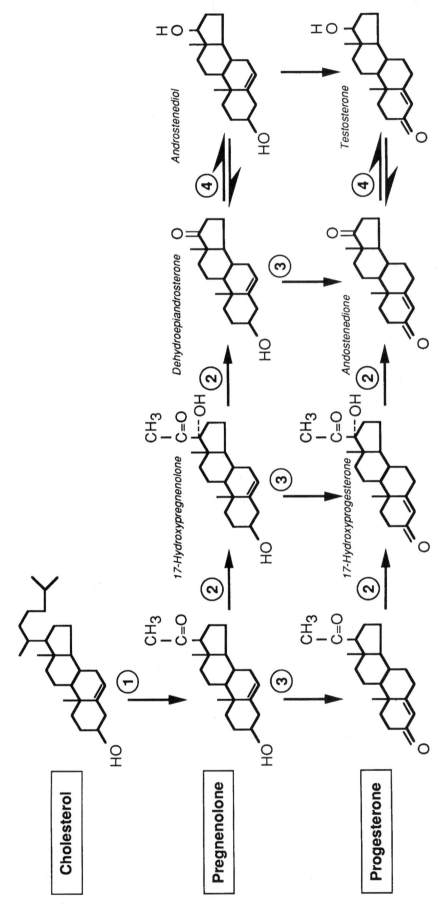

Fig. 10-1. Pathways of steroid synthesis involved in androstenedione and testosterone production. Enzymes: *1*, cholesterol side-chain cleavage enzyme; *2*, 17-hydroxylase, 17,20-lyase; *3*, 3β- hydroxysteroid dehydrogenase-isomerase; *4*, 17-ketosteroid oxidoreductase (17β-hydroxysteroid dehydrogenase).

Table 10-1. Secretion rate of major androgens from the adrenal and ovary in normally cycling women*

| Androgen | Secretion rate (mg/24h) | |
	Adrenal	Ovary
DHEAS	18	0
DHEA	<1	<1
A	1.5	1.5
T	0.02	0.05

*See references 26, 45, 46, and 55.

Table 10-2. Origin of testosterone in normally cycling women*

Origin of T	Production of T (mg/d)
Ovarian secretion	0.05
Adrenal secretion	0.02
Peripheral conversion	
A to T	0.13
DHEA to T	0.05
TOTAL	0.25

*See references 26, 35, 36, 45, 46, and 55.

doreductase enzyme.[78] The adrenal gland secretes DHEAS, DHEA, A, and a small amount of T. In contrast, the ovary secretes A and a small amount of T (Table 10-1).

Three types of reactions characterize the metabolism of all steroids: (1) Removal or addition of hydrogen occurs, as in the conversion of pregnenolone to progesterone. Enzymes in this class include the 3β-hydroxysteroid dehydrogenase-isomerase, the 17-ketosteroid oxidoreductase, and the 5α-reductase. (2) Monoxygenation (the addition of oxygen to the core cyclopentenophenanthrene ring) occurs, as occurs in the conversion of progesterone to 17-hydroxyprogesterone. Enzymes in this class include the CSCC enzyme; the 17-hydroxylase, 17,20-lase enzyme; the aromatase enzyme; and the 11-, 21-, and 18-hydroxylases. All of these monoxygenases utilize a cytochrome P-450 protein to cleave molecular oxygen, and insert a single oxygen atom into the carbon core of the steroid molecule. The cytochrome P-450–containing enzymes are susceptible to inhibition by pyridyl-containing compounds such as metyrapone and ketoconazole. (3) Conjugation reactions occur, such as sulfoconjugation and glucoconjugation.

Testosterone is a substantially more biologically effective androgen than is androstenedione. In normally cycling women, circulating T is derived from three major sources: (1) direct secretion from the ovary, (2) conversion of A secreted by the adrenal and ovary to T in the periphery, and (3) conversion of DHEA secreted by the adrenal to T in the periphery (Table 10-2).[35,36,45,46,55] In most hyperandrogenic states, the production rate of T is abnormally elevated because of an increase in ovarian secretion of T and an increase in ovarian and/or adrenal secretion of A, which is converted to T in the periphery.[35,45,55]

Androstenedione and testosterone can be converted to 5α-androstanedione and 5α-dihydrotestosterone (DHT), respectively, by the enzyme 5α-reductase (Fig. 10-2). DHT is not secreted by the normal ovary or adrenal.[39,54] DHT arises from the peripheral conversion of A, DHEA, and T.[39,54] The pilosebaceous unit contains the enzymes 5α-reductase and 17-ketosteroid oxidoreductase and is therefore an important source of DHT production in

women.[39,55,70] The 5α-reductase enzyme is induced by T and DHT. This regulatory feature creates a positive feedback loop whereby DHT stimulates the 5α-reductase enzyme, which results in more DHT production. The 5α-reduced androgens are metabolized to glucuronide and sulfate conjugates, which circulate at high concentrations.[54] For example, in hirsute women, the circulating concentrations of androsterone glucuronide and 3α, 5α-androstanediol sulfate are approximately 100 ng/mL and 50 ng/mL, respectively. In normally cycling women, these levels are approximately 40 ng/mL, respectively, In hirsute women, androsterone sulfate circulates at a concentration of 1 µg/mL (0.75 µg/mL in normally cycling women).[54]

Sources of androgens

As noted earlier, the major sites of androgen biosynthesis include the ovary, adrenal, and pilosebaceous unit. The ovarian stroma and theca are major sources of A and T synthesis.[56,57] In ovarian stroma and theca from normal ovaries, A and T are secreted at a ratio of approximately 4:1.[56,57] In ovarian stroma from some hyperandrogenic women, A and T are secreted at a ratio of approximately 1:1.[9,56] Androgen production in both theca and stroma is stimulated by LH and human chorionic gonadotropin (hCG).[56,57] Theca is more steroidogenically active than stroma per milligram of tissue,[56,57] but the mass of the ovarian stroma is far greater than the thecal mass in all ovaries, normal or hyperandrogenic. Consequently, the stroma is an important source of ovarian androgen secretion.

The organization of the adrenal gland is characterized by three major steroidogenic zones: zona glomerulosa, zona fasciculata, and zona reticularis. Although all three zones are capable of synthesizing androgens, the zona reticularis is the main source of adrenal androgen secretion. The adrenal secretes large quantities of the weak androgen DHEAS, significant amounts of A, and small quantities of T (Table 10-1). The pilosebaceous unit contains the 5α-reductase and the 17-ketosteroid oxidoreductase enzymes, and is a major site of DHT production.

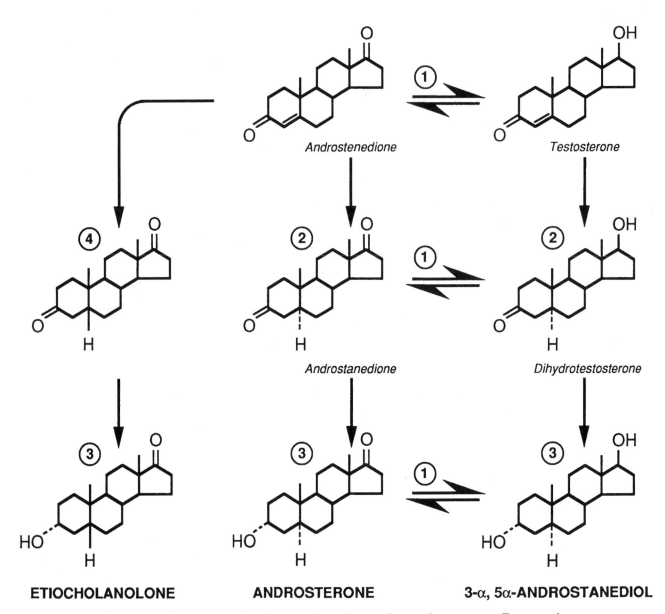

Fig. 10-2. Pathways involved in the reduction androstenedione and testosterone. Enzymes: *1, 17-ketosteroid oxidoreductase (17β-hydroxysteroid dehydrogenase); 2, 5α-reductase; 3, 3α- reductase; 4, 5β-reductase.*

Androgen transport

Testosterone and DHT are present in the circulation bound to sex hormone–binding globulin (SHBG), bound to albumin and as the free steroid. SHBG binds many C-18 and C-19 17β-hydroxysteroids (Table 10-3).[76] In normally cycling women at 37°C, circulating T is distributed in three phases: 1% is free, 30% is bound to albumin, and 60% is bound to SHBG.[62] Of interest, the affinity of SHBG for T is greater at 4°C than at 37°C, so that studies that examine the SHBG-T interaction at 4°C report that up to 90% of circulating T is bound to SHBG.[3]

Many factors control hepatic production of SHBG. Estradiol and high concentrations of thyroxine increase hepatic production of SHBG. Androgens and hyperinsuline-mia appear to decrease hepatic production of SHBG. In hyperandrogenic women, SHBG concentrations are clearly suppressed.[3,63,90,91] This results in an increase in the percentage of free T and albumin-bound T and a decrease in the SHBG-bound T.[90,91] Current data indicate that both free and albumin-bound T are capable of entering tissues and exerting an androgenic effect. The SHBG-bound T is unable to enter tissues and exert a biologic effect. The decrease in SHBG concentration in hyperandrogenic women results in more biologically available circulating T.

Androgen action

To exert their effects, circulating androgens must enter cells and bind to low-capacity, high-affinity intracellular

Table 10-3. Relative affinity of various steroids for SHBG*

Steroid	Affinity (%)
DHT	250
Androstane-3α,17β-diol	108
T	100
A (Δ⁵)	90
Estradiol	30

*Data are from reference 76.

androgen receptors. After binding to its receptor, the androgen (T or DHT) causes the receptor to change its conformation, resulting in the activation of a DNA-binding domain. The activated receptor binds to regulatory elements (steroid response elements [SREs]) of genes and activates (or suppresses) transcription and translation.[21] The SREs are at the 5′ end of genes and serve as DNA-binding sites for the activated steroid-receptor complex. The SREs typically are composed of two half-sites, located on complementary strands of DNA and pointing in opposite directions to form a palindrome.[21]

The androgen receptor has important structural domains that subserve three functions: (1) hormone binding (2) DNA binding, and (3) regulation of gene transcription.[50] The receptor domain that binds DNA consists of cysteine residues that are complexed into "zinc fingers." Each zinc finger contains one zinc ion complexed with four cysteine residues. Deletion of this domain markedly decreases receptor activity. Androgen receptors undergo posttranslational phosphorylation. The state of phosphorylation of the receptor appears to control, in part, affinity of the receptor for androgen.

Pilosebaceous unit physiology

The pilosebaceous unit is clearly both an androgen-dependent target organ and a site of androgen production and metabolism.[70] Sebum production is stimulated by T, and excess sebum production may play an important role in the development of acne. Androgens regulate many aspects of hair growth, especially in certain regions of the body. At birth, with the exception of the scalp and eyebrows, the body is covered by vellus hair, which is light-colored and has a very narrow diameter. Vellus hair can be transformed into terminal hair (dark, thick diameter) by the action of androgens (Fig. 10-3). The amount of androgen necessary to stimulate this transformation is dependent on many factors, including race, and the site of the hair follicle on the body. Hair whose growth is regulated by androgen includes the axillae, pubis, face, lower abdomen, thighs, chest, and breasts. At puberty, small quantities of adrenal and ovarian androgens are capable of stimulating the transformation of vellus hair on the pubic region and axillae

into terminal hair. Substantially larger amounts of androgen are required to stimulate the growth of a beard.

Terminal hair does not grow continuously but in a cyclic fashion, with periods of growth and quiescence. Androgen-dependent hair can be pushed into a growth phase (anagen) by exposure to an appropriate "dose" (concentration × time) of androgen. The length of hair is determined in part by the duration of anagen. At the termination of growth (catagen), the keratinized column and the bulb shrink and the resting state is achieved (telogen).

Androgen response hierarchy

The sensitivity of target organs to T varies significantly. Moderately elevated T production rates may result in increased facial and body hair. Greater degrees of T overproduction may result in oligoovulation or anovulation and the parallel endometrial responses of oligomenorrhea, menometrorrhagia or amenorrhea. To produce features of virilization—clitorimegaly, deepening of the voice, balding, or increased muscle mass—marked elevations in androgen production rate are required.

HYPERANDROGENISM: DISEASES AND SYNDROMES
Genetic causes of hyperandrogenism

A major goal of modern medicine is to identify gene defects that cause specific diseases. For most women with hyperandrogenism, a specific genetic cause cannot be identified. However, two major groups of genetic disorders that can result in a hyperandrogenic phenotype have been identified: genetic disorders of the insulin receptor gene and genetic disorders of enzymes responsible for adrenal steroid hormone synthesis. These genetic causes of hyperandrogenism are reviewed.

Genetic disorders of the insulin receptor gene. A unique opportunity to identify a specific molecular cause of hyperandrogenism is provided by recent clinical observations that suggest that there is a strong association between hyperinsulinemia and hyperandrogenism in women of reproductive age.[19] The "insulin hypothesis" is that chronic hyperinsulinemia stimulates the ovary to secrete excessive quantities of androgens, especially T.[13,14] The insulin hypothesis has been strengthened by the observation that mutations in the insulin receptor system can be associated with hyperandrogenism. To clarify the association between hyperinsulinemia and hyperandrogenism, hyperandrogenism (HA), insulin resistance (IR), and acanthosis nigricans (AN) (HAIR-AN) syndrome, and mutations in the insulin receptor gene reported in women with the HAIR-AN syndrome are reviewed.

The HAIR-AN syndrome. A unique opportunity to identify a specific etiologic cause of hyperandrogenism is provided by the HAIR-AN syndrome.[13,14] It is not possible to identify one specific investigator, or group of investigators, as the first to describe the HAIR-AN syndrome. Many

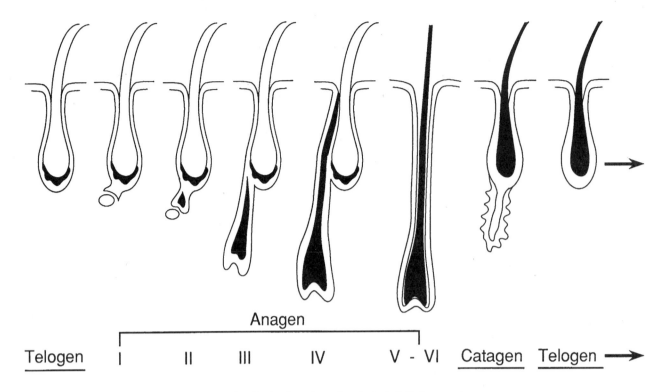

Anagen

Telogen | I | II | III | IV | V - VI | Catagen | Telogen →

Fig. 10-3. Growth cycle of a hair follicle.

fascinating accounts of "bearded diabetics" (Achard-Thiers syndrome), IR and AN, or hirsutism and AN have been reported since the turn of the century. However, it is only in the past decade that the full HAIR-AN syndrome has been clearly described. Until recently, the HAIR-AN syndrome was thought to be rare. In contrast, recent experience suggests that as many as 5% of hyperandrogenic women have the HAIR-AN syndrome.

In the HAIR-AN syndrome, the ovary is the primary source of androgen overproduction, and serum total T concentrations typically are greater than 1 ng/mL. In the HAIR-AN syndrome, the IR typically is due to a decreased number of insulin receptors, decreased functional activity of the receptor, or circulating anti–insulin receptor antibodies.[13,14] In the HAIR-AN syndrome, the primary pathologic derangement is the IR and compensatory hyperinsulinemia. The hyperinsulinemia, together with LH, stimulates ovarian stromal and thecal androgen production. The AN is a dermatologic epiphenomenon of severe hyperinsulinemia and hyperandrogenism.

Clinically, AN presents as a velvety, mossy, verrucous, hyperpigmented skin change that usually develops over the nape of the neck, in the axillae, on the vulva,[30a] beneath the breasts, and occasionally in other body folds (Fig. 10-4). Histologically, AN consists of hyperkeratosis, epidermal papillomatosis, and hyperpigmentation. Skin tags (acrochordons) are often found in, or near, areas of AN. Histocytochemistry has demonstrated the presence of excess quantities of glycosaminoglycans, especially hyaluronic

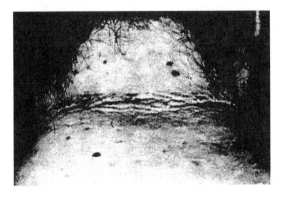

Fig. 10-4. Acanthosis nigricans on the neck of an obese, hyperandrogenic, insulin-resistant woman.

acid, in the papillary dermis of acanthotic lesions.[95] The factors that induce the lesion of AN have not been fully characterized. Insulin, insulin growth factor I (IGF-I), epidermal growth factor, and T have all been implicated as growth factors involved in the development of AN.

AN can occur in the setting of benign or malignant disease. When AN is associated with a malignancy, an adenocarcinoma is almost always present. Adenocarcinoma of the stomach is the most common tumor associated with AN. Obesity is one of the most common benign causes of AN. Many of the benign cases of AN occur in association with various endocrinopathies, including IR due to decreased insulin receptor function or anti–insulin receptor antibodies, acromegaly, diabetes, Addison disease, and Cushing disease.

From a clinician's viewpoint, careful attention to the entire neck, the axillae, the area under the breasts, and the groin provides adequate screening for AN. If AN is present in a young woman who does not have an associated malignancy, marked IR can be demonstrated to be present in more than 90% of cases.[14] Although the finding of AN is relatively specific for the presence of IR, it is not a sensitive marker of IR.[14] If AN is noted during the physical examination of the hirsute woman, the clinician should appreciate that the patient is at high risk for having or developing (1) severe IR; (2) ovarian stromal hyperthecosis; (3) major lipid abnormalities, including hypercholesterolemia; (4) non–insulin-dependent diabetes mellitus; and (5) essential hypertension.

Important clinical features of the HAIR-AN syndrome include the following: (1) In the HAIR-AN syndrome, ovarian stromal hyperthecosis is a common pathologic finding. (2) The severity of the IR is highly correlated with the severity of the AN. (3) Low-normal gonadotropin profiles are common in the HAIR-AN syndrome and suggest that a hormone or hormones (e.g., insulin) other than the gonadotropins are contributing to the stimulation of ovarian androgen production. (4) Gonadotropins play an essential role in the development of the HAIR-AN syndrome. Administration of combined estrogen-progestogen pills or gonadotropin-releasing hormone (GnRH) agonists results in a decrease in serum T. (5) Reduction in ovarian androgen overproduction by medical or surgical means does not improve the IR.[13,14]

Insulin resistance. Laboratory studies demonstrate that insulin stimulates androgen production in incubations of human ovarian stroma and theca obtained from women with the HAIR-AN syndrome.[10,12] In one study, insulin alone (500 ng/mL) and LH alone (25 ng/mL) stimulated A and T accumulation in incubations of human ovarian stroma from four hyperandrogenic women.[12] This concentration of insulin is similar to that observed in severely insulin-resistant women after a carbohydrate challenge. These studies suggest that insulin can regulate androgen synthesis in the human ovary.

Recent observations that some women with HAIR-AN syndrome have point mutations in the insulin receptor gene provide further support for the hypothesis that hyperinsulinemia causes hyperandrogenism. The biology of the insulin receptor is briefly reviewed. The insulin receptor is a high-molecular-weight (154 kd) heterotetrameric structure consisting of two alpha subunits and two beta subunits.[8] The α-subunits reside entirely on the extracellular surface and bind insulin. The β-subunits span the membrane and contain the intracellular tyrosine kinase domain (Fig. 10-5). Insulin binding to the receptor activates the tyrosine kinase activity of the receptor, resulting in autophosphorylation of tyrosine residues on the receptor and phosphorylation of other intracellular proteins. The activated insulin receptor appears to stimulate multiple serine/threonine kinases, S6 kinase, and protein-activated kinase II. Although protein phosphorylation is probably a critical component of insulin action, the precise molecular mechanisms by which insulin exerts its intracellular effects are unknown.[8]

Recent advances in molecular biology have made it possible to sequence the entire insulin receptor gene in women with ovarian hyperandrogenism and to identify the precise DNA changes that are associated with the HAIR-AN phenotype. To date, 10 women with the HAIR-AN syndrome have been demonstrated to have mutations in the insulin receptor gene (Table 10-4).* For example, Moller and Flier[59] studied the insulin receptor gene in a woman with the HAIR-AN syndrome. Complementary DNA (cDNA) prepared from fibroblast cell lines and lymphocyte cell lines was amplified by using the polymerase chain reaction (PCR) technique. Specific amplified DNA segments were cloned into M13 phage and sequenced. Amplified DNA from this patient revealed one important base change (from TGG to TCG) at codon 1200, which resulted in the replacement of tyrosine by serine. Codon 1200 is in a region of the β-subunit of the insulin receptor that is involved in expressing the tyrosine kinase activity of the receptor. It is likely that the base change at codon 1200 results in an insulin receptor that has lost part of its tyrosine kinase ability and is nonfunctional.[59] The loss of insulin receptor function results in severe IR and a compensatory hyperinsulinemia. In turn, it is our belief that the severe, chronic, hyperinsulinemia synergizes with LH to stimulate the ovarian androgen production, which was seen in this patient.

An important genetic principle is that if a phenotypic trait (such as the HAIR-AN syndrome) segregates in a family and is associated with a single gene, then that trait may be caused by the gene. Accili and colleagues[1] recently reported a linkage analysis of one pedigree with the HAIR-AN syndrome (Kahn type A diabetes), that included two affected daughters, three unaffected daughters, and one unaffected son. Insulin receptor cDNA cloned from one affected sister showed a single missense mutation in both alleles of the insulin receptor gene, resulting in the substitution of a valine for phenylalanine at position 382 of the α-subunit. Analysis of restriction fragment length polymorphism (RFLP) demonstrated that the two affected sisters are homozygous for this mutation, whereas the two parents and the unaffected siblings are heterozygous carriers. Using the homozygosity mapping method, a logarithm of the odds (LOD) score of 2.25 ($P < 0.01$) was calculated for this pedigree. The LOD score supports the hypothesis that the mutation in the insulin receptor gene is statistically associated with the HAIR-AN phenotype ($P < 0.01$). Of interest,

*References 1, 20, 42, 58, 59, 82, 87, 96.

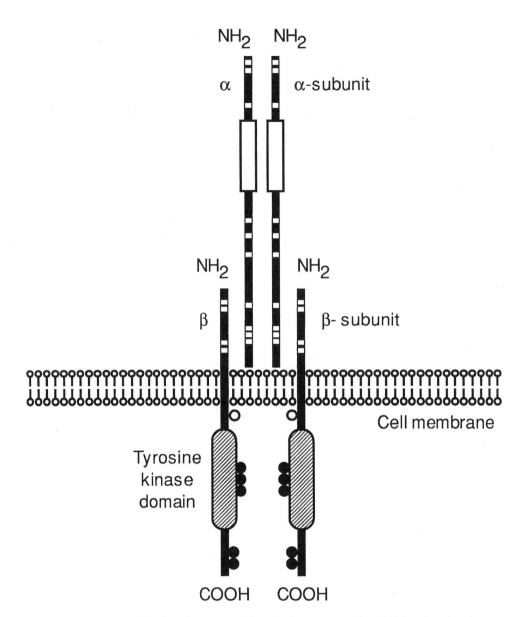

Fig. 10-5. Structure of the insulin receptor. Black circles represent identified tyrosine phosphorylation sites. (Modified from Harrison RM et al: In Rifkin H, LaPorte D, editors: *Diabetes mellitus,* Norwalk, Conn 1990, Appleton Lange.)

Table 10-4. Mutations in the insulin receptor gene reported in women with the HAIR-AN syndrome

Investigators	No. of alleles affected	Subunit affected	Codon and amino acid replacement	Inheritance
Moller and Flier[59]	1	Beta	1200, serine for tyrosine	Unknown
Taira et al.[87]	1	Beta	Deletion, exons 17 to 22	Unknown
Moller[58]	1	Beta	1134, Threonine for alanine	Dominant
Cama et al.[20]	1	Beta	1153, Isoleucine for methionine	Unknown
Shimada et al.[82]	1 or 2	Beta	Deletion, exon 14 (? compound heterozygote)	Recessive
Accili et al.[1]	2	Alpha	382, Valine for phenylalanine	Recessive, consanguineous parents
Kadowaki et al.[42]	2	Alpha	133, Stop codon 462, Serine for asparagine	Recessive
Yoshimasa et al.[96]	2	Processing site	735, Serine for arginine	Recessive, consanguineous parents

transfection of the mutant insulin receptor cDNA into NIH-3T3 cells demonstrated that the substitution of valine for phenylalanine at position 382 impairs post-translational processing and retards the transport of the insulin receptor to the plasma membrane.[1] The mutation may cause IR (and the HAIR-AN syndrome) by decreasing the number of insulin receptors on the cell surface.

The observation that mutations in the insulin receptor gene are associated with the HAIR-AN syndrome is important. It is the first example of a specific genetic cause of ovarian hyperandrogenism and should allow detailed genetic analysis of large pedigrees with familial ovarian hyperandrogenism. In the future, gene therapy may be available for women with HAIR-AN syndrome caused by insulin receptor mutations.

The precise mechanisms by which hyperinsulinemia causes ovarian hyperandrogenism are unclear. If a mutation in the insulin receptor gene results in severe IR, then the liver, muscle, ovary, and all other tissues should be insulin resistant. This creates a paradox: How can insulin induce ovarian hyperandrogenism in insulin-resistant states?[71] The definitive answer to this question remains to be determined. One possibility is that in insulin-resistant states, insulin may be able to stimulate ovarian androgen production by interacting with ovarian IGF-I receptors. Ovarian IGF-I receptors are known to be present in the human ovary, and they appear to regulate ovarian steroidogenesis.[12] Alternatively, insulin may stimulate ovarian steroidogenesis by acting through a "non-classic" insulin receptor–intracellular messenger pathway.

The observation that mutations in the insulin receptor gene that cause severe insulin resistance are often associated with ovarian hyperandrogenism raises the possibility that a causal link between obesity and the polycystic ovary syndrome (PCO) may be insulin resistance.[8,12-14] Women with PCO are often obese and/or insulin resistant. In women with PCO, the severity of the hyperinsulinemia and hyperandrogenism are positively correlated.[19] The pathophysiology of PCO is reviewed in greater detail in Chapter 11.

Genetic disorders of adrenal steroid hormone synthesis. Mutations in three separate enzymes necessary for cortisol synthesis can result in adrenal androgen overproduction. These three genetic disorders are reviewed below.

21-Hydroxylase deficiency. Adrenal 21-hydroxylase deficiency is one of the most common genetic disorders. Abnormal alleles for 21-hydroxylase may be carried by as many as 1 in 100 Caucasian women. The failure to synthesize a fully functional 21-hydroxylase enzyme results in a decrease in the conversion of 17-hydroxyprogesterone to 11-deoxycortisol, a relative decrease in cortisol production, a compensatory increase in ACTH secretion, and an increase in the production of 17-hydroxyprogesterone, A, and DHEA. If the defect in the 21-hydroxylase gene is severe (gene deletion), adrenal

androgen overproduction will be marked in utero, and the phenotype will be congenital adrenal hyperplasia (clitoromegaly, labioscrotal fusion, abnormal course of the urethra, and virilization). Salt wasting due to decreased mineralocorticoid production may occur in severe forms of the disease. If the defect in the 21-hydroxylase gene is mild, the phenotype will be adult-onset adrenal hyperplasia (hirsutism, menstrual irregularity, or infertility). Some women with mild gene defects have elevated circulating 17-hydroxyprogesterone concentrations but no clinical symptoms or signs (cryptic).

The 21-hydroxylase gene is on chromosome 6 within the human leukocyte antigen (HLA) region. The active 21-hydroxylase gene (*CYP21*) is located at the 3' end of the gene for complement C4a, and a pseudogene for the 21-hydroxylase enzyme (*CYP21P*) is located at the 3' end of the gene for complement C4b. The pseudogene for the 21-hydroxylase enzyme (*CYP21P*) contains mutations that render the gene nonfunctional. For most genetic disorders, many different gene defects can produce the same phenotype. The gene defects that cause adrenal hyperplasia have been examined by two techniques, RFLP[31] and PCR amplification.[64] Haglund-Stengler et al.[31] evaluated 43 patients with adrenal hyperplasia with the RFLP technique. Sixteen patients had point mutations in the 21-hydroxylase gene that rendered the gene nonfunctional. Eleven patients had deletions of major portions of the 21-hydroxylase gene. Two patients with the salt-wasting form of the disease had major deletions at the 5' end of *CYP21*. Seven patients had large gene conversions between the active *CYP21* gene and the *CYP21P* pseudogene, which resulted in the transfer of deleterious mutations from the *CYP21P* pseudogene to the *CYP21* gene. By using the PCR technique, Owerbach et al.[64] demonstrated abnormalities identified as gene deletion of the active *CYP21* gene, gene conversion, frame shift mutations in exon 3, mutations in intron 2 that caused abnormal mRNA splicing, and an abnormal stop codon in exon 8.

Approximately 3% to 10% of women with hyperandrogenism have 21-hydroxylase deficiency.[7] Although the prevalence is low, detection of women with 21-hydroxylase deficiency is of clinical value because specific treatment of this disorder is available (glucocorticoids) and prenatal genetic counseling may be of value. The two approaches with the greatest sensitivity for detecting 21-hydroxylase deficiency are measurement of the 8 AM serum 17-hydroxyprogesterone concentration during the follicular phase of the cycle or an ACTH stimulation test.[6] For women with 21-hydroxylase deficiency, 8 AM serum 17-hydroxyprogesterone concentrations are typically greater than 4 ng/mL in the follicular phase.[6] Most unaffected women have 8 AM follicular phase 17-hydroxyprogesterone concentrations less than 2 ng/mL. To detect 21-hydroxylase deficiency using an ACTH test, 0.25 mg of cosyntropin (synthetic ACTH; α 1-24-corticotropin) is administered

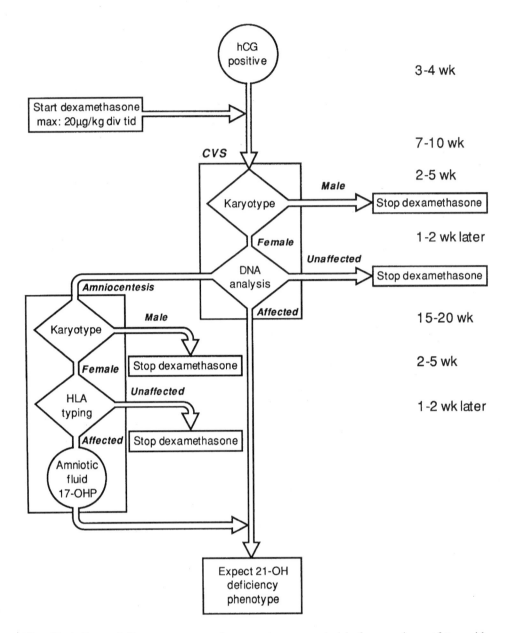

Fig. 10-6. Protocol for management of pregnant women at risk for carrying a fetus with 21-hydroxylase deficiency. (Redrawn with permission from Speiser PW et al: First-trimester prenatal treatment and molecular genetic diagnosis of congenital adrenal hyperplasia, *J Clin Endocrinol Metab* 70:838, 1990; © The Endocrine Society.)

intravenously at 8 AM. The serum 17-hydroxyprogesterone concentration is determined 60 minutes later, and values greater than 10 ng/mL demonstrate the presence of 21-hydroxylase deficiency.[6] Of note, measurement of DHEAS is of little value in screening for 21-hydroxylase deficiency.[83]

The discovery of the molecular causes of adrenal hyperplasia have paved the way for the prenatal diagnosis of this disorder. If a female fetus with congenital adrenal hyperplasia can be identified in utero, then the use of maternal glucocorticoid therapy may suppress fetal adrenal steroido-

genesis and prevent the phenotype of labioscrotal fusion, abnormal course of the urethra, and clitoromegaly. Speiser et al.[85] have described a protocol that may be effective in the prenatal treatment of adrenal hyperplasia (Fig. 10-6). Families at risk were identified, and the mother began to receive dexamethasone treatment (20 μg/kg) as soon as pregnancy was diagnosed. Chorionic villus sampling was performed between 8 and 10 weeks of gestation. If a male fetus was identified, therapy was discontinued. Chromosomal DNA was analyzed for defects in the 21-hydroxylase gene, using the RFLP technique. If an affected female fetus was identified, glucocorticoid treatment was continued for the entire pregnancy. By applying this protocol to 14 fetuses at risk, two affected female fetuses were successfully treated. Labioscrotal fusion and an abnormal course of the urethra were prevented, and the two children avoided genital reconstructive surgery. Maternal estradiol is derived from fetal adrenal precursors; therefore, maternal estradiol levels can be used to monitor the ability of maternal glucocorticoid therapy to suppress fetal adrenal steroidogenesis.

Pang et al.[65] reviewed the effects of prenatal glucocorticoid treatment on 15 female infants with congenital adrenal hyperplasia. Five infants responded completely and 10 infants responded partially. This heterogeneity in response could have been caused by unidentified genes that modify the phenotype, differences in bioeffectiveness of dexamethasone among patients, or the control of fetal adrenal steroidogenesis by factors other than ACTH.

11β-Hydroxylase deficiency. 11β-Hydroxylase deficiency results in a decrease in cortisol production, resulting in a compensatory increase in ACTH, and overproduction of 11-deoxycortisol, deoxycorticosterone (DOC), A, and DHEA. The diagnosis can be confirmed by observing an exaggerated elevation in DOC and/or 11-deoxycortisol after ACTH stimulation.[28] Women with mild forms of 11-hydroxylase deficiency can present as adults with oligoovulation, hirsutism, and (occasionally) hypertension. Although many women with hyperandrogenism have an exaggerated 11-deoxycortisol response to ACTH stimulation, less than 1% of hyperandrogenic women have an 11β-hydroxylase deficiency due to genetic mutation.

3β-Hydroxysteroid dehydrogenase-isomerase deficiency. Complete absence of 3β-hydroxysteroid dehydrogenase-isomerase (3-HSD) enzymatic activity results in a failure to produce estrogens and androgens and should produce a hypogonadal phenotype. However, women with partial 3-HSD deficiency may present with hirsutism and menstrual irregularity.[5,77] Diagnosis can be established by determination of 17 α hydroxypregnenolone levels, which are characteristically elevated after ACTH (cortrosyn) stimulation. The genetics of human 3-HSD deficiency is still poorly understood, and the number of hyperandrogenic women with genetic mutations in the 3-HSD gene(s) remains to be fully defined. Some authorities have hypothesized that there may be a very high incidence of mutations in the 3-HSD genes in women with hyperandrogenism.

In women with hirsutism and partial 3-HSD deficiency, adrenal overproduction of DHEA and DHEAS is the likely cause of the hyperandrogenism. An important inconsistency that requires resolution is, how can the peripheral tissues convert DHEA to A if the adrenal is deficient in 3-HSD because of a genetic mutation? The inconsistency may be resolved by recent reports that two 3-HSD genes exist in the human genome.[52,73] 3-HSD type I gene codes for a protein of 372 amino acids and is expressed in skin, placenta, and breast. 3-HSD type II gene codes for a protein of 371 amino acids with 94% homology with 3-HSD type I. Interestingly, 3-HSD type II gene is expressed only in adrenal, ovary, and testis. Conceivably a partial defect in 3-HSD type II gene is expressed only in adrenal, ovary, and testis. Conceivably also, therefore, a partial defect in 3-HSD type II gene could result in adrenal DHEA overproduction. The adrenal DHEA could then be metabolized to A (and ultimately to T and DHT) by a normal 3-HSD type I gene present in extraadrenal tissue, such as skin.[73]

Syndromes of androgen overproduction

A major goal of medical research is to identify those diseases that are caused by specific genetic defects. Hyperandrogenism can be caused by mutations in the insulin receptor gene, the 21-hydroxylase gene and the 11 β-hydroxylase gene. In addition to these genetic causes of hyperandrogenism, there are syndromes of androgen overproduction that do not yet have an identified genetic cause.

Hyperprolactinemia. Hyperprolactinemia is reviewed in Chapter 9. Controversy exists as to a possible relationship between hyperprolactinemia and elevated DHEAS concentration. Several studies have reported a positive correlation between hyperprolactinemia and elevated DHEAS.[34,47] However, other investigators have been unable to confirm an association.[18,66] Schiebinger and colleagues[79] investigated the DHEAS production rate (PR) and metabolic clearance rate (MCR) in hyperprolactinemic women before and after therapy (bromocriptine or microsurgery). Treatment of the hyperprolactinemia decreased the DHEAS PR from 27 mg/d to 17 mg/d, and increased the DHEAS MCR from 16 L/d to 21 L/d. Concomitant with these changes, serum DHEAS decreased from 2.5 μg/mL to 1.8 μg/mL. This detailed study does suggest that prolactin may play a role in the control of DHEAS PR and MCR.

Ovarian stromal hyperthecosis. Careful examination of most histologicically diagnosed "polycystic ovaries" reveals islands of "luteinized" steroidogenically active stromal cells (stromal hyperthecosis) that are not associated with follicular structures.[37] However, in extreme cases, diffuse and marked activation of stromal cells occurs, resulting in stromal hyperthecosis. In contrast to polycystic ovaries, hyperthecotic ovaries contain only small numbers of antral follicles. Women with stromal hyperthecosis can present with virilization, markedly elevated total T (>2.0 ng/mL), and low-normal LH and follicle-stimulating hormone (FSH) concentrations. IR, hyperinsulinemia, and AN are commonly observed in women with stromal hyperthecosis.[60] In cases of familial stromal hyperthecosis, mutations in the insulin receptor gene may be the cause of the stromal hyperthecosis.

Compared with women with PCO, women with stromal

hyperthecosis often fail to normalize levels of circulating T when treated with low-dose combination estrogen-progestin (E-P) contraceptives. In women with stromal hyperthecosis, treatment with GnRH analogues plus E-P combinations will often result in a normalization of ovarian androgen production.[2] A possible interpretation of this finding is that LH and FSH must be profoundly suppressed to decrease T secretion by the hyperthecotic ovaries. Low-dose E-P contraceptives probably do not suppress pituitary LH and FSH secretion as completely as do parenteral GnRH analogues or GnRH analogues plus E-P contraceptives.

Idiopathic hirsutism. Hirsutism in women with regular, ovulatory menstrual cycles and normal concentrations of circulating T is often called idiopathic hirsutism. In some cases this disorder may be due to excess 5α-reductase activity resulting in excessive conversion of T to DHT, and A to androstanedione (and then to DHT) (Fig. 10-2).[68,81] In women with idiopathic hirsutism, the circulating T level may be normal, but levels of 5α-reduced metabolites of A and T such as androsterone glucuronide, 5α-androstanediol sulfate, and 5α-androstanediol glucuronide are significantly elevated. The factors that control the overproduction of the 5α-reductase enzyme remain to be completely defined.[54]

Ovarian and adrenal tumors. Both ovarian and adrenal tumors may produce severe hyperandrogenism, resulting in the rapid onset of virilization.[38] Ovarian tumors that can cause hyperandrogenism include 1) Sertoli-Leydig cell tumors (androblastomas); (2) hilus cell tumors; (3) lipoid cell (adrenal rest) tumors; (4) occasionally, granulosa-theca cell tumors; and (5) rarely, ovarian stroma may overproduce androgens when stimulated by Krukenberg tumors, pseudomucinous cystoadenomas, Brenner tumors, and epithelial adenocarcinomas.

Sertoli-Leydig cell tumors typically are large and palpable (85%) on bimanual pelvic examination as a unilateral (95%) mass. These tumors tend to occur during the second to fourth decades of life. Many are associated with androgen overproduction, but some may be steroidogenically inactive or rarely may oversecrete estrogen. Most Sertoli-Leydig cell tumors are of low malignant potential. After surgical excision, the 5-year recurrence rate is less than 30%. Hilus cell tumors are often small (in the range of 1 cm in diameter), unilateral tumors that occur in perimenopausal or postmenopausal women. All hilus cell tumors are benign. Endometrial hyperplasia is often observed in association with hilus cell tumors. Women with Sertoli-Leydig cell tumors often have rapidly progressing symptoms of androgen excess. In contrast, many women with hilus cell tumors have slow progression of their symptoms and signs.

The onset of severe hyperandrogenism during pregnancy is often due to luteomas or hyperreactio luteinalis. Luteomas of pregnancy are benign unilateral or bilateral tumors that secrete large amounts of testosterone. In some cases, virilization of the fetus can occur. Hyperreactio luteinalis is probably caused, in part, by excess placental hCG secre-

tion. The ovaries are grossly enlarged and filled with multiple, small (<8 mm in diameter) follicular cysts. Hyperreactio luteinalis is never associated with virilization of the fetus. Both luteomas and ovaries affected by hyperreactio luteinalis regress or improve after delivery.

Adrenal carcinomas typically present with the rapid onset of virilization. DHEAS concentrations are often greater than 8 μg/mL, and 24-hour urinary 17-ketosteroid excretion is markedly increased (>30 mg/d). Many adrenal carcinomas have decreased 3-HSD activity, causing the relative overproduction of Δ^5 steroids. In this respect, adrenal carcinomas resemble the fetal zone of the adrenal. Adrenal carcinomas are extremely aggressive malignant tumors, and the 5-year survival rate is very low (<20%). Adrenal adenomas can contain the full complement of steroidogenic enzymes and be highly efficient producers of T, or they can be deficient in 3-HSD and resemble adrenal carcinomas in their steroidogenic pattern.

Women with virilization should be evaluated for the presence of an androgen-secreting ovarian or adrenal tumor. If the serum T level is greater than 1.5 ng/mL and the DHEAS level is normal, the androgen overproduction is probably from an ovarian source or a highly efficient adrenal adenoma. If the DHEAS level is greater than 8 μg/mL and the urinary 17-ketosteroid output is markedly elevated, an adrenal source of the androgen overproduction is likely. Pelvic ultrasound examination of the ovaries and magnetic resonance imaging of the adrenal glands are sensitive imaging techniques for identifying ovarian and adrenal tumors. In some cases, selective catheterization of the ovarian and adrenal veins may be necessary to localize the tumor.

Hyperandrogenism and menopause. In menopause, loss of all ovarian follicles results in decreased ovarian estradiol and inhibin secretion, producing a compensatory increase in FSH and LH secretion. The high circulating LH concentration activates ovarian stromal and hilus cell steroidogenesis. Of note, the stromal and hilus cells appear to be efficient at producing T, possibly because of increased activity of the 17-ketosteroid oxidoreductase enzyme.[9] Measurement of ovarian vein androgens and estrogens have demonstrated that the menopausal ovary is a major source of T, secretes moderate amounts of A, and produces little estradiol or estrone[40,41,61] (Fig. 10-7). This pattern of androgen secretion (T > A) contrasts markedly with the pattern of androgen secretion in the premenopausal ovary (A >> T).

As women become menopausal, the circulating concentrations of estradiol, A, and T decrease, but the magnitude of the decline in T concentration (20% decrease) is much less than the decline in estradiol (95% decrease) and A (50% decrease) concentrations.[40,41] This results in an altered androgen to estrogen ratio and may account for some of the signs and laboratory findings suggestive of androgen excess observed in the menopause. Wild et al[94] have

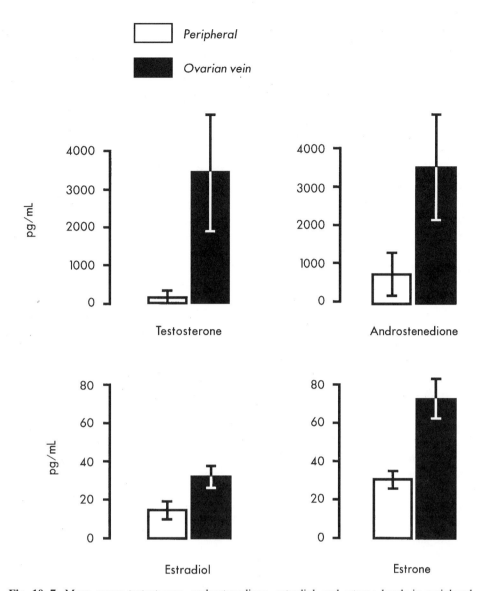

Fig. 10-7. Mean serum testosterone, androstenedione, estradiol, and estrone levels in peripheral serum and ovarian veins in 10 postmenopausal women. (Redrawn with permission from Judd HL et al: Endocrine function of the postmenopausal ovary: concentration of androgens and estrogens in ovarian and peripheral vein blood, *J Clin Endocrinol Metab* 39:1020, 1974; © The Endocrine Society.)

reported that in women older than 60 years of age there was a strong correlation among hirsutism, acne, upper-body-segment obesity, and coronary artery stenosis as demonstrated by cardiac catheterization. This raises the intriguing possibility that treatment of hyperandrogenism in menopausal women may decrease the risk of myocardial infarction.

Hyperandrogenism and cigarette smoking. Cigarette smoking is an extremely complex behavioral and pharmacologic process. Cigarette smoke contains more than 3000 chemical components, and many of these compounds are converted to multiple metabolites in vivo. Nicotine (a major alkaloid in cigarette smoke) and cotinine (a major metabolite of nicotine) contain pyridyl rings and share structural homology with inhibitors of cytochrome P-450, such as aminoglutethimide and metyrapone. Both nicotine and cotinine have been shown to inhibit the human adrenal 11β-hydroxylase[10] and the placental aromatase[11] by binding to the cytochrome P-450 portion of these enzyme systems. If nicotine and cotinine are inhibitors of the adrenal 11β-hydroxylase, then women who smoke might be expected to have increased concentrations of circulating adrenal androgens.

Friedman and colleagues[30] reported that women who smoke had elevated serum concentrations of A and T, compared with women who did not smoke. Similar observations have been made by Khaw and colleagues,[44] who also reported that there was a dose-dependent relationship between number of cigarettes smoked daily and the serum concentrations of A and DHEAS. In premenopausal women, Longcope and Johnstone[49] reported that A concentrations were elevated in women who smoked. These observations suggest that smoking may contribute to hyperandrogenism and that discontinuing smoking may result in a reduction in circulating androgens.

Hyperandrogenism in neurologic and psychiatric disorders. Although the incidence and mechanisms remain to be fully defined, preliminary reports suggest there may be a relationship between neuropsychiatric disorders and hyperandrogenism. For example, women with temporal lobe epilepsy have a high incidence of menstrual cycle abnormalities (amenorrhea 14%, oligomenorrhea 24%).[22,32,33] Herzog and colleagues[32,33] observed that women with left-sided lateralization of interictal epileptic discharges often had coexisting PCO. They postulated that limbic seizures may cause an increase in GnRH pulse frequency and/or amplitude that results in an increase in LH secretion, contributing to ovarian androgen overproduction. Alternatively, hyperandrogenic anovulation may predispose women to develop temporal lobe epilepsy. Greater understanding of the neuroendocrinology of PCO and neuropsychiatric disorders should help clarify the possible links between these two disorders.

Hirsutism due to drugs. Excessive hair growth has been definitely reported in association with the use of cyclosporine, minoxidil, diazoxide, and natural and synthetic androgens. In general, drug-induced hair growth is characterized by hair growth over all skin surfaces (not an androgen-dependent pattern) with minimal thickening of the hair shaft. This type of hair growth is called hypertrichosis. The molecular mechanisms by which cyclosporine, minoxidil, and diazoxide cause hypertrichosis are not known. As a rule, androgens are seldom prescribed to women. Exceptions to this rule include the treatment of endometriosis with androgens such as danazol, the treatment of menopausal women with methyltestosterone, and the treatment of lichen sclerosus with testosterone cream. In all these situations, hirsutism and other signs of hyperandrogenism can occur.

DIAGNOSTIC APPROACH TO HYPERANDROGENISM

Women with hirsutism, menstrual irregularity, infertility, or endometrial hyperplasia should be screened for hyperandrogenism. The history, physical examination, and select laboratory tests aid in the differential diagnosis of hyperandrogenism.

History

Key aspects in the history include the following: (1) Note the rate of progression of symptoms and signs. Ovarian and adrenal tumors that secrete androgens typically present with the rapid onset of hirsutism and signs of virilization. (2) Note the state of menstrual cycles. Regular, ovulatory, 28-day menstrual cycles are rarely associated with severe hyperandrogenic disorders; in women with hyperandrogenism, amenorrhea is a worrisome finding and should prompt a careful search for signs of virilization. (3) Inquire about ethnic origin. Moderate hirsutism in Asiatic or Scandinavian women is unusual and a cause for intensive investigation; moderate hirsutism in women of the Mediterranean basin is not unusual and often occurs in the absence of an identifiable hormone disorder; European and Eskimo women appear to carry genes for 21-hydroxylase deficiency at a high frequency. (4) Inquire about use of drugs. The surreptitious self-administration of androgens is rare but is typically a manifestation of a major psychiatric disorder or Munchausen syndrome.

Physical examination

Key aspects of the physical examination include the following: (1) Note any signs of virilization. If signs of virilization, such as deepening of the voice, balding, clitoromegaly, or increased upper body muscle mass, are present the physician must make an intensive and exceedingly complete attempt to identify the cause of the hyperandrogenism. (2) Evaluate the adnexa carefully. If an adnexal mass is present in a woman with hyperandrogenism, surgical removal of the mass may be necessary. (3) Note the presence of galactorrhea. Some women with hyperprolactinemia due to a pituitary tumor will present as a typical patient with PCO (hirsutism, oligomenorrhea, obesity). (4) Note any signs of Cushing disease. Objective signs of Cushing disease include osteoporosis, spontaneous ecchymoses, violescent striae greater than 1 cm, hypokalemia, central obesity, and weakness.

In women with hyperandrogenism, an important aspect of the physical examination is an objective assessment of the severity of the hirsutism. The Ferriman and Gallwey[29] system grades 11 sites and assigns a severity score (0, no terminal hair, to 4, severe hirsutism) at each site (Fig. 10-8). The scores for the 11 sites are summed to obtain a final score. Although somewhat cumbersome and time consuming, the methodology does allow for a quantitative comparison between patients and within a patient over time.

Laboratory evaluation

The goals of the laboratory evaluation of hyperandrogenism are to rule out tumors, assess severity, and evaluate the source of the hyperandrogenism: adrenal versus ovary. The laboratory tests that are most useful in the evaluation of

Site	Grade	Definition	Site	Grade	Definition
Upper lip	1	Few hairs at outer margin	Upper abdomen	1	Few midline hairs
	2	Small mustache at outer margin		2	Rather more, still midline
	3	Mustache extending halfway from outer margin		3 & 4	Half and full cover
			Lower abdomen	1	Few midline hairs
	4	Mustache extending to midline		2	Midline streak of hair
Chin	1	Few scattered hairs		3	Midline band of hair
	2	Scattered hairs with small concentrations		4	Inverted V-shaped growth
			Arm	1	Sparse growth affecting not more than one quarter of limb surface
	3 & 4	Complete cover, light and heavy			
Chest	1	Circumareolar hairs		2	More than this; cover still incomplete
	2	With midline hair in addition		3 & 4	Complete cover, light and heavy
	3	Fusion of these areas, with three-quarters cover	Forearm	1,2,3,4	Complete cover of dorsal surface; 2 grades of light and 2 of heavy growth
	4	Complete cover			
Upper back	1	Few scattered hairs	Thigh	1,2,3,4	As for arm
	2	Rather more, still scattered	Leg	1,2,3,4	As for arm
	3 & 4	Complete cover, light and heavy			
Lower back	1	Sacral tuft of hair			
	2	With some lateral extension			
	3	Three-quarters cover			
	4	Complete cover			

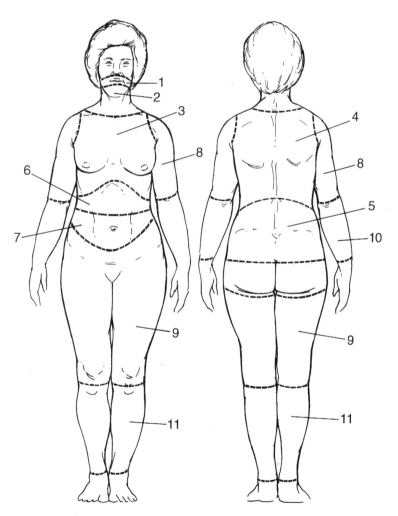

Fig. 10-8. Ferriman-Gallwey scoring system for quantitating hirsutism. The 11 sites are graded from 0 (no terminal hair) to 4 (severe hirsutism). (Redrawn with permission from Ferriman D, Gallwey JD: Clinical assessment of body hair growth in women, *J Clin Endocrinol Metab* 21:1440, 1961; © The Endocrine Society.)

hyperandrogenism include measurement of total T concentration; a screening test for 21-hydroxylase deficiency, DHEAS, and prolactin if oligomenorrhea or amenorrhea is present; and a screening test if Cushing disease is suspected (24-hour urinary free cortisol or the overnight 1-mg dexamethasone suppression test). If the total T concentration is greater than 2 ng/mL, the patient probably has ovarian stromal hyperthecosis or an adrenal or ovarian tumor. If the total T concentration is less than 1.5 ng/mL, an adrenal or ovarian tumor is unlikely to be present. An exception to this rule is that some menopausal women may have androgen-secreting adrenal or hilus cell tumors and circulating concentrations of T less than 1.5 ng/mL. Clinicians must be aware that some commercial T assays are not specific, and assay T, DHT, and other androgens. These assays typically report T results 50% to 100% higher than truly specific T assays.

As noted earlier, two sensitive screening tests for 21-hydroxylase deficiency are the 8 AM follicular phase 17-hydroxyprogesterone and the ACTH stimulation test.[6] DHEAS is largely of adrenal origin. A DHEAS level that is more than twice the upper limits of normal should raise the possibility of an adrenal tumor. Although DHEAS is largely of adrenal origin, most women with adult-onset adrenal hyperplasia do not have a markedly elevated DHEAS level.[83] In contrast, many women with PCO, an ovarian cause of hyperandrogenism, have an elevated DHEAS. This paradoxical situation limits the utility of the DHEAS measurement in identifying the source of the hyperandrogenism. Measurement of DHEAS may have special value in the evaluation of women with hyperandrogenism and infertility. In women with hyperandrogenism, infertility, and a DHEAS greater than 2 µg/mL, treatment with dexamethasone may improve the ovarian response to clomiphene and human menopausal gonadotropins.[25]

In selected cases of hyperandrogenism, structural studies of the ovary (transvaginal ultrasonography) or the adrenals (magnetic resonance imaging) may be required. Selective catheterization of the adrenal and ovarian veins is reserved for complex cases where a tumor is suspected.

MANAGEMENT OF HYPERANDROGENISM

Women with hyperandrogenism typically require treatment for one or more of the following problems: (1) hirsutism and/or acne; (2) anovulation; (3) endometrial hyperplasia or cancer; and (4) metabolic abnormalities, including IR, diabetes, hypertriglyceridemia-hypercholesterolemia, and hypertension.

Hirsutism and acne

Hirsutism and acne due to hyperandrogenism are best treated by simultaneously suppressing androgen production and androgen action. Strategies and pharmacologic agents that may be effective in the treatment of hirsutism include weight loss, cessation of smoking, E-P oral contraceptives, GnRH analogues, glucocorticoids, spironolactone, flutamide, cyproterone acetate, and ketoconazole.

Weight loss. In women with hyperandrogenism and obesity, weight loss can often result in a decrease in circulating T and A. For example, Bates and Whitworth[16] studied 18 obese women before and after a hypocaloric diet designed to result in the loss of 450 g of body weight per week. Before start of the hypocaloric diet, the mean weight for the study population was 77 kg. After dieting, the mean weight for the study population was 57 kg. The plasma A concentrations before and after weight loss were 2.95 and 1.79 ng/mL ($P < 0.001$), respectively. The plasma T concentrations before and after weight loss were 0.75 and 0.39 ng/mL ($P < 0.001$), respectively.

Pasquali et al.[67] evaluated the effects of weight loss on 20 women with obesity and hyperandrogenism. The 20 obese women had a body mass index of more than 26 kg/m^2 (mean 32.1 kg/m^2); at least 3 months of amenorrhea; and increased plasma concentrations of A, T, or DHEAS. All 20 women were treated for at least 6 months with a 1000 to 1500 kcal/d diet. Weight loss ranged from 4.8 to 15.2 kg (mean 9.7 kg). Multiple hormones, including insulin, LH, FSH, estradiol, estrone, T, free T, A, DHT, DHEAS, progesterone, and 17-hydroxyprogesterone were measured before and after weight loss. After weight loss, significant reductions in insulin, T, progesterone, and LH occurred. There were no significant changes in any of the other hormones measured. After weight loss, insulin decreased by 40%, T decreased by 35%, and LH decreased by 45%. Taken together, these studies clearly suggest that weight loss is associated with decreased circulating androgens in women with obesity and hyperandrogenism. In many obese women with anovulatory hyperandrogenism, weight loss will result in resumption of ovulation and pregnancies.

Estrogen-progestin therapy. Combined E-P therapy is relatively inexpensive, has few major deleterious side effects, and is moderately effective in suppressing ovarian (and adrenal) androgen production. E-P agents reduce LH and FSH secretion, thereby decreasing ovarian steroid production.[72] In addition, E-P agents increase hepatic production of SHBG, potentially resulting in a decrease in circulating free T concentrations. Finally, E-P agents decrease circulating DHEAS.[52]

The choice of which E-P agent to use remains controversial. Low-dose triphasic agents may not suppress LH and FSH as completely as monophasic agents. Our preferred E-P agent is ethinyl estradiol, 50 µg, plus ethynodiol diacetate, 1 mg daily (Demulen 1/50). The high ethinyl estradiol dose maximizes SHBG production and LH suppression. In addition, ethynodiol diacetate is probably less androgenic on a molar basis than norgestrel. Most clinicians prescribe E-P agents for 21 days with 7 days off therapy. This approach may allow LH and T production to increase during the 7 days off therapy, creating a pulse of androgens that may stimulate the pilosebaceous unit. Continuous E-P therapy for the first 3 to 6 months of therapy may prevent this phenomenon.

Gonadotropin-releasing hormone analogue therapy. For women with ovarian hyperandrogenism who fail to respond to E-P treatment, GnRH analogues are of value.[2] As noted earlier, GnRH analogues may produce more profound suppression of LH and FSH than do E-P contraceptives. In women with stromal hyperthecosis, profound suppression of LH and FSH may be necessary in order to fully suppress ovarian androgen secretion. Compared with normally cycling women, women with ovarian hyperandrogenism may require higher doses of GnRH analogue to fully suppress ovarian steroidogenesis.[4,74] Of note, Rittmaster[74] has reported that full suppression of ovarian androgen production requires higher doses of GnRH analogue than those required to suppress estradiol production. He reported that in women with PCO, leuprolide acetate in a 5-μg/kg subcutaneous injection daily suppressed estradiol to menopausal levels, but that a 15-μg/kg subcutaneous injection daily was required to fully suppress circulating T concentrations. Unlike uterine leiomyomas or endometriosis, ovarian hyperandrogenism is not an estrogen-dependent process. Therefore, it is possible to utilize combined GnRH analogue plus E-P therapy in the treatment of ovarian hyperandrogenism. Combined GnRH analogue plus E-P therapy prevents the osteopenia that can occur during therapy with GnRH analogue treatment.

Glucocorticoid therapy. In patients with ACTH-dependent adrenal androgen overproduction, treatment with glucocorticoids may be appropriate.[75] A major problem with exogenous glucocorticoid therapy is that it is difficult to completely suppress ACTH production without giving more glucocorticoid than would normally be produced by the adrenal. On a chronic basis, the need to treat with a "supraphysiologic" dose of glucocorticoid may result in the development of iatrogenic Cushing syndrome, including—in severe cases—the onset of diabetes and osteopenia. In addition, the corticotropin-releasing hormone–ACTH–cortisol axis may be sufficiently suppressed that the endogenous adrenal response to stress is blunted. One approach to this problem is to decide to suppress ACTH secretion only partially with low-dose or alternate-day glucocorticoids, and to employ antiandrogens simultaneously. This approach may decrease the risk of iatrogenic Cushing syndrome and minimize the number of patients with adrenal suppression.

Antiandrogen therapy. Antiandrogens such as spironolactone,[23,48] cyproterone acetate,[86] and flutamide[24] are important agents in the treatment of hirsutism. Approximately 50% of hirsute women treated with an antiandrogen will report improvement in their hair growth. In general, 3 to 6 months of treatment is needed to assess the efficacy of antiandrogen therapy. Successful treatment results in an initial decrease in the hair caliber and pigmentation and subsequently, in some women, a decrease in the rate of hair growth.

Spironolactone binds to the androgen receptor and acts as an androgen antagonist.[48] In addition, spironolactone inhibits androgen biosynthesis.[48] Spironolactone is effective in daily doses of 100 to 200 mg. A common starting dose is 50 mg twice daily. Spironolactone can cause irregular uterine spotting or bleeding, especially at a daily dose of 200 mg. No antiandrogen should be given to a pregnant woman because of the potential of blocking androgenization of a male fetus. In addition, because of its potassium-sparing actions, spironolactone should not be given to women with renal failure.

Flutamide is an antiandrogen approved for the treatment of prostate carcinoma. In one study, at doses of 250 mg twice daily, it was effective in the treatment of hirsutism.[24] Flutamide is significantly more expensive than spironolactone.

Cyproterone acetate is both an antiandrogen and a progestin. Cyproterone acetate may be given as 50 to 100 mg daily on days 5 to 15 of the menstrual cycle, combined with 35 to 50 μg of ethinyl estradiol on days 5 to 26. Cyproterone acetate therapy is limited to days 5 to 15 of the cycle to minimize the development of amenorrhea. Cyproterone acetate is not available in the United States, but is widely used in other countries.

Antiandrogens such as cyproterone acetate or spironolactone are often combined with estrogen to improve efficacy (simultaneous suppression of ovarian androgen production and peripheral androgen blockade) and control uterine bleeding. The relative efficacy of cyproterone acetate plus ethinyl estradiol-norgestrel was studied in a randomized trial by O'Brien et al.[63] Both cyproterone acetate plus ethinyl estradiol and spironolactone plus ethinyl estradiol-norgestrel were comparable in reducing total hair-shaft diameter (−17%) and medullary diameter of the hair (cyproterone acetate plus ethinyl estradiol, −32%; spironolactone plus ethinyl estradiol-norgestrel, −18%). Both combinations also reduced circulating T concentrations. The decrease in the diameter of the hair correlated with the decrease in testosterone (r - .49). Since cyproterone acetate is not available in the United States, the combination of spironolactone plus ethinyl estradiol-norgestrel could be considered as primary therapy for hirsutism.

The importance of antiandrogen therapy in the treatment of hirsutism must be emphasized. In some cases, antiandrogen treatment may be more effective than suppression of androgen production in the treatment of hirsutism. For example, Spritzer and colleagues[86] randomized 30 women with adrenal hyperplasia due to a 21-hydroxylase defect to receive hydrocortisone (20 mg/d) or cyproterone acetate plus percutaneous estradiol. This combined regimen consisted of administering the antiandrogen cyproterone acetate (50 mg/d) for days 5 through 25 each month and

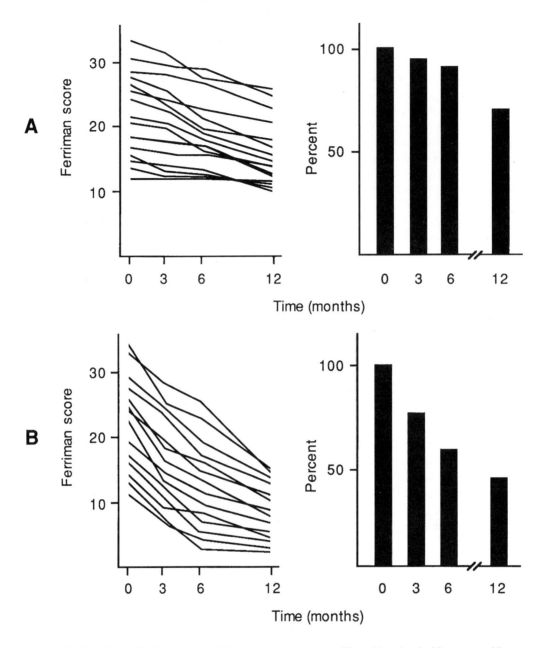

Fig. 10-9. Effects of hydrocortisone (**A**) or cyproterone acetate (**B**) on hirsutism in 30 women with adrenal hyperplasia. (Redrawn with permission from Spritzer P et al: Cyproterone acetate versus hydrocortisone treatment in late onset adrenal hyperplasia, *J Clin Endocrinol Metab* 70:642, 1990; © The Endocrine Society.)

percutaneous estradiol (3 mg/d), for days 16 through 25 each month. Therapeutic effects were assessed by using the Ferriman-Gallwey score[29] and measuring the circulating A and T levels. In hydrocortisone-treated patients, plasma androgens decreased to normal levels. Testosterone levels decreased from 3.05 nmol/L to 1.46 nmol/L, and A levels decreased from 13.6 nmol/L to 6.33 nmol/L. The cyproterone acetate regimen produced only minimal changes in circulating androgen levels. Testosterone levels decreased from 2.98 nmol/L to 2.29 nmol/L, and A levels decreased from 12.9 nmol/L to 9.86 nmol/L. Surprisingly, cyproterone

acetate therapy was superior to hydrocortisone therapy in the treatment of hirsutism (Fig. 10-9). In the cyproterone-treated patients there was a 54% decrease in the hirsutism score. In the hydrocortisone-treated patients there was only a 23% decrease in the hirsutism score. The authors concluded that peripheral receptivity to androgens is important in the clinical expression of hyperandrogenism. Peripheral antiandrogen therapy with cyproterone acetate may be more effective in the treatment of hirsutism in adult-onset adrenal hyperplasia than is conventional adrenal suppression with glucocorticoids.

Ketoconazole has received considerable attention as a novel agent for the suppression of hyperandrogenism.[69,89] Ketoconazole decreases androgen production by inhibiting an enzyme critical to androgen synthesis—cytochrome P-450–17α-hydroxylase, 17,20-lyase. In one study, ketoconazole (600 to 1000 mg/d) was administered to eight women with hyperandrogenism.[69] Ketoconazole treatment produced a 50% decrease in serum concentrations of T and a 50% decrease in the rate of hair growth.[69] In another study, 53 women with hirsutism were treated with ketoconazole at a dose of 400 mg daily.[89] This regimen produced decreases in circulating T, A, and DHEA concentrations, as well as decreases in rates of hair growth and hair-shaft diameter. Of the 53 women, 22 had no significant decrease in their hirsutism score. Acne improved in all women with this problem. Many side effects attributed to the ketoconazole therapy were reported, including nausea, hepatitis, and loss of scalp hair.[89] This study suggests that ketoconazole should not be used as a primary agent for the treatment of hirsutism.

Anovulation

The treatment of anovulation associated with hyperandrogenism is reviewed in Chapters 32, 33, and 34.

Endometrial hyperplasia

The anovulation and "hypoprogestinism" associated with states of hyperandrogenism increase the risk of developing endometrial hyperplasia and cancer. Atypical hyperplasia is associated with a high risk of developing endometrial cancer.[92] Women with hyperandrogenism and anovulation should be evaluated for cyclic or continuous progestin therapy in order to reduce the risk of developing hyperplasia or cancer.

Metabolic abnormalities

Metabolic abnormalities such as IR, diabetes, hypertriglyceridemia-hypercholesterolemia, and hypertension are common findings in women with hyperandrogenism.[93] A discussion of the clinical approach to these complex metabolic abnormalities is beyond the scope of this chapter. However, the major morbidity associated with hyperandrogenism is probably due to the accelerated atherosclerosis caused by these metabolic derangements.[94]

ACKNOWLEDGEMENT

This work was supported in part by Grant HD-24567.

REFERENCES

1. Accili D et al: A mutation in the insulin receptor gene that impairs transport of the receptor to the plasma membrane and causes insulin resistant diabetes, *EMBO J* 8:2509, 1989.
2. Adashi EY: Potential utility of gonadotropin releasing hormone agonists in the management of ovarian hyperandrogenism, *Fertil Steril* 53:765, 1990.
3. Anderson DC: Sex hormone binding globulin, *Clin Endocrinol* 3:69, 1974.
4. Andreyko JL, Monroe SE, Jaffe RB: Treatment of hirsutism with a gonadotropin releasing hormone agonist (nafarelin), *J Clin Endocrinol Metab* 63:854, 1986.
5. Axelrod LR, Goldzieher JW, Ross SD: Concurrent 3-beta-hydroxysteroid dehydrogenase deficiency in adrenal and sclerocystic ovary, *Acta Endocrinol* 48:392, 1965.
6. Azziz R, Zacur HA: 21-Hydroxylase deficiency in female hyperandrogenism: screening and diagnosis, *J Clin Endocrinol Metab* 69:577, 1989.
7. Azziz R et al: Abnormalities of 21-hydroxylase gene ratio and adrenal steroidogenesis in hyperandrogenic women with an exaggerated 17-hydroxyprogesterone response to acute adrenal stimulation, *J Clin Endocrinol Metab* 73:1327, 1991.
8. Barbieri RL: Hyperandrogenic disorders, *Clin Obstet Gynecol* 33:640, 1990.
9. Barbieri RL: Human ovarian 17-ketosteroid oxidoreductase: unique characteristics of the granulosa-luteal cell and stromal enzyme, *Am J Obstet Gynecol* 166:1117, 1992.
10. Barbieri RL, Friedman AJ, Osathanondh R: Cotinine and nicotine inhibit human fetal adrenal 11-beta-hydroxylase, *J Clin Endocrinol Metab* 69:1221, 1989.
11. Barbieri RL, Gochberg J, Ryan KJ: Nicotine, cotinine and anabasine inhibit aromatase in human trophoblast in vitro, *J Clin Invest* 77:1717, 1986.
12. Barbieri RL, Hornstein MD: Hyperinsulinemia and ovarian hyperandrogenism: cause and effect, *Endocrinol Metab Clin North Am* 17:685, 1988.
13. Barbieri RL, Ryan KJ: Hyperandrogenism, insulin resistance, acanthosis nigricans: a common endocrinopathy with unique pathophysiologic features, *Am J Obstet Gynecol* 147:90, 1983.
14. Barbieri RL, Smith S, Ryan KJ: The role of hyperinsulinemia in the pathogenesis of ovarian hyperandrogenism, *Fertil Steril* 50:197, 1988.
15. Barbieri RL et al: Insulin stimulates androgen accumulation in incubations of ovarian stroma obtained from women with hyperandrogenism, *J Clin Endocrinol Metab* 62:904, 1986.
16. Bates GW, Whitworth NS: Effect of body weight reduction on plasma androgens in obese infertile women, *Fertil Steril* 38:406, 1982.
17. Belisle S, Love EJ: Clinical efficacy and safety of cyproterone acetate in severe hirsutism: results of a multicenter Canadian study, *Fertil Steril* 46:1015, 1986.
18. Belisle S, Menard J: Adrenal androgen production in hyperprolactinemic states, *Fertil Steril* 33:396, 1980.
19. Burghen GA, Givens JR, Kitabchi AE: Correlation of hyperandrogenism with hyperinsulinemia in polycystic ovarian disease, *J Clin Endocrinol Metab* 50:113, 1980.
20. Cama A et al: A mutation in the tyrosine kinase domain of the insulin receptor associated with insulin resistance in an obese woman, *J Clin Endocrinol Metab* 73:894, 1991.
21. Carson-Jurica MA, Schrader WT, O'Malley BW: Steroid receptor family: structure and function, *Endocr Rev* 11:201, 1990.
22. Cogan PH, Antunes JL, Correl JW: Reproduction function in temporal lobe epilepsy: the effect of temporal lobectomy, *Surg Neurol* 12:243, 1979.
23. Crosby PDA, Rittmaster RS: Predictors of clinical response in hirsute women treated with spironolactone, *Fertil Steril* 55:1067, 1991.
24. Cusan L et al: Treatment of hirsutism with the pure anti-androgen flutamide, *J Am Acad Dermatol* 23:462, 1990.
25. Daly DC et al: A randomized study of dexamethasone in ovulation induction with clomiphene citrate, *Fertil Steril* 41:844, 1984.
26. Dorfman RI, Shipley RA: *Androgens,* New York, 1956, John Wiley & Sons.
27. Dunaif A: Acanthosis nigricans, insulin action and hyperandrogenism: clinical, histological and biochemical findings, *J Clin Endocrinol Metab* 73:590, 1991.

28. Ehrmann DA, Rosenfield RL: Hirsutism: beyond the steroidogenic block, *N Engl J Med* 323:909, 1990.

29. Ferriman D, Gallwey JD: Clinical assessment of body hair growth in women, *J Clin Endocrinol Metab* 21:1440, 1961.

30. Friedman AJ, Ravnikar VA, Barbieri RL: Serum steroid hormone profiles in postmenopausal smokers and nonsmokers, *Fertil Steril* 47:398, 1987.

30a. Grasinger CC, Wild RA, Parker IJ: Vulvar acanthosis nigricans: a marker for insulin resistance in hirsute women, *Fertil Steril* 59:583, 1993.

31. Haglund-Stengler R, Ritzen FM, Luthman H: 21-Hydroxylase deficiency: disease causing mutations characterized by densitometry of 21-hydroxylase specific deoxyribonucleic acid fragments, *J Clin Endocrinol Metab* 70:43, 1990.

32. Herzog AG et al: Temporal lobe epilepsy: an extra hypothalamic pathogenesis for polycystic ovary syndrome?, *Neurology* 34:1389, 1984.

33. Herzog AG et al: Reproductive endocrine disorders in women with partial seizures of temporal lobe origin, *Arch Neurol* 43:341, 1986.

34. Higuchi K et al: Prolactin has a direct effect on adrenal androgen secretion, *J Clin Endocrinol Metab* 59:714, 1984.

35. Horton R, Tait JF: Androstenedione production and interconversion rates measured in peripheral blood and studies on the possible sites of its interconversion to testosterone, *J Clin Invest* 45:301, 1966.

36. Horton R, Tait JF: In vivo conversion of dehydroepiandrosterone to plasma androstenedione and testosterone in man, *J Clin Endocrinol Metab* 27:79, 1967.

37. Hughesdon PE: Morphology and morphogenesis of the Stein Leventhal ovary and of so called "hyperthecosis," *Obstet Gynecol Surv* 37:59, 1982.

38. Ireland K, Woodruff JD: Masculinizing ovarian tumors, *Obstet Gynecol Surv* 31:83, 1976.

39. Ito R, Horton R: The source of plasma dihydrotesterone in man, *J Clin Invest* 50:1621, 1971.

40. Judd HL, Lucas WE, Yen SSC: Effect of oophorectomy on circulating testosterone and androstenedione levels in patients with endometrial cancer, *Am J Obstet Gynecol* 118:793, 1974.

41. Judd HL et al: Endocrine function of the postmenopausal ovary: concentration of androgens and estrogens in ovarian and peripheral vein blood, *J Clin Endocrinol Metab* 39:1020, 1974.

42. Kadowski T et al: Five mutant alleles of the insulin receptor gene in patients with genetic forms of insulin resistance, *J Clin Invest* 86:254, 1990.

43. Khan CR, White MF: The insulin receptor and the molecular mechanism of insulin action, *J Clin Invest* 82:1151, 1988.

44. Khaw KT, Tazuke S, Barrett-Connor E: Cigarette smoking and increased adrenal androgens in post menopausal women, *N Engl J Med* 318:1705, 1988.

45. Kirschner MA, Bardin CW: Androgen production and metabolism in normal and virilized women, *Metabolism* 21:667, 1972.

46. Kirschner MA, Jacobs JB: Combined ovarian and adrenal vein catheterization to determine the site(s) of androgen overproduction in hirsute women, *J Clin Endocrinol Metab* 33:199, 1971.

47. Lobo RA: Prolactin modulation of DHEAS secretion, *Am J Obstet Gynecol* 138:632, 1980.

48. Lobo RA et al: The effects of two doses of spironolactone on serum androgens and anagen hair in hirsute women, *Fertil Steril* 43:200, 1985.

49. Longcope C, Johnstone CC: Androgen and estrogen dynamics in pre- and postmenopausal women: a comparison between smokers and non-smokers, *J Clin Endocrinol Metab* 67:379, 1988.

50. Lubahn DB et al: Cloning of human androgen receptor complementary DNA and localization to the X chromosome, *Science* 240:327, 1988.

51. Luu-The V et al: Full length cDNA structure and deduced amino acid sequence of human 3-beta-hydroxy-5-ene steroid dehydrogenase, *Mol Endocrinol* 3:1310, 1989.

52. Madden JD et al: The effect of oral contraceptive treatment of the serum concentration of dehydroepiandrosterone sulfate, *Am J Obstet Gynecol* 132:380, 1978.

53. Mahaudeau JA, Bardin CW, Lipsett MB: The metabolic clearance rate and origin of plasma dihydrotesterone in man and its conversion to 5-alpha-androstanediol, *J Clin Invest* 50:1338, 1971.

54. Matteri RK et al: Androgen sulfate and glucuronide conjugates in non-hirsute and hirsute women with polycystic ovarian syndrome, *Am J Obstet Gynecol* 161:1704, 1989.

55. Mauvis-Jarvis P, Juttenn F, Mowszowicz I: *Hirsutism,* Berlin, 1981, Springer-Verlag.

56. McNatty KP et al: The intraovarian sites of androgen and estrogen formation in women with normal and hyperandrogenic ovaries as judged by in vitro experiments, *J Clin Endocrinol Metab* 50:755, 1980.

57. McNatty KP et al: Effects of luteinizing hormone on steroidogenesis by thecal tissue from human ovarian follicles in vitro, *Steroids* 36:53, 1980.

58. Moller DE: A naturally occurring mutation of insulin receptor A1A 1134 impairs tyrosine kinase function and is associated with dominantly inherited insulin resistance, *J Biol Chem* 265:14979, 1990.

59. Moller DE, Flier JS: Detection of an alternation in the insulin receptor gene in a patient with insulin resistance, acanthosis nigricans and the polycystic ovary syndrome, *N Engl J Med* 319:1526, 1988.

60. Nagamani M, Dinh TV, Kelver ME: Hyperinsulinemia in hyperthecosis of the ovaries, *Am J Obstet Gynecol* 154:384, 1986.

61. Nagamani M et al: Ovarian steroid secretion in postmenopausal women with and without endometrial cancer, *J Clin Endocrinol Metab* 62:508, 1986.

62. Nilsson B et al: Free testosterone levels during danazol therapy, *Fertil Steril* 39:505, 1983.

63. O'Brien RC et al: Comparison of sequential cyproterone acetate/estrogen versus spironolactone/oral contraceptive in the treatment of hirsutism, *J Clin Endocrinol Metab* 72:1008, 1991.

64. Owerbach D, Crawford YM, Draznin MR: Direct analysis of CYP21B genes in 21-hydroxylase deficiency using polymerase chain reaction amplification, *Mol Endocrinol* 4:125, 1990.

65. Pang S et al: Prenatal treatment of congenital adrenal hyperplasia due to 21-hydroxylase deficiency, *N Engl J Med* 322:111, 1990.

66. Parker LN, Chang S, Odell WD: Adrenal androgens in patients with chronic marked elevation of prolactin, *Clin Endocrinol* 8:1, 1978.

67. Pasquali R et al: Clinical and hormonal characteristics of obese and amenorrheic hyperandrogenic women before and after weight loss, *J Clin Endocrinol Metab* 68:173, 1989.

68. Paulson RJ et al: Measurements of 3-alpha, 17-beta-androstanediol glucuronide in serum and urine and the correlation with skin 5-alpha-reductase activity, *Fertil Steril* 36:222, 1981.

69. Pepper G, Brenner SH, Gabrilove JL: Ketoconazole used in the treatment of ovarian hyperandrogenism, *Fertil Steril* 54:438, 1990.

70. Pochi PE, Strauss JS: Endocrinologic control of the development and activity of the human sebaceous gland, *J Invest Dermatol* 62:191, 1974.

71. Poretsky L: On the paradox of insulin induced hyperandrogenism in insulin resistant states, *Endocr Rev* 12:3, 1991.

72. Raj GS et al: Normalization of testosterone levels using low estrogen containing oral contraceptive in women with polycystic ovary syndrome, *Obstet Gynecol* 60:15, 1982.

73. Rheaume E et al: Structure and expression of a new complementary DNA encoding the almost exclusive 3-beta-hydroxysteroid dehydrogenase-isomerase in human adrenals and gonads, *Mol Endocrinol* 5:1147, 1991.

74. Rittmaster RS: Differential suppression of testosterone and estradiol in hirsute women with the superactive gonadotropin releasing hormone agonist leuprolide, *J Clin Endocrinol Metab* 67:651, 1988.

75. Rittmaster RS, Loriaux DL, Cutler GB: Sensitivity of cortisol and adrenal androgens to dexamethasone suppression in hirsute women, *J Clin Endocrinol Metab* 81:462, 1985.

76. Rosenfield RL: Studies of the relation of plasma androgen levels to androgen action in women, *J Steroid Biochem* 6:695, 1975.

77. Rosenfield RL et al: Pubertal presentation of congenital 3-beta-hydroxysteroid dehydrogenase deficiency, *J Clin Endocrinol Metab* 51:345, 1980.

78. Ryan KJ, Smith OW: Biogenesis of steroid hormones in the human ovary, *Recent Prog Horm Res* 21:367, 1965.

79. Schiebinger RJ et al: The effect of serum prolactin on plasma adrenal androgens and the production and metabolic clearance rate of dehydroepiandrosterone sulfate in normal and hyperprolactinemic subjects, *J Clin Endocrinol Metab* 62:202, 1986.

80. Schuler LA et al: Regulation of de novo biosynthesis of cholesterol and progestins and formation of cholesterol ester in rat corpus luteum by exogenous sterol, *J Biol Chem* 254:8662, 1979.

81. Serafini P, Aflan R, Lobo RA: 5-Alpha-reductase activity in the genital skin of hirsute women, *J Clin Endocrinol Metab* 60:349, 1985.

82. Shimada F et al: Insulin-resistant diabetes associated with partial deletion of the insulin receptor gene, *Lancet* 335:1179, 1990.

83. Siegel SF et al: Adrenocorticotropic hormone stimulation tests and plasma dehydroepiandrosterone sulfate levels in women with hirsutism, *N Engl J Med* 323:849, 1990.

84. Smith S, Ravnikar VA, Barbieri RL: Androgen and insulin response to an oral glucose challenge in hyperandrogenic women, *Fertil Steril* 48:72, 1987.

85. Speiser PW et al: First trimester prenatal treatment and molecular genetic diagnosis of congenital adrenal hyperplasia, *J Clin Endocrinol Metab* 70:838, 1990.

86. Spritzer P et al: Cyproterone acetate versus hydrocortisone treatment in late onset adrenal hyperplasia, *J Clin Endocrinol Metab* 70:642, 1990.

87. Taira M et al: Human diabetes associated with a deletion of the tyrosine kinase domain of the insulin receptor, *Science* 245:63, 1989.

88. Tureck RW, Strauss JF III: Progesterone synthesis by luteinized human granulosa cells in culture: the role of de novo sterol synthesis and lipoprotein-carried sterol, *J Clin Endocrinol Metab* 54:367, 1982.

89. Venturoli et al: Ketoconazole therapy for women with acne and/or hirsutism, *J Clin Endocrinol Metab* 71:335, 1990.

90. Vermeulen A, Ando S: Metabolic clearance rate and interconversion of androgens and the influence of the free androgen fraction, *J Clin Endocrinol Metab* 48:320, 1979.

91. Vermeulen A, Stoica T, Verdonck L: The apparent free testosterone concentration and index of androgenicity, *J Clin Endocrinol Metab* 33:759, 1971.

92. Wentz WB: Progestin therapy in endometrial hyperplasia, *Gynecol Oncol* 2:362, 1974.

93. Wild RA et al: Lipoprotein lipid concentrations and cardiovascular risk in women with polycystic ovary syndrome. *J Clin Endocrinol Metab* 61:946, 1985.

94. Wild RA et al: Clinical signs of androgen excess as risk factors for coronary artery disease, *Fertil Steril* 54:255, 1990.

95. Wortsman J: Glycosaminoglycan deposition in the acanthosis nigricans lesion of the polycystic ovary syndrome, *Arch Intern Med* 143:1145, 1983.

96. Yoshimasa Y: Insulin-resistant diabetes due to a point mutation that prevents insulin proreceptor processing, *Science* 240:784, 1988.

Chapter 11

POLYCYSTIC OVARY SYNDROME

Ricardo Azziz, M.D.
and Howard A. Zacur, M.D., Ph.D.

Definition
Clinical and pathological features
    Hypothalamic-pituitary-ovarian axis disturbance
    Intrinsic ovarian abnormalities
    Obesity and polycystic ovary syndrome (PCOS)
    Insulin homeostasis in PCOS
    Adrenocortical dysfunction in PCOS
Long-term consequences of PCOS
    Obesity
    Diabetes mellitus
    Hypertension
    Lipid abnormalities and coronary artery disease
    Malignancy
    Increased bone mass
Therapy of PCOS
    Weight loss
    Ovulation induction
    Treatment of hirsutism
    Treatment of dysfunctional uterine bleeding
    Surgical therapy of PCOS
    Future treatments

In 1935, Stein and Leventhal described a condition of amenorrhea associated with bilateral polycystic ovaries in seven obese women who, in some instances, were also hirsute.[190] Cyst formation within the ovary was defined by these authors as "sufficient enlargement . . . to make it visible to the naked eye." Excessive, persistent, and progressive development of these cysts were believed by these authors to cause the ovary to become enlarged, adversely affecting ovarian function. Although the existence of sclerocystic ovaries was described some 100 years before 1932,[88] the term *Stein-Leventhal syndrome* was soon used to characterize all obese women with hirsutism, menstrual-cycle irregularity, and enlarged cystic ovaries.

The patients described by Stein and Leventhal appear to represent a select subset of the disorder that is defined as *polycystic ovary syndrome* (*PCOS*). The terms *polycystic ovarian disease* (*PCOD*) or *hyperandrogenic chronic anovulatory syndrome* have also been used, although it may be preferable to describe this disorder as *functional ovarian hyperandrogenism*. Clinicians unfamiliar with this disorder often describe the PCOS patient as obese, hirsute, oligomenorrheic, with a serum immunoreactive luteinizing hormone (LH) to follicle-stimulating hormone (FSH) ratio greater than 2:1 or 3:1, and with enlarged multicystic ovaries found upon surgery or sonography. Yet, as reported by Goldzieher and Green, it is quite clear that patients with this disorder are heterogeneous, and not all patients with polycystic ovaries have all the signs of the syndrome[43, 86] (Table 11-1).

DEFINITION

Defining PCOS is currently quite complicated. A syndrome is defined as a constellation of symptoms and signs that characterize a particular abnormality. Unfortunately, the clinical features of PCOS are variable and not ubiquitous. Furthermore, there appear to be several possible etiologies for the signs and symptoms observed in patients

Table 11-1. Signs and symptoms of patients with polycystic ovaries

Observation	Number of cases	Average incidence (%)	Range (%)
Infertility	296	75	35-94
Hirsutism	457	56	17-83
Amenorrhea	350	47	19-77
Obesity	344	33	16-49
Regular menses	253	16	7-28
Virilization	204	17	0-28

Modified from Goldzieher JW and Green JA: The polycystic ovary: clinical and histologic features, *J Clin Endocrinol Metab* 22:325, 1962.

with PCOS. Initially, it may be best to define PCOS by what it is not. It is clear that patients with adrenal or ovarian androgen-producing tumors, Cushing syndrome, hyperprolactinemia, and nonclassic (late-onset) adrenocortical deficiencies may present with hirsutism, acne, obesity, oligoamenorrhea, and polycystic ovaries. Considering these disorders, the diagnosis of PCOS becomes a diagnosis of exclusion.

As previously discussed, major clinical components of PCOS include oligoanovulation, polycystic ovaries, hirsutism, and obesity. Each of these aspects of the syndrome are discussed in more detail later in this chapter. Nevertheless, not all patients with PCOS demonstrate hirsutism,[86, 103, 121, 129] and those who do rarely present with virilization. With the syndrome defined endocrinologically or by ovarian pathology, approximately 60% of these patients are not obese and approximately 15% have regular menses.[86]

Pathologically, the ovarian cortex in patients with PCOS generally contains multiple intermediate sized (2-6 mm in diameter) and atretic follicles, giving the gonad its "polycystic" appearance. However, not all patients with the endocrinologically or clinically defined PCOS demonstrate polycystic ovaries, nor are all polycystic ovaries diagnostic for PCOS (Fig. 11-1).[64, 149, 162, 195]

In fact the presence of polycystic ovaries may be a clinical sign suggestive of the disorder, but is not diagnostic.[84] Recently, ultrasonography has been used to establish the presence of polycystic ovaries, defined as ovaries that are enlarged, possessing more than 10 follicles measuring between 2-8 mm in diameter, and demonstrating increased ovarian stroma.[1, 74, 151, 195] The ovarian size can be determined sonographically either by calculating the ovarian volume (ovarian volume = length × height × width × 0.5),

or by determining the cross-sectional area (cross-sectional area = length × width × π/4) (Fig. 11-2).

Nonetheless, patients with all the clinical stigmata of the syndrome have been found at surgery to have ovaries described as normal.[184] Some patients clinically identified as having PCOS also have not been found to have polycystic ovaries by sonographic criteria.[74] Furthermore, up to 40% of women suffering from inherited nonclassic adrenal hyperplasia also demonstrate polycystic ovaries upon ultrasound.[17] Conversely, normal women having regular menstrual cycles and no other stigmata of PCOS have been found to have polycystic ovaries by ultrasound. In fact, polycystic ovaries diagnosed by ultrasound have been reported in as many as 22% of women who otherwise considered themselves to be normal.[41, 162] This rate seems high when contrasted with autopsy data. For example, in one series of 740 autopsies performed consecutively in unselected women of all ages, bilateral polycystic ovaries were found in 26 individuals for a rate of only 3.5%.[186]

Signs and symptoms of the disorder most often appear at or shortly after puberty[166] and may even result in primary amenorrhea.[33, 189] In fact, one convincing sign of PCOS is a history of irregular menses since menarche. Zumoff et al. detected an abnormal LH hormonal profile in pubertal girls who went on to develop PCOS.[215] In his study, girls who experienced regular menses following puberty demonstrated LH elevations at night during early puberty, whereas girls with irregular menses since puberty, and who were later diagnosed with PCOS, demonstrated their LH elevations during the day. Although developing PCOS later in life appears to be unlikely, many young patients may demonstrate subtle signs or symptoms of the disorder, which is progressive. Some women with PCOS and regular menstrual cycles may eventually become anovulatory and pro-

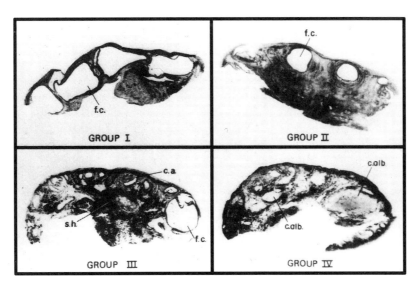

Fig. 11-1. The spectrum of histologic findings in polycystic ovary syndrome: f.c. refers to follicular cysts; s.h. to stromal hyperplasia; c.a. to corpora albicantia. (From Givens JR: *Sem Reprod Endocrinol* 2:271.)

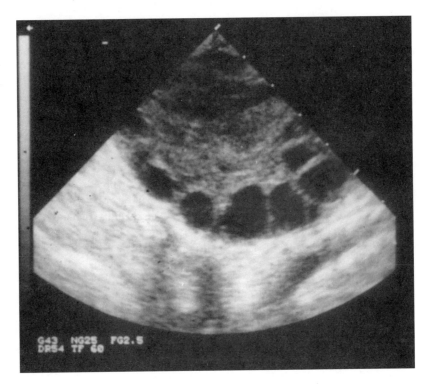

Fig. 11-2. Typical transvaginal sonographic appearance of a polycystic ovary (courtesy of Dr. Michael P. Steinkampf, The University of Alabama at Birmingham).

gressively hyperandrogenemic, particularly if they have gained a large amount of weight. For these women, a return to cyclic menstruation may be possible following weight loss.

Use of biochemical criteria as a means of diagnosing women with PCOS has also produced contradictory data. Endocrinologically, patients with PCOS usually demonstrate elevated circulating levels of free testosterone and lower levels of sex hormone-binding globulin (SHBG), accompanied by variable increases in total testosterone and androstenedione.[125, 174, 201] Approximately 50% of patients with PCOS also demonstrate an elevated dehydroepi-androsterone sulfate (DHEAS) level, although it is rarely above 6000 ng/ml (Fig. 11-3).[101] Although some patients with the disorder have been reported to have normal testosterone and androstenedione levels,[196] single androgen measurements may not be sufficient to identify androgen excess. In fact, hirsutism is better correlated with the production rate of these androgens, rather than with their isolated circulating values.[114, 115] The prolactin level is usually normal, although occasional PCOS patients may demonstrate mild elevations in the level of this hormone, but generally less than 80 ng/ml (depending on the assay), without apparent cause.[35, 123] The LH to FSH ratio is 3:1 or greater[111, 198, 209] in approximately 60% of these patients, although in some patients with PCOS the gonadotropin levels and ratios are normal (Fig. 11-4).[167] In addition measurements of single LH and FSH levels may fail to demonstrate the expected ratio due to the inherent pulsatility of these hormones, or to assay variation.

In general, PCOS can be viewed as a heterogeneous disorder in which ovarian, and possible adrenal, androgen excess is present. The etiology of the disorder remains unknown, but PCOS may result from a hypothalamic-pituitary-adrenal-ovarian axis dysfunction present at or before puberty. Hyperandrogenism in these patients results in the development of a combination of signs and symptoms, including acne, hirsutism, oligoamenorrhea, and possibly, abdominal obesity. Because some PCOS patients demonstrate hyperinsulinemia and insulin resistance, several investigators have suggested separating this disorder into two subsets.[7, 185] One group consists of patients with elevated LH and normal insulin levels, and who are usually not obese. A second group includes subjects with marked hyperinsulinemia and normal LH levels. These patients are more commonly obese and often demonstrate clinically or microscopically evident acanthosis nigricans.

Unfortunately, establishing a strict definition of the syndrome is not possible nor advisable at the present time. However, in spite of the clinical and endocrinologic ambiguities, patients with this disorder are readily recognized.

CLINICAL AND PATHOLOGICAL FEATURES
Hypothalamic-pituitary-ovarian axis disturbance

Absence of regular ovulation results in irregular menstrual-cycle intervals, amenorrhea, or dysfunctional uterine bleeding (DUB); these are prominent features of the patient with PCOS. The cause of irregular or absent ovulation in patients with PCOS remains unclear. Hypothalamic

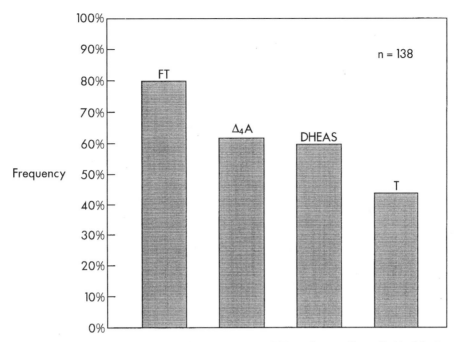

Fig. 11-3. The frequency with which free testosterone (FT), androstenedione (Δ_4A), dehydroepiandrosterone sulfate (DHEAS), and testosterone (T) were above normal in 138 women thought to have hyperandrogenism. (From Wild RA et al: *Am J Obstet Gynecol* 146:602, 1983.)

dysfunction manifested by an increased GnRH pulse frequency and amplitude, resulting in disordered gonadotropin release with a persistent elevation in LH in preference to FSH, has been suggested as one cause. This dysfunction may be the result of a primary and intrinsic disturbance of the hypothalamus, or may simply reflect the impact of an abnormality in peripheral stimulation.

While Stein and Leventhal theorized that an intraovarian defect results in mechanical crowding of follicle cysts, and interferes with normal maturation, they noted that the ovarian changes also may result from abnormal hormonal stimulation by the pituitary gland. Support for this latter thesis was presented by McArthur et al. in 1958. These investigators measured the levels of LH and FSH hormones in the urine of women with menstrual-cycle disturbances by bioassay, and concluded that the excretion of one or more of these gonadotropic hormones was abnormal in women with the Stein-Leventhal syndrome.[128] When specific serum radioimmunoassays for LH and FSH were later developed, Yen et al., in 1970, studied 16 patients with polycystic ovaries and demonstrated that the mean circulating LH concentrations are consistently higher than the mean FSH values. This finding is consistent with the hypothesis that a hypothalamic-pituitary disturbance in gonadotropin secretion is present in these patients.[209]

Initially it was suggested that the abnormal gonadotropin profile results from an increased amplitude in the hypothalamic GnRH pulses, a hormone stimulating the secretion of LH and FSH, rather than as a result of an increase in pulse frequency.[167] However, this hypothesis was not confirmed

in later studies, as increases in both LH-pulse frequency and amplitude were observed in these patients,[74, 112, 204] which suggests similar changes in GnRH-pulse characteristics. Differences in the assays used to measure circulating LH concentrations have been suggested as a possible source of the discrepancy in these study results. Imse et al. used five different assay systems (including immunoassays and a bioassay) to measure serum LH in PCOS patients, and while significant differences between bioassay and immunoassay measurements of this gonadotropin were documented, these investigators still concluded that both LH-pulse frequency and amplitude were increased in their PCOS patients.[107]

The intrahypothalamic regulation of GnRH release is mediated in part by catecholamines and opiates (see Chapter 3). A deficiency in hypothalamic dopaminergic activity and/or opioid tone has been suggested in women with PCOS.[46, 164] Because inhibition of hypothalamic GnRH release is believed to be mediated by opiates and the catecholamine, dopamine, an increase in GnRH release would be expected to be seen with lowered opioid tone. Nevertheless, when the serum concentration of one prominent opioid, β-endorphin, was measured in women with PCOS, it was found to be above, not below, normal.[3, 83, 208] However, the elevated circulating levels of this opiate may not solely reflect central nervous system (CNS) activity, but also peripheral secretion. The pancreas may be a likely source of extra CNS secretion because increased serum opioid levels have been noted following oral glucose ingestion.[37] Other investigators have concluded that no major alterations exist in central dopamine or opioid tone to account for the disordered gonadotropin profile seen in patients with PCOS.[21, 22]

As opposed to a primary disturbance within the hypothalamus, gonadotropin changes seen in this syndrome may reflect the response of the CNS to peripheral hormonal events, including androgen and estrogen excess, hyperprolactinemia, and inhibin deficiency. Yen has suggested that the discordant levels of LH and FSH seen in PCOS patients results from the priming of the hypothalamic-pituitary axis by the chronically elevated circulating estrogen levels frequently seen in this disorder.[211] In support of this hypothesis, increased release of LH after GnRH administration has been reported in some healthy women and in some women with PCOS given estrogen exogenously.[18, 180] In addition, a correlation between circulating estrone levels, but not estradiol, with the pulsatile LH release has been reported in hyperandrogenic, chronically anovulatory women.[89] Alternatively, the hypothalamic-pituitary axis of PCOS patients may escape negative inhibition by sex steroids, and the increased frequency and amplitude of LH pulses noted in PCOS patients may result from the inability of estradiol and progesterone to slow the pulsatile release of GnRH.[91]

Furthermore, because androgens are aromatized to estrogens within the CNS[137] and elsewhere, it has also been suggested that the increased estrogen stimulation of the hypothalamic-pituitary axis in PCOS may be the result of increased CNS aromatization of androgens. Surprisingly, no changes in LH levels were observed in normal women receiving testosterone implants.[51] In addition, other studies have failed to demonstrate an impact of an intravenous testosterone infusion in women with PCOS,[56] or the administration of an antiandrogen to normal women or patients with PCOS[45] on LH release. These findings, in addition to those studies noting that the administration of exogenous dihydrotestosterone (DHT) to normal women actually suppressed LH-pulse frequency,[200] suggest that androgens do not result directly in the hypothalamic-pituitary dysfunction noted in PCOS.

Prolactin is a pituitary hormone known to stimulate the release of hypothalamic dopamine.[80] This catecholamine is believed to suppress LH levels (see Chapter 3), thus one would predict that the LH level would be low in the presence of hyperprolactinemia. Since the incidence of hyperprolactinemia in PCOS patients is not greater than that of the general population[212] disordered prolactin release seems unlikely to cause the gonadotrophic dysfunction noted in this disorder.

Inhibin, a glycoprotein hormone secreted by the granulosa cells of ovarian follicles, can inhibit pituitary FSH secretion. Release of excessive ovarian inhibin could explain the lower levels of FSH, relative to those of LH, in patients with PCOS. When circulating serum inhibin levels have been measured, no differences were found between normal women and patients with PCOS.[28, 70]

Intrinsic ovarian abnormalities

Distinctive differences between the ovaries of women with eumenorrhea and the ovaries of women with PCOS have been observed since 1845.[88] Hughesden histologically evaluated ovarian sections taken at the time of wedge biopsies in patients with PCOS (n = 34) with ovarian sections taken from age-matched controls (n = 30).[106] Compared with the control ovaries, polycystic ovaries had twice the cross-sectional area; contained twice as many developing and atretic follicles; had a tunica albuginea that was 50% thicker; had a five-fold increase in subcortical stroma thickness; and demonstrated a four-fold increase in ovarian hilar cell nests.

For many years, there has been debate over whether the histological changes observed in the ovaries of PCOS patients represent an underlying disturbance within the ovary, or whether they simply reflect the impact of extraovarian factors. Stein and Leventhal initially postulated that an intraovarian defect results in mechanical crowding of the follicle cysts, interfering with normal maturation. Polycystic ovaries may be created de novo, however, as a result of exogenous androgen administration[4, 79, 150, 188] or secondarily to inherited adrenal androgen excess.[17] Abnormal follicle maturation or acceleration of follicular atresia has been reported in the presence of elevated intraovarian androgen levels.[66, 163] Therefore, intraovarian androgen excess resulting from either circulating hyperandrogenemia or an abnormality in ovarian steroidogenesis, may result in abnormal follicular development and a "polycystic" ovary.

A deficiency in the activity of aromatase was one of the earliest postulated intraovarian disturbances in steroidogenesis thought to cause PCOS.[181] Testosterone and androstenedione are converted to estradiol and estrone, respectively, by granulosa cell aromatase, and a decrease in the activity of this enzyme could be expected to result in increased ovarian androgen production. Granulosa cells taken from polycystic ovaries possess a relative lack of basal aromatase activity in comparison to control ovaries. However, ovaries from PCOS patients have similar levels of aromatase activity when stimulated by FSH compared with controls.[65] Thus, low intrafollicular FSH levels, rather than a constitutive ovarian defect, may account for the earlier experimental findings noting an aromatase deficiency in PCOS.

Most recently, it has been suggested that increased ovarian androgen production in women with PCOS results from "dysregulation" of the 17α-hydroxylase/17,20-lyase (desmolase) enzyme.[23, 62, 175] This cytochrome enzyme complex, known as P450c17α, converts the Δ^5 steroid pregnenolone to 17-hydroxypregnenolone, and then to dehydroepiandrosterone (DHEA) (Fig. 11-5). It also converts

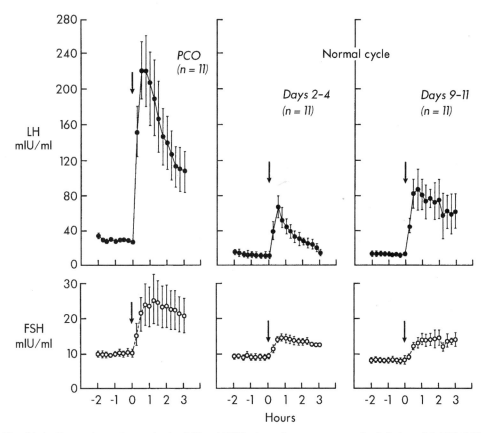

Fig. 11-4. Comparison of quantitative LH and FSH release in response to a single bolus of GnRH (150 μg) in polycystic ovary (PCO) syndrome patients and normal women during the early and late follicular phases of their menstrual cycle. Mean ± standard error are depicted. (From Rebar R et al: *J Clin Invest* 57:1320, 57:1320, 1976).

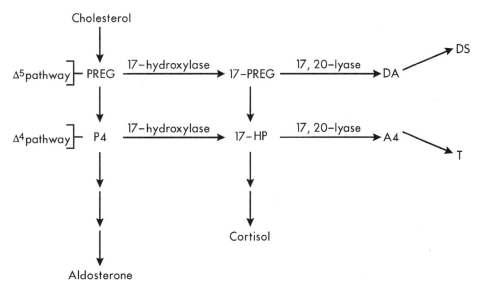

Fig. 11-5. Scheme of the adrenocortical steroidogenic cascade, highlighting the principal actions of 17-hydroxylase and 17,20-lyase. Both enzymatic activities are the product of a single enzyme, cytochrome P450c17α. Abbreviations are as follows: PREG, pregnenolone; 17-HPREG, 17-hydroxypregnenolone; P4, progesterone; 17-HP, 17-hydroprogesterone; DA, dehydroepiandrosterone; and A4, androstenedione.

the Δ^4 steroid progesterone to 17α-hydroxyprogesterone (17-OHP) and then to androstenedione. Barnes et al. suggest that the activities of both 17-hydroxylase and 17,20-lyase are increased in functional ovarian hyperandrogenism, but that the 17,20-lyase activity is increased to a lesser degree than 17-hydroxylase. The dysregulation in P450c17α activity was detected after acute endogenous LH release following GnRH agonist administration in women with PCOS and in normal males (Fig. 11-6).[23] Although the proposed 17-hydroxylase/17,20-lyase dysregulation appears to result in an increased production of 17-OHP, it is still unclear how the observed abnormality in steroidogenesis results in androgen excess.

The described dysregulation in P450c17α activity may result from desensitization of LH receptors within the ovary due to the chronic circulating LH excess.[175] Dysregulation of this enzyme may also arise through amplification of the action of LH by insulin or insulin-like growth factors (IGFs).[34] Alternatively, an unidentified cause for this dysregulatory process may exist, perhaps involving the active site of the enzyme. For example, it has been shown recently that serine, an amino acid found in putative residue 106 of the cytochrome p450c17α protein, is located at the enzyme's active site and may affect 17α-hydroxylase and 17,20-lyase activity.[120] Alteration of this and/or other key amino acids by genetic or acquired means could account for the dysregulation of p450c17α activity in PCOS patients. Clustering of polycystic ovarian cases within families,[96]

and linkage of some cases of PCOS with the inheritance of human leucocyte antigens,[146] suggests a genetic basis for the disorder.

Nonetheless, not all data support the concept of an inherited defect of cytochrome P450c17α action in PCOS. Although the same enzyme is involved in both ovarian and adrenal steroidogenesis, concordance between 17α-hydroxylase/17,20-lyase "dysregulation" detected in the ovary and the adrenal cortex appears to be poor.[62] Furthermore, we studied the adrenal response to acute ACTH (1–24) in 92 consecutive women with hirsutism and/or hyperandrogenic oligomenorrhea, and our findings suggested that 17α-hydroxylase/17,20-lyase dysregulation was an infrequent cause of adrenocortical hyperandrogenism in these women.[14] In fact the endocrine findings in this population most likely represented a generalized alteration of adrenocortical control or biosynthesis since 17α-hydroxylase precursors were also increased following ACTH stimulation. These data suggest that the abnormality observed by Barnes and colleagues[23] may not arise from an inherited defect of cytochrome P450c17α.

Obesity and PCOS

Obesity is the presence of excess body fat, a definition that requires a measurement of adiposity. Alternatively, *overweightness* denotes a body weight above some reference weight. The deviation of body weight in relationship to an arbitrary standard is referred to as *relative weight.*

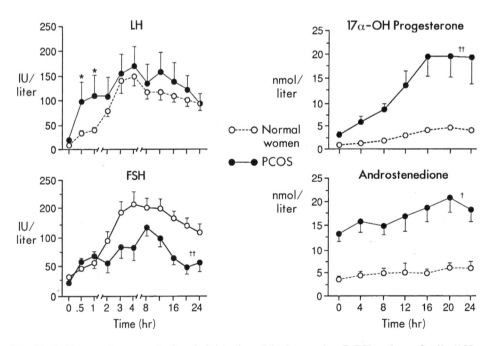

Fig. 11-6. Hormonal response to the administration of the long-acting GnRH analog nafarelin (100 υg subcutaneous) in nine normal women and five women with polycystic ovary syndrome (PCOS) after pretreatment with dexamethasone 2 mg/day for 4 days. An asterisk (*) indicates a P value of < 0.05 for comparison with the response of normal women. Two daggers (‡) indicates a P value of < 0.01, and one dagger (†) a P value of < 0.02 for comparison with the response of normal women. Depicted are the mean values ± standard error. (From Barnes et al: *N Engl J Med* 320:559, 1989.)

Excess body fat and overweightness do not necessarily correlate; this relationship is determined by variations in body build and muscle mass. The prevalence of obesity in a population entirely depends on the criteria used because the degree of adiposity represents a continuum. If a body weight above 20% of ideal body weight (IBW) is considered the lower end of obesity (using the 1959 Metropolitan Life Insurance Company standards) 40%, 46%, and 45% of women aged 40 to 49, 50 to 59, and 60 to 69 years are defined as obese, respectively.[75] If obesity is arbitrarily defined as a body mass index (BMI) over 30 kg/m^2, only 12% of females in the United States are considered obese.[26] Unfortunately, the proportion of obese women in the United States is steadily increasing.[97]

Bayer reported in 1939 that increased body weight and decreased glucose tolerance are associated with the frequency of menstrual disturbances.[25] Rogers and Mitchell noted that, of 100 patients with menstrual disorders, 43 were more than 20% overweight.[172] In a control group of eumenorrheic women, the incidence of obesity was only 13%. The association of corpulence and ovulatory disturbances has been confirmed in subsequent reports.[42, 139] The relationship between excess body fat and ovulatory disturbances appears to be strongest for early-onset obesity. Hartz et al. noted that the incidence of teenage obesity is greater among nulligravida, married women than for previously pregnant married females.[99] In this study, teenage obesity was also more frequent among women undergoing surgery for polycystic ovaries than for those having ovarian surgery for other reasons. In another report, 96% of women with the onset of obesity after menarche reported normal menses, as compared to 69% of women with a premenarchal onset of excess weight.[76] Alternatively, Combes et al. reported that juvenile-onset obesity is less likely to be associated with later menstrual disorders (31%) when compared with pubertal or adult-onset obesity (53% and 51%, respectively).[42] The relationship of peripubertal obesity and oligoovulation has been stressed by other investigators.[210]

Obesity has been associated with PCOS since the syndrome was initially described by Stein and Leventhal. In a review of the world literature of the time, Goldzieher and Axelrod noted that the incidence of obesity among patients with PCOS, diagnosed by ovarian pathology, ranged from 16-49%.[87] Goldzieher and Green reported from their study that, of 39 patients with surgically proven PCOS, at least half had a body weight within normal limits.[86] Raj et al. observed that 63% of 37 PCOS patients were non-obese.[165] In this study, the diagnosis of PCOS was non-established by a characteristic ovarian pathology associated with oligomenorrhea and other androgenic signs and symptoms. Shou-Qing et al. defined PCOS as the presence of menstrual disturbances in the face of an elevated LH to FSH ratio.[182] Of 87 patients, 75 (86%) demonstrated hirsutism and 22% were obese.

Overall, 20-50% of patients with PCOS are defined as obese; the incidence varies depending on the criteria used to define overweightness. However, the frequency of obesity among PCOS patients may not be much higher than in the general population of the United States, where obesity is defined as 20% above IBW (see above). Furthermore, the ovarian changes observed in women with morbid obesity do not appear to be similar to the pathological findings in PCOS[73] or to those seen following long-term androgen treatment.[4] These data suggest that while there is a relationship between obesity and anovulation, PCOS and obesity-related oligoovulation are not identical.

It is unclear whether obesity follows or precedes the development of hyperandrogenism. Patients with PCOS have more androgens available for peripheral aromatization, which can result in higher estrone and estradiol levels. Roncari and Van have noted that 17β-estradiol promotes human lipocyte replication in vitro.[173] Other investigators have noted that testosterone administration increases body weight in female rats.[177] It also increases food intake in oophorectomized animals, although a change in food intake is necessary for an increase in body weight. Thus, while obesity appears to predispose to the development of PCOS, the development of hyperandrogenemia may in turn encourage or aggravate overweightness.

Comparing obese and nonobese PCOS patients, many investigators have noted that circulating total testosterone, androstenedione, and DHEAS levels are not significantly different.[118, 126, 159, 178] Nevertheless, obese patients with PCOS have lower SHBG levels than their nonobese counterparts. Decreased SHBG levels lead to increased unbound and albumin-bound testosterone.[118, 126, 178] Furthermore, Hosseinian et al. observed that subjects with obesity and oligomenorrhea often had depressed SHBG levels, even in the absence of hirsutism.[103] In their patients, androgen levels were higher in obese oligomenorrheic women with mild hirsutism than in severely hirsute women who were not obese. These investigators suggest that obesity in hyperandrogenism may offer a slight protection against the development of hirsutism, and androgen excess should be suspected in oligomenorrheic obese women, even in the absence of hirsutism.

Laatikainen et al. studied the pattern of gonadotropin secretion in obese and nonobese patients with PCOS by sampling every 15 minutes for six hours.[118] These investigators noted that, in obese women, the mean LH levels were less elevated and pulse amplitudes were smaller than in nonobese women. Paradisi et al. also studied the gonadotropin secretion of PCOS patients and noted similar findings.[151] Furthermore, the LH response to GnRH stimulation was significantly less in obese PCOS patients than in nonobese PCOS women. No differences were found in the FSH response.

Some authors have suggested that increased estrone levels, resulting from increased peripheral aromatization of androgens, play a role in the amenorrhea of obese subjects.[122] However, comparisons between obese and non-obese patients with PCOS have not revealed any significant differences in circulating estrone or estradiol levels.[118, 160]

It is clear that weight loss re-establishes normal menstrual cycles in some obese oligoovulatory women. In the study by Mitchell and Rogers, there was no clear correlation between the amount of weight lost and the return of menses.[132] In another study, 13 obese, anovulatory women who experienced a reduction in body weight of more than 15% resumed regular menstrual function.[24] Ten of these women (77%) became pregnant without additional therapy. These observations have been confirmed by others.[98] Pasquali et al. studied the clinical and hormonal response to weight loss of 20 obese, amenorrheic, hyperandrogenic women.[156] Eight (40%) had significantly improved menstrual cyclicity. Hirsutism improved significantly in more than half of these women. The investigators concluded that weight loss is beneficial in all obese hyperandrogenic women, regardless of the presence of polycystic ovaries, the degree of hyperandrogenism, and the degree or distribution of obesity.

More important than the presence of overall obesity is the regional distribution of adiposity. Female adiposity occurs predominantly in the gluteal/femoral region, in contrast with the abdominal obesity preponderant in men. In women, abdominal obesity appears to be associated with the degree of androgenicity. Women with androgen excess have a higher mean waist-hip ratio (WHR) than euandrogenic controls. Plasma testosterone levels in PCOS are directly correlated with the WHR, but not obesity.[68] In premenopausal women a decrease in circulating SHBG and/or an increase in free testosterone is associated with an increasing WHR, independent of obesity level.[67, 116] Furthermore, SHBG and free testosterone are positively correlated with the size of abdominal, but not femoral, adipocytes.[67] Kirshner and colleagues observed that premenopausal women with upper body obesity had lower SHBG and higher total and free testosterone and estradiol levels, compared with women with lower body obesity (Fig. 11-7). Women with upper body obesity also had higher testosterone and DHT production rates.

In this study there was a significant correlation between the size of the adipocytes, various measures of androgenicity, and the insulin response to glucose loading,[67] which suggests that the distribution of fat in obese females (abdominal vs femoral) may hinge on the interactions of androgens and insulin.

Insulin homeostasis in PCOS

Although increased LH-dependent ovarian androgen production has been associated with PCOS, bioactive LH alone cannot account for the enhanced ovarian androgen production observed in this condition.[7, 52] By using potent analogues of GnRH (GnRHa) to suppress pituitary LH-

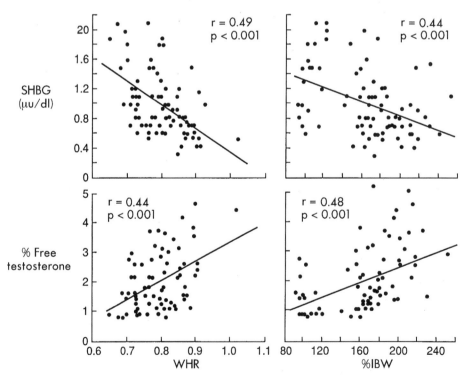

Fig. 11-7. Relationship of body fat topography and obesity level to sex hormone binding globulin (SHBG) and % free testosterone in 80 premenopausal women. (From Evans DJ et al: *J Clin Endocrinol Metab* 57:304, 1983.)

dependent ovarian androgen production, it has been demonstrated that markedly higher ratios of both serum testosterone and androstenedione to bioactive LH are observed in PCOS.[32, 52, 197] Additionally, enhanced ovarian testosterone production per unit of bioactive LH is observed in subjects with PCOS.[32] These findings suggest that some women with PCOS may have additional trophic factor(s) that potentiate LH-induced thecal and stroma cell androgen production, in particular insulin and its related growth factors.[19, 20, 109, 197]

Insulin resistance in women with PCOS is a well-recognized phenomenon (Fig. 11-8).[29, 38] The prevalence of insulin resistance in these women is comparable in the United States, Italy, and Japan.[36] Both hyperinsulinemia and insulin resistance have been reported in women with PCOS, regardless of weight.[31, 38, 58, 109] Although severe insulin resistance secondary to defects in insulin-receptor or postreceptor action has been reported in individuals with the HAIRAN syndrome (see Chapter 10), the cause of the more mild form of insulin resistance found in PCOS is less well explained. It is unclear whether the hyperinsulinemia observed in many subjects with PCOS is secondary to enhanced pancreatic insulin secretion, reduced catabolism, defective target-cell action, or a combination of these or other factors. However, it appears that insulin resistance in nonobese hyperandrogenic women is due to peripheral rather than hepatic resistance to insulin action,[157] and is associated with higher basal insulin-secretory rates.[148] De-

fects in insulin-signal transduction between the receptor kinase and glucose transport have been postulated as the mechanism of insulin resistance observed in some patients.[40] Defects in insulin signal transduction between the receptor kinase and glucose transport have been postulated as the mechanism of insulin resistance in some or most of these patients.[40, 61] Intrinsic defects of the insulin receptor gene appear to be relatively rare, but have been reported in a few women with PCOS.[133]

The hyperinsulinemia often observed in PCOS does not appear to be secondary to increased ovarian androgen production for several reasons. Several investigators have shown that suppression of ovarian androgens with long-acting GnRH analogues does not eliminate the insulin resistance in PCOS.[60, 82, 145] Bilateral oophorectomy does not improve the hyperinsulinemia of women with hyperthecosis.[138] Obese women with PCOS continue to have insulin resistance both after weight loss alone and weight loss combined with antiandrogen therapy.[155] Finally, normal men have markedly elevated testosterone levels compared to hyperandrogenic women, but do not have hyperinsulinemia or insulin resistance as a consequence.

Hyperinsulinemia does not alter gonadotropin secretion in PCOS.[57, 59] A reduction in serum testosterone values was observed in obese PCOS patients after short-term suppression of insulin release by diazoxide alone.[143] The administration of diazoxide to reduce pancreatic-insulin release, after suppression of pituitary gonadotropins with a long-

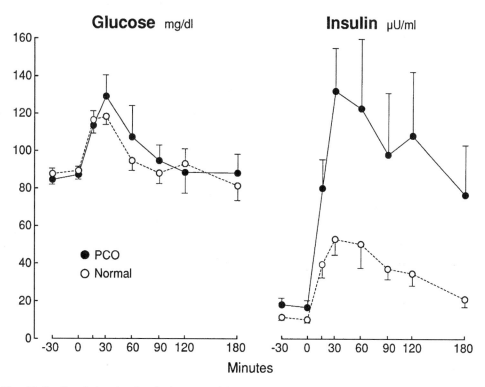

Fig. 11-8. Circulating levels of glucose and insulin in polycystic ovary (PCO) syndrome and control (normal) women in response to oral glucose administration. (From Chang JR et al: *J Clin Endocrinol Metab* 57:356, 1983.)

acting GnRH analogue, was unable to further reduce circulating testosterone levels in obese PCOS women.[145] These observations suggest that LH, rather than insulin, is the principal regulator of hyperandrogenemia in PCOS.

Hyperinsulinemia appears to induce androgen excess by direct stimulation of LH-dependent androgen biosynthesis. First, both LH and insulin stimulate androgen production in vitro using ovarian thecal and stroma cell cultures from hyperandrogenic women.[19, 144] Furthermore, in these studies, insulin and LH together enhanced androgen production more than LH alone. Second, suppressing circulating gonadotropin levels with a long-acting GnRH analogue in a patient with severe hyperandrogenemia, insulin resistance, and acanthosis nigricans resulted in a marked decrease in androgen levels in this patient, although circulating insulin levels did not change significantly.[10]

Hyperinsulinemia may further magnify androgen excess by decreasing the SHBG levels in PCOS.[59, 145] Gonadal sex steroids have been implicated as the principal regulators of SHBG levels, with elevated SHBG noted in the presence of estrogen and depressed levels of SHBG noted in the presence of androgens. This interaction between sex steroids and SHBG is complicated by recent in vivo and in vitro evidence of stimulatory, rather than suppressive, action of testosterone on SHBG levels.[158, 161] These observations suggest factors other than gonadal steroids may be the principal regulators of circulating SHBG in vivo. Current observations suggest insulin, insulin-like growth factor (IGF-1), and growth hormone may be important modulators of circulating SHBG concentrations.[203] Furthermore, in vitro experiments with a human hepatic cell line have shown that insulin reduces SHBG production.[160, 161]

In PCOS patients, reducing insulin production with diazoxide resulted in a significant rise in serum SHBG concentrations and a decline in circulating testosterone levels.[143] A similar suppression of serum insulin concentrations in healthy, nonobese, ovulatory women did not significantly alter either serum SHBG or testosterone levels.[144] In vivo studies in obese subjects with PCOS and in normal subjects have shown an inverse relationship between circulating insulin and SHBG levels.[67, 145] In obese PCOS women, this correlation was independent of serum sex steroids.[67] Furthermore, cross-sectional studies in Mexican-American women confirmed that the negative correlation between insulin and SHBG is independent of serum androgen concentrations or the degree of obesity.[95]

Elevated circulating levels of insulin could stimulate intraovarian receptors for IGF-1 and/or IGF-1-like peptides, which would augment androgen production. This, in turn, could lead to nested follicular development and formation of the "cystic ovary." Elevated insulin levels could also be responsible for the decreased sex hormone-binding globulin levels that are found in these patients.[161]

In summary, hyperinsulinemia is frequently observed in women with PCOS, independent of body mass or androgen levels. Elevated circulating insulin appears to directly enhance LH-stimulated androgen secretion from the ovary. Alternatively, insulin appears to have the opposite effect on adrenal androgens (see below), possibly because the insulin-resistance effect predominates over the hyperinsulinemia. Elevated insulin levels also serve to decrease circulating SHBG, resulting in higher levels of free androgens.

Adrenocortical dysfunction in PCOS

Although the majority of patients with hyperandrogenism demonstrate an ovarian source for their high androgen secretion, approximately half also have excessive adrenocortical production. Using selective catheterization of the adrenal and ovarian vessels, 12-42% of hyperandrogenic women demonstrate significant adrenal androgen hypersecretion, including androstenedione, DHEA, and Δ_5-androstenediol.[113, 130, 131] Others have observed a higher uptake of iodocholesterol by the adrenal gland of PCOS patients compared to normal subjects.[92] DHEAS, a metabolite of DHEA formed primarily by the adrenal cortex, was found to be elevated in over 50% of patients with PCOS.[152] As a result, some investigators have proposed the existence of an adrenal androgen-stimulating hormone (CASH or AASH), separate from adrenocorticotropic hormone (ACTH) but presumed to be derived from the same precursor molecule.[93, 153] Although it is possible that the adrenal androgen excess observed in some hyperandrogenic patients is secondary to increased pituitary secretion of a AASH, evidence for the existence of this hormone remains circumstantial.

Adrenal androgen excess may result from a generalized adrenocortical hyperreactivity to ACTH stimulation. Some investigators have observed an exaggerated secretion of adrenal androgens[119, 124] and cortisol[130] following ACTH administration. It has also been observed also that 40-50% of hyperandrogenic women demonstrate an exaggerated secretion of cortisol, 11-deoxycortisol, DHEA, and 17-hydroxypregnenolone to ACTH stimulation that correlates to the circulating DHEAS level (Fig. 11-9).[11, 12]

The exact etiology for the adrenocortical hyperreactivity in these patients is unclear. Circulating ACTH serum levels are not higher in women with PCOS than in normal women.[39, 102, 147] However, it is not known whether an increased sensitivity or responsivity of the adrenal cortex (or the cholesterol cleavage enzyme system) to ACTH stimulation is present in PCOS patients with adrenocortical hyperreactivity and/or androgen excess. Dysregulation of 11β-hydroxysteroid dehydrogenase within the adrenal gland has recently been proposed as one mechanism for adrenal hyperactivity observed in PCOS patients. Corroboration of these results by others is necessary.[171]

Many PCOS patients are obese, and overweightness has been shown to correlate with the responsivity of DHEA secretion to incremental doses of ACTH without altering

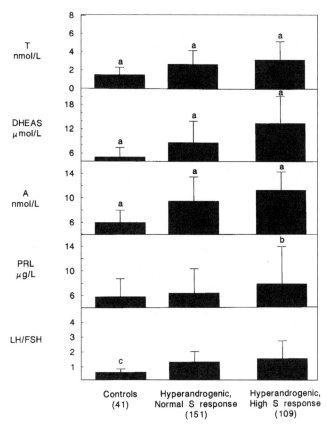

Fig. 11-9. Comparison of the basal levels of testosterone (T), dehydroepiandrosterone sulfate (DHEAS), androstenedione (A), prolactin (PRL) and the LH/FSH ratio, in control women and hyperandrogenic patients with a normal or an exaggerated 11-deoxycortisol (S) response to acute ACTH-(1-24) stimulation (1 mg). The number of women in each group is noted in parenthesis, and the mean plus standard deviation is depicted.

[a]All groups different from each other, P < 0.008.

[b]Hyperandrogenic patients with a high S response were significantly different from controls or hyperandrogenic women with an S response, P < 0.02.

[c]Controls were lower than hyperandrogenic patients, P < 0.0001.

the cortisol response.[117] The authors studied the effect of body weight on the adrenal response to acute ACTH stimulation in 57 healthy, normal, ovulatory women of varying weights. Adrenocortical steroidogenesis was not altered, although the increment in androstenedione with ACTH stimulation increased with body mass.[13]

Various investigators have demonstrated a negative correlation in women with PCOS between basal circulating DHEAS and fasting insulin, or the insulin response to an oral glucose-tolerance test (OGTT).[154, 179, 185] Furthermore, obesity appears to be associated with both hyperinsulinemia and decreased DHEAS concentrations.[9] Alternatively, Smith et al. noted a positive correlation between DHEAS and fasting insulin levels in healthy postpubertal children 17 years of age or younger.[183] There is also conflicting information concerning the relationship between basal DHEA and fasting insulin levels.[69, 71]

Using supraphysiologic insulin infusions, some investigators have observed an acute decrease in circulating DHEAS levels in normal women,[53, 140] normal men,[141] and one hyperandrogenic, insulin-resistant patient.[140] Nestler et al. noted a 39% drop in DHEAS levels following 12 hours of insulin infusion in five healthy women (mean insulin level of 13,144 ± 2095 pmol/L), and an 89% decrease at four hours in ten men (mean insulin of 12,390 ± 259 pmol/L).[141] Dunaif and Graf did not observe a decrease in circulating DHEAS during an eight-hour supraphysiological insulin infusion (mean insulin of 8997 ± 452 pmol/L) in ten hyperinsulinemic, insulin-resistant patients with PCOD, or five ovulatory women whose age and weight matched.[59]

The effect of physiologic increases in circulating insulin concentrations on DHEAS levels has not been well established. Diamond et al. noted a 16% decrease in DHEAS levels during a 100-minute, 1 mU/kg/minute insulin infusion in five normal women, and a 24% drop following a two-hour hyperglycemic infusion (125 mg/dl, [6.9 mmol/L] above baseline) in ten normal women.[53] Hubert et al. reported a significant decrease in DHEAS levels at two hours during an OGTT in seven healthy women.[105]

In five hyperandrogenic and eight normal ovulatory women, however, Elkind-Hirsch et al. reported an actual increase in DHEAS during a 180-minute modified intravenous glucose-tolerance test.[63] During a three-hour euglycemic insulin clamp achieving physiologic insulin levels (420 ± 35 pmol/L), Stuart and Nagamani observed no change in the circulating DHEAS level in oophorectomized women.[194] In that same study, an increase in the circulating levels of DHEA was noted in intact and castrate women. Alternatively, Falcone et al. reported a significant decline in circulating DHEA levels following a three-hour intravenous glucose tolerance test in nine healthy women and seven PCOS patients with normal insulin sensitivity, although no change in DHEA levels was observed in 12 PCOS women with reduced insulin sensitivity.[69] The authors have studied the acute changes in circulating DHEAS levels during endogenous insulin release in response to a two-hour oral glucose challenge, and did not observe a significant change in circulating DHEAS levels in either PCOS or control women, independent of the presence of obesity.[30]

The impact of chronic elevations in insulin is even less clear. Levels of androgens were compared between seven hirsute/oligomenorrheic women with chronic severe hyperinsulinemia (demonstrating a peak insulin level >500 µU/ml) during an OGTT, with nine hyperandrogenic normoinsulinemic patients and nine euandrogenic normoinsulinemic controls. The results of this unpublished study suggest that chronic severe hyperinsulinemia is not associated with an increase in circulating adrenal androgens (Azziz R: unpublished data).

As previously mentioned, dysregulation of cytochrome P450c17α has been proposed to lead to the exaggerated secretion of ovarian androgens in PCOS.[23] This enzyme demonstrates both 17-hydroxylase and 17, 20-lyase activity, and is expressed in both adrenocortical and ovarian tissue. An exaggerated adrenal secretion of 17-hydroxylated C_{21} steroids and C_{19} androgens in response to ACTH may also result from dysregulation (i.e., exaggerated activity) of this enzyme. Although the 17-hydroxylase and 17, 20-lyase activities appear to result from the action of a single gene product, it is unclear whether these activities are affected to the same degree in hyperandrogenemic women. Furthermore, there is a poor correlation between ovarian and adrenal 17-hydroxylase and/or 17, 20-lyase dysfunction.[62] We were unable to demonstrate a correlation between 17-hydroxylase and/or 17, 20-lyase dysregulation and adrenal androgen excess.[16]

Adrenocortical dysfunction in PCOS patients may represent an acquired defect secondary to defective ovarian secretion, particularly excessive testosterone secretion. Fruzzetti et al. determined the adrenal response to acute ACTH stimulation in hyperandrogenic women with normal (n = 14) or high circulating testosterone levels (n = 25).[77] Patients with high testosterone levels had higher 17-OHP, and higher 17-OHP to cortisol ratios following stimulation. Vermesh et al. studied the effect of a five-hour intravenous testosterone infusion on adrenal biosynthesis, as determined by the steroid response to ACTH, in normal women.[202] Their observations revealed very subtle inhibitions of 21-hydroxylase and/or 11β-hydroxylase activities, but no change in 17, 20-lyase or 3β-hydroxysteroid dehydrogenase (3β-HSD) activities. The authors prospectively studied the effect of three weeks of exogenous testosterone in healthy oophorectomized women, and did not observe a significant change in adrenocortical steroidogenesis, with the exception of an apparent increase in the metabolism of DHEA to DHEAS.[11] The DHEAS to DHEA ratio is also higher in men,[214] suggesting that circulating testosterone alters the sulfation rate of DHEA.

Suppression of gonadotropin and ovarian secretion can also be used to determine the role of gonadal steroids on adrenocortical function, and can be accomplished with the administration of a long-acting analogue of GnRH. A number of investigators have observed a normalization of testosterone and androstenedione serum levels following GnRH analogue treatment in PCOS.[6, 55, 77, 154, 169, 192] In spite of this decrease in ovarian androgens, little change in circulating DHEAS levels was observed. It does not appear that circulating androgen levels of ovarian origin play a significant role in the development of adrenal androgen excess in PCOS.

Although some of the adrenocortical/adrenal androgen abnormalities noted in some hyperandrogenic patients may be acquired, others may represent inherited defects of enzyme function. In the classic or congenital form of adrenal hyperplasia, the defect is severe enough to cause in utero virilization of the female fetus. In some newborns with classic adrenal hyperplasia, cortisol production is insufficient to sustain life, and death ensues unless the disease is rapidly recognized and corticosteroid replacement is begun immediately. In contrast, in nonclassic adrenal hyperplasia (NC-CAH) or late-onset adrenal hyperplasia, the deficiency is relatively mild and hyperandrogenic symptoms generally develop at or following puberty. The prevalence of this disorder varies according to the racial/ethnic distribution of the population being studied. Among the authors' hyperandrogenic patients, approximately 3% demonstrate either 21-hydroxylase, 11-hydroxylase or 3β-HSD deficiency.[8, 12, 15] However, among Ashkenazi Jewish patients, the prevalence of 21-hydroxylase deficiency can be as high as one in 27 patients.[187] It is interesting to note that patients with NC-CAH do not consistently demonstrate an elevation in circulating DHEAS levels, although they generally have high androstenedione and 17-OHP levels.[8] Overall, only a very small portion of the adrenal androgen abnormalities noted in hyperandrogenic women can be attributed to NC-CAH.

In summary, approximately 50% of patients with PCOS demonstrate elevated adrenal androgen levels. Many of these patients also demonstrate evidence of adrenocortical hyperactivity in response to ACTH. The exact etiology for this abnormality is unclear, but it does not appear to be related to circulating insulin levels, exogenous androgen production by the ovaries, or obesity. A very small percentage of adrenal androgen excess is due to NC-CAH. It is possible that the same factors that lead to ovarian hyperandrogenemia also stimulate adrenal androgen excess, although these factors remain to be defined.

LONG-TERM CONSEQUENCES OF PCOS
Obesity

It is unclear whether obesity precedes or follows the development of hyperandrogenemia. Although there is some animal data suggesting that androgens increase body weight,[159] many of the women who develop PCOS and hyperandrogenism are obese prior to the onset of puberty.

Diabetes mellitus

As noted previously, a number of authors have indicated that PCOS patients, regardless of weight, demonstrate increased plasma insulin levels, compared to controls. Insulin resistance in PCOS patients may predispose them to the development of diabetes mellitus. Dahlgren et al. noted that in a retrospective, cohort study, 15% of women with PCOS had been diagnosed with diabetes mellitus, compared to 2.3% of controls, after a follow-up period of 22-31 years.[49] In addition, hyperinsulinemia has also been associated with a high risk for the development of hypertension, hyperlipidemia, and coronary artery disease.[213]

Hypertension

In a transectional, retrospective, cohort, follow-up study of 33 women with PCOS, 22 to 31 years after diagnosis, 39%

were being treated for hypertension, compared to 11% of controls. Furthermore, nonobese PCOS patients had higher systolic and diastolic blood pressures compared with controls with equal body-fat mass.[100, 168]

Lipid abnormalities and coronary artery disease

Wild et al. noted that hyperandrogenemia in women results in higher mean serum triglycerides and very low-density lipoprotein levels (VLDL), but lower high-density lipoprotein cholesterol levels.[205] These investigators subsequently demonstrated that androgens and insulin have an independent and synergistic role in the development of the altered lipid profile in hyperandrogenic women.[207] In a study evaluating 102 women undergoing coronary artery catheterization, hirsutism was found more commonly in those women with confirmed coronary artery disease.[206] Furthermore, the presence of abdominal obesity was associated with the presence of hirsutism and coronary artery disease. As would be expected for a lesion that takes a number of years to develop, these associations were strongest in older women (aged 60 years or over).

Malignancy

Chronic anovulation is a well-known risk factor for the development of endometrial carcinoma.[44] More specifically, untreated PCOS is a significant risk factor for endometrial carcinoma. Jackson and Dockerty noted that 16 of 43 patients with Stein-Leventhal syndrome (37%) had malignant endometrial lesions.[108] A number of early investigations noted that almost 20% of women who developed endometrial cancer at 40 years of age or older had clinical evidence of PCOS.[108] More recently, seven of 10 patients with endometrial cancer, aged 15 to 25, had clinical characteristics of PCOS.[72] It appears that early diagnosis and follow-up of patients with this syndrome may reduce the risk of developing an endometrial malignancy. In the study of Dahlgren et al., 18 patients (of a total of 26 potential subjects) underwent an endometrial biopsy 22 to 31 years after ovarian wedge resection.[49] None demonstrated endometrial atypia or malignancy.

Increased bone mass

The presence of androgen excess appears to be protective against bone demineralization. A patient with amenorrhea secondary to PCOS had a higher bone density compared to amenorrheic patients who demonstrated normal ovaries by ultrasound.[54] Furthermore, Buchanan et al. demonstrated that superphysiological levels of endogenous estrogens in young women were associated with increased trabecular bone density, although cortical bone density was not different from controls.[27]

In conclusion, patients with PCOS are at higher risk for developing obesity, diabetes mellitus, hypertension, lipid abnormalities, coronary artery disease, and endometrial carcinoma. Alternatively, it is possible that their risk of

developing postmenopausal osteoporosis is reduced, due to a higher trabecular bone density, even in amenorrheic subjects.

THERAPY OF PCOS

Successful treatment for the patient with PCOS requires that the specific goal(s) of therapy first be established. Therapeutic goals include pregnancy, treatment of hirsutism and/or acne, and regularization of the menstrual cycle. Specific drug therapy is available for each treatment goal, but weight loss for those who are obese with this syndrome may be of help in all instances.

Weight loss

Although obesity is not believed to be the causal factor for PCOS, it may exacerbate the dysfunction. Loss of significant weight (e.g., greater than 15% of body weight) has been reported to result in lowered androgen levels and spontaneous resumption of ovulation in some women with PCOS. Increased sex hormone-binding globulin levels and reduced basal levels of insulin, as well as a reduced insulin response to glucose challenge, have been observed following weight reduction in these women.[112] In fact, weight loss appears to be of benefit in *all* obese hyperandrogenic women whether or not polycystic ovaries are present.[156]

Ovulation induction

For individuals with PCOS who do not ovulate or who ovulate irregularly, ovulation-inducing drugs may be provided alone or in conjunction with attempted weight loss for those wishing to conceive. Ovulation induction with clomiphene citrate therapy is usually attempted initially and is successful for approximately 80% of patients with PCOS. This treatment is discussed in detail in Chapter 32. Should clomiphene citrate fail to induce ovulation, administration of human menopausal gonadotropins alone or in conjunction with GnRH agonists may be provided. This therapeutic modality is discussed further in Chapters 33 and 34.

Treatment of hirsutism

A variety of medications have been used for the treatment of hirsutism and acne in women with PCOS, including oral-contraceptive pills, cyproterone acetate, gonadotropin-releasing hormone agonists, spironolactone, flutamide, cimetidine, and ketoconazole. These agents act by either increasing steroid-binding globulin levels, inhibiting androgen synthesis by the ovary and adrenal, or blocking androgen receptors or 5α reductase at target tissues. Dosages of administration, mechanisms of action, and side effects of these medications are fully discussed in Chapter 10.

Treatment of dysfunctional uterine bleeding

Anovulation in women with functional hyperandrogenism is a frequent occurrence. As a consequence, the endometrial lining of the uterus may be exposed to chronic, unopposed estrogen stimulation resulting in bleeding. This is usually treated with cyclical progestogen therapy or with contraceptive pills. This subject is discussed in detail in Chapter 8.

Surgical therapy of PCOS

In their original description, Stein and Leventhal advocated wedge resection of the ovaries as therapy for the PCOS because this treatment appeared to restore cyclic menstruation.[190] The etiology for the apparent success of this therapy in PCOS is not clear, although a reduction in the amount of androgen-producing ovarian tissue has been suggested. In 1965, Stein reviewed 108 cases and noted that 95% of women with PCOS resumed cyclic menstruation, and 85% of those who desired to conceive did so following wedge resection.[191] He also noted that this effect was permanent. However, other studies have reported that less than 10% of women resume cyclic menstruation, and only 13% conceive following wedge resection.[86] Furthermore, formation of periovarian and peritubal adhesions following wedge resection has been observed and is felt to aggravate the patients' infertility.[2, 199] As a consequence, bilateral ovarian wedge resection is no longer recommended as primary therapy for patients with PCOS, especially because comparable or better success of pregnancy can be obtained medically.

More recently, laparoscopic electrocautery of the ovarian surface was reported to result in regular menstrual cycles in 51 out of 62 women with PCOS.[85] A decline in circulating androgen levels was observed within four days of surgery,[90] which was similar to the fall in androgen levels produced after wedge resection.[110] Comparable results in resumption of ovulation and reduction in circulating androgens have been reported following laparoscopic ovarian vaporization using argon, carbon dioxide, or potassium-titanyl phosphate (KTP) lasers (Fig. 11-10).[50, 104, 176] Unfortunately, adhesion formation in 20-70% of ovaries has also been reported following either ovarian electrocauterization or laser drilling.[48, 94, 136] Naether et al. recently summarized the findings of 11 clinical studies involving 407 women who received electrocoagulation or laser therapy, and reported an ovulation rate of 77% and a pregnancy rate of 50%.[135] Because these success rates are so close to those obtained by medical therapy, the risk of ovarian adhesion formation must be carefully considered when deciding whether to recommend laparoscopic ovarian vaporization.

Future treatments

New drugs are being considered for the treatment of hirsutism and hyperinsulinemia related to PCOS. Flutamide is an antiandrogen primarily used for the treatment of prostatic cancer. Recent data suggest that 500-750 mg/day is effective for the treatment of hirsutism,[78] possibly more so than spironolactone given as 100 mg/day.[47] Terminal hair growth and sebaceous secretion depends to a large degree on the conversion of testosterone to the more androgenic steroid, dihydrotestosterone, within the hair follicle by 5α-reductase.[193] Finasteride is a 5α-reductase inhibitor currently approved for use only in the treatment of prostatic cancer. Nonetheless, it may also be useful for the treatment of hirsutism and/or acne. The side effects of finasteride, which have been reported in men, are generally related to altered sexual function, including decreased libido and impotence.[81] Little is known of the drug's side effects in women; it is not FDA approved for use in females due to concern that feminization of the external genitalia of a male fetus could occur if the drug is taken during an undiagnosed pregnancy. Five α-reductase appears to exist in two enzyme forms, Type I and Type II, encoded by two different genes. Type I 5α-reductase is expressed in skin and Type II 5α-reductase is expressed in genital tissue.[5, 134] Finasteride affects both enzymes, but is a more potent inhibitor of Type I. Perhaps in the future it will be possible to develop a specific Type I 5α-reductase inhibitor, reducing the risk of feminizing a male fetus. The mechanism of action and side effects of this drug have been reviewed recently.[170]

Defects in glucose transport have been suggested as a cause of insulin resistance in women with PCOS.[40] Drugs, such as metformin,[127] that improve glucose transport, allowing a decrease in circulating insulin levels, might be of benefit in treating hyperinsulinemic, hyperandrogenemic women. Suppression of serum insulin by diazoxide was previously shown to reduce testosterone levels in obese

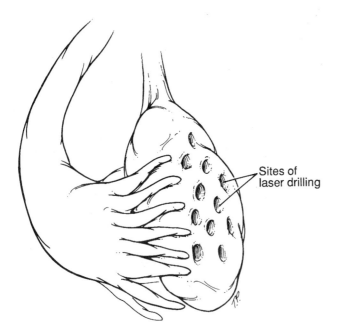

Sites of laser drilling

Fig. 11-10. Ovarian appearance following CO_2 laser "drilling." Drawn from a photograph. Note the width and depth of tissue vaporization.

women with PCOS,[142] although this drug has significant side effects.

REFERENCES

1. Adams J, Polson DW, Franks S: Prevalence of polycystic ovaries in women with anovulation and idiopathic hirsutism, *Br Med J* 293:355, 1986.
2. Adashi EY, Rock JA, Guzick D et al: Fertility following bilateral ovarian wedge resection: a critical analysis of 90 consecutive cases of the polycystic ovary syndrome, *Fertil Steril* 36:320, 1981.
3. Aleem FA, McIntosh T: Elevated plasma levels of β-endorphin in a group of women with polycystic ovarian disease, *Fertil Steril* 42:686, 1984.
4. Amirikia H, Savoy-Moore RT, Sundareson AS et al: The effects of long-term androgen treatment on the ovary, *Fertil Steril* 45:202, 1986.
5. Andersson S, Bishop RW, Russell DW: Expression cloning and regulation of steroid 5 alpha-reductase, an enzyme essential for male sexual differentiation, *J Biol Chem* 264:16247, 1989.
6. Andreyko JL, Monroe SC, Jaffe RB: Treatment of hirsutism with a gonadotropin-releasing hormone agonist (nafarelin), *J Clin Endocrinol Metab* 63:854, 1986.
7. Anttila L, Ding Y-Q, Ruutiainen K et al: Clinical features and circulating gonadotropin, insulin, and androgen interactions in women with polycystic ovarian disease, *Fertil Steril* 55:1057, 1991.
8. Azziz R, Zacur HA. 21-hydroxylase deficiency in female hyperandrogenemia: screening and diagnosis, *J Clin Endocrinol Metab* 69:577, 1989.
9. Azziz R: Reproductive endocrinologic alterations in female asymptomatic obesity, *Fertil Steril* 52:703, 1989.
10. Azziz R, Murphy AG: Long-acting GnRH analog treatment of severe hyperandrogenism associated with insulin resistance and acanthosis nigricans, *American Fertility Society* No P-079, 1990.
11. Azziz R, Gay F, Potter SR et al: Effect of prolonged hypertestosteronemia on adrenocortical biosynthesis in oophorectomized women, *J Clin Endocrinol Metab* 72:1025, 1991.
12. Azziz R, Boots LR, Parker Jr CR et al: 11-hydroxylase deficiency in hyperandrogenism, *Fertil Steril* 55:733, 1991.
13. Azziz R, Zacur HA, Parker Jr CR et al: Effect of obesity in the response to acute adrenocorticotropin (ACTH-124) stimulation in eumenorrheic women, *Fertil Steril* 56:427, 1991.
14. Azziz R, Bradley Jr EL, Potter HD et al: Adrenocortical hyperactivity and androgen excess hyperandrogenism: the role of 17-hydroxylase and 17,20 lyase dysregulation (submitted for publication).
15. Azziz R, Bradley Jr EL, Potter HD et al: Deficient 3β-hydroxysteroid dehydrogenase (3β-HSD) activity in hyperandrogenism, *Society for Gynecologic Investigation* No 167, 1991.
16. Azziz R, Bradley Jr EL, Parker Jr CR et al: Adrenocortical hyperactivity in hyperandrogenism: the role of 17-hydroxylase (17-OH) and 17,20-desmolase (17,20-D) dysfunction, *Society for Gynecologic Investigation* No 622, 1992.
17. Azziz R, DeWailly D, Owerbach D: Non-classical adrenal hyperplasia: current concepts, *J Clin Endocrinol 78:810, Metab* 78:810, 1994.
18. Barbarino A, DeMarinis L, Mancini A et al: Estrogen-dependent plasma prolactin response to gonadotropin-releasing hormone in intact and castrated men, *J Clin Endocrinol Metab* 78:810, 55:1212, 1982.
19. Barbieri RL, Makris A, Randall RW et al: Insulin stimulates androgen accumulation in incubations of ovarian stroma obtained from women with hyperandrogenism, *J Clin Endocrinol Metab* 62:904, 1986.
20. Barbieri RL, Smith S, Ryan KJ: The role of hyperinsulinemia in the pathogenesis of ovarian hyperandrogenism, *Fertil Steril* 50:197, 1988.

21. Barnes RB, Lobo RA: Central opioid activity in polycystic ovary syndrome with and without dopaminergic modulation, *J Clin Endocrinol Metab* 61:779, 1985.
22. Barnes RB, Mileikowsky GN, Cha KY et al: Effects of dopamine and metoclopramide in polycystic ovary syndrome, *J Clin Endocrinol Metab* 63:506, 1986.
23. Barnes RB, Rosenfield RL, Burstein S et al: Pituitary-ovarian responses to nafarelin testing in the polycystic ovary syndrome, *N Engl J Med* 320:559, 1989.
24. Bates GW, Whitworth NS: Effect of body-weight reduction on plasma androgens in obese, infertile women, *Fertil Steril* 38:406, 1992.
25. Bayer LM: Build in relation to menstrual disorders and obesity, *Endocrinology* 24:260, 1939.
26. Bray GA: Overweight is risking fate. In Wurtman RJ, Wurtman JJ, editors: *Human obesity,* New York, 1987, The New York Academy of Sciences.
27. Buchanan JR, Hospodar P, Myers C et al: Effect of excess endogenous androgens on bone density in young women, *J Clin Endocrinol Metab* 67:937, 1988.
28. Buckler HM, McLachlan RI, MacLachlan VB et al: Serum inhibin levels in polycystic ovary syndrome: basal levels and response to luteinizing hormone-releasing hormone agonist and exogenous gonadotropin administration, *J Clin Endocrinol Metab* 66:798, 1988.
29. Bughen GA, Givens JR, Kitabchi AE: Correlation of hyperandrogenism with hyperinsulinemia in polycystic ovarian disease, *J Clin Endocrinol Metab* 50:113, 1980.
30. Buyalos RP, Bradley Jr EL, Judd HL et al: No acute effect of physiological insulin increase on dehydroepiandrosterone sulfate in women with obesity and/or polycystic ovarian disease, *Fertil Steril* 56:1179, 1991.
31. Buyalos RP, Geffner ME, Bersch N et al: Insulin and insulin-like growth factor-I responsiveness in polycystic ovarian syndrome, *Fertil Steril* 57:796, 1992.
32. Calogero AE, Macchi M, Montanini V et al: Dynamics of plasma gonadotropin and sex steroid release in polycystic ovarian disease after pituitary-ovarian inhibition with an analog of gonadotropin-releasing hormone, *J Clin Endocrinol Metab* 64:980, 1987.
33. Canales ES, Zarate A, Castelazo-Ayala L: Primary amenorrhea associated with polycystic ovaries, *Obstet Gynecol* 37:205, 1971.
34. Cara JF, Rosenfield RL: Insulin-like growth factor 1 and insulin potentiate luteinizing hormone-induced androgen synthesis by rat ovarian thecal-interstitial cells, *Endocrinology* 123:733, 1988.
35. Carmina E, Rosato F, Maggiore M et al: Prolactin secretion in polycystic ovary syndrome (PCO): correlation with the steroid pattern, *Acta Endocrinol* (Copenh) 105:99, 1984.
36. Carmina E, Koyama T, Chang L et al: Does ethnicity influence the prevalence of adrenal hyperandrogenism and insulin resistance in polycystic ovary syndrome? *Am J Obstet Gynecol* 167:1807, 1992.
37. Carmina E, Ditkoff ED, Malizia G et al: Increased circulating levels of immunoreactive β-endorphin in polycystic ovary syndrome is not caused by increased pituitary secretion, *Am J Obstet Gynecol* 167:1819, 1992.
38. Chang RJ, Nakamura R, Judd HL et al: Insulin resistance in non-obese patients with polycystic ovarian disease, *J Clin Endocrinol Metab* 57:356, 1983.
39. Chang RJ, Laufer LR, Meldrum DR et al: Steroid secretion in polycystic ovarian disease after ovarian suppression by a long-acting gonadotropin-releasing hormone agonist, *J Clin Endocrinol Metab* 56:897, 1983.
40. Ciaraldi TP, El-Roeiy A, Madar Z et al: Cellular mechanisms of insulin resistance in polycystic ovarian syndrome, *J Clin Endocrinol Metab* 75:577, 1992.
41. Clayton RN, Ogden V, Hodgkinson J et al: How common are polycystic ovaries in normal women and what is their significance for the fertility of the population? *Clin Endocrinol* 37:127, 1992.

42. Combes R, Altomare E, Tramoni M et al: Obesity in menstrual disorders. In Mancini M, Lewis B, Contaldo F, editors: *Medical complications of obesity, serono symposi, vol 26,* New York, 1979, Academic.

43. Conway GS, Honour JW, Jacobs HW: Heterogeneity of the polycystic ovarian syndrome: clinical, endocrine and ultrasound features in 556 patients, *Clin Endocrinol* 30:459, 1989.

44. Coulam CB, Annegers JF, Kranz JS: Chronic anovulation syndrome and associated neoplasia, *Obstet Gynecol* 61:403, 1983.

45. Couzinet B, Thomas G, Thalabard JC et al: Effects of a pure antiandrogen on gonadotropin secretion in normal women and in polycystic ovarian disease, *Fertil Steril* 52:42, 1989.

46. Cumming DC, Reid RL, Quigley ME et al: Evidence for decreased androgenous dopamine and opioid inhibitory influences on LH secretion in polycystic ovary syndrome, *Clin Endocrinol* (Oxf) 20:643, 1984.

47. Cusan L, Dupont A, Gomez JL et al: Comparison of flutamide and spironolactone in the treatment of hirsutism: a randomized controlled trial, *Fertil Steril* 61:281, 1994.

48. Dabirushrafi H, Mohamad K, Behjatnia Y et al: Adhesion formation after ovarian electrocauterization on patients with polycystic ovarian syndrome, *Fertil Steril* 55:1200, 1991.

49. Dahlgren E, Johansson S, Lindstedt G et al: Women with polycystic ovary syndrome wedge resected in 1956 to 1965: a long-term follow-up focusing on natural history and circulating hormones, *Fertil Steril* 57:505, 1992.

50. Daniell JF, Miller W: Polycystic ovaries treated by laparoscopic laser vaporization, *Fertil Steril* 51:232, 1989.

51. Dewis P, Newman M, Ratcliffe WA et al: Does testosterone affect the normal menstrual cycle? *Clin Endocrinol* (Oxf) 24:515, 1986.

52. de Ziegler D, Steingold K, Cedars M et al: Recovery of hormone secretion after chronic gonadotropin-releasing hormone agonist administration in women with polycystic ovarian disease, *J Clin Endocrinol Metab* 68:1111, 1989.

53. Diamond MP, Grainger D, Laudano AJ et al: Effect of acute physiological elevations of insulin on circulating androgen levels in nonobese women, *J Clin Endocrinol Metab* 72:883, 1991.

54. Di Carlo C, Shoham Z, MacDougall J et al: Polycystic ovaries as a relative protective factor for bone mineral loss in young women with amenorrhea, *Fertil Steril* 57:314, 1992.

55. Dodson WC, Hughes CL, Whitesides B et al: The effect of leuprolide acetate on ovulation induction with human menopausal gonadotropins in polycystic ovary syndrome, *J Clin Endocrinol Metab* 65:95, 1987.

56. Dunaif A: Do androgens directly regulate gonadotropin secretion in the polycystic ovary syndrome? *J Clin Endocrinol Metab* 63:215, 1986.

57. Dunaif A, Mandeli J, Fluhr H et al: The impact of obesity and chronic hyperinsulinemia on gonadotropin release and gonadal steroid secretion in the polycystic ovary syndrome, *J Clin Endocrinol Metab* 66:131, 1988.

58. Dunaif A, Segal K, Futterweit W et al: Profound peripheral resistance independent of obesity in polycystic ovary syndrome, *Diabetes* 38:1165, 1989.

59. Dunaif A, Graf M: Insulin administration alters gonadal steroid metabolism independent of changes in gonadotropin secretion in insulin-resistant women with the polycystic ovary syndrome, *J Clin Invest* 83:23, 1989.

60. Dunaif A, Green G, Futterweit W et al: Suppression of hyperandrogenism does not improve peripheral or hepatic insulin resistance in the polycystic ovary syndrome, *J Clin Endocrinol Metab* 70:699, 1990.

61. Dunaif A, Segal KR, Shelley DR et al: Evidence for distinctive and intrinsic defects in insulin action in polycystic ovary syndrome, *Diabetes* 41:1257, 1992.

62. Ehrmann DA, Rosenfield RL, Barnes RB et al: Detection of functional ovarian hyperandrogenism in women with androgen excess, *N Engl J Med* 327:157, 1992.

63. Elkind-Hirsch KE, Valdes CT, McConnell TG et al: Androgen responses to acutely increased endogenous insulin levels in hyperandrogenic and normal cycling women, *Fertil Steril* 55:486, 1991.

64. El Tabbakh GH, Lotfy I, Azab I et al: Correlation of the ultrasonic appearance of the ovaries in polycystic ovarian disease and the clinical, hormonal, and laparoscopic findings, *Am J Obstet Gynecol* 154:892, 1986.

65. Erickson GF, Hsueh AJW, Quigley ME et al: Functional studies of aromatase activity in human granulosa cells from normal and polycystic ovaries, *J Clin Endocrinol Metab* 49:514, 1979.

66. Erickson GF, Magoffin DA, Dyer CA et al: The ovarian androgen producing cells: a review of structure/function relationships, *Endocr Rev* 6(3):371, 1985.

67. Evans DJ, Hoffmann RG, Kalkhoff RK et al: Relationship of androgenic activity to body-fat topography, fat-cell morphology, and metabolic aberrations in premenopausal women, *J Clin Endocrinol Metab* 57:304, 1983.

68. Evans DJ, Barth JH, Burke CW: Body-fat topography in women with androgen excess, *Int J Obes* 12:157, 1988.

69. Falcone T, Finegood DT, Fantus IG et al: Androgen response to endogenous insulin secretion during the frequently sampled intravenous glucose tolerance test in normal and hyper-androgenic women, *J Clin Endocrinol Metab* 71:1653, 1990.

70. Falcone T, Billrai R, Morris D: Serum inhibin levels in polycystic ovary syndrome: effect of insulin resistance and insulin secretion, *Obstet Gynecol* 78:171, 1991.

71. Farah MG, Givens JR, Kitabchi AE: Bimodal correlation between the circulating insulin level and the production rate of dehydroepiandrosterone: positive correlation in controls and negative correlation in the polycystic ovary syndrome with acanthosis nigricans, *J Clin Endocrinol Metab* 70:1075, 1990.

72. Farhi DC, Nosanchuk J, Silverberg SG: Endometrial adenocarcinoma in women under 25 years of age, *Obstet Gynecol* 68:741, 1986.

73. Fisher ER, Gregorio R, Stephan T et al: Ovarian changes in women with morbid obesity, *Obstet Gynecol* 44:839, 1974.

74. Franks S: Polycystic ovary syndrome: a changing perspective, *Clin Endocrinol* 31:87, 1989.

75. Frequency of overweight and underweight, *Stat Bull Metropol Life Insur* 41:4, 1960.

76. Friedman CI, Kim MH: Obesity and its effect on reproductive function, *Clin Obstet Gynecol* 28:645, 1985.

77. Fruzzetti F, Melis GB, Mais V et al: High testosterone levels in ovarian origin affect adrenal steroidogenesis: *J Clin Endocrinol Metab* 72:416, 1991.

78. Fruzzetti F, DeLorenzo D, Rici C et al: Clinical and endocrine effects of flutamide in hyperandrogenic women, *Fertil Steril* 60:806, 1993.

79. Futterweit W, Deligdisch L: Histopathological effects of exogenously administered testosterone in 19 female to male transsexuals, *J Clin Endocrinol Metab* 62:16, 1986.

80. Fuxe Y, Hokfelt T, Nilsson O: Factors involved in the control of the tuberoinfundibular neurons during pregnancy and lactation, *Neuroendocrinology* 5:257, 1969.

81.. Garnley GS, Stoner E, Bruskewitz RC et al: The effect of finasteride in men with benign prostate hyperplasia, *N Engl J Med* 327:1185, 1992.

82. Geffner ME, Kaplan SA, Bersch N et al: Persistence of insulin resistance in polycystic ovarian disease after inhibition of ovarian steroid secretion, *Fertil Steril* 45:327, 1986.

83. Givens JR, Wiedeman E, Andersen RN et al: β-endorphin and β-lipotropin plasma levels in hirsute women: correlations with body weight, *J Clin Endocrinol Metab* 50:975, 1980.

84. Givens JR: Polycystic ovaries—a sign, not a diagnosis, *Semin Reprod Endocrinol* 2(3):271, 1984.

85. Gjonnaess H: Polycystic ovarian syndrome treated by ovarian electrocautery through the laparoscope, *Fertil Steril* 41:20, 1984.

86. Goldzieher JW, Green JA: The polycystic ovary, I: clinical and histologic features, *J Clin Endocrinol Metab* 22:325, 1962.

87. Goldzieher JW, Axelrod LR: Clinical and biochemical features of polycystic ovarian disease, *Fertil Steril* 14:631, 1963.

88. Goldzieher JW: Polycystic ovarian disease, *Fertil Steril* 35:371, 1981.

89. Graf MA, Bidfeld P, Distler W et al: Pulsatile luteinizing hormone secretion pattern in hyperandrogenemic women, *Fertil Steril* 59:761, 1993.

90. Greenblatt E, Casper RF: Endocrine changes after laparoscopic ovarian cautery in polycystic ovarian syndrome, *Am J Obstet Gynecol* 156:279, 1987.

91. Grenman S, Ronnemaa T, Irjala K et al: Sex-steroid, gonadotropin, cortisol, and prolactin levels in healthy, massively obese women: correlation with abdominal fat-cell size and effect of weight reduction, *J Clin Endocrinol Metab* 63:1257, 1986.

92. Gross MD, Wortsman J, Shapiro B et al: Scintigraphic evidence of adrenal corticoid dysfunction in the polycystic ovary syndrome, *J Clin Endocrinol Metab* 62:197, 1986.

93. Grumbach MM, Richards GE, Conte FA et al: Clinical disorders of adrenal function and puberty: an assessment of the role of the adrenal cortex in normal and abnormal puberty in man and evidence for an ACTH-like pituitary adrenal androgen stimulating hormone. In James VHT, Giusti MS, Giusti G et al, editors: *The endocrine function of the human adrenal cortex, proceedings of the serono symposia, vol 18,* New York, 1978, Academic.

94. Gurgan T, Kisnisei H, Yarali H et al: Evaluation of adhesion formation after laparoscopic treatment of polycystic ovarian disease, *Fertil Steril* 56:1176, 1991.

95. Haffner SM, Katz MS, Stern MP et al: The relationship of sex hormones to hyperinsulinemia and hyperglycemia, *Metabolism* 37:683, 1988.

96. Hague WM, Adams J, Reedus ST et al: Familial polycystic ovaries: a genetic disease? *Clin Endocrinol (Oxf)* 29:593, 1988.

97. Harlan WR, Landis JR, Flegal KM et al: Secular trends in body mass in the United States, 1960-1980, *Am J Epidemiol* 128:1065, 1988.

98. Harlass FE, Plymate SR, Fariss BL et al: Weight loss is associated with correction of gonadotropin and sex-steroid abnormalities in the obese anovulatory female, *Fertil Steril* 42:649, 1984.

99. Hartz AJ, Barboriak PN, Wong A et al: The association of obesity with infertility and related menstrual abnormalities in women, *Int J Obes* 3:57, 1979.

100. Hauner H, Ditschuneit HH, Pal SB et al: Distribution of adipose tissue and complications of obesity in overweight women with and without hirsutism, *Dtsch Med Wochenschr* 112:709, 1987.

101. Hoffman DI, Klove K, Lobo RA: The prevalence and significance of elevated dehydroepiandrosterone sulfate levels in anovulatory women, *Fertil Steril* 42:76, 1984.

102. Horrocks PM, Kandeel FR, London DR et al: ACTH function in women with the polycystic ovarian syndrome, *Clin Endocrinol* 19:143, 1983.

103. Hosseinian AH, Kim MH, Rosenfield RL: Obesity and oligomenorrhea are associated with hyperandrogenism independent of hirsutism, *J Clin Endocrinol Metab* 42:765, 1976.

104. Huber J, Hosmann J, Spona J: Polycystic ovarian syndrome treated by laser through the laparoscope, *Lancet* 2:215, 1988.

105. Hubert GD, Schriock ED, Givens JR et al: Insulin suppression of adrenal androgen concentrations during glucose tolerance testing in normal women. (Abstr. 31) Presented at the 37th Annual Meeting of the Society for Gynecologic Investigation, St. Louis, Missouri, March 21 to 25, 1990. Published by the Society for Gynecologic Investigation, in Program and Abstracts, 1990.

106. Hughesden PE: Morphology and morphogenesis of the Stein-Leventhal ovary and of so-called hyperthecosis, *Obstet Gynecol Surv* 37:59, 1982.

107. Imse V, Holzapfel G, Hinney B et al: Comparison of luteinizing hormone pulsatility in the serum of women suffering from polycystic ovarian disease using a bioassay and five different immunoassays, *J Clin Endocrinol Metab* 74:1053, 1992.

108. Jackson RL, Dockerty MB: The Stein-Leventhal syndrome: analysis of 43 cases with special reference to association with endometrial carcinoma, *Am J Obstet Gynecol* 73:161, 1957.

109. Jialal I, Naiker P, Reddi K et al: Evidence for insulin resistance in nonobese patients with polycystic ovarian disease, *J Clin Endocrinol Metab* 64:1066, 1987.

110. Judd HL, Diggs LA, Andersen DC et al: The effects of ovarian wedge resection on circulating gonadotropin and ovarian steroid levels in patients with polycystic ovary syndrome, *J Clin Endocrinol Metab* 43:347, 1976.

111. Kazer RR, Kessel B, Yen SSC: Circulating luteinizing hormone pulse frequency in women with polycystic ovary syndrome, *J Clin Endocrinol Metab* 65:233, 1987.

112. Kiddy DS, Hamilton-Fairly D, Bush A et al: Improvement in endocrine and ovarian function during dietary treatment of obese women with polycystic ovary syndrome, *Clin Endocrinol* 36:105, 1992.

113. Kirschner A, Jacobs JB: Combined ovarian and adrenal vein catheterization to determine the site(s) of androgen over-production in hirsute women, *J Clin Endocrinol Metab* 33:199, 1971.

114. Kirschner MA, Bardin LW: Androgen production and metabolism in normal and virilized women, *Metabolism* 21:667, 1972.

115. Kirschner MA, Zucker IR, Jepersen D: Idiopathic hirsutism—an ovarian abnormality, *N Engl J Med* 294:637, 1976.

116. Kirschner MA, Samojlik E, Drejka M et al: Androgen-estrogen metabolism in women with upper-body versus lower-body obesity, *J Clin Endocrinol Metab* 70:473, 1990.

117. Komindr S, Kurtz BR, Stevens MD et al: Relative sensitivity and responsitivity of serum cortisol and adrenal androgens to α-adrenocorticotropin (1-24) in normal and obese nonhirsute, eumenorrheic women, *J Clin Endocrinol Metab* 63:860, 1986.

118. Laatikainen T, Tulenheimo T, Andersson B et al: Obesity, serum steroid levels, and pulsatile gonadotropin secretion in polycystic ovarian disease, *Eur J Obstet Gynecol Reprod Biol* 15:45, 1982.

119. Lachelin GCL, Barnett M, Hopper BR et al: Adrenal function in normal women and women with the polycystic ovary syndrome, *J Clin Endocrinol Metab* 49:892, 1979.

120. Lin D, Black SM, Nagahama Y et al: Steroid 17α hydroxylase and 17,20-lyase activities of p450c17: contributions of serine and p450-reductase, *Endocrinology* 132:2498, 1993.

121. Lobo RA, Goebelsmann U, Horton R: Evidence for the importance of peripheral tissue events in the development of hirsutism in polycystic ovary syndrome, *J Clin Endocrinol Metab* 57:393, 1983.

122. Loughlin T, Cunningham SK, Culliton M et al: Altered androstenedione and estrone dynamics associated with abnormal hormonal profiles in amenorrheic subjects with weight loss or obesity, *Fertil Steril* 43:720, 1985.

123. Luciano AA, Chapler FK, Sherman BM: Hyperprolactinemia in polycystic ovary syndrome, *Fertil Steril* 41:719, 1984.

124. Lucky AW, Rosenfield RL, McGuire J et al: Adrenal androgen hyperresponsiveness to adrenocorticotropin in women with acne and/or hirsutism: adrenal enzyme defects and exaggerated adrenarche, *J Clin Endocrinol Metab* 62:840, 1986.

125. Mathur RS, Moody LO, Landgrebe S et al: Plasma androgens and sex-hormone-binding globulin in the evaluation of hirsute females, *Fertil Steril* 35:29, 1981.

126. Mathur RS, Moody LO, Landgrebe SC et al: Sex-hormone-binding globulin in clinically hyperandrogenic women: association of plasma concentrations with body weight, *Fertil Steril* 38:207, 1982.

127. Matthaei S, Reibold JP, Hamann A et al: In vivo metformin treatment ameliorates insulin resistance: evidence for potentiation of insulin-induced translocation and increased functional activity of glucose transporters in obese (fa/fa) zucher rat adipocytes, *Endocrinology* 133:304, 1993.

128. McArthur JW, Ingersoll FM, Worcester J: The urinary excretion of interstitial-cell and follicle-stimulating hormone activity by women with diseases of the reproductive system, *J Clin Endocrinol Metab* 18:1202, 1958.

129. McKenna TJ, Loughlin T, Daly L et al: Variable clinical and hormonal manifestations of hyperandrogenemia, *Metabolism* 33:714, 1984.

130. Meikle AW, Worley RJ, West CD: Adrenal corticoid hyper-responsiveness in hirsute women, *Fertil Steril* 41:575, 1984.

131. Milewicz A, Silber D, Mielecki P: The origin of androgen synthesis in polycystic ovary syndrome, *Obstet Gynecol* 62:601, 1983.

132. Mitchell Jr GW, Rogers J: The influence of weight reduction on amenorrhea in obese women, *N Engl J Med* 249:835, 1953.

133. Moller DE, Flier JS: Detection of an alteration in the insulin-receptor gene in a patient with insulin resistance, acanthosis nigricans, and the polycystic ovary syndrome (Type A insulin resistance), *N Engl J Med* 319:1526, 1988.

134. Moore RJ, Wilson JD: Steroid 5 α-reductase in cultured human fibroblasts: biochemical and genetic evidence for two distinct enzyme activities, *J Biol Chem* 251:5895, 1976.

135. Naether OGJ, Fischer R, Weise HC et al: Laparoscopic electrocoagulation of the ovarian surface in infertile patients with polycystic ovarian disease, *Fertil Steril* 60:88, 1993.

136. Naether OGJ, Fischer R: Adhesion formation after laparoscopic electrocoagulation of the ovarian surface in polycystic ovary patients, *Fertil Steril* 60:95, 1993.

137. Naftolin F, Ryan KJ, Petro Z: Aromatization of androstenedione by the anterior hypothalamus of adult male and female rats, *Endocrinology* 90:295, 1972.

138. Nagamani M, Dinh TV, Kelver ME: Hyperinsulinemia in hyperthecosis of the ovaries, *Am J Obstet Gynecol* 154:384, 1986.

139. Nagata I, Kato K, Seki K et al: Ovulatory disturbances, *J Adolesc Health Care* 7:1, 1986.

140. Nestler JE, Clore JN, Strauss III JF et al: The effects of hyperinsulinemia on serum testosterone, progesterone, dehydroepiandrosterone sulfate, and cortisol levels in normal women and in a woman with hyperandrogenism, insulin resistance, and acanthosis nigricans, *J Clin Endocrinol Metab* 64:180, 1987.

141. Nestler JE, Usiskin KS, Barlascini CO et al: Suppression of serum dehydroepiandrosterone sulfate levels by insulin: an evaluation of possible mechanisms, *J Clin Endocrinol Metab* 69:1040, 1989.

142. Nestler JE, Clone JN, Blackard WG: The central role of obesity (hyperinsulinemia) in the pathogenesis of the polycystic ovary syndrome, *Am J Obstet Gynecol* 161:1095, 1989.

143. Nestler JE, Barlascini CO, Matt DW et al: Suppression of serum insulin by diazoxide reduces serum testosterone levels in obese women with polycystic ovary syndrome, *J Clin Endocrinol Metab* 66:1027, 1989.

144. Nestler JE, Singh R, Matt DW et al: Suppression of serum insulin level by diazoxide does not alter serum testosterone or sex-hormone-binding globulin levels in healthy, nonobese women, *Am J Obstet Gynecol* 163:1243, 1990.

145. Nestler JE, Powers LP, Matt DW et al: A direct effect of hyperinsulinemia on serum sex-hormone-binding globulin levels in obese women with the polycystic ovary syndrome, *J Clin Endocrinol Metab* 72:83, 1991.

146. Ober C, Weil S, Steck T et al: Increased risk for polycystic ovary syndrome associated with human leucocyte antigen DQA1*0501, *Am J Obstet Gynecol* 167:1803, 1992.

147. Ohel G, Katz M, Tobler C et al: Serum ACTH levels in patients with polycystic ovarian disease, *Clin Exp Obstet Gynecol* 12:29, 1985.

148. O'Meara N, Blackman JD, Ehrmann DA et al: Defects in B-cell function in functional ovarian hyperandrogenism, *J Clin Endocrinol Metab* 76:1241, 1973.

149. Orsini LF, Venturoli S, Lorusso R et al: Ultrasonic findings in polycystic ovarian disease, *Fertil Steril* 43:709, 1985.

150. Pache TD, Gooren LJG, Hop HCJ et al: Ovarian morphology in long-term androgen-treated female to male transsexuals. A human model for the study of polycystic ovarian syndrome, *Histopathology* 19:445, 1991.

151. Paradisi R, Venturoli S, Pasquali R et al: Effects of obesity on gonadotropin secretion in patients with polycystic ovarian disease, *J Endocrinol Invest* 9:139, 1986.

152. Parisi L, Ramanti M, Casciano S et al: The role of ultrasound in the study of polycystic ovarian disease, *J Clin Ultrasound* 10:167, 1982.

153. Parker LN, Odell WD: Control of adrenal androgen secretion, *Endocr Rev* 1:392, 1980.

154. Pasquali R, Casimirri F, Venturoli S et al: Insulin resistance in patients with polycystic ovaries: its relationship to body weight and androgen levels, *Acta Endocrinol* 104:110, 1983.

155. Pasquali R, Raffaella F, Venturoli S et al: Effect of weight loss and antiandrogenic therapy on sex hormone blood levels and insulin resistance in obese patients with polycystic ovaries, *Am J Obstet Gynecol* 154:139, 1986.

156. Pasquali R, Antenucci D, Casimirri F et al: Clinical and hormonal characteristics of obese amenorrheic hyperandrogenic women before and after weight loss, *J Clin Endocrinol Metab* 68:173, 1989.

157. Peiris AN, Aiman EJ, Drucker WD et al: The relative contributions of hepatic and peripheral tissues to insulin resistance in hyperandrogenic women, *J Clin Endocrinol Metab* 68:715, 1989.

158. Peiris AN, Sothmann MS, Aiman EJ et al: The relationship of insulin to sex-hormone-binding globulin: role of adiposity, *Fertil Steril* 52:69, 1989.

159. Plymate S, Fariss BL, Bassett ML et al: Obesity and its role in polycystic ovary syndrome, *J Clin Endocrinol Metab* 52:1246, 1981.

160. Plymate SR, Jones RE, Matej LA et al: Regulation of sex-hormone-binding globulin (SHBG) production in HEP G^2 cells by insulin, *Steroids* 52:339, 1988.

161. Plymate SR, Matej LA, Jones RE et al: Inhibition of sex-hormone-binding globulin production in the human hepatoma (Hep G2) cell line by insulin and prolactin, *J Clin Endocrinol Metab* 67:460, 1988.

162. Polson DW, Wadsworth J, Adams J et al: Polycystic ovaries—a common finding in normal women, *Lancet* 870, 1988.

163. Poretsky L: On the paradox of insulin-induced hyperandrogenism in insulin-resistant states, *Endocr Rev* 12(1):3, 1991.

164. Quigley ME, Rakoff JS, Yen SSC: Increased luteinizing sensitivity to dopamine inhibition in polycystic ovary syndrome, *J Clin Endocrinol Metab* 52:231, 1981.

165. Raj SG, Thompson IE, Berger MJ et al: Clinical aspects of the polycystic ovary syndrome, *Obstet Gynecol* 49:552, 1977.

166. Rao JK, Chihal HJ, Johnson CM: Primary polycystic ovary syndrome in a premenarchal girl, *J Reprod Med* 30:361, 1985.

167. Rebar R, Judd HL, Yen SC et al: Characterization of the inappropriate gonadotropin secretion in polycystic ovarian syndrome, *J Clin Invest* 57:1320, 1976.

168. Rebuffe-Scrive M, Cullberg G, Lundberg PA et al: Anthropometric variables and metabolism in polycystic ovarian disease, *Horm Metab Res* 21:391, 1989.

169. Rittmaster RS: Differential suppression of testosterone and estradiol in hirsute women with the superactive gonadotropin-releasing hormone agonist leuprolide, *J Clin Endocrinol Metab* 67:651, 1988.

170. Rittmaster RS: Finasteride, *N Engl J Med* 330:120, 1994.

171. Rodin A, Thakkar H, Taylor N et al: Hyperandrogenism in polycystic ovary syndrome, *N Engl J Med* 330:460, 1994.

172. Rogers J, Mitchell Jr GW: The relation of obesity to menstrual disturbances, *N Engl J Med* 247:53, 1952.

173. Roncari DAK, Van RLR: Promotion of human adipocyte precursor replication by 17-β-estradiol in culture, *J Clin Invest* 62:503, 1977.

174. Rosenfield RL: Plasma testosterone-binding globulin and indexes of the concentration of unbound plasma androgens in normal and hirsute subjects, *J Clin Endocrinol Metab* 32:717, 1971.

175. Rosenfield RL, Barnes RB, Cara JF et al: Dysregulation of cytochrome p450c17 as the cause of polycystic ovarian syndrome, *Fertil Steril* 53:785, 1985.

176. Rossmanith WG, Keckstein J, Spatzier K et al: The impact of ovarian laser surgery on the gonadotropin secretion in women with polycystic ovarian disease, *Clin Endocrinol* 34:223, 1991.

177. Rowland DL, Perrings TS, Thommes JA: Comparison of androgenic effects of food intake and body weight in adult rats, *Physiol Behav* 24:205, 1980.

178. Ruutiainen K, Erkkola R, Gronroos MA et al: Androgen parameters in hirsute women: correlations with body mass index and age, *Fertil Steril* 50:255, 1988.

179. Schriock ED, Buffington CK, Hubert GD et al: Divergent correlations of circulating dehydroepiandrosterone sulfate and testosterone with insulin levels and insulin-receptor binding, *J Clin Endocrinol Metab* 66:1329, 1988.

180. Shaw RW, Duignan MN, Butt WR et al: Modification by sex steroids of LHRH response in the polycystic ovary syndrome, *Clin Endocrinol* 5:495, 1976.

181. Short RV, London DR: Defective biosynthesis of ovarian steroids in the Stein-Leventhal syndrome, *Br Med J* 1:1724, 1961.

182. Shou-Qing L, Qin-Sheng G, Chun-Xia G et al: Diagnosis of polycystic ovary syndrome and preliminary studies on its mechanism, *Chin Med J* 98:95, 1985.

183. Smith CP, Dunger DB, Williams AJK et al: Relationship between insulin, insulin-like growth factor I, and dehydroepiandrosterone sulfate concentrations during childhood, puberty and adult life, *J Clin Endocrinol Metab* 68:932, 1989.

184. Smith KD, Steinberger E, Perloff WH: Polycystic ovarian disease, *Am J Obstet Gynecol* 193:994, 1965.

185. Smith S, Ravnikar VA, Barbieri RL: Androgen and insulin response to an oral glucose challenge in hyperandrogenic women, *Fertil Steril* 48:72, 1987.

186. Sommers SC, Wadman PJ: Pathogenesis of polycystic ovaries, *Am J Obstet Gynecol* 72:160, 1956.

187. Speiser PW, DuPont B, Rubinstein P et al: High frequency of nonclassical steroid 21-hydroxylase deficiency, *Am J Hum Genet* 37:650, 1985.

188. Spinder T, Spijkstra JJ, van den Tweel JG et al: The effects of long-term testosterone administration on pulsatile luteinizing hormone secretion and on ovarian histology in eugonadal female to male transsexual subjects, *J Clin Endocrinol* 69:151, 1989.

189. Stanhope R, Adams J, Brook CGD: Evolution of polycystic ovaries in a girl with delayed menarche, *J Reprod Med* 33:482, 1988.

190. Stein IF, Leventhal ML: Amenorrhea associated with bilateral polycystic ovaries, *Am J Obstet Gynecol* 29:181, 1935.

191. Stein IF: Duration of fertility following ovarian wedge resection—Stein-Leventhal syndrome, *Obstet Gynecol Surv* 20:124, 1965.

192. Steingold K, De Ziegler D, Cedars M et al: Clinical and hormonal effects of chronic gonadotropin-releasing hormone agonist treatment in polycystic ovarian disease, *J Clin Endocrinol Metab* 65:773, 1987.

193. Stoner E: The clinical development of a 5α-reductase inhibitor, finasteride, *J Steroid Biochem Molec Biol* 37:375, 1990.

194. Stuart CA, Nagamani M: Insulin infusion acutely augments ovarian androgen production in normal women, *Fertil Steril* 54:788, 1990.

195. Swanson M, Sauerbrei EE, Cooperberg PL: Medical implications of ultrasonically detected polycystic ovaries, *J Clin Ultrasound* 9:219, 1981.

196. Takai I, Tair S, Tahakura K et al: Three types of polycystic ovarian syndrome in relation to androgenic function, *Fertil Steril* 56:856, 1991.

197. Taylor SI, Dons RF, Hernandez E et al: Insulin resistance associated with androgen excess in women with autoantibodies to the insulin receptor, *Ann Intern Med* 97:851, 1982.

198. Taymor ML, Barnard R: Luteinizing hormone excretion in the polycystic ovary syndrome, *Fertil Steril* 13:501, 1962.

199. Toaff R, Toaff ME, Peyser MR: Infertility following wedge resection of the ovaries, *Am J Obstet Gynecol* 124:92, 1976.

200. Vermesh M, Silva PD, Lobo RA: Endogenous opioids modulate the inhibitory effects of androgen on the hypothalamic-pituitary axis of normal women, *J Clin Endocrinol Metab* 65:183, 1987.

201. Vermeulen A, Stoica T, Verdonck L: The apparent free testosterone concentration, an index of androgenicity, *J Clin Endocrinol Metab* 33:759, 1971.

202. Vermesh M, Silva PD, Rosen GF et al: Effect of androgen on adrenal steroidogenesis in normal women, *J Clin Endocrinol Metab* 66:128, 1988.

203. von Schoultz B, Carlstrom K: On the regulation of sex-hormone-binding globulin—a challenge of an old dogma and outlines of an alternative mechanism, *J Steroid Biochem* 32:327, 1989.

204. Waldstreicher J, Santoro N, Hall JE et al: Hyperfunction of the hypothalamic-pituitary axis in women with polycystic ovarian disease: indirect evidence for partial gonadotroph desensitization, *JCEM* 66:165, 1988.

205. Wild RA, Painter PC, Coulson PB et al: Lipoprotein lipid concentrations and cardiovascular risk in women with polycystic ovary syndrome, *J Clin Endocrinol Metab* 61:946, 1985.

206. Wild RA, Grubb B, Hartz A et al: Clinical signs of androgen excess as risk factors for coronary artery disease, *Fertil Steril* 54:255, 1990.

207. Wild RA, Applebaum-Bowden D, Demers LM, et al: Lipoprotein lipids in women with androgen excess: independent associations with increased insulin and androgen, *Clin Chem* 36:283, 1990.

208. Wortsman J, Wehrenberg WB, Gavin JR et al: Elevated levels of plasma β-endorphin and gamma 3-melanocyte-stimulating hormone in the polycystic ovary syndrome, *Obstet Gynecol* 63:630, 1984.

209. Yen SSC, Vela P, Rankin J: Inappropriate secretion of follicle-stimulating hormone and luteinizing hormone in polycystic ovarian disease, *J Clin Endocrinol Metab* 30:435, 1970.

210. Yen SSC, Chaney C, Judd HL: Functional aberrations of the hypothalamic-pituitary system in polycystic ovary syndrome: a consideration of the pathogenesis. In James VHT, Serio M, Guisti G, editors: *The endocrine function of the human ovary,* New York, 1976, Academic.

211. Yen SSC: The polycystic ovary syndrome, *Clin Endocrinol* 12:177, 1980.

212. Zacur HA, Foster GB: Hyperprolactinemia and polycystic ovarian syndrome, *Semin Reprod Endocrinol* 10:236, 1992.

213. Zavaroni I, Bonora E, Pagliara M et al: Risk factors for coronary artery disease in healthy persons with hyperinsulinemia and normal glucose tolerance, *N Engl J Med* 320:702, 1989.

214. Zumoff B, Rosenfeld RS, Strain GW et al: Sex differences in the twenty-four-hour mean plasma concentrations of dehydroisoandrosterone (DHA) and dehydroisoandrosterone sulfate (DHAS) and the DHA to DHAS ratio in normal adults, *J Clin Endocrinol Metab* 51:330, 1980.

215. Zumoff B, Freeman R, Coupey S et al: A chronobiologic abnormality in luteinizing hormone secretion in teenage girls with the polycystic-ovary syndrome, *N Engl J Med* 309:1206, 1983.

Chapter 12

THYROID DISEASES

David S. Cooper, MD
and Paul W. Ladenson, MD

Seventeenth-century British physicians believed that the purpose of the thyroid gland was to beautify the neck, particularly in women. Subsequent advances in the understanding of thyroid physiology and pathophysiology have led to an appreciation of the fact that almost all thyroid disorders are more common in women. In addition, important interactions between thyroid dysfunction and female reproductive endocrinology make knowledge of thyroid diseases and their diagnosis and management particularly important for physicians who care for women.

CLINICAL ANATOMY AND PHYSIOLOGY OF THE THYROID GLAND

Anatomy and embryology

The thyroid gland's normal position, anterior to the second through fourth tracheal rings, makes it a readily visible organ, particularly in women with slender necks. The gland is closely apposed to other structures in the neck, which can be affected by goitrous expansion or neoplastic invasion arising from the thyroid. Consequently, compression of the esophagus and trachea can produce dysphagia or dyspnea, respectively. The gland's intimate relationship to the recurrent laryngeal nerves may endanger vocal cord motion through tumor compression. Both these nerves and the adjacent parathyroid glands are at risk of injury during surgical treatment of thyroid disorders. Aberrant embryologic migration of thyroid tissue from its origin at the foramen caecum to the anterior neck may leave thyroglossal duct cysts or glandular remnants, which can be affected by thyroid diseases, anywhere between the tongue and the diaphragm.

Thyroid hormones

Action. The biologically active thyroid hormones, thyroxine (T_4) and triiodothyronine (T_3), express their actions in target tissues through binding to protein receptors.[66] Because T_3 binds to these receptors with higher affinity, it is considered the chief effector of thyroid hormone actions, whereas T_4 provides a stable circulating and intracellular reservoir for conversion to T_3. Although thyroid hormone-binding sites have been identified in the cytoplasmic membrane, cytosol, and mitochondria, the principal thyroid hormone receptor is widely believed to reside in the nucleus. T_3 receptors, which exist in several isoforms, are members of a receptor family that has structural homology to the protein encoded by the cellular homologue of the avian erythroblastosis virus oncogene, c-*erb* A. In addition to T_3 binding, these receptors bind to T_3 regulatory elements, specific nucleotide sequences in the regulatory regions of thyroid hormone-responsive genes. Most actions of thyroid hormone are currently attributed to altered expression of such genes (e.g., growth hormone, thyrotropin, and α-myosin heavy chain). The genes implicated in thyroid hormone regulation of female reproductive functions have yet to be identified.

Biosynthesis and transport. Thyroid epithelial cells possess two unique biologic properties that enable them to synthesize thyroid hormones: an incompletely characterized iodine-trapping mechanism and expression of the gene encoding the large protein thyroglobulin. Specific tyrosine residues within thyroglobulin are covalently linked to an oxidized iodine intermediate in a reaction catalyzed by the enzyme thyroid peroxidase to form monoiodotyrosines and diiodotyrosines. Coupling of two iodinated tyrosines, which is facilitated by the tertiary structure of thyroglobulin and catalyzed by thyroid peroxidase, results in formation of the iodothyronines T_4 and T_3. Thyroglobulin, to which the thyroid hormones remain linked, is secreted into the lumen of the follicle, a spheric arrangement of thyroid epithelial cells, where it is stored as colloid. Pinocytotic uptake of colloid and hydrolytic cleavage of T_4 and T_3 is followed by their secretion into the circulation. T_4 is the principal hormonal product of the human thyroid gland, synthesized in tenfold to fifteenfold excess of T_3.

Both iodothyronines circulate predominantly bound to plasma proteins.[73] T_4 is 99.97% bound to thyroxine-binding globulin (TBG, 75%), transthyretin (thyroxine-binding pre-albumin, 15%), and albumin (10%); whereas T_3 is somewhat less protein bound, 99.7%. In most tissues, only the small, free fractions of circulating thyroid hormones are available for intracellular exchange and hormone action. Changes in the quantity or binding avidity of these plasma proteins alter total serum thyroid hormone levels but do not affect tissue responsiveness or patients' clinical status. The most common form of protein-binding derangement, TBG excess, is particularly common in women, in whom endogenous or exogenous estrogens can alter the carbohydrate composition of the glycoprotein TBG.[1] This estrogen-induced increase in sialic acid residues on TBG results in a longer plasma half-life and higher circulating TBG concentrations. Congenital TBG excess, a rare X-linked dominant trait, is obviously more common in women, whereas more prevalent X-linked TBG deficiency is more common in men; heterozygous women are less severely affected. (See Thyroid Function Testing.)

Metabolism. T_4 is converted to T_3 in both the cytoplasm and nucleus of all thyroid hormone-responsive organs by outer ring or 5'-monodeiodination[86] (Fig. 12-1). Inner ring or 5-monodeiodination results in formation of biologically inactive reverse T_3. Subsequent deiodinative steps, deamination, and hepatic conjugation of iodothyronines all contribute to their metabolism. Enhanced thyroid hormone catabolism, due at least in part to the action of placental deiodinase, may increase the thyroxine dose requirement during pregnancy.[55]

The activities of the two distinct types of 5'-monodeiodinase, which catalyze the crucial process of T_4 to T_3 conversion, are diminished in a number of pathophysi-

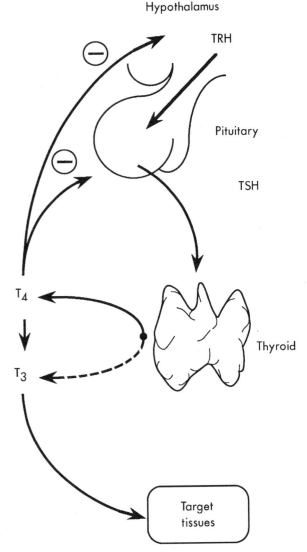

Fig. 12-1. Deiodinative metabolism of thyroid hormones. T_4 is enzymatically converted to more potent T_3 by outer-ring mono-deiodination in target tissues and thyroid. Inner-ring deiodination of T_4 yields reverse T_3, which is biologically inactive. (Redrawn from Ladenson PW et al: In *Principles and practice of medicine*, ed 22, Norwalk, Conn, 1988, Appleton & Lange.)

ologic states. Consequently, malnutrition and severe illnesses[47] (e.g., sepsis, malignancy, and hyperemesis gravidarum) are characterized by a low serum T_3 concentrations. Similarly, several pharmacologic agents, including propranolol and amiodarone, reduce T_4 to T_3 conversion. Occasionally, the resulting impaired T_4 clearance may result in a modestly elevated serum T_4 level under these same circumstances.[10] More often, however, nonthyroidal illnesses cause a low serum T_4 concentration.[97] This phenomenon remains incompletely understood, but it has been attributed variously to interference with plasma protein binding of T_4

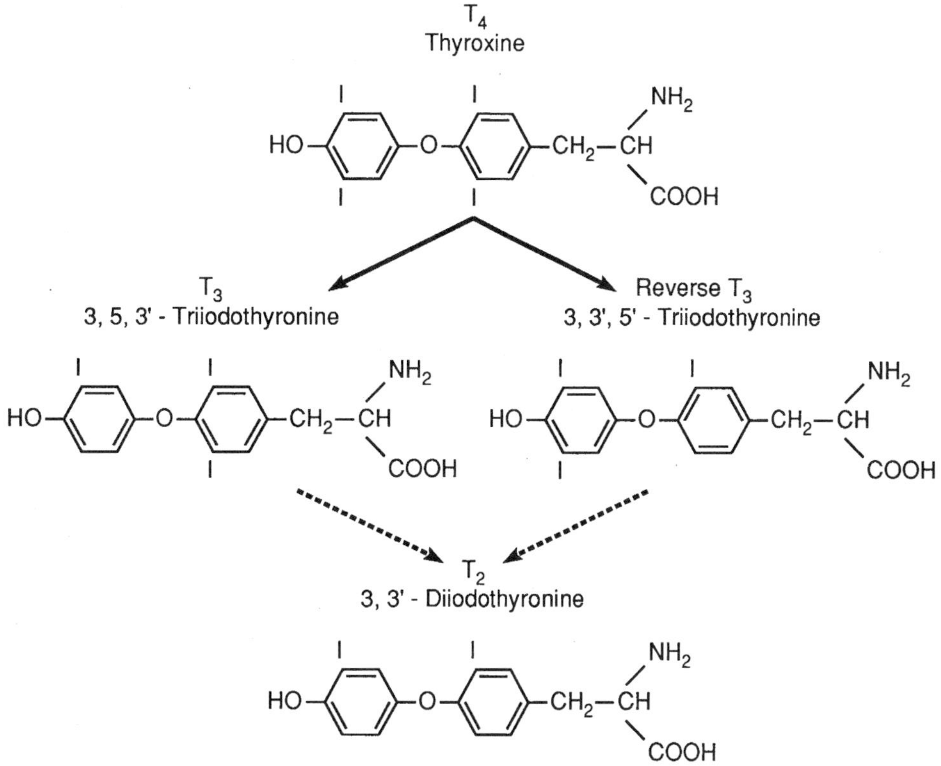

Fig. 12-2. Hypothalamic-pituitary-thyroid axis. Hypothalamic TRH stimulates pituitary thyrotropin production. TSH regulates thyroid gland growth and the biosynthesis and release of thyroid hormones (T_4 and T_3), which act on target tissues, including the pituitary, where negative feedback inhibits TSH production. (Redrawn from Ladenson PW et al: In *Principles and practice of medicine,* ed 22, Norwalk, Conn, 1988, Appleton & Lange,)

catabolism or to cytokine-induced alterations in thyroid cell function.[48] In the absence of disease, puberty, menopause, and aging per se are not associated with significant changes in thyroid function or circulating hormone concentrations.

Control of thyroid function

The chief regulator of thyroid gland growth and hormone biosynthesis is thyrotropin (thyroid-stimulating hormone [TSH]), a heterodimeric glycoprotein secreted by specialized anterior pituitary thyrotropic cells. The unique TSH β-subunit confers its biologic specificity, whereas the α-subunit is identical with those found in the gonadotropins: luteinizing hormone (LH), follicle-stimulating hormone (FSH), and human chorionic gonadotropin (hCG). TSH production is regulated by two factors: thyrotropin-releasing hormone (TRH) and negative feedback by the thyroid hormones (Fig. 12-2).

TRH is a tripeptide produced by specialized neurons in the anteromedial hypothalamus. It is transported by the hypothalamic-hypophysial venous portal system to the pituitary, where it binds to thyrotropic cell receptors linked to the inositol phosphate–intracellular calcium-signaling system. Both circulating T_3 and T_3 generated locally by the active intrapituitary deiodinase contribute to the intra-nuclear T_3 concentration in thyrotropic cells, in which T_3

suppresses expression of genes encoding both TSH subunits.[81] TRH synthesis is also negatively regulated by direct thyroid hormone feedback at the hypothalamic level.

TSH exerts its action on thyroid epithelial cells by binding to a specific membrane receptor, which activates the adenylate cyclase second-messenger system.[26] Thyroid-stimulating immunoglobulins directed against the TSH receptor, which develop more commonly in women, cause hyperthyroid Graves disease.[95] Less frequently, TSH receptor-blocking antibodies may be the cause of hypothyroidism.[101]

Iodine also plays a role in regulation of thyroid gland function. In the absence of sufficient dietary iodine intake (i.e., less than 50 ug/d), thyroidal uptake of iodine is enhanced and the gland enlarges. Although the North American diet provides an adequate iodine intake, it is estimated that 1 billion people in the world exist on a borderline or frankly low iodine diet, resulting in endemic goiter and cretinism. At the other end of the spectrum, pharmacologic iodine intake (i.e., > 1 mg/d) can also alter thyroid gland function. In individuals whose thyroid glands have an underlying iodine organification defect (e.g., autoimmune thyroiditis) iodine may cause hypothyroidism,[12] whereas iodine may provoke hyperthyroidism in patients with nodular goiter[92] (Jod-Basedow effect). Consequently,

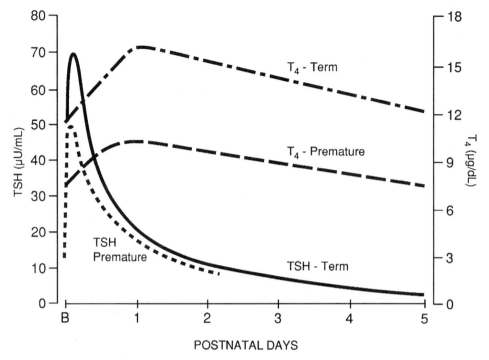

Fig. 12-3. Changes in serum TSH and T_4 concentrations in full-term and premature infants during the first 5 days of life. (Redrawn from Fisher DA, Klein AH: *N Engl J Med* 304:702, 1981. Reprinted by permission of the *New England Journal of Medicine.*)

women, who have higher prevalences of both autoimmune and nodular thyroid diseases, are at greater risk of iodine-induced thyroid dysfunction.

Fetal and neonatal thyroid function

Hypothalamic TRH, pituitary TSH, and iodine-concentrating thyroid epithelium all appear late in the first trimester of pregnancy.[69] Fetal thyroid development is normally independent of maternal pituitary or thyroid function. There is minimal transplacental transfer of maternal thyroid hormones, and their role in normal fetal development remains unclear. Consequently, maternal TSH or thyroid hormone deficiency per se is not associated with increased risk of neonatal hypothyroidism. Whether maternal hypothyroidism may be associated with subtle impairment of subsequent neuropsychologic performance in childhood remains controversial.[24] Furthermore, maternal L-thyroxine treatment in appropriate dosage is entirely safe during pregnancy and has no deleterious effects on the fetus. In contrast, the immunoglobulins that cause autoimmune thyroid diseases do cross the placenta and may produce transient thyroid dysfunction in the fetus and neonate.[101] (See Hyperthyroidism.) Furthermore, the fetus is exposed to all pharmacologic agents commonly used in treatment of hyperthyroidism, including the antithyroid drugs, radioactive and stable iodine, and β-adrenergic blocking agents.

Normal delivery is accompanied by surges in neonatal secretion of TSH and thyroid hormones[28] (Fig. 12-3). Birth is also accompanied by a rise in neonatal 5'-monodeiodinase activity,[99] which is low during fetal development, accounting for the low serum T_3 and elevated serum reverse T_3 concentrations in neonatal plasma. These physiologic changes and the effects of nonthyroidal illnesses in sick infants must be considered in the interpretation of neonatal thyroid function tests obtained routinely for detection of congenital hypothyroidism.

THYROID FUNCTION TESTING

Symptoms and signs of hypothyroidism and hyperthyroidism are nonspecific and easily confused with the clinical manifestations of other diseases and physiologic states, including normal pregnancy. It is fortunate that extremely accurate, safe, and relatively inexpensive tests can confirm or exclude the presence of thyroid diseases.

Serum thyroid function tests

There are two general strategies for diagnosing functional disorders of the thyroid: measuring the serum thyroid hormone concentrations themselves or quantifying the pituitary thyrotropic response to ambient thyroid hormone levels by measuring the serum TSH concentration.[50,51] Each approach has certain advantages and limitations.

Serum total T_4 and total T_3 concentrations are precisely quantified by immunoassays. Abnormal total thyroid hormone concentrations may reflect true derangements of thyroid hormone production, altered thyroid hormone-binding protein concentrations or binding affinities, or the presence of circulating substances that interfere with the interaction of thyroid hormones and plasma proteins. Because an increased serum TBG concentration is extremely common in women, who may have increased estrogen action due to pregnancy or exogenous hormonal replacement or contraceptive therapy, total serum thyroid hormone measurements are not the optimal way to screen women with potential thyroid dysfunction. In this patient population, an elevated serum total T_4 concentration is more likely to be due to physiologic or pharmacologic estrogen effects than to hyperthyroidism.

The common forms of potentially misleading plasma protein alterations are circumvented by direct measurement or indirect estimation of the serum free T_4 and free T_3 concentrations. The gold standard for free thyroid hormone quantitation, equilibrium dialysis, is a cumbersome technique with limited availability. Estimates of the free T_4 and free T_3 concentrations by immunoassay techniques or by calculation of the free T_4 index are adequate under most circumstances. The free T_4 index is generally calculated by multiplying the total T_4 concentration and the T_3 resin uptake (or thyroid hormone-binding ratio). The T_3 resin uptake is determined by incubating patient serum with radiolabeled T_3 and quantifying tracer activity that is not bound by plasma proteins. The residual resin-adsorbed T_3 tracer activity is inversely proportionate to the number of endogenously unoccupied thyroid hormone-binding sites (Fig.12-4). Thus, patients with hyperthyroidism have increased levels of both the serum total T_4 and the T_3 resin uptake, reflecting high occupancy of thyroid hormone-binding sites by endogenous hormone and yielding a high free T_4 index product. In contrast, patients with TBG excess also have a total T_4 elevation but a low T_3 resin uptake, reflecting the greater number of protein-binding sites and yielding a normal free T_4 index.

Serum free T_4 estimates usually provide reliable and economical information regarding a patient's thyroid status in most circumstances. However, in several settings, this parameter alone may be inaccurate. Rarer plasma protein-binding abnormalities may not be distinguished from hyperthyroidism (e.g., familial dysalbuminemic hyperthyroxinemia,[83] in which an albumin variant binds T_4 with greater affinity) and the presence of endogenous anti-T_4 antibodies. In patients with severe nonthyroidal illnesses, both the serum free T_4 radioimmunoassay and free T_4 index may be misleadingly low without true hypothyroidism. In other systemic illnesses (e.g., hyperemesis gravidarum[11] and acute psychosis[85], the serum free thyroxine may be increased. Furthermore, subtle derangements of thyroid function may be obscured by the relatively broad normal

ranges for free T_4 that are typical in most laboratories. Therefore, individuals with mild or subclinical thyroid dysfunction may not be recognized.

Serum TSH measurement is an extremely accurate alternate strategy to diagnose thyroid dysfunction, particularly in women who may have an elevated serum TBG concentration. In both overt and subclinical hypothyroidism due to primary thyroid disease, the serum TSH concentration is elevated. All common forms of hyperthyroidism are associated with a markedly decreased serum TSH level, less than 0.1 mU/L.[84] Serum TSH measurement also represents an extremely precise technique for the adjustment of prescribed L-thyroxine for either hypothyroidism or suppression of thyroid neoplasia. Quantitation of thyroid function by serum TSH concentration entirely avoids the potential for misdiagnosis due to alterations in plasma thyroid hormone–binding proteins.

There are, however, certain limitations in assessment of thyroid function based on the serum TSH alone. Some apparently healthy and euthyroid older persons may have serum TSH concentrations that are low but are detectable in highly sensitive assays. In patients with hypothyroidism secondary to hypothalamic or pituitary disease, the serum TSH concentration is typically low or normal. Conversely, rare patients with hyperthroidism due to TSH-secreting pituitary adenomas[31] have a normal or elevated serum TSH concentration. Individuals with familial thyroid hormone resistance also have normal or increased serum TSH levels, which are inappropriate for their elevated circulating free thyroid hormone concentrations. Occasionally, recent changes in thyroid hormone concentrations may not yet be reflected in pituitary TSH production (e.g., recent reversal of hyperthyroidism and intermittent noncompliance with replacement therapy for hypothyroidism). In most laboratories, the serum TSH assay is somewhat more expensive than estimates of the free T_4. The availability of highly sensitive TSH assays, which can detect concentrations less than 0.1 mU/L, have made TRH stimulation testing obsolete in almost all circumstances.

In summary, both the free T_4 and TSH measurement strategies have acceptable accuracy to evaluate patients in whom overt primary thyroid dysfunction is suspected. The serum TSH is more sensitive for detection of subtle thyroid disease. Serum TSH measurement is also preferred in the evaluation of patients with systemic illness. In the presence of possible hypothalamic or pituitary disease, serum free T_4 estimates should be obtained with the serum TSH.

Differential diagnosis of thyroid dysfunction

Once the diagnosis of hypothyroidism or hyperthyroidism has been established, additional tests may be useful to define the underlying cause of thyroid dysfunction. The vast majority of women with hypothyroidism not due to previous thyroid surgery or radiation have autoimmune

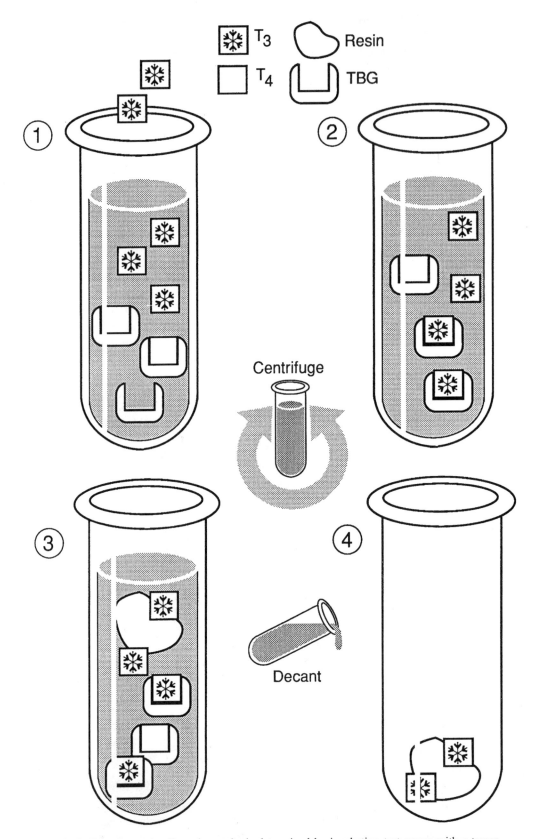

Fig. 12-4. T_3 resin uptake. T_3 resin uptake is determined by incubating test serum with a tracer quantity of radiolabeled T_3 ($*T_3$), which interacts with available binding sites on TBG. At equilibrium between bound and free $*T_3$, an insoluable resin is added and free $*T_3$ is adsorbed. Resin is separated from serum by centrifugation, and the resin-associated $*T_3$ activity is quantified. (Redrawn from Ladenson PW et al: In *Principles and practice of medicine,* ed 22, Norwalk, Conn, 1988, Appleton & Lange.)

thyroiditis (Hashimoto disease). This diagnosis can be established with greater certainty by screening serum for the presence of antithyroglobulin and antimicrosomal thyroid antibodies. The latter parameter is more sensitive and specific as a single test and is now known to reflect the presence of immunoglobulins directed against the crucial biosynthetic enzyme thyroid peroxidase.[45] Antithyroid antibody measurements are useful to define the probability of subsequent overt hypothyroidism in women with subclinical hypothyroidism[90] (i.e., an elevated serum TSH in the presence of a normal serum free T_4). In patients to whom L-thyroxine has previously been prescribed for unclear indications, antithyroid antibody screening may help clarify whether continued thyroid hormone therapy is appropriate (i.e., whether the patient has underlying autoimmune thyroiditis).

In most patients with hyperthyroidism, the cause is clinically obvious, that is, Graves disease. When a diffuse goiter and exophthalmos are absent, or when clinical findings suggest other disorders (e.g., postpartum thyroiditis or factitious hyperthyroidism), additional tests may be required to identify the underlying disorder. The fractional radionuclide uptake by the thyroid, using either iodine 123 or technetium Tc 99m pertechnetate, is increased in Graves disease and is usually elevated or high-normal in toxic nodular goiter. Radionuclide imaging can assist further by revealing the pattern of tracer distribution within the gland, which can assist in differentiating toxic nodular goiter from Graves disease in patients without ophthalmopathy or dermopathy. In contrast, glandular concentration of radioisotope is markedly decreased in subacute (de Quervain) and postpartum (lymphocytic) thyroiditis and in factitious (exogenous) hyperthyroidism.

Blood tests may also be useful in the differential diagnosis of hyperthyroidism. Although thyroid-stimulating immunoglobulin and TSH receptor-binding inhibition measurements are not usually needed to diagnose Graves disease, occasionally they may be useful to differentiate it from toxic nodular goiter and to estimate the risk of neonatal thyrotoxicosis in pregnant women with current or previously treated Graves disease.[100] The erythrocyte sedimentation rate typically is increased in subacute thyroiditis. The serum thyroglobulin is usually elevated in all types of endogenous hyperthyroidism, whereas it is suppressed when hyperthyroidism is due to exogenous thyroid hormone.[56]

Evaluation of goiter, thyroid nodules, and cancer

The fine-needle aspiration biopsy is the most accurate and cost-effective initial procedure to differentiate benign from malignant thyroid nodules.[36] Radionuclide scanning can identify the 5% of nodules that are "hot," that is, those that represent the only thyroid tissue concentrating tracer; These can be assumed to be benign. However, the majority of nodules, which function either relatively less ("cold" nodules) or equivalently ("warm" nodules) to the remainder of the gland require further investigation. Ultrasound examination of the thyroid can determine whether thyroid nodules are solid or cystic, but only small, simple cysts can be considered benign. Ultrasound can be useful to define the size of nodules precisely for serial comparison. The presence of antithyroid antibodies suggests that a diffuse goiter is attributable to autoimmune thyroiditis. Serum thyroglobulin measurement is useful in the follow-up of patients with treated thyroid malignancies but cannot distinguish between benign and malignant thyroid nodules.[93] The serum calcitonin concentration is an extremely useful tumor marker in patients with sporadic or familial medullary thyroid carcinoma.

HYPOTHYROIDISM

Thyroid hormone deficiency is among the most common diseases affecting women. Two percent of women suffer overt hypothyroidism and 5% develop subclinical hypothyroidism during their lives. An additional 6% of women have transient postpartum hypothyroidism.[6] Furthermore, complaints consistent with thyroid hormone deficiency (e.g., fatigue and weight gain) are common in euthyroid individuals and must be distinguished from actual thyroid dysfunction. Finally, clinical manifestations of hypothyroidism may include significant disturbances of reproductive physiology: both precocious and delayed puberty, menstrual dysfunction, and ovulatory disorders that can contribute to infertility.

Causes

Autoimmune thyroiditis. Autoimmune thyroiditis (Hashimoto disease), the chief cause of hypothyroidism, is tenfold more common in women than in men. There is a familial predisposition to autoimmune thyroiditis, but the precise genetic and environmental determinants of the disease are unknown.[94] Evidence in support of an autoimmune pathogenesis includes the presence of thyroid-specific cellular immunity, circulating immunoglobulins directed against thyroidal antigens, linkage with certain human leukocyte antigen (HLA) class I haplotypes, and associations with other endocrine and non–endocrine autoimmune diseases.

Autoimmune thyroiditis can occur at any age. It is rare in the first decade of life and affects 15% of women over age 65 years. The severity of hypothyroidism ranges from subclinical gland dysfunction to profound thyroid hormone deficiency with myxedema. The mildest degree of thyroid gland failure has been termed decreased thyroid reserve or subclinical hypothyroidism, although some patients in fact experience symptoms that are reversible by thyroid hormone therapy. The syndrome is biochemically characterized by an elevated serum TSH concentration in association with a normal serum T_4 level. Patients with autoimmune thyroiditis typically have a diffuse, firm, and painless goiter; although complete absence of palpable tissue, an asymmetrically enlarged gland, or a tender thyroid are occasionally encountered. Autoimmune thyroiditis is uncommonly associated with primary adrenal insufficiency (Schmidt's syndrome), hypoparathyroidism, primary ovarian failure, and type I diabetes mellitus. Vitiligo, prematurely gray hair, pernicious anemia, and rheumatoid arthritis are more common in individuals with this thyroid disease. The diagnosis of autoimmune thyroiditis is confirmed by the presence of primary hypothyroidism (i.e., an elevated serum TSH concentration) and the presence of circulating antithyroid antibodies.

Postablative hypothyroidism. Hypothyroidism frequently follows surgical or radioactive iodine treatment of hyperthyroidism, particularly Graves disease, in which the natural history of thyroid dysfunction itself may also lead to spontaneous thyroid gland failure. Even among patients who remain euthyroid in the year after subtotal thyroidectomy or iodine 131 therapy, approximately 3% develop thyroid gland failure each year. Patients with Graves disease previously treated only with antithyroid drugs also have a substantial prevalence of hypothyroidism, approximately 25% after a decade.[98] Irradiation of the thyroid gland incidental to treatment of head, neck, and upper mediastinal neoplasms (e.g., lymphoma) is also associated with high prevalences of both overt and subclinical hypothyroidism.[38]

Thyroiditis. Transient thyroid gland inflammation causes spontaneously resolving hypothyroidism in two diseases. Postpartum thyroiditis is a common disorder that affects at least 1 of 20 women after delivery.[6] (See Postpartum Thyroid Disease.) This idiopathic disorder is more common in women with a previous history of autoimmune thyroid disease or detectable serum antithyroglobulin antibodies during pregnancy. Patients usually have a small, painless goiter, reflecting its infiltration with lymphocytes. Thyroid hormone deficiency in the disorder typically has its onset 2 to 6 months postpartum and lasts from 2 to 10 weeks. Hypothyroidism may be preceded by or, rarely, followed by transient hyperthyroidism.

Subacute thyroiditis (de Quervain thyroiditis) is believed to be caused by viral infection of the thyroid. Clinical features of the disease include a viral prodrome; constitutional symptoms, including malaise and fever; severe thyroidal pain, which can radiate to the jaw or ear; and transient hyperthyroidism followed by hypothyroidism, both of which typically resolve completely.

Pituitary or hypothalamic diseases. Rarely, hypothyroidism is due to pituitary or hypothalamic diseases causing deficiency of biologically active TSH. Pituitary tumors and previous pituitary surgery or irradiation are the most common causes. Hypothalamic sarcoidosis, tumors, and vasculitis also may be responsible. In patients with central hypothyroidism, the serum free T_4 concentration is usually low-normal or modestly decreased in association with an undetectable or an inappropriately low or normal serum TSH level, as measured by immunoassay. The immunologically detected TSH in this setting has decreased biologic activity,[25] that is, diminished TSH receptor-binding or receptor-activating properties, or both. This alteration in biologic to immunologic activities has been attributed to defective posttranslational glycosylation of TSH.

Thyroid hormone resistance. Thyroid hormone resistance is a rare familial disorder in which there is defective expression of T_3 action in target tissues.[70] In several kindreds, the disease has been linked to mutations in the genes encoding the β_1 isoform of the T_3 receptor. Affected individuals may be hypothyroid or euthyroid in the face of elevated serum total and free T_4 and T_3 concentrations and an inappropriately normal or elevated circulating TSH level.

Clinical manifestations

The classic constitutional manifestations of hypothyroidism are fatigue, lethargy, cold intolerance, and weight gain despite poor appetite. The amount of weight gain typically is modest, 5 to 10 kg. Some hypothyroid patients, particularly the elderly, actually lose weight because of reduced caloric intake. Neuropsychiatric symptoms include impaired concentration and memory; depression; irritability; and, rarely, frank dementia, seizures, and coma. Other common manifestations include dry skin, hair loss, constipation, myalgias, and carpal tunnel syndrome. In addition to nonpitting subcutaneous edema, serous effusions can accumulate in the pericardium, pleural space, joints, and middle ear. Menstrual dysfunction is relatively common in hypothyroid women. Menorrhagia is the most frequent disorder and may provoke iron deficiency anemia. Amenorrhea is less frequently encountered. Related anovulation may cause infertility; however, thyroid hormone treatment is not useful for anovulatory euthyroid women. There is no convincing evidence that overt or subclinical hypothyroidism contributes to the development of premenstrual syndrome or that thyroid hormone treatment of premenstrual syndrome is more effective than placebo.[63]

Hypothyroidism can cause both isosexual precocious puberty and delayed puberty. In girls with juvenile hypothyroidism, who typically have extremely high serum TSH concentrations, premature menarche without preceding adrenarche occasionally occurs.[94] It has been postulated that TSH or a variant of normal TSH may bind and stimulate ovarian gonadotropin receptors, increasing estrogen production. With treatment of hypothyroidism, menses cease until normal puberty ensues. Hypothyroidism may also be associated with delayed puberty, which occurs in the context of growth retardation that accompanies juvenile hypothyroidism. Thyroid hormone replacement therapy restores normal pubertal potential and accelerates growth, although children with longstanding untreated hypothyroidism may never achieve their full predicted height, probably because of pubertal epiphyseal closure.

Hyperprolactinemia and galactorrhea are unusual manifestations of hypothyroidism. In patients with the syndrome of amenorrhea, galactorrhea, and modest hyperprolactinemia (i.e., serum prolactin 25 to 75 ng/mL), it is essential that the serum TSH concentration be assayed to differentiate primary hypothyroidism from a pituitary adenoma with secondary hypothyroidism. Furthermore, in younger women with primary hypothyroidism, pituitary imaging may be misleading because thyrotropic cell hyperplasia may cause symmetric pituitary enlargement.

Severe hypothyroidism or myxedema may be accompanied by severe, life-threatening derangements of organ function.[96] Thyroid hormone deficiency decreases myocardial contractility, potentially contributing to development of heart failure. Decreased ventilatory responsiveness to hypercapnia and hypoxia occur and may cause ventilatory failure or sleep apnea, or exacerbate depression of respiratory drive by depressant medications. Impaired renal free water excretion may lead to hyponatremia and hypoosmolality. Hypothermia and a blunted febrile response to sepsis may develop. Ultimately, profound and prolonged thyroid hormone deprivation and secondary metabolic complications may lead to myxedema coma, a syndrome of multisystem failure, which is associated with substantial mortality.

These morbid complications of hypothyroidism require postponement of elective surgical procedures in hypothyroid patients until replacement therapy has been instituted and, ideally, the serum TSH concentration has been normal for 1 month. When urgent surgery is required, perioperative L-thyroxine therapy, intravenously if necessary, can reduce some of the attendant risks.[52] General medical management of patients requiring surgery should focus particularly on detection and preemptive management of perioperative heart failure, sepsis, ileus, and neuropsychiatric complications.[53]

Clinical and biochemical features of hypothyroidism may be masked during pregnancy, when weight gain and fatigue may be attributed to gestation. Furthermore, the serum total thyroxine concentration may be maintained in the apparently normal range by the expected increase in TBG associated with pregnancy. Accurate diagnosis is ensured by serum TSH measurement. Prompt institution of L-thyroxine therapy is essential to minimize maternal symptoms, prepare the mother for an uncomplicated delivery, and ensure normal fetal development. The precise importance of maternal thyroid hormone in embryogenesis remains unclear. However, it is generally expected that children of hypothyroid mothers who are treated promptly will not suffer a higher risk of congenital anomalies or any readily discernible decrement in subsequent intellectual development.

Diagnosis and differential diagnosis

Because the clinical features of thyroid hormone deficiency are nonspecific, it is essential that the diagnosis of hypothyroidism be confirmed with thyroid function tests in every case. In patients with suspected hypothyroidism, serum TSH measurement is the most accurate single test, identifying patients with both overt and subclinical hypothyroidism, who have low or low-normal serum T_4 concentrations, respectively. Whenever central hypothyroidism due to pituitary or hypothalamic disease is suspected, the serum free T_4 concentration should also be measured. In patients with possible central hypothyroidism, measurement of the serum TSH concentration after administration of TRH (200 ug intravenously) is valuable in the diagnosis of patients who have serum T_4 concentrations in the lower half of the normal range.

In most cases, the underlying etiology of hypothyroidism is clinically obvious and is due to either autoimmune thyroiditis or postablative hypothyroidism. Autoimmune thyroiditis can be confirmed by the presence of circulating antimicrosomal or antithyroglobulin thyroid antibodies. Antimicrosomal antibodies, which are now known to be directed against the membrane-bound enzyme thyroid peroxidase, represent the more sensitive parameter. In patients with hypothyroidism due to postpartum thyroiditis, a low titer of antithyroid antibodies may be present as well. Individuals with subacute thyroiditis have an elevated erythrocyte sedimentation rate during the acute phase of their illness, which typically has resolved by the time hypothyroidism develops. Both forms of spontaneously resolving thyroiditis are also associated with a markedly decreased fractional thyroidal radionuclide uptake. Central hypothyroidism is characterized by a low or low-normal serum free T_4 concentration with an undetectable, low, or inappropriately normal serum TSH. Other hormonal or radiologic evidence of pituitary or hypothalamic disease should then be sought.

Treatment

Levothyroxine sodium (L-thyroxine) is the treatment of choice for sustained hypothyroidism, regardless of the underlying cause. By virtue of its conversion to T_3 in target tissues, L-thyroxine creates a physiologic milieu for thyroid hormone action, although the circulating T_4 concentration typically is slightly higher and the serum T_3 concentration minimally lower than in individuals with normal endogenous thyroid gland secretion.

L-Thyroxine is well absorbed, approximately 90% absorbed with contemporary formulations.[27] Only severe malabsorptive disorder or the simultaneous administration of cholestyramine or sucralfate interferes significantly with the medication's bioavailability. The L-thyroxine dose requirement is weight-related and age-related. In athyrotic patients, approximately 2 ug/kg is needed. Children have larger dose requirements, whereas the dose is lower in the older persons because of a decrease in metabolic clearance of L-thyroxine.[80] It is important to monitor the appropriateness of the L-thyroxine dose, clinically and by measuring the serum TSH concentration, every 1 to 2 years. Otherwise, a previously optimal dose may become excessive in older women, who are most susceptible to clinical consequences of even mild hyperthyroidism (e.g., osteoporosis and atrial dysrhythmias). Whenever precise regulation of thyroid hormone therapy is sought, administration of a single identifiable and refillable preparation will minimize potential variability in tablet formulation and drug bioavailability.

Because of its binding to plasma proteins, L-thyroxine has a conveniently long 7-day plasma half-life, permitting administration of a single daily dose. If necessary, patients can make up missed L-thyroxine doses the following day; and, in unusual circumstances where compliance is a problem, a larger medication dose may be administered under supervision 1 or 2 days per week.

L-Thyroxine metabolism is increased in approximately one third of women during pregnancy.[55] The increased dose requirement generally becomes evident during the first or second trimester and may necessitate an increase in dose by 25% to 100%. Consequently, the serum TSH concentration should be determined in all pregnant women with treated hypothyroidism during the second and fifth months of pregnancy. Another serum TSH measurement should then be obtained 1 month after adjustment of the L-thyroxine dose, to assure adequate treatment. Postpartum, the prepregnancy L-thyroxine dose can be resumed, although a serum TSH measurement should again be obtained after 1 month to confirm the appropriateness of this change. Other causes of enhanced L-thyroxine clearance include simultaneous administration of anticonvulsant drugs (e.g., diphenylhydantoin) and systemic nonthyroidal illnesses in some patients.

An excessive dosage of L-thyroxine predictably causes clinical thyrotoxicosis. In addition, subclinical hyperthyroidism due to less excessive L-thyroxine doses and producing serum T_4 concentrations at the upper limit of normal with an undetectable serum TSH may also be associated with subtle clinical complications. For example, excessive thyroid hormone therapy has been associated with significant cortical bone loss, even in premenopausal women.[68,78] Atrial fibrillation may develop in older patients whose sole manifestation of thyroid hormone excess is subnormal suppression of the serum TSH concentration. Consequently, in patients requiring thyroid hormone replacement therapy, the L-thyroxine dosage should be adjusted to maintain the serum TSH within the normal range. Putative allergies to available preparations of L-thyroxine have not been well documented. In patients reporting supposed hypersensitivity reactions, counseling, a lower L-thyroxine dose, and use

of multiples of uncolored tablets of 0.05-mg strength are appropriate approaches.

Biologic preparations of thyroid hormone (i.e., desiccated thyroid and thyroglobulin) and synthetic combinations of L-thyroxine and L-triiodothyronine are not physiologic. The combination of T_3 in the preparation and T_3 generated by endogenous deiodination of T_4 creates a state of absolute or relative T_3 excess. Furthermore, the short 1-day half-life of T_3 results in substantial fluctuations in the serum T_3 concentration throughout the day with single daily dosing. As a result, these thyroid preparations and T_3 itself are not appropriate for treatment of hypothyroidism and should be considered obsolete.

Three circumstances may justify L-thyroxine treatment of subclinical hypothyroidism (i.e., an elevated serum TSH elevation in association with a normal serum free T_4 level): (1) circulating antithyroid antibodies, which confer substantial risk of progression to frank hypothyroidism; (2) symptoms consistent with thyroid hormone deficiency, which have been shown to be benefited by L-thyroxine therapy more than by placebo[18]; and (3) elevated serum low-density lipoprotein cholesterol concentration, which may be caused or exacerbated by thyroid hormone deficiency.[5]

Myxedema coma, a rare life-threatening syndrome of multiple organ system failure,[29,96] is most common in elderly patients with profound and longstanding thyroid hormone deficiency. In patients who are obtunded or in whom gastrointestinal motility is impaired, intravenous L-thyroxine therapy, approximately 1 ug/kg, should be given in the absence of known atherosclerotic coronary artery disease. However, survival is equally dependent on anticipating, recognizing, and managing specific complications of severe hypothyroidism, including heart failure, hypoventilation, hyponatremia, ileus, hypothermia, and lack of a febrile response to sepsis. The depressant effects of sedatives and analgesics may be enhanced by impaired metabolic clearance of these drugs. Functional central adrenal insufficiency has been reported and should be treated by the simultaneous administration of glucocorticoids in maximal stress doses, for example, hydrocortisone hemisuccinate 300 mg/d or methylprednisolone 60 mg/d, in divided doses.

HYPERTHYROIDISM

Hyperthyroidism is a clinical and biochemical state produced when tissues are exposed to excessive circulating quantities of the thyroid hormones T_4 and T_3. Hyperthyroidism is far more common in women than in men, with an estimated annual incidence of 2 to 3/1000 women and a prevalence of 19/1000 women, compared with 1.6/1000 men.[90] Because of this difference, hyperthyroidism plays an important role in the reproductive lives of many women, with an impact on fertility, pregnancy management, and the postpartum period.

Causes

Hyperthyroidism is caused by the uncontrolled secretion or release of thyroid hormone into the blood stream or by the ingestion of excessive amounts of thyroid hormone. Causes of hyperthyroidism are

Graves disease
Toxic adenoma
Toxic multinodular goiter
Thyroiditis
    Subacute
    Painless (postpartum)
Iatrogenic, factitious
Rare causes
    Struma ovarii
    Trophoblastic tumors
    TSH-secreting pituitary tumors
    Iodine-induced hyperthyroidism (Jod-Basedow)

In Graves disease, the thyroid is stimulated to produce thyroid hormone by thyroid-stimulating autoantibodies. Rarely, other factors may stimulate the thyroid and cause hyperthyroidism (e.g., TSH secreted by a pituitary TSH-secreting tumor or hCG from a choriocarcinoma). Hyperthyroidism may be produced by benign thyroid neoplasia, as in patients with a toxic nodule or toxic multinodular goiter. It may also be produced by thyroid inflammation, with release of thyroid hormone into the blood stream from damaged follicles in the various forms of thyroiditis. Hyperthyroidism may also be produced by the ectopic secretion of thyroid hormones by ovarian teratomas (struma ovarii).

Patients may have elevated serum levels of T_4 and/or T_3 *without* being hyperthyroid, in situations of increased thyroid hormone binding by TBG or other proteins, altered peripheral conversion of T_4 to T_3 due to illness or certain drugs, and (rarely) congenital peripheral resistance to thyroid hormones.

Graves disease. Because of the great frequency of Graves disease in women of reproductive age, a brief overview of its pathophysiology and clinical manifestations is presented. Graves disease is a syndrome that includes toxic diffuse goiter, Graves eye disease (orbitopathy), and pretibial myxedema. The frequency of these physical findings is variable, depending on patient age, disease severity, and other unknown factors; and, in the case of eye disease, depending on the sensitivity of the diagnostic measures used to detect it. Goiter is present in more than 95% of younger women with Graves disease, but thyroid enlargement may be absent in as may as 50% of similarly affected elderly women.[64] Also, nodular thyroid glands are common in older patients who nevertheless have Graves disease. Typical eye findings of swelling, lid retraction, and exophthalmos develop in 30% to 40% of patients clinically, but subtle orbital changes can be found in more than 90% of

patients by orbital ultrasonography or computed tomography. As in the case of thyroid enlargement, clinically obvious eye disease is more frequent in younger patients. Pretibial myxedema, also called thyroid dermopathy, is quite uncommon, being present in less than 1% of patients. Orbital disease and, rarely, dermopathy can develop in patients who do not have hyperthyroidism, a disorder termed euthyroid Graves disease.

Graves disease is a multisystem disorder caused by an incompletely defined disturbance in immune surveillance.[20] The immunologic hallmark of Graves disease is the presence of circulating polyclonal immunoglobulin G (IgG) autoantibodies, termed thyroid-stimulating immunoglobulins (TSI), which are directed against the TSH receptor. After binding to the TSH receptor, these antibodies stimulate thyroidal growth and thyroid hormone synthesis and secretion. The presence of these serum antibodies can be detected in bioassays that have clinical utility in pregnant women with Graves disease. The precipitating factors that lead to the development of circulating TSI and Graves disease are unknown. One possibility is an abnormality of suppressor T lymphocytes, which allows for the expansion of normally suppressed B lymphocytes. In addition, there is evidence for activation of intrathyroidal helper T lymphocytes, in response to the abnormal expression of thyroid follicular cell antigens, perhaps caused by tissue injury or environmental factors. The increased tendency in women to develop Graves disease is also modified by genetic, hereditary (i.e., a higher frequency in *HLA-B8/DR-3*-positive individuals), and possibly hormonal influences.

Although the proximate cause of thyroid overactivity in Graves disease is the presence of autoantibodies to the TSH receptor, the pathogenesis of eye and skin manifestations is less clear. Most hypotheses invoke cross-reactivity between thyroid cellular surface antigens and antigens on extraocular muscle cell or fibroblast cell membranes. Recent studies have suggested an important role for retroorbital fibroblasts in the pathogenesis of Graves orbitopathy, with possible stimulation of collagen and glycosaminoglycan production by antifibroblast antibodies.

The tendency for symptoms of Graves disease to wax and wane over time is an important clinical consideration. Patients treated with antithyroid drugs may develop spontaneous remissions, perhaps caused in part by immunosuppressive effects of the antithyroid drugs themselves.[14] Remissions are characterized by a disappearance of TSI from the serum. Most remissions are not lifelong, however, and subsequent relapses are common, if not inevitable.[87] Some patients may develop hypothyroidism many years after having been hyperthyroid, and rarely a patient may become hyperthyroid after a period of typical hypothyroidism. These transitions illustrate the close relationship between Graves disease and autoimmune thyroiditis (Hashimoto disease). Like other autoimmune diseases, Graves disease tends to remit during pregnancy and has a tendency to recur in the postpartum period. These observations are important clinically and are discussed later in greater detail.

Thyroiditis

Subacute. Subacute thyroiditis, also called granulomatous or de Quervain thyroiditis, is most likely viral in origin. Hyperthyroidism is due to destruction of thyroid follicles with release of hormonal stores into the circulation. Clinical hyperthyroidism is present in less than half the cases. The symptoms are usually dominated by fever, malaise, and exquisite anterior neck pain and tenderness. An elevated erythrocyte sedimentation rate is present in virtually all patients, biochemical hyperthyroidism is present in most patients, and the radioiodine uptake is characteristically low. Therapy consists of aspirin or other nonsteroidal antiinflammatory agents for the local neck symptoms. A brief course of glucocorticoids is sometimes necessary, however. For symptomatic hyperthyroidism, which is self-limited, treatment with β-adrenergic blockers alone is indicated. Subacute thyroiditis characteristically follows a triphasic course, with the period of hyperthyroidism lasting 4 to 12 weeks, followed by a similar period of hypothyroidism that also resolves spontaneously, and finally ending with a return to the euthyroid state. Permanent thyroid failure after an episode of subacute thyroiditis is rare, and repeated bouts are also very unusual.

Painless. Painless thyroiditis has been described only within the last 20 years. Most patients with painless thyroiditis develop it in the postpartum period; hence the term *postpartum thyroiditis.* Painless thyroiditis is thought to be an autoimmune disease, because many patients have positive serum antithyroid antibodies and because a lymphocytic infiltration is present cytologically. Patients develop typical hyperthyroid signs and symptoms, as well as a painless, small goiter. The radioiodine uptake is low and the erythrocyte sedimentation rate is normal. Treatment with β-adrenergic blockers is indicated for symptomatic patients. The disease follows a triphasic course similar to that outlined for subacute thyroiditis. Unlike subacute thyroiditis, painless thyroiditis tends to recur, particularly after pregnancies. Painless thyroiditis evolves into permanent thyroid failure in approximately 25% of patients.

Rare causes

Thyrotropin-producing pituitary tumors. Patients with TSH-producing pituitary tumors present with typical symptoms of hyperthyroidism—diffuse goiter and an elevated radioiodine uptake. Thus they resemble patients with Graves disease. Occasionally patients have symptoms of a sellar mass lesion, and some patients have concomitant acromegaly or hyperprolactinemia. The diagnosis can be made only if a serum TSH determination is obtained when the hyperthyroidism is being evaluated. Frequently, the TSH level is within the normal range but inappropriate for the level of T_4 and T_3 in the serum. These patients also have elevated serum levels of the common α-subunit with an elevated molar ratio of α-subunit to intact TSH. In contrast, patients with generalized thyroid hormone resistance, who also have high T_4 and T_3 levels and inappropriate TSH levels, have serum α-subunit concentrations that are equimolar to TSH. Therapy consists of surgical extirpation of the pituitary neoplasm. Radiotherapy, dopamine agonists, and the somatostatin analogue octreotide have been used as adjunctive treatments.

Struma ovarii. The presence of histologically normal thyroid remnants in an ovarian teratoma is termed struma ovarii, *struma* being an archaic term for the thyroid gland. There have been approximately 400 cases of struma ovarii in the world's literature, with a reported frequency of hyperthyroidism of approximately 10%.[54] The diagnosis is made by noting hyperthyroidism without goiter, and a low radioiodine uptake over the thyroid gland. In several cases, abnormal radioiodine uptake in the pelvis has been described. An ovarian mass is palpable in the majority of patients, and ascites may be present. Therapy involves surgical removal of the teratoma. Rarely, papillary thyroid carcinoma has been found within ovarian thyroid tissue.

Choriocarcinoma. Trophoblastic tumors, including choriocarcinoma and hydatidiform mole, can cause hyperthyroidism by secreting a factor capable of stimulating the thyroid gland. Much evidence has accumulated that hCG is the thyrotropic factor, since hCG can stimulate thyroid cells in vitro when present in high concentrations and because there is a correlation between the degree of thyroid overactivity and the serum hCG concentration. The frequency of hyperthyroidism in gestational trophoblastic disease may be as high as 30%,[49] but patients are often undiagnosed because the hyperthyroidism is mild. Hyperthyroidism resolves with removal of the tumor.

Iodine-induced. Iodine-induced hyperthyroidism, also termed the Jod-Basedow phenomenon, typically is seen when populations residing in iodine-deficient areas of the world are exposed to increased quantities of iodine in the diet or to iodine-containing medications. However, this form of hyperthyroidism can also occur in iodine-sufficient areas, usually in patients who have an underlying nontoxic multinodular goiter.[91] Occasionally patients have no known preexisting thyroid abnormality. The hyperthyroidism is transient but is often severe and resistant to standard doses of antithyroid drugs. Radioiodine cannot be used, because the large circulating pool of iodide reduces the radioiodine uptake by the thyroid to low levels. In North America, iodine-induced hyperthyroidism has been associated with the use of expectorants containing potassium iodide, iodine-containing contrast dyes, and the iodine-containing antiarrhythmic drug amiodarone.

Clinical manifestations

The diagnosis of hyperthyroidism is made easily when patients complain of typical hypermetabolic and adrenergic symptoms, and when goiter, tremor, tachycardia, and, in the case of Graves disease, eye findings are present. There may be a paucity of symptoms and signs in patients with mild disease or in elderly patients, and the diagnosis may be easily overlooked. Most young women present with heat intolerance, nervousness, palpitations, fatigue, and weight loss; and they have thyroid enlargement, lid retraction, exophthalmos, tachycardia, and warm, moist skin on physical examination. In the elderly, the diagnosis may be elusive, but it should be suggested by unexplained weight loss or the development of new atrial fibrillation or angina pectoris. Because osteoporosis may be aggravated by hyperthyroidism, thyroid function should be evaluated in all patients with this common problem.

Effects on menstrual cycle and fertility. Although hyperthyroidism is a cause of oligomenorrhea and amenorrhea, most hyperthyroid patients continue to have regular menstrual cycles, but with lighter flow.[9] Amenorrhea occurs in less than 10% of patients, even among those with severe thyrotoxicosis.[9] Unfortunately, only a limited number of studies have examined the reproductive biochemical milieu in hyperthyroidism. Furthermore, interpretation of the observed changes in steroid hormone levels is clouded by the dramatic elevations in sex hormone-binding globulin (SHBG) levels induced by thyroid hormone.[3] Thus, although total estradiol and testosterone levels are increased in hyperthyroidism, changes in unbound or free hormone concentrations are less certain.

Effects on gonadotropin secretion. Plasma levels of LH are elevated throughout the cycle in menstruating hyperthyroid women, although the levels may actually be slightly lower during the midcycle surge in hypomenorrheic women.[4] Mean LH levels are also elevated in amenorrheic hyperthyroid women, compared with euthyroid, normally cycling controls, when the 3 days around the midcycle are excluded. Furthermore, mean LH levels are higher in postmenopausal hyperthyroid women than in euthyroid postmenopausal controls[4] (Fig. 12-5). These changes may be caused by diminished sensitivity of the negative feedback system to estrogenic compounds in hyperthyroid patients.[2] In premenopausal women, the LH response to gonadotropin-releasing hormone stimulation has been reported to be normal[21] or increased.[88] Hyperthyroid patients may have an exaggerated dopaminergic inhibition of LH secretion, suggesting enhanced sensitivity to dopaminergic stimuli in hyperthyroidism.[89] Thus the possibility exists that the elevated LH levels observed in hyperthyroidism may be due, in part, to reduced endogenous dopaminergic inhibition.

Plasma levels of FSH generally follow a pattern similar to that seen with LH: levels are elevated throughout the cycle in menstruating hyperthyroid women, compared with levels of controls.[4,88] The responses to gonadotropin-releasing hormone are variable.[21,88]

The changes in gonadotropin levels in hyperthyroidism are reversed rapidly with restoration of the euthyroid state.

Effects on sex steroids. The levels of total estradiol and testosterone are elevated twofold to threefold in hyperthyroid women because hepatic SHBG production is stimulated by thyroid hormone. Free estradiol levels in hyperthyroid women levels are within the range of normal.[89] The production rate of estradiol was found to be normal in most hyperthyroid subjects,[71,72] consistent with the concept that both glandular secretion and peripheral conversion from testosterone are normal. The conversion of estradiol to estrone is also normal in hyperthyroidism.[72] The metabolic clearance rate of estradiol is diminished in hyperthyroidism, probably because of increased binding by SHBG.

The mean serum levels of total testosterone are elevated in hyperthyroid women, and values may be well outside the normal range.[3,72] Androstenedione, which is not bound to SHBG, is normal.[72] Free androgen levels have not been studied systematically in hyperthyroid women.

Luteal phase progesterone levels in menstruating women, with or without hypomenorrhea, are normal. Thus it can be inferred that most menstruating hyperthyroid women are ovulatory, although no formal studies of fertility in such women exist. Infertility in hyperthyroidism is probably confined to the 10% of women with amenorrhea.

Diagnosis

The laboratory diagnosis of hyperthyroidism is usually straightforward. Most patients have elevated circulating levels of T_4 and T_3, and an elevated free thyroxine index or directly measured free T_4. In hyperthyroid patients with normal serum T_4 values, serum T_3 should be measured, since T_3 toxicosis is seen in 10% to 15% of hyperthyroid patients. The development of sensitive assays for TSH has simplified the ability to diagnose mild hyperthyroidism. All forms of hyperthyroidism, except for the rare forms of TSH-mediated hyperthyroidism, are associated with low or undetectable serum TSH concentrations. In the absence of severe illness or thyroxine ingestion, this finding should suggest the diagnosis. With the widespread availability of sensitive TSH assays, the TRH test—wherein the TSH response to a bolus of TRH is assessed—has become obsolete.

The 24-hour radioiodine uptake is not sensitive or specific for hyperthyroidism. It can be elevated in some patients with hypothyroidism due to Hashimoto thyroiditis; conversely, it can be low in hyperthyroid patients with subacute thyroiditis or painless thyroiditis (postpartum thyroiditis) and in patients with Graves disease with previous exposure to iodine-containing compounds. However, the 24-hour radioiodine uptake is useful in the differential diagnosis of hyperthyroidism, particularly to distinguish Graves disease that develops during the postpartum period from postpartum thyroiditis.

Assays for anti-TSH receptor antibodies are available commercially; the prevailing technique employs thyroid cell cultures to determine the cellular cyclic adenosine

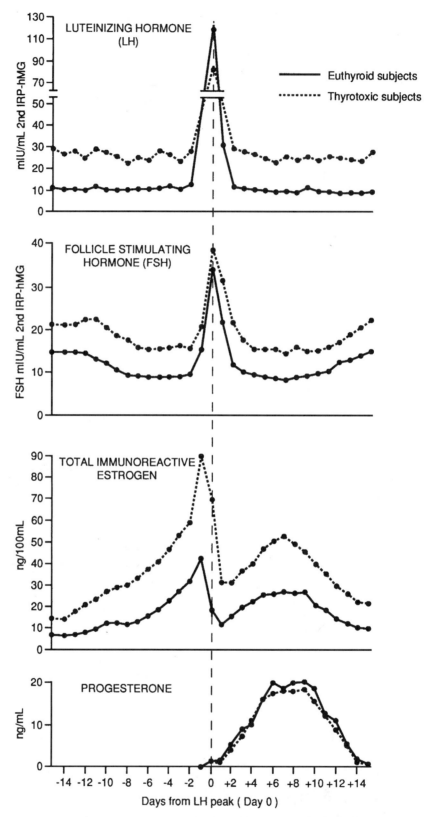

Fig. 12-5. Mean plasma LH, FSH, estradiol, and progesterone levels in 10 thyrotoxic women and 12 euthyroid controls. (Redrawn from Akande EO, Hockaday TDR: *Br J Obstet Gynaecol* 82:541, 1975, with permission of Blackwell Scientific Publications, Ltd.)

monophosphate response to the lgG fraction of the patient's serum. Another technique measures the degree to which the patient's lgG inhibits the binding of radiolabeled TSH to thyroid membranes, so-called TSH-binding inhibiting activity (TBI). However, the clinical utility of TSI or TBI assays is not great, since the diagnosis of Graves disease is generally quite simple and the cost of the assay is high. In Graves disease in pregnancy, however, TSI assays have greater importance, because high maternal titers may be predictive of neonatal Graves disease due to transplacental passage of the TSI.

Treatment

Before therapy of hyperthyroidism is undertaken, the precise cause of the condition should be ascertained. The vast majority of patients, both young and old, will have Graves disease, although the fraction of patients with toxic multinodular goiter increases with age. Together, these two diagnoses account for more than 90% of all cases of hyperthyroidism. It is particularly important to rule out the various forms of thyroiditis as a cause of hyperthyroidism, since they resolve spontaneously and require only symptomatic therapy. Pituitary TSH-secreting tumors, and thyrotoxicosis related to choriocarcinoma or struma ovarii require treatments directed at the underlying cause of the problem, rather than at the thyroid gland itself. Immediate, comprehensive treatment of hyperthyroidism is rarely necessary, and patients can be managed symptomatically with β-adrenergic blocking agents until a precise diagnosis is firmly established.

Since the underlying causes of the immunologic abnormalities in Graves disease are unknown, treatment centers around efforts to lessen thyroid hormone secretion. Although surgery historically was the first form of satisfactory therapy for Graves disease, antithyroid drugs and radioiodine are now the treatments of choice.[16] Both treatments are effective and safe, and provide a satisfactory outcome for most patients. Antithyroid drugs provide the opportunity for the patient to experience a spontaneous remission without lifelong medication. However, remissions are attained in less than 50% of patients, and continuous or repeated courses of antithyroid drug therapy usually are necessary. On the other hand, radioiodine is curative, but it has the disadvantage of causing hypothyroidism in virtually all patients. Nevertheless, the management of postablative hypothyroidism is simpler for most patients than long-term antithyroid drug therapy. Therefore, one should not consider radioiodine as a treatment that merely exchanges one thyroid problem for another.

The major controversy surrounding the use of radioiodine is the possible long-term carcinogenic or mutagenic effects of ionizing radiation. To date, however, despite numerous studies, there are no data to demonstrate that radioiodine therapy for hyperthyroidism is hazardous to the patient,[22,43,44] nor has it been shown that it affects subsequent fertility or reproductive outcome when given to women of childbearing age.[16] Thus radioiodine has emerged in the United States as the primary treatment for most women with hyperthyroidism.[82] The use of radioiodine in children and adolescents is more controversial, but it has replaced surgery in most clinics if antithyroid drugs fail because of drug allergy or poor compliance. Whatever the inclinations and biases of the physician, it is important to stress that the participation of the patient in the decision-making process is crucial, since all treatments have distinct advantages and disadvantages.

Antithyroid drugs. The thionamide antithyroid drugs propylthiouracil (PTU) and methimazole (Tapazole) are derivatives of thiourea and have as their major property the ability to inhibit thyroid hormone biosyntheses.[14] Thionamides block the utilization of trapped iodide at a step involving the binding of oxidized iodide to tyrosine residues to form monoiodotyrosine and diiodotyrosine. The coupling of these iodotyrosines to form T_4 and T_3 may also be inhibited by antithyroid drugs. In addition, PTU, but not methimazole, inhibits T_4 to T_3 conversion in peripheral tissues. Thionamides also may have immunosuppressive effects, which might explain why 30% of patients treated with these drugs undergo a period of remission.[16]

The starting dose of PTU is approximately 300 mg daily, given as two 50-mg tablets every 8 hours. PTU generally cannot be given as a single daily dose because of its relatively short duration of action. In contrast, methimazole can be given as a single daily dose. Since it is 10 to 50 times as potent as PTU, starting doses are approximately 5 to 30 mg/d. The time until a euthyroid state is achieved varies, depending on the underlying disease activity, the amount of stored thyroid hormone within the gland, and the dose of antithyroid drug. In general, it takes 4 to 6 weeks for methimazole and 6 to 12 weeks for comparable doses of PTU.[65] β-adrenergic blocking drugs are usually given as adjunctive therapy for adrenergic symptoms. Long-acting β-blockers such as metoprolol, atenolol, nadolol, and long-acting propranolol are preferable to propranolol, which has a short duration of action.

The side effects of antithyroid drugs include fever, rash, and arthralgias, which occur in 1% to 5% of patients; it is sometimes possible to switch to the other drug if a patient develops one of these minor side effects. The most dreaded reaction is agranulocytosis, which occurs in about 0.2% of patients. Typically, agranulocytosis develops within 90 days of starting thionamide therapy and is heralded by high fever and signs of infection, usually of the oropharynx.[17] Thus patients should be warned to discontinue their medication if they develop a fever or a sore throat, and to call their physician. If agranulocytosis is present, hospitalization and broad-spectrum antibiotic therapy is indicated. The white cell count usually normalizes within 7 to 10 days in most patients once the medication has been discontinued, and fatalities are extremely rare. Other major side effects include toxic hepatitis, vasculitis, and drug-induced lupus erythematosus.

Generally, antithyroid drugs are administered for a period of 6 to 24 months and are then tapered or discontinued in order to establish whether a remission has occurred. None of the numerous clinical and biochemical markers that have been proposed to assist the clinician in predicting which patients are more likely to achieve a remission has proven to have adequate sensitivity or specificity.[16] In general, remission rates are higher in patients with milder hyperthyroidism and smaller goiters, who are diagnosed earlier in their illness and who are treated for longer periods of time with antithyroid agents. There are several studies suggesting higher remission rates with higher antithyroid drug doses,[76] but because of a possible increase in side effects with higher doses,[17] this concept has not been widely put into practice. Recently it was suggested that the concomitant use of thyroxine and antithyroid drugs, and thyroxine alone for a period of 3 years after remission has been achieved, leads to a higher remission rate.[40]

Should a remission be achieved, lifelong follow-up is warranted, since most remissions are not permanent.[87] Relapses are particularly likely to occur in the postpartum period.[7] If a remission is not achieved, the patient is faced with the choice of a second course of antithyroid drug therapy or radioiodine. A minority of patients who remit with antithyroid drug therapy alone eventually develop spontaneous hypothyroidism. The frequency of this phenomenon is not known.

Radioiodine. Radioiodine has been in use as a therapy for hyperthyroidism for almost 50 years. It is the preferred treatment for most adults with Graves disease, toxic nodules, and toxic multinodular goiter. Radioiodine damages the thyroid largely via beta emissions, which have a path length of less than 2 mm. Because radiation damage occurs relatively slowly, a period of 1 to 6 months (sometimes longer) is needed for the full effects on thyroid function to be observed. Although the radiation dose delivered to the thyroid gland is high (5,000 to 15,000 rads), the radiation dose to the whole body is quite small. In women, it has been estimated that the dose to the ovaries, largely due to gamma radiation from radioiodine in the urinary bladder, is approximately 0.2 rad per administered millicurie of radioiodine.[74] Since a typical radioiodine dose in Graves disease is 5 to 10 mCi, the ovarian dose would be 1 to 2 rads. This is similar to that which might be obtained after several barium enemas or intravenous pyelograms. This is well within the range that is considered safe in terms of reproductive potential.

There are few immediate side effects of radioiodine therapy. Rarely, patients complain of anterior neck tenderness 7 to 10 days after therapy, consistent with radiation-induced thyroiditis, which is managed easily with salicylates. There is a potential for worsening hyperthyroidism

soon after administration of radioiodine, secondary to inflammation and release of stored thyroid hormone into the blood stream. For this reason, elderly patients and patients with cardiac disease are usually pretreated with thionamides before receiving radioiodine. Pretreatment with antithyroid agents is not necessary in otherwise healthy young and middle-aged adults, and symptoms can be controlled with β-adrenergic blocking agents. If it is considered necessary to normalize thyroid function rapidly, antithyroid drugs can be started, or restarted, several days after radioiodine administration.

The major adverse reaction from radioiodine is iatrogenic hypothyroidism. Indeed, this development is so characteristic that it is considered an inevitable consequence of therapy rather than a side effect. Hypothyroidism develops in at least 50% of patients within the first year after therapy, with a gradual 2% to 3% annual incidence thereafter. Thus within 10 to 20 years virtually all patients will have become hypothyroid. It is therefore mandatory that all radioiodine-treated patients receive lifelong follow-up, with close monitoring of thyroid function, especially the serum TSH level.

Hyperthyroidism in pregnancy

Although hyperthyroidism in pregnancy is relatively uncommon, affecting 1 in 500 to 1 in 2000 pregnant women, all physicians who care for women in the reproductive years should be familiar with the essentials of management.[13] Although there is no increase in maternal morbidity or mortality, it has been well documented that the risks of prematurity, low birth weight, neonatal mortality, and congenital abnormalities [19,58] are higher in untreated hyperthyroidism. Thus prompt and effective therapy is required, despite theoretic risks to the fetus of antithyroid drugs, β-adrenergic blocking agents, and, in rare instances, surgery.

Diagnosis. In most situations, the diagnosis of hyperthyroidism has been made before pregnancy, although the disease can certainly also be first recognized during pregnancy. The clinical diagnosis can be difficult, because many of the typical symptoms (e.g., heat intolerance, fatigue, and rapid pulse) are also found in normal pregnant women. Thus a high index of suspicion is required, and screening for hyperthyroidism should be performed for most nonspecific complaints, particularly if the patient fails to gain adequate amounts of weight or in the presence of a goiter. Although there may be a slight increase in thyroid size detectable ultrasonographically during pregnancy, the presence of definite thyroid enlargement during pregnancy should prompt a formal evaluation of thyroid function.[62]

Another presentation that should suggest hyperthyroidism during pregnancy is severe nausea and vomiting, also called thyrotoxic vomiting,[23] which may mimic hyperemesis gravidarum. Patients with hyperemesis gravidarum may have free T_4 levels that are slightly, but significantly, higher and serum TSH levels that are slightly, but significantly, lower than those of either nonpregnant women or pregnant women without nausea or vomiting.[60] In some patients with hyperemesis, the free T_4 may extend into the thyrotoxic range, and the serum TSH may actually be suppressed, suggesting the diagnosis of hyperthyroidism. Whether these changes are indicative of true hyperthyroidism in need of therapy or simply an exaggeration of the normal thyroid stimulation by hCG, the levels of which peak at 12 weeks of gestation,[34] is not clear. If hyperthyroidism is suggested by other findings (e.g., goiter, exophthalmos, or positive antithyroid antibody or TSI titers) treatment with antithyroid drugs is indicated. If, on the other hand, there is less clear-cut clinical or biochemical evidence of a thyroid problem, the use of antithyroid drugs is less well established.

The biochemical diagnosis of hyperthyroidism is relatively straightforward. Total T_4 and T_3 concentrations are normally elevated by 25% to 50% during pregnancy because of an estrogen-induced rise in serum TBG levels. Concentrations of free T_4 and free T_3 generally are normal throughout pregnancy, except for possible slight increases above normal early in pregnancy,[34] probably because of the thyroid-stimulating effects of placental hCG. TSH levels are unaltered during normal pregnancy. Therefore, a suppressed TSH level in a sensitive TSH assay is an extremely simple and cost-effective way of establishing the diagnosis of hyperthyroidism.

Of course, the radioiodine uptake test and scans are never used during pregnancy. The measurement of anti-TSH receptor antibodies during pregnancy is recommended as a predictor of neonatal Graves disease because of their transplacental passage. The test should not be ordered until 34 to 36 weeks of gestation, since the levels fall progressively throughout pregnancy and reach their nadir late in the third trimester. If the titers of anti-TSH receptor antibody remain high, an increased risk of neonatal Graves disease exists.[61,100] Women with a history of Graves disease in the past, who may be euthyroid or even hypothyroid during pregnancy, may still harbor anti-TSH receptor antibodies in their serum. Therefore, the presence of these antibodies should be assessed in all pregnant women with a history of Graves disease, regardless of the activity of the disease during pregnancy.

Treatment. Radioiodine is absolutely contraindicated, and surgery is relatively contraindicated during pregnancy. Antithyroid drugs are the treatment of choice for Graves disease, the most common form of hyperthyroidism, as well as for pregnant patients with toxic nodules and toxic multinodular goiter. After delivery, patients with these latter conditions are best treated with radioiodine, since, unlike patients with Graves disease, there is little possibility of a spontaneous remission.

Antithyroid drugs. Antithyroid drugs are the mainstay of therapy of hyperthyroidism during pregnancy. In the United States, PTU is the drug of choice for several

reasons. First, it has no known teratogenic effects. Second, because it is heavily protein bound, it crosses the placenta poorly. Third, it blocks peripheral T_4 to T_3 conversion, which may be of some clinical benefit in a severely thyrotoxic individual. In contrast, use of methimazole may be associated with a scalp deformity known as aplasia cutis congenita, although this association has been disputed.[92] Methimazole crosses the placenta well because it is non–protein bound. However, methimazole is used widely during pregnancy in other parts of the world, as is the methimazole precursor carbimazole, without obvious ill effects.

Doses of PTU or methimazole should be adequate to control the hyperthyroidism, and free T_4 levels should be maintained at or just above the upper end of normal to avoid overmedication and potential deleterious effects on fetal thyroid function.[59] For PTU this would be a dosage of 100 to 150 mg every 8 hours, whereas for methimazole the dosage would be 10 to 30 mg as a single daily dose. Even if large doses are necessary to control the hyperthyroidism, surgery is not indicated, since the potential for harm to the fetus from antithyroid drugs is low and not necessarily dose related. As soon as the hyperthyroidism has been adequately controlled biochemically, which usually requires about 8 weeks for PTU and less time for methimazole, the dose of antithyroid drug can be decreased by about 30% for maintenance therapy. In pregnancy, with TSI titers progressively diminishing in most patients throughout gestation, the dosage of antithyroid drug generally can be cut every 1 to 2 months, so that patients are taking little (e.g., 50 to 100 mg of PTU daily) or no drug during the last few weeks. It is important to continue to monitor thyroid function, however, since the degree of anticipated improvement in the hyperthyroidism varies greatly from person to person. Unfortunately, serum TSH levels may be of little value in this situation, since pituitary TSH secretion may remain chronically suppressed, despite the attainment of a euthyroid or even a hypothyroid state with antithyroid drugs. Therefore, free thyroxine indexes or the free T_4 levels are the most suitable parameters to follow.

The use of concomitant thyroxine therapy with antithyroid drugs is ill advised. First, the addition of thyroxine may lead to an unwitting increase in antithyroid drug dose. Second, thyroxine crosses the placenta so poorly that it will not protect the fetus from iatrogenic hypothyroidism. Clinicians should simply administer the least amount of drug that will satisfactorily control the patient's hyperthyroidism. Although transplacental passage of antithyroid drugs may lead to mild depression in neonatal thyroid function at birth, significant hypothyroidism or goiter is extremely rare. Several long-term follow-up studies have documented that children exposed to antithyroid drugs in utero are intellectually normal, compared with control populations of unexposed siblings or age-matched children.[13,57]

b-Adrenergic blocking agents. In nonpregnant women,

β-adrenergic blocker therapy is an important adjunct to the other, more definitive and specific, therapies of hyperthyroidism. However, β-blockers as sole therapy for thyrotoxicosis due to Graves disease is not advisable. First, spontaneous remissions occur only very infrequently. More important, β-blockers do not fully normalize the hypermetabolic state, so that heightened oxygen consumption and tissue catabolism continue. Despite this drawback, β-blockers are beneficial in alleviating tachycardia, tremor, and irritability until the antithyroid drugs have had a chance to normalize the patient's thyroid function. During pregnancy, the use of β-blockers as an adjunct to antithyroid drugs has been shown to be safe,[79] as long as the drug is not administered during the time of delivery, when neonatal bradycardia or hypoglycemia may result. Since most women will be euthyroid at term, β-blocker therapy should not be necessary in most instances.

Subtotal thyroidectomy. The only indications for thyroid surgery in the hyperthyroid pregnant woman are antithyroid drug sensitivity or nonremediable poor compliance. This is because of the small possibility of spontaneous abortion, as well as the maternal complications of recurrent laryngeal nerve palsy and hypoparathyroidism. Although these sequelae are unusual (2% frequency), they are lifelong and can be difficult to manage.

When necessary, surgery probably should be deferred until after the first trimester, although data on increased risk to the fetus in the first trimester are lacking. Before surgery, the patient must be prepared to avoid thyroid storm perioperatively. If surgery has been necessitated by allergy to antithyroid drugs, the patient can be prepared with β-blockers for 1 to 2 weeks until the pulse rate is normal, with the addition of potassium iodide for 10 days before surgery. The potassium iodide inhibits thyroid hormone synthesis (the Wolff-Chaikoff effect) and release, although T_4 and T_3 levels are not necessarily normalized. Long-term use of potassium iodide or iodide-containing compounds is contraindicated during pregnancy, because the fetal thyroid is more sensitive to the Wolff-Chaikoff effect, and large and potentially obstructive goiter can be the result. If poor compliance has been the problem that has led to surgery, the patient should be rendered euthyroid with antithyroid drugs in standard doses for pregnancy.

Neonatal Graves disease

If present in high titer, anti-TSH receptor antibodies can cross the placenta and stimulate the fetal thyroid gland. This situation is exceedingly rare, affecting fewer than 1% of all pregnancies associated with Graves disease.[13] It is important to reiterate that the mother need not be actively hyperthyroid but only need have a history of hyperthyroidism due to Graves disease. Fetal Graves disease can be diagnosed in utero by noting a fetal heart rate above 160 beats per minute and high maternal TSI titers. Fetal goiter may also be seen on ultrasonographic examination. If the

clinical suspicion is high, the fetus can be treated with antithyroid drugs via the mother, and continued after parturition. If the mother is herself euthyroid, she will require supplemental thyroxine therapy.

Neonatal Graves disease is characterized by extreme irritability, tachycardia, goiter, and, occasionally, congestive heart failure and premature craniosynostosis. If the mother has been treated with antithyroid drugs during the pregnancy, the diagnosis in the baby may not be apparent for 7 to 10 days after birth, until the inhibitory effects of the drug on the neonatal thyroid have dissipated. Indeed, if this is the case, the condition may be mistaken for colic or sepsis. Antithyroid drug therapy should be continued for 6 to 8 weeks, until the passively transferred antibodies have been cleared from the circulation.

Antithyroid drug therapy and lactation

Newer assays for antithyroid drugs have challenged the previous proscriptions against breast-feeding in postpartum women with hyperthyroidism. For PTU, the quantities of drug reaching the baby are approximately 0.025% of an administered dose, or about 100 µg after a 400-mg oral dose to the mother. Children exposed to PTU via breast milk for extended periods of time have maintained normal thyroid function.[15] The situation is slightly different for methimazole (and the methimazole precursor carbimazole), because methimazole freely crosses the breast epithelial barrier and appears in breast milk in concentrations equal to those in serum. Nevertheless, babies exposed to methimazole through breast milk have been shown to have normal thyroid function while nursing. Thus if a woman taking antithyroid drugs desires to nurse her child, it should be permitted as long as the mother is informed of the risks and benefits.[15] PTU is the preferred drug, but low doses of methimazole could also be used safely. It is recommended that the baby's thyroid function be checked periodically, preferably with serum TSH determinations.

Thyroid storm

Thyroid storm is a clinical diagnosis reserved for patients with severe hyperthyroidism accompanied by fever and mental status changes. Thyroid function testing does not reveal higher thyroid hormone levels in patients with thyroid storm than in hyperthyroid patients in general. The reasons for decompensation usually relate to stress (e.g., trauma, surgery, or childbirth). Often the diagnosis of hyperthyroidism has not been made previously, or if it has, the patient has been treated inadequately. Once the diagnosis has been made, therapy consists of large doses of antithyroid drugs and β-blockers. PTU is the preferred drug because of its ability to block peripheral T_4 to T_3 conversion; dosages of 200 to 400 mg every 6 hours are recommended. β-blocking drugs should be administered in doses adequate to lower the heart rate to below 90 beats per minute. If congestive heart failure is present, however, these agents should be used cautiously, unless the heart failure is clearly only rate related. Potassium iodide in dosages of 1 to 2 g intravenously over 24 hours, or as a saturated solution of potassium iodide 5 to 10 drops three or four times a day orally, is given to inhibit release of thyroid hormone from the gland. Iodide should be administered only after antithyroid drugs have been started. Recently, the iodinated contrast agents sodium ipodate (Oragraffin) and sodium iopanoate (Telepaque) have been used in the management of severe thyrotoxicosis. Both agents are potent inhibitors of T_4 to T_3 conversion and have the added benefit of undergoing spontaneous deiodination in the body, thereby liberating free iodide, which inhibits thyroid hormone release. The dose of both agents is 1 g daily. Other measures used in the management of thyroid storm include stress doses of glucocorticoids, strict attention to fluid and electrolyte balance, and administration of antipyretics.

POSTPARTUM THYROID DISEASE

In the last decade, a spectrum of autoimmune thyroid problems that develop in the postpartum period have been recognized. Of course, thyroid disease in the postpartum period can be due to hypopituitarism (Sheehan syndrome), recurrent Graves disease, a toxic thyroid nodule, or other conventional disorders. However, a specific form of thyroid inflammation, characterized by transient, painless hyperthyroidism or hypothyroidism, occurs almost exclusively in the first year after delivery. The prevalence of postpartum thyroid disease varies according to the ethnic group studied, the sensitivity of the detection methods for

thyroid disease, and the frequency and duration of follow-up. In studies from Japan, Scandinavia, the United Kingdom, Canada, and the United States, the prevalence has ranged from 1.9% to 16%, with an overall prevalence of approximately 5%.[30]

A number of clinical courses have been described in patients with postpartum thyroid disease, ranging from new-onset Graves disease to permanent hypothyroidism[8] (Fig. 12-6). However, the most typical sequence of thyroid dysfunction is transient hyperthyroidism followed by transient hypothyroidism, each phase lasting approximately 12 weeks. In patients first presenting with hypothyroidism without an antecedent period of hyperthyroidism, it is often impossible to know whether transient mild hyperthyroidism might have been missed clinically. In patients presenting with postpartum hyperthyroidism, another potential problem is distinguishing postpartum thyroiditis from recurrent or new-onset Graves disease. The presence of orbital involvement or serum anti-TSH receptor antibodies favors Graves disease. The radioiodine uptake also will distinguish the two entities, since it is elevated in Graves disease and low in postpartum thyroiditis. Although this test is contraindicated in lactating women, it can be performed safely with ^{123}I or ^{99m}Tc if breast-feeding is suspended for 2 days.[77]

Most patients with postpartum thyroiditis have positive antimicrosomal antibodies. In the general population of pregnant women, 10% will have antimicrosomal antibodies; of these, approximately 40% to 50% will develop some form of postpartum thyroid disease. Whether it is cost

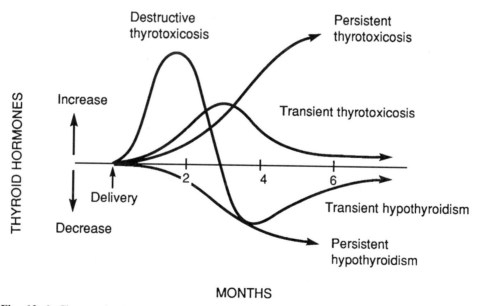

Fig. 12-6. Changes in thyroid function in various forms of postpartum thyroid disease. The numbers indicate months postpartum. (Redrawn from Amino N et al: In Walfish PG, Wall JR, Volpe R, editors: *Autoimmunity and the thyroid,* Orlando, Fla, 1985, Academic Press.)

effective to screen all pregnant women with antithyroid antibodies is controversial. If screening is performed, it should be done early during pregnancy, since titers of antithyroid antibodies tend to fall throughout gestation.[35] It does appear that women who develop postpartum thyroid disease, especially hypothyroidism, have a higher frequency of fatigue and depression than do euthyroid controls.[39] In addition, a recent long-term follow-up study of women who had had postpartum thyroiditis revealed a 23% prevalence of subsequent permanent hypothyroidism.[67] Women with positive antithyroid antibodies also have a higher rate of spontaneous abortion than do antibody-negative controls.[35]

THYROID NODULES AND THYROID CANCER

Thyroid nodules are extremely common, affecting more than 5% of women clinically and up to 50% of individuals studied ultrasonographically.[75] Most nodules thought to be solitary clinically can be shown subsequently to be part of a multinodular goiter. As with most forms of thyroid disease, women are afflicted with nodular thyroid disease more often than men. The vast majority (more than 90%) of thyroid nodules are histologically benign: follicular adenomas, areas of adenomatous hyperplasia, or autoimmune thyroiditis. However, thyroid malignancy is also threefold more common in women and must be excluded in most situations.

Most patients with a thyroid nodule are asymptomatic, and most nodules are discovered during a routine physical examination. Although the clinical clues of childhood head and neck irradiation, rapid growth, hoarseness, ipsilateral cervical lymphadenopathy, and firm consistency suggest malignancy, these findings are unusual. Thus most nodules require a diagnostic evaluation, since surgical removal of all nodules cannot be justified from a medical or an economic standpoint.

Thyroid function testing is indicated, since an elevated serum TSH level suggests the presence of autoimmune thyroid disease, whereas a suppressed or low TSH level suggests an autonomous nodule or toxic multinodular goiter. In the past, most patients would have undergone thyroid scanning, since hyperfunctioning ("hot") nodules are rarely, if ever, malignant, whereas nonfunctioning or hypofunctioning ("cold") nodules are potentially malignant and require further evaluation. However, because 95% of nodules are cold and hence require a tissue diagnosis, thyroid scanning is not a cost-effective diagnostic tool. Ultrasonography also is not worthwhile, since more than 90% of lesions are either solid or complex (having a mixture of cystic and solid elements) and also require a tissue diagnosis. Thus fine-needle aspiration biopsy has emerged as the diagnostic procedure of choice for patients with thyroid nodules. Fine-needle biopsy has been shown to have a high degree of specificity for malignant disease with an acceptable level of sensitivity. In a recent large series, the positive predictive value of fine-needle aspiration biopsy was 100%, with a false-negative rate of 0.7%.[37]

If the results of the biopsy are consistent with a benign process, a trial of suppression therapy with thyroxine is prudent for both therapeutic and diagnostic reasons. About 30% to 50% of nodules will decrease in size, and a decrease in size further confirms the impression that the lesion is benign. Doses of thyroxine of approximately 1 µg/lb of lean body mass will suppress the serum TSH level in most patients, promoting shrinkage of those nodules dependent on TSH for growth. Decreases in nodule size occur slowly and may take 1 to 2 years to be evident clinically. Because of recent concerns over possible skeletal calcium loss resulting from suppressive doses of thyroxine,[68] it is advisable to maintain the serum TSH concentration in the low-normal range after 12 to 24 months of TSH suppression. If there has been no change in the size of the nodule after 12 months of suppression therapy, the medication is discontinued, and a second fine-needle biopsy may be indicated. The fact that a nodule does not shrink is no cause for alarm; for example, benign colloid nodules seldom respond to thyroxine suppression therapy.[33]

Unfortunately, fine-needle biopsy cannot distinguish benign follicular adenomas from low-grade follicular carcinomas, since the pathognomonic feature of the latter is penetration of the thyroid capsule and vascular invasion, which can be recognized only histologically. Approximately 15% of nodules will thus be classified as "indeterminate" or "suggestive" by fine-needle biopsy. At surgery, about 20% of these nodules will actually prove to be malignant.[32] Thus surgery is indicated if a suggestive biopsy result is obtained, although a 3- to 6-month trial of thyroxine suppression is an acceptable alternative. Should the nodule fail to decrease in size, surgical excision should be performed.

When a suggestive biopsy specimen has been obtained, a thyroid scan should always be performed before consideration of surgery, since benign hot nodules can be quite cellular and thus have a cytologic appearance suggestive of malignancy. If such a nodule is hot, no additional therapy is indicated, provided that the patient's thyroid function is normal. Most patients with hot nodules are clinically and biochemically euthyroid, although the serum TSH level may be low or suppressed. Hyperthyroidism may develop during follow-up, particularly with nodules larger than 3 cm in diameter.

Papillary thyroid carcinoma accounts for 70% of thyroid cancer and has a very favorable prognosis. Patients under age 50 years with small (<4 cm) tumors and no evidence of extraglandular spread have a life expectancy that is similar to the life expectancy of the general population. The various controversies surrounding the extent of surgery, the routine ablation of thyroid remnants with radioiodine, the monitoring of serum thyroglobulin, and the follow-up of patients with thyroid cancer by radioiodine scanning are beyond the scope of this chapter and are detailed else-where,[41] as is a discussion of other, more unusual, forms of thyroid carcinoma.[46] In general, total thyroidectomy is recommended. This is usually followed by radioiodine ablation of remnants visualized on a subsequent scan done while the patient is hypothyroid. Lifelong therapy with suppressive doses of thyroxine is mandatory.

The diagnostic evaluation of a pregnant woman who is discovered to have a thyroid nodule should be identical with the strategy just outlined, except that thyroid scanning is contraindicated. If results of the biopsy are benign or suggestive, thyroxine suppression therapy is indicated. In the case of a suggestive nodule, surgery could be performed after delivery should the nodule fail to shrink. Limited data suggest that thyroid nodules may tend to enlarge during pregnancy,[35] but the impact of this observation on patient management is unclear. The major area of uncertainty is in the management of a pregnant patient who clearly has thyroid carcinoma according to fine-needle biopsy results. On the one hand, a case can be made for thyroid surgery in the second trimester, despite the small risk of fetal loss. On the other hand, given the lack of evidence of an adverse effect of pregnancy on thyroid tumor growth,[42] an equally strong argument could be made for suppression therapy with thyroxine until after the time of delivery, particularly if the tumor has a papillary histology.

REFERENCES

1. Ain KB, Mori Y, Refetoff S: Reduced clearance rate of thyroxine-binding globulin (TBG) with increased sialylation: a mechanism for estrogen-induced elevation of serum TBG concentration, *J Clin Endocrinol Metab* 65:689, 1987.
2. Akande EO: The effect of oestrogen on plasma levels of luteinizing hormone in euthyroid and thyrotoxic postmenopausal women, *J Obstet Gynaecol Br Commonw* 81:795, 1974.
3. Akande EO, Anderson DC: Role of sex-hormone-binding globulin in hormonal changes and amenorrhoea in thyrotoxic women, *Br J Obstet Gynaecol* 82:557, 1975.
4. Akande EO, Hockaday TDR: Plasma concentration of gonadotrophins: oestrogen and progesterone in thyrotoxic women, *Br J Obstet Gynaecol* 82:541, 1975.
5. Althaus BU et al: LDL/HDL-changes in subclinical hypothyroidism: possible risk factors for coronary artery disease, *Clin Endocrinol* 28:157, 1988.
6. Amino N et al: High prevalence of transient postpartum thyrotoxicosis and hypothyroidism, *N Engl J Med* 306:849, 1982.
7. Amino N et al: Aggravation of thyrotoxicosis in early pregnancy and after delivery in Graves' disease, *J Clin Endocrinol Metab* 55:108, 1982.
8. Amino N et al: Postpartum autoimmune thyroid syndromes. In Walfish PG, Wall JR, Volpe R, editors: *Autoimmunity and the thyroid,* Orlando, Fla, 1985, Academic Press.
9. Benson RC, Dailey Morris E: The menstrual pattern in hyperthyroidism and subsequent posttherapy hypothyroidism, *Surg Gynecol Obstet* 100:19, 1955.
10. Borst GC, Eil C, Burman KD: Euthyroid hyperthyroxinemia, *Ann Intern Med* 98:366, 1983.
11. Bouillon R et al: Thyroid function in patients with hyperemesis gravidarum, *Am J Obstet Gynecol* 143:922, 1982.
12. Braverman LE et al: Enhanced susceptibility to iodide myxedema in patients with Hashimoto's disease, *J Clin Endocrinol Metab* 32:515, 1971.
13. Burrow GN: The management of thyrotoxicosis in pregnancy, *N Engl J Med* 313:562, 1985.
14. Cooper DS: Antithyroid drugs, *N Engl J Med* 311:1353, 1984.
15. Cooper DS: Antithyroid drugs: to breast-feed or not to breast-feed, *Am J Obstet Gynecol* 157:234, 1987.
16. Cooper DS: Therapy of hyperthyroidism. In Braverman LE, Utiger RD, editors: *The thyroid,* Philadelphia, 1991, JB Lippincott.
17. Cooper DS et al: Agranulocytosis associated with antithyroid drugs, *Ann Intern Med* 98:26, 1983.
18. Cooper DS et al: L-Thyroxine therapy in subclinical hypothyroidism: a double-blind, placebo-controlled trial, *Ann Intern Med* 101:18, 1984.
19. Davis LE et al: Thyrotoxicosis complicating pregnancy, *Am J Obstet Gynecol* 160:63, 1989.
20. Degroot LJ, Qunitans J: The causes of autoimmune thyroid disease, *Endocr Rev* 10:537, 1989.
21. Distiller LA, Sagel J, Morley JE: Assessment of pituitary gonadotropin reserve using luteinizing hormone-releasing hormone (LRH) in states of altered thyroid function, *J Clin Endocrinol Metab* 40:512, 1975.
22. Dobyns BM et al: Functional and histologic effects of therapeutic doses of radioactiveiodine on the thyroid of man, *J Clin Endocrinol Metab* 13:548, 1953.
23. Dozeman R et al: Hyperthyroidism appearing as hyperemesis gravidarum, *Arch Intern Med* 143:2202, 1983.
24. Emerson CH: Thyroid disease during and after pregnancy. In Braverman LE, Utiger RD, editors: *The thyroid,* Philadelphia, 1991, JB Lippincott.
25. Faglia G et al: Thyrotropin secretion in patients with central hypothyroidism: evidence for reduced biological activity of immunoactive thyrotropin, *J Clin Endocrinol Metab* 48:989, 1979.
26. Field JB: Thyroid-stimulating hormone and cyclic adenosine 3'5'-monophosphate in the regulation of thyroid gland function, *Metabolism* 24:381, 1975.
27. Fish LH et al: Replacement dose, metabolism, and bioavailability of levothyroxine in treatment of hypothyroidism, *N Engl J Med* 316:764, 1987.
28. Fisher DA, Klein AH: Thyroid development and disorders of thyroid function in the newborn, *N Engl J Med* 304:702, 1981.
29. Gavin LA: Thyroid crises, *Med Clin North Am* 75:179, 1991.
30. Gerstein HC: How common is postpartum thyroiditis?, *Arch Intern Med* 150:1397, 1990.
31. Gesundheit N et al: Thyrotropin-secreting pituitary adenomas: clinical and biochemical heterogeneity. *Ann Intern Med* 111:827, 1989.
32. Gharib H et al: Fine-needle aspiration biopsy of the thyroid, *Ann Intern Med* 101:25, 1984.
33. Gharib H et al: Suppressive therapy with levothyroxine for solitary thyroid nodules, *N Engl J Med* 317:70, 1987.
34. Glinoer D et al: Regulation of maternal thyroid during pregnancy, *J Clin Endocrinol Metab* 71:276, 1990.
35. Glinoer D et al: Pregnancy in patients with mild thyroid abnormalities: maternal and neonatal repercussions, *J Clin Endocrinol Metab* 73:421, 1991.
36. Hamburger J, Kaplan MM, Husain M: Diagnosis of thyroid nodules by needle biopsy. In Braverman LE, Utiger RD, editors: *the Thyroid,* Philadelphia, 1991, JB Lippincott.
37. Grant CS et al: Long-term follow-up of patients with benign thyroid fine-needle aspiration cytologic diagnoses, *Surgery* 106:980, 1989.
38. Hancock SL, Cox RS, McDougall IR: Thyroid diseases after treatment of Hodgkin's disease, *N Engl J Med* 325:599, 1991.
39. Harris B et al: Transient post-partum thyroid dysfunction and postnatal depression, *J Affective Disord* 17:243, 1989.
40. Hashizume K et al: Administration of thyroxine in treated Graves' disease, *N Engl J Med* 324:947, 1991.

41. Hay ID: Papillary thyroid carcinoma, *Endocrinol Metab Clin North Am* 19:545, 1990.

42. Hill CS, Clark RL, Wolf M: The effect of subsequent pregnancy on patients with thyroid carcinoma, *Surg Gynecol Obstet* 122:1219, 1966.

43. Hoffman DA et al: Mortality in women treated with hyperthyroidism, *Am J Epidemiol* 115:243, 1982.

44. Holm L et al: Malignant thyroid tumors after iodine-131 therapy, *N Engl J Med* 303:188, 1980.

45. Iataka M et al: Comparison of measurements of in vitro production of antithyroid microsomal antibody versus anti-thyroid peroxidase antibody, *Reg Immunolul* 1:106, 1988.

46. Kaplan MM: Thyroid carcinoma, *Endocrinol Metab Clin North Am* 19:469, 1990.

47. Kaptein EM et al: Peripheral serum thyroxine, triiodothyronine, and reverse triiodothyronine kinetics in the low thyroxine state of nonthyroidal illnesses: a noncompartmental analysis, *J Clin Invest* 69:526, 1982.

48. Kasuga Y et al: Effects of recombinant human interleukin-2 and tumor necrosis factor-α with or without interferon-gamma on human thyroid tissues from patients with Graves' disease and from normal subjects xenografted into nude mice, *J Clin Endocrinol Metab* 72:1296, 1991.

49. Kennedy RL et al: Thyroid function in choriocarcinoma: demonstration of a thyroid stimulating activity in serum using FRTL-5 and human thyroid cells, *Clin Endocrinol* 33:227, 1990.

50. Ladenson PW: Diagnosis of hyperthyroidism. In Braverman LE, Utiger RD, editors: *The thyroid,* Philadelphia, 1991, JB Lippincott.

51. Ladenson PW: Diagnosis of hypothyroidism. In Braverman LE, Utiger RD, editors: *The thyroid,* Philadelphia, 1991, JB Lippincott.

52. Ladenson PW, Ridgway EC: Early peripheral responses to intravenous L-thyroxine in primary hypothyroidism, *Am J Med* 73:467, 1982.

53. Ladenson PW et al: Complications of surgery in hypothyroid patients, *Am J Med* 77:261, 1984.

54. Lazarus JH et al: Struma ovarii: a case report, *Clin Endocrinol* 27:715, 1987.

55. Mandel SJ et al: Increased need for thyroxine during pregnancy in women with primary hypothyroidism, *N Engl J Med* 323:91, 1990.

56. Marrioti S et al: Low serum thyroglobulin as a clue to the diagnosis of thyrotoxicosis factitia, *N Engl J Med* 307:410, 1982.

57. Messer PM et al: Antithyroid drug treatment of Graves' disease in pregnancy: long-term effects on somatic growth, intellectual development and thyroid function of the offspring, *Acta Endocrinol* 123:311, 1990.

58. Momotani N et al: Maternal hyperthyroidism and congenital malformation in the offspring, *Clin Endocrinol* 20:695, 1984.

59. Momotani J et al: Antithyroid drug therapy for Graves' disease during pregnancy, *N Engl J Med* 315:24, 1986.

60. Mori M et al: Morning sickness and thyroid function in normal pregnancy, *Obstet Gynecol* 72:355, 1986.

61. Mortimer RH et al: Graves' disease in pregnancy: TSH receptor binding inhibiting immunoglobulins and maternal and neonatal thyroid function, *Clin Endocrinol* 32:141, 1990.

62. Nelson M et al: Thyroid gland size in pregnancy, *J Reprod Med* 32:888, 1987.

63. Nikolai TF et al: Thyroid function and treatment in premenstrual syndrome, *J Clin Endocrinol Metab* 70:1108, 1990.

64. Nordyke RA, Gilbert FI, Harada ASM: Graves' disease: influence of age on clinical findings, *Arch Intern Med* 148:626, 1988.

65. Okamura K et al: Reevaluation of the effects of methylmercapitoimidazole and propylthiouracil in patients with Graves' hyperthyroidism, *J Clin Endocrinol Metab* 65:719, 1987.

66. Oppenheimer JH: Thyroid hormone action at the molecular level. In Braverman LE, Utiger RD, editors: *The thyroid,* Philadelphia, 1991, JB Lippincott.

67. Othman S et al: A long-term follow-up of postpartum thyroiditis, *Clin Endocrinol* 32:559, 1990.

68. Paul TL et al: Long-term L-thyroxine therapy is associated with decreased hip bone density in premenopausal women, *JAMA* 259:3137, 1988.

69. Pintar JE, Toran-Allerand CD: Normal development of the hypothalamic-pituitary-thyroid axis. In Braverman LE, Utiger RD, editors: *The thyroid,* Philadelphia, 1991, JB Lippincott.

70. Refetoff S: Thyroid hormone resistance syndromes. In Braverman LE, Utiger RD, editors: *The thyroid,* 1991, Philadelphia, JB Lippincott.

71. Ridgway EC, Longcope C, Maloof F: Metabolic clearance and blood production rates of estradiol in hyperthyroidism, *J Clin Endocrinol Metab* 41:491, 1975.

72. Ridgway EC, Maloof F, Longcope C: Androgen and oestrogen dynamics in hyperthyroidism, *J Endocrinol* 95:105, 1982.

73. Robbins JR: Thyroid hormone transport proteins and the physiology of hormone binding. In Braverman LE, Utiger RD, editors: *The thyroid,* Philadelphia, 1991, JB Lippincott.

74. Robertson JS, Gorman CA: Gonadal radiation dose and its genetic significance in radioiodine therapy of hyperthyroidism, *J Nucl Med* 17:826, 1976.

75. Rojeski MT, Gharib H: Nodular thyroid disease, *N Engl J Med* 313:428, 1985.

76. Romaldini JH et al: Comparison of effects of high and low dosage regimens of antithyroid drugs in the management of Graves' hyperthyroidism, *J Clin Endocrinol Metab* 57:563, 1983.

77. Romney BM et al: Radionuclide administration to nursing mothers: mathematically derived guidelines, *Radiology* 160:549, 1986.

78. Ross DS et al: Subclinical hyperthyroidism and reduced bone density as a possible result of prolonged suppression of the pituitary-thyroid axis with L-thyroxine, *Am J Med* 82:1167, 1987.

79. Rubin PC: Beta-blockers in pregnancy, *N Engl J Med* 305:1323, 1981.

80. Ruiz M et al: Familial dysalbuminemic hyperthyroxinemia: a syndrome that can be confused with thyrotoxicosis, *N Engl J Med* 306:635, 1982.

81. Sawin CT et al: Aging and the thyroid: decreased requirement for thyroid hormone in older hypothyroid patients, *Am J Med* 75:206, 1983.

82. Shupnik MA, Ridgway EC, Chin WW: Molecular biology of thyrotrophin, *Endocr Rev* 10:459, 1989.

83. Solomon B et al: Current trends in the management of Graves' disease, *J Clin Endocrinol Metab* 70:1518, 1990.

84. Spencer CA et al: Applications of a new chemiluminometric thyrotropin assay to subnormal measurements, *J Clin Endocrinol Metab* 70:453, 1990.

85. Spratt DI et al: Hyperthyroxinemia in patients with acute psychiatric disorders, *Am J Med* 73:41, 1982.

86. Sterling K, Brenner MA, Newman ES: Conversion of thyroxine to triiodothyronine in normal human subjects, *Science* 169:1099, 1970.

87. Sugrue E et al: Hyperthyroidism in the land of Graves: results of treatment by surgery, radioiodine and carbimazole in 837 cases, *Q J Med* 49:51, 1980.

88. Tanka T et al: Gonadotropin response to luteinizing hormone releasing hormone in hyperthyroid patients with menstrual disturbances, *Metabolism* 30:323, 1981.

89. Tourniaire J et al: Increased luteinizing hormone sensitivity to dopaminergic inhibition in Graves' disease, *Acta Endocrinol* 115:91, 1987.

90. Tunbridge WMG et al: The spectrum of thyroid disease in a community: the Whickham survey, *Clin Endocrinol* 7:481, 1977.

91. Vagenakis AG et al: Iodide induced thyrotoxicosis in Boston, *N Engl J Med* 287:523, 1972.

92. Van Dijke CP, Heydendael RJ, DeLkeine MJ: Methimazole, carbimazole and congenital skin defects, *Ann Intern Med* 106:60, 1987.

93. Van Herle AJ: Thyroglobulin. In Braverman LE, Utiger RD, editors: *The thyroid,* Philadelphia, 1991, JB Lippincott.

94. Van Wyk JJ, Grumbach MM: Syndrome of precocious menstruation and galactorrhea in juvenile hypothyroidism: an example of hormonal overlap in pituitary feedback, *J Pediatr* 59:416, 1960.

95. Volpe R: Immunology of human thyroid disease. In Volpe R, editor: *Autoimmunity in endocrine disease,* Boca Raton, Fla, 1990, CRC Press.

96. Wartofsky L: Myxedema coma. In Braverman LE, Utiger RD, editors: *The thyroid,* Philadelphia, 1991, JB Lippincott.

97. Wartofsky L, Burman KD: Alterations in thyroid function in patients with systemic illness: the "euthyroid sick syndrome," *Endocr Rev* 3:164, 1982.

98. Wood LC, Ingbar SH: Hypothyroidism as a late sequela in patients with Graves' disease treated with antithyroid agents, *J Clin Invest* 64:1429, 1971.

99. Wu SY et al: Alterations in tissue 5′-monodeiodinating activity in the perinatal period, *Endocrinology* 103:235, 1978.

100. Zakarija M, McKenzie JM, Hoffman WH: Prediction and therapy of intrauterine and late-onset neonatal hyperthyroidism, *J Clin Endocrinol Metab* 62:368, 1986.

101. Zakarija M, McKenzie LM, Eidson MS: Transient neonatal hypothyroidism: characterization of maternal antibodies to the thyrotropin receptor, *J Clin Endocrinol Metab* 70:1239, 1990.

Chapter 13

REPRODUCTION AND DISORDERS OF ADRENAL FUNCTION

James S. Prihoda, MD
and D. Lynn Loriaux, MD, PhD

Adrenal physiology and anatomy
Hypercortisolism
    Cushing syndrome
    Stress
Adrenal insufficiency
Congenital adrenal hyperplasia

Alterations in the serum concentrations of adrenal steroids can cause anovulation, amenorrhea, and infertility. Glucocorticoid excess occurs in Cushing syndrome and the "stress" disorders. Glucocorticoid insufficiency also can be associated with anovulation. Androgen excess characterizes the virilizing forms of congenital adrenal hyperplasia. Treatment of these disorders can restore normal ovulation and allow conception. In addition, early diagnosis and treatment of Cushing syndrome and adrenal insufficiency associated with pregnancy can decrease maternal and fetal morbidity.

ADRENAL PHYSIOLOGY AND ANATOMY

The adult adrenal gland is divided into cortical and medullary portions. Each has a different ontogeny and function. The cortex comprises 80% of the gland by weight. The cortex derives from mesoderm and the medulla derives from neuroectoderm. The adrenal medulla produces catecholamines, primarily epinephrine. The adult adrenal cortex is divided into three morphologic zones and two functionally distinct zones. The outermost zona glomeru-

James S. Prihoda is a recipient of the American Heart Association's Clinician Scientist Award.

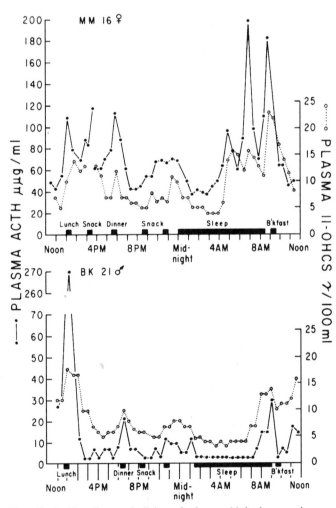

Fig. 13-1. Circadian periodicity of plasma 11-hydroxycorticosteroid (*11-OHCS*) and plasma ACTH levels over a 24-hour period. (From Krieger DT et al: with permission of Williams & Wilkins.)

losa comprises 5% of the cortex and is the source of aldosterone. The zona fasciculata and zona reticularis, the middle and inner zones, form a functional unit that secretes cortisol and the adrenal androgens.

HYPERCORTISOLISM

Cortisol secretion is regulated by adrenocorticotropin (ACTH). The acute effect of ACTH is to increase the conversion of cholesterol to pregnenolone. This is the initial and rate-limiting step in cortisol synthesis. An important chronic effect of ACTH is to increase the expression of the low-density lipoprotein receptor providing circulating cholesterol for subsequent steroid biosynthesis. ACTH and cortisol are secreted episodically in eight to ten pulses per day; most of these pulses cluster in the morning hours,

leading to a diurnal pattern of cortisol secretion (Fig. 13-1). ACTH secretion is largely regulated by corticotropin-releasing hormone (CRH) and arginine vasopressin. This hypothalamic-pituitary-adrenal (HPA) axis forms a feedback loop with cortisol that inhibits the synthesis and secretion of CRH in the hypothalamus and the action of CRH on the anterior pituitary gland.

The function of the HPA axis is altered in normal pregnancy. Total and free plasma cortisol and urinary free cortisol (UFC) increase to levels that can overlap those of established Cushing syndrome. Morning plasma cortisol levels rise from 15 µg/dL at 11 weeks to 35 µg/dL at 26 weeks of gestation[16] (Fig. 13-2). The UFC usually does not rise above 250 µg/d in normal pregnant women[68] (Fig. 13-3). In addition, exogenous corticosteroids do not suppress

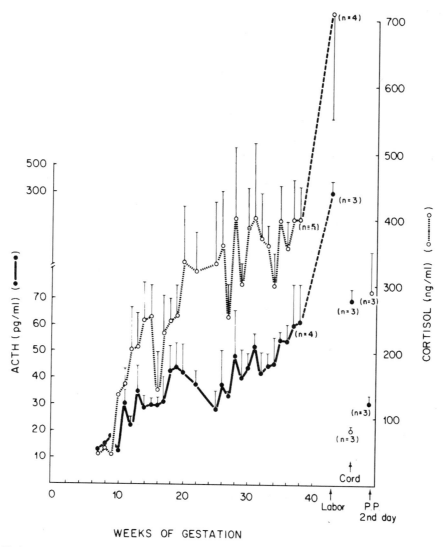

Fig. 13-2. Plasma concentrations of ACTH and cortisol during normal pregnancy. Blood samples were obtained weekly from five normal pregnant women and from three women during labor and on the second postpartum (*P.P.*) day. In addition, umbilical cord blood plasma was obtained from the newborn infants of three of these subjects. Data are presented as means ± SEM. (From Carr BR et al[16]: *Am J Obstet Gynecol* 139:416, 1981.)

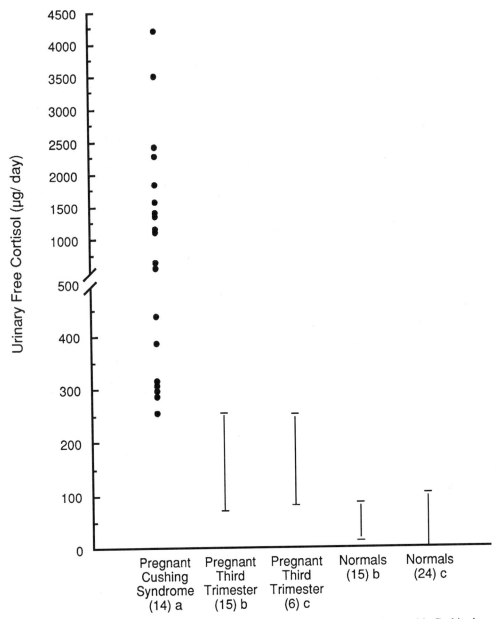

Fig. 13-3. Twenty-four-hour urinary free cortisol excretion in pregnant patients with Cushing's syndrome, normal pregnant patients, and nonpregnant subjects. Numbers of patients are shown in parentheses. *a*, Prihoda and Davis[68]; *b*, Lindholm and Schultz-Moller[52]; *c*, Rees et al.[70]

the axis normally[62] (Fig. 13-4). ACTH levels also rise during pregnancy, suggesting an altered cortisol feed-back set-point. The source of this ACTH may be the placenta[70] or the pituitary.[25] CRH produced by the placenta and fetal membranes may stimulate ACTH production, contributing to the increased plasma ACTH concentration.[39,44] Cortisol-binding globulin levels rise during the first two trimesters.[30] This increase accounts for some, but not all, of the rise in total cortisol concentration. The normal diurnal pattern of cortisol and ACTH secretion is maintained, although at a higher level (Fig. 13-5).[16]

Cushing syndrome

Pathophysiology. The syndrome of chronic hyperadrenalism was first described by Harvey Cushing in 1910.[24] Cushing syndrome can be classified as ACTH dependent and ACTH independent. Causes of the ACTH-dependent form include ACTH-secreting pituitary microadenoma and ectopic sources of ACTH such as a bronchial carcinoid. Causes of the ACTH-independent form include adrenal cancer, adrenal adenoma, primary adrenocortical nodular dysplasia, and iatrogenic or factitious processes.

Most patients with ACTH-dependent Cushing syn-

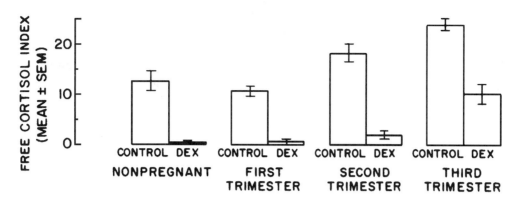

Fig. 13-4. Mean free cortisol indexes measured sequentially in seven women in each trimester of pregnancy and 3 months postpartum (nonpregnant) at 8 hours before (CONTROL) and on the morning after ingestion of a single nighttime dose of dexamethasone (DEX). (From Nolten WE et al[63]: *J Clin Endocrinol Metab* 51:466, 1980, with permission.)

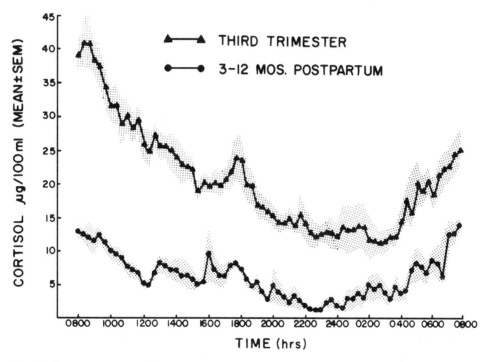

Fig. 13-5. Mean plasma cortisol concentrations measured at 20-minute intervals during a 24-hour period in seven third-trimester pregnant women and three nonpregnant women. (From Nolten WE, Rueckert PA[62]: *Am J Obstet Gynecol* 139:492, 1981.)

drome have a pituitary adenoma. Most of these tumors are less than 2 mm in diameter. These tumors secrete ACTH in a pulsatile fashion, but the usual diurnal variation is lost. The most common source of ACTH is small-cell carcinoma of the lung.

The common ACTH-independent causes of endogenous Cushing syndrome include adrenal carcinoma, adrenal adenoma, and primary adrenocortical nodular dysplasia. Adrenal carcinomas are large and often can be palpated through the anterior abdominal wall. Virilization in women,

feminization in men, hypokalemic alkalosis, and peripheral edema all suggest adrenal carcinoma. Adrenal adenomas usually produce only cortisol. They are smaller than adrenal carcinomas.[54]

In pregnancy, ACTH-dependent causes of Cushing syndrome account for half of the cases. Most of the remainder are caused by adrenal adenomas.[6]

Clinical manifestations. The diagnosis of Cushing syndrome in the setting of pregnancy can be delayed, since many of the normal physiologic changes of pregnancy

Table 13-1. Clinical features of Cushing syndrome

Feature	% of patients
Obesity	94
Facial plethora	84
Hirsutism	82
Menstrual disorders	76
Hypertension	72
Muscle weakness	58
Back pain	58
Striae	52
Acne	40
Psychologic symptoms	40
Bruising	36
Congestive heart failure	22
Edema	18
Renal calculi	16
Headache	14
Polyuria/polydipsia	10
Hyperpigmentation	6

Modified from Baxter JD, Tyrell JB: In Felig P et al, editors: *Endocrinology and metabolism,* ed 2, New York, 1987, McGraw-Hill.

mimic the manifestations of Cushing syndrome. Pregnant women can develop abdominal striae, weight gain, glucose intolerance, fluid retention, and hypertension.[8] Most of the reports of Cushing syndrome in pregnancy describe centripetal redistribution of fat over the clavicles, around the neck, on the trunk and abdomen, in the temporal fossae, and in the cheeks.[72] The striae associated with pregnancy and Cushing syndrome are similar. Ross and Linch[71] reported that the most common findings in nonpregnant patients with Cushing syndrome were ecchymoses, myopathy, and hypertension (Table 13-1). As in nonpregnant patients, hypercortisolism in pregnancy can lead to cutaneous ulceration, ecchymoses, insomnia, mood disturbance, depression, mania, and psychosis.[8] Hirsutism in Cushing syndrome can take two forms: increased lanugo hair growth by glucocorticoids and terminal hair growth from androgen stimulation. Mineralocorticoid excess is manifest as hypertension and hypokalemic alkalosis. Other laboratory findings include granulocytosis, lymphocytopenia, eosinopenia, and hypercalciuria.

The common maternal complications in pregnancy-related Cushing syndrome include hypertension (87% of cases) and gestational diabetes (61%).[5] Pulmonary edema has been seen in patients with adrenal adenoma.[5,46] In one review, 3 of 63 patients died of complications related to Cushing syndrome (disseminated aspergillosis, heart block, and adult respiratory distress syndrome).[5]

Diagnostic investigation. The most sensitive laboratory study for the diagnosis of glucocorticoid excess is the 24-hour UFC.[54] In nonpregnant patients, values below 100 μg/d are normal. Values above 250 μg/d are virtually diagnostic of Cushing syndrome. The normal range is increased by pregnancy, however, and can extend to 250

μg/d.[68] Since 1970 UFC levels have been reported in 18 pregnant patients with Cushing syndrome. These values have ranged between 255 and 4200 μg/d.[68] Thus in pregnancy the UFC discriminant between normal and cortisol excess is 250 μg/d. Overnight dexamethasone suppression has less utility during pregnancy because of an increased rate of false-positive tests in the second and third trimesters.[62] If the diagnosis of Cushing syndrome is in question, the loss of a normal diurnal rhythm favors the diagnosis. The normal circadian rhythm of cortisol production is maintained during pregnancy, but at a higher average level.[16, 62] Failure to double the average cortisol levels of three samples collected at 30-minute intervals between 2200 and 2400 (10 PM and midnight) and 0600 and 0800 (6 AM and 8 AM) suggests a blunting of the diurnal rhythm.[54]

The dexamethasone suppression test is the traditional tool for differentiating pituitary adenoma from the ectopic source of ACTH and ACTH-independent causes of Cushing syndrome. In the classic dexamethasone suppression test, a 50% decrease of Porter-Silber chromogens (mostly 17-hydroxycorticosteroids) suggests a pituitary adenoma. Flack et al.,[33] using more stringent criteria, showed that a 90% decrease in UFC and a 64% suppression of 17-hydroxysteroid excretion has 100% specificity for ACTH-secreting pituitary microadenomas. The dexamethasone suppression test must be interpreted with caution during pregnancy, since normal women in the third trimester can fail to exhibit suppression of serum cortisol[23,62] or UFC.[62,70]

A more contemporary and sensitive approach to the diagnosis is first to determine ACTH dependency or independency. Plasma ACTH values of greater than 10 pg/mL correlate well with ACTH dependency. In that case, eutopic versus ectopic secretion of ACTH can be determined with inferior petrosal sinus sampling (IPSS) for ACTH. To date, this test has a 100% sensitivity and specificity in defining the site of ACTH production. The test can "lateralize" the site of a pituitary adenoma in the majority of cases.[64] IPSS requires dye exposure, cranial radiation, and femoral vein catheterization. It has not been reported in pregnancy. Because of the serious consequences of Cushing syndrome in pregnancy, however, IPSS, when needed, seems justified.

Useful imaging modalities include ultrasound, magnetic resonance imaging (MRI), and, on occasion, computed tomography (CT) scanning. Adrenal ultrasound is safe but not as sensitive as MRI or CT. Of 11 patients with adrenal adenoma presenting during pregnancy, ultrasound revealed the mass in eight.[68] If an adrenal adenoma is suspected but not demonstrated by ultrasound, MRI is a safe alternative to CT.[82] CT scanning of the sella turcica has a sensitivity of 47% and a specificity of 74% for ACTH-secreting pituitary adenomas[45]; MRI is modestly better.[45] Neither test can replace biochemical studies, particularly since 12% to 27% of patients have an incidental pituitary adenoma. In other words, a mass demonstrated by imaging studies may not be

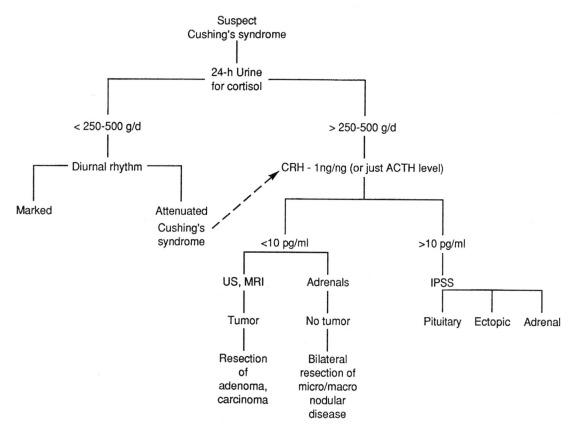

Fig. 13-6. Flow diagram of a potential diagnostic scheme for Cushing syndrome, *US*, Ultrasound. (See text for explanation.)

the source of ACTH.[64] Chest CT with fundal shielding or MRI can be useful for identifying ectopic sources of ACTH.[54,61]

There are inherent difficulties in summarizing a diagnostic strategy with a flow diagram. This is especially true in a rare combination such as pregnancy and Cushing disease. An attempt to do this, however, is shown in Fig. 13-6. If Cushing syndrome is suspected, the diagnosis can be provisionally confirmed if the UFC is greater than 250 g/d. If the clinical features strongly suggest hypercortisolism but the UFC is between 100 and 250 μg/d, a blunted diurnal cortisol rhythm is supportive of the diagnosis. ACTH dependence can be demonstrated by ACTH values in excess of 10 pg/mL. If the ACTH level is low (< 10 pg/mL), ultrasound imaging is appropriate; if that is negative, MRI of the adrenal glands is indicated. If the plasma ACTH concentration is not suppressed, IPSS can separate patients with pituitary sources of ACTH production from those with ectopic sources.

The fetus is profoundly affected by maternal Cushing syndrome. Of 72 reported cases, spontaneous abortions were described in 14. Of 52 live births, 38 infants were premature or required early cesarean delivery.[68] Several patients had spontaneous abortions before the diagnosis was made.[11] Intrauterine growth retardation occurs in

38%.[15] Although some maternal glucocorticoids cross the placenta, neonatal adrenal insufficiency is rare.[12,47] When present, it can be accompanied by hypoglycemia, seizures, circulatory collapse, fever, failure to thrive, hyperkalemia, and hyponatremia.[58] There are no reports of fetal masculinization.

Treatment. Medical and surgical treatments for hypercortisolism have been used during pregnancy. The results suggest that definitive therapy leads to a better outcome for mother and fetus.[15] If appropriately timed, transsphenoidal pituitary surgery for Cushing disease and unilateral adrenalectomy (via flank incision) for adrenal adenoma appear to be well tolerated.[5,15,66] Unilateral adrenalectomy has been performed with good results as late as 29 weeks into gestation. Definitive surgical treatment is recommended for most cases, even in the early third trimester.[11] Bilateral adrenalectomy is required for treatment of primary adrenocortical nodular dysplasia.[22]

Pharmacologic agents have been used in pregnancy to reduce the degree of hypercortisolism. The safety of these drugs for the fetus has not been established. Both aminoglutethimide and metyrapone cross the placenta. Aminoglutethimide has caused fetal virilization, and metyrapone has been associated with elevation of maternal 11-deoxycorticosterone levels and hypertension.[68] Ketoconazole was used successfully at 32 weeks of gestation in one woman with a female fetus. Ketoconazole crosses the placenta poorly but could block testosterone production,[3] causing incomplete masculinization of a male fetus. This result has not been reported. Cyproheptadine, a serotonin antagonist that reduces ACTH secretion, is effective in less than 50% of nonpregnant patients with Cushing disease. Although details were not given in all cases, cyproheptadine occasionally may be of benefit in Cushing syndrome associated with pregnancy.

The effects of surgical management of pregnant patients with Cushing syndrome on maternal and fetal morbidity and mortality are difficult to quantitate from the available literature. The rate of prematurity appears to decrease from 72% to 47%.[15] There is no clear-cut decrease in the perinatal death rate or in intrauterine growth retardation with definitive surgical treatment, but there are no reports of stillbirths in women so treated.[15]

A few investigators[11,67,81] have discussed the timing and the surgical approach. They generally recommend definitive surgery when Cushing syndrome is diagnosed, until the early third trimester, when prompt delivery of the baby followed by definitive therapy is advocated. Management of adrenal carcinoma is more difficult because the preferred transabdominal approach is compromised by the enlarging uterine fundus. Termination of pregnancy may be required to allow adequate visualization. Vaginal delivery, if possible, is preferred to reduce the rate of wound infection and dehiscence.[11]

Stress

Types. Stress can be partitioned, conceptually, into at least three types: starvation, work, and anxiety. Examples of these kinds of stress in semiisolation have been studied extensively in the forms of anorexia nervosa, aerobic exercise, and depression. Each of these conditions is associated with an increased incidence of amenorrhea. The incidence of amenorrhea in anorexia nervosa, for example, approaches 100%. Amenorrhea begins before the onset of weight loss in 20% of cases. It begins with the onset of weight loss in half of the cases and after weight loss has been established in the remainder.[34]

Athletic amenorrhea is a well-established cause of secondary amenorrhea. Elite marathon runners have an incidence of amenorrhea of about 19%.[36] Another study showed that the incidence of amenorrhea has a rough but direct relationship to the intensity of training. In runners, the incidence of amenorrhea varied between 5% at 5 miles per week and more than 40% at 70 miles per week.[31] Similar findings have been observed with other forms of exercise, in particular ballet.[84]

Psychologic stress leading to secondary amenorrhea has been referred to as "dormitory" amenorrhea or, as the circumstance allows, "war amenorrhea." The incidence of secondary amenorrhea in the general population is esti-

mated to be between 2% and 5%. Examples of amenorrhea associated with psychologic stress include an incidence of 6% in armed forces recruits,[75] 15% in postulants and novitiates entering the religious life,[26] 20% to 50% in concentration camp victims, and 100% in a group of prisoners on death row.[83]

Each of these examples of stress-related reproductive dysfunction is associated with increased activity of the HPA axis. The end result is an increased cortisol production rate. In most of these conditions, the cortisol production rate has not been measured directly but has been suggested by indirect measurements.[14,55,73] It is clear that primary disorders of cortisol excess such as the exogenous administration of glucocorticoids or Cushing syndrome of any cause are associated with a high incidence of reproductive dysfunction. It is less clear that activation of the HPA axis in response to stress is causally linked to reproductive dysfunction. Several recent studies, however, have suggested possible mechanisms for this effect. These are reviewed below.

Response. With the ability to monitor the activity of the adrenal cortex by measuring its products of secretion or the metabolites of these products of secretion came the discovery that adrenal secretory activity increases with stress. One of the earliest examples of this was the finding that 17-hydroxysteroid excretion doubled during attacks of experimentally induced tularemia.[9] How this occurs has been the object of intense study.

The hypothalamus, the pituitary gland, and the adrenal gland play essential roles in mediating the stress-associated rise in plasma cortisol concentration. The interactions between the hypothalamus and the pituitary gland were reviewed previously. In the stressed state, the secretory bursts of ACTH and cortisol become more numerous and of greater amplitude. "Regulatory" changes also occur. For example, basal secretion of cortisol can be inhibited by the exogenous administration of glucocorticoids, whereas the stress-mediated secretion of cortisol cannot. Since the action of CRH on pituitary ACTH secretion is blocked by exogenous glucocorticoid, other hypothalamic ACTH secretagogues such as vasopressin probably play an important role in the stress-mediated rise in ACTH and cortisol.[19] On the other hand, if CRH is not sufficient to explain the stress-mediated rise in cortisol, it is necessary, and its effects on reproductive function have been studied extensively. Studies in the rhesus monkey show that an intravenous infusion of CRH can completely suppress the releasing hormone gonadotropin (GnRH) pulse generator.[65] This effect cannot be reproduced by an infusion of ACTH,[32] but it can be blocked with naloxone.[35] These studies imply that CRH suppresses GnRH secretion through the intermediation of an opiate peptide. Hypogonadotropic hypogonadism results, a pattern of reproductive dysfunction that fits well with the known examples of stress amenorrhea.

Cortisol itself can modulate reproductive function. This

is best seen in the example of Cushing syndrome. Cushing syndrome is a constellation of clinical changes resulting from excess cortisol. One of these changes is amenorrhea. It was recognized as a prominent feature of the syndrome by Harvey Cushing in 1932.[24] The incidence of amenorrhea in Cushing syndrome approaches 100%. Unlike the examples of stress-induced amenorrhea outlined earlier, however, Cushing syndrome is associated with low or absent CRH synthesis and secretion. This is inferred from the observation that cure of Cushing syndrome leads to relative adrenal insufficiency that is long lasting and attributable to CRH deficiency.[7] Thus cortisol itself must have an effect on reproductive competence.

Cortisol can alter gonadal function directly. For example, women undergoing ovulation induction with human menopausal gonadotropins have an attenuated response to those hormones if they are treated concurrently with dexamethasone.[38] A similar effect has been observed in men treated with glucocorticoid for chronic obstructive pulmonary disease. Plasma testosterone concentrations fell by almost half in the absence of any change in circulating gonadotropin concentrations or changes in sex hormone-binding globulin binding capacity.[56] Similar findings have been reported in baboons in which the testicular response to luteinizing hormone has been shown to be attenuated in the presence of glucocorticoid.[74]

A primary effect of cortisol on the gonad, however, would result in a hypergonadotropic form of hypogonadism. This is not the case in Cushing syndrome. Like other forms of stress-induced reproductive dysfunction, the hypogonadism of Cushing syndrome is associated with normal or low gonadotropin concentrations. Thus cortisol also must have an effect on gonadotropin secretion. This effect has been demonstrated in castrated rhesus monkeys. Parenteral hydrocortisone acetate markedly suppressed circulating concentrations of luteinizing hormone and follicle-stimulating hormone. The gonadotropin concentrations were restored nearly to normal, however, with exogenous GnRH administration, supporting the hypothesis that cortisol can suppress GnRH synthesis or secretion.[27] This is supported further by the recent finding that the GnRH gene contains a glucocorticoid regulatory element 106 base pairs upstream of the TATA box, providing a potential biochemical mechanism for the effect of cortisol on GnRH elaboration.[69]

In summary, stress is associated with reproductive dysfunction. The primary abnormality seems to be at the level of hypothalamic secretion of GnRH. CRH plays an important role in the stress response and is a powerful modulator of GnRH secretion, probably through the intermediary action of an opiadergic mechanism. Cortisol can also inhibit the secretion of GnRH. It can, as well, interrupt gonadal function directly.

Why glucocorticoid levels rise in response to stress is unknown. Most experiments designed to probe this question have revealed no survival advantage associated with increased circulating concentrations of cortisol.[79] Worth considering is the possibility that a primary reason for the glucocorticoid rise in response to stress is to inhibit reproduction. In other words, the primary biologic effect of the stress response may be to prevent reproduction during times of environmental uncertainty. If so, it is not difficult to see how the trait has been selected for and amplified. As well, its role in the genesis of idiopathic infertility is not difficult to visualize.

ADRENAL INSUFFICIENCY

Adrenal insufficiency can be primary or secondary in nature. The most common cause of primary adrenal insufficiency (Addison disease) is idiopathic or autoimmune adenitis. The next most common cause is tuberculosis.[43] Autoimmune adenitis is associated with gonadal failure, autoimmune thyroid disease, vitiligo, hypoparathyroidism, and pernicious anemia (polyglandular failure).[53] With the advent of glucocorticoid replacement therapy, women with adrenal insufficiency become pregnant normally, and recent reviews suggest that these pregnancies do not deviate significantly from normal.[2,42]

The most common cause of secondary adrenal insufficiency is corticosteroid therapy for other medical reasons. Because aldosterone secretion is maintained, hyperkalemia is not a feature of secondary adrenal insufficiency. It is important to consider this entity in patients treated with corticosteroids during the previous year, since they may require supplemental glucocorticoids during stress.

New-onset adrenal insufficiency is more commonly diagnosed during the puerperium than during pregnancy. This is so, in part, because many symptoms of pregnancy (nausea, fatigue, anorexia, and hyperpigmentation) can occur in adrenal insufficiency.[2] Hyperpigmentation secondary to primary adrenal insufficiency can be differentiated from the chloasma of pregnancy by (1) bluish black discolorations on the lips, gums, and mucous membranes of the mouth, rectum, and vagina; (2) a diffuse tan; (3) hyperpigmentation of the exposed surfaces of the body, pressure points, scars, and lines on the palms of the hands; (4) multiple freckles; and (5) areas of vitiligo or leukoderma.[51] The diagnosis may not be suspected until adrenal crisis develops.

Patients with undiagnosed adrenal insufficiency can tolerate pregnancy, but they may decompensate with stress such as infection, trauma, surgery, labor, or dehydration due to vomiting and diarrhea. The clinical features of acute primary adrenocortical insufficiency include hypotension and shock, weakness, nausea, vomiting, anorexia, abdominal or flank pain, and hyperthermia. Electrolyte abnormalities include hyponatremia, hyperkalemia, mild azotemia, and metabolic acidosis. Hypoglycemia occurs rarely.[8] Secondary adrenal insufficiency should be considered in patients recently treated with glucocorticoids.

The diagnosis of adrenal insufficiency rests on the cortisol response to ACTH stimulation. The plasma cortisol concentration should be greater than 20 μg/dL 45 minutes after the intravenous administration of 250 μg of α^{1-24}-ACTH (cosyntropin). A plasma ACTH level usually will differentiate primary from secondary adrenal insufficiency. In Addison's disease the ACTH level is elevated; in secondary adrenal insufficiency it is normal or low.[10]

The treatment for acute adrenal insufficiency is hydrocortisone, 50 to 100 mg intravenously every 6 hours for 24 hours. This dose can be reduced by half when the patient shows improvement and can be changed to an oral maintenance dose in 4 to 5 days. Patients on chronic corticosteroid therapy should be given increased doses for infections and surgery, and during the stress of labor and delivery. In patients with primary adrenocortical insufficiency, 0.1 mg of fluorocortisol for mineralocorticoid replacement can be used for postural symptoms or hyperkalemia.[8,80] The cortisol production rate in mid-pregnancy to late pregnancy is not significantly greater than normal.[1,18,80] Thus replacement doses are similar to doses in nonpregnant patients, hydrocortisone 20 to 25 mg/d for most subjects.[80]

CONGENITAL ADRENAL HYPERPLASIA

There are five enzymatic steps between cholesterol and cortisol that, when attenuated, lead to specific syndromes of congenital adrenal hyperplasia (CAH). All are transmitted as autosomal recessive traits. The affected enzymes, in order from cholesterol to cortisol, are 20, 22-desmolase, 17-hydroxylase, 3β-hydroxysteroid dehydrogenase (3β-HSD), 21-hydroxylase, and 11-hydroxylase (Fig. 13-7). The most common abnormality is 21-hydroxylase deficiency. It accounts for about 85% of cases of CAH. 11-Hydroxylase deficiency and 3β-HSD deficiency account for most of the remainder.[85] A convenient way to categorize these disorders is to separate them into virilizing and feminizing forms. 21-Hydroxylase deficiency and 11-hydroxylase deficiency are virilizing forms; 20, 22-desmolase deficiency and 17-hydroxylase deficiency are feminizing forms. 3β-HSD deficiency is virilizing in females and feminizing in males. All forms of CAH can affect reproductive competency adversely by altering sex steroid synthesis and secretion.

The most common form of CAH is the 21-hydroxylase–deficient form of the disease. There are two 21-hydroxylase genes, designated A and B, located in the major histocompatibility (human leukocyte antigen [HLA]) region of the short arm of chromosome 6.[17,87] The B gene codes for the functioning 21-hydroxylase enzyme; the A gene contains a deletion of eight of the nine bases composing codons 110 to 112 and is considered to be a pseudogene for the 21-hydroxylase enzyme.[40,85] The B gene is in linkage disequilibrium with the *HLA-B* haplotype.[29,50]

21-Hydroxylase deficiency occurs in two major clinical forms, classic and attenuated. The classic form of 21-

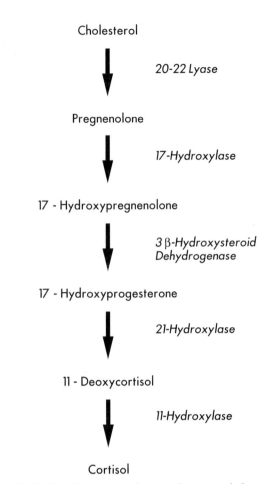

Fig. 13-7. The five enzymatic steps between cholesterol and cortisol that, when attenuated, lead to specific syndromes of congenital adrenal hyperplasia.

hydroxylase deficiency usually becomes manifest in neonatal life or in childhood. It has two clinical presentations roughly equally divided in prevalence: the simple virilizing form and the salt-wasting form.[13,86] The simple virilizing form of the disease is the most common cause of heterosexual precocious puberty in girls and the most common cause of isosexual precocity in boys. It frequently becomes manifest after the neonatal period. The salt-wasting form of the disorder occurs when the synthesis and secretion of both cortisol and aldosterone are impaired. This disorder in children is almost always discovered in the neonatal period because of failure to thrive. Female infants with both forms of the disease can have ambiguous genitalia. Several different mutations of the B gene have been associated with the classic form of 21-hydroxylase deficiency. These include gene deletions, gene conversion events, and point mutations.[4,41,57,86] The attenuated form of the disorder is usually detected in the peripubertal period. The usual manifestations are those of idiopathic hirsutism and the polycystic ovary syndrome. Hirsutism, oligomenorrhea, and infertility dominate the clinical picture. There is only one clinical form of this disorder, although there is great variability in severity. "Salt loss" is not a feature, but mild impairment of mineralocorticoid secretion can be demonstrated in most cases.[21] The disorder is frequently associated with the *HLA-B14* and the *HLA-DR1* haplotypes. In these cases, there is a single base change in the B gene.[78]

For practical purposes, the attenuated form of the disease is an important consideration in the list of adrenal disorders leading to infertility. The incidence of this abnormality varies widely, depending on the specific population under study. For example, it occurs in 1 in 27 Ashkenazi Jews, 1 in 53 Hispanics, 1 in 63 Yugoslavs, and 1 in 333 Italians.[28,76,77] Other studies show carrier rates ranging between 1% and 6%.[20,21,48]

The clinical complex associated with this biochemical lesion was first clearly described in 1980.[60] The disorder can vary in severity from hirsutism, oligomenorrhea, and infertility at one extreme[21] to phenotypically normal women at the other. These women would not be known to have the disorder except for the presence of the characteristic biochemical abnormality—an elevated plasma 17-hydroxyprogesterone concentration.[49] The disorder should be considered in all cases of hirsutism, oligomenorrhea, or unexplained infertility. A good guide to its presence is the plasma testosterone level. Infertility and hirsutism associated with plasma testosterone concentrations in the normal range are rarely caused by attenuated CAH. At the other extreme, virilization and plasma testosterone levels above 200 ng/dL are rarely associated with the attenuated forms of CAH. Measurement of 17-hydroxyprogesterone 45 minutes after the administration of 250 µg of synthetic β^{1-24}-ACTH is the appropriate test. Normal 17-hydroxyprogesterone levels will not exceed 350 ng/dL after an ACTH challenge. The 17-hydroxyprogesterone values are virtually always in excess of 1000 ng/dL in patients with attenuated CAH.

Treating the attenuated form of CAH is not difficult. The basic lesion is one of inefficient production of cortisol due to an altered 21-hydroxylase enzyme. To compensate for this inefficiency, the precursor pool of 17-hydroxyprogesterone is increased, maintaining a normal synthesis rate of cortisol at the expense of an increased rate of testosterone synthesis. The process can be reversed by supplying cortisol from an exogenous source. As in adrenal insufficiency, 20 to 25 mg of hydrocortisone by mouth, once daily, effectively reduces the increased testosterone production rate. In most instances, hirsutism improves and cyclic menses return.

REFERENCES

1. Adrogue HJ, Barrero J, Eknoyan G: Salutary effects of modest fluid replacement in the treatment of adults with diabetic ketoacidosis, *JAMA* 262:2108, 1989.
2. Albert E et al: Addison's disease and pregnancy, *Acta Obstet Gynecol Scand* 68:185, 1989.
3. Amado JA et al: Successful treatment with ketoconazole of Cushing's syndrome in pregnancy, *Postgrad Med J* 66:221, 1990.
4. Amor M et al: Mutation in the CYP21B gene causes steroid 21-hydroxylase deficiency, *Proc Natl Acad Sci U S A* 85:1600, 1988.
5. Aron DC, Schnall AM, Sheeler LR: Cushing's syndrome and pregnancy, *Am J Obstet Gynecol* 162:244, 1990.
6. Aron DC, Schnall AM, Sheeler LR: Spontaneous resolution of Cushing's syndrome after pregnancy, *Am J Obstet Gynecol* 162:472, 1990.
7. Avgerinos et al: The CRH test in the postoperative evaluation of patients with Cushing's syndrome, *J Clin Endocrinol Metab* 65:906, 1987.
8. Baxter JD, Tyrell JB: The adrenal cortex. In Felig P et al, editors: *Endocrinology and metabolism,* ed 2, New York, 1987, McGraw-Hill.
9. Beisel W: Adrenocortical responses during tularemia in human subjects, *J Clin Endocrinol Metab* 27:61, 1967.
10. Besser GM et al: Immunoreactive corticotropin levels in adrenocortical insufficiency, *Br Med J* 000:374, 1971.
11. Bevan JS et al: Cushing's syndrome in pregnancy: the timing of definitive treatment, *Clin Endocrinol* 27:225, 1987.
12. Bongiovanni AM, McFadden AJ: Steroids during pregnancy and possible fetal consequences, *Fertil Steril* 11:181, 1960.
13. Bongiovanni AM, Root AW: The adrenogenital syndrome, *N Engl J Med* 268:1283, 1963.
14. Boyar R: Cortisol secretion and metabolism in anorexia nervosa, *N Engl J Med* 296:190, 1977.
15. Buescher MA, McClamrock HD, Adashi EY: Cushing syndrome in pregnancy, *Obstet Gynecol* 79:130, 1992.
16. Carr BR et al: Maternal plasma adrenocorticotropin and cortisol relationships throughout human pregnancy, *Am J Obstet Gynecol* 139:416, 1981.
17. Carrol MC, Campbell RD, Porter RR: Mapping the steroid 21-hydroxylase genes adjacent to complement component C4 genes in HLA, the major histocompatibility locus in man, *Proc Natl Acad Sci USA* 82:521, 1985.
18. Charrier MJ: Syndrome de Cushing et grossesse: eniant vivant, *Soc Natl Gynecol Obstet Fr* 00:460, 1965.
19. Cheesman et al: Suppression of the preovulatory surge of luteinizing hormone and subsequent ovulation in the rat by arginine vasotocin, *Endocrinology* 101:1194, 1977.
20. Chetkowski RJ, DeFazio J, Shamonki I: The incidence of late onset congenital adrenal hyperplasia due to 21-hydroxylase deficiency among hirsute women, *J Clin Endocrinol Metab* 58:595, 1984.
21. Chrousos GP, Loriaux DL, Mann DL: Late-onset 21-hydroxylase deficiency mimicking polycystic ovarian disease, *Ann Intern Med* 96:143, 1982.
22. Cook, DJ, Riddell RH, Booth JD: Cushing's syndrome in pregnancy, *Can Med Assoc J* 141:1059, 1989.
23. Cousins L et al: Qualitative and quantitative assessment of the circadian rhythm of cortisol in pregnancy, *Am J Obstet Gynecol* 145:411, 1983.
24. Cushing H: The basophil adenomas of the pituitary body and their clinical manifestations, *Bull Johns Hopkins Hosp* 50:137, 1932.
25. Dörr HG et al: Longitudinal study of progestins, mineralocorticoids, and glucocorticoids throughout human pregnancy, *J Clin Endocrinol Metab* 68:863, 1989.
26. Drew F, Stifel E: Secondary amenorrhea among young women entering religious life, *Obstet Gynecol* 32:47, 1968.
27. Dubey A, Plant A: A suppression of gonadotropin secretion by cortisol in castrated male rhesus monkeys, *Biol Reprod* 33:423, 1985.
28. Dumic M, Brkljacic L, Speiser PW: An update on the frequency of non-classic deficiency of 21-hydroxylase in the Yugoslav population, *Acta Endocrinol* 122:703, 1990.
29. DuPont B, Oberfield SE, Smithwick EM: Close genetic linkage between HLA and congenital adrenal hyperplasia, *Lancet* 2:1309, 1977.
30. Evans JJ et al: Estrogen-induced transcortin increase and progesterone

and cortisol interactions: implications from pregnancy studies, *Ann Clin Lab Sci* 17:101, 1987.

31. Feicht CB: Secondary amenorrhea in athletes, *Lancet* 2:1145, 1978.

32. Ferin M: A role for endogenous opioid peptides in the regulation of gonadotropin secretion in the primate, *Horm Res* 28:119, 1987.

33. Flack MR et al: Urine free cortisol in the high-dose dexamethasone suppression test for the differential diagnosis of the Cushing syndrome, *Ann Intern Med* 116:211, 1992.

34. Freis H: Body image perception. In Vigersky R, editor: *Anorexia nervosa,* New York, 1989, Raven Press.

35. Gindoff PR, Ferin M: Endogenous opioid peptides modulate the effect of CRH on gonadotropin release in the primate, *Endocrinology* 121:837, 1987.

36. Glass AR, Deuster PA: Amenorrhea in Olympic athletes, *Fertil Steril* 48:740, 1987.

37. Gormley MJJ et al: Cushing's syndrome in pregnancy: treatment with metyrapone, *Clin Endocrinol* 16:283, 1982.

38. Grodin J, Loriaux L: Functional studies of ovarian responsiveness to human menopausal gonadotropins. In Amsterdam, 1972, Excerpta Medica.

39. Harris B et al: The hormonal environment of post-natal depression, *Br J Psychiatry* 154:660, 1989.

40. Higashi Y et al: Complete nucleotide sequence of two steroid 21-hydroxylase genes tandemly arranged in human chromosome: a pseudo-gene and a true gene, *Proc Natl Acad Sci U S A* 83:2841, 1986.

41. Higashi Y et al: Aberrant splicing and missense mutations cause steroid 21-hydroxylase deficiency in humans: possible gene conversion products, *Proc Natl Acad Sci U S A* 85:7486, 1988.

42. Hilden J, Ronnike F: On birth weight and gestation period in infants born to mothers with Addison's disease, *Dan Med Bull* 18:62, 1971.

43. Irvine WJ, Barnes EW: Adrenocortical insufficiency, *J Clin Endocrinol Metab* 00:549, 1972.

44. Jones SA, Challis JR: Steroid, corticotropin-releasing hormone, ACTH and prostaglandin interactions in the amnion and placenta of early pregnancy in man, *J Endocrinol* 125:153, 1990.

45. Kaye TB, Crapo L: The Cushing syndrome: an update on diagnostic tests, *Ann Intern Med* 112:434, 1990.

46. Koerten JM et al: Cushing's syndrome in pregnancy: a case report and literature review, *Am J Obstet Gynecol* 154:626, 1986.

47. Kreines K, DeVaux WD: Neonatal adrenal insufficiency associated with maternal Cushing's syndrome, *Pediatrics* 47:516, 1971.

48. Kuttenn F, Couillin P, Girard F: Late-onset adrenal hyperplasia in hirsutism, *N Engl J Med* 313:222, 1985.

49. Levine LS, DuPont B, Lorenzen F: Genetic and hormonal characterization of the cryptic form of 21-hydroxylase deficiency, *J Clin Endocrinol Metab* 53:1193, 1981.

50. Levine LS, Zachman M, New MI: Genetic mapping of the 21-hydroxylase deficiency gene within the HLA linkage group, *N Engl J Med* 299:911, 1978.

51. Levine SN, Loewenstein JE: Treatment of diabetic ketoacidosis, *Arch Intern Med* 141:713, 1981.

52. Lindholm J, Shultz-Moller N: Plasma and urinary cortisol in pregnancy and during estrogen-gestagen treatment, *Scand J Clin Lab Invest* 31:119, 1973.

53. Loriaux DL: Adrenocortical insufficiency. In Becker KL, editor: *Principles and practice of endocrinology and metabolism,* Philadelphia, 1990, JB Lippincott.

54. Loriaux DL: Cushing's syndrome. In Becker KL et al, editors: *Principles and practice of endocrinology and metabolism,* New York, 1990, JB Lippincott.

55. Luger A, Deuster P: Acute hypothalamic-pituitary-adrenal responses to the stress of treadmill exercise, *N Engl J Med* 316:1309, 1987.

56. MacAdams M et al: Reduction of serum testosterone levels during chronic glucocorticoid therapy, *Ann Intern Med* 104:648, 1986.

57. Matteson KJ, Phillips JA, Miller WL: P450XXI gene deletions are not found in family studies of congenital adrenal hyperplasia, *Proc Natl Acad Sci U S A* 84:5858, 1987.

58. Migeon CJ: Adrenal cortex. In Rudolph AM, Hoffman JIE, editors: *Pediatrics,* ed 18, Norwalk, Conn, 1987, Appleton & Lange.

59. Migeon CJ, Bertrand J, Wall PE: Physiological disposition of 4-C14-cortisol during late pregnancy, *J Clin Invest* 36:1350, 1957.

60. Migeon C, Rosenwaks Z, Lee PA: The attenuated form of congenital adrenal hyperplasia as an allelic form of 21-hydroxylase deficiency, *J Clin Endocrinol Metab* 51:647, 1980.

61. Miller DL, Doppman JL: Diagnostic imaging of the adrenal gland. In Becker KL, editors: *Principles and practice of endocrinology and metabolism,* New York, 1990, JB Lippincott.

62. Nolten WE, Rueckert PA: Elevated free cortisol index in pregnancy: possible regulatory mechanisms, *Am J Obstet Gynecol* 139:492, 1981.

63. Nolten WE et al: Diurnal patterns and regulation of cortisol secretion in pregnancy, *J Clin Endocrinol Metab* 51:466, 1980.

64. Oldfield EH et al: Petrosal sinus sampling with and without corticotropin-releasing hormone for the differential diagnosis of Cushing's syndrome, *N Engl J Med* 325:897, 1991.

65. Olster DH, Ferin M: CRH inhibits gonadotropin secretion in the ovariectomized rhesus monkey, *J Clin Endocrinol Metab* 65:262, 1987.

66. Pickard J et al: Cushing's syndrome in pregnancy, *Obstet Gynecol Surv* 45:87, 1990.

67. Pricolo VE et al: Management of Cushing's syndrome secondary to adrenal adenoma during pregnancy, *Surgery* 108:1072, 1990.

68. Prihoda JS, Davis LE: Metabolic emergencies in obstetrics, *Obstet Gynecol Clin North Am* 18:301, 1991.

69. Radowick S: Structural studies on the human GnRH gene. Paper presented at the Endocrine Society annual meeting, 1988 (abstract 192).

70. Rees LH et al: Possible placental origin of ACTH in normal human pregnancy, *Nature* 254:620, 1975.

71. Ross EJ, Linch DC: Cushing's syndrome—killing disease: discriminatory value of signs and symptoms aiding early diagnosis, *Lancet* 2:646, 1982.

72. Ross EJ, Marshall-Jones P, Friedman M: Cushing's syndrome: diagnostic criteria, *Q J Med* 138:149, 1966.

73. Sachar EJ et al: Cortisol production in depressive illness, *Arch Gen Psychiatry* 23:289, 1970.

74. Sapolsky R: Stress induced suppression of testicular function in the wild baboon: role of glucocorticoid, *Endocrinology* 116:2273, 1985.

75. Sher N: Causes of delayed menstruation and treatment: an investigation in women's auxiliary service, *Br Med J* 1:347, 1946.

76. Sherman SL, Aston CE, Morton NE: A segregation and linkage study of classical and non-classical 21-hydroxylase deficiency, *Am J Hum Genet* 42:830, 1988.

77. Speiser P, DuPont B, Rubenstein P: High frequency of non-classical steroid 21-hydroxylase deficiency, *Am J Hum Genet* 37:650, 1995.

78. Speiser PW, New MI, White PC: Molecular genetic analysis of non-classic steroid 21-hydroxylase deficiency associated with HLA-B14, DR1, *N Engl J Med* 319:19, 1988.

79. Udelsman R et al: Adaptation during surgical stress, *J Clin Invest* 77:1377, 1986.

80. Vagnucci A, Lee P: Diseases of the adrenal cortex in pregnancy. In Brody SA, Ueland K, Kase N, editors: *Endocrine disorders in pregnancy,* Norwalk, Conn, 1989, Appleton & Lange.

81. van der Spuy ZM, Jacobs HS: Management of endocrine disorders in pregnancy, part II: pituitary, ovarian and adrenal disease, *Postgrad Med J* 60:312, 1984.

82. Verdugo C et al: Sindrome de Cushing y embarazo con remision espontanea despues del parto, *Rev Med Chil* 110:584, 1982.

83. von Steive H: Nervos bedingte veranderungen an den geschlechtsorganen, *Dtsch Med Wochenschr* 66:925, 1992.

84. Warren MP: The effect of exercise on pubertal progression and reproductive function in girls, *J Clin Endocrinol Metab* 51:1150, 1980.

85. White PC, New MI, DuPont B: Structure of the 21-hydroxylase genes, *Proc Natl Acad Sci U S A* 83:5111, 1986.

86. White PC, New MI, DuPont B: Congenital adrenal hyperplasia, *N Engl J Med* 316:1580, 1987.

87. White PC et al: Two genes encoding steroid 21-hydroxylase are located near the genes encoding the fourth component of complement in man, *Proc Natl Acad Sci U S A* 82:1089, 1985.

Part **III**

CONTRACEPTION

Chapter 14

OVERVIEW OF CONTRACEPTION

Daniel R. Mishell, Jr., MD

An ideal method of contraception for all individuals is not now available and most probably will never be developed. However, a variety of very effective methods of contraception currently are available, each with certain advantages and disadvantages. This chapter presents an overview of the use and effectiveness of those methods, along with a description and advantages and disadvantages of each.

CONTRACEPTIVE USE IN THE UNITED STATES

Data from the 1988 National Survey of Family Growth[32] revealed that about one third of the 57.9 million women of reproductive age (15 to 44), or 19.2 million women, were not exposed to unwanted pregnancy because they were not having sexual intercourse; had had a hysterectomy for reasons other than sterility (noncontraceptively sterile); or were infertile, pregnant, or attempting to conceive. Of the remaining 38.7 million women who were exposed to the risk of pregnancy, all but 3.8 million (9.7%) used a method of contraception. Failure to use a contraceptive method was about twice as frequent in unmarried exposed women as in those who were married.

The remaining 35 million women, about 60% of women of reproductive age, were using a method of contraception in 1988. Sterilization was the most common method of preventing conception used by these women. A total of 13.7 million women (35% of those exposed to unwanted pregnancy) used sterilization of one member of the couple, 9.6 million women (17%) and 4.1 million men (7%), to prevent pregnancy. Use of sterilization among married women in the United States has increased dramatically in the past 25 years. In 1973 about one fourth of married women of reproductive age who practiced contraception used sterilization as their method of preventing pregnancy. By 1988 more than half of married women of reproductive age exposed to the risk of unwanted pregnancy were using sterilization.

Of the nonsurgical, reversible methods of contraception, oral contraceptives (OCs) were most popular, being used by 10.7 million women, 18.5% of all women in this age group. OCs were followed in frequency of use by condom, periodic abstinence, withdrawal, diaphragm, intrauterine device (IUD), and spermicides alone (Table 14-1). Overall, about one fourth of women of reproductive age exposed to unwanted pregnancy (27%) used OCs, about half of the exposed unmarried women and one fifth of exposed married women. More women using reversible contraceptive methods used OCs (50.4%) than all the other methods combined.

OCs were first marketed in the United States in 1960 and their use increased steadily until 1973. Pharmacy purchases of OCs began declining in the United States in 1975. Among married U.S. women practicing contraception, OC use peaked at 36% in 1977 but declined to 23% by 1982. However, after 1982 there was a reversal of the trend: by 1988, 27% of all women exposed to unwanted pregnancy used OCs. Condom use increased in the 6-year period between 1982 and 1988, mainly due to increased usage by unmarried women. During this time use of the IUD de-

Table 14-1. Contraceptive use of 57.9 million U.S. women 15 to 44 years old (1988 National Survey of Family Growth)

Exposure and contraceptive method	Number (millions)	% Exposed women	% All women aged 15-44
Exposed users	34.7	90.0	60.3
Sterilization	13.7	35.5	23.6
Female	9.6	24.9	16.6
Male	4.1	10.6	7.0
Oral contraceptive	10.7	27.7	18.5
Condom	5.1	13.2	8.8
Spermicide	0.3	0.7	0.6
Withdrawal	0.8	2.1	1.3
Diaphragm	2.0	5.2	3.5
Periodic abstinence	0.8	2.1	1.4
IUD	0.7	1.8	1.2
Douche	0.05	0.1	0.1
Exposed nonusers	3.8	9.8	6.5
Not exposed	19.2	49.6	33.2
TOTAL	57.9		

From Mosher WD, Pratt WF: *Contraceptive use in the United States, 1973-88,* vol 182, Washington, DC, 1990, National Center for Health Statistics.

Table 14-2. First-year contraceptive failure rates (%)

Method	Lowest (method)	Typical (use)
Combined oral contraceptive	0.1	3
IUD (Copper T 380A)	0.8	3
Norplant	0.04	0.04
Condom	2	12
Diaphragm	6	18
Sponge	6	18
Spermicides	3	21
Cap	6	18
Periodic abstinence (symptothermal)	2	20

Modified from Trussell J et al: *Stud Fam Plann* 21:51, 1990.

creased by about two thirds, diaphragm use declined among unmarried women but not among married women, and use of the other techniques remained relatively stable.

CONTRACEPTIVE EFFECTIVENESS

It is difficult to determine the actual effectiveness of various methods of contraception because of a large number of factors that affect contraceptive failure. The terms *method effectiveness* and *use effectiveness* (or *method failure* and *patient failure*) have been used to differentiate whether conception occurred while the contraceptive method was being used correctly or incorrectly. In general, methods used at the time of coitus—such as diaphragm, condom, spermicides, and withdrawal—have a much greater method effectiveness than use effectiveness. With use of the methods in which coitus-related activities are not needed, such as OCs and IUDs, there is less difference between method effectiveness and use effectiveness, and thus their overall effectiveness is greater than that of coitus-related methods.

The overall value of a contraceptive method as used by a couple (correctly or incorrectly) is determined by calculation of actual effectiveness as well as the continuation rate. To determine these rates, actuarial methods such as the log-rank life table method should be used instead of the less accurate Pearl index.

Even with the use of these excellent statistical techniques, it is difficult to determine the effectiveness of the various methods in actual practice. Most studies undertaken

to determine effectiveness of a contraceptive method are performed under carefully controlled clinical trials, during which frequent contact with supportive clinical personnel results in lower failure rates and higher continuation rates than occur in normal use. Furthermore, these clinical trials are infrequently performed in a comparative randomized manner, so clinicians cannot compare results of a trial of one type of contraceptive method with the results of a trial of another type.

Several other factors influence contraceptive failure rates. One of the most important is motivation of the couple. Contraceptive failure is more likely to occur in couples seeking to delay a wanted birth than in couples seeking to prevent any more births, especially for coitus-related methods. The woman's age has a strong negative correlation with the failure of a contraceptive method, as does the socioeconomic class and level of education. Thus one must consider many variables when evaluating the effectiveness of any method of contraception for an individual patient. In addition, failure rates of prospective studies are consistently lower than those of retrospective interview studies. Finally, for all methods failure rates are greater during the first year of use than in subsequent years; yet most studies report failure rates for only first-year use. Thus, many variables must be considered when evaluating the effectiveness of any method of contraception for an individual woman.

In 1987 Trussell and Kost[47] performed a comprehensive critical review of the existing scientific literature concerning effectiveness of the various contraceptive methods. After analyzing the entire data base they calculated the lowest expected (method) and typical (use) failure rates of the various contraceptive methods or during their first year of use. In 1990 Trussell et al.[48] published a revised estimate of first-year failure rates based on recently reported data. Oral contraceptives, IUDs, and Norplant had the lowest method and use failure rates (Table 14-2).

An analysis of failure rates during several years of use by motivated women was published by Vessey and col-

Table 14-3. Contraceptive failure rates with various methods

Method	Failure rate (per 100 woman-years)
Sterilization	
Male	0.02
Female	0.13
OCs	
<50 μg estrogen	0.27
50 μg estrogen	0.16
>50 μg estrogen	0.32
Progesterone only	1.2
IUD	
Copper T	1.2
Copper 7	1.5
Dalkon Shield	2.4
Loop A	6.8
Loop B	1.8
Loop C	1.4
Loop D	1.3
Saf-T-Coil	1.3
Not known	1.8
Diaphragm	1.9
Condom	3.6
Withdrawal	6.7
Spermicides	11.9
Rhythm	15.5

From Vessey M, Lawless M, Yeates D: *Lancet* 1:841, 1982.

leagues.[50] They reported failure rates of various contraceptive methods among the more than 17,000 women who were enrolled in the Oxford/Family Planning Association Contraceptive Study. This study enrolled only married women, 25 to 39 years of age, who had been using the diaphragm, IUD, or OCs for at least 5 months before enrollment. Most of the women were well educated and of higher socioeconomic status. This select population comprised women who were motivated to attend family planning clinics and who had been under observation for an average of 9.5 years. Failure rates per 100 woman-years were very low for several contraceptive methods. They were approximately 0.3 for OCs, 1.3 for IUDs, 1.9 for diaphragms, 3.6 for condoms, 11.9 for spermicides, and 15.5 for the rhythm method (Table 14-3). Failure rates declined with increasing age and increasing duration of use, especially for barrier methods and IUDs. However, with the exception of the diaphragm, there was no substantial difference in failure rates among women wishing to delay or prevent a pregnancy.

Further data from national surveys[49] indicate that 1-year continuation rates for the various contraceptive methods are highest for use of IUDs, which necessitates a visit to a health care facility to discontinue use, and lowest for diaphragms, condoms, and spermicides.

CONTRACEPTIVE METHODS
Nonhormonal contraception
Barrier methods
Spermicides: intravaginal sponge, foams, creams, and suppositories. Spermicides contain a surfactant, usually nonoxynol-9, which immobilizes or kills sperm on contact. The vehicle of delivery also provides a mechanical barrier and usually needs to be placed in the vagina before each coital act. The effectiveness of these agents, with the exception of the sponge, increases with increasing age of the woman and is similar to that of the diaphragm in all age and income groups.

The most popular spermicidal vehicle is the contraceptive sponge, which is a cylindric piece of soft polyurethane impregnated with 1 mg of nonoxynol-9. In contrast to other spermicidal methods, the sponge does not have to be inserted into the vagina before each act of intercourse and is effective for 24 hours. In large clinical trials, the 1-year failure rate for the sponge was slightly but significantly higher than that for the diaphragm, about 15%. A study by McIntyre and Higgins[28] indicated that the increased risk of pregnancy occurred only in women who has already had a child. In nulliparous women, the first-year failure rate was similar to that for the diaphragm, about 13%; in parous women with children the first-year failure rate with the sponge was 28%, more than twice as high as the rate for diaphragm users. The latest study by the original investigators, Edelman and North,[14] using the same data base, however, failed to confirm the differences in failure rates according to parity and has created some controversy.

The incidence of toxic shock syndrome appears to be slightly increased in users of the sponge, especially if it is used during the menses or the puerperium, or if it is left in place for more than 24 hours. Each of these risk factors contraindicates use of the sponge. The overall incidence of toxic shock syndrome in users of the sponge is low, estimated at 1 per 2 million sponges.

Although a few early studies linked the use of a spermicide at the time of conception with an increased risk of some congenital malformations, these studies were probably flawed by recall bias. Several well-performed studies by Linn et al.,[24] Louik et al.,[26] and Bracken and Vita[6] have shown no increased risk of congenital malformations in the newborns or karyotypic abnormalities in the spontaneous abortuses of women who conceived while using spermicides.

Diaphragm. A diaphragm must be carefully fitted by the physician or nursing personnel. The largest size that does not cause discomfort or undue pressure on the vaginal mucosa should be used. After the fitting, the patient should remove the diaphragm and reinsert it herself. She should then be examined to make sure the diaphragm is covering the cervix. The diaphragm should be used with contraceptive cream or jelly and be left in place for at least 8 hours after coitus. If repeated intercourse takes place or coitus occurs more than 8 hours after insertion of the diaphragm, additional contraceptive cream or jelly should be used. Although advisable, it may not be necessary to use a spermicide with the diaphragm, since it has not been conclusively demonstrated that pregnancy rates are lower when a spermicide is used with a diaphragm than when the diaphragm is used alone. The number of urinary tract infections in women who use diaphragms is significantly higher than that in nonusers, probably because of the mechanical obstruction of the outflow of urine by the diaphragm.

Diaphragm users should also be cautioned not to leave the device in place for more than 24 hours, because ulceration of the vaginal epithelium may occur with prolonged usage.

Data from the Oxford Family Planning Association Contraceptive Study[50] indicate that the diaphragm is an effective method of contraception in married motivated women and that failure rates decline with increasing age and increasing duration of use. In this cohort study of married women who had been using a diaphragm for more than 5 months before enrollment, the pregnancy rates were 4.1/100 woman-years for women 25 to 29 years of age and 1.1 for women 35 to 39 years of age. In a recent cohort study by Kovacs et al.[21] of both married and unmarried women in which most of the diaphragm users were young, however, the pregnancy rate at 1 year was 21% and it rose to 37% at 2 years, mainly because the women did not use the method consistently.

Cervical cap. The cervical cap, a cup-shaped plastic or rubber device that fits around the cervix, has been used as a barrier contraceptive for decades, mainly in Britain and other parts of Europe.

There has been a recent resurgence of interest in the use of this older method, since the cervical cap can be left in place longer than the diaphragm and is more comfortable. Each type of device is manufactured in different sizes and should be fitted to the cervix by a clinician. The cervical cap should not be left in place for more than 72 hours because of the possibility of ulceration, unpleasant odor, and infection.

The Prentif cavity-rim cervical cap was approved in 1988 for general use in the United States. Product labeling stipulates that the cap should be left on the cervix for no more than 48 hours and that a spermicide should always be placed inside the cap before use. The cap is manufactured in four sizes and requires more training, both for the provider in fitting it and for the user in placing it correctly, than does the diaphragm. Failure rates are similar to those observed with the diaphragm. In a large randomized clinical trial of the cap and diaphragm, 1-year pregnancy rates were 17.4% for the cap and 16.7% for the diaphragm. Of the pregnancies with the cap, one third were method failure and two thirds were user-related failures. In other studies,

pregnancy rates at 1 and 2 years with the use of the cervical cap ranged from 8% to 17% and 14% to 38%, respectively, with good continuation rates. Because of concern about a possible adverse effect of the cap on cervical tissue, the cervical cap should be used only by women with a normal cervical cytologic examination, and it is recommended that users have another cervical cytology examination 3 months after starting to use this method.

Condom. Use of the condom by individuals with multiple sexual partners should be encouraged. It is the contraceptive method most effective in preventing transmission of sexually transmitted diseases. The condom should not be applied tightly. The tip should extend beyond the end of the penis by about $\frac{1}{2}$ inch to collect the ejaculate. In the Oxford Study,[10] which is one of the largest for which findings of condom use have been published, all condom users had previously used another method, mainly OCs. During 12,497 woman-years of exposure, 449 unplanned pregnancies occurred, for a use-pregnancy rate of 3.6/100 woman-years. The pregnancy rate increased linearly over time, from 0.7/100 woman-years at 3 months to 8.4/100 woman-years at 24 months. Accidental pregnancy rates were slightly lower among women over age 35 years and among women who had completed their families, even when these factors were standardized for other characteristics. The results of this study are consistent with those of several older studies, which show a similar high level of effectiveness for the condom when used by strongly motivated couples.

Barrier techniques are effective methods of contraception in women aged 30 years or older. In the analysis by Trussell and Kost,[47] the first-year failure rates for condom use among women wishing no more pregnancy ranged between 3% and 6% when the woman was over age 30, but between 8% and 10% when the woman was under age 25.

Barrier techniques and sexually transmitted diseases. Barrier methods have the advantage of reducing the rate of transmission of sexually transmitted diseases. Several epidemiologic studies have shown that spermicides reduce the frequency of clinical infection with sexually transmitted diseases, both bacterial and viral. In vitro studies by Conant et al.[10] have demonstrated that condoms prevent the transmission of viruses, specifically herpesvirus and human immunodeficiency virus, as well as *Chlamydia trachomatis* bacteria, which is a frequent cause of salpingitis. Several epidemiologic studies, both case-control and cohort, indicate that the use of the condom or diaphragm protects both men and women from clinically apparent gonorrheal infection. An epidemiologic study by Cramer et al.[11] of women with infertility due to tubal obstruction found that the past use of barrier techniques protected women against tubal damage. The greatest protection occurred with the use of diaphragms or condoms with spermicides. The incidence of cervical neoplasia was also markedly diminished among women in couples using condoms or diaphragms, probably because of the decreased transmission of human papillomavirus. This antiviral action may be the reason why women who use spermicides are only one third as likely to have cervical cancer as members of a control group. Certain strains of this virus have been causally linked to the later development of cervical neoplasia. Unfortunately, the failure rates of users of the diaphragm or condom are highest for persons younger than age 25 years, those most likely to become infected with sexually transmitted diseases. Therefore, to prevent the transmission of these diseases as well as unwanted pregnancy in this age group, the use of a barrier technique together with the most effective reversible method, the OC, is advisable.

Periodic abstinence. The avoidance of sexual intercourse during the days of the menstrual cycle when the ovum can be fertilized is used by many highly motivated couples as a means of preventing pregnancy. Four techniques of periodic abstinence are now being used. The oldest of these is the calendar rhythm method, but in the past two decades, new techniques have been developed whereby women rely on physiologic changes during each cycle to determine the fertile period. The term *natural family planning* has been used instead of *rhythm* to describe these new techniques. They include the temperature method, the cervical mucus method, and the symptothermal method. Each of these techniques requires strong motivation as well as training. In most reports of use of these methods pregnancy rates are relatively high and continuation rates are low.

Calendar rhythm method. With the calendar rhythm method, the period of abstinence is determined solely by calculating the length of the individual woman's previous menstrual cycle. The rationale for the rhythm method is based on three assumptions: (1) the human ovum is capable of being fertilized for only about 24 hours after ovulation; (2) spermatozoa retain their fertilizing ability for only about 48 hours after coitus; and (3) ovulation usually occurs 12 to 16 days (14 ± 2 days) before the onset of the subsequent menses. According to these assumptions, after the woman records the lengths of her cycles for several months, she establishes her fertile period by subtracting 18 days from the length of her previous shortest cycle and 11 days from her previous longest cycle. Then, in each subsequent cycle, the couple abstains from coitus during this calculated fertile period. This method requires abstinence by the majority of women with regular menstrual cycles for nearly half the days of each cycle and cannot be used by women with irregular menstrual cycles. Although the calendar rhythm method is the most widely used technique of periodic abstinence, pregnancy rates are high, ranging from 14.4 to 47/100 woman-years, mainly because most couples fail to abstain for the relatively long periods required. The use of the calendar rhythm method by itself is currently not advocated or taught to couples who are interested in practicing periodic abstinence.

Temperature method. The temperature method relies on measuring basal body temperature daily. The woman is required to abstain from intercourse from the onset of the menses until the third consecutive day of elevated basal temperature. Because abstinence is required for the entire preovulatory period in ovulatory cycles and for the entire cycle in anovulatory cycles, the temperature method alone is no longer commonly used.

Cervical mucus method. The cervical mucus method requires that the woman be taught to recognize and interpret cyclic changes in the presence and consistency of cervical mucus; these changes occur in response to changing estrogen and progesterone levels. Abstinence is required during the menses and every other day after the menses ends, because of the possibility of confusing semen with ovulatory mucus, until the first day that copious, slippery mucus is observed. Abstinence is required every day thereafter until 4 days after the last day on which the characteristic mucus is present, called the "peak mucus day." In two well-designed randomized clinical trials by Medina et al.[29] and Wade et al.,[54] the pregnancy rates for new users of this method in the first year after they completed a 3- to 5-month training period were 20% and 24%, with the discontinuation rates between 72% and 74%. In a five-country study of 725 highly motivated couples, sponsored by the World Health Organization,[58, 59] the use failure rate during the first year after the completion of three cycles of training was 19.6% and the method failure rate was 3.5%. Most of the pregnancies (15.4% of the 19.6%) resulted from conscious deviation from the rules of the method. The mean length of the fertile period in this study was 9.6 days, and abstinence was therefore required for about 17 days in each cycle. In this study the continuation rate after 1 year was high, 64.4%.

Symptothermal method. The symptothermal method, rather than relying on a single physiologic index, uses several indexes to determine the fertile period, most commonly calendar calculations and changes in the cervical mucus to estimate the onset of the fertile period and changes in mucus or basal body temperature to estimate its end. Because several indexes must be monitored, this method is more difficult to learn than are the single-index methods, but it is more effective than the cervical mucus method alone. In the two large, randomized studies by Medina et al.[29] and Wade et al.[54] comparing these methods, the pregnancy rates at the end of 1 year of use, after the training phase, were 10.9% and 19.8% with the symptothermal method, compared with 20% and 24% with the cervical mucus method. In addition, the continuation rate among the women who used the symptothermal method in these studies was higher after 1 year (about 50% in each study) than that among the women who used the cervical mucus method (26% and 40%).

The major reason for the lack of acceptance of natural family planning, as well as the relatively high pregnancy rates among users of these methods, is the need to avoid having sexual intercourse for a large number of days during each menstrual cycle. To overcome this problem, many women use barrier methods or spermicides during the fertile period. In a study by Rogow et al.[38] of women who used the symptothermal method with barrier contraceptives or withdrawal during the fertile period, the failure rate during the first year was 9.9% and the discontinuation rate was 33%.

Since the use of any method of contraception other than abstinence is unacceptable to many couples, simple, self-administered tests to detect hormone changes have been developed to reduce the number of days of abstinence required in each cycle to a maximum of 7. Enzyme immunoassays for urinary estrogen and pregnanediol glucuronide have recently been developed that can easily be used at home at minimal cost and require minimal time to perform. Such tests must be performed by the woman about 12 days each month, but they should reduce the number of days of abstinence required.

Intrauterine devices. The main benefits of IUDs are (1) a high level of effectiveness, (2) a lack of associated systemic metabolic effects, and (3) the need for only a single act of motivation for long-term use. In contrast to other types of contraception, there is no need for frequent motivation to ingest a pill daily or to use a coitus-related method consistently. These characteristics, as well as the necessity for a visit to a health care facility to discontinue the method, account for the fact that IUDs have the highest continuation rate of all currently available reversible methods of contraception. Of course, it is desirable for all women to make at least annual visits to a health care facility, but in some areas of the world this is not possible.

Unlike other contraceptives, such as the barrier methods, which rely on frequent use by the individual for effectiveness and therefore have higher use failure rates than method failure rates, the IUD has similar method effectiveness and use effectiveness rates. First-year failure rates with copper-bearing IUDs have been reported to range from less than 1% to 3.7%. Pregnancy rates are related to the skill of the clinician inserting the device. With experience, correct high-fundal insertion occurs more frequently, and there is a lower incidence of partial or complete expulsion, with resultant lower pregnancy rates. Furthermore, the incidence of accidental pregnancy decreases steadily after the first year of IUD use. The incidence of all major adverse events with IUDs, including pregnancy, expulsion, or removal for bleeding and/or pain, also steadily decreases with increasing age. Thus the IUD is especially suited for older parous women who wish to prevent further pregnancies.

Mechanism of action. The IUD's main mechanism of contraceptive action in women is spermicidal, produced by a local sterile inflammatory reaction caused by the presence of the foreign body in the uterus. Moyer and Mishell[33] found a nearly 1000% increase in the number of leukocytes in washings of the human endometrial cavity 18 weeks after the insertion of an IUD, compared with washings obtained before insertion. Tissue breakdown products of these leukocytes are toxic to all cells, including spermatozoa and the blastocyst. Small IUDs do not produce as great an inflammatory reaction as larger ones do. Therefore, smaller IUDs have higher pregnancy rates than larger devices of the same design. The addition of copper increases the inflammatory reaction. Tredway et al.[46] found that sperm transport from the cervix to the oviduct in the first 24 hours after coitus was markedly impaired in women wearing IUDs. Because of the spermicidal action of IUDs, very few, if any, sperm reach the oviducts, and the ovum usually does not become fertilized.

Further evidence for this spermicidal action of IUDs was reported by Alvarez et al.[1] These investigators performed oviductal flushing in 56 women with IUDs and in 45 women using no method of contraception, who were sterilized by salpingectomy soon after ovulation and also had unprotected sexual intercourse shortly before ovulation. Normally cleaving, fertilized ova were found in the tubal flushings of about half of the women not wearing IUDs, whereas no eggs that had the microscopic appearance of a normally fertilized and developing preimplantation embryo were found in the oviducts of the women wearing IUDs.

After removal of both copper-bearing and non–copper-bearing IUDs, the inflammatory reaction rapidly disappears. Resumption of fertility after IUD removal is not delayed and occurs at the same rate as resumption of fertility after discontinuation of barrier methods of contraception, such as the condom and diaphragm. Vessey et al.[52] reported that at 1 and 2 years pregnancy rates of women who discontinued using IUDs were similar to those of women who discontinued barrier methods. The only exception was for women discontinuing IUDs for medical problems, including infection, who had a slightly lower pregnancy rate at these time intervals (Table 14-4).

Types of devices. In the past 25 years, many types of IUDs have been designed and used clinically. The devices developed and initially used in the 1960s were made of a plastic, polyethylene, impregnated with barium sulfate to make them radiographically visible. In the 1970s smaller plastic devices covered with copper wire, such as the copper T, were developed and widely used. In the 1980s devices bearing a larger amount of copper, including sleeves on the horizontal arm, such as the copper T 380A and the copper T 220C, were developed. These devices had a longer duration of high effectiveness, and thus had to be reinserted at less frequent intervals than the devices bearing a smaller amount of copper. Although many of all the types of IUDs developed are still available for use in Europe, Canada, and elsewhere, at present only the copper T 380A and a progesterone-releasing IUD are currently being marketed in the United States. Although the barium-impregnated plastic loop and the copper-bearing copper 7

Table 14-4. Fertility rates (mean % ± SE) of parous women remaining undelivered of live birth or stillbirth at given intervals after stopping contraception to plan pregnancy

Method of contraception stopped	Mean age (y)	% Women remaining undelivered by months since discontinuation					
		12	18	24	30	36	42
IUD	31.4	48.8 ± 2.4	18.1 ± 1.9	10.6 ± 1.6	9.3 ± 1.5	6.7 ± 1.4	6.3 ± 1.4
Oral contraceptive	30.6	60.7 ± 1.2	20.4 ± 1.0	10.8 ± 0.8	7.6 ± 0.7	5.4 ± 0.6	4.5 ± 0.6
Diaphragm	30.9	36.8 ± 1.5	13.8 ± 1.1	8.2 ± 0.9	6.2 ± 0.9	4.6 ± 0.8	4.2 ± 0.8
Other method	31.8	39.4 ± 1.5	16.2 ± 1.3	10.6 ± 1.1	7.8 ± 1.0	6.2 ± 0.9	5.0 ± 0.9
IUD users in past, stopped for medical reasons	32.7	49.3 ± 4.7	19.1 ± 4.1	13.6 ± 3.8			

From Vessey MP et al: *Br Med J* 286:106, 1983.

and copper T 200B are still approved by the Food and Drug Administration (FDA) for use in the United States, they are no longer being sold. Production and distribution of the shield device with a multifilament tail were discontinued in 1974. Because of the increased risk of infection reported with Dalkon shield IUDs, if any are still in place they should be removed. All IUDs now approved for distribution by the FDA have monofilament tails.

The T- and 7-shaped plastic devices are smaller than most non–copper-bearing types of IUDs. When T-shaped devices without copper underwent clinical trials, they were found to result in a much higher pregnancy rate than that of the larger loops and coils. With the addition of copper wire, the effectiveness of these IUDs was increased by the mechanism described earlier and was comparable to or higher than that of the nonmedicated IUDs.

Because of the constant dissolution of copper, which amounts daily to less than that ingested in the normal diet, all copper IUDs have to be replaced periodically. The copper T 380A is approved for use in the United States for 4 years. However, a large ongoing clinical trial by the World Health Organization[60] indicates that this device retains its contraceptive effectiveness for at least 7 years. At the scheduled time of removal, the device can be removed and another inserted during the same office visit.

Adding a reservoir of progesterone to the vertical arm also increases the effectiveness of the T-shaped devices. The currently marketed progesterone IUD releases 65 mg of progesterone daily. This amount is sufficient to prevent pregnancy by local action within the endometrial cavity, but it is not enough to cause a measurable increase in peripheral serum progesterone levels. The currently approved progesterone-releasing IUD needs to be replaced annually, because the reservoir of progesterone becomes depleted after about 18 months of use.

Unlike the medicated IUDs there is no need to change a nonmedicated plastic IUD unless the patient develops increased bleeding after it has been in place for more than 1 year. Calcium salts are deposited on the plastic over time, and their roughness can cause ulceration and bleeding of the endometrium. If increased bleeding develops after a non–copper-bearing IUD has been in the uterus for a year or more, the old IUD should be removed and a new device inserted.

Time of insertion. Although it is widely believed that the optimal time for insertion of an IUD is during menses, there are data indicating that if a woman is not pregnant, the IUD can be safely inserted on any day of the cycle. White et al.[56] analyzed 2-month event rates of about 10,000 women who had copper T 200s inserted on various days of the cycle. Rates of expulsion were lower when insertion occurred during the week after menses stopped, whereas rates of removal for bleeding and pain as well as pregnancy were higher with insertions after cycle day 18. However, the differences were small and of little clinical relevance.

It has also been recommended that IUDs not be inserted until more than 2 to 3 months have elapsed after completion of a term pregnancy. However, Mishell and Roy[30] analyzed event rates in their clinic among women who had copper T IUDs inserted between 4 and 8 weeks postpartum and more than 8 weeks postpartum. The 1- and 2-year event rates for all causes were similar for the two groups, indicating that copper T IUDs can be safely inserted at the time of the routine postpartum visit. No perforations occurred in this series, in which the withdrawal technique of insertion was used.

Although one report suggested that the perforation rate may be higher if the IUD is inserted when a woman is lactating,[9] this finding has not been confirmed in other studies. The effect of breast-feeding on performance of the copper T 380A IUD was evaluated from data obtained from a large multicenter clinical trial by Chi et al.[9] in which the device was inserted into 559 breast-feeding and 590 non–breast-feeding women, all of whom were at least 6 weeks postpartum. There were significantly fewer problems with pain and bleeding at the time of insertion in the group that was breast-feeding. The expulsion rate, which was low, and the continuation rate, which was high, were lower in the breast-feeding and non–breast-feeding groups 6 months after insertion.

Adverse effects. In general, in the first year of use, most IUDs have about a 2% pregnancy rate, a 10% expulsion rate, and a 15% rate of removal for medical reasons, mainly bleeding and pain. The incidence of each of these events, especially expulsion, diminishes steadily in subsequent years.

The copper T 380A IUD, which has copper on the horizontal arm as well as the vertical arm, has a higher rate of effectiveness. In a multicenter study performed in the United States the net cumulative pregnancy rate with this copper T device at the end of 4 years was reported by Sivin and Tatum[44] to be only 1.9%. In an ongoing World Health Organization study[60] of this device, termination rates for adverse effects continued to decline annually following the first year after insertion for each of the 7 years in which sufficient data have accumulated to date. In that study, the cumulative discontinuation rates for pregnancy, bleeding or pain, and expulsion at the end of 7 years were 1.6, 22.7, and 8.6, respectively (Table 14-5). Thus, the addition of copper on the horizontal arm of the T-shaped device appears to lower the pregnancy rate as well as increase the estimated duration of action to at least 7 years.

Uterine bleeding. The majority of women discontinuing this method of contraception do so for medical reasons. Nearly all the medical reasons accounting for IUD removal involve one or more types of abnormal bleeding: heavy and/or prolonged menses or intermenstrual bleeding. The IUD does not affect the pattern or level of circulating gonadotropins and steroid hormones during the menstrual cycle. The IUD, however, does exert a local effect on the endometrium, causing menses to be about 2 days earlier than normal, when steroid levels are higher than in control cycles. It is possible that this early onset of menses may be produced by a premature and increased rate of local release of prostaglandins, brought about by the presence of the intrauterine foreign body. The stimulation of uterine contractions by excessive levels of prostaglandins may prolong the duration of the menstrual flow, which is significantly longer in women wearing IUDs.

The exact mechanism whereby IUDs cause increased menstrual blood loss is not completely understood, despite extensive investigative efforts. Histologic studies of endometrium obtained by biopsy and hysterectomy have demonstrated two types of lesions in association with IUDs. Vascular erosions have been seen in areas of direct contact with the IUD, and evidence of increased vascular permeability has been found in areas not in direct contact with the IUD. Both types of lesions could cause increased menstrual blood loss as well as intermenstrual bleeding. Increased concentrations of proteolytic enzymes and plasminogenic activators that may lead to increased fibrinolytic activity have been found in the endometrial tissue adjacent to the device. This increase in fibrinolytic activity adversely affects hemostasis and increases menstrual blood loss.

Excessive bleeding in the first few months after IUD

Table 14-5. Cumulative discontinuation rate for copper T 380A IUD

Years since insertion	3	5	7
Event			
Pregnancies	1.0	1.4	1.6
Expulsions	7.0	8.2	8.6
Medical removals	14.6	20.8	25.8
Nonmedical removals	13.8	25.6	34.4
Loss to follow-up	10.2	15.5	22.1
All discontinuations	32.2	46.7	56.3
Woman-months	38,571	56,010	67,885

From World Health Organization (WHO): *Contraception* 42:141, 1990.

insertion should be treated with reassurance and supplemental oral iron. The bleeding may diminish with time, as the uterus adjusts to the presence of the foreign body. Excessive bleeding that continues or develops several months or more after IUD insertion may be treated by systemic administration of one of the prostaglandin synthetase inhibitors.

Mefenamic acid at a dosage of 500 mg three times daily during the days of menstruation has been shown by Anderson et al.[2] to reduce menstrual blood loss significantly in IUD users. If excessive bleeding continues despite this treatment, the device should be removed. After a 1-month interval, another type of device may be inserted if the patient still wishes to use an IUD for contraception. Consideration should be given to using a progesterone-releasing IUD, because this device is associated with less blood loss than are the copper-bearing IUDs.

Uterine perforation. Although uncommon, one of the potentially serious complications associated with use of the IUD is perforation of the uterine fundus. Perforation initially occurs at insertion. It can best be prevented by straightening the uterine axis with a tenaculum and then probing the cavity with a uterine sound before IUD insertion. Sometimes only the distal portion of the IUD penetrates the uterine muscle at insertion. Uterine contractions over the next few months then force the IUD into the peritoneal cavity. IUDs correctly inserted entirely within the endometrial cavity do not wander through the uterine muscle into the peritoneal cavity. The incidence of perforation is generally related to the shape of the device and/or amount of force used during its insertion, as well as the experience of the clinician performing the insertion.

Perforation rates for the copper 7 and the copper T200 were found to be about 1/1000 insertions. The clinician should always suspect perforation if a patient says she cannot feel the appendage but did not notice that the device was expelled. One should not assume that an unnoticed expulsion has occurred when the appendage is not visualized. Sometimes the IUD is still in its correct position in the uterine cavity but the appendage has been withdrawn into the cavity as the position of the IUD within the cavity has changed. In this situation, after pelvic examination has been performed and the possibility of pregnancy excluded, the uterine cavity should be probed.

If the device cannot be felt with a uterine sound or biopsy instrument, a pelvic sonogram or X-ray should be obtained. If the device is not visualized with pelvic ultrasonography, an X-ray visualizing the entire abdominal cavity should be performed, as IUDs that have been pushed through the uterus may be located anywhere in the peritoneal cavity—even in the subdiaphragmatic area.

Any type of IUD found to be outside the uterus, even if it is asymptomatic, should be removed from the peritoneal cavity, because complications such as adhesions and bowel obstruction have been reported. Both the copper IUDs and the shields have been found to produce severe peritoneal reactions. Therefore, it is best to remove these devices as soon as possible after the diagnosis of perforation is made. Unless severe adhesions have developed, most intraperitoneal IUDs can be removed by means of laparoscopy, avoiding the need for laparotomy.

Perforation of the cervix has also been reported with devices having a straight vertical arm, such as the copper T or copper 7. The incidence of downward perforation into the cervix has been reported to range from about 1/600 to 1/1000 insertions. When follow-up examinations are performed on patients with these devices, the cervix should be carefully inspected and palpated, because often perforations do not extend completely through the ectocervical epithelium. Cervical perforation is not a major problem, but devices that have perforated downward should be removed through the endocervical canal with uterine packing forceps. Their downward displacement is associated with reduced contraceptive effectiveness.

Infection. In the 1960s, despite great concern among clinicians that use of IUDs would markedly increase the incidence of salpingitis, or pelvic inflammatory disease (PID), there was little evidence that such an increase did occur. During that decade, IUDs were inserted mainly into parous women, and the incidence of sexually transmitted disease was not as high as occurred subsequently. In 1966, Mishell et al.[31] prepared aerobic and anaerobic cultures of homogenates of endometrial tissue obtained transfundally from uteri removed by vaginal hysterectomy at various intervals after insertion of the loop IUD. During the first 24 hours, the normally sterile endometrial cavity was consistently infected with bacteria. Nevertheless, in 80% of cases, the women's natural defenses destroyed these bacteria within the following 24 hours. In this study, the endometrial cavity, the IUD, and the portion of the thread within the cavity were consistently found to be sterile when transfundal cultures were obtained more than 30 days after insertion. These findings support the belief that development of PID more than 1 month after insertion of the loop IUD is

Table 14-6. Duration of current IUD use (excluding Dalkon shield) for women with PID and controls

Duration of use of current IUD (mo)*	Women with PID†	Controls†	Relative risk‡ (95% confidence limits)
≤1	27	17	3.8 (2.1–6.8)
2–4	22	32	1.7 (1.1–3.1)
5–12	33	90	1.1 (0.7–1.7)
13–24	32	81	1.2 (0.7–1.8)
25–60	23	62	1.2 (0.7–2.0)
>60	13	40	1.4 (0.7–2.7)
No method	250	763	1

From Lee NC et al: *Obstet Gynecol* 62:1, 1983. Reprinted with permission from The American College of Obstetricians and Gynecologists.
*IUD used in the 3 months before interview.
†Limited to women who reported no past history of PID.
‡Relative risk adjusted for age, marital status, and number of sexual partners within the previous 6 months.

due to infection with a sexually transmitted pathogen and is unrelated to the presence of the device.

These findings agree with the incidence of clinically diagnosed PID found in a group of 23,977 mainly parous women wearing non–copper-bearing IUDs.[23] When PID rates were computed according to the duration of IUD use, the rates were highest in the first 2 weeks after insertion and then steadily diminished. Rates after the first month were in the range of 1 to 2.5/100 woman-years.

The results of both of these studies indicate that an IUD should not be inserted into a patient who may have been recently infected with gonococci or chlamydia. Insertion of the device will transport these pathogens into the upper genital tract. If there is clinical suspicion of infectious endocervicitis, cultures should be obtained and the IUD insertion delayed until the results reveal that no pathogenic organisms are present. It does not appear to be cost effective to administer systemic antibiotics routinely with every IUD insertion, but the insertion procedure should be as aseptic as possible.

In 1983 investigators from the Centers for Disease Control and Prevention (CDC) reported results from a multicenter case-control study of the relationship of the IUD and PID.[23] They found the overall risk of PID in IUD users versus noncontraceptive users to be 1.9. The risk in shield users was 8.3; in other IUD users, it was only 1.6. When the risk of PID in IUD users (other than shield users) was correlated with duration of use, it was found that a significantly increased risk of PID with the loop and copper 7 was present only during the first 4 months after insertion (Table 14-6). Beyond 4 months of use, there was no significantly increased risk in IUD users other than those with shields. Thus, this report is in agreement with our bacteriologic study and the 1970 summary of 23,977 IUD users mentioned earlier. These data provide additional evidence that aside from the insertion process the IUD with monofilament tail strings does not itself alter the incidence of PID. Additional support for this statement is provided from results of an epidemiologic study investigating the incidence of tubal infertility among former IUD users. It was reported that nulliparous women with a single sexual partner who had previously used an IUD had no increased risk of tubal infertility, whereas women with multiple sexual partners who used an IUD did have an increased risk of tubal infertility (Table 14-6).

A more detailed analysis of data from the CDC study was published in 1988.[22] This analysis produced information about risk factors for developing PID, such as number of sexual partners and frequency of intercourse among IUD users and users of no method of contraception. These investigators found that married women were less likely to have more than one sexual partner in the previous 6 months before data were gathered than previously married or never-married women. Among women in each of these groups, as well as those cohabiting but not married, who reported having only one sexual partner, the risk of developing PID in women wearing an IUD was significantly increased only in the previously married or never-married group (Table 14-7). The authors postulated that this was probably due to the fact that the partners of such women had an increased risk of transmitting a pathogen responsible for PID. In the group of married or cohabiting women who had an IUD inserted more than 4 months earlier, the relative risk of developing PID compared to users of no method was 1.0 with confidence limits of 0.6 to 1.6, whereas those who had it inserted within 4 months had a nonsignificantly increased risk of developing PID of 1.8. Thus analysis of this large amount of data indicates that PID occurring more than a few months following insertion of loop or copper devices is due to a sexually transmitted disease and is not related to the IUD.

The populations at high risk for PID include those with a prior history of PID, nulliparous women under 25 years of age, and women with multiple sexual partners. The FDA has recommended that women with these characteristics be especially advised about the risk of developing PID during IUD use and the possibility of subsequent loss of fertility. They should be told to watch for the early symptoms of PID, so that treatment can be started before complications occur. These data, as well as those of two epidemiologic studies showing an increased risk of tubal causes of infertility in nulliparous women who had used an IUD, indicate that the clinician should avoid using IUDs in nulliparous women who may want to conceive in the future. The increased risk of impairment of future fertility from PID in the first few months after IUD insertion, as well as the possibility of ectopic pregnancy, must be considered when deciding whether to use an IUD in a nulliparous woman.

Symptomatic PID can usually be successfully treated with antibiotics—without removing the IUD—until the

Table 14-7. Risk of PID associated with IUD use versus no method, by marital status among women with only one recent sexual partner

Marital status	Relative risk (95% confidence interval)
Currently married	1.2 (0.7-1.9)
Cohabiting	1.0 (0.4-2.4)
Previously married	1.8 (1.0-3.2)
Never married	2.6 (1.6-4.3)

From Lee NC, Rubin GL: *Obstet Gynecol* 72:1, 1988.

patient becomes symptom free. In patients with clinical evidence of a tuboovarian abscess or with a shield in place, the IUD should be removed only after a therapeutic serum level of appropriate parenteral antibiotics has been reached, and preferably after a clinical response has been observed. An alternative method of contraception should be substituted in patients who develop PID with an IUD in place (or in those with a past history of PID).

There is evidence that IUD users may have an increased risk for colonizing actinomycosis organisms in the upper genital tract. The relationship of actinomycosis to PID is unclear, as many women without IUDs have actinomyces in their vaginas. If these organisms are identified on the routine annual cytologic smear of IUD users, their existence should be confirmed by culture because cytologic diagnosis of actinomycosis is not very precise. If the culture confirms the presence of actinomyces in the cervix, appropriate antimicrobial therapy should be used to eradicate the organisms, but the IUD does not have to be removed.

Complications of pregnancy.

Congenital anomalies. When pregnancy occurs with an IUD in place, implantation takes place away from the device itself, so the device is always extraamniotic. Although there is a paucity of published data, so far there is no evidence of an increased incidence of congenital anomalies in infants born with an IUD in utero. In a study by Poland[37] of spontaneously aborted tissue, 21% of the embryos conceived with an IUD in situ had evidence of abnormalities. This was considerably less than the 44% incidence of abnormalities in abortuses of women using no contraception and was similar to the incidence of embryonic abnormalities in abortuses of women having induced abortions. This suggests that the presence of an IUD has no influence on embryonic development and that the increased incidence of spontaneous abortion in IUD users is not due to a greater incidence of embryonic abnormalities.

Tatum and associates[45] reported that of 166 embryos conceived with an intrauterine copper T in place and large enough to permit adequate examination, only one had a congenital anomaly, a fibroma of the vocal cords. Guillebaud[17] reported that in a series of 167 pregnancies that reached viability with the copper 7 in place, 159 normal babies were born. No details were given regarding three infants in this series, and the other five had a variety of anomalies. Therefore the incidence of congenital defects, 3%, was similar to the usually expected rate. Thus there is no evidence from these studies to indicate that the presence of a copper IUD in the uterus exerts a deleterious effect on fetal development. Although relatively few infants have been born with a progesterone-releasing IUD in the uterus, careful examination of these infants has revealed no increased incidence of cardiac or other anomalies.

Spontaneous abortion. In all reported series of pregnancies with any type of IUD in situ, the incidence of fetal death was not significantly increased; however, a significant increase in spontaneous abortion has been consistently observed. Three studies indicate that if a patient conceives while wearing an IUD that is not subsequently removed, the incidence of spontaneous abortion is about 55%, approximately three times greater than would occur without an IUD.

After conception, if the IUD is spontaneously expelled, or if the appendage is visible and the IUD is removed by traction, the incidence of spontaneous abortion is significantly reduced. Of women who conceived with copper T devices in place, the incidence of spontaneous abortion was only 20.3% if the device was removed or spontaneously expelled. This figure is similar to the normal incidence of spontaneous abortion and significantly less than the 54.1% incidence of abortion reported in the same study among women retaining the devices in utero. Thus, if a woman conceives with an IUD in place and wishes to continue the pregnancy, the IUD should be removed if the appendage is visible. This will significantly reduce the chance of spontaneous abortion even if the appendage is not visible. Probing of the uterine cavity may increase the chance of abortion as well as sepsis. However, two recent reports indicate that with careful ultrasonography and meticulous techniques it is possible to remove intrauterine IUDs without a visible appendage during pregnancy and have a normal outcome of gestation.

Septic abortion. If the IUD cannot be easily removed, there is some evidence that suggests that the risk of septic abortion may be increased if the IUD remains in place. Most of the evidence is based on data from women who conceived while wearing the shield type of IUD. This device, with its multifilament tail, was widely used from 1971 to 1974. It has been shown that the structure of the shield's appendage allowed bacteria to enter the spaces between the filaments of the tail underneath the sheath. This contrasts with the inability of bacteria to enter the monofilament tails of other devices. During pregnancy, when the shield was drawn upward into the uterus as gestation advanced, the bacteria in the tail had the potential for causing a severe and sometimes fatal uterine infection, usually in the second trimester of pregnancy.

Although there is theoretic and actual evidence of an increased risk of septic abortion if a patient conceives with a shield IUD in place, there is no conclusive evidence of an increased risk if a patient conceives with a device other than the shield in place. In the Oxford study, there was no significant difference in the incidence of septic abortion among women who conceived with an IUD in place and those who conceived while using other methods. None of the women with septic abortions were seriously ill, and all responded promptly to treatment. In a study of 918 women who conceived with the copper T in situ, there were only two cases of septic abortion, both occurring in the first trimester. This evidence does not suggest an increase in sepsis in pregnancy due to the presence of an IUD, except that about 2% of all spontaneous abortions are septic, and IUDs increase the rate of spontaneous abortion.

Although there is no conclusive evidence of an increased incidence of sepsis with IUDs other than the shield, the patient should be informed of the possibility of a greater chance of sepsis and, if she wishes to continue the pregnancy, of the need to report symptoms of infection promptly. If an intrauterine infection does occur during pregnancy with an IUD in place, treatment should proceed in the same manner as if the IUD were absent. In such a situation, the endometrial cavity should be evacuated following a short interval of appropriate antibiotic treatment.

Ectopic pregnancy. As stated earlier, the IUD's main mechanism of contraceptive action is the production of a continuous sterile inflammatory reaction in the uterine cavity due to foreign body presence. As the large numbers of leukocytes stimulated to enter the uterine cavity by the inflammatory reaction are catabolized, their breakdown products exert a toxic effect on sperm and the ovaries. If the egg is fertilized, effects of this foreign body reaction act to prevent implantation of the embryo into the endometrium. Since inflammatory reaction is more prevalent in the endometrial cavity than in the oviducts, the IUD prevents intrauterine pregnancy more effectively than it prevents ectopic pregnancy.

If a patient conceives with an IUD in place, her chances of having an ectopic pregnancy range from 3% to 9%. This incidence is about 10 times greater than the reported ectopic pregnancy frequency of 0.3% to 0.7% of the total births in similar populations. In two large Population Council studies,[42] the ectopic pregnancy rate in IUD wearers was about 1.0 to 1.2/1000 woman-years.

Thus if a patient conceives with an IUD in place, ectopic pregnancy should be suspected. There appears to be a higher frequency of ectopic pregnancy with the progesterone-releasing IUD. Patients conceiving while wearing any type of IUD should have sonography performed early in gestation. In addition, the possibility of ovarian pregnancy should always be considered, as the incidence of ovarian pregnancy is greater in women conceiving with an IUD in place than in those conceiving while not wearing an IUD. IUD users with a clinical diagnosis of ruptured corpus luteum may, in fact, have an unrecognized ovarian pregnancy. If any patient with an IUD has an elective termination of pregnancy, the evacuated tissue should be examined histologically to be certain that the gestation was intrauterine.

The effect of the IUD on increased development of ectopic pregnancy while it is in place appears to be temporary and does not persist after removal of the IUD. In two large European studies,[27, 40] women wishing to conceive after they had an ectopic pregnancy had a much greater chance of having a successful intrauterine pregnancy if they were using an IUD at the time of their ectopic pregnancy than those who had an ectopic pregnancy without an IUD.

Prematurity. Several studies indicate that the rate of preterm delivery is higher if an IUD remains in the uterus throughout gestation. If a pregnant patient has an IUD in place and the device cannot be removed but the patient wishes to continue her gestation, she should be warned of the increased risk of prematurity as well as that of spontaneous abortion and ectopic pregnancy. She should also be informed of the possible increased risk of septic abortion and advised to report promptly the first signs of pelvic pain or fever. There is no evidence that pregnancies with IUDs in utero are associated with an increased incidence of other obstetric complications. There is also no evidence that prior use of an IUD results in a greater incidence of complications in pregnancies occurring after its removal.

Overall safety. Several long-term studies have indicated that the IUD is not associated with an increased incidence of endometrial or cervical carcinoma. Nevertheless, the IUD does produce morbidity that may result in hospitalization. The main causes of hospitalization among IUD users are complications of pregnancy, uterine perforation, and hemorrhage, as well as pelvic infection. Despite the increased morbidity with IUDs, the actual incidence of these problems is very low. IUDs are not being inserted in women at risk for developing PID, and physicians are aware of the potential complications associated with IUDs in pregnancy. The IUD is a particularly useful method of contraception for women who have completed their families and do not wish permanent sterilization and have contraindications to or do not wish to use OCs.

Hormonal contraception

Oral steroid contraceptives. Oral steroid contraceptives were initially marketed in the United States in 1960. Because of their extremely high rate of effectiveness and ease of administration they soon became one of the most widely used methods of reversible contraception in developing countries among both married and unmarried women. The initially marketed formulations of OCs contained 150 µg of the estrogen component, mestranol, and 9.85 mg of the progestin component, norethynodrel. The side effects produced by each of these steroids, such as

nausea, breast tenderness, and weight gain, were common and occasionally severe enough to cause discontinuation of use. During the past 30 years many other formulations have been developed and marketed with steadily decreasing dosages of both the estrogen and progestin component. All of the formulations initially marketed after 1975 contain less than 50 µg of ethinyl estradiol and 1 mg or less of several progestins. The use of these agents is associated with very low pregnancy rates, similar to those for formulations with higher doses of steroid, and a significantly lower incidence of adverse metabolic effects.

Data compiled by the FDA indicate that the use of formulations containing less than 50 µg of estrogen has steadily increased in the United States since they were first marketed in 1973, from about 10% of prescriptions in 1976 to 82% in 1988. There was a steady decrease in prescriptions for formulations with more than 50 µg of estrogen since 1964, and in 1988 only 1.6% of OC prescriptions were for these high-dose compounds. Because these higher-dose estrogen formulations are associated with a greater incidence of adverse effects without greater efficacy, they are no longer marketed for contraceptive use in the United States, Canada, and Great Britain.

Pharmacology. There are three major types of oral steroid contraceptive formulations: fixed-dose combination, combination phasic, and daily progestin. The combination formulations are the most widely used and most effective. They consist of tablets containing both an estrogen and a progestin given continuously for 3 weeks. The original sequential type, which is no longer marketed, provided a regimen of estrogen alone given for about 2 weeks, followed by 1 week of combination estrogen-progestin tablets. The combination phasic formulations contain two or three different amounts of the same estrogen and progestin. Each of the tablets containing one of these various dosages is given for intervals varying from 5 to 11 days during the 21-day medication period. These formulations have been described as multiphasic. The rationale for this type of formulation is that a lower total dose of steroid is administered without increasing the incidence of breakthrough bleeding. In the usual regimen for combination OCs, no medication is given for 1 week out of 4 to allow withdrawal bleeding to occur. The third type of contraceptive formulation, consisting of tablets containing a progestin without any estrogen, is designed to be taken daily without a steroid-free interval.

Oral contraceptives currently being used are formulated from synthetic steroids and contain no natural estrogens or progestins. There are two major types of synthetic progestins: (1) derivatives of 19-nortestosterone and (2) derivatives of 17α-acetoxyprogesterone. The latter group are C-21 progestins, consisting of such steroids as medroxyprogesterone acetate and megestrol acetate. In contrast to the 19-nortestosterone derivatives, when high dosages of the C-21 progestins were given to female beagle dogs, the animals developed an increased incidence of mammary cancer. Because of this carcinogenic effect, oral contraceptives containing these progestins are no longer being made.

All OC formulations now available in the United States consist of varying dosages of one of the following six 19-nortestosterone progestins: norethindrone, norethindrone acetate, ethynodiol diacetate, norgestrel, norgestimate, and desogestrel. The parent compound of norgestrel, *dl*-norgestrel, consists of two isomers, only one of which is biologically active. Currently most formulations produced contain only the active isomer of *dl*-norgestrel, levonorgestrel. Formulations containing the three progestins, desogestrel, gestodene, and norgestimate, which have greater progestational activity but are less androgenic than the currently used progestins, have been marketed in Europe for several years. Clinical testing with these formulations in the United States has been completed, and compounds containing norgestimate and desogestrel have received approval for use.

With the exception of two daily progestin-only formulations, the progestins are combined with varying dosages of two estrogens, ethinyl estradiol and ethinyl estradiol 3-methyl ether, also known as mestranol. All of the older higher-dosage formulations contained mestranol, and this steroid is still present in some 50-μg formulations. All formulations with less than 50 μg of estrogen contain the parent compound ethinyl estradiol. All the synthetic estrogens and progestins in OCs have an ethinyl group at position 17. The presence of this ethinyl group enhances the oral activity of these agents, because their essential functional groups are not as rapidly hydroxylated and then conjugated as they initially pass through the liver via the portal system, in contrast with what occurs when natural sex steroids are ingested orally. The synthetic steroids thus have greater oral potency per unit of weight than do the natural steroids.

The various modifications in chemical structures of the different synthetic progestins and estrogens also affect their biologic activity. Thus one cannot judge the pharmacologic activity of the progestin or estrogen in a particular contraceptive steroid formulation only by the amount of steroid present. The biologic activity of each steroid also has to be considered. By using established tests for progestational activity in animals, it was found that a given weight of norgestrel is several times more potent than the same weight of norethindrone. Studies in humans, using delay of menses or endometrial histologic alterations such as subnuclear vacuolization as end points, also have shown that norgestrel is several times more potent than the same weight of norethindrone. Norethindrone acetate and ethynodiol diacetate are metabolized in the body to norethindrone. The human studies, measuring progestational activity as described above, as well as other studies comparing the effects on serum lipids in humans, were summarized by Dorflinger,[13] who concluded that each of these three progestins had approximately equal potency per unit of

weight, whereas levonorgestrel is 10 to 20 times as potent. Thus, when considering which contraceptive to prescribe, the physician needs to consider both the dose and the potency of each steroid. The currently marketed triphasic contraceptive formulations with levonorgestrel contain about 10% as much progestin as triphasic formulations containing norethindrone and have similar effects on lipid and carbohydrate metabolism. Several fixed-dose monophasic formulations currently marketed in the United States have a lower total dose of norethindrone per treatment cycle than the triphasic formulations containing norethindrone.

The two estrogenic compounds used in OCs, ethinyl estradiol and its 3-methyl ether, mestranol, also have different biologic activity in women. To become biologically effective, mestranol must be demethylated to ethinyl estradiol, because mestranol does not bind to the estrogen cytosol receptors. The degree of conversion of mestranol to ethinyl estradiol varies among individuals; some are able to convert it completely, but others convert only a portion of it. Thus, in some women, a given weight of mestranol is as potent as the same weight of ethinyl estradiol, whereas in other women it is only about half as potent. Overall, it has been estimated that ethinyl estradiol is about 1.7 times as potent as the same weight of mestranol. This factor was determined by using human endometrial response and effect on liver corticosteroid-binding globulin production as end points. Thus, it is important to evaluate the biologic activity as well as the quantity of both steroid components when comparing potency of the various formulations.

Radioimmunoassay methods have been developed to measure blood levels of these synthetic estrogens and progestins. Peak plasma levels of ethinyl estradiol occur about 1 hour after ingestion, then rapidly decline. However, measurable amounts of ethinyl estradiol are still found in plasma 24 hours after ingestion. With mestranol, peak levels of ethinyl estradiol are lower than with ethinyl estradiol, and occur 2 to 4 hours after ingestion. This delay is due to the time necessary for mestranol to be demethylated to ethinyl estradiol in the liver.

When different doses of norgestrel were administered to women, Brenner et al.[7] found that the serum levels of levonorgestrel were related to the dosage. Peak serum levels were found $\frac{1}{2}$ to 3 hours after oral administration, followed by a rapid, sharp decline. However, 24 hours after ingestion, 20% to 25% of the peak level of levonorgestrel was still present in the serum. After 5 days of norgestrel administration, measurable amounts of levonorgestrel were present for at least the following 5 days.

Brenner et al.[7] measured serum levels of levonorgestrel, follicle-stimulating hormone (FSH), luteinizing hormone (LH), estradiol, and progesterone 3 hours after ingestion of a combination OC containing 0.5 mg of *dl*-norgestrel and 50 μg of ethinyl estradiol in three women during two consecutive cycles, as well as during the intervening pill-free interval. Daily levels of levonorgestrel rose during the first few days of medication, plateaued thereafter, and declined after ingestion of the last pill. Nevertheless, substantial amounts of levonorgestrel remained in the serum for at least the first 3 to 4 days after the last pill was ingested. These steroid levels were sufficient to suppress gonadotropin release; thus follicle maturation, as evidenced by rising estradiol levels, does not occur during the pill-free interval.

From these data, it seems reasonable to conclude that accidental pregnancies during OC use probably do not occur because of a failure to ingest one or two pills more than a few days after a treatment cycle is initiated, but rather because initiation of the next cycle of medication is delayed for a few days. Therefore, it is very important that the pill-free interval be limited to no more than 7 days. This is best accomplished by administering either a placebo or iron pill daily during the steroid-free interval (the so-called 28-day package). Alternatively, treatment may be started on the first Sunday after menses begins instead of the first or fifth day of the cycle. It is easier to remember to start the new package on a Sunday. Patients should be warned that the most important pill to remember to take is the first one of each cycle.

Physiology

Mechanism of action. The estrogen-progestin combination is the most effective type of OC formulation, because these preparations consistently inhibit the midcycle gonadotropin surge and thus prevent ovulation. Such formulations also act on other aspects of the reproductive process. They alter the cervical mucus, making it thick, viscid, and scanty, which thus retards sperm penetration. They also alter motility of the uterus and oviduct, thus impairing transport of both ova and sperm. Furthermore, they alter the endometrium, so that its glandular production of glycogen is diminished and less energy is available for the blastocyst to survive in the uterine cavity. Finally, they may alter ovarian responsiveness to gonadotropin stimulation. Nevertheless, neither gonadotropin production nor ovarian steroidogenesis is completely abolished, and levels of endogenous estradiol in the peripheral blood during ingestion of combination OCs are similar to those found in the early follicular phase of the normal cycle.

Contraceptive steroids prevent ovulation mainly by interfering with release of gonadotropin-releasing hormone (GnRH) from the hypothalamus. In rats, and in a few studies in humans, this inhibitory action of the contraceptive steroids could be overcome by the administration of GnRH. However, in most other human studies, most women who had been ingesting combination OCs had suppression of the release of LH and FSH following infusion of GnRH, indicating that the steroids had a direct inhibitory effect on the pituitary as well as on the hypothalamus.

It is possible, however, that when hypothalamic inhibition is prolonged, the mechanism for synthesis and release of gonadotropins may become refractory to the normal amount of GnRH stimulation. However, in a few OC users studied, after serial daily administration of GnRH, there was still a refractory response to a GnRH infusion. Thus, the combination OCs probably do have a direct inhibitory effect on the gonadotropin-producing cells of the pituitary, in addition to affecting the hypothalamus. This effect occurs in about 80% of women ingesting combination OC steroids. It is unrelated to the age of the patient or the duration of steroid use, but it is related to the potency of the preparations. The effect is more pronounced with formulations containing a more potent progestin and with those containing 50 μg or more of estrogen than with 30- to 35-μg formulations. It has not been demonstrated that the amount of pituitary suppression is related to the occurrence of postpill amenorrhea, but if there is a relationship, the lower-dose formulations should be associated with a lower frequency of this entity. Bracken et al.[5] reported that the delay in the resumption of ovulation following discontinuation of OC use is shorter in women ingesting preparations with less than 50 μg of estrogen than in those ingesting formulations with 50 μg of estrogen or more.

The daily progestin-only preparations do not consistently inhibit ovulation. They exert their contraceptive action via the other mechanisms discussed earlier, but because of the inconsistent ovulation inhibition, their effectiveness is significantly less than that of the combined type. Because a lower dose of progestin is used, it is important that they be taken consistently at the same time of day to ensure that blood levels do not fall below the effective contraceptive level.

No significant difference in clinical effectiveness has been demonstrated among the various combination formulations currently available in the United States (Table 14-8). Provided no tablets are omitted, the pregnancy rate is less than 0.2% at the end of 1 year with all combination formulations.

Metabolic effects. It is important to realize that OCs have metabolic effects in addition to the effects on the reproductive axis. The estrogenic component and progestin component have different, and sometimes opposite, metabolic effects. These metabolic effects can produce both the more common, less serious, side effects and the rare, potentially serious, complications. The magnitude of these effects is directly related to the dosage and potency of the steroids in the formulations. For a more in-depth discussion of the metabolic effects of OCs see Chapter 15.

Reproductive effects. The magnitude and duration of the delay in the return of fertility are greater for women discontinuing use of OCs with 50 μg of estrogen or more than with those containing lower doses of estrogen. However, Bracken et al.[5] reported that use of the low-dose formulations still resulted in a reduction in conception rates for at least the first six cycles after discontinuation. In

Table 14-8. Estrogen and progestin components of OCs

Manufacturer and product	Type	Progestin	Estrogen
Berlex			
Levlen	Combination	0.15 mg levonorgestrel	30 µg ethinyl estradiol
Tri-Levlen 6/	Comb-triphasic	0.05 mg levonorgestrel	30 µg ethinyl estradiol
Tri-Levlen 5/	Comb-triphasic	0.075 mg levonorgestrel	40 µg ethinyl estradiol
Tri-Levlen 10/	Comb-triphasic	0.125 mg levonorgestrel	30 µg ethinyl estradiol
Mead Johnson Laboratories			
Ovcon 35	Combination	0.4 mg norethindrone	35 µg ethinyl estradiol
Ovcon 50	Combination	1.0 mg norethindrone	50 µg ethinyl estradiol
Organon Desogen	Combination	0.15 mg desogestrel	0.030 mg ethinyl estradiol
Ortho Pharmaceutical			
Micronor	Progestin	0.35 mg norethindrone	
Modicon	Combination	0.5 mg norethindrone	35 µg ethinyl estradiol
Ortho-Cyclen	Combination	0.250 mg norgestimate	0.035 mg ethinyl estradiol
Ortho-Novum 1/35	Combination	1.0 mg norethindrone	35 µg ethinyl estradiol
Ortho-Novum 1/50	Combination	1.0 mg norethindrone	50 µg mestranol
Ortho-Novum 7/7/7	Comb-triphasic	0.5 mg norethindrone	35 µg ethinyl estradiol
Ortho-Tri-Cyclen	Combination	0.180 mg norgestimate	0.035 mg ethinyl estradiol
Ortho-Cept	Combination	0.15 mg desogestrel	0.03 mg ethinyl estradiol
Parke-Davis			
Loestrin 1/20	Combination	1.0 mg norethindrone acetate	20 µg ethinyl estradiol
Loestrin 1.5/30	Combination	1.5 mg norethindrone acetate	30 µg ethinyl estradiol
Roberts Pharmaceutical			
Norethin 1/35E	Combination	1 mg norethindrone	35 µg ethinyl estradiol
Norethin 1/50M	Combination	1 mg norethindrone	50 µg ethinyl estradiol
Searle			
Demulen 1/35	Combination	1 mg ethynodiol diacetate	35 µg ethinyl estradiol
Demulen 1/50	Combination	1 mg ethynodiol diacetate	50 µg ethinyl estradiol
Syntex			
Brevicon (Genora 0.5/35)	Combination	0.5 mg norethindrone	35 µg ethinyl estradiol
Norinyl 1+35 (Genora 1/35)	Combination	1 mg norethindrone	35 µg ethinyl estradiol
Norinyl 1+50 (Genora 1/50)	Combination	1 mg norethindrone	50 µg mestranol
Nor-Q D	Progestin	0.35 mg norethindrone	
Tri-Norinyl 7/	Comb-triphasic	0.5 mg norethindrone	35 µg ethinyl estradiol
9/	Comb-triphasic	1 mg norethindrone	35 µg ethinyl estradiol
5/	Comb-triphasic	0.5 mg norethindrone	35 µg ethinyl estradiol
Wyeth-Ayerst			
Lo/Ovral	Combination	3 mg norethindrone	30 µg ethinyl estradiol
Nordette	Combination	0.15 mg norethindrone	30 µg ethinyl estradiol
Ovral	Combination	0.5 mg norgestrel	50 µg ethinyl estradiol
Ovrette	Progestin	75 µg norgestrel	30 µg ethinyl estradiol
Triphasil 6/	Comb-triphasic	50 µg levonorgestrel	40 µg ethinyl estradiol
5/	Comb-triphasic	75 µg levonorgestrel	40 µg ethinyl estradiol
10/	Comb-triphasic	125 µg levonorgestrel	30 µg ethinyl estradiol

women stopping use of OCs in order to conceive, the probability of conception is lowest in the first month after stopping their use and increases steadily thereafter. There is little, if any, effect of duration of OC use on the length of delay of subsequent conception, but the magnitude of the delay to return of conception after OC use is greater among older premenopausal women.

Thus for 2 to 3 years after the discontinuation of contraceptives in order to conceive, the rate of return of fertility is lower for users of OCs than for women who have used barrier methods, but eventually the percentage of women who conceive after ceasing to use each of these contraceptive methods becomes the same. Thus the use of OCs does not cause permanent infertility.

Since the resumption of ovulation is delayed for variable periods after OCs are stopped, it is difficult to estimate the expected date of delivery if conception takes place before spontaneous menses return. For this reason, when women stop OCs in order to conceive, it is probably best that they use barrier methods for about 1 or 2 months until regular cycles resume. If conception occurs before resumption of spontaneous menses, gestational age should be estimated by serial sonography. Neither the rate of spontaneous abortion nor the incidence of chromosomal abnormalities in abortuses is increased in women who conceive in the first or subsequent months after ceasing to use OCs.

Several cohort and case-control studies of large numbers of babies born to women who stopped using OCs have been undertaken. These studies indicate that these infants have no greater chance of being born with any type of birth defect than infants born to women in the general population, even if conception occurred in the first month after the medication was discontinued. If these steroids are ingested during the first few months of pregnancy, a review by Bracken and Vita[6] of all the prospective epidemiologic studies with a control group of women not using OCs indicated that there was no increased risk of congenital malformations overall among the offspring of OC users. Furthermore, there was no increased risk of congenital heart defects or limb reduction defects in offspring of OC users. An increased risk of these anomalies had been reported in early case-control studies of women ingesting OCs after conception. However, the results could have been influenced by recall bias. A statement warning of a possible teratogenic effect of ingestion of OCs during pregnancy has been deleted from current product labeling for OCs.

Neoplastic effects. OCs have been used extensively for about 30 years and numerous epidemiologic studies, of both cohort and case-control design, have been performed to determine the relationship between use of these agents and the development of all types of neoplasms. This relationship is discussed in detail in Chapter 16.

Oral contraceptive use and overall mortality. In 1989 Vessey and colleagues[53] reported the cause of mortality through 1987 among OC users and nonusers enrolled in the Oxford Family Planning Association Cohort Study between 1968 and 1974. During this 20-year follow-up of 17,032 women there were 238 deaths. The overall risk of death among the OC users was 0.9 (confidence limits [CL] 0.7 to 1.2) compared with the women of similar age and socioeconomic status using a diaphragm or condom for contraception. The risk of death from breast cancer in OC users was 0.9 (CL 0.5 to 1.4); from cervical cancer, 3.3 (CL 0.9 to 17.9); and from ovarian cancer, 0.4 (CL 0.1 to 1.2). These cancer mortality rates are consistent with the other epidemiologic data discussed earlier. The death rate for circulatory disease was 1.5 (CL 0.7 to 3.0), and nearly all these deaths in OC users occurred in women who were also smokers. Thus the risk of death from circulatory disease was less than that reported for the first 10 years of the Royal College of General Practitioners' study[18] when higher-dose formulations were used and women with cardiovascular risk factors were using OCs. It thus appears that OC use has no appreciable risk on overall mortality. With exclusive use of low-dose formulations given to women without cardiovascular risk factors who have frequent cervical cytologic screening, an overall beneficial effect on mortality with OC use may be expected.

Contraindications to use of oral contraceptives. Oral contraceptives can be prescribed for the majority of women of reproductive age, because these women are young and generally healthy. However, there are certain absolute contraindications, including a present or past history of vascular disease, including thromboembolism, thrombophlebitis, atherosclerosis, and stroke; or systemic disease that may affect the vascular system, such as lupus erythematosus or hemoglobin SS disease. Cigarette smoking in women over age 35, hypertension, diabetes mellitus with vascular disease, and hyperlipidemia are also contraindications, because high-dose OC use in women with these disorders was reported to increase the risk of stroke or myocardial infarction. One of the contraindications listed by the FDA is cancer of the breast or endometrium, although there are no data indicating that OCs are harmful to women with these diseases.

Pregnant women should not ingest OCs because of the theoretic masculinizing effect of the 19-norprogestins on the external genitalia of female fetuses. As mentioned earlier, concerns that OCs might produce other deleterious fetal effects, such as limb reduction and heart defects, have not proven valid.

Patients with functional heart disease should not use OCs, because the fluid retention they produce could result in congestive heart failure. There is no evidence, however, that individuals with an asymptomatic prolapsed mitral valve should not use OCs. Patients with active liver disease should not take OCs, because the steroids are metabolized in the liver. However, women who have recovered from liver disease, such as viral hepatitis, and whose liver function test results have returned to normal can safely take OCs.

Relative contraindications to OC use include heavy cigarette smoking under age 35, migraine headaches, amenorrhea, and depression. Migraine headaches can be worsened by OC use, and patients who develop strokes have been reported to have an increased incidence of headaches of the migraine type, fainting, temporary loss of vision or speech, or paresthesias prior to the stroke. If any of these symptoms develop in an OC user, the use of OCs should be stopped.

Patients who are amenorrheic for a cause other than polycystic ovary syndrome should probably not take OCs, because a pituitary microadenoma may be present. Since OC use may mask the symptoms produced by a prolactin-secreting adenoma, amenorrhea and galactorrhea, amenorrheic patients should not receive OCs until the diagnosis for this symptom is established. If galactorrhea develops during OC use, OCs should be discontinued and after 2 weeks a serum prolactin level should be measured. If the level is elevated, further diagnostic evaluation is indicated. Patients with gestational diabetes can take low-dose OC formulations, because, as reported by Kjos et al.,[20] these agents do not affect glucose tolerance or accelerate the development of diabetes mellitus. Insulin-dependent diabetes without vascular disease is a relative contraindication to OC use.

Starting oral contraceptives

In adolescents. In deciding whether a sexually active pubertal girl should use OCs for contraception, the clinician should be more concerned about compliance with the regimen than about possible physiologic harm. Provided she has demonstrated maturity of the hypothalamic-pituitary-ovarian axis with at least three regular, presumably ovulatory, menstrual cycles, it is safe to prescribe OCs without concern that permanent damage to the reproductive process will result. It is probably best not to prescribe OCs for women of any age with oligomenorrhea, except those with polycystic ovary syndrome, because of their increased likelihood of developing postpill amenorrhea. Oligomenorrhea is more frequent in adolescence than in later life. Postpill amenorrhea that lasts for more than 6 months is not produced by OCs but becomes manifest after discontinuing OCs, because OCs mask the development of the symptoms of amenorrhea. It is not necessary to be concerned about accelerating epiphyseal closure in the postmenarcheal female. Endogenous estrogens have already initiated the process a few years before menarche, and the contraceptive steroids will not hasten it.

After pregnancy. There is a difference in the relationship of the return of ovulation and bleeding in the postabortal woman and one who has had a term delivery. The first episode of menstrual bleeding in the postabortal woman is usually preceded by ovulation. After a term delivery, the first episode of bleeding is usually, but not always, anovulatory. Ovulation occurs sooner after an abortion, usually between 2 and 4 weeks, than after a term delivery, when ovulation is usually delayed beyond 6 weeks but may occur as early as 4 weeks in a woman who is not breast-feeding.

Thus after spontaneous or induced abortion of a fetus of less than 12 weeks of gestation, OCs should be started immediately to prevent conception following the first ovulation. For patients who deliver after 28 weeks and are not nursing, the combination pills should be initiated 2 to 3 weeks after delivery. If the termination of pregnancy occurs between 21 and 28 weeks, contraceptive steroids should be started 1 week later. The reason for delay in the latter instances is that the normally increased risk of thromboembolism occurring postpartum may be further enhanced by the hypercoagulable state associated with contraceptive steroid ingestion. Because the first ovulation is delayed for at least 4 weeks after a term delivery, there is no need to expose the patient to this increased risk.

Since estrogen inhibits the action of prolactin in breast tissue receptors, the use of combination OCs (those containing both estrogen and progestin) diminishes the amount of milk produced by OC users who breast-feed their babies. Although the diminution of milk production is directly related to the amount of estrogen in the contraceptive formulation, only one study, by Lönnerdel et al.,[25] has been published in which the amount of breast milk was measured by breast pump in women using formulations with less than 50 μg of estrogen. In this study, the use of this low-dose estrogen reduced the amount of breast milk. Thus it is probably best for women who are nursing not to use combination OCs.

Women who are breast-feeding every 4 hours, including at nighttime, will not ovulate until at least 10 weeks after delivery and thus do not need contraception before that time. Since only a small percentage of full breast-feeding women ovulate as long as they continue full nursing and remain amenorrheic, either a barrier method or progestin-only OC can be used. The latter does not diminish the amount of breast milk and is effective in this group of women. Once supplemental feeding is introduced, ovulation can resume promptly and effective contraception is then needed.

For all patients. At the initial visit, after a history and physical examination have determined that there are no medical contraindications for OCs, the patient should be informed about the benefits and risks. For medicolegal reasons it is best to note on the patient's medical record that the benefits and risks have been explained to her.

Type of formulation. In determining which formulation to use, it is best initially to prescribe a formulation with less than 50 μg of ethinyl estradiol, as these agents are associated with less cardiovascular risk as well as fewer estrogenic side effects. It would also appear reasonable to use formulations with the lowest dosage of a particular progestin, as there would be fewer progestogenic metabolic and clinical adverse effects associated with their use. The development of multiphasic formulations has allowed the total dose of progestin to be reduced compared with some monophasic formulations without increasing the incidence of breakthrough bleeding. However, several monophasic formulations have a lower total dose of progestin per cycle than the multiphasic formulations.

The FDA has stated that the product prescribed should be one that contains the least amount of estrogen and progestin that is compatible with a low failure rate and the needs of the individual patient. Because few randomized studies have been performed comparing the different marketed formulations, until large-scale comparative studies are performed, the clinician must decide which formulation to use based on which formulations have the fewest adverse effects among patients in his or her practice. If estrogenic or progestogenic side effects occur with one formulation, a different agent with less estrogenic or progestogenic activity can be given.

The contraceptive formulations containing progestins without estrogen have a lower incidence of adverse metabolic effects than the combination formulations. Since the factors that predispose to thromboembolism are caused by the estrogen component, the incidence of thromboembolism in women ingesting these compounds is probably not increased. Furthermore, blood pressure is not affected, nausea and breast tenderness are eliminated, and milk production and quality are unchanged. Despite these advantages, these agents have the disadvantages of a high frequency of intermenstrual and other abnormal bleeding patterns, including amenorrhea, and a lower rate of effectiveness. The use failure rate of these preparations is higher than with the combined formulations, and a relatively high percentage of the pregnancies that do occur are ectopic. Since nursing mothers have reduced fertility and have amenorrhea, the major disadvantages of these preparations are minimized for these patients. Furthermore, since milk production and quality are unaffected in contrast to the changes produced by combination pills, the formulations with only a progestin may be offered to these women while they are nursing. However, small portions of these synthetic steroids have been detected in breast milk. The long-term effects (if any) of these progestins on the infant are not known, but none have been detected to date. A long-term follow-up study by Nilsson et al.[34] of breast-fed children whose mothers ingested 50 μg of estrogen-combined OCs while they were lactating revealed no difference in weight gain or height increase up to 8 years of age compared with breast-fed children whose mothers did not ingest OCs. There was also no difference in occurrence of disease or intellectual or psychologic behavior between the two groups.

Follow-up. If the patient has no contraindications to OC use, the only routine laboratory tests indicated are a complete blood count, urinalysis, and cervical cytology. At the end of 3 months, the patient should be seen again; at this time a nondirected history should be obtained and the blood pressure measured. After this visit the patient should be seen annually, at which time a nondirected history should

again be taken, blood pressure and body weight measured, and a physical examination (including breast, abdominal, and pelvic examination with cervical cytology) performed. It is important to perform annual cervical cytologic examinations on OC users, as they are a relatively high-risk group for development of cervical neoplasia. The routine use of other laboratory tests is not indicated unless the patient has a family history of diabetes or vascular disease. Routine use of these tests in women is not indicated because the incidence of positive results is extremely low. However, if the patient has a family history of vascular disease, such as myocardial infarction occurring in family members under the age of 50, it would be advisable to obtain a lipid panel before OC use is started, as hypertriglyceridemia may be present and OC use will further raise triglycerides. Since the low-dose formulations do not alter the lipid profile except for triglycerides, it is not necessary to measure lipids, other than the routine every-5-year cholesterol screening, in women without cardiovascular risk factors even if they are over age 35 years. If the patient has a family history of diabetes or evidence of diabetes during pregnancy, a 2-hour postprandial blood glucose test should be performed before OCs are started; if the glucose level is elevated, a glucose tolerance test should be performed. If the patient has a past history of liver disease, a liver panel should be obtained to make certain that liver function is normal before OCs are started.

Drug interactions. Although synthetic sex steroids can retard the biotransformation of certain drugs (e.g., phenazone and meperidine) as a result of substrate competition, such interference is not important clinically. Oral contraceptive use has not been shown to inhibit the action of other drugs. However, some drugs can clinically interfere with the action of OCs by inducing liver enzymes that convert the steroids to more polar and less biologically active metabolites. Certain drugs have been shown to accelerate the biotransformation of steroids in the human. These include barbiturates, sulfonamides, cyclophosphamide, and rifampicin. Back et al.[3] have reported a relatively high incidence of OC failure in women ingesting rifampicin, and these two agents should not be given concurrently. The clinical data concerning OC failure in users of other antibiotics (e.g., penicillin, ampicillin, and sulfonamides), analgesics (e.g., phenytoin), and barbiturates are less clear. A few anecdotal studies have appeared in the literature, but reliable evidence for a clinical inhibitory effect of these drugs, such as occurs with rifampicin, is not available. Until controlled studies are performed, it would appear prudent when both agents are given simultaneously to suggest use of a barrier method in addition to the OCs because of possible interference with OC action by the action of the antibiotic or the gut flora. In addition, women with epilepsy requiring medication possibly should be treated with 50-μg estrogen formulations because a higher incidence of abnormal bleeding has been reported in these women with the use of lower-dose estrogen formulations.

Noncontraceptive health benefits. In addition to being the most effective method of contraception, OCs provide many other health benefits. Some are due to the fact that the combination OCs contain a potent, orally active progestin as well as an orally active estrogen and there is no time when the estrogenic target tissues are stimulated by estrogens without a gestagen (unopposed estrogen).

Both natural progesterone and the synthetic progestins inhibit the proliferative effect of estrogen, the so-called antiestrogenic effect. Estrogens increase the synthesis of both estrogen and progesterone receptors, whereas progesterone decreases their synthesis. Thus one mechanism whereby progesterone exerts its antiestrogenic effects is by decreasing the synthesis of estrogen receptors. Relatively little progestin is needed to do this, and the amount present in OCs is sufficient. Another way progesterone produces its antiestrogenic action is by stimulating the activity of the enzyme, estradiol 17β-dehydrogenase, within the endometrial cell. This enzyme converts the more potent estradiol to the less potent estrone, reducing estrogenic action within the cell.

Antiestrogenic action of progestins. As a result of the antiestrogenic action of the progestins in OCs, the height of the endometrium is less than that in an ovulatory cycle, and there is less proliferation of the glandular epithelium. These changes produce several substantial benefits for the oral contraceptive user. One is a reduction in the amount of blood loss at the time of endometrial shedding. In an ovulatory cycle the mean blood loss during menstruation is about 35 mL, compared with 20 mL for women ingesting OCs. This decreased blood loss makes the development of iron deficiency anemia less likely. Data from the Royal College of General Practitioners' study[19] showed that OC users were about half as likely to develop iron deficiency anemia as were the controls. Moreover, the beneficial effect persisted to a similar degree in women who had previously used OCs and then stopped them, probably because of an increase in the iron stores that remained for several years after the drug was discontinued.

Since the OCs produce regular withdrawal bleeding, it would be expected that OC users would have fewer menstrual disorders than controls. The results of the Royal College of General Practitioners' study confirmed the fact that OC users were significantly less likely to develop menorrhagia, irregular menstruation, or intermenstrual bleeding. Since these disorders are frequently treated by curettage and/or hysterectomy, OC users require these procedures less frequently.

Because progestins inhibit the proliferative effect of estrogens on the endometrium, women who use OCs have been found to be significantly less likely to develop adenocarcinoma of the endometrium.

Several studies have shown that OCs reduce the incidence of benign breast disease, and two prospective studies by Ory[36] and Brinton et al.[8] have indicated that this reduction is directly related to the amount of progestin in the compounds.

Data from the Oxford Study[8] indicate that current users of OCs have an 85% reduction in the incidence of fibroadenomas and 50% reductions in chronic cystic disease and nonbiopsied breast lumps, compared with controls using IUDs or diaphragms. The risk of developing these three diseases decreased with increased duration of OC use and persisted for about 1 year following discontinuation of OCs, after which no reduction in risk was observed.

Inhibition of ovulation. Other noncontraceptive medical benefits of OCs result from their main action, inhibition of ovulation. Some disorders, such as dysmenorrhea and premenstrual tension, occur much more frequently in ovulatory cycles than in anovulatory cycles. In fact, inhibition of ovulation by exogenous steroids has been used as therapy for severe dysmenorrhea for decades. The Royal College of General Practitioners' study[19] showed that OC users had 63% less dysmenorrhea and 29% less premenstrual tension than controls. Another study by Warner and Bancroft[55] indicated that OC users were less likely to have variation in the degree of feeling of well-being throughout the cycle than non-OC users.

Another serious adverse effect of ovulatory menstrual cycles is the development of functional ovarian cysts—specifically, follicular and luteal cysts—that frequently require laparotomy because of enlargement, rupture, or hemorrhage. When ovulation is inhibited, functional cysts do not usually develop. In a survey performed by the Boston Collaborative Drug Surveillance Program,[51] less than 2% of women with a discharge diagnosis of functional ovarian cysts were taking OCs, in contrast to 20% of controls. However, 20% of women with nonfunctional cysts were taking OCs, an incidence similar to that observed in the controls. Although investigators in one small series postulated that the formation of functional ovarian cysts may be increased in users of multiphasic OCs, the rate of hospitalization for ovarian cysts in the United States has remained unchanged following the widespread use of multiphasic formulations.

Another disorder linked to incessant ovulation is ovarian cancer, and the development of ovarian cancer is significantly reduced in OC users with a duration-dependent decrease in risk.

Other benefits. Several European studies, including the Royal College of General Practitioners' study,[19] showed that the risk of developing rheumatoid arthritis in OC users was only about half that in controls. Another benefit is protection against salpingitis, commonly referred to as PID. There have been at least 11 published epidemiologic studies estimating the relative risk of developing PID among OC users. Seven of these studies compared OC use to nonuse of any other contraception. As summarized by Sennayake and

Kramer,[41] the relative risk of developing PID among OC users in most of these studies was about 0.5%. It has been estimated that between 15% and 20% of women with cervical gonorrheal infection will develop salpingitis. In a Swedish study by Rydén et al.,[39] all cases of suspected salpingitis were confirmed by laparoscopic visualization 1 day after hospital admission. Of these who used contraception other than IUDs and oral steroids, 15% developed salpingitis; only about half as many, 8.8%, of those who used OCs developed salpingitis. The results of this study indicate that OCs reduce the clinical development of salpingitis in women with gonorrhea. Although the incidence of cervical infection with *C. trachomatis* is increased in OC users compared with controls, Wølner-Hanssen et al.[57] reported that the incidence of chlamydial salpingitis in OC users was only half that of controls. This protection may be related to the decreased duration of menstrual flow, which permits a smaller number of organisms to ascend to the upper genital tract and allows the body's defenses to eliminate them more easily. One sequela of PID is ectopic pregnancy, an entity that has tripled in incidence in the last decade. OCs reduce the risk of ectopic pregnancy by more than 90% in current users and may reduce the incidence in former users by decreasing their chance of developing salpingitis.

Ory[36] estimated that of 100,000 women in the United States using OCs each year, OC use will prevent 320 from developing iron deficiency anemia, 32 from developing rheumatoid arthritis, and 450 from developing PID that does not require hospitalization. In addition, there will be 150 fewer women hospitalized for PID, 235 fewer hospitalized for breast disease, 35 fewer hospitalized for ovarian tumors, and 117 fewer hospitalized for tubal pregnancies (Table 14-9). Ory[36] estimated that each year about 1 of every 750 women taking OCs will not require hospitalization for a serious disease she would have developed if she had not taken this drug. He estimated that use of OCs prevents 500,000 women from being hospitalized in the United States each year. Although this study was based on data obtained with higher-dose formulations, since the lower-dose agents contain a progestin that inhibits estrogenic mitotic activity and also inhibits ovulation, the scope and magnitude of beneficial effects should be similar with all combination formulations currently marketed. It is unfortunate that the infrequent adverse effects of OCs have received widespread publicity, whereas the more common noncontraceptive health benefits have attracted little attention.

Long-acting contraceptive steroids

Injectable suspensions. Three types of injectable steroid formulations are currently in use for contraception throughout the world. These include (1) depo-medroxyprogesterone acetate (DMPA), given in a dose of 150 mg every 3 months; (2) norethindrone enanthate (NET-EN), given in a dose of 200 mg every 2 months, and

Table 14-9. Hospitalization prevented annually by OC use

Disease	Rate (per 100,000 pill users)	No. of hospitalizations*
Benign breast disease	235	20,000
Ovarian retention cysts	35	3,000
Iron-deficiency anemia†	320	27,200
Pelvic inflammatory disease (first episodes)		
Total episodes†	600	51,000
Hospitalizations	156	13,300
Ectopic pregnancy	117	9,900
Rheumatoid arthritis†	32	2,700
Endometrial cancer‡	5	2,000
Ovarian cancer‡	4	1,700

From Ory HW: The noncontraceptive health benefits from oral contraceptive use. *Fam Plann Perspect* 14:182, 1982.
*Except where noted, figures refer to hospitalizations prevented among the estimated 8.5 million current OC users in the United States.
†Episodes prevented regardless of whether hospitalizations occurred.
‡Based on the estimated 39 million U.S. women who have ever used OCs.

(3) several once-a-month injections of combinations of different progestins and estrogens. It is estimated that about 5 million women are currently using injectable steroid formulations, twice the number who used them in 1985.

Depo-medroxyprogesterone acetate. DMPA is the most widely used injectable contraceptive and also the most widely studied. It is estimated that more than 15 million women have used DMPA since it was first made available for contraceptive use in the mid-1960s, and currently there are about 3.5 million users in the world. More than 1000 scientific articles have been written about DMPA. DMPA is approved for use as a contraceptive in more than 90 countries, including Sweden, France, Germany, and the United Kingdom. In the United States, the drug, which had originally been approved only for the treatment of endometrial cancer, has recently been approved for contraception.

DMPA is extremely effective. The failure rates in various studies range from 0.0 to 1.2/100 woman-years. In a large World Health Organization multiclinic study of 1587 users of DMPA,[62] the failure rate at the end of 1 year was only 0.1%, and at the end of 2 years, 0.4% (Table 14-10).

DMPA is formulated as a crystalline suspension. It should be given by injection in the upper outer quadrant of the gluteal region. The area should not be massaged, so that the drug is released slowly into the circulation. Administering the drug by this method should result in a very low failure rate.

Ortiz et al.[35] found that for a few days after the injection, MPA levels in the serum ranged from 1.5 to 3 ng/mL and gradually declined thereafter, reaching 0.2 ng/mL during the sixth month, and became undetectable about $7\frac{1}{2}$ to 9 months after administration.

Table 14-10. Net termination rates per 100 women in WHO study of DMPA and NET-EN

Reasons for termination	1-Year net cumulative event rates			2-Year net cumulative event rates		
	DMPA	NET-EN 60	NET-EN 60/84	DMPA	NET-EN 60	NET-EN 60/84
Pregnancy	0.1	0.4	0.6	0.4	0.4	1.4
Amenorrhea	11.9	6.8	8.4	24.2	14.7	14.6
Bleeding	15.0	13.6	13.7	18.8	18.4	21.8
Medical	11.8	13.7	12.7	15.0	16.0	16.7
Personal	20.7	24.5	22.8	38.8	42.6	40.2
TOTAL	51.4	49.7	50.3	73.5	70.7	72.4

From World Health Organization Expanded Programme of Research, Development and Research Training in Human Reproduction Task Force on Long-acting Systemic Agents for the Regulation of Fertility: *Contraception* 28:1, 1983.

Serum estradiol levels remained at early follicular phase levels for 4 to 6 months after the DMPA injection. When serum levels of MPA fell below 0.5 ng/mL, estradiol rose to preovulatory levels. Ovulation, however, as evidenced by elevated serum progesterone levels, did not occur, apparently because the LH peak was suppressed by inhibition of the positive feedback of estrogen upon its release. When serum MPA levels fell below 0.1 ng/mL, about 7 to 9 months after the injection, cyclic ovulatory ovarian function resumed. Thus the delay in ovulation after receiving injections of DMPA is due to prolonged MPA release and persists until serum levels of MPA become very low. The time required for the drug to disappear from the circulation after the last of several injections should be approximately the same as that following a single injection, because MPA is rapidly cleared from the blood stream. The prolonged presence in serum is related to the slow release from the injection site.

MPA acts by inhibiting the midcycle gonadotropin surge. Levels of LH and FSH remain in the follicular-phase range and are not completely suppressed. Mean estradiol levels remain relatively constant, about 40 pg/mL, for up to 5 years of treatment. These estradiol levels are higher than menopausal levels, and patients receiving DMPA do not develop signs or symptoms of estrogen deficiency such as vaginal atrophy, hot flushes, or decreased bone density. As a result of the high progestin and low estrogen levels, the endometrium becomes low lying and atrophic. The glands are narrow and widely spaced with deciduoid stroma. With this atrophic type of endometrium, most women treated with DMPA develop amenorrhea.

After treatment with DMPA is discontinued, about half of the women resume a regular cyclic menstrual pattern within 6 months, and about three fourths have regular menses within 1 year. When bleeding does resume after the effect of the last injection is dissipated, it is initially regular in about half the women and irregular in the remainder.

Additional side effects include slight weight gain; and, because of the long duration of action of the drug, there is a delay in return of fertility. Fertility rates have been calculated for fertile couples discontinuing various methods of contraception other than DMPA in order to conceive. At the end of 3 months, about 50% of these women are pregnant; at the end of a year, about 90% are pregnant. For DMPA users, the curve is shifted to the right, so the 50% pregnancy rate does not occur until after about a year, a delay of about 9 months compared with women discontinuing barrier methods.

Therefore, use of DMPA does not cause sterility, but causes a temporary period of infertility. A major benefit of the prolonged effect of the drug is that when patients do not return for their scheduled injections on time, but delay for 1 or 2 months, pregnancy rates remain very low. The incidence of failure to conceive and the interval to conception after stopping DMPA were similar among women who had used DMPA for various periods of time and received many or few injections of the drug.

Because DMPA does not increase liver globulin production as does the estrogen component of OCs (ethinyl estradiol), no alteration in blood clotting factors or angiotensinogen levels is associated with its use. Thus, unlike OCs, DMPA has not been associated with increases in hypertension or thromboembolism. A World Health Organization study[62] reported that blood pressure measurements were unchanged in DMPA users after 2 years of injections.

When glucose tolerance tests were performed on long-term DMPA users, a slight, statistically significant but clinically insignificant, impairment in glucose tolerance was observed when compared with that of a control group of women.

In a long-term cross-sectional study, Deslypere et al.[12] reported that long-term DMPA users have altered levels of serum lipids. Levels of triglycerides and high-density lipoprotein cholesterol but not total cholesterol were significantly lower in long-term users compared with controls of similar age. However, there was no significant difference in low-density lipoprotein cholesterol levels.

Concern has also been raised that DMPA may be associated with an increased incidence of abnormal cervical cytology. In a multinational case-control study conducted by the World Health Organization,[61] the adjusted relative risk for cervical cancer among women who had ever used DMPA compared with users of no contraception was 1.2 with confidence intervals of 0.4 to 1.5. This insignificantly increased risk showed no trend of increasing with increasing duration of use of DMPA, as has been observed in several studies of the relationship of OC use and cervical neoplasia. Thus the increased incidence of abnormal cervical cytology reported among DMPA users appears to be related to confounding factors, such as failure to use a diaphragm or sexual activity with many partners, because there is no evidence that the drug itself causes an increase in cervical dysplasia or carcinoma.

DMPA has been associated with an increased incidence of two types of carcinoma in animals but not in humans. When given in high doses to beagle dogs, it is associated with an increase in mammary cancer; however, beagles are poor models for study of steroid action in humans, because progestins are metabolized differently in the two species. Beagles develop a high incidence of breast carcinoma after receiving various types of progestins. After 25 years of study with this agent in humans, there is no evidence of an increased incidence of breast carcinoma. In the large World Health Organization study mentioned earlier, the relative risk of developing breast cancer among ever users of DMPA was 1.0.

In long-term monkey studies, two monkeys developed adenocarcinoma of the endometrium when treated with high doses of DMPA for 10 years; however, there is no evidence that DMPA produces endometrial cancer in humans. DMPA produces an atrophic endometrium, and actually is used to treat metastatic endometrial carcinoma. In the World Health Organization study the relative risk of developing endometrial cancer was 0.3. Nevertheless, concern about carcinogenicity in the animal studies prevented approval of this drug for use as a contraceptive in the United States for many years, despite the fact that it appears to have several noncontraceptive health benefits, similar to OCs. These benefits include a reduction in menstrual blood loss, and thus anemia; a probable decreased incidence of developing salpingitis, as most users are amenorrheic; and a decreased risk of developing endometrial and ovarian cancer, as DMPA is progestational and inhibits ovulation.

Norethindrone enanthate. NET-EN is an injectable progestogen that has been approved for contraceptive use in more than 40 countries, but not in the United States. It is administered in an oily suspension, and thus has pharmacodynamics different from those of DMPA.

Goebelsmann et al.[16] measured levels of norethindrone, FSH, LH, estradiol, and progesterone in a group of women for 6 months after a single injection of 200 mg of NET-EN. About 1 week after the injection, peak serum levels of norethindrone of 12 to 17 ng/mL were reached. These high serum levels lasted for about 3 weeks and decreased thereafter, first precipitously and then gradually. Serum levels of norethindrone of 4 ng/mL or more suppressed gonadotropin levels and follicular development. Norethindrone levels in this range persisted for approximately 1 to 2 months after the injection. With a further fall in norethindrone levels, follicular maturation, as determined by estradiol peaks, occurred. Nevertheless, these peaks were not followed by ovulation, because of inhibition of the positive feedback of estrogen as long as the serum norethindrone levels stayed above 1.8 ng/mL. Ovulation occurred at variable intervals in the subjects, when their norethindrone concentrations ranged from 0.1 to 1.8 ng/mL. Thus, a variability in the amount of norethindrone levels as well as inhibition of positive feedback was observed among different women. These findings indicate why some women conceive in the last few weeks of NET-EN therapy with an injection interval of 12 weeks.

Furthermore, if the woman does not return exactly when scheduled for a subsequent injection, the possibility of pregnancy increases greatly. In a comparative study done by the World Health Organization in 10 centers around the world in 1977,[61] at the end of 1 year the pregnancy rate with DMPA treatment was 0.7%, whereas that with NET-EN given every 12 weeks was 3.6%, significantly higher. Because the rate of discontinuation of therapy was higher with DMPA than with NET-EN, mainly because of amenorrhea, it was decided to administer the latter drug at more frequent intervals in an attempt to lower the pregnancy rate.

In a subsequent comparative study using DMPA and NET-EN, NET-EN was given every 60 days to one group of subjects; a second group received NET-EN every 60 days for the first 6 months, followed by every 84 days thereafter (Table 14-10). With both these regimens, at the end of 1 year the pregnancy rates with NET-EN were more comparable to the 0.1% rate found with DMPA: 0.4% for the 60-day regimen and 0.6% for the 60/84-day regimen. At the end of 2 years, the pregnancy rate for the 60-day regimen was still 0.4%, the same as with DMPA, whereas with the 60/84-day regimen it was 1.4%. For this reason, it is now recommended that NET-EN be given every 60 days for at least the first 6 months and no less often than every 12 weeks thereafter. The World Health Organization recommends that the drug be given at intervals no shorter than 46 days and no longer than 74 days.

NET-EN is also associated with irregular menstrual bleeding and few systemic effects other than weight gain. In the World Health Organization study, mean weight gain with both DMPA and NET-EN was approximately 1.8 kg at the end of 1 year and 3.3 kg at the end of 2 years. Fewer NET-EN users than DMPA users became amenorrheic and, at the end of 1 year, more women discontinued the use of DMPA for this reason than discontinued NET-EN. About 55% of DMPA users were amenorrheic at 1 year and 62% at 2 years, in contrast with about 30% and 40% of NET-EN users after the same periods. Nevertheless, total discontinuation rates for the two methods were similar at the end of 1 and 2 years, about 50% and 75%, respectively.

Progestin-estrogen injectable formulations. Various injectable combinations of estrogen and progestogens have been investigated. The two formulations most widely studied have been dihydroxyprogesterone acetophenide, 150 mg, with estradiol enanthate, 10 mg (Deladroxate, Perlutal); and medroxyprogesterone acetate, 50 or 25 mg, with estradiol cypionate, 10 or 5 mg (Cyclo-Provera). All of these formulations have an extremely high rate of effectiveness with no pregnancies being reported in nearly 23,000 cycles of use of the former formulation. These formulations cause less abnormal bleeding than do the injectable contraceptives without estrogen; however, not all subjects have regular cycles, and irregular bleeding and amenorrhea occur in some. Because of concerns about the toxicity of high doses of estrogen, as well as the need for monthly injections, these formulations are not available for use in most countries; however, they are widely used in Mexico and some other countries in Latin America. It is reported that other monthly injectable formulations, including one with 250 mg of 17α-hydroxyprogesterone caproate and 5 mg of estradiol valerate, are used in the People's Republic of China.

Subdermal implants. Subdermal implants of capsules made of polydimethylsiloxane (Silastic) containing levonorgestrel have been developed and patented by the Population Council as Norplant. Clinical trials of this long-acting, effective, reversible method of contraception were initiated in 1975. To date Norplant has been used by more than 500,000 women in 45 countries. It is currently approved for use by regulatory agencies of 15 countries and approval by the U.S. FDA was granted in 1991. As with all steroid-containing Silastic devices, the rate of steroid delivery is directly proportional to the surface area of the capsules, whereas duration of action depends on the amount of steroid within the capsules. To produce effective blood levels of norgestrel, it was found necessary to use six capsules filled with crystalline levonorgestrel. The cylindric capsules are 3.4 cm long and 2.4 mm in outer diameter with the ends sealed with Silastic medical adhesive. Each capsule contains 36 mg of crystalline levonorgestrel for a total amount of 216 mg in each six-capsule set.

Insertion is performed in an outpatient area, and the entire procedure takes about 5 minutes. After infiltration of the skin with local anesthesia, a small (3 mm) incision is made with a scalpel, usually in the upper arm, although the lower arm and the inguinal and gluteal regions have also been used. The capsules are implanted into the subcutaneous tissue in a radial pattern through a large (10- to 12-gauge) trocar, and the incision is closed with adhesive. Stitches are not necessary. Because polydimethylsiloxane is not biodegradable, the capsules have to be removed through another incision when desired by the user or at the end of 5 years, which is the duration of maximal contraceptive effectiveness.

After insertion, blood levels of levonorgestrel rise rapidly to reach levels between 400 and 500 pg/mL in 24 hours. The serum levels remain relatively constant during the first year of use, with a mean of about 400 pg/mL, which is usually sufficient to inhibit ovulation. When the amount of steroid was measured in capsules removed from patients after various times, it was found that the rate of release was fairly constant during the first year of use, averaging about 50 μg of levonorgestrel per day from the six-capsule set. From about the end of the first year of use until 8 years of use, daily release rates decline to about 30 μg/d, but remain constant during this time interval. Mean serum levels of levonorgestrel also decline slightly beyond the third year of use and average about 300 pg/mL.

With this low level of levonorgestrel, gonadotropin levels are not completely suppressed, and follicular activity results in periodic peaks of estradiol. Since the level of circulating levonorgestrel is usually sufficient to inhibit the positive feedback effect of these estradiol peaks upon LH release, LH levels are lower, even in Norplant users with regular cycles, and ovulation occurs infrequently.

The major side effect of Norplant use is the irregular pattern of uterine bleeding. Other alterations in uterine blood flow involve changes in duration and volume, with most bleeding episodes being scanty in amount. About half the bleeding episodes can be characterized as fairly regular, with the interval between bleeding episodes ranging between 21 and 35 days; about 40% as irregular, with intervals outside this range; and about 10% as amenorrheic, with no bleeding for more than a 3-month interval. Because of the high incidence of bleeding irregularities, potential Norplant users must be thoroughly counseled about this potential problem prior to insertion. Bleeding episodes tend to be more prolonged and irregular during the first year of use, after which there is greater frequency of a more regular pattern occurring. The mean number of days of bleeding also declines steadily with time from 54.3 days in the first year to 44.1 days in the fifth year. Mean total blood loss in Norplant users is about 25 mL/mo, slightly less than the average monthly blood loss of normally cycling women. Several clinical studies have shown that the mean hemoglobin concentration in the first 3 years of Norplant use tends to rise slightly. Sivin[43] reported that even women who stop using the method because of bleeding problems have been found to have an increase in hemoglobin levels. When pregnancies occur in Norplant users they nearly always occur in women with a recent history of regular cyclic uterine bleeding. Thus women who are amenorrheic or have infrequent episodes of uterine bleeding do not need to be monitored by periodic pregnancy tests.

Other problems associated with this method of contraception include infection, local irritation, or painful reaction at the insertion site. Occasionally expulsion of a capsule occurs, usually in association with infection. The incidence of insertion site infection is less than 1%. Headache is the single most frequent medical problem causing removal of the implants, accounting for about 30% of the medical reasons for removal. Weight gain was a common reason for medical removal in U.S. studies, whereas weight loss was more common in the Dominican Republic. Other medical problems among Norplant users include acne, mastalgia, and mood changes, including anxiety, depression, and nervousness. Since ovarian follicular development without subsequent ovulation is common among Norplant users, adnexal enlargement due to persistent unruptured follicles has been noted during routine biannual pelvic examination of many Norplant users. These enlarged follicles, which may reach 5 to 7 cm in diameter, usually regress spontaneously in 1 to 2 months without therapy.

The removal process, like the insertion procedure, is performed in the clinic area using local anesthesia and a small skin incision. Removal of Norplant is more difficult than insertion because fibrous tissue develops around the implant and must be cut before removing it. It is important that the capsules be inserted superficially to enhance the ease of removal. Deeply implanted capsules are more difficult to remove.

After removal of the implant the incision is closed without stitches and a pressure dressing is applied for about 24 hours after removal. If the woman wishes to continue use, another set of capsules can be inserted through the same incision or in the opposite arm. If another set of capsules is not inserted after removal, the steroid is cleared rapidly from the circulation and serum levels of norgestrel fall rapidly, reaching nearly undetectable levels in 96 hours. If pregnancy is desired, return of ovulation is prompt and is similar to that in women discontinuing nonhormonal methods of reversible contraception, reaching 50% at 3 months and 86% at 1 year.

Continuation rates with the Norplant method of contraception are very high, ranging from 76% to 99% at 1 year in different countries and from 33% to 78% at 5 years. These high continuation rates are similar to those observed with IUDs and are due in large part to the fact that in order to discontinue use these methods require the user to return to the clinic. This is the main reason why Norplant implants and IUDs have the highest continuation rates of any methods of contraception in use today.

Postcoital contraception

Estrogen compounds. Various estrogenic compounds have been used for postcoital contraception (PCC), or what is commonly referred to as the "morning-after pill." The estrogen compounds that have been most commonly used by various investigators for this purpose include diethylstilbestrol (DES), 25 to 50 mg/d; ethinyl estradiol, 5 mg/d; and conjugated estrogens, 30 mg/d. Treatment is continued for 5 days. If it is begun within 72 hours after an isolated midcycle act of coitus, its effectiveness is very good. If more than one episode of coitus occurred, or if treatment is initiated later than 72 hours after coitus, the method is much less effective.

Table 14-11. Observed and expected pregnancies according to various methods of postcoital contraception

Treatment	No. of studies	Total no. of patients considered	No. of observed pregnancies	Pregnancy rate (%)
Ethinyl estradiol: high dosage	4	3168	19	0.6
Other estrogens: high dosage	2	975	11	1.1
Ethinyl estradiol + *dl*-norgestrel	11	3802	69	1.8
Danazol	3	998	20	2.0
IUD	9	879	1	0.1

From Fasoli M et al: *Contraception* 39:459, 1989.
χ_4^2 for heterogeneity = 35.31; $P < .001$.

Fasoli et al.[15] performed a comprehensive literature review in 1989 and summarized the results of the 21 articles published in English, Italian, and French between 1975 and 1977 on the subject of PCC. In the six studies of high-dose estrogen, 4143 women were included and the majority, 3168, received ethinyl estradiol. Pregnancy rates among the women treated with ethinyl estradiol were 0.6%; DES, 0.7%; and conjugated estrogen, 1.6% (Table 14-11). None of these rates were significantly different from the overall mean failure rate of 0.7%. None of the trials included a control group, but it has been estimated that the clinical pregnancy rate after midcycle coitus is about 7%. Thus high-dose estrogen is an effective method of PCC.

Antiprogestins. A few years ago Baulieu[4] synthesized a progestogenic steroid compound that had weak progestational activity but marked affinity for progesterone receptors in the endometrium. This compound, called RU 486 or mefisterone, because of its high receptor affinity prevented progesterone from binding to its receptors and thus had an antiprogesterone action. In clinical trials it was found that, if a single 600-mg dose of RU 486 was administered orally in early pregnancy, prior to 6 weeks after the onset of the last menses, about 85% of the pregnancies were terminated spontaneously. When this treatment was combined with administration of a prostaglandin 36 to 48 hours later, the efficacy of pregnancy termination increased to 96%. However, side effects include nausea, vomiting, and abdominal pain. The main disadvantage of this method is prolonged and sometimes heavy vaginal bleeding that on occasion can cause anemia, necessitating a blood transfusion and possibly curettage. The mean duration of bleeding after administration of this drug is about 12 days when administered alone, and 9 days when used with a prostaglandin. Currently distribution of this drug is limited to France, but compounds with similar activity or steroid enzyme inhibitors that prevent progesterone synthesis are also being studied.

STERILIZATION

In 1988 in the United States sterilization of one member of a couple was the most widely used method of preventing pregnancy. The popularity of sterilization was greatest if (1) the wife was over age 30 years, (2) the couple had been married for more than 10 years, and (3) the couple desired no additional children. In contrast to the other methods of contraception, which are reversible or temporary, sterilization should be considered permanent. Although anastomosis after vasectomy or tubal ligation is possible, the reconstructive operation is much more difficult than the original sterilizing procedure, and the results are variable. Pregnancy rates after anastomosis of the vas range from 45% to 60%, whereas those following oviduct anastomosis range from 50% to 80%, depending on the amount of tissue damage associated with the original procedure, as well as technical competency.

Voluntary sterilization is legal in all 50 states, and the decision to be sterilized should be made solely by the patient in consultation with the physician. Since all currently available sterilization procedures require surgical techniques, patients who request sterilization should be counseled regarding both the risks and the irreversibility of the procedures. It is advisable to fully inform the patient, and the spouse if possible, of the benefits and risks of these surgical procedures. In addition, it is useful to have more than one counselor when sterilization is requested by a woman younger than age 25 years, as well as a woman under age 40 years without any children.

The rational of such careful scrutiny of younger candidates for sterilization is that they tend to change their minds more often, their attitudes may be less fixed, and they face a longer period of reproductive life during which divorce, remarriage, or death among their children can occur. About 1% of sterilized women subsequently request reversal. In the United States approximately 7000 women request reversal each year.

The most effective, least destructive method of tubal occlusion is the most desirable in younger patients, since ovarian dysfunction and adhesion formation are diminished, whereas the incidence of successful reversal procedures is increased. The effective laparoscopic band techniques or the modified technique should be used in patients who are younger than age 25 years. Reversal after this method of sterilization is followed by pregnancy in about 75% of cases, a rate that is higher than that reported after most laparoscopic fulgurations, when more tube is destroyed.

Male sterilization

Sterilization of men is performed by vasectomy, an outpatient procedure that takes about 20 minutes and requires only local anesthesia. The vas deferens is isolated and cut. The ends of the vas are closed, either by ligation or by fulguration; they are then replaced in the scrotal sac, and the incision is closed. Complications of vasectomy include hematoma (in up to 5% of subjects), sperm granulomas (inflammatory responses to sperm leakage), and spontaneous anastomosis (if this is to occur, it usually does so within a short time after the procedure). Hematoma is best prevented by ligating all small vessels in the scrotal wall. The occurrence of sperm granuloma is minimized by cauterizing or fulgurating the ends of the vas instead of ligating them. After the procedure the man is not considered sterile until two sperm-free ejaculates have been produced. Semen analysis should be performed 1 and 2 months after the procedure. It usually requires about 15 to 20 ejaculations after the operation before the man is sterile. Although in the United States requests range from 6% to 7%, vas anastomosis is a difficult and meticulous procedure that has a success rate of about 50%.

Female sterilization

Sterilization of women is more complicated, requiring a transperitoneal incision and, usually, general anesthesia. Postpartum sterilization is performed by making a small infraumbilical incision and performing either a Pomeroy or modified Irving-type of tubal ligation. These simple and rapid procedures can be performed either in the delivery room immediately after delivery or in the operating room the following day without prolonging the patient's hospital stay. The same operative techniques can be used for female sterilization at times other than the puerperium, but additional techniques are also used for what has been termed interval sterilization. Ligation of the oviducts by the Pomeroy technique can be performed easily and rapidly through a small abdominal incision. The latter has been termed minilaparotomy. On occasion a colpotomy incision may also be used, but this incision is associated with a higher incidence of postoperative infection.

The development of fiberoptic light sources has made laparoscopy a popular gynecologic operative technique. By using various accessories, in addition to the laparoscope, the operator can fulgurate and cut the oviducts without making an intraperitoneal incision other than one or two small punctures. Most gynecologists find the two-puncture technique for laparoscopic sterilization easier to learn and perform than the single-puncture technique. General anesthesia is usually used for laparoscopic sterilization, but overnight hospitalization is unnecessary. The failure rate with this technique is about 1/1000 procedures. Because the pregnancy rate after fulguration and transection is similar to that after fulguration alone, it is now recommended that the oviducts not be cut after fulguration. The incidence of complications after laparoscopic fulguration ranges from 1% to 6%; major complications (hemorrhage, puncture, or cautery of bowel) occur in about 0.6% of cases.

In an attempt to eliminate the problem of bowel injury, bipolar forceps were developed to replace the unipolar apparatus, which has a grounding plate attached to the patient through which the current passes. In the bipolar system, the current passes from one prong of the forceps, through the tissue, to the other prong, thus producing a limited coagulation with destruction of a small segment of the oviduct. After coagulation, if division is to be performed, scissors are introduced to cut the oviduct. If division is not to be performed, some operators perform a coagulation of two or three contiguous burns on each oviduct to ensure adequate obliteration of the lumen. When the unipolar apparatus is used, a single 1-cm burn on each oviduct is sufficient. However, even with this small amount of coagulation, damage is extensive and attempts at anastomosis have a very low rate of success. Because bipolar coagulation not only is safer but also is associated with a higher success rate after reversal of sterilization, this technique is now preferred.

Because of the problems of electrocoagulation, efforts have been made to develop safer methods that destroy less tissue. Nonelectrical tubal occlusion techniques that may be performed through the laparoscope are those using the tantalum, plastic, spring-loaded clips, and the Silastic band (Falope ring). All of these techniques require a modification of the conventional laparoscope, as well as specialized training in their use. The failure rate for the clip and band technique is about 2/1000 procedures, with a range of 1 to 6/1000.

INDUCED ABORTION

Induced abortion is one of the most common gynecologic operations performed in the United States and in many other countries. As determined by the landmark *Roe v. Wade* Supreme Court decision, states may not interfere with the practice of abortion in the first trimester. In the second trimester, states may regulate abortion services in the interest of preserving the health of the woman. However, restrictions limiting the performance of second-trimester abortions to a hospital have been declared unconstitutional.

From 1973 through 1980, the number of legal abortions performed annually in the United States increased steadily, but has remained relatively stable since then. The annual variation has been less than 3% each year from 1980 to 1988. In 1988 there were an estimated 1.6 million elective abortions performed in the United States. The abortion ratio (number of abortions per 100 pregnancies) was 28.8 and the abortion rate (number of abortions per 1000 women of reproductive age) was 27.3. About one third of abortions are performed in women under age 20 years, another third in women aged 20 to 24 years, and the remaining third among women aged 25 and older. Only one fourth of abortions are obtained by married women. Ninety percent of abortions are performed within the first 12 weeks of pregnancy, and about 50% of abortions are performed during the first 8 weeks of pregnancy.

Methods

Three principal methods are used for elective abortion: transcervical evacuation, induction of labor, and major operations. Suction curettage is the predominant method of performing abortion in the United States, accounting for about 85% of all abortion procedures; the remainder are performed by dilation and evacuation (D&E) (curettage techniques in the second trimester), induction of labor, and major operations.

Transcervical evacuation

Vacuum aspiration. Curettage by vacuum aspiration is the predominant method of performing abortion in the first trimester. Very early in pregnancy, endometrial aspiration, also termed menstrual extraction, can be done with a small, flexible plastic cannula without dilation or anesthesia. Abortions performed 8 weeks or more after the last menstrual period generally require dilation of the cervix and some type of anesthesia, either local or general.

Dilation of the cervix can be facilitated by use of osmotic dilators. These are usually placed in the cervical canal for several hours to overnight to produce gradual dilation. The traditional method has been use of *Laminaria japonica*—seaweed sticks. Synthetic osmotic dilators include a polyvinyl alcohol sponge impregnated with magnesium sulfate and a hygroscopic plastic polymer. Use of such osmotic dilators in nulliparous women substantially reduces the risk of uterine trauma such as perforation and cervical injury.

Dilation and evacuation. D&E is the predominant method of abortion used beyond the first trimester. Since larger cervical dilation is usually needed, osmotic dilators are usually inserted for a period of several hours or several days prior to the procedure. Although recent data are lacking, early studies suggested that D&E was substantially safer than induction of labor or major operations for abortions at 13 to 16 weeks of gestation. For later abortions, D&E and induction of labor appear to have comparable risks of morbidity and mortality, although the range of complications varies by technique. Disadvantages of D&E include the greater technical expertise required, the emotional burden for participating physicians and medical personnel, and possible long-term effects on the cervix. Advantages include less emotional stress for the patient, avoidance of the need for hospitalization, greater convenience, and lower cost.

Induction of labor. Second-trimester abortion is also performed by induction of labor. One technique involved instillation of hypertonic solutions into the amniotic cavity. The solution most commonly used was hypertonic saline (200 mL of 20% saline), although hypertonic glucose and urea were also used. Labor usually started within 12 to 24 hours, and abortion occurred within a few hours thereafter. Use of ancillary agents such as *Laminaria* or oxytocin facilitate the procedure; however, instillation of hypertonic solutions is used infrequently today.

Two prostaglandin compounds have been used increasingly for inducing labor in the second trimester. One, prostaglandin E_2, is administered as a vaginal suppository; the other, 15-methyl prostaglandin $F_{2\alpha}$, is administered as an intramuscular injection. Both techniques have the advantage of easy administration. Each compound is given at 2- to 3-hour intervals until evacuation of the gestational material is achieved. Disadvantages include gastrointestinal side effects and—with the prostaglandin E_2 suppositories—fever and chills.

Major operations. Hysterotomy and hysterectomy are infrequently used for performing abortion in the United States. Both procedures have a much higher risk of morbidity and mortality than the alternative methods. Hysterectomy should be reserved for those situations in which preexisting gynecologic pathology, such as carcinoma in situ of the cervix or large leiomyomas, also exists.

Ancillary techniques

Pregnancy tests should be performed on all patients before abortion is carried out unless there is ultrasound evidence of pregnancy. Performing a qualitative pregnancy test 2 weeks after the procedure will ensure that the pregnancy has been successfully aborted. In the first trimester, ultrasound is usually reserved for determining gestational age when a substantial discrepancy occurs between menstrual history and clinical examination or when other uterine pathology, such as leiomyomas, is present. Routine preoperative ultrasound before second-trimester abortions has avoided the problem of misestimation of gestational age, which is an important cause of complications. Performing ultrasonography during D&E may facilitate the procedure.

Complications

Elective abortion in the United States is a very safe operation. Complications are infrequent, and the overall mortality rate is less than 1/100,000 procedures. Two important determinants of complications are the gestational age and method of abortion chosen. Abortions at 6 weeks and less have slightly higher complication rates than do abortions at 7 to 10 weeks. Thereafter, abortion complication rates increase progressively with gestational age. Suction curettage is the safest method of abortion, followed by D&E, induction of labor, and major operations.

The most common complication is infection, and the routine use of preoperative antibiotic prophylaxis has proven to be effective in reducing this risk. Other complications include hemorrhage, the consequences of uterine perforation, and anesthetic hazards.

CONCLUSION

When giving advice about contraception, the clinician should explain to partners of the couple the advantages and disadvantages of each method, so that they will be fully informed and can rationally choose the method most suitable for them. Because no contraceptive method other than use of the condom or vasectomy has as yet been developed for the male partner, the contraceptive provider generally counsels the female partner; he or she should inform her if there are medical reasons that contraindicate the use of certain methods and offer her alternatives.

REFERENCES

1. Alvarez F et al: New insights on the mode of action of intrauterine contraceptive devices in women, *Fertil Steril* 49:768, 1988.
2. Anderson ABM et al: Reduction of menstrual blood loss by prostaglandin synthetase inhibitors, *Lancet* 1:774, 1976.
3. Back DJ et al: The effects of rifampicin on the pharmacokinetics of ethinylestradiol in women, *Contraception* 21:135, 1980.
4. Baulieu EE: Contraception with RU 486: a new approach to postovulatory fertility control, *Acta Obstet Gynecol Scand Suppl* 149:5, 1989.
5. Bracken MB, Hellenbrand KG, Holford TR: Conception delay after oral contraceptive use: the effect of estrogen dose, *Fertil Steril* 53:21, 1990.
6. Bracken MB, Vita K: Frequency of non-hormonal contraception around conception and association with congenital malformations in offspring, *Am J Epidemiol* 117:281, 1983.
7. Brenner PF et al: Serum levels of d-norgestrel, luteinizing hormone, follicle-stimulating hormone, estradiol, and progesterone in women during and following ingestion of combination oral contraceptives containing d-norgestrel, *Am J Obstet Gynecol* 129:133, 1977.
8. Brinton LA et al: Risk factors for benign breast disease, *Am J Epidemiol* 113:203, 1981.
9. Chi I-c et al: Performance of the copper T-380A intrauterine device in breastfeeding women, *Contraception* 39:603, 1989.
10. Conant MA, Spicer DW, Smith CD: Herpes simplex virus transmission: condom studies, *Sex Transm Dis* 11:94, 1984.
11. Cramer DW et al: Tubal infertility and the intrauterine device, *N Engl J Med* 312:941, 1985.
12. Deslypere JP, Thiery M, Vermeulen A: Effect of long-term hormonal contraception on plasma lipids, *Contraception* 31:633, 1985.
13. Dorflinger L: Relative potency of progestins used in oral contraceptives, *Contraception* 31:557, 1985.
14. Edelman DA, North BB: Updated pregnancy rates for the Today contraceptive sponge, *Am J Obstet Gynecol* 157:1164, 1987.
15. Fasoli M et al: Post-coital contraception: an overview of published studies, *Contraception* 39:459, 1989.
16. Goebelsmann U et al: Serum norethindrone (NET) concentrations following intramuscular NET enanthate injection: effect upon serum LH, FSH, estradiol and progesterone, *Contraception* 19:283, 1979.
17. Guillebaud J: Copper IUDs and pregnancy, *Br J Fam Plann* 7:88, 1981 (letter).
18. Kay CR: Progestins and arterial disease: evidence from the Royal College of General Practitioners' study, *Am J Obstet Gynecol* 142:762, 1982.
19. Kay CR: The Royal College of General Practitioners' Oral Contraception Study: some recent observations, *Clin Obstet Gynaecol* 11:759, 1984.
20. Kjos SL et al: Effect of low-dose oral contraceptives on carbohydrate and lipid metabolism in women with recurrent gestational diabetes: results of a controlled randomized prospective study, *Am J Obstet Gynecol* 163:1882, 1990.
21. Kovacs GT et al: The contraceptive diaphragm: is it an acceptable method in the 1980's?, *Aust N Z J Obstet Gynaecol* 26:76, 1986.
22. Lee NC, Rubin GL: The intrauterine device and pelvic inflammatory disease revisited: new results from the women's health study, *Obstet Gynecol* 72:1, 1988.
23. Lee NC et al: Type of intrauterine device and the risk of pelvic inflammatory disease, *Obstet Gynecol* 62:1, 1983.
24. Linn S et al: Lack of association between contraceptive usage and congenital malformations in offspring, *Am J Obstet Gynecol* 147:923, 1983.
25. Lönnerdel B, Forsum E, Hambraeus L: Effect of oral contraceptives on composition and volume of breast milk, *Am J Clin Nutr* 33:816, 1980.

26. Louik C et al: Maternal exposure to spermicides in relation to certain birth defects, *N Engl J Med* 317:474, 1987.

27. Makinen JI et al: Encouraging rates of fertility after ectopic pregnancy, *Int J Fertil* 34:46, 1989.

28. McIntyre SL, Higgins JE: Parity and use-effectiveness with the contraceptive sponge, *Am J Obstet Gynecol* 155:796, 1986.

29. Medina JE et al: Comparative evaluation of two methods of natural family planning in Colombia, *Am J Obstet Gynecol* 138:1142, 1980.

30. Mishell DR Jr, Roy S: Copper intrauterine contraceptive device event rates following insertion 4 to 8 weeks postpartum, *Am J Obstet Gynecol* 143:29, 1982.

31. Mishell DR Jr et al: The intrauterine device: a bacteriologic study of the endometrial cavity, *Am J Obstet Gynecol* 96:119, 1966.

32. Mosher WE, Pratt WF: *Contraceptive use in the United States, 1973–88,* United States Department of Health and Human Services, National Center for Health Statistics, US Public Health Service Pub No. 90-1250, Washington, DC, 1988, US Government Printing Office.

33. Moyer DL, Mishell DR Jr: Reactions of human endometrium to the intrauterine foreign body, II: long-term effects on the endometrial histology and cytology, *Am J Obstet Gynecol* 111:66, 1971.

34. Nilsson S et al: Long-term follow-up of children breast-fed by mothers using oral contraceptives, *Contraception* 34:443, 1986.

35. Ortiz A et al: Serum medroxyprogesterone acetate (MPA) concentrations and ovarian function following intramuscular injection of depo-MPA, *J Clin Endocrinol Metab* 44:32, 1977.

36. Ory HW: The noncontraceptive health benefits from oral contraceptive use, *Fam Plann Perspect* 14:182, 1982.

37. Poland B: Conception control and embryonic development, *Am J Obstet Gynecol* 106:365, 1970.

38. Rogow D, Rintoul EJ, Greenwood S: A year's experience with a fertility awareness program: a report, *Adv Plann Parent* 15:27, 1980.

39. Rydén G et al: Do contraceptives influence the incidence of acute pelvic inflammatory disease in women with gonorrhoea?, *Contraception* 20:149, 1979.

40. Sandvei R, Ulstein M, Wollen A-L: Fertility following ectopic pregnancy with special reference to previous use of an intra-uterine contraceptive device (IUCD), *Acta Obstet Gynecol Scand* 66:131, 1987.

41. Sennayake P, Kramer DG: Contraception and the etiology of pelvic inflammatory disease: new perspectives, *Am J Obstet Gynecol* 138:852, 1980.

42. Sivin I: Copper T IUD use and ectopic pregnancy rates in the United States, *Contraception* 19:151, 1979.

43. Sivin I: International experience with Norplant® and Norplant®-2, *Stud Fam Plann* 19:81, 1988.

44. Sivin I, Tatum HJ: Four years of experience with the T Cu 380A intrauterine contraceptive device, *Fertil Steril* 36:159, 1981.

45. Tatum HJ, Schmidt FH, Jain AK: Management and outcome of pregnancies associated with the copper T intrauterine contraceptive device, *Am J Obstet Gynecol* 126:869, 1976.

46. Tredway DR, Umezaki CU, Mishell DR Jr: Effect of intrauterine devices on sperm transport in the human being: preliminary report, *Am J Obstet Gynecol* 123:734, 1975.

47. Trussell J, Kost K: Contraceptive failure in the United States: a critical review of the literature, *Stud Fam Plann* 18:237, 1987.

48. Trussell J et al: Contraceptive failure in the United States: an update, *Stud Fam Plann* 21:51, 1990.

49. Vessey M, Lawless M, Yagi J: Contraceptive failure in the United States: estimates from the 1982 National Survey of Family Growth, *Fam Plann Perspect* 18:200, 1986.

50. Vessey M, Lawless M, Yeates D: Efficacy of different contraceptive methods, *Lancet* 1:841, 1982.

51. Vessey M et al: Ovarian neoplasma, functional ovarian cysts, and oral contraceptives, *Br Med J* 294:1518, 1987.

52. Vessey MP et al: Fertility after stopping use of intrauterine contraceptive device, *Br Med J* 286:106, 1983.

53. Vessey MP et al: Mortality among oral contraceptive users: 20 year follow up of women in a cohort study, *Br Med J* 299:1487, 1989.

54. Wade ME et al: A randomized prospective study of the use-effectiveness of two methods of natural family planning. Paper presented at the International Federation for Family Life Promotion Second International Congress, Navan, Ireland, Sept 24-Oct 1, 1980.

55. Warner P, Bancroft J: Mood, sexuality, oral contraceptives and the menstrual cycle, *J Psychosom Res* 32:417, 1988.

56. White MK et al: Intrauterine device termination rates and the menstrual cycle day of insertion, *Obstet Gynecol* 55:220, 1980.

57. Wølner-Hanssen P et al: Laparoscopic findings and contraceptive use in women with signs and symptoms suggestive of acute salpingitis, *Obstet Gynecol* 66:233, 1985.

58. World Health Organization: A prospective multicentre trial of the ovulation method of natural family planning, II: the effectiveness phase, *Fertil Steril* 36:591, 1981.

59. World Health Organization: A prospective multicentre trial of the ovulation method of natural family planning, III: characteristics of the menstrual cycle and of the fertile phase, *Fertil Steril* 40:773, 1983.

60. World Health Organization [WHO]: The TCu220C, multiload 250 and Nova T IUDs at 3, 5, and 7 years of use: results from three randomized multicentre trials, *Contraception* 42:141, 1990.

61. World Health Organization Expanded Programme of Research, Development and Research Training in Human Reproduction Task Force on Long-Acting Systemic Agents for the Regulation of Fertility: Multinational comparative clinical evaluation of two long-acting injectable contraceptive steroids: norethisterone enanthate and medroxyprogesterone acetate, I: use-effectiveness, *Contraception* 15:5, 1977.

62. World Health Organization Expanded Programme of Research, Development and Research Training in Human Reproduction Task Force on Long-Acting Systemic Agents for the Regulation of Fertility: Multinational comparative clinical evaluation of two long-acting injectable contraceptive steroids: norethisterone enanthate and medroxyprogesterone acetate: final report, *Contraception* 28:1, 1983.

Chapter 15

METABOLIC EFFECTS OF ORAL CONTRACEPTIVES

Howard A. Zacur M.D., Ph.D.
and Edward E. Wallach, M.D.

Since the introduction of the combination oral-contraceptive pill in the 1960s, millions of women worldwide have used and continue to use this medication to prevent pregnancy. When the pill (Enovid) was introduced in 1960, it contained 150 µg of the estrogen, mestranol, and 9.85 mg of the progestogen, norethynodrel. Publications suggesting that use of the combination contraceptive pill could result in thrombosis and thromboembolism, causing cerebrovascular accidents,[15, 54] preceded efforts to reduce the estrogen component of the pill by 76-80%. The well-known increased risk of thrombosis during pregnancy, coupled with a documented increase in the plasma concentrations of blood-clotting factors following pill administration, focused attention on the estrogenic component of the pill. However, lowering the estrogen content of the combi-

nation pill to reduce side effects needed to be balanced against the risk that this could cause contraceptive failure. The resulting efforts to create a contraceptive pill for the general population that maximized pill benefits while minimizing risks have been quite successful. However, it is still not entirely possible to identify who, among "normal" women, might be at risk of complications from contraceptive pill use. When different "normal" individuals ingest the same formulation of an oral-contraceptive pill, vast differences exist in measured plasma levels of steroids contained in the pill among these subjects.[99] Only 28% of this variation among users can be explained by such variables as day of cycle, race, age, weight, height, blood pressure, and cigarette or alcohol use.[99] It is the intent of this chapter to review the pharmacology of oral-contraceptive pill use and to discuss in some detail the metabolic consequences of pill use on coagulation, and lipid and carbohydrate metabolism. This is to improve the understanding of the specific components that might cause adverse reactions in patients who use this medication.

METABOLISM OF CONTRACEPTIVE-PILL STEROIDS

Virtually all contraceptive pills prescribed today contain ethinyl estradiol as the estrogen. Mestranol (the 3-methyl ether of ethinyl estradiol), the estrogen contained in the original pill prototypes (e.g., Enovid, Ortho-Novum), can be found in some brands today (see Chapter 14 and Fig. 15-1). Mestranol itself has limited biological activity and must first be metabolized within the body to achieve biological activity. Both mestranol and ethinyl estradiol possess an ethinyl group at the C-17 position of the steroid molecule (see Fig. 15-1). Existence of this chemical moiety facilitates absorption while inhibiting hydroxylation at C-16, a step that increases the solubility of the molecule and thus, its excretion. When mestranol is taken orally, it must be demethylated at C-3 to become biologically active. Hydrolysis of the methyl ethyl group at the C-3 position converts mestranol into ethinyl estradiol. Rates of conversion of mestranol molecules into ethinyl estradiol mol-

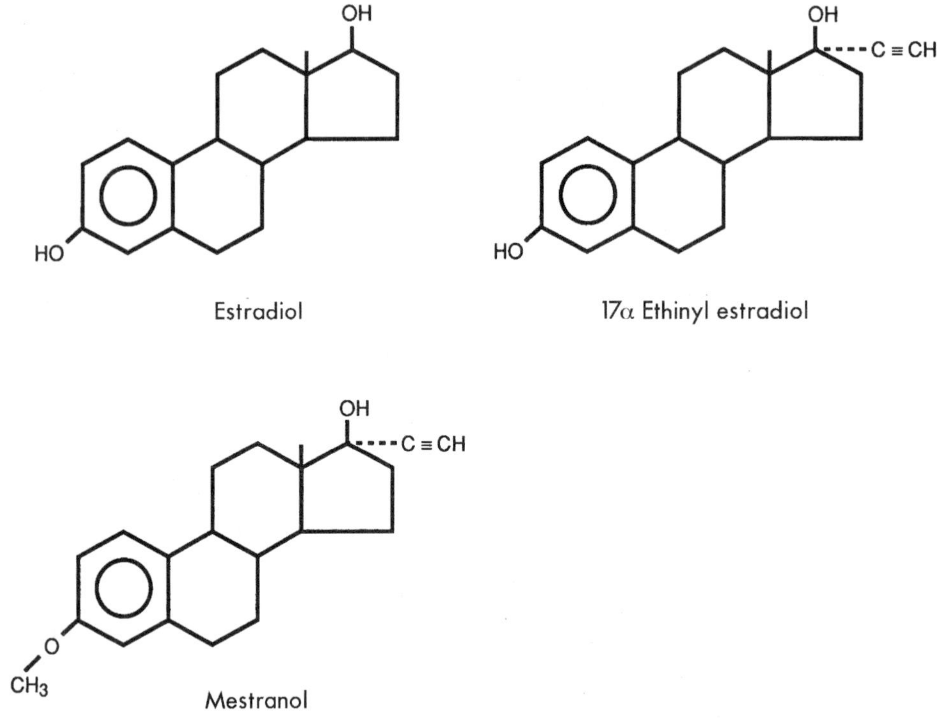

Estradiol

17α Ethinyl estradiol

Mestranol

Fig. 15-1. The structures of the estrogens ethinyl estradiol and mestranol contained in combination oral contraceptive pills compared with estradiol.

ecules within the human body have been reported to range from 50-97%.

Mestranol was initially included in the manufacture of the first oral-contraceptive pills by virtue of an inadvertent occurrence. Early pill formulations utilizing norethynodrel as the progestational agent resulted in less breakthrough bleeding because of an "impurity" formed during its synthesis, namely mestranol.[85] Only later did it become apparent that mestranol was a weaker estrogen than ethinyl estradiol.[28] Until that discovery was made, mestranol was consistently incorporated as the estrogen in pill formulations. When taken orally, ethinyl estradiol is rapidly absorbed by the upper gastrointestinal (GI) tract. This site of absorption is reflected by the comparison of plasma contraceptive steroid levels found in women who have undergone an ileostomy[45] with women who have not. The ethinyl estradiol molecule is absorbed as a free steroid, or may undergo initial conjugation with a sulfate group at the C-3 position (Fig. 15-2). Rapid uptake into the portal bloodstream occurs following absorption by the GI tract with quick transit to the liver, where any remaining free steroid may undergo conjugation to a sulfate or a glucuronide group, which increases solubility and allows the steroid to be excreted in urine. Orally administered estradiol undergoes similar metabolism, and ultimately, most of the orally administered estradiol is rapidly excreted in the urine, with little steroid excreted into the feces. In contrast to estradiol, orally administered ethinyl estradiol is metabolized more slowly; consequently, more of it is excreted in the feces. Presence of the 17α-ethinyl group creates steric hindrance,

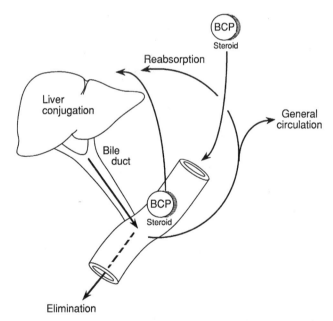

Fig. 15-2. Absorption of steroids contained in oral contraceptive pills illustrating how the steroids may be absorbed and conjugated, excreted and reabsorbed.

preventing conjugation of the hydroxyl group at C-16, or conversion of the hydroxyl group to a keto group (estradiol to estrone conversion). This increases the "potency" of ethinyl estradiol; it has been estimated that 30-50 µg ethinyl estradiol is comparable to 4 mg of estradiol administered orally.[2]

Following absorption, estradiol is assumed to be bound to albumin and sex hormone-binding globulin (SHBG), with only about 2% remaining free in the circulation.[83] Protein-binding patterns of ethinyl estradiol are similar to those of estradiol, with most steroid bound to albumin and little bound to SHBG.[77] Controversy exists about the ability of SHBG to bind and transport estradiol. Some authors report that the binding affinity of estradiol to SHBG is almost 1/20 that of testosterone.[105] This lack of significant binding to SHBG is consistent with the absence of changes in the metabolic clearance rate of estradiol found in conditions where SHBG levels may be elevated (e.g., liver disease and hyperthyroidism). Controversy also exists as to whether or not biological activity is possible with only free steroid or steroid bound to SHBG.[70, 80, 94] When some sex hormones are bound to smaller molecules, biological action is possible. Conjugated estrogens (i.e., estrone sulfate or equilin sulfate) exhibit biological activity with potencies dependent upon the assay system utilized.[10] This point is significant because it is now becoming apparent that not all estrogens affect target tissues in a similar manner, and differences may exist between estrogens in their abilities to be active whether or not they are bound to other molecules. One type of estrogen may affect the liver and not the uterus, while another may do the opposite.[109]

Relationships between total and free estradiol concentration and the influence of binding to SHBG may be quite important in improving the understanding of certain diseases, such as breast cancer. For example, it has been reported that free fatty acids are capable of increasing the free estrogen concentration by displacing estradiol from SHBG in vitro.[18, 90] Lower levels of free fatty acids are present in the luteal phase compared to the follicular phase of the menstrual cycle, and free fatty acid levels are higher after oophorectomy, but can be lowered by giving estrogen therapy.[79] Although the dynamics of binding between SHBG, estradiol, and free fatty acids may have been flawed in previous in vitro studies due to albumin that was also present in test solutions,[73] the changes in estradiol and free fatty acids observed in the in vivo studies remain to be explained.

Hydroxylation of the A ring of the free or conjugated estradiol or ethinyl estradiol steroid nucleus is also a component of the metabolic process. Within the liver, a specialized family of cytochrome P-450 mixed-function oxidases exists. One of these enzymes, cytochrome P-450 NF (so named because of its activity in oxidizing the calcium channel blocker, nifedipine), is believed to be responsible for causing hydroxylation of ethinyl estradiol and estradiol. This enzyme has also been termed cytochrome P-450 III A4.[47, 48] Its activity is induced by barbiturates and certain antibiotics.[110] Inhibition of its activity results from exposure to the progestogen, gestodene.[49] It appears that 2-hydroxylation resulting from mixed-function oxidase activity is the major initial step in the metabolism of ethinyl estradiol.[13] Following its formation, 2-OH-ethinyl estradiol is methylated and excreted in the urine as 2-methoxy-17α-ethinyl-estradiol after conjugation to a sulfate or glucuronide group (Fig. 15-3). In contrast to ethinyl estradiol, metabolism of estradiol proceeds with 2-hydroxylation, but the enzyme usually responsible for this is cytochrome P-450 III A5, a mixed-function

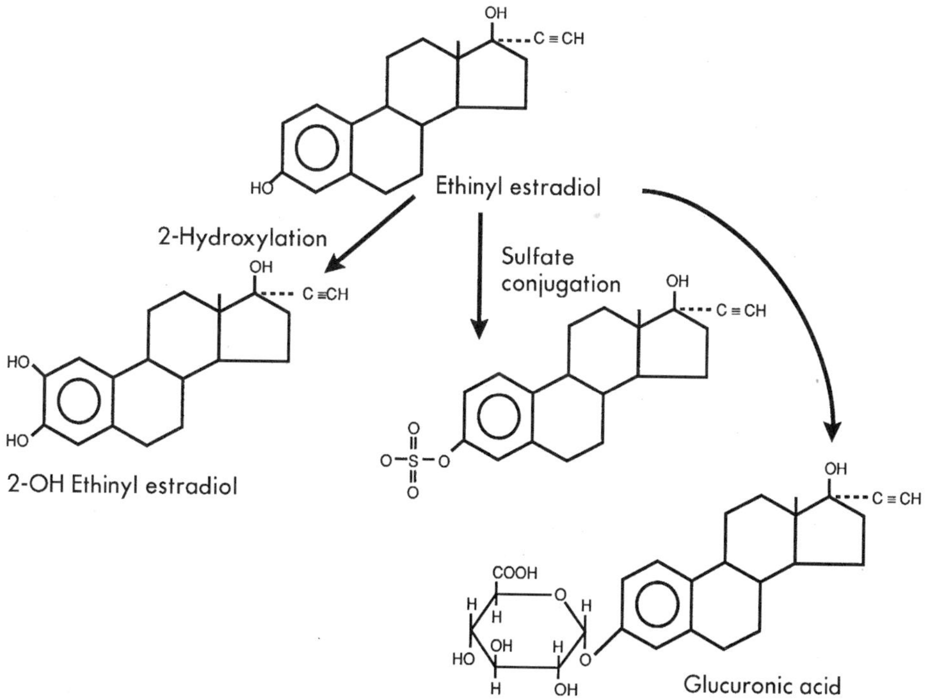

Fig. 15-3. Metabolism of ethinyl estradiol.

oxidase that does not catalyze 2-hydroxylation of ethinyl estradiol.[111] Formation of a 2-hydroxyl estradiol moiety results in a loss of biological activity. Another hepatic enzyme capable of catalyzing the 2-hydroxylation step of estradiol is cytochrome P-450 I A2, which can be induced by cigarette smoking.[71] This property may be responsible for certain "antiestrogenic" activities observed in cigarette smokers, such as a reduced incidence of endometrial cancer.[67] However, cigarette smoking does not appear to significantly influence 17-α ethinyl estradiol metabolism.[25]

Other agents that can inhibit the cytochrome P-450 III A4 hydroxylase enzyme involved in ethinyl estradiol metabolism include the histamine antagonist, cimetidine,[63] the flavonoid, naringin (present in grapefruit juice), as well as the progestogen, gestodene.[48] Cimetidine usage has been reported to raise estradiol levels in male volunteers,[39] but its ability to alter plasma ethinyl estradiol levels in human volunteers has not been reported. Similarly, no studies on the ability of naringin to alter plasma ethinyl estradiol levels in humans have been reported. Jung-Hoffman and Kuhl reported in 1989 that pill users taking gestodene with ethinyl estradiol exhibited higher peak levels of ethinyl estradiol, as well as increased area-under-the-curve (AUC) measurements of this steroid, when compared to pill users taking ethinyl estradiol and desogestrel.[57] This feature was thought to be a consequence of inhibition of steroid hydroxylation, leading the German government to issue a warning that gestodene-containing contraceptive pills could result in elevated ethinyl estradiol levels and pose a potential risk for thromboembolic events.[89] Following this initial report, additional studies have failed to confirm higher ethinyl estradiol levels in users of pills containing gestodene.[30,78]

When ethinyl estradiol is taken orally, it passes across the intestinal wall as either free steroid, or steroid conjugated to a sulfate group after being acted upon by an intestinal sulfatase enzyme (see Fig. 15-3). Interference with intestinal sulfatase activity can result in alterations in the metabolism of ethinyl estradiol. For example, ascorbic acid is also metabolized by intestinal sulfatase. Competition for intestinal sulfatase activity by ascorbic acid in oral contraceptive users could result in increased absorption of unconjugated ethinyl estradiol, resulting in higher free hormone levels. This finding was reported by Back et al.,[5] but recently, not confirmed by Zamah et al.[114] Acetaminophen (paracetamol) is also metabolized by intestinal sulfatase activity, and higher ethinyl estradiol levels have also been observed in acetaminophen users.[6] Whether or not these observed changes in the metabolism of ethinyl estradiol result in an increased risk of an adverse clinical event remains hypothetical, and reports of adverse reactions from drug interaction between contraceptive pills and ascorbic acid, cimetidine, acetaminophen, or gestodene do not exist. However, it is clear that many factors can influence the availability of estrogen and progestogen

preparations once these are ingested, including concomitant use of other pharmacological agents. Awareness of this interaction might lead to the identification of clinically significant events.

In interpreting pharmacological studies of the oral-contraceptive pill, the term *bioavailability* is used. This term refers to the amount of measurable drug in the circulation. Administration of the same dosage of contraceptive steroid by the oral or intravenous route results in different plasma concentrations of the hormones when measured over time. Plasma levels of contraceptive steroid following oral administration, when compared to those following intravenous administration, are typically lower, reflecting what is called the *first-pass effect*. This term implies that, after its intestinal absorption following oral administration, the steroid passes into the portal circulation and is shunted to the liver. The steroid then undergoes conjugation and 2-hydroxylation, followed by excretion into the bile. The amount of steroid that is measured in the plasma following oral administration can be compared to the plasma level following intravenous administration of the same dose of the drug and it is expressed as a percentage. This percentage is termed the *bioavailable drug*. For example, plasma levels of ethinyl estradiol following oral administration are 40% of the levels observed after intravenous administration of a similar dose. Thus, 40% of the drug is bioavailable, while the remaining 60% is presumed to be retained in the hepatic system, undergoing metabolism. This is described as the first-pass effect.[4] Different percentages for first-pass effects are possible, depending upon rates of intestinal absorption and metabolism of the steroids. Progestogens, for example, exhibit less of a first-pass effect than estrogens.

Following conjugation in the liver with excretion into the bile, ethinyl estradiol may be hydrolyzed within the gut lumen, allowing free steroid to be reabsorbed across the gut wall. Reabsorbed steroid may then proceed again to the liver via the portal circulation, and be recirculated into the bloodstream or reexcreted into bile. This "enterohepatic loop" of drug metabolism may produce fluctuations or "peaks" in steroid drug levels,[113] complicating attempts to compare steroid hormone levels between subjects ingesting the same pill dose (Fig. 15-4, **A, B**). Food ingestion[76] and the use of medications that could alter the intestinal processing of steroids may also play a role in affecting steroid hormone drug absorption. Alteration in the intestinal environment might result from changing the bacterial flora, an event believed to occur following the administration of some antibiotics.

Progestogens

Only two estrogens, ethinyl estradiol and mestranol, are found in current oral-contraceptive pills, in contrast to a larger number of progestogens. Use of the term *progestin* should be limited to describing steroid molecules derived

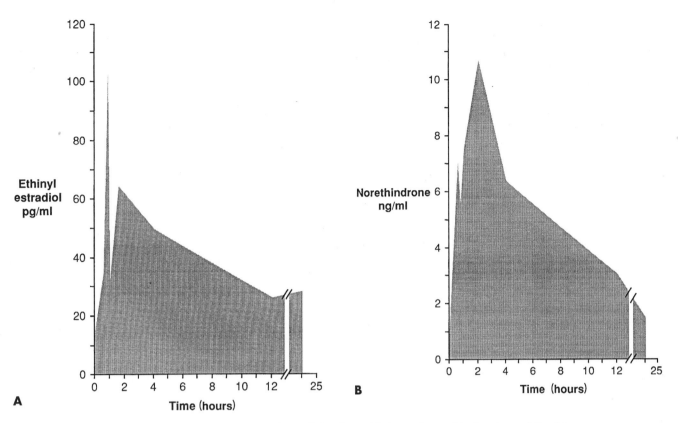

Fig. 15-4. Concentrations of ethinyl estradiol and norethindrone observed in the plasma following oral administration of a single pill containing 35 mg ethinyl estradiol (**A**) and 1 mg norethindrone (**B**). (From Zacur H et al: *J Clin Endocrinal Metab* 75:1268, 1992.)

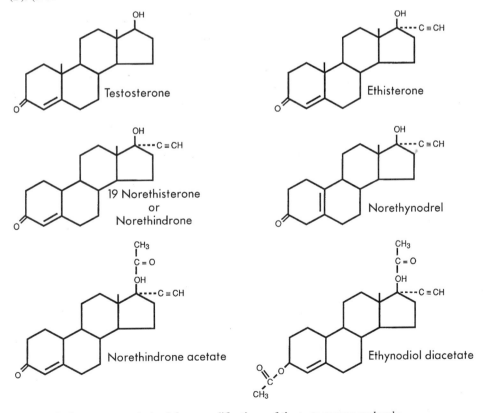

Fig. 15-5. Progestogens derived from modifications of the testosterone molecule.

from the corpus luteum, such as progesterone; the terms *progestogen* or *gestagen* should be used to describe steroid hormones that produce a progesterone-like effect within the uterine endometrium. Only certain progestogens are found in combination oral-contraceptive pills. Progestogens may be divided into three general groups: pregnanes, estranes, and gonanes.[26] Pregnanes are progestogenic compounds derived from the progesterone steroid nucleus, altered by the addition of a methyl group at the C-6 position. Medroxyprogesterone acetate (Provera) and megestrol acetate (Megace) are two examples. Neither of these progestogens are found in today's commercially available combination-type oral-contraceptive pills. These progestogens are taken without estrogens, either to induce withdrawal bleeding or for treatment of endometrial neoplasia. Medroxyprogesterone has been used in the past in a combined oral-contraceptive formulation marketed as Provest.

Estranes refer to progestogens derived from testosterone. If an ethinyl group is added to the C-17α position of testosterone, it improves absorption and prolongs metabolic half-life (Fig. 15-5). This new molecule is called *ethisterone*. If C-19 is removed from ethisterone, the resulting product is called *norethisterone* (*nor* means "without" in German), also known as *norethindrone,* a progestogen present in many of today's combination oral-contraceptive pills. Removal of C-19 eliminates almost all androgenic

activity of this molecule. Norethindrone contains a 4-5 double bond in the A ring of the steroid nucleus. Repositioning of this double bond to the 5-10 position of the steroid nucleus results in the formation of norethynodrel, which is another progestogen found in some birth-control pill preparations. If an acetate group is added to the hydroxyl group at C-17 of norethindrone, another progestogen, norethindrone acetate, is formed. If another acetate is added to the C-3 keto group of this molecule, ethynodiol diacetate is formed. Following oral ingestion, norethindrone acetate and ethynodiol diacetate are both metabolized to norethindrone. Thus, in the estrane group of progestogens, norethindrone is the predominant steroid formed after ingestion of the compound.

The third group of progestogens, gonanes, is derived from norgestrel (Fig. 15-6). This progestogen is formed when a methyl group is added at the C-18 position of norethindrone. Norgestrel's biologically active molecular configuration is known and is similar to that of D-glyceraldehyde. As a result, D-norgestrel is the biologically active parent molecule. D-norgestrel is also optically active and capable of rotating light toward the left, or l or (−), for levorotatory. Light rotation to the right, dextrorotatory or (+), produces a biologically inactive molecule. Thus, the correct term for describing biologically active norgestrel molecules is D-*(1) norgestrel* or D*(−) norgestrel,*

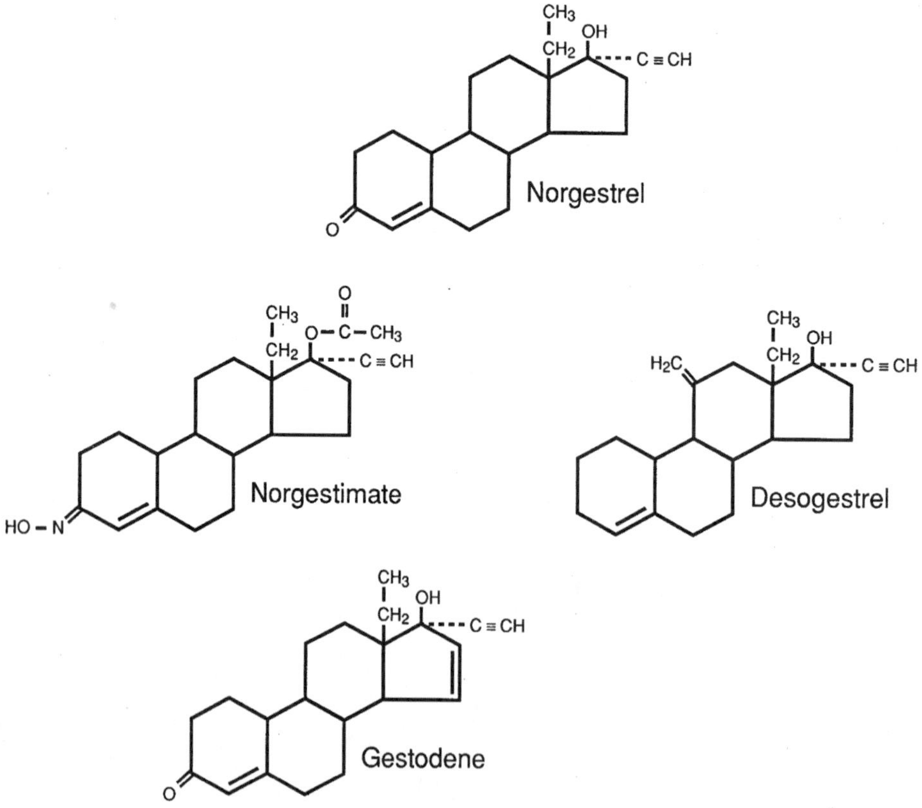

Fig. 15-6. Progestogens derived from modification of the norgestrel molecule.

while the inactive form of norgestrel is known as *D-(d) norgestrel* or *D(+) norgestrel*. Some pill formulations containing norgestrel utilize the racemic mixture of norgestrel (i.e., dl norgestrel), while others contain only the levorotatory biologically active form, called *levonorgestrel*.[100]

NEW PROGESTOGENS

Recent modifications of the levonorgestrel molecule have resulted in certain new progestogens. These modifications were made to lower the total progestogen dosage required for contraceptive efficacy, and to reduce the risk of progestogen-associated side effects. These new compounds include norgestimate, desogestrel, and gestodene. Addition of an oxime at C-3 and an acetate at C-17 to the levonorgestrel molecule results in norgestimate (see Fig. 15-6). Addition of a methylene group at C-11 and absence of a keto group at C-3 distinguishes desogestrel from levonorgestrel (refer to Fig. 15-6). Gestodene differs from norgestrel by a 15-16 double bond in ring D (see Fig. 15-6). The metabolism of desogestrel and norgestimate is similar to that of norgestrel, and norgestrel itself is formed in small amounts during metabolism of these progestogens. Interestingly, very little, if any, gestodene is metabolized to norgestrel. Desogestrel and norgestimate are now available in contraceptive-pill products in the United States, but gestodene has not yet been approved by the United States Food and Drug Administration (FDA). All three progestogens are available in Europe.

Following oral administration, the metabolism of progestogen molecules is similar to that of the estrogens, with some exceptions. There is greater bioavailability of the orally administered progestogen than of oral estrogens. This property implies either greater intestinal absorption of the progestogen or a smaller first-pass effect. Progestogens undergo hydroxylations at multiple positions within the steroid nucleus, particularly at the 3 and 5 positions. Glucuronide and sulfate conjugation of these molecules occurs as well. Knowledge of the metabolism of progestogens is limited compared with that of estrogens.[100]

PHARMACOKINETICS

Following administration of a single pill at 0700 hours, mean ethinyl estradiol and norethindrone levels peak within 1-2 hours and gradually decline, with very low levels above background detected 24 hours later (Fig. 15-7).[113] This pattern of hormone levels yields marked variation among individuals with multiple peaks in the drug observed in some users, thus reflecting inherent differences in enterohepatic recirculation (see Fig. 15-4). Fluctuating steroid levels of oral-contraceptive components expose the hypothalamic pituitary axis, as well as other organ systems, to only very low levels of contraceptive steroid hormones after 24 hours of pill use. Oral contraceptive pills are ingested for 21 days, followed by a 7-day pill-free interval, during which no pills are taken or placebo pills are used. This medication-free

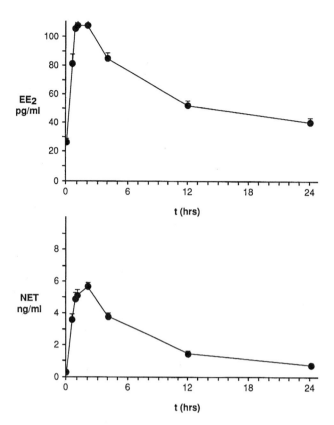

Fig. 15-7. Ethinyl estradiol and norethindrone concentrations measured in 60 women taking a single combination oral contraceptive pill containing 25 mg of ethinyl estradiol and 1 mg norethindrone. (From Zacur H. et al: *J Clin Endocrinol Metab* 75:1268, 1992.)

period, known as the *pill-free interval,* was recommended many years ago as a means of mimicking the natural menstrual cycle by leading to withdrawal bleeding at monthly intervals.[50] Because pill steroid levels are barely detectable 24 hours after ingestion, very little contraceptive steroid is present in the circulation during this 7-day window. The abrupt decline in contraceptive-pill steroid levels mimics the fall in steroids observed during the menstrual cycle, triggering withdrawal bleeding during the pill-free interval. If endogenous gonadotropins and steroids are measured during this time, it is evident by the 7th pill-free day that rises in hormones are taking place. Thus, the initial rapid withdrawal in contraceptive steroids, followed by a gradual rise in endogenous hormones, may be responsible for some side effects observed during the pill-free interval.[50]

DRUG INTERACTIONS

Drugs that interact with oral-contraceptive steroids may do so by altering absorption or metabolism, or by affecting the site of steroid action. GI absorption may be altered, as previously mentioned, by use of ascorbic acid or acetaminophen, agents that compete for intestinal sulfatase activity and result in increased transport of free steroid across the intestinal wall.

Drugs that affect the liver's mixed-function oxidase system can affect the metabolism of oral-contraceptive steroids, as previously mentioned. Stimulation of mixed-function oxidase activities in liver microsomal enzyme systems may increase the metabolism of pill steroids, resulting in reduced contraceptive efficacy, while inhibition of these enzymes may increase steroid levels and heighten the potential for adverse side effects.

Phenytoin, primidone, barbiturates, carbamazepine, ethosuximide, and methsuximide can induce liver microsomal-enzyme activity and thus, cause contraceptive failure.[3] Rifampicin therapy induces hepatic microsomal enzyme activity and lowers ethinyl estradiol levels, causing breakthrough bleeding and contraceptive failure.[12, 91] Griseofulvin may also cause breakthrough bleeding and contraceptive failure in oral-contraceptive pill users through a similar mechanism.[104]

Interference with enterohepatic recirculation by preventing reabsorption of steroid excreted in the bile could lower plasma contraceptive steroid levels and reduce contraceptive-pill efficacy. This could occur by altering the enteric bacterial flora with antibiotics. Pregnancies have been reported in women using ampicillin and tetracycline,[7, 31] but studies in humans have failed to demonstrate reduced plasma contraceptive steroid levels in women using these two antimicrobials.[35, 74]

Although patients frequently inquire about the effect of contraceptive steroids on *other* medications, only limited data are available to provide an informed response. As previously mentioned, intestinal sulfatase activity is responsible for sulfate conjugation of acetaminophen; as a result, acetaminophen may compete for absorption with ethinyl estradiol. As high levels of acetaminophen may adversely affect absorption of ethinyl estradiol, high levels of ethinyl estradiol may reduce the absorption of acetaminophen.[72] What effect this may have on the efficacy of acetaminophen therapy remains to be determined.

The use of oral-contraceptive pills in conjunction with the antibiotic troleandomycin, or the immune suppressive agent cyclosporin A, have been reported to cause reversible cholestatic hepatitis.[34, 66] It has been suggested that this may have resulted from increased levels of these drugs "induced" by the pill. Because an adverse hepatic effect is not uncommon when troleandomycin or cyclosporin A are taken alone, it is difficult to incriminate the oral-contraceptive pill as an accelerant of this process.

Oral-contraceptive pills are capable of inhibiting hepatic microsomal enzymes, which could result in decreasing the metabolic clearance rate of other drugs. The use of oral-contraceptive pills may also accelerate hepatic metabolism of certain drugs, increasing their clearance rate. Elevated levels of the antidepressant imipramine have been reported in women taking 50 μg of ethinyl estradiol.[86] Decreased metabolic clearance of chlordiazepoxide, diazepam, nitrazepam, and alprazolam, and increased clearance of lorazepam, oxazepam, and temazepam, have been noted with oral-contraceptive pill use. Inhibition of hepatic microsomes for the former drugs, and acceleration of glucuronide conjugation for the latter drugs, have been suggested.[33] Reduced plasma clearance has also been reported for theophylline[92] and caffeine,[81] but no reports exist documenting clinically adverse events from these changes. A decreased rate of ethanol metabolism has been demonstrated in women taking oral contraceptives in one study.[55] In another investigation, 30 μg or more of ethinyl estradiol did not affect the pharmacokinetics of alcohol in light or moderate drinkers.[52]

Reduced clearance of corticosteroids has also been reported during oral-contraceptive pill use.[11] Because glucocorticoids and oral-contraceptive pills are used separately to treat women with hirsutism, it is wise not to use the two medications together.

CONTRACEPTIVES AND LIPIDS

Numerous reports published in gynecological literature are devoted to alterations in lipid and lipoprotein levels following oral-contraceptive pill use. To respond appropriately to the questions raised by patients, and to be able to interpret the evolving data on this subject, it is essential to understand lipoprotein physiology and the effects of oral-contraceptive steroids on lipid metabolism. Many excellent reviews have been presented on this subject, and readers are referred to these citations for more detailed information.[32, 41, 46, 65, 103]

Following ingestion of a meal containing fat (triglyceride) and cholesterol, these lipids are absorbed across the small intestine and taken up by the lymphatic system as chylomicrons, which are eventually secreted into the bloodstream via the thoracic duct. The surface of the chylomicron can be viewed as a "sphere of lipid" that acquires on its surface proteins synthesized in intestinal cells. These proteins are termed *apoproteins*. The protein apo C-II has special significance because when it is present on the surface of a chylomicron, it allows the chylomicron to be recognized and activated by the enzyme, lipoprotein lipase. Lipoprotein lipase is present in the cells of many tissues, including adipose and muscle. Lipoprotein lipase hydrolyzes triglycerides within chylomicrons to free fatty acids, which may then be oxidized as a fuel source in some tissues or esterified and stored as fat in others (e.g., adipose tissue). As the chylomicron loses its triglyceride during its encounter with lipoprotein lipase, it becomes a smaller particle known as a *chylomicron remnant,* which is cleared from the circulation by the liver (see Fig. 15-7).

In addition to being absorbed from the intestine, triglycerides can also be synthesized by the liver. Common fatty acids synthesized in the liver include palmitic acid, stearic acid, and oleic acid. After these fatty acids are formed, they are esterified to glycerol and released by the liver into the circulation in the lipoprotein, VLDL (very low-density lipoprotein). The VLDL particle has triglycerides at its center, but also contains some cholesterol. These particles also acquire protein molecules on their surface that are made by the liver and include the protein apo C-II. Lipoprotein lipase is then capable of being activated by the VLDL particle, which will stimulate its release of triglycerides for fuel consumption or storage in fat. As triglycerides are removed from the VLDL particle, the particle becomes smaller, forming a specialized remnant called IDL (intermediate-density lipoprotein). Once IDL is formed, it too can interact with lipoprotein lipase, causing the release of additional triglycerides and formation of a new, even smaller and denser particle called LDL (low-density lipoprotein). This particle has had almost all of its triglyceride removed and contains mostly cholesterol.

The LDL particle has apoproteins on its surface, such as apo B-100 or apo E, that allow this particle to be recognized by special receptors in the cells of tissues. When LDL reacts with these receptors, it is allowed to donate its cholesterol to those tissues. For example, LDL may donate its cholesterol to steroid-forming cells in the adrenal or ovary. However, the bulk of the cholesterol in the LDL particles is returned to the liver. The importance of LDL to the understanding of hypercholesterolemia was made quite clear by the Nobel Prize-winning work of Brown and Goldstein.[17] In brief, the ability of the liver or other tissues to synthesize cholesterol is determined by the amount of cholesterol in the circulation, by processes involving LDL and the LDL receptor. When LDL receptors of the liver are occupied by LDL, synthesis of cholesterol within the liver

is reduced. When LDL receptors on the surface of liver cells are reduced in number, LDL cannot bind to them. This means that if additional cholesterol is added to the circulation from the diet and more LDL particles are formed, these will not be as readily cleared by the liver. As a consequence, this excess cholesterol in the form of LDL will enter certain cells of the body by a process independent of the LDL receptor, which can ultimately result in abnormal disposition of cholesterol. This is believed to occur in coronary artery atheromata formation.

Before their conversion to LDL, the VLDL and IDL particles can act as "cholesterol donors" for a special particle called HDL_3, which is synthesized in the liver. HDL stands for *high-density lipoprotein,* a particle that has a cholesterol-rich inner core, the surface of which is covered by an apoprotein of the A class. As a group, these particles may be divided into the subclasses, HDL_3 and HDL_2. HDL_3 particles are immature, nascent, or "empty" particles that accept cholesterol supplied by IDL and VLDL. As HDL_3 receives more cholesterol, it enlarges and acquires more apoproteins and becomes an HDL_2 particle. Once formed, HDL_2 is allowed to return its cholesterol to the liver. This process is described as the *reverse cholesterol pathway.* When HDL_2 donates its cholesterol to the liver, a hepatic enzyme, hepatic lipoprotein lipase, converts the HDL_2 to an HDL_3 particle by releasing its cholesterol (Fig. 15-8).

The preceding review of lipoprotein physiology has particular significance in understanding relationships between lipids, atherosclerosis, and contraceptive pills. First,

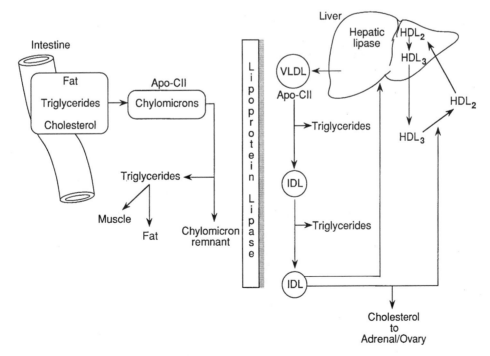

Fig. 15-8. Lipoprotein metabolism illustrating the exogenous (ingestion of cholesterol) and endogenous (synthesis) pathways.

relationships between lipoproteins and coronary artery disease have been noted in many epidemiological studies. In general, these studies have observed an increased risk of death from heart disease as the level of serum cholesterol increases. It is believed that this risk is secondary to the formation of atheromata, or fatty fibrinous plaques, in the coronary arteries of the heart. Although all of the steps leading up to formation of a fatty fibrous plaque within a coronary artery remain unknown, many have been identified. This has resulted in the prevailing view of atherosclerosis that is briefly summarized below. A more detailed explanation is available elsewhere.[37, 38]

Endothelial cells lining the coronary artery become injured. The type of injury that these cells experience may or may not result in morphological changes of the endothelial cells. After injury, monocytes (macrophages) are attracted to the site. These cells ingest cholesterol provided by LDL and become "foam" cells that cover the damaged endothelium (Fig. 15-9 **A-D**). Platelets are also attracted to the site of vessel injury and adhere there. Macrophages and platelets then release cytokines, including growth factors

that attract smooth muscle cells. Migration of these smooth muscle cells from the media of the vessel wall covers the injury site and produces collagen, thus forming a fibrous plaque blanketing the foam cells. Eventually the foam cells undergo necrosis and release their cholesterol esters, which precipitate at the site. This results in the formation of a fatty fibrinous plaque.

It is believed that the formation of foam cells is more likely to occur when LDL levels are high. It is certainly clear that when LDL levels are elevated, the risk of coronary artery disease is greater. Increased levels of LDL are more likely to be found when liver LDL receptors are not available to clear LDL from the circulation. This occurs when the liver has been continually exposed to cholesterol and saturated fat in the diet. Cholesterol may be cleared from the circulation and returned to the liver by HDL_2 particles (the reverse cholesterol pathway). Descriptive population data have indicated that the risk for coronary artery disease is less in those individuals with a low LDL level and a high HDL_2 level.

Changes in lipoprotein levels following administration

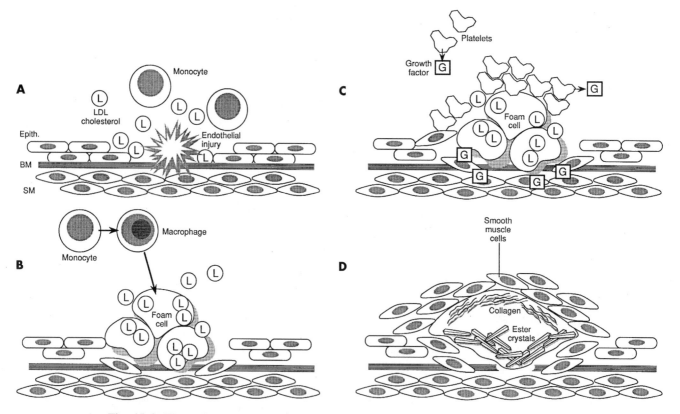

Fig. 15-9. The pathogenesis of atherosclerosis illustrating **A**, endometrial injury that attracts monocytes and cholesterol; **B**, monocytes become macrophagic and penetrate the vessel wall; macrophages ingest cholesterol and become "foam cells"; **C**, platelets are attracted that release growth factors stimulating smooth muscle cells that cover the foam cells; **D**, necrosis of foam cells results in release of cholesterol esters and formation of cholesterol crystals. (From Gotto AM: Clinician's Manual Cholesterol Education Program sponsored by American Health Association and Sandoz Pharmaceuticals Science Press, 1991, London, United Kingdom.)

of oral-contraceptive pills have produced changes in the concentrations of lipids that may be viewed as worrisome based on this epidemiological data. Following oral-contraceptive pill administration, a rise in total cholesterol, LDL, and triglycerides is observed, with a fall in HDL cholesterol. How does this happen? Estrogen is believed to stimulate the hepatic production of VLDL. Because LDL is derived from VLDL, a corresponding increase in LDL would not seem surprising under these circumstances. Hepatic lipase in the liver converts HDL_2 to HDL_3 and estrogen inhibits hepatic lipase activity. As a result, a rise in HDL_2 would be expected to occur in women given estrogen, and this has been reported in menopausal women receiving "estrogen-only" hormone replacement. Although elevated HDL levels are associated with beneficial cardiac outcomes, inhibition of hepatic lipase by estrogen under these circumstances would not appear to be beneficial because it would prevent the donation of HDL_2 cholesterol to the liver. Estrogen increases the hepatic uptake of free fatty acids,[62] however, and will decrease lipolysis in adipocytes.[82] These actions would be expected to be cardioprotective and may counteract the previously mentioned adverse events.

Lipoprotein responses from combination oral contraceptive pills must also be viewed from the perspective of progestogens, in particular, those derived from androgens. In general, androgen ingestion is associated with lowered levels of HDL and higher levels of LDL, which are worrisome lipoprotein changes. Because hepatic lipase is stimulated by androgens, conversion of HDL_2 to HDL_3 is enhanced, leading to lower HDL levels. Progesterone-derived progestins do not appear to have a similar effect. From these observations, the decline in HDL_2 levels following progestogen use may be due to donation of cholesterol by HDL to the liver, which should decrease the risk of coronary artery disease. However, in contrast to estrogens, progestogens appear to increase free fatty acid levels and antagonize insulin activity—actions that may not be cardioprotective.

Thus, a combination oral-contraceptive pill's effects on coronary artery disease may be influenced by its progestogen component, as well as its estrogen component. In a recent study the authors performed, three different combination pill preparations were given to three different groups of women who were matched for variables known to affect lipoproteins. Each pill preparation contained ethinyl estradiol and norethindrone, but in different amounts. In this study, all groups experienced an increase in cholesterol of 2.7-9.2% over nine months, with a 59.1-67% increase in triglycerides, and a 21.1-23.9% increase in LDL. A significant increase in HDL was seen only for the pill preparation containing 0.5 mg norethindrone, the other two preparations contained 1 mg.[19, 20]

Despite early concerns with contraceptive pills containing higher doses of contraceptive steroids, and the adverse changes in lipoproteins observed in current low-dose pill users, a significant risk of heart disease in past and current pill users does not exist independently of variables, such as smoking. This situation is surprising in view of the lipoprotein changes discussed above, and the effects of the pill on coagulation, which are discussed later. An explanation for this discrepancy may be that estrogen and progesterone have vascular effects independent of those caused by lipoproteins. For example, estrogen, even when given with progestogen, may protect against coronary artery atheroma formation. Studies in monkeys have revealed an absence of coronary artery atheroma formation when these animals were given combination oral contraceptive pills in conjunction with a high-cholesterol diet. When a high-cholesterol diet was given to the monkeys without oral contraceptives, coronary artery disease ensued. It has been postulated that estrogens affect the vessel endothelium "directly," preventing atheroma formation even in the presence of elevated lipids.[22,23]

EFFECT OF CONTRACEPTIVES ON COAGULATION

After the introduction of the oral contraceptive pill, early reports indicated a risk of pulmonary venous and cerebral thrombosis or embolism with increasing dosages of estrogen, suggesting an adverse effect of the pill on blood coagulation.[54] When initially raised, this concern did not seem surprising in view of the risk of venous thrombosis that occurs during pregnancy, a physiological state in which elevated levels of both estrogen and progesterone are found. An extensive review of the clotting system is beyond the scope of this chapter, but a brief review is provided below. More detailed information can be obtained through the following references.[1, 9, 16, 21, 29, 36, 51, 68, 69, 75, 108]

A thrombus may form in either a vein or an artery following activation of the clotting system. Activation of the clotting cascade occurs in response to a variety of stimuli. The concentration of clotting factors at any given moment within the circulation is far in excess of the amount of clotting-factor protein consumed to form a small venous or arterial thrombus.

Initiation of the hemostatic system within a vessel is usually prompted by an injury to the endothelium that exposes cell membrane proteins. Platelets bind to these proteins assisted by a circulating plasma protein, von Willebrand's factor, that serves as a tissue glue. Platelets are normally kept from binding to the vessel wall because of the flow of blood, absence of vessel wall injury, and release of prostacyclin from the vessel endothelium, which discourages platelet activity while promoting vasodilation. Following the arrival of platelets at the endothelium, plasma fibrinogen is converted to a fibrin clot at the site of injury, and activation of the coagulation system is required to accomplish this step.

Activation of the clotting cascade occurs intrinsically

with activation of factor XII (Hageman factor) or extrinsically by activation of factor VII. The distinction between extrinsic or intrinsic clotting systems may be artificial. In vivo, activation of factor VII (tissue factor) results in activation of factor IX (which is part of the intrinsic pathway), as well as activation of factor X (classical extrinsic pathway) (Fig. 15-10). When prothrombin is converted to thrombin, fibrinogen is enzymatically attacked, releasing the A and B fibrinopeptides. This alteration in fibrinogen allows it to polymerize to form the fibrin clot.

The clotting process can be regulated by adjusting the activity of thrombin, as well as by degradation of the fibrin clot. In the former, circulating levels of antithrombin III serve as an alternative substrate for thrombin and activated factor Xa. When thrombin or activated factor X interact with antithrombin III, the clotting enzymes are "trapped" and thus, are unable to stimulate further conversion of fibrinogen to fibrin. Heparin accelerates this trapping process.

When thrombin is formed, it may establish a complex with the protein, thrombomodulin, which exists on the surface of the endothelial cell. Activation of thrombomodulin in turn can activate the circulating proenzyme, protein C, which requires a cofactor, protein S, for full activation (Fig. 15-11). Once protein C is activated, it begins enzymatically to degrade activated clotting factors VIIIa and Va, preventing them from further stimulating the clotting process.

A fibrin clot, once formed, may be degraded by the enzyme, plasmin, which is formed from the precursor, plasminogen. The conversion of plasminogen to plasmin is stimulated by release of tissue plasminogen activator from endothelial cells. These endothelial cells also can release prostacyclin, preventing further thrombosis formation.

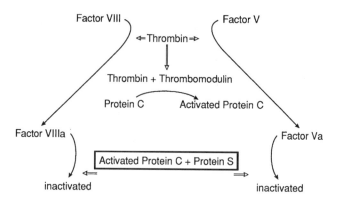

Fig. 15-11. Protein C anticoagulant pathway.

Studies of oral contraceptive pill users have usually focused on measuring the concentration of clotting factors within the circulation following pill administration. Increased levels of clotting factors are presumed to reflect hepatic synthesis of these suspect proteins by hormones contained within the pill. However, because concentrations of clotting factors already exist in excessive amounts in the circulation, a further increase does not appear to explain thrombosis in pill users.

Other studies of pill users have also demonstrated a 30-40% decline in antithrombin III levels.[21] Although this change would seem to predispose to clot formation, this may not be true. For example, in families with congenital antithrombin III deficiency, many family members have a 40-50% decline in antithrombin III levels, and these individuals do not experience thromboembolism.

Some studies have demonstrated that the use of the oral-contraceptive pill is associated with increased tissue plasminogen activator levels. Thus, even if a hypercoagulable state exists following oral-contraceptive pill use, a balance might be present due to the increased activity of the fibrinolytic system.

These observations suggest that the risk of coagulation following the use of current low-dose oral contraceptive pills should not be high, a concept that appears to be substantiated by current observations. Earlier studies of thrombosis formation in pill users may not have adequately been controlled for the adverse consequences of smoking. It has been suggested, for example, that noxious substances in cigarettes may be responsible for causing endothelial damage that could initiate clot formation. In addition, the higher concentration of steroids contained in the older pill preparations may have resulted in an increased thrombotic risk.

ORAL CONTRACEPTIVES AND CARBOHYDRATE METABOLISM

Following the introduction of oral contraception, impairment of glucose tolerance was reported as a possible side effect.[106] As a consequence, investigations were initiated to address several key questions: (1) if oral contraceptive pills affect carbohydrate metabolism, how soon after beginning

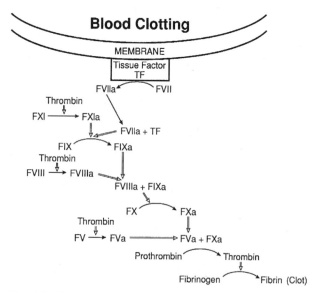

Fig. 15-10. Depiction of the clotting cascade. Activation of factors is designated by use of the lower case "a".

pill use do changes occur? (2) If there is an adverse effect on carbohydrate metabolism, is it progressive for the duration of use of the contraceptive preparation? (3) If carbohydrate metabolism is impaired during pill use, does the impairment remain following cessation of use? (4) Are women who experience glucose impairment during pregnancy at increased risk for altered carbohydrate metabolism when taking the pill? (5) If the pill impairs carbohydrate metabolism, is this effect a consequence of estrogen, progestogen, or both? (6) Can adjustment of steroids in the pill affect impairment in carbohydrate intolerance if it exists?

Agreement upon the effect of combination oral contraceptive pills on carbohydrate metabolism has been difficult to reach. This is true in large part because of the different parameters used in studies to define glucose tolerance. For example, it is difficult to compare results between studies when oral glucose tolerance testing (OGTT) is used in one study and intravenous glucose tolerance is used in another. Many individual differences are found in peripheral glucose and insulin levels in response to a glucose challenge. This feature has particular relevance to users of oral contraceptives. Current testing schemes are satisfactory for detecting the frankly diabetic individual, but interpretation becomes difficult when "mild glucose impairment" is sought, particularly when marked individual variation may already exist. For example, large variations in glucose levels have been reported for the same normal individual when tested on numerous separate occasions.[96]

Despite these limitations, a consensus does exist that combination-type oral contraceptive pill use may cause mild impairment in glucose intolerance during the very first cycles of use. This impairment does not cause frank diabetes in users of current low-dose pills, but may cause 6% of users to become frankly diabetic when combination pills containing 50 μg or more of ethinyl estradiol are taken.[58]

Deterioration in glucose tolerance

Deterioration in glucose tolerance over a 36-month interval was reported by Wynn for subjects using a pill containing 30 μg ethinyl estradiol and 150 μg levonorgestrel. Conclusions were based on results using AUC analysis. Surprisingly, insulin increased for the first three months of pill use in this study, but did not increase thereafter. When a similar study by the same investigators was performed using norethindrone as the progestogen, progressive deterioration in glucose tolerance was not seen over time.[112] In contrast, Spellacy et al. reported that in subjects using 0.075 mg mestranol and 5 mg norethynodrel, changes in glucose and insulin were not observed in OGTT after 32 months of pill use.[97] However, Spellacy did note that some individuals (12.5% of the study group) exhibited worsening of carbohydrate tolerance after three years of pill use.

Persistence of impairment in glucose tolerance

Widespread agreement exists that the impairment in glucose tolerance observed in pill users is reversible and does not persist following cessation of pill use. A return to normal glucose metabolism has been noted within three months of discontinuation of the pill.[56] No persistent discernible difference in glucose response appears to exist between past users of the combination pill and those who never used it, regardless of the duration of pill use or the interval following discontinuation.[84]

Effect of gestational diabetes

Previous history of gestational diabetes appears to place individuals at risk for impairment in glucose tolerance when taking oral contraceptive pills.[44, 87, 101] This effect seems to be dose dependent, with lower-dose pills less likely to cause adverse changes in glucose concentration.[8] Nevertheless, an increase in insulin in response to glucose remains in these individuals.[95]

Duration of use and age

Duration of oral contraceptive pill use, as well as the age of the user, may affect carbohydrate metabolism. Women under the age of 35 who used triphasic pill preparations for 12 months demonstrated an increase in AUC for insulin and glucose as compared with controls. However, all increases in glucose and insulin levels among these subjects fell within the normal range for the laboratory.[40] A positive correlation between age and elevation of serum triglyceride levels in long-term pill users (greater than two years) has been mentioned in a recent review. No interaction of age on glucose or insulin responses was reported in this study.[43]

Progestogen or estrogen effect

Clinical studies, conducted to determine whether the pill steroid components of oral contraceptives given alone or in combination to intact or oophorectomized volunteers over short and long intervals to affect carbohydrate metabolism, have produced conflicting results. Estrogens administered alone can increase glycogen deposition,[107] inhibit glycogenolysis,[102] suppress gluconeogenesis, and improve muscle uptake of glucose.[59] Pancreatic islet cell hypertrophy and hyperinsulinemia[53, 59] also can occur as a result of estrogen administration.

Progesterone can produce pancreatic islet cell hypertrophy and increase insulin secretion. However, it can also block cortisol-induced hyperglycemia and suppress hepatic gluconeogenesis.[60] Responses to the progesterone-like components of the oral contraceptive pill may be more variable than those caused by estrogen simply by virtue of the various progesterone derivatives available. For example, pregnanes may exert effects on carbohydrate metabolism that are different from those of the estrane or gonane classes of progestogens.

Effects of both estrogen and progesterone components of the pill may also be due to drug dosage and duration of action. Newer generations of oral contraceptive pills containing the progestogens—desogestrel, gestodene, and norgestimate—may produce less adverse effects on carbohydrate metabolism than their higher-dosage predecessors.[98]

Importance of insulin

Although the effect of oral contraceptives on changes in glucose levels has received widespread attention, less notice has been paid to the compensatory hyperinsulinemic response that these drugs cause. Recent studies have suggested that hyperinsulinemia itself may play a significant role in the pathogenesis of hypertension and atherosclerotic cardiovascular disease.[27, 88] It is beyond the scope of this chapter to review in detail the consequences of hyperinsulinemia, as this is addressed in the cited reviews, but a brief summary is offered.

Hyperinsulinemia may be responsible for renal sodium retention ultimately producing hypertension. Insulin can also stimulate sympathetic nervous system activity, causing hypertension. Hyperinsulinemia can stimulate the liver to increase VLDL production and decrease HDL concentrations, increasing the risk of atherogenesis. In view of these concerns, changes in insulin in response to oral contraceptive pill use deserve special consideration.

Insulin and oral contraceptives

Following administration of low-dose, combination oral contraceptive pills (30 µg ethinyl estradiol and 150 µg levonorgestrel) and using a glucose clamp technique, Kasdorf and Kalkhoff demonstrated insulin resistance during the six months of pill use that was studied.[61] One cause of insulin resistance may be related to the ethinyl estradiol component of the pill, as suggested by Kojima et al., who used an insulin tolerance test with normal volunteers who were given ethinyl estradiol in different dosages.[64] These results confirmed the insulin resistance of low-dose, oral-contraceptive pills studied by Godsland et al., who used an intravenous glucose tolerance test and concluded that not only did estrogen induce insulin resistance, but the progestogen component in the pill reduced the metabolic clearance of insulin.[42] Using the euglycemic hyperinsulinemic glucose clamp technique, Scheen et al., using a contraceptive containing 35 µg ethinyl estradiol and 2 mg cyproterone acetate, found that insulin sensitivity was not altered and the metabolic clearance of insulin was felt to be increased.[93] Thus, it can be seen that differences in conclusions may result from different methods used to assess changes in carbohydrate metabolism.

OTHER METABOLIC EFFECTS OF ORAL CONTRACEPTIVE PREPARATIONS

It is well recognized that the effect of estrogen in increasing binding globulins is not confined to SHBG. Estrogen also increases transcortin, the cortisol-binding globulin; thus, the increase in plasma cortisol derived from oral contraceptive use largely reflects cortisol bound to globulin and not the biologically active free component. The adrenal cortex responds normally to adrenocorticotropic hormone (ACTH) stimulation and to stress. These findings parallel changes in maternal plasma cortisol levels during normal pregnancy.

Similarly, thyroxine-binding globulin (TBG) increases as a result of estrogen use. Consequently, total plasma thyroxine levels rise in women taking oral contraceptive preparations. Measurement of free thyroxine and TSH substantiate normal thyroid function during the use of oral contraceptives.

SUMMARY

The pharmacology and pharmacokinetics of combination oral contraceptive pills have been reviewed in this chapter. This has been followed by a discussion of the effects of various drugs and medications on the metabolism of the contraceptive pill, and has concluded with observations of the effect of the pill on coagulation, as well as lipoprotein and carbohydrate metabolism. Knowledge of the metabolic consequences of oral-contraceptive pill use should allow physicians to be most reassuring to their patients when discussing the risks and benefits of oral contraceptive pill use.

REFERENCES

1. Alving BM, Comp PC: Recent advances in understanding clotting and evaluating patients with recurrent thrombosis. *Am J Obset Gynecol* 167:1184, 1992.
2. Astedt B, Sianberg L, Jeppsson S, et al: The natural estrogenic hormone estradiol as a new component of combined oral contraceptives, *Br Med J* 1:269, 1977.
3. Back DJ, Bates M, Dowden A, et al: The interaction of phenobarbital and other anticonvulsants with oral contraceptive steroid therapy, *Contraception* 22:495, 1980.
4. Back DJ, Breckenridge AM, Crawford FE, et al: Interindividual variation and drug interactions with hormonal steroid contraceptives, *Drugs* 21:46, 1981.
5. Back DJ, Breckenridge AM, MacIver M, et al: Interaction of ethinyl estradiol with ascorbic acid in man, *Br Med J* 282:1516, 1981.
6. Back DJ, Orme MLE: Pharmacokinetic drug interaction with oral contraceptives, *Clin Pharmacokinet* 18:472, 1990.
7. Bacon JF, Shenfield GM: Pregnancy attributable to interaction between tetracycline and oral contraceptives, *Br Med J* 1:293, 1980.
8. Beck WN: Update on oral contraception, *Clin Obstet Gynecol* 24:867, 1981.
9. Beller FK, Ebert C: Effects of oral contraceptives and blood coagulation: a review, *Obstet Gynecol Surv* 40:425, 1985.
10. Bhavnani BR: The saga of the ring B unsaturated equine estrogens, *Endocr Rev* 9:396, 1988.
11. Boekenoogen SJ, Szefler SJ, Jusko WJ: Prednisone disposition and protein binding in oral contraceptive users, *J Clin Endocrinol Metab* 56:702, 1983.
12. Bolt HM, Kappus H, Bolt M: Effect of rifampicin treatment on the metabolism of oestradiol and 17-α-estradiol by human liver microsomes, *Eur J Clin Pharmacol* 8:301, 1975.
13. Bolt HM: Metabolism of estrogens—natural and synthetic, *Pharmacol Ther* 4:155, 1979.
14. Bolt HM, Kappus H, Kashohrer R: Metabolism of 17α-

ethynylestradiol by human liver microsomes in vitro aromatic hydroxylation and irreversible protein binding of metabolites, *J Clin Endocrinol Metab* 39:1072, 1974.

15. Bottiger LE, Boman G, Eklund G, et al: Oral contraceptives and thromboembolic disease: effects of lowering estrogen content, *Lancet* 1:1097, 1980.

16. Bonnar J: Coagulation effects of oral contraceptives, *Am J Obstet Gynecol* 157:1042, 1987.

17. Brown MS, Goldstein JL: A receptor-mediated pathway for cholesterol homeostasis, *Science* 232:34, 1986.

18. Bruning PF, Bonfer JMG: Free fatty acid concentrations correlated with the available fraction of estradiol in the human plasma, *Cancer Res* 46:2606, 1986.

19. Burkman RT, Zacur HA, Kimball AW, et al: Oral contraceptives and lipids and lipoproteins. I: variations in the mean levels by oral contraceptive type, *Contraception* 40:553, 1989.

20. Burkman RT, Zacur HA, Kimball AW, et al: Oral contraceptives and lipids and lipoproteins. II: relationship to plasma steroid levels and outlier status, *Contraception* 40:676, 1989.

21. Burkman RT, Bell WR, Zacur HA, et al: Oral contraceptives and antithrombin III: variations by dosage and ABO blood group, *Am J Obstet Gynecol* 164:1453, 1991.

22. Clarkson TB, Adams MR, Kaplan JR, et al: From menarche to menopause: coronary artery atherosclerosis and protection in cynomolgus monkeys, *Am J Obstet Gynecol* 160:1280, 1989.

23. Clarkson TB, Shively CA, Morgan TM, et al: Oral contraceptives and coronary artery atherosclerosis of cynomolgus monkeys, *Obstet Gynecol* 75:217, 1990.

24. Comp PC, Zacur HA: Contraceptive choices in women with coagulation diseases, *Am J Obstet Gynecol* 168:1990, 1993.

25. Crawford FE, Back DJ, Orme MLE, et al: Oral contraceptive steroid plasma concentrations in smokers and nonsmokers, *Br Med J* 282;1829, 1981.

26. Creatsas G: Progestogens in reproductive endocrinology, *J Obstet Gynecol Reprod Biol* 41:28, 1991.

27. DeFronzo RA, Ferrannini E: Insulin resistance: a multifaceted syndrome responsible for NIDDM, obesity, hypertension, dyslipidemia, and atherosclerotic heart disease, *Diabetes Care* 14:173, 1991.

28. Delforge JP, Ferin J: A histometric study of two estrogens: ethinyl estradiol and its 3-methyl ether derivative (mestranol): their comparative effect upon the growth of the human endometrium, *Contraception* 1:57, 1970.

29. Demers C, Ginsberg JS, Hirsh J, et al: Thrombosis in antithrombin-III deficient persons, *Ann Intern Med* 116:754, 1992.

30. Dibbelt L, Knuppen R, Jutting G, et al: Group comparison of serum ethinyl estradiol, SHBG and CBG levels in 83 women using two low-dose oral contraceptives for three months, *Contraception* 43:1, 1991.

31. Dossetor J: Drug interactions with oral contraceptives, *Br Med J* 4:467, 1975.

32. Eckel RH: Lipoprotein lipase, *N Engl J Med* 320:1060, 1989.

33. Fazio A: Oral contraceptive drug interactions: important considerations, *South Med J* 84:997, 1991.

34. Fevery J, Steenberger W, VanDesmet V, et al: Severe intrahepatic cholestasis due to the combined intake of oral contraceptives and triacetyloleandomycin, *Acta Clin Belg* 38:242, 1983.

35. Friedman CI, Huneke AL, Kim MH, et al: The effect of ampicillin on oral contraceptive effectiveness, *Obstet Gynecol* 55:33, 1980.

36. Furie B, Furie BC: Molecular and cellular biology of blood coagulation, *N Engl J Med* 326:800, 1992.

37. Fuster V, Badimon L, Badimon JJ, et al: The pathogenesis of coronary artery disease and the acute coronary syndromes. (First of two parts), *N Engl J Med* 326:242, 1992.

38. Fuster V, Badimon L, Badimon JJ, et al: The pathogenesis of coronary artery disease and the acute coronary syndromes. (Second of two parts), *N Engl J Med* 326:310, 1992.

39. Galbraith RA, Michnovicz JJ: The effects of cimetidine on the oxidative metabolism of estradiol, *N Engl J Med* 321:269, 1989.

40. Gillespy M, Notelovitz M, Ellingsan AB, et al: Effect of long-term triphasic oral contraceptive use on glucose tolerance and insulin secretion, *Obstet Gynecol* 78:108, 1991.

41. Ginsberg HN: Lipoprotein physiology and its relationship to atherogenesis, *Endocrinol Metab Clin North Am* 19:211, 1990.

42. Godsland IF, Walton C, Felton C, et al: Insulin resistance, secretion and metabolism in users of oral contraceptives, *J Clin Endocrinol Metab* 74:64, 1991.

43. Godsland IF, Crook D, Wynn V: Clinical and metabolic considerations of long-term oral contraceptive use, *Am J Obstet Gynecol* 66:1955, 1992.

44. Goldman JA, Eckerling B: Blood glucose levels and glucose tolerance in women with subclinical diabetes receiving an oral contraceptive, *Am J Obstet Gynecol* 107:325, 1970.

45. Grimmer SF, Back DJ, Orme MLE, et al: The bioavailability of ethinyl estradiol and levonorgestrel in patients with an ileostomy, *Contraception* 33:51, 1986.

46. Grundy SM: Cholesterol and coronary heart disease: a new era, *Science* 256:2849, 1986.

47. Guengerich FP: Oxidation of 17α-ethynylestradiol by human liver cytochrome P-450, *Mol Pharmacol* 35:500, 1988.

48. Guengerich FP: Metabolism of 17α-ethynylestradiol in humans, *Life Sci* 47:1981, 1990.

49. Guengerich FP: Inhibition of oral contraceptive steroid-metabolizing enzymes by steroids and drugs, *Am J Obstet Gynecol* 163:2159, 1990.

50. Guillebaud J: The forgotten pill and the paramount importance of the pill-free week, *Br J Fam Planning* 12 (suppl): S35, 1987.

51. Hirsh J: Heparin, *N Engl J Med* 324:1565, 1991.

52. Hobbes J, Boutagy J, Shenfield GM: Interaction between ethanol and oral contraceptive steroids, *Clin Pharmacol Ther* 38:371, 1985.

53. Houssay BA, Foghia VG, Rodriguez RR: Production or prevention of some types of experimental diabetes by estrogens or corticosteroids, *Acta Endocrinol* 17:146, 1954.

54. Inman WHW, Vessey MP, Westerholm B, et al: Thromboembolic disease and the steroidal content of oral contraceptives: a report to the committee on safety of drugs, *Br Med J* 2:203, 1970.

55. Jones MK, Jones BM: Ethanol metabolism in women taking oral contraceptives, *Clin Exp Res* 8:24, 1984.

56. Joshi VM: The effects of oral contraceptives on carbohydrate, lipid, and protein metabolism in subjects with altered nutritional status and in association with lactation, *J Steroid Biochem* 11:483, 1979.

57. Jung-Hoffman C, Kuhl H: Interaction with the pharmacokinetics of ethinyl estradiol and progestogens contained in oral contraceptives, *Contraception* 40:299, 1989.

58. Kalkhoff RK: Effects of oral contraceptive agents on carbohydrate metabolism, *J Steroid Biochem* 6:949, 1975.

59. Kalkhoff RK: Effects of oral contraceptive agents and sex steroids on carbohydrate metabolism, *Am Rev Med* 23:429, 1972.

60. Kalkhoff RK: Metabolic effects of progesterone, *Am J Obstet Gynecol* 142:735, 1982.

61. Kasdorf G, Kalkhoff RK: Prospective studies of insulin sensitivity in normal women receiving oral contraceptive agents, *J Clin Endocrinol Metab* 66:846, 1988.

62. Kenagy R, Weinstein I, Heimberg M: The metabolism of free fatty acid by perfused livers from normal female and ovariectomized rats, *Endocrinology* 8:1613, 1981.

63. Knodell RG, Browne DG, Gwozdz GP, et al: Differential inhibition of individual human liver cytochromes P-450 by cimetidine, *Gastroenterology* 101:1680, 1991.

64. Kojima T, Lindheim SR, Duffy DM, et al: Insulin sensitivity is decreased in normal women by doses of ethinyl estradiol used in oral contraceptives, *Am J Obstet Gynecol* 169:1540, 1993.

65. Krauss RM, Burkman RT: The metabolic impact of oral contraceptives, *Am J Obstet Gynecol* 167:1177, 1992.

66. Leimenstoll G, Jessen P, Zabel P, et al: Drug-induced liver damage related to the combined use of cyclosporin A and a contraceptive, *Dtsch Med Wochenschr* 109:1989, 1984.

67. Lesko SM, Rosenberg L, Kaufman DW, et al: Cigarette smoking and the risk of endometrial cancer, *N Engl J Med* 313:593, 1985.

68. Loscalzo J, Braunwald E: Tissue plasminogen activator, *N Eng J Med* 319:925, 1988.

69. Mammen EF: Oral contraceptives and blood coagulation: a critical review, *Am J Obstet Gynecol* 142:781, 1982.

70. Mendel CM: The free hormone hypothesis: a physiologically based mathematical model, *Endocr Rev* 10:232, 1989.

71. Michnovicz JJ, Hershcope RJ, Naganuma H, et al: Increased 2-hydroxylation of estradiol as a possible mechanism for the anti-estrogenic effect of cigarette smoking, *N Engl J Med* 315:1305, 1986.

72. Mitchell MC, Hanew T, Meredith CG, et al: Effects of oral contraceptive steroids on acetaminophen metabolism and elimination, *Clin Pharmacol Ther* 34:48, 1983.

73. Murai JT, Mendel CM, Siiteri PK: Free fatty acids do not influence the concentrations of free steroid hormones in serum under physiological conditions, *J Clin Endocrinol Metab* 72:137, 1991.

74. Murphy AA, Zacur HA, Charache P, et al: The effect of tetracycline on levels of oral contraceptives, *Am J Obstet Gynecol* 164:28, 1991.

75. Nachman RL, Silverstein R: Hypercoagulable states, *Ann Intern Med* 119:819, 1993.

76. Nakajima ST, Gibson M: The effect of a meal in circulating steady-stage progesterone levels, *J Clin Endocrinol Metab* 69:917, 1989.

77. Orme ML'E, Back DJ, Breckenridge Am: Clinical pharmacokinetics of oral contraceptive steroids, *Clin Pharmacokinet* 8:95, 1983.

78. Orme M, Back DJ, Ward S, et al: The pharmacokinetics of ethynylestradiol in the presence and absence of gestodene and desogestrel, *Contraception* 43:305, 1991.

79. Pansini F, Bonaccorsi G, Genovesi F, et al: Influence of estrogens on serum free fatty acid levels in women, *J Clin Endocrinol Metab* 71:1387, 1990.

80. Pardridge WM: Serum bioavailability of sex steroid hormones, *J Clin Endocrinol Metab* 15:259, 1986.

81. Patwardhan RV, Desmond PV, Johnson RF, et al: Impaired elimination of caffeine by oral contraceptive steroids, *J Lab Clin Med* 95:603, 1980.

82. Pecquery R, Leneveu MC, Givdicelli Y: Estradiol treatment decreases the lipolytic responses of hamster white adipocytes through a reduction in the activity of the adenylate cyclase catalytic subunit, *Endocrinol* 118:2210, 1986.

83. Philip A, Murphy BEP: Does sex hormone-binding globulin play a role in the transport of estradiol in vivo? *Am J Obstet Gynecol* 148:643, 1984.

84. Phillips N, Duffy T: One-hour glucose tolerance in relation to the use of contraceptive drugs, *Am J Obstet Gynecol* 116:91, 1973.

85. Pincus G: *The control of fertility,* New York, 1965, Academic Press.

86. Prange AJ: Estrogen may well affect response to antidepressant, *JAMA* 219:143, 1972.

87. Radbert T, Gustafsan A, Skryten A, et al: Metabolic studies in gestational diabetic women during contraceptive treatment: effects on glucose tolerance and fatty acid composition of serum lipids, *Gynecol Obstet Invest* 12:17, 1982.

88. Reaven GM: Role of insulin resistance in human disease, *Diabetes* 37:1595, 1988.

89. Rebar RW, Zeserson K: Characteristics of the new progestogens in combination oral contraceptives, *Contraception* 44:1, 1991.

90. Reed MJ, Cheng RW, Noel CT, et al: Plasma levels of estrane, estrone sulfate and estradiol and the percentage of unbound estradiol in postmenopausal women with and without breast cancer, *Cancer Res* 43:3940, 1983.

91. Reimers D, Jezek A: The simultaneous use of rifampicin and other antitubercular agents with oral contraceptives, *Prax Klin Pneumonol* 25:255, 1971.

92. Roberts RK, Grice J, McGuffie C, et al: Oral contraceptive steroids impair the elimination of theophylline, *J Lab Clin Med* 101:821, 1983.

93. Scheen AJ, Jondrain BJ, Humblet DMP, et al: Effects of a 1-year treatment with a low-dose combined oral contraceptive containing ethinyl estradiol and cyproterone acetate on glucose and insulin metabolism, *Fertil Steril* 59:797, 1993.

94. Siiteri PK, Murai JT, Hammond GC, et al: The serum transport of steroid hormones, *Recent Prog Horm Res* 38:457, 1982.

95. Skkouby SO, Molsted-Pedersen L, Kuhl C: Low-dosage oral contraception in women with previous gestational diabetes, *Obstet Gynecol* 59:325, 1982.

96. Spellacy WN, Buhi WC, Spellacy CE, et al: Glucose insulin, and growth hormone studies in long-term users of oral contraceptives, *Am J Obstet Gynecol* 106:173, 1970.

97. Spellacy WN, Bendel RP, Buhi WC, et al: Insulin and glucose determinations after two and three years of use of a combination-type oral contraceptive, *Contraception* 20:892, 1969.

98. Speroff L, DeCherney A: Evaluation of a new generation of oral contraceptives, *Obstet Gynecol* 81:1034, 1993.

99. Stadel BV, Steinthal PM, Schlesselman JJ, et al: Variation of ethinyl estradiol blood levels among healthy women using oral contraceptives, *Fertil Steril* 33:257, 1980.

100. Stanczyk FA, Roy S: Metabolism of levonorgestrel, norethindrone and structurally related contraceptive steroids, *Contraception* 42:67, 1990.

101. Szabo AJ, Cole HS, Grimaldi RD: Glucose tolerance in gestational diabetic women during and after treatment with a combination-type oral contraceptive, *N Engl J Med* 282:646, 1976.

102. Thomas JA: Modification of glucagon-induced hyperglycemia by various steroidal agents, *Metabolism* 12:207, 1963.

103. Tikkanen MJ, Nikkila EA: Regulation of hepatic lipase and serum lipoprotein by sex steroids, *Am Heart J* 113:562, 1987.

104. VanDijke CPH, Weber JCP: Interaction between oral contraceptives and griseofulvin, *Br Med J* 288:1125, 1984.

105. Vigersky RA, Kono S, Saver M, et al: Relative binding of testosterone and estradiol to testosterone-estradiol-binding globulin, *J Clin Endocrinol Metab* 49:879, 1979.

106. Waine H, Frieden EH, Caplan HI, et al: Metabolic effects of Enovid in rheumatoid patients, *Arthritis Rheum* 6:796, 1963.

107. Walaas O: Effect of estrogens on the glycogen content of the rat liver, *Acta Endocrinol* 10:193, 1952.

108. Ware JA, Heistad D: Platelet-endothelium interactions, *N Engl J Med* 328:628, 1993.

109. Washburn SA, Adams MR, Clarkson TB, et al: A conjugated equine estrogen with differential effects with uterine weight and plasma cholesterol in the rat, *Am J Obstet Gynecol* 169:251, 1993.

110. Watkins PB, Wrighton SA, Maurel P, et al: Identification of an inducible form of cytochrome P-450 in the human liver, *Proc Natl Acad Sci USA* 82:6310, 1985.

111. Wrighton SA, Brian WR, Sari MA, et al: Studies on the expression and metabolic capabilities of human liver cytochrome P-450IIIA5 (HLP$_3$), *Mol Pharmacol* 38:207, 1990.

112. Wynn V, Godsland I: Effects of oral contraceptives on carbohydrate metabolism, *J Reprod Med* 31:892, 1986.

113. Zacur HA, Burkman RT, Kimball AW, et al: Existence of multiple peaks in plasma ethyl estradiol and norethindrone after oral administration of a contraceptive pill, *J Clin Endocrinol Metab* 75:1268, 1992.

114. Zamah NM, Humpel M, Kuhnz W, et al: Absence of an effect of high vitamin dosage on the systemic availability of ethinyl estradiol in women using a combination oral contraceptive, *Contraception* 48:377, 1993.

Chapter 16

ORAL CONTRACEPTIVES AND NEOPLASIA

George R. Huggins, MD,
Kathryn F. McGonigle, MD,
and Peter K. Zucker, MD

Combined estrogen-progestogen oral contraceptives (OCs) have been available in the United States since 1960. The first compound approved contained 10 mg of norethynodrel and 150 µg of mestranol. Current estimates of worldwide use are approximately 55 million and in the United States use is estimated at 8 million to 10 million women. Clearly, to justify such wide use of potent drugs, the risk-benefit ratio must weigh substantially in favor of the drug benefits. In the past 26 years more than 40 brands of combined OCs have been sold in the United States. Today, they contain one of the five synthetic progestogens (all derived from 19-nortestosterone and one of two estrogens). Most women are

now using combined OCs with 0.3 to 1 mg of progestogen and 20 to 50 µg of estrogen.[28] Since 1970 all of the newly introduced compounds have used ethinyl estradiol (EE_2) as the estrogen fraction.

Few issues evoke as much concern and controversy as does the suspected association between OC use and the development of cancer. Isolated case reports and preliminary findings may give rise to overwhelming pressure to discontinue use of the drug with little attempt to weigh its possible risk-benefit ratios (Fig. 16-1). This response is not confined to evidence among women. Suspicion of carcinogenicity in any animal species has raised similar concerns and evoked the same demand for drug withdrawal.

PROBLEMS OF INVESTIGATION

Investigation of the association of OC use and the development of cancer is confounded by several problems: (1) there is no suitable animal model in most cases; (2) there is generally a long lag time (approximately 15 years) after exposure to a carcinogen until the development of overt malignancy[29]; (3) there is a low incidence of malignant disease in the young female population; and (4) there are multiple etiologic influences, such as genetic, cultural, geographic, and environmental exposure to many possible carcinogens.

Each steroid formulation used for contraception undergoes extensive testing in several animal species before investigative use in women. These animal studies provide only presumptive evidence of carcinogenic potential within a single species and sometimes within a single strain of that species.

Extrapolation of conclusions from one species to another has dubious validity. Neither positive nor negative results with animal exposure to suspected carcinogens can be used with any degree of certainty in relation to women.

INVESTIGATIVE METHODS

The principal investigative methods in women include various epidemiologic approaches.[59] The methodologies most frequently used are (1) case reports (tumor registries), (2) disease rates and trends, (3) case-control studies, and

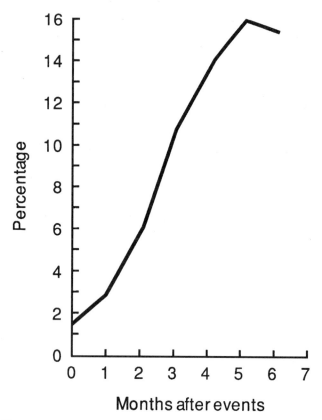

Fig. 16-1. OC discontinuation rates as a function of time elapsed after selected news events. (Redrawn from Grimes DA: In Mann RD, editor: *Oral contraceptives and breast cancer,* Park Ridge, NJ, 1989, Parthenon Publishing Group.)

(4) cohort studies. Each of these approaches provides a specific piece of a very complex puzzle. None of these methods taken by itself will provide a definitive answer as to causal relationships between exposure to an environmental carcinogen and the occurrence of disease. Needless to say, one would be unrealistic to ignore increasing and consistent evidence that is confirmed by these multiple approaches.

ORAL CONTRACEPTIVES AND BREAST DISEASE

The incidence of breast cancer in women has been rising since the mid-1940s, but the mortality rate has increased minimally. Most of this rise has occurred since 1980. Breast cancer incidence increased by about 4.5% per year between 1982 and 1986.[49] There are many theories as to why this increase is occurring. Reasons often cited can only partially explain this increase and include delayed childbearing, less breast-feeding, and increased mammographic screening. Improved treatment modalities and earlier detection may explain the relatively stable mortality rate despite the increasing incidence.

Most of the data fail to support a contribution of OCs to this rise. However, any commonly used drug that may change the risk of benign or malignant breast diseases would have significant public health implications. OCs have always been under great scrutiny as to what potential adverse effects on the breast they may have. Recently because of a few studies suggesting a positive association, this scrutiny has increased.

Breast physiology: endogenous and exogenous hormones

There is a paucity of data on the physiology of the human breast and the effects of endogenous and exogenous hormones. If OCs exert an adverse effect for cancer of the breast, it is not clear whether it is the estrogen component, the progestogen component, or an interaction of both components that is most significant.

Although the physiology of growth, differentiation, and hormonal control of the human breast are not fully understood, some information is available. The development of the female breast depends on an ideal progesterone (P) to estradiol (E_2) balance in conjunction with prolactin and other endogenous hormones. Before complete differentiation of breast epithelial ductal cells, the cells may be highly susceptible to the action of a carcinogen. Full development of the mammary gland is completed only at the end of the first pregnancy.[47] Thus there is concern that OCs may increase the risk of breast cancer with use before a first term pregnancy or with use at a very young age.

The effect of the changing levels of endogenous hormones during the menstrual cycle on proliferative activity of breast intralobular epithelium may be important. The greatest proliferative activity occurs during the second half of the menstrual cycle, and the peak proliferative activity declines with increasing age.

Potten et al.[61] studied the effect of age and menstrual cycle on proliferative activity of normal human breast intralobular epithelium, using tritiated thymidine. They noted that proliferative activity was highly variable and was highest on day 21.5 and lowest on day 7.5 of a 28-day menstrual cycle. Anderson et al.[3] studied proliferative activity of normal breast epithelial cells, using morphologic identification of mitosis. They also found a peak in proliferative activity during the second half of a 28-day menstrual cycle, with a peak in mitotic index on day 25. When the authors examined the data by subgroups of age between ages 15 and 45 years, they found that all subgroups showed significant cyclic variation in proliferative activity throughout the menstrual cycle but that the youngest group showed the greatest fluctuation. The differences between the age groups were not significantly different. When the authors examined their data on the basis of parity, they found that the degree of fluctuation for mitosis was slightly greater for the nulliparous groups.

The peak of proliferative activity in the breast during the second half of the menstrual cycle is opposite to that seen in the endometrium, where the peak proliferation occurs during the first half of the menstrual cycle. These studies demonstrate that peak proliferative activity in the breast occurs at a time in the menstrual cycle when endometrial proliferation is at its lowest, a time of relatively higher endogenous P levels.

No difference has been found between the proliferative rates of terminal ductal cells of benign breast tissues and fibroadenomas of OC users versus nonusers. However, a study by Anderson et al.[2] suggested that the nulliparous breast may be more susceptible to the adverse effects of exogenous hormones. There was a differential effect for OCs on parous breasts versus nulliparous breasts for proliferative activity. For OC users nulliparous breasts showed a significant increase in proliferative activity, compared with controls and parous breasts. When the data were analyzed for OC type for nulliparous breasts, the progestogen-only pills showed the greatest overall activity. These data are preliminary, and whether an increase in breast epithelial proliferative activity precedes the development of malignancy is unknown.

Progestogens and breast cancer risk

Most studies suggest that progestogens are protective against benign breast disease. Whether progestogens are protective for breast cancer is less clear. Because of the paucity of breast tissue studies, many of the data suggesting a protective effect of progestogens on the breast have been extrapolated from endometrial data, which may not be valid. In the endometrium, unopposed estrogens exert an adverse effect and progestogens are protective against endometrial cancer. The studies just discussed on breast epithelial proliferative activity during the menstrual cycle suggest that the effects of endogenous hormones on breast tissue are different from those on endometrium. Furthermore, if exogenous progestogens are protective against cancer, preliminary studies suggest that the mechanism differs from that for endometrium.[72,83] Progestogens are thought to decrease endometrial cancer by (1) down-regulating estrogen receptors[84] and (2) increasing 17β-E_2 dehydrogenase (E_2DH) activity, an enzyme that converts E_2 to biologically less active estrone.[26] Neither of these mechanisms occurs in preliminary studies of breast cancer tissues.[72,83]

Shinzaburo et al.[72] evaluated the effect of high-dose oral medroxyprogesterone acetate on estrogen and progestogen receptors in breast cancer tissues. Progestogen receptors but not estrogen receptors were reduced. Furthermore, Teulings et al.[83] evaluated patients with progressive metastatic breast cancer. E_2DH activity was measured at baseline and after megestrol acetate treatment. No increase in E_2DH activity after treatment with megestrol acetate was seen. Thus it appears that the mechanisms by which progestogens affect breast cancer vary substantially from those on endometrial cancer and benign endometrial tissues. Although progestogens down-regulate estrogen receptors and increase E_2DH activity in endometrial cancer and benign endometrial tissues, these preliminary data suggest that they fail to do so in breast cancer tissue. Accordingly, data on endometrial tissue should not be extrapolated to breast tissue. If progestogens are protective against breast cancer the effect may be due to other, indirect, mechanisms, such as by decreasing gonadotropin and adrenocorticotropic hormone levels and decreasing estrogen synthesis from the ovaries and the adrenals.[72]

Preliminary data do not suggest an adverse effect of progestogen on the risk of developing breast cancer. Clearly, however, more basic breast tissue studies and epidemiologic studies are needed to elucidate the effects of endogenous and exogenous hormones on benign and malignant breast tissues.

Benign breast disease

Association with risk of subsequent breast cancer. Benign breast disease is associated with an increased risk of subsequent breast cancer.[31] Benign breast disease is not a single well-defined disease, making this hypothesis difficult to evaluate. The histologic diagnoses are sometimes confusing and inconsistent. Fibrosis, fibrocystic disease, fibroadenoma, cystic mastitis, adenosis, hypermetaplastic disease, and intraductal papillomas are terms used in discussion of benign breast disease.[36] Because there is no standard terminology for benign proliferative breast disorders, direct comparisons among various studies are difficult.

Despite this confusion, an attempt to analyze benign breast disorders as to risk of subsequent development of breast cancer has been made.[31] Studies have demonstrated that proliferative epithelial lesions affecting the small ducts and terminal ductal lobular units confer an excess risk for breast cancer.[31] A consensus conference jointly sponsored by the College of American Pathologists and the American Cancer Society convened in 1985 to determine the risk relationship between benign lesions and breast cancer.[21] Risks were determined and categorized by pathologic examination. The most common symptomatic benign breast conditions are lobular hyperplasia, cystic duct dilation, fibroadenoma, and sclerosing adenosis. These conditions were not associated with an increased risk of breast cancer. Only those patients with significant hyperplasia showed an increased risk of breast cancer (1.5 to 5 times).[21]

Epidemiologic studies. A number of studies have demonstrated that OC use is associated with significantly decreased risks of benign breast disease.[12,68,89] Relative risks generally have been found to be 0.3 to 0.7 those of non–OC users. Most studies do not include women with biopsy-proven benign breast disease, making the data less clear-cut.

There are excellent data to support the hypothesis that the high-progestogen-dose OCs used before the mid-1970s protected against most forms of benign breast disease. However, the data are unclear whether OCs protect against

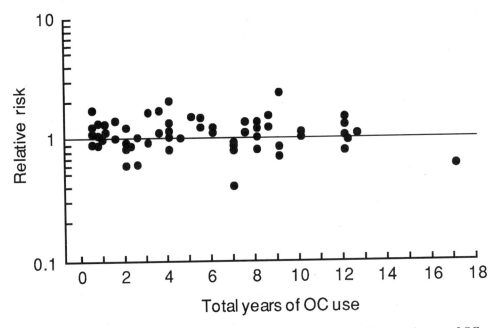

Fig. 16-2. Breast cancer in women younger than age 60 years: relative risk by total years of OC use in 17 studies. (Redrawn from Schlesselman JJ: *Contraception* 40:1, 1989, with permission of Butterworth-Heinemann, Stoneham, Mass.)

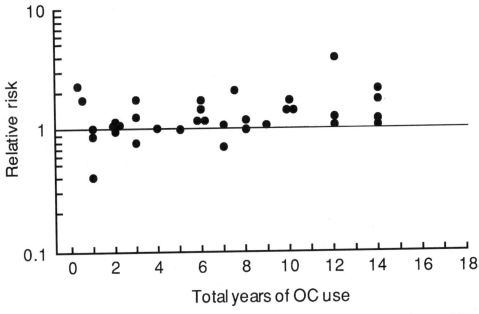

Fig. 16-3. Breast cancer in women younger than age 45 years: relative risk by total years of OC use in nine studies. (Redrawn from Schlesselman JJ: *Am J Obstet Gynecol* 163:1379, 1990.)

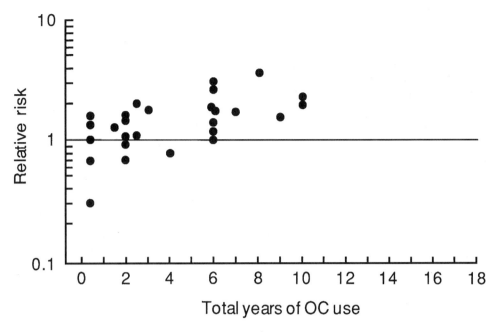

Fig. 16-4. Breast cancer in women younger than age 45 years: relative risk by total years of OC use before first term pregnancy in nine studies. (Redrawn from Schlesselman JJ: *Am J Obstet Gynecol* 163:1379, 1990.)

those forms of benign breast disease associated with a decreased or increased risk of subsequent breast cancer, based on histologic or mammographic studies. Furthermore, it is unclear whether current low-progestogen-dose OCs will confer the same protection. Accordingly, the beneficial effects of OCs on benign breast disease may be much less than early estimates. Further studies are necessary to clarify this issue.

Breast cancer

Epidemiologic studies. Immense amounts of data have been published concerning the relationship between OC use and the risk of breast cancer in women. Studies that have shown a protective effect of OCs against benign breast disease have failed to show the same protection against breast cancer. Fig. 16-2 summarizes the results of 17 case-control studies published during the 1980s. These studies evaluated the risk for the cohort of women under age 60 and overall failed to show an association between breast cancer and increasing duration of OC use.[70]

However, as data accumulated in the 1980s, several studies suggested that OCs may increase the risk of breast cancer before age 45. Fig. 16-3 summarizes the results of nine case-control studies for the development of breast cancer before age 45 based on years of OC use.[70] Overall there appears to be an increase in risk with increased duration of OC use. Furthermore, some studies have suggested that use before a first term pregnancy may be a significant risk factor for this cohort. Fig. 16-4 summarizes the results of nine case-control studies based on OC use

before a first full-term pregnancy for the development of breast cancer before age 45.[70] Again there appears to be a subtle increase in risk with increased duration of OC use. Because of these preliminary data, most recent studies have separately analyzed a cohort of women for development of breast cancer at a young age and have also evaluated other subgroups. Investigators have focused on those subgroups of patients that are independently at an increased risk of breast cancer. Several of these recent studies have identified a possible association of increased risk of early-occurring breast cancer and long-term use of high-dose combination OCs used in the 1960s and 1970s, sometimes only in a particular subgroup.

Association with age. For the cohort of women developing breast cancer under age 60, almost all studies published in the last 10 years have failed to identify a positive association between OCs and breast cancer.[65] During this time period, data from two studies, Ravnihar et al.[63] and the World Health Organization (WHO) Collaborative Study,[97] suggested an increased risk with increased duration of use for this group. Ravnihar et al.[63] found the risk for OC users of developing breast cancer between the ages of 24 and 54 was about 1.6-fold that of never-users. The risk increased with increasing duration of OC use. The highest risk was in those who used OCs for more than 7 years, with a statistically significant test for trend with increased duration. The WHO Collaborative Study[97] found an increased relative risk (RR = 1.15) for breast cancer in women less than age 60 who had ever used OCs. The risk was of borderline statistical significance. A statistically significant trend of increasing risk with years of use was found. For more than 8 years of use the relative risk was 1.56.

When the cohort is limited to women developing breast cancer before age 45, a positive association emerges in some studies. Several of these studies have noted this increase only in certain subgroups of this cohort. The WHO Collaborative Study[97] found no significant difference overall in evaluating risks for women under age 35 versus those over age 35. Relative risks for both groups were not statistically increased (RR = 1.26 and 1.12, respectively). In contrast, Wingo et al.,[93] in the Centers for Disease Control analysis of the Cancer and Steroid Hormone Study data, found a differential effect for the risk of breast cancer based on age at presentation. For breast cancer presenting between ages 20 and 34 years the risk was increased (RR = 1.4), whereas for breast cancer diagnosed between ages 45 and 54 years the risk was slightly decreased (RR = 0.9) for those who had used OCs. Both risks were of borderline statistical significance, and there was no trend of increasing or decreasing cancer risks with increased duration of use. Other studies have failed to identify an increased risk of breast cancer in young women under age 45 even when examining subgroups.[35,88,92]

Before age 45 years. For several groups, early analyses of data failed to reveal an increased risk. Only after further accumulation of data and/or further statistical analyses of subgroups did an increased risk emerge for the cohort of women under age 45 at diagnosis. These include the Cancer and Steroid Hormone Study analyses,[76,93] the study by Miller et al.,[45] and the Royal College of General Practitioners (RCGP) study.[35] Before the 1988 analysis, the Cancer and Steroid Hormone Study consistently failed to find an increased risk of breast cancer in young women with OC use.[15,18,71,78] Stadel et al.,[78] in the 1985 analysis of the Cancer and Steroid Hormone Study data, found no statistical change in the risk of breast cancer for women under age 45, but they did find that with start of OC use between ages 30 and 34, the risk increased slightly with duration of use (RR = 1.3 for 13 to 48 months of use and 1.5 for more than 48 months of use); however, the statistical test for trend was not significant. Schlesselman et al.,[71] in a later analysis of the Cancer and Steroid Hormone Study data, found no increased risk of breast cancer for women aged 20 to 44 with increased length of OC use, even with 10 to 14 years of use. On the contrary, Stadel and Lai,[76] in an even later analysis of the Cancer and Steroid Hormone Study data, found an increased relative risk of breast cancer before age 45 only in nulliparous women who had had menarche before age 13 and who had used OCs for more than 8 years. For this group, the risk increased with increasing duration of OC use, from 2 to 3 years of use to more than 12 years of use, but statistical significance was not reached until 8 or more years of use. The relative risk for more than 8 years of use was 3.8. In contrast, in an analysis of the Centers for

Disease Control data performed independently of that by Stadel and Lai,[76] Wingo et al.[93] found that, among women aged 20 to 34 years at diagnosis, ever-users had a slightly increased risk of breast cancer (RR = 1.4), compared with never-users, that was of borderline statistical significance. There were no statistically significant trends of increasing risk with increasing duration of use. However, the youngest women consistently had elevated risks. Unlike the analysis by Stadel and Lai[76] of the Cancer and Steroid Hormone Study, the increased risk for this age cohort was identified in all subgroups.

Miller et al.,[44] in a hospital based, case-control study, found no increased risk with increasing length of use. In a later study conducted in the same manner, Miller et al.[45] found a statistically significant increased risk for breast cancer before age 45 with OC use of more than 5 years (RR = 3.3) for women aged 25 to 34 and for women aged 35 to 44 (RR = 2.4). There was a statistically significant increased risk with increased length of use. Interestingly, in this study, the increased risk pertained to women using OCs for less than 3 months, which is biologically unlikely.

In an early report from the RCGP prospective cohort study,[69] no overall increased risk for breast cancer was found. A nonsignificant increased risk (RR = 2.81) was found for women diagnosed with breast cancer before age 35. For women aged 30 to 34 at diagnosis, the risk (RR = 3.33) was of borderline statistical significance. In a later analysis of the ongoing data, Kay and Hannaford[35] found a statistically significant increased risk of developing breast cancer for women aged 30 to 34 (RR = 3.33) compared with never-users, but the trend of increasing risk with increased duration of use was not significant.

Each of these studies has demonstrated an increased risk for the development of breast cancer before age 45. Although the increased risk often occurs in somewhat different subgroups of women, there is a suggestion that long-term use of high-dose OCs confers an increased risk for the development of breast cancer at a young age.

Association with parity and use before first term pregnancy. Most studies have found no association with OC use before a first term pregnancy[71] for the cohort of women under age 60 diagnosed with breast cancer. However, many of these studies did not separately analyze this risk factor for development of breast cancer at a young age.

When the evaluation is limited to those women developing breast cancer before age 45, more data are available and several studies have identified an increased risk of breast cancer for this cohort with increasing OC use before a first term pregnancy. In a recent analysis of the Cancer and Steroid Hormone Study data, Stadel and Lai[76] identified significantly elevated risk (RR = 3.8) of breast cancer before age 45 in women using OCs for more than 8 years who had had menarche before age 13 but only for nulliparous women. This association was not found for women whose menarche occurred after age 13 or with use less than 8 years. The relative risk for 8 to 11 years of use was 2.7 and for more than 12 years of use was 11.7. Paul et al.[56] attempted to replicate the Cancer and Steroid Hormone Study analysis in their case-control study. They found a nonstatistically significant increased risk (RR = 1.2) for nulliparous women under age 45 who had had menarche before age 13, and with 12 or more years of OC use. There was no trend in risk with increased duration of use.

Romieu et al.[64] performed a meta-analysis to summarize data on OC use and breast cancer. Study results were pooled, using a model that accounted for both interstudy and intrastudy variability. Romieu et al. found an increased risk of breast cancer for women under age 45 exposed to OCs for prolonged durations. This risk was significantly elevated among women who had used OCs for at least 4 years before their first term pregnancy (RR = 1.72). On the contrary, Miller et al.[45] found an increased risk of breast cancer before age 45 for women using OCs for more than 5 years. The risk was no greater for use before a term pregnancy. Overall, Paul et al.[56] failed to identify an association between OC use and breast cancer risk before age 45 at diagnosis; however, they found that for nulliparous women and parous women, OC use before a first term pregnancy was associated with a decreased risk of breast cancer before age 45 with increasing duration of OC use, but the trend was not statistically significant.

Overall, the data are suggestive of a slightly increased risk of breast cancer before age 45 with increasing length of high-dose OC use before a first term pregnancy. However, there are significant inconsistencies in the studies, making any definitive conclusions difficult.

At young ages. The question of whether early start of OC use and/or prolonged use at a young age is an important determinant of risk has been addressed by many studies. Most studies define use at a young age to be use either before age 20 or before age 25. Olsson et al.,[52] in a case-control study from Sweden, found that women starting OCs before age 20 had a nearly six-fold increased risk for developing breast cancer. For women using OCs for more than 5 years before age 25, there was a fivefold increased risk. The trends for increased risk with duration of use before age 25 and with earlier starting ages were significant. The study by Olsson et al. has been criticized because the interviews may have been biased.[79] In the 1985 analysis of the Cancer and Steroid Hormone Study data,[78] Stadel and Lai[76] found no association with OC use before age 20. In an analysis of the Cancer and Steroid Hormone Study data by subgroups, Stadel and Lai[76] found that for women developing breast cancer before age 45, with menarche before age 13 and for use of more than 8 years, there was an increased risk with use before age 20 (RR = 5.6) relative to use after age 20 (RR = 2.6). No mention was made as to whether these two numbers were significantly different. On

the contrary, in the recent Centers for Disease Control analysis of the Cancer and Steroid Hormone Study data by Wingo et al.,[93] among women aged 45 to 54 years, there was a statistically significant trend of decreasing breast cancer risk with decreasing age at first use. The protective effect was most pronounced among women who first used OCs before age 25 (RR = 0.5).

Most studies failed to find an increased risk of breast cancer with duration of OC use at a young age[74] or with early start of OC use. Overall, the largest and best-conducted studies evaluating risk based on age at first use and prolonged use at a young age have failed to identify an association with breast cancer and OC use for this group, suggesting that these are not significant risk factors. However, in view of a few studies suggesting some association, more data are required.

Association with hormone content. Several studies have evaluated the effect of OC formulation on the risk of breast cancer. Although a few studies suggest that one formulation or another may be associated with an increased risk, there is no consensus. Because most of the data are based on retrospective analyses, there is the problem of recall, which makes the quality of data questionable. Overall, on the basis of these studies there is no particular formulation or hormone type that is associated with an increased risk of breast cancer.

There are few data specifically analyzing the effect of estrogen dose. However, a recent study by the UK National Case-Control Study Group[85] found that OCs containing less than 50 μg of estrogen present a lower risk than do higher-dose pills. They also found that progestogen-only pills may have some protective effect with use over 12 months. These findings suggest that there may be a dose-response effect based on estrogen content and that the current lower-dose-estrogen contraceptives and progestogen-only OCs may confer a lower risk.

Association with history of benign breast disease. Several studies have evaluated the risk of breast cancer with OC use in women with a history of benign breast disease. Unfortunately, many of these studies have failed to confirm the diagnosis of benign breast disease by a history of previous biopsy. Fasal and Paffenbarger[23] found a significantly increased risk (RR = 11.2) for women with a history of benign breast disease who had used OCs for more than 6 years. Stanford et al.[80] found a twofold increased risk of breast cancer for OC users with a history of two or more breast biopsies.

Numerous other studies have found no increased risk. An analysis of the Cancer and Steroid Hormone Study data[18] demonstrated a significantly decreased risk (RR = 0.7) for women with a history of OC use and surgery for benign breast disease relative to non–OC users with a history of surgery for benign breast disease. Based on the inconsistent study designs and data, Stadel and Schlesselman[77] published a review assessing the overall risk of women with *existing* benign breast disease and OC use. They pointed out that the designs of many studies failed to exclude clearly the possibility that some patients included developed benign breast disease subsequent to the initiation of OCs. They concluded that there is insufficient evidence to show that OC use increases the risk of breast cancer in women with a preexisting history of benign breast disease and made a plea for inclusion of only women with documented benign breast disease before OC use when evaluating this risk factor.

Association with family history of breast cancer. Studies have varied considerably as to their conclusions about the risk of breast cancer in an OC user with a family history of breast cancer. Ravnihar et al.[63] found that patients who had used OCs and had a positive family history had a relative risk of 7.36 compared with OC users with no family history of breast cancer (RR = 1.54). Black et al.[10] found that women with a positive family history for breast cancer (grandmother or aunt) had an increased risk for developing breast cancer before age 45 with usage of OCs. However, they also found that OC use with a negative family history was associated with a significantly decreased risk of breast cancer (RR = .4 for current users and .58 for ever-users). In a recent analysis of the data from the UK National Case-Control Study Group,[86] although women with a family history of breast cancer had a slightly greater risk associated with OC use than those without, the difference in trends was not significant.

A recent analysis of the Cancer and Steroid Hormone Study data[48] failed to identify a positive association between OC use and family history of breast cancer. In fact, among women with a first-degree family history, a significantly decreased risk (RR = 0.4) occurred for women who had used OCs for 73 to 96 months. However, there was no pattern of increasing or decreasing risk by duration of use. Other studies have similarly failed to find a positive association. Although the data are not clear, the largest and best-conducted studies thus far suggest that women with a family history of breast cancer are not at increased risk of breast cancer because of OC use.

Association with disease at presentation and prognosis. There are very few data evaluating whether OCs change the "type" of breast cancer that occurs after exposure to OCs. Data on unopposed estrogen exposure for postmenopausal women suggest that estrogen use is associated with a well-differentiated, early-stage, and often easily treatable type of endometrial cancer. Preliminary data do not suggest that OC exposure results in a more curable type of breast cancer.

An evaluation of the histopathology of breast cancer tissue in women with a history of OC use demonstrated no significant difference from breast cancer tissue in controls.[46] Similarly, Spencer et al.[75] found no differences in the histologic features of tumor or extent of axillary node disease in patients with breast cancer who had taken OCs compared with those who had never taken OCs. Rosner et al.[66] found no difference between OC users and nonusers for extent of disease at presentation, histologic features of tumor or axillary node involvement, or disease-free interval or survival. The WHO Collaborative Study[97] failed to identify a difference in tumor size at presentation for OC users versus non–OC users.

Several studies have found that a history of OC use results in a more favorable prognosis in women with breast cancer. Matthews et al.[41] found that tumors in women who had used OCs had more favorable clinical and histologic features than did tumors of control subjects. Vessey et al.[88] found that women who had used OCs presented with less advanced tumors than did women who had not been using OCs during the year before detection of the cancer. Furthermore, they found that recent OC users had a lower mortality than did past users, who had a lower mortality than did never-users. The differences were not statistically significant. The UK National Case-Control Study Group[85] found that patients who had ever used OCs were more likely to have a lower clinical stage and less likely to have cancer-positive axillary nodes than never-users.

On the contrary, several studies have associated a history of OC use with poor prognostic factors. Olsson et al.[53] found that women who had used OCs at an early age (under age 20) had decreased survival with breast cancer. Those patients presented at more advanced stages, compared with women who had never used OCs or those who had started use at age 20 or later. Kay and Hannaford[35] found that in women under age 35 at diagnosis, a not-statistically-significant increased number of women had more invasive (grade III) tumors than did control women. Similarly, for this group, the 5-year survival rate was significantly lower than that of controls (37% versus 100%). Romieu et al.[65] found no difference between past users and non–OC users in the frequency of histologic type, tumor size, or lymph node involvement. However, they found that current users tended to have tumors that were larger and more likely to be metastatic at diagnosis. Because of the inconsistent data, it is unclear whether a history of OC use changes the stage at presentation or the prognosis of breast cancer.

Association with receptor status. Several groups have examined estrogen or progestogen receptor status in relationship to history of OC use. Romieu et al.[65] found that breast cancers diagnosed in women who were past OC users were more likely to be positive for estrogen receptors than were those diagnosed in women who had never used OCs. No relationship was noted between OC use and the progestogen receptor status. In contrast, in a prospective study of women with breast cancer,[54] OC use and family history of breast cancer were examined with reference to their effects on estrogen receptor status. Among premenopausal and perimenopausal women, those patients with a family history of breast cancer in only a first-degree relative showed a borderline significant association between previous OC usage and subsequent tumor estrogen receptor protein expression. Lesser et al.[38] found that women taking OCs at the time of diagnosis of breast carcinoma had lower median estrogen receptor binding levels; they suggested that current OC hormone use may cause spuriously low estrogen receptor protein levels. Stanford et al.[81] demonstrated that women who had ever taken OCs had a 22% increased relative risk for receptor-negative cancer compared with nonusers. A history of prolonged OC use (more than 6 years) was associated with a 70% increased relative risk of receptor-negative cancer.

Based on these data, there is a suggestion that current or past OC use may influence the subsequent receptor status of breast cancer by decreasing the amount of estrogen receptor tumor protein in breast cancers. The effect of OCs on progestogen receptor status is less clear. Because of the paucity of data and some inconsistencies, more data are required to answer these questions.

Clinical implications. Despite the fact that large amounts of data are available on the relationship between OCs and breast cancer, significant controversy still remains. Although there are some consistencies, many of the data are conflicting and confusing. Epidemiologists use five criteria to evaluate the evidence: (1) strength of association, (2) temporal sequence, (3) dose-response relationships, (4) biologic plausibility, and (5) consistency of results. The first criterion, strength of association or magnitude by which the risk of a disease is changed, is significant only in some studies and usually just for a very small fraction of OC users. The second criterion, temporal sequence, is present in each study. Women were exposed to OCs before the development of breast cancer. The third criterion, dose-response relationship, is demonstrated in several studies. Studies that demonstrate a trend of increasing relative risk with increased duration of OC use (dose) are more convincing than those in which there is an increased relative risk without an associated trend. The fourth criterion, biologic plausibility, also is demonstrated in most of the studies. However, in the study by Miller et al.[45] an increased risk was found after only 3 months of OC use. This is not biologically plausible. The fifth criterion, consistency of results, is the biggest problem with the data. For example, consider recent studies evaluating breast cancer in women under age 45: The analysis by Stadel and Lai[76] of the Cancer and Steroid Hormone Study found an increased risk in nulliparous women who had had menarche before age 13 with long-term use. In contrast, a recent analysis of the Centers for Disease Control Cancer and Steroid Hormone Study data[93] suggests a borderline increased risk for women aged 20 to 34 at diagnosis and a protective effect of women aged 45 to 54 years at diagnosis that was more pronounced for use of OCs at a young age. The RCGP study[35] found independent increased risks for women of para 1 and for women aged 30 to 34 at diagnosis, whereas

the UK National Case-Control Study[85] found an increased risk for parous and nulliparous women under age 36. Meirik et al.[42] found use before a first term pregnancy to be significant, whereas Olsson et al.[52] found use at a young age and early age at start of use to be most significant. Thus with five different studies and two different analyses of the same study, there are six somewhat different findings. The one most consistent finding is an increase in risk for breast cancer at a young age.

The apparent inconsistencies in epidemiologic findings are perplexing, and investigators have analyzed their study designs for an explanation. Skegg[74] noted that case-control studies may be influenced by bias through (1) the selection of cases and controls that are not truly compatible; (2) the potential differences in recall of information by patients with breast cancer, compared with controls; and (3) a difference in surveillance for breast cancer for OC users versus controls, that is, more frequent breast examination of women using OCs can result in earlier diagnosis and an apparent excess of cases in the younger age group who have used OCs.

Despite some inconsistencies in the data, one cannot ignore the fact that so many of the major epidemiologic studies have identified an increased risk in one subgroup or another for the development of breast cancer at a young age. Stadel et al.[51] have suggested that this may represent a promotional effect associated with long-term use of the discontinued, high-dose OC formulations in subgroups of women. If so, an increased incidence of breast cancer in young women may be associated with a concurrent decreased incidence in older women. In such case, the lifetime risk of breast cancer would not be increased, but the disease would occur at younger ages. This theory is supported by an analysis of the Cancer and Steroid Hormone Study data, in which the increased risk found in nulliparous women aged 20 to 44 is followed by an apparently decreased risk in women aged 45 to 54.[51] Similarly, the RCGP study[35] found an increased risk for women aged 30 to 34 at diagnosis but failed to find an increased risk in other age categories.

Present studies do not evaluate the risk of breast cancer for OC exposure in women currently over age 60, those women with the highest underlying risk. Because of the significantly higher baseline incidence of disease in this population, an increase or decrease in relative risk would be quite significant. The Centers for Disease Control Cancer and Steroid Hormone Study analysis[93] found that women aged 45 to 54 who had used OCs had a 10% decreased risk of breast cancer. If such a decrease in risk continues to be seen in even older women, a significant number of the aging population would actually be protected from breast cancer. There are significant data indicating that premenopausal and postmenopausal breast cancers are quite different diseases. They differ in biologic behavior, hormone receptor expression, and risk factors. It is reasonable to expect that there may also be a differential effect of OCs on the breast for the development of premenopausal versus postmenopausal breast cancer.

Furthermore, it is important to evaluate what an increased risk means to a given population. In the Cancer and Steroid Hormone Study analysis[76] in which an increased risk of breast cancer before age 45 was found only for nulliparous women who had had menarche before age 13 and had used OCs for more than 8 years, only 1.3% of the cases of breast cancer occurred in the "at risk group" (39 women). Furthermore, for the RCGP study[35] in which a 40% to 70% increased risk was found for all subgroups, the authors calculated that the absolute excess risk is about 1 in 7000 ever-users per year for those under age 35. Given how inconsistent the data from various studies are, it is likely that the risk, if present, even for subgroups of women, is small. In terms of evaluating the risk to current OC users it is important to remember that these data are based on the use of the high-dose formulations used in the 1960s to 1970s. It is reasonable to expect that the current lower-dose formulations carry even less risk, as is suggested by data from the UK National Case-Control Study Group in which combination OCs with a lower dose of estrogen conferred less risk.

The etiology of the rising incidence of breast cancer is largely unexplained. However, it is unlikely that OCs have contributed significantly to the increasing incidence of breast cancer: (1) The increase began in the mid-1940s, long before the introduction of OCs. (2) The increased incidence is noted in all age groups. The rise is greatest for older women (over age 50), who were less commonly exposed to OCs. Furthermore, the aggregate data suggest that if there is an increased risk of OCs for breast cancer, it is in women less than age 45 at diagnosis. (3) The data suggest that a very small number of women are affected, if any may have developed breast cancer as a result of OC exposure. Accordingly, national incidence data would unlikely be affected.

Based on all the evidence, authoritative bodies in the United States, Great Britain, and other countries independently came to similar conclusions in 1989. These include the United States Food and Drug Administration's Fertility and Maternal Health Drugs Advisory Committee, the American College of Obstetricians and Gynecologists, the United Kingdom Committee on the Safety of Medicines, the Swedish national drug authorities, the WHO, and the International Planned Parenthood Federation. Each agency has recommended no change in OC labeling, prescribing, or use.[1,51] However, in August 1990 the manufacturers of OCs in the United Kingdom, as a result of discussions with the United Kingdom Medicines Control Agency, inserted a statement in the OC leaflets about the possible association between the prolonged use of OCs and breast cancer in young women.[32]

ORAL CONTRACEPTIVES AND CERVICAL NEOPLASIA

The epidemiologic factors responsible for the development of cervical dysplasia and subsequent progression to carcinoma in some patients are complex and poorly understood. One of the major epidemiologic factors in carcinoma of the cervix seems to be age at first intercourse. Others, such as human papillomavirus, multiparity, frequency of intercourse, multiple sexual partners, and low socioeconomic status, may also relate to early age at the time of first intercourse.

Conclusions derived from a number of epidemiologic studies of cervical neoplasia vary considerably. A number of factors contribute to this variability: (1) The histologic interpretation of degrees of dysplasia and carcinoma in situ may vary from one pathologist to another. (2) The most important risk factors (age at first intercourse, frequency of intercourse, and number of sexual partners) are difficult to determine accurately. Despite the large numbers of both case-control and cohort studies, only one study before 1975 specifically analyzed the issues of age at first intercourse and contraceptive choice.[43] (3) There is a tendency for women using steroidal contraception to avail themselves of medical care more frequently than noncontraceptive users. As a result, certain disease processes may be underreported in populations not using contraceptives. (4) There is a confounding influence of sexually transmitted carcinogens. The carcinogenic effect of human papillomavirus is an important risk factor for cervical neoplasia. Epidemiologic studies must be designed to detect the incidence of this disease in their cases and controls. Analysis must also control adequately for this factor and other sexually transmitted diseases. Unfortunately, the authors of the most recent, sophisticated case-control studies of OC use and risk of cervical cancer have not been able to accomplish these ends. There are major problems in obtaining an accurate history of specific sexually transmitted diseases. Many patients cannot or will not relate a history of a specific sexually transmitted disease.

Most case-control studies before 1977 indicated no increased risk of cervical neoplasia associated with OC use.[11,98] The early analysis from the cohort studies was also reassuring. In their 1976 report Vessey et al.[89] found no cases of cervical dysplasia among 4217 diaphragm users. The incidences of dysplasia among 3162 intrauterine device (IUD) users and 9653 OC users were similar (0.28 and 0.31/1000 woman-years, respectively). There were only 12 cases recorded, and no valid statistical analysis was possible with so few cases. The RCGP reported on only "malignant neoplasm of cervix uteri" in 1974.[68] Two cases were observed in OC takers, two cases among "ex-takers," and four cases among the non–OC takers. These numbers were too small for statistical analysis. The Walnut Creek study[62] involving 17,942 women observed for 37,373 woman-years initially reported a statistically significant association between carcinoma in situ and duration of OC use. This analysis involved only 34 cases of carcinoma in situ and did not include analysis of age at first term birth or sexual activity and number of sexual partners. A later analysis of their data in 1977[57] confirmed the significance of these preliminary findings.

In a 1983 update Vessey et al.[91] reported on the incidence of biopsy-proven cervical neoplasia among 6838 parous women taking OCs who had been followed for 10 years in the Oxford Family Planning Association study. The control group consisted of 3145 parous women who entered the study while using an IUD. "Cervical neoplasia" in this study includes biopsy-proven dysplasia, carcinoma in situ, and invasive cancer. All 13 cases of invasive cervical cancer occurred in the OC group ($P < .05$). The aggregated data for all forms of cervical neoplasia showed a significant association with duration of OC use. The risk for OC users rose from 0.8/1000 woman-years to 2.2/1000 woman-years, whereas the risk among IUD users remained relatively constant at approximately 1/1000 woman-years. This study has been criticized in part for the lack of data on age at first intercourse and number of sexual partners.

The RCGP updated in 1988 its earlier report on genital tract malignancies.[8] Ever-users of OCs had an excess of invasive cervical cancer and of carcinoma in situ of the cervix. Furthermore, the incidence of both invasive and in situ lesions increased significantly with increasing duration of OC use. After more than 10 years of use the incidence was more than four times that in never-users. When incidence and number of previously normal cervical smears were examined, incidence tended to decline with the number of previous smears.

Several large studies reported after 1979 have attempted to determine age at first intercourse, age at first term birth, number of sexual partners, incidence of sexually transmitted disease, and other factors thought to be important in evaluating the relationship between risk of cervical cancer and OC use. Harris et al.[27] conducted one of the first case-control studies on the risks of cervical dysplasia and carcinoma in situ in which there was ascertainment of age at first intercourse and number of sexual partners. Significant risk factors were age at first intercourse, multiple sexual partners, and use of OCs. Statistically significant ($P < .05$) linear relationships were seen for length of use of OCs and risk of severe dysplasia and carcinoma in situ. These associations remained significant after adjusting for number of sexual partners.

The National Cancer Institute (NCI) undertook a large case-control study in five metropolitan areas in the United States[13] to examine this problem further. Analysis found that a number of risk factors were significantly correlated with the probability of exposure to OCs. The most significant confounding variable was interval since last Papanico-

laou smear. This variable exerted a substantially negative confounding result because those with a limited screening history were at extremely low risk for never having used OCs and at extremely high risk for invasive cervical cancer (fivefold to sixfold excess risk for those never having a cervical smear in the 10 years preceding diagnosis). The number of sexual partners, age at first intercourse, and history of a nonspecific genital infection or a genital sore acted as positive confounders. After adjusting for pertinent confounding variables, the risk associated with ever-use of OCs was 1.49 (95% confidence interval 1.1 to 2.1). In addition, there was a significant linear increase in risk ($P = .003$) with increasing duration of OC use.

Another large multicenter case-control study of cervical cancer and combined OCs was carried out under the auspices of the WHO.[94] To address some of the deficiencies of previous studies the data collection and analysis considered 23 variables of sexual behavior or access to medical care that might have been confounding variables. Included were data on gynecologic and obstetric history, sexual relationships, age at first intercourse, contraceptive history, and prior Papanicolaou smears. Among women who had ever used OCs the relationship to invasive cervical cancer showed a relative risk of 1.19 (95% confidence interval 0.99 to 1.44). When data were analyzed by duration of use, the relative risk rose in a linear trend and become significant for those patients who had no history of cervical smears. When duration of use was categorized in the same manner as that of Vessey et al.,[91] a similar trend was evident, and a relative risk of 1.63 (95% confidence interval 1.03 to 2.59) was observed in women who had used OCs for more than 8 years. The patients in this study were taken from populations quite different from those of the Oxford Family Planning Association study[91] or the NCI study[13] in the United States.

The Oxford prospective study[91] analyzed white, married British women. The NCI study[13] analyzed hospitalized women at both rural and urban settings in the United States. The WHO study[94] examined women who were from diverse geographic, racial, and socioeconomic backgrounds. These recent reports, like all other epidemiologic studies, suffer from methodologic problems. However, the consistency of their results adds weight to the concern that long-term OC use is associated with an increased risk of cervical dysplasia. Further studies involving diverse patient populations continue to show a slight increased risk of both in situ and invasive cervical cancer among long-term OC users. It is quite clear that most of this slight excess risk can be avoided by regular cervical cancer screening.

ORAL CONTRACEPTIVES AND OVARIAN CANCER

Since 1977 more than 10 studies have evaluated the risk of ovarian cancer and OC use. All have shown a protective effect of OCs. The largest study is the Cancer and Steroid Hormone Study.[17] The results published in 1983, based on a preliminary analysis of data, revealed that (1) the use of OCs reduced the risk of ovarian cancer, (2) the risk decreased as the duration of use increased, and (3) the effect persisted long after OCs had been discontinued. An update of the 1983 study[20] confirmed the initial findings and elaborated further on this protective effect of OCs. Women who had ever used OCs had a relative risk for ovarian cancer of 0.6, compared with those with no history of use. This reduced risk became apparent after only 3 to 6 months of use and was decreased further after 5 or more years of cumulative use. The protection was found to continue for 15 years after discontinuation of OC use. Furthermore, although both the duration of use and interval since first use appeared to be important variables, users of OCs compared with nonusers had a lowered risk of epithelial ovarian cancer, regardless of the time interval since most recent use. Additionally, this beneficial effect was noted to be independent of the specific OC formulation and unrelated to histologic type of epithelial ovarian cancer. These findings are supported by the RCGP OC cohort study of 47,000 women[8] demonstrating that ovarian cancer was responsible for 18% of invasive genital cancers in ever-users versus 35% in never-users.

The public health implications of this protective effect are significant. It is estimated that in the United States there were 18,000 new cases and 11,400 attributable deaths from ovarian cancer in 1983. Investigators estimate that more than 1700 cases of ovarian cancer are averted each year by past and current OC use among women in the United States.[20] If the current trend of increasing numbers of older contraceptors using OCs continues, the number of averted cases of ovarian cancer will increase substantially.

ORAL CONTRACEPTIVES AND GESTATIONAL TROPHOBLASTIC DISEASE

The potential for persistent trophoblastic proliferation after the initial evacuation of a hydatidiform mole is well documented. The successful evaluation and treatment of gestational trophoblastic disease depends on meticulous serial measurement of serum human chorionic gonadotropin (hCG) titers.[6] It may take as long as 100 days for serum hCG levels to disappear after termination of the molar gestation. Pregnancy should be avoided for at least 6 months after negative hCG levels are obtained.

The effect of OCs on the course of resolving gestational trophoblastic disease has been studied extensively. An earlier study by Stone and colleagues[82] found that administration of OCs to patients before the decline in postmolar hCG levels to normal resulted in a twofold risk of trophoblastic disease requiring chemotherapy. In addition, OCs were also found to inhibit the decline in hCG levels even in those not needing chemotherapy. Berkowitz et al.[9] analyzed

two groups of patients followed after molar pregnancy to determine the effects of OCs on the incidence of trophoblastic disease. Patients were comparable in age, gravidity, tumor histology, pretreatment hCG titers, and exposure to prophylactic chemotherapy. Of these patients, 11 of 58 (18.9%) using OCs and 6 of 42 (14.3%) using barrier methods developed post-molar pregnancy trophoblastic disease. These differences were not significantly different, and the authors concluded that OCs do not increase the risk of post-molar pregnancy trophoblastic disease. They recommended their use during the entire interval of gonadotropin monitoring. They further reported no significant difference in the mean hCG regression time regardless of whether a hormonal or nonhormonal contraceptive was used.

The conflicting conclusions of the two studies just discussed prompted further investigation. Yuen and Burch[99] prospectively studied 194 patients with pathologically confirmed molar pregnancies. Postpartum there was no significant difference in the β-hCG-positive interval among women who used barrier methods, IUDs, or combined OCs. The most recent report on the role of contraception in the development of post-molar pregnancy gestational trophoblastic tumor demonstrated a significantly lower risk for OC users than for noncontraceptors and a lower, but not statistically significant, difference for barrier and IUD contraception.

On the basis of the few available studies, use of combination OCs that contain 50 μg or less of EE_2 after evacuation of a hydatidiform mole appears to be safe and effective. Further studies are necessary to elucidate the relationship between high estrogen dose and persistent trophoblastic disease.

ORAL CONTRACEPTIVES AND PITUITARY TUMORS

Recognition of the complex relationship between serum estrogen concentration and potential augmentation of serum prolactin (PRL) release via effects on hypothalamic-pituitary sensors has led to scrutiny of the role that combination OCs might have in altering these neuroendocrine interactions. It has been speculated that OC-mediated stimulation of pituitary lactotropes by estrogen may cause excessive PRL secretion. Continued uncontrolled estrogenic influence might then lead to hypertrophy and hyperplasia of the lactotrope with possible formation of a pituitary PRL-secreting adenoma.

An awareness of these relationships, coupled with a reported rise in the incidence of pituitary adenomas among women of childbearing age, resulted in study of the relationship between the use of combination OCs and pituitary adenomas. Annegers et al.[4] reviewed the incidence of pituitary adenomas among various age-adjusted and sex-adjusted populations in Olmsted County, Minnesota, during 1935–1977. A dramatic increase in the mean annual incidence of these lesions was found in women aged 15 through 44 when data after 1969 were compared with those of earlier years. This observation led the authors to conduct a case-control study to determine whether OCs were associated with this increased incidence of pituitary adenomas. A decreased relative risk (0.5) was found for pituitary tumors in OC users. The authors concluded that the apparent rise in the incidence of pituitary tumors among women was due to improved diagnostic capabilities, including advances in radiologic technique and endocrinologic assays. This study involved only nine cases. Coulam et al.[22] noted that although several studies had reported a high prevalence of previous OC use by patients with pituitary adenomas (70% to 84%), the frequency of OC use in the general population frequently was unknown.

Because of the paucity of data on this important issue, the Pituitary Adenoma Study Group was established. This group undertook a large multicenter case-control investigation to analyze further the relationship between OCs and PRL-secreting pituitary adenomas.[58] Three groups consisting of 212 women with adenomas, 119 hyperprolactinemic patients with amenorrhea and/or galactorrhea with normal or equivocal tomograms, and 205 normoprolactinemic women with amenorrhea and/or galactorrhea were matched with neighborhood control subjects. No association was found between OC use and the development of pituitary adenomas within any of the three study groups.

On the basis of current available data there appears to be no increased risk of developing a pituitary adenoma in normal patients taking OCs. The question of whether women with menstrual irregularity taking OCs represent a high-risk group for these lesions remains unresolved.

ORAL CONTRACEPTIVES AND ENDOMETRIAL NEOPLASIA
Effects of estrogen and progesterone on endometrium

The endometrium is a hormonally responsive tissue layer whose histologic appearance is directly dependent on intrinsic steroid receptor-mediated activity. The interaction of estrogen and progesterone with their cytoplasmic protein receptors results in endometrial growth effects. Estrogenic influence results in cellular proliferation and further increase in the content of estrogen and progesterone receptors. As estrogen exerts its biologic effects via receptors, an increase in progesterone receptors facilitates the establishment of an estrogen-responsive milieu. Progesterone administration operates in reverse by decreasing levels of estrogen receptors, which results in diminished uterine estrogen response.

Unopposed estrogenic stimulation is believed to be responsible for these increased endometrial receptor levels and for the production of hyperplasia. Conversely, progesterone administration in patients with endometrial hyperplasia has been found to decrease hormone receptor con-

tent, with the more pronounced effect on progesterone receptors. There is convincing evidence that unopposed estrogen exposure leads to a spectrum of endometrial hyperplastic alterations that can progress to carcinoma.

Exposure of the normal estrogen-primed endometrium to progesterone converts the tissue to the typical secretory type seen during the luteal phase of the menstrual cycle. This cyclic effect of progesterone prevents the progression of normal proliferative endometrium to hyperplasia. Progesterone has been used therapeutically to convert a spectrum of hyperplastic lesions to normal histology. It is apparent that the delicate balance between circulating estrogen and progesterone levels and their interaction with endometrial cell receptor systems can have profound effects on endometrial growth.

Sequential oral contraceptives

Sequential OCs were first marketed in the United States in 1963. Their use was prompted in part by an effort to simulate more closely the natural sequence of estrogen only followed by estrogen-progesterone as found during the normal menstrual cycle. The scheme of administration involved estrogen (80 to 100 µg) alone for 14 to 16 days followed by an estrogen-progesterone combination for 5 or 6 days. The progestogen content varied from 2 to 25 µg.[1]

Silverberg and Makowski[73] and Lyon[39] in 1975 first reported the occurrence of endometrial carcinoma in young women taking sequential OCs. These reports were quickly followed by others. Because of the lack of a population-based registry, these authors were unable to establish whether endometrial carcinoma was more common in women using sequential agents than in the general population, or whether the incidence was merely decreased in users of combined agents. Further epidemiologic analysis of this problem in the United States by case-control or cohort studies was not possible. In 1976 the sequential OCs were voluntarily removed from the market by the manufacturers.

Combination oral contraceptives

Currently used combination OCs differ from their "sequential" predecessors in administration, composition, and dosage. The addition of a progestogen of higher potency to every pill taken per cycle has the effect of sufficiently opposing the stimulatory effect of estrogen and preventing hyperplastic growth patterns. All combined estrogen and progestogen OC pills exert a progestin or suppressive effect on endometrial growth. Several recent case-control studies found that users of combination OCs have approximately half the risk of developing endometrial carcinoma than do women who had never used these preparations.[30,34] This protective effect is evident after 1 year of continuous use.[34] Kaufman et al.[34] found the magnitude of protection to be directly proportional to the duration of use of combination

OCs, with a peak of protection at 3 years and beyond. Similarly, Hulka et al.[30] found that the risk of endometrial carcinoma was reduced further with 5 or more years of combination OC use.

The Centers for Disease Control analyzed data from its Cancer and Steroid Hormone Study to assess the relationship between use of combination OCs and the risk of endometrial cancer.[16,19] This report includes a case group larger than any previously reported. Ever-users of combination OCs had a relative risk of 0.6 of development of endometrial cancer, compared with never-users, which became apparent after 12 to 23 months of use. Reduction in risk was found to persist for at least 15 years after discontinuation. Protection appeared to be higher in women with parity less than 5 and maximal among nulliparous women. This study estimated that in 1982 approximately 2000 cases of endometrial cancer were averted by OC use in the United States. The WHO Collaborative Study of Neoplasia and Steroid Contraceptives[95] found a reduced relative rate for endometrial carcinoma in ever-users of combination OCs similar to that in the Cancer and Steroid Hormone Study.

The protective effect of OCs against endometrial cancer has significant public health implications, although disagreement exists regarding the duration and magnitude of the protective effect after the discontinuation of OCs. Several studies have observed a persistent effect for 5 to 15 years,[16,19] whereas others have noted a loss of this protective effect within 3 years.[30] As with ovarian cancer, increased OC use by older women will avert significantly more cases of endometrial cancer.

ORAL CONTRACEPTIVES AND LIVER TUMORS
Benign tumors

The first descriptions of a relationship between OC use and the development of benign hepatic lesions were reported in the early 1970s. The histopathologic diagnosis of benign liver tumors has been variously reported as focal nodular hyperplasia, adenoma, hamartoma, benign hepatoma, solitary hyperplastic nodule, and focal cirrhosis. Lesions of chief concern are hepatic adenoma and focal nodular hyperplasia. Subsequently, the relationship between usage of OCs and the development of hepatic adenoma has been well documented. The association between OC use and the appearance of focal nodular hyperplasia is less clear.

The Hepatic Branch of the Armed Forces Institute of Pathology and the Family Planning Evaluation Division, Bureau of Epidemiology, Centers for Disease Control in 1977 showed an increasing risk with increased duration of use.[5] In addition to duration of use, the study suggested that women aged 27 years and older who had used "high hormonal potency" pills for 7 or more years were at greatest risk for development of hepatocellular adenoma.

In an attempt to determine more carefully the extent of the problem, the National Cancer Advisory Board requested the American College of Surgeons' Commission on Cancer to conduct a national survey of the extent of primary benign and malignant liver tumors.[87] Four hundred seventy-seven hospitals in the United States searched their tumor registries and reported all primary benign and malignant liver tumors diagnosed from 1970 to 1975 in male and female patients aged 15 to 45 years. A total of 543 cases were uncovered, 378 in women and 165 in men. These cases were analyzed as to histologic type, age distribution, and contraceptive use. Analysis of malignant tumors revealed that the frequency increased with age. This finding mirrors the reported distribution in the general population. However, the frequency of benign lesions showed a large peak in the 26- to 30-year-old group. This peak corresponds to increased use of OCs in this age group. This large increase in benign lesions in the 26- to 30-year-old group is true only for OC users and only for benign lesions. However, the survey found no dose-response relationship and no association with duration of use. Forty percent of tumors were diagnosed in women exposed for 5 years or less. Hemorrhage was most frequently associated with adenomas and almost exclusively confined to the OC users. Although the risk of benign adenoma is elevated, these lesions are extremely rare and occur in less than 1/500,000 patients.

Focal nodular hyperplasia. Focal nodular hyperplasia is a benign liver tumor that is found most commonly in women of reproductive age. Histologic examination reveals that these tumors consist of proliferating nodules of normal-appearing hepatocytes separated by fibrous bands that contain large vessels and proliferating bile ducts. Because most patients do not experience symptoms, the lesion is usually discovered incidentally at laparotomy or in the course of evaluation of an unrelated condition.

Estimated incidence. Baum and associates[7] estimated an incidence of liver tumors of 1/500,000 to 1/1,000,000. Garcia and colleagues[25] suggested an incidence of 0.04/1,000,000 women. These low estimates of occurrence rates were confirmed by Vessey and colleagues.[89] They searched the records of patients enrolled in the RCGP OC study (116,000 woman-years of exposure to OCs) and the Oxford Family Planning Association follow-up study of women using different methods of contraception (more than 83,000 woman-years of exposure), and no case of benign or malignant liver tumor was found. In addition, the records of the Oxford linkage study were searched. This study covered the hospital admissions and deaths in a population of more than 1 million. No benign liver tumors were found in women of childbearing age from 1970 through 1975.[90] In a search of the Scottish National Diagnostic Index for the years 1968 through 1974, one case of benign liver tumor was found in a 23-year-old woman taking OCs for 2 years.[89] The system covered hospital admissions and deaths for a population of approximately 5 million people.

Clinical aspects. Although benign, hepatic tumors may

be life threatening because of their tendency to hemorrhage spontaneously, causing death. The patient at highest risk for spontaneous hemorrhage seems to be an OC user who has a hepatic cell adenoma larger than 3 cm who has taken a high-dose combination pill for more than 4 years. Adenoma size is the major risk factor for bleeding. The management of tumors determined to be focal nodular hyperplasia are managed similarly, although the chance of a hemorrhage is significantly less.

A hepatic adenoma can first present as an asymptomatic mass, but the majority of patients initially complain of epigastric or right upper quadrant abdominal pain. Unfortunately, a significant number of these patients also present with signs of intraperitoneal hemorrhage and shock. Timing may be significant in that some of these lesions seem most prone to rupture at or about the time of menstruation.[7]

The standard blood liver function tests are of little value in diagnosing these lesions because no consistent abnormalities are found. Computed tomography, ultrasonography, angiography, and sulfur colloid scintigraphy offer the most precise diagnostic approaches. Hepatic scintigraphy with sulfur colloid-labeled tracer may yield crucial information in assessing the nature of hepatic tumors with a benign computed tomographic and angiographic appearance. Correlation of roentgenographic and scintigraphic characteristics of primary hepatic tumors may in some cases establish a diagnosis. The need for confirming tissue diagnosis must be weighed against the risk of hemorrhage caused by needle or open biopsy. Hepatic lesions are extremely vascular, and biopsy alone is attendant with significant risk. Several deaths have occurred after attempts at resection.

There is evidence that these tumors will regress spontaneously after OC use is stopped. Pregnancy, with the resultant high levels of sex steroids, may have a particularly stimulating effect and increase the propensity of these lesions to hemorrhage. The best and safest course of management for asymptomatic lesions would be to discontinue the OCs, urge the patient to avoid pregnancy, and await spontaneous resolution of the lesion. Marks and colleagues[40] emphasized the importance of maintaining vigilance until these tumors have resolved completely. They reported three cases in which hepatic adenomas failed to regress after discontinuation of OCs. Importantly, they recommend excision of tumors larger than 5 cm in diameter that have persisted for longer than 6 months.

Malignant tumors

Investigation of the possible relationship between OCs and liver cancer has provoked considerable controversy. Synthetic sex steroids are believed to potentiate cholestasis, hypervascularity, microsomal enzyme induction, thrombogenesis, and blood vessel wall thickening, thereby facilitating tumor development. Additionally, steroids can induce hepatic neoplasia in mice and in patients receiving anabolic steroids.

Porter and colleagues[60] studied tissue specimens obtained from five female patients with diseased livers to identify the presence of estrogen receptors. Estrogen-binding proteins with the characteristics of receptor were found in the cytosol and nuclei from both normal human liver and neoplastic lesions containing focal nodular hyperplasia and hepatic adenoma. Significantly higher levels of nuclear estrogen receptor were found in neoplastic tissue than in adjacent normal liver and were believed to represent enhanced hormone sensitivity at these sites. Similarly, Carbone and Vecchio[14] verified the presence of progesterone receptors in two young women with hepatic adenomas, only one of whom had a previous history of OC use. These studies imply that hepatic tissues of different composition may respond variably to altered hormonal milieus.

Estrogens have been implicated in the development of hepatocellular carcinoma through a role that is postulated to be either a direct hepatocarcinogenic effect or by potentiation of some other known factors that cause liver cancer. In 1986 Neuberger and associates[50] reviewed a series of 26 women under age 50 diagnosed with hepatocellular carcinoma in noncirrhotic liver to determine whether OCs had an etiologic role. These investigators found that although short-term pill use was not associated with an increased risk of tumor development, there was a 4.4-fold increased risk ($P < .01$) for 8 or more years of use. They concluded that although the overall risk for development of a hepatocellular cancer appeared to be very low, the association should be recognized, particularly in long-term users of OCs. Similarly, Forman and colleagues[24] conducted a case-control study to investigate this issue. They looked specifically at women aged 20 to 44 who had died of liver cancer between 1979 and 1982. Analysis of the data showed that ever-use of OCs was associated with a relative risk of 3.8 for hepatocellular carcinoma. The relative risk rose to 20.1 (95% confidence interval 2.3 to 175.7) after 8 or more years of use. OC use did not appear to increase significantly the risk of cholangiocarcinomas. The authors recognized various methodologic problems with their study. The validity of these conclusions has been challenged by some investigators, who have underlined problems with interpretation of the data, the limited numbers of patients, the study design, and data collection between 1978 and 1983.

Three additional recently reported case-control studies, one from the United States and two internationally based, have provided results that elaborate further on the association of OCs and liver cancer. The WHO Collaborative Study of Neoplasia and Steroid Contraceptives[96] found a relative risk of 0.71 (95% confidence interval 0.4 to 1.2) for women who had ever used combination OCs. The average duration of use was 38.0 months among the 25 "exposed" cases versus 71.8 months for the controls ($P = .05$). The investigators concluded that no significant association could be demonstrated between the ever-use of combined OCs and liver cancer as an aggregate or specifically for hepatocellular carcinoma or cholangiocarcinoma. They recognized the positive association reported by the investigators noted earlier and suggested two possible explanations for the difference: (1) The WHO study population was composed of women from areas where hepatitis B virus (HBV) is endemic and the rate of liver cancer is relatively high as compared with the study groups of others.[96] They theorized that (1) if OCs have an effect on incidence of liver cancer that is independent of HBV infection or if they affect only women without previous HBV infection, then the effect on relative risk in women from areas where HBV is endemic would be small and (2) the increased relative risk detected in other studies was most pronounced in long-term users, whereas most of the women in the study had used OCs on a short-term basis.

In the study by LaVecchia et al.[37] from the greater Milan area, a relative risk of 1.8 (95% confidence interval 0.4 to 9.2) was found for use of OCs for 5 years or less, increasing to 8.3 (95% confidence interval 1.4 to 48.7) for exposure beyond 5 years. Demonstration of an association between OCs and hepatocellular carcinoma in this study group from Italy is particularly interesting because they are derived from a population where epidemiologically the incidence of primary liver cancer is higher than that in northern European and American countries.

Palmer et al.[55] conducted a hospital-based case-control study in five U.S. cities between 1977 and 1985. Among 12 patients with liver cancer, 8 of the 9 women with hepatocellular carcinoma had used OCs (89%), compared with 16 (36%) of 45 control subjects. The estimated relative risk for 2 to 4 years of OC use, compared with less than 2 years of OC use, was 20 (95% confidence interval 2.0 to 190); the relative risk for 5 or more years of use was also 20 (95% confidence interval 1.6 to 250). OCs had been stopped for 8 or more years before the interview by 71% of the study patients and 69% of control subjects. The authors interpret their findings to suggest that usage of OCs increases the risk for hepatocellular carcinoma in young women who apparently are without other risk factors for this disease. They raise the possibility that OCs may play a role in the initiation of this tumor rather than in its promotion, because most of the patients in the study had discontinued use in the distant past.

Review of the above reports suggests an association of OCs in the development of hepatocellular carcinoma that may be influenced by duration of use. It is of greater concern that this increased risk for hepatocellular carcinoma is possibly related to ever-use and may persist indefinitely after discontinuation of OCs. The incidence of these tumors, however, is extremely rare. Although there have been anecdotal reports of benign adenomas progressing to malignancy, a cause-effect relationship has not been established.

Reports of the development of hepatocellular carcinoma in patients with previously resolved "contraceptive-steroid-induced" hepatic adenomas are of particular concern and suggest the need for long-term follow-up using ultrasonography to exclude recurrent disease. The persistent conflicting data require further definitive studies.

ORAL CONTRACEPTIVES AND UTERINE LEIOMYOMAS

Estrogens seem to have an association with leiomyomas. Leiomyomas rarely occur before menarche, tend to regress after menopause, and may enlarge rapidly during pregnancy or during exogenous estrogen administration. During the early years of OC use, it was feared that leiomyomas might grow under the stimulation of estrogen contained in the OCs. The presence of leiomyomas has been considered by some to be a relative contraindication for OC use, and many physicians are reluctant to use OCs in patients who have a leiomyoma of any type or size.

At present, there is little objective evidence in the literature to support this concern. The RCGP[68] study found a slightly decreased risk of developing uterine leiomyomas in users as opposed to nonusers. Vessey and associates[89] in their original report found no significant difference in occurrence rates among OC, diaphragm, or IUD users. None of the patients in either of these studies was taking medication containing more than 50 μg of estrogen.

Ross and colleagues[67] in 1983 updated the analysis of risk factors for uterine fibroids using data from the Oxford Family Planning Association study. As of July 1985, 538 women in the cohort study had had pathologically confirmed fibroids. The study found a significant decrease in risk of leiomyomas with increasing number of pregnancies (relative risk 1.00 with first pregnancy, 0.47 with second pregnancy, and 0.24 with fifth pregnancy). The risk decreased significantly with increasing duration of OC use (relative risk 0.80 at 2 years and 0.54 at 145 months). The risk of developing leiomyomas was decreased by 31% in women who had used OCs for 10 years. Data from this series were obtained from women who were using OCs containing 50 μg of EE_2, but with varying amounts of progestogen. There was some suggestion that the higher the dose of progestogen, the more protective the OC. Should these data be confirmed by other studies, the presence of leiomyomas should not be considered a relative contraindication to use of OCs.

REFERENCES

1. Alan Guttmacher Institute: FPA panel examines link between breast cancer, pill, says more research needed, Washington memo W-3:3, New York, 1989, The Institute.
2. Anderson TJ, Ferguson DJP, Raab GM: Cell turnover in the "resting" human breast: influence of parity, contraceptive pill, age and laterality, *Br J Cancer* 46:376, 1982.
3. Anderson TJ et al: Oral contraceptive use influences resting breast proliferation, *Hum Pathol* 20:1139, 1989.

4. Annegers JF et al: Pituitary adenoma in Olmsted County, Minnesota, 1935–1977, *Mayo Clin Proc* 53:641, 1978.

5. Armed Forces Institute of Pathology, Hepatic Branch, and Centers for Disease Control, Bureau of Epidemiology, Family Planning Evaluation Division: Increased risk of hepatocellular adenoma in women with long-term use of oral contraceptives, *MMWR* 26:293, 1977.

6. Bagshawe KD: Trophoblastic disease. In Caplan RM, Sweeney WJ, editors: *Advances in obstetrics and gynecology,* vol 3, Baltimore, 1978, Williams & Wilkins.

7. Baum JK et al: Possible association between benign hepatomas and oral contraceptives, *Lancet* 2:926, 1973.

8. Beral V, Hannaford P, Kay C: Oral contraceptive use and malignancies of the genital tract: results from the Royal College of General Practitioners' Oral Contraceptive Study, *Lancet* 2:1331, 1988.

9. Berkowitz RS et al: Oral contraceptives and postmolar trophoblastic disease, *Obstet Gynecol* 58:474, 1981.

10. Black MM et al: Family history, oral contraceptive usage, and breast cancer, *Cancer* 51:2147, 1983.

11. Boyce JG et al: Oral contraceptives and cervical carcinoma, *Am J Obstet Gynecol* 128:761, 1977.

12. Brinton LA et al: Risk factors for benign breast disease, *Am J Epidemiol* 113:203, 1981.

13. Brinton LA et al: Long term use of oral contraceptives and risk of invasive cervical cancer, *Int J Cancer* 38:339, 1986.

14. Carbone A, Vecchio FM: Presence of cytoplasmic receptors in hepatic adenomas: a report of two cases, *Am J Clin Pathol* 85:325, 1986.

15. Centers for Disease Control-Cancer and Steroid Hormone Study: long-term oral contraceptive use and the risk of breast cancer, *JAMA* 249:1591, 1983.

16. Centers for Disease Control-Cancer and Steroid Hormone Study: oral contraceptive use and the risk of endometrial cancer, *JAMA* 249:1600, 1983.

17. Centers for Disease Control-Cancer and Steroid Hormone Study: oral contraceptive use and the risk of ovarian cancer, *JAMA* 249:1596, 1983.

18. Centers for Disease Control and National Institute of Child Health and Human Development: The Cancer and Steroid Hormone Study: oral-contraceptive use and the risk of breast cancer, *N Engl J Med* 315:405, 1986.

19. Centers for Disease Control and National Institute of Child Health and Human Development: The Cancer and Steroid Hormone Study: combination oral contraceptive use and the risk of endometrial cancer, *JAMA* 257:796, 1987.

20. Centers for Disease Control and National Institute of Child Health and Human Development: The Cancer and Steroid Hormone Study: the reduction in risk of ovarian cancer associated with oral-contraceptive use, *N Engl J Med* 316:650, 1987.

21. Consensus conference: Is fibrocystic disease of the breast precancerous?, *Arch Pathol Lab Med* 110:171, 1986.

22. Coulam CB et al: Pituitary adenoma and oral contraceptives: a case-control study, *Fertil Steril* 31:25, 1979.

23. Fasal E, Paffenbarger RS: Oral contraceptives as related to cancer and benign lesions of the breast, *J Natl Cancer Inst* 55:767, 1975.

24. Forman D, Vincent TJ, Doll R: Cancer of the liver and the use of oral contraceptives, *Br Med J* 292:1357, 1986.

25. Garcia CR, Gordon J, Drill VA: Contraceptive steroids and liver lesions, *J Toxicol Environ Health* 3:197, 1977.

26. Gurpide E, Tseng L, Gusberg SB: Estrogen metabolism in normal and neoplastic endometrium, *Am J Obstet Gynecol* 129:809, 1977.

27. Harris RWL et al: Characteristics of women with dysplasia or carcinoma in situ of the cervix uteri, *Br J Cancer* 42:359, 1980.

28. Hatcher RA et al: *Contraceptive technology,* New York, 1986, Irvington Publishers.

29. Hueper WC: Environmental cancer. In Homburger F, editor: *The physiopathology of cancer,* ed 2, New York, 1959, Hoeber.

30. Hulka BS, Chambless LE, Kaufman DG: Protection against endometrial carcinoma by combination-product oral contraceptives, *JAMA* 247:475, 1982.

31. Hutchinson WB et al: Risk of breast cancer in women with benign breast disease, *J Natl Cancer Inst* 65:13, 1980.

32. Information on oral contraceptives, *Lancet* 336:498, 1990.

33. Jick SS et al: Oral contraceptives and breast cancer, *Br J Cancer* 59:618, 1989.

34. Kaufman DW, Shapiro S, Slone D: Decreased risk of endometrial cancer among oral contraceptive users, *N Engl J Med* 303:1045, 1980.

35. Kay CR, Hannaford PC: Breast cancer and the pill: a further report from the Royal College of General Practitioners' oral contraception study, *Br J Cancer* 58:675, 1988.

36. Kodlin D et al: Chronic mastopathy and breast cancer, *Cancer* 39:2603, 1977.

37. La Vecchia C, Negri E, Parazzini F: Oral contraceptives and primary liver cancer, *Br J Cancer* 59:460, 1989.

38. Lesser ML et al: Estrogen and progesterone receptors in breast carcinoma: correlations with epidemiology and pathology, *Cancer* 48:299, 1981.

39. Lyon FA: The development of the endometrium in young women receiving long-term sequential oral contraception: report of four cases, *Am J Obstet Gynecol* 123:299, 1975.

40. Marks WH, Thompson N, Appleman H: Failure of hepatic adenomas (HCA) to regress after discontinuance of oral contraceptives, *Ann Surg* 208:190, 1988.

41. Matthews PN, Millis RR, Hayward JL: Breast cancer in women who have taken contraceptive steroids, *Br Med J* 282:774, 1981.

42. Meirik O et al: Breast cancer and oral contraceptives: patterns of risk among parous and nulliparous women-further analysis of the Swedish-Norwegian material, *Contraception* 39:471, 1989.

43. Merritt CG et al: Age at first coitus and choice of contraceptive method: preliminary report on a study of factors related to cervical neoplasia, *Soc Biol* 22:255, 1975.

44. Miller DR et al: Breast cancer risk in relation to early oral contraceptive use, *Obstet Gynecol* 68:863, 1986.

45. Miller DR et al: Breast cancer before age 45 and oral contraceptive use: new findings, *Am J Epidemiol* 129:269, 1989.

46. Miller N et al: Histopathology of breast cancer in young women in relation to use of oral contraceptives, *J Clin Pathol* 42:387, 1989.

47. Moolgavkar SH, Day NE, Stevens RG: Two-stage model for carcinogenesis: epidemiology of breast cancer in females, *J Natl Cancer Inst* 65:559, 1980.

48. Murray PP, Stadel BV, Schlesselman JJ: Oral contraceptive use in women with a family history of breast cancer, *Obstet Gynecol* 73:977, 1989.

49. National Cancer Institute: *Annual cancer statistics review, including cancer trends: 1950–1985,* Bethesda, Md, 1989, National Institutes of Health.

50. Neuberger J et al: Oral contraceptives and hepatocellular carcinoma, *Br Med J* 292:1355, 1986.

51. OCs and breast cancer: a round table discussion, *Dialogues Contraception* 2:1, 1989.

52. Olsson H. Möller TR, Ranstam J: Early oral contraceptive use and breast cancer among premenopausal women: final report from a study in southern Sweden, *J Natl Cancer Inst* 81:1000, 1989.

53. Olsson H et al: Early oral contraceptive use as a prognostic factor in breast cancer, *Anticancer Res* 8:29, 1988.

54. Osborne MP et al: The relationship between family history, exposure to exogenous hormones, and estrogen receptor protein in breast cancer, *Cancer* 51:2134, 1983.

55. Palmer JR et al: Oral contraceptive use and liver cancer, *Am J Epidemiol* 130:878, 1989.

56. Paul C, Skegg DCG, Spears GFS: Oral contraceptives and risk of breast cancer, *Int J Cancer* 46:366, 1990.

57. Peritz E et al: The incidence of cervical cancer and duration of oral contraceptive use, *Am J Epidemiol* 106:462, 1977.

58. Pituitary Adenoma Study Group: Pituitary adenomas and oral contraceptives: a multicenter case-control study, *Fertil Steril* 39:753, 1983.

59. Population Reports: *Oral contraceptives: update on usage, safety, and side effects,* Baltimore, 1979, Population Information Program, Johns Hopkins University.

60. Porter LE et al: Hepatic estrogen receptor in human liver disease, *Gastroenterology* 92:735, 1987.

61. Potten CS et al: The effect of age and menstrual cycle upon proliferative activity of the normal human breast, *Br J Cancer* 58:163, 1988.

62. Ramcharan S: *The Walnut Creek contraceptive drug study: a prospective study of the side-effects of oral contraceptives,* vol 1, Dept Health, Education and Welfare Publication, Washington, DC, 1974, US Government Printing Office.

63. Ravnihar B et al: A case-control study of breast cancer in relation to oral contraceptive use in Slovenia, *Neoplasma* 35:109, 1988.

64. Romieu I, Berlin JA, Colditz G: Oral contraceptives and breast cancer: review and meta-analysis, *Cancer* 66:2253, 1990.

65. Romieu I et al: Prospective study of oral contraceptive use and risk of breast cancer in women, *J Natl Cancer Inst* 81:1313, 1989.

66. Rosner D, Lane WW, Brett RP: Influence of oral contraceptives on the prognosis of breast cancer in young women, *Cancer* 55:1556, 1985.

67. Ross RK et al: Risk factors for uterine fibroids: reduced risk associated with oral contraceptives, *Br Med J* 293:359, 1983.

68. Royal College of General Practitioners: *Oral contraceptives and health,* New York, 1974, Pitman Publishing.

69. Royal College of General Practitioners: Breast cancer and oral contraceptives: findings in Royal College of General Practitioners' study, *Br Med J* 282:2089, 1981.

70. Schlesselman JJ: Oral contraceptives and breast cancer, *Am J Obstet Gynecol* 163:1379, 1990.

71. Schlesselman JJ et al: Breast cancer risk in relation to type of estrogen contained in oral contraceptives, *Contraception* 36:595, 1987.

72. Shinzaburo N et al: Inability of medroxyprogesterone acetate to down regulate estrogen receptor level in human breast cancer, *Cancer* 65:1375, 1990.

73. Silverberg SG, Makowski EL: Endometrial carcinoma in young women taking oral contraceptives, *Obstet Gynecol* 46:503, 1975.

74. Skegg DCG: Potential for bias in case-control studies of oral contraceptives and breast cancer, *Am J Epidemiol* 127:205, 1988.

75. Spencer JD, Millis RR, Hayward JL: Contraceptive steroids and breast cancer, *Br Med J* 1:1024, 1978.

76. Stadel BV, Lai S: Oral contraceptives and premenopausal breast cancer in nulliparous women, *Contraception* 38:287, 1988.

77. Stadel BV, Schlesselman JJ: Oral contraceptives and breast cancer in young women with a "prior" history of benign breast disease, *Am J Epidemiol* 123:373, 1986.

78. Stadel BV et al: Oral contraceptives and breast cancer in young women, *Lancet* 2:970, 1985.

79. Stadel BV et al: Oral contraceptives and breast cancer in young women, *Lancet* 1:436, 1986.

80. Stanford JL, Brinton LA, Hoover RN: Oral contraceptives and breast cancer: results from an expanded case-control study, *Br J Cancer* 60:375, 1989.

81. Stanford JL et al: A case-control study of breast cancer stratified by estrogen receptor status, *Am J Epidemiol* 125:184, 1987.

82. Stone M et al: Relationship of oral contraceptives to development of trophoblastic tumor after evacuation of a hydatidiform mole, *Br J Obstet Gynaecol* 83:913, 1976.

83. Teulings FAG et al: Estrogen, androgen, glucocorticoid, and progesterone receptors in progestin-induced regression of human breast cancer, *Cancer Res* 40:2557, 1980.

84. Tseng L, Gurpide E: Effects of progestins on estradiol receptor levels in human endometrium, *J Clin Endocrinol Metab* 41:402, 1975.

85. UK National Case-Control Study Group: Oral contraceptive use and breast cancer risk in young women, *Lancet* 1:973, 1989.

86. UK National Case-Control Study Group: Oral contraceptive use and breast cancer risk in young women: subgroup analyses, *Lancet* 1:1507, 1990.

87. Vana J et al: Primary liver tumors and oral contraceptives: results of a survey, 238:2154, 1977.

88. Vessey MP, McPherson K, Doll R: Breast cancer and oral contraceptives: findings in Oxford-Family Planning Association contraceptive study, *Br Med J* 282:2093, 1981.

89. Vessey MP et al: A long-term follow up study of women using different methods of contraception: an interim report, *J Biosoc Sci* 8:375, 1976.

90. Vessey MP et al: Oral contraceptives and benign liver tumors, *Br Med J* 1:1064, 1977.

91. Vessey MP et al: Neoplasia of the cervix uteri and contraception: a possible adverse effect of the pill, *Lancet* 2:930, 1983.

92. Weiss NS, Szekely R, Austin DF: Increasing incidence of endometrial cancer in the United States, *N Engl J Med* 294:1259, 1976.

93. Wingo PA et al: Age-specific differences in the relation between oral contraceptive use and breast cancer, *Am J Epidemiol* 132:769, 1990 (abstract).

94. WHO Collaborative Study of Neoplasia and Steroid Contraceptives: Invasive cervical cancer and combined oral contraceptives, *Br Med J* 290:961, 1985.

95. WHO Collaborative Study of Neoplasia and Steroid Contraceptives: Endometrial cancer and combined oral contraceptives, *Int J Epidemiol* 17:263, 1988.

96. WHO Collaborative Study of Neoplasia and Steroid Contraceptives: Combined oral contraceptives and liver cancer, *Int J Cancer* 143:254, 1989.

97. WHO Collaborative Study of Neoplasia and Steroid Contraceptives: Breast cancer and combined oral contraceptives: results from a multinational study, *Br J Cancer* 61:110, 1990.

98. Worth AG, Boyes DA: A case control study into the possible effects of birth control pills on pre-clinical carcinoma of the cervix, *J Obstet Gynaecol Br Common*

99. Yuen BHO, Burch P: Relationship of oral contraceptives and the intrauterine contraceptive devices to the regression of concentrations of the beta subunit of human chorionic gonadotropin and invasive complications after molar pregnancy, *Am J Obstet Gynecol* 145:214, 1983.

Chapter 17

EXPANDING CONTRACEPTIVE CHOICES FOR MEN AND WOMEN

Sheldon J. Segal, PhD

The world has experienced a contraceptive revolution over the past 35 years. Modern science has produced an array of new methods that have become widely accepted not only in economically advanced nations but also in many developing countries.

Worldwide there has been a tenfold increase in the number of couples using methods of fertility control, and the research community is working on a new wave of innovations. In the developing world, the number of contraceptive users has increased from under 30 million before 1960 to almost 400 million in 1994.[31] Contraceptive prevalence—percent of couples in the reproductive age group using contraception—has increased from 8% to more than 50% and is continuing to rise in most regions of the developing world (Fig. 17-1).

Consequently, fertility in the developing world has been steadily declining over the past 30 years. The total fertility rate—the number of children a woman will have in her lifetime—has gone from more than six in the 1960s to fewer than four in 1993, more than halfway to the replacement level of 2.1 (Fig. 17-2). Most industrialized countries are at, or even below, replacement levels of fertility.

Global demographic and health surveys over the past 20 years have demonstrated the strong correlation between the use of contraceptives and total fertility rate, and they have also provided detailed information on the methods that people choose.[30]

There are country-by-country differences in patterns of methods chosen, but in most countries, contraception is practiced chiefly by women. In the United States, female methods account for more than two thirds of contraceptive use. Surgical sterilization, primarily tubal ligation, ranks first among methods chosen by American couples.[15] Combination oral contraception is the most widely used reversible method. In other countries the pattern is different. In Sweden, the intrauterine device (IUD) is the preferred reversible method. Modern hormonal methods for women are not openly available in Japan; the predominant method used is the condom. Only 10% of couples use methods classified as female methods. Japanese reliance on a male-initiated method, however, is more apparent than real. The actual practice in Japan is the use of the condom, a relatively ineffective male method, backed up by women's resorting to surgical abortion, usually performed under general anesthesia, when faced with contraceptive failure. It is estimated that only one third of surgical abortions in Japan are registered, and that about 50% of all pregnancies are terminated.[53] Whether registered or unregistered, legal abortion is done almost always early in the first trimester of pregnancy, keeping the surgical risks to a minimum. (See Chapter 14.)

In Latin America and Africa, male use of contraception is negligible. In India, on the other hand, where surgical sterilization is the chief method used to prevent pregnancy, the percentages of male and female sterilization operations

Percent users

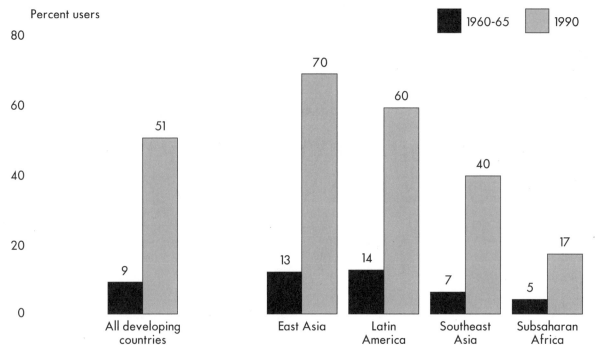

Fig. 17-1. Trends in percentages of couples of reproductive age using contraceptives, 1960–1990. (Data from Ross JA, Mauldin WP, Miller VC: *Family planning and population: a compendium of international statistics,* New York, 1993, The Population Council; ISBN: 0-87834-080-7; Library of Congress catalog number 93-93706.)

Births per woman

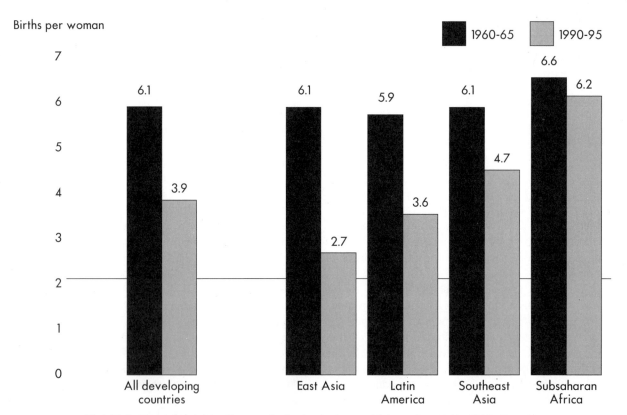

Fig. 17-2. Trends in total fertility rates in the developing world, by region, 1960–1990. (Data from Segal SJ: *Ann Med* 25:51, 1993.)

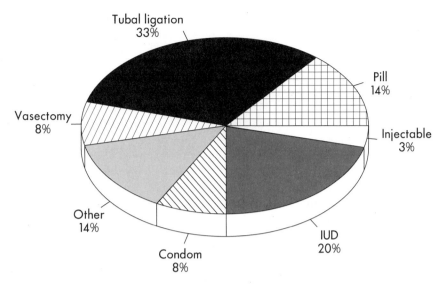

Fig. 17-3. Contraceptive use, worldwide, 1993, by percentages of all contraceptive users of each method, based on country surveys conducted 1980–1993. Methods for women comprise approximately 75%. (Data from Ross JA, Mauldin WP, Miller VC: *Family planning and population: a compendium of international statistics,* New York, 1993, The Population Council; ISBN: 0-87834-080-7; Library of Congress catalog number 93-93706.)

are equal. Consequently, Indian men account for about half of the contraceptive prevalence that has climbed in recent years to about 43% of eligible couples. Some provinces of China also rely heavily on vasectomy. Nevertheless, in the developing world as a whole, as in most industrialized countries, about 75% of couples who wish to prevent pregnancies adopt methods that are used by women (Fig. 17-3).

In countries in which abortion is illegal and done under unsafe conditions, when a contraceptive method fails to protect against unwanted pregnancy, it is the woman's health that is placed at risk. Contraceptive failure is not a rare event. For a discussion of methods of contraception currently available, see Chapter 14. Even surgical sterilization by tubal ligation, usually assumed to be the most reliable of methods, does not always succeed. During the first year postoperatively, one or two women per thousand will learn by having a pregnancy that the operation was not successful. Among reversible methods, failure rates for 1 year of typical use are lowest with copper-carrying IUDs, contraceptive implants, or injectable progestins (in each case, less than 1%). The contraceptive pill and plastic IUDs fail at a rate of about 3%. Failure rates with use of condoms, vaginal sponges or spermicides, cervical caps, diaphragms, periodic abstinence, and withdrawal range from 12% to 21%.

It is a simple matter to calculate the number of pregnancies that result from contraceptive failure by multiplying the number of users of each method by its annual failure rate. Of the approximately 6 million pregnancies that occur annually in the United States, more than 3 million are unintended and about one half of these occur while couples are using a method of contraception and did not plan to conceive during the month of conception. These pregnancies, over 1.5 million, can be attributed to contraceptive failure. Studies show that about half of these are carried to term and the other half are terminated by abortion.[21] Of all abortions done in the United States, 50% are carried out consequent to a conception that occurred during a month when couples believed that they were taking measures to prevent pregnancy. There is no surer way to reduce the number of abortions in the United States and throughout the world than by improving the effectiveness of contraception.

RECENT ADVANCES IN CONTRACEPTION

Since 1973 some major advances have been made in contraceptive technology, resulting in far fewer unplanned pregnancies and abortions. Most notable have been the copper-bearing IUDs, a 5-year contraceptive implant, and injectable progestins.

The copper T380A, the most effective of IUDs, was developed by research sponsored by The Population Council of New York,[57, 58] but, because of concern about legal problems stemming from a product no longer in use (the Dalkon Shield), IUDs are used only to a limited extent in the United States. But intrauterine contraception is the method of choice in many other countries, representing a range of different cultures. It is used by 30% of contracept-ing women in Sweden and by more than half of all couples using reversible contraception in China and Cuba. Its appeal is based on simplicity of use, absence of systemic side effects, low cost, and remarkable effectiveness. A World Health Organization study found that the cumulative 7-year pregnancy rate for the Copper T380A, the device that is available in the United States, is 1.6.[71] This averages to about 2 pregnancies per 1000 women per year, an effectiveness rate equivalent to that of surgical sterilization, with a method that is reversible by simply removing the device.

Norplant contraceptive implants have been available in the United States since 1991. The subdermal silastic implants, also a product of Population Council research,[38, 50] slowly release the synthetic progestin levonorgestrel, establishing a blood level above the threshold required to inhibit ovulation or to provide a contraceptive effect by the secondary mechanism of preventing sperm passage through a thickened cervical mucus. An effective blood level of levonorgestrel can be maintained for at least 5 years.[51] Norplant contraception is another reversible method that is in the range of effectiveness experienced with surgical sterilization. The main side effect is irregular vaginal bleeding.[56] By 1994 Norplant had been registered in 26 countries and used by more than 2 million women in 44 countries.

Contraceptive preparations, based on injectable forms of synthetic progestins, are not new but have experienced a revival of interest in recent years. Depo-Provera, a 3-monthly depot injection of medroxyprogesterone acetate, was approved for use as a contraceptive in the United States in 1992, after having been in use in more than 40 other countries for decades. It was first proposed as a contraceptive in 1966, when a Brazilian investigator reported that doses of 150 mg administered intramuscularly trimonthly caused reversible sterility by inhibiting ovulation.[6] The same investigator, Elsimar Coutinho, reported 2 years later that conception control, with less disturbance of menstrual bleeding, can be achieved by monthly injections of the same progestin combined with a long-acting estrogen.[5] The combination injectable product was reintroduced recently in Mexico and Indonesia, under the trade name Cyclofem, after extensive research that was sponsored by the World Health Organization.[43]

FEMALE CONTRACEPTION
New contraceptive implants

Even as use of Norplant implants begins to widen, research is progressing with other implant contraceptives, including a new version of the Norplant system itself,[55] biodegradable implants,[12] and single-implant contraceptives that can be used for 1 year or 2 years. One of these, Uniplant,[4] employs the silastic matrix used in Norplant and another, Implanon,[16] is made of ethylene vinyl acetate, a polymer approved for some medical applications but not

previously used subdermally. Both of these investigational new products utilize synthetic progestins found in established products administered orally, so that extensive clinical pharmacology and toxicity data are accumulated. Another single-implant contraceptive, which uses a progestin (ST1435) not active orally, is being developed.[9, 22] It may have special advantages for use by lactating women.

Two additional methods of contraception are based on the release of steroid hormones from a polymeric matrix. One is a progestin-releasing IUD that has the effectiveness and long duration of action characteristic of Norplant. Based on the slow release of levonorgestrel, this product is now available in Scandinavia and has been studied extensively in many other countries.[29] The other is a vaginal ring that a woman can insert and remove herself, eliminating the disadvantage of clinic dependency that is associated with intrauterine and subdermal contraception.[34]

Vaginal contraceptive pill

Another approach to hormonal contraception by the vaginal route is the use of a combination progestin-estrogen pill per vaginum. Since steroids are readily absorbed across the vaginal mucosa, this method of administration can bypass gastrointestinal absorption and avoid the bolus effect of first pass of the entire dosage to the liver, where metabolic side effects of steroids can be initiated.[8] Combination pills, containing either levonorgestrel or desogestrel and ethinyl estradiol, have been tested as vaginal pills[10] and found to be equally effective whether given vaginally or given orally.[11]

Pill to terminate early pregnancy

Progesterone support is a condition sine qua non for the establishment and maintenance of an intrauterine pregnancy. Compounds that occupy progesterone-receptor sites, without acting as an agonist, prevent the natural hormone from carrying out its progestational role and are, therefore, contragestational.[52] The first of these progesterone antagonists is RU 486 (mifepristone). It was synthesized in 1980[67] and by 1994 had been registered as an approved drug for medical abortion in France, China, Sweden, and the United Kingdom and used successfully by more than a quarter of a million women.

Mifepristone has high affinity for progesterone receptors, but it is not a pure antagonist. In the absence of progesterone it can act as a partial progestin agonist, which may account for some of its observed biologic effects that do not fit the pattern of progesterone antagonism. In postmenopausal women receiving only estrogen, for example, mifepristone has biochemical and morphologic effects on the endometrium similar to those of progesterone.[18] Mifepristone also has antiglucocorticoid activity.[40]

Abortion induction has been the first clinical application of this important new class of drugs. The first study used mifepristone alone.[24] The success rate in women with established pregnancies confirmed by human chorionic gonadotropin (hCG) determinations, who had amenorrhea for less than 7 weeks, ranged from 64% to 85%. The lack of response in some women was most likely due to inadequate uterine contractility required to expel the products of conception. The combination of a mifepristone dose of 600 mg, with prostaglandin given 48 hours later by intramuscular injection,[2] by vaginal suppository,[25] or orally,[39] has resulted in a rate of complete abortion approaching 100%. The oral route, using misoprostol in combination with mifepristone, has become the therapy of choice and is highly effective in women who have had amenorrhea for up to 9 weeks.

Several approaches have been studied to use mifepristone as a contraceptive. Clinical studies have revealed promising prospects for its use in the preovulatory period, to prevent luteinizing hormone (LH) surge,[28] and in the late luteal phase, to induce menses, whether or not a fertilization has occurred.[3] Mifepristone has also been used as a postcoital contraceptive within 72 hours of unprotected intercourse. In a randomized study, 402 women received a single dose of 600 mg of mifepristone, and 398 women received a conventional emergency contraceptive regimen (levonorgestrel and ethinyl estradiol at total doses of 2 mg and 200 μg, respectively, in 24 hours). None of the women who received mifepristone became pregnant, as compared with four who received the progestin-plus-estrogen therapy. Even more impressive was the absence of side effects among the mifepristone users.[17]

Political opposition to introducing mifepristone in the United States has prevented its availability as a medical abortifacient and has impeded progress on the investigation of its use for a number of other indications in endocrinology, obstetrics, gynecology, and oncology.[13]

Contraceptive vaccine

The most comprehensive program toward the development of a contraceptive vaccine is based on the use of hCG as the antigenic component. The underlying rationale is to develop antibodies that will interfere with or prevent the action of hCG, which is essential for the establishment and maintenance of an early pregnancy. The gene for its production is one of the first to be activated in a newly fertilized egg. Without the luteotropic action of hCG, the endometrium would lose its progestational support and, at the time of the next expected menses, endometrial sloughing and a menstrual flow would occur, whether or not the preceding ovulatory cycle had been fertile.

There are two approaches to the development of an hCG-inhibiting vaccine. Both utilize the principle of coupling a haptenic group derived from the native hCG molecule to a carrier protein that acts as an immunogen stimulator. In both cases, this is usually tetanus toxoid or diphtheria toxin chain B macromolecules, that have proven to be as safe as vaccines in large-scale use in human

populations. Work done primarily in India, sponsored by that country's National Institute of Immunology, utilizes the beta subunit of hCG linked to the alpha subunit of ovine LH, in order to create a tertiary structure closely resembling that of hCG itself.[64] This heterodimer is then linked to the tetanus or diphtheria macromolecule by carbodiimide coupling. A study of contraceptive effectiveness was completed in India in 1992. One conception in over 1200 cycles was recorded in fertile women exposed to pregnancy, who developed antibody titers that exceeded the threshold of 50 ng of hCG-equivalent neutralizing capacity per milliliter.[66]

To avoid the potential of immunologic cross-reaction with human LH when using the entire β-subunit as an antigen, the second line of investigation, sponsored primarily by the World Health Organization, uses as the primary immunogen the 37–amino acid C-terminal peptide of β-hCG.[62] Each vaccine has been investigated sufficiently to establish the feasibility of the approach, but both present problems that remain to be solved if an acceptable product is to be developed. In the case of the entire-subunit vaccine, cross-reaction occurs with LH, and, even though this has not been demonstrated to interfere with menstrual regularity, the biologic consequences of this cross-reaction needs continued surveillance. Rhesus monkeys immunized for 7 years with a comparable vaccine did not develop pathologic changes in the pituitary gland or other organs.[68] The C-terminal vaccine develops a weak antibody response but, based on studies in baboons, it is postulated that this may be sufficient to prevent pregnancy by acting locally to prevent implantation.[61] This theory will have to be tested in clinical studies of effectiveness.

Both vaccines induce a temporary immunization of short duration, so that frequent booster shots are required in order to maintain antibody levels above the threshold required for effective hCG neutralization. This feature is sometimes overlooked by critics who are concerned about the potential irreversibility of an hCG vaccine. Work toward developing an adjuvant that would permit a feasible and acceptable schedule for temporary—but longer—periods of immunization is necessary and now in progress.

Research on the development of contraceptive vaccines has become socially and politically controversial. Feminist groups and human rights advocates have expressed grave concern about the potential for misuse of an antifertility vaccine, by its involuntary application in order to sterilize women forcibly.[69] Given this perceived potential for abuse, they question the ethics of developing contraceptive vaccines and call for restraint on the part of scientists and organizations that support scientific research.

Past experience has shown that medically and scientifically acceptable technology, such as surgical sterilization, can be used unethically or injudiciously as instruments of punishment or social engineering. In the United States, all legislative or judicial efforts to require forced sterilization of either men or women have been deemed unconstitutional,[59] and the same would probably be the fate of similar proposals for the coercive application of a contraceptive vaccine.

In developing countries, the temporary nature of the vaccines being studied would make them less likely to be singled out as an instrument of abuse than the irreversible methods that have been forcibly applied in some countries in the past. Scientists involved in contraceptive research have joined in the condemnation of the unethical use of technology that is intended to enhance the rights and health of women.[54]

MALE CONTRACEPTION

These contraceptive innovations and others of the recent past, such as the classic pill itself and the variations of it that have followed, have been in the category of methods that are used by women. This would have delighted the early fighter for women's reproductive rights, Margaret Sanger, who was frequently imprisoned for demanding that women be given control over their own reproduction. Yet many contemporary feminists and women's health advocates, concerned that women are required to take the health risks they believe to be associated with systemic use of hormones or other contraceptive interventions, urge that greater attention and resources be devoted to developing methods that would be used by men.[72] The present contraceptive research agenda reflects the success of this advocacy.

A contraceptive pill for men, hormonal implant systems for men, vaccines that could suppress sperm production or fecundability, and new techniques for occlusion of the vas deferens are all under serious investigation by researchers in the United States and elsewhere.

Contraceptive pill

The most extensive clinical experience with a systemic male contraceptive has been accumulated with a pill tested mostly in China, but also investigated in other countries. It consists of gossypol, the phenolic aldehyde that is the yellow pigment found in cottonseed. First tested as a male contraceptive in the 1970s by a team of Chinese investigators, the idea for its use sprang from the serendipitous observation that uncooked cottonseed oil had been responsible for an epidemic of infertility in a rural area in China.

More than 10,000 Chinese men were enrolled in studies employing several dose levels of gossypol. The initial countrywide study reported a success rate of 99.4% for suppressing spermatogenesis to levels believed to be incompatible with fertility, with a dosage schedule that started with 20 mg daily for approximately 3 months and was then reduced to every other day to maintain spermatogenic arrest.[37] This antifertility effect was achieved without lowering plasma testosterone levels so that, unlike other approaches to male contraception, hormone replacement therapy to maintain libido and other secondary sexual characteristics was not required.

In this study, hypokalemia at the dosage of gossypol used arose as an issue of concern, and this matter has clouded subsequent attitudes toward the potential use of gossypol as a male contraceptive. Some of the collaborating centers reported no instances of reduction in serum potassium levels, where as other centers reported that up to 6% of cases fell below 3.5 mEq/L, the cutoff level in the study protocol, or experienced symptoms of hypokalemia, including transient paralysis. Without adequate controls, it was not possible to gauge the association of gossypol to this change in blood chemistry, but it has been found subsequently that the average serum potassium levels in Chinese men are lower than those found elsewhere[44] and that fluctuations tend to be associated with diet.[19]

Although several studies have attempted to establish an animal model or a mechanism of action for the imputed hypokalemic effect of gossypol, these have not been definitive. When gossypol has been tested as a contraceptive in countries other than China, no evidence of hypokalemia has been reported.[7] Doses higher than those for the male contraceptive regimen, used in the United States for the treatment of adrenal cancer, failed to cause hypokalemia.[14] In yet another study, human immunodeficiency virus (HIV)-positive men in Mexico received continuously, for up to 20 months, gossypol treatment exceeding the dose required for contraception without experiencing drug-related side effects. Semen analysis revealed azoospermia and reduction in HIV-P24 antigen. Monthly evaluations revealed no significant changes in serum potassium levels.[41] The progression of the underlying disease was not affected by the oral administration of gossypol.

The usefulness and acceptability of gossypol as a male contraceptive will be determined by its reversibility. It appears that the chance for reversal decreases with dose and duration of use.[32] Even though some men who use gossypol for 1 year or longer are able to resume spermatogenesis after cessation of treatment, it will not be possible to assure an individual patient that fertility will return. The implication of this is that gossypol, if proven to be safe and effective as a male contraceptive, would have application as a medical alternative for men seeking surgical vasectomy rather than as a reversible method. An international, multicenter trial is in progress to test the use of gossypol for this purpose. All clinical studies undertaken since the original Chinese work have confirmed the observation that gossypol treatment does not reduce the production of testosterone by testicular Leydig cells.

Contraceptive implant system

If gossypol is the product of serendipity, the other main line of work toward a reversible male method is the result of sophisticated fundamental research that earned Nobel prizes for two American biochemists. In 1971, after an intensive search, they announced independently the structure of gonadotropin-releasing hormone (GnRH), the 10–amino acid polypeptide produced in the hypothalamus that regulates the production of pituitary gonadotropins.[35, 46] By regulating the release of LH and follicle-stimulating hormone (FSH), the decapeptide controls the production of both sperm and testicular androgens. Both agonists and antagonists to GnRH were synthesized soon thereafter,[45] and it was quickly learned through animal studies that either type of analogue can interfere with the action of endogenous GnRH, resulting in suppression of spermatogenesis, with a concurrent suppression of testicular hormone production.

Early contraceptive research focused on the use of the paradoxical inhibitory effect of GnRH agonists and revealed problems such as an initial endogenous-androgen burst effect and erratic results in maintaining spermatogenic arrest, so attention shifted to the use of releasing hormone analogues that acted as antagonists. Unexpectedly, it was observed that the first antagonists bound to mast cells, causing a release of histamine that created a severe local allergic reaction, thus making them unacceptable for clinical use.[49]

More recently, GnRH antagonists have been synthesized that do not evoke histamine release and appear to be long-acting when administered by subcutaneous injection.[27] The availability of GnRH antagonists, free of undesirable side effects and with increased biologic half-life, is a positive step toward a contraceptive based on the principle of GnRH inhibition.

The discovery of delivery forms that could be acceptable for male contraception remains a serious obstacle. Unlike the extensive experience with polymeric release of steroids and other lipid-soluble compounds for long-acting delivery systems such as implants or depot injectables, there is no similar technology from which to borrow to create a delayed-release system for water-soluble peptides. To be practical, several criteria must be met. The delivery system, whether or not it is biodegradable, must employ materials that can be used clinically without causing a local or systemic foreign-body reaction or toxic effect; it must be possible to achieve sufficient storage of an adequate amount to ensure a significant period of effectiveness; release rate of the peptide from the vehicle must be slow and steady enough to provide a reasonably constant blood level over the period of use. Hydrogel, a methyl acrylate polymer, may meet these requirements.[26] It is similar in structure to the polymer widely used for soft contact lenses, which rarely initiates a foreign-body reaction when placed in proximity to the epithelium of the cornea. The diffusibility of peptidic compounds in this material has been known for many years, but the polymer has not been used clinically as the basis for a long-acting drug-delivery system.

A male contraceptive method based on GnRH will need to meet another requirement. Since the releasing hormone controls both the gamete-producing and the hormone-producing functions of the testis, men treated with an antagonist or agonist to suppress spermatogenesis would require androgen replacement therapy to maintain libido,

potency, and other secondary male sexual characteristics. The development of suitable hormone replacement therapy for men is complicated by the fact that concurrent testosterone treatment can interfere with the inhibitory effect of GnRH analogues on spermatogenesis.[33] Because the stimulatory effect of testosterone is species-specific, animal models may not be helpful in resolving this matter, so that the evaluation of the stability of spermatogenic arrest caused by a combination of a GnRH analogue and replacement androgen may have to depend on trials involving a substantial number of men.

Potential toxicity and metabolic issues further complicate the development of appropriate androgen replacement therapy. Unlike estrogens and progestins, orally active androgens are not available. When androgen therapy is used for the treatment of sexual dysfunction or hypogonadism, frequent intramuscular injections are required, usually using long-acting esters such as testosterone enanthate.[60] Although studies with delivery systems such as pellets or microspheres suitable for steroids suggest that injectable preparations that would last for 6 months may be feasible,[20] this work is not yet definitive, and no such preparations are commercially available.

Androgens with high potency may hold even greater promise for overcoming the problem of a suitable sustained-release form for androgen replacement therapy, not only for GnRH analogue contraception but for other therapies, as well.[70] 7α-Methylnortestosterone is a highly potent androgen that can be prepared in a silastic matrix implant that has a life span of at least 1 year.[63] Used in conjunction with a GnRH analogue-releasing implant, this development has considerable promise for solving the many problems that have confronted researchers striving to develop a practical male contraceptive over the past several decades. An implant form of male contraception would avoid major obstacles, such as compliance requirements of a continuous-use method or the acceptability and logistic problems of a frequent-schedule injectable regimen.

Injectable contraceptive

Although reports continue to appear from time to time on the use of injections of androgens, progestins, or androgen-progestin combinations for the suppression of spermatogenesis,[73] it is unlikely that these research activities will lead to the development of an acceptable and practical system for male contraception. They are, however, interesting in demonstrating that spermatogenic arrest can be reversible and in establishing information on the clinical pharmacology of continuous androgen therapy.

It has been more than 35 years since steroidal suppression of gonadotropins was proposed as an approach to male contraception,[23] and some of the same basic uncertainties remain today. In 1978 a published summary of results of clinical trials with many steroid formulations revealed that unacceptably high failure rates occurred. Some men did not respond sufficiently, and others experienced breakthrough spermatogenesis after having responded initially.[47] The daunting challenge when using an androgenic steroid to suppress gonadotropins is to establish a dose that would remain within normal limits for all men, without reaching hyperandrogenic levels in some. Given individual variability that can be expected in absorption, metabolic clearance rates, and hepatic function, this may be difficult to achieve. Any method that risks exceeding physiologic blood levels would be viewed with skepticism, because of the critical role of androgens in cardiovascular events and prostatic pathology.

Contraceptive vaccine

As scientists, armed with the powerful tools of molecular biology and dramatic advances in understanding the immune system, attempt to develop an array of new vaccines to combat disease, they have included the exploration of potential immunologic means to suppress male fertility.

One line of research is based on the principle of GnRH inhibition, similar to the use of antagonist analogues described previously. The decapeptide itself is too small a molecule to be significantly antigenic, but coupling it to a carrier protein enhances antigenicity substantially.[65] With a vaccine based on this principle, spermatogenesis would be inhibited by GnRH-neutralizing antibodies, and androgen replacement therapy would ensure normal male secondary sexual characteristics and functions. A few men with prostate cancer have been immunized with a GnRH vaccine in order to achieve androgen suppression. These preliminary studies are useful in establishing the feasibility of immunologic suppression of GnRH in men, but they have not dealt with an essential requirement for a GnRH vaccine that would be used to control fertility in normal men, the issue of androgen replacement.

To avoid the need for androgen replacement, FSH can be used as an antigen in order to generate antibodies that would neutralize the endogenous hormone and suppress spermatogenesis, without interfering with testosterone production. Testicular Leydig cells derive their gonadotropic support from LH, not FSH. Studies in male bonnet monkeys have established the feasibility of the FSH vaccine,[36] but clinical trials have not been attempted.

Other vaccine possibilities are based on advances in the isolation of sperm or ovum surface proteins or receptors that are involved in the process of sperm-ovum interaction or penetration of the sperm through the outer coats to the ovum membrane.[42] These are at early stages of research, and the potential for clinical application is not predictable.

Criticism, cited earlier, that has been leveled against research toward the development of a contraceptive vaccine for women, on which work is more advanced, would presumably apply to research toward a male vaccine, as well.

Percutaneous vasectomy

Simplification of the operative procedure may enhance the popularity of vasectomy. There are short-term complications with the conventional operation that include hematoma in approximately 1% of cases, infection, epididymitis, and spontaneous recanalization of the vas deferens. A recent development, perfected and utilized by surgeons in China, has been popularized as the "no-scalpel" vasectomy. The scrotal skin is punctured at the midline with a sharpened forceps, and the vas is grasped and visualized through the small puncture hole. The advantages are to minimize bleeding and other side effects. No sutures are required to close the entry site. In China, more than 15 million vasectomies have been performed with this procedure, and it is now being adopted by American urologists.[48]

CONCLUSION

In this era of acquired immunodeficiency syndrome, discussion of contraceptive choices must emphasize the need for methods that women can use to protect themselves from sexually transmitted disease, including HIV. The vaginal sheath (female condom), vaginal virucidal creams or gels, medicated condoms, or other means to reduce the potential of transinfection of women by infected men now urgently need greater attention than ever before. Some explorations are in progress,[1] but this line of research is not receiving the attention it should have.

There is no perfect method to meet the changing contraceptive needs in the reproductive life-cycle of a woman or couple, or to accommodate the world's cultural diversity. Providing a greater choice of safe and effective methods can help ensure that, throughout the world, all couples can select an appropriate and acceptable means to regulate their fertility voluntarily without jeopardizing the health of either partner.

REFERENCES

1. Anderson DJ, Voeller B: AIDS and contraception. In Shoupe D, Haseltine FP, editors: *Contraception (Clinical perspectives in obstetrics and gynecology* series), New York, 1993, Springer-Verlag.
2. Bygdeman M, Swahn ML: Progesterone receptor blockage: effect on uterine contractility and early pregnancy, *Contraception* 32:45, 1985.
3. Croxatto HB et al: Late luteal phase administration of RU 486 for three successive cycles does not disrupt bleeding patterns of ovulation, *J Clin Endocrinol Metab* 65:1272, 1987.
4. Coutinho EM: One year contraception with a single subdermal implant containing nomegestrol acetate (Uniplant), *Contraception* 47:97, 1993.
5. Coutinho EM, De Souza JC: Conception control by monthly injections of medroxyprogesterone suspension and a long-acting oestrogen, *J Reprod Fertil* 15:209, 1968.
6. Coutinho EM, De Souza JC, Csapo AI: Reversible sterility induced by medroxyprogesterone injections, *Fertil Steril* 17:261, 1966.
7. Coutinho EM et al: Antispermatogenic action of gossypol in men, *Fertil Steril* 42:424, 1984.
8. Coutinho EM et al: Conception control by vaginal administration of pills containing ethinylestradiol and dl-norgestrel, *Fertil Steril* 42:478, 1984.

9. Coutinho EM et al: Contraception with single implants and mini-implants of ST-1435. In Zatuchni GI et al, editors: *Long-acting contraceptive delivery systems,* Philadelphia, 1984, Harper & Row.

10. Coutinho EM et al: Comparative study on the efficacy and acceptability of two contraceptive pills administered by the vaginal route: an international multicenter clinical trial, *Clin Pharmacol Ther* 53:65, 1993.

11. Coutinho EM et al: Comparison of oral and vaginal administration of levonorgestrel as a contraceptive pill, *Clin Pharmacol Ther* 54:540, 1993.

12. Dhall GI, Krishna U, Sivaraman R: Phase II clinical trial with biodegradable subdermal contraceptive implant Capronor (4.0-cm single implant), *Contraception* 44:409, 1991.

13. Donaldson MS, Dorflinger L, Brown SS, editors: *Clinical applications of mifepristone (RU 486) and other antiprogestins: assessing the science and recommending a research agenda,* Washington, DC 1993, National Academy Press.

14. Flack MR et al: Oral gossypol in the treatment of metastatic adrenal cancer, *J Clin Endocrinol Metabol* 76:1019, 1992.

15. Forrest JD, Fordyce RR: Women's contraceptive attitudes and use in 1992, *Fam Plann Perspect* 25:175, 1993.

16. Geelen JAA et al: Release kinetics of 3-keto-desogestrel from contraceptive implants (Implanon) in dogs: comparison with in vitro data, *Contraception* 47:215, 1993.

17. Glasier A et al: Mifepristone (RU 486) compared with high-dose estrogen and progestogen for emergency postcoital contraception, *N Engl J Med* 327:1041, 1992.

18. Gravinis A et al: Endometrial and pituitary responses to the steroidal antiprogestin RU 486 in postmenopausal women, *J Clin Endocrinol Metab* 60:156, 1985.

19. Gu Z, Segal S, Reidenberg MM: Low serum potassium in normal men in Shanghai, *J Clin Chem* 40:340, 1994.

20. Handelsman DJ, Conway AJ, Boylan LM: Pharmacokinetics and pharmacodynamics of testosterone pellets in man, *J Clin Endocrinol Metab* 71:216, 1990.

21. Harlop S, Kost K, Forrest JD: *Preventing pregnancy, protecting health,* New York, 1991, Alan Guttmacher Institute.

22. Haukkamaa M et al: Contraception with subdermal implants releasing the progestin ST-1435: a dose-finding study, *Contraception* 45:49, 1992.

23. Heller CG et al: Effects of progestational compounds on the reproductive process of the human male, *Ann N Y Acad Sci* 71:649, 1958.

24. Hermann W et al: Effet d'un steroide anti-progesterone chez la femme, *C R Acad Sci* 294:933, 1982.

25. Hill NCW, Ferguson J, MacKenzie IZ: The efficacy of oral mifepristone (RU 38,486) with a prostaglandin E_1 analog vaginal pessary for the termination of early pregnancy: complications and patient acceptability, *Am J Obstet Gynecol* 162:414, 1990.

26. Kuzma P, Moro D, Quandt H: U.S. patent no. 5266325. Washington, DC, November 30, 1993, U.S. Patent Office.

27. Leal JA et al: Prolonged duration of gonadotropin inhibition by a third generation GNRH antagonist, *J Clin Endocrinol Metab* 67:1325, 1988.

28. Ledger WL et al: Inhibition of ovulation by low-dose mifepristone (RU 486), *Hum Reprod* 7:945, 1992.

29. Luukkainen T et al: Effective contraception with the levonorgestrel-releasing intrauterine device: twelve-month report of a European multicenter study, *Contraception* 36:169, 1987.

30. Mauldin WP, Ross JA: Family planning programs: efforts and results, 1982–89, *Stud Fam Plann* 22:350, 1991.

31. Mauldin WP, Segal SJ: Prevalence of contraceptive use: trends and issues, *Stud Fam Plann* 19:335, 1988.

32. Meng GD et al: Recovery of sperm production following the cessation of gossypol treatment: a two center study in China, *Int J Androl* 11:1, 1988.

33. Michel E et al: Failure of high-dose sustained release luteinizing hormone releasing hormone agonist (buserelin) plus oral testosterone to suppress male fertility, *Clin Endocrinol* 23:663, 1985.

34. Mishell DR et al: Clinical performance and endocrine profiles with contraceptive vaginal rings containing a combination of estradiol and d-norgestrel, *Am J Obstet Gynecol* 130:55, 1978.

35. Monahan J et al: Synthese totale par phase solide d'un decapeptide qui stimule la secretion des gonadotropines hypophysaires LH et FSH, *C R Acad Sci* 273:508, 1971.

36. Moudgal NR et al: Development of oFSH as a vaccine for the male—a status report on the recent researches carried out using the bonnet monkey (M. radiata). In: Talwar GP, editor: *Immunological approaches to contraception and promotion of fertility (Reproductive biology* series), New York, 1986, Plenum Press.

37. National coordinating group on male antifertility agents: gossypol: a new antifertility agent for males, *Chin Med J* 4:417, 1978.

38. *Norplant levonorgestrel implants: a summary of scientific data,* New York, 1990, The Population Council.

39. Peyron R et al: Early termination of pregnancy with mifepristone (RU 486) and the orally active prostaglandin misoprostol, *N Engl J Med* 328:1509, 1993.

40. Philibert D: Ru 38486: an original multifaceted antihormone in vivo. In: Agarwal MK, editor: *Adrenal steroid antagonism,* Berlin, 1984, Walter de Gruyter.

41. Ponce de León S et al: Gossypol suppresses P24AG in semen. Presented at the VIII International Conference on AIDS, Amsterdam, July 1992.

42. Primakoff P, Lathrop W, Woolman L: Fully effective contraception in male and female guinea pigs immunized with the sperm protein PH-20, *Nature* 335:543, 1988.

43. Program for Appropriate Technology in Health, Seattle, Washington: Cyclofem: a new once-a-month injectable contraceptive, *Outlook* 9:1, 1992.

44. Reidenberg MM et al: Regional differences in serum potassium concentrations in normal men, *J Clin Chem* 39:72, 1993.

45. Schally AV, Coy DH, Arimura A: LH-RH agonists and antagonists, *Int J Gynecol Obstet* 18:318, 1980.

46. Schally AV et al: Isolation and properties of the FSH and LH-releasing hormone, *Biochem Biophys Res Commun* 16:392, 1971.

47. Schearer SB et al: Hormonal contraception for men, *Int J Androl* (suppl 2):680, 1978.

48. Schlegel PN, Goldstein M: Vasectomy. In: Shoupe D, Haseltine FP, editors: *Contraception (Clinical perspectives in obstetrics and gynecology* series), New York, 1993, Springer-Verlag.

49. Schmidt F et al: [Ac-D-Nal(2)^1, 4F-D-Phe^2, D-Trp^3, D-Arg^6]-LHRH, a potent antagonist of LHRH, produces transient edema and behavioral changes in rats, *Contraception* 29:283, 1984.

50. Segal SJ: Contraceptive subdermal implants. In: Mishell DR Jr, editor: *Advances in Fertility Research,* New York, 1982, Raven Press.

51. Segal S: A new delivery system for contraceptive steroids, *Am J Obstet Gynecol* 157:1090, 1987.

52. Segal SJ: Mifepristone (RU 486), *N Engl J Med* 322:691, 1990 (editorial).

53. Segal SJ: The role of technology in population policy, *Populi* 18:5, 1991.

54. Segal SJ: The uses of Norplant *Baltimore Sun,* Feb 18, 1993 (letters to the editor).

55. Sivin I: International experience with Norplant and Norplant-2 contraceptives, *Stud Fam Plann* 19:81, 1988.

56. Sivin I: Norplant contraceptive implants. In: Shoupe D, Haseltine FP, editors: *Contraception (Clinical perspectives in obstetrics and gynecology* series), New York, 1993, Springer-Verlag.

57. Sivin I, Tatum HJ: Four years of experience with the TCu 380A intrauterine contraceptive device, *Fertil Steril* 36:159, 1981.

58. Sivin I et al: *The Copper T 380 intrauterine device: a summary of scientific data,* New York, 1992, The Population Council.

59. *Skinner v. State of Oklahoma* (316 U.S. 535): 62 Supreme Court Reporter:1110–1116, 1942.

60. Snyder PJ, Lawrence DA: Treatment of male hypogonadism with testosterone enanthate, *J Clin Endocrinol Metab* 51:1335, 1980.

61. Stevens VC: Immunization of female baboons with haptencoupled gonadotropins, *Obstet Gynecol* 42:496, 1973.

62. Stevens VC: Immunological contraception. In: Shoupe D, Haseltine FP, editors: *Contraception (Clinical perspectives in obstetrics and gynecology* series), New York, 1993, Springer-Verlag.

63. Sundaram K, Kumar N, Bardin CW: 7α-Methyl nortestosterone (MENT): the optimal androgen for male contraception, *Ann Med* 25:199, 1993.

64. Talwar GP et al: Isoimmunization against human chorionic gonadotropin with conjugates of processed beta-subunit of the hormone and tetanus toxoid, *Proc Natl Acad Sci U S A* 73:218, 1976.

65. Talwar GP et al: Vaccines against LHRH and hCG. In: Naz RK, editor: *Immunology of reproduction,* part III, New Delhi, 1993, CRC Press.

66. Talwar GP et al: A vaccine that prevents pregnancy in women, *Proc Natl Acad Sci U S A* (in press).

67. Teutsch G: Analogues of RU 486 for the mapping of the progestin receptor: synthetic and structural aspects. In: Baulieu EE, Segal SJ, editors: *The antiprogestin steroid RU 486 and human fertility control,* New York, 1985, Plenum Press.

68. Thau RB et al: Long-term immunization against the beta-subunit of ovine luteinizing hormone (oLH beta) has no adverse effects on pituitary function in rhesus monkeys, *Am J Reprod Immunol* 15:92, 1987.

69. Various (232) organizations: Call for a stop of research on antifertility "vaccines" (immunological contraceptives). Open letter sponsored by Women's Global Network for Reproductive Rights, Amsterdam, November 8, 1993.

70. Weinbauer GF, Marshall GR, Nieschlag E: New injectable testosterone ester maintains serum testosterone of castrated monkeys in the normal range for two months, *Acta Endocrinol* 113:128, 1986.

71. World Health Organization: The TCu 380A, TCu 220C, Multiload 250 and Nova T IUDs at 3, 5 and 7 years of use—results from three randomized multicentre trials, *Contraception* 42:141, 1990.

72. World Health Organization: Creating common ground: women's perspectives on the selection and introduction of fertility regulation technologies. Report of a meeting between women's health advocates and scientists, held in Geneva, Feb 1991 [WHO/HRP/ITT/91]), Geneva, 1991, World Health Organization.

73. World Health Organization Task Force on Methods for the Regulation of Male Fertility: Contraceptive efficacy of testosterone-induced azoospermia in normal men, *Lancet* 336:955, 1990.

Part IV

INFERTILITY EVALUATION

Chapter 18

EVALUATION OF THE INFERTILE COUPLE

Raphael Jewelewicz, MD
and Edward E. Wallach, MD

The urge to reproduce and preserve the species is an inherent part of life. Since time immemorial, family and children have been the basis of human society. This is most beautifully expressed in the Bible: "For thou shalt eat the labour of thine hands: happy shalt thou be, and it shall be well with thee. Thy wife shall be as a fruitful vine by the sides of thine house: thy children like olive plants round about thy table" (Psalm 128). The majority of couples getting married aspire to have a family and raise children. When pregnancy does not happen within a certain period of time, the couple becomes alarmed and distressed. Infertility is one of the most common reasons for couples of child-bearing age to seek medical advice. Spurred by a decline in the number of babies available for adoption and the development of new reproductive technology that offers the possibility of attaining parenthood in situations in which a generation ago it would have been unimaginable, the demand for infertility investigation and treatment has increased dramatically, from approximately 600,000 physician visits in 1968 to over 2 million in the early 1980s.[92] With the increased demand, fertility clinics, services, counseling, and treatment centers have multiplied.[9] This chapter reviews and updates the procedures used to investigate infertility in the 1990s.

PREVALENCE OF INFERTILITY

Infertility is defined as failure to conceive after 1 year of regular coitus without contraception. This definition is based on evidence showing monthly conception rates of 20% to 25% in normal young couples actively attempting pregnancy.[52] In 1956, Guttmacher reported that 85% of normal couples conceived after 1 year of trial, and 93% after 2 years.[92] More recently, Page[73] surveyed 250 couples by mail and found that of the 82% who responded to his inquiry, 20% to 35% took longer than 1 year to conceive. At present in the United States, approximately 10% to 20% of couples are infertile.[8,52,92] It is not clear whether these figures represent an increase in infertility in the last generation, more heightened frequency of diagnosis because of a more open society, or better and easier access to medical care.

ETIOLOGY OF INFERTILITY

Conception and pregnancy leading to a live birth depend on complete, interdependent integration of anatomic, physiologic, and immunologic factors acting in concert. In addition to anatomic integrity of her reproductive tract, the woman requires a functionally intact hypothalamic-pituitary-ovarian axis, regular ovulatory cycles, normal folliculogenesis and ovulation, and an effective luteal phase. The man requires normal spermatogenesis, intact reproductive anatomy, and appropriate sexual function in order to deposit an adequate number of morphologically normal and motile spermatozoa in the upper vagina. For the ovum and spermatozoa to unite in the fallopian tube, the spermatozoa must initially penetrate periovulatory cervical mucus, and the fallopian tube must be adequately mobile and functional to pick up and transport the ovum. Once fertilization has occurred, the preembryo is transferred to the uterus, where successful implantation depends on a hormonally primed endometrium maintained by a functional corpus luteum. Any element of dissociation in this chain of events can cause infertility.

A male factor is responsible for infertility in 40% to 50% of cases, and a female factor for most of the balance. The leading causes of infertility are ovulatory dysfunction, uterine or tubal disease, cervical problems, immunologic factors, and infectious diseases. The incidence of any individual factor as a cause of infertility can only be estimated, and varies with the study population.[52] For instance, sexually transmitted diseases, infections, and tubal disease are more common among lower socioeconomic groups and drug abusers.

In many couples infertility has multiple etiologies. However, in approximately 20% of infertile couples no cause can be identified. The prevalence of unexplained infertility has been said to range from 6% to 60% in various studies.[18]

EPIDEMIOLOGY OF INFERTILITY

Many epidemiologic factors contribute to infertility, but the most common in both sexes is genital tract infection. The incidence of gonorrhea and other sexually transmitted diseases increased in the past decade. About 2 million cases of gonorrhea occur each year in the United States. The consequences of genital infection by sexually transmitted pathogens range from minor discomfort to impaired reproductive performance, manifest as infertility, ectopic pregnancy, recurrent spontaneous abortion, stillbirth, and neonatal death.

Of women with untreated endocervical gonorrhea, 10% to 17% will develop salpingitis, and 20% of those women will be infertile after one or more infections. Infection with other sexually transmitted pathogens, such as chlamydia, mycoplasma, and herpesvirus and other viruses, can have the same outcome as gonorrhea. In addition, use of intrauterine devices increases the risk of pelvic inflammatory disease (PID) and infertility.[64]

In general, the risk of infertility becomes greater with each repetitive episode of PID.[69,102] It is estimated that about 35% of infertile women have postinflammatory sequelae involving the fallopian tubes or surrounding peritoneum.[22] Chronic inflammation of the cervix and endometrium are also associated with infertility. In men, infection can cause deficient spermatogenesis and blockage. A detailed discussion of infections of the genital tract and their management is presented in Chapter 25.

Age-related infertility has been seen increasingly in the last decade. It is a major factor in women who delay childbearing for social or economic reasons. Fertility rates have been shown to decline with age of spouse and duration of marriage, presumably because of a decrease in sexual activity.[64] Advancing age also increases the risk of other medical problems that may affect fertility, such as endometriosis, sexually transmitted diseases and their sequelae, PID, and general medical diseases. Physical exercise and dieting, when practiced judiciously, are very important to physical and emotional well-being, but excessive dieting or overstrenuous exercise can lead to menstrual abnormalities and decreased fecundity.[42] A considerable number of women who participate in strenuous sports experience oligomenorrhea or amenorrhea. When strenuous exercise results in low weight for height, gonadotropin and gonadal hormone production may be affected adversely, culminating in menstrual and ovulatory dysfunction and infertility.[5,42]

Cigarette smoking and use of alcohol and illicit or "recreational" drugs have been associated with infertility in both men and women. Approximately 30% of women smoke.[69] An epidemiologic study of affluent, well-educated women uncovered a lower pregnancy rate per cycle among smokers than among nonsmokers (0.22 versus 0.32, respectively).[4] In experimental animals, exposure to nicotine, cigarette smoke, and polycyclic aromatic hydrocarbons blocks spermatogenesis, alters sperm morphology, and leads to testicular atrophy. The Oxford Family Planning Association contraceptive study showed a consistent and significant trend of decreasing fertility with increasing numbers of cigarettes smoked.[51] When smoking was discontinued, fecundity improved. Thus, cessation of smoking may increase the chances of conception.[93] A number of studies have indicated adverse effects of nicotine and other components of tobacco smoke on the reproductive system. Smoking may result in decreased estrogen levels and altered tubal ciliogenesis and cervical mucus. Nicotine and cotinine, a nicotine metabolite, are present in cervical mucus of smokers and may be toxic to sperm.[75] Some human and animal studies point to the possibility of alterations in tubal physiology, motility, and oocyte transport.[75,93] Experimental evidence supports the hypothesis that nicotine and polycyclic aromatic hydrocarbons result in oocyte and follicle destruction.[93]

Some clinical studies have shown impairment of sperm density, motility, and morphology in male smokers as compared with nonsmokers. However, others found no statistically significant effect of smoking on these parameters in healthy men.[51,98]

Chronic alcohol use has been associated with infertility and menstrual disorders and may have severe consequences for the fetus. Approximately 5% of women of childbearing age drink at least two alcohol-containing beverages per day. In men, alcohol affects testicular synthesis and secretion of testosterone and can result in abnormal sperm morphology and sexual dysfunction; chronic alcoholism can lead to permanent impotence.

Drug abuse is another cause of infertility. Approximately 20% of young adults use marijuana more than five times per month.[69] Animal studies clearly show that Δ^9-tetrahydrocannabinol, the principal psychoactive ingredient in marijuana, inhibits the secretion of luteinizing hormone (LH), follicle-stimulating hormone (FSH), and prolactin (PRL), thereby inhibiting ovulation at the hypothalamic level.[86] In women, marijuana use has been associated with shorter menstrual cycles and shorter luteal phases. However, one study revealed development of tolerance with regular use and subsequent return to normal hormone levels and cycles.[86] In men, use of marijuana caused a transient decrease in sperm count.

Other illicit drugs such as heroin, cocaine, and crack cocaine have more deleterious effects. Illicit use of narcotics, which act on the central nervous system, can modify hypothalamic-pituitary control of gonadotropins and PRL. Subsequent effects on the physiology of the reproductive process include changes in libido and sexual dysfunction.

Exposure to certain noxious agents in the environment or workplace may have adverse effects on fertility. A case-control study in Denmark demonstrated an increased risk of idiopathic infertility in women occupationally exposed to noise, dry cleaning chemicals, mercury, cadmium, and textile dyes.[69] Exposure of men to heat, vibration, ionizing radiation, and numerous chemicals has been associated with alterations in sperm morphology and a decrease in sperm production.[69]

EVALUATION OF INFERTILITY

History and physical examination

History. The infertility evaluation begins with elicitation of a comprehensive medical, surgical, family, and social history from both partners. Specific questions for the female partner include menstrual, pregnancy, and sexual history and contraceptive use. It is important to inquire about coital frequency and timing, sexual dysfunction, and use of lubricants that may be spermicidal. An endocrinologic etiology may be suggested by menstrual irregularity, galactorrhea, weight fluctuations, acne, oiliness of skin and hair, frontal balding, or hirsutism. Hirsutism may not be apparent on physical examination because of the patient's ethnic origin or use of electrolysis or depilatory agents. The male partner's sexual history should also be elicited, including past fertility. Any evidence of exposure to environmental or occupational toxins needs to be considered. Because many of the questions are very personal and the answers may not be known to the spouse, great care and tact should be used. The initial visit, by virtue of objectivity, provides the ideal opportunity to inquire about all issues of lifestyle that can influence fertility. In many cases, the full answers will be given at later visits when a good rapport develops between patient and physician.

Finally, the history must include any prior work-up or treatment for infertility. Pertinent records should be obtained. If they are available, pathology reports, endometrial biopsy slides, films of previous hysterosalpingograms, and tapes of endoscopic procedures should be reviewed.

Physical examination. The initial physical examination should be complete, because the obstetrician-gynecologist is usually the woman's primary care physician and the physical examination may uncover coexisting medical problems. Findings on the initial physical examination often define the extent and sequence of the infertility work-up. Special attention should be directed at height and weight (lean mass), arm span, breast development and size, presence of galactorrhea or acne, hair distribution, and abdominal or other surgical scars.

The pelvic examination will reveal anatomic or pathologic abnormalities, including masses, infections, and suggestive evidence of pelvic adhesions or endometriosis. In addition to a Papanicolaou smear, appropriate cervical smears for culture of mycoplasma, ureaplasma, and chlamydia are taken routinely. Cultures for gonorrhea and Venereal Disease Research Laboratories serology screen are done when indicated. A random aspirate of cervical mucus at the first visit may substitute for a subsequent postcoital test, if numerous motile spermatozoa are observed under the microscope.

An examination of the male external genitalia is necessary if there is reason to suspect an abnormality. The examination includes testicular size, consistency, position of urethral opening, and identification of a possible varicocele.

Before initiating further diagnostic evaluation, the menstrual cycle, fertile period, and reproductive anatomy and physiology should be outlined briefly for the couple so that they understand the importance and timing of the diagnostic tests and can ask questions. Knowledgeable patients are more cooperative and less frustrated. The work-up should be individualized, targeted, and not prolonged. Tests should be performed expediently but should allow adequate time for conception after certain procedures. Many tests not only are diagnostic but can be therapeutic.

The history and physical examination findings may indicate the need for a thorough endocrine investigation. A full discussion is beyond the scope of this chapter; however, a few basic concepts are reviewed. If the patient has galactorrhea, amenorrhea, or irregular cycles, a serum PRL measurement is needed to rule out hyperprolactinemia. In view of daily and cyclic fluctuations in PRL levels, an elevated level warrants another test. The samples should be obtained in the morning after a quiet period, and in the absence of a preceding high-protein meal.[80] Thyroid function should also be evaluated. If virilization, hirsutism, or acne is noted, androgen production needs investigation. Some recent studies even suggest that determination of androgens is indicated in the initial evaluation of all infertile women.[77] Hyperandrogenism may impair folliculogenesis and cause anovulation[27] or prevent conception.[77] Latent, cryptic, or adult-onset congenital adrenal hyperplasia may cause hyperandrogenism.[59] The gene for this disorder, nonclassic 21-hydroxylase deficiency, is prevalent. Jews of Ashkenazi descent have a 1 in 30 chance of having it; Hispanics, a 1 in 40 chance; and Yugoslavs, a 1 in 50 chance.[92] Its importance for infertility is currently under investigation.

Semen analysis

Cooperation of the male partner is mandatory for a proper infertility investigation. The male factor as a cause of infertility is reported in 50% of cases. In 20% to 25% of cases, both the man and the woman have reproductive abnormalities.[29] Therefore, knowledge of male reproductive physiology and results of the male partner's diagnostic infertility work-up is essential. This requirement calls for close cooperation and coordination of care with the andrologist and/or urologist.[1,2,29]

To determine adequacy of the spermatozoa, the man must submit a semen sample for analysis. A history of paternity or an adequate postcoital test does not eliminate the need for a semen analysis. After 3 to 7 days of sexual abstinence,[1] the sample is obtained by masturbation and collected in a clean glass or plastic jar. If masturbation is impossible because of religious or personal reasons, silicone condoms can be used to obtain specimens through intercourse. Latex condoms are to be avoided because they are spermicidal.[8] Ideally, the sample should be produced in the laboratory so that it is fresh. If it is produced elsewhere, the sample must be kept warm and delivered to the laboratory within 1 hour. A laboratory should be selected on the basis of its experience and expertise in performing semen analyses. The interpretation by inexperienced personnel in a laboratory that performs semen analysis infrequently is often meaningless.

The basic semen analysis assesses the physical characteristics of the spermatozoa, their density, motility, and morphology. Table 18-1 defines the 1987 World Health Organization criteria for normal values of semen variables.[105] Numerous studies have shown that conception can occur with abnormal semen parameters,[32] although the chances are better when all parameters fall within the normal range.

Sperm density has been investigated extensively. Nelson and Bunge[71] correlated the concentration of sperm in the ejaculate with the relative risk of infertility (Table 18-2). There is a decrease in fertility with sperm counts of less than 20×10^6/mL. The larger the decrement, the higher the incidence of infertility. Nevertheless, 20% to 25% of fertile men have sperm counts of less than 20×10^6/mL.

Normal motility is generally accepted as 50% or more motile sperm. Dunphy et al.[32] graded sperm motility on the basis of progression, linearity, and velocity. Slow linear or nonlinear motility appeared to be the superior form of spermatozoal motion. Dunphy et al.[32] hypothesized that rapid movements may be less effective and may be associ-

Table 18-1. Normal values of semen variables

Variable	Normal value
Volume	2.0 mL or greater
pH	7.2 to 7.8
Sperm concentration	20×10^6/mL or greater
Total sperm count	40×10^6 or greater
Motility	50% or more with forward progression of 25% or greater with rapid linear progression within 60 min after collection
Morphology	50% or more with normal morphology
Viability	50% or more live
White blood cells	$<1 \times 10^6$/mL
Zinc (total)	2.4 μlmolI or more per ejaculate
Citric acid (total)	52 μlmolI (10 mg) or more per ejaculate
Fructose (total)	13 μlmolI or more per ejaculate
Mixed antiglobulin test	<10% spermatozoa with adherent particles
Immunobead test	<10% spermatozoa with adherent beads

Modified from World Health Organization: *WHO laboratory manual for the examination of human semen and semen-cervical mucus interaction,* ed 2, Cambridge, UK, 1987, Press Syndicate of the University of Cambridge.

Table 18-2. Relative risk of infertility according to sperm count*

Sperm count	Relative risk	Significance
<10	10.3	$<10^{-9}$
10–19	5.2	$<10^{-5}$
20–39	3.1	<0.001
40–59	1.7	<0.02
60–159	1.0	
160–199	1.3	NS†
200+	1.5	NS

Modified from Nelson CMK, Bunge R: *Fertil Steril* 4:10, 1953, and DeCherney AH: In Kase NG, Weingold AB, editors: *Principles and practice of clinical gynecology,* New York, 1983, Churchill Livingstone.
*Unit risk is that obtained for counts of 60 to 159 × 10⁶/mL.
†NS, not significant.

ated with decreased survival and decreased fertilizing capacity. As for morphology, an in vitro study revealed enhanced fertilization with a greater degree of normal morphology.[29]

Since numerous variables can affect the quality of semen, it is important to evaluate more than one sample, as well as a postcoital test. Artificially poor samples can occur secondary to stress, lack of adequate stimulation, or loss of part of the ejaculate when it is obtained and collected.[2] Abnormal semen can arise from changes in hormone levels, genetic or congenital abnormalities (including retrograde ejaculation), exposure to occupational and environmental toxins, infections, surgical sequelae, and drug use.

Variables that may affect spermatogenesis include frequent and prolonged hot baths, wearing tight underwear, and use of certain medications and recreational drugs, including alcohol and tobacco.[44] Since a full cycle of spermatogenesis entails approximately 74 days, plus another 2 weeks for sperm to pass through the testis and epididymis, the effect of avoidance of harmful factors may not be apparent for 3 to 4 months. Similarly, a retrospective history of illness or drug exposure is required from a man whose semen analysis is abnormal.

In the presence of persistent oligospermia or azoospermia, an endocrine evaluation is required, which should include measurement of testosterone, FSH, and PRL levels. If these hormone levels are normal and there is a suspicion of retrograde ejaculation, a postejaculatory urinalysis may reveal spermatozoa in the urine, which have entered the bladder. A vasogram and a testicular biopsy are performed to evaluate the ductal system and testicular abnormalities. Current technology makes it possible to remove live spermatozoa retrograde to an obstruction and use them for intrauterine insemination (IUI) or in vitro fertilization (IVF).

The relevance of a varicocele to infertility is highly controversial. A varicocele is present in 8% to 23% of men and in 17% of men with proven fertility.[74] Of men attending infertility clinics, 19% to 41% had a varicocele.[74] Some investigators advocate a spermatic vein ligation when a varicocele is associated with infertility and the presence of oligospermia, azoospermia, or teratospermia.[65] They speculate that the reason for abnormal sperm may be diminished oxygenation of the testis, increased scrotal temperature, and influence of catecholamines and steroids from the left adrenal gland. A positive effect of varicocelectomy was first reported by Tulloch in 1952, but subsequent studies have produced contradictory results.[65,74]

Assessment of ovulation and luteal phase

Ovulation disorders account for about 20% of all infertility.[92] However, as pointed out earlier, the incidence of ovulatory disturbance depends on the patient mix and the specific expertise of the clinic or physician. Definitive proof of ovulation is established only by pregnancy or recovery of an ovum from the oviduct. In the absence of definitive parameters the physician usually relies on presumptive evidence of ovulation, which is generally determined by charting the basal body temperature (BBT), steroid or gonadotropin hormone assays, cervical mucus changes, changes in the vaginal smear, endometrial biopsy, and, recently, pelvic ultrasound. Ovulation should be evaluated in several cycles using different methods.

In assessing ovulation, the history can be helpful. A woman who experiences regular monthly menstruation (regardless of cycle length), premenstrual symptoms, and dysmenorrhea is probably ovulatory. The old dictum *nulla dysmenorrhea sine ovulatione* is probably still valid, since when dysmenorrhea becomes incapacitating, inhibiting ovulation almost always relieves pain.

Basal body temperature. The BBT is a simple, noninvasive, cost-effective means to determine retrospectively that ovulation has occurred, although it does not permit immediate detection of ovulation, and it is not an accurate predictor of ovulation.[17,58,60] Ovulation has been reported to occur in association with 3% to 20% of monophasic BBT curves, and conversely may be absent in a small number of biphasic curves.[8,17] Nevertheless, the basal body temperature is reliable when properly taken by the patient on awakening, before any physical activity, and recorded on a BBT graph to the closest tenth of a degree. Patients are also asked to mark on the BBT graph any episodes of staining or bleeding, and when intercourse occurs. From the chart, it is possible to determine the probable occurrence and time of ovulation, and the frequency of intercourse and its relation to the cycle. The BBT chart also may be helpful in the timing and interpretation of various diagnostic tests, such as an endometrial biopsy or postcoital test. Factors that may influence the day-to-day variability of the BBT include accuracy of reading, cycle variability, illness, medication, and alterations in sleeping pattern.[60] The nadir, or dip, in the curve has been thought to signal the approach of ovulation. The temperature at the nadir should be at least 0.1°F (0.06°C) lower than that of the 6 previous days.[60] A sharp rise of 0.4°F to 0.6°F (0.22°C to 0.33°C) between 2 consecutive days indicates ovulation. The temperature elevation is a function of the thermogenic effect of progesterone on the hypothalamus.[67] However, the temperature shift measures less than 0.4°F (0.22°C) in up to 39% of BBT charts.[60]

Several studies have demonstrated the inaccuracy of the nadir in the BBT for predicting ovulation. For instance, using vaginal ultrasound and hormone assays, Vermesh et al.[97] reported that ovulation occurred on the day of the nadir in 10%, 1 day after in 20%, and within the following 3 days in the remaining 70%. In another study, Quagliarello and Arny[76] measured LH levels and blindly read BBT charts of 21 patients for 60 cycles and found that the BBT indicated ovulation occurring from 2 to 3 days on either side of the LH surge.

Luteinizing hormone surge. Ovulation occurs 16 to 48 hours after the onset of the LH surge,[106] defined as a threefold increase in LH over the average LH level of the 3 previous days.[58] Although the midcycle LH surge is the most reliable predictor of ovulation, it is not practical to measure LH because of the need for frequent blood sampling and the expense of the radioimmunoassays.

A urine test for LH is available that is noninvasive, rapid, convenient, self-administered, and less expensive than blood tests. Urinary LH kits are reliable and can be obtained in any pharmacy. Their intelligent use can be helpful when attempting pregnancy or insemination, but the results can be affected by the patient's ability to read and follow instructions correctly. Determination of the LH surge is not essential for the basic fertility work-up. Ovulation can be detected by the BBT and endometrial biopsy.

Endometrial biopsy. The endometrial biopsy provides histologic evidence of endometrial development and acts as an in vivo bioassay for estrogen and progesterone production.[62,99] In effect, the biopsy also evaluates the adequacy of the luteal phase. Endometrial histology can also detect unsuspected pathology such as polyps or endometritis,[95] which also may impair fertility. To allow for full endometrial development, the biopsy should be performed 2 to 3 days before the subsequent menses.[99] A combination of menstrual history and BBT patterns aids in determining the appropriate time for the biopsy. A urinary LH kit has also been used as a reference point.

The histologic characteristics of the endometrial biopsy are dated according to the criteria established by Noyes et al.[72] The tissue should be obtained from the anterior or posterior wall of the fundus rather than from the less vascularized lower uterine segment, where the tissue may not be in phase.[101,103]

The endometrial biopsy is a simple office procedure with minimal risks. An analysis of 774 patients who underwent endometrial biopsies for infertility revealed a complication rate of 3.6%.[29] Complications included difficulty in obtaining the biopsy secondary to cervical stenosis,[51] excessive bleeding,[73] uterine perforation,[9] and interruption of pregnancy.[24,92]

The risk of performing an endometrial biopsy in a cycle of conception is 3% to 5%. The overall incidence of interrupting a pregnancy is 0.067%, when less than 2% of the implantation site is sampled.[101] Wentz et al.[101] studied patients who had an endometrial biopsy performed in the cycle of conception and concluded that the procedure did not appear to increase fetal wastage. Patients who are concerned about the possibility of interrupting an early pregnancy should abstain from coitus, use a barrier contraceptive method in the biopsy cycle, or have a very sensitive pregnancy test carried out just before the biopsy specimen is taken.

Whether an endometrial biopsy is necessary has been questioned. Driessen et al.[31] reported that biopsy findings had no effect on the diagnosis or outcome of infertility, whereas others have shown that diagnosis of an inadequate luteal phase and its treatment resulted in improved reproductive outcome.[49,99,100] In either event, the opportunity to detect endometritis is best achieved by biopsy sampling; in this way procedures that entail lavage of the tubes (e.g., hysterosalpingography, chromoperturbation) can be delayed until after appropriate antibiotic therapy has been instituted to avoid eliciting a pelvic infection.

Luteal phase defects. Diagnosis and treatment of luteal phase defects (LPD) remains controversial. Some authors define LPD as endometrium that is 2 or more days out of phase in two successive cycles,[25,81,83] whereas others define it as endometrium more than 2 days out of phase.* Second, there is the problem of cycle date. Endometrial biopsies are dated on a 28-day idealized cycle, with day 28 defined as the first day of the subsequent cycle. Some investigators believe that prospective dating of the endometrium corresponds more accurately to subsequent endometrial maturation.[43] They claim that the LH surge or ultrasound follicular assessment defines more accurately the day of ovulation and onset of the luteal phase.[43,85,107]

As determined by customary methods, the luteal phase is inadequate in up to 30% of cycles in normal women. The incidence of recurrent LPD in infertile women ranges from 3% to 14%.[28,84,90,92,101] Factors associated with an increase in LPD include the extremes of reproductive age, hyperprolactinemia, use of ovulation-inducing drugs,[6] and recurrent pregnancy wastage.[28,99] However, in 50% of patients with LPD none of these factors is present.[99]

LPD may be caused by inadequate progesterone secretion by the corpus luteum or a defect in the endometrial response to hormonal stimulation.[72] The defect may occur in the follicular, preovulatory, or luteal phase. It may initially happen at the time of folliculogenesis,[25,43,50] or it may be inherent in the endometrium.[23,43,62,82] Postulated and proven causes[62] of LPD are as follows:

Neuroendocrine
    Increased LH pulse frequency
    Deficient follicular phase FSH levels
    Inadequate LH surge
    Abnormal follicular phase LH:FSH ratio
    Mild hyperprolactinemia
    Deficient luteal phase LH levels
Ovarian
    Reduced number of primordial follicles
    Accelerated luteolysis
Uterine
    Inadequate endometrial steroid (progesterone)
      receptors
    Endometritis
Other
    Physiologic changes (postpartum, postmenarcheal, premenopause)
    Chronic hypoxia
    Drugs (e.g., clormiphene citrate, human menopausal gonadotropin)
    Chronic systemic disease (e.g., renal or hepatic failure)
    Thyroid disease
    Overweight or underweight
    Exercise
    Psychosocial stress

*References 20, 25, 30, 72, 84, 90, 91, 99, 100.

A detailed discussion of LPD is found in Chapter 24. The most reliable method of evaluating the luteal phase is a well-timed endometrial biopsy. Other methods include mid-luteal phase progesterone levels, cervical mucus changes, and the BBT graph. Most women with LPD have normal BBT graphs.[62] Persistent elevation of temperature for 11 days or less usually correlates with LPD.[62] An abbreviated thermal shift on the BBT chart suggests LPD, but the diagnosis must be documented by objective means.

A randomly measured serum progesterone level is insufficient evidence, since progesterone is released in a pulsatile fashion and the range may vary considerably. A single serum progesterone level of 3 ng/mL or less in the luteal phase is presumptive evidence of ovulation.[46] Some clinicians advocate a level of 12 to 13 ng/mL in the midluteal phase, or a sum of more than 15 ng/mL for three samples obtained on alternate days in the midluteal phase.[20,62] In the presence of an equivocal BBT graph, the progesterone level can be used to ascertain whether ovulation has occurred before performing an endometrial biopsy to consider LPD.

Finally, recording of alterations in the amount, physical characteristics, and chemical constituents of cervical mucus has been used successfully to detect and predict ovulation.[67] These changes are regulated by, and reflect, changes in ovarian steroids. Cervical mucus is clinically apparent on cycle days 8 to 10 and is most profuse at ovulation, when the peak in estradiol levels results in production of large amounts of thin, watery, alkaline, acellular cervical mucus with ferning, spinnbarkeit and maximal sperm receptivity. Ovulation can occur from 3 days before to 3 days after peak mucus output.[67] After ovulation occurs, progesterone inhibits secretory activity of the cervical epithelium. The cervical mucus becomes scant, viscous, cellular, and impenetrable to sperm with minimal spinnbarkeit and no ferning.[67] (See Chapter 19.) This change is presumptive evidence that ovulation has occurred.

Assessment of cervical factors

A cervical factor accounts for 5% to 10% of infertility. Sperm receptivity of the cervical mucus is of prime importance. (See Chapter 19.) Normal, midcycle mucus facilitates passage of normal motile spermatozoa and acts as a filter restricting entry of morphologically abnormal spermatozoa.[40] The cervical crypts are filled with mucus and provide storage for live spermatozoa, which are gradually released into the uterus and fallopian tubes over a period of 48 to 72 hours after coitus. The first stage of sperm capacitation probably also occurs in the endocervical crypts.[79] The postcoital test (PCT) assesses the cervical mucus and sperm-mucus interaction and provides concrete evidence of coital adequacy. Although the PCT is generally accepted as an integral part of the infertility work-up, controversy exists concerning its standardization, interpretation, reliability, and correlation with pregnancy.[10]

The PCT should be performed near the time of ovulation, as predicted by the BBT, changes in cervical mucus, the LH surge (as determined by a commercial urine kit), or by assessment of follicular development by ultrasound. The couple is instructed to abstain from intercourse for 48 hours before the test. The optimal time after intercourse for a PCT is debatable. Several investigators report no decrease in the number of spermatozoa after 24 hours, whereas others report a decrease after 8 hours.[92] Some clinicians advise performing the PCT within 2 hours after intercourse—a difficult condition with which to comply—whereas others advise 12 to 18 hours. It should be noted that complement-dependent reactions that immobilize sperm require 8 to 10 hours. Thus performing a PCT earlier than 8 to 10 hours after intercourse may not detect this potential problem.[12] A time span of at least 8 hours after intercourse is recommended prior to performance of the PCT.

After wiping the external os, the mucus is obtained with a fenestrated or polyp forceps or aspirated with a pipette and rubber ball. The mucus is placed on a clean, dry slide, covered with a coverslip, and examined under a microscope. Because sperm distribution is uniform throughout the cervical canal, there is no need for selective sampling.[92] Grossly, the quantity, quality, color, and viscosity are assessed. Mucus should be clear and abundant. Spinnbarkeit is assessed by stretching the mucus between the blades of the forceps, between the cervical os and forceps, or between the slide and coverslip, and measuring it in centimeters before the thread of mucus breaks. Eight to ten centimeters of spinnbarkeit is normally found at midcycle. The microscopic examination assesses cellularity, debris, white blood cells, and number and motility of spermatozoa. Cellular elements and/or a typical fern pattern indicate possibly underlying cervicitis.[79] If cervicitis is suspected, cultures are obtained and treatment with a course of doxycycline or other appropriate antibiotic may improve the results of a subsequent PCT.[34]

The number of motile sperm considered adequate in a PCT remains debatable.[54,92] According to Speroff et al.,[92] 5 motile sperm per high-power field (HPF) is adequate. Others have different criteria: 7 motile sperm per HPF progressing purposefully; $10 sperm per HPF with $50% showing purposeful motility; $10 sperm per HPF with directional motility[39,67,105]; >20 sperm per HPF; a single active sperm per HPF.

Jette and Glass[54] examined the relationship of the quality of mucus to pregnancy and found pregnancy rates of 53.8% and 37% for good and consistently poor mucus, respectively. Clear, watery mucus without white blood cells was considered good; thick, tenacious, cloudy mucus with many white blood cells was considered poor. A correlation between the concentration of sperm in the semen and the number of spermatozoa in cervical mucus also has been reported. More than 20 spermatozoa per HPF has been associated with sperm counts greater than $20 \times 10^6/mL$.[12] Nevertheless, a semen analysis is still necessary to evaluate morphology.[54]

The correlation between PCT results and pregnancy rates is controversial. Some investigators report a good correlation, whereas others report no correlation.[16,29,92] An abnormal PCT does not preclude pregnancy. Aspirates obtained during laparoscopy have revealed live spermatozoa in the cul-de-sac up to 28 hours after an abnormal PCT.[23]

Despite its shortcomings, the PCT is valuable in assessing coital technique and hostile cervical mucus, and raising the possibility of antisperm antibodies. When the PCT reveals satisfactory mucus but no sperm or only immotile sperm, the use of spermicidal lubricants must be ruled out.[92] Egg white or vegetable oil is not spermicidal and can be used if a lubricant is needed as an adjuvant for intercourse.

The most common reason for inadequate cervical mucus is inappropriate timing of the PCT. Other reasons include hyporesponsiveness of the cervix to estrogens, inadequate estrogen levels, vaginal or cervical infection, acid mucus, or presence of antisperm antibodies. Previous cervical surgery (cone biopsies, for example), or in utero exposure of the patient to diethylstilbestrol can also affect mucus production.[17] Finally, treatment with clomiphene citrate may have a negative effect on cervical mucus. In such cases supplementary estrogens in the late follicular phase may improve the PCT results and be therapeutic.

When cervical mucus is acidic, alkalinization of the vaginal environment and the cervical mucus by douching with sodium bicarbonate (baking soda, 2 tablespoons per quart of water) 30 to 60 minutes before intercourse may improve the PCT. This is a simple, inexpensive procedure that may be therapeutic. The possible mechanisms of the action of a baking soda douche include alteration of vaginal pH; alteration of cervical mucus pH; alteration of cervical mucus electrolytes; removal of excess vaginal discharge; and reduction of pathogenic organisms.[3]

The presence of white blood cells in the cervical mucus may indicate an underlying infection even if cervical cultures are negative. The importance of microbial colonization for sperm-mucus interaction and the benefit of antibacterial therapy in asymptomatic couples with negative cultures is controversial.

Sperm antibody testing may be informative when the PCT reveals no sperm, nonmotile sperm, or shaking sperm with poor progression in the presence of satisfactory mucus and a normal sperm count.[92] Table 18-3 summarizes the etiologies of abnormal sperm-cervical mucus interaction.[32] Intrauterine insemination with washed sperm is a therapeutic possibility for cervical factor infertility.

Assessment of tubal, uterine, and peritoneal factors

Tubal factors. Tubal disease may be a factor in 30% to 50% of infertility.[70] The patient's history will alert the

physician to possible tubal or peritoneal factors. A history of complicated appendicitis, especially with a ruptured appendix, PID, septic abortion, previous pelvic or tubal surgery, ectopic pregnancy, or use of an intrauterine device (IUD) should raise the index of suspicion. Patients with tubal disease generally are older, are of lower socioeconomic status, are more likely to be smokers or to abuse drugs, and have more sexual partners.[19] However, about half of patients with tubal damage or pelvic adhesions have a negative history of PID. This is especially true with chlamydial infection, which is customarily silent yet produces tubal and peritubal damage. According to Westrom's data,[102] the incidence of infertility after one episode of salpingitis is 11% to 12%; after two episodes, 23%; and after three episodes, 54%. Epidemiologic studies link the use of IUD with increased risk of PID and tubal infertility.[19] The relative risk of tubal infertility is 2.6-fold greater for women who ever used an IUD compared with those who never used one.[21] The actual relative risk varied with the type of IUD used. It was highest for the Dalkon Shield, which was discontinued, and lowest (only slightly elevated compared with controls) for the copper IUD.[21] Women who reported having only one sexual partner had no increased risk of primary tubal infertility associated with IUD use.[19]

Mueller et al.[70] showed no excess risk of tubal infertility associated with a simple uncomplicated appendectomy, but

Table 18-3. Etiologic classification of abnormal sperm-cervical mucus interaction

Female-related causes	Male-related causes
Inappropriate timing	Deposition problems
Ovulatory disorders	Impotence
Anovulation	Retrograde ejaculation
Subtle anomalies of	Hypospadias
ovulatory process	
Deposition problem	Semen abnormalities
Dyspareunia	Low sperm concentration
Prolapse	Low sperm motility
Congenital and anatomic	High percentage of
anomalies	abnormal forms
Anatomic and organic causes	High volume (>8 mL)
Amputation or deep	Low volume (<1 mL)
conization of the cervix	
Deep cauterization or	Nonliquefying semen
cryotherapy	
Tumors: polyps,	Antisperm antibodies in
leiomyomas	serum or seminal plasma
Severe stenosis	
Endocervicitis	
Hostile cervical mucus	
Increased viscosity	
Increased cellularity	
(infection)	
Acid mucus	
Presence of sperm	
antibodies	

From Moghissi K: *Obstet Gynecol Clin North Am* 14:893, 1987.

a ruptured appendix was associated with a relative risk of 4.8% for nulligravidas and 3.2% for multiparous women. Tubal obstruction and/or disease is usually diagnosable by hysterosalpingography, although the gold standard for detection of tubal patency and tubal and peritubal disease (e.g., endometriosis, adhesions) is laparoscopy and lavage.[87] At present, diagnostic laparoscopy may be extended as a therapeutic procedure.

Uterine and peritoneal factors. Uterine abnormalities are responsible for infertility in about 2% of cases. Gross deformities of the uterus, whether congenital or acquired, may be a cause of infertility. One of most common findings is leiomyomas, which may enlarge and distort the uterine cavity, causing interference with sperm transport or abnormal endometrial vascularity sufficient to interfere with implantation. Intrauterine synechiae (Asherman syndrome) also may block sperm transport and interfere with implantation. In extreme cases, the uterine cavity can be completely obliterated. (See Chapter 39.)

The hysterosalpingogram is the simplest method for initial evaluation of the uterine cavity, tubal patency, and peritubal adhesions.[89] The procedure should be performed in the early follicular phase after menses has stopped. At this stage, the endometrium is at its thinnest and least likely to distort the image. A pregnancy will not be interrupted if the procedure is carried out in the preovulatory phase of the cycle.

When there is a suspicion of infection because of tenderness on pelvic examination or presence of adnexal masses, an erythrocyte sedimentation rate (ESR) and white count are determined. If either is elevated, cultures should be obtained and the hysterogram postponed until the patient is treated. In high-risk populations an ESR should be performed on all patients. The chance of infection is less than 1% in low-risk populations and 3% in high-risk populations.[92] Anaerobic bacteria are responsible for the majority of infections.

Prophylactic use of antibiotics for hysterosalpingography is controversial. Some physicians prescribe antibiotics, but others do not.[94] A prostaglandin inhibitor, such as ibuprofen or an analgesic, administered orally 30 to 60 minutes before the procedure, decreases discomfort. Under fluoroscopy, the dye is slowly injected through a cervical cannula so that filling of the uterine cavity and tubes can be observed directly. Although rare, injection of the contrast material may induce localized uterine or tubal spasm, giving the false impression of tubal (cornual) obstruction. Spasm can be prevented by counseling the patient before injection to reduce tension, and by injecting the dye slowly and steadily.[35] If tubal spasm occurs, administration of 10 mg of glucagon followed by a 5-minute delay before continuing the dye injection has been reported to result in relief of tubal spasm in 80% of instances.[57] Generally tubal spasm is rarely encountered when the procedure is performed by experienced personnel. (See Chapter 27.)

Complications of hysterography include uterine perforation, hemorrhage, hypersensitivity to iodine, exacerbation of PID, and pain. Current techniques of hysterosalpingography have about 75% correlation with laparoscopy and hysteroscopy. A hysterogram still provides valuable information even if the patient ultimately undergoes laparoscopy and hysteroscopy. The permanent record delineating the uterine contour is useful in interpreting hysteroscopic and laparoscopic findings.

Two types of contrast medium are used in hysterosalpingography, oil-soluble and water-soluble media. The oil-soluble medium provides a sharper film image, flows more slowly, and is claimed to fill in contours of the uterine cavity and tubes more extensively. It is less irritating to the peritoneal cavity and associated with less pain than when water-soluble dye is used. Because oil-soluble dye is absorbed more slowly, it requires a delayed film to detect and define hydrosalpinx and peritubal adhesions.[7,89] Disadvantages of an oil-soluble medium include the risk of granuloma formation (because of the slow absorption), additional irradiation to the gonads because of delayed films, and intravasation.[7,89] The prevalence of granuloma after use of an oil-soluble medium is unknown. Intravasation of the contrast medium occurs in 0% to 6.3% of cases and has a 1.1% risk of embolization. In most instances embolization has been innocuous[7]; however, lipoid pneumonia and death have been associated with the use of oil-contrast media. If intravasation is detected during the procedure, injection of the contrast medium is immediately stopped and the patient observed for undesirable side effects. Advocates of water-soluble contrast media report nearly as good a radiographic image as with an oil medium, but without the potential for serious adverse effects.[89]

Use of oil-soluble contrast media has been associated with higher pregnancy rates.[7,89,92] This presumed therapeutic effect may be related to the hydrotubation itself, with mechanical lavage that breaks fine intratubal and peritoneal adhesions, to a bacteriostatic effect of the iodine, or to enhancement of ciliary action. Ethiodized oil (Ethiodol), the contrast material most commonly used, has been shown in vitro to decrease phagocytosis of peritoneal macrophages, which may imply a possible in vivo decrease in phagocytosis of spermatozoa.[92] Since hysterosalpingography may be therapeutic in addition to being diagnostic, time should be set aside for such effects to occur.

Hysteroscopy and laparoscopy are the final diagnostic procedures of the basic infertility work-up. (See Chapter 28.) Improvement in instrumentation, distention media, and education of residents and clinicians has resulted in increased interest in and use of hysteroscopy.[35] Hysteroscopy should be performed in the early follicular phase, immediately after menses. Bleeding, infection, and pregnancy are contraindications. The procedure can be done in the office under light analgesia. Possible complications include uterine perforation, bleeding, infection, and risks associated with use of distention media. Carbon dioxide as a distending agent carries the risk of gas intravasation with acidosis and possible embolus. In the United States, the most commonly used medium is high-molecular-weight dextran, which has the risk of cardiovascular overload if an excess amount is given and there is extravasation. Other agents include sorbitol and glycine. Because hysteroscopy provides direct visualization, one can identify the nature of intrauterine lesions or anomalies suspected from the hysterogram.[9,35] When the possibility of transcervical surgery is anticipated, hysteroscopy should be done in a well-equipped operating room under general anesthesia by an experienced gynecologist who can perform an operative procedure if indicated.

When laparoscopy is performed toward the end of the infertility work-up, it is usually combined with hysteroscopy and tubal hydrotubation. Since there is a likelihood of detecting endometriosis or pelvic adhesions, a laser or operative laparoscope should be readily available.

UNEXPLAINED INFERTILITY

Criteria for the diagnosis of unexplained infertility include infertility of at least 2 years' duration; normal history and physical examination; adequate coital frequency; three normal semen analyses; regular monthly menstrual cycles with biphasic BBT and luteal phase of 12 or more days; adequate cervical mucus and a normal PCT; normal levels of LH, FSH, PRL, progesterone, and testosterone; and normal results of hysterosalpingography and laparoscopy.[57] Additional parameters include negative results for bacteriologic cultures, immunologic tests, sperm penetration tests, major histocompatibility complex analyses, and ultrasound studies.[45] (See Chapter 25.)

Infection

Over the past 30 years, subclinical infections due to several microorganisms have been implicated in infertility. Two types of mycoplasma (microorganisms the size of large viruses having no cell wall), *Mycoplasma hominis* and *Ureaplasma urealyticum,* have been recovered from the genital tract.[38] Several studies have reported a greater prevalence of genital mycoplasma in cervical mucus and semen of infertile couples than in normal controls.[14,36,38,92] There are also reports that sperm of men with semen cultures positive for ureaplasma tend to have increased abnormal morphology and poor motility. After successful treatment with antibiotics, the quality of sperm improved.[14,38] Increased pregnancy rates after eradication of *Ureaplasma* also have been reported.[38] However, other studies have found no significant effect of genital mycoplasma in infertile couples.[33,48,88] Furthermore, positive genital mycoplasma cultures have been found in up to 50% of normal men.[63]

Although the correlation of genital mycoplasma with male or female unexplained infertility is controversial, a positive culture for genital mycoplasma warrants treatment with doxycycline or tetracycline. Invasive procedures should be delayed until repeated cultures are negative.

Immunologic factors

Immunologic factors have been found in 5% to 17% of infertile couples[29] and in up to 40% of couples with unexplained infertility.[68] Immunologic factors should be considered when the sperm count is normal, yet sperm are immotile or show shaking movements without progression; when a vasectomy has been reversed; when spontaneous spermagglutination occurs on semen analysis; or when there is a long history of unexplained infertility.[11,68]

How immune factors affect fertility is not well understood. (See Chapter 21.) Immune infertility could result from depletion or destruction of gametes, inhibition of transport of sperm in the female genital tract, inhibition of gamete interaction, or prevention of embryo cleavage or implantation.[13,29]

In men, infection, vasectomy, testicular torsion, or trauma may result in breakdown of the blood-testis barrier, resulting in an immunologic reaction and subsequent formation of antisperm antibodies. In women, sexual activity involving intravaginal ejaculation results in exposure to the antigenic stimuli of spermatozoa and seminal plasma that may cause development of antisperm antibodies. Infection or inflammation may also increase the probability that sperm will interact with systemic immune system components and form antisperm antibodies.[104]

There are no standard methods for detection of antisperm antibodies or for interpreting test results.[37] Several studies have shown discordance between results of sperm antibody tests in matched serum and sperm samples.[61] There is no accepted treatment. Proposed treatments include abstinence; use of condoms to decrease contact between the vaginal mucus and semen, and thus decrease repeated sensitization; use of corticosteroids; in vitro manipulation of semen; and IVF with possible micromanipulation of oocytes.[13,29] The clinical significance of immune factors in infertility remains in dispute. It has been suggested that immune infertility is an intermittent phenomenon.[13,29]

Fertilizing capacity of sperm

A functional test of the fertilizing capacity of sperm was described in 1926 by Uehera and Yanagimachi.[96] Human spermatozoa are added to hamster eggs after removal of the zona pellucida by enzymatic dissection with trypsin. The eggs are then examined for sperm penetration. Neither standards nor normal ranges have been established for the assay,[29] and its clinical significance remains controversial. Human IVF and pregnancy have occurred when results of the hamster egg test were poor or negative.[1,8,18,29]

Histocompatibility leukocyte antigens

A role for histocompatibility leukocyte antigens (HLA) in infertility is suggested by a negative association between certain haplotype combinations and infertility, as well as an increased frequency of the *HLA-B5* locus in women with unexplained infertility. Furthermore, homozygosity at the B locus has been shown to occur more frequently in couples with unexplained infertility than in controls. However, several studies have shown no significant distribution of HLA antigens, or increased sharing, in couples with unexplained infertility.[18] The value of HLA tests in an infertility investigation is unknown.

Luteinized unruptured follicle syndrome

In luteinized unruptured follicle (LUF) syndrome the follicle does not collapse after the LH surge and actually may increase in size during the luteal phase.[92] Although the pathophysiology of LUF syndrome is not known, women with diagnosed LUF syndrome should not take prostaglandin synthetase inhibitors because prostaglandins appear to be required for follicular wall rupture.[55]

There are several reports claiming an increased incidence of LUF syndrome in women with unexplained infertility, endometriosis, or pelvic adhesions, and after clomiphene citrate therapy.[56,92] The overall incidence of LUF syndrome is unknown, but it has been reported in 5% to 18% of cycles in infertile women.[18,41,53,56] Several studies found an even higher incidence in women with unexplained infertility or endometriosis.[53] However, LUF syndrome has been detected in 5% to 11% of cycles in normal fertile women,[53,78] and pregnancy has occurred during cycles with LUF syndrome.[55]

On vaginal ultrasound, follicular rupture presents the following features: (1) partial or total collapse or disappearance of the follicle, (2) development of internal echoes, and (3) increased fluid in the cul-de-sac.[47] In addition to ultrasound, diagnostic methods to evaluate LUF syndrome include early luteal phase laparoscopy to identify ovulation stigmata, and comparison of estrogen and progesterone levels in early luteal phase peritoneal fluid with plasma levels of the hormones.[55]

The LUF syndrome may be a variation of normal follicular development because it is rarely recurrent. Inappropriate luteinization could result from LUF syndrome or from development of multiple small follicles causing premature luteinization.

Coulam et al.[18] followed 57 couples with unexplained infertility and found LUF syndrome in 5%, antisperm antibodies in 5%, low sperm penetration in 11%, and HLA-locus homozygosity in 37%. Thus, in the hands of Coulam's group, use of immunologic tests (sperm antibodies, histocompatibility antigen testing), ultrasound monitoring of follicular development, and the sperm penetration assay reduced the diagnosis of unexplained infertility by about 60%.

Various treatments have been used empirically in patients with unexplained infertility, including gonadotropins, clomiphene citrate, antibiotics, thyroid hormones, danazol, and mucolytic agents.[68] Since none of these treatments have been proven effective in controlled studies, they should not be advocated.

CONCLUSION

Pregnancy rates are independent of treatment for infertility. Pregnancy has occurred in patients with unexplained infertility, in women with "blocked" fallopian tubes, and in patients whose male partners were severely infertile.[15] According to life table analysis, 64% of women with primary unexplained infertility and 79% with secondary infertility will conceive within 9 years.[38] This does not mean that the physician should wait 9 years before doing an infertility work-up and starting treatment, but the decision to initiate investigation should be individualized.

The tests and treatments for infertility are very expensive, and success rates remain relatively low. Since infertile patients are usually anxious and eager and will do almost anything to have a child, care must be taken to avoid exploitation of their hopes with unnecessary procedures and treatments.

The role of the infertility specialist is not only to evaluate and treat but to counsel. The specialist can offer realistic advice about the use of assisted reproductive technology, adoption, and other alternatives, and direct couples to the various social support systems available.

REFERENCES

1. Acosta AA et al: Assisted reproduction in the diagnosis and treatment of the male factor, *Obstet Gynecol Surv* 44:1, 1988.
2. American College of Obstetricians and Gynecologists: Technical Bulletin #142: *Male infertility,* Washington, DC, June 1990, The College.
3. Ansari AH, Gould KG, Ansari VM: Sodium bicarbonate douching for improvement of the postcoital test, *Fertil Steril* 33:608, 1980.
4. Baird DD, Wilcox AJ: Cigarette smoking associated with delayed conception, *JAMA* 253:2979, 1985.
5. Baker ER: Menstrual dysfunction and normal status in athletic women: a review, *Fertil Steril* 36:691, 1981.
6. Balasch J, Creus M, Vanrell JA: Luteal function after delayed ovulation, *Fertil Steril* 45:342, 1986.
7. Bateman BG et al: Utility of the 24-hour delay hysterosalpingogram film, *Fertil Steril* 47:613, 1987.
8. Blackwell RF, Steinkampf MP: Infertility: diagnosis and therapy. In Soules MR, editor: *Controversies in reproductive endocrinology and infertility,* New York, 1989, Elsevier.
9. Blackwell RF et al.: Are we exploiting the infertile couple?, *Fertil Steril* 48:735, 1987.
10. Blasco L: Clinical approach to the evaluation of sperm-cervical mucus interactions, Fertil Steril 28:1133, 1977.
11. Bronson RA, Cooper GW, Rosenfeld DL: Correlation between regional specificity of antisperm antibodies to the spermatozoan surface and complement-mediated sperm immobilization, *Am J Reprod Immunol* 2:222, 1982.
12. Bronson RA, Cooper GW, Rosenfeld DL: Autoimmunity to spermatozoa: effect in sperm penetration of cervical mucus as reflected by postcoital testing, *Fertil Steril* 41:609, 1984.

13. Bronson R, Cooper G, Rosenfeld D: Sperm antibodies: their role in infertility, *Fertil Steril* 42:171, 1984.

14. Cassell GH et al: Microbiologic study of infertile women at the time of diagnostic laparoscopy-association of *Ureaplasma urealyticum* with a defined subpopulation, *N Engl J Med* 308:502, 1983.

15. Collins JA et al: Treatment-independent pregnancy among infertile couples, *N Engl J Med* 309:1201, 1983.

16. Collins JA et al: The postcoital test as a predictor of pregnancy among 355 infertile couples, *Fertil Steril* 41:703, 1984.

17. Corson SL: Ovulation prediction in the treatment of infertility, *J Reprod Med* 31(suppl):739, 1986.

18. Coulam CB, Moore SM, O'Fallon W: Investigating unexplained infertility, *Am J Obstet Gynecol* 158:1374, 1988.

19. Cramer DW et al: Tubal infertility and the intrauterine device, *N Engl J Med* 312:941, 1985.

20. Crosignani PG: The defective luteal phase, *Hum Reprod* 3:157, 1988.

21. Daling JR et al: Primary tubal infertility in relation to the use of an intrauterine device, *N Engl J Med* 312:937, 1985.

22. Daling JR et al: Tubal infertility in relation to prior induced abortion, *Fertil Steril* 43:389, 1985.

23. Daling JR et al: Post-coital test abnormalities in relation to contraceptive use, *Int J Fertil* 32:436, 1987.

24. Davidson BJ, Thrasher TV, Seraj IM: An analysis of endometrial biopsies performed for infertility, *Fertil Steril* 48:770, 1987.

25. Davis OK et al: The incidence of luteal phase defect in normal, fertile women, determined by serial endometrial biopsies, *Fertil Steril* 51:582, 1989.

26. DeCherney AH: Infertility: general principles of evaluation. In Kase NG, Weingold AB, editors: *Principles and practice of clinical gynecology,* New York, 1983, Churchill Livingstone.

27. Diamond MP: Hyperandrogenism in infertility, *J Reprod Med* 34:10, 1989.

28. Dizerega GS, Hodgen GD: Luteal phase dysfunction infertility: a sequel to aberrant folliculogenesis, *Fertil Steril* 35:489, 1981.

29. Dodson MC, Joshi PN: Male factor infertility and the gynecologist, *Am J Gynecol Health* 3:9, 1989.

30. Downs KA, Gibson M: Basal body temperature graph and the luteal phase defect, *Fertil Steril* 40:466, 1983.

31. Driessen F et al: The significance of dating an endometrial biopsy for the prognosis of the infertile couple, *Int J Fertil* 25:112, 1980.

32. Dunphy BC, Neal LM, Cooke ID: The clinical value of conventional semen analysis, *Fertil Steril* 51:324, 1989.

33. Eggert-Kruse W et al: Influence of microbial colonization on sperm-mucus interaction in vivo and in vitro, *Hum Reprod* 2:301, 1987.

34. Eggert-Kruse W et al: Effects of antimicrobial therapy in sperm-mucus interaction, *Hum Reprod* 3:861, 1988.

35. Fayez JA, Mutie G, Schneider PJ: The diagnostic value of hysterosalpingography and hysteroscopy in infertility investigation, *Am J Obstet Gynecol* 156:558, 1987.

36. Fowlkes DM, MacLeod J, O'Leary WM: T-Mycoplasmas and human infertility: correlation of infection with alterations in seminal parameters, *Fertil Steril* 26:1212, 1975.

37. Franco JG et al: Reproducibility of the indirect immunobead assay for detecting sperm antibodies in serum, *J Reprod Med* 34:259, 1989.

38. Friberg J: Mycoplasmas and ureoplasmas in infertility and abortion, *Fertil Steril* 33:351, 1980.

39. Galle PC et al: Sperm washing and intrauterine insemination for cervical factor oligospermia, immunologic infertility and unexplained infertility, *J Reprod Med* 35:116, 1990.

40. Gonzales J, Jezequel F: Influence of the quality of the cervical mucus on sperm penetration: comparison of the morphologic features of spermatozoa in 101 postcoital tests with those in the semen of the husband, *Fertil Steril* 44:796, 1985.

41. Graf MJ, Kase N: The luteinized unruptured follicle syndrome: an update, *Postgrad Obstet Gynecol* 6:1, 1986.

42. Green BB et al: Exercise as a risk factor for infertility with ovulatory dysfunction, *Am J Public Health* 76:1432, 1986.

43. Grunfeld L et al: Luteal phase deficiency after completely normal follicular and periovulatory phases, *Fertil Steril* 52:919, 1989.

44. Hammond KR et al: Performance anxiety during infertility treatment: effect on semen quality, *Fertil Steril* 53:337, 1990.

45. Hammond MG, Talbert LM: *Infertility: a practical guide for the physician,* ed 2, Oradell NJ, 1985, Medical Economics.

46. Healy DL et al: Pulsatile progesterone secretion: its relevance to clinical evaluation of corpus luteum function, *Fertil Steril* 41:114, 1984.

47. Hecht BR, Hoffman DI: The use of ultrasound in infertility, *Clin Obstet Gynecol* 32:541, 1989.

48. Hellstrom WJ et al: Is there a role for Chlamydia trachomatis and genital mycoplasma in male infertility?, *Fertil Steril* 48:337, 1987.

49. Hill GA et al: Comparisons of late luteal phase endometrial biopsies using the Novak curette or pipelle endometrial suction curette, *Obstet Gynecol* 73:443, 1989.

50. Hodgen GD: The dominant ovarian follicle, *Fertil Steril* 38:281, 1982.

51. Howe G et al: Effects of age, cigarette smoking and other factors in fertility: findings in a large prospective study, *Br Med J* 290:1697, 1985.

52. Jacobs LA: Initial clinical survey of the infertile couple, *Prim Care* 15:575, 1988.

53. Janssen-Caspers HAB et al: Diagnosis of luteinized unruptured follicle by ultrasound and steroid hormone assays in peritoneal fluid: a comparative study. Fertil Steril 46:825, 1986.

54. Jette NT, Glass RH: Prognostic value of the postcoital test, *Fertil Steril* 23:29, 1972.

55. Katz E: The luteinized unruptured follicle and other ovulatory dysfunctions, *Fertil Steril* 50:839, 1988.

56. Kerin JF et al: Incidence of the luteinized unruptured follicle phenomenon in cycling women, *Fertil Steril* 40:620, 1983.

57. Lewinthal D et al: Subtle abnormalities in follicular development and hormonal profile in women with unexplained infertility, *Fertil Steril* 46:833, 1986.

58. Luciano AA et al: Temporal relationship and reliability of the clinical, hormonal, and ultrasonographic indices of ovulation in infertile women, *Obstet Gynecol* 75:412, 1990.

59. Mani P et al: Screening study for partial adrenal enzyme defects in infertile subjects. Paper presented at the 73rd Annual Meeting of the Endocrine Society, Washington, DC, June 19–22, 1991 (abstract 1671).

60. McCarthy JJ, Rockette HE: Prediction of ovulation with basal body temperature, *J Reprod Med* 31:742, 1986.

61. McClure RD et al: Sperm check: a simplified screening assay for immunological infertility, *Fertil Steril* 52:650, 1989.

62. McNeely MJ, Soules MR: The diagnosis of luteal phase deficiency: a critical review, *Fertil Steril* 50:1, 1988.

63. Megory E et al: Infections and male infertility, *Obstet Gynecol Surv* 42:283, 1987.

64. Menken J, Trussel J, Larsen U: Age and infertility, *Science* 233:1389, 1986.

65. Model N et al: Spermatic vein ligation as treatment for male infertility, *J Reprod Med* 35:123, 1990.

66. Moghissi K: Cervical and uterine factors in infertility, *Obstet Gynecol Clin North Am* 14:893, 1987.

67. Moghissi KS: Cervical mucus changes and ovulation prediction and detection, *J Reprod Med* 31:748, 1986.

68. Moghissi KS, Wallach EE: Unexplained infertility, *Fertil Steril* 39:5, 1983.

69. Mueller BA, Daling JR: Epidemiology of infertility. In Soules MR, editor: *Controversies in reproductive endocrinology and infertility,* New York, 1989, Elsevier.

70. Mueller BA et al: Appendectomy and the risk of tubal infertility, *N Engl J Med* 315:1506, 1986.

71. Nelson CMK, Bunge R: Semen analysis: evidence for changing parameters of male fertility potential, *Fertil Steril* 4:10, 1953.

72. Noyes RW, Hertig A, Rock J: Dating the endometrial biopsy, *Fertil Steril* 1:3, 1950.

73. Page H: Estimation of the prevalence and incidence of infertility in a population: a pilot study, *Fertil Steril* 51:571, 1989.

74. Peng BCH, Tomashefsky P, Nagler HM: The cofactor effect: varicocele and infertility, *Fertil Steril* 54:143, 1990.

75. Phipps WR et al: The association between smoking and female infertility as influenced by cause of the fertility, *Fertil Steril* 48:377, 1987.

76. Quagliarello J, Arny M: Inaccuracy of basal body temperature charts in predicting urinary luteinizing hormone surges, *Fertil Steril* 45:334, 1986.

77. Rantala ML, Stenman UH, Koskimies AI: Serum androgens in infertile women with ovulatory dysfunction, *Hum Reprod* 3:437, 1988.

78. Ritchie WG: Ultrasound in the evaluation of normal and induced ovulation, *Fertil Steril* 43:167, 1985.

79. Roland M: Pitfalls of the post-coital test, *Int J Fertil* 30:29, 1985.

80. Scott MG, Ladenson JH: Hormonal evaluation of female infertility and reproductive disorders (Washington University case conference), *Clin Chem* 35:620, 1989.

81. Scott RT et al: The effect of interobserver variation in dating endometrial histology on the diagnosis of luteal phase defects, *Fertil Steril* 50:888, 1988.

82. Seif MW, Aplin JD, Buckley CH: Luteal phase defect: the possibility of an immunohistochemical diagnosis, *Fertil Steril* 51:273, 1989.

83. Shangold M, Berkely A, Gray J: Both midluteal serum progesterone levels and late luteal endometrial histology should be assessed in all infertile women, *Fertil Steril* 40:627, 1983.

84. Sharma SC, Ray RC, Sen S: Luteal phase deficiency–an important cause of female infertility, *J Obstet Gynaecol India* 39:74, 1989.

85. Shoupe D et al: Correlation of endometrial maturation with four methods of estimating day of ovulation, *Obstet Gynecol* 73:88, 1989.

86. Smith CG, Asch RH: Drug abuse and reproduction, *Fertil Steril* 48:355, 1987.

87. Snowden EU, Jarrett JC, Dawood MY: Comparison of diagnostic accuracy of laparoscopy, hysteroscopy, and hysterosalpingography in evaluation of female infertility, *Fertil Steril* 41:709, 1984.

88. Soffer Y et al: Male genital mycoplasmas and Chlamydia trachomatis culture: its relationship with accessory gland function, sperm quality, and autoimmunity, *Fertil Steril* 53:331, 1990.

89. Soules MR, Spadoni L: Oil versus aqueous media for hysterosalpingography: a continuing debate based on many opinions and few facts, *Fertil Steril* 38:1, 1982.

90. Soules MR et al: The diagnosis and therapy of luteal phase deficiency, *Fertil Steril* 28:1033, 1977.

91. Soules MR et al: Luteal phase deficiency: characterization of reproductive hormones over the menstrual cycle, *J Clin Endocrinol Metab* 69:804, 1989.

92. Speroff L, Glass RH, Kase NG: *Clinical gynecologic endocrinology and infertility,* ed 4, Baltimore, 1989 Williams & Wilkins.

93. Stillman RJ, Rosenberg MJ, Sachs BP: Smoking and reproduction, *Fertil Steril* 46:545, 1986.

94. Stumpf PG, March CM: Febrile morbidity following hysterosalpingography: identification of risk factors and recommendations for prophylaxis, *Fertil Steril* 33:487, 1980.

95. Sugkraroek P, Chaturachinoa K: Endometrial biopsy in the evaluation of infertility: a 15 year review at Ramathibodi Hospital, *J Med Assoc Thai* 71:118, 1988.

96. Uehera T, Yanagimachi R: Microsurgical injection of spermatozoa into hamster eggs with subsequent transformation of sperm nuclei into male pronuclei, Biol Reprod 15:467, 1976.

97. Vermesh M et al: Monitoring techniques to predict and detect ovulation, *Fertil Steril,* 47:259, 1987.

98. Vogt HJ, Heller WD, Borelli S: Sperm quality of healthy smokers, ex-smokers, and never-smokers, *Fertil Steril* 45:106, 1986.

99. Wentz AC: Endometrial biopsy in the evaluation of infertility, *Fertil Steril* 33:121, 1980.

100. Wentz AC: Diagnosing luteal phase inadequacy, *Fertil Steril* 37:334, 1982.

101. Wentz AC et al: Cycle of conception endometrial biopsy, *Fertil Steril* 46:196, 1986.

102. Westrom L: Effect of acute pelvic inflammatory disease on infertility, *Am J Obstet Gynecol* 121:707, 1975.

103. Wild RA, Sanfilippo JS, Toledo AA: Endometrial biopsy in the infertility investigation: the experience at two institutions, *J Reprod Med* 31:954, 1986.

104. Witkin SS, Chaudhury A: Relationships between circulating antisperm antibodies in women and autoantibodies on the ejaculated sperm of their partners, *Am J Obset Gynecol* 161:900, 1989.

105. World Health Organization: *WHO laboratory manual for the examination of human semen and semen-cervical mucus interaction,* ed 2, Cambridge, UK, 1987, Press Syndicate of the University of Cambridge.

106. World Health Organization Task Force Investigators: Temporal relationships between ovulation and defined changes in the concentration of plasma estradiol-17β, luteinizing hormone, follicle-stimulating hormone and progesterone, *Am J Obstet Gynecol* 138:383, 1980.

107. Ying Y et al: Ultrasonographic monitoring of follicular growth for luteal phase defects, *Fertil Steril* 48:433, 1987.

Chapter 19

CERVICAL FACTOR IN INFERTILITY

Kamran S. Moghissi, MD

An important step in the investigation of infertility is the evaluation of cervical factor and sperm–cervical mucus interaction. Abnormalities of the cervix and its secretion are believed to be responsible for infertility in approximately 5% to 10% of women. This chapter deals with the functional role of the cervix in human reproduction.

ANATOMY OF THE CERVIX

The cervix represents the terminal portion of the uterus and separates the vagina from the uterine cavity. It is a thick-walled, cylindric structure that tapers at its inferior extremity. The canal of the cervix is 2.5 to 3 cm long, is fusiform, and is flattened in its posterior; its middle third is slightly dilated. The average transverse diameter at its widest point is 7 mm. The external os is the opening in the portio vaginalis that connects the cervical canal with the vagina.

Histologically the cervix differs from the corpus uteri. The pars vaginalis of the cervix is lined with stratified squamous epithelium similar to that lining the vagina, and it normally shows no cornification. The epithelial cells of the endocervix comprise different types of nonciliated secretory and ciliated cells that are tall and columnar, resemble picket cells, rest on the thin basement membrane, and form a single layer; their nuclei are oval and are located basally. Secretory cells are covered by microvilli and contain massive numbers of cytoplasmic granules and clear droplets of mucus. Some ciliated cells have been observed with both transmission and scanning electron microscopy. Columnar epithelium from the ectocervix has very few ciliated cells, whereas endocervical epithelium has many nonciliated cells.[31]

There are no true glands in the cervix. The basic epithelial structure of the cervical mucosa is an intricate system of crypts or grooves which, grouped together, give an illusory impression of glands. These crypts may run in an oblique, transverse, or longitudinal direction. They never cross one another, although they may bifurcate or extend downward. The arrangement of crypts in the endocervical canal resembles the trunk and branches of a tree, and occasionally the crypts are referred to as the "arbor vitae." There is considerable variation in the size of the crypt openings. The smallest openings are 40 to 50 μm and the largest range from 300 to 600 μm.[10]

The junction of columnar epithelium and squamous epithelium is known as the squamocolumnar junction. Unless active metaplasia is present, the junction is very sharp.

Insler et al.[27] studied the number of cervical crypts at different levels of the endocervical canal under different hormonal conditions. The upper and lower segments of cervices removed at surgical operation were cut into serial slices of 6-μm thickness, starting from the distal end. Every tenth slice was taken for evaluation and counting. Crypts with a demonstrable opening into the cervical canal and with their entire length clearly traceable were counted and their circumference was measured using a cartograph. The crypts were then classified into four sizes, as measured on the enlargement screen. In uterine cervices of women pretreated with estrogen or gestagen, the mean number of crypts per slice was 5.04. There were more crypts in estrogen-pretreated cervices than in gestagen-pretreated cervices, and in the latter, the lower segment contained significantly more crypts than the upper segment. In both estrogen-pretreated and gestagen-pretreated specimens the majority of crypts were medium to large; there were few giant crypts. On the basis of these data, Insler et al.[27] calculated that the mean total number of crypts per cervix was 28,000 for estrogen-pretreated cervices and about 23,000 for gestagen-pretreated cervices. This finding is in contrast to the figure reported by Odeblad,[59,60] who suggested there were approximately 100 mucus-secreting, glandlike units (crypts) in the cervical canal.

Cyclic changes in the shape and diameter of the cervix have been described. In the immediate premenstrual period and during menstruation, the isthmus of the cervix (the narrow part of the canal between the endocervix and endometrial cavity) is short, wide, and atonic. Isthmic tone gradually increases during the follicular phase. In the luteal phase, progressive lengthening and narrowing of the isthmus result in a hypertonic, tubular appearance that persists until the immediate premenstrual phase.

The embryology of the cervix has been the subject of many investigations. The cervix, like the rest of the uterus, is clearly derived from the female or müllerian ducts. However, its epithelial lining is continuous with that of the vagina, and there is some controversy about when the two epithelia (i.e., squamous and cylindric) normally join, both prenatally and postnatally.

BLOOD AND NERVE SUPPLY OF THE CERVIX

The blood supply of the cervix is derived primarily from the uterine artery; the azygous arteries of the vagina and ascending branches of the vaginal arteries also contribute. The venous drainage parallels arterial vessels and communicates with the vascular network of the bladder neck. Veins from the cervix join the uterine and ovarian venous plexuses and empty finally into the hypogastric veins. Zinser[87] has demonstrated that the major source of blood supply to mucus-producing endocervical epithelia is from the first branches of the uterine arteries as they descend along the body of the cervix.

The nerve supply of the cervix is derived from three plexuses of the pelvic autonomic system: the superior, middle, and inferior hypogastric plexuses. The pelvic plexus contains sympathetic (inferior hypogastric fibers) and parasympathetic (nervi erigentes) components. The sensory components, which are visceral for the most part, are found in the nervi erigentes. There are apparently a number of sensory fibers in the sympathetic component as well.

Giro[17] studied the terminal nerve supply to the endocervical crypts in rodents and women. He found numerous nerve fibers following the vascular network in the submucosa and, independent of the vascular system, in the endocervix of women. Collateral branches of these terminal nerves were in contact with endocervical crypts. Other nerve fibers were found to traverse the submucosa of the cervical crypts and to form a dense network around the epithelial invagination. These fibers were in intimate contact with glandular epithelium and actually appeared to enter into these columnar cells. Nerve endings bordering the epithelial covering of the cervical canal were perpendicular to the base of the epithelial cells but did not make contact with them.

Nerve fibers positive for cholinesterase-specific staining are most numerous in relation to cervical crypts, arterial vessels, and strands of smooth muscle. These nerve fibers are more abundant in the cervix. Rodin and Moghissi[65] used a differential staining technique to distinguish adrenergic (sympathetic) from cholinergic (parasympathetic) fibers. They demonstrated an extensive adrenergic network at the internal os, where smooth muscle is abundant, and throughout the cervix in relation to blood vessel walls. The distribution of cholinergic fibers was much the same, although the cholinergic supply was less profuse. The extensive network of nerve fibers was not present in postmenopausal cervices.

The precise function of this neural network is unclear. Clinical observations, however, indicate that these nerves may be involved in pain perception resulting from the stretching of the endocervix, particularly the internal os. Adrenergic and cholinergic nerve fibers may also play a role, directly or indirectly, in the secretory function of the epithelial cells through their action on blood vessels.

CERVICAL MUCUS

Cervical mucus is a complex secretion produced constantly by the secretory cells of the endocervix. A small amount of endometrial, tubal, and possibly follicular fluid may also contribute to the cervical mucus pool. Cellular debris from uterine and cervical epithelia and leukocytes is also present. Secretory units of the cervix produce mucus at the rate of 20 to 60 mg/day in normal women of reproductive age. During midcycle, the amount increases 10- to 20-fold and may reach up to 700 mg/d.[52] Cyclic variation in the amount, physical properties, and chemical content of the cervical mucus constituents has been reported.

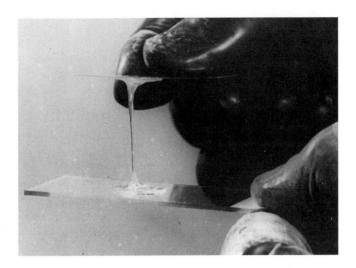

Fig. 19-1. Technique for determining spinnbarkeit (fibrosity) of cervical mucus.

Physical properties

Cervical mucus is a heterogeneous secretion with a number of rheologic properties, including viscosity, flow elasticity, spinnbarkeit, plasticity, and tack or stickiness.[45]

Viscosity. Since cervical mucus is not a true fluid or a homogeneous substance, its viscosity (consistency) cannot be measured with any degree of accuracy. *Anomalous viscous behavior* is the general term applied to secretions such as cervical mucus.

Flow elasticity. The property of cervical mucus whereby it resumes its original shape after deformation caused by external pressure or stress is referred to as flow elasticity, or retraction. When a material showing flow elasticity is caused to flow along a tube and the pressure is suddenly released, the material recoils to regain its original position.

Spinnbarkeit. The capacity of liquids to be drawn into threads is known as spinnbarkeit (fibrosity). To measure spinnbarkeit a sample of mucus is stretched between a glass slide and a coverslip. An estimate of spinnbarkeit is made by measuring the length (in centimeters) of the thread before it breaks (Fig. 19-1).

Plasticity. Plasticity allows a material to be deformed continuously and permanently without rupture. Cervical mucus plasticity is observed predominantly during pregnancy.

Tack. Tack refers to the stickiness of the mucus and is measured by quickly drawing away a coverslip from a sample of mucus on a slide. The mucus does not form long threads but adheres to the coverslip and can be drawn only 1 to 2 cm away from the glass slide.[45] All samples of cervical mucus exhibit stickiness, but only during pregnancy does mucus show this property to a marked degree.

Rheologic properties of cervical mucus are known to change during the menstrual cycle. From the termination of menstruation to the time of ovulation, viscosity and flow elasticity progressively decrease and spinnbarkeit increases. After ovulation and during the luteal phase, spinnbarkeit decreases and flow elasticity and viscosity markedly increase (Fig. 19-2).

The specific density of cervical mucus is close to that of a 0.8% saline solution of the same temperature.[45] The osmotic pressure of cervical mucus remains unchanged during the menstrual cycle. The optical transparency of cervical mucus is high at ovulation and low premenstrually and postmenstrually, when diffuse light scattering is considerably increased. The index of refraction is about 1.336 at midcycle and 1.338 to 1.346 at other phases of the menstrual cycle.[45] Static samples of cervical mucus do not exhibit birefringence.

Physical properties of cervical mucus such as spinnbarkeit, consistency, and flow elasticity are of clinical value in (1) determining the time of ovulation, (2) determining the optimal time for induction of ovulation, (3) determining the optimal time for artificial insemination, (4) recognizing anovulation, (5) diagnosing pregnancy, and (6) diagnosing ovarian dysfunction.[49]

Ferning. Cervical mucus, when spread on a slide and allowed to dry, exhibits an intriguing pattern of arborization with crystallization (Fig. 19-3). The phenomenon of arborization with crystallization, also termed ferning, occurs particularly at ovulation and has been used extensively for

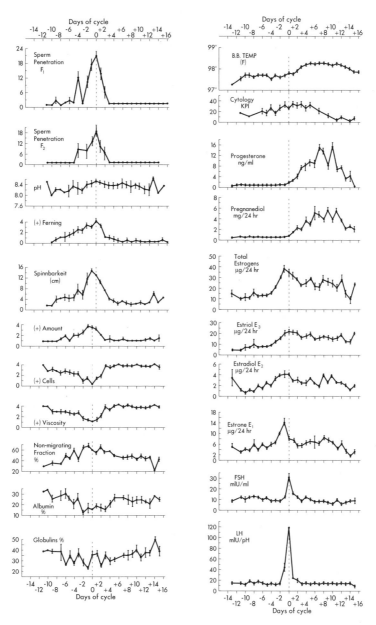

Fig. 19-2. Composite profile of serum gonadotropin and progesterone; urinary estrogens and pregnanediol; basal body temperature (B.B. TEMP); karyopyknotic index (*KPI*) of vaginal cells; and cervical mucus properties throughout the menstrual cycle in 10 normal women. Day 0, day of LH peak (*broken vertical line*). Vertical bars represent one standard error of the mean. F_1 and F_2 indicate the number of sperm in the first and second microscopic fields (×200) from interface, 15 minutes after the start of the in vitro sperm–cervical mucus penetration test.[54]

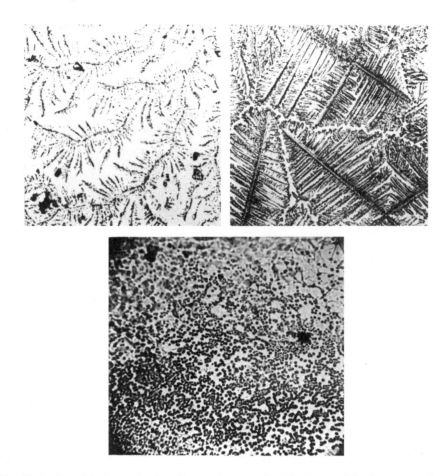

Fig. 19-3. Crystallization or ferning of cervical mucus. *Top left,* 1+; *top right,* 4+; *bottom,* absence of ferning.

detecting ovulation and as an index of circulating estrogen level in clinical medicine. Ferning results when true crystals of sodium and potassium chloride form around a small and optimal amount (1% to 1.5%) of organic matter.[45] Arborization with crystal formation is not specific for cervical mucus and may occur in any protein or colloid solution that contains electrolytes. If the protein content is too high (4% to 6%), as seen in mucus during pregnancy, ferning does not occur.

Ferning appears between days 8 and 10 of a typical cycle in women and reaches its peak at ovulation. Immediately after ovulation it decreases or disappears completely. Serial evaluations of ferning correlated with basal body temperature, vaginal cytology, estrogen and progesterone excretion, midcycle rise of luteinizing hormone (LH) and follicle-stimulating hormone (FSH), and other properties of cervical mucus indicate a high degree of accuracy by the crystallization pattern in predicting the peak of estrogenic activity and the onset of ovulation (Fig. 19-2). Postovulatory mucus and the mucus of pregnancy do not crystallize.

Biochemical properties

Human cervical mucus usually is about 92% to 94% water. At ovulation, when the mucus is most abundant, the water content rises to 98%.[45] Human cervical secretions contain 1% inorganic salts, of which the principal constituent is sodium chloride (0.7%). Traces of potassium, magnesium, calcium, copper, zinc, iron phosphates, sulfates, and bicarbonate are also present.[45] The mucus is isotonic with saline throughout the cycle. The salt content of dry mucus, however, shows an increase coinciding with the time of ovulation. Since the concentration of salt remains constant while the gross amount changes cyclically, the water content of the mucus must change in the same proportion as the salt to maintain a constant concentration. In other words, there is a relative increase in the secretion of water and salt and a decrease in the amount of organic material in the dry weight of the midcycle mucus, which incidentally favors the occurrence of the ferning phenomenon. The osmotic pressure of cervical mucus remains the same throughout the cycle. Ascorbic acid has been detected in cervical mucus and is lowest in concentration at midcycle.[45]

Low-molecular-weight organic compounds in cervical mucus include the free simple sugars (glucose, maltose, mannose), lipids, and free amino acids.

High-molecular-weight components. Ultracentrifugation of the mucus results in two fractions: the supernatant, which contains the soluble macromolecules (polysaccharides, enzymes, and serum-type proteins), and the sediment (gel), which consists mainly of high-molecular-weight glycoproteins (mucins).

Glycogen is the principal polysaccharide of cervical secretion. Amylase, an enzyme capable of reducing glycogen to utilizable glucose, has been found in the mucus. In addition to amylase, cervical mucus contains a large number of enzymes, including alkaline phosphatase, esterase, aminopeptidase, lactate dehydrogenase, and guaiacol peroxidase. These enzymes show a marked preovulatory decrease and postovulatory rise in response to progesterone in the luteal phase. It has been suggested that assay of some of the enzymes that exhibit preovulatory decline and postovulatory rise may be used to predict or detect ovulation.[49,50]

Pooled human cervical mucus contains about 1% to 3%[45] protein in two basic forms, soluble proteins and mucin. The major components of soluble proteins consist of albumin and gamma globulin (immunoglobulin G [IgG]). By immunodiffusion and immunoelectrophoretic studies of human cervical mucus, 15 additional proteins, including lactoferrin, secretory IgA, and α_1-antitrypsin, have been identified. Cyclic variation in the amount of several proteins in cervical mucus has been described. In general, there appears to be a preovulatory decrease and a postovulatory increase in the amount of albumin, alpha$_1$-antitrypsin, and immunoglobulins.[45,67,68] Most serum-type proteins in the cervical mucus probably originate in blood serum.[40] Soluble proteins such as secretory IgA and lactoferrin obviously are synthesized by cervical epithelium, since they are absent in blood.

Mucins comprise 45% of proteins in the cervical mucus. Mucin is a special class of glycoprotein that is rich in carbohydrates and is responsible for the distinctive viscoelastic properties of cervical mucus. Mucin plays an important role in sperm transport.

Detailed structural analyses of the protein moiety of human cervical mucin are lacking, but the close analogy between human cervical mucin and other well-defined epithelial mucins with respect to size and chemical composition strongly suggests adherence to the generally accepted model of mucin structure in which the polypeptide is segregated into two major physical and functional domains. The major portion of mucins is a carbohydrate-rich, protease-resistant hydrophilic domain of extended β structure enriched in serine, threonine, and proline residues. The second domain, often referred to as "naked peptide," is a protease-sensitive, carbohydrate-deficient region enriched in glutamic acid, aspartic acid, leucine, lysine, and cystine residues and is responsible for intramolecular and intermolecular interactions via disulfide linkages and hydrophobic bonding.[79,82,84-86] Several models have been proposed for the supramolecular organization of cervical mucin in the gel phase of cervical mucus. Earlier proposals of a relatively ordered micellar structure based on nuclear magnetic resonance studies[59,61] have been challenged by an alternative model based on laser light–scattering data suggesting a random network of entangled mucin molecules, a structure similar to that of raw rubber.[35,36] The latter model possesses a conceptual advantage because of the ease with which it correlates known ovarian phase–dependent changes in mucus hydration with corresponding changes in the viscoelasticity and sperm transport potential of cervical mucus. However, a functional role of intermolecular cross-links has not been excluded and is likely to be of importance.

Cervical mucin and the reproductive cycle. Several groups have studied the temporal relationship of cervical mucin composition and changes in cervical mucus rheology and sperm transport during the reproductive cycle. Despite earlier reports to the contrary, recent studies clearly demonstrate that the overall amino acid and carbohydrate composition of human cervical mucin remains unchanged during the menstrual cycle.[79,82] Although these results do not exclude more subtle changes in the mucin molecule, such as cyclic changes in structures of the oligosaccharide chains, demonstrated for monkey cervical mucin, the data to date do not implicate variation in human cervical mucin structure as the direct causative factor of changes in cervical mucus rheology or physiology. The changes are more readily correlated with well-defined variations in the water content of cervical mucus obtained at different phases of the menstrual cycle or in response to the use of certain contraceptive steroids.

pH of cervical mucus. In assessing the pH of cervical mucus it is important to distinguish between the values obtained on mucus from the vaginal pool and those obtained on mucus from the external cervical os and endocervix. The pH gradient increases toward the cervical canal; this is due to the acidity of vaginal secretions, which partially contaminate cervical mucus discharged in the vagina. Endocervical secretion is generally alkaline during the entire menstrual cycle.[37,44,45] The range of pH reported is between 6.3 and 8.5. Serial determinations have revealed an increase in alkalinity at midcycle (Fig. 19-2). The optimal pH for sperm penetration is also in the range of 7 to 8.5.[53]

Antibacterial activity and bacteriology

Cervical mucus has bacteriostatic and bactericidal properties against certain strains of bacteria. Various bacteria are unable to migrate in a capillary tube filled with ovulatory cervical mucus. However, aerobic and anaerobic bacteria obtained from semen specimens or added to semen could easily penetrate the cervical barrier when active spermatozoa were present. No bacterial migration could be demonstrated when luteal phase of pregnancy cervical mucus was used.[77] Similarly, mucus collected from women taking oral contraceptives showed only minimal penetration by spermatozoa and bacteria. The conclusion drawn from these in vitro observations is that microorganisms migrate through the cervical mucus with moving spermatozoa. The importance of these observations relative to the protective effect of cervical mucus against bacterial invasion of the upper reproductive tract is clear.

Martin et al.[39] demonstrated that cervical mucus from uninfected healthy women converted gonococci susceptible to killing by fresh human serum to a resistant state after 3 hours of incubation at 37°C. This serum resistance could play an important role in vivo in the survival of gonococci in the initial stages of urogenital infection. Bactericidal activity of the human cervical mucus is present during all phases of the menstrual cycle but is least pronounced at ovulation.[9]

Normal cervical mucus has been found to be sterile in one third of women examined; the remaining two thirds show scanty flora. Lactobacilli, diphtheroids, coagulase-negative staphylococci, nonhemolytic streptococci, *Escherichia coli,* and yeasts were the most important organisms.[72]

Chronic cervicitis has been incriminated as a factor contributing to infertility in women. Certain bacteria such as *E. coli,* alpha-hemolytic streptococci (*Streptococcus viridans*), *S. hemolyticus,* aerobacter, and others have been found to have spermicidal properties in vitro. The bacteria most commonly cultured from the cervices of women with chronic cervicitis have included *Staphylococcus aureus, Aerobacter aerogenes, S. faecalis, S. viridans, E. coli,* and *Proteus vulgaris.* The spermicidal action of these bacteria does not appear to be an absolute deterrent to sperm transport and fertility, since conception can and does occur frequently in women who have chronic cervicitis. However, in a study of 350 infertile patients, Sobrero[72] found that treatment of chronic cervicitis significantly increased the subsequent chance of the women to conceive.

Cyclic changes and their relation to ovulation

The secretion of cervical mucus is regulated by ovarian hormones. Estrogen stimulates the production of copious amounts of watery mucus, whereas progesterone inhibits the secretory activity of cervical epithelial cells. The physical properties and certain chemical constituents of cervical mucus show cyclic variations, and their determination may be used to evaluate indirectly the amount of circulating sex hormones, which can then be used to detect the occurrence of ovulation. Cyclic alterations in the constituents of cervical mucus may also influence sperm penetrability, nutrition, and survival. Fig. 19-2 shows serial determinations of important properties of human cervical mucus, tested during a normal menstrual cycle in 10 women, in relation to pituitary and ovarian hormone secretion and in vitro sperm penetration. These data clearly demonstrate that optimal changes of cervical mucus properties, such as greatest increase in quantity, spinnbarkeit, ferning, pH, and decrease in viscosity and cell content, occur immediately before ovulation and are reversed after ovulation. Preovulatory mucus is most receptive to sperm penetration.[54] The pro-

portion of saline in cervical secretion directly determines the consistency of the mucus and the rate of sperm penetration.

SPERM MIGRATION THROUGH CERVICAL MUCUS

For many years reproductive biologists and clinicians have attempted to elucidate factors responsible for the passage of spermatozoa through the human cervix and to the upper reproductive tract. Studies in animal species, in which the cervix and its secretions are similar to those in the human, provide much useful information. Caution should be exercised, however, when extrapolating animal data to humans. Ethical and experimental considerations preclude the performance of critical studies to confirm the results of many animal experiments in women.

Information on the mechanism of sperm migration and survival in the human female reproductive tract is derived from clinical observations and indirect data. Approximately 50 million to 500 million sperm are deposited on the cervix and posterior vaginal fornix during a normal coitus. Human semen coagulates immediately after ejaculation and traps most sperm cells until seminal proteolytic enzymes bring about liquefaction. The first portion of the ejaculate usually contains three fourths of the sperm, which, under favorable conditions, quite promptly penetrate the cervical secretion.[38] Because sperm are quickly destroyed by vaginal acidity, their entrapment in the coagulum until liquefaction takes place may be considered a protective device to prevent demise.

In vitro studies have shown that nonliquefying semen samples are lysed when treated with an acid buffer. Thus it is possible that vaginal acidity enhances liquefaction of the seminal coagulum. Indeed, complete liquefaction of the seminal clot in the vagina appears to occur somewhat faster after ejaculation.[74] In women, the vaginal content is usually acid, with a pH of about 3 to 5. However, cervical secretions coating the upper part of the vagina and its fornices considerably increase the alkalinity of the vaginal milieu. They provide a favorable medium for sperm survival and appear to promote their motility and longevity.

Seminal plasma, an alkaline fluid, has a buffering effect on the vaginal acidity and changes the vaginal pH, thus smoothing the transition of sperm from the semen into the cervical mucus. Fox et al.[12] measured vaginal pH continuously during coitus by telemetry and observed that 8 seconds after ejaculation the pH of the vagina rose from 4.3 to 7.2.

Sperm migration through the cervix involves three distinct but interrelated factors: the ability of sperm to penetrate the mucus by their intrinsic motility; the fibrillar structure of cervical mucin, which enables it to participate actively in the process of sperm transport; and the morphologic configuration of cervical crypts, which contributes to the storage and preservation of sperm in the cervical canal and to their sustained and prolonged release to the upper tract. Various studies have shown that there is an excellent correlation among sperm density, percentage of the normal forms (oval sperm), and sperm motility and the ability of sperm to penetrate the cervical mucus. Sperm motility and normal morphology appear to be the most important factors.

Spermatozoa are highly active cells possessing the enzymes required to carry out the biochemical reactions of the Embden-Meyerhof pathway, tricarboxylic acid cycle, fatty acid oxidation, electron transport system, and, perhaps, the hexose monophosphate shunt. The metabolic and glycolytic enzymes apparently are located in the tail portion, and the respiratory enzymes are confined to the mitochondria. Despite assistance the spermatozoa may derive from uterine contractions during their ascent in the female reproductive tract, their own motility is essential for reproductive performance.

Spermatozoa are capable of metabolizing a variety of exogenous and some endogenous substrates. Because they possess only a negligible reserve of endogenous glycogen, they must depend on extracellular carbohydrates for energy under anaerobic conditions and during their passage through the mucus. Glucose is the major fuel used by human spermatozoa in the female reproductive tract. Fructose and mannose also are rapidly utilized in vivo by spermatozoa. Fructose is the sugar found in largest quantity in human semen (average, 300 mg/dL). However, the affinity constant for glucose utilization by spermatozoa is nearly 30 times greater than that for fructose.

Cervical mucus contains reducing substances throughout the cycle in, at times, amounts comparable to those reported for semen. These include glycogen, glucose, mannose, and maltose. Amylase, an enzyme capable of reducing glycogen to glucose, is also found in cervical mucus.

Human seminal plasma contains a proteolytic enzyme called seminin (a chymotrypsin-like enzyme). Spermatozoa also show seminin activities similar to those of seminal plasma. In addition, a trypsinlike enzyme (acrosin), hyaluronidase (a corona-penetrating enzyme), and adenosine triphosphatase activity have been demonstrated in the sperm acrosome. Seminin is either localized in the soluble crytoplasmic portions of the sperm or, more likely, absorbed from the seminal plasma by the sperm cell. Proteolytic enzymes may be involved in the process of sperm migration. The impression gained from a number of in vitro observations is that proteolytic enzymes may increase the initial invasion of sperm into cervical mucus.

To determine whether acrosin actually has a major role in sperm penetration through cervical mucus, Beyler and Zaneveld[3] pretreated human spermatozoa with low-molecular-weight acrosin inhibitors and observed their effect on the penetration process. At inhibitor concentrations far exceeding those necessary for the inhibition of human acrosin, there was no effect on spermatozoal penetration

into or through cervical mucus in vitro. These findings suggested that in humans, under normal circumstances, acrosin activity is neither necessary nor facilitative to sperm penetration of cervical mucin.

In other experiments, Overstreet et al.[62] showed that more of the collusions between spermatozoa and mucus resulted in successful penetration in tests in which the sperm were suspended in whole seminal plasma than in tests in which they were suspended in seminal plasma diluted with Tyrode's solution. These observations indicate that components of the seminal plasma, possibly proteolytic enzymes (seminin), are important for efficient entry of human spermatozoa into cervical mucus and for overcoming the initial resistance (surface tension) of cervical secretion.

CERVICAL CRYPT AS A SITE FOR SPERM STORAGE

Cervical crypts play an important role in the process of sperm penetration and storage in the cervix (Fig. 19-4). Mattner[41,42] was the first to demonstrate that the sperm in the cervices of ruminants following mating are not uniformly distributed within the lumen but tend to aggregate at or near the mucosa. According to Mattner, under natural conditions, the line of strain (mucin fibrils) originate at the mucus-secreting epithelium and passes through to the anterior portion of the vagina. On entering the mucus, sperm are constrained to follow these pathways and pass to the

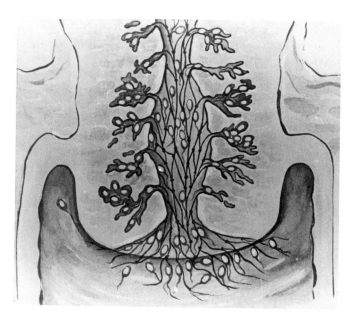

Fig. 19-4. Schematic representation of current concept of sperm transport through the cervix. Note long mucus filaments, sperm penetration along the molecular line of strains, and aggregation of spermatozoa in the crypts and clefts of the cervical canal.[45] (From Moghissi KS: In Grepp R, editor: *Handbook of physiology,* vol 2, part 2, *Endocrinology,* Washington, DC, 1973, American Physiological Society.)

mucosa of the cervix rather than penetrate directly to the uterus. Return of sperm along strain lines to the vagina is prevented by a series of intervening strain lines, each tending to reorient the sperm back toward the crypts.

Such a process could cause aggregation of a large number of sperm in the crypts of cervical mucosa, where they are stored and released at a constant rate into the uterus. Spermatozoa are thus retained in the cervix, despite the continued flagellation and drainage of mucus from the cervix into the vagina. In support of this theory, Mattner[41,42] has demonstrated that only motile sperm accumulate in the crypts of the cervical canal, where, in addition, they are protected from phagocytosis. The presence of sperm in the genital tract results in an increased number of leukocytes in the lumen of the uterus and cervix. In the cervix, the majority of leukocytes are found in the central mass of the mucus. The resulting separation of sperm and leukocytes in the cervix is, according to Mattner,[42] an important factor in the survival of an adequate population of sperm in the cervix. Dead sperm cells also are confined to the central portion of the lumen and are eliminated from the cervix. Similar observations have been made on secretions from subhuman primates in our laboratories.[28] Certain similarities between the epithelial structures of the human cervix and cervical mucus and those of subhuman primates suggest that an identical or closely related process may also be operative in women.

Some clinical reports lend further support to the concept of the cervix as a site of sperm storage. For example, in some studies, spermatozoa have been recovered for as long as 48 hours from the cervices of women who were artificially inseminated.[22,78] In another study, Insler et al.[27] examined histologically specimens from cervices of women who were treated with estrogen, inseminated, and subjected to hysterectomy for various gynecologic indications. Cervical crypts were carefully identified, classified, and counted, and the numbers of sperm-containing crypts and spermatozoa present within each crypt were recorded. The results of these observations indicated that in estrogen-treated women, the percentage of cervical crypts that were colonized with spermatozoa increased nine times, compared with crypts in cervices of subjects treated with gestagens. Similarly, the sperm density in the crypts was also greater in estrogen-treated cervices. Insler et al.[27] estimated the numbers of sperm stored in cervical crypts to be 15,000, 18,000, and 53,250 at 2, 24, and 48 hours after insemination.

Sperm penetrability of human cervical mucus begins approximately on the ninth day of a normal cycle and increases gradually to a peak at ovulation. It is usually inhibited within 1 to 2 days after ovulation but may persist to a lesser degree for a longer period.[44,54] In some women, sperm penetrability occurs only during a limited period of the menstrual cycle. Individual variations are common.[44,54] Familiarity with this process is of considerable importance, since inappropriate timing of sperm migration studies may lead to erroneous interpretations.

Two phases of sperm migration through the cervix have been recognized: (1) a rapid phase, during which within a few minutes the leading spermatozoa penetrate the central portion of the cervical canal and advance in a line parallel to mucin fibrils originating in the vicinity of the internal os, and (2) a delayed phase. During the delayed phase, spermatozoa enter the cervical mucus around the periphery of the central core and are oriented by mucin fibrils originating from the crypts and colonize them.[48] The latter process is responsible for the storage of sperm in the cervical crypts and their gradual release over an extended period into the uterus and oviducts (Fig. 19-4).

SUCTION THEORY OF SPERM MIGRATION

It has been suggested that during coitus the muscular activity of the uterus or respiratory effort causes a sucking in of semen, and in this way sperm migration is aided.[12] A number of in vitro and in vivo studies have failed to confirm these suggestions. Noyes et al.[58] could not demonstrate aspiration of radiopaque oil in the reproductive tract of rabbits. Sobrero[73] was unable to observe any movement of the cervical plug in more than 100 women during the fertile period, in the course of forcible inhalation and exhalation. In another series of experiments, he fit a group of women with snug cervical caps containing water-soluble opaque material or normal semen mixed with an opaque medium. Pelvic radiography before and after masturbation and/or coitus with and without female orgasm failed to show evidence of any radiopaque material beyond the vagina.

Postcoital tests as early as 1.5 to 3 minutes after ejaculation have not shown any mixture of cervical mucus and semen or the presence of male urethral epithelial cells or vaginal epithelial cells in the mucus.[74] Furthermore, in these tests, the distribution of sperm in cervical mucus has been found to be uniform and in lower concentrations than in the vaginal pool, indicating an orderly and uniform sperm penetration, rather than en bloc insemination.

Masters[40] did not observe any displacement of the cervical plug during coitus, nor was he able to demonstrate the entry of radiopaque fluid from a cervical cap into the uterus after coitus or clitoral stimulation. The only definitive response of the cervix to sexual stimulation appears to be minimal dilatation of the external os. The strongest argument against the suction theory is that artificial insemination in women, with deposition of semen in the vagina or on the cervix, is followed by a high rate of pregnancy. Orgasmic reaction and seminal aspiration could hardly be implicated under these conditions. However, there must be other mechanisms at work that would allow the rapid transport of spermatozoa through the cervix, since sperm velocity alone cannot explain the rapidity with which spermatozoa gain access to the upper reproductive tract.

SPERM SURVIVAL AND CAPACITATION IN THE CERVICAL CANAL

Longevity of sperm in the female genital tract is an important factor in fertility. A distinction should be made between the duration of motility and fertilizing potential. Sperm motility is not necessarily a criterion of fertilizing potential. Live sperm have been found in the vagina up to 12 hours after coitus.[14] Kremer[34] found that the motility of human spermatozoa that have remained in the vagina longer than 35 minutes is so compromised that their ability to penetrate cervical secretion is lost. Contamination with mucus at times alters the pH of the posterior fornix of the vagina and prolongs the survival of ejaculated sperm. A clear relationship between the pH of the intravaginal seminal pool and the motility of spermatozoa has been established. When the pool pH is higher, appreciable numbers of motile sperm are encountered in the vagina.

The viability of sperm in vitro is related to the glucose concentration of cervical mucus. There is normally an increase in glucose in the cervical mucus at ovulation. During the fertile period, cervical mucus contains 200 mg/dL or more of glucose. A decrease in glucose concentration in the cervical mucus has been found in many infertile patients. On postcoital tests, sperm viability was depressed in women with a low glucose content of cervical mucus. Unexplained cervical hostility may then reflect a deficient glucose content in cervical mucus.

In human cervical mucus, motile sperm have been found 2 to 8 days after coitus[47] and 7 days after artificial insemination. In the human uterus and oviducts, live sperm cells have been recovered up to 84 hours after sexual intercourse.[1,69]

Capacitation of sperm has been defined broadly as the physiologic changes in sperm that must take place as prerequisites for the acrosome reaction. Capacitation of sperm before fertilization in a number of mammalian species has been established. This phenomenon seems to exist in men as well. Cervical secretion may play a role in the process of capacitation. Overstreet et al.[63] have demonstrated that human spermatozoa achieve capacitation during migration through a column of human cervical mucus contained within a capillary tube. Other studies have shown that sperm that were allowed to reside and migrate out of cervical mucus and into a culture medium did not immediately acrosome react in response to biologic stimulus, but an acrosome reaction was observed when the sperm were challenged after 6 hours of incubation. These findings suggest that there is conservation of sperm function in the cervix.

SPERM VELOCITY IN CERVICAL MUCUS AND OTHER MEDIA

Spermatozoa readily penetrate a number of physiologic solutions and blood serum. However, with the exception of blood serum and normal saline, the progression rate of human sperm in these media is less than that in cervical mucus. Sperm cells perish instantly in distilled water.

The rate of sperm progression in cervical mucus has been determined by several investigators who used the capillary tube technique. The speed of penetration in human mucus varies during the menstrual cycle from 1.5 to 50 μm/s and is greatest in preovulatory mucus.[34] The extent and depth of sperm penetration in a given sample of cervical mucus are directly related to sperm density and motility. Higher sperm density and greater motility are associated with more massive penetration into the mucus. Dead or immotile spermatozoa do not penetrate cervical mucus. Broer et al.[5] have shown that Y chromatin-positive spermatozoa penetrate more readily into cervical mucus, in which their relative number is greater in samples collected postcoitally than in the ejaculate.

Temperature affects the rate of sperm motility and metabolism. Higher temperatures increase the metabolic rate and correspondingly decrease the life span. However, in vitro sperm migration tests performed at 22°, 30°, and 37° C have yielded similar results.

RELATION OF MOLECULAR STRUCTURE OF MUCUS TO SPERM TRANSPORT

Although spermatozoa appear to move at random in the cervical secretion, they may move along strands of cervical mucus (Fig. 19-4). Tampion and Gibbons[75] suggested that bull sperm travel in threads of bovine mucus by following the path of least resistance and are oriented along the lines of strain, that is, parallel with the direction of elongation of the molecules. It is readily apparent that the shape of the sperm cell would favor its movement through mucus in this manner rather than by passing across the molecular network. According to Gibbons and Mattner,[15] when progression of a spermatozoon in mucus is impeded, the sperm cell usually resumes its forward course with a sudden deflection onto a parallel path, as if it had broken obliquely through the laterally restraining glycoprotein strands. In vitro studies using human spermatozoa and cervical mucus confirmed this phenomenon.[34]

Odeblad[59,61] has suggested that, at midcycle, human cervical mucus is composed of flexible, threadlike molecules (micelles) of cross-linked glycoprotein networks. This model implies that the micelles have a diameter of about 0.5 μm. The intermicellar spaces, averaging 3 μm, are filled with a complex cervical plasma. The micelles are regarded as harmonic oscillators. It has been suggested that spermatozoa swim into these spaces and are assisted in their forward progression by the thermal modulations of the macromolecules, which cause the cavities with low-viscosity water to expand and contract more or less rhythmically. The expanded regions propagate in the mucus, conveying the swimming spermatozoa through the cervical canal with a minimum of energy expenditure.[60,61] During the luteal phase, or in women receiving progestogens, the

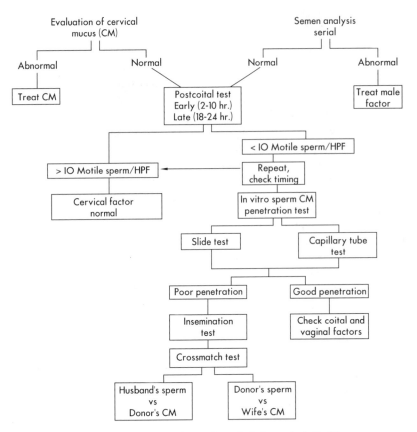

Fig. 19-5. Steps in evaluation of cervical factor in infertility.

number of cross-linkages increases, some water is lost, and the mucin assumes an arrangement of a much more dense network—a most effective barrier to a sperm transport. Studies of cervical mucus with the scanning electron microscope lend some support to this hypothesis. Lee et al.,[35,36] on the basis of laser light–scattering and cinematographic studies, found that midcycle cervical mucus is composed of an ensemble of entangled, randomly coiled macromolecules rather than a fibrillar system. This model suggests that cyclic variation in the viscoelastic properties of cervical mucus is dependent on the amount of fluid in which the glycoproteins are entangled. High-speed cinematography, according to these investigators, indicates that the pioneering spermatozoa reorient the local molecular arrangement and allow the following sperm to move forward with much less inhibition. These observations differed from those of Katz et al.,[32] who found that vanguard spermatozoa actually swam more efficiently in cervical mucus than did the spermatozoa that followed. They attributed this to an alteration in the properties of the mucus rather than to a difference in the vigor of the two sperm populations.

INVESTIGATION OF CERVICAL FACTOR IN INFERTILITY

Spermatozoa are at all times suspended in a fluid medium. The interaction of spermatozoa with fluids of the female reproductive tract is of critical importance for survival and function of spermatozoa (Fig. 19-5). Unfortunately, there is no practical method for evaluation of human uterine and tubal fluids and the study of their effect on sperm. Cervical mucus, however, is readily available for sampling and studies. Evaluation of sperm-cervical mucus interaction must, therefore, be included in infertility investigation. A stepwise plan for the evaluation of the cervical factor in infertility is shown in Fig. 19-5. Semen analysis and examination of cervical mucus should precede postcoital tests and more specific in vitro studies.

Information regarding semen volume and appearance; liquefaction time; sperm density; immediate and delayed motility; quality of motility; viability (eosin stain); percentage of different morphologic types (seminal cytology); and the presence of pus cells, agglutination, and other changes must appear on every report.

Evaluation of cervical mucus

The condition of cervical mucus greatly influences sperm receptivity; therefore, it should be evaluated accurately before a postcoital test is performed. Preovulatory mucus receptive to sperm penetration is profuse, thin, clear, acellular, and alkaline. It exhibits 4+ ferning (crystallization) and high spinnbarkeit. Fig. 19-6 shows a scoring system that we have devised to evaluate the quality and

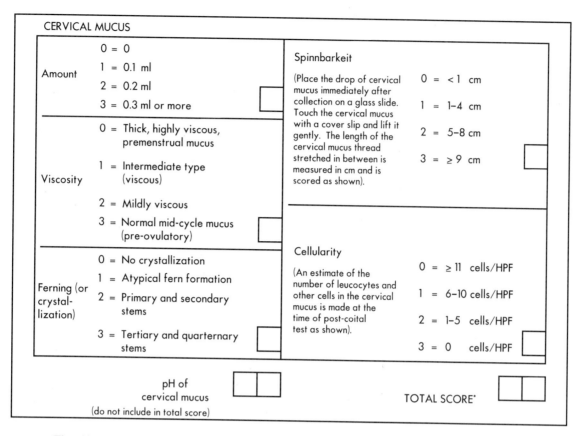

Fig. 19-6. Cervical score. A composite of the amount, spinnbarkeit, ferning, viscosity, and cellularity of cervical mucus. Maximum score is 15; scores less than 10 represent unfavorable mucus and less than 5, hostile cervical secretion.

adequacy of cervical mucus. This system takes into account five important properties of cervical mucus that are known to affect cervical mucus by sperm: amount, spinnbarkeit, ferning, viscosity, and cellularity. Each item receives a score of 0 to 3. A score of 3 represents optimal changes. A maximum score of 15 indicates preovulatory cervical mucus that is receptive to sperm penetration. A score of less than 10 is associated with relatively unfavorable cervical secretion, and a score of less than 5 represents hostile cervical mucus usually impenetrable by the sperm.[47,83]

Several techniques for collection of cervical mucus have been described. Methods most commonly used consist of aspiration with a tuberculin syringe (without needle), pipette, or polyethylene tube, or sampling with a mucus forceps. Cervical mucus should be collected and studied as close to the time of ovulation as possible as determined by basal body temperature or urinary LH surge. Clinical examination of cervical mucus includes determination of amount, viscosity, cellularity, pH, ferning, spinnbarkeit, and cultural studies, if infection is suspected. Ferning is performed by spreading cervical mucus on a glass slide and allowing it to dry. It is customarily graded from 0 to 4+, depending on the extent of crystal formation. Spinnbarkeit is measured by placing an adequate amount of cervical mucus on a microscope slide, covering it with a coverslip, and drawing the mucus between slide and coverslip. An estimate of spinnbarkeit (in centimeters) is made by measuring the length of the thread before it breaks (Fig. 19-1). The pH of cervical mucus should be measured in situ or immediately after collection. Care should be taken to assay the pH of endocervical mucus correctly, since the pH of the exocervical pool is always lower than that of the endocervical canal.

Postcoital test

The postcoital test (Sims-Huhner test) was first described by Sims in 1866, who also recognized the importance of sperm motility and timing of the test. Sims performed immediate postcoital tests on many women, and found sperm in cervical mucus within a few minutes after coitus. He further observed the presence of live spermatozoa in the cervix 36 to 48 hours after intercourse. To Huhner, however, goes the credit for popularizing the test as an index of cervical mucus–sperm interaction. The Sims-Huhner test is now considered an integral part of infertility investigation; but, despite its popularity, there is a lack of standardization, and disagreement remains on how to interpret the results.

Timing. Postcoital tests (Fig. 19-5) should be performed as closely as possible to the time of ovulation, as determined by usual clinical means (basal body temperature, cervical mucus changes, and urinary LH surge). Each couple is instructed to abstain from sexual intercourse for 2 days before the test, which is performed approximately 6 to 10 hours after intercourse (standard test). If the initial test result is satisfactory, the test may be repeated at a longer interval of 18 to 24 hours (delayed test) when infertility persists. When the initial test yields poor results, the second test is planned 1 to 3 hours after coitus (early test).

On the basis of cervical mucus examination after artificial insemination, Tredway et al.[78] have suggested that the most appropriate time to perform a postcoital test is 2.5 hours after intercourse, since they found the largest sperm population in the mucus at this time. The purpose of a postcoital test is not only to determine whether there is a sufficient number of active spermatozoa in the cervical mucus, but also to evaluate sperm survival and behavior many hours after coitus (reservoir role). Therefore, 6 to 10 hours after coitus is a balanced time to determine both sperm density and longevity. Earlier timing may be reserved for subjects who have negative or abnormal tests.

Techniques. A nonlubricated speculum is inserted into the vagina and a sample of the posterior vaginal fornix pool is aspirated with a tuberculin syringe (without needle), a mucus syringe, pipette, or polyethylene tube. Samples of cervical mucus are obtained from the exocervix and endocervical canal. These are placed on separate glass slides, covered with a coverslip, and examined under a microscope at ×200 and ×400. If exocervical mucus is covered with cells, debris, and vaginal content, the area should be wiped dry with cotton before obtaining the endocervical specimen. Whenever possible, the quality of the mucus should be evaluated immediately after collection (Fig. 19-6).

Interpretation. Interpreting the postcoital test requires an understanding of cervical function and sperm transport. Cervical mucus protects sperm from the hostile environment of the vagina and from being phagocytosed. The mucus also may supplement the energy requirements of sperm, act as a filter to retain abnormal and sluggish sperm, and provide the proper milieu for sperm capacitation.

The function of the cervix as a sperm reservoir is of considerable importance in fertility. Only rarely does coitus occur at ovulation. In most instances, the union of gametes depends on a constant supply of sperm at the site of fertilization for some hours before and after ovulation. After coitus, a gradient is established within the cervix that is entirely time dependent. With increasing intervals between coitus and examination, there is an orderly progression of sperm population from the lower to the upper part of the canal. With these facts in mind, postcoital tests may be

interpreted on a rational basis, as follows:

1. *Vaginal pool sample:* Spermatozoa are usually destroyed in the vagina within 2 to 4 hours and lose their fertilizing ability within a few hours.[14] The purpose of examining the vaginal pool sample, therefore, is to ensure that semen have actually been deposited in the vagina.

2. *Exocervical sample:* The number of sperm in the lower part of the cervical canal varies with time elapsed after coitus. Within 2 to 3 hours after intercourse there is a large accumulation of sperm in the lower part of the cervical canal.[7,46,78] In a normal woman, after coitus with a fertile man, more than 25 motile sperm per high-power field (with 2 to 3+ motility) is considered satisfactory. Less than 5 sperm per high-power field, particularly when associated with sluggish or circular motion, is an indication of oligoasthenospermia or abnormality of cervical mucus.[8]

Sperm motility in cervical mucus is graded from 0 to 3, as follows: 0, immotile; 1, in situ motility; 2, sluggish motility; and 3, vigorous forward motility.

Causes of a negative test. One negative postcoital test has little clinical value and must be repeated. Controversy continues as to the significance of sperm found in cervical secretions several hours after coitus. Some investigators have suggested that they consist mainly of sperm populations of poor quality, which have failed their passage to the uterus. This conclusion is not supported by animal and human studies.

Grant[18] compared the results of postcoital tests and endometrial aspirations in 920 women and found that motile spermatozoa were present in the uteri in the cervical mucus. An explanation of this finding may be that, in cases of oligospermia or when cervical mucus is relatively hostile, the more vigorous and healthier spermatozoa penetrate the cervix and reach the uterine cavity shortly after coitus (rapid phase of transport). Other spermatozoa, which normally are stored in cervical crypts and mucus, do not survive long enough to be detected (disturbed delayed phase of transport).

Most investigators believe that persistently negative postcoital tests indicate either a mucus abnormality or oligoasthenospermia. Recently the importance of the movement characteristics exhibited by the spermatozoa have been emphasized. It was shown that the concentration of motile spermatozoa with a linear velocity and rolling mode of progression as determined by time exposure photomicrography or computer-assisted semen analysis influence the number of spermatozoa penetrating the mucus.[2]

Hostile cervical mucus. The most common cause of a negative or abnormal postcoital test is inappropriate timing (see box on opposite page). Tests performed too early or too late in the cycle may be negative in an otherwise fertile woman. In some women the test may be positive for only 1 or 2 days in the entire menstrual cycle. When ovulation cannot be timed with a reasonable degree of accuracy, an LH home kit may be used to identify the LH surge. Alternatively, serial postcoital tests may be performed. In women with absent mucorrhea or persistent hostile cervical mucus an artificial cycle might be induced by administration of ethinyl estradiol, 50 µg daily, beginning on day 5 of a normal menstrual cycle and continuing for 3 weeks. The postcoital test may be performed 7 to 14 days after ingestion of ethinyl estradiol has begun. Postcoital tests are usually negative or abnormal in anovulatory cycles. Subtle anomalies of the ovulatory process, such as inadequate follicular maturation with low-level preovulatory estrogen production, may also adversely affect cervical secretion and postcoital test results. Roumen et al.[66] found that repeated abnormal postcoital tests in a group of presumably ovulating infertile women were associated with lower preovulatory serum estradiol levels and higher serum FSH and prolactin levels. Similarly, Sher and Katz[70] evaluated a group of patients with idiopathic infertility and inadequate cervical mucus. Hormone investigation revealed that some of these women had low sex steroid profiles despite apparent ovulation. Treatment with ovulation-inducing agents was attempted to produce "controlled" ovarian hyperstimulation and an improved cervical mucus and was followed by pregnancy in four of six patients. These data indicate that an optimal amount of circulating estrogen during a determined period of time before ovulation is required to stimulate adequate quantity and quality of cervical secretion. Under normal circumstances the rise in the preovulatory estradiol level is sufficient to trigger the surge of LH and ovulation and to stimulate cervical mucus secretion. However, it is possible that in some instances the midcycle increase in estrogen level would be sufficient to induce ovulation without causing concomitantly optimal cervical mucus secretion.

Consistency and cell content of cervical mucus. The consistency (viscosity) of cervical mucus is the greatest barrier to sperm penetration. There is no resistance to sperm migration in thin mucus, but viscous mucus, such as that observed during the luteal phase, pregnancy, and in progestogen-treated women, forms an impenetrable barrier. Increased cervical mucus viscosity may also be induced occasionally as a result of treatment with clomiphene citrate. Viscous mucus diluted artificially with normal saline or 5% dextrose is more readily penetrated by sperm than is undiluted mucus.[53]

Some relatively viscous samples of cervical mucus present a high degree of surface tension and thus appear to be initially impenetrable by sperm. When these samples are mixed with semen, sperm invasion may occur. This in vitro mixing test (M test) is a useful device to determine the ability of sperm to penetrate the mucus in vivo, particularly when it is realized that during coitus such mixing of

---

Etiologic classification of abnormal sperm–cervical mucus interaction

Female-related causes
1. Inappropriate timing
2. Ovulatory disorders
   —Anovulation
   —Subtle anomalies of ovulatory process
3. Deposition problems
   —Dyspareunia
   —Prolapse
   —Congenital and anatomic anomalies
4. Anatomic and organic causes
   —Amputation or deep conizacion of the cervix
   —Deep cauterization or cryotherapy
   —Tumors: polyps, leiomyomas
   —Severe stenosis
   —Endocervicitis
5. Hostile cervical mucus
   —Increased viscosity
   —Increased cellularity (infection)
   —Acid mucus
   —Presence of sperm antibodies

Male-related causes
1. Deposition problems
   —Impotence
   —Retrograde ejaculation
   —Hypospadias
2. Semen abnormalities
   —Low concentration
   —Low motility
   —High percentage of abnormal form
   —High volume (>8 mL)
   —Low volume (<1 mL)
   —Nonliquifying semen
3. Antisperm antibodies in semen and/or seminal plasma

---

cervical mucus and semen commonly takes place.

Cleanliness of the cervical mucus appears to be a factor favoring sperm migration. Cellular debris and leukocytes impede the progress of spermatozoa in mucus. Severe endocervicitis has been associated with reduced fertility. The precise relationship of mycoplasma infection to the postcoital test and to infertility remains to be determined.

Effect of pH of cervical mucus. Spermatozoa are susceptible to changes in the pH of cervical mucus. Acid mucus immobilizes spermatozoa, whereas alkaline mucus enhances their motility. Excessive alkalinity of cervical mucus (over 8.5) may also adversely affect the viability of spermatozoa. The optimal pH for sperm migration and survival in cervical mucus is between 7 and 8.5.[44,53,54] The pH ranges of normal midcycle cervical mucus have been reported to be between 6.3 and 8.5 (Fig. 19-2).

Effect of immune antibodies. Human cervical mucus contains IgA, secretory IgA, and occasionally traces of IgM. IgG is the most constant constituent and is found in almost all samples. The presence of IgG, IgA, and IgM in the luminal contents of cervical crypts and basement membrane and in the interstitium has been demonstrated by immunologic studies. Biosynthesis of IgG and IgA in the uterine, cervical, and vaginal tissues of rabbits and cervical tissues of women has been reported. Also agglutinating and immobilizing sperm antibodies are known to occur in cervical mucus. These antibodies may be found in the cervical mucus independent of those in the serum or may be associated with circulating antibodies. Postcoital tests in most patients who have cervical mucus antibodies are either negative or grossly abnormal.[51] When sperm antibodies are found in the cervical mucus or on the surface of sperm the ability of sperm to penetrate cervical mucus is impaired and the sperm lose their progressive movements and show a local shaking motion. The sperm–cervical mucus contact test readily elicits this shaking phenomenon.

The presence of antisperm antibodies on the sperm head may also prevent its penetration into otherwise normal-appearing cervical mucus and be associated with a negative or poor postcoital test.[20] Interestingly, antibodies of similar isotype, when directed against the sperm tail, may not impair mucus penetration.[81]

Anatomic and organic causes. Amputation or deep conization of the cervix may result in total destruction of secretory epithelial cells lining the endocervix and cervical crypts and in an impairment of mucus production. The condition of "dry cervix" is usually associated with considerable impairment of fertility, since normal insemination and sperm migration cannot take place. Similar consequences may follow extensive cauterization or cryotherapy of the endocervix. The presence of a tumor (i.e., cervical leiomyoma or polyp) may also cause a disturbance of mucus secretion. Cervical stenosis is usually secondary to previous operative procedures. When cervical stenosis is pronounced, no vaginal pool of mucus exists, and there is interference with the discharge of cervical secretion. This may have a deleterious effect on sperm survival in the vagina and sperm penetration in cervical mucus. Finally, in endocervicitis, because of the presence of numerous leukocytes, exogenous proteins, and bacterial toxins in cervical mucus, sperm migration in the mucus may be impeded.

Miscellaneous causes. Poor coital techniques, vaginismus, and dyspareunia may occasionally be associated with a negative postcoital test. A markedly anteflexed cervix may not come in contact with the semen pool (particularly when the volume of semen is scanty) and may be a cause of infertility. Vaginal infections and infestations are an uncommon cause of negative or abnormal postcoital tests.

Male-related causes. A positive postcoital test results only when semen of good quality is deposited in the vagina. Conditions that prevent ejaculation, intromission, or full penetration of the penis into the vagina are associated with a negative postcoital test. These include premature or retrograde ejaculation, operations on the prostate gland and bladder neck, hypospadias, and impotence. A common cause of a negative postcoital test is abnormal semen. Oligospermia, asthenospermia, a large number of morphologically abnormal spermatozoa, and delayed or abnormal liquefaction are known to be associated with absence of inadequate sperm penetration into cervical mucus.

The presence of sperm antibodies in the serum or semen also may be associated with an abnormal postcoital test. In these cases the sperm is coated with antibodies and may be unable to penetrate cervical mucus.

Significance of the postcoital test. Soon after ejaculation, spermatozoa are transferred from seminal plasma to female genital tract fluid, in which they are suspended. Migration, survival, and fertilizing potential of spermatozoa depend, to a large extent, on how they can adapt themselves to this new environment. The postcoital test provides valuable information on sperm–cervical mucus interaction.

A survey of published reports on postcoital tests indicates a great deal of controversy. Most investigators believe that postcoital tests correlate well with sperm concentration, morphology and motility in the semen, and in vitro studies.[7] Substantial variance in all semen measures over an extended period in humans has been observed. These changes affect the results of postcoital tests performed at different times.[64] Motile sperm have been observed in samples of cervical mucus obtained from the cervical os and canal 1.5 to 3 minutes after ejaculation and as long as 7 days after coitus.[74] Under normal conditions, the percentages of motile and morphologically normal spermatozoa are usually higher in cervical mucus than in semen.[13,21]

Serial postcoital tests have shown that the increased fluidity and spinnbarkeit of preovulatory cervical mucus coincides with a greater number of motile sperm being observed in mucus samples. After ovulation the mucus becomes thick, and few—if any—live sperm cells are found in it. Combined postcoital tests and endometrial aspirations have demonstrated that the greatest numbers of sperm in the endometrial cavity are found at or near the time of ovulation. Very few were found to be present in the uterus during the luteal or early follicular phases of the cycle.

Other studies have shown that the number of sperm in cervical mucus and the uterine cavity correlates well with that in the oviducts and pouch of Douglas.[1] The greatest number of progressively motile sperm in these locations has been observed in the presence of a mature follicle in the ovaries. A significant decrease in the motile sperm population has been seen when ovaries contained corpora lutea. However, once the sperm reach the uterine cavity their further progression to the oviduct may not be influenced by the stage of the ovarian cycle. The presence of sperm in the uterus correlates directly with high sperm density of the cervical mucus approximately 25 to 41 hours after coitus.

Attempts have been made to correlate the results of postcoital tests with pregnancy. Some studies show a positive relationship, whereas others do not. Generally, in carefully performed studies that have excluded other causes of infertility, a positive postcoital test with at least 10 sperm per high-power field (HPF) (×200) in cervical mucus is associated with a higher pregnancy rate.[25] Jett and Glass[29] found that the pregnancy rate in 555 infertile women was significantly higher in the presence of favorable cervical mucus and when there were more than 20 sperm per HPF in the mucus as demonstrated in postcoital tests. Giner et al.,[16] however, were unable to demonstrate such a relationship.

Moghissi[48] performed a fractional postcoital test as a part of a complete infertility survey in 208 infertile women. The results of the best postcoital tests of 58 women who became pregnant was compared with those of 143 who did not. Excluded from the study were all women who had a definite impediment to fertility that could not be corrected and tests that were not timed to coincide with ovulation. Cervical scores were not significantly different in the two groups. Significantly larger numbers of sperm were found in postcoital tests of women who achieved pregnancy than in those who remained infertile. Since cervical scores in the two groups were comparable, the data indicated that the greater number of sperm in cervical mucus was associated with a greater chance of pregnancy.

In other studies, Hanson and associates[21,22] analyzed the relationship of the number of motile sperm seen in cervical mucus 48 hours after artificial insemination with donor semen (AID) with subsequent fertility. They demonstrated a significant association between the occurrence of conception after AID and sperm survival for 48 hours in the cervical mucus. Examination of their data suggested that when spermatozoa were consistently present in the mucus there was a significantly higher probability of conception in that insemination cycle.

The lack of correlation of postcoital test results with the occurrence of pregnancy has also been documented in some studies. For example, Harrison[23] in a study of 423 couples found that the postcoital test was not a good indicator of fertility potential, since 24.5% of 98 women who had persistently negative postcoital tests achieved pregnancy. To evaluate the validity of the postcoital test, Griffith and Grimes[19] reviewed the English literature and found that the test suffers from a lack of standard methodology, lack of uniform definition of normal, and unknown reproducibility. Unfortunately, this effort was based on the premise that the postcoital test is of value only if it can predict pregnancy, rather than assessing sperm transport. Griffith and Grimes also compared studies using different methodology and criteria for normalcy rather than standards recommended by the World Health Organization (WHO).[83]

The findings of these studies could easily be explained and should not invalidate the usefulness of postcoital tests.

It is now well recognized that sperm concentration, motility, and morphology of most men are subject to considerable changes when serial semen analyses are performed.[64,83] These alterations will be reflected in the results of postcoital or in vitro sperm–cervical mucus tests. Furthermore, timing of the tests, technical variation, and other variables may alter the test results. Finally, it should be realized that pregnancy results only when various factors involved in the reproductive process, in addition to sperm–cervical mucus interaction, are in optimal functioning order.

In vitro studies

Cervical mucus–sperm penetration tests. Negative or abnormal postcoital tests are indications for in vitro cervical mucus–sperm penetration tests. Two different techniques have been used for in vitro investigation of sperm penetration of cervical mucus: the slide method and the capillary tube system. A good correlation has been found between the results obtained by these techniques.[34] The results of in vitro sperm–cervical mucus penetration tests also compare fairly well with sperm concentration, motility, and percentage of normal morphology in semen samples.[26,33] Mortimer et al.[57] found that both the concentration of progressively motile spermatozoa and their movement characteristics are significant factors determining the outcome of homologous tests of human sperm–cervical mucus interaction. Finally, there is a significant correlation between the results of postcoital tests, in vitro tests, and semen analysis findings.[22] The slide method, as originally described by Miller and Kurzrok, has been altered to provide quantitative results[53] (Fig. 19-7).

Slide method. In in vitro studies by the slide method a sharp boundary is observed separating human cervical mucus placed in juxtaposition to semen on a microscopic slide[53] (Fig. 19-7). At the interface, fingerlike projections or phalanges of seminal fluid develop within a few minutes and penetrate the mucus. Spermatozoa usually fill these canals before entering the mucus. Most spermatozoa penetrate the apex of the phalangeal canal and enter the mucus. In most instances a single spermatozoon appears to lead a column of sperm into the mucus. After the initial resistance has been overcome by the leading sperm, others follow without difficulty. Once in the cervical mucus, sperm fan out and move at random. Some return to the seminal plasma layer, but most migrate deep into the cervical mucus until they meet with resistance from cellular debris or leukocytes. They then either stop or change direction. Both phalanx and interface formations appear to be physical phenomena resulting from the contact of two biologic fluids of differing viscosities and surface tensions.

To quantitate the test, the first microscopic field from the interface, called F_1, is counted at various time intervals. The suggested times are 5 and 15 minutes after initiation of the test. This is scored at ×200 and ×400 magnification. To study the depth of penetration, the second microscopic field

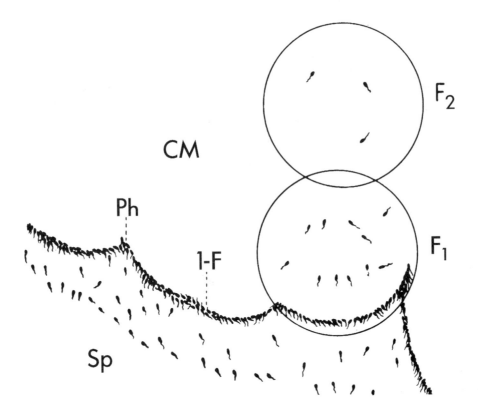

Fig. 19-7. Schematic representation of in vitro sperm–cervical mucus penetration test by quantitative slide method. *CM,* Cervical mucus; *Sp,* sperm; *I-F,* interface; *Ph,* phalanges; *F₁,* first microscopic field; *F₂,* second field adjacent to F₁. (From Moghissi KS: Cyclic changes of cervical mucus in normal and progestin-treated women, *Fertil Steril* 17:663, 1966. Reproduced with permission of the publisher, The American Fertility Society, Birmingham, Ala.)

adjacent to the first one (i.e., F_2) and the third (F_3) can also be evaluated and the number of spermatozoa in these fields can be counted and recorded. In good tests at least 15 motile sperm per HPF in F_1, and at least 20 sperm per HPF in F_2 are recorded.

Capillary tube system. The capillary tube system measures the ability of spermatozoa to penetrate a column of cervical mucus in a flat capillary tube (Fig. 19-8). Sperm penetration in the capillary tube is assessed at 10 minutes, 30 minutes, or 3 hours, or at other intervals depending on the type of study. Both linear penetration and density of penetration should be recorded. A scoring system for the evaluation of sperm penetrability has been devised.[83] The capillary tube system is particularly useful for evaluation of midcycle cervical mucus and to study depth of penetration.[34] The slide method is applicable to a variety of cervical mucus samples, including those too viscous or too scanty to be studied by the tube technique. When both in vivo and in vitro tests are negative, normal donor sperm may be tested in vitro against the wife's cervical mucus, and preovulatory mucus obtained from a fertile donor should be tested with the husband's sperm. This crossmatch test will determine whether the sperm or cervical mucus is

responsible for abnormal results. With the introduction and popularity of modern techniques of intrauterine insemination (IUI) fewer in vitro tests are being performed by clinicians. These tests continue, however, to be an important research tool.

Use of bovine estrous cervical mucus. Bovine estrous cervical mucus may be used as a substitute for human midcycle mucus.[56] Bovine cervical mucus (BCM) is biochemically and functionally similar to human mucus. The viscoelastic and rheologic properties of the two secretions are also remarkably alike. Human spermatozoa can enter BCM readily in vitro and maintain good motility and viability for several hours. Moghissi et al.[56] demonstrated that the pattern and depth of sperm penetration in human cervical mucus (HCM) and BCM were very similar. Human sperm appeared to migrate somewhat more slowly in BCM than in HCM. Highly significant correlation was found between the depth of sperm penetration in HCM and BCM, particularly when both were of optimal quality. As expected, sperm count and motility showed significant correlation with the rate of sperm migration in both HCM and BCM. Greater sperm concentration and higher sperm motility were associated with greater depth of penetration in

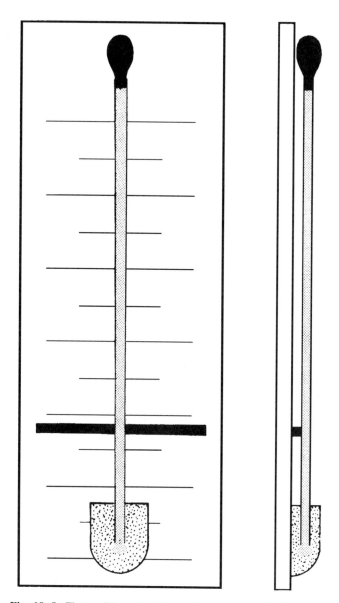

Fig. 19-8. Flat capillary tube for in vitro sperm–cervical mucus penetration test. The tube is filled with cervical mucus, sealed at the top, and placed in a sperm reservoir (*bottom*). The entire system is mounted on a graduated slide. (From Kremer J: *The in vitro spermatazoal penetration test in fertility investigation,* thesis, Groningen Netherlands, 1968, Rijksuniversiteit Groningen.)

both HCM and BCM. However, BCM was more discriminating with regard to sperm form. Spermatozoa from ejaculates containing a higher percentage of abnormal cells did not migrate through the BCM as rapidly as they did in HCM.

In another study, Hayes et al.[24] compared the results of in vitro sperm penetration tests in HCM and BCM in 35 couples with the results of postcoital tests. Postcoital test results correlated significantly with in vitro sperm penetration. Furthermore, the concentration of morphologically normal motile sperm per ejaculate also correlated positively with the sperm penetration test and correlated more significantly with the postcoital test.

The results of these and several other studies indicate that BCM may indeed be used as a substitute for HCM to test in vitro sperm–cervical mucus interaction whenever difficulties are experienced in securing sufficient amounts of human material. Commercially prepared capillary tubes containing standardized samples of bovine mucus have now become available.* The use of bovine estrous mucus can considerably facilitate the testing of the ability of spermatozoa from a given man to penetrate normal cervical mucus and provides a new dimension by which to evaluate the etiology of abnormal sperm–cervical mucus interaction.

Postinsemination test

When results of postcoital tests are consistently negative but in vitro tests show adequate sperm penetration in cervical mucus obtained from the wife, use of the postinsemination test may be considered. In this test the couple is instructed to abstain from intercourse for a period of 2 days and to report at the time of anticipated ovulation of the wife. The husband is required to provide a semen sample obtained by masturbation. The ejaculate is allowed to liquefy and the wife is artificially inseminated with this sample, using the intracervical technique of insemination. Approximately 1 to 2 hours later, samples of mucus from the exocervix and the endocervix are obtained and the concentration and quality of sperm are observed and recorded, using the technique described for postcoital tests. In cases where large semen volume, oligospermia, or liquefaction defects have been observed in the process of semen analysis, the first portion (or better portion) of a split ejaculate may be used for this purpose.

The results of postinsemination tests are interpreted in a manner similar to those of postcoital tests. If the postinsemination test shows at least 10 vigorously motile sperm per HPF, one should suspect the presence of factor(s) in the vagina, or alterations of buffering capacity of seminal plasma and/or cervical mucus that contribute to early obstruction of sperm in the vagina. This situation may be encountered particularly when the volume of the ejaculate is small and cervical mucus is scanty. The results of postinsemination tests may also be used as a guide for the management of the patient. If the result is favorable one may expect a good prognosis for achieving pregnancy with the use of homologous artificial insemination.

TREATMENT OF CERVICAL INFERTILITY

Functional disorders

A negative or abnormal postcoital test result may be due to male factors (inadequacy of the semen or abnormal sperm deposition) or vaginal or cervical diseases. Fig. 19-9

*Pentrak Kit, Sorono Laboratories, Randolph, Mass.

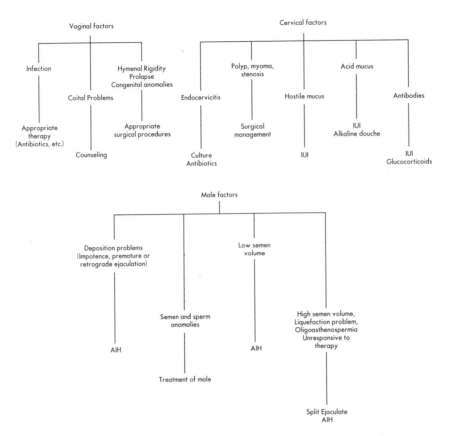

Fig. 19-9. Management of cervical factors in infertility.

shows the principles of management of cervical mucus–sperm interaction abnormalities. In all cases of infertility associated with an abnormal or negative result on the Sims-Huhner test, the male factor and sperm abnormalities should be thoroughly investigated and excluded. If cervical mucus abnormality is established, treatment should be directed toward improving the physiochemical properties and sperm receptivity of the mucus. In the past, viscous and hostile cervical mucus was treated with small doses of estrogen. Poor cervical mucus may be a manifestation of anovulation or inadequate follicular development. Small doses of clomiphene citrate (i.e., 50 mg/d for 5 days, beginning on day 5 of the cycle) may be effective. If clomiphene does not induce mucorrhea, administration of human menopausal gonadotropin (hMG) should be considered. hMG improves the ovulatory process and ovarian estrogen output and induces excellent mucorrhea.

Satisfactory treatment for infertility resulting from sperm antibody in cervical mucus has not been established. Although preliminary data suggested that the use of condoms may be successful, controlled studies have not supported these claims.[30,55] Similarly, treatment with glucocorticoids has not received adequate and controlled clinical studies and needs to be explored further.[71]

Persistent viscosity or acidity of cervical mucus will require intrauterine insemination (IUI). IUI may also be used when deep cauterization or conization has entirely destroyed the mucus-producing cells. The goal of sperm preparation for IUI is to optimize the concentration of motile spermatozoa, capacitating them and removing the seminal plasma. Sperm is separated from the seminal plasma by centrifugation, washed and suspended in a buffer solution (e.g., Ham's F-10), and introduced directly inside the uterus at ovulation via a polyethylene tube, and slowly injected. In properly selected cases of cervical factor infertility, IUI has been found to be highly successful.[6,76]

Organic disorders

Anatomic and neoplastic conditions of the cervix should be treated appropriately. Endocervicitis requires bacteriologic studies and specific antibiotic therapy. Hot cauterization of the endocervix should be avoided. Destruction of secretory epithelium by other means, such as cold conization, laser, and deep cryosurgery, may have a similar adverse effect. These procedures, sometimes performed in young women without clear-cut indications, can lead to the condition of "dry cervix" and impairment of fertility. Cervical amputation similarly destroys cervical function with respect to sperm transport and storage and may cause cervical incompetence, leading to abortion, even if pregnancy occurs.

Effect of ovulation-inducing agents on cervical mucus

Clomiphene citrate, a synthetic ovulation-inducing compound, has a marked antiestrogenic effect on cervical secretion. During the administration of this medication, cervical mucus becomes viscous, turbid, and cellular and exhibits little or no spinnbarkeit and ferning.[80] Sperm penetration through the mucus may be inhibited. About 5 to 10 days after the termination of clomiphene therapy, however, a rebound mucorrhea develops in most subjects and sperm penetrability is restored. In some women, the rebound mucorrhea may not develop and normal sperm–cervical mucus interaction may be impaired.

Vander Merwe[80] analyzed 157 menstrual cycles in 50 patients receiving clomiphene citrate (doses of 50 and 100 mg) for ovulation induction. There was a significant inhibition of cervical mucus production with both dosages of clomiphene, as determined by cervical score as well as ferning and spinnbarkeit. The inhibition of mucorrhea occurred despite hypersecretion of endogenous estradiol and was not corrected with exogenous conjugated estrogen therapy.

Treatment with hMG usually produces increasing amounts of endogenous estrogen; this stimulates the secretion of preovulatory-type cervical mucus, which is receptive to sperm penetration.[80]

The administration of human chorionic gonadotropins, if followed by ovulation, brings about progestational changes with inhibition of sperm migration.

Bromocriptine, a dopamine agonist, does not have a direct effect on the secretory activity of cervical epithelia. However, in optimal doses, the drug is successful in inducing ovulation and adequate preovulatory mucorrhea in hyperprolactinemic patients.

Administration of gonadotropin-releasing hormone (GnRH) in pulsatile fashion to appropriately selected anovulatory women produces follicular development and ovulation. The preovulatory rising levels of estrogen are, as expected, associated with mucorrhea, allowing sperm penetration to occur. On the contrary, the chronic use of GnRH again results in suppression of ovulation and disappearance of mucorrhea, as well as alteration of cervical mucus, characteristics associated with anovulation and hypoestrogenism.

OVULATION PREDICTION AND THE PERIODIC ABSTINENCE METHOD OF CONTRACEPTION

Changes in cervical mucus during the menstrual cycle have been used to determine the time of ovulation for the purpose of the sexual abstinence method of family planning. The cervical mucus method relies on self-observation and perception of midcycle mucorrhea for ovulation timing. Five phases of the cervical mucus pattern are recognized: phase 1, dry days; phase 2, early preovulatory days; phase 3, wet days; phase 4, postovulatory days; and phase 5, late postovulatory days. The fertile or unsafe period is presumed to start on the first day in which postmenstrual mucus is observed (phase 2), and to continue until the fourth day after the clear lubricative cervical mucus (peak day) appears—a period that can last from 7 to 14 days. All subsequent days are considered infertile and safe for intercourse.

Billings et al.[4] have claimed a high degree of effectiveness in well-motivated couples who have been adequately trained. Others have been less enthusiastic. In a randomized, prospective study performed in the Los Angeles area during the year after formal entry into the study, 36.6% of users withdrew from the program and 24.8% became pregnant. This rate is similar to the pregnancy rates reported by other investigators.[43]

To improve on the objectivity of the cervical mucus method and to narrow the number of days when abstinence needs to be practiced, attempts have been made to use one of the constituents of cervical mucus, such as an enzyme (alkaline phosphatase, guaiacol peroxidase), as a marker to be detected by the patient with a simple colorimetric or dipstick method. Preliminary experiments along these lines, however, have not met with overwhelming success.

CONCLUSION

The uterine cervix may be likened to a biologic valve that, at certain periods during the reproductive cycle, allows the entry of sperm into the uterus and at other times bars their admission. It is by no means a passive organ; it is an active participant in the process of sperm migration. Most of the physiologic functions of the cervix are effected by the secretion of the cervical epithelium. Despite species variations, the cervix uteri presents certain anatomic and histologic structures common to most mammalian species.

From a functional point of view, the following properties may be ascribed to the cervix and its secretions: (1) receptivity to sperm penetration at or near ovulation and impedance of entry at other times, (2) action as a sperm reservoir, (3) protection of sperm cells from the hostile environment of the vagina and from phagocytosis, (4) supplementation of the energy requirements of sperm, (5) filtration effect, and (6) possible capacitation of sperm. Current data indicate that ejaculated sperm rapidly enter midcycle cervical mucus. The mucus is a favorable medium for sperm survival and capacitation and probably provides sperm cells with energy substances required for their motility.

Evaluation of cervical factors and sperm–cervical mucus interaction must be an integral part of the studies done on infertile couples and should be initiated before more invasive procedures are contemplated. The postcoital test determines the adequacy of sperm and receptivity of cervical mucus. It is the only test that evaluates the interaction between the sperm and the female genital tract fluids. Since cervical mucus accurately reflects the ovarian cycle, the postcoital test is also a useful indicator of endocrine preparation of the female reproductive tract. When the postcoital test is abnormal, in vitro sperm–cervical mucus tests may assist the clinician in determining whether the sperm or the cervical mucus is responsible for abnormal results.

REFERENCES

1. Ahlgren M et al: Sperm transport and survival in women with reference to the fallopian tube. In Hafez ESE, Thibault CG, editors: *Biology of spermatozoa: transport, survival, and fertilizing ability,* Basel, Switzerland, 1975, S Karger.

2. Atkin RJ, Warner PE, Reid C: Factor influencing the success of sperm-cervical mucus interaction in patients exhibiting unexplained infertility, *J Androl* 7:3, 1986.

3. Beyler SA, Zaneveld LJD: The role of acrosin in sperm penetration through human cervical mucus, *Fertil Steril* 32:671, 1979.

4. Billings EL et al: Symptoms and hormonal changes accompanying ovulation, *Lancet* 1:282, 1972.

5. Broer KH et al: Frequency of Y-chromatin-bearing spermatozoa in intracervical and intrauterine postcoital tests, *Int J Fertil* 21:181, 1976.

6. Confino E et al: Intrauterine inseminations with washed human spermatozoa, *Fertil Steril* 46:55, 1986.

7. Davajan V, Kunitake G: Fractional in vivo and in vitro examination of postcoital cervical mucus in the human, *Fertil Steril* 20:197, 1969.

8. Elstein M et al: Cervical mucus: present state of knowledge. In Elstein M, Moghissi KS, Borth R, editors: *Cervical mucus in human reproduction,* Copenhagen, 1973, Scriptor.

9. Enhorning G et al: Ability of cervical mucus to act as a barrier against bacteria, *Am J Obstet Gynecol* 106:532, 1970.

10. Fluhmann CF: *The cervix uteri and its disease,* Philadelphia, 1961, WB Saunders.

11. Fox CA et al: Measurement of intravaginal and intrauterine pressure during human coitus by radio-telemetry, *J Reprod Fertil* 22:243, 1970.

12. Fox CA et al: Continuous measurement by radio-telemetry of vaginal pH during human coitus, *J Reprod Fertil* 33:69, 1973.

13. Fredricsson B, Bjork G: Morphology of postcoital spermatozoa in the cervical secretion and its clinical significance, *Fertil Steril* 28:841, 1977.

14. Frenkel DA: Sperm migration and survival in the endometrial cavity, *Int J Fertil* 6:285, 1961.

15. Gibbons RA, Mattner PE: The chemical and physical characteristics of the cervical secretion and its role in reproductive physiology. In Sherman A, editor: *Pathways to conception,* Springfield, Ill, 1971, Charles C Thomas.

16. Giner J et al: Evaluation of the Sims-Huhner postcoital test in infertile couples, *Fertil Steril* 24:145, 1974.

17. Giro C: Contribution a l'etude du système nervaux terminaux des glandes cervicals des rongeurs et de la femme. In *Les fonctions du col uterin,* Paris, 1964, Masson et Cie.

18. Grant A: Cervical hostility, *Fertil Steril* 9:321, 1982.

19. Griffith CS, Grimes DA: The validity of the postcoital test, *Am J Obstet Gynecol* 162:615, 1990.

20. Haas GG: The inhibitory effect of sperm-associated immunoglobulins on cervical mucus penetration, *Fertil Steril* 44:334, 1986.

21. Hanson FW, Overstreet JW: The interaction of human spermatozoa with cervical mucus in vivo, *Am J Obstet Gynecol* 140:173, 1981.

22. Hanson FW, Overstreet JW, Katz DF: A study of the relationship of motile sperm numbers in cervical mucus 48 hours after artificial insemination with subsequent fertility, *Am J Obstet Gynecol* 143:85, 1982.

23. Harrison MF: The diagnostic and therapeutic potential of the postcoital test, *Fertil Steril* 36:71, 1981.

24. Hayes MF et al: Comparison of the in vitro sperm penetration test using human cervical mucus and bovine estrus cervical mucus with the postcoital test, *Int J Fertil* 29:133, 1984.

25. Hull MG, Savage PE, Bronham DR: Prognostic value of the postcoital test: prospective study based on time-specific conception rate, *Br J Obstet Gynaecol* 89:299, 1982.

26. Insler V et al: Correlation of seminal fluid analysis with mucus penetrating ability of spermatozoa, *Fertil Steril* 32:316, 1979.

27. Insler V et al: Cervical crypts and their role in storing spermatozoa. In Insler V, Bettendorf G, editors: *Advances in diagnosis and treatment of infertility,* New York, 1981, Elsevier-North Holland.

28. Jaszczak S et al: Effects of prostaglandins $F_{2\alpha}$ on sperm transport in the reproductive tract of female macaques (M. fascicularis), *Arch Androl* 4:17, 1980.

29. Jette NT, Glass RH: Prognostic value of the postcoital test, *Fertil Steril* 23:29, 1972.

30. Jones WR: The use of antibodies developed by infertile woman to identify relevant antigens, *Acta Endocrinol* 78:376, 1975.

31. Jordan JA: Scanning electron microscopy of the physiological epithelium. In Jordan JA, Singer A, editors: *The cervix,* Philadelphia, 1976, WB Saunders.

32. Katz D et al: Alteration of cervical mucus by vanguard human spermatozoa, *J Reprod Fertil* 65:171, 1982.

33. Keel BA, Webster BW: Correlation of human sperm motility characteristics with an in vitro cervical mucus penetration test, *Fertil Steril* 49:138, 1988.

34. Kremer J: The in vitro spermatozoal penetration test in fertility investigation, thesis, Groningen, Netherlands, 1968, Rijksuniversiteit Groningen.

35. Lee W et al: Laser light-scattering studies of cervical mucus. In Insler V, Bettendorf G, editors: *The uterine cervix in reproduction,* Stuttgart, 1977, Georg Thieme Verlag.

36. Lee WI et al: Molecular arrangement of cervical mucus: a re-evaluation based on laser light-scattering spectrometry, *Gynecol Invest* 8:254, 1977.

37. MacDonald RR, Lumley IB: Endocervical pH measured in vivo through the normal menstrual cycle, *Obstet Gynecol* 35:202, 1970.

38. Macleod J, Hotchkiss RS: Distribution of spermatozoa and certain chemical constituents in the human ejaculate, *J Urol* 48:225, 1942.

39. Martin PMV et al: Induction in gonococci of phenotypic resistance to killing by human serum by human genital secretions, *Br J Vener Dis* 58:363, 1982.

40. Masters WH: The sexual response cycle of the human female, I: gross anatomic considerations, *West J Surg* 68:57, 1960.

41. Mattner PE: Spermatozoa in the genital tract of the ewe, II: distribution after coitus, *Aust J Biol Sci* 16:688, 1963.

42. Mattner PE: The distribution of spermatozoa and leucocytes in the female genital tract in goats and cattle, *J Reprod Fertil* 17:253, 1968.

43. Medina J et al: Comparative evaluation of two methods of natural family planning in Colombia, *Am J Obstet Gynecol* 138:1142, 1980.

44. Moghissi KS: Cyclic changes of cervical mucus in normal and progestin-treated women, *Fertil Steril* 17:663, 1966.

45. Moghissi KS: Composition and function of cervical secretion. In Gripp R, editor: *Handbook of physiology, vol 2, part 2, Endocrinology,* Washington, DC, 1973, American Physiological Society.

46. Moghissi KS: Sperm migration through the human cervix. In Elstein M, Moghissi KS, Borth R, editors: *Cervical mucus in human reproduction,* Copenhagen, 1973, Scriptor.

47. Moghissi KS: Significance and prognostic value of postcoital test. In Insler V, Bettendorf G, editors: *The uterine cervix in reproduction,* Stuttgart, 1977, Georg Thieme Verlag.

48. Moghissi KS: Sperm migration through the human cervix. In Insler V, Bettendorf G, editors: *The uterine cervix in reproduction,* Stuttgart, 1977, George Thieme Verlag.

49. Moghissi KS: Prediction and detection of ovulation, *Fertil Steril* 34:89, 1980.

50. Moghissi KS: The function of human cervix in reproduction, *Curr Probl Obstet Gynecol* 7:1, 1984.

51. Moghissi KS, Sacco AG, Borin KS: Immunologic infertility, I: cervical mucus antibodies and postcoital test, *Am J Obstet Gynecol* 136:941, 1980.
52. Moghissi KS, Syner FN: Cyclic changes in the amount of sialic acid of cervical mucus, *Int J Fertil* 21:246, 1976.
53. Moghissi KS et al: Mechanism of sperm migration, *Fertil Steril* 15:15, 1964.
54. Moghissi KS et al: A composite picture of the menstrual cycle, *Am J Obstet Gynecol* 114:405, 1972.
55. Moghissi KS et al: Immunologic infertility: pregnancies in patients with sperm antibodies. In Insler V, Bettendorf G, editors: *Advances in the diagnosis and treatment of infertility,* New York, 1981, Elsevier-North Holland.
56. Moghissi KS et al: In vitro sperm-cervical mucus penetration: studies in human and bovine cervical mucus, *Fertil Steril* 37:823, 1982.
57. Mortimer D, Pandya J, Sawers RS: Relationship between human sperm motility characteristics and sperm penetration to human cervical mucus in vitro, *J Reprod Fertil* 78:93, 1986.
58. Noyes RW et al: Transport of spermatozoa into the uterus of the rabbit, *Fertil Steril* 9:288, 1958.
59. Odeblad E: Micro-NMR in high permanent magnetic fields, *Acta Obstet Gynecol Scand* 45:127, 1966.
60. Obeblad E: The functional structure of human cervical mucus, *Acta Obstet Gynecol Scand* 47:59, 1968.
61. Obeblad E, Rudolfsson C: Types of cervical secretions: biophysical characteristics. In Blandau RJ, Moghissi KS, editors: *The biology of the cervix,* Chicago, 1973, University of Chicago Press.
62. Overstreet JW et al: The importance of seminal plasma for sperm penetration of human cervical mucus, *Fertil Steril* 34:569, 1980.
63. Overstreet JW et al: In vitro capacitation of human spermatozoa after passage through a column of cervical mucus, *Fertil Steril* 34:604, 1980.
64. Polan ML et al: Variation of semen measures within normal men, *Fertil Steril* 94:396, 1985.
65. Rodin M, Moghissi KS: Intrinsic innervation of the human cervix: a preliminary study. In Blandau RJ, Moghissi KS, editors: *The biology of the cervix,* Chicago, 1973, University of Chicago Press.
66. Roumen FJME et al: Hormonal patterns in infertile women with a deficient postcoital test, *Fertil Steril* 38:42, 1982.
67. Schumacher GFB: Biochemistry of cervical mucus, *Fertil Steril* 21:697, 1970.
68. Schumacher GFB, Pearl MJ: Alpha$_1$-antitrypsin in cervical mucus, *Fertil Steril* 19:91, 1968.
69. Settlage DSF et al: Sperm transport from the vagina to the fallopian tubes in women. In Hafez ESE, Thibault CG, editors: *Biology of spermatozoa: transport, survival, and fertilizing ability,* Basel, Switzerland, 1975, S Karger.
70. Sher G, Katz M: Inadequate cervical mucus: a cause of idiopathic infertility, *Fertil Steril* 27:886, 1976.
71. Shulman JF, Shulman S: Methylprednisone treatment of immunologic infertility in the male, *Fertil Steril* 38:591, 1982.
72. Sobrero AJ: Bacteriological findings in the midcycle endocervical mucus in infertile women, *Ann N Y Acad Sci* 97:591, 1962.
73. Sobrero AJ: Sperm migration in the human female. In Westin B, Wiqvist N, editors: *Proceedings of the Fifth World Congress on Fertility and Sterility,* New York and Amsterdam, 1967, Excerpta Medica.
74. Sobrero AJ, Macleod J: The immediate postcoital test, *Fertil Steril* 13:184, 1962.
75. Tampion D, Gibbons RA: orientation of spermatozoa in mucus of the cervix uteri, *Nature* 194:381, 1962.
76. teVeld ER, van Koox RJ, Waterreus JJ: Intrauterine insemination with washed husband's spermatozoa: a controlled study, *Fertil Steril* 51:182, 1989.
77. Toth A et al: Evidence for microbial transfer by spermatozoa, *Obstet Gynecol* 59:559, 1982.
78. Tredway DT et al: Significance of timing for postcoital evaluation of cervical mucus, *Am J Obstet Gynecol* 121:387, 1975.
79. Van Kooij RJ et al: Human cervical mucus and its mucous glycoprotein during the menstrual cycle, *Fertil Steril* 34:226, 1980.
80. Vander Merwe JV: The effect of clomiphene citrate and conjugated estrogens on cervical mucus, *S Afr Med J* 60:347, 1981.
81. Wang C et al: Interaction between human cervical mucus and sperm surface antibodies, *Fertil Steril* 44:484, 1985.
82. Wolf DP et al: Composition and function of human cervical mucus, *Biochim Biophys Acta* 630:545, 1980.
83. World Health Organization: *Laboratory manual for examination of human semen and semen-cervical mucus interaction,* WHO, 1987, Geneva.
84. Yurewicz EC, Moghissi KS: Purification of human midcycle cervical mucin and characterization of its oligosaccharides with respect to size, composition, and microheterogeneity, *J Biol Chem* 256:11895, 1981.
85. Yurewicz EC et al: Structural characterization of neutral oligosaccharides of human midcycle cervical mucin, *J Biol Chem* 257:2314, 1982.
86. Yurewicz EC et al: Structure of sialylated oligosaccharides of human cervical mucin, *Fed Proc* 41:887, 1982.
87. Zinser HK: La vascularization du col uterin. In *Les fonctions due col uterin,* Paris, 1964, Masson et Cie.

Chapter 20

MALE FACTOR INFERTILITY

Glenn R. Cunningham, MD

The past two decades have brought remarkable advancements in our understanding of the factors that regulate spermatogenesis and the Leydig cells, the biology of the accessory sex glands, sperm capacitation, and fertilization. Unfortunately, the molecular causes for impaired spermatogenesis and impaired sperm motility, for most infertile males, are still poorly understood. Furthermore, our ability to prevent or to reverse infertility is in most cases ineffective.

Two major developments have had a significant effect on the general problem of male factor infertility. First, there is a much greater awareness of the male problem, and there are many more andrologists (urologists and endocrinologists) who are interested and qualified to evaluate and treat infertile men. As a result, several scientific trials have documented the ineffectiveness of empirical therapy. This information helps us to focus on new strategies. Second, there now are a large number of reproductive biologists who possess the skills required to assist the clinician in performing assisted reproduction for oligospermic and/or asthenospermic childless men. These techniques offer many previously infertile men a reasonable chance of having children.

Studies in England indicate that 24% of women aged 25 to 44 years who attempted to conceive experienced subfertility at some time in their reproductive lives.[48] Thirteen percent noted this when attempting to conceive their first child and 17% when attempting to conceive a subsequent pregnancy. Of women 3% were involuntarily childless, and 6% of parous women were not able to have as many children as they desired.

When the subfertile couple requests medical advice, the woman and the man should undergo evaluation by individuals with expertise in reproductive disorders. Duration of infertility, age of the man, sperm morphology, and sperm motility contribute significantly to the fertilizing potential.[14,38]

It is important to recognize that a normal reproductive system in one spouse may overcome what would appear to be significant abnormalities in the partner. This interaction has prompted some clinicians to observe that subfertility may be manifested by a longer time to achieve conception.[119] Although it is unlikely, fertility can occur in the presence of very severe oligoasthenospermia. Sokol and Sparkes[116] documented a pregnancy by a man with less than 0.5 million sperm per milliliter and less than 10% sperm motility.

PHYSIOLOGY OF MALE REPRODUCTION

The reproductive process in the man depends on gonadotropic stimulation of the testes, and paracrine and probably autocrine and cell-to-cell–mediated regulation of spermatogenesis and spermiogenesis. Spermatozoa normally undergo maturation in the epididymides. They are ejaculated through the vasa deferentia and urethra with contributions of seminal fluid at the time of ejaculation from the seminal vesicles, prostate, and bulbourethral glands. Much has been learned about these processes, but additional insights will be required before most aberrations can be treated effectively.

Initiation of human spermatogenesis normally is dependent on both follicle-stimulating hormone (FSH) and luteinizing hormone (LH). The testes remain immature in individuals who have a complete congenital deficiency of gonadotropin-releasing hormone (GnRH). As is detailed later in this chapter, pulsatile administration of GnRH or parenteral administration of LH and FSH-like hormones will stimulate spermatogenesis. The process of spermatogenesis involves differentiation of spermatogonia into spermatocytes, spermatids, and spermatozoa.[21] Several mitotic events, as well as meiosis, serve to expand greatly the number of germ cells during this process, which takes 74 ± 5 days in man.[54] Initiation of spermatogenesis has been reported in a few prepubertal-aged boys who have had a Leydig cell tumor of the testis.[120] In such patients testosterone alone has been thought to be responsible for stimulating spermatogenesis; however, it is possible that other locally produced factors also are involved. Precocious puberty has been observed in the absence of either a testicular tumor or a detectable rise in serum or urinary gonadotropins.[102,106,133] This syndrome is not gonadotropin dependent, but there is hyperplasia of the Leydig cells. It has been postulated to arise on the basis of hypersecretion of paracrine factors.

Maintenance of qualitative or complete spermatogenesis in gonadotropin-deficient men has been observed in hypophysectomized men and in normal men who have been treated with gonadotropins. Spermatogenesis can be maintained in individuals who are hypophysectomized and treated immediately with human chorionic gonadotropin (hCG).[43] In the absence of treatment, spermatogenesis is arrested before meiosis.[70,118] If the testis is allowed to regress to this stage for a prolonged period, it may be necessary to add human menopausal gonadotropin (hMG), which has FSH-like properties, in order to restore quantitative spermatogenesis. We reported a patient with a large FSH-secreting pituitary tumor who had undetectable serum levels of testosterone.[29] His seminiferous tubules contained Sertoli cells that morphologically were essentially normal. Spermatogonia through pachytene spermatocytes were present in good numbers, but there were very few early or late spermatids. Although studies in hypophysectomized men are limited, Bremner and Matsumoto have conducted a series of studies using weekly injections of testosterone enanthate to suppress gonadotropin secretion and secondarily spermatogenesis.[15,75-78] In this model, qualitative spermatogenesis can be achieved with administration of either hCG or hMG, but quantitative spermatogenesis requires both hCG and hMG. Since this model has normal or somewhat elevated serum levels of testosterone, one cannot conclude that FSH alone is able to maintain qualitative spermatogenesis.

Studies in nonhuman primates support the observations in rodents and indicate that it is possible to maintain qualitative but not quantitative spermatogenesis with large doses of testosterone enanthate in rhesus monkeys that have undergone sectioning of the pituitary stalk and regression of the testes before treatment.[73] Additional evidence that FSH is important in the maintenance of quantitative spermatogenesis in nonhuman primates is found in studies using passive immunization to FSH. Sperm production was reduced, but azoospermia was not observed.[132]

Most experimental studies of spermatogenesis have been carried out in rats. Not only are rats readily available and relatively inexpensive, but spermatogenesis in rats is much easier to study than it is in primates. In this species FSH and LH are required for the initiation of spermatogenesis, but administration of large doses of testosterone to hypophysectomized or intact adult rats is able to maintain testicular weight and daily sperm production at 65% to 93% of that in intact, untreated animals.[118,122] It may be that one could maintain spermatogenesis equally well in primates if comparable amounts of testosterone were administered.

Studies during the past two decades have focused on the cells and the mechanisms by which FSH, LH, and testosterone exert their effects on the testes (Fig. 20-1). The interstitial spaces contain macrophages, Leydig cells, and capillaries. The outer portion of the seminiferous tubules is lined with myoid cells, which are separated by a basement membrane from the base of the Sertoli cells, the spermatogonia, and preleptotene spermatocytes. These germ cells are separated from differentiating spermatocytes and spermatids by tight junctions that are formed between Sertoli cells. Thus cells in the adluminal compartment are totally dependent on the Sertoli cells for their nourishment.

It is likely that the spermatogenic capacity of the testis is determined by the population of both Sertoli cells and spermatogonia. The undifferentiated spermatogonia retain the capacity to repopulate the germinal epithelium, but this is not true for the Sertoli cells. In rodents, Sertoli cells stop dividing before age 20 days. The mitotic activity of the Sertoli cells appears to be mediated by FSH. Hemicastration of rats before 20 days of age results in an increase in serum FSH and hypertrophy of the remaining testis.[30] Hypertrophy is observed in germ cell–depleted testes, indicating that Sertoli cells undergo hypertrophy or hyperplasia, or both. Compensatory hypertrophy does not occur if mature rats undergo hemicastration.

This constancy of germ cell associations provides the basis for assignment of stages to the spermatogenic process. At any one time the types of germ cells associated with a Sertoli cell are predictable. Although there are interspecies differences, this principle is maintained in all animals. In man one may observe more than one stage within a cross-section of a tubule. In the rat and mouse one may observe lengthy segments of a tubule at the same stage of development. This fact has enabled Parvinen and associ-

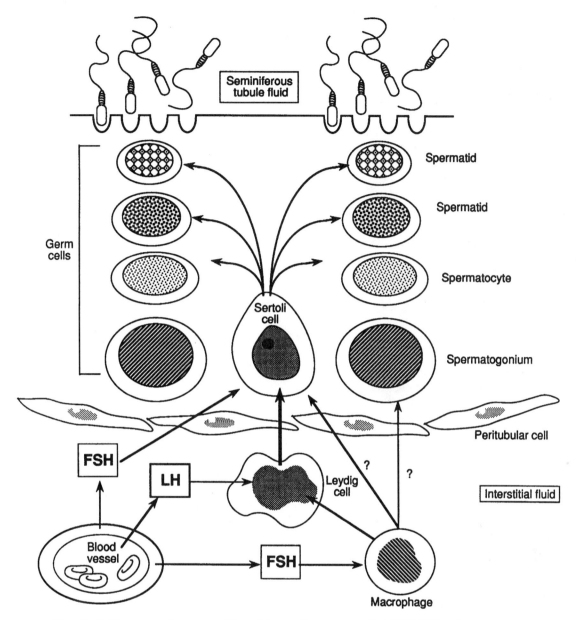

Fig. 20-1. Diagrammatic representation of the mechanisms by which FSH, LH, and testosterone exert their effects on the testes.

ates[93,94] to transilluminate unstained tubules and to identify stage-specific characteristics. This technique has permitted analysis of factors unique to a given stage.

It has been possible to identify target cells for FSH, testosterone, and paracrine factors induced by these hormones.[33,67,103,112] Evidence has accumulated to indicate that the Sertoli cells and probably intratesticular macrophages are target cells for FSH. Both cell types posses specific receptors for and respond to FSH. It is likely that macrophages secrete factors that can affect both Leydig and Sertoli cells. Sertoli cells and the peritubular myoid cells contain androgen receptors and respond to androgen. FSH

and testosterone are thought to affect spermatogenesis indirectly by stimulating the production of factors that act in a paracrine manner. The Sertoli cells secrete a large number of factors, and in some studies coculturing Sertoli cells with peritubular cells augments the secretion of some of these factors. It also has been possible to demonstrate that FSH induces the Sertoli cells to secrete a factor that augments LH-stimulated secretion of testosterone by the Leydig cells. This is consistent with clinical observations. Finally, Leydig cells secrete factors that have autocrine and paracrine effects.

In rats, responsiveness of the Sertoli cells to both FSH

and testosterone depends on the stage of the spermatogenic cycle.[93,94] Evidence is accumulating that the neighboring germ cells are responsible for the variability in the responsiveness of the Sertoli cells. It is not known whether this effect is mediated by paracrine factors or by cell-cell contact. Additionally, both FSH and testosterone stimulate stage-specific factors. At this time it is not known with certainty how most of these factors affect spermatogenesis. It is likely that these processes that have been observed in rodents are applicable to men and that altered secretion of some of these factors results in defective spermatogenesis in men. For example, a meiosis-inducing substance (MIS) and a meiosis-preventing substance (MPS) have been identified in humans.[49] It is quite possible that a reduction in the MIS:MPS ratio could result in arrested spermatogenesis at the spermatocyte level of development.

EVALUATION

The man must be evaluated by a physician who is knowledgeable about the conditions that can impair his reproductive potential. One might argue that this is not necessary if the results of routine analysis of semen are entirely normal on at least two occasions. Even under this condition, involvement of the man in the couple's problem is important.

History

Many factors can result in male infertility. Usually the history is more informative than is the physical examination. Historical information that should be obtained during the initial interview include the following:

1. Fertility history
   - Previous fertility
   - Duration of infertility
   - Frequency of intercourse
   - Coital techniques
   - Libido and impotence
   - Timing of intercourse
   - Wife's evaluation
   - Previous evaluation or treatment
2. History of use of drugs and physical agents
   - Alcohol
   - Marijuana
   - Anabolic steroids
   - Sulfasalazine
   - Chemotherapeutic agents
   - Irradiation
   - Excessive heat
3. Past history
   - Mumps
   - Bronchitis
   - Cryptorchidism
   - Scrotal or inguinal surgery
   - Sexually transmitted diseases
   - Epididymitis
   - Orchitis
   - Testicular trauma
   - Hypospadias or transurethral resection of the prostate
   - Autonomic neuropathy
4. Family history
   - Sexual infantilism
   - Anosmia or hyposmia
   - Colorblindness
   - Infertility
   - Cystic fibrosis
5. Occupational history
   - Exposure to pesticides
   - Exposure to lead
6. History of systemic diseases
   - Hemochromatosis
   - Chronic renal insufficiency
   - Chronic liver disease
   - Lymphoma
   - Hyperthyroidism
   - Hypothyroidism
   - Chronic bronchitis
   - Cystic fibrosis

It is important to know whether either the patient or his partner has had previous pregnancies and to know the duration of infertility. As previously noted, the ages of the individuals and the duration of infertility are negatively correlated with their chances of fertility. One should obtain information about libido, potency, the frequency of intercourse, coital techniques, and the timing of intercourse in relation to the woman's menstrual cycle. The details of previous evaluations and treatment for both the man and the woman are important.

The possibility of infertility arising as a result of use of drugs or physical agents should be examined by specific questions. Excessive alcohol intake is known to have direct as well as indirect effects on the testes. Marijuana has been observed to reduce sperm motility. Anabolic steroids will suppress gonadotropins and secondarily spermatogenesis. The degree and duration of suppression seem to be related to the dose and duration of anabolic steroid use. Sulfasalazine, which is used chronically to treat individuals with ulcerative colitis, has been observed to reduce sperm motility and to cause infertility. Potent chemotherapeutic agents, especially the alkylating agents, affect mitotically active spermatogonia. These cells also are sensitive to the effects of irradiation. In both cases recovery of the germinal epithelium is related to the dose and duration of exposure. Finally, excessive heat as experienced by individuals taking very hot baths may impair Sertoli cell function and spermatogenesis.[65]

The past history may reveal failure to undergo puberty at the expected time and the necessity for hormone treatment to achieve virilization. Patients with isolated gonadotropin deficiency also may have anosmia or hyposmia, colorblindness, or congenital deafness. A history of mumps after age 12, a sexually transmitted disease, epididymitis, orchitis, or testicular torsion or trauma can provide a rationale for semen abnormalities. A history of cryptorchidism is important even if orchiopexy were performed at an early age, since there frequently is evidence of testicular abnormalities. Other scrotal or inguinal surgery can be associated with testicular damage. Occasionally a patient may have had a transurethral resection of the prostate that results in retrograde ejaculation. Retrograde ejaculation also can be observed in some diabetics who have an autonomic neuropathy. Younger men with chronic bronchitis who are nonsmokers should be considered as candidates for Young's syndrome. These men have motility abnormalities that affect both the cilia of the respiratory epithelium and spermatozoa. They, as well as those with cystic fibrosis, may have obstructive azoospermia due to secretory plugs in the epididymides. Patients with Klinefelter syndrome may present with loss of libido or gynecomastia as well as infertility.

Occupational exposure to pesticides such as dibromochloropropane can cause severe testicular damage. Exposure to lead also has been reported to impair fertility. It is likely that this list will expand, so it is important to take detailed histories regarding the work environment. Available evidence is not convincing that use of tobacco impairs spermatogenesis.

Systemic diseases such as hemochromatosis, chronic renal insufficiency, chronic liver disease, lymphoma, or hyperthyroidism can impair testicular function and cause infertility.

Physical examination

Usually the physical examination helps to confirm abnormalities suggested by the history. It is of particular importance to examine the scrotal contents carefully for evidence of testicular atrophy ($<4.0 \times <2.0$ cm), a varicocele, and epididymal induration or tenderness. Varicoceles are best detected by having the patient perform a Valsalva maneuver while upright. Usually varicoceles are on the left, but recent reports have emphasized more frequent involvement of the right side than previously suspected.

Laboratory examination

Laboratory evaluation of the man begins with the examination of a semen specimen collected by masturbation after 2 to 4 days of abstinence. The specimen should be kept at body temperature and examined for sperm motility within 2 hours. It is essential that the clinician observe a wet preparation of the semen within 2 hours of the time it was collected. Allowing the patient to view the specimen with the clinician provides him with a better understanding of the problem. (See Chapter 29 for semen evaluation.)

It is useful to measure the serum for FSH, since values more than two times the normal range usually indicate severe, irreversible testicular disease. A low or normal FSH

level in a patient with small testes suggests hypothalamic or pituitary disease. Androgen deficiency is unusual in the individual who presents with infertility, normal libido and potency, and no abnormalities on physical examination. Therefore, the routine measurement of testosterone probably is not cost effective. When the total testosterone level is in an equivocally low range, measurement of testosterone that is not bound to testosterone-estradiol–binding globulin is useful. It is now thought that both free and albumin-bound testosterone are available to peripheral tissues. LH levels must be measured in men with low testosterone levels in order to determine whether the androgen deficiency is due to testicular or pituitary or hypothalamic disease. The serum concentration of prolactin should be determined in all androgen-deficient men who have low or normal LH and FSH levels. Chromosomal studies are indicated in individuals with primary hypogonadism unless it clearly has resulted from cryptorchidism, trauma, or a toxin. An elevated LH level in the presence of a normal or a high serum testosterone value suggests the possibility of hyperthyroidism or androgen resistance. Verification of androgen resistance requires analysis of the androgen receptor in fibroblasts cultured from a scrotal skin biopsy specimen. Since no effective therapy currently is available for this condition, only a relatively small number of infertile men have been evaluated in detail.

The possibility of antisperm antibodies is suggested by the findings of impaired sperm motility, clumping of sperm in a wet preparation, impaired postcoital test, impaired sperm migration test, or an abnormal hamster egg penetration test. (See Chapter 22 for discussion of evaluation and treatment of antisperm antibodies.)

DIAGNOSTIC CONSIDERATIONS

A large number of conditions have been associated with male infertility. Specific etiologies account for only a small percentage of the currently recognized conditions. The frequency of these conditions is illustrated in Table 20-1. It has been estimated that 15% of men have a varicocele; however, only one third of them present with infertility. Some fertile men with varicoceles have been observed to have impairment in semen quality, but many do not. Varicocele and idiopathic disease comprise approximately 80% of the infertile population. Recognition of the precise mechanisms that cause infertility in these patients should lead to improvements in therapy.

AZOOSPERMIA/OLIGOSPERMIA

The presence of azoospermia or oligospermia on repeated semen analyses necessitates further evaluation. It is useful to classify patients further according to the serum FSH level. FSH secretion by the pituitary is dependent on GnRH stimulation. Testosterone and its metabolites estradiol and dihydrotestosterone exert inhibition on FSH secretion at the level of both the hypothalamus and the pituitary. Inhibin, which is secreted by the Sertoli cells in the testis,

Table 20-1. Relative frequency of conditions associated with male infertility in 1041 men

Condition	Frequency (%)
Idiopathic	38.9
Varicocele (medium and large)	25.0
Varicocele (small)	15.3
Cryptorchidism	6.4
Possible obstruction	4.5
Epididymal or vas deferens obstruction	4.1
Klinefelter's syndrome	1.9
Mumps orchitis	1.6
Hypogonadotropic hypogonadism	0.6
Nonmotile sperm	0.6
Irradiation/chemotherapy	0.5
Coital disorders	0.5
Androgen resistance	0.1
	100.0

Modified from Baker HWG et al: In Santen RJ, Swerdloff RS, editors: *Male reproductive dysfunction,* New York, 1986, Marcel Dekker, p 341.

inhibits FSH secretion at the level of the pituitary gland. Since severe primary testicular disease is thought to cause impaired secretion of inhibin by the Sertoli cells, one might ask why patients are not classified by their inhibin level. Since a low inhibin level could result from inadequate FSH or from abnormal Sertoli cell function, serum FSH levels provide a more reliable means for diagnosing primary and secondary hypogonadal states.

Hypogonadotropic

Gonadotropin-releasing hormone deficiency or luteinizing hormone and follicle-stimulating hormone deficiency. Combined LH and FSH deficiency can result from either hypothalamic deficiency of GnRH or from destructive lesions that directly affect the gonadotropes within the pituitary. Congenital lesions are nearly always due to deficiency of GnRH, whereas acquired conditions can involve either the hypothalamus or pituitary. Acquired hypogonadotropic hypogonadism in men usually is caused by anatomic lesions in the hypothalamus or pituitary. Pituitary tumors, extrasellar tumors, hypothalamic tumors, surgical trauma, basilar skull fractures, and infiltrative diseases account for most of these lesions. Recent reports, especially of studies of women, have emphasized the importance of functional defects. Efforts to demonstrate psychologic or exercise-induced androgen deficiency and impaired spermatogenesis in men have brought conflicting reports. Transient androgen deficiency has been reported to be caused by psychologic and physical stress, but semen studies are lacking. Prolonged physical exercise has been associated with reductions in total and free testosterone levels in some men,[9] but other investigators have found that most conditioned marathon runners have normal total test-

osterone levels and semen studies.[10] In one study there was some reduction in LH pulse amplitude and frequency, and sensitivity to Gn-RH was reduced.[66] Total and free testosterone levels were normal.

These patients must have a thorough evaluation of pituitary function and anatomic evaluation with magnetic resonance imaging or computed tomography scanning. Either GnRH or hCG alone or in combination with hMG can be used to treat hypothalamic abnormalities. The availability of GnRH and the recognition that it must be given in a pulsatile manner have resulted in several studies of sufficient size and duration to provide guidelines for treatment of patients with hypothalamic deficiency. Patients who have a loss of gonadotropes must be treated with hCG alone or in combination with hMG.

Treatment is most effective when a patient has testicular volume in excess of 4 mL and no history of cryptorchidism. Experience has taught that the dose of GnRH required to achieve normal serum levels of testosterone varies greatly among patients.[130] Adequate pulsatile stimulation will achieve normal testosterone levels in essentially all patients.

Spermatogenesis was induced successfully in 34 of 51 GnRH-deficient men.[130] Of the 17 patients who did not respond, 2 were cryptorchid, 3 discontinued therapy before there was significant testicular growth, 3 discontinued treatment while they were still azoospermic (8 to 18 months), 3 did not submit semen specimens, and 6 had been treated for less than 6 months. The size of the testis before treatment was correlated positively with the time before the first appearance of sperm in the ejaculate, which ranged from 18 to 139 weeks. Eight of the nine patients desiring fertility achieved a pregnancy (Table 20-2). The unsuccessful patient had a history of cryptorchidism. Morris and colleagues[84] treated 10 patients with congenital GnRH deficiency with 15 μg of GnRH every 90 minutes for 1 to 18 months. Four patients achieved sperm in the ejaculate, and three fathered children. Shargil[111] has reported that pulsatile administration of GnRH (25 ng/kg) every 90 minutes is more effective than the administration of 500 μg of GnRH twice a day. Of 12 patients treated with the pump, 10 fathered children, compared with 8 of 18 treated by injections.

Several centers have used gonadotropin therapy for many years to treat hypogonadotropic men (Table 20-3). Patients who developed hypopituitarism after puberty respond more quickly and more completely to gonadotropin therapy. hCG alone may induce adequate spermatogenesis in patients with acquired hypopituitarism and in those with partial GnRH deficiency (testicular volume >4.0 mL).[17] Nine of eleven men with partial GnRH deficiency produced from 0.1 to 44.4 million sperm per milliliter, and seven wives conceived during treatment with only hCG. Fertility frequently is achieved even if the patient is oligospermic. Burris et al.[18] noted that 71% of pregnancies occurred when

Table 20-2. Treatment of hypogonadotropic hypogonadism with GnRH

Investigator	Congenital, no. of patients	Acquired,* no. of patients	Dose	Frequency (h)	Duration (mo)	↑ Testosterone, no. of patients	↑ Count, no. of patients	Sperm count (× 10^6)	Fertility, no. of patients
Whitcomb and Crowley[130]	9		25-600 ng/kg	2	<45	9	9	1-68/mL	8
Morris and co-workers[84]	10		15 µg	1.5	1-18	4	4	5.7-26	3
		5	15 µg	1.5	1-18	3	2	<0.1-100	

*Postpubertal.

Table 20-3. Treatment of hypogonadotropic hypogonadism with hCG and hMG

Investigator	Congenital, no. of patients	Acquired,* no. of patients	Dose (IU)	Frequency	Duration (mo)	↑ Testosterone, no. of patients	↑ Count, no. of patients	Sperm count (× 10^6)	Fertility, no. of patients
Ley and Leonard[62]	10	1 pre	hCG, 2000,	3/wk	6-24	11	3	1.1-6.5/mL	
			+ hMG, 75	3/wk	4-11		10	0.1-59/mL	
		2 post	hCG, 4000,	3/wk	3-5	2	0		
			+ hMG, 75	3/wk	9		2	7.4-64/mL	2
Finkel and co-workers[43]	15		hCG, 2000,	3/wk	>6	15	3	1-45	
			+hMG, 75,	3/wk	4				
			or +hMG, 150	3/wk	4		9	10-120	9
Okuyama and co-workers[90]	13	6 post	hCG, 2000	3/wk	>6	6	6	50-170	
			hCG, 3000						
			+hMG, 75	2/wk	24-48	3	5	1-10/mL	
		5 pre	hCG, 3000						
			+hMG, 75	2/wk	24-48	5	5	8-35/mL	3

*Prepubertal or postpubertal.

GnRH-deficient men had less than 20 million sperm per milliliter in the ejaculate.

Liu and colleagues[63] treated eight men with isolated hypogonadotropic hypogonadism with GnRH after they had received maximal benefit from hMG and hCG. Only four men had normal testosterone levels with GnRH pulses (up to 286 ng/kg) every 2 hours for 18 months. These men had a 53% increase in testicular size, but there was little change in sperm density. Liu et al. concluded that treatment with GnRH was not superior to treatment with hCG and hMG.

Isolated follicle-stimulating hormone deficiency. Isolated FSH deficiency has been reported rarely in infertile men.[85,98] Since FSH and LH are secreted by the same pituitary cell under stimulation by GnRH, there may be a change in sensitivity to GnRH or in the regulation of FSH secretion at the level of the pituitary. It is known that both GnRH pulse frequency and dose affect the FSH:LH ratio.[50] Treatment with both hMG and hCG has been reported to increase sperm density and to result in pregnancy in a patient with isolated FSH deficiency.[7]

Isolated luteinizing hormone deficiency. Isolated LH deficiency (fertile eunuch syndrome) presents with normal-sized testes in the presence of a eunuchoid habitus and lack of virilization.[80,95] These patients have normal serum and urinary levels of FSH but reduced serum LH and testosterone values. It has been suggested that this syndrome represents an incomplete form of GnRH deficiency. Presumably the low LH levels in the presence of normal serum levels of FSH are adequate to increase intratesticular testosterone levels that stimulate spermatogenesis. Virilization has been achieved by the administration of hCG or exogenous testosterone. Usually the initial semen volume and the sperm count are low and increase during treatment with hCG.[41]

Prolactinoma. The incidence of hyperprolactinemia in 3 series of men comprising 635 patients who presented with infertility was 5.2%[51,57,110] Since many conditions can cause mild to moderate hyperprolactinemia, it is important that these patients be carefully evaluated. Surgical cures and restoration of libido, potency, spermatogenesis, and fertility have been reported for microadenomas.[97] However, macroadenomas account for 90% of the prolactinomas that are diagnosed in men.[83] One would expect permanent gonadotropin deficiency in many men who undergo surgical treatment of macroadenomas. Murray and co-workers[86] examined eight patients 6 to 13 months after serum prolactin levels were reduced by surgery and/or drug therapy. Testosterone levels increased into the normal range for five men, but only two men achieved sperm counts greater than 20 million per milliliter. Mancini and colleagues[69] studied nine patients who remained hyperprolactinemic after surgery. Eight had less than 10 million sperm per milliliter, and seven had low LH values and testosterone levels less than 3 ng/mL. After treatment for 90 days with bromocriptine (7.5 mg/d) prolactin levels fell, testosterone levels were greater than 3 ng/mL in six patients, and sperm counts rose more than fivefold (exceeding 20 million/mL) in five men. One man fathered a child.

Hemochromatosis and thalassemia. Hypogonadism can be caused by iron deposition in the pituitary or hypothalamus.[36] This can be due to hemochromatosis or to iron overload from transfusions, as is seen in patients with thalassemia major. Phlebotomy alone has been reported to restore libido, potency, spermatogenesis, and fertility in patients with hemochromatosis.[113] Chelation therapy can be used to treat iron overload due to transfusion. If this is ineffective, most patients will respond to hCG and hMG.[35,128]

Lead toxicity. Lead has been shown to affect the hypothalamus and to decrease testosterone levels in rats.[115] Presumably this is the mechanism for the impairment of spermatogenesis that has been reported in men.[28]

Anabolic steroids. A significant number of male athletes use anabolic steroids at some time during their athletic careers. Usually the dose of androgen greatly exceeds a replacement dose, and it is common to use more than one agent at a time. Although carefully controlled, double-blind trials with these agents have not been conducted in athletes, testosterone enanthate and 19-nortestosterone have been evaluated as potential male contraceptives. Higher doses suppress gonadotropins and spermatogenesis in most men, but azoospermia is not achieved in everyone. Similar findings have been reported in body builders.[58] Of 19 men who had taken anabolic steroids for 3 to 12 months, 14 had sperm counts of less than 20 million/mL. Seven men were azoospermic. Of the 11 men who had been off anabolic steroids for more than 4 months, 3 had sperm counts of less than 5 million/mL and 1 had less than 20 million/mL. Men who are well virilized with low gonadotropin levels should be considered as candidates for anabolic-suppressed testicular function. Serum testosterone levels vary depending on which anabolic agent is used. Recovery of spermatogenesis in contraceptive studies usually occurred within 3 months, but up to 12 months was required in the minority of subjects.

Adrenal syndromes. Three adrenal syndromes have been associated with hypogonadotropic hypogonadism. The hypogonadism that may accompany the X-linked form of congenital adrenal hypoplasia has responded to pulsatile administration of GnRH.[92] Cortisol secretion is impaired in patients with a partial deficiency of 21-hydroxylase, and corticotropin levels are increased. The adrenals are stimulated to produce excessive amounts of androgens, which suppress FSH and LH secretion. Testicular production of testosterone and spermatozoa is impaired in some patients.[13,31,124] Suppression of corticotropin secretion by replacement doses of glucocorticoids may result in normal testicular function. Although partial deficiency of 21-hydroxylase appears to account for 5% of the patients with hirsutism,[16] this abnormality does not appear to be a common cause of male infertility.[89,125] It may be that the diagnosis would be made more frequently by measurement of 21-deoxycortisol, a more reliable indicator of this condition than 17α-hydroxyprogesterone.[42] Decreased libido or impotence has been reported in 8 of 122 men with Cushing syndrome.[64] The majority of these men had subnormal testosterone and LH levels, and some had an abnormal response to GnRH. Semen studies have not been reported.

Eugonadotropic

Most men with azoospermia or oligospermia have normal serum levels of FSH and testosterone. A normal FSH level in patients having impaired spermatogenesis suggests that testicular factors that regulate FSH secretion are intact. This is consistent with the view that differentiated germ cells do not influence the secretion of inhibin by Sertoli cells. The majority of these men have impaired spermatogenesis, but obstruction in the epididymides or vasa deferentia and retrograde ejaculation are seen in a small, but significant, number. Identification of the correct etiology in the latter groups can lead to specific and effective therapy.

Obstruction of the epididymides or vasa deferentia. The finding of normal-sized testes, azoospermia, and a normal FSH level suggests the possibility of obstruction in the epididymides or vasa deferentia. Frequently these patients have a history of epididymitis, and one may detect induration of the epididymis on physical examination. Congenital atresia or agenesis of a portion of the epididymis and previous inflammatory diseases are the most common etiologies. Usually exploration of the scrotum will identify the site of obstruction. (See Chapter 40.) A testicular biopsy specimen will reveal normal spermatogenesis. Recent reports of pregnancies after sperm from the proximal caput epididymides were used for in vitro fertilization indicate that maturation of sperm in the more distal caput epididymis is not an absolute requirement for fertility.[26,114] Of course, men who have undergone a vasectomy will have this constellation of findings. Restoration of fertility is possible for the majority of these men (See Chapter 40.)

Retrograde ejaculation. Retrograde ejaculation is an important cause of low ejaculate volume. The diagnosis can be established by finding a large number of sperm in the centrifugate of a urine specimen obtained immediately after ejaculation. Retrograde ejaculation is caused by incompetence of the internal sphincter of the bladder. It is a well-known complication of a transurethral prostatectomy and of diabetic autonomic neuropathy. Patients with a neurogenic etiology can be treated with ephedrine (25 or 50 mg orally four times daily), phenylpropanolamine (50 or 75 mg twice daily), or imipramine (25 or 50 mg/d). Brompheniramine, an H_1 antihistamine with strong anticholinergic activity, has been reported to be effective in some men when used in a dose of 8 mg three times daily.[107] Usually it is necessary to centrifuge a postejaculation urine specimen to retrieve the sperm, and then to inseminate them artificially. A full bladder may enable some patients to have antegrade ejaculation with minimal contamination by urine.[27] Alkalinization of the urine before ejaculation and washing the sperm with isoosmotic medium containing albumin immediately after voiding have been demonstrated to enhance sperm viability and motility.[105,138] Of course, timing of insemination is critical for a successful outcome.

Varicocele. Many patients with unilateral or bilateral varicoceles have oligospermia and normal serum FSH levels. The causes for the impairment of spermatogenesis that may accompany the varicocele still remain poorly understood. Using a nonhuman primate model, Harrison et al.[53] observed that sperm motility was depressed and that it improved after varicocelectomy. Sperm concentration was affected less. Although most urologists believe that the potential for fertility is improved by elimination of large varicoceles,[37,104] some studies have suggested that varicocele ligation does not increase fertility for patients with sperm counts of more than 20 million/mL or for those with less than 10 million/mL. sperm/ml.[1,99,127] Attempts to use the sperm penetration assay to determine who should undergo varicocele ablation have not been useful[96]; however, Rogers et al.[100] reported improved sperm penetration

assays in 23.7% of men who underwent varicocele ligation, compared with 10% in the nonsurgical group. There is a need for a study in which a large number of patients are evaluated carefully before randomization into treatment and nontreatment groups and then followed for at least 2 years. It also has been suggested that fertility rates are higher when patients with sperm counts of less than 10 million/mL are given hCG after correction of the varicocele.[37] This, too, needs to be studied.

Idiopathic. The large numbers of patients with idiopathic azoospermia or oligospermia and their intense desire to have children have prompted clinicians to try a large number of empirical therapies. Several carefully conducted trials have failed to prove the efficacy of the agents that have been used most commonly. A large number of empirical therapies remain that have not undergone carefully controlled, randomized trials, but there is little evidence that any of these agents has significant benefit. Most approaches have attempted to utilize hormonal manipulation in an effort to improve semen quality.

Clomiphene citrate. Clomiphene citrate has been the most commonly used treatment for idiopathic oligospermia. It increases serum levels of LH, FSH, and testosterone. Since clomiphene citrate is given orally, it is much easier and less expensive to use than hCG and hMG, which must be given parenterally. The studies in Table 20-4 were randomized and placebo controlled. Patients were treated for 3 to 12 months. In each study the wives had undergone appropriate gynecologic evaluation and the results were thought to be normal. Although a statistical increase in sperm concentration over that observed during the control period was noted with several of the studies, the differences were not significant when the treatment and placebo groups were compared.

Table 20-4. Treatment of eugonadotropic azoospermia/oligospermia with clomiphene citrate

| Investigator | Treatment | No. of patients | Sperm count ($\times 10^6$/mL) | | Pregnancies (%) |
			Pretreatment	Posttreatment	
Ronnberg[101]	50 mg/d	27	13.3	28.7*	11.4
	Placebo	29	17.3	17.3	3.4
Abel et al.[3]	50 mg/d	98	30 (0-99)		17
	Vitamin C	86	30 (0-92)		13
	50 mg/d	10	<20		5
	Vitamin C	14	<20		0
Wang et al.[129]	25 mg/d	11	8.8	15.3*	36.4
	50 mg/d	18	7.1	10.9*	22.2
	Placebo	7	8.2	8.3	0
Sokol et al.[117]	25 mg/d	11	17.8	30.2	9.1
	Placebo	9	17.5	21.6	44.4

*Statistically significant increase in sperm concentration.

Tamoxifen citrate. Tamoxifen citrate, another antiestrogen, is thought to have less intrinsic estrogen activity than clomiphene citrate. There are reports that it may improve sperm concentration and perhaps pregnancy rates, but randomized, placebo-controlled studies with this compound cannot be found.

Aromatase inhibitor. Estradiol has a direct adverse effect on the germinal epithelium independent of its ability to suppress gonadotropin secretion. It has been postulated that the germinal epithelium of patients with idiopathic oligospermia might be exposed to increased concentrations of estradiol, and that inhibition of aromatase, the enzyme that converts testosterone to estradiol, might enhance spermatogenesis in these patients. Clark and Sherins[20] randomized 25 men into two groups. Patients were treated with placebo or testolactone (2 g/d) for 8 months and were crossed over to the other regimen for an additional 8 months. Testolactone had no significant effect on sperm density, and there were no pregnancies.

Testosterone suppression. There have been two rationales for using an exogenous androgen to treat azoospermic or oligospermic infertile men. First, it has been proposed that suppression of FSH and LH with an exogenous androgen can suppress spermatogenesis and azoospermia and that after stopping testosterone there will be a rebound in spermatogenesis. Second, suppression of spermatogenesis might be useful in men who have antibodies directed toward antigens on developing spermatids. Wang and colleagues[129] randomized seven patients into a placebo group and nine patients into a group that received testosterone enanthate (250 mg every 2 weeks for 4 months) and then followed them for at least 5 months with no therapy. The mean sperm count was 0.16 million/mL at the end of 4 months in the treated group. Post-treatment sperm density was not increased over the control period, and there were no pregnancies in either group.

Bromocriptine. The possibility that normal or minimally elevated serum levels of prolactin might impair spermatogenesis has been evaluated. Glatthaar and colleagues[46] conducted a double-blind, crossover study in five azoospermic and five oligospermic men. Bromocriptine (2.5 mg orally three times daily) was given for 4 months. Prolactin levels fell, but there was no improvement in sperm density. In a similar study, AinMelk and co-workers[6] administered 5 mg of bromocriptine per day for 4 months to 17 infertile oligospermic men. There was no improvement in sperm density, motility, or morphology. There was one pregnancy in each group 4 and 6 weeks after cessation of therapy.

Miscellaneous agents. Initially, it was hoped that treatment of eugonadotropic men with hCG plus hMG might stimulate spermatogenesis.[71,88] The expense, the necessity of giving both agents intramuscularly for several months, and lack of evidence that these agents were more effective than clomiphene citrate have discouraged investigators from conducting large, randomized, placebo-controlled trials. One study in a limited number of men failed to demonstrate a beneficial effect.[59]

Pentoxifylline, a methylxanthine, was used in the randomized study by Wang and colleagues.[129] Patients received 400 mg four times daily for 4 months. There was no improvement in sperm density, and there were no pregnancies.

The nonsteroidal antiinflammatory agent indomethacin has been evaluated by Barkay and co-workers[12] in a placebo-controlled, nonrandomized, open study. They reported that 25 mg/d and 75 mg/d, but not 100 mg/d resulted in more than a twofold increase in sperm density when compared with the control period and 35% and 30% pregnancy rates as compared with 8% for the placebo group. These results have not been confirmed.

Other agents that have been tried and reported in the medical literature to have some effect on semen quality include ionized zinc, captopril, and some neurotransmitters. Patients who have prostatitis have been observed to be deficient in zinc, and therapy with zinc has been reported to improve sperm density.[72] Captopril, which inhibits conversion of kininogen to kinin, has been used on the theoretic basis that kinin adversely affects reproductive function.[91] The combination of an α_1-adrenergic inhibitor and a β-adrenergic agonist has been reported to improve sperm density.[136] To date, there have been no reported randomized, placebo-controlled studies with any of these agents.

Hypergonadotropic

A twofold or greater elevation in the concentration of FSH has been considered an indication that the testes have been irreversibly damaged and that no medical or surgical treatment would be of benefit. Usually FSH values more than two times normal are associated with some degree of testicular atrophy. Most of these patients have normal serum testosterone values, but LH values frequently are increased.

Congenital syndromes. Elevated serum FSH levels may be seen in patients who have cryptorchid testes or who have had orchiopexy for unilateral or bilateral cryptorchid testes. Patients with Klinefelter syndrome usually present with infertility, small testes, variable degrees of androgen deficiency, azoospermia, and elevated FSH levels. This syndrome occurs with a frequency of approximately 1 in 600 male births. Patients with the vanishing testes syndrome have had functional testes during the early phases of gestation but are born without detectable testes. As previously noted, patients with a varicocele and unilateral testicular atrophy may have an elevated FSH level.

Patients with myotonic dystrophy have elevated FSH levels during the third and fourth decades of life, although they usually are fertile during their early reproductive years. Later in life they develop androgen deficiency. At this time there is no means for preventing the testicular disease associated with this syndrome.

Infections. Patients who have had bacterial or viral orchitis can present with oligospermia/azoospermia and elevated serum FSH levels. Preventive or early therapy of individuals who are at risk for developing mumps orchitis has received some attention. The practice of immunization for mumps virus during early childhood has greatly reduced the incidence of mumps orchitis. A recent study suggests that treatment with interferon-α2B during acute mumps orchitis may prevent late sequelae.[40]

Toxins. Several environmental, nutritional, industrial, and medical compounds are recognized to impair androgen action or to be testicular toxins. Drugs that have antiandrogen effects such as cimetidine, spironolactone, and flutamide can reduce testicular and accessory sex gland function. Chronic alcoholism is known to cause liver disease and secondarily testicular atrophy. Alcohol also can impair spermatogenesis by direct effects on the testes in the absence of liver disease.[126] The pesticide dibromochloropropane causes testicular damage that may be reversible, depending on the extent and duration of exposure.[60] Several antibiotics, including nitrofurans and aminoglycosides, impair spermatogenesis in lower species.[109] Chemotherapeutic agents such as cyclophosphamide, busulfan, methotrexate, and chlorambucil may cause reversible or irreversible damage, depending in part on the dose and duration of therapy.[32,108] FSH levels more than two times normal usually indicate irreversible damage, but moderate elevation may be transient. Unfortunately, neither suppression of spermatogenesis with an exogenous androgen nor with a long-acting GnRH agonist has been able to provide protection from these agents. These chemotherapeutic agents act directly on the spermatogonia, which are mitotically active even when gonadotropins are suppressed.

Unilateral orchiectomy. Patients who have had unilateral orchiectomy for testicular torsion, cryptorchidism, trauma, or tumor frequently have an elevated FSH even when the semen quality is within the normal range. FSH levels tend to be higher and there tends to be compensatory hypertrophy of the remaining testis when orchiectomy occurs before or during puberty. Many of these patients are fertile.

Idiopathic. Finally, some patients with idiopathic azoospermia/oligospermia are included in this group. Some patients have tubular sclerosis, an arrest of spermatogenesis at the spermatogonia or spermatocyte stage or germinal cell aplasia, but others have only hypospermatogenesis. The possibility has been raised that some of these patients have abnormal pulsatile secretion of GnRH rather than irreversible testicular disease as a primary cause for the increase in serum FSH level. In one study involving 14 men with elevated FSH levels and normal LH and testosterone levels, patients were treated with 4 μg of GnRH every 120 minutes for 6 months. FSH levels were decreased to normal and mean LH levels increased, but testosterone levels were not

changed. Sperm density was increased in eight men, and three pregnancies occurred during treatment.[8] Bals-Pratsch and co-workers[11] treated six men with sperm density less than 5 million/mL and three azoospermic men with 5 μg of GnRH every 90 minutes for 24 weeks and noted no improvement. In a preliminary study involving seven men with selective elevation of FSH levels, Matsumoto and colleagues[79] administered 5 μg of GnRH every 90 minutes for a minimum of 6 months. LH levels and pulse frequency were increased, FSH levels tended to fall, and testosterone values increased. The five azoospermic men remained azoospermic. Neither of the oligospermic men had a significant improvement in semen quality, but one man impregnated his wife during treatment. Although there is a suggestion that there may be some patients with oligospermia and selective elevation of FSH levels who might benefit from chronic pulsatile GnRH, the studies are very limited and uncontrolled.

ASTHENOSPERMIA

Many patients have a sperm count of more than 10 million/mL of ejaculate but poor sperm motility. The sperm are able to exclude dye, indicating that they are viable. It is tempting to think that the seminal plasma is deficient in a motility factor or perhaps there is an inhibitory factor; however, donor seminal plasma rarely improves sperm motility.[68] Frequently, asthenospermia is associated with abnormal sperm morphology. The availability of technology that permits more precise measurement of motility offers the investigator an opportunity to study conditions associated with asthenospermia in much greater detail. It is to be hoped that carefully conducted studies in the near future will address conditions associated with asthenospermia.

Varicocele

Clinicians have reported for many years that improvement in sperm motility is the most consistent change in semen quality that follows varicocelectomy. Interestingly, this observation is supported by the studies in the primate model for varicocele.[53] The reports of enhanced fertility rates after varicocelectomy usually are associated with improvements in sperm motility and sperm penetration.[100]

Infection of accessory sex glands

The possibility that infection of the accessory sex glands impairs fertility, primarily by reducing sperm motility, has been evaluated. Male accessory sex gland infection was diagnosed in 1.6% of 2871 infertile couples who were evaluated at seven centers using a World Health Organization protocol.[25] The diagnosis was based on (1) a history of recurrent infections of the genitourinary system; (2) the presence of 40 white blood cells or a positive bacterial culture in expressed prostatic fluid; (3) the presence of peroxidase-positive white blood cells (more than 1 million/

mL) in the ejaculate; (4) uniform growth of 10^3 or more pathogens or 10^4 or more nonpathogens per milliliter of semen; or (5) abnormal biochemical parameters such as low fructose levels, low acid phosphatase levels, abnormal seminal pH, increased viscosity after liquefaction, or the presence of mucus threads. Patients and their partners were observed for 1 to 3 months before being randomly assigned to receive placebo or doxycycline for 30 days. Signs of infection disappeared in both groups and sperm motility increased in both groups. Doxycycline treatment did not improve sperm motility or pregnancy rates when compared with placebo treatment.

Antisperm antibodies

Antibodies to sperm have been shown to reduce sperm motility and the ability of sperm to penetrate cervical mucus and zona-free hamster eggs. Infection with *Chlamydia trachomatis* has been reported to increase spermagglutinating antibodies in serum, but the presence of antibody to *C. trachomatis* was not associated with a significant change in semen quality.[22] Vasectomy usually results in the development of antibodies to sperm. There is evidence that the presence of immunoglobulin A and the titer of antibody in the serum are inversely correlated with fertility rates in men who undergo vasectomy reversal.[82] Most patients who present with idiopathic asthenospermia and antisperm antibodies in the serum or seminal plasma or on ejaculated sperm do not have a documented infection of the genitourinary system. Pregnancies associated with immunosuppressive therapy have been reported, but there are few controlled studies. Immunosuppressive therapy does carry some risk. A recent report by Hendry et al.[55] involved 43 subfertile men who were given prednisolone (20 mg twice daily) in a double-blind, crossover study. There were nine pregnancies during treatment with prednisolone, compared with two with placebo. (See Chapter 22.) Suppression of spermatogenesis with an exogenous androgen might reduce antibodies directed toward antigens on developing spermatids; however, there is no scientific evidence that this approach is beneficial.

Drugs

Three antibiotics have been reported to reduce sperm motility. Sulfasalazine, a drug that is used chronically to treat ulcerative colitis, has been reported to reduce sperm motility and sperm counts. Erythromycin and chlortetracycline, two agents that may be used on a chronic basis, have been reported to impair sperm motility.[131] There is little evidence that the latter agents cause infertility.

Intrinsic structural abnormalities

The sperm tails from patients with Young syndrome have fewer central pair microtubules, radial spokes, and inner dynein arms. The cilia of their respiratory tracts also contain fewer dynein arms.[134] These men may have chronic sinopulmonary infection. Patients with Kartagener syndrome have immotile sperm and radial spoke or dynein arm defects.[39,121]

Idiopathic

Asthenospermia in the majority of men is not associated with any of the previously discussed entities. Since understanding of sperm motility is advancing rapidly, it is likely that many patients who currently are classified as having idiopathic asthenospermia will have specific defects of the motility apparatus or metabolic deficiencies that impair motility. It is likely that patients with reduced but not absent sperm motility have fewer severe structural abnormalities.

Asthenospermia has been treated empirically with exogenous androgen. It has been reasoned that exogenous androgen might have a direct effect on accessory sex glands to improve sperm motility and maturation. Mesterolone and testosterone undecanoate have been best studied.

Mesterolone (1α-methyl-5α-androstan-17β-ol-3-one) has been used primarily in Europe in an attempt to improve sperm motility. This agent does not cause much suppression of FSH, even at a dose of 150 mg/d[45]; but this dose does cause some suppression of LH and testosterone. Four randomized studies with mesterolone have been published.[2,45,52,135] There was no consistent improvement in sperm motility or in sperm density. Pregnancy rates were not improved by treatment with mesterolone.

Testosterone undecanoate is an oral androgen that is used in countries other than the United States. It has been demonstrated to be a more potent androgen in men than is mesterolone. The undecanoate side chain causes testosterone undecanoate to be taken up by the intestinal lymphatics, enabling it to escape immediate metabolism by the liver. It still has a short half-life, which requires dosing three or four times a day. Comhaire[24] treated 20 men with 240 mg of testosterone undecanoate per day. They were randomly assigned to 3 months of active drug or to placebo and then crossed over to the other regimen. Neither LH nor FSH levels were consistently suppressed. There was no significant improvement in sperm concentration, viability, motility, or morphology. Two pregnancies occurred early in the study and were not attributed to treatment.

ASSISTED REPRODUCTION

Artificial insemination

Artificial insemination using husband's sperm (AIH) is thought to be useful for a limited number of conditions associated with infertility. Patients with severe hypospadias, retrograde ejaculation, low ejaculate volume, neurologic impotence, and sexual dysfunction refractory to counseling may be candidates for AIH. Evidence that intravaginal insemination is effective for treating idiopathic oligospermia is less convincing. Nachtigall and colleagues[87] reviewed this topic and reported a pregnancy rate of 18% with AIH in 408 couples, compared with 14% in controls.

Intrauterine insemination (IUI) for male factor infertility also has been reported to result in a pregnancy rate of 18%. (See also Chapters 41 and 42.)

IUI currently uses techniques that select sperm with progressive motility. In a recent report, 81 couples underwent IUI for male factor infertility.[44] Altogether, 18 pregnancies resulted over 276 cycles (6.5% per cycle). Martinez and co-workers[74] have compared timed natural intercourse with IUI in 40 infertile men and their mates who had either spontaneous or clomiphene citrate–induced ovulation. There were five pregnancies in cycles treated with clomiphene citrate and IUI and three pregnancies in spontaneous cycles with IUI. Only one pregnancy was associated with timed intercourse in a stimulated cycle. IUI also has been compared by Hewitt and colleagues[56] with in vitro fertilization (IVF) in 50 couples. Pregnancies occurred in 4.7% of cycles treated by IUI and 21.2% of cycles treated by IVF.

Gamete intrafallopian transfer

Gamete intrafallopian transfer (GIFT) has proven to be an effective approach for treating male factor infertility. GIFT was used for male factor infertility in 578 transfer cycles in the 1989 U.S. Registry of centers conducting IVF–embryo transfer and related techniques.[81] Pregnancies resulted in 31% of the transfers.

Zygote intrafallopian transfer

The use of zygote intrafallopian transfer (ZIFT) has been used much less often than either GIFT or IVF for male factor infertility. Whereas one cannot determine whether failure is due to lack of fertilization or to failure to implant when GIFT is used, ZIFT permits better identification of the problem. Patients treated with ZIFT for male factor infertility were not identified in the 1989 Registry.

In vitro fertilization

IVF now offers men with poor semen quality more than just hope for achieving fertility. In the 1989 U.S. Registry, 23.4% of the 9911 stimulated cycles were for male factor abnormalities.[81] Eggs were retrieved in 82% of the cycles, but embryos were transferred in only 42.5% of the cycles in which eggs were available for fertilization. This compares with 74.5% of cycles in which tubal factors were the indication for IVF. The clinical pregnancy rate per cycle and the live delivery rate per cycle of 20% and 15%, respectively, were similar to those with other conditions. De Kretser and colleagues[34] have emphasized the detrimental effects of multiple sperm abnormalities. Acosta and colleagues[4] have noted very poor fertilization rates when there were less than 1.5 million motile sperm after using the swim-up technique to improve semen quality. They also have noted a fertilization rate of 49.5% when less than 14% of sperm exhibited normal morphology, whereas specimens with more than 14% normal sperm morphology had a fertilization rate of 88.3%. The impaired fertilization rate could be overcome by increasing the ratio of sperm per milliliter to egg from 50,000 to 500,000.

At this time several approaches are being undertaken to improve the fertilization rate and the live birth rate per cycle. Treatment of the men with FSH for 3 months did not improve semen parameters, but the fertilization rate and the rate of live births per cycle were improved in one limited study.[5] It may be possible to increase the number of motile sperm by obtaining two ejaculates at 2-hour intervals,[123] by using prolonged incubation,[19] or by adding pentoxifylline to the ejaculate.[137] Other techniques being evaluated include the use of smaller droplet size, microinjection of sperm under the zona pellucida,[61] and microdrilling into the zona.[47] Interestingly, the latter technique has been reported to increase the pregnancy rate by facilitating implantation.[23]

SUMMARY

Recent years have witnessed significant advancements in our understanding of the biology of spermatogenesis and of the accessory sex glands, sperm capacitation, and fertilization. To date this knowledge has most affected patients in the area of assisted reproduction. While there are good reasons to believe that there will continue to be technological breakthroughs in assisted reproduction, it is also likely that information gained from basic research will begin to expand diagnostic and therapeutic considerations in the clinical management of subfertile males.

REFERENCES

1. Aafjes JH, van der Vijver JCM: Fertility of men with and without a varicocele, *Fertil Steril* 43:901, 1985.
2. Aafjes JH et al: Double-blind crossover treatment with mesterolone and placebo of subfertile oligospermic men: value of testicular biopsy, *Andrologia* 15:531, 1983.
3. Abel BJ et al: Randomised trial of clomiphene citrate treatment and vitamin C for male infertility, *Br J Urol* 54:780, 1982.
4. Acosta AA et al: Assisted reproduction in the diagnosis and treatment of the male factor, *Obstet Gynecol Surv* 44:1, 1988.
5. Acosta AA et al: Possible role of pure human follicle-stimulating hormone in the treatment of severe male-factor infertility by assisted reproduction: preliminary report, *Fertil Steril* 55:1150, 1991.
6. AinMelk Y et al: Bromocriptine therapy in oligozoospermic infertile men, *Arch Androl* 8:135, 1982.
7. Al-Ansari AA-K et al: Isolated follicle-stimulating hormone deficiency in men: successful long-term gonadotropin therapy, *Fertil Steril* 42:618, 1984.
8. Aulitzky W, Frick J, Hadziselimovic F: Pulsatile LHRH therapy in patients with oligozoospermia and disturbed LH pulsatility, *Int J Androl* 12:265, 1989.
9. Ayers JWT et al: Anthropomorphic, hormonal, and psychologic correlates of semen quality in endurance-trained male athletes, *Fertil Steril* 43:917, 1985.
10. Bagatell CJ, Bremner WJ: Sperm counts and reproductive hormones in male marathoners and lean controls, *Fertil Steril* 53:688, 1990.
11. Bals-Pratsch M et al: Pulsatile GnRH-therapy in oligozoospermic men does not improve seminal parameters despite decreased FSH levels, *Clin Endocrinol* 30:549, 1989.
12. Barkay J et al: The prostaglandin inhibitor effect of antiinflammatory drugs in the therapy of male infertility, *Fertil Steril* 42:406, 1984.

13. Bonaccorsi AC, Adler I, Figueiredo JG: Male infertility due to congenital adrenal hyperplasia: testicular biopsy findings, hormonal evaluation, and therapeutic results in three patients, *Fertil Steril* 47:664, 1987.

14. Bostofte E et al: Fertility prognosis for infertile men: results of follow-up study of semen analysis in infertile men from two different populations evaluated by the Cox regression model, *Fertil Steril* 54:1100, 1990.

15. Bremner WJ et al: Follicle-stimulating hormone and human spermatogenesis, *J Clin Invest* 68:1044, 1981.

16. Brodie BL, Wentz AC: Late onset congenital adrenal hyperplasia: a gynecologist's perspective, *Fertil Steril* 48:175, 1987.

17. Burris AS et al: Gonadotropin therapy in men with isolated hypogonadotropic hypogonadism: the response to human chorionic gonadotropin is predicted by initial testicular size, *J Clin Endocrinol Metab* 66:1144, 1988.

18. Burris AS et al: A low sperm concentration does not preclude fertility in men with isolated hypogonadotropic hypogonadism after gonadotropin therapy, *Fertil Steril* 50:343, 1988.

19. Chan Y-M, Chan SYW, Tucket MJ: Successful pregnancies resulting from the use of prolonged-incubation human spermatozoa in gamete intrafallopian transfer, *Fertil Steril* 54:730, 1990.

20. Clark RV, Sherins RJ: Treatment of men with idiopathic oligozoospermic infertility using the aromatase inhibitor, testolactone, *J Androl* 10:240, 1989.

21. Clermont Y: The cycle of the seminiferous epithelium in man, *Am J Anat* 112:35, 1963.

22. Close CE et al: The relationship of infection with *Chlamydia trachomatis* to the parameters of male fertility and sperm autoimmunity, *Fertil Steril* 48:880, 1987.

23. Cohen J et al: Impairment of the hatching process following IVF in the human and improvement of implantation by assisting hatching using micromanipulation, *Hum Reprod* 5:7, 1990.

24. Comhaire F: Treatment of idiopathic testicular failure with high-dose testosterone undecanoate: a double-blind pilot study, *Fertil Steril* 54:689, 1990.

25. Comhaire FH, Rowe PJ, Farley TMM: The effect of doxycycline in infertile couples with male accessory gland infection: a double blind prospective study, *Int J Androl* 9:91, 1986.

26. Cooper TG: In defense of a function for the human epididymis, *Fertil Steril* 54:965, 1990.

27. Crich JP, Jequier AM: Infertility in men with retrograde ejaculation: the action of urine on sperm motility, and a simple method for achieving antegrade ejaculation, *Fertil Steril* 30:572, 1978.

28. Cullen MR, Kayne RD, Robins JM: Endocrine and reproductive dysfunction in men associated with occupational inorganic lead intoxication, *Arch Environ Health* 39:431, 1984.

29. Cunningham GR, Huckins C: An FSH and prolactin-secreting pituitary tumor: pituitary dynamics and testicular histology, *J Clin Endocrinol Metab* 44:248, 1977.

30. Cunningham GR et al: Mechanisms for the testicular hypertrophy which follows hemicastration, *Endocrinology* 102:16, 1978.

31. Cutfield RG, Bateman JM, Odell WD: Infertility caused by bilateral testicular masses secondary to congenital adrenal hyperplasia (21-hydroxylase deficiency), *Fertil Steril* 40:809, 1983.

32. Damewood MD, Grochow LB: Prospects for fertility after chemotherapy or radiation for neoplastic disease, *Fertil Steril* 45:443, 1986.

33. de Kretser DM: Germ cell-Sertoli cell interactions, *Reprod Fertil Dev* 2:225, 1990.

34. de Kretser DM, Yates C, Kovacs GT: The use of IVF in the management of male infertility, *Clin Obstet Gynecol* 12:767, 1985.

35. De Sanctis V et al: Induction of spermatogenesis in thalassemia, *Fertil Steril* 50:969, 1988.

36. Diamond T, Stiel D, Posen S: Osteoporosis in hemochromatosis: iron excess, gonadal deficiency, or other factors?, *Ann Intern Med* 110:430, 1989.

37. Dubin L, Amelar RD: Varicocelectomy: twenty-five years of experience, *Int J Fertil* 33:226, 1988.

38. Ducot B et al: Male factors and the likelihood of pregnancy in infertile couples, II: study of clinical characteristics—practical consequences, *Int J Androl* 11:395-404, 1988.

39. Eliasson R et al: The immotile-cilia syndrome: a congenital ciliary abnormality as an etiologic factor in chronic airway infections and male sterility, *N Engl J Med* 297:1, 1977.

40. Erpenbach KHJ: Systemic treatment with interferon-α2B: an effective method to prevent sterility after bilateral mumps orchitis, *J Urol* 146:54, 1991.

41. Faiman C et al: The "fertile eunuch" syndrome: demonstration of isolated luteinizing hormone deficiency by radioimmunoassay technique, *Mayo Clin Proc* 43:661, 1968.

42. Fiet J et al: Comparison of basal and adrenocorticotropin-stimulated plasma 21-deoxycortisol and 17-hydroxyprogesterone values as biological markers of late-onset adrenal hyperplasia, *J Clin Endocrinol Metab* 66:659, 1988.

43. Finkel D, Phillips JL, Snyder PJ: Stimulation of spermatogenesis by gonadotropins in men with hypogonadotropic hypogonadism, *N Engl J Med* 313:651, 1985.

44. Friedman AJ et al: Life table analysis of intrauterine insemination pregnancy rates for couples with cervical factor, male factor, and idiopathic infertility, *Fertil Steril* 55:1005, 1991.

45. Gerris J et al: Placebo-controlled trial of high-dose mesterolone treatment of idiopathic male infertility, *Fertil Steril* 55:603, 1991.

46. Glatthaar C et al: Pituitary function in normoprolactinaemic infertile men receiving bromocriptine, *Clin Endocrinol* 13:455, 1980.

47. Gordon KW et al: Fertilization of human oocytes by sperm from infertile males after zona pellucida drilling, *Fertil Steril* 50:68, 1988.

48. Greenhall E, Vessey M: The prevalence of subfertility: a review of the current confusion and a report of two new studies, *Fertil Steril* 54:978, 1990.

49. Grinsted J, Byskov AG: Meiosis-inducing and meiosis-preventing substances in human male reproductive organs, *Fertil Steril* 35:199, 1981.

50. Gross K et al: Increased frequency of pulsatile luteinizing hormone-releasing hormone administration selectively decreases follicle-stimulating hormone levels in men with idiopathic azoospermia, *Fertil Steril* 45:392, 1986.

51. Hargreave TB et al: Searching for the infertile man with hyperprolactinemia, *Fertil Steril* 36:630, 1981.

52. Hargreave TB et al: Randomised trial of mesterolone versus vitamin C for male infertility, *Br Med J* 56:740, 1984.

53. Harrison RM, Lewis RW, Roberts JA: Pathophysiology of varicocele in nonhuman primates: long-term seminal and testicular changes, *Fertil Steril* 46:500, 1986.

54. Heller CG, Clermont Y: Kinetics of the germinal epithelium in man, *Recent Prog Horm Res* 20:545, 1964.

55. Hendry WF et al: Comparison of prednisolone and placebo in subfertile men with antibodies to spermatozoa, *Lancet* 335:85, 1990.

56. Hewitt J et al: Treatment of idiopathic infertility, cervical mucus hostility, and male infertility: artificial insemination with husband's semen or in vitro fertilization?, *Fertil Steril* 44:350, 1985.

57. Jequier AM, Crich JC, Ansell ID: Clinical findings and testicular histology in three hyperprolactinemic infertile men, *Fertil Steril* 31:525, 1979.

58. Knuth UA, Maniera H, Nieschlag E: Anabolic steroids and semen parameters in bodybuilders, *Fertil Steril* 52:1041, 1989.

59. Knuth UA et al: Treatment of severe oligospermia with human chorionic gonadotropin/human menopausal gonadotropin: a placebo-controlled, double blind trial, *J Clin Endocrinol Metab* 65:1081, 1987.

60. Lantz G et al: Recovery of severe oligospermia after exposure to dibromochloropropane (DBCP), *Fertil Steril* 35:46, 1981.

61. Lanzendorf S et al: Fertilizing potential of acrosome-defective sperm following microsurgical injection into eggs, *Gamete Res* 19:329, 1988.

62. Ley SB, Leonard JM: Male hypogonadotropic hypogonadism: factors influencing response to human chorionic gonadotropin and human menopausal gonadotropin, including prior exogenous androgens, *J Clin Endocrinol Metab* 57:1041, 1983.

63. Liu L et al: Comparison of pulsatile subcutaneous gonadotropin-releasing hormone and exogenous gonadotropins in the treatment of men with isolated hypogonadotropic hypogonadism, *Fertil Steril* 49:302, 1988.

64. Lutton JP et al: Reversible gonadotropin deficiency in male Cushing's disease, *J Clin Endocrinol Metab* 45:488, 1977.

65. Lynch R et al: Improved seminal characteristics in infertile men after a conservative treatment regimen based on the avoidance of testicular hyperthermia, *Fertil Steril* 46:476, 1986.

66. MacConnie SE et al: Decreased hypothalamic gonadotropin-releasing hormone secretion in male marathon runners, *N Engl J Med* 315:411, 1986.

67. Maddocks S et al: Regulation of the testis, *J Reprod Immunol* 18:33, 1990.

68. Magnus O et al: Effects of seminal plasma from normal and asthenozoospermic men on the progressive motility of washed human sperm, *Int J Androl* 14:44, 1991.

69. Mancini A et al: Bromocriptine in the management of infertile men after surgery of prolactin secreting adenomas, *J Androl* 5:294, 1984.

70. Mancini RE et al: Effect of testosterone in the recovery of spermatogenesis in hypophysectomized patients: hormones and antagonists, *Gynecol Invest* 2:98, 1971.

71. Margalioth EJ et al: Treatment of oligoasthenospermia with human chorionic gonadotropin: hormonal profiles and results, *Fertil Steril* 39:841, 1983.

72. Marmar JL et al: Semen zinc levels in infertile and postvasectomy patients and patients with prostatitis, *Fertil Steril* 26:1057, 1975.

73. Marshall GR et al: Stimulation of spermatogenesis in stalk-sectioned rhesus monkeys by testosterone alone, *J Clin Endocrinol Metab* 57:152, 1983.

74. Martinez AR et al: Intrauterine insemination does and clomiphene citrate does not improve fecundity in couples with infertility due to male or idiopathic factors: a prospective, randomized, controlled study, *Fertil Steril* 53:847, 1990.

75. Matsumoto AM, Bremner WJ: Stimulation of sperm production by human chorionic gonadotropin after prolonged gonadotropin suppression in normal men, *J Androl* 6:137, 1985.

76. Matsumoto AM, Karpas AE, Bremner WJ: Chronic human chorionic gonadotropin administration in normal men: evidence that follicle-stimulating hormone is necessary for the maintenance of quantitatively normal spermatogenesis in man, *J Clin Endocrinol Metab* 62:1184, 1986.

77. Matsumoto AM, Paulsen CA, Bremner WJ: Stimulation of sperm production by human luteinizing hormone in gonadotropin-suppressed normal men, *J Clin Endocrinol Metab* 55:882, 1984.

78. Matsumoto AM et al: Reinitiation of sperm production in gonadotropin-suppressed normal men by administration of follicle-stimulating hormone, *J Clin Invest* 72:1005, 1983.

79. Matsumoto AM et al: The luteinizing hormone-releasing hormone pulse generator in men: abnormalities and clinical management, *Am J Obstet Gynecol* 163:1743, 1990.

80. McCullagh EP, Beck JC, Schaffenberg CA: A syndrome of eunuchoidism with spermatogenesis, normal urinary FSH and low or normal ICSH: ("fertile eunuchs"), *J Clin Endocrinol Metab* 13:489, 1953.

81. Medical Research International: In vitro fertilization-embryo transfer (IVF-ET) in the United States: 1989 results from the IVF-ET registry, *Fertil Steril* 55:14, 1991.

82. Meinertz H et al: Antisperm antibodies and fertility after vasovasostomy: a follow-up study of 216 men, *Fertil Steril* 54:315, 1990.

83. Melmed S et al: Pituitary tumors secreting growth hormone and prolactin, *Ann Intern Med* 105:238, 1986.

84. Morris DV et al: The response of patients with organic hypothalamic-pituitary disease to pulsatile gonadotropin-releasing hormone therapy, *Fertil Steril* 47:54, 1987.

85. Mozaffarian GA, Highley M, Paulsen CA: Clinical studies in an adult male patient with "isolated follicle stimulating hormone (FSH) deficiency," *J Androl* 4:393, 1983.

86. Murray FT, Cameron DF, Ketchum C: Return of gonadal function in men with prolactin-secreting pituitary tumors, *J Clin Endocrinol Metab* 59:79, 1984.

87. Nachtigall RD, Faure N, Glass RH: Artificial insemination of husband's sperm, *Fertil Steril* 32:141, 1979.

88. Namiki M et al: Testicular follicle stimulating hormone receptors and effectiveness of human menopausal gonadotropin-human chorionic gonadotropin treatment of infertile men, *Clin Endocrinol* 25:495, 1986.

89. Ojeifo JO, Winters SJ, Troen P: Basal and adrenocortocotropic hormone-stimulated serum 17α-hydroxyprogesterone in men with idiopathic infertility, *Fertil Steril* 42:97, 1984.

90. Okuyama A et al: Testicular responsiveness to long-term administration of hCG and hMG in patients with hypogonadotropic hypogonadism, *Horm Res* 23:21, 1986.

91. Parsch E-M, Schill W-B: Captopril: a new approach for treatment of male subfertility?, *Andrologia* 537, 1988.

92. Partsch C-J, Sippell WG: Hypothalamic hypogonadism in congenital adrenal hypoplasia, *Horm Metab Res* 21:623, 1989.

93. Parvinen M: Regulation of the seminiferous epithelium, *Endocr Rev* 3:404, 1982.

94. Parvinen M, Vihko KK, Toppari J: Cell interactions during the seminiferous epithelial cycle, *Int Rev Cytol* 104:115, 1986.

95. Pasqualini RQ, Bur G: Hypoandrogenic syndrome with spermatogenesis, *Fertil Steril* 6:144, 1955.

96. Plymate SR et al: The use of sperm penetration assay in evaluation of men with varicocele, *Fertil Steril* 47:680, 1987.

97. Pont A et al: Prolactin-secreting tumors in men: surgical cure, *Ann Intern Med* 91:211, 1979.

98. Rabinowitz D et al: Isolated follicle-stimulating hormone revisited, *N Engl J Med* 300:126, 1979.

99. Rodriguez-Rigau LJ, Smith KD, Steinberger E: Relationship of varicocele to sperm output and fertility of male partners in infertile couples, *J Urol* 120:691, 1978.

100. Rogers BJ et al: Monitoring of suspected infertile men with varicocele by the sperm penetration assay, *Fertil Steril* 44:800, 1985.

101. Ronnberg L: The effect of clomiphene citrate on different sperm parameters and serum hormone levels in preselected infertile men: a controlled double-blind cross-over study, *Int J Androl* 3:479, 1980.

102. Rosenthal SM, Grumbach MM, Kaplan SL: Gonadotropin-independent familial sexual precocity with premature Leydig and germinal cell maturation (familial testotoxicosis): effects of a potent luteinizing hormone-releasing factor agonist and medroxyprogesterone acetate therapy in four cases, *J Clin Endocrinol Metab* 57:571, 1983.

103. Saez JM et al: Paracrine regulation of testicular function, *J Steroid Biochem* 27:317, 1987.

104. Saypol DC: Varicocele, *J Androl* 2:61, 1981.

105. Scammell GE et al: Retrograde ejaculation: successful treatment with artificial insemination, *Br J Urol* 63:198, 1989.

106. Schedewie HK et al: Testicular Leydig cell hyperplasia as a cause of sexual precocity, *J Clin Endocrinol Metab* 52:271, 1981.

107. Schill W-B: Pregnancy after brompheniramine treatment of a diabetic with incomplete emission failure, *Arch Androl* 25:101, 1990.

108. Schilsky RL et al: Gonadal dysfunction in patients receiving chemotherapy for cancer, *Ann Intern Med* 93:109, 1980.

109. Schlegel PN, Chang TSK, Marshall FF: Antibiotics: potential hazards to male fertility, *Fertil Steril* 55:235, 1991.
110. Segal S, Polishuk WZ, Ben-David M: Hyperprolactinemic male infertility, *Fertil Steril* 27:1425, 1976.
111. Shargil AA: Treatment of idiopathic hypogonadotropic hypogonadism in men with luteinizing hormone-releasing hormone: a comparison of treatment with daily injections and with the pulsatile infusion pump, *Fertil Steril* 47:492, 1987.
112. Sharpe RM: Paracrine control of the testis, *Clin Endocrinol Metab* 15:185, 1986.
113. Siemons LJ, Mahler CH: Hypogonadotropic hypogonadism in hemochromatosis: recovery of reproductive function after iron depletion, *J Clin Endocrinol Metab* 65:585, 1987.
114. Silber SJ et al: Congenital absence of the vas deferens, *N Engl J Med* 323:1788, 1990.
115. Sokol RZ: The effect of duration of exposure on the expression of lead toxicity on the male reproductive axis, *J Androl* 11:521, 1990.
116. Sokol RZ, Sparkes R: Demonstrated paternity in spite of severe idiopathic oligospermia, *Fertil Steril* 47:356, 1987.
117. Sokol RZ et al: A controlled comparison of the efficacy of clomiphene citrate in male infertility, *Fertil Steril* 49:865, 1988.
118. Steinberger E: Hormonal control of mammalian spermatogenesis, *Physiol Rev* 51:1, 1971.
119. Steinberger E, Rodriguez-Rigau LJ: The infertile couple, *J Androl* 4:111, 1983.
120. Steinberger E et al: The role of androgens in the initiation of spermatogenesis in man, *J Clin Endocrinol Metab* 37:746, 1973.
121. Sturgess JM et al: Cilia with defective radial spokes. *N Engl J Med* 300:53, 1979.
122. Sun Y-T et al: The effects of exogenously administered testosterone on spermatogenesis in intact and hypophysectomized rats. *Endocrinology* 125:1000, 1989.
123. Tur-Kaspa I et al: Pooled sequential ejaculates: a way to increase the total number of motile sperm from oligozoospermic men, *Fertil Steril* 54:906, 1990.
124. Uehling DT: Adrenal rest tumors of the testis: a case report of fertility following treatment, *Fertil Steril* 29:583, 1978.
125. Urban MD, Lee PA, Migeon CJ: Adult height and fertility in men with congenital virilizing adrenal hyperplasia, *N Engl J Med* 299:1392, 1978.
126. Van Thiel DH et al: Alcohol-induced testicular atrophy in the adult male rat, *Endocrinology* 105:888, 1979.
127. Vermeulen A, Vandeweghe M: Improved fertility after varicocele correction: fact or fiction?, *Fertil Steril* 42:249, 1984.
128. Wang C, Tso SC, Todd D: Hypogonadotropic hypogonadism in severe β-thalassemia: effect of chelation and pulsatile gonadotropin-releasing hormone therapy, *J Clin Endocrinol Metab* 68:511, 1989.
129. Wang C et al: Comparison of the effectiveness of placebo, clomiphene citrate, mesterolone, pentoxifylline, and testosterone rebound therapy for the treatment of idiopathic oligospermia, *Fertil Steril* 40:358, 1983.
130. Whitcomb RW, Crowley WF Jr: Clinical review, 4: diagnosis and treatment of isolated gonadotropin-releasing hormone deficiency in men, *J Clin Endocrinol Metab* 70:3, 1990.
131. White IG: The toxicity of some antibacterials for bull, ram, rabbit and human spermatozoa, *Aust J Exp Biol Med Sci* 32:41, 1954.
132. Wickings EJ et al: The role of follicle stimulating hormone in testicular function of the mature rhesus monkey, *Acta Endocrinol* 95:117, 1980.
133. Wierman ME et al: Puberty without gonadotropins, *N Engl J Med* 312:65, 1985.
134. Wilton LJ et al: Young's syndrome (obstructive azoospermia and chronic sinobronchial infection): a quantitative study of axonemal ultrastructure and function, *Fertil Steril* 55:144, 1991.
135. World Health Organization Task Force on the Diagnosis and Treatment of Infertility: Mesterolone and idiopathic male infertility: a double-blind study, *Int J Androl* 12:254, 1989.
136. Yamamoto M et al: Successful treatment of oligospermic and azoospermic men with α_1-blocker and β-stimulator: new treatment for idiopathic male infertility, *Fertil Steril* 46:1162, 1986.
137. Yovich JM et al: Influence of pentoxifylline in severe male factor infertility, *Fertil Steril* 53:715, 1990.
138. Zavos PM, Wilson EA: Retrograde ejaculation: etiology and treatment via the use of a new noninvasive method, *Fertil Steril* 42:627, 1984.

Chapter 21

IMMUNOLOGIC INFERTILITY

Warren R. Jones, MD

OVERVIEW

In the past decade or so, understanding of the mechanisms involved in both naturally occurring and experimentally induced immunologic inhibition of fertility has advanced considerably. The major practical interest in immunologic infertility undoubtedly lies in the mechanisms and clinical significance of immunity to spermatozoa in the man and the woman. (See Chapter 22.)

However, experimental models—both contrived and natural—in laboratory animals and in humans and the pathogenesis of certain clinical disorders inform us that immunologic processes may disrupt the reproductive process at several levels from its hormonal controls, through gametogenesis and fertilization to implantation and early placental and embryonic development. These disorders and their immunopathology form the substance of this chapter.

AUTOIMMUNITY INVOLVING THE ANTERIOR PITUITARY GLAND, ITS HORMONES, AND THEIR RECEPTORS

There are intriguing, but mostly anecdotal, reports in the literature suggesting that autoimmunity to the anterior pituitary gland, its hormones, and their receptors may contribute to, or result from, pathologic processes in reproduction. Pituitary autoimmunity is a recognized phenomenon,[6,63] but its clinical significance in most instances remains to be fully defined. Circulating autoantibodies directed against gonadotropes and other pituitary cell populations have been reported in patients with polyendocrine diseases,[63] diabetes mellitus,[59] and postpartum pituitary insufficiency.[29,31,38] The autoantibodies in postpartum women are likely to be a sequel to, rather than a cause of, overt or occult pituitary necrosis as part of Sheehan and Simmonds syndromes.

Circulating antigonadotropin cell antibodies have also been described in a proportion of boys with cryptorchidism and may be associated with the complex endocrine abnormalities comprising this disorder. Serum reactivity against pituitary cells is also found occasionally in a normal adult population[6,25] and was demonstrated in several normal women (including control subjects) undergoing a clinical trial of a contraceptive vaccine.[48] The clinical significance of these findings is unclear. There is also a more general problem dictating caution in assessing reports of pituitary autoimmunity based on serologic findings. This relates to the considerable methodologic difficulties in the standardization and interpretation of antibody-localization techniques using pituitary tissue substrates derived both from laboratory animals and from human cadavers.

There is now a well-established association of autoantibodies directed against hormone receptors with several endocrine disorders, including Graves disease, myasthenia gravis, and insulin-resistant diabetes mellitus. It is attractive, therefore, to consider that some categories of gonadal failure might have their genesis in autoimmune reactions to gonadotropin or prolactin receptors. Animal models have been described involving autoimmunity to these receptors,[5,54] but there is little evidence that similar mechanisms operate in clinical disorders in humans.

The resistant ovary syndrome described by Jones and Ruehsen[45] in 1969 comprises amenorrhea, elevated serum gonadotropin levels, and arrested ovarian follicular development. It requires differentiation from other, somewhat more intractable, causes of ovarian failure in which follicles are either mysteriously absent (idiopathic premature menopause) or have been destroyed (autoimmune ovarian failure), although the therapeutic implications deriving from such a differential diagnosis are probably illusory (see later). Lucky et al.[55] and Koninckx and Brosens[50] first suggested that the features of the resistant ovary syndrome were consistent with the presence of antibodies directed against gonadotropin receptors in the ovary. Evidence has accumulated for and against this hypothesis,[2,16,56,74] but the matter remains unresolved.

There is experimental evidence in nonhuman primates that immunization against follicle-stimulating hormone (FSH) will suppress spermatogenesis.[80] Antibodies to the FSH receptor have been described in association with primary gonadal failure in a man with polyostotic fibrous dysplasia and an immunoglobulinopathy.[25] There is no evidence from the literature, however, to suggest that gonadotropin receptor antibodies play a role in any of the less esoteric causes of male infertility.

Antigonadotropic activity was demonstrated in the urine of 52% of 50 women with the polycystic ovary (PCO, Stein-Leventhal) syndrome,[49] but it is unclear whether this was antibody related or due to metabolic inhibition. No subsequent evidence has appeared to support the interesting notion that the PCO syndrome might involve tonic ovarian stimulation by luteinizing hormone in the presence of autoantibodies to the hormone or its receptor molecule.

OVARIAN AUTOIMMUNITY

Although much less common in clinical practice than sperm immunity, there is now clear evidence that a proportion, perhaps 10%, of cases of premature ovarian failure belong to a spectrum of autoimmune diseases involving, primarily, endocrine glands. In a review of mechanisms whereby autoimmunity may cause abnormalities of ovarian function and other reproductive processes, Gleischer and El-Roeiy[36] coined the descriptive term *reproductive autoimmune failure syndrome.* (Additional information on premature ovarian failure is found in Chapter 54.)

It is of interest that much of the knowledge in this area has derived initially from clinical studies and "experiments of nature" rather than from animal experiments. However, just as a murine model for autoimmune orchitis can be established by neonatal (day 3) thymectomy in male animals (see above), a similar model of experimental autoimmune oophoritis has been described in female mice.[60] Lymphoid infiltration of the ovaries became intense about the time of puberty and was followed by progressive follicular destruction and ovarian atrophy. The serum contained autoantibodies against the zona pellucida, the theca cells, and the ooplasm of oocytes in secondary and tertiary follicles (i.e., growing), but not in primordial follicles. Levels of these antibodies diminished significantly at the end stage of ovarian atrophy when follicles had disappeared. This raised the question whether the absence of circulating antibodies to ovarian components excludes a diagnosis of autoimmune ovarian failure in the clinically occult situation, in which no other features of autoimmune disease are present. In any event, mice with autoimmune oophoritis demonstrated antibodies against gastric parietal and thyroid epithelial cells, in association with gastritis and thyroiditis.

Women with premature ovarian failure of autoimmune origin present within the clinical group of patients defined as having premature menopause. Up to 30% of such women exhibit organ-specific autoantibodies, which react with ovarian granulosa and theca cells.[23,66] Their serum may also contain antibodies reactive with steroid-producing cells in the testis, adrenal gland, and placenta.[3,42,43,66] There is also a serologic clinical association of this syndrome with other autoimmune disorders. This was first recognized because of a striking incidence of primary and secondary ovarian failure in women with Addisonian adrenal disease: 23% in one study[77] and 8% in another.[43] The premature ovarian failure tends to precede the adrenal failure by some years.[77,79] This finding has been confirmed by others, who recommend routine testing of adrenal reserve in all patients with premature ovarian failure, even though the yield may be low.[1,22,64]

Although it is now generally accepted that autoimmune abnormalities can cause ovarian failure, there is, however, a poor correlation with circulating antiovarian antibodies.[41] They are present in up to 100% of cases when ovarian and adrenal failure coexist[71] but were detected in only 1 of 45 cases when Addison disease was absent.[41]

In a report of 24 cases of premature ovarian failure, Mignot et al.[58] found serologic evidence of other autoimmune disorders in 22 (92%). Apart from Addison disease, the strongest serologic and clinical associations of autoimmune ovarian failure are with Hashimoto thyroiditis, Graves disease, and hypoparathyroidism.[1,20,66,79] Overall, the incidence of concomitant autoimmune disease has been reported, variously, as 55%,[66] 39%,[1] and 20%.[20] Other autoimmune associations reported in lower incidence include diabetes mellitus,[9] pernicious anemia, autoimmune thrombocytopenic purpura, autoimmune hemolytic anemia, Crohn disease, ulcerative colitis, rheumatoid arthritis, myasthenia gravis, alopecia, and vitiligo.*

It has been accepted clinical practice to perform ovarian biopsy at open laparotomy in women with secondary amenorrhea and increased FSH levels to differentiate premature menopause from the resistant ovary syndrome, in which primordial follicles are normal. On occasion, when an autoimmune cause exists, lymphocytic infiltration can be demonstrated.[21,37,43] Although in most cases of autoimmune premature ovarian failure (particularly those associated with other autoimmune diseases) ovarian biopsy fails to demonstrate primordial follicles, occasionally when the pathologic process is incomplete, follicles may be present.[20] Such patients may respond to glucocorticoid[21,42] or, rarely, may recover follicular activity spontaneously and menstruate.[75]

---

*References 1, 18, 20, 51, 66, 79, 82.

In practical terms, however, an increased FSH level denotes a poor prognosis for fertility whether the diagnosis is premature menopause or resistant ovary syndrome, and the value of ovarian biopsy has been questioned. This is reinforced by the fact that, although the presence of ovarian follicles in these patients may raise theoretic hopes for ovulation induction, the results of such treatment have been extremely poor. The advent of assisted reproductive techniques with the use of donor oocytes or embryos has offered real hope for childbearing in women with premature ovarian failure.

Autoimmune ovarian failure and its concomitants may present as primary amenorrhea in chromosomally normal girls.[20] The association of autoimmunity with cases of both primary and secondary amenorrhea underlines the fact that these two syndromes, although often clinically discrete, may merge imperceptibly to form a spectrum in which similar etiologic factors may operate. Vasquez and Kenny[79] describe two sisters who exemplified this fact. Both sisters had failure of adrenal, thyroid, and parathyroid function, with a family of tissue autoantibodies, including reactivity against ovarian follicles. One girl had primary amenorrhea and sexual infantilism, and the other menstruated for a short time before developing premature menopause.

In addition to the association of primary ovarian failure (pure ovarian dysgenesis) with autoimmunity, there have been a number of reports of the coexistence of Turner syndrome and other chromosomally determined cases of ovarian dysgenesis with autoimmune disease.[30,68,81] An abnormal incidence of tissue autoantibodies (notably against the thyroid gland) has been demonstrated in such patients by some investigators.[27,33,78]

It is an intriguing fact that ovarian embryogenesis is initially normal in Turner syndrome but that the primordial follicles disappear at some time during fetal and prepubertal development. (See Chapter 7.) There may be an immunologic basis for this phenomenon, but this possibility remains to be examined comprehensively by histologic and immunologic study of appropriate fetal and childhood material.

Ovarian participation in mumps virus infection is a rare but well-recognized occurrence. It is likely that this involvement, as well as causing primary tissue destruction, may also provoke an autoimmune reaction similar to that seen in mumps orchitis and in the (apparently) very rare condition of mumps adrenalitis.[19]

The zona pellucida (ZP) and its antigens have been investigated as potential targets for a contraceptive vaccine.[46] The possibility that naturally occurring autoantibodies to ZP may contribute to "unexplained" infertility has also attracted interest.[67,70] Difficulties in controlling and interpreting results for anti–ZP antibody assays have contributed to confusing data on the biologic significance of these antibodies, and at best any association with infertility would appear to be tenuous.[7,15,26]

EARLY PREGNANCY FAILURE

Although the spectrum of causes of reproductive failure in early pregnancy is covered in Chapter 49, it is pertinent to include here a brief account of these phenomena when they may be assumed (but not yet proved) to be relevant to occult periimplantation loss and therefore to infertility. The rationale for this incursion into pregnancy loss is that preclinical abortion appears to be at least as common as its clinically obvious counterpart.

Immunology of the mother-conceptus relationship

Before considering the ways in which the earliest stages of pregnancy may be disrupted by immunologic factors, it is important to summarize current knowledge and theory about the immunologic relationship between the mother and her conceptus. In 1953 Medawar[57] proposed three mechanisms to explain the immunologic paradox of placentation:

1. Anatomic separation of mother and fetus
2. Antigenic immaturity of the fetus
3. Immunologic unresponsiveness of the mother

Each component of this classic triad of theories is now known to be intrinsically incorrect. This knowledge, however, has been gained only through the efforts of a generation of scientists who have been stimulated by Medawar's writings to pursue the central questions in reproductive immunology.

Two clear statements may now be made about the immunologic paradox of mammalian pregnancy:

1. The allogeneic conceptus is not normally rejected by the mother.
2. Maternal immune recognition of the conceptus is essential to the success of pregnancy.

The components of maternal recognition and immunomodulation in pregnancy are summarized in the box below. The placenta can no longer be considered to be a mechanical barrier to immunologic contact between the mother and her allogeneic conceptus. Rather, the trophoblast plays a sophisticated role in modulating recognition and effector mechanisms while serving its biologic function of controlled invasion of the maternal host. At its point of contact with the maternal host, the syncitiotrophoblast lacks major histocompatibility complex (MHC) class II antigens. It acts as a dynamic functional barrier to immune effector mechanisms while permitting afferent recognition by the mother of the conceptus, and it is manifestly resistant to immune attack. Despite recognition of these essential components of the immunophysiology of pregnancy, the ways in which their abrogation might lead to reproductive failure remain obscure.

Immunology of spontaneous and recurrent abortion

Circumstantial clinical, histologic, and serologic evidence,[11,39,44] together with data from experimental ani-

---

Immunologic components of the mother-conceptus relationship

Afferent mechanisms

1. Decidual suppressor cells
2. Soluble immunomodulatory factors from decidua, embryo, and trophoblast
   - Maternal interleukins
   - Embryo-derived "messages"
   - Locally acting cytokines

Efferent mechanisms

1. Blocking antibodies
2. Other blocking factors
3. Hormones
4. Other suppressive factors

---

mals,[17] suggest that immunologic factors may be operative in a proportion of patients with spontaneous and recurrent abortion. These factors may operate in two circumstances. One is relatively well defined and involves a maternal autoimmune pathogenesis embodied in the condition known as the lupus obstetric or antiphospholipid syndrome, an established cause of reproductive failure throughout pregnancy. The other is ill-defined and is thought to be due to an abrogation of physiologic protective immune recognition and response mechanisms in the mother that mediate a successful pregnancy. This, in turn, is postulated to result in the immunologic rejection and disruption of implantation and placentation.

Antiphospholipid autoimmunity. Autoimmune connective tissue disorders, particularly systemic lupus erythematosus (SLE), may complicate reproduction in several ways, including maternal nephritis and hypertension; abortion and fetal death; and neonatal syndromes such as discoid LE, congenital complete heart block (CCHB), and neonatal systemic disease (reviewed by Gatenby[34]). It has also been recognized for some time that there is a high degree of reproductive wastage in SLE and related disorders, even in the preclinical phase of disease. This wastage includes spontaneous abortion and intrauterine fetal death, and may rise as high as 35% in the absence of overt maternal disease manifestations.

The term *lupus obstetric syndrome* was coined to encompass the reproductive failure in these cases. Its main associations are with pathologic autoantibodies directed against phospholipids.[53,62] These may be detected in vitro as so-called lupus anticoagulant (LA) activity or by more specific assays such as the enzyme-linked immunosorbent assay and radioimmunoassay.

Lupus anticoagulant is so named because its assay depends on the prolongation of phospholipid-dependent coagulation tests without inhibiting the activity of specific coagulation factors. LA activity is detected in plasma by using tests that reflect the conversion of prothrombin to thrombin, such as the activated partial thromboplastin time (APTT), the Russell viper venom time (RVVT), the kaolin clotting time (KCT), and the prothrombin time (PT). Coagulation factor deficiency is excluded by retesting the plasma after admixture with an equal volume of normal plasma; clotting times will not correct to normal if LA is present.

Quantitative assays for antiphospholipid antibodies involve the use of cardiolipin or other phospholipids such as phosphatidylserine as substrates. Anticardiolipin antibodies are similar to, but not identical with, those involved in LA activity. Antibodies detected by both tests are probably responsible for some of the biologic false-positive results seen in standard tests for syphilis.

High levels of anticardiolipin antibodies, particularly in the immunoglobulin G (IgG) class, together with LA activity, are significant markers of the antiphospholipid syndrome, which comprises a high prevalence of thrombosis, reproductive loss, thrombocytopenia, and Coombs' positivity. The component of this spectrum of pathologic process that relates to recurrent abortion and intrauterine fetal death is known as the lupus obstetric syndrome.

Significant levels of antiphospholipid antibodies and/or LA activity are found in 10% to 15% of women with recurrent fetal loss. The reproductive wastage in patients with LA or high titers of anticardiolipin antibodies is substantial. Of 242 reported cases of untreated pregnancies in 65 women with LA, 91% were lost as spontaneous abortions or fetal deaths.[8] The reproductive loss associated with the lupus obstetric syndrome may occur at any period of gestation to give this cumulative poor prognosis. Gatenby[34] summarized three collected series totaling 153 pregnancies and found a 61% loss before 20 weeks of gestation and a 29% loss after 20 weeks. It is also of note in the context of this chapter that antiphospholipid antibodies have been reported in association with unexplained infertility,[76] and they have been found in the follicular fluid of patients undergoing in vitro fertilization.[28]

The pathogenic mechanism of the reproductive wastage associated with antiphospholipid antibodies is unknown but has attracted several hypotheses.[53,62] It has been proposed that the autoantibodies bind to phospholipids in endothelial cell membranes to block arachidonic acid release and thereby decrease prostacyclin production. The agonist thromboxane would then predominate and cause vasoconstriction, platelet aggregation, and intravascular thrombosis. Other possibilities are decreased thrombomodulin-dependent activation of protein C, inhibition of fibrinolysis, or a primary effect on the platelet membrane. The pathologic end result, the thrombotic process, is a decidual vasculopathy with disruption of placentation.

There is evidence that the poor prognosis of the lupus obstetric syndrome can be modified by treatment, but less so in recurrent abortion than in cases of fetal loss in later pregnancy. Treatment indications and strategies are controversial.[53,62] Agents used have included low-dose aspirin (75 to 100 mg), high-dose prednisone (40 to 60 mg), heparin, dipyridamole, intravenous immunoglobulin, plasmapheresis, and azathiaprine. High-dose corticosteroids given throughout pregnancy cause severe and barely acceptable side effects, and corticosteroids and heparin enhance the endogenous osteoporotic effects of pregnancy.

A rational, but by no means exclusive, plan of management in women entering pregnancy with antiphospholipid antibodies has been suggested by Out et al.[62]:

- In primigravidae or women with previous successful pregnancies: no treatment or low-dose aspirin
- In women with previous relevant fetal loss: low-dose aspirin or heparin
- In women previously treated unsuccessfully with low-dose aspirin or heparin: low-dose aspirin plus high-dose prednisone, or possibly plasmapheresis or intravenous immunoglobulin

Disordered immune response to pregnancy. Early studies of the disordered immune response to pregnancy sought evidence of increased histoincompatibility between reproductive partners and of classic allograft rejection phenomena as proof of immunologically determined abortion.[47] Reports in the literature of normal pregnancies in recurrent aborters after a change in partner also suggested that there was a significant immunogenetic component in successful reproduction.

With the more recent comprehensive realization that maternal immune recognition, rather than suppression, is essential to the establishment of normal pregnancy, evidence for a breakdown in these recognition (protective) mechanisms was sought in human populations of recurrent aborters.[4,11,32,39,44] The following phenomena have been described and proposed either as pathogenic mechanisms in abortion or as selection and monitoring markers for immunotherapy, using allogenic leukocytes from the male partner or third parties:

- Excessive human leukocyte antigen (HLA) sharing between partners
- Decrease in blocking factors, antipaternal leukocytotoxic antibodies, and decidual suppressor cells in the female partner
- Decreased mixed lymphocyte reactivity (MLR) between partners
- Altered cellular immune responses in the female partner

There is little evidence, however, to support a role for these immunologic phenomena in otherwise unexplained recurrent abortion, its treatment, or prognosis.* Despite these uncertainties, the treatment of recurrent abortion by

*References 12, 13, 35, 44, 65, 69, 73.

Table 21-1. Immunotherapy of recurrent abortion in controlled trials

Authors	Successful pregnancy (%)	
	Test cases	Controls
Mowbray et al.[61] (1985)	77	37*
Carp et al.[10] (1990)	72	34*
Cowchock et al.[24] (1990)	58	39*
Ho et al.[40] (1990)	76	66
Cauchi et al.[14] (1991)	62	76

*The low success rates in the control groups in these studies is at variance with the majority of reports in the literature of outcome in untreated patients with unexplained recurrent abortion.

immunotherapy has achieved an almost irresistible momentum. Historically, properly conducted controlled trials of treatments for unexplained recurrent abortion have been few and far between, and immunotherapy is no exception (Table 21-1). These results raise very real questions about the efficacy of immunotherapy, and clinicians should retain an open mind on this issue until the results of further (multicenter) controlled trials are available.

In the final analysis it is salutary to reflect that we are still uncertain whether immunologic mechanisms can cause abortion; if they do, we do not know how to identify them. In addition, we do not know whether immunotherapy is successful; if it is, we do not know how it works or which patients might benefit from it. It is also difficult to contemplate how immunotherapy can compete with the success rates of greater than 60% reported in unexplained recurrent aborters exposed to almost any treatment modality, including psychologic support,[52,72] or left untreated. The only clear prognostic factors in these patients, regardless of treatment, are length of history of recurrent abortion, number of abortions, interval since most recent abortion, and length of infertility history.[13] It is the last of these that potentially unites the possible immunologic etiology of recurrent abortion with that of infertility.

REFERENCES

1. Alper MM, Garner PR: Premature ovarian failure: its relationship to autoimmune disease, *Obstet Gynecol* 66:27, 1985.
2. Austin GE, Coulam CB, Ryan RJ: A search for antibodies to luteinizing hormone receptors in premature ovarian failure, *Mayo Clin Proc* 54:394, 1979.
3. Anderson JR et al: Immunological features of idiopathic Addison's disease: an antibody to cells producing steroid hormones, *Clin Exp Immunol* 3:107, 1968.
4. Beer AE: Immunopathologic factors contributing to recurrent spontaneous abortion, *Am J Reprod Immunol* 4:182, 1983.
5. Bohnet HG et al: In vivo effects of antisera to prolactin receptors in female rats, *Endocrinology* 102:1657, 1978.
6. Bottazzo GF, Doniach D: Pituitary autoimmunity: a review, *J R Soc Med* 71:433, 1978.
7. Bousquet D et al: Zona pellucida antibodies in a group of women with idiopathic infertility, *Am J Reprod Immunol* 2:73, 1982.
8. Branch DW: Immunologic disease and fetal death, *Clin Obstet Gynecol* 30:295, 1987.

9. Camperhout J, van Antaki A, Rasio E: Diabetes mellitus and thyroid immunity in gonadal dysgenesis, *Fertil Steril* 24:1, 1973.

10. Carp HJA et al: Immunization by paternal leukocytes for prevention of primary habitual abortion, *Gynecol Obstet Invest* 29:16, 1990.

11. Carp HJA et al: Recurrent miscarriage: a review of current concepts, immune mechanisms and results of treatment, *Obstet Gynecol Surv* 45:657, 1990.

12. Cauchi MN et al: Immunogenetic studies in habitual abortion, *Aust N Z J Obstet Gynaecol* 27:52, 1987.

13. Cauchi MN et al: Predictors of pregnancy success in repeated miscarriage, *Am J Reprod Immunol Microbiol* 26:72, 1991.

14. Cauchi MN et al: The treatment of recurrent aborters by immunization with paternal cells: controlled trial, *Am J Reprod Immunol Microbiol* 25:16, 1991.

15. Caudle MR, Shivers C, Wild RA: Clinical significance of naturally occurring anti-zona pellucida antibodies in infertile women, *Am J Reprod Immunol Microbiol* 15:119, 1987.

16. Chiauzzi V et al: Inhibition of follicle stimulating hormone receptor binding by circulating immunoglobulins, *J Clin Endocrinol Metab* 54:1221, 1982.

17. Clark DA: What do we know about spontaneous abortion mechanisms?, *Am J Reprod Immunol* 19:28, 1989.

18. Collen RJ, Lippe BM, Kaplan SA: Primary ovarian failure, juvenile rheumatoid arthritis and vitiligo, *Am J Dis Child* 133:598, 1979.

19. Colls BM: Addison's disease, autoimmunity and mumps, *N Z Med J* 66:314, 1967.

20. Coulam CB: The prevalence of autoimmune disorders among patients with primary ovarian failure, *Am J Reprod Immunol* 2:63, 1983.

21. Coulam CB, Kempers RD, Randall RV: Premature ovarian failure: evidence for an autoimmune mechanism, *Fertil Steril* 36:238, 1981.

22. Coulam CB, Lujkin EC: Absence of adrenal failure in the polyglandular failure syndrome with primary ovarian failure, *Fertil Steril* 35:365, 1981.

23. Coulam CB, Ryan RJ: Prevalence of circulating antibodies directed toward ovaries among women with premature ovarian failure, *Am J Reprod Immunol Microbiol* 9:23, 1985.

24. Cowchock FS et al: Paternal mononuclear cell immunization therapy for repeated miscarriage: predictive variables for pregnancy success, *Am J Reprod Immunol* 22:12, 1990.

25. Dias JA, Gates SA, Reichard LE: Evidence for the presence of follicle stimulating hormone receptor antibody in human serum, *Fertil Steril* 38:330, 1982.

26. Deitl J, Knop G, Mettler L: The frequency of serological anti-zona pellucida activity in males, females and children, *J Reprod Immunol* 4:123, 1982.

27. Doniach D, Roitt IM, Polani PE: Thyroid antibodies and sex-chromosome anomalies, *Proc R Soc Med* 61:278, 1968.

28. El-Roeiy A et al: Correlation between peripheral blood and follicular fluid autoantibodies and impact on in vitro fertilization, *Obstet Gynecol* 70:163, 1987.

29. Engelberth O, Jezkova Z: Autoantibodies in Sheehan's syndrome, *Lancet* 2:1194, 1965.

30. Engle E, Forbes AP: An abnormal medium-sized metacentric chromosome in a woman with primary gonadal failure, *Lancet* 2:1004, 1961.

31. Etzrodt H et al: Immunohypophysitis, a cause of hypopituitarism?, *Acta Endocrinol* 264:137, 1984.

32. Faulk WP: Idiopathic spontaneous abortions, *Am J Reprod Immunol* 3:48, 1983.

33. Fialkow PJ: Autoantibodies and chromosomal abortions, *Lancet* 1:1106, 1967.

34. Gatenby PA: Systemic lupus erythematosus and pregnancy, *Aust N Z J Med* 19:261, 1989.

35. Gatenby PA et al: Treatment of recurrent spontaneous abortion by immunization with paternal lymphocytes: correlates with outcome, *Am J Reprod Immunol* 19:21, 1989.

36. Gleischer N, El-Roeiy A: The reproductive autoimmune failure syndrome, *Am J Obstet Gynecol* 159:223, 1988.

37. Glover E, Hurlimann J: Autoimmune oophoritis, *Am J Clin Pathol* 81:105, 1984.

38. Goudie RB, Pinkerton PH: Anterior hypophysitis and Hashimoto's disease in a young woman, *J Pathol Bacteriol* 83:584, 1962.

39. Hill JA: Immunological mechanisms of pregnancy maintenance and failure: a critique of theories and therapy, *Am J Reprod Immunol* 22:33, 1990.

40. Ho HN et al: A control study of lymphocyte immunotherapy for unexplained recurrent spontaneous abortion, *Am J Reprod Immunol* 22:86, 1990.

41. Ho PC et al: Immunologic studies in patients with premature ovarian failure, *Obstet Gynecol* 71:622, 1990.

42. Irvine WJ: Autoimmunity in endocrine disease, *Proc R Soc Med* 67:548, 1974.

43. Irvine W et al: Immunological aspects of premature ovarian failure associated with idiopathic Addison's disease, *Lancet* 2:883, 1968.

44. Johnson PM, Ramsden GH: Recurrent miscarriage. In Johnson PM, editor: *Immunological disease in pregnancy*, London, 1988, Bailliere Tindall.

45. Jones GES, Ruehsen MdeM: A new syndrome of amenorrhea in association with hypergonadotropism and apparently normal ovarian follicular apparatus, *Am J Obstet Gynecol* 104:597, 1969.

46. Jones WR: Immunization against the oocyte. In *Immunological fertility regulation*, Oxford, 1982, Blackwell Scientific.

47. Jones WR: Immunological factors in pregnancy. In MacDonald RR, editor: *Scientific basis of obstetrics and gynaecology*, London, 1985, Churchill Livingstone.

48. Jones WR et al: Phase I clinical trial of a World Health Organization birth control vaccine, *Lancet* 1:1295, 1988.

49. Kolarov R et al: Antigonadotrophins in some reproductive disorders in man. In Bratonov K et al, editors: *Immunology of reproduction*, Sofia, 1973, Bulgarian Academy of Science Press.

50. Koninckx PR, Brosens IA: The gonadotropin resistant ovary syndrome as a cause for secondary amenorrhea and infertility, *Fertil Steril* 28:926, 1977.

51. Kuki S, Morgan RL, Tucci JR: Myasthenia gravis and premature ovarian failure, *Arch Intern Med* 141:1230, 1981.

52. Liddell HS, Pattison NS, Zanderigo A: Recurrent miscarriage: outcome after supportive care in early pregnancy, *Aust N Z J Obstet Gynaecol* 31:320, 1991.

53. Lockshin MD, Qamar T, Levy RA: In Scott JS, Bird HA, editors: *Anticardiolipin and related antibodies: thrombosis and fetal death*, Oxford, 1990, Oxford University Press.

54. Luborsky JL, Behrman HR: Antiserum against rat leuteinizing hormone (LH) receptors, *Biochem Biophys Res Commun* 90:1407, 1979.

55. Lucky AW et al: Pubertal progression in the presence of elevated serum gonadotrophins in girls with multiple endocrine deficiencies, *J Clin Endocrinol Metab* 45:673, 1977.

56. Maxson WR, Wenz AC: The gonadotrophin resistant ovary syndrome, *Semin Reprod Endocrinol* 1:147, 1983.

57. Medawar PB: Some immunological and endocrinological problems raised by the evolution of viviparity in vertebrates, *Symp Soc Exp Biol* 7:320, 1953.

58. Mignot MH et al: Premature ovarian failure, I: the association with autoimmunity, *Eur J Obstet Gynecol Reprod Biol* 30:67, 1989.

59. Mirakian R et al: Autoimmunity to anterior pituitary cells and the pathogenesis of type 1 (insulin-dependent) diabetes mellitus, *Lancet* 2:755, 1982.

60. Miyake T et al: Acute oocyte loss in experimental autoimmune oophoritis as a possible model of premature ovarian failure, *Am J Obstet Gynecol* 158:186, 1988.

61. Mowbray JF et al: Controlled trial of treatment of recurrent spontaneous abortion by immunization with paternal cells, *Lancet* 1:941, 1985.

62. Out HJ et al: Anti phospholipid antibodies and pregnancy loss, *Hum Reprod* 6:889, 1991.

63. Pouplard A: Pituitary auto immunity, *Horm Res* 16:289, 1982.

64. Rebar RW, Erickson GF, Yen SSC: Idiopathic premature ovarian fail-

ure: clinical and endocrine characteristics, *Fertil Steril* 37:35, 1982.

65. Redman CWG: Immune factors and recurrent abortion: a review, *Am J Reprod Immunol* 4:179, 1983.

66. Ruehsen MdeM et al: Autoimmunity and ovarian failure, *Am J Obstet Gynecol* 112:693, 1979.

67. Sacco AG, Moghissi KS: Anti zona pellucida activity in human sera, *Fertil Steril* 31:503, 1979.

68. Salmon MA, Ashworth M: Association of auto-immune disorders and sex-chromosome anomalies, *Lancet* 2:1085, 1970.

69. Sargent IL, Wilkins T, Redman CWG: Maternal immune responses to the fetus in early pregnancy and recurrent miscarriage, *Lancet* 2:1099, 1988.

70. Shivers C, Dunbar BS: Autoantibodies to zona pellucida: a possible cause for infertility in women, *Science* 197:1082, 1977.

71. Sotsion F, Bottazzo GF, Doniach D: Immunofluorescence studies on autoantibodies to steroid-producing cells and to germ line cells in endocrine disease and infertility, *Clin Exp Immunol* 39:97, 1980.

72. Stay-Pedersen B, Stay-Pedersen S: Etiologic factors and subsequent reproductive performance in 195 couples with a prior history of habitual abortion, *Am J Obstet Gynecol* 148:140, 1984.

73. Stirrat GM: Recurrent abortion: a review, *Br J Obstet Gynaecol* 90:881, 1983.

74. Talbert LM et al: Endocrine and immunologic studies in a patient with resistant ovary syndrome, *Fertil Steril* 42:741, 1984.

75. Tan SL et al, Autoimmune premature ovarian failure with polyendocrinopathy and spontaneous recovery of ovarian follicular activity, *Fertil Steril* 45:421, 1986.

76. Taylor PV, Campbell JM, Scott JS: Presence of autoantibodies in women with unexplained infertility, *Am J Obstet Gynecol* 161:377, 1989.

77. Turkington RW, Lebovitz HE: Extra-adrenal endocrine deficiencies in Addison's disease, *Am J Med* 43:499, 1967.

78. Vallotton MB, Forbes AR: Autoimmunity in gonadal dysgenesis and Klinefelter's syndrome, *Lancet* 1:648, 1967.

79. Vasquez AM, Kenny FM: Ovarian failure and antiovarian antibodies in association with hyperparathyroidism moniliasis, and Addison's and Hashimoto's diseases, *Obstet Gynecol* 41:414, 1973.

80. Wickings EJ, Nieschlag E: Suppression of spermatogenesis over two years in rhesus monkeys actively immunized with follicle stimulating hormone, *Fertil Steril* 34:269, 1980.

81. Williams ED, Engle E, Forbes AP: Thyroiditis and gonadal dysgenesis, *N Engl J Med* 270:805, 1964.

82. Williamson HO et al: Myasthenia gravis, premature menopause and thyroid autoimmunity, *Am J Obstet Gynecol* 137:893, 1980.

Chapter 22

SPERM ANTIBODIES

Gilbert G. Haas, Jr., MD

Antisperm antibodies in women
Antisperm antibodies in men
In vivo effects of antisperm antibodies
Tests for antisperm antibodies
Importance of circulating versus locally-produced antisperm antibodies
Clinical findings that suggest antisperm antibodies
Therapy for antisperm antibodies
Summary

The foundation for the acceptance of antibody-mediated infertility as a diagnosis has been strengthened by several recently defined tenets: (1) Antibodies are made by most individuals sensitized by sperm to internal or surface sperm antigens, but only the antibody population reactive to sperm surface antigens interferes with sperm function; hence only assays that use antigens found on living, intact sperm are adequate for antibody assessment. (2) Only certain immunoglobulin (Ig) isotypes (IgG and secretory IgA) are commonly found in the male and female reproductive tracts; therefore it is important to use assays that are capable of distinguishing individual isotypes of immunoglobulin in order to ignore trivial sperm antibodies (i.e., circulating IgM antibodies), which are not commonly found in the same body compartments as those inhabited by sperm. (3) Antisperm antibodies exert their deleterious effects on reproduction primarily by interfering with sperm function after their attachment to the surface of the sperm, rather than initiating complement-mediated or macrophage-mediated events. (4) Clinically important antisperm antibodies should be searched for on the sperm or in the secretions of the female genital tract. Some deductions about antibody-mediated infertility in women can be made by measuring serum IgG antisperm antibodies, since these immunoglobulins can transude into cervical mucus and follicular fluid.[36]

The purpose of this chapter is to substantiate and expand these premises by allusion to relevant recent substantive research advances in the field.

ANTISPERM ANTIBODIES IN WOMEN

It is common knowledge that most couples do not share sufficient numbers of tissue or blood group antigens to forestall immunologic rejection of a graft from the male partner to his spouse. For this reason it seems logical that spermatozoa deposited in the female genital tract would share the same dismal fate of rejection that would befall a skin graft from the male partner. However, careful analysis of the pertinent factors reveals that a woman's response to spermatozoal antigens may not mirror the events that are expected to follow a poorly cross-matched organ transplant.

The spermatozoal plasma membrane does not express class I major histocompatibility antigens (MHC; HLA-A, HLA-B, or HLA-C).[66] There is disagreement as to whether class II MHC antigens (HLA-D or HLA-DR) are totally absent[66] or whether they are only minimally expressed on the sperm surface.[17] Since the MHC antigens are the primary mediators of both transplantation rejection and microbiologic antigen recognition,[2] their absence on the sperm surface would mollify the usual mechanisms for antigenic stimulus by spermatozoal surface antigens.

Approximately one fifth of the human population can be labeled as "secretors."[42] Secretors express their blood group antigens in certain glandular products (e.g., saliva), but blood group antigens are not found in the secretions of the majority of individuals ("nonsecretors"). A, B, and O blood group antigens are found only in the seminal plasma and secondarily coated on the sperm of secretors.[59] However, these antigens are not important mediators of reproductive events, since the fertility of a couple is unaffected by the blood types of the two partners.[45] Because of the lack of MHC and blood group antigen expression, it is apparent that spermatozoa may be deficient in the classically accepted stimuli for an antibody response to xenogeneic antigens. In light of these facts, the principal instigator of an immune response to sperm antigens is elusive.

Failure to produce antibodies to minor histocompatibility antigens found on the trophoblast (trophoblast/lymphocyte cross-reacting antigens) has been associated with pregnancy wastage.[44] These potentially important antigens have been identified on developing spermatozoa within the testis; they have not been identified on mature spermatozoa,[9] although they have been alleged to occur in seminal plasma.[102] Seminal plasma–coating antigens can become integrally associated with the sperm membrane.[171] This process is reminiscent of the incorporation of antigenic material into and onto the sperm surface during epididymal transport.[16] Recent research in this area has investigated the ability of seminal plasma constituents to act as potential immunosuppressants,[98] although they may provide a reservoir of antigens that are critical to the instigation of an antisperm immune response.

Regardless of our inability to identify the broad category of putative antigens that mediate an antibody response, spermatozoa can reproducibly and predictably elicit an antibody response when they are inoculated systemically in either women[15] or female animals.[131] Baskin[15] reported in a 1932 article that women who received injections of untreated human semen subsequently mounted an immune response to spermatozoal antigens that was associated with infertility. Although a patent was eventually awarded for this early form of immunocontraception, it was never widely used. However, the report is important because it demonstrated that, like female animals, women mount an antibody response against sperm antigens when exposed to these antigens at sites distant from the female reproductive tract. These experiments firmly established that it was not a sperm's deficient antigenicity that limited a woman's immune response to her partner's gametes.

Nor does it seem that the female genital tract is bereft of immune affectors and effectors when challenged with a locally applied inoculum. Several studies have shown that a variety of antigens placed in the vagina, cervix, or uterus can elicit both a systemic and a local immune response.[94,169] The characteristics of the immune response depend primarily on the antigen used, rather than the site of inoculation. However, in general, application of provocative antigens within the female genital tract usually stimulates a local antibody response (mediated by secretory IgA immunoglobulins), and systemic inoculation stimulates circulating IgG and/or IgM antibodies, the former of which can transude in a limited manner into the genital tract secretions.[125]

From the preceding two paragraphs it can be deduced that the factors that inhibit the formation of antisperm antibodies in most women cannot be explained by either a lack of human spermatozoal immunogenicity or a deficient capability of a woman's genital tract to mount an immune response to putative antigens placed there. The increased incidence of antisperm antibodies in prostitutes[153] implies a possible correlation between the amount and variety of sperm antigen stimulation and the chance of a secondary immune response. Whether this is due to an overwhelming inoculum of spermatozoal and seminal plasma antigens or to an adjuvant effect of venereal infections is unknown.

Another explanation for why some women develop sperm antibodies is that the antigens on their husbands' spermatozoa may be uniquely capable of eliciting an antibody response. This hypothesis is supported by the discovery that a small percentage of women with antibody-mediated infertility produce antibodies specific for their husbands' sperm.[180] Unlike women who have antibodies against antigens common to all spermatozoa, donor insemination would be a viable therapeutic alternative for women in this situation. Although antibody reactivity to specific sperm donors has been reported,[116] this is most likely a problem arising from the use of fixed sperm as an antigen, which results in exposure to the assayed serum of internal sperm antigens.

Witkin[174] has proposed several mechanisms by which women minimize the possibility of an immune response to spermatozoal antigens after coitus: (1) retardation of spermatozoal antigen absorption by the thick, stratified, squamous epithelium of the vagina; (2) rapid reduction of the sperm antigen load after coitus; (3) active suppression of an immune response by spermatozoa themselves via the activation of suppressor T lymphocytes; (4) adsorption of antisperm antibodies by leukocytes due to the partial antigenic cross-reactivity between spermatozoa and lymphocytes; and (5) immunosuppression by seminal plasma factors. Factors that might predispose to an antisperm immune response include the following: (1) inability of a woman's suppressor T lymphocytes to be activated by semen, (2) idiopathic decline in the quantity of suppressor T lymphocytes in the cervix, and (3) an increased potential for an evoked immune response in women whose husbands are positive for antisperm antibodies because of the presence of immunoglobulin molecules on their sperm.

The mechanisms by which a woman's cell-mediated immune system responds to the deposition of spermatozoa in her genital tract have been summarized by Anderson and Hill.[8] Initially there is an infiltration of leukocytes, possibly due to chemotactic factors found in seminal plasma. Increases in certain subpopulations of these cells have been noted in women with infertility, as well as in women with endometriosis. These sequestered leukocytes potentially could secrete a variety of substances (lymphokines or monokines) that might adversely affect human sperm motility and the events surrounding fertilization. Whether these leukocytes are the initiators of an antisperm antibody reaction is not known.

It is possible that the presence of antisperm antibodies in the female partner may be due to abnormalities in the idiotype–antiidiotype immune network.[24] This network provides the basis for the body's control of the immune system. If it were not present, an uncontrolled overgrowth of antibody-producing cells might follow each exposure to a foreign antigen. After an antigen has elicited an antibody response, the new antibody itself becomes an antigen that is foreign to the host and can itself stimulate a second antibody response. This second antibody response (antiidiotype) dampens and controls the primary response (idiotype). The sequential formation of idiotype and antiidiotype antibodies prevents the excessive production of antibodies and antibody-producing plasma cells during each antibody response. If the formation of antisperm antibodies is normally damped by a robust antiidiotype response, the deficiency of this immune regulation could result in the formation of sperm antibodies sufficient to cause reproductive impairment.

ANTISPERM ANTIBODIES IN MEN

Most physicians can readily conceptualize the potential for sperm antibody formation in women who are repeatedly challenged with spermatozoal antigens after coitus. It is underemphasized that spermatozoal antigens are antigenically as foreign to a man as they can be to a woman. Postpubertally mature spermatozoa appear several years after the process of immune self-recognition. The process of immunologic self-recognition is an antigen inventory that occurs during fetal life and results in the deletion of lymphocyte clones that could produce antibodies against self (in this case the male host).[2] Since mature spermatozoa (and certain of their precursors) do not appear until puberty, they are viewed as foreign cells by the host and are potential targets for an immune response. If spermatozoa were present during the self-recognition process, it is presumed that the incidence of antisperm antibodies in men would be greatly reduced, because sperm would no longer be antigenically foreign. Although the descriptive term *autoimmunity* has been used to describe the presence of antisperm antibodies in men, it is a misnomer. In fact, production of antisperm antibodies in men is precisely parallel to processes that evoke antibodies against any other foreign antigen such as might occur after an inappropriately matched organ transplant or a microbial infection. Because an antibody response against a man's own gametes is obviously genocidal, biologic processes had to evolve to limit the possibility of an immune reaction against the foreign sperm antigens.

The primary mechanism for the prevention of antisperm antibody activity in men was long thought to be sequestration of the male gametes (spermatozoa) within the male genital tract.[39] During meiotic maturation, cohorts of developing sperm migrate toward the lumen of the seminiferous tubules.[135] As an integral part of this process, tight junctions form behind the maturing gametes between the adjacent Sertoli cells to isolate the developing sperm from the extratubular environment.[149] The sequestration theory became less plausible after the identification of potential sites of immunoglobulin leakage into the male genital tract and sites of sperm egress into the circulation.[8] A breakdown in sperm antigen sequestration seemed most obvious within the rete testis and ductuli efferentes. Apologists for the sequestration theory suggested that suppressor T lymphocytes were often located within these regions of the male genital tract and that these cells might suppress an immune response to leaked antigenic material.[4] However, the human testis is not entirely impregnable to circulating immune effectors. For instance, after the induction of experimental orchitis in animals, circulating immunoglobulin molecules can be found within the seminiferous tubules to the level of the spermatocytes.[187] (As spermatogonia mature, they migrate from the basal to the adluminal compartments of the seminiferous tubules; the most mature spermatozoa are found closest to the center of the tubules.[149]) The most convincing evidence that the male genital tract is not completely sequestered has been derived from the guinea pig experimental allergic orchitis model. It has been reported that the passive transfer of testis antigen-activated leukocytes reproducibly results in active orchitis in the recipient.[166] This reaction is first noted in the rete testis,[164] one of the potential sites of sperm antigen leakage. This successful passive transfer of immune activity has suggested that the male genital tract is not totally segregated from its environment, because in order for the leukocytes to be activated, they would first have to be exposed to sperm antigens. Mononuclear infiltration of the seminiferous tubules and rete testis can be treated effectively with corticosteroids.[89]

Mahi-Brown et al.[118] noted in a review of the literature that it was necessary for the blood-testis barrier to be breached by an insult (trauma, infection, etc.) for immune effectors to have access to all of the potentially foreign testicular antigens. However, despite the tight junctions of the blood-testis barrier, the fact that injected immunoglobulins can enter the rete testis[164] even though junctional complexes exist there suggested that sperm antigens that could elicit an autoantibody antisperm response were in potential communication with circulating immune mediators. In addition, some spermatozoal autoantigens that are potentially immunogenic to their host are located outside the blood-testis barrier within the seminiferous tubule.[117] This suggested that some type of active immunosuppression must be occurring to inhibit an antibody response to these developing sperm.[163] The only satisfactory explanation for the ability to incite orchitis by transfer of leukocytes[167] is that, although the blood-testis barrier assists in protecting the male gametes from immune attack, active suppression of an immunologic response to the foreign testicular antigens must be occurring or the blood-borne mediators of orchitis would not be transferable.

Although helper T lymphocytes predominate in the interstitial tissue surrounding the male genital tract, the lymphocytes most intimately adherent to the adluminal surface of the genital epithelium are predominantly suppressor T cells.[40] This ratio of suppressor lymphocytes to helper lymphocytes is important in determining the cell-mediated immune reaction to antigenic material that transudes from the male genital tubules. When this ratio is elevated, antigenic leakage results in suppression rather than activation of an immune response. Investigators have also noted that suppressor lymphocytes predominate in the basal layer of the testicular epithelium.[40] These suppressor cells are also apparent in the epithelium of the epididymis, vas deferens, and prostate gland.[4] Similarly, suppressor T cells predominate in semen, unlike the situation in peripheral blood, where most T cells are of the helper T/inducer type.[183] This ratio is reversed in the genital secretions of previously vasectomized men who undergo vasovasostomy and subsequently develop antisperm antibodies.[177] This suggests that when helper T/inducer cells predominate in the genital tract, an antibody-mediated response to sperm may occur, although there are exceptions.[13] The numbers of B lymphocytes that would mediate an immunoglobulin response to sperm are limited in the male genital tract,[145] as are leukocytes in general.[105]

Acknowledging that suppressor lymphocytes mediate sperm immunosuppression, Witkin[174] has hypothesized three possible mechanisms for sperm antibody formation in men: (1) a decrease in the quantity or activity of genital tract suppressor cells, (2) a decline or absence of factors in male genital tract fluids that recruit suppressor cells, or (3) an altered sperm antigenicity that results in an inadequate suppression of immune responses to sperm. To this it might be added that any event or insult that would provide an overwhelming inoculum of spermatozoal antigens could override the mechanisms of immunosuppression. The most common events in men that have been noted to increase the risk of antisperm antibodies are vasectomy, trauma, torsion, cancer, infection, obstruction of the male genital tract, cryptorchidism, varicocele, testicular biopsy, receptive anal intercourse in homosexuals, and genetic predisposition.[56] Because most antibody-positive men do not recall any of these events in their medical history, it is usually presumed that the majority of men who develop antisperm antibodies either have been inoculated with an antigen from a cross-reactive ubiquitous microorganism or have experienced an event that resulted in a large inoculum of sperm antigens that overrode the immunosuppressive mechanisms. It should be emphasized that there is not a 1:1 correlation between a history of these predisposing events and the occurrence of antisperm antibodies; however, there is an increased risk that antisperm antibodies can occur after these events. When one of the predisposing historic factors is found during the initial evaluation of the male partner, antisperm antibodies might be appropriately assessed in the male partner at an early stage of the couple's infertility evaluation.

Spermatozoal antigens may themselves be immunosuppressive, since animals preexposed to spermatozoa without adjuvant are inhibited from developing experimental allergic orchitis.[91,92,99] This inhibitory effect can be blocked by pretreatment with an immunosuppressant such as cyclophosphamide at the time of the sperm inoculation, which would normally induce suppressor T cell activation.[92]

Thymectomized animals are rendered incapable of immune interactions mediated by suppressor T cells and do not undergo sperm-induced immunosuppression, implying that the immunosuppression is mediated by suppressor T cells.[160] It is not known whether the suppressor T cells in close proximity to the male genital tract develop as a direct response to peripubertal development of spermatozoal antigens.

Antisperm antibodies may adversely affect reproductive success in vasectomized men after a surgically successful vasovasostomy. However, sperm antibody testing is not a reliable predictor of pregnancy success for men who undergo a surgically successful vas anastomosis. Measurement of circulating antisperm antibodies, except when high titers are noted, has not been predictive.[180] In men with high serum titers of antisperm antibodies, there is an increased transudation of antibodies into the male genital tract, which can subsequently impair sperm function.[113] Even assay of antibodies on the man's spermatozoa after vasovasostomy does not correlate with subsequent pregnancy success.[133] It is known that seminal plasma from vasectomized men is frequently devoid of antisperm antibodies, despite the fact that the majority of vasectomized men are known to have circulating sperm antibodies.[112] Contrariwise, vasovasostomized men frequently have antisperm antibodies in their seminal plasma.[112] This implies that anastomosis of the vas deferens permits the site of antisperm antibody formation in vasectomized men to contribute to the makeup of the ejaculate. Linnet and Fogh-Anderson[112] reported that antisperm antibodies in the fluid from the testicular side of the vasectomy site collected at the time of vasovasostomy may predict impaired postvasovasostomy fertility. If the majority of sperm antibodies are produced at this location in vasectomized men, it will prove difficult to predict preoperatively whether a vasectomized man will have difficulty in achieving a pregnancy in his partner postvasovasostomy because of antibody-mediated hindrances to his fertility. If the presence of antibodies on the testicular side of the vasectomy site is the only specific predictor of antibody mediators to fertility postvasovasostomy, only a preoperative transcrotal sampling technique can identify antibodies within the testis or epididymis that might impair fertility after the vas anastomosis. Assay for sperm-associated antibodies after a vasovasostomy is predictive of subsequent fertility if 100% of sperm are coated with IgA (sperm-associated IgG levels are not predictive of fertility) and there is a high (1:256) serum agglutination titer.[130]

In summary, the prevailing evidence suggests that the mechanism by which a man coexists with the potentially foreign antigens on his gametes is active suppression of a potentially detrimental immune response to his sperm.

IN VIVO EFFECTS OF ANTISPERM ANTIBODIES

The majority of circulating antibodies against cellular or microbiologic antigens attach to their putative target cell and then either sequentially activate the nine components of the complement cascade or opsonize (or activate) macrophages, which then aggregate, phagocytose, and eliminate the antibody-coated cell from the circulation. Circulating complement components provide the raw material for complement-mediated immune destruction. Circulating macrophages or the cells of the reticuloendothelial system are the source of phagocytes that remove antibody-bound cells from the blood stream. The presence of a single IgM molecule or two IgG molecules that are spatially adjacent is required to activate the complement cascade. Secretory IgA is incapable of activating the classic complement pathway, although an alternative pathway can be initiated by this group of locally secreted immunoglobulins.

In the typical situation, the organisms attacked by the host's antibody-mediated immune response are potentially harmful to the host because of the sequelae of an infection. These microbiologic agents do not have complex functions to perform; they simply live, metabolize, and damage the host cells. The success of the immune response against these invading organisms can be defined arbitrarily as to whether the host survived. Spermatozoa are decidedly different from these sedentary microbiologic invaders because they have complex functions they must perform, including motility, mucus penetration, capacitation, zona binding, acrosomal loss, zona penetration, oolemma binding and fusion, fertilization, and genetic contribution to cell division. An immune response that results in the death of sperm in the female genital tract would meet the criteria for an immune response to sperm; however, it is reasonable to presume that an immune response that could perturb any step in reproductive function, even though the response did not result in cell death, could also be considered detrimental to reproductive function. This modified definition of the success of an immune response becomes particularly important when it is considered that the environment to which sperm are exposed during their passage through both the male genital tract and certain regions of the female genital tract contains limited amounts of complement[68,142] and variable macrophages.[186] Moreover, seminal plasma is an inhibitor of phagocytosis by macrophages[157] and complement-mediated sperm cytolysis.[32] Macrophage ingestion of human sperm has been confirmed in in vivo systems[35]; the role of this phenomenon in vitro is unclear.

Antibody-laden human sperm are capable of initiating phagocytosis by human macrophages if the antibody on the sperm surface is capable of activating complement; antibody-free sperm or sperm with bound antibodies incapable of activating complement cannot induce phagocytosis.[33,35] This phagocytosis is associated with the release of oxidative radicals at the point of contact between the sperm and polymorphonuclear leukocyte surfaces only when an antisperm antibody capable of activating complement is present on the sperm's surface[33]; such release can usually be detected in the fluid surrounding the leukocytes and the cell to be ingested (bacteria, etc.), and it is usually not limited to such a local presence. Follicular fluid is the only

fluid in the male or female genital tract that has been found to contain amounts of complement sufficient to achieve complement-dependent sperm cytotoxicity.[34] Since sperm-bound antibodies are capable of activating the entire complement cascade,[34] it is possible that complement-mediated sperm cytotoxicity could occur after exposure to sperm antibody-positive follicular fluid either in vivo or during in vitro fertilization (IVF). The consequences of activation of complement on the sperm surface are morphologically reminiscent of the effect of exposure of sperm to a hypoosmotic solution.[35] Thus antibodies capable of activating complement when bound to sperm are capable of initiating cytolysis and phagocytosis; it remains to be seen whether conditions exist in vivo to support these phenomena (i.e., adequate amounts of complement and adequate numbers of macrophages). One of the two predominant subclasses (IgG1 and IgG3) of circulating antisperm IgG (IgG3) can activate the complement cascade.[62]

It is important to identify those steps in sperm function that can be detrimentally affected by the presence of antisperm antibodies. The "chicken or the egg" dilemma quickly becomes apparent.[52] Should infertile couples first be tested by functional assays, and if a functional deficit is found, should tests for antisperm antibodies be performed? Or should infertile couples first be tested for sperm antibodies, and if they are positive for antibodies, should functional assays that are hindered by the antibodies be performed? The usual first step is to establish whether an antisperm antibody is present in the male or female genital tract that could come in contact with sperm. This is followed by determination of which step in sperm function is affected by the presence of the antibody.

TESTS FOR ANTISPERM ANTIBODIES

Many of the available assays for antisperm antibodies test for isotypes of serum antisperm antibodies that may not be found within the male or female genital tract. The large pentameric IgM molecule does not transude readily into the reproductive tract[148,152]; circulating IgA molecules do not mirror the locally produced secretory IgA immune response of mucosal surfaces.[161] For these reasons it is appropriate to assess antisperm antibodies that can be found in the passages through which sperm travel from the testis to the ampulla of the fallopian tube. As in any good murder mystery, if a suspect could not have been present at the scene of the crime, he or she should be dropped from the list of potential criminals. Thus antibodies that, because of their size (i.e., IgM) or origin (i.e., circulating IgA), would not be normally found in the male or female genital tract should not be assessed.

After the acrosome reaction, antigens on the acrosomal membrane are exposed. This is the only time when antibodies that bind to antigens not on the sperm plasma membrane may be clinically important. However, in general, the criterion for acceptance of an assay for antibody-mediated infertility is the ability to measure antibodies against antigens on the intact plasma membrane of living human spermatozoa.[20] These antibodies should be capable of being adsorbed by living sperm, and the assay should remain positive if a motility-enhanced (swim-up) sperm population is used as an antigen. The use of a highly motile sperm population achieved by swim-up ensures the presence of plasma membrane–intact sperm as the antigen in the assay. Although the question can be posed in a variety of ways, the important proposition in choosing an assay for antibody-mediated infertility is, does the antibody being measured diminish the chance that living, motile sperm (sperm that are capable of fertilizing eggs) will achieve their goal of fertilization? One exception to this dictum may be the possibility that women can form antibodies against only the plasma membrane of capacitated sperm,[48] which could present antigens different from those of uncapacitated sperm.[138] There are detractors to this possibility.[172]

In general, experiments using fixed sperm, sperm membrane preparations, whole sperm extracts, or air-dried sperm antigen preparations should be carefully scrutinized for the possibility of false-positive results.[72] These techniques have often been used to devise solid-phase assay systems (assays in which an antigen is affixed to a test tube, glass bead, or another solid surface for ease of testing), but in many cases the results of these assays have not correlated with the fertility status of the patient tested.[45] Antigens attached to a solid phase have the advantage that they can be stored indefinitely and can be sold as a kit that can be shipped anywhere. It will be possible to formulate acceptable solid-phase assay systems only when sperm antigens have been isolated whose putative antibody has been shown to disturb consistently a particular step in reproductive function. Solid-phase assays with purified antigens from the sperm plasma membrane would eliminate the complicating effects of antibodies against trivial internal or chemically altered sperm antigens, so the possibility of a false-positive test result would be minimized.

The use of polyacrylamide beads (immunobeads) as probes has demonstrated that in many instances 100% of motile sperm are found to be positive for sperm-associated immunoglobulin. The use of fluorescein-labeled antibody probes has failed to find that a majority of all spermatozoa (motile plus immotile) in a single ejaculate were coated with Ig molecules.[58] These disparate results imply that immotile sperm may not be associated with sperm antibodies because possibly they express different antigen determinants on their surfaces after cell death (as manifested by their immotility). We have recently reported that antisperm antibodies are usually formed by infertile patients against both surface and internal sperm antigens.[63]

Many verbal and written arguments have been made justifying or theorizing which particular label for immunoglobulin-specific assays is most useful or appropriate. Perhaps a more important consideration would be which sperm antigen or antigens should be used in an assay

for antisperm antibodies.[63] Radiolabeled and immunobead tests give very similar results when sperm surface antibodies attached in vivo to the sperm surface are assessed.[73] This is because the antibody attached to the living sperm when the sperm plasma membrane was intact and undamaged. Most indirect assays that identify serum or cervical mucus antibodies that associate with the sperm surface in vitro must employ intact, unfixed, and live sperm if a valid assay result is to occur. In an indirect sperm antibody assay, a fluid (serum, cervical mucus, etc.) is assayed for sperm antibodies. Many laboratories have attempted to utilize disrupted, treated, fixed, or mechanically pulverized spermatozoa as an antigen because this material can be refrigerated or stored for prolonged intervals of time and therefore is always available for use. Unfortunately, although it may be possible for a man to make antibodies against internal sperm antigens,[63] with the exception of the inner acrosomal membrane after the acrosome reaction, the only antigens exposed on spermatozoa capable of successful reproductive function are the antigens on the intact sperm plasma membrane. Thus assays of antibodies against antigens other than those found on the sperm plasma membrane may be inappropriate and may give erroneous results when related to the clinical situation.[72,100] This may explain why some antisperm antibody assays using nonsurface antigens as a target do not compare favorably with the more traditional functional assays[18]—immunoglobulin-specific assays using living, intact sperm[63]—nor with the state of fertility of the individual assessed.[165] Although fixatives do not affect immunoglobulin already attached to the sperm surface (i.e., antibodies attached to a man's sperm in vivo), sperm fixation can markedly affect the gross morphology of spermatozoa and the antigenicity of the sperm plasma membrane.[72] Assays using fixed spermatozoa must be carefully evaluated to determine whether the results should be accepted as relevant to the in vivo situation in which unfixed, living sperm pass through the male and female genital tracts. Although certain fixatives may maintain the morphologic integrity of spermatozoa, the antigenic integrity of spermatozoal antigens may still be compromised after such treatment.[72]

The discordance in the literature regarding the label that is most appropriate for immunoglobulin-specific assays can usually be reconciled if the same antigen is used in the comparison.[63] With the exception of sensitivity, there is little difference between assay results when different antibody labels (immunobeads, radioisotopes, or fluorochromes) are compared[63] if living, intact sperm are used in all of the assays. Although results with the immunobead assay suggest the location of the sperm antibody, a better definition of antibody binding beyond head/tail/tail-tip cannot be inferred. Utilization of an immunofluorescent assay system that maintains the antigenic integrity of the plasma and acrosomal membranes has proven useful in our laboratory to obtain a clear delineation of the location of antibody binding.[54] Assays utilizing enzymes or radioisotopes as sperm antibody probes are more quantitative than the immunobead assay; however, with these assays no information is available about the location of the antibody-binding site.

In summary, when reviewing an article in the field of antibody-mediated infertility, a quick check of the "Materials and Methods" section should be made to determine what antigen was used in the sperm antibody assay. If the assay does not fulfill the requirement of assessing only antibodies that can attach to the intact plasma membrane (or perhaps the inner acrosomal membrane after acrosomal loss or the plasma membrane of capacitated sperm), the conclusions of the study may not be supported by the results presented.

Antibodies that attach to the sperm surface either are selective in which steps in reproductive function they perturb or may perturb all steps. Knowledge of the particular step(s) in reproductive function that are altered is important in planning a strategy for therapy. To date clinicians have not attempted to preselect infertile individuals with antisperm antibodies who would be candidates for a particular therapy (such as intrauterine insemination) by assessing which step(s) in reproductive function are disturbed by the antibody. If it could be shown that an antibody population that inhibited mucus penetration did not disturb any of the terminal events in reproduction (zona binding and penetration, oolemma binding and fusion, etc.), then intrauterine insemination, gamete intrafallopian transfer (GIFT), or zygote intrafallopian transfer (ZIFT) would be appropriate therapies because the hindrance to cervical mucus penetration and/or transport would be successfully bypassed. More precise knowledge of the steps surrounding fertilization is necessary to define what therapy might best overcome the effects of a particular population of sperm antibodies. Chemical or physical zona drilling might relieve the problem of antibody-mediated hindrances to zona binding. Microinjection of sperm into the perivitelline space or ooplasma might treat antibody-mediated interferences to zona penetration or oolemma fusion, respectively. Alternative instigators of acrosomal loss (such as heat shock, follicular fluid constituents, and progesterone exposure[184]) might be utilized when acrosomal loss is perturbed by the presence of sperm antibodies.

Although more examples could be given, it is clear that just as the label "antisperm antibody assay" is insufficient to include that particular test in a physician's diagnostic armamentarium, the diagnostic result "positive for antisperm antibodies" is insufficient to finalize the diagnosis of antibody-mediated infertility.

With improvements in assays for antibody-mediated infertility, problems of insensitivity have been replaced by potential problems of specificity. It may be possible by using the newer immunoglobulin-specific assays to detect such low levels of sperm antibodies that the antibody level is insufficient to interdict reproductive function. The cutoff for a positive result in a sperm antibody assay is often arbitrarily established on the basis of observed differences between fertile and infertile populations. However, the absence of a particular level of antisperm antibodies in a fertile population does not necessarily imply that a slightly (albeit statistically significant) higher level of antisperm antibodies will always result in infertility. This dilemma may be insolvable, since the number of antibody molecules on each sperm's surface and the number of motile sperm in an ejaculate that bind the required number of immunoglobulin molecules may prove difficult to quantitate.[60]

A perfect assay to detect antisperm antibodies should be able to locate the site of antigen-antibody binding; be quantitative, reproducible, sensitive, and specific; require few special pieces of equipment; measure antibody binding to living intact sperm; and be capable of being performed on sperm shipped for analysis to a central laboratory. In general, the indirect assays in which living, intact donor sperm are preincubated with the reproductive fluid or serum to be tested and the sperm are washed and incubated with a labeled second antibody probe are the most acceptable. The most popular probe has been polyacrylamide beads, although radioisotopes, enzymes, or fluorescein molecules have been used. A variation on this theme occurs in the indirect mixed antiglobulin reaction (MAR),[127] in which red blood cells or plastic beads are coated with purified IgG or IgA. These cells or beads are mixed with unprepared semen, and anti-IgG or anti-IgA is added to the mixture. If IgG or IgA is on the surface of the sperm, the anti-Ig will agglutinate the cells or beads to the sperm. The MAR test has the advantage of not requiring additional preparation of the semen sample. The immunobead assay[20] requires a motility-enhanced sperm sample to assist in identifying the binding of the polyacrylamide beads coated with anti-IgG or anti-IgA to the motile sperm. Newer variations on the immunobead theme include the use of latex beads of uniform size, which further clarifies the identification of bead binding to the sperm.[126] Both the MAR and the immunobead assay are available in commercial kits.[83,126]

All of these immunoglobulin-specific "sandwich" assays can be used in a direct testing method to assay for the presence of sperm-associated immunoglobulin placed in vivo on a man's sperm. Comparison of the direct immunobead assay and the MAR test shows correspondence in the identification of sperm-associated IgG but not IgA.[129] Some investigators have suggested that the MAR test may be more sensitive than the immunobead assay.[83]

One test that has gained favor in the European literature and can be performed with modest laboratory support is the sperm–cervical mucus contact test. The sperm–cervical mucus contact test involves mixing a small drop of semen from the male partner with a small drop of cervical mucus from the female partner.[107] The presence of sperm that are shaking in situ indicates that the man or woman (or both) have antisperm antibodies. During the sperm–cervical mucus contact test, the sperm and cervical mucus are physically intermixed, and the spermatozoa are mechanically placed in contact with the cervical mucus micellular structure. Even though antisperm antibodies placed in vivo on the man's sperm usually prevent cervical mucus penetration at the time of postcoital testing, if the sperm are forced into the cervical mucus by mechanical mixing during the sperm–cervical mucus contact test, the in situ shaking will occur. The source of the shaking phenomenon is thought to be an interaction between the Fc portion of the sperm-associated immunoglobulin molecule and the micellular structure of the mucus. It has been difficult to define how this interaction occurs, since Fc receptors are not likely to be present in a mucous secretion.

We have recently confirmed the hypothesis that if living, intact sperm are used as the antigen in an immunoglobulin-specific assay, any label can be used as a probe on the secondary antihuman immunoglobulin.[63] Variations in results that occur with the immunoglobulin-specific assays almost always occur because different antigens were used in the assays[26] or the assays had different sensitivities.

The traditional agglutination and immobilization assays are suspect as a sperm antibody assay, even though some immobilization assays have a high degree of specificity.[95] IgM antisperm antibodies can immobilize sperm; however, if a serum is tested in an immobilization assay and is found to be positive, this does not guarantee that an IgM antibody found in the serum could ever be found in the female or male genital tract,[148,152] since IgM does not easily transude into those compartments. Because two closely adjacent IgG molecules (or a single IgM molecule) are required to effect complement-mediated sperm immobilization, a large number of IgG molecules must be present for a positive immobilization test to occur; thus immobilization assays can lack sensitivity. Sperm immobilization assays have also been used to assess cervical mucus antibodies[58]; the potential for nonspecific sperm immobilization by nonimmunoglobulin mucus constituents has not been thoroughly investigated and must be borne in mind.

Agglutination assays can be positive because of the presence of immunoglobulins of the IgG, IgM, or IgA isotypes. If serum is tested with these assays, the possibility of a positive IgM result not reflecting antibodies that could be found in the genital tract must be considered. Several agglutination assays have been falsely shown to be positive in the presence of nonspecific agglutinins.[81] Both the agglutination assay and the immobilization assay are subjectively interpreted and may not be reproducible, and neither immobilization nor agglutination assays can assess immunoglobulins that are placed on the surface of a man's sperm.

IMPORTANCE OF CIRCULATING VERSUS LOCALLY PRODUCED ANTISPERM ANTIBODIES

Because men deposit their gametes into the female, only sperm that carry on their surface a man's antibody against sperm can be detrimental to subsequent reproductive events.[12] Thus it is important to determine whether antibodies have attached to a man's sperm, independent and regardless of whether the antibodies are in his blood or seminal plasma. Although sperm antibodies can hinder sperm maturation or decrease a man's sperm count by harming the developing sperm within the testicular environs, this does not commonly occur (i.e., autoimmune orchitis is rare in men). Moreover, if an adequate number of antibody-free sperm are ejaculated, it makes little difference that some of the developing sperm may have been adversely affected by an antibody-mediated phenomenon. The exception to this rule occurs when antibodies bound to a man's sperm cannot be assayed because a man has azoospermia or severe oligospermia. The deficiency of motile sperm in these men makes it difficult to obtain adequate numbers of sperm to perform a direct assay for antibodies on the sperm surface. These men should be assayed for circulating levels of IgG antisperm antibodies (the only immunoglobulin isotype that can transude into the male genital tract) or seminal plasma antisperm IgG or secretory IgA. Serum IgG antibodies may be found concomitantly in semen (in seminal plasma and on sperm), but secretory IgA when found in seminal plasma[173] and on sperm is often not present in serum.[128]

In the woman a more complex picture exists. Secretory IgA can be produced locally within the female genital tract from the endocervix to the fallopian tube without the parallel formation of circulating antisperm antibodies.[152] A small fraction (approximately 1%) of circulating IgG can transude into the female genital tract, particularly into cervical mucus and to a greater extent into follicular fluid[34] (the latter is basically an ultrafiltrate of serum[154]). Passively infused sperm antibodies will inhibit female fertility but will do so to a lesser extent in men.[111] This implies a greater transudation of circulating immunoglobulins in women than in men. Whether sperm antibodies of peritoneal fluid origin contaminate secretions of the fallopian tube is unknown. However, antisperm antibodies are not found in the peritoneal fluid of women with endometriosis.[49] Testing for cervical mucus antisperm IgG should identify the vast majority of women with biologically significant levels of circulating IgG antibodies against sperm, and similar assays for cervical mucus IgA should identify locally produced antibodies.[61] Circulating IgM antibodies against sperm do not transude into either the male or female genital tract and can be ignored.

In the female genital tract, the largest number of plasma cells capable of producing secretory IgA are fortuitously also in the region of the female genital tract that is most available for sampling, the endocervix.[144] Plasma cells beneath the cervical mucosal surface produce the monomeric IgA molecules, two of which are joined by the epithelial mucosal cells using secretory piece and the J-chain as a biologic weld.

Human cervical mucus undergoes marked alterations in the concentrations of its constituents during the menstrual cycle. Although human immunoglobulins found in the cervical mucus are at their highest concentrations during the early proliferative and the entire secretory phase of the menstrual cycle, the quantity of mucus that is available for sampling at these times is limited. Leukocyte contamination and the increased viscoelasticity of nonovulatory mucus hinder the ability to use cervical mucus in assays for antisperm antibodies. During the periovulatory interval, cervical mucus is easier to collect because of the increased volume, the decreased viscoelasticity, and the decreased contamination by white blood cells. However, the concentrations of immunoglobulins during this interval are at a nadir, since the production and transudation of immunoglobulins remain relatively constant throughout the menstrual cycle and only the volume of diluent (water) fluctuates.[67] However, the influx of water during the periovulatory interval results in a decline in the concentration of mucus immunoglobulins.

CLINICAL FINDINGS THAT SUGGEST ANTISPERM ANTIBODIES

A litany of potential deficits in reproductive physiology exists that can occur secondary to antisperm antibodies. Some abnormalities are readily accessible to testing by all clinicians (e.g., postcoital testing[132]); others may be relegated to testing by research laboratories (e.g., effect of antisperm antibodies on computer-monitored sperm motility characteristics[3]).

Since immunoglobulins can agglutinate cells, it has been suggested that spermagglutination at the time of semen analysis is a harbinger of sperm antibodies. Several investigators have reported, however, that spermagglutination in many instances may not be antibody-mediated but may be due to an association of bacteria or other organisms to the sperm's surface.[81] Alternatively, the agglutination may be due to alterations in the biochemical milieu of the seminal plasma. Even if autoagglutination of sperm is an antibody-mediated phenomenon, there almost always are a number of nonagglutinated spermatozoa swimming free in the ejaculate that are able to penetrate the cervical mucus and reach the upper levels of the female genital tract.

As has been mentioned, one of the functions of most circulating antibodies is to clear antibody-bound cells by the process of complement activation or macrophage engulfment. Considering this usual fate of antibody-bound cells, it might be predicted that oligozoospermia or asthenozoospermia would be the sequela of antisperm antibody

formation in men. Nonetheless, it has been difficult to demonstrate an association between any semen analysis abnormality and the presence of sperm antibodies.[68] This lack of correlation may be due to the low levels of seminal plasma complement[142,158] or the reported anticomplement activity of seminal plasma.[141] Limited numbers of macrophages in the male genital tract[186] may limit the role of this sequela to antibody binding to sperm.

Inhibition of cervical mucus penetration at the time of postcoital testing is a common consequence of antisperm antibody activity in both men and women. It has been reported that antisperm antibodies[21,25,55] on the sperm inhibit the sperm's entry into periovulatory mucus. This impairment in mucus penetration is found only with antibodies against the sperm plasma membrane and is not present if sperm are preincubated with antibodies against internal sperm antibodies.[20] The inhibition of sperm crossing the seminal plasma–cervical mucus interface occurs even though the cervical mucus appears perfectly normal during the periovulatory interval and even though there may be adequate numbers of spermatozoa within the man's ejaculate. We have found that approximately 50% of men whose partners have this type of postcoital test (abundant, clear, watery, and leukocyte-free cervical mucus with very few or no sperm present) will be found to have either IgG or IgA (or both) on their sperm.[55] This can be a useful clinical clue to determining when a man should be assayed for sperm-associated antibodies based on the results of a postcoital test.

When women have antisperm antibodies in their mucus, penetration of sperm into the mucus may be adequate (a quite different situation from that described earlier, when the man has sperm-associated antibodies), but sperm transport through the mucus is impeded. In these cases, a large number of nonmotile or shaking sperm are seen at the time of postcoital testing. It is believed that the Fc portion of the immunoglobulin molecule becomes entangled with the mucin molecule of the mucus and tethers the sperm, which results in a characteristic shaking phenomenon.[69] The presence of this shaking phenomenon can be monitored by the sperm–cervical mucus contact test.[96]

Antisperm antibodies do not in themselves cause abnormalities of the quality of a woman's periovulatory cervical mucus. The vast majority of postcoital tests associated with abnormal mucus are due to inadequate periovulatory estrogen production or an abnormal response of the endocervix to estrogen. In other words, the problem of abnormal mucus relates to an abnormal balance of hormonal stimulation and endocervical response and *not* to an antibody-mediated problem. Increased endogenous or exogenous estrogen stimulation or intrauterine insemination to bypass the abnormal mucus may prove to be an effective therapy in these situations. Although it is possible that the combination of an abnormality of cervical mucus production and an antibody-mediated problem can occur concomitantly, this is uncommon.

There may be an increased incidence of antisperm antibodies in the female partners of men who have antisperm antibodies on their sperm surface.[176] Sperm-associated immunoglobulins conceivably could influence the response of the female genital tract to the potentially foreign spermatozoal antigens. Thus situations can arise in which both partners have potentially detrimental sperm antibodies. It will not be easy to prove that a woman has antibodies against the sperm of her antibody-positive partner, since the immunoglobulins placed on the sperm by the man will be difficult to differentiate from any antibodies placed on the sperm by the woman during an indirect testing procedure. Thus donor sperm should be used as the antigen in a sperm antibody assay if the man has sperm-associated antibodies.

Some women may produce antibodies against antigens unique to their husbands' sperm.[123,181] If this proves to be the case, donor insemination is a valid therapy for these couples. Considering the dearth of individual-specific antigens that have been found on the sperm surface, careful analysis of this phenomenon must be made before it can be accepted unreservedly.

The most likely site of sperm capacitation and initiation of hyperactivated sperm motility (the hallmark of successfully capacitated human sperm) is within the cervical mucus.[136] Even if other influences can initiate capacitation, such as follicular fluid within the cumulus cells, it is possible that antisperm antibodies could bind to the sperm surface "receptor"[19] that activates capacitation and thus interfere with the process.

Acrosomal loss in humans may not occur until the sperm has bound to the zona pellucida.[184] We reported that antisperm antibodies placed on the sperm may result in premature acrosomal loss.[109] Sperm that have undergone acrosomal loss have a limited span of time during which fertilization can occur.[14] After this time interval has elapsed, despite the continuation of sperm motility, fertilization can no longer occur. The ability of acrosome-reacted hamster sperm to fertilize hamster ova may last only a few hours.[79] If human sperm that have undergone acrosomal loss prematurely are capable of attaching to the zona, these acrosome-reacted sperm should be brought into contact with the zona soon after ejaculation if fertilization is to occur. This observation and hypothesis may affect treatment regimens for antibody-mediated infertility, since it may be important to expedite spermatozoal contact with the target eggs.

Murine monoclonal antibodies have been developed that interfere with only a single step in the final events of the fertilization process.[150,151] These monoclonal antibodies uniquely can interfere with zona binding but not with oolemma penetration, or vice versa. The possibility that antibodies that block both or either of these steps in

reproductive function could develop spontaneously in infertile couples seems plausible. The possibility that the final steps in fertilization could be impaired while cervical mucus penetration remains adequate in sperm antibody-positive patients implies that antisperm antibody testing may not necessarily be limited to couples with an abnormal postcoital test. The ability to monitor sperm hypermotility (indicating successful capacitation[3]) to assess the acrosomal reaction using monoclonal antibodies[182] or plant lectins[31] and to determine the ability of human sperm to penetrate the oolemma of hamster ova[43,69,70] may allow a precise dissection of which of the final steps in reproduction are being affected by sperm antibodies.

It is unclear at present whether the results of the zona-free hamster egg assay can accurately monitor sperm antibody-mediated interference with oolemma binding. It may be that human IVF is in truth the only valid method by which to determine any detrimental effects of antisperm antibodies on fertilization. It has been reported that there is a greater incidence of antisperm antibodies in couples with unexplained infertility undergoing IVF than in couples with tubal factor infertility.[29] The choice in antibody-positive patients of an assisted reproductive technology that allows fertilization to occur in vitro may be important (IVF–embryo transfer, ZIFT, etc.), since this may be the only way to determine whether the antibody interferes with fertilization. In the antibody-positive man who fails the GIFT procedure it is unclear whether the failure was due to failed fertilization or another problem, although GIFT using antibody-bound sperm has been successful.[170] In IVF or ZIFT, antibodies from the female partner can be prevented from interfering with fertilization by utilizing a protein source other than the wife's serum in the incubation medium and by carefully washing the ova free of follicular fluid before insemination.[29] Elimination of maternal antisperm antibodies from the site of fertilization is not possible with the GIFT procedure.

Sperm antibodies in animals may interfere with postfertilization events and result in abortion, presumably because of the conservation of sperm antigens on the surface of the developing embryo.[134] Another possibility is that sperm antibodies may stimulate interferon-γ, which may increase the presentation of paternal MHC antigens on the trophoblast and result in immune rejection.[174] It does not appear that women with antisperm antibodies who become pregnant after successful therapy have an increased risk of pregnancy wastage. One large study found that an assay that assessed antisperm antibodies against sperm plasma membrane antigens was positive in less than 2% of women with three or more first-trimester pregnancy losses.[71] However, another study has shown an association between IgG tail-directed antibodies and recurrent spontaneous abortion.[175]

The couple with an abnormal postcoital test or unexplained infertility or the man with an abnormal semen analysis or autoagglutination of sperm are candidates for antisperm antibody testing. In addition, the incidence of antisperm antibodies is increased in men with a history of several diseases.[57] Of all potential causes of antisperm antibodies in men, vasectomy has been the most carefully studied.[1] After ligation of the vas deferens, all animal species studied, including man, have been noted to have an increased incidence of antisperm antibodies. Depending on the assay employed, approximately 50% to 80% of vasectomized men will have circulating antisperm antibodies. The factors that influence the formation of antisperm antibodies after vasectomy are multiple. Prospective studies have investigated the incidence of antibodies on the sperm of vasovasostomized men and compared these with the pregnancy rates achieved after a vasovasostomy; the correlation has been disappointing.[133] The incidence of seminal plasma antisperm antibodies in vasectomized (but not vasovasostomized) men is low.[112] Although extensively examined, it has been difficult, using assays for serum antisperm antibodies, to predict fertility after vasovasostomy except when a very high serum antibody titer is present, in which case a pregnancy is unlikely to occur.[147,159]

Witkin et al.[179] have found that sperm antigens associated with circulating immune complexes can be detected in vasectomized men in the first few months after vasectomy. Antibodies bound in these immune complexes cannot be detected by most assays for antisperm antibodies. For this reason the incidence of postvasectomy antisperm antibody formation may be greater than the 50% to 80% that has been reported. In general, the incidence of antisperm antibodies decreases from an immediate postvasectomy peak 6 to 12 months after the procedure[11,82] to a level of approximately 30% several years thereafter.[140] Antisperm antibodies can be found as early as 2 months or as late as 20 years after vasectomy.[108] Sotolongo[156] has hypothesized that 100% of vasectomized men do not initiate an antisperm antibody response because of genetic variables or an inhibition of the immune response to sperm antigens by the men's high levels of testosterone. Although the cell-mediated response to sperm antigens has not been well characterized,[162,186] delayed hypersensitivity skin reactions to sperm antigens in vasectomized men have been reported by Alexander and Anderson.[4]

It has been hypothesized that the formation of a sperm granuloma after vasectomy increases the risk of antisperm antibody formation. The granulomas are composed of leukocytic infiltrates arising as an immune response to sperm antigens that have leaked into the tissues surrounding the incised vas deferens. The relationship between sperm granulomas and antisperm antibody activity, however, has not been well defined,[6] and several men with large granulomas have not had detectable antisperm antibodies.

Alexander and Clarkson[5] reported accelerated atheroma formation in vasectomized monkeys, compared with non-vasectomized controls; both groups of animals were fed comparable high-cholesterol diets. Long-term studies, however, indicate that this complication does not occur in vasectomized men.[114]

Several studies reported in the literature have investigated the incidence of antisperm antibodies in men with unilateral or bilateral obstruction to the male genital tract, a congenital or acquired condition that might mimic vasectomy,[78,86,103] although there have been dissenting reports of this association.[139] Hendry et al.[86] reported that 26 (81%) of 32 men with unilateral obstruction of the proximal genital tract were found to have agglutinating sperm antibodies in their serum. Girgis et al.[51] reported that 10 (71%) of 14 men with bilateral congenital absence of the vas deferens had sperm agglutinating or immobilizing sperm antibodies. It is interesting to note that in this report no immunoglobulin of any class was detectable in the semen of these men with obstructed genital tracts. This implies that the source of the seminal plasma immunoglobulin is not transudation via the prostate gland, but may be a result of production or transudation of immunoglobulin from more proximal regions of the male genital tract. We have reported that the acquired obstruction of the genital tracts of men with cystic fibrosis is sometimes associated with the formation of antisperm antibodies.[36] In summary, the continued spermatogenesis that occurs in men with congenital or acquired genital tract obstruction can result in sperm antigen leakage and subsequent inoculation of these men's immune systems with spermatozoal antigens.

A testicular biopsy possibly may initiate the formation of sperm antibodies, since this procedure obviously could breach the protective mechanisms of the blood-testis barrier. Hjort et al.[90] reported that 6 (17%) of 35 men who underwent a testicular biopsy developed a weak titer of serum agglutinating sperm antibodies; 5 of these 6 men had previously undergone a testicular biopsy. The implication of this report was that multiple insults to the testis portends a greater possibility of an immune reaction against sperm.

One report[1] of an association between benign and malignant prostatic lesions and the presence of antisperm antibodies suggested a lack of specificity of antibodies to sperm. However, since antibodies to a solubilized sperm preparation were used in this study, the problem of internal versus plasma membrane sperm antigens arises and severely jeopardizes the conclusions of the experiments.

Although genital trauma or injury has been found to be associated with an increased risk of sperm antibodies[37,74,143] some studies have failed to confirm this association.[46] Testicular torsion is a form of trauma to the male genital tract that has been intensely studied.[47,80] The suggestion has been made that, if the injured testis is not removed at the time of the torsion in postpubertal animals, an immune response, presumably against spermatozoal antigens, will permanently damage the retained testis. It has proven difficult to document post-torsion antisperm antibody formation in the serum or on the sperm surface in men,[47] although damage to the contralateral testis (sympathetic orchiopathy) and decreased fertility after torsion occur.[82] The process of sympathetic orchiopathy is prevented by the administration of adrenocorticotropic hormone.[104] The lack of a sperm antibody response after prepubertal torsion[84] is presumably due to the absence of antigens from mature spermatozoa, which are necessary to excite an immune response that could be detrimental to subsequent fertility. Thus in instances of prepubertal torsion it appears that more consideration should be given to ischemia of the torsive testis than to the potential formation of sperm antibodies.

Cryptorchidism is another clinical situation that could increase the risk for formation of antisperm antibodies. Interest regarding the sequelae of cryptorchidism stems from the fact that 10% of men with unilateral disease are infertile when treatment for the undescended testis occurs late in childhood; 70% to 80% of cryptorchid men are infertile if the disease is bilateral. Koskimies and Hovatta[106] found that 3 (13%) of 23 cryptorchid men had agglutinating sperm antibodies in their serum. Two of three men also had seminal plasma antibodies at a titer of 1:4 or greater. It is not clear whether the additional 20 men were negative for antisperm antibodies or were not assessed for them.

Varicocele has been associated with infertility, and some investigators have considered that this condition might be associated with an increased incidence of antisperm antibodies. Ozen et al.[137] found that 16 (25%) of 65 men with palpable unilateral varicoceles had antisperm antibodies by an indirect immunofluorescent assay using methanol-fixed, air-dried sperm. As has been mentioned, a positive result with fixed sperm may be of little clinical significance. Golomb et al.[53] reported that 29 (91%) of 32 men with palpable varicoceles were found to have antisperm antibodies by an enzyme-linked immunosorbent assay (ELISA) using glutaraldehyde-fixed sperm. It is interesting that there was no correlation between the class of Ig in the men's seminal plasma and the class of Ig on the sperm surface. This may have been due to the fact that in the seminal plasma assay, fixed sperm were used as the antigen before the immunochemical assay; in the assay for sperm-associated antibody, the antibodies would have attached to the men's sperm in vivo before exposure of the sperm to fixatives. Sperm-bound antibodies also appear to have an increased risk of occurring in men with varicoceles.[50]

Several investigators have found an increased incidence of serum antisperm antibodies in men who have a positive history for genital tract infections. Andrada et al.[10] demonstrated a positive correlation between mumps orchitis and serum agglutinating or immobilizing sperm antibodies. No such relationship has been found between genital mycoplasma infections in men and serum or seminal plasma sperm antibodies.[77] Hargreave et al.[79] and Witkin and Toth[178] have reported conflicting results of the effect of

genital infections in men and the subsequent risk of formation of antisperm antibodies. Hargreave et al.[79] noted an incidence of positive agglutination and immobilization assays for antisperm antibodies among 217 men attending a sexually transmitted disease clinic similar to that among 151 fertile men. This finding implied that genital tract infections did not increase the risk of serum sperm antibodies. Witkin and Toth,[178] however, using an ELISA employing glutaraldehyde-fixed sperm, found that men with genital tract infections had a high incidence of seminal plasma antisperm antibodies. Because the importance of antibodies against glutaraldehyde-fixed sperm is unknown, it is difficult to access adequately the importance of genital infections on the formation of antisperm antibodies in men.

Despite the suggestive data, a 1:1 correspondence between any of these clinical entities and the presence of antisperm antibodies does not exist. Since many men develop antisperm antibodies without any of these factors, a genetic influence may play a role. Hancock et al.[76] and Law et al.[110] have reported an association between sperm antibodies with the HLA antigen A28; Marsh et al.[121] failed to demonstrate this relationship.

Male homosexuals who participate in recipient anal intercourse have an increased incidence of antisperm antibodies.[185] Some investigators have reported that the formation of antisperm antibodies in this group of men could play a role in the development of the acquired immunodeficiency syndrome (AIDS).[124,146,155] Some monoclonal antibodies against helper lymphocytes can cross-react with human sperm plasma membrane antigens.[183] Whether oral heterosexual intercourse can increase the risk of antisperm antibodies is unknown, but an increased risk has been reported in some animal models.[7] Contrariwise, oral administration of sperm antigens has been proposed as a therapy for sperm antibodies by some investigators.[30] The incidence of antisperm antibodies in heterosexual couples who engage in anal intercourse is unknown.

We have characterized 1452 men assayed for antisperm antibodies by a radiolabeled antiglobulin assay.[54] Of these men 12.5% were positive for plasma IgG antisperm antibodies (plasma IgA and IgM were not assessed), and 11% of the 288 men tested were found to have IgG on their sperm; 11% had sperm-associated IgA. Ninety percent of the men had primary infertility of an average duration of 5.0 years. The average age of the men with sperm antibodies was 33.7 years. There was no association between any semen abnormality and the presence of sperm antibodies. Only 20% of the poor postcoital tests of men with sperm-associated Ig could be attributed to hostile periovulatory mucus; the remainder of the tests were abnormal because of limited sperm penetration into normal periovulatory mucus.

THERAPY FOR ANTISPERM ANTIBODIES

The most appropriate therapy for a particular individual's antisperm antibodies depends on the secondary reproductive deficits that are present. The logic of discovering the problem caused by the antibodies and overcoming this problem was discussed earlier. It is obvious that if virtually all events associated with fertility are impaired, only therapies such as corticosteroid immunosuppression can lower the total antibody complement and be effective. The efficacy of corticosteroids in double-blind studies has been controversial,[38,65] although long-term, placebo-controlled studies suggest cumulative pregnancy rates of 30% with these drugs.[87,88] Many individuals cannot tolerate a long therapeutic exposure to corticosteroids. Since pregnancy can occur in placebo-treated groups independent of a diminution of sperm-associated Ig, spontaneous fluctuations of sperm-associated antibody levels probably occur. This phenomenon underscores the necessity of placebo-controlled trials.

The risk of corticosteroids cannot be overestimated. Bilateral aseptic hip necrosis occurs in 21% to 27%[93] of individuals who have undergone kidney transplantation because of the common usage of corticosteroids as immunosuppressive agents in these patients. Many patients in the United States have come to this author's attention after the administration of corticosteroids for antibody-mediated infertility had been associated with hip problems.[85] Extreme care must be taken in obtaining an informed consent from these patients. A signed and witnessed informed consent, perhaps approved by the local institutional review board, may be the most appropriate way to provide the patient with a truly informed consent while ensuring the medical-legal protection of the physician. Care must be taken in interpreting the literature reviewing the results of corticosteroid therapy, since in the majority of the reports, men were selected for corticosteroid therapy because of the presence of circulating antisperm antibodies. The possibility that these antibodies (especially if they were of the IgM isotype) did not enter the male genital tract and had no effect on sperm function must be considered. The efficacy of corticosteroids in this instance would be fallacious, since these individuals might not have had antibody-mediated infertility.

The pregnancy rate after intrauterine insemination of the husband's swim-up, antibody-positive sperm is less than 20% even when four treatment cycles are undertaken.[122] Similarly low pregnancy rates (13%) may occur when women with antibody-mediated infertility are treated with intrauterine insemination; however, the use of clomiphene citrate or human menotropins along with intrauterine insemination results in pregnancy rates of 30% and 39%, respectively.[120] When men have antisperm antibodies, substitution of antibody-free donor sperm is a viable therapeutic possibility. When intrauterine insemination is undertaken, the primary sperm capacitator and reservoir for sperm in the cervix are bypassed. For this reason, the coincidence of ovulation and insemination may be critical to success. This may necessitate either frequent monitoring of serum or urine luteinizing hormone levels or triggering of ovulation with clomiphene or menotropins and human chorionic gonadotropin. The increased pregnancy rates associated with the use of ovulation-inducing agents combined with insemination of antibody-free sperm may be due to the precise coincidence of ovulation and insemination that is possible with these regimens. There does not appear to be an increased incidence of sperm antibodies induced by intrauterine insemination, although intraperitoneal insemination may incite the formation of sperm antibodies.[115] Low pregnancy rates after intrauterine insemination for an abnormal postcoital test are not affected by whether sperm-associated antibodies were on the inseminated sperm.[122]

Although some series report that fertilization is inhibited by sperm-associated antibodies on the male partner's sperm, pregnancy rates remain adequate with IVF, ZIFT, or GIFT.[138] In one large series, a low fertilization rate of 27% occurred when the male partner had sperm-associated antibodies, and pregnancies did not occur in the antibody-positive group.[28]

Although IVF has been successfully employed in couples in whom the man had sperm-associated Ig,[28] only a 14% pregnancy rate[57] was reported. Fertilization rates can be as low as 24% to 27% in men with both IgG *and* IgA on their sperm surface, but embryo cleavage appears to proceed normally if fertilization is successful.[27,101] These low fertilization rates are particularly apparent when the antisperm antibody–positive men are also oligozoospermic.[28] Surprisingly, there does not appear to be a close association between the location of antibody binding to the sperm surface (as assessed by immunobead binding) and whether impaired fertilization occurs[28]; however, antisperm antibodies that attach to the sperm head may be particularly detrimental to women undergoing IVF for unexplained infertility.[119] Increasing the number of antibody-free motile sperm in the insemination medium to greater than 50,000 appears to be more effective than attempting to separate unbound from antibody-bound sperm in vitro.[75]

Attempts to remove the sperm-associated antibody by repeated washes have proven futile.[64] Attempts to remove sperm-associated IgA1 with specific proteases has been reported to be successful in vitro,[23] but the pregnancy rate after insemination of sperm treated with this protease is not known. When a woman with antisperm antibodies undergoes IVF, the use of a protein source other than her serum in the insemination medium can raise the fertilization and pregnancy rate to levels expected in women without a sperm antibody problem.[29] In general, because fertilization may be impaired if antibodies are present on the male partner's sperm, IVF or ZIFT may be preferable to the GIFT procedure when the man has sperm-associated antibodies, since it is important to determine whether failed fertilization was the cause of an unsuccessful cycle. Donor insemination when the woman has antibody-mediated infertility is not usually efficacious, since her antisperm antibodies are not against novel antigens on her husband's sperm but are against antigens common to all sperm. As has been mentioned, donor sperm insemination is appropriate when the male partner is found to have sperm-associated antibodies. This is true except in those cases in which the woman is making antibodies against unique antigens found only on her husband's sperm.[180] The additional complicating effect of oligozoospermia or asthenozoospermia must be taken into account when considering IVF as therapy for antibody-mediated infertility. The roles of micromanipulation, zona drilling, and perivitelline space sperm insertion by microinjection in antibody-mediated infertility await additional study. Another therapy requiring additional study includes frequent ejaculation to exhaust the immunoglobulins within the male genital tract that could attach to the sperm surface. It has been proposed that collecting the ejaculate in large volumes of sperm antigen-containing medium might effectively inhibit the attachment of sperm antibody molecules to the sperm surface.[22,41] Attempts have been made to separate antibody-bound sperm from antibody-free sperm,[46] but no controlled trials of the efficacy of this therapy have been reported. Multicenter studies are needed to investigate the therapeutic efficacy of these investigative treatment alternatives in large groups of antibody-positive couples as well as in carefully delineated subgroups.

The cautions regarding systemic corticosteroid therapy may not be relevant when these drugs are administered locally to the female genital tract. It has been noted that the intravaginal administration of corticosteroids diminishes the number of plasma cells beneath the cervical epithelium.[97] A pilot study has shown that local treatment with intravaginal corticosteroid suppositories diminishes secretory IgA sperm antibodies in the cervical mucus.[168] The squelched antibody level has been associated with an increased pregnancy rate with few side effects. Obviously, large-scale studies are necessary, but the possibility of using intravaginal foams or suppositories containing corticosteroids that are directly applied to the site of antibody production is intriguing.

It is hoped that this review will justify the appropriateness of the diagnosis of antibody-mediated infertility. In addition, it is this author's hope that the continued use of proven immunologic precepts will impart a better understanding of this interesting malady to both researchers and clinicians.

SUMMARY

Literature support of the four tenets mentioned at the beginning of the chapter can place antibody-mediated infertility as a well-substantiated diagnosis that can be effectively treated by the clinician who is aware of the immune events leading to this phenomenon.

ACKNOWLEDGMENT

The patient and talented secretarial assistance of Ms. Lisa Harris is gratefully acknowledged.

REFERENCES

1. Ablin RJ, Kulikauskas V, Gonder MJ: Antibodies to sperm in benign and malignant diseases of the prostate in man: Incidence, disease-associated specificity and implications, *Am J Reprod Immunol Microbiol* 16:42, 1988.
2. Adams DD: Autoimmune mechanisms. In Davies TF, editor: *Autoimmune endocrine disease,* New York, 1983, John Wiley & Sons.
3. Adeghe AJ-H et al: Antisperm antibodies and sperm motility: a study using timed exposure photomicrography, *Int J Androl* 12:281, 1989.
4. Alexander NJ, Anderson DJ: Vasectomy: consequences of autoimmunity to sperm antigens, *Fertil Steril* 32:253, 1979.
5. Alexander NJ, Clarkson TB: Vasectomy increases the severity of diet-induced atherosclerosis in *Macaca* fascicularis, *Science* 201:538, 1978.
6. Alexander NJ, Schmidt SS: Incidence of antisperm antibody levels and granulomas in men, *Fertil Steril* 28:655, 1977.
7. Allardyce RA: Effect of ingested sperm on fecundity in the rat, *J Exp Med* 159:1548, 1984.
8. Anderson DJ, Hill JA: Cell-mediated immunity in infertility, *Am J Reprod Immunol Microbiol* 17:22, 1988.
9. Anderson DJ, Michaelson JS, Johnson PM: Trophoblast/leukocyte-common antigen is expressed by human testicular cells and appears on the surface of acrosome-reacted sperm, *Biol Reprod* 41:285, 1989.
10. Andrada JA et al: Immunological studies in patients with mumps orchitis, *Andrologia* 9:207, 1977.
11. Ansbacher R et al: Vas ligation: humoral sperm antibodies, *Int J Fertil* 21:258, 1976.
12. Asch RH, Balmaceda J, Pauerstein CJ: Failure of seminal plasma to enter the uterus and oviducts of the rabbit following artificial insemination, *Fertil Steril* 28:671, 1977.
13. Barratt CLR et al: Antisperm antibodies and lymphocyte subsets in semen—not a simple relationship, *Int J Androl* 13:50, 1990.
14. Barros C, Fujimoto M, Yanagimachi R: Failure of zona penetration of hamster spermatozoa after prolonged preincubation in a blood serum fraction, *J Reprod Fertil* 35:89, 1973.
15. Baskin MJ: Temporary sterilization by the injection of human spermatozoa: a preliminary report, *Am J Obstet Gynecol* 24:892, 1932.
16. Bedford JM, Calvin H, Cooper GW: The maturation of spermatozoa in the human epididymis, *J Reprod Fertil Suppl* 18:199, 1973.
17. Bisbara A et al: Human leukocyte antigens (HLA) class I and class II on sperm cells studied at the serological, cellular, and genomic levels, *Am J Reprod Immunol Microbiol* 13:97, 1987.
18. Boettcher B et al: Auto- and iso-antibodies to antigens of the human reproductive system, I: results of an international comparative study, *Clin Exp Immunol* 30:173, 1977.
19. Boettger H et al: Effects of in vitro incubation on a zona binding site found on murine spermatozoa, *J Exp Zool* 249:90, 1989.
20. Bronson RA, Cooper GW: Effects of sperm-reactive monoclonal antibodies on the cervical mucus penetrating ability of human spermatozoa, *Am J Reprod Immunol Microbiol* 14:59, 1987.
21. Bronson RA, Cooper GW, Rosenfeld DL: Autoimmunity to spermatozoa: effect on sperm penetration of cervical mucus as reflected by postcoital testing, *Fertil Steril* 41:609, 1984.
22. Bronson R, Cooper G, Rosenfeld D: Rapid semen dilution as a means to diminish post-ejaculatory sperm-antibody binding, *Fertil Steril* 41:40S, 1984 (abstract).
23. Bronson RA et al: Effect of IgA$_1$ protease on immunoglobulins bound to the sperm surface and sperm cervical mucus penetrating ability, *Fertil Steril* 47:985, 1987.
24. Carron CP, Mathias A, Saling PM: Anti-idiotype antibodies prevent antibody binding to mouse sperm and antibody-mediated inhibition of fertilization, *Biol Reprod* 40:153, 1989.

25. Clarke GN: Immunoglobulin class and regional specificity of anti-spermatozoal autoantibodies blocking cervical mucus penetration by human spermatozoa, *Am J Reprod Immunol Microbiol* 16:135, 1988.

26. Clarke GN: Lack of correlation between the immunobead test and the enzyme-linked immunosorbent assay for sperm antibody detection, *Am J Reprod Immunol Microbiol* 18:44, 1988.

27. Clarke GN, Elliott PJ, Smaila C: Detection of sperm antibodies in semen using the immunobead test: a survey of 813 consecutive patients, *Am J Reprod Immunol Microbiol* 7:118, 1985.

28. Clarke GN et al: Effect of sperm antibodies in males on human in vitro fertilization (IVF), *Am J Reprod Immunol Microbiol* 8:62, 1985.

29. Clarke GN et al: In vitro fertilization results for women with sperm antibodies in plasma and follicular fluid, *Am J Reprod Immunol* 8:130, 1985.

30. Congleton L, Potts W, Mathur S: Oral immunization with sperm antigens: possible therapy for sperm antibodies, *Fertil Steril* 52:106, 1989.

31. Cross NL et al: Two simple methods for detecting acrosome-reacted human sperm, *Gamete Res* 15:213, 1986.

32. D'Cruz OJ, Haas GG Jr: Lack of complement activation in the seminal plasma of men with antisperm antibodies associated *in vivo* on their sperm, *Am J Reprod Immunol* 24:51, 1990.

33. D'Cruz OJ, Haas GG Jr: Phagocytosis of IgG and C3-bound human sperm by human polymorphonuclear leukocytes is not associated with the release of free oxidative radicals, *Am J Reprod Immunol* 25:55, 1991 (abstract).

34. D'Cruz OJ, Haas Jr GG, Lambert H: Evaluation of antisperm complement-dependent immune mediators in human ovarian follicular fluid, *J Immunol* 144:3841, 1990.

35. D'Cruz OJ et al: Activation of human complement by IgG antisperm antibody and the demonstration of C3 and C5b-9-mediated immune injury to human sperm, *J Immunol* 146:611, 1991.

36. D'Cruz OJ et al: Occurrence of serum antisperm antibodies in men with cystic fibrosis, *Fertil Steril* 56:519, 1991.

37. Daugaard G et al: Sequelae to genital trauma in torture victims, *Arch Androl* 10:245, 1983.

38. De Almeida M et al: Steroid therapy for male infertility associated with antisperm antibodies: results of a small randomized clinical trial, *Int J Androl* 8:111, 1985.

39. Dym M, Fawcett DW: The blood-testis barrier in the rat and the physiological compartmentalization of the seminiferous tubule, *Biol Reprod* 3:308, 1970.

40. El-Demirey MIM et al: Lymphocyte sub-populations in the male genital tract, *Br J Urol* 57:769, 1985.

41. Elder KT, Wick KL, Edwards RG: Seminal plasma antisperm antibodies and IVF: the effect of semen sample collection into 50% serum, *Hum Reprod* 5:179, 1990.

42. Ernst C et al: Monoclonal antibody localization of A and B isoantigens in normal and malignant fixed human tissues, *Am J Pathol* 117:451, 1984.

43. Falk RM et al: Establishment of TEST-yolk buffer enhanced sperm penetration assay limits for fertile males, *Fertil Steril* 54:121, 1990.

44. Faulk WP, McIntyre JA: Immunological studies of human trophoblast: markers, subsets and functions, *Immunol Rev* 75:139, 1983.

45. Fernandez-Collazo E, Thierer E: Action of ABO antisera on human spermatozoa, *Fertil Steril* 23:376, 1972.

46. Foresta C, Varotto A, Caretto A: Immunomagnetic method to select human sperm without sperm surface-bound autoantibodies in male autoimmune infertility, *Arch Androl* 24:221, 1990.

47. Fraser I et al: Testicular torsion does not cause autoimmunization in man, *Br J Surg* 72:237, 1985.

48. Fusi F, Bronson RA: Effects of incubation time in serum and capacitation on spermatozoal reactivity with antisperm antibodies, *Fertil Steril* 54:887, 1990.

49. Gentry WL: Failure to demonstrate significant antisperm antibodies in peritoneal fluid of patients with endometriosis, *Fertil Steril* 52:949, 1989.

50. Gilbert BR, Witkin SS, Goldstein M: Correlation of sperm-bound immunoglobulins with impaired semen analysis in infertile men with varicoceles, *Fertil Steril* 52:469, 1989.

51. Girgis SM et al: Sperm antibodies in serum and semen in men with bilateral congenital absence of the vas deferens, *Arch Androl* 8:301, 1982.

52. Gocial B et al: Correlations between results of the immunobead test and the sperm penetration assay, *Am J Reprod Immunol Microbiol* 16:37, 1988.

53. Golomb J et al: Demonstration of antispermatozoal antibodies in varicocele-related infertility with an enzyme-linked immunosorbent assay (ELISA), *Fertil Steril* 45:397, 1986.

54. Haas GG Jr: Evaluation of sperm antibodies and autoimmunity in the infertile male. In Santen RJ, Swerdloff RS, editors: *Male reproductive function,* New York, 1986, Marcel Dekker.

55. Haas GG Jr: The inhibitory effect of sperm-associated immunoglobulins on cervical mucus penetration, *Fertil Steril* 46:334, 1986.

56. Haas GG Jr: Antibody-mediated causes of male infertility, *Urol Clin North Am* 14:539, 1987.

57. Haas GG Jr: Male fertility and immunity. In Lipshultz LI, Howards SS, editors: *Infertility in the male,* ed 2, St Louis, 1991, Mosby–Year Book.

58. Haas GG Jr, Cunningham ME: Identification of antibody-laden sperm by cytofluorometry, *Fertil Steril* 42:606, 1984.

59. Haas GG Jr, D'Cruz OJ: ABH blood group antigens in human semen, *Am J Reprod Immunol Microbiol* 16:28, 1988.

60. Haas GG Jr, D'Cruz OJ: Quantitation of immunoglobulin G on human sperm, *Am J Reprod Immunol* 20:37, 1989.

61. Haas GG Jr, D'Cruz OJ: A radiolabeled antiglobulin assay to identify human cervical mucus immunoglobulin (Ig) A and IgG antisperm antibodies, *Fertil Steril* 52:474, 1989.

62. Haas GG Jr, D'Cruz OJ, DeBault LE: The predominance of IgG1 and IgG3 subclass antisperm antibodies in infertile patients with IgG-mediated auto- and iso-immunity to human sperm. Poster presented at the 46th annual meeting of The American Fertility Society, Washington, DC, October 15-18, 1990.

63. Haas GG Jr, D'Cruz OJ, DeBault LE: Comparison of the indirect immunobead radiolabeled and immunofluorescence assays for serum antibodies to human sperm, *Fertil Steril* 55:377, 1991.

64. Haas GG Jr, D'Cruz OJ, Denum BM: Effect of repeated washing on sperm-bound immunoglobulin G, *J Androl* 9:190, 1988.

65. Haas GG Jr, Manganiello P: A double-blind, placebo-controlled study of the use of methylprednisolone in infertile men with sperm-associated immunoglobulins, *Fertil Steril* 47:295, 1987.

66. Haas GG Jr, Nahhas F: Failure to identify HLA ABC and Dr antigens on human sperm, *Am J Reprod Immunol* 10:39, 1986.

67. Haas GG Jr, Nicosia SV, Wolf DP: Influence of estrogens on vascular transudation and mucus production in the rabbit endocervix, *Fertil Steril* 48:1036, 1987.

68. Haas GG Jr, Schreiber AD, Blasco L: The incidence of sperm-associated immunoglobulins and C3, the third component of complement, in infertile men, *Fertil Steril* 39:542, 1983.

69. Haas GG Jr, Sokoloski J, Wolf DP: The interfering effect of human IgG antisperm antibodies on human sperm penetration of zona-free hamster eggs, *Am J Reprod Immunol* 1:40, 1980.

70. Haas GG Jr et al: The effect of immunoglobulin occurring on human sperm in vivo on the human sperm/hamster ova penetration assay, *Am J Reprod Immunol Microbiol* 7:109, 1985.

71. Haas GG Jr et al: Circulating antisperm antibodies in recurrently aborting women, *Fertil Steril* 45:209, 1986.

72. Haas GG Jr et al: The effect of fixatives and/or air-drying on the plasma and acrosomal membranes of human sperm, *Fertil Steril* 50:487, 1988.

73. Haas GG Jr et al: Comparison of the direct radiolabeled antiglobulin assay and the direct immunobead binding test for detection of sperm-associated antibodies, *Am J Reprod Immunol* 22:130, 1990.

74. Haensch R: Spermatozoen-Autoimmunphaenomene bei genitaltraumen und verschlubbazoospermie, *Andrologia* 5:147, 1973.

75. Hamilton F, Gutlay-Yeo AL, Meldrum DR: Normal fertilization in men with high antibody sperm binding by the addition of sufficient unbound sperm in vitro, *J In Vitro Fert Embryo Transfer* 6:342, 1989.

76. Hancock RJT et al: Anti-sperm antibodies, HLA antigens, and semen analysis, *Lancet* 2:847, 1983 (letter).

77. Hargreave TB et al: Isolation of Ureaplasma urealyticum from seminal plasma in relation to sperm antibody levels and sperm motility, *Andrologia* 14:223, 1982.

78. Hargreave TB et al: Studies of testicular and epididymal damage in relation to the occurrence of antisperm antibodies, *Br J Urol* 54:769, 1982.

79. Hargreave TB et al: Serum agglutinating and immobilising sperm antibodies in men attending a sexually transmitted diseases clinic, *Andrologia* 16:111, 1984.

80. Harrison RG et al: Mechanism of damage to the contralateral testis in rats with an ischaemic testis, *Lancet* 2:723, 1981.

81. Hekman A, Rumke P: Seminal antigens and autoimmunity, In Hafez ESE, editor: *Human semen and fertility regulation in men,* St. Louis, 1976, CV Mosby.

82. Hellema HWJ, Rumke P: Sperm autoantibodies as a consequence of vasectomy, I: within 1 year post-operation, *Clin Exp Immunol* 31:18, 1978.

83. Hellstrom WJG et al: A comparison of the usefulness of SpermMar and Immunobead test for the detection of antisperm antibodies, *Fertil Steril* 52:1027, 1989.

84. Henderson IV JA et al: The effect of unilateral testicular torsion on the contralateral testicle in prepubertal Chinese hamsters, *J Pediatr Surg* 20:592, 1985.

85. Hendry WF: Bilateral aseptic necrosis of femoral heads following intermittent high-dose steroid therapy, *Fertil Steril* 38:120, 1982 (letter).

86. Hendry WF et al: The diagnosis of unilateral testicular obstruction in subfertile males, *Br J Urol* 54:774, 1982.

87. Hendry WF et al: Cyclic prednisolone therapy for male infertility associated with autoantibodies to spermatozoa, *Fertil Steril* 45:249, 1986.

88. Hendry WF et al: Comparison of prednisolone and placebo in subfertile men with antibodies to spermatozoa, *Lancet* 1:85, 1990.

89. Hendry WF et al: Testicular obstruction: clinicopathological studies, *Ann R Coll Surg Engl* 72:396, 1990.

90. Hjort T, Husted S, Linnet-Jepsen P: The effect of testis biopsy on autosensitization against spermatozoal antigens, *Clin Exp Immunol* 18:201, 1974.

91. Hurtenbach U, Morgenstern F, Bennett D: Induction of tolerance in vitro by autologous murine testicular cells, *J Exp Med* 151:827, 1980.

92. Hurtenbach U, Shearer GM: Germ cell-induced immune suppression in mice: effect of inoculation of syngeneic spermatozoa on cell-mediated immune response, *J Exp Med* 155:1719, 1982.

93. Ibels LS et al: Aseptic necrosis of bone following renal transplantation: experience in 194 transplant recipients and review of the literature, *Medicine* 57:25, 1978.

94. Ingerslev HJ: Antibodies against spermatozoal surface-membrane antigens in female infertility, *Acta Obstet Gynecol Scand Suppl* 100:1, 1981.

95. Isojima S, Li TS, Ashitaka Y: Immunological analysis of sperm-immmobilizing factor found in sera of women with unexplained infertility, *Am J Obstet Gynecol* 101:677, 1968.

96. Jager S et al: The significance of the Fc part of antispermatozoal antibodies for the shaking phenomenon in the sperm-cervical mucus contact test, *Fertil Steril* 36:792, 1981.

97. Jalanti R, Isliker H: Immunoglobulins in human cervico-vaginal secretions, *Int Arch Allergy Appl Immunol* 53:402, 1977.

98. James K, Szymaniec S: Human seminal plasma is a potent inhibitor of natural killer cell activity in vitro, *J Reprod Immunol* 8:61, 1985.

99. Jassim A, Festenstein H: Immunological and morphological characterisation of nucleated cells other than sperm in semen of oligospermic donors, *J Reprod Immunol* 11:77, 1987.

100. Jones R et al: Surface and internal antigens of rat spermatozoa distinguished using monoclonal antibodies, *Gamete Res* 8:255, 1983.

101. Junk SM et al: The fertilization of human oocytes by spermatozoa from men with antispermatozoal antibodies in semen, *J In Vitro Fert Embryo Transfer* 3:350, 1986.

102. Kajino T et al: Trophoblast antigens in human seminal plasma, *Am J Reprod Immunol Microbiol* 17:19, 1988.

103. Kay DJ et al: Antispermatozoal antibodies in three men with infertility due to congenital aplasia of the vasa deferentia, *Am J Reprod Immunol Microbiol* 17:48, 1988.

104. Kearney SE, Lewis-Jones DI: Effect of ACTH on contralateral testicular damage and cytotoxic antisperm antibodies after unilateral testicular ischaemia in the rat, *J Reprod Fertil* 75:531, 1985.

105. Kormano M, Reijonen K: Microvascular structure of the human epididymis, *Am J Anat* 145:23, 1976.

106. Koskimies AL, Hovatta O: Hypothalamo-pituitary-gonadal axis and sperm-agglutinating antibodies in infertile men treated for cryptorchidism, *Arch Androl* 8:181, 1982.

107. Kremer J, Jager S: The sperm-cervical mucus contact test: a preliminary report, *Fertil Steril* 27:335, 1976.

108. Kremer J, Jager S, Kuiken J: Treatment of infertility caused by antisperm antibodies, *Int J Fertil* 23:270, 1978.

109. Lansford B et al: Effect of sperm-associated antibodies on the acrosomal status of human sperm, *J Androl* 11:532, 1990.

110. Law HY et al: The immune response to vasectomy and its relation to the HLA system, *Tissue Antigens* 14:115, 1979.

111. Lee C-Y G et al: Sex difference of antifertility effect by passively immunized monoclonal sperm antibodies, *Am J Reprod Immunol Microbiol* 13:9, 1987.

112. Linnet L, Fogh-Anderson P: Vasovasostomy: sperm agglutinins in operatively obtained epididymal fluid and in seminal plasma before and after operation, *J Clin Lab Immunol* 2:245, 1979.

113. Linnet L, Hjort T, Fogh-Anderson P: Association between failure to impregnate after vasovasectomy and sperm agglutinins in semen, *Lancet* 1:117, 1981.

114. Linnet L et al: No increase in arteriolosclerotic retinopathy or activity in tests for circulating immune complexes 5 years after vasectomy, *Fertil Steril* 37:798, 1982.

115. Livi C et al: Does intraperitoneal insemination in the absence of prior sensitization carry with it a risk of subsequent immunity to sperm, *Fertil Steril* 53:137, 1990.

116. Lynch DM, Howe SE: Antibody binding specificity to donor sperm in sera from infertile patients, *Am J Reprod Immunol Microbiol* 13:104, 1987.

117. Mahi-Brown CA, Yule TD, Tung KSK: Adoptive transfer of murine autoimmune orchitis to naive recipients with immune lymphocytes, *Cell Immunol* 106:408, 1987.

118. Mahi-Brown CA, Yule TD, Tung KSK: Evidence for active immunological regulation in prevention of testicular autoimmune disease independent of the blood-testis barrier, *Am J Reprod Immunol Microbiol* 16:165, 1988.

119. Mandelbaum SL, Diamond MP, DeCherney AH: Relationship of antibodies to sperm head to etiology of infertility in patients undergoing in vitro fertilization/embryo transfer, *Am J Reprod Immunol* 19:3, 1989.

120. Margalloth EJ et al: Intrauterine insemination as treatment for antisperm antibodies in the female, *Fertil Steril* 50:441, 1988.

121. Marsh JA, O'Hern P, Goldberg E: The role of an X-linked gene in the regulation of secondary humoral response kinetics to sperm-specific LDH-C4 antigens, *J Immunol* 126:100, 1981.

122. Martinuzzi K, Haas GG Jr: The effect of sperm-associated antibodies

on the success of intrauterine insemination with husband's sperm. Paper presented at the 15th annual meeting of the American Society of Andrology, Columbus, SC, April 6-9, 1990.

123. Mathur S et al: Special antigens on sperm from autoimmune men, *Am J Reprod Immunol Microbiol* 17:5, 1988.

124. Mavligit GM et al: Chronic immune stimulation by sperm alloantigens: support for the hypothesis that spermatozoa induce immune dysregulation in homosexual males, *JAMA* 251:237, 1984.

125. McAnulty PA, Morton DB: The immune response of the genital tract of the female rabbit following systemic and local immunization, *J Clin Lab Immunol* 1:255, 1978.

126. McClure RD et al: SpermCheck: a simplified screening assay for immunological infertility, *Fertil Steril* 52:650, 1989.

127. Meinertz H: Indirect mixed antiglobulin reaction (MAR) as a screening procedure for antisperm antibodies, I: methodological studies, *Am J Reprod Immunol Microbiol* 14:129, 1987.

128. Meinertz H: Indirect mixed antiglobulin reaction (MAR) as a screening procedure for antisperm antibodies, II: clinical studies, *Am J Reprod Immunol Microbiol* 15:101, 1987.

129. Meinertz H, Bronson R: Detection of antisperm antibodies on the surface of motile spermatozoa. Comparison of the immunobead binding technique (IBT) and the mixed antiglobulin reaction (MAR), *Am J Reprod Immunol Microbiol* 18:120, 1988.

130. Meinertz H et al: Antisperm antibodies and fertility after vasovasostomy: a follow-up study of 216 men, *Fertil Steril* 54:315, 1990.

131. Menge AC: Immune reactions and infertility, *J Reprod Fertil Suppl* 10:171, 1970.

132. Moghissi KS, Sacco AG, Borin K: Immunologic infertility, I: cervical mucus antibodies and postcoital test, *Am J Obstet Gynecol* 136:941, 1980.

133. Newton RA: IgG antisperm antibodies attached to sperm do not correlate with infertility following vasovasostomy, *Microsurgery* 9:278, 1988.

134. Nishioka D, Gorman EA, Ward RD: Changing localizations of site-specific sperm surface antigens during sea urchin fertilization, *J Exp Zool* 251:74, 1989.

135. Overstreet JW: Human sperm function: acquisition in the male and expression in the female. In Santen RJ, Swerdloff RW, editors: *Male reproductive function*, New York, 1986, Marcel Dekker.

136. Overstreet JW et al: In vitro capacitation of human spermatozoa after passage through a column of cervical mucus, *Fertil Steril* 34:604, 1980.

137. Ozen H et al: Varicocele and antisperm antibodies, *Int Urol Nephrol* 17:97, 1985.

138. Palermo G et al: Assisted procreation in the presence of a positive direct mixed antiglobulin reaction test, *Fertil Steril* 52:645, 1989.

139. Patrizio P et al: Low incidence of sperm antibodies in men with congenital absence of the vas deferens, *Fertil Steril* 52:1018, 1989.

140. Phadke AM, Padukone K: Presence and significance of autoantibodies against spermatozoa in the blood of men with obstructed vas deferens, *J Reprod Fertil* 7:162, 1964.

141. Price RJ et al: Anticomplementary activity in human semen and its possible importance in reproduction, *Am J Reprod Immunol* 6:92, 1984.

142. Quinlaven WLG, Sullivan H: Antispermatozoal effects of human seminal plasma—an immunologic phenomenon, *Fertil Steril* 27:1194, 1976.

143. Rapaport FT et al: Immunological sequelae of experimental thermal injury to the testis, *Surg Forum* 20:503, 1969.

144. Rebello R, Green FHY, Fox H: A study of the secretory immune system of the female genital tract, *Br J Obstet Gynaecol* 82:812, 1975.

145. Ritchie AWS et al: Intra-epithelial lymphocytes in the normal epididymis: a mechanism for tolerance to sperm auto-antigens, *Br J Urol* 56:79, 1984.

146. Romrell LJ, O'Rand MG: Capping and ultrastructural localization of sperm surface isoantigens during spermatogenesis, *Dev Biol* 63:76, 1978.

147. Royle MG et al: Reversal of vasectomy: the effects of sperm antibodies on subsequent fertility, *Br J Urol* 53:654, 1981.

148. Rumke P: The origin of immunoglobulins in semen, *Clin Exp Immunol* 17:287, 1974.

149. Russell L: Movement of spermatocytes from the basal to the adluminal compartment of the rat testes, *Am J Anat* 148:313, 1977.

150. Saling PM: Mouse sperm antigens that participate in fertilization, IV: a monoclonal antibody prevents zona penetration by inhibition of the acrosome reaction, *Dev Biol* 117:511, 1987.

151. Saling PM, Irons G, Waibel R: Mouse sperm antigens that participate in fertilization, I: inhibition of sperm fusion with the egg plasma membrane using monoclonal antibodies, *Biol Reprod* 33:515, 1985.

152. Schumacher GFB: Humoral immune factors in the female reproductive tract and their changes during the cycle. In Dhindsa DS, Schumacher GFB, editors: *Immunological aspects of infertility and fertility regulation*, New York, 1980, Elsevier/North-Holland.

153. Schwimmer WB, Ustay KA, Behrman SJ: Sperm-agglutinating antibodies and decreased fertility in prostitutes, *Obstet Gynecol* 30:192, 1967.

154. Shalgi R et al: Proteins of human follicular fluid: the blood follicle barrier, *Fertil Steril* 24:429, 1973.

155. Sonnabend J, Witkin SS, Purtilo DT: Acquired immunodeficiency syndrome, opportunistic infections, and malignancies in male homosexuals, *JAMA* 249:2370, 1983.

156. Sotolongo JR Jr: Immunological effects of vasectomy. *J Urol* 127:1063, 1982.

157. Strzemienski PJ: Effect of bovine seminal plasma on neutrophil phagocytosis of bull spermatozoa, *J Reprod Fertil* 87:519, 1989.

158. Sullivan H, Quinlivan WLG: Immunoglobulins in the semen of men with azoospermia, oligospermia, or self-agglutination of spermatozoa, *Fertil Steril* 34:465, 1980.

159. Sullivan MJ, Howe GE: Correlation of circulating antisperm antibodies to functional success in vasovasostomy, *J Urol* 117:189, 1977.

160. Taguchi O, Nishizuka Y: Experimental autoimmune orchitis after neonatal thymectomy in the mouse, *Clin Exp Immunol* 46:425, 1981.

161. Tomasi Jr TB: The secretory immune system. In Dhindsa DS, Schumacher GFB, editors: *Immunological aspects of infertility and fertility regulation*, New York, 1980, Elsevier/North-Holland.

162. Tumbo-Oeri AG: Cell-mediated immunity to spermatozoal antigens after vasectomy: recent developments, *East Afr Med J* 62:372, 1985.

163. Tung KSK: Autoimmunity of the testis. In Dhindsa DS, Schumacher GFB, editors: *Immunological aspects of infertility and fertility regulation*, New York, 1980, Elsevier/North-Holland.

164. Tung KSK, Unanue ER, Dixon FJ: Pathogenesis of experimental allergic orchitis, II: the role of antibody, *J Immunol* 106:1463, 1971.

165. Tung KSK et al: Human sperm antigens and antisperm antibodies, II: age-related incidence of antisperm antibodies, *Clin Exp Immunol* 25:73, 1976.

166. Tung KSK et al: Distribution of histopathology and Ia positive cells in actively induced and passively transferred experimental autoimmune orchitis, *J Immunol* 138:752, 1987.

167. Tung KSK et al: Murine autoimmune orchitis, epididymoorchitis, and gastritis induced by day 3 thymectomy: immunopathology, *Am J Pathol* 126:293, 1987.

168. Ulcova-Gallova Z et al: Local hydrocortisone treatment of sperm-agglutinating antibodies in infertile women, *Int J Fertil* 33:421, 1988.

169. Vaerman J-P, Ferin J: Local immunological response in the vagina, cervix and endometrium. In Diczfalusy E, Diczfalusy A, editors: *Immunological approaches to fertility control*, Stockholm, 1974, NSKA Institute.

170. van der Merwe JP et al: Treatment of male sperm autoimmunity by using the gamete intrafallopian transfer procedure with washed spermatozoa, *Fertil Steril* 53:682, 1990.

171. Weil AJ: The spermatozoa-coating antigen (SCA) of the seminal vesicle, *Ann N Y Acad Sci* 124:267, 1965.

172. Witkin SS: Suppressor T-lymphocytes and cross-reactive sperm antigens in human semen, *AIDS Res* 1:339, 1984.

173. Witkin SS: Mechanisms of active suppression of the immune response to spermatozoa, *Am J Reprod Immunol Microbiol* 17:61, 1988.

174. Witkin SS: Scope and limitations of immunobead testing, *Fertil Steril* 55:852, 1991 (letter).

175. Witkin SS, Chaudhry A: Association between recurrent spontaneous abortion and circulating IgG antibodies to sperm tails in women, *J Reprod Immunol* 15:151, 1989.

176. Witkin SS, Chaudhry A: Relationship between circulating antisperm antibodies in women and autoantibodies on the ejaculated sperm of their partners, *Am J Obstet Gynecol* 161:900, 1989.

177. Witkin SS, Goldstein M: Reduced levels of suppressor/cytotoxic lymphocytes in semen from vasovasostomized men: relationship to sperm antibodies, *J Reprod Immunol* 14:288, 1988.

178. Witkin SS, Toth A: Relationship between genital tract infections, sperm antibodies in seminal fluid, and infertility, *Fertil Steril* 40:805, 1983.

179. Witkin SS et al: Demonstration of 11S IgA antibody to spermatozoa in human seminal fluid, *Clin Exp Immunol* 44:368, 1981.

180. Witkin SS et al: Sperm-related antigens, antibodies, and circulating immune complexes in sera of recently vasectomized men, *J Clin Invest* 70:33, 1982.

181. Witkin SS et al: Heterogeneity of antigenic determinants on human spermatozoa: relevance to antisperm antibody testing in infertile couples, *Am J Obstet Gynecol* 159:1228, 1988.

182. Wolf DP: Acrosomal status quantitation in human sperm, *Am J Reprod Immunol* 20:106, 1989.

183. Wolf DP et al: Acrosomal status evaluation in human ejaculated sperm with monoclonal antibodies, *Biol Reprod* 32:1157, 1985.

184. Wolff H, Anderson DJ: Immunohistologic characterization and quantitation of leukocyte subpopulations in human semen, *Fertil Steril* 49:497, 1988.

185. Wolff H, Schill W-B: Antisperm antibodies in infertile and homosexual men: relationship to serologic and clinical findings, *Fertil Steril* 44:673, 1985.

186. Wolff H et al: Leukocytospermia is associated with poor semen quality, *Fertil Steril* 53:528, 1990.

187. Yule T et al: Murine testis autoantigens are not immunologically sequestered, *Ann N Y Acad Sci* 513:523, 1987.

Chapter 23

DIAGNOSIS OF OVULATORY DISORDERS

Roger J. Pepperell, MD

Etiology of ovulatory disorders
    Secondary amenorrhea
    Primary amenorrhea
Assessment of the patient with an ovulatory disorder
    Clinical and hormonal assessment of ovarian function
    Ultrasound assessment of ovarian function
Management after initial evaluation
    Further investigation of patients with elevated FSH levels
    Further investigation of patients with elevated LH levels
    Further investigation of patients with elevated PRL levels
    Further investigation of patients with abnormal thyroid function
    Further investigation of patients with abnormal androgen levels
    Further investigation of patients with normal or subnormal FSH, LH, and PRL levels

Disorders of ovulation are present in 15% to 25% of couples presenting with infertility. In many of these women the disorder of ovulation is obvious, as there is a complete lack of menstruation (primary or secondary amenorrhea); however, in others menstruation may be occurring irregularly (oligomenorrhea with cycles every 6 weeks to 6 months) or even regularly every 28 days, yet a disorder of ovulation is present. Because women with cycles of longer than 6 weeks have a reduced number of ovulations per year (if they are ovulating at all), they are usually investigated and treated along the same lines as those with a complete lack of menstrual periods.

Of all the causes of infertility, an ovulatory disorder is the most important to recognize because, with appropriate treatment, pregnancy can usually be achieved. Evaluation of all infertile patients should thus aim to confirm the presence and adequacy of ovulation. When an ovulatory disorder is identified, the initial investigations performed assist the physician to determine the cause of the disorder, additional investigations that might be required, and the therapy most likely to achieve satisfactory ovulation.

ETIOLOGY OF OVULATORY DISORDERS

The basic causes of amenorrhea are shown in Fig. 23-1, with the primary ones due to ovulatory disturbances and presenting as primary and secondary amenorrhea being clearly identified.

Secondary amenorrhea

With the exception of ovarian failure, which occurs in virtually all women who reach ages 55 to 60 years but is also seen in 10% of women with amenorrhea under age 30 years, the most common causes of anovulation associated with secondary amenorrhea act at the level of the hypothalamus.

The approximate frequency distribution of the various causes of secondary amenorrhea at age 30 years is shown in Table 23-1. Knowledge of this distribution clearly influences the clinician in determining the investigations performed and the advice offered to the patient.

Obesity is associated more with oligomenorrhea than with secondary amenorrhea; but severe weight loss, particularly when combined with other features of anorexia nervosa, is associated with amenorrhea. Under the latter circumstances the hypothalamic disturbance can be so profound that the amenorrhea may persist for 12 months or longer after ideal body weight has been restored.

Approximately 1% of women will have at least 12 months of secondary amenorrhea after cessation of the oral contraceptive pill (OCP), even when the menstrual cycles had been perfectly regular before commencement of the OCP regimen. This incidence is markedly increased when the cycles were previously irregular. Although this effect of the OCP was originally thought to be due to hypothalamic

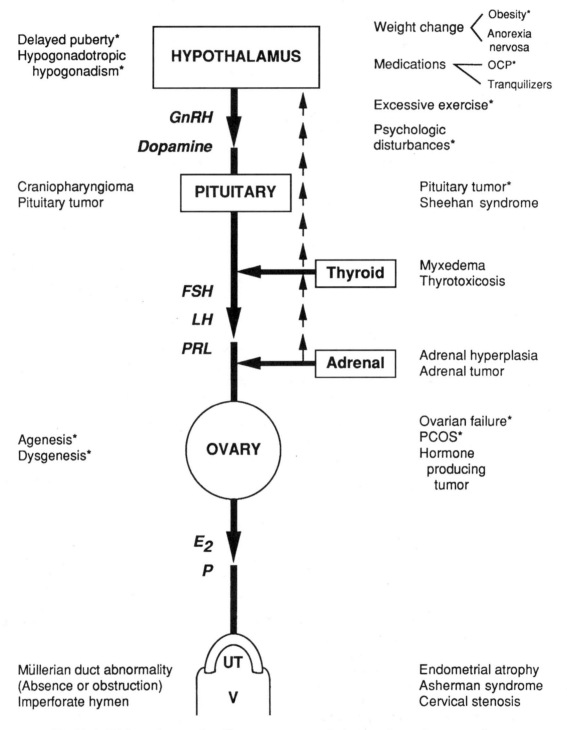

Fig. 23-1. Etiology of amenorrhea. The common causes of primary and secondary amenorrhea are marked with an asterisk on the left and right sides, respectively. Some of the causes of secondary amenorrhea may, when they occur before puberty, produce primary amenorrhea. *GnRH,* Gonadotropin-releasing hormone; *FSH,* follicle-stimulating hormone; *LH,* luteinizing hormone; *PRL,* prolactin; *E₂,* estradiol; *P,* progesterone; *UT,* uterus; *V,* vagina; *OCP,* oral contraceptive pill; *PCOS,* polycystic ovary syndrome.

Table 23-1. Approximate frequency distribution of the causes of secondary amenorrhea at age 30 years

Cause of secondary amenorrhea	Frequency
Hypothalamic dysfunction	50%-70%
Pituitary tumor (predominantly microprolactinoma)	5%-10%
Ovarian failure	5%-10%
Polycystic ovary syndrome	5%-30%*
Hypothyroidism	1%
Others	4%

*This incidence depends on the method used to make this diagnosis. If ultrasound assessment alone is the method of diagnosis, the incidence of polycystic ovary syndrome is much higher and the incidence of hypothalamic dysfunction is lower.

Table 23-2. Approximate frequency distribution of the causes of primary amenorrhea

Cause of primary amenorrhea	Frequency
Delayed puberty	15%-25%
Hypogonadotropic hypogonadism	15%-25%
Pituitary tumor or craniopharyngioma	5%-10%
Ovarian agenesis	5%-10%
Ovarian dysgenesis	20%-25%
Absent or obstructed müllerian duct	5%-10%

suppression from its hormonal constituents, it is now clear that many patients with "postpill" amenorrhea have other hypothalamic factors acting as well, such as weight change, psychologic disturbances, or excessive exercise. Tranquilizers result in secondary amenorrhea by inhibiting dopamine secretion by the hypothalamus, with the resultant hyperprolactinemia producing reduced hypothalamic gonadotropin-releasing hormone (GnRH) production and/or secretion, thence oligomenorrhea or secondary amenorrhea.

Excessive exercise, such as is commonly seen in very competitive athletes (particularly long-distance swimmers and runners) and ballet dancers, probably acts by a combination of effects, including extent of exercise, weight loss, and psychologic stress. Reduction in training schedules will often restore cyclic ovarian function.

Psychologic disturbances (particularly change of employment, family stress, scholastic examinations, or overseas travel) are also commonly associated with disturbed hypothalamic function and secondary amenorrhea.

Pituitary tumors can result in secondary amenorrhea due to production of prolactin (PRL), which reduces hypothalamic dopamine secretion; production of adrenocorticotropic hormone (ACTH), resulting in adrenal cortex overactivity; local pressure on gonadotropin-producing cells in the anterior hypophysis; or disturbance of the hypothalamic-hypophysial–portal vein system by pressure on the pituitary stalk. By far the most common of these manifestations is PRL production by a tumor, called a microprolactinoma if it is 1 cm or less in diameter and a macroprolactinoma if it exceeds 1 cm in diameter. Sometimes this tumorous PRL production is accompanied by production of other hormones, as well (such as growth hormone [GH]), but many patients with acromegaly due to GH excess have only minimal elevation of their PRL levels, this presumably being due to a local pressure rather than a tumor hormone production effect.

Although the diagnosis of congenital adrenal hyperplasia is commonly made at birth or shortly thereafter, it should

not be forgotten that some patients with apparent polycystic ovary syndrome (PCOS) will be shown to have late-onset congenital adrenal hyperplasia (LOCAH) by appropriate investigations. It is particularly important that the correct diagnosis be made because the treatments of LOCAH and PCOS are obviously very different.

PCOS, initially described in terms of clinical features[21] and later found to be associated with distinct hormonal parameters (increased serum luteinizing hormone [LH], decreased serum follicle-stimulating hormone [FSH], increased LH:FSH ratio, increased serum testosterone), is a common cause of secondary amenorrhea, occurring in at least 10% of such patients. The demonstration of polycystic ovaries by ultrasound (see later in this chapter) has led to increased numbers of patients being deemed to have PCOS.

Primary amenorrhea

Many of the causes of secondary amenorrhea can result in primary amenorrhea if they occur before the menarche; however, the common causes of primary amenorrhea, defined as no evidence of menstruation by the age of 16 years, are shown with an asterisk in Fig. 23-1 and the approximate frequency distribution of these causes is detailed in Table 23-2.

Hypogonadotropic hypogonadism is a disorder associated with an apparent lack of production of GnRH. Usually this is an isolated hypothalamic hormone production problem, although a combined deficiency of both GH-releasing hormone (GHRH) and GnRH is found occasionally.

Basal investigations often will not enable clear differentiation between delayed puberty and hypogonadotropic hypogonadism, and many patients have been described with an apparent lack of GnRH at ages 16 to 18 years, yet who menstruate spontaneously some years later—even up to age 25 years.

Craniopharyngioma is a tumor involving the pituitary stalk that often results in a combination of gonadotropin and GH deficiency. Other pituitary hormones can also be disturbed.

Patients with ovarian agenesis who have a chromosome complement of 46,XX have no identifiable ovarian tissue. This is in contrast to ovarian dysgenesis, in which streak gonads are present and the chromosome complement may be 46,XY, 45,XO, or a large variety of mosaic forms such as 45,XO/46,XX, 45,XO/47,XXX, and 45,XO/46,XY. Dysgenetic gonads in a phenotypic female are prone to the development of a dysgerminoma or gonadoblastoma if a Y chromosome line is present; this complication is rare before the age of puberty but becomes more common with older age and reaches approximately 50% by age 50 years.

Müllerian duct obstruction or absence, or imperforate hymen, does not cause an ovulatory defect but results in primary amenorrhea because the menstrual loss is hidden (cryptomenorrhea) or there is no endometrium to respond to normal ovarian hormone production.

ASSESSMENT OF THE PATIENT WITH AN OVULATORY DISORDER

Clinical and hormonal assessment of ovarian function

The basic initial evaluation of women with secondary amenorrhea or oligomenorrhea should include a skull X-ray and measurement of serum FSH, LH, PRL, thyroxine (T_4), triiodothyronine resin uptake, and thyroid-stimulating hormone (TSH) levels. In the past it was also common to measure estradiol (E_2) and progesterone levels in these patients or to assess the possibility of withdrawal bleeding after progestogen administration. These assessments are probably not required, however, as they are of little use in establishing the exact diagnosis or determining the most appropriate therapy.

Patients with primary amenorrhea should have all of the aforementioned tests performed but should, in addition, have a chromosome analysis. If there is any doubt concerning the presence of a uterus, a pelvic ultrasound examination should also be performed.

Although a single blood sample does not provide a completely accurate value for the integrated serum FSH or LH levels over a 12- to 24-hour time interval, single samples provide valid information under most circumstances. If the FSH level is elevated, this hormone assessment should be repeated on at least two more occasions before the patient is informed of the likely diagnosis. The investigation should also be repeated when the initial serum PRL level is found to be elevated. In these circumstances, subsequent serum specimens should be collected in the late morning or early afternoon, with the patient rested both physically and emotionally.

For the clinician making decisions about patient management, stimulatory tests with GnRH or thyrotropin add little further information to that provided by the basal FSH, LH, and PRL values and are thus usually unnecessary.

When there is clinical evidence of hirsutism or virilization, serum testosterone, androstenedione, and dehydroepiandrosterone sulfate levels should also be measured. In the absence of hirsutism or virilization, these investigations are not required. This subject is dealt with in more detail in Chapter 10.

For the patient with primary or secondary amenorrhea or oligomenorrhea, the results of these investigations usually will enable the clinician to clearly define the cause of anovulation, what further investigations are required, and which treatment, if any, is indicated.

Pelvic ultrasound has also become an important investigation in many of these patients, and the current use of ultrasound in the assessment of ovarian function and the uterus is detailed later in this chapter.

When the patient does not have an obvious disorder of ovulation, it is important to assess whether ovulation is occurring, because approximately 5% to 10% of such women are found to be anovulatory when assessed appropriately. In the past this assessment was commonly made by having the patient keep a basal body temperature (BBT) chart, wherein a temperature shift of 0.5°F to 1°F could be expected soon after ovulation and for the duration of the luteal phase. This assessment was often incorrect in defining the presence or absence of ovulation and was unable to determine, even where ovulation had occurred, whether the hormone levels were adequate. Assessment of ovulation by hormonal methods has thus replaced the use of the BBT chart, the most common being the measurement of plasma progesterone or urinary pregnanediol levels in the midluteal phase of the cycle, values greater than 10 ng/mL and 2 mg/24 h, respectively, being indicative of ovulation.[7,14] Provided the plasma or urine specimen is collected 4 to 10 days before the onset of the menstrual period, the values are an accurate reflection of the presence or absence of ovulation. When anovulation is proven, the investigations are the same as those described earlier for the patient with secondary amenorrhea.

When the adequacy of corpus luteum function needs to be assessed, however, more than one plasma or urine specimen may be necessary; samples are often collected every third day during the entire luteal phase for measurement of E_2 and progesterone levels, or an endometrial biopsy is performed 2 or 3 days before the expected time of menstruation. There is a lack of agreement with regard to both the relevance of the deficient corpus luteum in infertile patients and what is the best treatment for this alleged condition when it is diagnosed.[3,20] However, this is discussed in more detail in Chapter 24.

Ultrasound assessment of ovarian function

The initial assessment of ovarian changes during the menstrual cycle, as seen by transabdominal ultrasound, described the growth rate of the dominant follicle as being 2 mm/d, with follicles reaching 20 to 25 mm in diameter before rupture occurred. Confirmation that ovulation occurred was then made by detection of previously nonexistent fluid in the cul-de-sac, decrease in size or collapse of a follicle, the development of intrafollicular echoes, and the classic appearance of the corpus luteum.[6]

Transvaginal ultrasound has now virtually replaced

transabdominal ultrasound. It obviates the need for a full bladder as an acoustic window, reduces scanning time, and has increased patient compliance. Because the transducer is much closer to the pelvic organs, very small structures such as follicles only 2 to 3 mm in diameter can be readily observed, whereas with transabdominal scans follicles cannot be seen reliably until they exceed 5 mm in diameter.[8]

Transvaginal ultrasound is thus of great use to the practicing gynecologist because it allows recognition of normal or abnormal organs, or physiologic structures within organs, and certainly assists the physician in making a diagnosis of the clinical problem and treating it appropriately. It is thus indicated as a baseline investigation in many infertile subjects and, as its use increases and is evaluated further, it may well become one of the routine evaluations in all patients with infertility irrespective of the cause.

When cyclic ovarian function is occurring, multiple transvaginal ultrasound evaluations may be required; but in the presence of amenorrhea of more than 2 months' duration, more than one evaluation during the diagnostic phase is not usually necessary. The following conditions can be recognized on transvaginal ultrasound examination:

Normal follicular development and ovulation. As mentioned earlier, a number of follicles of 2 to 3 mm in diameter are seen early in the cycle, with one being selected as a dominant follicle on day 6 to day 8 (at about 8 to 10 mm in diameter), following which the follicle grows at a rate of about 2 mm/d until rupture occurs at a diameter of 20 to 25 mm.[6,11]

Follicles rupturing at a small size or abnormal follicular growth. Both of these findings have been described in patients with alleged luteal phase defect. Because of the lack of association between premenstrual endometrial biopsy findings, hormone profiles, and fertility, there is currently considerable debate about this condition and the treatment modalities offered, but this topic is considered in much more detail in Chapter 24.

Luteinized unruptured follicle syndrome. Luteinized unruptured follicle syndrome will be diagnosed if the ultrasound examination has failed to provide evidence of follicular rupture yet the biochemical and biopsy parameters are indicative of ovulation.[9] There has been considerable controversy about this diagnosis, and the general consensus now is that this condition may occur occasionally in perfectly normal fertile women, but it is rarely seen in repetitive cycles; treatment for this condition alone, therefore, is usually not required.

Ovarian cysts. Ovarian cysts are cystic structures of greater than 2 to 3 cm in diameter.[17] The cyst may be a simple follicular cyst (rarely >6 cm in diameter), an endometriotic cyst, a dermoid cyst, or a benign or malignant neoplasm. Specific appearances enable the ultrasonographer to suggest a likely diagnosis, although laparoscopy, laparotomy, or transvaginal aspiration under ultrasound guidance may be necessary before the final diagnosis can be made.

Multiple follicular cystic structures in the ovaries. As outlined previously, multiple small follicular structures (2 to 3 mm in diameter) are seen in the early follicular phase; however, once the dominant follicle has been selected, only one or two follicles continue to grow to maturity and rupture unless the patient is being treated with ovarian stimulants. If large numbers of small cystic structures are seen within the ovaries on repeated scans, or on a single scan in a patient with oligomenorrhea or amenorrhea, one of the two forms of ovarian cystic "disease" should be defined.[5]

In PCOS, 15 or more cystic structures 2 to 10 mm in diameter should be visible in the subcapsular portion of each ovary, which itself is often moderately enlarged, and a prominent, highly echogenic stroma should be visible. (See Fig. 23-2.) Many of these patients will have the classic clinical features described by Stein and Leventhal,[21] and polycystic ovaries have been observed ultrasonically in 26% of women with secondary amenorrhea, in 87% of those with oligomenorrhea, and in more than 90% of women with hirsutism but regular ovulatory cycles.[1] Others will have the classic clinical features of PCOS discussed earlier in this chapter, and in up to 90% of patients the ultrasound diagnosis is supported by at least one of these hormonal features.[1]

The polycystic changes have also been described in 20% of apparently normal women,[16] so the functional significance of ultrasound-diagnosed PCOS has yet to be determined.

The other form of multiple follicular cystic ovarian disease has been described as "multifollicular" in type, to clearly differentiate it from the polycystic variety.[2] For this multifollicular diagnosis to be made, six or more cystic structures 4 to 10 mm in diameter should be found scattered throughout normal-sized ovaries showing no evidence of increased ovarian stroma. These women often have had a recent episode of weight loss, are not hirsute, their LH levels and other biochemical parameters are not those associated with PCOS, and they are often estrogen deficient. Treatment with clomiphene citrate may not be effective, but treatment with GnRH or human menopausal gonadotropin (hMG) is usually successful. This is in contrast to patients with PCOS, who often respond well during treatment with clomiphene citrate but are more difficult to treat with GnRH or hMG.

Uterine pathology. Uterine fibroids may be visible within the myometrium or projecting into the endometrial cavity, a uterine malformation such as a bicornuate or subseptate uterus may be present, or occasionally intrauterine adhesions or polyps may be seen. Many of these findings will need confirmation by hysterosalpingography or hysteroscopy before a decision is made regarding the need for any definitive treatment.

Endometrial thickness. The endometrium is usually clearly defined from the underlying myometrium in trans-

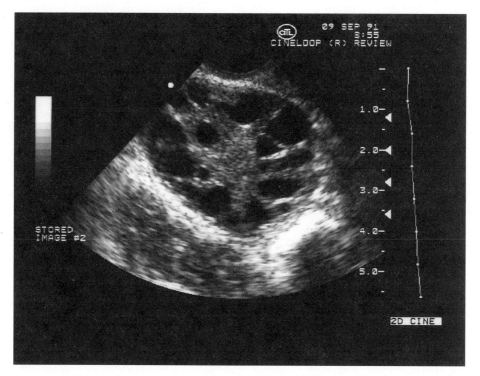

Fig. 23-2. Classic findings of PCOS, with 16 cystic structures 2 to 10 mm in diameter evident in the subcapsular portion of the ovary and a prominent echogenic stroma in the middle of the ovary.

vaginal ultrasound examination. Because the thickness of the endometrium increases during the menstrual cycle, an assessment of this thickness provides valuable information to the clinician concerning the stage of the cycle and the possible hormone levels at the time.

The endometrial thickness is usually measured as the total anteroposterior width between the junction of myometrium and endometrium on the anterior and posterior uterine walls, respectively, and therefore the endometrial cavity is included in this measurement. Under normal circumstances this "cavity" is only a potential cavity because the anterior and posterior endometrial surfaces are virtually in contact.

At the time of menstruation the total anteroposterior width is 1 to 4 mm; this increases to 4 to 8 mm during the follicular phase and to 8 to 16 mm during the luteal phase.[4] No correlation has been found between endometrial thickness and plasma E_2 levels in the periovulatory period; therefore, it cannot be used as an assessment of likely plasma E_2 levels at the time. This applies during both spontaneous cycles and those in which ovarian hyperstimulation is being achieved. It possibly does reflect a more "functional" maturity of the follicular phase of the cycle, however, if a progressive increase in width has been demonstrated and has reached 8 to 9 mm. This fact has been used by some clinicians in their management of patients during treatment within an in vitro fertilization (IVF) program.[19]

Endometrial width assessment has also been used to predict estrogen status in amenorrheic patients and may well supplant the use of a progestogen withdrawal test in such patients. When the endometrial width is 4 mm or less, plasma E_2 levels are low (<40 pg/mL) and withdrawal bleeding usually does not follow 5 days of treatment with medroxyprogesterone acetate (Provera). When the width is 5 mm or more, withdrawal bleeding usually occurs.[18]

MANAGEMENT AFTER INITIAL EVALUATION

When the initial investigations have been completed, analysis of the hormonal results usually allows the patients to be clearly separated into six distinct categories: those with elevated FSH levels; those with elevated LH levels; those with elevated PRL levels; those with thyroid function disorders; those with abnormal androgen levels; and those in whom FSH, LH, PRL, and thyroid hormone levels are all normal or low.

Further investigation of patients with elevated FSH levels

When the serum FSH level is persistently elevated to values above those seen at the midcycle peak of the normal menstrual cycle, the diagnosis in a patient with secondary amenorrhea or oligomenorrhea is either premature menopause or the resistant ovary syndrome. These conditions can only be differentiated by the passage of time and ovarian biopsy, and neither of these is absolutely reliable.

Patients who show a return of ovarian function and associated menstruation obviously do not have ovarian failure, but the duration of continued cyclic ovarian function cannot be predicted. Ovarian biopsy is often difficult because the biopsy specimen should be about 1 cm in diameter and should include deeper portions of the ovary in order to reliably diagnose the lack of ovarian follicles seen in ovarian failure. Open laparotomy is often required to obtain such a biopsy specimen, especially when the ovaries are small and damage to the hilar region (with resulting hemorrhage) may follow a biopsy done laparoscopically.

Even when follicles have not been observed in such a large biopsy specimen and the patient has been labeled as having "premature menopause," fertility has still been reported. One patient in our group who conceived spontaneously, with twins, 2 years after having an ovarian biopsy performed as an open procedure, in which half of each ovary was removed and in which no graafian follicles were identified despite serial sectioning of all the ovarian tissue obtained. The conception occurred after 6 years of secondary amenorrhea and was not preceded by any apparent evidence of returning ovarian activity.

Because of the lack of absolute predictive value of the ovarian biopsy and the fact little, if anything, can be done to achieve release of ova even where they are shown to be present, ovarian biopsy is now rarely performed. When fertility is required, however, the patient is given advice that about 50% of patients with elevated gonadotropin levels will menstruate again and 10% will conceive, and that ovulation induction therapy does not improve these figures.[12] Recently there have been reports alleging a benefit from the administration of low-dose hormone replacement therapy; however, these reports need confirmation. Certainly the best chance of achieving pregnancy would be with the use of ovum donation within an IVF program.

It should not be forgotten, however, that in patients with secondary amenorrhea, premature ovarian failure can be associated with chromosome abnormalities, other autoimmune diseases, and previous cytotoxic therapy or irradiation. It is therefore appropriate to assess the chromosome status of the patient if she is less than 35 years of age and to look for evidence of hypoparathyroidism (measure calcium and phosphorus levels), thyroiditis (thyroid antibodies in addition to thyroid function tests), adrenal insufficiency (cortisol) or rheumatic processes (antinuclear factor, rheumatoid factor, etc.). In primary amenorrhea, in addition to chromosome abnormalities and ovarian agenesis or dysgenesis, galactosemia also needs to be considered.

Further investigation of patients with elevated LH levels

When the LH level is elevated, consideration of the FSH level will usually allow a correct evaluation to be made. Elevation of both FSH and LH levels is usually associated with premature ovarian failure or ovarian resistance, whereas an elevated LH level associated with an upper-normal FSH level is usually indicative of midcycle peaks of these hormones consistent with spontaneous cure of the anovulatory disorder. When the LH level is markedly elevated but the FSH level is in the low-normal range, an early pregnancy should be suspected, because most LH assays show significant cross-reactivity between LH and human chorionic gonadotropin; when the FSH level is normal but the LH level is mildly elevated, PCOS is often found. The FSH and LH levels in the latter condition are also often observed in obese patients without evidence of PCOS and in women in whom the anovulatory problem is about to be resolved spontaneously.

Clarification of the status of the ovary, if PCOS is suspected, is best achieved by transvaginal ultrasound examination, as described earlier in this chapter.

When ovulation induction is indicated and clomiphene citrate or gonadotropin therapy is used, extreme care should be exercised if the LH level is moderately elevated, because hyperstimulation commonly occurs if an excessive dose of either agent is given.

It should also not be forgotten that congenital adrenal hyperplasia (especially LOCAH) may be associated with all of the clinical, laboratory, and ultrasound features of PCOS. LOCAH can usually be excluded by the finding of normal levels of 17-hydroxyprogesterone levels during the follicular phase of the cycle; however, sometimes an ACTH stimulation test is required to rule out this diagnosis completely.

Further investigation of patients with elevated PRL levels

The incidence of hyperprolactinemia in subjects with secondary amenorrhea is 23% and in subjects with oligomenorrhea, 8%.[13] It is less commonly encountered in patients with primary amenorrhea or those with regular ovulatory or anovulatory cycles.

Approximately 20% to 30% of amenorrheic women with elevated PRL levels can be shown to have a pituitary tumor when sophisticated radiologic techniques such as computed axial tomography (CAT) or nuclear magnetic resonance (NMR) are used in the assessment. There is now general agreement that one of these procedures should be performed when the simple X-ray is abnormal or when the PRL level is markedly elevated (more than six-fold normal.) Our own data clearly indicate that patients at risk of tumor progression are those in whom the PRL levels are only minimally elevated (less than four-fold normal) and in whom the PRL elevation is due to local pressure from a non–hormone-producing adenoma, which itself will usually not be reduced in size by dopamine agonist therapy. For these reasons, we now perform CAT scans during the initial diagnostic evaluation in *all* patients shown to have persistent hyperprolactinemia, irrespective of the degree of PRL elevation, except in those patients receiving long-term tranquilizer therapy and in whom this is assumed to be the cause of the PRL elevation.

The association of hyperprolactinemia with acromegaly requires the clinician to consider this latter diagnosis when an adenoma is defined and the PRL level is only moderately elevated. In many instances there will be clinical evidence of acromegaly (enlargement of hands, feet, jaw, and tongue, and evidence of diabetes); however, in some instances there is no evidence of acromegaly despite elevated GH levels being demonstrated.[15] It is therefore necessary to measure fasting GH levels in patients with pituitary adenomas; when these are elevated (>10 ng/mL) or when they are normal but there is clinical evidence of acromegaly, confirm that suppression to normal (<5 ng/mL) during a glucose tolerance test does not occur.[10]

Management of hyperprolactinemic patients is considered in detail in Chapter 9.

Further investigation of patients with abnormal thyroid function

Approximately 1% of patients with ovulatory disorders will be found to have abnormal thyroid function. Where this is the case, thyroid antibodies should be sought and appropriate therapy given. Further sophisticated evaluation is rarely required.

Further investigation of patients with abnormal androgen levels

If the serum testosterone is markedly elevated, pelvic ultrasound, CAT scanning, or NMR assessment should be performed in an attempt to localize the probable ovarian tumor prior to its removal. Laparoscopy is of little value in this assessment because the ovary may not be enlarged and the tumor itself is often deep within the ovarian tissue and not visible on the surface of the ovary.

If the DHEAS level is markedly elevated, attention should be directed towards the adrenal gland with assessment of glucocorticoid levels (cortisol) in addition to CAT scanning or NMR evaluation. If an adenoma or carcinoma is discovered, surgical removal is usually indicated. Selective venous catheterization procedures are rarely required today to localize the site of the tumor.

Minimal elevation of one or more of testosterone, androstenedione, or dehydroepiandrosterone sulfate is commonly seen in PCOS, and the only further evaluation necessary is the performance of a transvaginal ultrasound scan if this has not been performed as part of the initial evaluation. Again, the possibility of LOCAH should not be forgotten.

Further investigation of patients with normal or subnormal, FSH, LH, PRL, and thyroid hormone levels

No further investigations are usually required in such patients; however, factors that adversely affect hypotha-

lamic function (excessive weight, excessive thinness, psychologic stress, tranquilizer therapy, excessive exercise) should be corrected, when possible, before proceeding with drug therapy.

REFERENCES

1. Adams J, Polson DW, Franks S: Prevalence of polycystic ovaries in women with anovulation and idiopathic hirsutism, *Br Med J* 293:355, 1986.
2. Adams J et al: Multifollicular ovaries: clinical and endocrine features and response to pulsatile GnRH, *Lancet* 2:1375, 1985.
3. Davis OK et al: The incidence of luteal phase defect in normal fertile women, determined by serial endometrial biopsies, *Fertil Steril* 51:582, 1989.
4. Fleischer AC et al: Transvaginal scanning of the endometrium, *J Clin Ultrasound* 18:337, 1990.
5. Fox R et al: Oestrogen and androgen status in oligoamenorrheic women with polycystic ovaries, *Br J Obstet Gynaecol* 98:294, 1991.
6. Hackeloer BJ et al: Correlation of ultrasonic and endocrinologic assessment of human follicular development, *Am J Obstet Gynecol* 135:122, 1979.
7. Israel R et al: Single luteal phase serum progesterone assay as an indicator of ovulation, *Am J Obstet Gynecol* 112:1043, 1972.
8. Itskowitz J et al: Transvaginal ultrasonography in the diagnosis and treatment of infertility, *J Clin Ultrasound* 18:248, 1990.
9. Janssen-Caspers HAB et al: Diagnosis of luteinized unruptured follicle by ultrasound and steroid hormone assays in peritoneal fluid, *Fertil Steril* 46:823, 1986.
10. Melmed S et al: Pituitary tumors secreting growth hormone and prolactin, *Ann Intern Med* 105:238, 1986.
11. O'Herlihy C, deCrespigny LJCh, Robinson HP: Monitoring ovarian follicular development with real-time ultrasound, *Br J Obstet Gynaecol* 87:613, 1980.
12. O'Herlihy C, Pepperell RJ, Evans JH: The significance of FSH elevation in young women with disorders of ovulation, *Br Med J* 281:1447, 1980.
13. Pepperell RJ: Clinical investigation and assessment of amenorrhea. In Proceedings of the Sixth Asian and Oceanic Congress of Endocrinology, Singapore, January 1978, p 389.
14. Pepperell RJ et al: The investigation of ovarian function by measurement of urinary oestrogen and pregnanediol excretion, *Br J Obstet Gynaecol* 82:321, 1975.
15. Pestell R et al: Growth hormone excess and galactorrhoea without acromegalic features, *Br J Obstet Gynaecol* 98:92, 1991.
16. Polson DW et al: Polycystic ovaries—a common finding in normal women, *Lancet* 1:870, 1988.
17. Rottem S et al: Classification of ovarian lesions by high frequency transvaginal sonography, *J Clin Ultrasound* 18:359, 1990.
18. Shulman A et al: Ultrasonic assessment of the endometrium as a predictor of oestrogen status amenorrhoeic patients, *Hum Reprod* 4:616, 1989.
19. Smith W et al: Ultrasonic assessment of endometrial changes in stimulated cycles in an in-vitro fertilization and embryo transfer program, *J In Vitro Fert Embryo Transfer* 1:233, 1984.
20. Soules MR: Luteal phase deficiency—foreword, *Clin Obstet Gynecol* 34:123, 1991.
21. Stein IF, Leventhal ML: Amenorrhea associated with bilateral polycystic ovaries, *Am J Obstet Gynecol* 29:181, 1935.

Chapter 24

LUTEAL PHASE DEFICIENCY
Diagnosis, Pathophysiology, and Treatment

**John R. Brumsted, MD
and Daniel H. Riddick, MD, PhD**

The latter half of the primate menstrual cycle is characterized by the function of the corpus luteum. This structure is formed through the actions of luteinizing hormone (LH) on the granulosa cells of the dominant follicle. The midcycle surge of LH is the physiologic signal that initiates both the process leading to ovulation and the formation of the corpus luteum.[61] Progesterone is the predominant hormone product of this endocrine organ, which, in the absence of pregnancy, has a life span of 13 ± 2 days. Since progesterone production is a prerequisite to secretory transformation of the endometrium and the maintenance of early pregnancy, normal function of the corpus luteum is essential for successful human reproduction.

In 1949 Jones[27] proposed that abnormal function of the corpus luteum, manifested by insufficient progesterone production, could cause recurrent pregnancy loss and infertility in some women. Although few practitioners doubt the existence of luteal phase deficiency (LPD), the etiology, appropriate method(s) of detection, true incidence, and standard therapy all remain controversial. The confusion surrounding LPD can be explained by the probability that this is a heterogenous disorder and not a single pathologic entity. This implies that a single diagnostic criterion may not be sufficient to define all possible luteal phase abnormalities. Furthermore, appropriate therapy may depend on precise definition of the underlying pathophysiology in each case of suspected LPD. This chapter details current understanding of the diagnosis, pathophysiology, and therapy of LPD.

DIAGNOSIS OF LUTEAL PHASE DEFECT

The infertility and recurrent pregnancy loss associated with a deficient luteal phase presumably are the result of either abnormal progesterone secretion or an insufficient response of the endometrium to normal progesterone levels. In either case, the endometrium should reflect this abnormal progesterone secretion or action in a measurable way. Noyes et al.[40] described the sequential changes that occur in endometrium during the normal luteal phase allowing for a histologic date to be ascribed to any endometrial sample. The secretory transformation of the endometrium, determined from a sample obtained late in the luteal phase, represents a bioassay of the cumulative effect of progesterone in a given menstrual cycle. Thus by comparing the histologic date of the endometrium to the ideal cycle day during which it was obtained, a measure of the adequacy of the luteal phase can be achieved. Although the histologic dating of an endometrial biopsy from late in the luteal phase has become the gold standard, several other measures of corpus luteum function have been described. These alternative criteria include determination of the length of the luteal phase by basal body temperature (BBT) and by measurement of serum progesterone concentration.

Endometrial biopsy

Classically, the adequacy of the luteal phase is determined by performing an endometrial biopsy late in the luteal phase and assigning a histologic date based on the criteria of Noyes et al.[40] The day of onset of the next menstrual period is, by convention, chronologic day 28. By counting back from the day of next menses to the day the biopsy was obtained, the chronologic date of the endometrial sample is determined. This convention assumes that the luteal phase is consistent in duration with ovulation occurring 14 days before the next menses. The ideal chronologic date and the histologic date are then compared. When the two dates agree, the function of the corpus luteum is normal. However, a discrepancy, expressed by a lag in histologic development relative to the chronologic date, represents an abnormal luteal phase. The diagnosis of LPD is made if a lag in the histologic development of the endometrium is documented in two cycles.[28]

Variability in endometrial dating. The preceding discussion implies uniform agreement in the use of endometrial sampling to confirm the diagnosis of LPD. This is clearly not the case as; the accuracy of endometrial dating, the number of days of lag, and the appropriate chronologic reference point in the cycle are all currently areas of controversy. The accuracy of histologic dating of the endometrium has been questioned relative to four potential sources of variability: (1) variability between observers (interobserver variability), (2) variability between separate observations by the same reader (intraobserver variability), (3) variation in endometrial maturation in different sites in the same uterus, and (4) variation between cycles.

Interobserver variability. The interobserver variability in dating secretory endometrium was first described by Noyes and Haman,[39] who concurrently, but independently, assigned a histologic date to more than 1000 biopsies. The two observers, dating the same sample of endometrium, agreed exactly in 29% of cases. There was agreement within 1 day in 63% of the observations and within two days in 81.5% of cases. In this study, the interobserver correlation coefficient was $r = 0.71$. A more recent study[49] described the interobserver variation among five pathologists independently dating 62 endometrial samples. The mean variation in all observations was 0.96 days, less than that found by Noyes and Haman.[39]

Intraobserver variability. The intraobserver variability in endometrial dating, using the criteria of Noyes et al.,[40] has recently been described.[34] The histologic dates assigned by a single observer reading the same endometrial sample on two separate occasions have significant correlation with

each other ($r = 0.91$). In this study, the two readings differed by more than 2 days in only 6 of 63 cases (9%). There was a tendency for greater consistency to be evident in endometrial samples obtained during the first half of the luteal phase.

Variation in endometrial maturation. The extent of histologic variation secondary to the location in the uterus from which the endometrial sample is obtained is small, as long as the lower uterine segment is avoided. Observations from 100 uteri, each sampled in four different fundal sites, found a high degree of uniformity in the histologic date. The standard deviation of the difference in dating within the uterus was noted to be only 0.7 days.[38] These findings have been corroborated by others.[11] Therefore, although interobserver and intraobserver variability may be clinically important, the site of endometrial sampling does not appear to be significant.

Variation between cycles. The presumption that endometrial dating is a clinically relevant marker of adequacy of the luteal phase depends on minimal variability between cycles in an individual. In fact, there is considerable between-cycle variability in the secretory transformation of the endometrium such that LPD may be identified sporadically in fertile women.[3] To be considered a relevant factor in a couple's infertility, LPD must be a consistent finding. Several investigators have noted a highly significant tendency for a second endometrial biopsy to disagree with the result based on an initial biopsy.[8,34] When three biopsies are obtained and the first two agree, the third is concordant 95% of the time. When the first two biopsies disagree, the third biopsy is normal in 53% of cases.[8] On the basis of these findings, two endometrial biopsies should be obtained on all patients irrespective of the result of the first sample. A third biopsy should be performed if the results of the first two are discordant.

Degree of discrepancy between histologic dating and chronologic dating. Central to the concept that the adequacy of the luteal phase can be determined through the use of endometrial histology is the degree to which a discrepancy between the histologic and chronologic date must exist to define LPD. Early reports required a lag in endometrial development of *greater than 2 days* (at least 3 days out of phase), occurring in two cycles.[28] However, more recent literature suggests that a histologic delay of *2 or more days* noted in two cycles is adequate for the diagnosis of LPD.[8,66] The error inherent in histologic dating, due to interobserver and intraobserver variability, can result in a discrepancy of up to 2 days in approximately 20% of cases.[39] Therefore, to ensure an accurate diagnosis, the earlier definition should be universally adopted and consistently applied.

Traditionally, endometrial dating determined by histology has been compared with the date of the next menstrual period to assess luteal phase adequacy. This implies that in a normal cycle the histologic date of the luteal phase

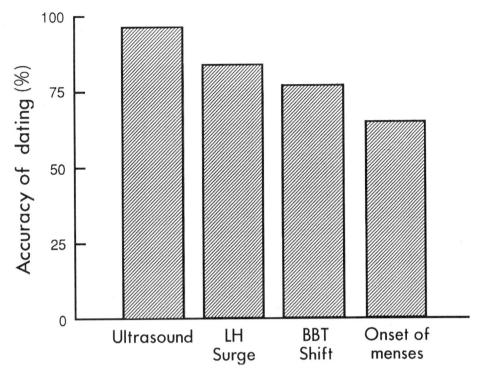

Fig. 24-1. Percentage of endometrial biopsy interpretations that correlated within 2 days using four different methods of ovulation prediction. Onset of menses: $P < .05$ compared with ultrasound. (Redrawn from Shoupe et al: *Obstet Gynecol* 73:88, 1989, with permission of The American College of Obstetricians and Gynecologists.)

endometrium is correlated with, and predictive of, the day of onset of the next menses. In fact, data from a variety of sources fail to support this contention. Noyes et al.[40] observed that menstruation occurred within 1 day of the predicted date in only 60% of cycles. Endometrial histology was found to be a more accurate predictor of the presumed day of ovulation as determined by the shift in basal body temperature (BBT). The failure of endometrial histology to predict the date of menstruation is most likely explained by the inherent variability in luteal phase length. Since the date of onset of the next menstrual period is poorly correlated with histologic dating of the endometrium, it appears that the use of this reference point to measure the adequacy of the luteal phase may need to be reevaluated.

A number of investigators have found endometrial histology to be highly correlated with the day of ovulation as determined by the shift in BBT, the LH surge, or follicular rupture.[28,32,55,64] Shoupe et al.[55] directly compared the correlation of the shift in BBT, the LH surge, ultrasound evidence of follicular rupture, and the date of the next menstrual period with histologic endometrial dating. Ovulation determined by ultrasound evidence of follicular rupture was found to be most highly correlated with endometrial histology, followed by the LH surge and the shift in the BBT (Fig. 24-1). In 35% of the endometrial biopsy readings, the onset of menses occurred more than 2

days later than the time predicted. The correlation between the day of ovulation and endometrial histology may be further enhanced by more sophisticated morphologic methods of dating.[33] If dating of the endometrium by any histologic method is used to determine the adequacy of the luteal phase, data strongly indicate that ovulation should be used as the point of reference, not the onset of the next menses.

Serum progesterone concentration

The term *luteal phase defect* implies abnormal function of the corpus luteum. Since progesterone is the principal, unique hormonal product of the corpus luteum, logic dictates that the diagnosis of LPD should be confirmed by abnormal serum progesterone concentrations. Consistent with this reasoning, Jones et al.[29] observed that the area under the curve defined by daily serum progesterone levels (the "integrated" progesterone concentration) was significantly smaller in women with LPD diagnosed by abnormal endometrial histology. However, the inconvenience and expense of daily venipunctures and progesterone determinations was believed to limit severely this method of diagnosis.

Radwanski and Dwyer[42] attempted to discriminate between normal and abnormal luteal function on the basis of a single serum progesterone concentration obtained in the mid–luteal phase. Among women with unexplained infertility, 60% demonstrated mid–luteal phase progesterone concentrations of less than 10 ng/mL. However, women with anatomic or male factor infertility had levels of less than 10 ng/mL in only 10% of cases. These investigators concluded that a mid–luteal phase progesterone concentration of 10 ng/mL or greater was indicative of normal luteal function. The observations of others have failed to confirm the usefulness of a single progesterone determination.[29,45]

Efforts have been made to improve the accuracy of progesterone values without resorting to daily measurement. Abraham et al.[1] noted that the sum of three serum progesterone levels, obtained 4 to 11 days before subsequent menstruation, was consistently greater than 15 ng/mL in normal cycles, whereas abnormal cycles were always below this level. Unfortunately, this study failed to include endometrial histology as a criterion in the definition of a normal cycle. When three pooled progesterone levels have been found to be in the normal range, endometrial histology is still abnormal in greater than 20% of cases.[7,73] In a unique application of a single progesterone value, Wu and Minassian[71] used the progesterone concentration obtained on a known day of the luteal phase to calculate an approximation of the total integrated luteal phase progesterone. A calculated integrated progesterone level in the normal range was highly correlated with a normal endometrial biopsy. However, in 50% of subjects with an abnormally low value the endometrial histology was found to be in phase.

To date, an acceptable method of detecting LPD based solely on the use of progesterone concentrations has not been described. This failure is explained by the frequent finding of abnormal endometrial development despite "normal" mid–luteal phase progesterone concentrations.[51,73] In a large cohort of women with abnormal endometrial histology associated with spontaneous abortion and infertility, Balasch and Vanrell[5] observed normal mid–luteal phase serum progesterone levels of 86% and inadequate progesterone levels in only 14%. Since the identification of individuals with inadequate mid–luteal phase serum progesterone concentrations may have therapeutic ramifications, thorough evaluation of the luteal phase should include both an endometrial biopsy and progesterone determinations.

Basal body temperature

Most investigations have been able to detect a significant shortening in the mean duration of the luteal phase in women with histologically confirmed LPD.[7,29,55] However, the overlap between the normal and abnormal populations diminishes the usefulness of luteal phase length as a diagnostic tool. The exception may be in women with a luteal phase that is noted to be less than 11 days in duration by BBT.[20] By using this criterion, Downs and Gibson[20] observed that 6 of 20 women with biopsy-proven LPD and

0 of 20 normal control subjects had an abbreviated luteal phase. It must be emphasized that a luteal phase length of more than 11 days according to BBT does not imply that the luteal phase is normal. Thus the BBT chart may be used as a simple initial screening tool to identify women with a significantly shortened secretory phase but must never be used as the only diagnostic modality.

PATHOPHYSIOLOGY OF LUTEAL PHASE DEFECT

The normal menstrual cycle is the result of complex interactions among the central nervous system, pituitary gland, and the reproductive organs. A multitude of physiologic events and environmental factors can influence reproductive function. It is therefore not surprising that a single, consistent cause of LPD has failed to be identified. What has emerged is a general description of abnormalities in gonadotropin secretion that are associated with deficient corpus luteum function and delayed endometrial maturation. In addition, abnormal endometrial patterns may result from altered end-organ responsiveness to sex steroids or variations in the dynamics of progesterone production.

Abnormalities of gonadotropin secretion

During initial investigations of the normal menstrual cycle, Strott et al.[63] identified a subset of women with a short luteal phase. Further characterization of these cycles revealed unusually low follicle-stimulating hormone (FSH) levels and elevated LH levels during the follicular phase, resulting in a significantly depressed mean FSH:LH ratio. The function of the corpus luteum was disrupted as manifested by significantly lower peak progesterone concentrations and shortened luteal phase duration. Subsequent studies in the rhesus monkey confirmed the observation that changes in the FSH:LH ratio could alter the dynamics of the luteal phase.[69] These early investigations made an important contribution to the understanding of LPD by confirming that abnormalities of gonadotropin secretion during the follicular phase could result in deficient function of the corpus luteum.

The pattern of gonadotropin secretion during the follicular phase in women with biopsy-proven LPD has been well described. When single daily serum samples are obtained during the early and mid–follicular phase, the mean FSH concentration and FSH:LH ratio are consistently depressed whereas the mean LH level is significantly elevated.[15,54,57] The selective lowering of FSH concentration during the early follicular phase in both monkeys and women results in depressed luteal phase estradiol and progesterone secretion.[53,62] These data make it difficult to refute the contention that altered follicular phase gonadotropin secretion, resulting in abnormal folliculogenesis, is at least one of the mechanisms leading to LPD.

Pituitary gonadotropins are secreted in a pulsatile fashion, with LH and FSH each having a characteristic pattern of pulse frequency and amplitude. The relative amounts of gonadotropins vary throughout the normal menstrual cycle. The complexity of gonadotropin production can mask abnormalities in this dynamic process when conclusions are drawn from single, daily, blood samples. In women with biopsy-proven LPD, frequent blood sampling during the early follicular phase reveals a significant increase in LH pulse frequency and a decrease in amplitude, compared with values in control subjects.[57] As a consequence, mean serum LH levels are significantly elevated, producing the characteristic lowering of the FSH:LH ratio. Soules et al.[58] tested directly the implied hypothesis that an increase in gonadotropin-releasing hormone (GnRH) pulse frequency in the early follicular phase is an etiologic factor in LPD. GnRH was administered intravenously with a supraphysiologic pulse frequency to normal volunteers during the follicular phase. In the study cycles, the FSH:LH ratio was depressed, the length of the luteal phase was significantly shortened, and the integrated serum progesterone levels were decreased. Thus artificially increasing follicular phase GnRH pulse frequency resulted in cycles with all of the characteristics of LPD.

With further scrutiny of the menstrual cycle in women with LPD, a picture has emerged of deranged follicular phase and periovulatory gonadotropin secretion, leading to a corpus luteum incapable of normal hormone production. Additional follicular phase abnormalities include subnormal plasma inhibin levels and decreased immunoreactive and bioactive LH release during the LH surge.[59] The subsequent luteal phase is characterized by low integrated serum progesterone and estradiol concentrations and decreased pituitary production of bioactive LH.[59,60] The subnormal integrated progesterone production classically found in this condition has been shown to be the result of decreased progesterone pulse amplitude with normal pulse frequency.[60] The theory that infertility and pregnancy loss related to LPD are ultimately the result of abnormalities of follicular phase gonadotropin secretion or aberrant follicular development (or both) is supported by the bulk of current evidence (Table 24-1).

Abnormalities of endometrial response

Theoretically, delayed endometrial maturation could result either from abnormal progesterone production or a lack of endometrial response to normal concentrations of sex steroids. Keller et al.[31] described a woman with infertility and persistent out-of-phase endometrial histology despite normal estradiol, FSH, LH, and progesterone production (based on daily serum determinations). Further investigation revealed that the endometrium contained progesterone receptors with normal affinity for substrate but in markedly reduced concentration. The inability of supplemental progesterone to correct the endometrial delay confirmed the presence of a defect in end-organ responsiveness.

Subsequent studies have attempted to document de-

Table 24-1. Abnormal endocrine parameters in women with LPD

Cycle phase and investigators	Parameter	Abnormality
Follicular phase		
Strott et al.[63]	Mean FSH:LH	Decreased
Soules et al.[57]	LH pulse frequency	Increased
	LH pulse amplitude	Decreased
Soules et al.[59]	Bioactive LH	Decreased
	Inhibin	Decreased
Luteal phase		
Jones[28]	Integrated serum progesterone	Decreased
	Integrated serum estradiol	Decreased
	Mean luteal phase length	Decreased
Soules et al.[60]	Progesterone pulse amplitude	Decreased
	Progesterone pulse frequency	Normal

creased levels of endometrial progesterone receptors as a significant factor in the pathogenesis of LPD. The data are mixed, but the most appropriately controlled investigations fail to confirm consistent abnormalities in progesterone receptor content.[22,26,46] If women with LPD lacked normal progesterone receptors, progestin-dependent biochemical events in the endometrium should be impaired. In fact, the amounts of prolactin produced in vitro by normal and defective luteal phase endometrium of the same histologic date were not different.[18,72] Other biochemical markers of progesterone action are also similar in normal subjects and patients with LPD when the data are corrected for the histologic date of the endometrium.[22,36] Although a lack of endometrial responsiveness rarely may cause clinically apparent LPD, in the majority of instances the endometrium is capable of responding if it is exposed to adequate amounts of progesterone. Therefore, the available data lead to the conclusion that the pathogenesis of LPD is most commonly related to altered corpus luteum function and not defective endometrium.

CONDITIONS ASSOCIATED WITH LUTEAL PHASE DEFECT

The diagnosis of LPD is usually made during a routine evaluation for infertility or repetitive pregnancy loss. However, in selected clinical settings, LPD may be caused by readily identified predisposing factors. For example, women routinely engaging in strenuous exercise may exhibit endocrinologic patterns consistent with LPD.[10,52] Menstrual disturbance may be particularly prevalent during the first several months of training or if exercise is associated with weight loss.[12,48] In addition, dieting in the absence of strenuous exercise can produce subtle ovulatory disturbances leading to LPD.[41,47] Whenever the diagnosis of LPD is entertained, historical information concerning eating and exercise habits should be obtained routinely.

A common cause of secondary amenorrhea is hyperprolactinemia. However, a slight elevation in serum prolactin concentration may result in LPD rather than rendering the patient completely anovulatory.[35,50] This association has been firmly established by the observation that LPD can be produced experimentally by administering a dose of metoclopramide sufficient to induce mild hyperprolactinemia.[30] The mechanism through which prolactin interferes with ovulation is unclear but probably involves alteration of gonadotropin secretion or direct interference with steroidogenesis by the luteinized granulosa cells.[2] The complete evaluation of a patient with LPD should include a serum prolactin determination.

In certain patients LPD may be iatrogenic, arising in association with the use of ovulation-enhancing agents or after follicular manipulation. When human menopausal gonadotropins are used either empirically or in women with anovulation, delayed endometrial maturation occurs in up to 27% of cycles.[2] Ovulation induction combined with follicle aspiration during in vitro fertilization cycles may also be associated with LPD.[43] In these clinical settings luteal support may be required frequently. Several investigators have reported the finding that use of clomiphene citrate (CC) in ovulatory women can be associated with the development of LPD.[4,16,68] The antiestrogenic effect of CC may interfere with the normal development of endometrial sex steroid receptors, resulting in delayed maturation.

TREATMENT OF LUTEAL PHASE DEFECT

Many different treatment regimens have been described for women with infertility or recurrent pregnancy loss associated with LPD. Unfortunately, no prospective, controlled data are currently available that confirm the efficacy of any of the commonly prescribed therapeutic agents. The initial therapy is frequently chosen at random, as objective findings, which would lead to a specific choice, often are not sought. Despite these shortcomings, a rational approach toward women with LPD, identified by rigorously applied diagnostic criteria, is possible. Since the original description by Jones et al.[29] of lowered integrated progesterone during the luteal phase in women with LPD, progesterone supplementation has been a primary mode of therapy. However, treatment with CC, human menopausal gonadotropins (hMG), and human chorionic gonadotropin (hCG) have also gained acceptance in specific clinical settings. The effectiveness of any therapy must be determined by repeated evaluation in an initial treatment cycle in order to ensure an optimal outcome.

Progesterone therapy

Progesterone supplementation can be administered through a variety of routes. The most common method involves the use of suppositories containing 25 to 50 mg of progesterone placed in either the vagina or the rectum twice daily.[29] As an alternative, progesterone in oil has been used in a dose of 12.5 mg administered by intramuscular injection daily during the luteal phase.[29,65] Either regimen will result in serum progesterone concentrations consistent with those of a normal luteal phase.[37] Micronized progesterone taken orally can also produce normal luteal phase serum levels but this route of administration has failed to gain widespread acceptance.[13] Supplemental progesterone should be provided throughout the luteal phase and up to the eighth week of gestation, should pregnancy occur. It is most convenient and appropriate to begin treatment 2 to 3 days after either the LH surge is detected in the urine or the temperature shift is noted by BBT monitoring. Care must be taken not to initiate therapy before ovulation.

In women with well-documented LPD receiving supplemental progesterone, abnormal endometrial maturation will be corrected in 65% to 80%.[6,68] The failure of progesterone treatment to result consistently in a normal luteal phase reaffirms the necessity of obtaining an endometrial biopsy early in the course of therapy. However, even adequate treatment based on a normalization of the endometrial biopsy does not guarantee success in the form of a viable pregnancy. Soules et al.[56] observed a 50% crude pregnancy rate in 16 women with infertility associated with LPD treated with progesterone. A similar rate of success was noted in a subsequent study in which 9 of 13 women achieved pregnancy while receiving progesterone therapy and 7 of 13 subjects (54%) delivered at term.[44] Wentz et al.[68] reported the outcome of progesterone treatment of LPD in women with infertility or recurrent pregnancy loss. A total of 54 women with infertility were treated; 23 conceived and 19 delivered viable infants (35%). In the subset of women with recurrent pregnancy loss, 10 of 17 women conceived while receiving treatment, and 8 of 10 (80%) delivered at term. Balasch and Vanrell[5] treated 14 women with recurrent pregnancy loss associated with LPD, and all delivered at term. Although these data are encouraging, controlled trials comparing progesterone supplementation to no therapy have not been completed. Thus the true efficacy of progesterone in the treatment of LPD has yet to be established.

Clomiphene citrate therapy

Since progesterone therapy is not uniformly successful, alternate treatments of LPD have been described. Agents that enhance ovulation, such as CC, have been widely used. The rationale supporting CC use follows from the observation that LPD may be the result of an abnormal follicular phase. Thus the positive influence of CC on follicular phase dynamics may produce a corpus luteum capable of normal endocrine function. (See Chapter 32 for further comments on CC use.)

Despite the potential negative effects of CC, several investigators have reported on its use. Hammond and Talbert[24] administered CC to infertile women with low mid–luteal phase progesterone concentrations. The dosage was increased until the serum progesterone concentration

Table 24-2. Treatment outcome in LPD

			Outcome	
Investigators	**Diagnosis***	**Treatment***	**Pregnancy**	**Spontaneous abortion**
Soules et al.[56]	Infertility (bx)	PVS 25 mg bid	8/16 (50%)	—
Rosenberg et al.[44]	Infertility (bx)	PVS 25 mg bid	9/13 (74%)	2/9 (22%)
Wentz et al.[68]	Infertility (bx)	Mixed P or CC	23/54 (43%)	4/23 (17%)
Wentz et al.[68]	Pregnancy loss (bx)	PVS 25 mg bid	10/17 (59%)	2/10 (20%)
Balasch and Vanrell[5]	Pregnancy loss (bx)	PVS 25 mg bid	14/14 (100%)	0/14
Hammond and Talbert[24]	Infertility (P)	CC	31/69 (45%)	—
Downs and Gilbert[21]	Infertility (bx)	CC	18/44 (41%)	3/18 (17%)

*bx, Endometrial biopsy diagnosis; P, progesterone; PVS, progesterone vaginal suppositories.

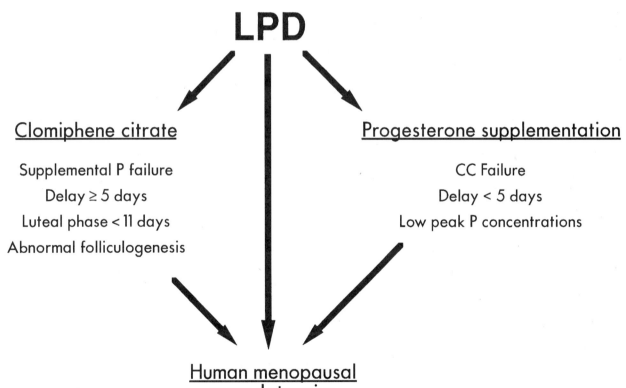

Fig. 24-2. Treatment options for LPD.

was noted to be at least 20 ng/mL on cycle day 21. With this regimen, 31 of 69 women conceived, for a crude pregnancy rate of 45%. CC therapy in women with LPD diagnosed by endometrial biopsy has been shown to yield a pregnancy rate of approximately 40% over six cycles of treatment. In a subset of women with a delay in endometrial maturation of 5 days or more, the pregnancy rate may be as high as 79%.[21] Other investigators have also reported on the efficacy of CC therapy, particularly when there is ultrasound evidence of abnormal folliculogenesis.[14,23] These data imply that, in certain specific clinical settings, CC may be the treatment of choice for LPD. As is the case with progesterone therapy, an endometrial biopsy should be obtained early in the course of treatment.

Gonadotropin therapy

Direct stimulation of the corpus luteum with luteal phase injections of hCG and follicular phase administration of gonadotropins has been reported as a treatment option for LPD. (See Chapter 33 for further comments on hMG therapy.) The results with hCG injections, in the absence of other ovulation-enhancing medications, have been uniformly poor.[17,29] However, the use of gonadotropins during the follicular phase has been associated with a pregnancy rate of 33% to 40% in appropriately selected cases.[9,17,25] This therapy is expensive and has a greater potential for complications than does any other treatment for LPD. Therefore, despite the effectiveness of gonadotropin therapy, this approach should be selected only after other methods have failed to achieve pregnancy (Table 24-2).

Selection of therapeutic agents

With a number of treatment options available, the woman with a well-defined LPD is best served by a systematic approach to her disorder. The primary goal is to correct the underlying defect in endometrial maturation. Therapy may be initiated with either CC or supplemental progesterone. If the endometrial biopsy in the initial treatment cycle is normal, therapy is continued for six cycles. Should pregnancy not be achieved, the alternate therapy can be used, again for six cycles. If both treatments fail, a trial of hMG ovulation induction is indicated. By using this stepwise approach, a pregnancy rate of 80% can be expected.[19]

Specific observations made during the infertility evaluation may be useful in directing therapy. For example, when the endometrial biopsy is more than 4 days out of phase or reveals asynchronous development of the glands and stroma, CC may be more effective than progesterone.[21,70] When ultrasound observation documents abnormalities of follicular development, ovulation-enhancing agents are the preferred therapy.[14,23] As with any other therapy for infertility or recurrent pregnancy loss, treatment should never be initiated until a thorough evaluation has completely ruled out other etiologic factors (Fig. 24-2).

SUMMARY

Among practitioners caring for couples with infertility and pregnancy loss, no diagnosis generates more controversy than LPD. The most appropriate methods of diagnosis and therapy, the pathophysiology, and the very existence of the disorder all remain topics for heated debate.[67] And yet, as these same practitioners use a variety of methods to scrutinize more closely every aspect of the menstrual cycle, it is clear that subtle derangements in folliculogenesis, ovulation, and corpus luteum function are relatively common in infertile women. It is within this complex of heterogeneous abnormalities that LPD exists. What remains is to define how specific findings may affect conception and early pregnancy survival. Clarification of the issues involved in the diagnosis and treatment of LPD will be achieved only through further basic investigation.

REFERENCES

1. Abraham GE, Maroulis GB, Marshall JR: Evaluation of ovulation and corpus luteum function using measurements of plasma progesterone, *Obstet Gynecol* 44:522, 1974.
2. Adashi EY, Resnick CE: Prolactin as an inhibitor of granulosa cell luteinization: implications for hyperprolactinemia-associated luteal phase dysfunction, *Fertil Steril* 48:131, 1987.
3. Aksel S: Sporadic and recurrent luteal phase defects in cyclic women: comparison with normal cycles, *Fertil Steril* 33:372, 1980.
4. Aksel S et al: Effects of clomiphene citrate on cytosolic estradiol and progesterone receptor concentrations in secretory endometrium, *Am J Obstet Gynecol* 155:1219, 1986.
5. Balasch J, Vanrell JA: Corpus luteum insufficiency and fertility: a matter of controversy, *Hum Reprod* 2:557, 1987.
6. Balasch J et al: Dehydrogesterone versus vaginal progesterone in the treatment of the endometrial luteal phase deficiency, *Fertil Steril* 37:751, 1982.
7. Balasch J et al: Luteal phase in infertility: problems of evaluation, *Int J Fertil* 27:60, 1982.
8. Balasch J et al: The endometrial biopsy for diagnosis of luteal phase deficiency, *Fertil Steril* 44:699, 1985.
9. Balasch J et al: Early follicular phase follicle-stimulating hormone treatment of endometrial luteal phase deficiency, *Fertil Steril* 54:1004, 1990.
10. Beitins IZ et al: Exercise induces two types of human luteal dysfunction: confirmation by urinary free progesterone, *J Clin Endocrinol Metab* 72:1350, 1991.
11. Bryn F et al: Sources of variability in a duplicate endometrial biopsy. Paper presented at the 42nd Annual Meeting of the American Fertility Society, Toronto, Sept 1986.
12. Bullen BA et al: Induction of menstrual disorders by strenuous exercise in untrained women, *N Engl J Med* 312:1349, 1985.
13. Chakmakjian ZH, Zachariah NY: Bioavailability of progesterone with different modes of administration, *J Reprod Med* 32:443, 1987.
14. Check JH et al: Pelvic sonography to help determine the appropriate therapy for luteal phase defects, *Int J Fertil* 29:156, 1984.
15. Cook CL, Rao Ch V, Yussman MA: Plasma gonadotropin and sex steroid hormone levels during early, midfollicular, and midluteal phases of women with luteal phase defects, *Fertil Steril* 40:45, 1983.
16. Cook CL et al: Induction of luteal phase defect with clomiphene citrate, *Am J Obstet Gynecol* 149:613, 1984.
17. Cooke ID et al: Some clinical aspects of pituitary-ovarian relationships in women with ovulatory infertility, *J Reprod Fertil* 51:203, 1977.
18. Daly DC et al: Prolactin production by luteal phase defect endometrium, *Am J Obstet Gynecol* 140:587, 1981.

19. Daly DC et al: Endometrial biopsy during treatment of luteal phase defects is predictive of therapeutic outcome, *Fertil Steril* 40:305, 1983.

20. Downs KA, Gibson M: Basal body temperature graph and the luteal phase defect, *Fertil Steril* 40:466, 1983.

21. Downs KA, Gibson M: Clomiphene citrate therapy for luteal phase defect, *Fertil Steril* 39:34, 1983.

22. Gravanis A et al: The "dysharmonic luteal phase" syndrome: endometrial progesterone receptor and estradiol dehydrogenase, *Fertil Steril* 42:730, 1984.

23. Guzick DS, Zeleznik A: Efficacy of clomiphene citrate in the treatment of luteal phase deficiency: quantity versus quality of preovulatory follicles, *Fertil Steril* 54:206, 1990.

24. Hammond MG, Talbert LM: Clomiphene citrate therapy of infertile women with low luteal phase progesterone levels, *Obstet Gynecol* 59:275, 1982.

25. Huang K, Muechler EK, Bonfiglio TA: Follicular phase treatment of luteal phase defect with follicle-stimulating hormone in infertile women, *Obstet Gynecol* 64:32, 1984.

26. Jacobs MH et al: Endometrial cytosolic and nuclear progesterone receptors in the luteal phase defect, *J Clin Endocrinol Metab* 64:472, 1987.

27. Jones GES: Some newer aspects of the management of infertility, *JAMA* 141:1123, 1949.

28. Jones GS: The clinical evaluation of ovulation and the luteal phase, *J Reprod Med* 18:139, 1977.

29. Jones GS, Aksel S, Wentz AC: Serum progesterone values in the luteal phase defects, *Obstet Gynecol* 44:26, 1974.

30. Kauppila A et al: Metoclopramide-induced hyperprolactinemia impairs ovarian follicle maturation and corpus luteum function in women, *J Clin Endocrinol Metab* 54:955, 1982.

31. Keller DW et al: Pseudocorpus luteum insufficiency: a local defect of progesterone action on endometrial stroma, *J Clin Endocrinol Metab* 48:127, 1979.

32. Koninckx PR et al: Accuracy of endometrial biopsy dating in relation to the midcycle luteinizing hormone peak, *Fertil Steril* 28:443, 1976.

33. Li T: A new method of histologic dating of human endometrium in the luteal phase, *Fertil Steril* 50:52, 1988.

34. Li T: How precise is histologic dating of endometrium using the standard dating criteria?, *Fertil Steril* 51:759, 1989.

35. Mahgoub SE: Galactorrhea and the defective luteal phase of the menstrual cycle, *Int J Gynaecol Obstet* 16:124, 1978.

36. McRae MA, Blasco L, Lyttle CR: Serum hormones and their receptors in women with normal and inadequate corpus luteum function, *Fertil Steril* 42:58, 1984.

37. Nillius SJ, Johansson EDB: Plasma levels of progesterone after vaginal, rectal, or intramuscular administration of progesterone, *Am J Obstet Gynecol* 110:470, 1971.

38. Noyes RW: Uniformity of secretory endometrium, *Fertil Steril* 7:103, 1956.

39. Noyes RW, Haman JO: Accuracy of endometrial dating, *Fertil Steril* 4:504, 1953.

40. Noyes RW, Hertig AT, Rock J: Dating the endometrial biopsy, *Fertil Steril* 1:3, 1950.

41. Pirke KM et al: The influence of dieting on the menstrual cycle of healthy young women, *J Clin Endocrinol Metab* 60:1174, 1985.

42. Radwanski E, Dwyer GM: Plasma progesterone estimation in infertile women and in women under treatment with clomiphene and chorionic gonadotropin, *J Obstet Gynaecol Br Commonw* 81:107, 1974.

43. Reshef E et al: Endometrial inadequacy after treatment with human menopausal gonadotropin/human chorionic gonadotropin, *Fertil Steril* 54:1012, 1990.

44. Rosenberg SM, Luciano AA, Riddick DH: The luteal phase defect: the relative frequency of, and encouraging response to, treatment with vaginal progesterone, *Fertil Steril* 34:17, 1980.

45. Rosenfeld DL, Chudow S, Bronson RA: Diagnosis of luteal phase inadequacy, *Obstet Gynecol* 56:193, 1980.

46. Saracoglu OF et al: Endometrial estradiol and progesterone receptors in patients with luteal phase defects and endometriosis, *Fertil Steril* 43:851, 1985.

47. Schweiger U et al: Diet-induced menstrual irregularities: effects of age and weight loss, *Fertil Steril* 48:746, 1987.

48. Schweiger U et al: Caloric intake, stress, and menstrual function in athletes, *Fertil Steril* 49:447, 1988.

49. Scott RT et al: The effect of interobserver variation in dating endometrial histology on the diagnosis of luteal phase defects, *Fertil Steril* 50:888, 1988.

50. Seppälä M, Hirvonen E, Ranta T: Hyperprolactinaemia and luteal insufficiency, *Lancet* 1:229, 1976.

51. Shangold M, Berkeley A, Gray J: Both midluteal serum progesterone levels and late luteal endometrial histology should be assessed in all infertile women, *Fertil Steril* 40:627, 1983.

52. Shangold M et al: The relationship between long-distance running, plasma progesterone, and luteal phase length, *Fertil Steril* 31:130, 1979.

53. Sheehan KL, Casper RF, Yen SSC: Luteal phase defects induced by an agonist of luteinizing hormone-releasing factor: a model for fertility control, *Science* 215:170, 1982.

54. Sherman BM, Korenman SG: Measurement of serum LH, FSH, estradiol and progesterone in disorders of the human menstrual cycle: the inadequate luteal phase, *J Clin Endocrinol Metab* 39:145, 1974.

55. Shoupe O et al: Correlation of endometrial maturation with four methods of estimating day of ovulation, *Obstet Gynecol* 73:88, 1989.

56. Soules MR et al: The diagnosis and therapy of luteal phase deficiency, *Fertil Steril* 28:1033, 1977.

57. Soules MR et al: Abnormal patterns of pulsatile luteinizing hormone in women with luteal phase deficiency, *Obstet Gynecol* 63:626, 1984.

58. Soules MR et al: Corpus luteum insufficiency induced by a rapid gonadotropin-releasing hormone-induced gonadotropin secretion pattern in the follicular phase, *J Clin Endocrinol Metab* 65:457, 1987.

59. Soules MR et al: Luteal phase deficiency: characterization of reproductive hormones over the menstrual cycle, *J Clin Endocrinol Metab* 69:804, 1989.

60. Soules MR et al: Luteal phase deficiency: abnormal gonadotropin and progesterone secretion patterns, *J Clin Endocrinol Metab* 69:813, 1989.

61. Speroff L, Glass RH, Kase NG: *Clinical gynecologic endocrinology and infertility*, ed 4, Baltimore, 1989, Williams & Wilkins.

62. Stouffer RL, Hodgen GD: Induction of luteal phase defects in rhesus monkeys by follicular fluid administration at the onset of the menstrual cycle, *J Clin Endocrinol Metab* 51:669, 1980.

63. Strott CA et al: The short luteal phase, *J Clin Endocrinol* 30:246, 1970.

64. Tredway DR, Mishell DR Jr, Moyer DL: Correlation of endometrial dating with luteinizing hormone peak, *Am J Obstet Gynecol* 117:1030, 1973.

65. Wentz AC: Treatment of luteal phase defects, *J Reprod Med* 18:159, 1977.

66. Wentz AC: Endometrial biopsy in the evaluation of infertility, *Fertil Steril* 33:121, 1980.

67. Wentz AC, Kossoy LR, Parker RA: The impact of luteal phase inadequacy in an infertile population, *Am J Obstet Gynecol* 162:937, 1990.

68. Wentz AC et al: Outcome of progesterone treatment of luteal phase inadequacy, *Fertil Steril* 41:856, 1984.

69. Wilks JW, Hodgen GD, Ross GT: Luteal phase defects in the rhesus monkey: the significance of serum FSH:LH ratios, *J Clin Endocrinol Metab* 43:1261, 1976.

70. Witten BI, Martin SA: The endometrial biopsy as a guide to the management of luteal phase defect, *Fertil Steril* 44:460, 1985.

71. Wu CH, Minassian SS: The integrated luteal progesterone: an assessment of luteal function, *Fertil Steril* 48:937, 1987.

72. Ying YK: Prolactin production by explants of normal, luteal phase defective, and corrected luteal phase defective late secretory endometrium, *Am J Obstet Gynecol* 151:801, 1985.

73. Zorn JR et al: Delayed endometrial maturation in women with normal progesterone levels: the dysharmonic luteal phase syndrome, *Gynecol Obstet Invest* 17:157, 1984.

Chapter 25

UNEXPLAINED INFERTILITY

Edward E. Wallach, MD

Failure to establish the reasons for infertility after a thorough evaluation is frustrating for both patient and physician. The term *unexplained infertility* has been applied to such a situation. This term is preferable to *idiopathic infertility* and *the normal infertile couple,* both of which designations have been used interchangeably with unexplained infertility. Unexplained infertility implies that a diagnostic evaluation has been completed but has failed to reveal any specific etiologic factor responsible for an inability to conceive.

OBJECTIVES IN SYSTEMATIZING AN APPROACH TO UNEXPLAINED INFERTILITY

The approach to unexplained infertility requires that the physician review the elements that should have been cov-

ered within the diagnostic evaluation of the couple, consider entities that may have been overlooked as potential causes of infertility, and evaluate the usefulness of various diagnostic tests and therapeutic approaches in the management of unexplained infertility.

The entity of unexplained infertility implies that the couple has already been subjected to a thorough diagnostic evaluation. With the data from this evaluation as background, the clinician should pursue four objectives:

1. Determine whether the diagnostic evaluation of the infertile couple has been complete with respect to current accepted diagnostic standards.
2. Reevaluate the findings of all preceding diagnostic studies to confirm that they were interpreted appropriately.
3. Keep in mind that any specific factor considered normal and consistent with fertility at the onset of the diagnostic evaluation may become abnormal during the course of a protracted work-up.
4. Consider that many of the processes necessary for fertility defy evaluation by current techniques.

INCIDENCE OF UNEXPLAINED INFERTILITY

In approximately 15% of infertile couples the basis for infertility will remain unexplained. The incidence of unexplained infertility varies among reported studies. The thoroughness of the evaluation also varies among different centers and is related to a combination of the expertise of the physician(s), the availability and quality of laboratory facilities, and the perseverance of the patients concerned. The more detailed the diagnostic evaluation, the greater is the probability of uncovering factors to which infertility may be attributed.

BASIC INFERTILITY EVALUATION
Detailed interview

As reviewed in Chapter 18, the infertility evaluation should begin with a detailed interview consisting of medical, surgical, and family history; past use of contraceptive techniques; exposure to pregnancy and time of occurrence and outcome of any previous pregnancies. The physician should not be reluctant to raise pertinent leading questions regarding sexual habits; coital patterns, satisfaction, and frequency; status of the marital relationship; emotional stability; and motivation. The physician should elicit a history of possible exposure to toxic agents or use of drugs that could adversely affect either male or female fertility.

Physical and pelvic examinations

Thorough physical and pelvic examinations should be directed at detecting evidence of systemic disease and reproductive tract disorders. The occurrence and regularity of ovulation and the characteristics of the postovulatory phase must be evaluated. The appraisal should consider not only semen quality as judged by semen analysis, but also adequacy and timing of sperm deposition at the cervix and sperm-cervical mucus interaction. The uterine cavity and endometrium must be assessed for abnormalities that may adversely influence this environment (e.g., neoplasia, infection, anomalous development). The adnexa should be observed directly to appraise the anatomic relationship of fallopian tube and ovary on each side, to detect evidence of endometriosis and/or periadnexal adhesions, and to determine oviductal patency. Basic studies must include investigation of the male factor; evaluation of cervical, uterine, tubal, peritoneal, and ovarian factors; determination of possible immunologic factors; and assessment of coital techniques and patterns. The degree of motivation of the couple should be appraised, and the emotional status of both partners needs to be sensitively assessed and factored into the management plan.

Infertility studies

Basic studies. The following studies should be incorporated into the basic infertility evaluation:

- Basal body temperature (BBT) recordings, for detection and timing of ovulation; for correlation with specific studies that require appropriate timing (postcoital test, endometrial biopsy); for supplementation of other data in evaluation of the luteal phase
- Postcoital test, performed in the immediate preovulatory phase
- Endometrial biopsy, performed in the late postovulatory phase
- Semen analysis
- Hysterosalpingography
- Laparoscopy and tubal lavage

If any of these studies have been performed elsewhere previously, the consultant should personally review the results. For example, the endometrial biopsy slides(s) and the BBT record during the cycle in which it was obtained should be requested and reinterpreted; the hysterosalpingogram should be obtained and reviewed; and the operative note from a laparoscopy should be scrutinized

for details regarding tuboovarian relationships, evidence of endometriosis, the presence of adhesions, and other subtle abnormalities. It is advisable to repeat a postcoital test, since interpretation of the test tends to be highly subjective.

Additional studies. Additional studies that might be performed on specific indication include the following:

- Cervical culture for *Ureaplasma urealyticum* and *Chlamydia trachomatis*
- Immunologic studies in the man, the woman, or both
- Tests of fertilizing capacity of spermatozoa (e.g., zona-free hamster ovum penetration test (See Spermatozoal Factors.)
- Tests of migrating capacity of spermatozoa, e.g., using bovine cervical mucus (Penetrak test) or cul-de-sac washings after sperm deposition at the cervix

REPETITION OF STUDIES
Postcoital test

Assuming that the couple fulfills the criteria for the diagnosis of unexplained infertility, a postcoital test should have been performed and considered normal. Postcoital testing is simple and inexpensive, and it provides significant information regarding adequacy of coital placement of sperm at the cervix, sperm-mucus interaction, and sperm concentration. The test should be repeated under the following circumstances:

- The results of the previous postcoital test were imprecisely reported (e.g., if the report states "many sperm seen," but no comment was made as to their location, the percentage and quality of motility, or the characteristics of the cervical mucus).
- The results of the previous test suggest borderline concentration, morphology, or motility of spermatozoa.
- The interpretation of the previous observer is in doubt.
- Significant time has elapsed since the previous postcoital examination.
- A significant discrepancy exists between results of the semen analysis and findings on postcoital testing.

Endometrial biopsy

The endometrial biopsy may also need to be repeated. Since examination of endometrial histology provides cumulative evidence of the sequential effects of estradiol and progesterone on the endometrial tissue, a biopsy affords insight into the degree and duration of corpus luteum function as well as the ability of the endometrium to respond appropriately. The endometrial biopsy will also provide an opportunity to determine the presence or absence of endometritis. Ideally the biopsy should be carried out as late as possible in the postovulatory phase and the dating correlated with time of ovulation as judged by the

BBT record and/or a urinary ovulation indicator, and with date of onset of subsequent menses and drop in BBT. Endometrial biopsy should be repeated if

- The previous biopsy was performed without correlation with times of BBT shift, onset of the premenstrual BBT drop, and time of subsequent menstruation
- There is a possibility of endometritis (e.g., previous use of an intrauterine device or history of intrauterine manipulation)
- Patterns of menstrual cycles have changed; or
- BBTs now suggest a luteal phase defect

Laparoscopic examination

Of all the basic diagnostic studies employed in the infertile couple, laparoscopy is the most invasive. However, a laparoscopic examination is essential for enabling direct visualization of the fallopian tubes and ovaries and revealing the anatomic relationships between the two structures. It can aid in determining tubal patency by carrying out concomitant chromopertubation and in disclosing the presence of gross or subtle lesions that may impair tubal transport of gametes (e.g., adhesions, endometriosis, uterine or ovarian neoplasia, hydatid cysts). If laparoscopy has been performed previously, the decision to repeat the procedure is often difficult for the patient, the physician, and the referring physician. Nonetheless, laparoscopy is such a vital aspect of the infertility evaluation that there is frequently good reason for repeating the procedure. The following circumstances represent instances in which a repeat laparoscopy is justified:

- The interpretation of the previous laparoscopist is in question or the previous laparoscopist lacked experience in identifying subtle anatomic abnormalities associated with infertility.
- The previous laparoscopist identified peritubal or periovarian abnormalities but did not at the time consider the lesions to be significant.
- The patient has experienced some relevant pelvic disorder in the interval between previous laparoscopy and the current evaluation (e.g., salpingitis, pelvic surgery, recent onset of pelvic pain, history compatible with disruption of an ovarian cyst).
- The patient has a condition associated with a high likelihood of progression (e.g., endometriosis).
- The patient has undergone reconstructive adnexal surgery but pregnancy has not occurred after an interval of approximately 2 years; second-look laparoscopy may be necessary to determine the effectiveness of the previous surgery in restoring patency or in recreating normal anatomic relationships.
- The patient has received a course of hormonal therapy for minimal endometriosis but pregnancy has not occurred for 12 months thereafter.

FACTORS INVOLVED IN INFERTILITY

Cervical or pelvic infection

If cervical or pelvic infection is suspected, samples from the cervix or uterine cavity (or both) may be cultured for several organisms that have been associated with reduced fertility, although the yield of positive results is frequently low.

Ureaplasma urealyticum. *Ureaplasma urealyticum* has been associated with both infertility and repeated spontaneous abortion. Friberg[14] and Gnarpe and Friberg[15] reported that 85% of men and 91% of women in a selected group of infertile couples harbored *U. urealyticum* in sperm and cervical mucus. In contrast, in a control group of pregnant women and their consorts this organism was found in only 22% and 23%, respectively. Stray-Pederson et al.[31] also reported significantly higher percentages of *Ureaplasma*-positive cultures among couples with unexplained infertility than among fertile controls. In men, the organism may be associated with decreased sperm motility or abnormal sperm morphology.[14] Although after treatment conception rates of 17% to 46% have been reported for couples with unexplained infertility,[14] double-blind studies using doxycycline, placebo, and no treatment have failed to demonstrate any significant differences in conception rates among these three groups.[21] Routine culture of the cervix for *Ureaplasma* in all infertile patients is hardly justifiable. On the other hand, as controversial as the subject may seem at present, samples for *Ureaplasma* culture should be obtained from the woman with unexplained infertility; if the culture is positive, a course of treatment is indicated for both her and her partner. Antimicrobials of choice include tetracycline (500 mg four times daily for 10 days) or doxycycline (100 mg twice daily for 10 days). Culture-positive evidence of infection should usually be documented before antimicrobial therapy is initiated. However, exceptions to this general principle are reasonable for couples with longstanding unexplained infertility when specific culture capability is unavailable or prohibitively expensive.

Chlamydia trachomatis. *Chlamydia trachomatis* has been recognized as a major etiologic agent in pelvic infections. The initial infection notoriously occurs in the absence of customary symptoms of salpingitis. In certain Scandinavian countries the organism has been isolated in 40% to 60% of cases of acute salpingitis.[24,33] The incidence of acute chlamydial infection in the United States may be lower, but it has become a formidable cause of pelvic inflammatory disease in this country. Chlamydial organisms may colonize the endocervical columnar epithelial cells. From this point they may extend to the endometrium, causing endometritis, or to the endosalpinx, giving rise to salpingitis. Infertility may result from associated tubal disease or endometritis. Identification requires tissue cell culture of infected material or serologic testing using a direct microimmunofluorescence test for fluorescent antibodies. A cytobrush technique recently introduced appears to be superior to a swab for optimal collection of endocervical specimens.

Immunologic factors

Immunologic factors are rarely involved in the etiology of unexplained infertility. However, antigenicity of spermatozoa and other components of the ejaculate has been recognized for many years. Under certain circumstances, including trauma to the male ductal system (e.g., after vas ligation), men may produce autoantibodies against seminal components. (See Chapters 21 and 22.) Among infertile couples approximately 5% to 10% of men have been found to demonstrate autoimmunity to sperm. Of those with antisperm antibodies found in serum, 85% will also have antibodies on sperm. Such antibodies may result in impairment of sperm motility through the female reproductive tract, as reflected by altered sperm motion in cervical mucus (postcoital testing, failed penetration of cervical mucus). Spermagglutination observed in seminal fluid may also alert the physician to the possibility of sperm autoantibodies. In women, the presence of antibodies to seminal components may compromise spermatozoal penetration of cervical mucus of sperm transport through the uterine cavity and fallopian tubes. Antibody-labeled spermatozoa may also demonstrate dysfunction in their zona-penetrating or egg-penetrating ability. Experimental evidence also points to the possibility of antibodies to the zona pellucida, the gelatinous layer surrounding the oocyte. Immunologic phenomena at this level could interfere with sperm penetration of the zona pellucida, thus preventing fertilization. The role of autoantibodies to the zona in human infertility is not yet clear.

When to consider immunologic factors. Because of controversial data regarding antisperm antibodies, studies should not be carried out routinely in every infertile couple. However, immunologic factors should be considered under certain circumstances:

- In the man with previous vas ligation prior to reversal or after reversal if infertility persists
- In the woman when postcoital testing or post–artificial insemination testing consistently demonstrates immotile spermatozoa despite normal motility in a freshly ejaculated specimen
- When spermatozoa consistently demonstrate a "shaking" movement rather than forward motion in the endocervical canal at the time of postcoital testing
- In the investigation of any couple in whom no factor has been found to explain infertility despite normal results of semen analysis and postcoital testing (The yield of positive findings, however, in such cases will be small.)

Tests for immunologic factors. Since appropriate treatment depends on an accurate diagnosis of an immunity to

sperm, the availability of specific testing is critical. Until relatively recently, spermagglutination, complement-dependent sperm immobilization, or indirect immunofluorescence formed the basis for antisperm antibody testing. Because of deficiencies in these tests, they have been replaced by radioimmunoassays and by an immunobead binding test.[4] The latter assay involves plastic microspheres coupled with anti-human antibodies. These antibodies on the surface of the immunobeads bind to any human antibodies present on the surface of spermatozoa. The binding to antibodies on the sperm surface can be visualized microscopically. The test can also be carried out indirectly for detecting serum antibodies. In this case the absence of sperm surface antibodies is first confirmed, after which sperm are incubated with various dilutions of serum, washed, and retested to detect antibodies acquired on the sperm surface from the serum.[4]

Historically, immunologic factors have been sought by using one or a combination of the following tests:

- Microagglutination tests
- Macroagglutination tests
- Sperm immobilization tests (Isojima et al.[22])
- Immunobead binding (Bronson[4])
- Anti-human globulin immunoassay (Haas et al.[18])

The first two tests assess agglutination of spermatozoa (head to head, tail to tail) on exposure to serum from men or women. The sperm immobilization test of Isojima et al.[22] utilizes the loss of motility of sperm in response to serum as a positive end point and appears to be more reliable than agglutination tests. Serum titers of sperm antibodies do not necessarily indicate the presence and concentration of local antibodies in the female reproductive tract. Immunobead binding is currently the most widely used test.

Spermatozoal factors

Fertilizing capacity. The functional capacity of spermatozoa takes into consideration their ability to exist in the female reproductive tract and their fertilizing capacity. Transport of the gamete to the site of fertilization can be surmised only indirectly. Ovum transfer to the lumen of the fallopian tube cannot be assessed by current conventional techniques. Most tests of sperm behavior in the female genital tract are based on in vivo or in vitro observations of the interaction of spermatozoa and cervical mucus. The ability of such tests to predict the ability of sperm to reach the site of fertilization is limited. Templeton and Mortimer[32] described a clinical approach to assessing sperm migration using sperm recovered from the pelvis by laparoscopy after coitus or artificial insemination, with partner's sperm, during the immediate preovulatory interval. The pregnancy rate in patients with successful sperm recovery was significantly higher than that in patients with negative recovery.

Tests for fertilizing capacity. Tests for the fertilizing capacity of spermatozoa have been sought by many investigators for several years. In 1976 Yanagimachi et al.[38] demonstrated that human spermatozoa can penetrate zona-free hamster ova and thereby established the basis for potential development of a standardized test for assessing the fertilizing capacity of human spermatozoa. The virtue of this approach is that it raises the possibility of detecting defective sperm function in the face of normal semen parameters using conventional standards for semen analysis. Such an approach has special application in evaluating couples with unexplained infertility. Aitken et al.,[1] using the zona-free hamster egg system, reported that approximately one third (34.1%) of 85 men from a group with unexplained infertility had subnormal (<10%) fertilizing capacity. Rogers et al.[30] investigated in vitro penetration of zona-free hamster eggs by both fertile and infertile semen donors and found penetration rates significantly lower in the semen samples from the infertile men; however, the percentage of penetration did not correlate with sperm concentration or motility. Trounson et al.[34] used human ova and investigated fertilization and cleavage as an end point after exposure to human sperm. A decreased incidence of fertilization and normal cleavage was found in patients classified as having unexplained infertility as compared with controls. A third approach, reported by Overstreet et al.,[28] employs a combination of zona-free hamster ova and freeze-preserved human zonae pellucidae. These authors also reported defective sperm function in infertile patients, including failure of sperm to bind to the zona pellucida, binding to the zona with penetration, incomplete zona penetration, and penetration with poor entry into the ooplasm. A hypoosmotic swelling test permits evaluation of the integrity of the sperm membrane. The test is relatively simple to perform, and correlates best with sperm viability.[7]

Of the approaches just described, only the zona-free hamster egg penetration test has been used extensively in the United States.[37] Although the significance of the test is still incompletely understood, further data attempting to correlate the ability of sperm to penetrate zona-free hamster eggs with standard parameters for semen analysis, immunologic studies, and fertility status of the couple are certain to clarify the ultimate role of this procedure in the infertility evaluation. At present, if such a system is readily available, it should be applied to the study of the couple with unexplained infertility. Its use possibly may aid in identifying couples in whom the fertilizing capacity of the man's spermatozoa is defective. Such couples might benefit from donor insemination.

The methodology for performing the zona-free hamster egg penetration test is associated with a number of pitfalls.[5] Among them are variations in sperm capacitation times. The World Health Organization protocol recommends a preincubation time of 18 to 24 hours and a sperm-egg co-incubation period of 3 hours. The sperm concentration during co-incubation also must be standardized (3.5×10^6

motile spermatozoa per milliliter). As with any other test of sperm function, this test may also be influenced by interval of sexual abstinence before obtaining the reference specimen. Bronson and Rogers[5] have clearly pointed out the variable egg-penetration frequencies of the sperm from the same known fertile donor depending on the source of serum albumin as a protein additive to the culture medium. Whether capacitation and the acrosome reaction in vitro are comparable to those occurring in situ within the fallopian tube is still unresolved. Basically, the cutoff at 10% of zona-free eggs penetrated was established in the first description of the test[38] as the figure below which sperm were considered abnormal with respect to penetrating ability.

In the final analysis, the zona-free egg penetration assay has the following advantages:

- Sperm must undergo the acrosome reaction to allow fusion with the plasma membrane of the ovum.
- It tests fusion/decondensation, thus pronuclear formation.
- Multiple penetrations permit use of a "sperm penetration index."
- It tests sperm chromosomal complement.
- It is a relatively simple test.
- Hamster eggs are readily available for testing.

Potential problems of the zona-free egg penetration assay are obvious when one considers interspecies tests. Others include the following:

- "Natural inducers" of the acrosome reaction are removed.
- The test results can vary greatly depending on conditions.
- The test does not study zona pellucida binding or penetration.

Since unexplained infertility has become a leading indication for in vitro fertilization (IVF), gamete intrafallopian transfer (GIFT), or zygote intrafallopian transfer (ZIFT), a ready opportunity exists to assess homologous fertilizing capacity of sperm and fertilizability of eggs. The fertilized eggs can be replaced in the same cycle during which they were obtained or cryopreserved and replaced in a subsequent cycle. There are other rarely used approaches to study sperm fertilizing ability, each of which shows some promise:

- Ultrastructure of spermatozoa (Zamboni[39])
- "Hemizona" assay, which uses control sperm and the sperm to be studied
- Competitive mixed-insemination penetration assay
- Measurement of sperm acrosin concentration

Specific factors

Peritoneal abnormalities. Peritoneoscopy is essential in the infertility investigation. An infertility investigation cannot be considered complete without direct visualization

Table 25-1. Laparoscopic findings in patients with unexplained infertility

Investigators	No. of patients	% with endometriosis	% with periadnexal adhesions
Peterson and Behrman[29]	204	33	20
Drake et al.[13]	24	46	29
Goldenberg and Magendantz[16]	64	26	18
Broekhuizen et al.[3]	25	60	12
Audebert[2]	70	23	23

of the pelvic structures by endoscopy. Although hysterosalpingography provides a simple evaluation of the contour of the uterine cavity and the oviducts, it is unable to demonstrate the anatomic relationship between the tubal ostium and the ovary or to identify periadnexal adhesions and peritoneal disease. Laparoscopy is the most widely used technique for pelvic endoscopy. Table 25-1 summarizes five studies reported in the early days of the introduction of laparoscopy to the infertility evaluation that support the concept that laparoscopy can bring to light abnormalities in roughly 50% to 75% of women with unexplained infertility. In these reports, endometriosis was found in approximately one third and periadnexal adhesions in one fifth of women whose infertility could not be explained before development of this diagnostic procedure.

Periadnexal adhesions may interfere with fertility through several mechanisms. Peritubal and periovarian adhesions may arise from any pelvic or peritoneal insult, including previous pelvic or abdominal surgery, pelvic inflammation, endometriosis, inflammatory bowel disease, or adnexal accidents such as torsion or cyst rupture. The location of adhesions is more significant in leading to infertility than is the extent of adhesions. They may create a barrier to transfer of the ovum from the follicle to the tubal ostium, restrict fimbrial activity and function by achieving coaptation of fimbriae, deflect the fimbriated end of the tube, or interfere with normal oviductal motility. Surgical lysis of periadnexal adhesions in management of infertility has been reported to result in delivery of term or nearly term viable infants in 57% and 45% of patients in two series reported from Pennsylvania Hospital.[6,35] Adhesiolysis may be performed at the time of the laparoscopy, thus converting a diagnostic to a combined diagnostic-therapeutic procedure.

Endometriosis. The causal relationship between endometriosis and infertility varies depending on location and extent of endometriosis. In some cases, peritubal and periovarian adhesions associated with peritoneal endometriotic implants may impair ovum transport, as described earlier. Although ovarian function is usually maintained, luteinization of unruptured follicles has been related to endometriosis, as have luteal phase defects. One of the most perplexing problems associated with endometriosis is

why patients with mild endometriosis who have only scattered implants, but no anatomic distortion of adhesions, have decreased fertility. The possible association of luteal phase defects and endometriosis was raised in 1966 by Grant,[17] who reported 45% of 96 patients with suggestive luteal phase dysfunction. The syndrome of ovum entrapment and luteinization of unruptured follicles is difficult to document; it can be suggested only through the inability to identify a corpus hemorrhagicum or ovulatory stigma at the time of laparoscopy performed in the presumed postovulatory phase of the cycle. At present, the significance of nonvisualization of these structures is dubious. Validation of this syndrome and its relationship to endometriosis would depend on consistency of this finding in successive cycles in the same patient as well as exclusion of this finding in normal patients during fertile cycles. In reviewing how mild endometriosis causes infertility, Muse and Wilson[26] raised a number of other intriguing possibilities, including hyperprolactinemia, autoimmune phenomena, altered prostaglandin secretion, increase in early spontaneous abortions, and genetic factors.

Components of peritoneal fluid have been implicated in the pathogenesis of endometriosis. Recently the role of activated peritoneal macrophages has gained in popularity as a potential etiologic factor in the pathophysiology of endometriosis, especially with regard to associated disturbances in fertility.[19,27] These cells secrete growth factors that may stimulate and support the growth of ectopic endometrial implants. Studies have described a relationship between peritoneal fluid from patients with endometriosis and sperm phagocytosis, human sperm penetration of zona-free hamster eggs, and ovum transfer into the tubal ostium via the fimbriae. Olive et al.[27] have demonstrated a high aggregate number of peritoneal macrophages in patients with mild endometriosis (implants only) without mechanical causes for infertility. They also showed that elevated numbers of macrophages are not exclusive to women with endometriosis but can be found in patients with unexplained infertility. Thus women with high peritoneal leukocyte counts may represent a distinctive type of infertility of which women with minimal endemetriosis represent a subset. In view of the frequent reports that mild endometriosis may be the only explanation for infertility, therapy for endometriosis under such circumstances seems warranted. A course of danazol or gonadotropin-releasing hormone analogue therapy, fulguration of implants, or even surgical excision appears justifiable after all other recognizable causes for infertility have been excluded in patients with mild endometriosis. The choice of approach should depend on extent and location of implants. (See Chapters 37 and 38.)

Luteal phase defect. The term *luteal phase defect* refers to abnormal ovarian function leading to inadequate progesterone production during the postovulatory phase of the cycle. Luteal phase defect has been associated with both infertility and recurrent early pregnancy loss. (See Chapter 24.) The diagnosis of luteal phase defect can be established by using several parameters of corpus luteum function, including BBT recordings and patterns, endometrial histology, and serum progesterone levels. Correlation among three parameters is essential. The simplest and most accurate diagnostic method is through interpretation of endometrial histology correlated with the point of rise in BBT and/or urinary LH peak testing. The biopsy should be obtained as close to the onset of the next menstrual period as possible in order to assess the cumulative effect of corpus luteum secretion on the endometrium. BBT recordings tempt overinterpretation. Certainly an abbreviated thermal shift is highly suggestive of defective luteal function; however, the physician should resist reliance on BBT patterns alone and perform an endometrial biopsy, possibly supplemented by measurement of serum progesterone levels. The combination of three luteal phase progesterone determinations or a mid–luteal phase progesterone level of greater than 15 ng/mL has been considered evidence of normal corpus luteum function, but these values do not signify luteal phase length.

TREATMENT APPROACHES

With these considerations as background, what then should be the approach to the couple with unexplained infertility? As described in Objectives, the physician should reevaluate the initial work-up to ensure that no essential studies were omitted and that those already performed were interpreted properly. Studies will have to be repeated if the validity of the previous interpretation is in doubt or if significant time has elapsed since performance of the original study.

Further diagnostic studies

When reevaluation of the initial work-up and repeated basic studies have failed to provide an explanation for infertility, consideration should be given to immunologic studies and tests of gamete transport and fertilizing capacity of spermatozoa. Bacteriologic studies should be conducted, especially for *U. urealyticum,* which appears to have a possible etiologic relationship to infertility. The luteal phase needs to be thoroughly investigated. Additional studies conducted may thus include

- *U. urealyticum* culture
- Follicle tracking by ultrasound
- Cul-de-sac aspiration for spermatozoa
- Testing for antisperm antibodies
- Zona penetration (human ova)
- Zona-free hamster egg penetration

Therapy

From a therapeutic standpoint, a specific diagnosis is essential before initiation of any specific treatment. Empirical treatment of the couple with unexplained infertility is inappropriate and may be intrinsically dangerous or even emotionally damaging by raising expectations of the couple without a logical or scientific basis. Although thyroid medications, bromocriptine, danazol, and mucolytic agents have in the past been suggested as efficacious in unexplained infertility, their effectiveness is still unproved and their empirical use should be avoided. Likewise there is no logical reason for the administration of ovulation-inducing agents such as clomiphene citrate or gonadotropins in a normally ovulating woman with a normal postovulatory phase.

Superovulation and intrauterine insemination. Controlled ovarian stimulation using ovulation-inducing agents with or without intrauterine insemination (IUI) has been advocated to treat couples with unexplained infertility. Clomiphene citrate in conjunction with IUI resulted in 14 pregnancies during 148 treated cycles (fecundity = 0.095) compared with 5 pregnancies in 150 untreated cycles (fecundity = 0.033) in a randomized, prospective study involving 67 couples with either unexplained infertility or surgically corrected endometriosis. There was no difference in fecundity between couples with unexplained infertility and those with endometriosis, but treatment significantly increased fecundity.[11]

Dodson et al.[12] have associated superovulation with human menopausal gonadotropin (hMG)/human chorionic gonadotropin (hCG) and IUI in patients with "refractory infertility" (Table 25-2). Likewise, Welner et al.[36] carried out empirical hMG/hCG therapy in patients with longstanding

Table 25-2. Superovulation and intrauterine insemination

Cycle no.	No. of pregnancies	No. of patients	Conception rate (%)
1	12	85	14
2	12	51	24
3	0	0	0
4	0	0	0
TOTAL	24	148	16

Modified from Dodson WC et al: *Fertil Steril* 48:441, 1987.

infertility of unknown etiology while they were awaiting IVF (Table 25-3). Twelve conceptions (12.4%) and eight (8.2%) term births occurred in their study group as compared with 1% in controls. On this basis the authors suggest a 4-month empirical trial of hMG/hCG in patients with unexplained infertility.

The approach of gonadotropin treatment for ovulatory patients was introduced in 1987 by Haney et al.[20] and in 1988 by Welner et al.[36] as an intermediary step for treatment of certain infertile women before IVF. At Johns Hopkins, patients with unexplained infertility and with early endometriosis treated with a combination of superovulation and IUI have achieved pregnancy in rates of 35% and 38%, respectively. The rationale for this approach is based on (1) a theoretic means for improving fecundity, (2) high costs associated with IVF and GIFT, and (3) pressures placed on the physician. In contrast, drawbacks need to be considered when resorting to a combination of controlled ovarian stimulation and IUI. Empirical therapy should not be considered as state of the art. There is ample evidence to suggest a significant spontaneous pregnancy rate in such patients. Results therefore need to be weighed against a spontaneously achieved pregnancy rate in couples with unexplained infertility as a control group. Controlled ovarian hyperstimulation with IUI also entails risks. The multiple pregnancy rate is high (25% to 30%). Severe hyperstimulation requires hospitalization; it occurs in approximately 1% of women undergoing superovulation with gonadotropins. Intrauterine cannulation for insemination is associated with pelvic infection, and the ectopic pregnancy rate (5%) is also high. With respect to cost factors, the cost of IVF is reducible, especially taking into consideration cryopreservation of embryos and extension of a number of potential transfer cycles thereby. A reasonable plan in unexplained infertility would be to consider a limited course of controlled ovarian hyperstimulation with IUI (e.g., three cycles) before proceeding to IVF or GIFT. In considering alternative therapy for the infertile couple, the bottom line in the decision-making process must include effectiveness, cost, and safety, as well as the rational use of treatment modalities.

In vitro fertilization and embryo transfer. In couples who have demonstrated immunologic hindrance of gamete transport or defective spermatozoal fertilizing capacity, IVF and embryo transfer may offer a reasonable approach to treatment. In the review by Lopata[23] of indications for IVF and embryo transfer during 1981, 32 of 229 patients underwent the procedure with an indication of unexplained infertility. This figure is higher today because overall results with IVF have improved. GIFT has also been used successfully in patients with unexplained infertility. Finally, one should realize that many of the processes responsible for fertility are currently beyond diagnostic reach and defy direct evaluation. This concept should be shared with the couple for whom the basis for infertility cannot be determined.

SUMMARY

To put the problem of unexplained infertility into perspective, Collins et al.[8] reported that of 597 infertile couples, 41% conceived after medical or surgical therapy, or both. In contrast, 191 of 548 untreated controls (35%) became pregnant. Seventy-five additional patients conceived 6 months or more after surgical therapy or at least 3 months after cessation of medical treatment. Collins and associates[9] also reported that 40% of couples with unexplained infertility followed for up to 3 years ultimately established pregnancy. In addition, Miller et al.[25] reported on 197 patients during 623 cycles in which 152 pregnancies occurred. Of these, 43% (64) resulted in pregnancy loss. Only 14 of the 64 losses were recognized as spontaneous abortions; the other 50 patients had positive urinary hCG levels, but no other evidence of pregnancy. Finally, Coulam

Table 25-3. Empirical hMG/hCG therapy

Cycle no.	No. of conceptions	Successful conceptions (%)
1	4	33
2	1	8
3	3	25
4	4	33
TOTAL	12/97 couples	12.4

Modified from Welner S, DeCherney AH, Polan ML: *Am J Obstet Gynecol* 158:111, 1988.

Table 25-4. Infertility investigations in 57 couples

Testing modality	Diagnosis	Patients No.	%
Ultrasound	Luteinized unruptured follicle syndrome	3	5
Sperm antibody	Antibodies present	11	5
Sperm penetration assay	Penetration	11	11
Human leukocyte antigen (HLA)	HLA homozygosity	21	37

Modified from Coulam CB, Moore SB, O'Fallon W: *Am J Obstet Gynecol* 158:1374, 1988.

and coworkers[10] have improved the yield from investigational studies for unexplained infertility. Their findings are summarized in Table 25-4.

Evaluation of any treatment for couples with unexplained infertility requires demonstration that the improvement is indeed treatment related. In the absence of a defined factor for infertility in couples with unexplained infertility, spontaneous conception can occur in the absence of treatment. In order to evaluate the effectiveness of any modality of treatment in these couples, a comparison with an untreated group should be included in the study design.

REFERENCES

1. Aitken RJ et al: An analysis of sperm function in cases of unexplained infertility: conventional criteria, movement characteristics, and fertilizing capacity, *Fertil Steril* 38:212, 1982.
2. Audebert AJ: The place of laparoscopy in unexplained infertility, *Acta Eur Fertil* 11:269, 1980.
3. Broekhuizen FF, Hanning RV Jr, Shapiro SS: Laparoscopic findings in twenty-five failures of artificial insemination, *Fertil Steril* 34:351, 1980.
4. Bronson RA: Sperm antibodies: problems in infertility, *Postgrad Obstet Gynecol* 11(20):1, 1991.
5. Bronson RA, Rogers BJ: Pitfalls of the zona-free hamster egg penetration test: protein source as a major variable, *Fertil Steril* 50:851; 1988.
6. Bronson RA, Wallach EE: Lysis of periadnexal adhesions for correction of infertility, *Fertil Steril* 28:613, 1977.
7. Coetzee K et al: Hypoosmotic swelling test in the prediction of male fertility, *Arch Androl* 23:131, 1989.
8. Collins JA et al: Treatment independent pregnancy among infertile couples, *N Engl J Med* 309:1201, 1983.
9. Collins JA et al: Clinical factors affecting pregnancy rates among infertile couples, *Can Med Assoc J* 130:269, 1984.
10. Coulam CB, Moore SB, O'Fallon W: Investigating unexplained infertility, *Am J Obstet Gynecol* 158:1374, 1988.
11. Deaton JL et al: A randomized, controlled trial of clomiphene citrate and intrauterine insemination in couples with unexplained infertility or surgically corrected endometriosis, *Fertil Steril* 54:1083, 1990.
12. Dodson WC et al: Superovulation with intrauterine insemination in the treatment of infertility: two possible alternatives to gamete intrafallopian transfer and in vitro fertilization, *Fertil Steril* 48:441, 1987.
13. Drake T et al: Unexplained infertility: a reappraisal, *Obstet Gynecol* 50:644, 1977.
14. Friberg J: Mycoplasmas and ureaplasmas in infertility and abortion, *Fertil Steril* 33:351, 1980.
15. Gnarpe H, Friberg J: Mycoplasma and human reproductive failure, I: the occurrence of seven different mycoplasmas in couples with reproductive failure, *Am J Obstet Gynecol* 114:727, 1972.
16. Goldenberg RC, Magendantz HG: Laparoscopy and the infertility evaluation, *Obstet Gynecol* 47:410, 1976.
17. Grant A: Additional sterility factors in endometriosis, *Fertil Steril* 17:514, 1966.
18. Haas GG Jr, Cines DB, Schreiber AD: Immunologic infertility: identification of patients with antisperm antibody, *N Engl J Med* 303:772, 1980.
19. Halme JK et al: Altered maturation and function of peritoneal macrophages: possible role in pathogenesis of endometriosis, *Am J Obstet Gynecol* 156:783, 1987.
20. Haney AF et al: Treatment-independent and treatment-associated pregnancies after additional therapy in a program of in vitro fertilization and embryo transfer, *Fertil Steril* 47:634, 1987.
21. Harrison RF et al: Doxycycline treatment and human infertility, *Lancet* 1:605, 1975.
22. Isojima S et al: Further studies on sperm-immobilizing antibody found in sera of unexplained cases of sterility in women, *Am J Obstet Gynecol* 112:199, 1972.
23. Lopata A: Concepts in human in vitro fertilization and embryo transfer, *Fertil Steril* 40:289, 1983.
24. Mårdh PA et al: *Chlamydia trachomatis* infections in patients with salpingitis, *N Engl J Med* 296:1377, 1977.
25. Miller JF et al: Fetal loss after implantation, *Lancet* 2:554, 1980.
26. Muse KN, Wilson EA: How does mild endometriosis cause infertility?, *Fertil Steril* 38:154, 1982.
27. Olive DL, Weinberg JB, Haney AF: Peritoneal macrophages and infertility: the association between cell number and pelvic pathology, *Fertil Steril* 44:772, 1985.
28. Overstreet JW et al: Penetration of human spermatozoa into the human zona pellucida and the zona-free hamster egg: a study of fertile donors and infertile patients, *Fertil Steril* 33:534, 1980.
29. Peterson EP, Behrman SJ: Laparoscopy of the infertile patient, *Obstet Gynecol* 36:363, 1970.
30. Rogers BJ et al: Analysis of human spermatozoal fertilizing ability using zona-free ova, *Fertil Steril* 32:431, 1980.
31. Stray-Pedersen B, Eng J, Reikvan TM: Uterine T mycoplasma colonization in reproductive failure, *Am J Obstet Gynecol* 130:307, 1978.
32. Templeton AA, Mortimer D: The development of a clinical test of sperm migration to the site of fertilization, *Fertil Steril* 37:410, 1982.
33. Treharne JD et al: Antibodies to *Chlamydia trachomatis* in acute salpingitis, *Br J Vener Dis* 55:26, 1979.
34. Trounson AO et al: The investigation of idiopathic infertility by *in vitro* fertilization, *Fertil Steril* 34:431, 1980.
35. Wallach EE, Manara LR, Eisenberg E: Experience with 143 cases of tubal reconstructive surgery, *Fertil Steril* 39:609, 1983.
36. Welner S, DeCherney AH, Polan ML: Human menopausal gonadotropins: a justifiable therapy in ovulatory women with long-standing idiopathic infertility, *Am J Obstet Gynecol* 158:111, 1988.
37. Yanagamachi R: Zona-free hamster eggs: their use in assessing fertilizing capacity and examining chromosomes of human spermatozoa, *Gamete Res* 10:187, 1984.
38. Yanagimachi R, Yanagimachi H, Rogers BJ: The use of zona-free animal ova as a test system for the assessment of fertilizing capacity of human spermatozoa, *Biol Reprod* 15:471, 1976.
39. Zamboni L: The ultrastructural pathology of the spermatozoon as a cause of infertility: the role of electron microscopy in the evaluation of semen quality. In Wallach EE, Kempers RD, editors: *Modern trends in infertility and conception control,* vol 4, Chicago, 1988, Year Book Medical Publishers.

SUGGESTED READINGS

Moghissi KS, Wallach EE: Unexplained infertility. In Wallach EE, Kempers RD, editors: *Modern trends in infertility and conception control,* vol 3, Chicago, 1985, Year Book Medical Publishers.

Wallach EE, Moghissi KS: Unexplained infertility. In Behrman SJ, Kistner RW, Patton GW, editors: *Progress in infertility,* Boston, 1987, Little, Brown.

Chapter 26

BEYOND CONCEPTION

The Psychologic Dilemmas of Infertility and Assisted Reproductive Technology

Patricia Payne Mahlstedt, EdD
and Susan Macduff Wood, MA

Gilda Radner, the popular comedienne from "Saturday Night Live," finished her book *It's Always Something* before she knew the outcome of her medical treatment for ovarian cancer. She reflected that she had always wanted to write a book about her life that had a happy ending before there even *was* an ending. She wanted to predict, and thus control, the outcome. However, as her work on the book reached closure and her health continued to decline, she recognized the limits of that dream:

Now I've learned, the hard way, that some poems don't rhyme, and some stories don't have a clear beginning, middle and end. Like my life, this book has ambiguity. Like my life, this book is about not knowing, having to change, taking the moment and making the best of it, without knowing what's going to happen next.*

*From Radner G: *It's always something,* New York, 1989, Simon & Schuster, p. 268. Copyright © 1989 by Gilda Radner. Reprinted by permission of Simon & Schuster, Inc.

Ambiguity, having to change, not knowing what is going to happen next might also describe the experience of infertile couples who are trying to define and resolve the dilemmas created by their infertility, to develop ways to cope with the uncertainty that it creates, and, at the very least, to make decisions about treatment that will be in the best interests of their marriage and their hoped-for children. Physicians who specialize in reproductive medicine and their staffs are also having to live with the frustrations of not knowing what is going to happen next or how they should respond to patients' needs for answers to the psychosocial questions that the technology poses. It appears that all participants in assisted reproductive technology live each day with hope that their medical goals will be achieved, with uncertainty about the duration and ramifications of their treatment decisions, and with the desire to create a happy ending for all involved.

Creating a happy ending might be seen as a metaphor for effectively resolving the emotional dilemmas created by infertility, as well as for making good decisions about treatment options, ones with which all involved will be satisfied in the future. *The impact of these decisions and the manner in which they are made will be felt long after conception or the termination of treatment.* In an attempt to fulfill infertile couples' need for parenthood, reproductive medicine has created a technology whose primary focus is pregnancy. For those who conceive, however, pregnancy is only the beginning. Life continues after treatment with the baby of their dreams and a marriage stressed by infertility's demands, dilemmas, and choices. Those patients who do not conceive also have to live with the decisions they make during treatment. For them the end of treatment is the beginning of a life without the biologic child of their dreams. They, too, deserve a happy ending. For this to happen, patients and physicians alike must broaden their focus beyond the medical goal of conception to include the emotional needs that arise naturally from the stresses of infertility and its treatment.

The goals of this chapter are twofold: (1) to present an

overview of the major psychologic issues of infertility and to recommend ways in which physicians and their staffs can help patients deal with these issues, and (2) to discuss emotional factors associated with specific assisted reproductive technologies and to recommend ways in which physicians and their staffs can help patients deal openly with the issues created by these technologies.

EMOTIONAL ISSUES OF INFERTILITY

When you absolutely cannot have children, it's called sterility. When it seems to be taking an awfully long time but you still hope, it's called infertility.

Infertility is worse.*

The process of diagnosing and treating infertility has a profound impact on the lives of those couples who experience it, arousing conflict in the most stable marriage or exacerbating existing problems between the partners. Even though this impact is usually greater when the treatment process is prolonged or unsuccessful, the emotional component begins to develop when the partners of a couple realize they are not conceiving as they had planned. They begin to worry, have doubts, become frustrated, and wonder why they cannot do something as natural as conceiving.

Day-to-day life changes significantly for infertile couples after medical treatment begins, exacting a heavy toll on the quality of life and affecting in some way the emotional, social, physical, occupational, intellectual, and even spiritual well-being of those it touches. Independence and flexibility are lost as their lives begin to revolve around the physician's plans for conception: medications, injections, ultrasound examinations, surgeries. Their attention becomes focused on this singular failure, and other goals and needs are neglected. Often this focus has a negative impact on their self-esteem, health, relationships, security, and even their ambitions. Each month contains hope for 2 weeks and despair for the next 2 weeks. A never-ending roller coaster ride is created, with hope on the upside and depression, anger, and guilt on the downside.[7]

Depression

Losses occurring in adulthood that have been found to be of the greatest importance as etiologic factors in depression are as follows: (1) loss of a relationship, (2) loss of health, (3) loss of status or prestige, (4) loss of self-esteem, (5) loss of self-confidence, (6) loss of security, (7) loss of a fantasy or the hope of fulfilling an important fantasy, and (8) loss of something or someone of great symbolic value.[15] Any one of these losses could precipitate a depressive reaction in an adult. In varying degrees, the experience of infertility involves them all.

Loss of a relationship. Depression often follows loss of a relationship with an emotionally important person be-

*From Office of Technology Assessment: *Infertility: medical and social choices,* Washington, DC, 1988, U.S. Government Printing Office, p. 131.

cause of death, divorce, the waning of affection, or separation. Infertility sometimes serves to emotionally isolate the infertile person from his or her fertile spouse, parents, siblings, in-laws, and friends, who are often unaware of the infertile person's need for support or uncertain how to demonstrate this support. Although well-meaning, these individuals may inadvertently make remarks such as "don't try so hard" or "just relax," which can be a source of tremendous frustration and pain. Such comments imply that the infertile couple is somehow at fault for not conceiving or that the medical treatment is not working because the couple is sabotaging it. Tension develops within the relationship. The infertile couple feels misunderstood, unloved, and unacceptable. Afraid of further alienating their friends and family by telling them how these remarks hurt, the infertile couple withdraws. One patient expressed this isolation:

My sister doesn't understand what is happening with me. I want to be close to her and her kids, like we used to be. Now I feel so envious and self-conscious whenever she tells me about their family activities. I'd rather not be around them.

Couples may fear loss of important relationships because of lack of information about the causes of infertility. They may wonder if this is punishment for a transgression earlier in life or about their responsibility for the outcome of the treatment. The partners themselves may experience a loss of closeness because infertility affects them differently or because they cope differently. In general, the potential loss of fertility is more threatening for women, whose core identity is fundamentally tied in with becoming a mother. Men, whose primary identity is not dependent on fatherhood, are less affected by that potential loss. Not understanding this basic difference, women often feel unloved or abandoned when their husbands do not experience the same emotional pain during the infertility crisis.

Further aggravating the stress is the common difference in coping styles between men and women. Typically, men cope with their pain by keeping it to themselves and focusing on their wives. Women manage their pain by talking at length about it with their husbands, who, unable to take away the pain, often stop listening. As women escalate their complaints to get their husbands involved, the husbands pull away and may even stop participating in the treatment process. In this case, both partners feel inadequate in their responses to each other's behavior. Furthermore, feelings of guilt for being infertile, disrupting the lives of others, depleting savings to pay for treatment, and for being unable to relieve a partner's frustrations can cause fear that the relationship will not survive:

My husband deserves so much more than I have given during the last three years of infertility treatment. I have spent so much money, been upset a lot, needed sex at a certain time, and all for nothing. Sometimes he seems so distant that I'm afraid he doesn't love me anymore.

Loss of health. Loss of health, important body functions, or physical attractiveness due to disease, injury, aging—in other words, loss of an acceptable self-image or body image—can cause depression. A positive body image is related to an individual's feeling attractive, normal, and acceptable to others, both inwardly and outwardly. Most couples entering treatment for infertility are in good health and have positive body images and self-images. They are accustomed to engaging in challenging situations and being successful, thereby reinforcing a positive self-image. However, the treatment process often seems to assault these images. Patients relinquish control of their bodies to medications that may have physically debilitating side effects, their sexual spontaneity to demands for performance frequency and timing prescribed by the physician, their time to the necessities of physician appointments, and even their consciousness to surgical procedures. The discovery of a physical defect such as infertility may threaten a patient's positive body image. Persons accustomed to feeling in control of their bodies or physical health may suddenly come to view themselves as defective, unable to perform the most fundamental task of life—reproduction:

I have always thought of myself as a healthy person. I exercise regularly, and I eat healthy foods. Infertility has changed that perception. Taking drugs, having surgeries, and going to the doctor so often has made me feel physically defective. I sometimes wonder if I will ever feel whole again.

Furthermore, for couples who are confused or ill-informed about their diagnostic and treatment plans, compliance with the regimen feels like "sick role" behavior. Couples surrender control of their reproductive activities (from the timing of sexual relations to the timing of ovulation) to the physician with highly sophisticated and abstract procedures. The physician, in turn, will accomplish the goal of creating a pregnancy. One woman expressed her feelings of loss of control:

You'd think I had a life-threatening condition and needed a doctor in charge of my life! I'm told to take my temperature at a certain time every morning, have sex on certain days, see the doctor so many days after my period starts and, within a certain time of having intercourse, report to the lab on certain days, and on and on. It's like my period proves that I'm sick and need someone to take care of me.

The medical problem, invisible to others, is experienced as if it were obvious to all. As is true of other emotional responses to infertility, this reaction seems to come spontaneously, almost overnight. Men and women enter treatment feeling strong and hopeful and soon find themselves physically and emotionally debilitated—all for an "illness" they do not understand. The rush and depth of emotional responses to infertility cannot be overemphasized.

Among men for whom fertility and virility are emotionally linked, a diagnosis of infertility may be devastating.

Infertile men often exhibit a pattern of impotence and depression coupled with hostility and guilt. The need to produce semen specimens for regular analysis is threatening and degrading:

Being infertile has damaged my sense of self in a profound way. As a man, I was not aware of the power of fertility until now. What is worse is that no one will discuss it with me. Doctors stay on the technical, friends who know avoid the subject, and even my wife doesn't know what to say. It is a very lonely experience.

Another aspect of this loss is the loss of sexual spontaneity and privacy. Because treatment often requires scheduled sexual intercourse, sexual relations are viewed as "sex for doctor" or "sex for baby," not "sex for love." Moreover, the medical treatment itself requires evaluation of a couple's sexual life, specifically, timing and frequency of intercourse. This alone violates a deep sense of privacy that surrounds this intimate aspect of marriage and affects sexual pleasure and potency.

Loss of status or prestige. Infertility can lead to perception of loss of status or prestige in the eyes of others, however real. Society places great value on parenthood. Because others expect married adults to have children, an inevitable question on meeting someone is "How many children do you have?" Such questions leave infertile couples feeling different, abnormal, less acceptable. They feel as though they are unable to meet the expectations of others and thereby suffer a social stigma attached to the inability to produce children[7]:

I feel like I don't belong, like a second-class citizen with no place to go. Without a child, I don't belong in the group with kids who play in the park. Without a child, my husband and I don't fit in with our friends who do.

Others may feel that their sexual identities are inextricably linked to fathering a child or assuming the role of mother. They believe that anything less than fulfillment of these roles threatens their value to the group (society or the family). Often real things happen to reinforce these perceptions. Feeling awkward about their own children, friends and relatives may avoid infertile couples and isolate them more. Couples who felt appreciated and well-liked by their friends before awareness of their infertility lose the confidence that others appreciate them. Attention and respect seem to be given to those who have children.

Loss of self-esteem. Loss of self-esteem or pride in oneself leads to a sense of failure. The definition of infertility (failure to conceive after trying for at least 1 year or failure to carry a pregnancy to a live birth) is the description of a failing. As a result, for some persons, making the decision to consult an infertility specialist is similar to making the decision to see a psychologist or psychiatrist. Before making that decision, a person must acknowledge that there is a problem.[8] Something is the matter with the self. One woman said:

I can't emphasize how devastating infertility is to one who has spent a lifetime basing her self-esteem on "what I can do." When you can't have children—the most natural and important aspect of life—none of your previous accomplishments seem important. They are overshadowed by this supreme failure.

The creation of a biologic family is the stated goal of infertility therapy. Those patients who are accustomed to taking responsibility for getting what they need and want often feel that they themselves are responsible and, thus, are failures. How could they be unable to accomplish such a simple task? Being infertile is an assault on their self-esteem.

Social myths about infertility and its causes also erode the infertile couples' self-confidence. For example, stories about couples who adopt and subsequently conceive are used to support the advice to "adopt and then you will conceive." This type of advice undermines the need for medical intervention and a couple's emotional, physical, and financial commitment to it. Moreover, it is not true. The reality is that only 5% of couples who adopt subsequently conceive. Because infertile couples are often unsure about the reality of the myth, they do not know how to respond. They want to feel good about what they are doing in response to their medical problem, not what they may not be doing. But myths like this make it difficult.

The emotional responses to infertility are very strong and come as a surprise to many couples. Their self-esteem erodes as they become aware of the extent to which emotions seem to rule their lives as never before. There are periods of calm and hope followed by explosions of underlying distress as monthly menstruation or the curve of the temperature chart reminds couples of their failure. Their self-respect and pride get lost in that vicious cycle, leading some to wonder whether they are good enough to be parents. Such negative thoughts are often followed by a sense of hopelessness and despair.

Loss of self-confidence. Failure to conceive often causes loss of self-confidence or loss of an adequate sense of competence or control. Loss of control is a major theme in the frustration of infertility patients. Immersion in infertility treatment involves surrendering control of many aspects of everyday life, such as decisions about when to go on vacation or business trips, job changes, career problems, or work schedules. Infertile couples have difficulty in concentrating on these and other important matters because they are controlled by the details of trying to conceive. Despite significant investments of time, money, and self, there is no baby.

Many patients feel that even the treatment regimen is out of their control. Some believe that they do not understand nor are they consulted regarding the intended treatments. In their powerless state of mind, they may be reluctant to speak up on their own behalf for fear the physician will become angry:

The most painful part of today's doctor visit was when he saw tears streaming down my cheeks after the exam and he said, "Why are you crying?" It sounded as if he didn't think his comments should warrant such a response. If he could just say, "I'm sorry you feel bad," I'd feel more like a person.

Infertility also involves many decisions concerning medical options that might include the use of powerful drugs for inducing ovulation, in vitro fertilization, the use of donor gametes, or the various forms of surrogacy. Couples struggle with important questions for which there are no definitive answers. This creates uncertainty about judgment and insecurity about making the "right" decision. The result is often procrastination or termination of treatment before all possible options have been tried.

The process of trying to conceive consumes the infertile person's life, eliminating the sense of self-confidence, competence, and control that comes from familiarity with and success in accomplishing a particular challenge.

Loss of security. The time and expense involved in infertility treatment can result in loss of occupational, financial, social, and cultural security. Occupational security and financial security are threatened when infertility treatment is prolonged, and frequent visits, medications, and diagnostic and surgical procedures take one away from work or create a financial burden. Many insurance companies provide only partial coverage for infertility treatment procedures. Job performance and relationships with co-workers may be jeopardized as the emotional impact of infertility interferes with the ability to concentrate. Social or cultural security is jeopardized as the infertile couple continues to feel like the "odd man out" among family and friends whose lives center to a large degree on their children.

The most significant loss of security by infertile couples is the loss of the belief in the fairness and predictability of life. The saying "No one gets out of here alive" develops real meaning as infertile couples come to terms with their vulnerability. As one man said:

My wife and I feel so depressed about the unfairness of it all. We have both been conscientious people, have done what others and we thought was right. We are afraid if this could happen, so could anything else.

Loss of a fantasy or the hope of fulfilling an important fantasy. Being a parent is both a lifelong dream and a developmental need of most people. It is so much taken for granted that most people do not realize its significance. For many, having a child is synonymous with achieving adulthood both in their own eyes and in the eyes of their parents. Moreover, many adult friendships are formed through the activities of children. These experiences are not available to the infertile couple.

Infertility interrupts the natural cycle of life: leaving home, starting a career, getting married, having children.

Infertile couples have the same expectations and fantasies about what their lives will be as any other couple. Without children, they cannot accomplish a very important life task—parenthood—and thus, in their own eyes, be normal. They fear that they will miss so much: being pregnant and giving birth, preparing for baptism, watching a child learn a sport, attending a graduation. Being a part of a child's life is a part of one's perception of an idealized adult. Losing that perception causes great emotional pain.

Loss of something or someone of great symbolic value. Infertile couples generally have examined carefully their reasons for wanting children. They can identify many of the taken-for-granted philosophic values of having children: links to the future; sources of pleasure, pride, and challenge; meaning in life. They yearn for the child who may never be and mourn the child who never was. The loss is as real to the infertile couple as if the child had been born, lived, and died.

Because there is no tangible loss for all to see, it is difficult for family and friends to truly comprehend the loss. Even the partners of a couple have trouble articulating their experience, but they feel wounded, and their wounds are reopened often. Children everywhere remind them that they are infertile. Pregnant women remind them of the pregnancy they may never experience. Toddlers on television commercials, birth announcements from friends, and families with children in Sunday services are salt in the wounds of infertile couples. They long for the sense of family that children represent.

The multiple losses associated with infertility are not, of course, mutually exclusive. A single belief, such as the common notion that one is responsible for his or her infertility or the outcome of the treatment, may trigger any or all of the losses. Because so many losses deplete couples of the psychologic energy needed to cope effectively, common emotional responses to this life experience are depression, anger, and guilt. The grief and sadness associated with infertility are similar to the grief and sadness caused by death and divorce. For some, the pain and loss of infertility will be with them throughout their lives. It may never end.

Anger

The loss of control over the basic desire for procreation is enraging for many infertility patients. The unanswerable question of "why?" plagues them while their anger is being fed by conflicting demands of work and treatment and the perceived insensitivity of friends, family, and even physicians. What is a routine procedure in the medical community is not so to the uninitiated infertility patient. The emotionally drained patient commonly experiences physical and/or emotional pain during diagnostic procedures the physician may believe to be relatively benign:

The doctor told me that the test he was doing was routine, that it takes 10 or 15 minutes and wouldn't hurt. Well, that was wrong.

It did hurt and he and the assistant were poking me for longer than I had expected. I felt humiliated and I was angry!

Patients will take extraordinary measures to cover their distress and anger with physicians. They are afraid that they will sabotage the treatment if the secret of their distress is discovered.

Anger due to a loss of control is very difficult to handle. At whom does one get mad? In the absence of an appropriate venue, anger may be channeled into the most important relationships (as between partners, who then fight), or it may be repressed and appear as depression only to be unleashed on the unfortunate individual available at the time the emotion is overwhelming.

Guilt

Patients may also feel guilt for being infertile, for letting down the spouse and other loved ones and for feeling so miserable. They believe that they have caused their infertility and, at the very least, should be able to control their responses to it. Guilt is a frustrated attempt to gain control of the question "why?" If there were an understandable reason, many would feel less depressed, less angry, less guilty.

Summary

As a major crisis, infertility blocks the way to the life goal of parenthood. It poses a problem that often is insolvable because it is beyond traditional problem-solving methods. Like a chronic illness, infertility overtaxes the existing resources of the persons involved. Similar to other crises, infertility brings up and magnifies unresolved issues from within the marriage. Moreover, it creates a psychologic disequilibrium that elicits common emotional reactions and proceeds to either an adaptive or maladaptive resolution.

The crisis of infertility shatters dreams at a time when people are most hopeful. If not worked through, the losses and subsequent wounds impede emotional growth for the individual and the couple, as well as any children eventually born. The Chinese symbol for crisis is composed of two words: danger and opportunity. Infertility is a crisis that involves many personal risks, and yet for some it becomes an opportunity for growth. Those who grow are probably surrounded by medical personnel, family, and friends who do what they can to support the partners of the couple and to help them through the crisis. They are also people who see conflict and suffering as a part of life that can enable one to grow: "What matters above all is the attitude we take toward suffering. Suffering ceases to be suffering in some way the moment it finds a meaning."[5]

A complete resolution of the infertility crisis is not absolute. As in loss due to death, the issue continues to reverberate and can be revived even though essentially it may have been resolved. However, by working through the multiple problems created by this crisis, many couples get to know each other in deeper ways than may have occurred if they had not been infertile. For these couples, infertility can be seen as a painful life experience that, because of their commitment and hard work, provided an opportunity for them to grow. For them, there will be a happy ending.

Recommendations

Develop an awareness of the emotional impact of infertility. Physicians can be a part of the opportunity for growth in a number of ways. First they should develop an awareness of the many ways in which infertility and its treatment intrude on and disrupt all infertile couples' lives. Talking with their patients early in treatment about the normalcy of sadness and frustration enables couples to integrate these feelings into their lives, to respect each other's responses, and to respond to medical recommendations more easily.

Encourage both partners to participate in treatment. All medical staff can and should encourage both partners to participate in the treatment procedures whenever possible. Joint participation doubles the patients' power to learn from the physician, to ask questions, and to help each other. It also prevents one person from feeling that he or she is the cause of the problem and the one responsible for fixing it—a heavy burden. Another strategy that helps couples feel more competent is the manner in which medical information is shared. Communicating *in writing* all medical, psychologic, and legal issues enables couples to discuss what they need to do, review the instructions and expectations at home, and make informed choices.

Encourage couples to talk about and be experts on each other's emotional responses to infertility. Couples often need to be reminded that they must pay attention to their emotional needs as well. Physicians can encourage couples to talk about and be experts on each other's emotional responses to infertility, acknowledging that men and women usually respond differently to the problem of infertility. A couple is two individuals. To expect both to feel the same way about infertility or to express their feelings in the same way causes considerable stress. Couples must be urged to identify and resolve any problems that may have developed during infertility treatment. This type of process enables them to make good decisions about future treatment and to incorporate both the gains and losses that the infertility experience has brought to their lives into a positive concept of themselves as individuals and as a couple.

As physicians listen to what patients say, and respect and accept reluctance to continue treatment—whatever the reason—they should discourage any notion that stopping treatment means that the partners are quitters or failures. Recommending support groups such as Resolve* and refer-

ring to mental health professionals with an expertise in infertility are helpful strategies during all decision-making periods during treatment.

Broaden the definition of successful treatment. Finally, physicians need to broaden the definition of *success* in medical treatment. While conception is one definition of success, another is satisfaction with the ways in which emotional pain was processed and decisions were made during treatment. In her book, *Give Us a Child*, Lynda Stephenson redefines success:

> Can there be a happy ending to an infertility story without a baby? Beyond what I may feel now and then, I think the answer is a definite, hope-filled yes. Because the conviction I feel deepest is that our happy endings must come from ourselves, if they are to come at all.
>
> I wish for you a baby. But more than that—above everything—I wish for you a happy ending.*

EMOTIONAL ISSUES ASSOCIATED WITH NONCOITAL METHODS OF REPRODUCTION

Not all infertile couples want to participate in the new technologic procedures of reproductive medicine. In general, those who do are a special group. They are well-integrated individuals whose personal resources have been stretched thin, whose marriages have withstood and sometimes have been strengthened by their infertility struggle, and whose determination to conceive is great. And, above all, they are willing to risk. They are gambling on something in which the stakes are high, the stress is great, the support from others is minimal, and the stated goal probably will not be achieved. Why will they do this? Because they desperately want a child, and they still hope.

In the prologue to the book *Our Miracle Called Louise*, Leslie Brown describes the kind of hope these couples feel:

> I never gave up hope of having a baby of my own, even though it was to take fourteen years. When a doctor told me, years ago, that it was a one-in-a-million chance that I'd ever have a child, I still kept trying.
>
> Crazy as it sounds, even when Mr. Steptoe, the gynecologist, warned me that a baby had never been successfully conceived outside the womb, I still wouldn't believe him. It was my last chance. It had to work for me. "Think pregnant," Mr. Steptoe now tells women like me, who would go through anything to have a child. That's how I thought. And the result was our miracle called Louise Lesley Brown.†

So hopeful couples such as Leslie and her husband decide to gamble. They commit their time, their money, their bodies, and their hopes to procedures that probably will not achieve their primary goal. Will they lose all that they committed? Will they try to place blame on each other and thus weaken their marriage? After the procedure, will

---

*Resolve, Inc., P.O. Box 474, Belmont, MA 02178; Telephone (617) 484-2424. Offers counseling and support to persons with problems of infertility through workshops, training sessions, and consultations.

*From Stephenson, L.: *Give us a child,* New York, 1987, Harper & Row, p. 225.
†From Brown L, Brown J: *Our miracle called Louise: a parents' story,* New York, 1979, Paddington Press (prologue).

they feel abandoned by the medical staff with whom they have worked so closely, in the same way that they often felt forgotten by family and friends during their infertility? Will they feel foolish for taking the risk? Will the medical staff understand the emotional significance of these medical procedures? DeCherney cautioned: "Technological parenthood may have the trappings of a business; but it is not a business. It is the answer to someone's most personal prayers. So it should be seen and handled."[3]

In other words, the answers to the prayers of infertile couples for new ways to make babies have the potential to be very, very good—and very, very bad. These alternatives are so packed with questions of one kind or another that ignoring them may just be asking for trouble later. As much as it may go against their personal need for a child, couples must, with help, carefully examine the pros and cons of each alternative. The integrity of their marriage and the emotional well-being of their potential offspring are at stake.

In vitro fertilization

In vitro fertilization (IVF) procedures are less complicated in terms of potential emotional loss to the adults or children than other noncoital means of reproduction. In most cases, IVF procedures involve the genetic material from both partners, so the emotional risk lies in either or both spouses' not being emotionally prepared for the process. If they are not prepared, couples may regret having tried IVF or may see themselves as failures if conception does not occur. The task, then, is to identify the emotional risks and to prepare couples for handling them prior to the beginning of an IVF cycle.

Emotional risks of in vitro fertilization. The primary emotional risks involved in IVF include the following:

1. Couples will feel like failures or regret having tried IVF if they do not conceive.
2. Couples will not know how to be involved in the process of IVF conception as a couple. They might see IVF as something the women do primarily alone.
3. Couples will not feel adequate support during the procedure.
4. Couples will be forgotten after they leave the program.
5. Couples will not adequately discuss cryopreservation; specifically, they may not consider alternate plans for frozen embryos if they do not use them.
6. Couples will not feel finished with the process; they may feel that they do not have enough medical information to make the next decision.
7. Couples will not be given necessary referrals to specialists and mental health professionals.

To avoid the feelings of regret or failure if conception does not occur, couples might broaden their expectations of the IVF experience by setting realistic, therapeutic goals.

Couples' goals for in vitro fertilization. There are actually four psychologic and medical goals for couples undergoing IVF: (1) to become closer emotionally as a couple; (2) to learn more about their reproductive systems; (3) to have the feeling that they have done everything they could do to achieve a biologic pregnancy; and (4) to conceive a child. If couples and the IVF team are working well together, and if couples do their homework, three out of four of these goals definitely can be achieved. Only the fourth—conceiving a child—is out of their control. While working on these four goals, couples will be avoiding the emotional risks just listed and moving toward a sense of competence about the challenges of IVF.[10]

Achieving the first goal—becoming closer emotionally as a couple—begins as the partners prepare for IVF. Couples should become experts on how each partner has been affected by the infertility experience. As they express their pain and feel understood, share ways in which each can support the other, and anticipate what they will do if they do not conceive, they begin to learn what the experience of IVF means to them both and what each person's needs and fears are. They will feel closer emotionally, know how to be involved as a couple, and understand the type of support each needs.

Many infertile couples go through IVF to determine the causes of their infertility, the second goal for IVF. For them, the detailed medical process might pinpoint an area of dysfunction that had not been identified before the IVF cycle. Even learning that everything works well can provide comfort and a feeling of success about IVF.

Achieving the third goal—having the feeling that they have done everything they could do to realize a biologic pregnancy—occurs as couples begin and progress through the IVF cycle. Couples who complete the entire procedure are more likely to achieve this goal, but those who are canceled should be helped to define their experience in a positive way, to know that they are not to blame for the cancellation. The preparation before treatment should include a discussion of both what they will do if cancellation occurs and how they will cope if conception does not occur. Planning for these potential outcomes enables couples to feel more competent and in control of their responses, thus lessening the emotional distress that both outcomes naturally create.

A small percentage of patients will achieve their goal of pregnancy. Surprisingly, they often fear that they will lose the baby if they do not do everything right, and so need immediate support and guidance.

For many couples, IVF is the last chance. The purpose of the preparation process is to enable all couples to be glad that they took the chance and to feel successful in whatever they accomplished in terms of the four goals of IVF.

Recommendations

Use a team approach in in vitro fertilization. Physicians and other members of the IVF team are very important in helping couples achieve feelings of success and satisfaction after IVF, whether or not they conceive. Often a team approach is used in the preparation process to prepare and support couples during three phases of IVF: before the procedure begins, during the procedure, and after the procedure. The physician, nurse coordinator, mental health professional, and program director may meet with all new patients to discuss medical, emotional, financial, and logistic aspects of the IVF procedure. From the initial consultation, the staff must create an environment in which patients feel free to express their emotions, knowing that acceptance and support will be given. Couples' fear that they will be rejected if their anxiety and apprehension are noticed should be alleviated.

Discuss emotional stresses of in vitro fertilization. Discussion with the couple of the emotional stresses of IVF should begin weeks before the woman actually starts taking ovulation medication. This process may be started in a consultation with a mental health professional or the nurse coordinator. The goals of this consultation are (1) to broaden the focus of the emotional experience of IVF so that couples can "succeed" at achieving certain goals besides conception and (2) to identify specific stresses besides failure to conceive for which they can develop specific coping strategies.

Involve husbands in every aspect of in vitro fertilization. Another important aspect of the psychologic consultation lies in helping husbands to be involved in every element of IVF. Since conception is something that is supposed to involve them, they can give injections, come for blood studies and ultrasound, and be there for surgery and recovery. In this way, they will be able to have a concrete image of where their child's conception took place and, if that does not occur, they will be able to process the experience more easily as they and their wives grieve. This type of involvement also enhances the experience for the woman and personalizes it for both partners.

Plan for disposition of frozen embryos. Another important part of the preparation process involves the medical staff's helping couples to plan for the disposition of frozen embryos if cryopreservation is chosen. Although couples do not anticipate conflict in this area and, in most cases, plan to use all embryos themselves, this question should be resolved before cryopreservation. At the time of cryopreservation, couples should sign an agreement indicating the disposition they desire in case of dispute, divorce, or unavailability.[14]

Plan for follow-up. It is important to begin plans for follow-up during the initial consultation. This includes suggestions for coping if there is no pregnancy, discussion about future IVF cycles, and resources for adoption and other alternatives. Planning for these contingencies helps couples feel better prepared to go on if conception does not occur. All patients should be contacted after they leave the program, regardless of why they left. Even those who

conceive will need continued support, because often they fear that they will lose the baby if they do not do everything right. Guidance and education about the pregnancy should be given immediately.

Couples who do not achieve a pregnancy when transfer has occurred generally experience grief reactions similar to those experiencing spontaneous abortion; severe disappointment and depression are common responses. They are often isolated from support, and a follow-up telephone call from the physician, nurse, or mental health professional on the team would reassure them about the appropriateness of their feelings. This is a critical time for an IVF program to demonstrate its commitment to serving the needs of the patients; it confirms that they have not been forgotten.

Use of donor gametes

Emotional risks of use of donor gametes. By the time most couples consider procedures that use donor gametes, they are willing to do almost anything to conceive. Because very little is known about long-term psychologic ramifications of such techniques and because legal and social guidelines for these procedures are inconsistent, neither couples nor physicians feel compelled to address the complex questions that surround them: Does biologic relatedness influence one's ability to love a child or to accept a child's limitations? What should potential parents know about an anonymous donor? Is it acceptable to use a known donor? A relative? Who should be told about the donor? Will the child's means of conception be a stigma? What will the child want to know about the donor? If the child knows (about) the donor, will the knowledge be enlightening or confusing? Will the child be accepted by grandparents, aunts, and uncles?[9]

Many physicians respond to these types of questions by assuring the couple that donor conception "will be the same as having your own," that "once conception occurs, you will forget how it happened," and that "no one needs to know."[11] Although comforting, assurances such as these often inhibit open discussion of both the impact of infertility on the marriage and the long-term ramifications of donor conception.

Experts in reproductive medicine must (1) acknowledge the possibility that using donor gametes is psychologically different from using the biologic gametes of both parents in conceiving a child and (2) stop pretending that, once a child is born, couples will not give another thought to how it all happened. Conceiving with donor sperm is not the same as conceiving with husband sperm; someone else's eggs are not the same as one's own. Couples who have tried for years to conceive a child biologically related to both partners know this.

Because couples cannot keep the means of conception a secret from each other, they need to begin donor gamete procedures with confidence as a couple that they are doing the right thing. Couple acceptance of the means of conception is imperative for a positive adjustment for the child.

Patient preparation. Patient preparation for the use of donor gametes should precede the treatment and should focus on two main processes: (1) identifying and resolving the specific ways in which infertility and infertility treatment have affected patients individually and as a couple and (2) discussing the specific issues involved in the treatment that they have chosen and developing ways of coping with these issues. Couples must allow several months of time to deal with these concerns.[9]

The major issues to be discussed prior to treatment include secrecy, donor anonymity, "multiple" parents, and social and religious attitudes about the use of donor gametes. A brief explanation of these issues follows.

Secrecy. It is very important for couples to discuss whether or not they plan to tell the child of his or her genetic heritage. Does the child have a right to know? Do the parents have the right to keep the secret? Under what circumstances is it important for the child to know? How and when should the child be told? Whatever they decide, couples must be helped to understand that both keeping a secret and sharing the means of conception require thoughtful discussion and planning. Keeping a secret requires a great deal of emotional energy and maintenance of innumerable lies over a long period of time. Sharing the information is a sensitive, somewhat awkward process that may occur many times over a child's lifetime and that requires skill, patience, and love. Whatever the choice, couples should make a joint decision about whether or not to tell the child as well as the ways in which they will discuss that choice over a lifetime.

Donor anonymity. Anonymity implies "no identity." How can the biologic father or mother of a child have no identity? Whether or not the actual names of biologic parents are known, donors can be known by their recipient families as real people with specific interests, skills, and family histories. There is a growing trend toward more openness in the use of donor gametes, as donors are interested in providing information to recipient families and families are more secure with having social, educational, and medical histories that they can later share with their children.[9]

Multiple parents. Because the parent-child relationship is the most significant of human bonds, clarity about the meaning of genetic parent and social parent is essential, especially for the social parent. The reality in the use of donor gametes is that there are more than two "parents" involved in the conception. Although this reality may be kept a secret from others, it cannot be changed or denied by the couple nor, in some cases, by the (known) donor. Therefore, when discussing donor conception, couples must acknowledge that there is a third "parent" whose "presence" will always represent a unique loss to each of them and, at times, pique their curiosity, but whose psychologic significance is not really understood. Although thoughts of that loss will not be a daily occurrence, unexpected events will remind each parent of the loss. At such times, each must feel free to express those feelings and receive comfort and support from the other.[9]

Social and religious attitudes about use of donor gametes. Our society loves children and places a high value on parenthood, but it is still ambivalent about creating families in nontraditional ways. Orthodox Judaism and Roman Catholicism forbid their practitioners from using donor gametes in the conception of their children. Therefore, overcoming negative social and religious attitudes and developing a sense of confidence about the choice of donor conception are overriding goals of patient preparation.

What about egg donation? Although the procedures are similar to those of IVF and sperm donation, the use of donor eggs in reproduction is medically more risky and psychologically more complex. In particular, there is greater concern about the long-term impact on the egg donor herself than on the sperm donor. Moreover, egg donation has unique problems because of its separation of female genetic and gestational parentage and the relative scarcity and inaccessibility of oocytes.[13] Other issues include the impact on offspring, on recipients, and on the family because of rearing arrangements that separate female genetic and gestational parentage, and questions of consent, risk, and commercialization in procuring donor eggs.

Questions about long-term impact on offspring are similar to those posed by the use of donor sperm. Parental response to and acceptance of the process before its beginning are very significant. Questions about impact on donor vary somewhat because the sources of egg donors are different. Anonymous egg donors are recruited from IVF patients, patients undergoing other surgery, and the general public. The psychologic stability of egg donors and the impact of such an action are ethical concerns. Should infertile women be egg donors for other infertile women? Should they be told if a conception occurs? What type of psychologic screening is necessary for egg donors? Is screening different if couples bring in their own donor? What constitutes an acceptable medical risk to the donor's fertility or life? Should the donor's spouse be a part of the screening process?

Although these questions require further consideration, there will never be a universally accepted answer to any of them. All couples who consider egg donation must examine their own needs, anticipate the long-term needs of their potential offspring, and decide what type of donor they want. Programs should explain options and provide legal and psychosocial guidelines. There should be room for choice.

Recommendations
Encourage couples to grieve for their infertility before use of donor gametes. Couples who are knowledgeable

about the psychologic issues in the use of donor gametes can make decisions in this area about which they will feel at peace in the future. Physicians are very important providers of information and can do so in a number of ways. First of all, they must encourage both partners of couples to take time for grieving their infertility before initiating procedures that use donor gametes and to examine the psychologic issues in the decision to use donor gametes. It is often tempting to rush into the process, especially when couples want to avoid examining their doubts. However, long-term acceptance is dependent on their grieving the initial loss that precipitated the choice of donor gametes and their discussing the complex emotional ramifications. Couples should be encouraged to examine the four long-term issues discussed earlier: secrecy, anonymity, multiple parents, and negative social and religious attitudes.

Determine the nonidentifying medical and psychologic information the couple needs about the donor. The medical staff must determine the amount of nonidentifying medical and psychologic information that the couple needs to know about an anonymous donor. Such information should be provided in written form on conception. If couples indicate at that time that they do not want this information, the medical staff should collect and store in-depth, nonidentifying information about all donors, which would be available on request at a later date.

Recommend written material and support groups dealing with infertility and donor conception. A final helpful strategy for physicians and their staffs is to recommend books and articles on the topics of infertility, donor conception, local and national support groups, and mental health professionals in the community. Although the physician provides suggestions for support, couples are responsible for making these types of decisions. They are the ones who will have to live with their choices after conception occurs.

Traditional surrogacy and gestational carrier

The practice of one woman's carrying a baby for another dates back to the Biblical story of Abraham and Sarah. When they were unable to conceive, Abraham turned to a concubine, Hagar, to bear his child. Since then, many couples have become parents with the help of surrogates.

Controversies of surrogacy. The use of surrogacy today—both traditional and gestational surrogacy—is the most controversial of all applications of biotechnology. Although the intention of all surrogacy agreements is to create or enhance a family, those who oppose this practice believe its inadvertent effect may be to inflict pain on the surrogate and her family. Because there appear to be class, economic, and educational differences between surrogates and infertile couples, there is concern that surrogacy for a fee encourages the exploitation of poor women. Because early studies revealed that a majority of traditional surrogates had limited psychosocial resources and prior repro-

ductive loss, there is concern that these women are high-risk obstetric patients.[12] And because there is little social support or legal certainty for surrogacy, infertile couples and surrogates alike are vulnerable to tragic consequences.

An essay, "Baby M.—Emotions for Sale," conveys the essence of these concerns:

> But the bargain struck in the Baby M. case seems to have been wrongheaded from the start because it involved a set of emotions, mainly on the part of Whitehead but Stern's as well, that were either unanticipated or uncomprehended.
>
> On the surface, Whitehead was paid to incubate another family's child. In fact, she was paid to experience maternal love, the forced cessation of that love, and a whole range of feelings in the process that are not ordinarily put up for sale. Those emotions, not Baby M., were the real, if hidden, commodity in the transaction. And the transaction fell through because neither buyer nor seller had a grasp of the commodity in the first place.
>
> Whatever Stern and Whitehead thought their pact was about, they were trafficking in goods too elusive to package and too universal for personal property. What you do not own, you cannot sell.*

Because emotions cannot be sold, promised, or predicted, the surrogate arrangement is much more than a medical/legal contract. To deny that is to deny major responsibility to infertility patients.

Recognition of the pitfalls of surrogacy and the risks to all involved is only part of the physician's task. It is also important to be sensitive to the reality that surrogacy is a happy ending for many couples. Perhaps attention should also be focused on those couples for whom surrogacy works, whose infertility struggle is resolved through a surrogate with whom they develop a positive relationship, whose child through surrogacy is a miracle. As one woman shared after the birth of her daughter:

> The experience of surrogacy has taught me that miracles can happen. It's hard to believe that after eight years of infertility tests and treatment, we are so blessed.

In February 1991, a 42-year-old South Dakota woman agreed to serve as a surrogate for her daughter, who was born without a uterus. She conceived twins. A medical ethicist of the Hastings Center, James Nelson, said that this case appeared to be an ideal case, and 86% of 1670 respondents to a *Houston Post* poll indicated that they believed that it was ethical for a woman to serve as a surrogate mother for her own daughter.[16]

This whole new arena of surrogate parenting is begging for acceptance and respect from a public with varied religious and cultural backgrounds. Whatever one's position, there is no denying that the surrogacy arrangement is highly emotional. Instead of a simple solution, it is a process whose complications are infinite and infinitely

---

*From Rosenblatt R: *Essay: Baby M.—emotions for sale, Time,* p. 88, April 6, 1987. Reprinted with permission of Time Inc., New York.

surprising; they are not predictable nor under anyone's control.

Ethical and legal considerations in surrogacy. In November 1990, the Ethics Committee of the American College of Obstetricians and Gynecologists published its ethical guidelines for surrogate motherhood. In the summer of 1991, six highly respected experts in the field of reproductive medicine published responses to these guidelines. Even though each commentary reflected in-depth analysis; sophisticated familiarity with the legal, moral, and social issues; sensitivity to the needs of both infertile couples and surrogates; and common sense, their views were highly divergent, ranging from recommending surrogacy to making it illegal. Despite such divergency, surrogacy in both its forms is legal in some but not all states in the United States; therefore, guidelines must be developed to protect those who choose this option. The Ethics Committee of the American Fertility Society supports such a recommendation:

In a country that gives to childbearing decisions a legal protection of magnitude unparalleled in the rest of the world, professional guidelines must not casually accede to restrictions on reproductive technologies that offer enhanced options. Rather, as this report attempts to do, guidelines should be set out that detail how the technologies may be offered with safety and ethical appropriateness, while giving due consideration to individual rights.*

When motherhood itself is split between genetics and gestation, genes, contracts, and biology alone cannot determine the status of "mother" and child. Moreover, it is impossible not only to anticipate with certainty how a surrogate will feel after the birth of a baby but also to make a plan that is risk free. Ultimately and unfortunately, all of the cases that result in a change of heart on the part of the surrogate will most likely be resolved in courts.[2] However, in a well-run surrogacy program, psychologic screening and counseling will be required and expert legal counsel will be provided for both surrogates and infertile couples to minimize the risks for all involved.

Physicians must examine their own beliefs and make a decision about whether or not to provide surrogacy, either traditional or gestational. The American College of Obstetricians and Gynecologists has published guidelines that acknowledge the complexity of the legal and psychosocial issues and has stated that a physician may justifiably decline to participate in initiating surrogate arrangements while not breaching the standards of quality care espoused by the College.[1]

Recommendations. Physicians who provide surrogacy can develop an ethical program that speaks to the emotional needs of both the surrogate and the recipient couple by incorporating the following suggestions into the surrogacy program.

Offer surrogacy only for refractory infertility or other major need. The physician should employ both types of surrogacy only in the case of refractory infertility or other major need. When that criterion has been met, the physician should encourage couples to acknowledge the losses experienced before making the choice to parent through surrogacy. Doing so enables them to integrate these losses into a positive perspective of this most unique, but unconventional, way of becoming parents.

View the surrogate as a high-risk patient from a psychosocial and legal perspective. The physician needs to see the surrogate as a high-risk patient, from a psychosocial and legal perspective, who is in need of careful health screening and ongoing psychologic counseling throughout the course of the childbearing experience. A psychologic consultation would help all involved to be clear about the goals, risks, and expectations of the surrogacy agreement. Current surrogacy programs require psychologic counseling for surrogates through the pregnancy and after the delivery. Ongoing legal counsel should formulate contingency plans and address emotional sequelae that might arise from this treatment choice.[4]

All of the medical staff must be sensitive to the surrogate's vulnerable position in this procedure. Since she has not been a patient, she will be unfamiliar with the "rules of the game," vulnerable to insensitive medical personnel accustomed to working with sophisticated infertility patients, and fearful of what the medical intervention will be like. The medical staff must also remember that couples who choose surrogacy are in a lonely position. Often reluctant to share their experience, couples are besieged with criticism from media, women's groups, religious groups, lawyers, and family and friends. They need support.

Recommend surrogacy support groups. A very important responsibility of the medical team is to recommend surrogacy support groups. Until 6 years ago, parents through surrogacy received peer support through adoptive parents' groups. In 1987, the Organization of Parents through Surrogacy was founded to "advocate, support, and protect the birth rights of all children and to keep open the options made available by advances in reproductive technology to those unable to have children in the conventional manner."[6]

Be aware of the emotional pitfalls of surrogacy. Physicians and their staffs must be familiar with the emotional pitfalls of the surrogacy experience in order to help couples discuss and resolve them. Some questions that might be posed to the surrogate and the couple include the following:

Surrogate
1. What are your expectations for yourself? How will you know when you have met them?
2. Have you experienced a reproductive loss such as

---

*From American Fertility Society: Ethical considerations of the American Fertility Society, Birmingham, Ala, 1991, The Society.

abortion, miscarriage, or stillbirth? How was your decision to be a surrogate tied in with that experience?

3. What do you expect from the couple during the pregnancy? After the baby is born? Do you want to be appreciated/thanked? How can the couple do this? What will it be like for you when you are no longer "the center of attention"?

4. What will your relationship with the baby be during pregnancy and after the birth? Are you distancing yourself during the pregnancy? Do you see yourself as his or her mother?

5. If you have children of your own, how do you think they will see this? If you don't have children, how do you know the ways in which being a surrogate might be harmful emotionally?

6. What do your friends/husband/parents think of your being a surrogate? How do you plan to deal with the criticism/harassment you will receive? Who will support you during the experience? After the baby is born and given to the parents?

7. What type of couple do you expect to carry for?

Couple

1. What type of relationship do you wish to have with the surrogate?

2. How will you view the surrogate during the pregnancy?

3. Why have you chosen this option instead of adoption?

4. Does your family know? Are you planning to tell your child the nature of his or her conception? Why or why not? Is this plan realistic?

5. How do you feel about your infertility?

6. How do you plan to deal with others' criticism of your decision to use a surrogate?

7. How will your marriage be stressed by this choice? Will you acknowledge your fears during the pregnancy, your tendency to distance yourself from the child?

8. How will you respond if the surrogate changes her mind and refuses to give you the child?

The mere process of asking and answering these questions will bring up problems that the couple or surrogate might not have faced and will facilitate communication between the surrogate and the couple. All involved are often relieved because so many fears are not named, and this process helps name them and provides a means of coping with them. Communication among all of the parties, including the surrogate's husband and children, is the foundation for any surrogate arrangement. The pitfall is that these issues will not come up until after conception or delivery. Then multiple tragedies occur.

Another way to provide support lies in developing ways to involve both spouses in all procedures leading to conception. When the efforts at conception involve only one spouse, the other spouse may feel left out, isolated, useless. Finally, those involved in providing this type of treatment need to foster research efforts aimed at the scientific scrutiny of the psychosocial health risks of the surrogate, the infertile couple, and the resulting offspring.

CONCLUSION

The bottom-line psychologic dilemmas created by the new reproductive technologies are relatively simple to conceptualize but are very difficult to predict or control. They include the following:

1. Does my spouse approve of my feelings, my needs for having a baby? Will he or she love me if I make a decision that he or she doesn't like or agree with?

2. Can I provide the support that my spouse will need to go through this procedure? Am I enough?

3. Will family and friends accept us and our child conceived in this manner?

4. Will I be able to bond with our baby? Will my spouse be able to do so?

5. What is the significance of being genetically related to a child? What does it actually mean?

6. Will I see our means of becoming a family as the reason for our child's problems or differences?

7. Will our marriage survive the stresses of all of these decisions and treatments? Will our sex life ever be the same? Can we go on to a normal life?

When assisted reproductive technology achieves its goal of conception, many of the dilemmas of "what is going to happen next" continue. Since there is uncertainty about the psychologic outcome for all concerned, all must be aware that parental attitude toward a child's means of conception and genetic makeup has a great impact on the child's perception of self. Children whose parents experienced infertility will be affected by their parents' subsequent adjustment to it. Parents who have resolved the issues created prior to their child's birth will face the challenges of parenting effectively and will not connect personality and behavior problems to the means of conception. Throughout treatment, physicians should encourage couples to identify and resolve the specific ways in which infertility has affected them individually and as a couple, thus enabling them to make decisions about treatment that will maintain the integrity of the marriage and the emotional well-being of their children. This is the happy ending that all involved in reproductive medicine desire.

Gilda Radner understood the importance of parent adjustment for a child's "happy ending" when she shared the following story:

When I was little, my nurse Dibby's cousin had a dog, just a mutt, and the dog was pregnant. I don't know how long dogs are pregnant, but she was due to have her puppies in about a week. She was out in the yard one day and got in the way of the lawn mower, and her two hind legs got cut off. They rushed her to the vet and he said, "I can sew her up, or you can put her to sleep if you want, but the puppies are OK. She'll be able to deliver the puppies."

Dibby's cousin said, "Keep her alive."

So the vet sewed up her backside, and over the next week, the dog learned to walk. She didn't spend any time worrying, she just learned to walk by taking two steps in the front and flipping up her backside, and then taking two steps and flipping up her backside again. She gave birth to six little puppies, all in perfect health. She nursed them and then weaned them. And when they learned to walk, they all walked like her.*

*Radner G: *It's always something,* New York, 1989, Simon & Schuster, p. 268. Copyright © 1989 by Gilda Radner. Reprinted by permission of Simon & Schuster, Inc.

REFERENCES

1. Bulfin MJ: Surrogate motherhood, *Women's Health Issues* 1:140, 1991.
2. Crocker SL: New surrogacy fight begins in California, *Fertil News* 25:18, 1991.
3. DeCherney AH: Doctored babies, *Fertil Steril* 40:724, 1983.
4. English MEE, Mechanick-Braverman A, Corson SL: Semantics and science: the distinction between gestational carrier and traditional surrogacy options, *Women's Health Issues* 1:155, 1991.
5. Frankl V: *Will to meaning,* New York, 1969, World Publishing.
6. Glazer ES: *The long-awaited stork,* Lexington, Mass, 1990, Lexington Books, p. 194.
7. Mahlstedt PP: The psychological component of infertility, *Fertil Steril* 43:335, 1985.
8. Mahlstedt PP: The crisis of infertility: an opportunity for growth. In Weeks GR, Hof L, editors: *Integrating sex and marital therapy,* New York, 1987, Brunner/Mazel.
9. Mahlstedt PP, Greenfeld DA: Assisted reproductive technology with donor gametes: the need for patient preparation, *Fertil Steril* 52:908, 1989.
10. Mahlstedt PP, Macduff S, Bernstein J: Emotional factors and the in vitro fertilization and embryo transfer process, *J In Vitro Fert Embryo Transfer* 4:232, 1987.
11. Mahlstedt PP, Probasco KA: Sperm donors: their attitude toward providing medical and psychosocial information for recipient families, *Fertil Steril* 56:747, 1991.
12. Reame NE: The surrogate mother as a high-risk obstetric patient, *Women's Health Issues* 1:151, 1991.
13. Robertson JA: Ethical and legal issues in human egg donation, *Fertil Steril* 52:354, 1989.
14. Robertson JA: Divorce and disposition of cryopreserved pre-embryos, *Fertil Steril* 55:681, 1991.
15. White RB, Davis HK, Cantress WA: Psychodynamics of depression: implications for treatment. In Usdin G, editor: *Depression: clinical, biological, and psychological perspectives,* New York, 1977, Brunner/Mazel.
16. Wilson DJ: Eighty-six percent of callers support woman pregnant with daughter's twins, *Houston Post,* p. A6, Aug 7, 1991.

Chapter 27

HYSTEROSALPINGOGRAPHY

Alvin M. Siegler, MD, DSc

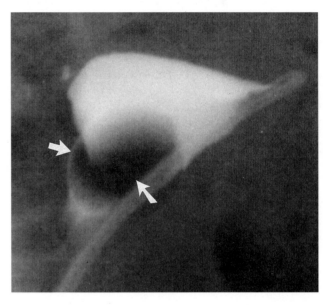

Fig. 27-1. The balloon catheter (*arrows*) occupies the lower uterine segment while its tip extends into the left horn.

Despite the advent of modern diagnostic gynecologic techniques, including laparoscopy, hysteroscopy, ultrasonography (US), and magnetic resonance imaging (MRI), hysterosalpingography (HSG) still serves as a relatively painless, simple, nonoperative, screening procedure. It is one of the basic tests to perform before undertaking surgical correction of pelvic causes of infertility. Although this examination does not define the extent of certain conditions such as endometriosis and periadnexal adhesions, it does reveal the shape of the uterine cavity and certain characteristics of the tubal lumina other than their patency.

This chapter reviews the fundamentals for performing proper HSG and discusses the interpretation of some uterine and tubal abnormalities encountered. Careful performance and interpretation are essential so that the radiologic findings can be correlated with endoscopic examinations. Abnormal shadows should be interpreted in association with the history and pelvic examination. When results of a properly performed HSG are interpreted as normal, it is unusual to find significant intrauterine abnormalities at hysteroscopy. With normal fill and spill of the contrast material from both fallopian tubes, it is uncommon for the laparoscopic examination to detect significant tubal disease.

INSTRUMENTS

Although various cervical cannulas have been described, the Jarcho metal type remains the preferred one to use. It has an adjustable steel collar and a rubber acorn. The rubber acorn is fixed securely with a set screw in the metal collar, and the tip of the acorn is positioned about 0.5 cm from the perforated end of the cannula.

The balloon catheter is an alternate device used for HSG.[29] It is inflated with about 2 mL of sterile water or air after the catheter has been inserted with a long dressing forceps through the endocervical canal. The contrast material is instilled through one port, and appropriate films are taken. The major disadvantage of this catheter is that it can obscure the lower uterine segment and may make the detection of intrauterine lesions more difficult (Fig. 27-1). To avoid the use of a tenaculum, some investigators have used a Swedish vacuum cannula in which the cup adheres

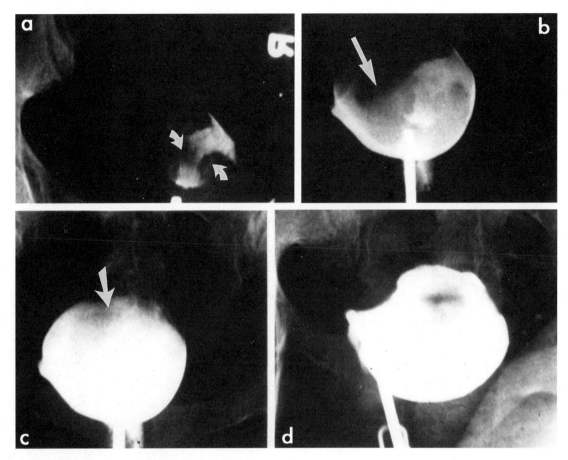

Fig. 27-2. The presence of a submucous tumor (*arrows*) can be ascertained by the distorted and enlarged cavity (**a** to **d**). No tubal filling is noted.

to the cervix by means of suction as the contrast medium is instilled through the cannula.[11] This technique enables complete observation of the endocervical canal and lower uterine segment. The disadvantages include the frequent loss of suction during manipulation of the uterus and the need for a suction apparatus with different-sized cups.

A scout film is indicated if a previous pelvic radiographic study had been done in which contrast material was used. For proper monitoring, spot films are taken at propitious intervals during television fluoroscopy. Four exposures can be recorded on one 10- by 12-inch film (Figs. 27-2 and 27-3). A drainage or follow-up film is essential to evaluate the dispersion of the contrast material.

MEDIA

Many contrast media have been used in HSG since the procedure was first described in 1910 by Rindfleisch,[18] who injected bismuth solution into the uterine cavity. An iodized oil-based medium (Lipiodol) was developed in 1921, later to be superseded by ethiodized oil (Ethiodol). The use of water-based contrast media (WBCM) with various viscous

additives avoids the risks of oil embolism and granuloma formation. In a comparative study between a low-osmolality contrast medium and conventional media (WBCM), no differences were noted concerning the incidence of abdominal pain or allergic reactions, or in the ability to make a radiologic diagnosis.[3,16]

All media used for HSG contain iodine; some are soluble in water and others are soluble in oil. Both types have certain advantages and disadvantages, and the physician should be familiar with their characteristics because the type of medium can influence the technique of the examination and the interpretation of the films. WBCM pass through the uterus and tubes more quickly, and greater amounts of it are needed. With WBCM, rugal folds evidenced by longitudinal dark lines can be detected. In distally obstructed tubes, a dark line often is visible clearly when the endosalpinx is not damaged severely. An oil-based contrast medium (OBCM) will not mix with the fluid in a hydrosalpinx, so that pearly clusters form in it. The proponents of the OBCM claim that this medium gives a clearer, sharper image, less pain is encountered after peri-

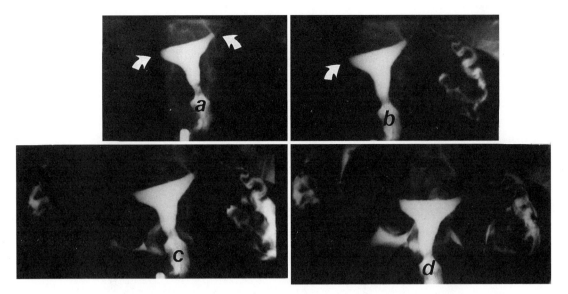

Fig. 27-3. Four spot films (**a** to **d**) show gradual filling of both fallopian tubes. Arrows point to rounded cornua in **a.** Nonfilling of the right tube (*arrow*) persists in **b.** Additional fluid shows bilateral tubal patency (**c** and **d**).

toneal spill, and peritubal disease can be detected more accurately by a delayed radiograph. Both types of contrast media have evolved to the point of reliably providing information about the uterine and tubal lumina, with minimal sequelae.

TECHNIQUE

Many hysterosalpingograms cannot be interpreted, principally because of failure to attend to the relatively simple details of proper performance. The best pictures with fewest complications can be obtained by gaining the confidence and cooperation of the patient through gentle pelvic manipulation of the instruments. A tranquilizer may be used for a very apprehensive patient. Tubal occlusion caused by uterotubal spasm can result from stress or from irritation caused by the contrast material. No medication has been successful in reducing spasm of the myosalpinx that envelops the interstitial tubal segment.[28]

The time in the cycle chosen for HSG varies according to the patient's clinical condition, although most procedures are done in the first week after menses. The search for an incompetent isthmus probably should be done premenstrually, however, when physiologic contraction of the lower uterine segment is greatest. The cannula is filled with contrast material to flush out the air, since artifacts in the uterus can be caused by air bubbles. After a tenaculum is fixed on the anterior cervical lip, the cannula is inserted into the external cervical os and the two instruments are held together by the properly gowned (lead apron) physician. Small increments of contrast material are instilled as spot films are taken. If the corpus is displaced, traction on the tenaculum corrects the abnormal position. Failure to correct

a uterus that is either flexed anteriorly or retrodisplaced prevents adequate examination of the lower uterine segment and proper evaluation of the uterine cavity (Fig. 27-4). Manometric control is not needed, because pressure on the fluid-filled syringe is satisfactory. The end point of the examination occurs when tubal filling and spilling are observed or when the patient complains of increasing abdominal pain during the injection. A follow-up, or drainage, film is essential to observe the dispersions of the liquid medium (Figs. 27-5 to 27-7). It should be taken about 30 minutes after removal of the instruments from the cervix if a water-soluble material is used. With oil-based substances, it is advisable to delay the drainage film until the following day, because this medium does not disperse as rapidly in the peritoneal cavity.[5]

Excessive contrast material exposes the patient needlessly to risk of mucosal or peritoneal irritation and prevents proper interpretation of the films. Insufficient fluid results in an incomplete study (Fig. 27-8).

ADVERSE EFFECTS

To minimize exposure to radiation, other HSG methods have been described, including modern 100-mm fluorography; low-dose, scanning-beam HSG; and color Doppler ultrasound HSG. Some adverse effects from HSG have been caused by faulty selection of patients and poor technique, but morbidity and sequelae occasionally result despite careful use.[10] Complications of HSG are related either to the medium or to the instrumentation. HSG can exacerbate pelvic inflammatory disease, leading to peritonitis, a pelvic abscess, and even death. The patients at increased risk for such an infection are those with a history

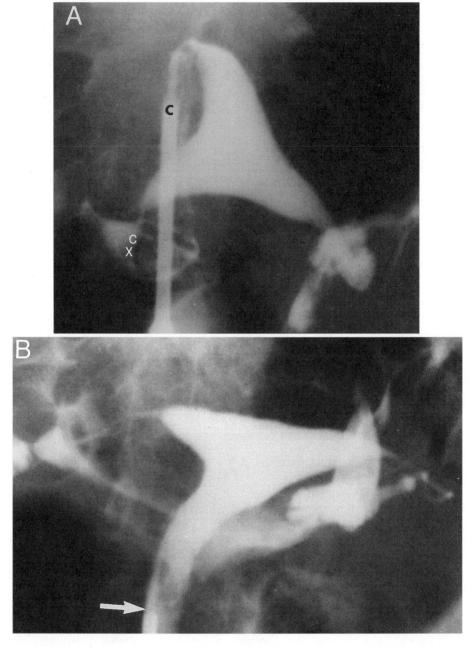

Fig. 27-4. A, Displaced uterine cavity is seen with the cannula (*c*) in the lower uterine segment. The outline of the cervical canal (*cx*) is noted. **B,** Traction on the tenaculum has corrected the displacement; arrow indicates the tip of the cannula.

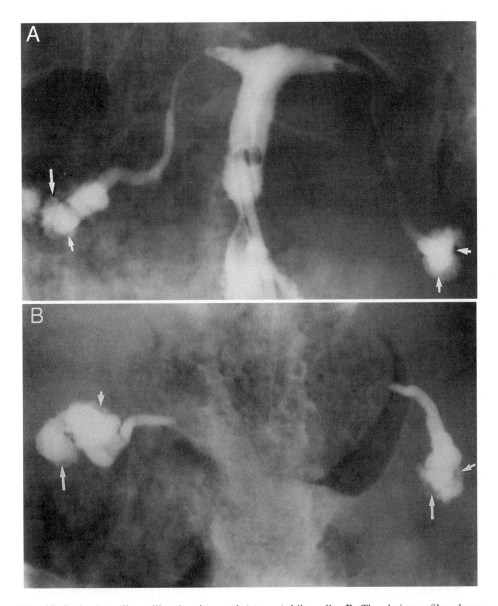

Fig. 27-5. A, Ampullary dilatation is noted (*arrows*) bilaterally. **B,** The drainage film shows localization of contrast material, indicating bilateral distal tubal obstruction. The irregular borders (*arrows*) suggest fibrosis and advanced disease.

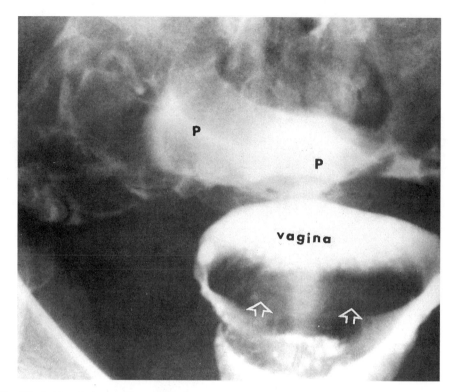

Fig. 27-6. The drainage film shows contrast fluid in the vagina and some dispersed in the peritoneal cavity (*p*). The dark area (*arrows*) is caused by the cervix.

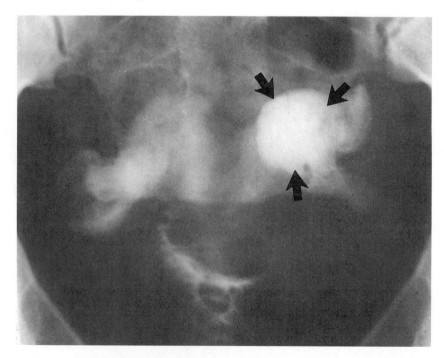

Fig. 27-7. Localization of contrast fluid (*arrows*) with some spillage of contrast material in the peritoneal cavity indicates peritubal adhesions or fimbrial phimosis.

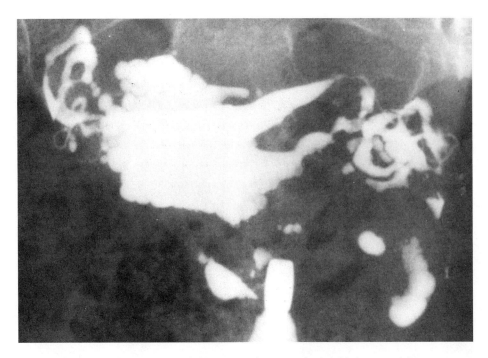

Fig. 27-8. Excessive contrast fluid prevents interpretation of this hysterosalpingogram.

of pelvic inflammatory disease. The incidence and severity of the pelvic peritonitis does not appear to be influenced by the type of medium, and no protective effects from prophylactic antibiotics have been shown.

The potential for hypersensitivity reactions to iodine exists with any of the HSG media, but allergic reactions are rare. Uterine perforation and postexamination hemorrhage are also a possibility. Some lower-abdominal pain and discomfort are commonly experienced by women undergoing HSG and are caused by placement of the tenaculum, insertion of the cannula, and instillation of the contrast material. Diminution of these symptoms is often related to the skill and patience of the physician. Other types of complications include granuloma formation and vascular intravasation (Figs. 27-9 to 27-11). The effects of vascular intravasation can be minimized by observation of the onset of the event during the fluoroscopic examination and promptly stopping the procedure.

The risk from pelvic irradiation, although real, is quite small. The total radiation dose to the ovaries depends on the following:

- Radiation output from the particular radiologic equipment
- Size and shape of the patient and the composition of her tissues
- Fluoroscopic dose plus the dose from the permanent radiographs
- Number of radiographic exposures made per patient. The range appears to be between two and six expo-

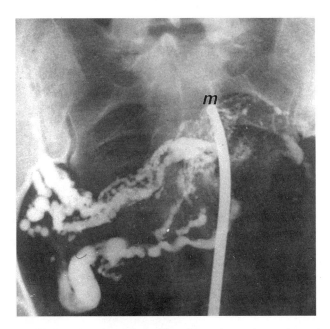

Fig. 27-9. When the cannula slipped into the uterine cavity and penetrated the myometrium (*m*), vascular intravasation resulted after instillation of the contrast agent.

sures per study. The objective is to minimize the radiation exposure with all diagnostic radiographic procedures.

INTERPRETATION OF RESULTS

Always begin the evaluation of the HSG by viewing the endocervical canal (Fig. 27-12). Its serrated borders are

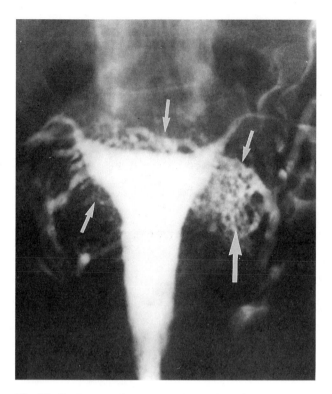

Fig. 27-10. Intravasation (*arrows*) is noted, but it is not possible to differentiate lymphatic penetration from venous intravasation.

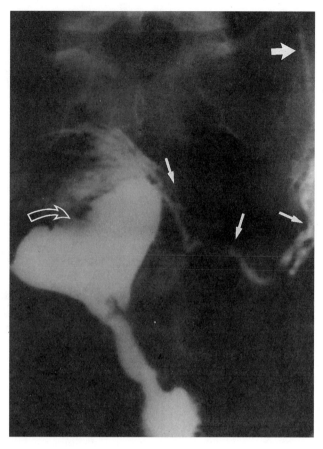

Fig. 27-11. Venous intravasation is seen (*solid arrows*) originating from a fundal defect (*open arrow*) caused by a submucous leiomyoma.

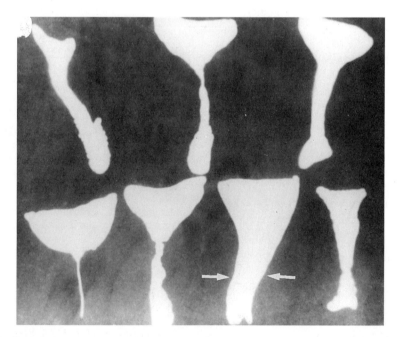

Fig. 27-12. Schematic representation of the endocervical canal, lower uterine segment, and normal uterine cavity. One of the lower segments is unusually wide and represents an incompetent os (*arrows*).

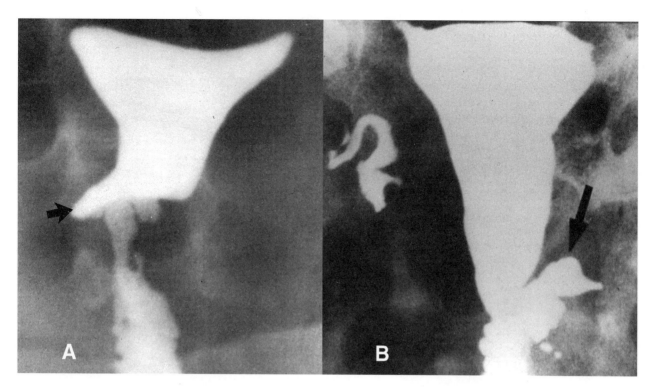

Fig. 27-13. **A** and **B,** Two examples of diverticula (*arrows*) in the lower segment caused by scars from previous cesarean deliveries.

caused by anatomic plicae palmatae. Abnormalities of the endocervical canal detectable by HSG include polyps and adhesions, which cause filling defects. The normal lower-uterine segment has parallel borders that are usually smooth. This segment may be unusually wide (>1 cm in an incompetent os). Outpouchings or spicular or wedge-shaped diverticula can occur from a previous cesarean operation (Fig. 27-13). The normal uterine cavity has a triangular appearance with smooth borders. The upper border, the fundus, may be convex or saddle shaped, and the cornua are generally pointed. Physiologic alterations may cause various indentations along the lateral borders of the uterine shadow, but their persistence on sequential films suggests an organic defect rather than a contraction (Fig. 27-14).

Peritoneal spill from normal HSG is identified easily (Fig. 27-15, **A**). The dispersion of the agent in the pelvis depends on

- The type and amount of medium used
- The degree of tubal patency
- The presence or extent of significant periadnexal adhesions

Collections of medium lateral to the uterus should not be mistaken for centrally placed fluid retained within the uterine canal or vagina (Fig. 27-15, **B** and **C**). The interpretation of small, localized pelvic collections of contrast material caused by significant peritubal adhesions, fimbrial phimosis, or even hydrosalpinges can be difficult. Contrast material coming from one patent tube may obscure the configuration of the contralateral oviduct. When an oily material is used, it may be difficult to be certain whether the "pearly clusters" are in the cul-de-sac fluid or enclosed in a hydrosalpinx. Some tubal configurations look normal initially, but the follow-up or drainage film may disclose localization of the contrast material. Sharply defined borders suggest that the contrast medium is confined within the tube, whereas a halo configuration indicates periadnexal adhesions that allow some of the fluid to surround and outline the tubal wall.

VISUALIZATION OF STRUCTURES
Congenital malformations

The HSG is a screening procedure that gives the initial clue to the possibility of a uterine anomaly. Since the types

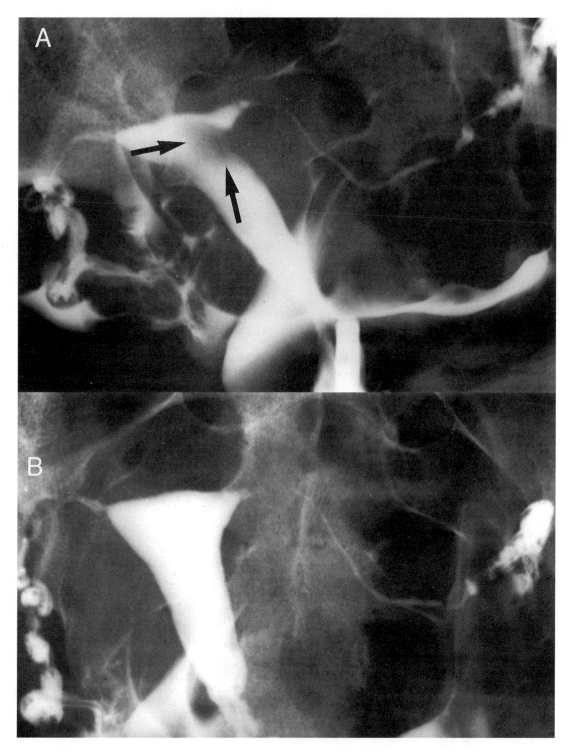

Fig. 27-14. A, "Filling defect" (*arrows*) in left horn caused by myometrial contraction. **B,** Same uterus moments later reveals that the "defect" is no longer present.

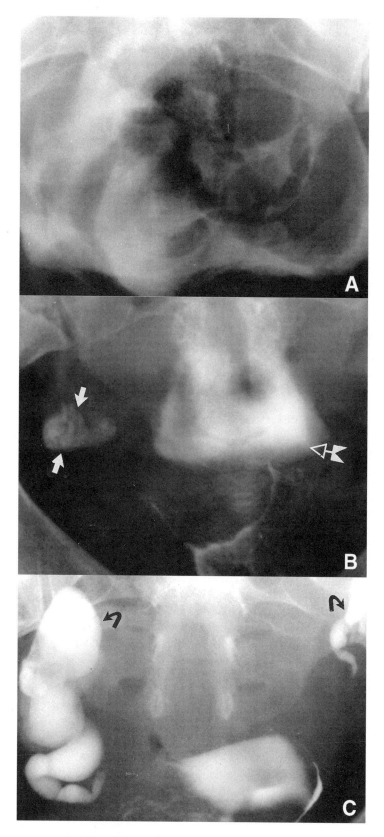

Fig. 27-15. A, Normal drainage film shows good dispersion of the contrast material in the pelvis. **B,** Localized collection in the right lower quadrant suggests fimbrial occlusion (*solid arrows*). Central opacified area represents the vagina and a tampon (*open arrow*). **C,** Bilateral distal tubal obstruction (*curved arrows*) is seen.

of malformations have different reproductive prognoses and clinical management, a precise diagnosis is important. It is necessary to know the configuration of the uterine serosal surface as well as the shape of the uterine cavity. US and MRI also have been used with this objective. Fedele et al.[8] examined 18 infertile women with MRI after an HSG diagnosis of a uterine anomaly. All of the patients had a subsequent laparoscopy or laparotomy to evaluate the capability of the MRI to discriminate among the types of uterine anomalies. The technique identified both women with bicornuate uteri correctly, both women with didelphic uteri, nine of 12 patients with septate uteri, and both women who had complete septa. Compared with laparoscopy, MRI is less expensive and less invasive, but it cannot provide information about tubal patency or the existence of endometriosis. Transvaginal US performed in the second half of the cycle, when the endometrium is thicker and more hyperechogenic, can improve the sonographic contrast, offering optimal observation of the uterine cavity. On the basis of the HSG findings alone, Reuter et al.[17] noted a diagnostic accuracy of only 55%. However, when the diagnostic protocol included US with HSG for evaluating müllerian defects, the accuracy improved to 90%.

Uterine anomalies result from failure of the müllerian ducts to canalize, failure of one or both ducts to develop, failure of proper fusion, or failure to reabsorb the midline septum. (See Chapter 61.) Ashton and co-workers[4] performed HSG in 840 women to evaluate tubal closure after the use of methyl 2-cyanoacrylate. They identified 16 congenital malformations, for an incidence of 1.9%. Almost all of the malformations were either bicornuate or septate. Some malformations cause complications at menarche, during pregnancy, or during labor. Although malformed uteri do not prevent implantation and most pregnancies proceed to term without difficulty, anomalies do increase the frequency of obstetric sequelae. A logical classification was proposed by the American Fertility Society.[2]

Hypoplasia/aplasia. In women with vaginal, cervical, fundal, or combined aplasia, hysterography is not possible. In patients who do not have tubes, a hysterogram will demonstrate a normal uterine shadow and only the intramural tubal segments. The hypoplastic uterine cavity measures no more than 5 cm in length, two-thirds cervix and one-third corpus, and the volume of contrast material needed to fill the uterine cavity and both fallopian tubes is often 1 mL or less.

Unicornuate uterus. A unicornuate uterus is an uncommon anomaly that results from failure to develop one müllerian duct. Approximately 75% of rudimentary horns do not communicate with the normal hemiuterus and consequently will not opacify on the hysterogram. Since these anomalies are frequently associated with either ipsilateral renal agenesis or a pelvic kidney, an intravenous pyelogram is essential in the work-up.

A unicornuate uterus should be suspected whenever the uterine shadow appears oval with its upper pole pointing either to the left or right. It should be differentiated from an incompletely filled cavity, an intense spasm of one horn, blockage of an opposite horn by severe synechiae, or an artifact caused by uterine torsion. In these instances a lateral film can be helpful. Hysteroscopy can substantiate the diagnosis, and laparoscopy can detect the presence of a rudimentary horn.

Uterus didelphys. Duplications of the uterus and vagina are caused by a failure of fusion of the müllerian ducts. This type of anomaly is associated with a vaginal septum in 75% of women. Although infertility does not seem to be a problem, there is an increased frequency of twins. Independent radiologic study of each horn will show the characteristic shadow of the unicornuate uterus. In such cases the Foley uterine catheter technique has an advantage because the vaginal canal sometimes cannot accommodate two sets of instruments, that is, cannulae and tenacula. Such uteri can be distinguished readily by ultrasound.

Bicornuate uterus. Incomplete or partial fusion of the fundal segments leaves paired uterine horns and one cervix. The division may be partial or complete, and the external uterine surface reflects the character of this division.

The bicornuate uterus cannot be differentiated from the septate uterus by HSG or hysteroscopy, because the crucial diagnostic point lies in the configuration of the serosal uterine surface. Ultrasonography, MRI, and laparoscopy will enable a more precise diagnosis. Although infertility is not a problem with these patients, spontaneous abortion, premature labor, and abnormal presentation are increased.

Septate uterus. The septate uterus is either completely or partially divided by a longitudinal, intrauterine, central septum. The length and width of the septum will cause different shadows on the HSG and, if complete, two separate, usually symmetric cavities are formed. A cannula inserted beyond the internal os can prevent adequate observation of one of the horns. Women with a septate uterus are about twice as likely to abort as those with a bicornuate uterus. Both conditions must be differentiated from a fundal submucous leiomyoma.

Hysteroscopic metroplasty is the ideal operation for this type of uterine anomaly.[21] The hysteroscopic examination should enable a panoramic view of the septum and both horns and uterotubal ostia. The septum is divided at its apex and the dissection is continued until the base of the septum is reached. The postoperative results are as good as those obtained previously from an abdominal metroplasty. The main advantages of hysteroscopic metroplasty are as follows:

- The operation can be performed on an outpatient basis.
- No abdominal or uterine scar results.
- Postoperative morbidity is minimal.

- No reduction in the volume of the uterine cavity results.
- Pregnancy may be attempted after postoperative results of either hysteroscopy or hysterography are normal.
- Vaginal delivery is typical.

Arcuate uterus. The arcuate uterus is a minor malformation in which the fundus appears concave, although the depth of the depression is less than 1.5 cm. The diagnosis is presumed if a line drawn from one cornu to the other, and another perpendicular to it and extending to the depth of the concavity, measures between 1 and 1.5 cm, and the fundus appears saddle shaped. The uterine cavity has smooth contours and symmetric horns. The hysterographic appearance can be verified hysteroscopically.

Diethylstilbestrol-related malformations. Another type of congenital uterine malformation has been described in some women who were exposed to diethylstilbestrol in utero. The uterus appears hypoplastic and T-shaped with indentations on its lateral borders (Fig. 27-16). On hysteroscopic examination these radiologic changes can be explained by structural alterations within the myometrium that resemble submucous leiomyomas. Bulbous cornual extensions often arise from the upper end of the uterine cavity. Cervical abnormalities, including hypoplasia, hoods, collars, and pseudopolyps, are seen in many of these women, almost 90% of whom also have hysterographic abnormalities. No characteristic findings are evident on the HSG in the fallopian tubes of these women, although "withered" tubes have been described in one report at laparoscopy. These findings consisted of foreshortened, sacculated tubes with pinpoint fimbrial ostia and constricted fimbriae.[6]

Intrauterine adhesions

Other terms used to describe intrauterine adhesions (IUA) include traumatic amenorrhea, adhesive endometritis, endometrial sclerosis, and uterine synechiae. More than 90% of patients with IUA have had a pregnancy-related curettage. Adhesions occasionally develop after a metroplasty, myomectomy, or diagnostic curettage or in association with tuberculous endometritis. A history of amenorrhea or hypomenorrhea after a uterine surgical procedure should lead to the suspicion of IUA. As a rule the pelvic examination fails to disclose any abnormalities. Suspicion of cervicoisthmic adhesions may be confirmed easily by attempting to pass a uterine sound.

HSG is the definitive screening procedure because a normal uterine shadow can be used to exclude the diagnosis (Fig. 27-17). The radiographic abnormalities vary from mild cases with multiple, linear, centrally placed defects with minimal distortion of the uterine outline to severe lesions with a disorganized uterine shadow associated with vascular intravasation or tubal occlusion, or both. The defects can be single or multiple, variable in size and shape, or central or marginal, and tend to persist on sequential

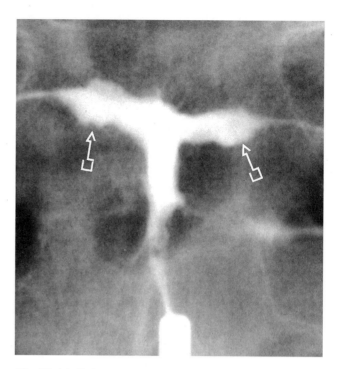

Fig. 27-16. T-shaped uterine cavity is noted with its characteristic bulbous horns (*arrows*).

films. Too much contrast material can obliterate these abnormal shadows. HSG tends to overdiagnose rather than miss the presence of IUA. Vascular intravasation associated with multiple filling defects and a distorted but not enlarged uterine shadow in a patient with a history of repeated early abortion and postabortal curettage followed by hypomenorrhea is diagnostic of IUA. The defects must be differentiated from those caused by polyps, leiomyomas, septa, and artifacts caused by air bubbles. With hysteroscopy the surgeon can ascertain the size and location of the adhesions and evaluate the surrounding endometrium. On US the adhesions are echogenic rather than sonolucent, and usually are located asymmetrically, not centrally, in the normal uterine cavity (Fig. 27-18).

The selection of patients for adhesiolysis should be based on hysteroscopic confirmation of the radiologic findings. Therapeutic principles include restoration of the normal uterine architecture, prevention of recurrence of the adhesions, and the promotion of endometrial regeneration. The generally accepted sequence of events is the hysteroscopic division of the adhesions, introduction of an intrauterine device (IUD), and sequential hormonal therapy.[26] After 2 to 3 months the IUD is removed and HSG or hysteroscopy is repeated to evaluate the state of the uterine cavity. It should always be remembered that pregnancies in women having had treatment for IUA are potentially hazardous and should therefore be regarded as high-risk pregnancies. The American Fertility Society[2] has proposed a classification of IUA based on the hysteroscopic findings of

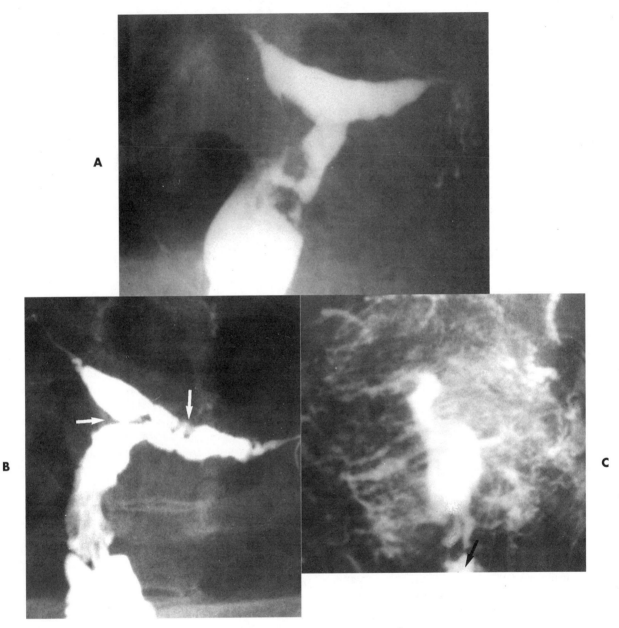

Fig. 27-17. A and **B**, Various types of intrauterine adhesions were the cause of these filling defects. **C**, The most advanced lesions predispose the patient to vascular intravasation.

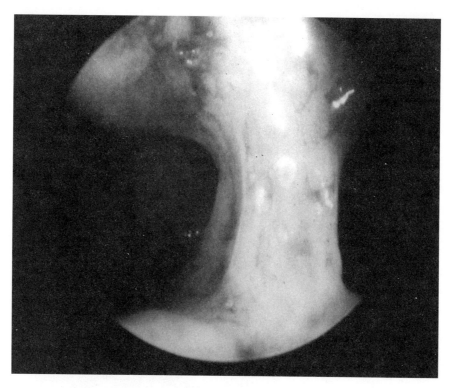

Fig. 27-18. Centrally placed, thick adhesion divides the cavity into two parts.

the extent of the cavity involved, the type of adhesions, and the menstrual pattern. Points are given for each stage of the disease (mild, moderate, or severe) and their summation provides a score. The adoption of this classification could result in standardized reports so that more meaningful comparisons could be made.

Uterine tumors

Endometrial polyps. When intrauterine lesions are suspected, the contrast medium should be instilled in fractional, small amounts so as not to overfill the cavity and obscure a lesion. This fact emphasizes the need for fluoroscopic control with spot films taken at appropriate moments of uterine filling. Endometrial polyps may be large or small, single or multiple, or pedunculated or sessile Fig. 27-19). A single polyp does not distort the triangular shape of the cavity, but multiple polyps producing larger defects cause some loss of the normal uterine outline. A defect along the outline of the uterine shadow corresponds to the pedicle of the polyp; it appears narrow in the pedunculated type and broad in the sessile types. An inner radiolucent area can be seen if the polyp is partially coated with medium. Other intrauterine abnormalities to be differentiated from polyps on HSG include submucous leiomyomas, IUA, air bubbles, and functional uterine changes (i.e., contractions). Disclosure of a polyp radiographically indicates the need for

confirmation and then a polypectomy under hysteroscopic control.

Leiomyomas. Leiomyomas are benign growths that tend to distort the normal uterine shadow in proportion to their size and location (Fig. 27-20). Submucosal and intramural leiomyomas often enlarge and distort the shape of the uterine cavity, and these tumors cause filling defects not easily obliterated by increments of the medium. Serosal or pedunculated leiomyomas are revealed radiologically only if they are calcified. Leiomyomas may occlude the tubal ostia and cause abnormal uterine bleeding and spontaneous abortion. Leiomyomas in the lower uterine segment or isthmus cause a ballooning of this region. Submucous tumors are among the predisposing causes of vascular intravasation. HSG can detect these tumors and test tubal patency, but the X-ray picture cannot show the size of the growth or its precise location. Ultrasonography and MRI are useful for documenting the growth of a myomatous uterus over extended periods.

When the diagnosis of submucous leiomyomas was made preoperatively in 103 hysterograms, it was incorrect in 21 instances; confusing abnormal shadows were caused by endometrial hyperplasia in 8 patients; endometrial polyps in 4 patients; a septate uterus, products of conception, and synechiae in each of 3 patients; blood clots in the uterine cavity in 2 patients; and no explanation for the error

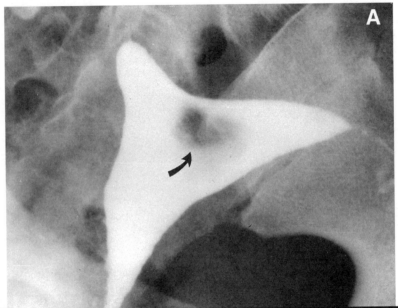

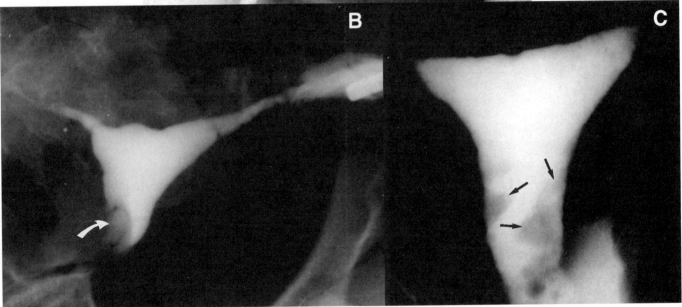

Fig. 27-19. Endometrial polyps (*arrows*) can be single (**A** and **B**) or multiple (**C**) and usually do not enlarge the cavity.

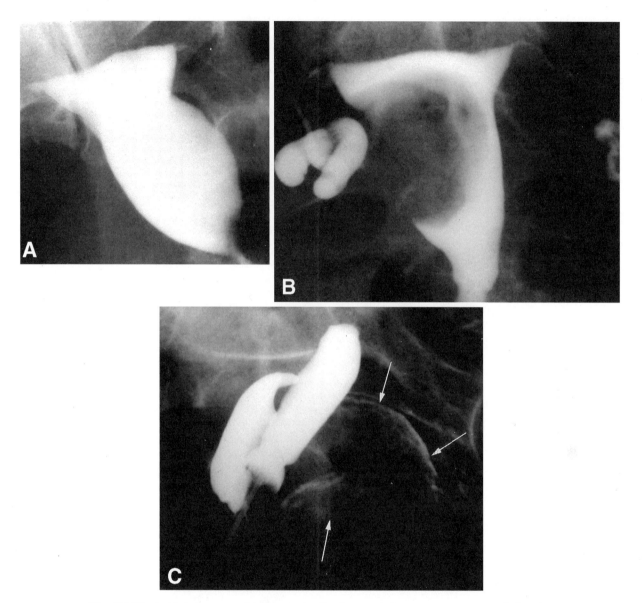

Fig. 27-20. A, A submucous leiomyoma in the lower uterine segment causes a ballooning configuration. **B,** Large intracavity filling defect resulted from a submucous leiomyoma in the uterine fundus. **C,** Combination of submucous and calcified leiomyomas (*arrows*) is seen.

in 4 patients.[27] A review of 829 hysterosalpingograms of patients operated upon for leiomyomas revealed that the cavity was enlarged in the hysterosalpingograms of 448 (54%), mucosal changes were observed in 232 (28%), and a deformed cavity was seen in 50 (6%). The operative and hysterographic findings were similar in 88% of patients.[14]

For women who wish to preserve their childbearing capacity and in whom the symptoms or sizes of the leiomyomas require surgery, preoperative HSG is important. It can demonstrate the presence of a submucous tumor and indicate the need to explore the endometrial cavity before the uterine repair is concluded. The radiographic findings can disclose the status of the fallopian tubes so that a prognosis can be given in regard to future potential fertility. Hysteroscopy can reveal the gross characteristics of the leiomyomas, and a decision can be made concerning their possible resection hysteroscopically.

Adenomyosis. The preoperative diagnosis of adenomyosis is difficult, since circumscribed adenomyomas are uncommon and endometrial sampling is not diagnostic. On HSG, diverticula seem to branch out into the myometrium from the uterine cavity outlined by contrast material if the abnormally located endometrial glands communicate with the endometrial lining (Fig. 27-21). The intramural outpouchings may cause a honeycombed configuration or appear as spicular structures ending in small sacs. Multiple asymmetrically distributed outpouchings perpendicular to the border of the cavity are characteristic. Hysteroscopic examination can reveal small openings along the endometrial surface to explain these outpouchings seen on HSG. Adenomyosis can be distinguished from salpingitis isthmica nodosa, the latter being confined more or less to the isthmic tubal segment. The narrow channels should be differentiated from vascular and lymphatic intravasation. Vascular intravasation can resemble adenomyosis, but the subsequent outlines of the uterine and ovarian vessels or lymph nodes soon become evident on later films.

Endometrial hyperplasia. HSG is not reliable for demonstrating endometrial hyperplasia, and it cannot differentiate cystic from atypical endometrial hyperplasia. On hysteroscopy polypoid hyperplasia shows scattered, rounded, endometrial elevations, whereas cystic hyperplasia exhibits blue-gray translucent cysts.

Endometrial cancer. Careful injection of contrast material under fluoroscopic control is not likely to disseminate tumor cells. Fractional instillation under fluoroscopic control reduces the chances of tubal filling and lessens the possibility of retrograde extension. Besides, doubt exists that tumor cells shed in the peritoneal washings are capable of independent metastasis. A study of 5-year survival rates in patients in whom HSG was performed in the management of endometrial adenocarcinoma failed to demonstrate any difference between women who had positive washings

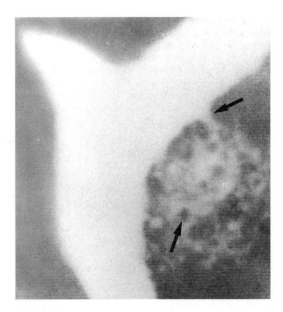

Fig. 27-21. Adenomyosis (*arrows*) causes a honeycombed, circumscribed shadow that appears to originate from the walls of the uterine cavity.

after HSG and those who did not.[23] However, a detailed discussion of this topic is not relevant to this text.

The fallopian tubes

HSG is an important procedure for evaluating the fallopian tubes and, occasionally, peritoneal causes of infertility. Its advantages include the ability to show proximal and distal occlusion and some cornual lesions and to assess the intratubal architecture. The limitations of HSG are its inability to disclose endometriosis and its inability consistently to detect significant periadnexal adhesions; false-positive diagnoses of proximal tubal obstruction can occur. Therefore, HSG and laparoscopy should be complementary, not competitive, investigative procedures.

In the search for tubal patency, the end point of the HSG is either tubal filling and spilling or increasing abdominal pain. If the tubes are not opacified on the HSG it is important to know the following:

1. Whether the cervix was occluded adequately
2. The amount of contrast agent used
3. The reason for discontinuation of the procedure before tubal filling

Proximal tubal obstruction. To differentiate cornual spasm from organic disease, the intramural segment should appear to be filled. It is uncommon to see proximal tubal obstruction caused by organic disease in the intramural segment. The radiologic differentiation of isthmic from intramural obstruction on HSG can be difficult because the myometrial width cannot be discerned radiographically.

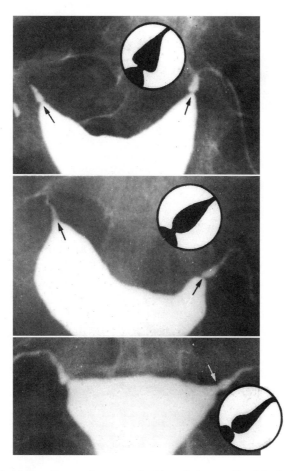

Fig. 27-22. Pretubal bulges (*arrows*) are noted with variations outlined in the insets.

The intramural section originates from the uterine cornu and extends as a fine line for about 1.5 to 2 cm, sometimes containing an ampulla-like dilation, a pretubal bulge. It may be helpful to remember the so-called thumb sign; if the thumb is placed at the cornu its width will approximate that of the myometrium, the tubal shadow underneath the thumb representing the intramural segment (Figs. 27-22 and 27-23).

Ostial or selective salpingography with tubal cannulation is a technique used in patients who have proximal tubal obstruction diagnosed from a properly performed and adequately interpreted HSG and a confirmatory laparoscopy during which multiple attempts to overcome the obstruction by chromopertubation were made. This interventional radiographic procedure is advisable before an attempt at tubocornual anastomosis. Under fluoroscopic control a 5.5 Fr (1.8 mm) catheter is wedged into the cornu with a *J* guide wire. After the guide wire is withdrawn, 2 to 5 mL of a water-soluble contrast material is inserted through the catheter and into the uterotubal ostium. The indications for stopping the procedure are increasing abdominal pain, intravasation, uterine perforation, or tubal filling and spilling. If the obstruction persists after selective salpingography, an attempt is made at recanalization with a guide wire passed through a 3 Fr (1 mm) nylon catheter. Once the wire is seen to pass into the isthmic segment, the wire is removed and the catheter over it is passed into the area. About 2 to 3 mL of contrast medium is injected to test for tubal patency.[13]

Occlusion caused by fibrosis and salpingitis isthmica nodosa (SIN) is the most common cause of proximal tubal obstruction. A previous tubal ligation, chronic salpingitis, tubal tuberculosis, and intraluminal debris are other causes of proximal tubal obstruction. One group of investigators found no histologic evidence of cornual obstruction in 16 women undergoing tubocornual anastomosis to restore patency. Based on these observations, the investigators performed tubal cannulation and lavage with the aid of a hysteroscope. They were able to establish tubal patency in all patients, and one had a successful pregnancy after the procedure.[24] The differential diagnosis can be made by observing the intramural and isthmic segments carefully to search for diverticula, filling defects, and luminal continuity.

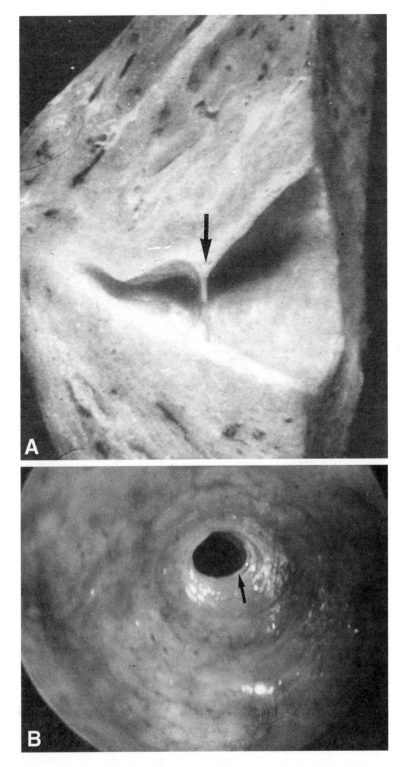

Fig. 27-23. A, The cause of the apparent separation is a membrane (*arrow*) that divides the endometrial cavity from the intramural tubal segment. **B,** This membrane (*arrow*) has been noted at hysteroscopy.

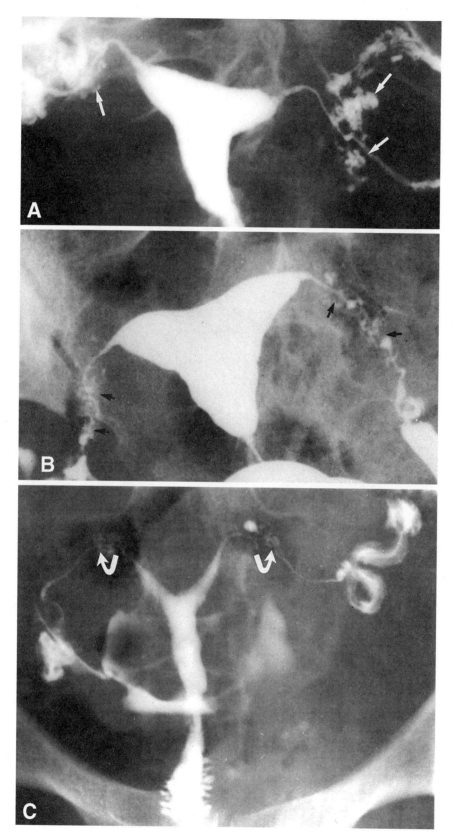

Fig. 27-24. A, B, and **C,** Salpingitis isthmica nodosa (*arrows*) is seen in these films.

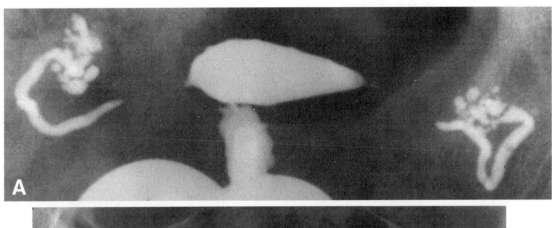

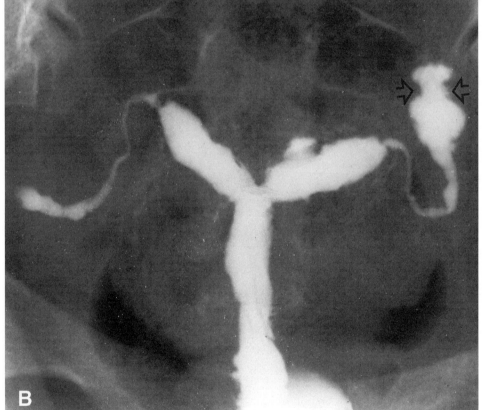

Fig. 27-25. **A** and **B,** Tubal tuberculosis with characteristic strictured "stiff" ampullary segments.

Salpingitis isthmica nodosa has a characteristic honeycombed appearance (Fig. 27-24). On HSG, whenever the luminal continuity of the isthmic segment is interrupted by white flecks of contrast material above or below the area of the expected tubal shadow, SIN should be suspected. On the drainage film the flecks of contrast material often persist as white stippled areas. Various theories have been advanced to explain its etiology and pathogenesis. The lesion cannot be felt on pelvic examination. Grossly, SIN appears as nodular thickenings in the isthmic tubal segment. During chromopertubation the blue dye seems to penetrate into these canals, which extend to the tubal serosa. The diverticula usually affect both tubes and predispose patients to tubal pregnancy. A patient with bilateral SIN and infertility is a candidate for tubal reconstructive surgery because the localized nature of the disease makes it amenable to resection and anastomosis. The dissection must be carried out to the intramural segment because the disease can extend into that area.

Although tuberculous salpingitis affects both the proximal and the distal tubal segments, its radiologic picture can be confused with SIN. The findings on HSG are often the first clue to the diagnosis of pelvic tuberculosis. The finely jagged or ragged tubal contours show numerous strictures and bulges. The occluded ampulla is often tufted and with less dilatation than other types of distally obstructed tubes (Fig. 27-25). The club-shaped appearance and rigid pipestem contours are caused by connective tissue scarring that constrict the lumen. Strictured tubes represent the oldest lesions. The gaps in the contrast material seen in the tubal lumen are caused by hypertrophic villi surrounded by areas of destroyed rugae. Calcifications appearing in the tubes, ovaries, and lymph nodes associated with uterine deformities are diagnostic of pelvic tuberculosis (Fig. 27-26).

Since the tubes are affected initially, almost half of the uteri seen on HSG appear normal. Advanced endometrial tuberculosis can cause uterine synechiae and predispose the patient to vascular intravasation; with sufficient endometrial destruction, amenorrhea is possible (Fig. 27-27).

Hysterosalpingography has sometimes been used as a guide to therapy, as some tubes become patent after antimicrobial treatment. However, the reproductive performances of these patients are poor. In one review of 7000 instances of genital tuberculosis, only 155 women had term pregnancies, 67 had spontaneous abortions, and 125 had tubal pregnancies. Histologic or bacteriologic confirmation was available in only 31 of the 155 women with term pregnancies.[19] Attempts to reconstruct tubes occluded because of tuberculosis are inevitably unsuccessful.

Tubal polyps create oval shadows in the intramural segment as the contrast fluid flows in a thin line above or below them. The remainder of the tube is normally patent in most patients, and it is doubtful that these tumors cause infertility. Sometimes they are seen at hysteroscopy; some have been excised at laparotomy through a small tubal incision. In most instances the diagnosis is made by HSG in the course of an infertility study.

Distal tubal obstruction. Ampullary opacification indicates that the proximal tube is patent, although not necessarily normal. Although distally obstructed tubes sometimes have small, club-shaped ends, they can reach as much as 4 to 5 cm in diameter, accommodating large amounts of fluid (Figs. 27-28 and 27-29). Linear dark shadows seen within the lumen obtained with WBCM are formed by the rugae, and their presence portends a better prognosis after neosalpingostomy than if they are not evident. Distal tubal obstructions have been classified into four groups based on HSG findings described by Donnez and Casanas-Roux.[7] A

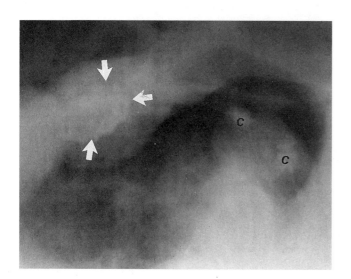

Fig. 27-26. Calcification (*arrows*) is seen in the uterine cavity and in the ovary (*c*).

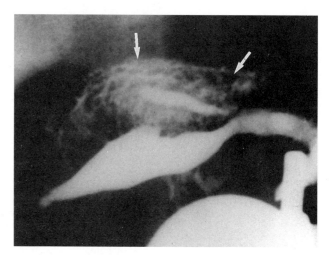

Fig. 27-27. Another cause of vascular intravasation (*arrows*) is endometrial tuberculosis.

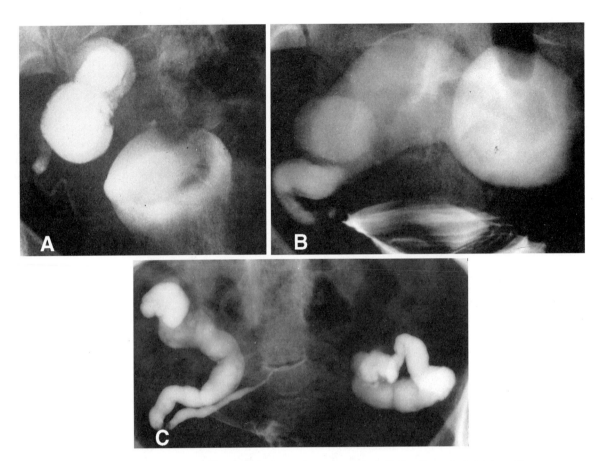

Fig. 27-28. Various types of distal tubal obstruction are noted. **A,** A distally occluded tube with a central localization of contrast material contained in the vagina. **B,** A very large hydrosalpinx. **C,** Bilateral distal tubal obstruction with poor prospects for a successful repair because of irregular borders and absence of rugal markings.

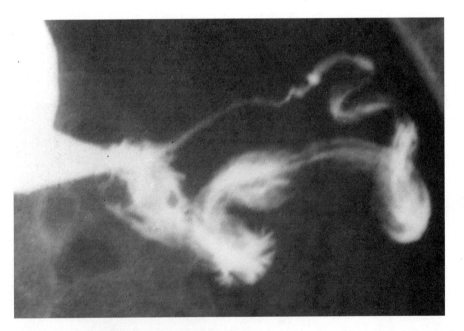

Fig. 27-29. The normal ampulla is seen with spill of the contrast agent. Note the dark line in the medium caused by rugal folds.

modified definition of their classification according to degree of involvement is as follows:

Degree I: Conglutination of the fimbrial folds (phimosis) with tubal patency

Degree II: Complete distal occlusion with normal ampullary diameter

Degree III: Complete distal occlusion with ampullary dilation of 15 to 25 mm in diameter

Degree IV: Occlusion with ampullary distention larger than 25 mm; also called hydrosalpinx simplex

One of the prognostic factors following neosalpingostomy, besides thickness of the tubal wall, the percentage of ciliated cells, and the morphologic condition of the tube, is the degree of ampullary dilatation ascertained with HSG. The use of a salpingoscope or tuboscope has recently been introduced to observe the endosalpinx for the purposes of ascertaining the extent of tubal abnormalities, establishing a prognostic index, and perhaps treating some intratubal conditions (Fig. 27-30). In the ampulla there are major and minor folds, 4 mm and 1 mm in height, respectively.[9] The larger folds can be seen on HSG as dark lines more or less in the center of the tubal lumen. Complete loss of these folds is a poor prognostic sign. Henry-Suchat et al.[9] examined 231 tubes salpingoscopically at the time of tubal microsurgery. If the endosalpinx appeared normal by HSG, endoscopy confirmed this finding in 58% of patients. In the other 42%, intratubal adhesions and loss of the rugal pattern (flattened mucosa) were not detected at HSG. Puttemans and co-authors[15] noted false-negative HSGs in 35%, whereas 48% of the tubal examinations by salpingoscopy were abnormal despite a normal HSG.

Many studies have described and compared the findings by laparoscopy and by HSG. The radiologic study seems to overdiagnose proximal tubal obstruction and miss significant periadnexal adhesions. With proper technique and careful interpretation concordant results should be obtained in 70% of cases. It is more usual to have normal HSG findings followed by significant peritubal adhesions laparoscopically than to have abnormal HSG findings followed by normal laparoscopic findings. Other techniques have been used to ascertain tubal patency and configuration, including the use of human serum microspheres labeled with technetium Tc 99m applied directly to the cervical mucosa.[12] These spheres will migrate from the vagina to the ovaries when the tubes are patent. Transvaginal higher-frequency transducer probes can produce pictures of a higher resolution, thus enabling imaging of the fallopian tube. Timor-Tritsch and Rottem[25] presented a report on sonographic pictures of normal and abnormal tubes by this method; they could delineate the tubal lumen, its walls, and its content as well as location and mobility.

THERAPEUTIC EFFECTS OF HYSTEROSALPINGOGRAPHY

HSG often has been claimed to have a therapeutic as well as a diagnostic function in infertility. A few investigators have purported to show a fertility-enhancing effect of OBCM in a group of patients with infertility of unknown cause.[20,22] Some of the beneficial effects attributed to HSG include the following:

- Expulsion of inspissated mucus or blood from the tubal lumen
- Ability to straighten kinks at the uterotubal junction or to stretch peritubal adhesions
- Dilation of tubes in patients with fimbrial phimosis
- Creation of a favorable effect on the tubal epithelium because of the iodine content of the contrast material
- Stimulation of tubal contractility from a bolus of fluid
- Effects on the immune milieu in the posterior cul-de-sac

Although Alper et al[1] reported data of a prospective, randomized study that demonstrated no difference in pregnancy rates between OBCM and WBCM, other retrospective studies suggested that OBCM may enhance fertility in patients with idiopathic or unexplained infertility. The occurrence of pregnancy within 6 months of such treatment might be considered treatment-dependent and suggest a beneficial effect of OBCM.

STERILIZATION AND HYSTEROSALPINGOGRAPHY

HSG has been performed as part of sterilization protocols because of the variable results in predicting tubal closure with some methods. Whenever a test is evaluated, the diagnosis of proximal tubal closure should be made cautiously. As a general rule, transcervical methods result in intramural obstruction so that no part of the tube is identifiable on the HSG. In patients who have been sterilized by laparotomy or laparoscopy, however, postoperative HSG usually reveals at least 2 cm of the proximal segment.

Before attempting reversal of sterilization, HSG and laparoscopy should be considered to evaluate the length and characteristics of the proximal tubal segment and to gain information about the uterine cavity. Some of the abnormalities encountered in the proximal tubal segment after tubal sterilization performed with unipolar electrosurgery include proximal hydrosalpinx, endometriosis, and fistula formation.

INTRAUTERINE DEVICES AND HYSTEROSALPINGOGRAPHY

Hysterography can demonstrate a possible or probable uterine perforation by an IUD. It can reveal an IUD extending beyond the outline of the uterine cavity delin-

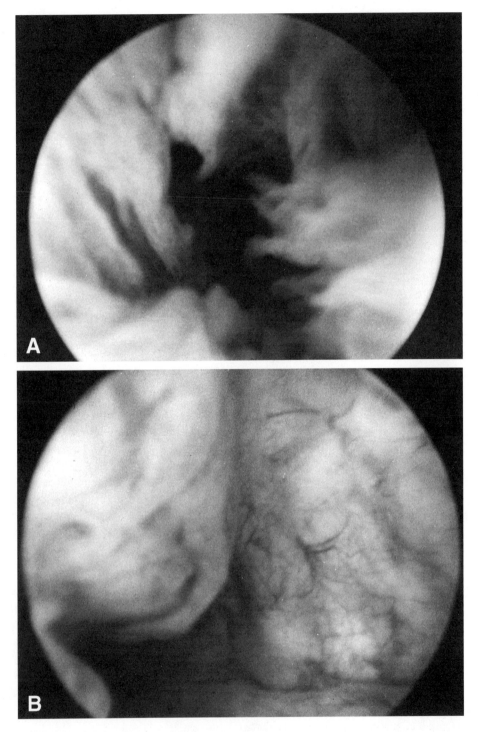

Fig. 27-30. **A,** Salpingoscopic examination of a normal endosalpinx. **B,** Salpingoscopic examination of a distally occluded tube after salpingoneostomy. Note the absence of rugal folds. (Courtesy Camran Nezhat, MD.)

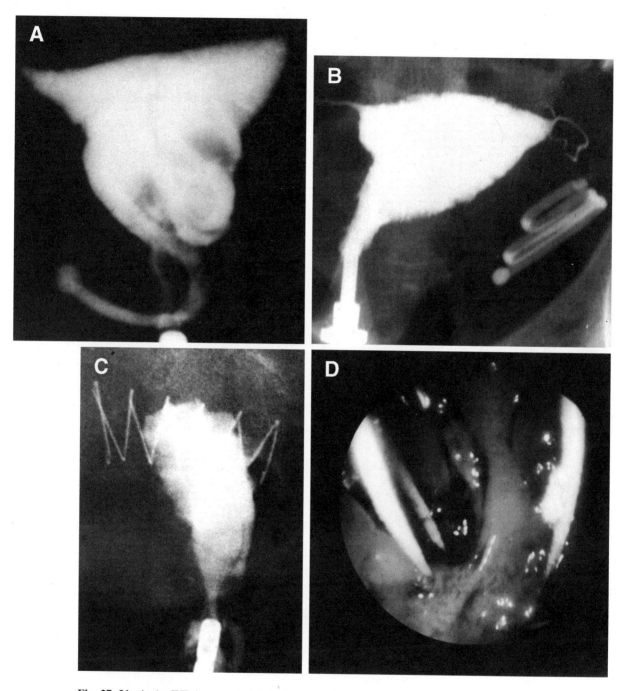

Fig. 27-31. A, An IUD has penetrated the lower uterine segment. **B,** Extrauterine position of this IUD is obvious. **C,** An IUD is seen penetrating the myometrium. **D,** Hysteroscopic examination shows penetration of the springs of this IUD into the myometrium.

eated with contrast material. The speculum should be removed before the radiographs are taken so as to avoid obscuring the lower uterine segment, an area of possible perforation. HSG can show an extrauterine position of the IUD (Fig. 27-31).

Despite some of the aforementioned advantages of HSG in regard to locating a missing or occult IUD, other diagnostic procedures such as hysteroscopy and imaging techniques have replaced HSG for this purpose.

SUMMARY

This review of the technique and interpretation of HSG was prepared to stress the most important aspects of the performance and the evaluation of the results of such studies. Despite the continued use of this procedure, a need remains for amplification and clarification of abnormal findings. Hysterosalpingography is a basic part of the infertility investigation and in many instances the results give the physician the first clue to the presence of an intrauterine or tubal abnormality. Technically unsatisfactory or poorly interpreted hysterosalpingograms are not uncommon, so that it appears justified to offer suggestions to improve skills in performance and interpretation.

REFERENCES

1. Alper MM et al: Pregnancy rates after hysterosalpingography with oil- and water-soluble contrast media, *Obstet Gynecol* 68:6, 1986.
2. American Fertility Society: The American Fertility Society classifications of adnexal adhesions, distal tubal occlusion, tubal occlusion secondary to ectopic pregnancy, müllerian anomalies and intrauterine adhesions, *Fertil Steril* 49:944, 1988.
3. Andrew E et al: Amipaque (metrizamide) in vascular use and use in body cavities: a survey of the initial clinical trials, *Invest Radiol* 16:455, 1981.
4. Ashton D et al: The incidence of asymptomatic uterine anomalies in women undergoing transcervical tubal sterilization, *Obstet Gynecol* 72:28, 1988.
5. Bateman BG et al: Utility of the 24 hour delay hysterosalpingogram film, *Fertil Steril* 47:613, 1987.
6. DeCherney AH, Cholst I, Naftolin F: Structure and function of the fallopian tubes following exposure to diethylstilbestrol (DES) during gestation, *Fertil Steril* 36:741, 1981.
7. Donnez J, Casanas-Roux F: Prognostic factors of fimbrial microsurgery, *Fertil Steril* 46:200, 1986.
8. Fedele L et al: Magnetic resonance evaluation of double uteri, *Obstet Gynecol* 74:844, 1989.
9. Henry-Suchat J et al: Endoscopy of the tube (=tuboscopy): its prognostic value for tuboplasties, *Acta Eur Fertil* 16:139, 1985.
10. Hunt RB, Siegler AM: *Hysterosalpingography: techniques and interpretation,* St. Louis, 1990, Mosby-Year Book.
11. Malstrom T: A vacuum uterine cannula, *Obstet Gynecol* 18:773, 1961.
12. McCalley MG et al: Radionuclide hysterosalpingography for evaluation of fallopian tube patency, *J Nucl Med* 26:868, 1985.
13. Novy MJ et al: Diagnosis of cornual obstruction by transcervical fallopian tube cannulation, *Fertil Steril* 50:434, 1988.
14. Pietla K: Hysterography in the diagnosis of uterine myoma: roentgen findings in 829 cases compared with the operative findings, *Acta Obstet Gynecol* 48:1, 1969.
15. Puttemans P et al: Salpingoscopy versus hysterosalpingography in hydrosalpinges, *Hum Reprod* 2:535, 1987.
16. Rapoport S et al: Experience with metrizamide in patients with severe anaphalactoid reactions to ionic contrast agents, *Radiology* 143:321, 1982.
17. Reuter KL, Daly DC, Cohen SM: Septate versus bicornuate uteri: errors in imaging diagnosis, *Radiology* 172:749, 1989.
18. Rindfleisch W: Darstellung des Cavum uteri, *Klin Wochenschr* 4:780, 1910.
19. Schaefer G: Full-term pregnancy following genital tuberculosis, *Obstet Gynecol Surv* 19:81, 1964.
20. Schwabe MG, Shapiro SS, Haning RV Jr: Hysterosalpingography with oil contrast medium enhances fertility in patients with infertility of unknown etiology, *Fertil Steril* 40:604, 1983.
21. Siegler AM et al: *Therapeutic hysteroscopy: indications and techniques,* St. Louis, 1990, Mosby-Year Book.
22. Soules MR, Spadoni LR: Oil versus aqueous media for hysterosalpingography: a continuing debate based on many opinions and few facts, *Fertil Steril* 38:1, 1982.
23. Stock RJ, Gallup DG: Hysterography in patients with suspected uterine cancer: radiographic and histologic correlations and clinical implications, *Obstet Gynecol* 69:872, 1987.
24. Sulack PJ et al: Hysteroscopic cannulation and lavage in the treatment of proximal tubal obstruction, *Fertil Steril* 48:493, 1987.
25. Timor-Tritsch IE, Rottem S: Transvaginal ultrasonographic study of the fallopian tube, *Obstet Gynecol* 70:424, 1987.
26. Valle RF, Sciarra JJ: Intrauterine adhesions: hysteroscopic diagnosis, classification, treatment, and reproductive outcome, *Am J Obstet Gynecol* 158:1459, 1988.
27. Wist A, Tahti E: Errors in roentgenological diagnosis of submucous myomas, *Ann Chir Gynaecol Fenn* 57:159, 1968.
28. World Health Organization: A new hysterographic approach to the evaluation of tubal spasm and spasmolytic agents, *Fertil Steril* 39:105, 1983.
29. Yoder IC: *Hysterosalpingography and pelvic ultrasound in infertility and gynecology,* Boston, 1988, Little, Brown.

Chapter 28

DIAGNOSTIC AND THERAPEUTIC LAPAROSCOPY

L. Michael Kettel, MD
and Ana A. Murphy, MD

Seldom has a surgical procedure had as much impact in a medical discipline as laparoscopy has had in the field of gynecology. The development of new instruments and technology has allowed the practicing gynecologist to accomplish in an ambulatory setting what once required an abdominal incision, several days of hospitalization, and an extended interval of recuperation. Despite the obvious advantages to this surgical approach, operative laparoscopy had not, until recently, been widely endorsed by the specialty. Although reports of operations performed laparoscopically were published in the early 1900s, many surgical procedures still remain to be accomplished through a traditional abdominal laparotomy.

HISTORY

It has been nearly 100 years since Jacobaeus visualized the human abdominal cavity with a primitive optical instrument.[13] This event was followed by a series of improvements in technique and instrumentation and an evolution of terminology. Carbon dioxide (CO_2) replaced air as the gas of choice for laparoscopy in 1924,[39] followed by the first use of laparoscopic cautery to divide adhesions in 1933.[7] By 1937 reports appeared concerning the use of laparoscopy to diagnose ectopic pregnancy[12] and perform tubal sterilization.[2] Further developments in the ability to perform laparoscopic procedures followed the introduction of fiberoptics in 1952 and safe intraabdominal electrocautery in 1963.[9]

In the field of gynecology, endoscopic procedures were originally described for evaluation of uterine and pelvic abnormalities. Laparoscopy is now firmly entrenched in the armamentarium of the gynecologist for visualization of pelvic pathology. However, laparoscopy can also be used to accomplish therapeutic procedures.

The first widely used operative application of laparoscopy was to perform tubal sterilizations. This remains the leading indication for laparoscopy, and mastery of this technique has become an essential part of training for every gynecologist. Operative laparoscopy, outside of tubal sterilization, had its beginnings on the coattails of diagnostic laparoscopy. In 1963 the development of an automatic insufflator to maintain pneumoperitoneum[3] heralded the beginning of the field of operative laparoscopy as it is known today. In the 1970s, Semm[31] reported on operative techniques to accomplish several traditional abdominal procedures laparoscopically. Continued evolution of new instrumentation and pioneering work by Reich and associates,[28,29] Gomel,[10] and others has brought operative laparoscopy and its inherent advantages into the forefront of clinical gynecologic practice.

INDICATIONS

Diagnostic laparoscopy

Diagnostic laparoscopy is used whenever there is need to visualize the intraabdominal cavity directly. It is an invaluable tool for the evaluation of a woman with acute or chronic pelvic symptoms. It can be used to establish the diagnosis of endometriosis or pelvic adhesions in a woman complaining of pelvic pain and is indispensable in the work-up of potential ectopic pregnancy. Additionally, evaluation of peritoneal surfaces, tuboovarian architecture, and external uterine contour can be useful in an infertile patient. In a woman presenting to the emergency department with acute onset of lower abdominal pain, laparoscopy can usually differentiate between adnexal or intestinal sources and can establish a diagnosis of infectious salpingitis. Other indications for laparoscopy include the evaluation of pelvic masses or other adnexal pathology. In rare circumstances laparoscopy may be used to establish anatomy in patients who present with müllerian tract anomalies or primary amenorrhea. The use of laparoscopy in the diagnosis, treatment, and surveillance of patients with pelvic malignancies is uncertain and at best probably plays a limited role.

Operative laparoscopy

Indications for operative laparoscopy depend to a great extent on the skill and experience of the surgeon. There are now reports describing the laparoscopic performance of almost all gynecologic procedures. Limitations on the types of procedures performed depend on the individual anatomy of the patient and on the instruments and training of the laparoscopist. Because operative laparoscopy is a field still in evolution, the success, recurrence, and complications of many of these procedures remain to be determined.

CONTRAINDICATIONS

Before any operative procedure is performed the patient must have a full understanding of the nature of the surgery involved as well as the potential risks, complications, and alternatives. It is important to emphasize to the patient that although her abdominal incision may be minuscule there is still significant potential for surgical complications. It is also important that the patient realize that this procedure is limited in its diagnostic and therapeutic scope. She should be apprised of the potential for laparotomy should unexpected injury to vital structures occur as well as the potential for additional surgery should the original procedure be aborted because of unexpected pathology or anatomy.

Contraindications to laparoscopy can be separated into absolute and relative categories, as follows:

- Absolute contraindications
  1. Bowel obstruction
  2. Ileus/bowel distention
  3. Severe cardiorespiratory disease
- Relative contraindications
  1. Advanced intrauterine pregnancy
  2. Massive obesity
  3. Large abdominal mass
  4. Inflammatory bowel disease
  5. Multiple previous abdominal procedures
  6. Severe abdominal adhesive disease
  7. Peritonitis
  8. Intraperitoneal hemorrhage

The conditions that lead to most of the absolute contraindications include diseases that make potential damage to the gastrointestinal tract unacceptably high or cardiopulmonary diseases that preclude the establishment of an effective pneumoperitoneum. Relative contraindications include circumstances that would raise the risk of laparoscopic complication. Although the benefit of surgery may outweigh the risk of complication in certain disease processes, this decision must be made on an individual basis. As more and more surgeons become comfortable with the laparoscopic techniques, the circumstances in which laparoscopy is not warranted become increasingly rare. The patient who is massively obese deserves special consideration before laparoscopy. Several instruments are available in long sizes that allow the technique to be performed; however, the thick anterior abdominal wall can make manipulation of intraabdominal instruments almost impossible. Additionally, the exceptionally thin patient deserves special mention. Because of the close proximity of vital intraabdominal structures to the anterior abdominal wall, the instruments must be inserted into the peritoneal cavity in an almost parallel fashion to avoid complication. Patients with previous abdominal surgery or a history of abdominal adhesions must be approached carefully. In some circumstances the placement of the trocar can be accomplished through an "open" technique to minimize the chances of bowel injury. Most important, it must be emphasized that bowel injury has been observed with both techniques.

OPERATIVE TECHNIQUES

Once the decision to proceed with laparoscopy has been reached, a complete history is taken, a physical examination is performed, and informed consent is obtained. Although there is some experience with laparoscopic procedures performed under local anesthesia, general anesthesia is preferred for most routine diagnostic and operative laparoscopic surgical procedures. The relaxation of the anterior abdominal wall and control over ventilation that can be achieved with general anesthesia are invaluable in performing laparoscopic surgery. The patient should be intubated to avoid accumulation of air within the stomach and to minimize the chances of intestinal complication with insertion of laparoscopic instruments.

Once the patient is asleep on the operating table she should be positioned to allow the surgeon easy access to the abdominal wall. To allow as much maneuverability as possible, most surgeons prefer that the patient's arms be tucked and not extended on arm boards. The legs should be placed in knee stirrups with footrests (Allen stirrups) and only slightly flexed to allow access to the perineum and vagina while keeping the legs and knees from the surgeon's operative field. The patient's buttocks should extend to the end of the table such that instruments that are placed in the vagina can be fully manipulated. If extensive operative procedures are anticipated, venous compression devices may be placed on the lower extremities preoperatively.

Once the patient is appropriately positioned on the operating table her urinary bladder should be emptied. If an extended surgical procedure is anticipated, continuous gravity drainage should be accomplished. The patient's stomach should be emptied by nasogastric suction before placement of any abdominal instrumentation. A pelvic examination to assess uterine size, shape, and contour, as well as adnexal pathology, is performed before insertion of uterine instruments. The patient's abdomen and perineum are then prepared with a suitable antiseptic, and the patient is draped in a sterile fashion with both the perineum and anterior abdominal wall exposed.

The basic instruments required to place the laparoscope are illustrated in Fig. 28-1. A pneumoperitoneum generally is created by inserting a Verres needle through a subumbilical incision into the peritoneal cavity. After elevation of the anterior abdominal wall, the needle is directed toward the sacral hollow and between the bifurcation of the aorta and uterine fundus. Placement of the needle within the peritoneal cavity can be confirmed by aspiration and easy flow of sterile fluids through the lumen of the Verres needle. The "hanging drop" test is performed by placing a drop of sterile saline on the top of the Verres needle and elevating the anterior abdominal wall. If the tip of the needle is correctly located within the peritoneal space, the suction created will draw the drop down the lumen of the needle. The insufflation tubing should then be attached and 2 to 3 L of CO_2 insufflated. Intraperitoneal pressures should not exceed 20 mm Hg and typically range between 7 and 12 mm Hg throughout the insufflation process. Symmetric distention of the abdominal cavity and tympany over the liver are additional signs of correct intraperitoneal placement of the Verres needle. After an appropriate pneumo-

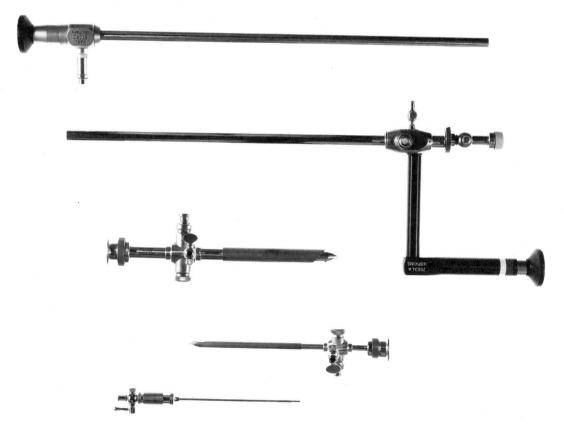

Fig. 28-1. Basic instruments for laparoscopy. *Top to bottom,* 10-mm straight laparoscope, 10-mm operating laparoscope, 10-mm trocar and sleeve, 5-mm ancillary trocar and sleeve, Verres needle. (Karl Storz Co., Tuttlingen, Germany)

peritoneum has been achieved, the Verres needle is withdrawn. Again, the anterior abdominal wall is elevated and the laparoscopic trocar with sleeve is placed at the same angle as the Verres needle. Placement of the trocar can be confirmed by the rapid outflow of gas once the trocar has been removed from the sleeve. The laparoscope is then placed through the trocar sleeve to confirm placement within the intraperitoneal space. A suprapubic manipulating probe is commonly required for thorough inspection of the pelvis. This is usually placed through a smaller (5 mm) incision, two fingerbreadths above the pubic bone, and insertion of the trochar and sleeve is observed through the laparoscope to minimize complication.

With these two instruments placed, diagnostic inspection of the pelvis can be undertaken. The uterus should be anteflexed and retroflexed with a uterine manipulation cannula, and the ovaries should be inspected on all sides with the aid of the manipulating probe. If there is fluid within the posterior cul-de-sac, it should be aspirated before the diagnostic survey is completed. If infection is suspected, the fluid may be sent for culture. The patency of the fallopian tubes can be assessed by injecting colored sterile fluid (indigo carmine) through the cervix with visualization of dye emanating from each fimbria. Absence of tubal fill may be secondary to tubal obstruction, tubal spasm, or an inadequate seal of the instrument at the cervix. Placement of an endometrial balloon can be used to secure an adequate seal around the cervix. Inspection of the upper abdominal structures, including the liver, gallbladder, and appendix, completes the diagnostic survey.

Pelvic or abdominal pathologic processes frequently can obscure visualization of the structures important to evaluate. Frequently, adhesions must be divided to gain access to all components of the pelvis. If operative laparoscopic procedures are performed it is frequently necessary to place second, third, or even fourth ancillary trocars to manipulate, cut, or ablate abnormal tissue. Generally the puncture sites are made in a radial fashion along an imaginary transverse line in the lower abdominal wall (Fig. 28-2). Transillumination of the proposed site from below can often reveal vascular structures to be avoided. One should keep in mind the course of the inferior epigastric vessels, which come over the semicircular fold of Douglas and enter the rectus sheath. Additionally, a 3.5-inch spinal needle can be inserted through the skin at the proposed site to allow laparoscopic visualization of the anticipated ancillary port.

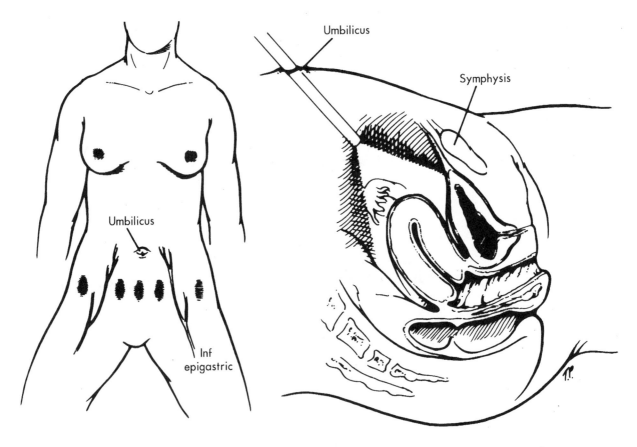

Fig. 28-2. *Left,* Potential sites for ancillary ports (*shaded areas*) approximately 2 cm above the pubic symphysis. The course of inferior epigastic vessels must be noted before placement of instruments. *Right,* Relationship of the laparoscope placed through the umbilicus to pelvic contents and the symphysis pubis.

Careful assessment of the procedure to be performed within the confines of the anatomy of the patient is essential before placement of ancillary trocars in order to facilitate surgery in a safe and effective fashion.

The use of video camera attachments to the laparoscope has greatly aided surgical assistants and operating room staff in facilitating the surgeon in laparoscopic procedures. By providing all members of the operating team a real-time view of the procedure, team members can much more effectively assist and anticipate the surgeon's needs. The role of the laparoscopic surgical assistant includes stabilizing instruments, holding structures in place, elevating the uterus, irrigating tissue, and using ancillary instrumentation.

Operative laparoscopy is not a procedure for the novice but for a well-trained gynecologic or reproductive surgeon. Laparoscopic surgery should not be attempted until the surgeon has mastered the basic skills required for diagnostic laparoscopy and sterilization procedures and has received special training in the technique. A preceptorship is the best way to achieve surgical laparoscopic competence. The inexperienced surgeon should begin with fairly simple cases and proceed with increasingly difficult cases.

EQUIPMENT

Basic laparoscopy

Diagnostic laparoscopes are available in several different styles and sizes. Most laparoscopes range from 10 to 12 mm in diameter and may include an operating channel (Fig. 28-1). The larger laparoscopes have operating channels (5 to 7 mm) that can accommodate larger instruments. Optical quality is dependent on the size of the lens, the quality of the fiberoptic cable, and the light source. For procedures performed with use of video cameras, the largest lens and strongest light source available will provide the finest image. Straight laparoscopes without operating channels provide the best image and have become increasingly popular. However, operative procedures performed with this laparoscope require additional ancillary ports. The slight compromise in lens size and therefore image quality in laparoscopes with operating channels must be weighed against the advantage of placing instruments directly through the operating channel of the instrument and minimizing the number of ancillary ports required.

Verres needles and trocars are available in reusable and disposable models. All Verres needles are designed to reduce the chances of accidental damage to intraabdominal structures by containing a spring-loaded obturator, which releases to cover the sharp tip once the needle has traversed the abdominal wall. A similar mechanism is available in some models of disposable trocars. The disposable instruments have the advantages of being sharp and readily available but are much more expensive. The "safety shields" on the trocar and Verres needle probably protect intraabdominal structures from inadvertent damage, but structures that are fixed or held by adhesions are not

protected. The potential advantages of the safety shields incorporated into the disposable devices have not been demonstrated in any controlled trials.

Insufflation of the peritoneal cavity requires a pump to deliver a controlled supply of CO_2. Laparoscopic surgery requires an adequate pneumoperitoneum, and the insufflator and the speed with which the insufflation occurs are critical in operative procedures that require multiple puncture sites and frequent loss of intraperitoneal gas. Most insufflators produce a flow of approximately 0.5 to 2.0 L/min. High-flow insufflators designed for operative procedures are now available and are capable of flows of up to 15 L/min. In most circumstances, an insufflation rate of 4 to 6 L/min is adequate. Although other gases have been used for creation of the pneumoperitoneum, CO_2 is preferable because it is inert, readily absorbed, and nonflammable and does not lead to intestinal distention.

Laparoscopy depends on a reliable and powerful light source. If video laparoscopy is performed, a xenon light source is preferable because of the high intensity achieved. However, halogen light sources are adequate for simple diagnostic procedures and simple operative procedures such as tubal sterilization. Light cables are equally important to achieving a high-quality image. Fiberoptic cables, composed of multiple coaxial quartz fibers, transmit light from the source to the endoscope with relatively little heat conducted to the end of the cable. The fibers range from 10 to 25 μm in diameter and with repeated use may break, resulting in less and less light transmission. The cables should be inspected before each use by looking at the end of the illuminated cable for black dots that represent broken filaments. When a substantial number of fibers have broken the cable should be replaced. New liquid-light cables have been developed that minimize this problem, but they are more expensive and leak if punctured.

Ancillary instruments

A wide variety of instruments are now available for the laparoscopic surgeon. Instruments are available in either reusable or disposable varieties and in several styles, lengths, and diameters. The surgeon should be acquainted with a variety of instruments and use the instruments that most appropriately accomplish the task at hand.

Probes. The most commonly used ancillary instrument is the atraumatic probe. This is a metal rod with calibrated 1-cm markings that can be used to manipulate intraabdominal structures to accomplish visualization and diagnosis. The atraumatic probe may also be used to stabilize structures and retract bowel, ovaries, or other organs or provide improved operative visibility.

Forceps. Many types of forceps are available (Fig. 28-3). Atraumatic forceps have delicate tips and are designed to grasp structures such as the fallopian tube, ovary, or intestine (Fig. 28-4). The surgeon must be cautioned against so-called atraumatic forceps with locking jaws,

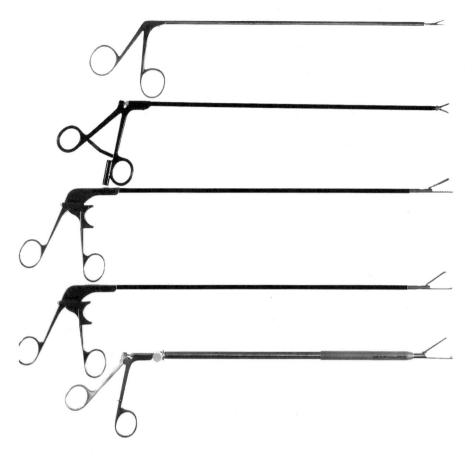

Fig. 28-3. Laparoscopic grasping forceps. *Top to bottom*, 5-mm atraumatic micrograsper, 5-mm sliding lock traumatic grasper, 10-mm claw forceps. (Karl Storz Co., Tuttlingen, Germany, and Davis and Geck, Wayne, NJ)

which may inadvertently crush tissue. This is especially important when performing microsurgical procedures. Traumatic grasping forceps are available in several varieties that can hold structures adequately for further surgical manipulation. These forceps are most applicable to structures that ultimately will be removed, such as diseased ovaries or fallopian tubes or pathologic processes of these organs.

Scissors. Many kinds of scissors are available to the laparoscopist (Fig. 28-5), including hook scissors, microscissors, and serrated scissors. It is imperative that scissors be sharp so that they cut instead of avulse tissue. Many scissors are available with cautery attachments such that ablative and hemostatic surgery can be performed with the same instrument. Disposable scissors are now available but are very expensive and have no inherent advantage over a set of sharp, reusable scissors. Unfortunately, in many operating rooms, it is difficult to maintain a set of sharp, reusable scissors.

Aspirators/irrigators. Just as in conventional abdominal surgery, endoscopic surgery can result in bleeding. The ability to irrigate and aspirate the surgical field to provide visualization is essential, especially for extensive operative procedures performed through the laparoscope. There are many devices now available, both reusable and disposable, that can accomplish both of these tasks. The instruments typically combine two ports, one for aspiration and another for irrigation. Irrigating fluid, usually saline or lactated Ringer's solution, is instilled under pressure through a cannula controlled with a trumpet valve. The instillation pressure can be regulated by either an electronic pump or wall nitrogen pressure. The use of irrigating fluids under high pressure for aquadissection is a simple technique for separating tissue planes in areolar spaces when performing operative procedures. Suction through the same cannula can be accomplished by attaching a separate port controlled by a trumpet valve to wall suction. The aspiration/irrigation cannulas have either straight or fenestrated tips to provide choices in the type of suction to be accomplished. These instruments should be available and set up before initiating an operative laparoscopic procedure. Should unexpected bleeding occur during the course of the surgery, the aspirator/irrigator is invaluable in identifying the source of bleeding and ensuring hemostasis.

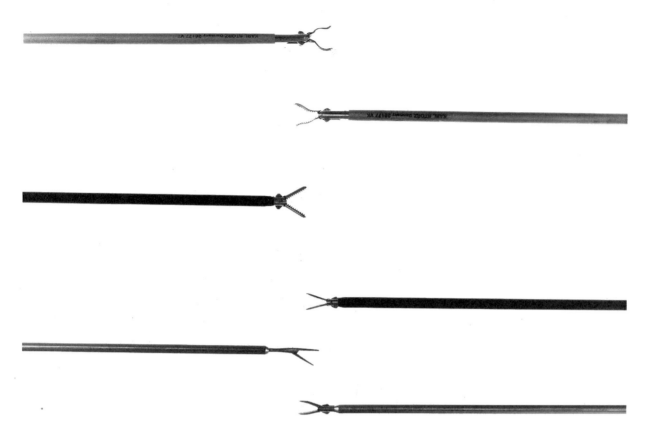

Fig. 28-4. Laparoscopic atraumatic grasping forceps. *Top to bottom,* 5-mm ampullary dilator, 5-mm micrograsper, 5-mm fine serrated grasper, 5-mm heavy serrated grasper, 5-mm serrated tubal grasper, 5-mm smooth tubal grasper. (Karl Storz Co., Tuttlingen, Germany)

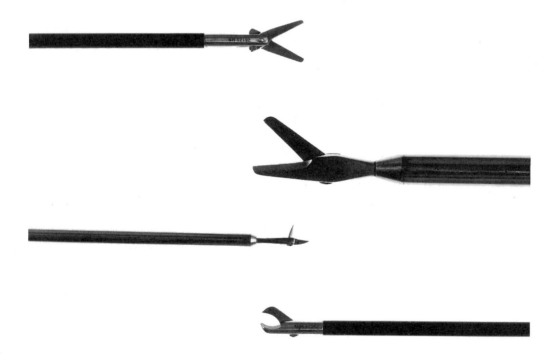

Fig. 28-5. Laparoscopic scissors. *Top to bottom,* 5-mm straight scissors, 10-mm strong scissors, 5-mm microscissors, 5-mm hook scissors. (Karl Storz Co., Tuttlingen, Germany)

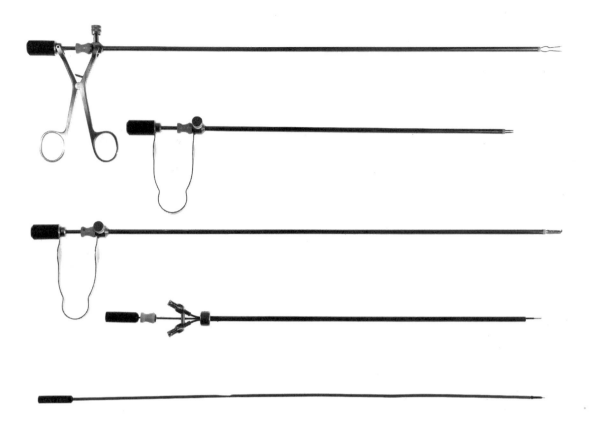

Fig. 28-6. Laparoscopic cautery instruments. *Top to bottom,* 5-mm smooth bipolar coagulating forceps, 5-mm microbipolar coagulating forceps, 5-mm bipolar grasping forceps, 5-mm Corson aspiration-irrigation cannula with monopolar needle-tip electrode, 3-mm knife-tip monopolar cautery electrode. (Karl Storz Co., Tuttlingen, Germany, and Richard Wolf Medical Instruments Corporation, Rosemont, Ill)

HEMOSTATIC TECHNIQUES

Multiple modalities are available to achieve hemostasis during the course of laparoscopic surgery. No one technique is ideal, and the laparoscopic surgeon should be familiar with all of them.

Electrosurgery

Electrosurgery is probably the most commonly used technique to obtain hemostasis. Modern electrosurgical units are available in most operating theaters and can deliver current in either a monopolar or bipolar mode. There are laparoscopic instruments available that can utilize either of these modalities (Fig. 28-6). When monopolar cautery is applied, the electrical current travels from the generator, through the instrument, into the target tissue, and back through a ground plate (which is attached to the patient) to the generator. With bipolar cautery, current is passed between two paddles contained within the same instrument. The tissue between the paddles is desiccated and completes the circuit. Each of these techniques has advantages.

Monopolar cautery can be attached to a variety of different instruments and allows the simultaneous performance of cutting and grasping with hemostasis. Needle-tip

electrosurgery is an accurate and inexpensive alternative to laser (see later). The variety of instruments available with monopolar cautery attachments allows for flexible and precise application of current.

Bipolar cautery is limited to areas in which the tissue can be either grasped or placed between the two paddles. However, an important advantage to bipolar cautery is that current does not pass through the body, and this limits potential for complication. Moreover, control of bleeding can be more quickly achieved with an instrument that can grasp and occlude an open vessel.

Current can be delivered in cutting or coagulating forms. Cutting currents provide a constant high-energy output, whereas coagulation wave forms create initial high voltage that then quickly dissipates and results in desiccation of the outer layer of tissue with corresponding increases in tissue resistance. It is important that the surgeon be aware that tissue damage can be seen as far as 2 to 3 cm away from the area of coagulation. This is especially true for monopolar cautery. It is important that the tip of the instrument remain within the surgeon's view at all times. The current should be applied by the operating surgeon and not by an assistant. Each manufacturer of electrosurgical devices uses a different numerical notation of power applied to the operating instrument. It is essential that the surgeon be familiar with the settings of the particular generator in use and the power output tested before actual operative use.

Thermocoagulation

Developed in 1962, thermocoagulation acquires hemostasis by coagulating tissue through heat convection.[32] An electrical current heats the tip of a thermocoagulator to 100° to 120°C, which then can be placed on the tissue. As the temperature in the tissue rises, its color changes and desiccation takes place. Because this unit works by local application of heat, no electrical current passes into the patient. It is important to realize that the tip of the thermocoagulating unit does not cool instantly once current is turned off and that injury is possible if tissue is touched inadvertently. As with electrosurgery, several types of instruments are available with thermocoagulating tips. However, all tips are large and therefore not applicable to microsurgical work.

Lasers

Lasers have achieved widespread use throughout clinical medicine and are particularly helpful in operative laparoscopic procedures. Laser is a device that produces and amplifies light energy into a coherent electromagnetic beam. The laser beam can be either reflected or carried through fiberoptic cables. This allows the operative laparoscopist to aim the laser light source precisely to pinpoint areas of tissue for destruction. By varying time of exposure, spot size, wattage, and wavelength the laser can be used to achieve several different effects, including cutting, coagulation, and desiccation.[3]

There are several types of lasers commonly used endoscopically. The CO_2 laser is the most commonly used laser for gynecologic procedures and is the only reflected beam laser used. Recent advances in laser technology have allowed laser light to be transmitted through fiberoptic cables. Argon, potassium titanyl phosphate (KTP), and neodymium:yttrium-aluminum-garnet (Nd:YAG) are the three most commonly used fiberoptic lasers. These lasers differ in their wavelength, depth of tissue penetration, and clinical uses.

The CO_2 laser is used primarily to vaporize tissue. The laser energy is generated in the infrared spectrum and is preferentially absorbed by tissue with a high water content. When focused to a fine beam (high-power density), the laser can be used for cutting and then defocused (low-power density) for coagulation. The fiberoptic lasers have greater coagulative effects and their cutting ability can be improved by passing them through fibers with sapphire tips, which focus the laser beam. The CO_2 laser is passed through an articulating arm and coupled to either the laparoscope or an ancillary instrument. The beam is then focused and power setting determined. By limiting the time

in which the laser energy is applied, the degree of tissue vaporization can be minimized; CO_2 laser models are available that deliver short pulses of energy (0.05- to 0.1-second duration). Because CO_2 laser light is preferentially absorbed by water, it cannot be transmitted through a fluid medium. This limits its utility in obtaining hemostasis and performing hysteroscopic procedures.

As stated previously, the argon, KTP, and Nd:YAG lasers can be carried through flexible fiberoptic fibers. This allows for easier setup, increased versatility, and convenience for the surgeon and the operating room staff. The argon and KTP laser light energy is in the visible spectrum and is preferentially absorbed by red pigmented tissues rich in hemoglobin, hemosiderin, or melanin. This quality makes these lasers ideal for treatment of endometriosis or obtaining hemostasis. They have limited ability to incise tissue, require special electrical connections and cooling systems, and are considerably more expensive. The Nd:YAG laser will pass through fluid medium and has a fairly great degree of tissue penetration, making it more suitable for hysteroscopic applications. It is less readily absorbed by heme-rich tissues. Unlike argon or KTP units, Nd:YAG laser units are available that are air-cooled, so that expensive water-cooling systems are not necessary. Sapphire tips are available for the fiberoptic cables. These tips control the scatter of laser energy as it escapes from the fiber and focus it for improved cutting and depth of penetration.

All of these lasers have been used to treat pelvic pathology through the laparoscope, most often endometriosis.[4,16,19] There are few comparative studies between different lasers and, more important, no prospective, blinded trials comparing laser surgery with electrosurgery. Whether laser surgery offers any real advantage over simple electrosurgery is debatable and at this point unresolved. Laser units are very expensive and must be maintained by experienced operating room personnel. Surgeons who choose to use lasers must be trained in laser technology and be familiar with the specific limitations and complications of the laser they have selected.

Suture, clips, and staples

Securing tissue for reconstruction, hemostasis, or support with suture has been an integral dimension of abdominal surgery since its inception. Techniques to place suture ligatures through the laparoscope have evolved such that the skilled laparoscopic surgeon no longer needs to compromise or limit the desired operative procedure. When fine sutures are used, the ligature can be secured with an instrument tie done inside the peritoneal space (intracorporeally). Laparoscopic needle holders are available in several different varieties to provide flexibility in suture and needle selection. If heavier-gauge suture material is required, it can be cumbersome to tie the ligature intracorporeally. Techniques have been developed for extracorporeal knot tying. These techniques require that the needle and suture be

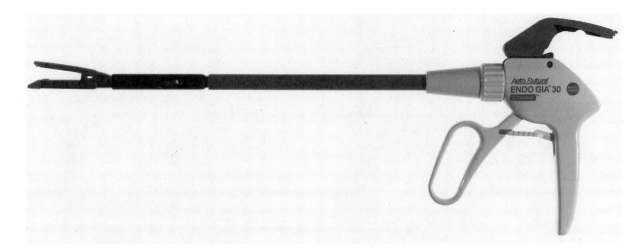

Fig. 28-7. Multifire ENDO GIA 30 disposable laparoscopic stapler. (Auto Suture Co., Norwalk, Conn)

placed through a port, leaving a long tail outside of the body. The needle is then placed through the tissues and withdrawn through the same port. The knot is tied and slipped down the ligature to secure the tissues together. In addition, there are several proprietary devices in which preformed loops, or lassos, are packaged and allow the laparoscopist a convenient tool by which to secure a pedicle. These devices are pretied Roeder loops that can be placed into a sleeve. The sleeve is then inserted through an ancillary port and the device is extended to expose the loop inside the abdomen. The appropriate tissue is then snared, and the knot is slipped down the ligature to secure the tissue.

Devices to place hemostatic clips or staples have been used for intraabdominal surgery for many years. Recently, several devices have been designed to accomplish the same tasks laparoscopically (Fig. 28-7). Such a device allows the laparoscopist to place a line of staples or a single staple or clip to a bleeding vessel. It is now possible to secure large vessels (e.g., infundibulopelvic ligament) easily with these devices, which opens new possibilities for extirpative surgery.

OPERATIVE PROCEDURES

The performance of gynecologic laparoscopic surgery requires an expert familiarization with the anatomy of the female pelvis. Many laparoscopic surgical complications arise because of failure to recognize the anatomical adjacencies of important pelvic structures such as the ureter, branches of the internal iliac artery, and sigmoid colon. The surgeon must be able to identify and trace the path of the ureter from the pelvic brim, along the pelvic sidewall, and under the uterine artery. The operative laparoscopist should be prepared to perform a retroperitoneal dissection of the sidewall should the anatomic relationships of these structures not be clear.

Ectopic pregnancy

Laparoscopy has provided a pivotal role in the diagnosis of ectopic pregnancy for many years. It is now possible to extend the application of the laparoscope to both diagnosis and treatment. Conservative and radical procedures can be performed through the laparoscope. As always, the hemodynamically unstable patient is not a candidate for laparoscopy. Several studies have now confirmed the feasibility of laparoscopic surgery for ectopic pregnancy.[27, 29] The investigators reported subsequent pregnancy rates historically comparable to those of patients who had undergone laparotomy and served as controls. In addition, Vermesh and colleagues[38] and Murphy and colleagues[21] have demonstrated a significant reduction in hospital stay, cost, and delay of return to normal activity.

Salpingectomy. Removal of the fallopian tube is still the treatment of choice for ectopic pregnancy in the patient who does not desire future fertility. Salpingectomy can be performed in patients with either a ruptured or unruptured ectopic pregnancy and is accomplished by dividing the mesosalpinx after achieving hemostasis with either electrosurgery or mechanical devices such as staples (Fig. 28-8). A suture loop may be used to secure the final pedicles. Removal of the fallopian tube can be accomplished in several ways. The tube can be morcellated intraperitoneally and removed in small pieces, cut on alternating sides to decrease the diameter of the tube, or removed through a minilaparotomy or colpotomy.

Conservative procedures. In a patient with an unruptured ectopic pregnancy who desires future fertility, it is preferable to conserve the fallopian tube by removing the products of conception alone. The patient must be prepared to return for serial human chorionic gonadotropin (hCG) titers to ensure resolution of the pregnancy and be counseled of the risk for possible future therapy or surgery should there prove to be persistent trophoblastic tissue (5%

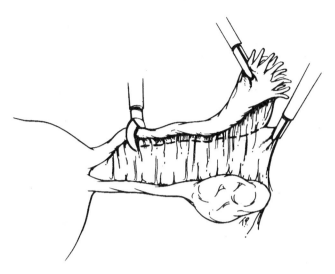

Fig. 28-8. Laparoscopic salpingectomy. The mesosalpinx is divided (*broken line*) by using bipolar cautery and hook scissors to achieve tissue coagulation and hemostasis before surgical division.

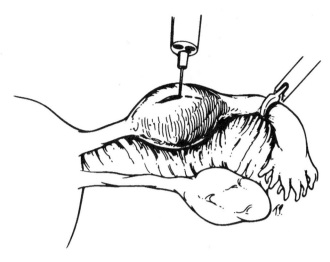

Fig. 28-9. Laparoscopic linear salpingostomy. The fallopian tube is stabilized with an atraumatic grasper. The salpingostomy is created with monopolar cautery, using a needle-tip electrode.

to 15%).[27] Recent reports have explored the usefulness of intramuscular methotrexate for the treatment of ectopic pregnancy.[34] In the case of a persistent hCG titer following endoscopic surgery, methotrexate may be useful to avoid subsequent surgery.

Salpingostomy. Unruptured ampullary and isthmic ectopic pregnancies should be treated with linear salpingostomy. With a needle-tip monopolar cautery or laser, a salpingostomy is created over the distended portion of tube containing the ectopic pregnancy (Fig. 28-9). In most cases, once the tube is opened the products of conception will extrude from the salpingostomy. They can then be teased away from the tube with grasping forceps; hemostasis is achieved as previously described. Occasionally, aquadissection or use of traumatic forceps is necessary to remove the ectopic conception. The salpingostomy incision usually is not closed. Fistula formation postoperatively is possible but fortunately is a rare event.

Partial salpingectomy. Should the ectopic pregnancy not lend itself to linear salpingostomy because of extensive tubal damage secondary to rupture, failure to remove trophoblastic tissue adequately, or uncontrolled hemorrhage, a partial salpingectomy can be performed. This results in either a fimbriectomy or a segmental resection of the fallopian tube (Fig. 28-10). After removal of a portion of the fallopian tube, subsequent tubal anastomosis offers potential salvage of fertility. If restoration of tubal function will not be possible, such as after fimbriectomy, strong consideration should be given to performing a complete salpingectomy. The vessels running within the mesentery of the fallopian tube must be secured before removal of any portion of the tube. A variation on this technique would be to apply electrosurgery or thermocoagulation in a fashion similar to tubal sterilization throughout the segment of tube

containing the ectopic pregnancy. Unfortunately, when this technique is used no specimen can be submitted for pathologic examination. Alternatively, a knuckle of tube containing the ectopic pregnancy can be secured with a loop suture and excised, similar to a Pomeroy tubal ligation technique.

Endometriosis

Endometriosis is one of the most common gynecologic disorders for which laparoscopy has been used for diagnosis and treatment. It is essential that the implants of this disease process be visualized to secure the diagnosis. The laparoscopic surgeon should be familiar with the many different appearances of endometriosis.[20] It is now possible to provide excellent surgical treatment through the laparoscope at the time of diagnosis. Laparoscopy is ideally situated for excision, ablation, or vaporization of endometriotic implants. In addition, laparoscopes provide a low degree of magnification that can aid the surgeon in identifying abnormalities of the peritoneal surface.

Peritoneal ablation. Peritoneal endometriotic implants can be ablated with electrosurgery, thermocoagulation, or laser. None of these techniques has been shown to be better than the other, although few comparative trials have been performed. Electrosurgery is simple to use, safe, and readily available in most operating rooms. By using delicate microtip electrodes, it is possible to obtain pinpoint accuracy. Thermocoagulation is an effective means to destroy endometriotic tissue, but needle-tip thermocoagulation instruments are not available. Laser has the potential advantages of extreme accuracy, versatility of spot size, and limited tissue destruction. Argon laser, specifically, has the advantage of being selectively absorbed by hemoglobin-pigmented lesions.[15] Whether these advantages justify the tremendous cost of laser equipment is debatable. If peritoneal endometriosis is situated overlying important struc-

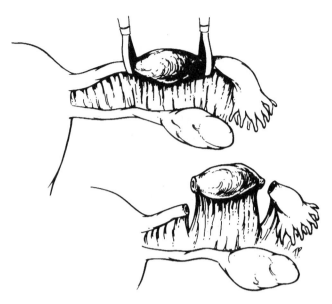

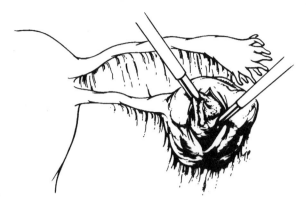

Fig. 28-11. Laparoscopic excision of an ovarian endometrioma. The endometrioma is opened, drained, and irrigated. The cyst wall is then separated from the ovary by stabilizing the edge of the ovary and peeling the cyst wall from within. The base of the excised endometrioma is then coagulated.

Fig. 28-10. Laparoscopic partial salpingectomy (segmental resection). The fallopian tube is coagulated on either side of the ectopic pregnancy by using bipolar cautery. The ectopic pregnancy is then elevated from the remaining tube and the mesosalpinx is coagulated and divided, using bipolar cautery and hook scissors.

tures in the pelvic sidewall, the peritoneum can usually be retracted off the underlying structure with grasping forceps or displaced from the underlying structures with aquadissection before applying ablative therapy.

In its severest forms endometriosis can involve bowel, bladder, and ureters. Implants can also be situated in areas immediately adjacent to large blood vessels. Under these circumstances judicious use of laparoscopic techniques for ablation should be emphasized. In some instances, severe disease might be better approached at the time of laparotomy.

Ovarian endometriomas. Ovarian endometriomas are managed according to size and location. If small collections of disease are encountered (<5 mm), simple ablation is corrective. However, if larger endometriomas are found they should be managed by incision, drainage, and dissection of the cyst wall.[28] The endometrioma is first identified and the ovary cleared of adhesive disease (if possible). The ovary is then fixed with a grasper, and an incision is made over the endometrioma in the axis of the ovary at its most dependent point. The "chocolate" fluid is then drained, and the cyst and peritoneal space are copiously irrigated. The cyst wall of the endometrioma should be removed to prevent recurrence (Fig. 28-11). This is done by gently teasing the lining away from the ovarian capsule with two atraumatic graspers. After this dissection any remaining portions of the endometrioma cyst wall should be coagulated. Although the relationship has been poorly studied, suturing the ovarian defect may be associated with an increase in postoperative adhesion formation; therefore, the ovary should be left open. Simple incision and drainage of endometriomas should be avoided because the recurrence rate is high.

Treatment results. Success in laparoscopic treatment for endometriosis can be measured in terms of pregnancy rates or pain relief. Pain relief is difficult to measure, and few randomized comparative trials have been performed. However, when compared with medical treatments or laparotomy, laparoscopic therapy appears to be at least equal to, if not better than, those forms of therapy.[1]

Pregnancy success in the infertile patient with endometriosis is often a frustrating end point to measure. The literature is replete with studies describing pregnancy rates ranging from 24% to 92% after laparoscopic therapy. To a large extent these studies were poorly controlled, and life table analysis was not performed to allow the reader some reference point by which to interpret the numbers. A few studies have been reported that utilized life table analysis; these studies have demonstrated that results of laparoscopic treatment of endometriosis are equal to results of medical therapy or laparotomy in patients with mild to moderate disease and may even be better in patients with severe disease.[22, 23]

Tubal disease

In many ways the treatment of tubal disease has been revolutionized by advances in laparoscopic surgery. It is now possible to address severe adhesive disease, hydrosalpinges, and other tubal pathologic processes through the laparoscope. This avoids the need for both diagnostic and operative procedures and allows most patients the opportunity to go home the same day they have surgery.

Adhesive disease. Laparoscopic adhesiolysis has been performed for many years. In some reports, results of adhesiolysis performed laparoscopically have been comparable to results of adhesiolysis performed at laparotomy.[10] It should be emphasized that laparoscopic surgery is performed under magnification and that, in effect, microsurgical techniques are used. As always, precise hemostasis and minimal tissue handling remain important.

Adhesions should be incised at both ends and the tissue removed from the abdominal cavity. This is best achieved by placing the adhesion on tension with grasping forceps and dividing the adhesion with any of a variety of instruments. Before dividing any adhesion, it is important that the surgeon identify bowel, bladder, ureter, and blood vessels to avoid unanticipated injury.

Tubal reconstruction and infertility. Neosalpingostomy and fimbrioplasty may be performed laparoscopically. Microsurgical techniques must be used and the adhesions must be completely excised and not simply divided. The same techniques that apply to corrective tubal surgery when performed under magnification at the time of an exploratory laparotomy apply to laparoscopic tubal reconstruction. In performing a fimbrioplasty the distal portion of the tube must first be freed of adhesions. The perifimbrial adhesions are then removed with delicate atraumatic grasping forceps. Stabilization of the fallopian tube laparoscopically can be a challenge because of the need to avoid potential tubal damage when rigid instruments are used. Often the adjacent ovary or tuboovarian ligament can be fixed to aid in the stabilization necessary to work on the tube itself. Caution must be exercised when directly grasping any portion of the tube. Once the adhesions are removed, it may be necessary to dilate the ampullary end of the tube. By placing an atraumatic grasping instrument into the tubal ostium and opening its jaws gently, any fimbrial agglutination that may be present usually can be reversed. The fimbria should be examined closely for interfimbrial adhesions which, if present, should be carefully taken down. Intrauterine pregnancy rates after laparoscopic fimbrioplasty[6] have been favorably compared with those obtained after microsurgical fimbrioplasty performed via laparotomy.[25] Unfortunately, published studies have used historical controls, and whether the results would be comparable to those of a prospective randomized trial is as yet unknown.

Laparoscopic neosalpingostomy is also performed by using traditional microsurgical techniques. After freeing the tube of adhesions, the dilated distal end of the tube is inspected. In most cases, a whitish scar is apparent where tubal agglutination has occurred. This marks the area where the tube should be reopened. The phimotic fimbriated end of the tube is opened sharply. The underlying tubal mucosa should be evaluated and stellate incisions made to expose the fimbria completely. Defocused laser beams, electrosurgery, or fine sutures can be used around the neosalpingostomy to evert the tubal ostium and prevent reclosure. It is unknown whether laparoscopic tubal reconstruction yields results similar to those of more traditional microsurgical reconstruction at the time of laparotomy. Certainly there are several reports of successful laparoscopic neosalpingostomies yielding pregnancy rates similar to those of historical controls.[5] To date, no prospective trial of laparoscopy versus microsurgical laparotomy has been reported.

Second-look laparoscopy

Pelvic surgery is often performed in women who desire preservation (or enhancement) of fertility. Procedures such as myomectomy, ovarian wedge resection, and tubal reconstruction commonly are complicated by extensive postoperative adhesion formation. These newly formed (reformed) adhesions may impede future fertility.

Prevention of adhesion formation or recurrence after pelvic reconstructive surgery or adhesiolysis can be facilitated by early second-look laparoscopy performed 1 to 12 weeks postoperatively. Division and excision of filmy adhesions before fibrosis and neovascularization may result in an improved end result. There are only limited data to assess the effectiveness of second-look laparoscopy. However, some studies have found that at least 50% of adhesions lysed at the time of second-look laparoscopy do not re-form.[14, 36, 37] These results are encouraging; however, the ultimate therapeutic benefit of second-look laparoscopy remains to be established.

Ooophorectomy/adnexectomy

Adnexal surgery can be performed laparoscopically. Whether the surgeon elects to remove the entire adnexa (tube and ovary) or perform a limited dissection, such as an ovarian cystectomy, techniques and instrumentation are available to accomplish these procedures laparoscopically. Certainly there are many instances in which the tissue to be excised is obviously benign and a laparoscopic approach is preferred to shorten hospital stay, improve recuperative time, and limit costs. However, the management of a potentially malignant ovarian or adnexal mass laparoscopically must be approached with caution. Laparoscopic surgical intervention in malignant disease may cause delays in diagnosis, errors in diagnosis, unintentional spread of disease, or the need for additional surgical procedures. There are reports of malignant disease found in tissue excised laparoscopically that was believed to be benign at the time of surgery.[18] Alternatively, in a well-designed pilot study, Park and Berek[24] described the successful removal of selected cystic adnexal masses through the laparoscope. All of the patients had been rigorously screened prospectively and were believed to have benign disease. In none of these patients was malignancy encountered. Until more information is available, the management of suggestive adnexal masses through the laparoscope must be approached with caution.

Removal of the ovary or adnexa can be accomplished laparoscopically by securing the infundibulopelvic and

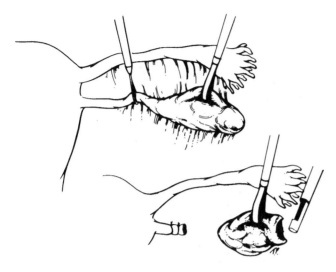

Fig. 28-12. Laparoscopic oophorectomy. In this example, the uteroovarian ligament is divided by using bipolar cautery and hook scissors. The pedicle is then secured (if necessary) with Roeder loops. The infundibulopelvic ligament is then secured with three Roeder loops and the ovary excised. The ovary can then be morcellated into small pieces and removed.

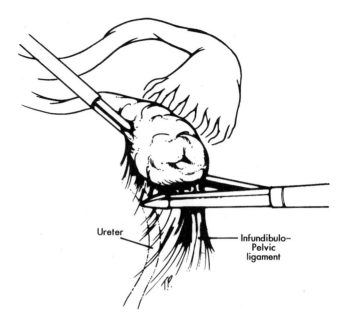

Fig. 28-13. Laparoscopic oophorectomy. In this example, the infundibulopelvic ligament is secured and divided, using the Multifire ENDO GIA 30 stapler (Auto Suture Co., Norwalk, Conn). The course of the ureter must be established before firing the device, to avoid accidental injury.

uteroovarian ligaments and dividing the mesoovaria or mesosalpinx (Fig. 28-12). The most commonly used technique involves placement of three Roeder loops around the ovary (or adnexa). Recent advances in instrumentation have allowed the placement of a hemostatic staple line through the support structures both to divide the ligaments and to obtain hemostasis (Fig. 28-13). Removal of the adnexa from the abdomen can be accomplished through morcellation, minilaparotomy, or colpotomy.

Laparoscopic neurectomy

Laparoscopic uterosacral nerve ablation (LUNA) is a modification of the technique described by Doyle in 1955. Since most uterine sensory nerve fibers run through the uterosacral ligaments, the division of these structures results in significant pain relief in selected patients. The technique for interrupting the uterosacral ligaments is relatively straightforward and can be accomplished with either laser or bipolar coagulation followed by sharp division. The ligament should be divided approximately 1 cm from its insertion onto the uterus and the depth of the division carried down to approximately 1 cm. Because a coalescence of nerves occurs between the uterosacral ligaments, this area is commonly ablated with either defocused laser energy or electrosurgical coagulation. It is imperative that the surgeon be fully aware of the course of the ureter and its adjacency to the uterosacral ligament before performing this procedure.

Approximately 50% to 70% of patients with primary dysmenorrhea have experienced pain relief lasting at least 1 year after LUNA.[17] When dysmenorrhea was combined with endometriosis, Feste[8] reported a 71% response to LUNA. Obviously, more studies are necessary to determine the long-term efficacy of this procedure. At this point, this procedure should be reserved for patients who have failed more conservative treatments.

Presacral neurectomy has been performed since the late 1800s for the relief of pelvic pain. This procedure has remained controversial since then, and controlled studies evaluating its true effectiveness are sparse. In a recent prospective study Tjaden et al.[35] reported very encouraging results after presacral neurectomy in well-selected patients. Patients with central pelvic pain, not adnexal pain, who have failed other therapies may be considered candidates for this procedure. Patients with back pain or dyspareunia may respond poorly.

As for many other pelvic procedures, instruments and techniques have evolved to accomplish neurectomy laparoscopically.[26] This is a procedure that requires a great deal of surgical skill and should not be attempted by surgeons who are not familiar with the retroperitoneal anatomy of the presacral space. The potential for vascular and ureteral complications, as well as incomplete resection of the presacral nerve plexus, should be discussed with the patient preoperatively. Long-term follow-up is not available for this procedure.

The retroperitoneal space should be opened and the boundaries of the dissection identified. The presacral nerves should be completely excised from the bifurcation of the aorta inferiorly to the division of the nerve plexus into its right and left bundles at the first sacral vertebra. Laterally the dissection should extend from the right internal iliac artery/ureter to the inferior mesenteric artery/superior hemorrhoidal artery on the left. The presacral nerve is isolated from the avascular space between the nerve and the periosteum. Care should be taken to recognize and avoid the middle sacral artery and vein, the left common iliac vein, and the ureters bilaterally. The superior portion of the nerve bundle is then grasped and coagulated. Either electrosurgical needles or lasers may be used to accomplish this, but care must be taken to ensure hemostasis. For this reason the CO_2 laser is probably not a good choice for this procedure, and the contact Nd:YAG laser with a sapphire-tip fiber is more appropriate. Electrosurgical needles work very nicely and may be used with a combination of coagulating, cutting, or blending currents. Once the nerve bundle has been divided superiorly it is gently retracted and divided approximately 3 to 4 cm caudad from where the nerve was transected.

The efficacy of laparoscopic presacral neurectomy has not been established, but it appears to be comparable to that of open procedures.[26] Common reasons for failure include poor patient selection and incomplete resection of the presacral nerve. It should be emphasized that this procedure is not recommended for relief of lateral pelvic pain and should be performed by surgeons with experience in this procedure.

Myomectomy

Pedunculated leiomyomas are easily resected through the laparoscope. The leiomyoma can then be removed through morcellation, minilaparotomy, or colpotomy. Subserosal, intramural, and submucosal leiomyomas also can be removed endoscopically. Subserosal and intramural leiomyomas are resected by coagulating the overlying serosa and creating an incision with either scissors or laser. The edges are held open with atraumatic forceps, and the leiomyoma is grasped and traction applied. Enucleation followed by cauterization of vessels completes the procedure. Once hemostasis has been obtained, the defect can be reapproximated with suture techniques previously described or left open to close primarily. Submucosal leiomyomas should be resected through the hysteroscope; resection should not be attempted laparoscopically.

There is some controversy surrounding the appropriate resection of uterine leiomyomas through the laparoscope. Certainly pedunculated leiomyomas can be resected quite easily. Whether or not intramural myomectomy should be attempted through the laparoscope is controversial. One can imagine that small fibroids are left unnoticed when this procedure is done laparoscopically, and the risk of incomplete resection is quite high. In addition, adhesion formation after laparoscopic myomectomy has not been assessed. There are no reports evaluating the effects of laparoscopic myomectomy on infertility, pregnancy wastage, pain, or abnormal bleeding. There is no information on operative complications, recurrence of leiomyomas, or adhesion formation. Until the role of this procedure is more adequately studied, its usefulness must be considered carefully. (See Chapter 39.)

Laparoscope assisted hysterectomy

The laparoscope can be an invaluable tool in diagnosis and therapy of disease processes that might influence the way in which hysterectomy is performed. Traditionally, the abdominal approach has been reserved for patients with known or suspected adhesive disease, pain, endometriosis, uterine leiomyomas, or the desire to remove the adnexa. If this surgery could be accomplished vaginally, the advantages of reduced hospital stay and rapid recovery from vaginal hysterectomy could be maximized. Techniques are now available for laparoscopic correction of pathologic conditions, which would then allow for a vaginal approach to hysterectomy. In our opinion, this procedure should not replace vaginal hysterectomy but would allow the surgeon who otherwise would consider an abdominal hysterectomy an option to complete the procedure vaginally.

This relatively new technique is a procedure in evolution. In experienced hands, the entire procedure can be performed via the laparoscope. However, a more judicious use of the laparoscope would envision treatment of associated pathology laparoscopically (e.g., ablation of endometriosis, lysis of adhesions, removal of pedunculated fibroids) followed by division of the upper support structures through the laparoscope. This part of the procedure can be accomplished with cautery and scissors or endoscopic stapling devices. The anterior leaf of the broad ligament can be opened laparoscopically and the remainder of the surgery completed in the usual fashion for vaginal hysterectomy. Some surgeons prefer to create the anterior and posterior colpotomies laparoscopically as well. Extirpated adnexa, leiomyomas, or other pathology can be removed through the colpotomy.

As with laparoscopic myomectomy, this procedure has not been well evaluated. Data on operative complications are lacking, and experience with this procedure is limited. Certainly the patient without suspected intraabdominal pathology has little to gain from laparoscopy and should continue to be treated with straightforward vaginal hysterectomy.

Laparoscopic appendectomy

Diagnostic laparoscopy has been used to aid in the diagnosis of appendicitis.[33] Historically, the diseased appendix was removed through a small laparotomy and the patient was hospitalized for 2 to 4 days. Removal of the appendix through the laparoscope would allow for shorter patient recovery, improved cosmetics, and, by combining a diagnostic and therapeutic procedure, potentially shorter operating time. There is a report describing the results of laparoscopic appendectomy.[11] In that report, only 12% of appendixes were histologically normal, and that percentage compares favorably to the rate observed with appendectomy via laparotomy. It was necessary to convert the operative approach to laparotomy only 3% of the time.

The technique of performing a laparoscopic appendectomy is similar to that when appendectomy is approached at laparotomy. The appendix is grasped with an atraumatic grasping forceps, and the mesoappendix is coagulated and divided with bipolar current and hook scissors. Once the appendix is free of its mesentery, two or three loops of absorbable suture can be placed around the base of the appendix and the appendix amputated between the loops. Alternatively, a hole can be placed through the base of the mesentery and a laparoscopic stapler used to divide the mesentery in one bite and amputate the appendix in another. Once the appendix is free within the abdominal cavity it should be placed within a latex sac to prevent spillage of fecal material into the peritoneal cavity. There are proprietary devices available for this, but a finger cut from a size 8 surgeon's glove works quite well. The sac is held closed with a grasping forceps, and the sac is removed through a large-bore trocar (10 to 12 mm) or through a small incision in the skin. Postoperatively the patient may remain in the hospital until normal bowel function is restored. Some groups place patients on a clear liquid diet and send them home on the day of surgery.

COMPLICATIONS OF LAPAROSCOPY

The complications of laparoscopy are well known and are shared by many other abdominal procedures. Complications may result from accidental injury to bowel, bladder, blood vessels, ureters, or other structures within the abdominal cavity. Some complications, such as those associated with the "blind" insertion of the trocar, are unavoidable.

Inadvertent penetration of viscera or blood vessels can occur with either the Verres needle or the trocar. Most complications of laparoscopy are associated with trocar insertion. It is essential that the patient's bladder be emptied before placement of any laparoscopic instrument and that a nasogastric tube be used to empty the stomach if there is any suspicion of distention. Use of a syringe to test placement of the Verres needle is somewhat helpful in determining whether a viscus has been penetrated. Most Verres needle injuries do not require laparotomy. These patients should be admitted to the hospital and followed closely. However, should a trocar injury occur, surgical correction should be performed immediately. If the trocar enters the intestine, it should be left in place to limit peritoneal spill and facilitate localization of the injured bowel. Puncture, penetration, or laceration of blood vessels invariably requires intervention. Injury to major vessels usually requires immediate laparotomy, transfusion, and vascular repair. Injury to smaller vessels may be controlled with bipolar cautery or other techniques of hemostasis. The inferior and superficial epigastric vessels and their branches may be injured with placement of secondary trocars in the lower abdomen. Transillumination of the abdominal wall with the laparoscope before placement of instruments can often identify these vessels, thereby limiting the potential for accidentally damaging these vessels.

Extraperitoneal insufflation of CO_2 can occur. When the misplacement is recognized, the CO_2 is released and the instruments are reinserted. In case of preperitoneal insufflation, the gas may extend into the mediastinum and the anesthetist may experience difficulty in ventilating the patient. Pneumothorax is a very rare complication, and emphysema of the omentum is usually a self-limited problem.

When performing operative procedures around the adnexa or pelvic sidewall, the ureter must be visualized in order to avoid injury. The ureter usually can be identified as it crosses the pelvic brim and runs under the peritoneum parallel to the iliac vessels. In some circumstances it will be necessary to open the sidewall to identify the ureter, especially in conditions with severe adnexal pathology such as endometriosis, pelvic inflammatory disease, or dense adhesions. The surgeon must always keep in mind that electrosurgery-induced damage extends beyond the actual area of "burn" and that the ureter may be susceptible to injury even though it is not immediately adjacent to these areas. Other electrosurgical injuries include skin burns, intestinal burns, and operator burns. Occult extension of tissue coagulation can cause injury to distant sites and subsequent necrosis that may not be evident immediately. Such "accidents" were more often reported with the use of older electrosurgical units. Laser beams can pass through target tissue, especially filmy adhesions, and cause damage beyond the desired area. Additionally, the beams can be reflected off metallic instruments that may be holding tissues and cause damage in areas quite distant from the operative target.

Bleeding accounts for almost half of the complications associated with laparoscopy. Damage to major blood vessels can occur and may result in life-threatening hemorrhage. The operating room staff must be prepared to deal with these emergencies and have instrumentation available for immediate laparotomy. Most bleeding complications fortunately require only simple electrosurgery. Before any operative procedures are performed it is essential that there is a functional bipolar cautery unit on the surgical field. Hematomas can occur in the abdominal wall secondary to instrument placement. The surgeon must survey the trocar sites and, if active bleeding continues, be prepared to open the skin to ligate the bleeding vessels.

SUMMARY

Diagnostic and therapeutic laparoscopic procedures are safe when guidelines are observed and the surgeon is aware of the limitations of the techniques. The benefits of laparoscopy, including reduced morbidity, short hospitalization, and decreased expense, have been well delineated. Laparoscopic surgery has advanced in great steps recently and in all likelihood will continue to become a more and more commonly applied technique. As experience with this technique increases and more applications are investigated, so will the ability to establish guidelines for appropriate procedures in which to perform laparoscopic surgery. It is becoming more and more obvious that laparoscopic procedures will replace many procedures traditionally performed by laparotomy. It is essential that the well-trained gynecologist keep abreast of the changes within this field and that future training emphasize the importance of laparoscopy in the armamentarium of the operating gynecologist.

REFERENCES

1. Adamson GD, Lu J, Suback LL: Laparoscopic CO_2 laser vaporization of endometriosis compared to traditional treatments, *Fertil Steril* 50:704, 1988.
2. Anderson ET: Peritoneoscopy, *Am J Surg* 35:36, 1937.
3. Buyalos RP: Principles of endoscopic laser surgery. In Azziz R, Murphy AA, editors: *Practical manual of operative laparoscopy and hysteroscopy,* New York, 1992, Springer-Verlag.
4. Corson SL et al: Laparoscopic laser treatment of endometriosis with the Nd:YAG sapphire probe, *Am J Obstet Gynecol* 160:718, 1989.
5. Donnez J, Casana-Roux F: Prognostic factors of fimbrial microsurgery, *Fertil Steril* 46:200, 1986.
6. Fayez JA: An assessment of the role of operative laparoscopy in tuboplasty, *Fertil Steril* 39:476, 1983.
7. Fervers C: Die Laparoskopie mit dem Cystoskop: ein Beitrag zur Vereinfachung der Technik and zur endoskopischen Strangdurchtrennung in der Bauchhohle, *Med Klin* 29:1042, 1933.
8. Feste JR: Laser laparoscopy: a new modality, *J Reprod Med* 30:413, 1985.
9. Frangenheim H: Tubal sterilization under visualization with the laparoscope, *Geburtshilfe Frauenheilkd* 24:470, 1964.
10. Gomel V: Salpingo-ovariolysis by laparoscopy in infertility, *Fertil Steril* 40:607, 1983.
11. Gotz F, Pier A, Bacher C: Modified laparoscopic appendectomy in surgery: a report on 388 operations, *Surg Endosc* 4:6, 1990.
12. Hope RB: The differential diagnosis of ectopic gestation by peritoneoscopy, *Surg Gynecol Obstet* 64:229, 1937.
13. Jacobaeus HC: Uber die Moglichkeit, die Zystoskopie bei Untersuchung seroser Hohlungen anzuwenden, *Muench Med Wochenschr* 57:2090, 1910.
14. Jansen RPS: Early laparoscopy after pelvic operations to prevent adhesions: safety and efficacy, *Fertil Steril* 49:26, 1988.
15. Keye WR Jr, Dixon J: Photocoagulation of endometriosis by the argon laser through the laparoscope, *Obstet Gynecol* 62:383, 1983.
16. Keye WR Jr et al: Argon laser therapy of endometriosis: a review of 92 consecutive patients, *Fertil Steril* 47:208, 1987.
17. Lichten EM, Bombard J: Surgical treatment of primary dysmenorrhea with laparoscopic uterine nerve ablation, *J Reprod Med* 32:37, 1987.
18. Maiman M, Seltzer V, Boyce J: Laparoscopic excision of ovarian neoplasms subsequently found to be malignant, *Obstet Gynecol* 77:563, 1991.
19. Martin DC: CO_2 laser laparoscopy for endometriosis associated with infertility, *J Reprod Med* 31:1089, 1986.
20. Martin DC et al: Laparoscopic appearance of peritoneal endometriosis, *Fertil Steril* 51:63, 1989.
21. Murphy AA et al: Operative laparoscopy vs. laparotomy in the management of ectopic pregnancy: a prospective trial, *Fertil Steril* 57:1180, 1992.
22. Nezhat C, Crowgey SR, Nezhat F: Videolaseroscopy for the treatment of endometriosis associated infertility, *Fertil Steril* 51:237, 1989.
23. Olive DL, Martin DC: Treatment of endometriosis-associated infertility with CO_2 laser laparoscopy: the use of one- and two-parameter exponential models, *Fertil Steril* 48:18, 1987.
24. Parker WH, Berek JS: Management of selected cystic adnexal masses in postmenopausal women by operative laparoscopy: a pilot study, *Am J Obstet Gynecol* 163:1574, 1990.
25. Patton GW: Pregnancy outcome following microsurgical fimbrioplasty, *Fertil Steril* 37:150, 1982.
26. Perez JJ: Laparoscopic presacral neurectomy: results of the first 25 cases, *J Reprod Med* 35:625, 1990.
27. Pouly MA et al: Conservative laparoscopic treatment of 321 ectopic pregnancies, *Fertil Steril* 46:1093, 1986.
28. Reich H, McGlynn F: Treatment of ovarian endometriosis using laparoscopic surgical techniques, *J Reprod Med* 31:577, 1986.
29. Reich H et al: Laparoscopic treatment of 109 consecutive ectopic pregnancies, *J Reprod Med* 33:885, 1988.
30. Semm K: Das Pneumoperitoneum mit CO_2. In Demiling L, Ottenjann RS, editors: *Edoskopie-Methoden, Ergebnisse,* Munich, 1967, Banaschewski.
31. Semm K: New methods of pelviscopy for myomectomy, ovariectomy, tubectomy and adnexectomy, *Endoscopy* 11:85, 1979.
32. Semm K, Mettle L: Technical progress in pelvic surgery via operative laparoscopy, *Am J Obstet Gynecol* 138:121, 1980.
33. Spirtos NM et al: Laparoscopy: a diagnostic aid in cases of suspected appendicitis, *Am J Obstet Gynecol* 156:90, 1987.
34. Stovall TG et al: Single dose methotrexate for treatment of ectopic pregnancy, *Obstet Gynecol* 77:754, 1991.
35. Tjaden B et al: The efficacy of presacral neurectomy for the relief of midline dysmenorrhea, *Obstet Gynecol* 76:89, 1990.
36. Trimbos-Kemper TCM, Trimbos JB, van Hall EV: Adhesion formation after tubal surgery: results of the eight-day laparoscopy in 188 patients, *Fertil Steril* 43:395, 1985.
37. Tulandi T, Falcone T, Kafka I: Second-look operative laparoscopy 1 year following reproductive surgery, *Fertil Steril* 52:421, 1989.
38. Vermesh M et al: Management of unruptured ectopic gestation by linear salpingostomy: a prospective randomized clinical trial of laparoscopy vs. laparotomy, *Obstet Gynecol* 73:400, 1989.
39. Zollikoffer R: Uber Laparoskopie, *Schweiz Med Wochenschr* 104:264, 1924.

Chapter 29

SEMEN EVALUATION

Anibal A. Acosta, MD,
Mahmood Morshedi, PhD,
and Gustavo Doncel, MD, PhD

Evaluation of semen in the clinical male factor
  Obtaining the semen sample
  Physical parameters of semen
  Quantitative and qualitative analysis of sperm
  Other cellular components of semen
  Investigation of seminal fluid
Evaluation of semen in assisted reproduction
  Basic semen analysis
  Immunologic investigation
  Bacteriologic screening
  Tests of spermatozoal function
  Hamster egg–human sperm penetration assay
  Human hemizona–sperm attachment assay
Evaluation of semen after cryopreservation
  History and background
  Cryopreservation techniques
  Use of cryopreserved semen samples in assisted reproduction
Evaluation of semen after electroejaculation
Evaluation of sperm after microscopic epididymal sperm aspiration
Potential areas for basic and clinical research

Under normal conditions in men, semen is the end result of testicular function within a normal hypothalamic-pituitary-testicular axis and of the secretion of post-testicular excretory and glandular systems.

Although it is not in the scope of this review, the final assessment of semen needs to be preceded by careful clinical evaluation of the man, followed by endocrine assessment in order to interpret findings at the sperm level and to try to determine the possibilities of systemic medical therapy, surgical treatment, or laboratory enhancement of sperm quality. Evaluation of semen and interpretation of results may be different when dealing with a clinical male factor and the goal is to try to achieve pregnancy through natural reproduction, rather than when assisted reproduction will be attempted. Furthermore, interpretation of results may also be different after spermatozoa have been subjected to cryopreservation or have been obtained by electroejaculation or epididymal aspiration. Finally, as a result of recent developments in spermatology, new areas of research have opened and new diagnostic tests are being developed. Accordingly, our review comprises (1) evaluation of semen in the clinical male factor, (2) evaluation of semen in assisted reproduction, (3) evaluation of semen after cryopreservation, (4) evaluation of semen after electroejaculation, (5) evaluation of sperm after microscopic epididymal sperm aspiration, and (6) potential areas for basic and clinical research.

EVALUATION OF SEMEN IN THE CLINICAL MALE FACTOR

The evaluation of semen in the clinical arena is a very important part of the decision-making process in approaching the male factor in infertility, but it must be interpreted in the context of a full andrologic consultation, including the patient's history, physical examination, and endocrine evaluation. The semen analysis must be comprehensive and needs to include information about the sperm and the seminal fluid; it is required that the semen analysis include (1) background information, (2) physical data, (3) quantitative and qualitative analysis, (4) biochemical analysis, and (5) functional tests.[107]

Obtaining the semen sample

The semen sample should be collected in the laboratory; but in special circumstances it can be obtained outside the facility, provided that clear written instructions are given to the patient about obtaining, handling, and transporting the material. A standardized abstinence time is highly recommended to eliminate one of the possible variables that modify sperm characteristics; most laboratories agree that an abstinence interval of 2 to 7 days is acceptable, and the majority suggest a 3-day abstinence before collection. A shorter period of abstinence decreases the sperm count, mainly in the male factor patient, and a longer abstinence decreases motility and acrosine content.

The most common method of obtaining the sample is by masturbation, making sure that no lubrication is used. It has been proposed that a specimen obtained after normal sexual intercourse, which includes foreplay and arousal, is better and more representative, but the majority of laboratories still use masturbation as the main method for collection. Patients who have problems obtaining a semen sample by masturbation can utilize a vibrator, a special plastic condom (Mylex), or a seminal collection device (HDC Corporation, Mountainview, Calif.) to provide a specimen after intercourse. The ideal container, which should be provided by the laboratory, is a 60- 100-mL wide-mouth jar made of polypropylene with a screw cap that fits tightly to prevent loss of semen during transportation.

In terms of the number of samples to be analyzed, if the first specimen is completely within normal limits, the analysis does not need to be repeated. On the other hand, if the specimen is abnormal, at least one more sample is required; under ideal conditions, three samples should be obtained at intervals of 3 to 5 weeks. Each specimen should be accompanied by a form with all the necessary background information and the type of service requested. (See Appendix 29-A, pp. 550-551.) This form is extremely important because it provides the laboratory with all the necessary identification data, the specimen collection details, and the type of analysis requested (Appendix 29-A). If the specimen is not collected in the laboratory it should be delivered, under carefully controlled conditions to avoid temperature shock, within 30 minutes of collection. It is good practice, mainly when a microbiologic investigation is going to be performed, for the patient to wash his hands and penis before collection.

Because of the potential risk to personnel working in an andrology laboratory when they handle specimens that may have come from patients with sexually transmitted diseases, safety guidelines must be carefully followed.[162]

Physical parameters of semen

Volume. The normal volume, according to the World Health Organization (WHO), is 2 mL or more.[162] Volumes less than 1 mL are considered abnormal and can be due to loss of a portion of the sample during collection, obstruction of the genital tract, or retrograde ejaculation.

Color. Normal semen is opaque and is of grayish color; it tends to turn yellow in cases of increased abstinence or infection (pyospermia). It may be of brownish color when red blood cells are present.

Odor. Semen has a strong, characteristic odor that may be caused by oxidation of spermine secreted by the prostate gland.

pH. The normal pH is between 7.2 and 8. Acute infections increase the pH and chronic infections decrease the pH. A pH of less than 7 in azoospermic patients may indicate agenesis of the excretory ducts and accessory glands.

Coagulation. Semen, which is in a liquid state at ejaculation, is rapidly transformed into a coagulum because of the presence of the enzyme protein kinase from the seminal vesicles. Congenital absence of seminal vesicles or severe impairment of function due to chronic infection can be associated with absence of coagulation.

Liquefaction. Liquefaction is produced by proteolytic enzymes secreted by the prostate gland and fibrinogenase and aminopeptidase. Coagulated semen should liquefy within 10 to 20 minutes, certainly within 1 hour. Lack of liquefaction requires laboratory treatment in order to be able to perform the basic semen analysis, mainly by mechanical disruption of the viscous material or exposure to enzymatic substances (bromelain, 1 g/L; plasmin, 0.35 to 0.50 casein units/mL; or chymotrypsin, 150 USP/mL). Immediately after liquefaction is completed, the sample is ready for examination.

Viscosity. Normal semen is slightly viscous, and the presence of a chronic infection (prostatitis, vesiculitis) can increase viscosity. Viscosity can be reduced mechanically by repeated gentle aspiration and ejection, using a small pipette.

Quantitative and qualitative analysis of sperm

Concentration. Analysis of sperm concentration (sperm density), expressed as millions per milliliter, can be done in several different ways: by use of an erythrocyte-counting chamber with a known dilution of the specimen after immobilization of the sperm with 1% formalin, using a micropipette or a glass tuberculin syringe to make the dilution; by use of a special sperm-counting chamber (Makler, Microcell), which allows counting spermatozoa in the undiluted specimen, again after immobilization of the spermatozoa; or by computer-assisted sperm analysis (CASA), which is gaining popularity especially in busy laboratories where saving of technician time is highly desirable.

Different values for a normal count have been proposed in the literature. The WHO[162] proposes 20×10^6 or more spermatozoa per milliliter as the normal figure; and, as always, the efficiency of such a sperm concentration will very much depend on the other sperm characteristics, namely, motility, morphology, agglutination, viscosity, and presence or absence of antisperm antibodies (Table 29-1).

Motility. Sperm motility depends mostly on the anatomic and functional integrity of the sperm midpiece and tail, and also on the efficiency of the sperm energy-generating system (see later). Motility must be judged according to the number of motile sperm; their moving characteristics (speed of progression); the number of immotile, live sperm; and the duration of motility in the in vitro

Table 29-1. Tests and normal values for semen and sperm analysis[162]

Test	Normal value
Standard tests	
Volume	2.0 mL or more
pH	7.2–8.0
Sperm concentration	20×10^6/mL or more
Total sperm count	40×10^6 spermatozoa per ejaculate or more
Motility	50% or more with forward progression or 25% or more with rapid progression within 60 minutes of ejaculation
Morphology	30% or more with normal forms*
Vitality	75% or more live (i.e., excluding dye)
White blood cells	Fewer than 1×10^6/mL
Immunobead test	Fewer than 20% spermatozoa with adherent particles
MAR† test	Fewer than 10% spermatozoa with adherent particles
Optional tests	
α-Glucosidase (neutral)	20 mU or more per ejaculate
Zinc (total)	2.4 μmol or more per ejaculate
Citric acid (total)	52 μmol or more per ejaculate
Acid phosphatase (total)	200 U or more per ejaculate
Fructose (total)	13 μmol or more per ejaculate

*Although no clinical studies have been completed, experience in a number of centers suggests that the percentage of normal forms should be adjusted downward when more strict criteria are applied. An empirical reference value is suggested to be 30% or more with normal forms.
†Mixed antiglobulin reaction.

laboratory system observation. The duration of motility can be judged while the spermatozoa are still in seminal fluid, which is not a physiologic environment; after the spermatozoa are placed in either ovulatory human cervical mucus or bovine cervical mucus; or when the spermatozoa are placed in special culture media. Under any of these conditions, a rapid decay of sperm motility may indicate impaired performance after seminal fluid is deposited in the female genital tract by natural or artificial insemination, but clear interpretation of survivability values has not been proposed. Therefore, unless it is definitely abnormal, other minor departures from the norm cannot be interpreted properly and applied to the clinical decision-making process.

Several classifications have been proposed to describe the types of movement of spermatozoa, mostly by arbitrary-scale systems rating 0 to 4, 1 to 5, or 0 to 10, in which the lowest number means immotile sperm and the highest number indicates normal, aggressive forward movements. Motility is expressed as a percentage in each of the following categories: rapid progressive motility, slow or sluggish progressive motility, in situ movement, and immotility. The results can also be expressed in terms of total sperm motility or total sperm progressive motility. The normal values recommended by the WHO[162] are 50% or more with forward progression, or 25% or more with rapid progression, within 60 minutes of ejaculation (Table 29-1). The use of CASA allows the determination of other param-

eters, such as straight-line velocity (VSL), equal to or greater than 25 μm/s; curvilinear velocity (VCL), greater than 45 μm/s; average path velocity (VAP); linearity (LN), greater than 59 μm/s; amplitude of lateral head displacement (ALH); and mean angular displacement (MAD). These values of normality are tentative, and application of these interpretations to the clinical arena is still uncertain.

The presence of poor motility (asthenospermia) can be due to inadequate collection involving toxic agents at any time during the process (lubricants, regular condoms, inadequate or dirty containers, mixing with vaginal secretions, exposure of the sample to very low or very high temperatures, improper manipulation of the sperm in the laboratory, etc.).

In severe asthenospermia, mainly when combined with teratospermia, electron microscopic investigation of the sperm can detect anatomic abnormalities that certainly are not correctable by treatment and therefore may indicate a permanent condition. Functional abnormalities, mainly in the energy-generating process, can be suspected when low values of adenosine triphosphate (ATP), creatine kinase, or some of the isozymes are found; furthermore, anomalies of the membranes, as detected by the hypoosmotic swelling (HOS) test may indicate abnormal permeability of the membranes, allowing the loss of the components of the energy-generating system. Certainly, abnormalities of sperm maturation (intratesticular or post-testicular) and other pathologic conditions (varicocele, chromosomal abnormalities, infections, and presence of abnormal substances) may also disturb normal motility. The immotile cilia syndrome and the short tail or absent tail syndrome are extreme manifestations of sperm abnormalities determining severe problems with the sperm movement.

Morphology. To be able to judge sperm morphology properly, the laboratory should follow stringent procedures regarding sperm handling and preparation. High-quality smears and stains allow a better evaluation of the sperm morphologic characteristics. Several different stains are used, mainly Papanicolaou, Giemsa, Bryan-Leischman, Shorr, or Diff-Quik. Between 100 and 200 spermatozoa should be screened and studied. Criteria for normality are determined by using normal fertile donor sperm, obtained after interaction with cervical mucus (upper part of the endocervical canal), after interaction with the entire female genital tract (sperm in peritoneal fluid), or after interaction with oocytes (sperm on the surface of the zona pellucida). All of these physiologic mechanisms select for normal sperm morphology, therefore the physical characteristics of the sperm under these conditions can be considered as evidence of sperm normality. The criteria for normal morphology have been defined by the WHO,[162] which has adopted strict criteria for evaluation of semen in assisted reproduction. According to the WHO, the normal head should be oval, and its size after shrinkage due to fixation and staining should be 4.0 to 5.5 μm long and 2.5 to 3.5 μm wide, with a length to width ratio of 1.5:1.75. The acrosomal region should comprise 40% to 70% of the head area. No neck, midpiece, or tail defects should be visualized, and no cytoplasmic droplets more than one third the size of the normal sperm head should be observed. All borderline forms should be considered abnormal. This classification adopted by the WHO is very close to the strict criteria detailed under evaluation of semen in assisted reproduction in this chapter (see later). For details on the morphologic abnormalities of sperm, refer to the *WHO Laboratory Manual for the Examination of Human Semen and Sperm Cervical Mucus Interaction,*[162] and for strict criteria to *Atlas of Human Sperm Morphology* by Menkveld et al.[109]

The predictive value of sperm morphology in natural fertilization has not been clearly addressed in the literature, and it is certainly controversial. van Zyl et al.[156] found a linear relationship between normal sperm morphology and natural fertilization, with a critical threshold of around 4% normal forms, below which the pregnancy rate drops dramatically and more steeply than the linear relationship present over that interval. Despite this dramatic decline (only 11.5% of natural fertilization occurred in this group), pregnancies can still occur, and the authors suggest that extremely good motility can compensate for that. In our experience, the group with excellent count and motility is the one that makes the exception in terms of the poor prognosis for this group.

A computerized system to evaluate morphology by strict criteria has been designed[91] and has shown excellent sensitivity, specificity, reproducibility, and therefore correlation with the results obtained by an experienced technician and with the prediction of fertilization rates.

Normal sperm morphology, according to the WHO,[162] should be 30% or higher. More detailed evaluation of sperm morphology is given later in this chapter.

Viability. The use of supravital staining (eosin, eosin-nigrosin) allows the laboratory to distinguish live immotile sperm from dead sperm. The abnormal permeability of the sperm membranes after death allows the supravital stain to enter the cell, and therefore the cell takes up the particular stain utilized. By using this technique and counting 100 to 200 spermatozoa, the normal semen should not contain more than 25% dead sperm. A higher percentage allows the clinician to diagnose necrospermia; when the condition is severe, no treatment is available.

Other cellular components of semen

The presence of leukocytes (WBC) is very common in semen specimens, most of them being neutrophils. An excess number of leukocytes (greater than 1×10^6/mL) indicates leukospermia. Leukospermia may be due to an infection in the male excretory duct system, mainly in the accessory glands, which must be investigated by history, clinical examination, and bacteriologic analysis of semen and prostatic fluid after prostatic massage and ultrasonography. It is also good practice to do a simultaneous bacteriologic investigation of urine to detect urinary tract infections, either isolated or concomitant. Some of the infections of the male genital tract may be subclinical and therefore asymptomatic. In prostatic fluid obtained by prostatic massage, the number of WBC should not exceed 15 per high-power field (HPF). Between 15 and 40 WBC/HPF is a gray zone, and with more than 40 WBC/HPF, prostatic inflammation is very likely.[162] If prostatic fluid cannot be obtained, urine should be examined after prostatic massage. The presence of WBC can be demonstrated by peroxidase staining, which is a very simple laboratory procedure. The diagnosis of infection in the male genital tract should be followed by adequate antibiotic treatment (e.g., doxycycline, clotrimazole, difloxacin, norfloxacin). These treatments are not very effective in restoring fertility. The presence of leukocytes can cause deterioration of sperm by generating reactive oxygen species (see later), with subsequent damage to sperm membranes, or by the production of cytotoxic cytokines.

If all of these examinations are negative, noninfectious leukospermia is diagnosed, indicating abnormal permeability of the male genital tract to passage of WBC through the walls. Other round cells that may be present in the specimen are immature cells of the spermatogenic line and epithelial cells from the urethra and bladder.

Investigation of seminal fluid

Seminal fluid is a mixture of components from epididymal and ampullary secretions (7% to 10%), seminal vesicles (last portion of ejaculate, 70% to 80% contribution), prostate gland (first portion, 15% to 20% contribution), and urethral glands (3% to 5% contribution). Evaluation of markers for each one of these areas can be performed to detect the level of obstruction, when present, or inflammatory conditions, which usually decrease the level of the markers.

Glycerophosphorylcholine originates mainly from the head of the epididymis and carnitine originates from the caudal portion; both markers have been used to detect impaired function and occlusions. Recently α-glucosidase determination has replaced determination of the other two markers in most laboratories because of its simplicity and equal efficiency.

For the seminal vesicles, the most widely used substance is fructose, produced by the vesicles under the influence of testosterone and dehydrotestosterone. Congenital anomalies, including absence of the seminal vesicles, or obstructions beyond that level (ejaculatory ducts), may prevent fructose from reaching the ejaculate, and therefore may be an indication of the pathology involved. Chronic inflammatory processes of the seminal vesicles (vesiculitis) may also decrease the level of fructose in the ejaculate.

Zinc, citric acid, γ-glutamyl transpeptidase, and acid phosphatase are indicators of prostatic function and can be used to monitor prostatic secretions.

Normal values for semen variables as recommended by the WHO[162] are given in Table 29-1.

EVALUATION OF SEMEN IN ASSISTED REPRODUCTION

The criteria established by the WHO in the 1992 modification[162] have been developed by using mainly pregnancy as an end point, therefore introducing another variable—female fertility—which cannot be evaluated accurately in all instances. Men whose semen quality fulfills the criteria of the WHO are considered fertile and those with semen parameters below those criteria are classified as subfertile, although pregnancy is known to occur with semen values well below those proposed by the WHO. The *subfertile male,* therefore, is the one with semen parameters below the thresholds proposed by the WHO who cannot establish a pregnancy in his female partner; nevertheless, it is possible that, if the same male had sexual intercourse with a female of higher fertility, normal pregnancy could occur. Male subfertility therefore is not an absolute diagnosis, and it certainly has no clearly defined boundaries in the semen analysis. Assisted reproduction in its multiple modalities (intracervical insemination [ICI] or intrauterine insemination [IUI] using natural or stimulated cycles, in vitro fertilization [IVF] and embryo transfer [ET], gamete intrafallopian transfer [GIFT], and zygote intrafallopian transfer

[ZIFT] has been proposed for the treatment of the male factor when all other treatment options have been unsuccessful or when the quality of the sperm is so poor that it is obvious that natural fertilization will not happen. The success rate using therapeutic intrauterine insemination (TII) and ovarian stimulation in women with male factor may produce a clinical pregnancy rate that varies between 3% and 15%,[75-77] with a term pregnancy rate that, in general, is below 10% per insemination cycle in most of the series published.[75-77] It is therefore admissible to use such an empirical treatment before assisted reproduction of higher complexity is utilized. We confine this discussion to the use of IVF and ET in the treatment of male factor.

One of the main problems that is still unresolved is the definition of a male factor in assisted reproduction.[2] In this situation, the end points to judge sperm efficiency are primarily the total fertilization rate and the normal fertilization rate, as well as the implantation, spontaneous abortion, and term pregnancy rates per cycle (retrieval). Series reporting results in the male factor in assisted reproduction by total clinical pregnancy rate per transfer are clearly misleading, because they ignore the patients who do not reach transfer because of lack of fertilization, as well as the potential higher spontaneous abortion rates in pregnancies established by abnormal sperm.[2]

In order to define normal fertilization rates, each embryology laboratory should determine the performance of normal gamete interaction. In the Norfolk program (1989-1991), this point was investigated by using oocytes from women participating in the IVF program who had a pure tubal factor, who had a normal follicle-stimulating hormone (FSH)-luteinizing hormone (LH) ratio on day 3 of the menstrual cycle, who produced three or more preovulatory oocytes at retrieval, and who were inseminated with sperm of normal laboratory characteristics. In 173 cycles producing 1305 oocytes, the total fertilization rate (total number of oocytes fertilized/total number of oocytes inseminated) was 89.3% ± 20.3% (mean ± SD), and the normal fertilization rate (total number of oocytes with normal fertilization/total number of oocytes inseminated) was 78.7 ± 22.3% (mean ± SD). The minimum total fertilization rate that can be considered normal in the Norfolk program (mean − 2 SD) is therefore 48.7% and the minimum normal fertilization rate is 34.1%. Similar figures in the University of Stellenbosch program (59 cycles, 589 oocytes) revealed a total minimum fertilization rate of 55% and a minimum normal fertilization rate of 37%, almost identical with the Norfolk figures. In other words, fertilization values below 50% and 35%, respectively, should be considered abnormal, and in the presence of normal stimulation and morphologically normal oocytes with sperm abnormalities detected, it should be ascribed to a *male factor in assisted reproduction.*

The introduction of corrective measures may improve low fertilization rates, but they seldom, if ever, will reach the fertilization efficiency of normal gametes.[115] Except for a poor prognosis pattern of morphology (P-pattern), as described later, no other sperm parameters allowed us to identify sperm with low fertilizing ability, unless extreme deteriorating conditions were present in the other sperm parameters; therefore IVF becomes the final test for sperm efficiency in the male factor.

These definitions do not represent pure semantics; spermatozoa that are classified as subfertile according to the WHO criteria but that fertilize normally in the IVF system cannot be considered to represent a male factor in assisted reproduction. If this kind of patient is included, the results would improve substantially and they would be significantly better in those cases.

Although in the majority of cases with no fertilization either a sperm factor or an oocyte factor can be identified, there are some with no detectable abnormalities of the gametes; in such cases, whenever possible, a cross-match test should be performed, allowing sperm from the husband and a fertile male donor to interact with the oocytes of the wife and a female donor, until the first evidence of fertilization is present (two pronuclei). At that time, the fertilized oocytes should not be allowed to continue development, or they can be transferred later, according to patient's desire. Immature oocytes matured in vitro from the patient and from another consenting patient treated on the same day can be utilized, together with the husband's sperm and fertile donor sperm from the sperm bank. Usually a final diagnosis can be made if this type of in vitro test is utilized.[2] Being able to determine the gamete at fault not only is reassuring but allows the proposal of a better therapeutic plan. In the event that a cross-match test cannot be performed, careful observation of the sperm attachment to the zona pellucida in the in vitro system and evaluation of the sperm-zona interaction by the hemizona assay may give further information on the nature of the problem.

As the male factor becomes progressively more severe, it may reach a point when the sperm quality will not allow fertilization. This type of problem should be recognized, because the patient may need systemic treatment, special laboratory preparation techniques, or micromanipulation assistance (assisted fertilization) in order to achieve fertilization.

The clinical male factor is usually treated empirically by medical means (gonadotropins, androgens, antiestrogens, or aromatase inhibitors) or by surgery, according to the etiologic factors presumptively involved, in an attempt to improve sperm quality to achieve pregnancy naturally. The male factor in assisted reproduction can also be treated empirically, not with the idea of normalizing sperm characteristics, but trying to improve them or stabilizing their quality in patients providing very different samples, to provide better sperm for the embryology laboratory to work with. The intractable severe male factor leaves no option but assisted fertilization (micromanipulation).

The criteria for semen normality, according to the

WHO,[162] should be determined by each laboratory using information obtained from men whose partners recently achieved pregnancy, preferably within 12 months of female interruption of contraception. The normal values recommended by the WHO in 1992 are described in Table 29-1. In the Norfolk program, we suspect the possibility of a male factor in assisted reproduction when the sperm density is less than 20×10^6 sperm per milliliter, when the sperm total progressive motility is less than 30%, when the sperm normal morphology is less than 14%, and when the total recovered sperm motile fraction after swim-up is less than 5×10^6. It becomes severe, and therefore fertilization is considered doubtful, when the sperm morphology is less than 4% (poor prognosis pattern), sperm density is less than 5×10^6/mL, motility is less than 10%, and the total motile fraction recovered after swim-up is less than 1.5×10^6. A hemizona index of less than 36% may indicate no fertilization in 75% of the cases.

The same semen evaluation methodologies indicated for the clinical male factor can be used for evaluation of semen in assisted reproduction, namely, basic semen analysis; bacteriologic and immunologic investigation; characteristics of sperm recovered after using some of the separation procedures and tests of sperm function, such as acrosin activity and ATP and creatinine kinase (CK) content; sperm cervical mucus penetration assay; HOS test, acrosome reaction test, hamster zona–free penetration assay, and hemizona assay. Despite all these investigations, the definitive test is IVF in a well-established laboratory.

Basic semen analysis

The general requirements for semen collection have already been described. The general characteristics of semen, coagulation, liquefaction, and viscosity, if grossly abnormal, should be reported to the embryology laboratory to alert it of possible difficulties in semen processing. Volume, unless it is extremely low, should not represent a problem for the embryology laboratory.

Sperm density. In the Norfolk experience, when the sperm density is below 20 million per milliliter, a clear effect on fertilization rate can be seen, with a decrease in fertilization rate to around 60% but no impact in pregnancy rate; when the sperm density is less than 10 million, the fertilization rate drops below 50% and the pregnancy rate is impaired; with a density below 5 million, there is a further drop to 30% and the term pregnancy rate is also decreased. Sperm density below 1 million represents a very severe male problem, and fertilization most likely will not occur. Unfortunately, sperm density, as any one of the other parameters, cannot be judged as an isolated factor, because it is usually combined with modifications of motility and morphology, which makes overall evaluation more difficult.

Sperm motility plays a secondary role in the IVF results, and even samples with slightly less than 10% progressive motility still are able to fertilize as long as the other parameters are acceptable. Nevertheless, specimens with less than 10% progressive motility should be considered as severe male factor in assisted reproduction, mainly when abnormalities are present in the other parameters.

Patients with poor sperm density and motility should be treated empirically to try to improve these characteristics and provide the embryology laboratory with a better specimen. A similar approach can be taken with patients who deliver sperm samples with extremely variable parameters; systemic treatment can stabilize the count and motility in some of these cases.

Computer-assisted sperm analysis. The introduction of automated assessment of the sperm by CASA allows determination of several different characteristics of sperm motility that cannot be determined manually. A pattern of motility, including mean velocity, mean linearity, fertility index, curvilinear velocity, and amplitude of lateral head displacement, introduced a kinematic approach to the sperm motility evaluation that may help in prediction of fertilization. Barlow et al.[11] reviewed the correlation of fertilizing ability of sperm with several different parameters evaluated by manual and computer-assisted methods, both in fresh semen and in preparations after swim-up, and found a significant correlation among sperm concentration, motility, velocity, vitality, and normal morphology in both types of specimens. They propose a predictive function to calculate the potential fertilization rate for a patient by using the post–swim-up motility and the normal sperm morphology in the fresh sample. There are several CASA systems on the market that allow investigation of these parameters.

Sperm motility. Evaluation of hyperactivated motility can also be added to the prediction armamentarium; this type of motility is one of several expressions of sperm capacitation. It was described originally in laboratory animals (hamsters) by Yanagimachi,[164] and currently efforts are being made to define similar changes in human sperm.[25,26,113] Hyperactivated motility can be evaluated by high-speed videomicrography with slow-motion analysis or by standard videomicrography with time-exposure analysis. Several patterns of hyperactivation have been identified: circling, high curvature, thrashing, helical, and star-spin.[26] Three criteria have been proposed to automatically determine hyperactivated motility[26]: linearity ≥ 65 μm, velocity ≥ 100 mm, and head displacement ≥ 7.5 mm. Wang et al.[159] investigated this type of motility in fresh and post–swim-up specimens, as well as in specimens 24 hours after incubation. Hyperactivated motility reached a peak at 1 hour and plateaued at 3 hours, and no correlation was found between the presence of hyperactivated motility and the sperm penetration assay in the hamster system. In the abnormal samples, the incidence of hyperactivated motility and the percentage with star-spin at 3 hours were significantly lower. Wang et al.[159] believe that hyperactivated motility may be useful as an early indicator of capacitation abnormalities in human spermatozoa that are not measured by the sperm penetration test (SPA). Murad et al.[114] concluded that the expression of hyperactivated motility requires interdependent changes at the axonemal and cytosolic levels, and determined that the highest percentage of hyperactivation was induced by decomplemented fetal cord serum in the medium.

We are still in need of a simplified method of evaluation of hyperactivated motility and a clear demonstration of a correlation with the fertilization ability of the sperm in order to be able to incorporate hyperactivated motility into the clinical arena. The complicated and expensive equipment needed, the difficulties in studying a large number of sperm by this method, the discrepancies in the descriptions and interpretation of sperm hyperactivated patterns in men, the change in pattern of motility in the same sperm with time, the lack of sufficient studies showing a positive correlation between this type of sperm motility and fertilization in vitro or fertilizability in vivo, and the small number of sperm detected in the hyperactivated state in some reports indicate that this method will not be available in the clinical evaluation of sperm parameters for quite some time.

Agents modifying conditions of sperm to induce better motility and hyperactivated motility have been tried in the human in vitro system. One of these agents is the steroid-rich fraction of human follicular fluid,[106] due to the presence of progesterone and 17-hydroxyprogesterone, which stimulate the calcium flux[18] and therefore improve motility. When the calcium ionophore is used, the number of hyperactivated sperm is significantly reduced[65] and the presence of a cumulus oophorus or a solubilized cumulus intercellular matrix induces a linear high-velocity motility different from the hyperactivated one that is reduced.[146] Other agents have also been used to improve the ability of the sperm to move adequately. Imoedemhe et al.,[73] who studied normal human spermatozoa that had been exposed to different concentrations of caffeine, were able to demonstrate a significant improvement in the various motility parameters in a dose-dependent manner, but such improvement did not lead to improvement in the fertilization rates; high concentrations adversely affected the fertilization rate, and embryonic development was also retarded. Imoedemhe et al. do not recommend, for the time being, the use of this stimulant in assisted reproduction programs. The same investigators[74] had used 2-deoxyadenosine for the same purposes in asthenospermic males. The sperm motility pattern was significantly improved, as well as the number of sperm recovered, and the fertilization rates were also enhanced, with a higher number of embryos being replaced. The pregnancy rate was comparable to the historic pregnancy rates for the group, so Imoedemhe et al. do not believe that 2-deoxyadenosine has an adverse effect on embryonic development, although they have not been able to assess actual preembryos. Lacham,[92] using the mouse model, demonstrated that 2-deoxyadenosine produced significant embryonic arrest between the two-cell and four-cell stage. In the human, 2-deoxyadenosine induced 80% blockage. Pentoxifylline showed a similar effect, but it was not statistically significant. Adenosine is a very potent blocker of the G-1 or G-2 phase of the cell cycle. Pentoxifylline, on the other hand, seems to have the advantage of reducing production of superoxide anions by human spermatozoa.[61] Chao et al.[32] have also used human follicular fluid to stimulate sperm motility and velocity. The amplitude increase in motility peaked at 12 hours, and the amplitude increase in curvilinear velocity also peaked at 12 hours after sperm washing in phosphate-buffered saline. They believe that there is a nondialyzable and heat-stable factor with a molecular weight of around 50,000 in human follicular fluid that improved and maintained the motility and velocity of washed human sperm.

Sperm morphology. The last crucial parameter to be investigated in semen analysis is morphology, using either the WHO[162] or Dusseldorf guidelines,[68] or the strict criteria for head and neck normality as proposed by the University of Stellenbosch and modified by Norfolk, which allows better reproducibility, predictability of fertilization, and/or pregnancy outcome.[88] A high number of sperm morphologic abnormalities seem to be characteristic of men; however, spermatozoa selected by cervical mucus screening after ejaculation in the vagina, recovered from the peritoneal cavity, or attached to the surface of the zona pellucida show morphologic characteristics that are normal, and the population's morphology is homogenous. The characteristics of these populations can be used to determine the criteria for normal morphology.

The classification used in our laboratory is a modification of the methods of MacLeod and Gold[99] and Eliasson,[51] taking into account the total morphologic characteristics of the sperm. Normal, ideal spermatozoa, according to strict criteria, should have a well-defined acrosome comprising between 40% and 70% of the sperm-head area and a small, perfectly oval head or one that tapers slightly at the level of the postacrosomal region. The head length should be between 3 and 5 μm and the width should be between 2 and 3 μm when Papanicolaou staining is used; the head length should be 5 to 6 μm and the width should be 3 to 4 μm when Diff-Quik[92] staining is used. No abnormalities in the neck, midpiece, or tail should be present. The midpiece should be slender, axially attached, and less than 1 μm in width; the length should be approximately 1.5 times the head length. No cytoplasmic droplets larger than half the area of the sperm head should be present. The tail should be uniform, slightly thinner than the mid-piece, uncoiled, and approximately 45 μm in length. Trivial variations in head morphology may still be considered normal, but borderline-normal heads are classified in a different category: slightly abnormal forms.

Acrosomal abnormalities can be classified as secondary when changes in the sperm membranes are determined by external factors or when there is loss of acrosome content due to damage or aging; in some of these cases the abnormalities may be reversible. The term *primary acrosomal abnormalities* is used when the changes occur during development and differentiation of the spermatozoa, and may be caused by abnormal formation, distribution, or attachment of the acrosome. Head abnormalities that may be considered major may affect size, shape, and the presence of vacuoles. Elongated or tapered heads may be caused by environmental factors or stress. Minor head abnormalities are of unknown significance.

Midpiece anomalies involve mitochondria, centrioles, microtubular formation, and/or retention of abnormally large cytoplasmic droplets. This type of abnormality may occur in an isolated fashion or may be present simultaneously with both head and tail defects. Tail abnormalities are characterized by various degrees of coiling with an intact plasma membrane, duplication, angulations, and other variations.

Using these criteria, a population with normal fertilization rates in IVF shows more than 14% normal forms; figures below 14% indicate progressive deterioration of sperm morphology and, consequently, of function. Two subgroups have been identified within this abnormal group: patients who have between 5% and 14% normal forms are considered to have a good prognosis pattern (G-pattern), and patients with 4% or less normal forms are considered to have a poor prognosis pattern (P-pattern) and show the worst performance in IVF.[90] This type of evaluation should be carried out in at least 200 sperm cells per slide.

The normal male population having more than 14% normal sperm forms has a morphology index (summation of normal forms plus slightly abnormal forms) of more than 40%; patients with a P-pattern have a morphology index well below 30%, and the G-pattern subgroup constitutes an intermediate category whose prognosis is more difficult to establish, and is perhaps in between that of the other two groups; its morphology index is between 30% and 40%. When a discrepancy is found between the percentage of abnormal morphology and the morphology index, the former seems to be a more reliable parameter for prediction.

The G-pattern must be judged according to its characteristics. All those that are very close to the P-pattern should be considered as having a poor prognosis; those that are close to the normal pattern should be considered as having a much better function.

Performance of each sperm group and subgroup is clearly different in IVF.[2] When insemination was performed using the regular 50,000 to 100,000 sperm per milliliter per egg in 3 mL, as is done in our laboratory, patients with normal sperm morphology had a fertilization rate of 88.3%. Meanwhile, patients with less than 14% normal forms showed a fertilization rate of 49.5%. The pregnancy rate per retrieval or per transfer was also significantly lower in this group. Patients with a G-pattern, on the other hand, had a fertilization rate of 63.9%, and patients with a P-pattern showed only 7.6% fertilization capacity.[90]

The fertilization decrease in the P-pattern can be corrected, partially, by a fivefold to tenfold increase in the number of sperm used at insemination (500,000 to 1,000,000 sperm per milliliter per egg). When these corrective measures are used, the fertilization rate improves to 63.6%, or up to 89.8% as demonstrated in the original work.[115] The spontaneous abortion rate may be high; therefore the ongoing term pregnancy rates per cycle and per transfer are much lower. In a more recent evaluation of a larger number of patients in Norfolk (1988-1989),[2] in terms of fertilization rate of preovulatory oocytes in 381 cycles performed using sperm of normal characteristics with a concentration at insemination of $120.6 \pm 26.5 \times 10^5$ (mean $\pm$ SD) sperm per milliliter per egg, a fertilization rate of 92.6% and subsequent total pregnancy rates per cycle and per transfer of 26.1% and 28.0% were achieved, respectively, and term/ongoing pregnancy rates of 17.3% and 18.5% were obtained. In the P-pattern group, using $1.3 \pm 0.1 \times 10^6$ sperm per milliliter per egg as sperm concentration at insemination, the fertilization rate was 55.6%, the total pregnancy rates per cycle and per transfer were 17.1% and 23.2%, and the term/ongoing pregnancy rates per cycle and per transfer were 7.8% and 10.7%, respectively, in a total of 76 cycles examined. Meanwhile, in the G-pattern subgroup, using a $6.4 \pm 0.5 \times 10^5$ sperm concentration at insemination, the fertilization rate was quite satisfactory (85.2%), the total pregnancy rates per cycle and per transfer were 22.4% and 24.0%, but the term/ongoing pregnancy rates per cycle and per transfer decreased to 11.2% and 12.0%. The abortion rate in the normal sperm population group was 34%, in the G-pattern it was 50%, and in the P-pattern it was 53%. These figures seem to indicate a severe impairment of results in terms of IVF when abnormal spermatozoa are used with both the G-pattern and P-pattern, although the P-pattern continues to show the poorest outcome. The results in male factor treatment by assisted reproduction accordingly should be reported as term pregnancy rate by cycle of aspiration in order to express the real efficiency of the sperm in establishing term pregnancies.

On the other hand, as in any biologic system, there are exceptions to these rules. Patients with a P-pattern of morphology but excellent sperm density and motility may behave in a completely different fashion, and even spontaneous pregnancies are possible in this category.

This information obtained in the human IVF system can be confirmed in the heterologous hamster SPA and in the homologous hemizona assay, as is seen later in this chapter. We therefore propose that, using these criteria for morphology diagnosis, severely dysmorphic spermatozoa will perform poorly; therefore the prognosis for those patients is not even close to the prognosis for patients with a normal sperm population. Similar results were obtained by Enginsu et al.,[52] who also found the strict criteria much more useful in predicting fertilization than the HOS test and the WHO criteria.

Sperm separation procedures. Despite all the efforts to determine the sperm fertilizing ability by the close scrutiny of each one of the parameters, there is something else that cannot be assessed properly by them. If spermatozoa are put under stress by some laboratory procedures, it can be demonstrated that their performance is worse than could be predicted by studying the fresh sample. For instance, if a sperm separation procedure is performed by using a swim-up technique, this seems to give an overall evaluation of the effect of each and every abnormality found in the specimen in the final quality and potential efficiency of the sperm. Early in the Norfolk program it was determined that when the double-wash, double-swim-up technique was used, less than 1.5×10^6 total motile sperm were recovered from the specimen, and results of fertilization were greatly decreased.[155] Reinvestigation of this matter during the years 1988-1989 revealed very few exceptions, even when insemination in a microtiter dish was performed. When the motility before and after swim-up was compared in 73 cases, 41.1% improvement was obtained, with highly significant differences between motility before and after swim-up.[3] One should remember that the selection of the highly motile fraction is achieved after losing a high proportion of sperm that will never be available for utilization in the actual process of insemination, unless the pellet is resuspended and utilized. Only 10% to 30% of the motile sperm present are recovered by this procedure. Similar considerations could be made for morphologic characteristics of the sperm recovered.[3] A significant increase is obtained in the percentage of normal forms and the morphology index in the post–swim-up specimen at the expense of losing a tremendous amount of sperm.

In terms of separation of the motile sperm fraction for therapeutic purposes at the time of IVF insemination, different methodologic procedures can be used. In very poor specimens with borderline parameters (severe male factor in assisted reproduction by Norfolk criteria), simple washing by dilution and centrifugation can be utilized. Sperm-washing techniques do not remove dead sperm cells, which according to results in zona-free hamster eggs decrease and impair the process of sperm fusion with hamster oocytes.[125] The regular swim-up procedure in those cases will diminish substantially the number of sperm available and therefore the chances of fertilization. Unfortunately, damage to the sperm mainly in abnormal samples has been reported with this technique, due either to the centrifugation process itself or to oxidative stress (hydrogen peroxide generation), which impairs lipid quality at the sperm membrane level.[6] These mechanisms of oxidative stress most likely are caused by sedimentation of the sperm, together with other cellular and particulate matters, although spermatozoa themselves, mainly when they are abnormal, produce oxidation substances that can stimulate lipid peroxidation and modify the membranes. Aitken and Buckingham[7] have utilized 7-dimethylaminonaphthalin-1,2-dicarbolic acid hydrazide, a luminol analogue, in combination with horseradish peroxidase to enhance the detection of reactive oxygen species produced by human spermatozoa. DeLamirande and Gagnon,[44] using Percoll-separated spermatozoa treated with hydrogen peroxide or the combination xanthine and xanthine oxidase, noticed a progressive decrease leading to complete arrest in sperm flagellar beat frequency; partial recovery could be obtained if the spermatozoa were demembranated in a medium containing magnesium-ATP; the recovery was transient. The most damaging effect came from hydrogen peroxide, but oxygen and hydroxy radicals also played a role. ATP depletion, according to those authors,[44] induced by reactive oxygen species generation, was responsible for the effects observed in the sperm. Kobayashi et al.[86] used superoxide dismutase to try to inhibit lipid peroxidation, which causes loss of motility in human spermatozoa. The addition of exogenous superoxide dismutase to the sperm suspension significantly decreased the loss of motility and increased the concentration of malonodialdehyde in spermatozoa, suggesting the possibility of using this agent to improve the situation. Other less popular migration procedures are the migration into albumin or into an intraviscous hyaluronate layer.

Another way to recover a more efficient sperm motile fraction is to use gradient or column separation procedures. The best known one utilizes silicone particles coated with polyvinyl pyrrolidone (Percoll) in continuous or discontinuous gradients. This avoids the oxidation stress referred to previously and allows the recovery of a proportion of sperm cells similar to or higher than that recovered by swim-up. Furthermore, it seems to favor capacitation and membrane fusion.

A trial was made in the Norfolk program to compare the effect of the swim-up separation in spermatozoa from patients with G-patterns and P-patterns of morphology.[117] The only difference found in the fresh specimen before processing was a significantly less mean velocity in the P-pattern; after swim-up, the percentage motility was also significantly lower in that group, and the velocity and linearity were decreased, although the decrease did not reach statistical significance. As a final result, a recovery rate of 42.0% ± 4% (mean ± SD) in the G-pattern group, versus 19% ± 2.8% in the P-pattern group, was observed. This seemed to indicate that, although minor differences can be found in terms of motility, a more significant difference is seen after swim-up in terms of total motile recovery fraction and recovery rate.

Immunologic investigation

Although immunologic infertility and sperm antibodies are discussed in Chapters 21 and 22, we review briefly the sperm antibody investigation in the male with reference to IVF. The majority of the publications trying to establish the correlation between antisperm antibodies (ASA) and IVF results have concluded that fertilization rates were impaired,[33,34,41,83,84] but very few have focused on the pure impact of ASA when all other semen parameters are kept constant. Furthermore, the presence of ASA has been associated with lower sperm motility in the majority of the reviews,[12,104] some found no correlation, and a single report noted an improvement in motility characteristics.[166]

There are several methodologic difficulties in interpreting these results. A review of our material at Norfolk[4] indicated that, even when sperm density and motility are kept constant and the morphology pattern is taken into consideration, the presence of ASA has a clear impact on the fertilization rate. The fertilization rates in the control group with no ASA and in the study group with ASA were 77.9% and 41.8%; in the G-pattern group without ASA the fertilization rate was 82.8%, and with ASA it was 52.2%; in the P-pattern group without ASA it was 67.8% versus 18.5% when ASA were present. All of these differences were highly significant. The total pregnancy rates per transfer and per cycle in the control group (60% and 65%, respectively) were significantly higher than those in the study group (23.5% and 21%), as well as the term pregnancy rates per transfer and per cycle (48% and 52% in the control group and 14.7% and 13.1% in the study group). These differences may be due to problems with implantation, because the spontaneous abortion rates were not significantly different. The measure proposed to improve this situation was to increase sperm concentration at insemination in an effort to ensure at least 50,000 unbound sperm around the oocyte[66]; this procedure is similar to that which our group has suggested in cases with abnormal morphology, with sperm collection into medium containing 50% maternal serum or albumin fraction.[50] Franken et al.,[59] using the hemizona assay, found a significant reduction in the average number of spermatozoa tightly bound to the zona pellucida in the patients with positive ASA, as characterized by the direct immunobead test. Seven of the nine couples involved eventually had success with fertilization using IUI or GIFT, and one couple conceived with natural coital insemination.

Bacteriologic screening

Bacteriologic screening should be carried out not only in those specimens that show high concentration of WBC (leukospermia), but also as a routine investigation in patients who are candidates for IVF. It is imperative to search for the presence of *Neisseria gonorrhoeae* and mycoplasma strains, including *Ureaplasma urealyticum* and *Chlamydia trachomatis,* using monoclonal antibodies labeled with fluorescein that are specific to the main membrane protein of the parasite, as well as to investigate the general flora in the specimen. The presence of infection in the semen used for insemination at the time of IVF has proved detrimental to fertilization; therefore any active process should be properly treated before the IVF attempt.

Tests of spermatozoal function

Adenosine triphosphate and creatine kinase system in sperm. Since the recognition that a semen sample is composed of a heterogenous sperm population, the shortcomings of the basic semen analysis have been apparent, one being the inability of that test to be of accurate diagnostic and prognostic value in assisted reproduction. New approaches based on biochemical and molecular markers of sperm function have been pursued. However, no single evaluation has been developed as yet to predict the sperm fertilizing ability.

Many sperm functions are energy-requiring processes, and the evaluation of biochemical markers of sperm energy metabolism seems to be a logical approach. Among them, the determination of sperm ATP content and the activity of phosphocreatine kinase (CK) and sperm-specific lactate dehydrogenase (LDH-C4, LDH-X) are typical examples. The most commonly accepted viewpoint is that sperm cells are able to synthesize the energy-source ATP needed by utilizing a variety of exogenous substrates such as glucose, fructose, pyruvate, and lactate. This is accomplished via the glycolytic pathway or the oxidative phosphorylation in sperm mitochondria. More than 45 years ago Ivanov et al.[78] suggested that the ATP thus formed diffuses in the sperm flagellum and is used by the sperm to maintain its important energy-requiring functions. In several recent investigations it has been suggested that ATP alone may not be the only factor involved in the subcellular biochemical energy accumulation of the sperm.[40,137,142,152] Saks et al.,[132] in their studies of cardiac muscle cells, reported that, although ATP utilization occurs in muscle contractions, the use of ATP cannot be detected. The implication is that the ATP pool is kept at a constant level at the expense of another energy source. Another energy supply at the sperm level is the phosphocreatine (creatine phosphate) system. ATP produced is converted to phosphocreatine in mitochondria, giving rise to ADP for further ATP synthesis. Phosphocreatine diffuses out from the site of production to the sites of utilization, where it can be dephosphorylated to produce ATP. Under normal conditions, this mechanism allows the immediate energy source, ATP, to be kept at an adequate level while the reserve source, phosphocreatine, is synthesized, transferred, accumulated, and utilized as needed.

Several investigators have reported the existence of a similar mechanism in sperm.[81,137,142] It is believed that via this "shuttle system" ATP is transferred from the site of synthesis to the sites of utilization, namely, the sperm membranes and the dynein arms of the flagellum (Fig. 29-1).

The enzyme responsible for the reversible conversion of ATP to phosphocreatine is ATP:creatine *N*-phosphotransferase (creatine kinase, CK). Since the equilibrium constant for the conversion is low and the ATP production from phosphocreatine is kinetically favorable, there must be different types of CK to direct this reversible reaction toward the desired direction. In mitochondria, a mitochondrial type of CK converts ATP to phosphocreatine, and at the site of utilization another CK subtype catalyzes the reverse reaction. In the sea urchin, the CK of the sperm head is in the conventional range of 40 kd, whereas the flagellar type has been identified to be 145 kd.[150,161] Specific inhibition of CK by low levels of 1-fluoro-2,4-dinitrobenzene attenuates flagellar beating, indicating that the energy shuttle involves CK and that it is essential for normal flagellar motion. CK was reported to be associated with the flagellar axonemes and may bind directly to polarize flagellar microtubules.[149,161] There are three CK subtypes (isoenzymes) identified in humans: CK-MM, CK-MB, and CK-BB. With high-voltage electrophoresis, these isoenzymes can further be subdivided to six isoforms as they exist in the body. Isoforms of CK-MM and CK-BB have been detected in human sperm and are believed to be involved in the proposed phosphocreatine shuttle system.

LDH, on the other hand, found in many organs, has five major isoenzymes. A sixth isoenzyme, LDH-C4 (LDH-X), is found specifically in ejaculated sperm.[21,62] Its gene locus is on chromosome 11 and it is initially expressed in primary spermatocytes. Since it is unique to sperm, autoimmunity against it may occur spontaneously or can be stimulated to try to develop a contraceptive method.[53] LDH catalyzes interconversion of lactate and pyruvate, two important energy substrates for sperm. Its evaluation may be useful in some instances. The locations of these isoenzymes have been reported to be in the sperm cytosol and in mitochondrial matrix.

The relative value of ATP, CK, or LDH-C4 determinations in assisted reproduction has been reported by several investigators. Calamera et al.[29] and Comhaire et al.[36,37] found a close relationship between sperm ATP content and sperm motility and fertilizing potential in a therapeutic insemination program. Our own limited study of samples used for IVF showed a good negative correlation ($P < .001$) between the sperm ATP content in the swim-up sample and the pregnancy outcome. Swim-up samples with ATP levels below 40 pmol/10^6 sperm showed no pregnancies.[111] Chan and Wang[31] determined ATP levels in whole semen and found no correlation with penetration in the hamster zona-free oocyte system. Methodologic differences may very well be the reason for such discrepancies. There have been several reports of

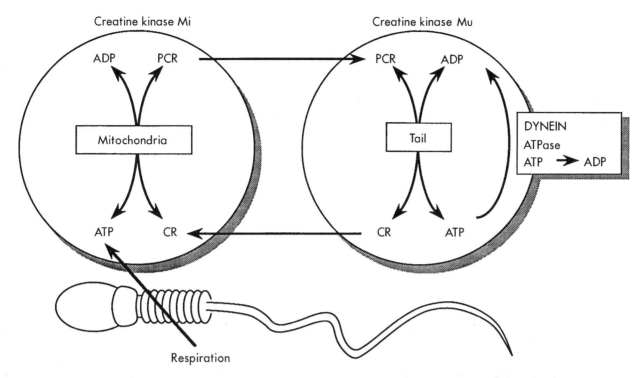

Fig. 29-1. The sperm creatine phosphate shuttle model. The sperm mitochondria and tail are the sites of the ATP production (respiration) and ATP consumption (dynein ATPase). The creatine phosphate/creatine system and the mitochondrial and muscle type creatine kinase isoenzymes facilitate the energy transfer between the two compartments. Creatine is phosphorylated by the mitochondrial creatine kinase and the creatine phosphate diffuses to the sperm tail. The high-energy phosphate is used for the rephosphorylation of ADP to ATP by the muscle type flagellar creatine kinase. The creatine is then available for a further phosphorylation cycle in the mitochondrion. *PCR,* Creatine phosphate; *Mi* and *Mu,* mitochondrial and muscle type creatine kinase. (Redrawn with permission from Tombes RM, Shapiro BM: *Cell* 41:325, 1985; Copyright 1985, Cell Press, Cambridge, Mass.)

close association between the sperm total CK content and the rate CK-MM/CK-BB plus CK-MM in samples used in assisted reproduction with the fertilization rate.[69-72] It has also been reported that oligospermic patients have much higher total CK per sperm and much lower CK-MM than do normospermic patients.[71] Higher total CK values have been correlated with a higher incidence of the presence of sperm cells with cytoplasmic droplets in oligospermic samples. The presence of higher CK-MM as compared with CK-BB is an indication of sperm maturity.

The role of LDH-C4 evaluation in assisted reproduction has not been investigated fully. Simultaneous determination of ATP, CK, and LDH-C4 perhaps will be of value diagnostically and prognostically. Since the process of sperm and egg interaction and fertilization is very complex, it is likely that problems can emerge at different steps of that process; therefore no single test, biochemical parameter, or marker can be accurate in all patients.

The WHO designed a prospective study to evaluate sperm characteristics and ATP content to try to predict the occurrence of pregnancy in infertile couples. Neither the common sperm parameters nor ATP content were good predictors.[161]

The levels of ATP have been reported to be lower in patients with good motility in terms of both mean sperm ATP concentration and ATP concentration per living spermatozoa, the implication being that highly motile spermatozoa consume more ATP than do sperm with impaired motility.[64] DeLamirande and Gagnon[44] have proposed that reactive oxygen species induce ATP depletion in the sperm, resulting mainly in loss of sperm motility due to axonemal damage induced by the depletion of ATP. All these studies, although very significant in understanding sperm physiology and some aspects of sperm pathophysiology, do not allow us to propose ATP determination as a routine test in evaluating sperm.

Reactive oxygen species. Human sperm can generate reactive oxygen species (ROS), mainly superoxide anion and hydrogen peroxide. Cells present in semen, especially WBC, have similar properties. The higher the number of WBC present and the lower the quality of the sperm cells, the higher the generating capacity and the levels of ROS, which in turn have an uncanny ability to damage the sperm plasma membrane. Special systems are present in semen to reduce the concentration of ROS.

Measurements of ROS have been proposed as a way to determine dangerous levels that may indicate the need for different sperm laboratory manipulation to reduce their damaging effects, for instance, use of Percoll gradient separation techniques instead of the routine swim-up procedure. The chemiluminescence technique of enhanced sensitivity is used to measure these substances in sperm.[7] Peroxidation damage of the cell membrane and the axonemes[43] impairs the ability of sperm to bind as well as to move. DeLamirande and Gagnon[44] concluded that the axoneme damage is due to ATP depletion. Determination of the presence of ROS and ROS measurement tests should be a goal of all well-equipped andrology laboratories in order to be able to detect those samples that are at high risk for ROS damage.

Acrosine determination. Sperm acrosine is a serum proteinase with the ability of cleaving peptide bonds containing arginine or lysine amino acid residues. Although it is one of the many enzymes contained within the acrosome, it has also been described on the surface of the sperm, perhaps by permeating through the sperm membranes.[145] Acrosine is involved in enhancing the acrosome reaction after it is triggered by sperm binding to ZP-3 on the surface of the zona pellucida, as well as in the sperm penetration of the zona.[129] Proacrosine, an inactive zymogen, is the precursor, and the total activity of the proacrosine-acrosine system needs to be evaluated in the sperm analysis.

Total acrosine activity was measured in the Norfolk andrology laboratory by a variation of the method proposed by Goodpasture et al.[63] There have been contradictory results in the literature with regard to the acrosine value in predicting IVF results. Liu and Baker[95] did not find that acrosine levels and the proportion of spermatozoa with normal intact acrosomes in semen were significantly related to the fertilization rate in vitro. Tummon et al.[154] found a good correlation between IVF and acrosine levels. Mahony et al.[101] in our laboratory reevaluated the program by using a commercially available kit Accu-Sperm; OEM Concepts, Toms River, N.J., which is used at present. The results obtained with this kit showed a positive correlation with the method described by Kennedy and associates.[84] The Accu-Sperm kit is valuable because it requires a minute amount of semen (100 μL) to complete the assay. Of 57 couples evaluated, 7 showed poor fertilization rates in IVF (<50%), 6 of whom had an acrosine activity index in the potentially subfertile or infertile range according to manufacturer's guidelines. A significant relationship was found between fertilization rate and acrosine activity. However, a 9% false-negative rate in which patients with good fertilization showed poor acrosine activity makes the value of the test doubtful in this preliminary investigation. Furthermore, the accuracy of the test depends on the accurate determination of sperm concentration; therefore the procedure becomes

difficult in specimens that are very viscous, for instance. Liu and Baker,[96] in a more recent review of several tests of sperm function to predict fertilization in vitro, did not list acrosine activity as one of the reliable tests. Jeyendran et al.[79] have suggested that several sperm populations are present in the ejaculate and that the best fraction is characterized by more sperm with progressive motility and increased acrosine content, as well as a positive HOS test and SPA. Nevertheless, the relationship with fertilization rate in vitro is not established. Francavilla et al.[54] studied bioactive and immunoreactive acrosine and found the content to be inversely correlated with the percentage of spermatozoa with an abnormal head. The authors proposed that a lower sperm acrosine activity in teratospermic ejaculates is due to an intrinsic defect of the immunogenic and functional domains of the protein. Meanwhile, a low sperm acrosine activity in infertile males with normal semen parameters results from a possible functional defect of the enzyme. Topfer-Petersen et al.[151] proposed that acrosine is a multifunctional enzyme having catalytic, hydrophobic, and carbohydrate binding sites, which allow acrosine to bind to the zona, digest the zona, and release sperm from the zona for further penetration. Blackwell and Zaneveld[19] reported that the sperm acrosine values decrease after prolonged abstinence, so in that regard, long abstinence periods may impair sperm acrosomal function. Senn et al.[135] studied the distribution of actin, acrosine, dynein, tubulin, and hyaluronidase by indirect immunofluorescence in sperm preparations from fertile donors and IVF patients; the presence of acrosine and tubulin yielded the most useful information on sperm function, structural status, and fertilizing ability.

Hamster egg–human sperm penetration assay

The hamster egg–human SPA measures several functions of the sperm, namely, capacitation, acrosome reaction, membrane fusion capability, incorporation into the ooplasm, and ability to decondense under these experimental conditions. The capability of the sperm to penetrate the cellular and matrix layers surrounding the oocytes and to penetrate the zona pellucida are not estimated by this test, nor can the expression of the sperm genome in the development of the preembryo after fertilization be evaluated. Conflicting results have been reported by different investigators when trying to find a correlation between conventional semen parameters, fertility, results of human IVF, and the SPA. Overall motility (mainly quality) and especially morphology seem to be the parameters with better correlation.[129] Rogers and Parker[128] established that both the sperm count and morphology were significant predictors of the SPA results, but the HOS test did not improve the predictive results. The SPA predicted fertilization with a high negative (74%) and positive (82%) predictive rate and good specificity (0.96%); it was concluded that the SPA correlated better with fertilization rate than did sperm count and motility, but not morphology. Chan and Tredway[30] have suggested a positive association between sperm nuclear decondensation and the fertilizing ability of sperm as judged by the SPA. Bronson et al.[24] have proposed a microwell SPA technique to study severely oligospermic patients using a single zona-free hamster egg and as few as 10,000 spermatozoa. With identical purposes, Johnson et al.[80] proposed a micro-SPA using only 25,000 sperm and found that the micro-SPA could accurately test 100% of the samples. Wang et al.[159] tried to establish a correlation between human sperm hyperactivated motility and the zona-free hamster oocyte SPA. No direct correlations were found between the two tests.

Correlations between SPA results and results of human IVF have been inconsistent, to say the least. Belkien et al.[14] concluded that the SPA is of limited value in predicting fertilization in an IVF program in the male factor. Ausmanas et al.[8] found good correlation between the results of the test and fertilization in the human system, but they were unable to establish a threshold for sperm fertilizing ability; fertilization, cleavage, and pregnancy occurred with sperm showing low penetration in the hamster assay. Margalioth et al.[102] found only 46% specificity in male factor IVF and 63% sensitivity, and concluded that the bioassay should not be relied upon for predicting IVF outcome in male subfertility, which is the area in which the predicting capabilities are needed most. Vasquez-Levin et al.[158] found no predictive value of the test for failures in IVF or for results after zona drilling, when the zona pellucida is bypassed and sperm–oocyte membrane fusion is facilitated, a step that the SPA is designed to measure. In our hands, the test showed a good correlation with the results of IVF when it was normal ($>10\%$ penetration). When it was abnormal ($<10\%$ penetration), 65% of those patients fertilized in the human system, and even when zero penetration occurred, IVF fertilization occurred in 66% of cases. So the prediction potential in our laboratory seems to be doubtful, mainly when the test is abnormal.

The enthusiasm for this test for the prediction of IVF fertilization results has tempered substantially lately, mainly in view of the fact that similar results can be obtained with simpler tests.

Human hemizona–sperm attachment assay

By using normal zonae pellucidae, this internally controlled bioassay is designed to measure and evaluate sperm tight-binding to the outer surface of one half of the zona, while the other half serves as a control using normal sperm of known, good, tight-binding capacity.[27] This test has a good application in research to determine one of the main functions of sperm that is not measured by the hamster egg–human SPA; it is too complex to be used routinely in the evaluation of sperm samples. Nevertheless, in our department, it is used for specific cases requiring elucidation of unexplained lack of fertilization or in cases with borderline capability of fertilization according to other test

batteries. The zonae pellucidae are obtained from oocytes collected from ovarian tissue postmortem or after surgical removal, or from immature or mature oocytes donated in IVF programs. The cutting of the zona pellucida in half requires micromanipulation in order to obtain hemizonae that are within 10% of each other in terms of external surface. The attachment capacity of the hemizona after micromanipulation and elimination of the oocyte is not significantly different from the entire zona pellucida that has not been micromanipulated. The inner aspect of the zona that is now exposed also has the ability to bind sperm, but that capacity is negligible compared with the outer surface of the zona. When the kinetics of binding is studied, maximal tight-binding occurs at approximately 4 hours, and reproducibility is high.[57] The hemizona assay index is calculated as number of sperm bound from the test sample $\times$ 100/number of sperm bound from the normal control.

When normal sperm are used, increasing the concentration of sperm does not increase the binding until a concentration of 100,000 sperm is obtained; after this, a dramatic increase in tight-binding occurs up to the maximum concentration used in the experiment (2 million sperm/mL),[58] validating the policy established in our division of increasing the number of sperm at insemination when low fertilization ability is predicted mainly by morphologic evaluation. It is interesting to note that prophase I oocytes obtained from nonstimulated ovaries provided zonae pellucidae that bound to sperm tightly in a concentration similar to metaphase II oocytes (41.6 ± 2.5 vs. 50.1 ± 11.8, mean $\pm$ SD); therefore prophase oocytes can be used effectively for these tests. On the other hand, prophase I oocytes obtained from IVF patients who had received gonadotropin stimulation and had been allowed to mature in vitro provided zonae pellucidae that had a much lower binding capacity (17.4 ± 2.2), very similar to that of prophase I oocytes cultured in vitro that did not mature because germinal vesicle breakdown did not occur (21.6 ± 3).[118] It seems that prophase I oocytes that have been exposed to exogenous gonadotropins during the process of ovulation stimulation have a different tight-binding pattern than prophase I oocytes from nonstimulated ovaries.

Patients with severe morphology problems (P-pattern) when compared with normal controls in the hemizona assay show significantly lower binding (72.2 ± 17.6 vs. 16.7 ± 5, mean $\pm$ SD), with a hemizona index that is also significantly reduced (124.5 ± 23.2 vs. 59.2 ± 13.0).[116] Similar results were obtained in IVF patients with failed fertilization due mainly to morphology problems (P-pattern). They showed significantly lower binding than did a group of normal patients who fertilized within the normal range for our laboratory (10.4 ± 3.6 vs. 3.61 ± 61.8 tightly bound sperm),[59] indicating that sperm with predominantly dysmorphic characteristics and secondary dyskinetic problems are also dysfunctional when fertilization is measured both by the hemizona assay and the human IVF system.

When the hemizona assay was used to try to detect populations with normal fertilization rates in the human IVF system (>55%) but low actual fertilization rates (<55%), the positive predictive value was 68% and the negative predictive value was 81%, with a sensitivity of 75% and a specificity of 75% (unpublished data). The hemizona index was significantly lower when no fertilization occurred in the in vitro system (18.4 ± 22) than when low fertilization was observed (35.7 ± 38) or when normal fertilization occurred (48.1 ± 65), but there is good amount of overlapping in the distribution of these patients; therefore there is no clear-cut threshold value for hemizona index that can be used with certainty to judge fertilization.

The hemizona index can also be used for other research purposes, as is discussed later in this chapter.

EVALUATION OF SEMEN AFTER CRYOPRESERVATION

After having exhausted the whole power of life in the production of heat, they froze; but that life was gone could not be known till we thawed them, which was done gradually. But their flexibility . . . they did not recover action, so that they were really dead . . . Till this time I had imagined that it might be possible to prolong life to any period by freezing a person in the frigid zone . . . Like other schemers, I thought I should make my fortune by it, but this experiment undeceived me.
—Hunter, his experiment with carp, early 1820s[60]

History and background

Since the early days of civilization, mankind has been aware of the methods of preserving biologic systems and the contribution of factors such as salting and low temperatures. The scientific and written aspects of cryopreservation began with Boyle's famous treatise, "New Experiments and Observations Touching Cold," in 1663.[60] More than a century later, in 1776, Lazaro Spallanzani reported the effects of cryopreservation on human semen. Later, in the 1820s, Hunter, one of the pioneers of modern cryobiology, expanded on Boyle's original work and experimented with the idea of cryopreserving complex biologic systems. Some of his ideas remain valid today. Ninety years after Spallanzani's report on human semen, Paolo Montegazza suggested the establishment of a sperm bank for veterinary use and, in addition, for human use to produce legitimate offspring after a husband's death on the battlefield.[152] In the early 1940s it became known that some spermatozoa could survive after freezing, and cryopreservation of spermatozoa became possible when Rostand discovered the cryoprotective role of glycerol (1,2,3-propanetriol, an alcohol) and propanediol for biologic structures.[81] Later, in 1949, the fundamental discovery by Polge et al.[137] that glycerol can be used to protect spermatozoa of several species was reported. The Polge protocol was rapidly used to breed domestic animals, especially bulls, but application to humans was not undertaken until 1953, when Sherman ob-

served that human spermatozoa frozen in dry ice (− 78°C) and later thawed were able to fertilize and induce normal embryonic development and a live birth. In the following years only 27 births were reported in the United States and Japan after inseminations with the cryopreserved sperm. The report of sperm cryopreservation using the nitrogen vapor technique (− 130° to − 140°C) in 1962-1963, and the first four births after freezing of human sperm with glycerol in nitrogen vapor, gave cryopreservation techniques a tremendous boost.[137]

Human sperm cryopreservation and the concept of sperm banking did not become a matter of routine until the 1970s. The greatest impact on the accelerated development of sperm cryopreservation occurred in the mid-1980s, when concerns heightened about sexually transmitted diseases, such as infections with human immunodeficiency virus type I (HIVI) and hepatitis B and later HIV-II and hepatitis C. Sperm cryopreservation then became widely known to the general public and to many health professionals who had not been aware of the availability of such a service. Since then, apart from sperm cryopreservation for the purpose of therapeutic donor insemination (TDI), many other categories of patients have benefited from the availability of the procedure.

Nowadays sperm cryopreservation is readily available to cancer patients before initiation of therapy, to men undergoing vasectomy, to husbands who will be absent at the time of the wife's therapeutic inseminations, to paraplegics, and to a variety of other patients with conditions and treatments that may affect the male reproductive system. The idea of sperm cryopreservation and its relevance to safety, convenience, and fertility is unquestionable. Along with the embryo/oocyte cryopreservation program, sperm banks are now an integral part of many rapidly developing centers for assisted reproduction and have contributed to the development and modification of many of these advanced technologies. Theoretically, sperm functional integrity should not change with time when stored at − 196°C; however, some questions remain concerning the influence that long-term storage may have on sperm. At this temperature, background ionizing radiation, which under normal circumstances is not significant, is the only source of damage to cells. It has been reported that it takes about 32×10^3 years for cells cryopreserved in 10% dimethyl sulfoxide (DMSO) to accumulate lethal and chromosomal damage equal to that inflicted by one acute dose of X-irradiation at 22°C. One report[142] indicates a significant decline in sperm motility in a specimen thawed after 3 years in storage; other reports[38,101] indicated no major change in post-thaw motility of samples stored for more than 10 years. Our experience with samples stored for up to 9 years shows no indication of major change in the quality of cryopreserved samples as assessed by post-thaw analysis of motility. There is no evidence of genetic damage to spermatozoa by cryopreservation, and risks of spontaneous abortion or malformation are not higher with cryopreserved than with fresh sperm.[81] The longest period of time a husband's semen sample was kept cryopreserved and resulted in a pregnancy after thawing remains at almost 19 years. This period for a donor sample resulting in a pregnancy is now 15 years.[137]

Cryopreservation techniques

Long-term storage and preservation of biologic systems such as spermatozoa require the arrest of cellular and metabolic activities while maintaining the integrity of the structures necessary to restore normal cell function during storage and after thawing. This can be accomplished by removing (or reducing) the water content of the cell and storage at ultralow temperatures. How that can be accomplished without killing cells is the heart of the science of cryobiology. Of course, the response of different systems to cryopreservation depends on a variety of factors: method of cryopreservation, type of cryoprotectant used, species, type and quality of the cells, and stage of development of the cells. For example, microtubules of oocytes, but not of spermatozoa, are sensitive to cold shock. Oocytes are depolymerized upon cooling and cryopreservation, leading to clumping or spreading of chromosomes and poor survival of the female gametes. Pig embryos do not survive chilling even to 0°C.[60] Late morula and blastocyst stages of bull embryos can be cryopreserved more successfully than the earlier stages.[105] How these developmental differences influence the outcome of cryopreservation and what factors within cells are responsible for these differences remain to be elucidated. Since cryopreservation of semen samples with poor quality is not always successful, one wonders whether certain developmental/structural differences in spermatozoa from patients with poor quality might be the reason. The cryoprotectant DMSO is toxic to sperm,[137] whereas it can be used to cryopreserve a variety of other cells.[81]

Use of cryopreserved semen samples in assisted reproduction

Despite reports indicating that cryopreservation may inflict damage to spermatozoa, the value of cryopreserved spermatozoa in assisted reproduction is unquestionable. There have been conflicting reports on the efficacy of cryopreserved spermatozoa in therapeutic inseminations (ICI, IUI) and other assisted reproductive techniques. Based on available information, it appears reasonable to conclude that, in the absence of female factor(s), the cumulative pregnancy rate using cryopreserved spermatozoa is comparable to that of fresh samples.[22,45,112] This rate has been reported to be about 65% to 76%.[160] It also may not be unreasonable to state that the monthly pregnancy rate may be different with cryopreserved semen versus fresh semen. This would indicate that, with cryopreserved semen samples, more inseminations may be required to achieve pregnancies.

Preliminary evaluation of our pregnancies resulting from IUI and ICI during the last 7 years indicates that 164 of 205 pregnancies (80%) reported occurred within the first six cycles of insemination. Thirty-nine pregnancies (19%) occurred within the first 12 cycles and two pregnancies (1%) occurred beyond 12 cycles. These preliminary data indicate that, besides other female factors, the factors contributing most to success were the age of the female and the total number of motile sperm used for inseminations. Females younger than 30 had the highest rates and those older than 40 had the lowest pregnancy rates. Inseminations with 25 to 40 million motile sperm appeared to be more successful for ICI. Higher pregnancy rates were observed when more than 8 million motile sperm were used for IUI. Similarly, in another study[136] evaluating 443 patients undergoing 2998 cycles of ICI, female age (<30) was found to be the most important factor contributing to success. Franco-Junior et al.[55] reported that a minimum of 0.4 mL of prepared sample was needed to ensure that the uterus and tubes were reached by that volume. Kahn et al.[82] used 4 mL of prepared (washed) cryopreserved donor samples (using an Allis clamp on the cervix to prevent reflux) to allow complete perfusion of fallopian tubes (fallopian tube sperm perfusion). Forty-five women underwent 172 treatment cycles and had a pregnancy rate per cycle of 27.9% and a cumulative pregnancy rate of 49.5%. The pregnancy rate for the first attempt in the study was 34.1% and declined to 14.3% for the fourth attempt. The pregnancy rate per treatment cycle has been reported to be between 3.8% and 10%, compared with 9% and 27% for fresh samples.[141] The pregnancy rate per cycle for our patients is about 10% for cervical inseminations, compared with the reported range of 3.9% to 14.6%.[82]

More advanced techniques such as IVF and GIFT have increased the chances of couples who otherwise have failed to achieve pregnancies; these methods, however, are relatively expensive and require special arrangements. More cost-efficient procedures, such as ICI and IUI, are usually the first methods of choice for the couples seeking therapeutic insemination using cryopreserved semen samples. One question remains: how to counsel patients and provide them with a realistic prognosis in terms of duration and outcome of treatment. As data just presented indicate, the pregnancy rate per treatment cycle after insemination with cryopreserved samples is dependent on many factors, such as the reproductive status of the female, the timing of ovulation and insemination, ovarian stimulation, number of motile spermatozoa inseminated, the volume of sample used, and the technique used (IUI, ICI, IVF, or GIFT).[28,49,82,103] Generally, the pregnancy rates for cryopreserved samples used in ICI have been reported to range from 3.9%[28] to 14.6%.[82] The rate for IUI has been reported to be about 9.7%[28] for unstimulated cycles; the rate for stimulated cycles ranges from 15.5% to 27.9%.[82]

A knowledge of the quality of the cryopreserved sample

(either husband's or donor's) and the relationship between this quality and the pregnancy outcome using a particular procedure is needed. In evaluation of the relationship between the pregnancy outcome and the semen quality, one should pay special attention to the post-freeze characteristics of the sample rather than those of the fresh ejaculate before cryopreservation. As related to the sample, the number of motile sperm and the motility of post-thaw and washed samples have been shown to be important predictors of success with IUI and ICI.* In one study,[76] it was found that cervical inseminations with 40×10^6 motile sperm resulted in a better pregnancy rate. Marshburn et al.,[103] in their retrospective study of 1147 IUI cycles using cryopreserved donor samples, found that the most significant predictors of the pregnancy outcome were curvilinear velocity and straight-line velocity of the post-freeze and washed spermatozoa, and the total number of motile sperm inseminated. In the same study, in evaluation of donor samples and their degree of fertility, it was found that spontaneous acrosome reaction in samples was negatively correlated with the pregnancy outcome from those samples. Maintenance of motility of washed samples at 37°C for 6 hours was positively correlated with the pregnancy outcome, whereas the hamster SPA for those samples gave no predictive value. For IVF techniques, cryopreserved spermatozoa have proven to give equal (if not better) fertilization and pregnancy rates.[112]

Pregnancy rates with cryopreserved samples from patients with malignancies are reported to be variable.[16,81,85,133,134] In one study, fertilization was reported to occur when swim-up recovered a mean of $1.8 \pm 0.5 \times 10^6$ motile spermatozoa per milliliter and when insemination was performed with at least 500,000 spermatozoa per oocyte per milliliter of medium.[85] Others have reported that no pregnancy could be achieved with cryopreserved semen when the sperm concentration was under 40% or 55% of the initial ejaculate.[81] In a study of the relationship between the number of motile spermatozoa from cancer patients recovered after cryopreservation and the pregnancy rate, it was found that with recoveries below 0.5×10^6, no pregnancy resulted from 106 cycles. Three pregnancies (159 cycles) resulted from samples with 0.5 to 2×10^6 motile cells recovered and 11 (267 cycles) from samples with more than 2×10^6 motile cells.[81]

Similar to other assisted reproductive methods, sperm cryopreservation techniques continue to improve as knowledge of the basic science of cryobiology is increased. Gradually, sperm cryobanks may become involved in the cryopreservation of male germ cells for patients who are to become sterile or for a transfer to a heterologous host. Undoubtedly patients will benefit and pregnancy rates will increase by attempts of cryobanks to improve techniques of

cryopreservation and recovery rates for the poor-quality samples. We may soon be able to cryopreserve several samples of severely oligozoospermic patients and have them combined after thawing for use in an assisted reproductive technique, and to develop more accurate methods of assessing the success and the damage of cryopreservation protocols. This will eventually guide us toward developing appropriate remedies for cryodamage and modifying techniques to achieve better success with cryopreserved samples. Design and implementation of various methods of cryopreservation matching different samples will eventually become a matter of routine.

EVALUATION OF SEMEN AFTER ELECTROEJACULATION

Patients suffering from anejaculation or retrograde ejaculation due to neurologic problems (spinal cord injury, diabetic neuropathy, damage to the sympathetic-parasympathetic system due to retroperitoneal lymph node dissection, use of pharmacologic substances, or unexplained causes) can be treated medically by using sympathomimetic agents or by physical/electrical stimulation through the rectum (electroejaculation). The most commonly used sympathomimetic agents are phenylpropanolamine hydrochloride (75 mg twice daily), pseudoephedrine hydrochloride (60 mg four times daily), ephedrine sulfate (25 to 50 mg four times daily), and imipramine hydrochloride (25 mg twice daily or 50 mg at bedtime).

If antegrade ejaculation is not achieved, the protocol for preparation and recovery of the sperm from the bladder is utilized. In patients with retrograde ejaculation, the protocol that can be recommended is as follows:

1. The patient should have sexual intercourse 4 to 7 days before the actual test or sperm recovery for IUI.
2. Urine should be neutralized during the 3 days before sperm collection by having the patient take two tablets of sodium bicarbonate (0.32 grain/tablet) six times daily (for instance, at 9, 11, 13, 15, 17, and 19 hours).
3. The patient should drink two large glasses of water with the tablets, and during the 3 days of preparation, he should avoid alcohol and other toxic substances.
4. The day of the test, the patient should urinate 1 hour before the test, and urine pH and osmolality should be measured. The pH should be around 7 or above, and osmolality should be between 200 and 300 mOsm/L, considering that the semen osmolality is around 366 ± 16 mOsm/L. The patient should drink 500 mL of water after the urine has been tested. If the osmolality is between 180 and 300 mOsm/L, the patient can try to collect semen; if the osmolality is less than 180 mOsm/L, the patient should wait for

*References 49, 76, 81, 82, 103, 141.

30 minutes and then try to ejaculate; and if the osmolality is more than 380 mOsm/L, the patient should again drink 200 mL of water, wait for 30 minutes, and deliver another urine sample to check the pH and osmolality.

5. The patient should try to collect a semen sample. If there is a small amount of antegrade ejaculation, it should be recovered. After 5 minutes, the patient should empty his bladder into a container. If there was no antegrade ejaculation, he should collect the urine 5 minutes after orgasm.

6. If there was antegrade ejaculation, basic semen analysis should be done on it. The urine should be distributed in centrifuge tubes and centrifuged at 280g for 10 minutes.

7. The supernatant is recovered and kept.

8. The pellets are resuspended in Tyrode's solution plus 4% human serum albumin or in Ham's F-10 plus 15% fetal cord serum (total volume 2.0 mL).

9. Volume pH and osmolality of the urine postejaculation are controlled.

10. Basic semen analysis is performed on the resuspended pellets.

11. If the semen will be used for IUI, the sperm suspension is centrifuged at 280g for 5 minutes in 15-mL polypropylene tubes.

12. The supernatant is discarded and the pellet is resuspended in a minimal volume of the same medium.

13. The pellet is carefully overlaid with 0.2 mL of Tyrode's solution with 4% human serum albumin or with Ham's F-10 plus 15% fetal cord serum.

14. The mixture is incubated for 2 hours at 37°C in 5% CO_2 in air.

15. The supernatant is retrieved. Count and motility are determined and the specimen is sent for IUI.

After electroejaculation, usually three portions of semen are sent to the laboratory: (1) antegrade ejaculation; (2) retrograde ejaculation, obtained by bladder washings; and (3) urine obtained by catheterization. These specimens are processed separately. Our laboratory uses Ham's F-10 for the collection of antegrade ejaculation and the bladder washing.

On arriving at the laboratory, the specimens are centrifuged, the supernatants are discarded, pellets are resuspended in Ham's F-10, and evaluation of count and motility is performed. If spermatozoa are present in all samples, they are centrifuged and resuspended in 250 μL of medium and sent for IUI.

Electroejaculation has also been used in combination with IVF and gamete micromanipulation for the treatment of anejaculatory male infertility.[148]

Most of the specimens show a low sperm count, low motility, and low morphology, with a considerable amount of non–sperm cells (red blood cells, white blood cells, and debris).

IUI and IVF combined with electroejaculation have produced pregnancies,[15] but the success rate is still low.

EVALUATION OF SPERM AFTER MICROSCOPIC EPIDIDYMAL SPERM ASPIRATION

Since the original publication of Silber et al.[140] and the possibility of using epididymal sperm in patients with congenital absence of the vas deferens for IVF, experience has multiplied with varying results. An attempt to predict the quality of the sperm available in the epididymis at the time of retrieval by doing testicular biopsies, which are useful in patients with nonobstructive problems, did not demonstrate efficiency in patients with chronic obstructions; in these patients, poor sperm recovery is due mainly to epididymal and preepididymal microscopic obstructive disease caused by intratubular hypertension and extravasation with a subsequent chronic inflammatory process at the interstitial level.[139] Bladou et al.[20] attempted this procedure in 23 patients (8 with vasal agenesis and 14 with secondary prolonged vasal obstruction), and obtained adequate sperm in terms of count in 13.8% of retrievals and in terms of motility in 15.5%. Five embryo transfers were performed and two couples had an early pregnancy loss. The authors believe that spermatozoa aspirated from the proximal epididymis originated a high rate of embryo degeneration after transfer.

Rojas et al.[130] found good correlation between the SPA and human IVF when sperm aspirated from the epididymis was used, suggesting that the SPA may be a good bioassay to test laboratory experimental conditions, trying to improve the fertilizing capacity of human epididymal sperm. Patrizio et al.,[123] studying the presence of antisperm antibodies on epididymal sperm and in epididymal fluid by the immunobead binding technique, found 35% positivity in sperm, 16% in epididymal fluid, and 29% in serum. Neither the fertilization rate nor the pregnancy rate seemed to be impaired, even in the presence of a high concentration of antisperm antibodies.

Ord et al.[121] summarized the experience of their laboratory in the preparation of epididymal sperm for assisted reproductive technologies. They confirmed that human epididymal sperm had severely impaired motility, progression, and morphology as compared with ejaculated sperm, and that the count was also usually much lower. Spermatozoa were contaminated in most cases with red blood cells, debris, macrophages, and degenerated sperm. Epididymal aspirates were diluted with 1 mL of 4-(2-hydroxyethyl)-1-piperazinepropanesulfonic acid (HEPES)-buffered human tubal fluid supplemented with 0.5% human serum albumin. An aliquot was examined for the presence of motile sperm. The aspirates were pooled, trying to keep together all the samples with the best quality. Best results were obtained by using the mini-Percoll technique with the addition of 3 mmol of pentoxifylline and 3 mmol of deoxyadenosine, which yielded an overall 35% fertilization rate and a rate of 58% if only the patients who fertilized were taken into consideration. Fifty-seven percent of patients achieved fertilization with this treatment, and the cleavage rate was between 96% and 98%. Excess embryos of 63% of patients were frozen. Despite the better performance of the sperm in the group treated this way, the pregnancy rate from fresh preembryo transfer was not different from the rate achieved with sperm prepared by wash and resuspension, by the swim-up or sedimentation technique, or by mini-Percoll alone (15%, 20%, and 14%, respectively, clinical pregnancy rate per patient).

POTENTIAL AREAS FOR BASIC AND CLINICAL RESEARCH

Several studies have clearly demonstrated that standard semen parameters such as sperm concentration, motility, and gross morphology have limited clinical value in predicting both natural and assisted fertilization.[13,25,31] Since the basic semen analysis does not appropriately address sperm function, numerous assays have been developed with this additional parameter in mind. Computer-assisted motion analysis, the HOS test, acrosomal and nuclear maturity assessments, the hamster egg penetration test, and zona binding penetration assays are part of today's armamentarium.

Although primarily intended as a therapy, IVF represents the ultimate assay to evaluate sperm-oocyte interactions and provides a significantly valuable end point. Therefore, almost all of the above-mentioned sperm function tests have been correlated with fertilization rates in vitro and their predictive values determined.[22] It is important to note, however, that work-ups for the initial screening of a presumptive clinical male factor patient and a male factor patient being studied for IVF are substantially different.[2,7] Tests with good prognostic value in one situation may not be so useful in the other.

Sperm function assays, both clinical and experimental, are focused mainly on processes undergone by the spermatozoon once it is in the egg investments. In revising the physiology of this interaction, two elements on the part of sperm appear to play a crucial role: they are the receptors for zona pellucida glycoproteins and the plasma membrane.

A variety of proteins from mammalian spermatozoa have been implicated as possible zona-binding receptors. Galactosyltransferase,[33] mannosidase,[36] 95-kd protein,[21] rabbit sperm autoantigens,[29] and galactose-binding lectins[1] are some of those proteins.

Expression of functional receptors and plasma membrane fluidity are two conditions intimately related to sperm-zona binding. Evaluation of sperm-binding capacity is now possible[6,24] and has proved to be significantly related to IVF success rates.[14,23] This high association probably arises from the zona pellucida property to select normal spermatozoa. It has been demonstrated that, according to strict criteria, 70% of spermatozoa bound to the zona are normal, at least morphologically.[26]

Morphology and plasma membrane structure, including receptors, are cast during spermatogenesis and maturation in the male reproductive organs. This may be the reason why sperm morphology, most probably as an epiphenomenon, is highly associated with sperm zona binding[28] and IVF rates.[19]

In a process called capacitation, sperm structure and metabolism are modified during transit along the female genital tract. Pieces of factual evidence indicate that such a process does not occur in all spermatozoa at the same time.[3] This, together with possible intrinsic differences generated at origin, results in the existence of sperm subpopulations within the semen. They are structurally and functionally different. For instance, spermatozoa undergoing the acrosome reaction far away from the oocyte will be unable to fertilize it; however, they might serve another purpose. During in vitro capacitation, receptor expression and stimulation thresholds, as well as membrane modifications, appear at different times in different subpopulations. This is an important concept to have in mind when interpreting any type of sperm assay.

After spermatozoa bind to the oocyte, zona pellucida glycoproteins acting as multivalent ligands aggregate surface sperm receptors. This phenomenon activates guanine nucleotide-binding regulatory proteins (G proteins), which, in turn, transduce the signal internally. Several intracellular mechanisms, such as protein phosphorylation, are triggered, ultimately leading to changes in motion parameters (hyperactivation), release of hydrolytic enzymes, and exposure of secondary binding receptors (acrosome reaction).[17,34]

A cyclic mechanism consisting of binding to and degradation of the zona pellucida ensures sperm penetration. Once in the perivitelline space, binding to oolemma, oocyte activation, and cytoplasmic engulfment of sperm occur very rapidly. Subsequently, chromatin decondensation takes place and the zygote evolves until the amphimixis marks the end of the fertilization process.

Current sperm function assays attempt to determine potential alterations of the sperm's capacity to undergo some of the aforementioned fertilization events. Tests have been developed to study zona binding/penetration ability: binding ratio,[24] acrosomal status (fluorescent lectin on antibodies,[8] acrosomal and cytoplasmic enzymes [acrosin,[39] hyaluronidase,[15] creatine phosphokinase,[39] lactate dehydrogenase,[20] energy substrates (ATP)]),[39] hyperactivation (computer-assisted analysis),[5] membrane integrity (dye exclusion[27] and HOS test),[16] and nuclear maturity (acridine orange,[35] acidic aniline blue,[9] sodium dodecyl sulfate-induced decondensation).[4]

However, using logistic regression analysis (a powerful statistical tool to correlate the binary probability of a given event [fertilization] to occur or not) and multiple potentially causative variables, only strict morphology, acrosomal status, mean linearity (one of the computerized motion parameters), and binding to the zona pellucida were significantly related to fertilization rates in vitro.[22] But even these assays are not able to predict fertilization in all cases, nor are they free from technical pitfalls. For instance, zona-binding tests utilize human oocytes, which are largely unavailable, at least in the amounts needed to allow the assays to become part of routine sperm evaluation. Strict morphology assay is technically simple and possesses a good correlation with IVF rates; however, its performance requires well-trained technicians, and the subjectivity involved makes interlaboratory standardization very difficult. Assessment of acrosome status may provide additional information, particularly in men with high proportions of spermatozoa with abnormal morphology. Nevertheless, in the way it is currently performed, it fails to examine inducibility of the acrosome reaction and, with that, a dynamic process that plays a crucial role in fertilization.

Keeping in mind that it is very unlikely that a single test will be able to predict sperm fertilizing ability with total accuracy, several evaluation trends can be anticipated for the near future. In an initial screening, assessment of semen samples with computer-assisted analysis of morphology, motility, and acrosomal status will provide information about sperm quality and, ultimately, spermatogenesis and maturation. These processes rationally will soon become the target of male factor therapy.

Sperm motion analyzers (e.g., Cell Soft, Hamilton-Thorn) providing detailed information about sperm movement characteristics have pioneered the introduction of computers in semen analysis. Better resolution and improved software are constantly appearing on the market.

Taking advantage of the same digital technology and in an attempt to avoid the subjectivity problem, computer-assisted morphology analyzers have just been marketed. There appears to be good correlation with man-generated data and IVF rates.[18] The status of the acrosome can be visualized with a cytochemical technique using specific antibodies or lectins conjugated with fluorochromes. These molecules will fluoresce upon illumination with monochromatic or ultraviolet light. This feature has not yet been included in the above-mentioned systems.

Within the context of assisted reproduction, several assays are being developed to assess sperm fertilizing potential after separation/enrichment techniques (such as swim-up, Percoll, glass wool) have been performed.

To study the presence and distribution of zona receptors on human sperm, specific antibodies and zona pellucida proteins may be used. It has been demonstrated[12] that antigalactosyltransferase and anti-p97 monoclonal antibodies, porcine ZP3, and a mannose-containing neoglycoprotein are able to significantly inhibit human sperm-zona interaction, being potential biomarkers for sperm receptors. Since the human ZP3 gene has been cloned,[10] the possibility exists that in the future a mammalian-expressed recombinant molecule would also be used as a biomarker. Antibodies and zona proteins can be labeled and fluorescent or colorimetric reactions developed. Solid substrates, such as silica beads, have been tried with mouse sperm[37] and remain an option; however, assay sensitivity should be addressed further.

To study the functionality of zona sperm receptors, synthetic zona pellucida proteins or putative substitutes (e.g., antireceptor antibodies) can be utilized as inducers in a liquid-phase or solid-phase assay. Binding, acrosome reaction, and redistribution of sperm receptors—primary and secondary—could be assessed. An assay employing an immobilized zona pellucida matrix has been described for rabbit sperm.[17] Evaluation of acrosin activity and sperm penetration through the zona is also possible with this type of assay.

Activation of intracellular mechanisms, such as protein phosphorylation, is a receptor-mediated function and therefore suitable for study. It has been reported that phosphotyronine-containing proteins, in both humans[11] and mice,[21] are involved in sperm-zona interaction. Antiphosphotyronine antibodies are available and represent an appropriate tool to be used in the above-mentioned assays.

The expression of receptors and the ability of the plasma membrane to allow their functions depend on the time and experimental conditions of the in vitro sperm incubations. Consequently, it may be convenient to perform the assays at least two different times.

After the sperm nucleus is incorporated in the oocyte, chromatin decondensation has to occur to enable a normal fertilization and, ultimately, the integration of paternal genes into the embryo's genome. Physiologic and consistent "decondensation" tests can be anticipated, possibly by using recombinant decondensation factors. Once this methodology is achieved, or even artificially decondensing the chromatin, chromosome and gene structural abnormalities will be identifiable on the sperm. Techniques such as fluorescent in situ hybridization could be used and, in turn, might be coupled to cell sorting to separate normal from abnormal spermatozoa.

All those assays in which localization and quantification of sperm molecules are end points will certainly benefit from digitalization and computer-assisted analysis of the generated images.

Current treatment of male factor patients is focused on bypassing the fertilization events that could be altered. Future therapies, however, will certainly be more etiologic, repairing processes, such as spermatogenesis and maturation, that control sperm quality. Finally, it is worth remembering that in order for this to happen, new screening methodology will first have to become a reality.

ACKNOWLEDGMENT

Portions of this paper were adapted from an earlier work by one of the authors (A.A.A.), "Male Factor in Assisted Reproduction", first published in *Infertility and Reproductive Clinics of North America*, Vol 3, No 2, pp. 487-503 (April 1992); adapted with permission.

REFERENCES

1. Abdullah M, Widgren ED, O'Rand MG: A mammalian sperm lectin related to rat hepatocyte lectin 2/3: purification from rabbit testes—an identification as a zona binding protein, *Mol Cell Biochem* 103:155, 1991.

2. Acosta AA: Male factor in assisted reproduction, *Infertil Reprod Med Clin North Am* 3:487, 1992.

3. Acosta AA et al: Assisted reproduction in the diagnosis and treatment of the male factor, *Obstet Gynecol Surv* 44:1, 1989.

4. Acosta AA et al: The real impact of male antisperm antibodies (ASA) in the results of in-vitro fertilization (IVF) needs to be re-evaluated, Manuscript submitted for publication, 1993.

5. Agrawal P, Magargee SF, Hammerstedt RH: Isolation and characterization of the plasma membrane of rat cauda epididymal spermatozoa, *J Androl* 9:178, 1988.

6. Aitken J: Molecular basis of sperm improvement in vitro. In Proceedings of the Seventh World Congress of in Vitro Fertilization and Medically Assisted Procreation, Paris, June 30-July 3, 1991.

7. Aitken RJ, Buckingham D: Enhanced detection of reactive oxygen species produced by human spermatozoa with 7-dimethyl aminonaphthalin-1,2-dicarbonic acid hydrazide, *Int J Androl* 15:211, 1992.

8. Ausmanas M et al: The zona-free hamster egg penetration assay as a prognostic indicator in a human in vitro fertilization program, *Fertil Steril* 43:433, 1985.

9. Bacetti B, editor: *Comparative spermatology 20 years after,* Serono Symposia Publications, New York, 1991, Raven Press.

10. Ballas SK: Red cell membrane protein changes caused by freezing and the mechanisms of cryoprotection by glycerol, *Transfusion* 21:203, 1981.

11. Barlow P et al: Predictive value of classical and automated sperm analysis for in-vitro fertilization, *Hum Reprod* 6:1119, 1991.

12. Barratt CLR et al: The poor prognostic value of low to moderate levels of sperm surface-bound antibodies, *Hum Reprod* 7:95, 1992.

13. Bedford JM, Best MJ, Calvin H: Variations in the structural character of nuclear chromation in morphologically normal human spermatozoa, *J Reprod Fertil* 33:19, 1973.

14. Belkien L et al: Prognostic value of the heterologous ovum penetration test for human in vitro fertilization, *Int J Androl* 8:275, 1985.

15. Bennett CJ et al: Electroejaculation of paraplegic males followed by pregnancies, *Fertil Steril* 48:1070, 1987.

16. Bergman S, Howard S, Sanger W. Practical aspects of banking patients' semen for future artificial insemination, *Urology* 13:408, 1979.

17. Bernard AG: Freeze preservation of mammalian reproductive cells. In Fuller BJ, Grout BWW, editors: *Clinical applications of cryobiology,* Boca Raton, Fla, 1991, CRC Press.

18. Blackmore PF et al: Progesterone and 17α-hydroxyprogesterone: Novel stimulators of calcium, *J Biol Chem* 265:1376, 1990.

19. Blackwell JM, Zaneveld LJ: Effect of abstinence on sperm acrosin, hypoosmotic swelling and other semen variables, *Fertil Steril* 58:798, 1992.

20. Bladou F et al: Epididymal sperm aspiration in conjunction with in vitro fertilization and embryo transfer in cases of obstructive azoospermia, *Hum Reprod* 6:1284, 1991.

21. Blanco A, Zimkhim WH: Lactate dehydrogenase in human testes, *Science* 139:601, 1963.

22. Bordson BL et al: Comparison of fecundability with fresh and frozen semen in therapeutic donor insemination, *Fertil Steril* 46:466, 1986.

23. Brockbank KGM, Carpenter JF, Dawson PE: Effects of storage temperature on viable bioprosthetic heart valves, *Cryobiology* 29:537, 1992.

24. Bronson RA, Ovla L, Bronson SK: A microwell sperm penetration assay, *Fertil Steril* 58:1078, 1992.

25. Burkman LJ: Characterization of hyperactivated motility by human spermatozoa during capacitation: comparison of fertile and oligozoospermic sperm populations, *Arch Androl* 13:153, 1984.

26. Burkman LJ: Discrimination between non-hyperactivated and classical hyperactivated motility patterns in human spermatozoa using computerized analysis, *Fertil Steril* 55:363, 1991.

27. Burkman LJ et al: The hemizona assay (HZA): development of a diagnostic test for the binding of human spermatozoa to human hemizona pellucida to predict fertilization potential, *Fertil Steril* 49:688, 1988.

28. Byrd W et al: A prospective randomized study of pregnancy rates following intrauterine and intracervical insemination using frozen donor sperm, *Fertil Steril* 53:521, 1990.

29. Calamera JC, Brugo S, Vilar O: Relation between motility and adenosine triphosphate (ATP) in human spermatozoa, *Andrologia* 14:239, 1982.

30. Chan PJ, Tredway DR: Association of human sperm nuclear decondensation and in vitro penetration ability, *Andrologia* 24:77, 1992.

31. Chan SYW, Wang C: Correlation between semen adenosine triphosphate and sperm fertilizing capacity, *Fertil Steril* 47:717, 1987.

32. Chao HT et al: Human follicular fluid stimulates motility and velocity of washed human sperm in vitro, *Andrologia* 24:47, 1992.

33. Clarke GN et al: Effect of sperm antibodies in males on human in vitro fertilization (IVF), *AJRIM* 8:62, 1985.

34. Clarke GN et al: Sperm antibodies and human in vitro fertilization, *Fertil Steril* 49:1018, 1988.

35. Comhaire FH: An approach to the management of male infertility, *Baillieres Clin Endocrinol Metab* 3:487, 1992.

36. Comhaire F, Thiery M: Methods of improvement of the success rate of artificial insemination with donor semen, *Int J Androl* 9:14, 1985.

37. Comhaire F et al: Adenosine triphosphate in human semen: a quantitative estimate of fertilizing potential, *Fertil Steril* 40:500, 1983.

38. Critser JK et al: Cryopreservation of human spermatozoa, I: effects of holding procedure and seeding on motility, fertilizability, and acrosome reaction, *Fertil Steril* 47:656, 1987.

39. Cross NC, Meizel S: Methods for evaluating the acrosomal status of mammalian sperm, *Biol Reprod* 41:635, 1989.

40. Dadoune JP, Mayaux MJ, Guihard-Moscato ML: Correlation between defects in chromatin condensation of human spermatozoa stained by aniline blue and semen characteristics, *Andrologia* 20:211, 1988.

41. DeAlmeida M et al: In-vitro processing of sperm with autoantibodies and in-vitro fertilization results, *Hum Reprod* 4:49, 1989.

42. Dean J et al: Developmental expression of ZP3—a mouse zona pellucida gene, *Proc Clin Mol Biol* 294:21, 1989.

43. DeLamirande E, Gagnon C: Reactive oxygen species and human spermatozoa, I: effects on the motility of intact spermatozoa and on sperm axonemes, *J Androl* 13:368, 1992.

44. DeLamirande E, Gagnon C: Reactive oxygen species and human spermatozoa, II: depletion of adenosine triphosphate plays an important role in the inhibition of sperm motility, *J Androl* 5:379, 1992.

45. DiMarzo SJ et al: Pregnancy rates with fresh versus computer-controlled cryopreserved semen for artificial insemination by donor in a private practice setting, *Am J Obstet Gynecol* 162:1483, 1990.

46. Doncel GF et al: In search of biomarkers for zona receptors in human sperm. Presented at the annual meeting of the American Society of Andrologists, Tampa, Fla, April 1993 (abstract).

47. Doncel GF et al: Potential biomarkers for zona receptors in human sperm, *Andrology in the nineties,* International Symposium, Belgium, April, 1993 (abstract).

48. Dunphy B, Neal NL, Cooke ID: The clinical value of conventional semen analysis, *Fertil Steril* 51:324, 1989.

49. Edvinson A et al: Factors in the infertile couple influencing the success of artificial insemination with donor sperm, *Fertil Steril* 53:81, 1990.

50. Elder KT, Wick KL, Edwards RG: Seminal plasma anti-sperm antibodies and IVF: the effect of semen sample collection in 50% serum, *Hum Reprod* 5:179, 1990.

51. Eliasson R: Standards for investigation of human semen, *Andrologia* 3:49, 1971.

52. Enginsu ME et al: Comparison between the hypo-osmotic swelling test and morphology evaluation using strict criteria in predicting in vitro fertilization (IVF), *J Assist Reprod Genet* 9:259, 1992.

53. Evrev TI: Auto antigenicity of LDH-X isoenzymes. In Markert CL, editor: *Isoenzymes, vol 2, physiological function,* New York, 1975, Academic Press.

54. Francavilla S et al: Sperm acrosine activity and fluorescence microscopic assessment of proacrosin/acrosin in ejaculates of infertile and fertile men, *Fertil Steril* 57:1311, 1992.

55. Franco-Junior JG et al: Radiologic evaluation of incremental intrauterine instillation of contrast material, *Fertil Steril* 58:1065, 1992.

56. Franken DR et al: The hemizona assay (HZA): a predictor of human sperm fertilizing potential in in vitro fertilization (IVF) treatment, *J In Vitro Fert Embryo Transfer* 6:44, 1989.

57. Franken DR et al: The hemizona assay using salt-stored human oocytes: evaluation of zona pellucida capacity for binding human spermatozoa, *Gamete Res* 22:15, 1989.

58. Franken DR et al: Hemizona assay and teratozoospermia: increasing sperm insemination concentrations to enhance zona pellucida binding, *Fertil Steril* 54:497, 1990.

59. Franken D et al: Assisted reproductive technologies may obviate apparent immunologic infertility, *Andrologia* 23:291, 1991.

60. Fuller BJ: The effects of cooling on mammalian cells. In Fuller BJ, Grout BWW, editors: *Clinical applications of cryobiology,* Boca Raton, Fla, 1991, CRC Press.

61. Gavella M, Liporac V: Pentoxifylline-mediated reduction of superoxide anion production by human spermatozoa, *Andrologia* 24:37, 1992.

62. Goldberg E. Lactic and malic dehydrogenases in human spermatozoa, *Science* 139:602, 1963.

63. Goodpasture J, Polakoski KL, Zaneveld LYS: Acrosin, proacrosin and acrosin inhibitor of human spermatozoa: extraction, quantitation and stability, *J Androl* 1:16, 1980.

64. Gottlieb C, Svanborg K, Bjdgeman M: Adenosine triphosphate (ATP) in human spermatozoa, *Andrologia* 23:421, 1991.

65. Grunert JH, DeGeyter C, Nieschlag E: Objective identification of hyperactivated human spermatozoa by computerized sperm motion analysis with the Hamilton-Thorn sperm motility analyzer, *Hum Reprod* 5:593, 1990.

66. Hamilton F, Gutlay-Yeo AL, Meldrum DR: Normal fertilization in men with high antibody sperm binding by the addition of sufficient unbound sperm in vitro, *J In Vitro Fert Embryo Transfer* 6:342, 1989.

67. Hirayama T, Hasegawa T, Hiroi M: The measurement of hyaluronidase activity of human spermatozoa by substrate slide assay and its clinical application, *Fertil Steril* 51:330, 1989.

68. Hofmann N, Haider SG: Neue Ergebnisse Morphologisher Diagnostik der Spermatogenesestorungen, *Gynaekologe* 18:70, 1985.

69. Huszar G, Corrales M, Vigue L: Correlation between sperm creatine phosphokinase activity and sperm concentrations in normospermic and oligospermic men, *Gamete Res* 19:67, 1988.

70. Huszar G, Vigue L: Serial sperm CPK measurements in oligospermic and normospermic patients. Presented at the Fifth World Congress on in Vitro Fertilization and Embryo Transfer, Norfolk, Va, April 5-10, 1987 (poster no 79, program supplement).

71. Huszar G, Vigue L: Spermatogenesis-related changes in the synthesis of the creatine kinase B-type and M-type isoforms in human spermatozoa, *Mol Reprod Dev* 25:258, 1990.

72. Huszar G, Vigue L, Morshedi M: Sperm creatine phosphokinase ratios and fertilizing potential of men: a blind study of 84 couples treated with in vitro fertilization, *Fertil Steril* 57:882, 1992.

73. Imoedemhe DA et al: The effect of caffeine on the ability of spermatozoa to fertilize mature human oocytes, *J Assist Reprod Genet* 9:155, 1992.

74. Imoedemhe DA et al: Successful use of the sperm motility enhancer 2-deoxyadenosine in previously failed human in vitro fertilization, *J Assist Reprod Genet* 9:53, 1992.

75. Irianni FM et al: Therapeutic intrauterine insemination (TII): controversial treatment for infertility, *Arch Androl* 25:147, 1990.

76. Irianni FM et al: Therapeutic donor insemination (TDI): the Norfolk clinical experience, *Assist Reprod Technol Androl (S): 35,* 1992.

77. Irianni FM et al: Therapeutic intrauterine insemination (TII) improves with gonadotropin ovarian stimulation, *Arch Androl,* 1993 (in press).

78. Ivanov II, Kassavina BS, Fomenko LD: Adenosinetriphosphate in mammalian spermatozoa, *Nature* 158:624, 1946.

79. Jeyendran RS et al: Fertilizing capacity of various populations of spermatozoa within an ejaculate, *J Assist Reprod Genet* 9:32, 1992.

80. Johnson A et al: The microsperm penetration assay: development of a sperm penetration assay suitable for oligospermic males, *Fertil Steril* 56:528, 1991.

81. Jouannet P et al: Cryopreservation and infertility. In Seibel MM, editor: *Infertility, a comprehensive text,* Norwalk, Conn, 1990, Appleton & Lange.

82. Kahn JA et al: Fallopian tube sperm perfusion used in a donor insemination programme, *Hum Reprod* 7:806, 1992.

83. Karow AM: Biophysical and chemical considerations in cryopreservation. In Karow AM, Pegg DE, editors: *Organ preservation for transplantation,* New York, 1981, Marcel Dekker.

84. Kennedy WP et al: A simple clinical assay to evaluate the acrosin activity of human spermatozoa, *J Androl* 10:221, 1989.

85. Khalifa E et al: Successful fertilization and pregnancy outcome in in vitro fertilization using cryopreserved/thawed spermatozoa from patients with malignant diseases, *Hum Reprod* 7:105, 1992.

86. Kobayashi T et al: Protective role of superoxide dismutase in human sperm motility: superoxide dismutase activity and lipid peroxide in human seminal plasma and spermatozoa, *Hum Reprod* 6:987, 1991.

87. Kopf GS, Gerton GL: The mammalian sperm acrosome and the acrosome reaction. In Wassarman PM, editor: *The biology and chemistry of mammalian fertilization,* CRC Uniscience Series, Boca Raton, Fla, 1990, CRC Press.

88. Kruger TF et al: Sperm morphologic features as a prognostic factor in in vitro fertilization, *Fertil Steril* 46:1118, 1986.

89. Kruger TF et al: A quick reliable staining technique for human sperm morphology, *Arch Androl* 18:275, 1987.

90. Kruger TF et al: Predictive value of abnormal sperm morphology in in vitro fertilization, *Fertil Steril* 49:112, 1988.

91. Kruger TF et al: A new computerized method of reading sperm morphology (strict criteria) is as efficient as technician reading, *Fertil Steril* 59:202, 1993.

92. Lacham O: Immobilized sperm motility stimulation and embryo development. In *Advances in assisted reproductive technology for the infertile male,* Serono International Clinical Meeting, Adelaide, Australia, November 30-December 1, 1992.

93. Lee CYG et al: Enzyme inactivation and inhibition by gossypol, *Mol Cell Biochem* 47:65, 1982.

94. Leyton J, Sailing P: 95Kd sperm proteins bind ZP3 and serve as tyrosine kinase substrates in response to zona binding, *Cell* 57:1123, 1989.

95. Liu DY, Baker HWG: Relationships between human sperm acrosin acrosomes, morphology and fertilization in vitro, *Hum Reprod* 5:298, 1990.

96. Liu DY, Baker HWG: Test of human sperm function and fertilization in vitro, *Fertil Steril* 58:465, 1992.

97. Liu DY et al: A human sperm-zona pellucida binding test using oocytes that failed to fertilize in vitro, *Fertil Steril* 50:782, 1988.

98. Liu DY et al: A sperm-zona pellucida binding test and in vitro fertilization, *Fertil Steril* 52:281, 1989.

99. MacLeod J, Gold RZ: The male factor in fertility and infertility, IV: sperm morphology in fertile and infertile marriage, *Fertil Steril* 2:394, 1952.

100. Mahadevan MM, Trounson AO: The influence of seminal characteristics on the success rate of human in vitro fertilization, *Fertil Steril* 42:400, 1984.

101. Mahony MC et al: Role of spermatozoa cryopreservation in assisted reproduction. In Acosta AA, Kruger TF, editors: *Human spermatozoa in assisted reproduction,* Baltimore, 1989, Williams & Wilkins.

102. Margalioth EJ et al: Correlation between the zona-free hamster egg sperm penetration assay and human in vitro fertilization, *Fertil Steril* 45:665, 1986.

103. Marshburn PB et al: Spermatozoal characteristics from fresh and frozen donor semen and their correlation with fertility outcome after intrauterine insemination, *Fertil Steril* 58:179, 1992.

104. Mathur S et al: Motion characteristics of spermatozoa from men with cytotoxic sperm antibodies, *AJRIM* 12:87, 1986.

105. Mazur P: Stopping biological time: the freezing of living cells, *Ann N Y Acad Sci* 541:514, 1988.

106. Mbizvo MT, Burkman LJ, Alexander NJ: Human follicular fluid stimulates hyperactivated motility in human sperm, *Fertil Steril* 54:708, 1990.

107. Menkveld R, Kruger TF: Basic semen analysis. In Acosta AA et al, editors: *Human spermatozoa in assisted reproduction,* Baltimore, 1990, Williams & Wilkins.

108. Menkveld R, Kruger TF: Laboratory procedures: review and background. In Acosta AA et al, editors: *Human spermatozoa in assisted reproduction,* Baltimore, 1990, Williams & Wilkins.

109. Menkveld R et al: *Atlas of human sperm morphology,* Baltimore, 1991, Williams & Wilkins.

110. Menkveld R et al: Sperm selection capacity of the human zona pellucida, *Mol Reprod Dev* 30:346, 1991.

111. Morshedi M: Andrological methods of predicting the pregnancy outcome of an IVF program, doctoral thesis, Norfolk, Va, 1989, Eastern Virginia Medical School/Old Dominion University.

112. Morshedi M et al: Cryopreserved/thawed semen for in vitro fertilization: results from fertile donors and infertile patients, *Fertil Steril* 54:1093, 1990.

113. Mortimer D et al: Human sperm motility after injection and incubation in synthetic media, *Gamete Res* 9:131, 1984.

114. Murad C, deLamirande E, Gagnon C: Hyperactivated motility is coupled with interdependent modifications at axonemal and cytosolic levels in human spermatozoa, *J Androl* 13:323, 1992.

115. Oehninger S et al: Corrective measures and pregnancy outcome in in vitro fertilization patients with severe sperm morphology abnormalities, *Fertil Steril* 50:283, 1988.

116. Oehninger S et al: Hemizona assay: assessment of sperm dysfunction and prediction of in vitro fertilization outcome, *Fertil Steril* 51:665, 1989.

117. Oehninger S et al: Relationship between morphology and motion characteristics of human spermatozoa in semen and in swim-up fractions, *J Androl* 11:446, 1990.

118. Oehninger S et al: Human preovulatory oocytes have a higher sperm binding ability than immature oocytes under hemizona assay (HZA) conditions: evidence supporting the concept of "zona maturation," *Fertil Steril* 55:1165, 1991.

119. Oettle EE et al: Ultrastructural parameters of fertile cryopreserved human sperm, *Arch Androl* 29:151, 1992.

120. O'Rand MG, Widgren ED, Fisher SJ: Characterization of the rabbit sperm autoantigen, RSA, as a lectin-like zona binding protein, *Dev Biol* 129:231, 1988.

121. Ord T et al: The role of the laboratory in the handling of epididymal sperm for assisted reproductive technologies, *Fertil Steril* 57:1103, 1992.

122. Overstreet JW et al: Penetration of the human spermatozoa into the human zona pellucida and the zona-free hamster egg: a study of fertile donors and infertile patients, *Fertil Steril* 33:534, 1980.

123. Patrizio P et al: Relationship of epididymal sperm antibodies to their in vitro fertilization capacity in men with congenital absence of the vas deferens, *Fertil Steril* 58:1006, 1992.

124. Polansky FF, Lamb EJ: Do the results of semen analysis predict future fertility?: a survival analysis, *Fertil Steril* 49:1059, 1988.

125. Rana N et al: Glass wool-filtered spermatozoa and their oocyte penetrating capacity, *J In Vitro Fert Embryo Transfer* 6:280, 1989.

126. Richardson RT et al: Localization of rabbit sperm acrosin during the acrosome reaction induced by immobilized zona matrix, *Biol Reprod* 45:20, 1991.

127. Rogers BJ, Bentwood BJ: Capacitation, acrosome reaction and fertilization. In Zaneveld LJD, Chatterton RJ, editors: *Biochemistry of mammalian reproduction,* New York, 1982, John Wiley & Sons.

128. Rogers BJ, Parker RA: Relationship between the human sperm hypo-osmotic swelling test and sperm penetration assay, *J Androl* 12:152, 1991.

129. Rogers BJ et al: Sperm morphology assessment as an indicator of human fertilizing capacity, *J Androl* 4:119, 1983.

130. Rojas RJ et al: Penetration of zona-free hamster oocytes using human sperm aspirated from the epididymis of men with congenital absence of the vas deferens: comparison with human in vitro fertilization, *Fertil Steril* 58:1000, 1992.

131. Sailing PM: How the egg regulates sperm function during gamete interaction: factors and fantasies, *Biol Reprod* 44:246, 1991.

132. Saks VA et al: Role of creatine kinase in cellular function and metabolism, *Can J Physiol Pharmacol* 65:691, 1978.

133. Sanger WG, Armitage JO, Schmidt MA: Feasibility of semen cryopreservation in patients with malignant disease, *JAMA* 244:789, 1980.

134. Scammel GE et al: Cryopreservation of semen in men with testicular tumors of Hodgkin's disease: results of artificial insemination of their partners, *Lancet* 2:31, 1985.

135. Senn A, Germond M, DeGrandi P: Immunofluorescence study of actin, acrosin, dynein, tubulin and hyaluronidase and their impact on in vitro fertilization, *Hum Reprod* 7:841, 1992.

136. Shenfield F et al: Effects of age, gravidity and male infertility status on cumulative conception rates following artificial insemination with cryopreserved donor semen: analysis of 2998 cycles of treatment in one centre over 10 years, *Hum Reprod* 8:60, 1993.

137. Sherman JK: Cryopreservation of human semen. In Kee BA, Webster BW, editors: *Handbook of the laboratory diagnosis and treatment of infertility,* Boca Raton, Fla, 1990, CRC Press.

138. Shur BD, Hall NG: A role for mouse sperm surface galactosyltransferases in sperm binding to the egg zona pellucida, *J Cell Biol* 95:574, 1982.

139. Silber SJ, Patrizio P, Asch RH: Quantitative evaluation of spermatogenesis by testicular histology in men with congenital absence of the vas deferens undergoing epididymal sperm aspiration, *Hum Reprod* 5:89, 1990.

140. Silber SJ et al: New treatment for infertility due to congenital absence of the vas deferens, *Lancet* 2:850, 1987.

141. Silva PD, Meisch J, Schauberger CW: Intrauterine insemination of cryopreserved donor semen, *Fertil Steril* 52:243, 1987.

142. Smith K, Steinberger E: Survival of spermatozoa in a human sperm bank. *JAMA* 223:774, 1973.

143. Subak LL, Adamson GD, Boltz NL: Therapeutic donor insemination: a prospective randomized trial of fresh versus frozen sperm, *Am J Obstet Gynecol* 166:1597, 1992.

144. Tejada RI et al: A test for the practical evaluation of male fertility by acridine orange (AO) fluorescence, *Fertil Steril* 42:87, 1984.

145. Tesarik J et al: Acrosin activation follows its surface exposure and precedes membrane fusion in human sperm acrosome reaction, *Development* 110:391, 1990.

146. Tesarik J, Mendoza Oltras C, Testart J: Effect of the human cumulus oophorus on movement characteristics of human capacitated spermatozoa, *J Reprod Fertil* 88:665, 1990.

147. Thachil J, Jewett MAS: Preservation techniques for human semen, *Fertil Steril* 35:546, 1981.

148. Toledo AA et al: Electroejaculation in combination with in vitro fertilization and gamete micromanipulation for treatment of anejaculatory male infertility, *Am J Obstet Gynecol* 167:322, 1992.

149. Tombes RM, Shapiro BM: Metabolic channeling: a phosphorylcreatine shuttle to mediate high energy phosphate transport between mitochondrion and tail, *Cell* 41:325, 1985.

150. Tombes RM, Shapiro BM: Enzyme termini of a phosphocreatine shuttle: purification and characterization of two creatine kinase isoenzymes from sea urchin sperm, *J Biol Chem* 262:1, 1987.

151. Topfer-Petersen E et al: Cell biology of acrosomal proteins, *Andrologia* 22:110, 1990.

152. Triana V: Artificial insemination and semen banks in Italy. In Daniel G, Price W, editors: *Human artificial insemination and semen preservation,* New York, 1980, Plenum Press.

153. Tulsiani DRP, Skudlarek MD, Orgebin-Crist MC: Novel α-D-mannosidase of rat sperm plasma membranes: characterization and potential role in sperm-egg interactions, *J Cell Biol* 109:1257, 1989.

154. Tummon I et al: Acrosin activity correlates with fertilization in vitro. In Programs and Abstracts of the 16th Annual Meeting of the American Society of Andrology, Montreal, April 1991 (abstract).

155. van Uem JF et al: Male factor evaluation in IVF: Norfolk experience, *Fertil Steril* 44:375, 1985.

156. van Zyl JA, Kotze VW, Menkveld R: Predictive value of spermatozoa morphology in natural fertilization. In Acosta AA et al, editors: *Human spermatozoa in assisted reproduction,* Baltimore, 1990, Williams & Wilkins.

157. Vazquez MH, Phillips DM, Wassarman PM: Interaction of mouse sperm with purified sperm receptors covalently linked to silica beads, *J Cell Sci* 92:713, 1989.

158. Vasquez-Levin et al: The predictive value of zona-free hamster egg sperm penetration assay for failure of human in vitro fertilization and subsequent successful zona drilling, *Fertil Steril* 53:1055, 1990.

159. Wang C et al: Evaluation of human sperm hyperactivated motility and its relationship with the zona-free hamster oocyte sperm penetration assay, *J Androl* 12:253, 1991.

160. Wolf DP, Patton PE: Sperm cryopreservation: state of the art, *J In Vitro Fert Embryo Transfer* 6:325, 1989.

161. World Health Organization: Adenosine triphosphate in semen and other sperm characteristics: their relevance for fertility prediction in men with normal sperm concentration, *Fertil Steril* 57:877, 1992.

162. World Health Organization: *WHO laboratory manual for the examination of human semen and sperm cervical mucus interaction,* ed 3, Cambridge, UK, 1992, Cambridge University Press.

163. Wothe DD, Charbonneau H, Shapiro BM: The phosphocreatine shuttle of sea urchin sperm: flagellar creatine kinase resulted from a gene triplication, *Proc Natl Acad Sci USA* 87:5203, 1990.

164. Yanagimachi R: In vitro capacitation of hamster spermatozoa by follicular fluid, *J Reprod Fertil* 18:275, 1969.

165. Yanagimachi R, Yanagimachi H, Rogers BJ: The use of zona-free animal ova as a test system for the assessment of the fertilizing capacity of human spermatozoa, *Biol Reprod* 15:471, 1976.

166. Zaneveld LJD, Leyendran RS: Biochemical analysis of seminal plasma and spermatozoa. In Keel BA, Webster BW, editors: *CRC handbook of the laboratory diagnosis and treatment of infertility,* Boca Raton, Fla, 1990, CRC Press.

167. Zovari R, DeAlmeida M, Feneux D et al: In vitro effect of spermatozoal antibodies on human sperm movement, *J Reprod Immunol,* vol 16(S), July 1989 (abstract no 60).

Appendix 29-A

Sample Patient Information Form to Accompany Semen Specimen

PATIENT INFORMATION FORM
EVMS/ODU ANDROLOGY LABORATORY
The Jones Institute for Reproductive Medicine
Second Floor, 601 Colley Avenue
Norfolk, Virginia 23507-1912
(804) 446-5737

PATIENT TELEPHONE NUMBERS

Home:_____ Work:_____
Address:_____
_____

Specimen No._____
                         (lab use only)
Patient:_____   _____   _____
            last name   first name   spouse's name
Physician:_____
                   address to receive lab report
Appointment Date:_____ Appointment Time:_____
Husband's Birthdate:_____ Social Security No.:_____
Wife's Birthdate:_____ Social Security No.:_____
New patient or repeat patient (circle one)   Private or in Vitro patient (circle one)
Type of specimen: semen, cervical mucus, blood serum (circle one):
Other (explain):_____
Time specimen collected:_____ Time specimen arrived in lab:_____
Location of specimen collected: Was specimen collection complete?_____
                                                                                                      yes or no
If collection was incomplete, was loss from first or last part? (circle one)
Date of last ejaculation, intercourse, or emission:_____

HEALTH PLAN/ATTACHMENTS		INSTITUTIONAL/MORPHOLOGY BY MAIL ACCOUNTS	
☐ Patient Pay	☐ Consent Form	☐ Naval Hospital - 88983	☐ Univ. of Colo - 176160
☐ Optima	☐ Referral Form	☐ Oceana Base - 102457	☐ Kevin Winslow - 176161
☐ Sentara Health	☐ Lab Slip	☐ Ganty SRC Murty - 89036	☐ Maryview - Hemo Lab - 178509
☐ Cigna	☐ APS Form	☐ Dr. C. Ann Mashchak - 138816	
☐ Bill Patient	☐ Other_____	☐ Sentara Ref. Lab - 113646	

ANDROLOGY LAB SERVICES

☐ MALE - 606.9
☐ FEMALE - 628.9
☐ BLOOD DRAWN - 36415 (5.00)

		PROCEDURE	CPT	FEE	
1	☐	BASIC SEMEN ANALYSIS	89320		
2	☐	SEMEN MICROBIOLOGY (UREAPLASMA)	87109		
3	☐	CERVICAL MUCUS MICROBIOLOGY	87109		
4	☐	COUNT ONLY - SEMEN	89310		
5	☐	MORPHOLOGY ONLY - SEMEN	88161		
6	☐	MAR TEST ANTIBODIES ON SPERM	89325		
7	☐	DIRECT IMMUNOBEAD ANTIBODIES ON SPERM	(C 89325		
9	☐	ANTISPERM ANTIBODIES - MALE SERUM	(C 89325		
10	☐	ANTISPERM ANTIBODIES - FEMALE SERUM	(C 89325		
12	☐	SPERM/CERVICAL MUCUS COMPATIBILITY TEST	89328		
13	☐	SPERM/CERVICAL MUCUS PENETRATION TEST	89329		
14	☐	COMBINED SPERM/CERVICAL MUCUS COMP/PENE	89330		
16	☐	HAMSTER OVA/HUMAN SPERM PENETRATION TEST	(C 89329		
17	☐	ELECTRON MICROSCOPY OF SPERM	(C 89399		
18	☐	PREPARATION OF SPECIMEN FOR AIH	(C 89399		
19	☐	SEPARATION OF MOTILE SPERM FRACTION	(C 89399		
20	☐	EVALUATION SPECIMEN RETROGRADE PATIENT	(C 89399		
21	☐	SEPARATION OF MOTILE SPERM ANTISPERM AUTOIMMUNE	(C 89399		
22	☐	HYPOOSMOTIC SWELLING TEST (HOS)	89370		

15 BIOCHEMICAL EVALUATION (SEMEN)

PROCEDURE & C	CPT	FEE
☐ Total Protein	84999	
☐ Fructose	84999	
☐ Citric Acid	84999	
☐ Acid Phosphatase	84999	
☐ Glycerylphosphoric	84999	
☐ Zinc	84999	
☐ Copper	84999	
☐ Acrosin	84999	
☐ ATP	84999	

8 INDIRECT IMMUNOBEAD TEST

PROCEDURE (C	CPT	FEE
☐ Male Serum	89325	
☐ Female Serum	89325	
☐ Follicular Fluid	89325	

11 INDIRECT MAR TEST

PROCEDURE (C	CPT	FEE
☐ Male Serum	89325	
☐ Female Serum	89325	
☐ CERVICAL MUCUS	89325	

☐ **ELOCTROEJACULATION**

PROCEDURE (C	CPT	FEE
☐ Basic Semen	89320	
☐ Swim - up & C	89399	

PATIENT PAYMENT $_____

Specimen Collection

1. For assays involving semen we strongly recommend collection in our private facilities. Most of these assays necessitate the use of a fresh specimen to ensure accurate determinations of sperm motility and viability. If it is impossible to collect the specimen in the Lab's facilities, then the sample must be collected in a **proper** collection container (provided by the Lab) and delivered to the Lab within 30-45 minutes after emission.

2. In order to ensure that the semen specimen is clinically useful, the following procedures should be employed:

   a. A period of sexual abstinence (no emission) of no more than 5 and no less than 3 days should be observed before collection of the ejaculate being tested.

   b. The specimen should be collected by manual masturbation, without the use of lubricants, condoms or oral sex. If masturbation is not possible, a SPECIAL SEMEN CONDOM will be provided by the Lab.

   c. The specimen should be collected in a container provided by the Lab or provided to the physician by the Lab.

   d. Avoid contamination of the inside of the collection container both before and after collection. (Note: the container is sterile until opened.)

   e. Collect the entire ejaculate and note on PATIENT INFORMATION form if any portion (first or last) of the ejaculate misses that container or if spillage occurs.

   f. During transport the specimen should not be subject to extreme heat or cold, nor to direct sunlight. We recommend that the container be carried in an inside pocket next to your body so that body temperature is maintained.

Part V

THERAPY OF INFERTILITY

Chapter 30

INDUCTION OF OVULATION
General Concepts

Edward E. Wallach, MD

Ovulation is the physiologic process whereby the female gamete is released from the ovarian follicle into a new environment in which fertilization may occur. This process normally occurs at monthly intervals from puberty to menopause; it is interrupted physiologically only by pregnancy and postpartum lactation. Although accompanied by significant and characteristic hormonal events, ovulation is directed exclusively toward procreation. When the ovulatory process fails to take place, intervention is required to achieve pregnancy. Fertilization and the earliest stages of embryonic development normally occur within the lumen of the fallopian tube after transfer of the ovum into the tubal ostium.

DEFINITION OF TERMS
Ovulation versus oocyte retrieval

The term *ovulation* must be distinguished from *oocyte retrieval,* in which the stimulated ovarian follicle is artificially punctured to aspirate the enclosed oocyte. The oocyte then undergoes fertilization either in vitro (IVF) or within the fallopian tube after artificial transfer (gamete intrafallopian transfer [GIFT]). Protocols used for ovulation induction and those for oocyte retrieval are technically distinct, and each requires its own set of diagnostic and therapeutic guidelines. For ovulation to be effective, the extruded oocyte must be mature, fertilizable, and capable of full embryonic development. To this end follicle rupture and oocyte maturation are coordinated by specific gonadotropic stimuli. After ovulation, the follicle undergoes rapid conversion into a corpus luteum capable of producing sufficient quantities of progesterone to ensure implantation and maintenance of early pregnancy.

Periovulatory interval

The periovulatory interval refers to that period bracketed by the gonadotropin surge and the development of an effective corpus luteum. The events that take place within the periovulatory interval include growth of the preovulatory follicle(s) and its contents, meiotic maturation and cytoplasmic changes in the oocyte necessary for fertilization and early embryonic development, follicle wall disruption (ovulation), and transformation of each ruptured follicle into a functioning corpus luteum (Fig. 30-1). Local ovarian factors operating within the periovulatory interval influence (1) the occurrence and timing of follicle wall disruption, (2) the maturational status of the oocyte and its postfertilization embryonic potential, and (3) the establishment of an effective corpus luteum. These three sequelae of follicular development are essential to achieve unassisted reproduction. To maximize the likelihood of conception in any given cycle, follicle rupture must be synchronized with meiotic and cytoplasmic maturation of the oocyte, and those factors responsible for conversion of a follicle into a corpus luteum should be intact.

Therapeutic ovulation induction

Therapeutic ovulation induction attempts to mimic a naturally occurring process that culminates in ovulation of a single follicle. However, in certain circumstances stimulation of multiple follicles is desirable, such as in controlled ovarian hyperstimulation, a technique often used in conjunction with intrauterine insemination. Likewise, in IVF, GIFT, and related therapeutic technologies for correction of infertility, the desired objective is to stimulate many follicles. Hyperstimulation in such instances is intentionally geared to facilitate the recovery of a large number of fertilizable oocytes, some of which, after fertilization, may be cryopreserved for future transfer. The oocyte is capable of maturation in vitro after it has been liberated from inhibitory influences exerted by the early preovulatory follicle. This capability, first reported in 1937 by Pincus and Enzmann,[47] forms the basis for retrieval of oocytes from their follicles before they have achieved full maturation and is in contradistinction to the course of events when ovulation occurs naturally and oocytes mature in vivo.

PHYSIOLOGY AND ENDOCRINOLOGY OF OOGENESIS

Primordial germ cells

The full complement of primordial germ cells arrives at the gonadal ridge early in embryonic life. Migration of these germ cells from the yolk sac endoderm begins during the fifth week of embryonic life. During their migration process and once they have been established in the ovary, the germ cells undergo mitotic replication and differentiation into oogonia. Mitotic division ceases by the seventh month of fetal life, at which time the total germ cell population has been achieved, and the germ cells are subsequently termed oocytes. Oocytes then enter into the first meiotic (reduction) division, and are arrested in prophase of this process. Subsequent decline in oocyte population occurs through one of two physiologic mechanisms: ovulation or follicular atresia.

Primordial follicles

When the germ cells initially reach the ovary, they become surrounded by a single layer of spindle-shaped follicular cells, thus forming individual units referred to as primordial follicles. The maximal number of germ cells within the fetal ovary has been estimated at between 6 million and 7 million, but this population declines rapidly during late embryonic life to approximately 2 million oocytes by the time of birth and 400,000 at menarche.[4] The original follicular cells eventually differentiate into granulosa and theca cells, which are vital to the production of ovarian steroid hormones and nonsteroidal factors that influence and protect the oocyte. The oocyte is the focal point of each follicular unit and as such communicates bidirectionally with the surrounding follicular cells. The primary oocyte remains in prophase of the first meiotic division until shortly before ovulation, at which time meiosis resumes under the influence of the preovulatory surge of luteinizing hormone (LH). In the immediate preovulatory interval, the membrane of the nucleus, also known as the germinal vesicle, undergoes dissolution (germinal vesicle breakdown) and its absence is readily verified cytologically by light microscopy. Ultimately the first polar body is formed; at this time the oocyte completes metaphase of the first meiotic division and is termed a secondary oocyte.

Ovulation

In the physiologic sequence of events, the oocyte surrounded by cumulus cells is extruded from the follicle at the time of ovulation. Penetration of the oocyte by a spermatozoon triggers completion of the meiotic process, yielding a haploid ovum and a second polar body. The fusion of male and female pronuclei during fertilization endows the newly formed zygote with a diploid complement of chromosomes.

Follicular atresia

Follicular atresia continues to occur from intrauterine life through menopause. Atresia is an ongoing process that occurs in utero, before menarche, during natural cycles and during oral contraceptive use, and throughout pregnancy and lactation. This process involves regression of follicles at each stage of development, from primordial to graafian follicles, and is the fate of 99.99% of the 400,000 follicles present at menarche. Loss of the remaining 0.01% of ovarian follicles is accounted for through the process of ovulation. Although follicular atresia is a major factor in limiting multiple gestations in women, the mechanism(s) responsible for the atretic process is poorly understood. Primordial follicles are able to progress to primary follicles independent of follicle-stimulating hormone (FSH). Once menarche has been established, cyclic gonadotropin production results in appropriate sequential ovarian stimulation.

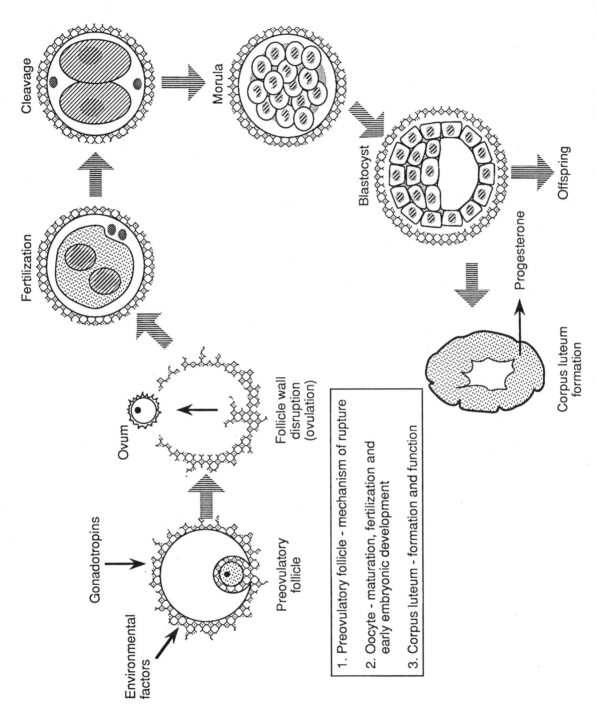

Cleavage

Morula

Blastocyst

Fertilization

Offspring

Progesterone

Ovum

Corpus luteum
formation

Follicle wall
disruption
(ovulation)

Gonadotropins

Preovulatory
follicle

Environmental
factors

1. Preovulatory follicle - mechanism of rupture

2. Oocyte - maturation, fertilization and
   early embryonic development

3. Corpus luteum - formation and function

Fig. 30-1. The periovulatory interval. This interval is the time period between the preovulatory gonadotropin surge and development of an effective corpus luteum.

Selection of the dominant follicle

At the beginning of each cycle, FSH stimulates the recruitment and growth of a cohort of follicles in both ovaries. By the sixth or seventh day of an ovulatory cycle one follicle of this cohort has been selected to be the dominant follicle.[25] Growth of the dominant follicle continues with replication of granulosa cells, accumulation of antral fluid, and increased estradiol production, all of which are under the influence of FSH. The remaining follicles in that cohort, located in both ovaries, undergo regression and degeneration. Stimulation by FSH results not only in granulosa cell replication, but also in enhanced aromatase activity in the granulosa cells. The aromatase enzyme converts androstenedione, a weak androgen produced by the theca cells and delivered to the granulosa cells, to estradiol. Simultaneously, FSH stimulates the appearance of LH receptors on the surface membrane of the granulosa cells.

Although LH is secreted in relatively low levels throughout almost the entire cycle, increasing production of estradiol from the dominant follicle of the cohort (the follicle destined to ovulate) leads to a rapid and evanescent increase in the pituitary production of LH, the gonadotropin ultimately responsible for provoking disruption of the follicle wall and ovulation. It has been estimated that 3 months are required from the time a follicle emerges from the primordial stage until its attainment of preovulatory status.[36] This observation has particular significance in therapeutic ovulation induction, since the follicle that responds to 10 days of stimulation with exogenous gonadotropins has probably undergone preliminary growth in previous cycles. In contrast, prolonged stimulation is required to induce ovulation in women who have not shown evidence of ovarian activity for many years.

Before follicle rupture, progesterone is secreted in small, but increasing, quantities. It is only after follicle wall disruption and oocyte expulsion have occurred that follicular production of progesterone begins to escalate significantly. Once ovulation has occurred and the follicle wall collapses, new vessels invade the follicle wall, a process termed neovascularization. Capillaries and fibroblasts rapidly penetrate the basement membrane separating theca and granulosa layers and enter the heretofore avascular granulosa layer of the follicle. These vessels vascularize the mural granulosa cells, surrounded by fibroblasts and theca cells.

Corpus luteum development

Early in corpus luteum development, the granulosa cells begin to assume a characteristic morphologic appearance, a process termed luteinization. On a per-unit weight basis, the corpus luteum has the greatest blood supply of any organ in the body.[9] The vasculature of the corpus luteum carries substrate in the form of low-density lipoprotein cholesterol to the luteinized cells, provides oxygenation, and delivers progesterone (the end product of corpus luteum steroid synthesis) to the systemic circulation. The corpus luteum normally functions for approximately 14 days, during which time its major secretory product, progesterone, prepares the endometrium for implantation and provides it with the hormonal support required for early pregnancy maintenance until the trophoblast assumes this responsibility at approximately 7 weeks of gestation. In the event that pregnancy does not occur, the corpus luteum begins to regress by approximately 12 days after ovulation and is ultimately transformed into a corpus albicans, a fibrotic structure that gradually becomes incorporated with the stromal tissue.

Establishment of pregnancy provides the trophoblastic signal in the form of chorionic gonadotropin (CG), which sustains the corpus luteum throughout early pregnancy. In addition to an adequate blood supply and LH or CG support, functional/structural well-being of the corpus luteum is dependent on the quality of the preovulatory follicle from which it was derived. The process of folliculogenesis preceding ovulation must result in the production of an appropriate number of granulosa cells endowed with an optimal complement of LH receptors to ensure the production and secretion of appropriate levels of progesterone after ovulation. The LH receptor content of granulosa cells is dependent on stimulation by FSH in the preovulatory phase, as noted above.

PURPOSES OF PROVIDING BACKGROUND ON OVARIAN FUNCTION

The use of exogenous substances to stimulate follicle development and to achieve ovulation requires an appreciation of the factors controlling normal physiologic ovarian function. Since ovulation-inducing agents can function at each compartment of the hypothalamic-pituitary-ovarian complex, understanding the site(s) of action of each agent, its mode of action, and the hazards of overstimulation or inappropriate stimulation calls for a thorough understanding of ovarian function. The remainder of this chapter is devoted to a description of the regulation of ovarian function at both central and ovarian levels, the various agents available for follicular maturation and ovulation induction, and the monitoring techniques to be used with each. Chapters 32, 33, and 34 provide specific details regarding each agent used for follicle stimulation and ovulation induction.

PHYSIOLOGIC CONTROL OF OVULATION

The process of ovulation integrates four distinct compartments that, when functioning normally, result in the cyclic development of ovarian follicles and the release of at least one mature ovum during each cycle (Fig. 30-2). Each of the four compartments is unique in its anatomic characteristics, as well as in the nature of its secreted hormone(s). The compartments include (1) the ovaries, (2) the anterior

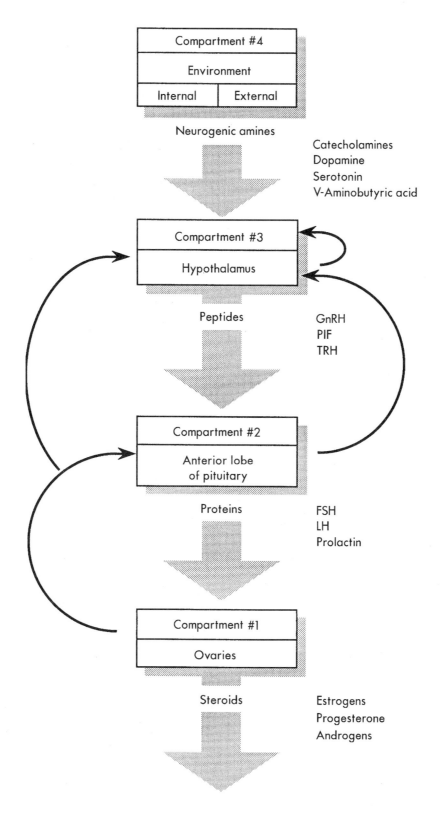

Fig. 30-2. The four compartments that participate in the ovulation process and their interrelationships. *PIF,* Prolactin-inhibiting factor; *TRH,* thyrotropin-releasing hormone.

lobe of the pituitary gland (hypophysis), (3) the hypothalamus, and (4) the environment.

Regulation by the ovaries

The ovaries produce steroid hormones (estrogens, progestogens, and androgens). For the most part, estrogens are produced by granulosa cells, progesterone by theca and granulosa cells, and androgens by theca cells and by enzymatically active stromal cells. Although the premenarcheal ovary possesses the capacity for steroid production, controlling mechanisms at the level of the anterior lobe of the pituitary gland and hypothalamus do not provide the appropriate level of stimulation to effect significant ovarian steroidogenesis until just before menarche.

Regulation by the anterior lobe of the pituitary gland

The anterior lobe of the pituitary gland produces protein hormones (FSH, LH, and prolactin) that are instrumental in regulating ovarian function. FSH and LH influence ovarian folliculogenesis and steroid hormone secretion via direct action on the ovary. Although the influence of prolactin on ovarian function is primarily indirect through modulation of gonadotropin release, there is also strong evidence for a direct ovarian action of prolactin.[23] Staining of the glycoprotein moieties of FSH and LH enables histologic identification of granules containing these hormones in the gonadotropes. Through this property, histochemical techniques and immunocytochemical methods have demonstrated that LH and FSH are individually produced largely by distinct gonadotropes, but to a lesser extent are secreted by the same cells.[46] The observation that both gonadotropins can arise from common cells may explain why a midcycle surge of FSH release accompanies the preovulatory LH surge. Prolactin-secreting cells are identifiable histologically by similar staining techniques. These distinct cells, termed lactotropes, are more laterally situated in the hypophysis than are the gonadotropes.[45] The first few days of the ovulatory cycle are characterized by a predominance of FSH secretion. In contrast, the midcycle surge of gonadotropins brought about by gonadotropin-releasing hormone (GnRH) is dominated by LH; the concomitant rise in FSH level is of lesser magnitude. After ovulation, serum levels of LH and FSH decline to their preovulatory range.

Regulation by the hypothalamus

The elaboration of LH and FSH, as well as other hypophysiotropic hormones, is regulated in large measure by the central nervous system, specifically the peptide hormones elaborated by the third compartment, the hypothalamus. The peptides involved in the regulation of ovarian function include GnRH (a decapeptide); prolactin-inhibiting factor (either a dopamine-like substance or dopamine itself); and thyrotropin-releasing hormone (a tripeptide), which stimulates thyrotropin release while concomitantly serving as a prolactin-stimulating factor. These hypothalamic peptides stimulate the synthesis and secretion of hormones by the anterior lobe of the pituitary gland. Early on in the evolution of knowledge about hypothalamic gonadotropic releasing factors, GnRH was thought to be exclusively related to LH secretion and consequently was originally termed LH-releasing factor (LRF). However, it is now apparent that secretion of both FSH and LH is dependent on this hypothalamic factor. The change in nomenclature from LRF to GnRH reflects this peptide's dual control over both gonadotropins and also emphasizes that this factor fulfills the criteria necessary to be identified as a hormone. No discrete FSH-releasing substance has been identified. Two important characteristics of hypothalamic control over gonadotropic secretions include (1) a varying responsiveness of the pituitary gonadotropin secreting cells to GnRH throughout the cycle and (2) the pulsatile release of gonadotropins in response to episodic elaboration of GnRH into the hypothalamic-hypophysial portal vasculature system. The pulses of GnRH vary in their frequency and amplitude. The sensitivity of these cells to GnRH depends on the steroid hormonal milieu, which in turn varies with time in the cycle.

Regulation by the environment

The fourth compartment may be arbitrarily termed the environment. This component of the superstructure that regulates ovarian function is not anatomically defined, as are the other three compartments. The environmental compartment consists of a wide array of heterogeneous factors that ultimately influence hypothalamic function. These factors are as disparate as diet, climate, light-dark cyclicity, level of stress, and the functional status of other endocrine structures. This spectrum of environmental features—internal and external—is translated into input recognizable by the hypothalamus via their biochemical conversion to neurochemical transmitters, included among which are norepinephrine, dopamine, epinephrine, serotonin, and γ-aminobutyric acid (GABA). Catecholamine and serotonin neuron innervation of the median eminence is particularly important in regulating secretions of the hypothalamic nuclei that control pituitary-ovarian function. In addition to monamines and amino acids, peptides appear to play a modulating role. The vasculature of the hypothalamus and pituitary is unique in that the blood flow is tridirectional,[5,44] with flow toward (1) the systemic circulation, (2) the anterior pituitary, and (3) the brain. This vascular arrangement gives rise to the possibility of both short and ultrashort feedback relationships acting between the hypothalamus and the hypophysis.

A number of peptide hormones are produced by the neurons in an area of the median eminence that terminates in capillary loops. These products, neurohormones, are released into the hypothalamic-hypophysial portal system. Opioid peptides such as β-endorphins and enkephalins also play a major role in the regulation of hypothalamic-pituitary function. Opioid receptors have been identified in the hypothalamus as well as in other regions of the central nervous system. Administration of opiates and enkephalin analogues results in inhibition of LH secretion and an increase in prolactin release.[49] Opioids exert an inhibitory effect on LH secretion by inhibiting GnRH neurons in the arcuate nucleus. Catecholamines also appear to regulate the elaboration of GnRH; dopamine inhibits LH secretion, and norepinephrine may stimulate LH release.[54]

The pulsatile release of GnRH by the hypothalamus has been well recognized since the pioneering work of Knobil,[30] carried out in rhesus monkeys. These classic studies revealed that the secretion of LH and FSH exhibits periodicity, with pulsatile release at approximately 90-minute intervals in response to the episodic release of GnRH. The continuous infusion of GnRH down-regulates the pituitary gland and results in failure of gonadotropin secretion. The use of long-acting analogues of this decapeptide also inhibits gonadotropin production. Thus the intervals between either physiologic episodes of GnRH elaboration or pulses of exogenous GnRH delivered by an infusion pump allow the pituicyte to recover its responsiveness to GnRH, thereby replenishing GnRH receptors. The ultimate elaboration of gonadotropins results from a multitude of factors, primarily an appropriate program of GnRH pulses with varying amplitude and frequency delivered to the hypophysis via the hypothalamic-hypophysial portal system. Modulating this mechanism are catecholamines, neuropeptides, opioids, and feedback signals originating at all four compartments.

Feedback mechanisms

The secretions elaborated by the four compartments just described (ovaries, hypophysis, hypothalamus, and environment) act in an integrated fashion to regulate the two major ovarian functions—ovulation and steroid production—via feedback mechanisms (Fig. 30-2).

For normal function, the basic system depends on pulsatile elaboration of GnRH by the arcuate nucleus in the medial basal hypothalamus. The elaboration of the decapeptide GnRH represents a final common pathway regulated by norepinephrine (positive effect) and dopamine (negative effect), modulated by endogenous opiates (negative effect). Catecholestrogens, synthesized from estrogens in the brain, may also play a role in modulating the influence of catecholamines on GnRH elaboration.[17] Circulating estradiol inhibits FSH secretion directly by suppressing hypothalamic GnRH release. Increasing levels of estradiol simultaneously act at the hypothalamus to facilitate the preovulatory surge of LH in response to GnRH. Progesterone, produced by the preovulatory follicle just before ovulation and by the corpus luteum after ovulation, acts in concert with estradiol to inhibit hypothalamic pulsations of GnRH, as well as to facilitate the preovulatory surge of LH and FSH. The interrelationships between the ovarian steroid

hormones estradiol and progesterone and pituitary gonadotropin elaboration constitute a *long* loop feedback system. A *short* loop feedback mechanism is exemplified by the negative effect exerted by gonadotropins on their own release via an inhibitory influence on hypothalamic elaboration of GnRH. An *ultrashort* loop has also been postulated to explain the theoretic ability of hypothalamic secretions to regulate their own release through local actions. This level of regulation of the hypothalamic-pituitary-ovarian axis is mediated via catecholamines, norepinephrine, dopamine, serotonin, and endorphins, as well as by various other peptides that have been postulated to act as neurotransmitters in the central nervous system, such as vasoactive intestinal peptide, cholecystokinin, neurotensin, and GABA.

The episodic elaboration of LH by the pituitary in response to GnRH also exhibits alterations in amplitude and frequency. For example, LH pulse mean amplitude is maximal in the early and mid–luteal phase and low in the follicular and late luteal phases. LH pulse mean frequency is maximal in the follicular phase, declines in the luteal phase, and is lowest in the late luteal phase.[18] These alterations in LH release correlate somewhat with FSH patterns, even though FSH is less responsive to GnRH than is LH. The ultimate elaboration of LH and FSH by the anterior lobe of the pituitary gland results in ovarian steroid secretion, folliculogenesis, follicular rupture, and corpus luteum formation and maintenance.

LOCAL EVENTS WITHIN THE OVARY LEADING TO FOLLICLE WALL DISRUPTION AND OVULATION

A number of local processes intercede between the preovulatory gonadotropin stimulus and ovulation. In a wide range of mammalian species, hormones, enzymes, smooth muscle cells, prostaglandins (PGs), histamines, and catecholamines participate locally to prepare the follicle for ovulation.[67] (Fig. 30-3).

Follicular morphology

Cumulus cells in the developing follicle are intimately attached to the oocyte by long microvilli that penetrate the vitelline membrane into the oocyte.[70] Granulosa cells are also physically associated with one another and are in contact with the antral fluid and cumulus cells. An abundance of gap junctions among granulosa cells, as well as between granulosa cells and the oocyte membrane, provide the mechanism for exchange of molecules between cumulus cells and the oocyte during follicular development.[22] Before ovulation, the intimacy of the cumulus-oocyte relationship diminishes.[38] The mechanisms responsible for the breakdown of intercellular communication are complex and as yet largely unknown, but they probably involve loss of gap junctions.[31] This dissociation of cells may lead to remodeling of the follicular architecture, yielding a weak-

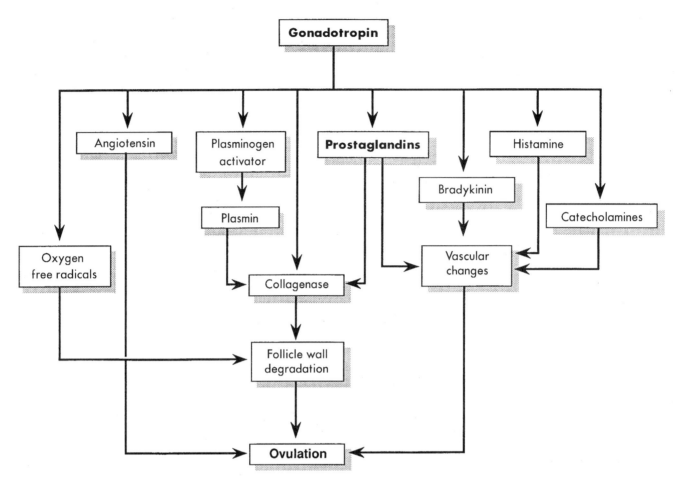

Fig. 30-3. The various processes that follow the gonadotropin surge and lead to disruption of the follicle wall.

ened follicle wall as well as liberation of the oocyte from specific biochemical factors that, before this point, had prevented its resumption of the meiotic process.

Perifollicular vascular changes in rabbit ovaries during the periovulatory interval have been examined by scanning electron microscopy (SEM) of microcorrosion casts.[28] These casts are prepared by injecting a resin directly into the ovarian artery and then digesting the ovarian tissue with potassium hydroxide, leaving a mold of the follicular microvasculature. Dilated vessels, extravasation of resin from weakened vessels, and filling defects are observed sequentially at the apex of the follicles in both in situ and in vitro perfused rabbit ovaries stimulated to ovulate with exogenous gonadotropin. Extravasation of resin is associated with increased vascular permeability. The presence of filling defects suggests areas of avascularity at the apical region, which may weaken the follicle wall, facilitating its disruption.

Progressive degeneration and decomposition of ovarian surface epithelial cells have been suggested as significant events leading to disruption of underlying connective tis-

sue.[6] Morphologic studies[62] clearly demonstrate disappearance of the surface epithelial cells at the apex of rabbit ovarian follicles perfused with gonadotropin in vitro, simulating observations made in vivo.[6]

Ovarian smooth muscle activity

The detection of ovarian smooth muscle tissue and demonstration of its contractility[40,50,59] form the basis for the hypothesis that autonomic nerves within the ovary may influence ovarian smooth muscle contractions at the time of ovulation and assist in achieving follicle rupture and ovum expulsion. Although ovarian smooth muscle contractions accompany the process of ovulation, and many agents that suppress ovarian contractions also inhibit ovulation,[60] the role of ovarian contractions in the ovulation process is not yet clear. These smooth muscle contractions may simply accompany ovulation but not play a causative role. Weiner et al.[64] have demonstrated the occurrence of ovulation and subsequent pregnancy in rabbits mating after ovarian denervation,[63] suggesting that autonomic innervation of the ovary is not essential for ovulation.

Proteolytic enzyme activity

Proteolytic enzymes appear to play a significant role in the process of mammalian ovulation. Lytic substances have been shown to originate from the surface epithelium at the apical region of the follicle,[51] and collagenolytic enzymes have been detected in ovarian follicles of various species.[13,26] Proteases have been shown to promote disruption of the follicle wall in the rabbit.[14] Ultrastructural studies of the tunica albuginea and theca externa of the apical region of rabbit graafian follicles before ovulation demonstrate progressive edema, fragmentation of collagen fibrils in the tunica, and dissociation of fibroblasts in the theca interna.[8] Structures identified as lysosomes appear in the surface epithelium immediately before follicle rupture.[7] These dense bodies in the apical surface epithelium are thought to represent a source of lysosomal enzymes that weaken the underlying follicle wall. Their presence is also associated with progressive dissociation of cumulus cells from one another, as well as from the oocyte, in response to gonadotropin stimulation. The involvement of collagenase in ovulation is supported by the observation that pectin, a microbial collagenase inhibitor, blocks ovulation in explanted ovaries.[26] Collagenase produced in granulosa cells of preovulatory human follicles is rapidly transported to the site of collagen degradation in the apical wall of the follicle.[20]

Plasminogen is present in follicular fluid, whereas plasmin, the product of the interaction of plasminogen activator and plasminogen, can weaken the follicle wall.[56] In addition to gonadotropins, certain PGs and cyclic adenosine monophosphate (cAMP) effectively stimulate granulosa cells to produce plasminogen activator. Under the influence of plasminogen activator, the ovum is dislodged from the granulosa cell layer and floats free in the follicular fluid; ultimately the tunica and theca are degraded. These changes follow the increase in gonadotropin and PG levels within the follicle. Although the secretion of plasminogen activator has been reported to be specifically responsive to FSH, Martinat and Combarnous[35] and Reich et al.[48] established that the preovulatory LH surge stimulates plasminogen activator activity. Canipari and Strickland[10] have reported that both FSH and LH can induce plasminogen activator secretion by granulosa cells, although the response to FSH is more immediate.

The relationship between PGs and proteolytic enzymes in the process of ovulation is not clear. Although PGs may be involved in the release or activation of collagenolytic enzymes within the follicle wall, blockade of PG synthesis does not inhibit plasminogen activator secretion.[15,48] Nonetheless, indomethacin, a PG synthase inhibitor, prevents ovarian collagen breakdown associated with ovulation in gonadotropin-treated rats.[48]

Prostaglandin activity

PGs have been implicated in the mechanism of ovulation in several species. Levels of PGE and PGF rise within developing rabbit ovarian follicles in response to LH or human CG (hCG).[33] PGE and PGF metabolites increase in the effluent of in vitro perfused rabbit ovaries before ovulation.[52] The increases in follicular PG content after gonadotropin treatment are blocked by administration of the PG synthase inhibitor indomethacin.[66] Indomethacin delays or inhibits ovulation in rats, rabbits, and monkeys.[2,11,42,57,61] It has been suggested that indomethacin alters ovulation by inducing the retrograde release of eggs from follicles through "misplaced" stigmata.[43] In rabbits, intrafollicular injection of either indomethacin or antiserum specific for F series PGs has also been shown to prevent ovulation in injected follicles without inhibiting ovulation in adjacent, untreated follicles.[3] These observations suggest that PGs influence ovulation locally at the ovarian level, but the precise nature of their role in the process of ovum expulsion has yet to be defined. $PGF_{2\alpha}$ can induce ovulation in the perfused rabbit ovary in the absence of gonadotropin.[29]

Although several of the periovulatory events within the follicle, including resumption of oocyte meiosis, steroidogenesis, and luteinization, are correlated with local levels of PG, these activities can proceed undisturbed despite blockade of PG synthesis. Follicle rupture, however, is the exception, and ovulation can be prevented by administration of PG synthase inhibitors or PG antibody. Espey[12] has likened ovulation to an inflammatory process with PG serving as a mediator (Fig. 30-4). Many other factors, however, are elaborated during inflammation and may be instrumental in regulating follicle rupture. In achieving ovulation, PGs may mediate a cascade of proteolytic activity in the follicle and/or give rise to vasodilation. Ultrastructural studies of ovarian capillaries in rabbits treated with indomethacin suggest that PGs increase the permeability of perifollicular capillaries that normally precedes ovulation.[41] Vasodilation of the microvasculature of preovulatory follicles after $PGF_{2\alpha}$ perfusion has also been demonstrated by SEM examination of vascular casts.[28] The perifollicular vascular changes stimulated by PGF_2 and PGI_2 are identical with those seen after gonadotropin treatment.

Other humoral factors

Simulating an acute inflammatory reaction, the ovulatory process is preceded by the local release of histamine,[65] PGs[58] and plasminogen activator,[24] and oxygen free radicals.[37] These substances appear to be produced by ovarian follicles in response to gonadotropic hormones (See Fig. 30-3). In addition, exposure of ovaries to exogenous histamine, PGs, and serine proteases similar to plasminogen activator can induce follicle rupture in the absence of gonadotropin. The inflammatory agent bradykinin also may be involved in the ovulation process.[12,55] This concept is supported by recent evidence of a significant increase in ovarian kinin-generating activity during the ovulation process in the rat.[16] More recently, bradykinin has been shown to induce

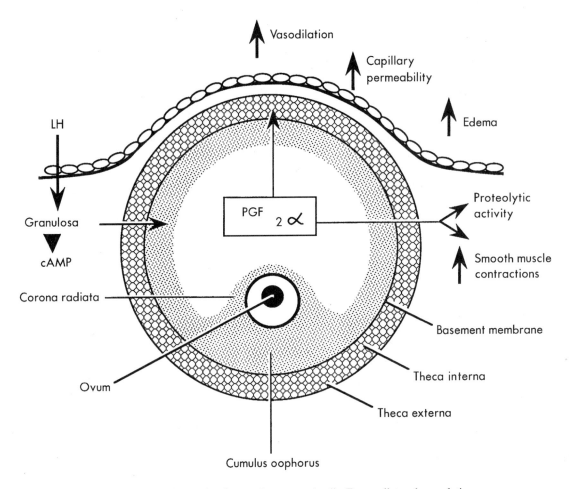

Fig. 30-4. Mechanisms whereby ovarian prostaglandin $F_{2\alpha}$ mediates the ovulation process.

rupture of mature follicles and to stimulate PG biosynthesis in in vitro perfused rabbit ovaries.[68] The mechanical process of ovulation that follows the preovulatory gonadotropin stimulus appears to involve numerous intermediaries acting in concert. PGs may thus act at several levels in this process (see Fig. 30-3).

AGENTS USED FOR OVULATION INDUCTION
Human menopausal gonadotropin

Human menopausal gonadotropin (hMG) (menotropins; Pergonal) is a potent preparation used for ovarian stimulation either to induce ovulation or to effect follicle maturation before oocyte retrieval for IVF or GIFT. The use of hMG was first described by Lunenfeld et al.[34] shortly after the 1958 report by Gemzell et al.[21] of successful pregnancy after ovulation induction with human pituitary gonadotropin. The preparation is a purified form of gonadotropins extracted from pooled urine specimens obtained from postmenopausal women, consisting of 75 or 150 IU each of FSH and LH per ampule. The gonadotropic preparation is administered by intramuscular injection, followed by hCG. hMG is used to stimulate follicle development, whereas

hCG is administered to simulate a preovulatory surge of LH when a single follicle or multiple follicles are deemed to have achieved preovulatory status.

Because it acts directly on the ovary, hMG does not require a functioning hypothalamus or pituitary to be effective. Without the benefit of internal feedback controls that are present during normal spontaneous gonadotropin secretion, however, the risk of ovarian hyperstimulation during the use of hMG is significant, and careful monitoring of folliculogenesis is mandatory. The dose of hMG required for follicular maturation must be individualized and titrated for each patient and even for different cycles in the same patient. An initial dose of 75 to 150 IU/d is customary, and treatment is usually continued for 7 to 12 days, with each daily dose of gonadotropin determined by indirect parameters of follicular response, using a combination of ultrasound monitoring and serial determinations of serum estrogen.

Adverse reactions to hMG include ovarian hyperstimulation, ovarian enlargement, abdominal discomfort, pain, bloating, pulmonary and vascular complications, multiple pregnancies, and occasional sensitivity reactions to the preparation itself. hMG is highly effective, and, provided that anovulation is not due to primary ovarian failure, approximately 90% of patients may be expected to respond with ovulation; pregnancy rates approach 70%. The rate of multiple gestation is high, occurring in 15% to 30% of gonadotropin-induced pregnancies. Details of administration of gonadotropins and management of ovarian hyperstimulation syndrome are provided in Chapters 33 and 35.

Human chorionic gonadotropin

hCG (A.P.L.; Follutein; Profasi; Pregnyl) is derived from human placentas. This preparation is generally used to achieve ovulation in patients whose ovaries have undergone preliminary stimulation with hMG to produce follicular maturation. The dosage customarily used is 5,000 to 10,000 U administered by intramuscular injection approximately 24 hours after the last dose of hMG. The timing of hCG administration is predicated upon a combination of ultrasound monitoring and serum estradiol levels and is based on the establishment of one or more mature, preovulatory follicles, usually approximately 15 to 20 mm in diameter. The usual upper level of serum estradiol attained just before hCG administration is 1500 pg/mL. Because the serum estradiol level at any given point cannot always be predicted by extrapolation from the rate of rise of the estradiol level, significantly higher levels occasionally are reached at the time of hCG administration. The higher the level of serum estradiol at the time hCG is administered, the greater is the risk of ovarian hyperstimulation. If a significant risk of ovarian hyperstimulation is suspected based on the estradiol level, hCG should be withheld.

Ultrasound monitoring does not completely preclude the possibility of hyperstimulation. The more follicles observed by ultrasound, however, the greater the risk of hyperstimulation, multiple ovulation, and/or multiple pregnancy. Women with polycystic ovaries, high serum estradiol levels before hCG administration (greater than 4000 pg/mL), multiple follicles in response to hMG, younger age, and lean body habitus are at heightened risk for ovarian hyperstimulation.[39] Ovulation should be induced with hCG only when there are no more than three or four follicles approximately 15 to 18 mm in diameter. More follicles may be desirable if the medication is being administered for follicle stimulation before oocyte retrieval for IVF or GIFT.

Purified follicle-stimulating hormone

Purified FSH (urofollitrophin; Follitropin; Metrodin) is separated from LH in hMG by chromatographic means. The final preparation consists of 75 IU of FSH per ampule and contains negligible LH activity. Purified FSH has been recommended for ovulation induction in patients with polycystic ovary disease who have an elevated LH:FSH ratio and have failed to ovulate in response to clomiphene citrate.[53] This preparation is also used in conjunction with hCG or hMG and hCG to achieve follicle maturation in an IVF cycle. Administration and monitoring measures are similar to those with hMG/hCG. Ovarian hyperstimulation syndrome with ovarian enlargement, ovarian cyst formation, multiple pregnancy, vascular effects, and gastrointestinal symptoms can also complicate the use of purified FSH. As with hMG, the ovary is the direct target for purified FSH. It is likely that newer forms of this preparation will be available soon. Such a preparation may be predicted to be more reliable, standardized, and free of systemic complications.

Clomiphene citrate

Clomiphene citrate (Clomid; Serophene) is a triphenylethylene derivative bound with citric acid, chloride, and an acetoxy group. This nonsteroidal agent consists of a mixture of two isomers: a *cis*-isomer, also termed zuclomiphene, and a *trans*-isomer, or enclomiphene. Cisclomiphene is the active moiety. It is weakly estrogenic and has antiestrogenic properties. Administered daily for 5 days beginning on the third, fourth, or fifth cycle day, clomiphene is highly effective in inducing ovulation, by virtue of competing with endogenous estrogen for hypothalamic estrogen receptors in patients who demonstrate evidence of follicular function (e.g., spontaneous anovulatory cycles or progestin-induced uterine bleeding). If ovulation fails to occur at this dose, increasing the daily dose to 100 mg and/or combining it with hCG (10,000 IU) administered approximately 1 week after the last dose of clomiphene may be effective. Alternatively, the duration of clomiphene administration may be extended. The lowest effective dose necessary to achieve ovulation is desirable to minimize antiestrogenic effects. If ovulation occurs but pregnancy is not established in a given clomiphene cycle, the same dose may be administered in subsequent cycles.

Because clomiphene acts primarily at the hypothalamic compartment, a functioning hypothalamus and pituitary gland are prerequisites for a satisfactory response. Clomiphene may also yield its pharmacologic effects at target tissues other than the hypothalamus (e.g., pituitary, ovary, endometrium, cervix, fallopian tube) inasmuch as the preparation binds to estrogen receptors. Generally 70% to 80% of well-selected patients may be expected to ovulate in response to clomiphene; however, pregnancy rates are generally considerably lower, in the range of approximately 40%. Approximately 75% of clomiphene-related pregnancies are achieved within three cycles of treatment.

Although multiple pregnancy is less likely with clomiphene than with gonadotropic preparations, the incidence is higher than that following spontaneous ovulation. Side effects occasionally encountered with clomiphene include vasomotor phenomena (hot flushes), abdominal discomfort, ovarian enlargement, and blurring of vision. No increase in birth defects has been detected among offspring when the drug has been administered to initiate ovulation. Clomiphene acts primarily through provoking the release of endogenous pituitary FSH and LH. Follicular maturation and concomitant ovarian estrogen production follow stimulation by endogenous gonadotropins. The rising levels of estrogen are responsible for an endogenously activated LH surge.[1]

Gonadotropin-releasing hormone

GnRH is a decapeptide synthesized by cells in the hypothalamus and released into the hypothalamic-hypophysial portal system. Its structure has been established and used for the synthesis of analogues with long-lasting effects. In the region of the median eminence, the decapeptide is secreted into the capillaries of the portal system. The observations that GnRH is produced intermittently and that this pulsatile exposure to GnRH is required by pituicytes for stimulation of gonadotropin release clarify (1) the poor success of GnRH in inducing ovulation when it is administered continuously and (2) the successful inhibition of pituitary gonadotropin production and release during the use of long-acting analogues of GnRH.

GnRH (Factrel; gonadorelin; Lutrepulse) is a synthetic decapeptide with a molecular weight of 1182 and possessing a chemical composition and structure identical with that of the substance that was originally extracted and isolated from porcine and ovine hypothalami. Although GnRH has been approved for clinical use only to evaluate the functional capacity of the anterior lobe of the pituitary and responsiveness of the gonadotropes in patients with pituitary dysfunction, GnRH has been used extensively to induce ovulation in patients with hypothalamic dysfunction. For ovulation induction, it is administered parenterally in an intermittent fashion. Intravenous or subcutaneous doses given at 60- to 120-minute intervals meet the dual requirement of a parenteral route and pulsatile administration. The preparation is available in the form of a lyophilized powder of the hydrochloride in vials containing 100 µg or 500 µg. Each vial is accompanied by an ampule containing 2 mL of sterile diluent (2% benzyl alcohol in sterile water). The solution is prepared immediately before use with the actual dilution based on the calculated dose per pulse. Favorable results have been achieved in patients with secondary amenorrhea who have failed to respond to clomiphene.[69]

In order for GnRH to achieve the desired effect it must be delivered by a pulsatile system; several types of pumps are commercially available (Autosyringe; Zyklomat; Pulsamat). The delivery system that has been primarily used in the United States is the Lutrepulse (Ortho Pharmaceutical Corporation), which is identical to the Zyklomat (Ferring GmbH, Germany). The pumps are small and can be reused repetitively. Although overdosage is unlikely, multiple pregnancies occur with GnRH-induced ovulation. The intravenous route is preferred over subcutaneous administration by some groups because of greater effectiveness.[19]

The starting pulsed dose for intravenous administration is 5 µg administered at 90- to 120-minute intervals. Larger doses, in the range of 5 µg to 25 µg per pulse, are required during subcutaneous use. To support corpus luteum function, pulsatile GnRH administration may be continued after ovulation; as an alternative, hCG can be administered for luteal support, enabling the pump to be discontinued. The advantages of continuing the pump after ovulation are twofold: (1) the lack of interference with pregnancy test interpretation by exogenous hCG and (2) the availability of the pump for subsequent cycles, if necessary, without requiring its reestablishment. In contrast, administration of hCG and progesterone supplementation are less expensive and more convenient means of providing luteal phase support after ovulation induced via GnRH than is the continued use of the GnRH pump.

Monitoring folliculogenesis is not as complex during GnRH administration as it is with hMG therapy. Serial ultrasound examinations of the ovaries may be helpful but are not essential, nor are measurements of serum estradiol levels required during the use of GnRH administration. Urinary LH testing and/or basal body temperature recordings, however, may help to identify the approximate time of ovulation and thus serve as a guide for determining when to initiate luteal phase support. Success in the treatment of hypogonadotropic amenorrhea due to GnRH deficiency (e.g., Kallmann's syndrome) is predictably high. Patients with lesser degrees of hypothalamic dysfunction also respond to GnRH therapy (80% to 90% ovulatory rate per cycle), but multiple pregnancies are more likely in these patients than in those with hypogonadotropic amenorrhea because of excessive folliculogenesis in the former group. Patients with polycystic ovaries tend not to respond as favorably to GnRH therapy as do other anovulatory patients, probably by virtue of preexisting elevated LH levels.[27] An ovulatory rate of 40% to 50% using pulsatile GnRH in patients with polycystic ovaries is an optimistic estimate, with expected pregnancy rates in the range of 16%. Filicori et al.[19] have reported improved outcomes with GnRH therapy for patients with polycystic ovaries by pretreating them with a GnRH analogue for 6 to 8 weeks to achieve a hypogonadotropic condition in preparation for pulsatile GnRH therapy.

Side effects are unusual with pulsatile GnRH administration. Local irritation at the insertion site and occasional phlebitis are among the more frequent adverse effects. Overdosage is rare, although multiple pregnancies are known to occur after successful ovulation induction with GnRH.

CONCLUSION

This chapter summarizes factors involved in the ovulation process. It is intended to serve as a guide to physiologic principles that should be applied to the pharmacologic principles used in ovulation induction. The four compartments that represent the superstructure of the regulatory process are described, as well as the manner in which they interact. The nature and production of hormones (steroids, proteins, peptides) and other humoral factors regulating ovarian function are discussed; the roles of other central nervous system compounds, including opiates, β-endorphins, and neurochemical transmitters in the ovulation process are emphasized. The periovulatory interval is a continuum beginning with the final stages of follicle selection and maturation, spanning follicle rupture and oocyte maturation, and concluding with establishment of the corpus luteum. The diverse local ovarian factors and events involved in achieving follicle wall rupture are critical in understanding how gonadotropins initiate ovulation and what extraneous substances may interfere with ovulation. Finally, features of the specific agents used for ovulation induction are discussed with emphasis on monitoring and appropriate usage.

REFERENCES

1. Adashi EY: Clomiphene citrate: mechanism(s) and site(s) of action—a hypothesis revisited, *Fertil Steril* 42:331, 1984.
2. Armstrong DT et al: Blockade of spontaneous and LH-induced ovulation in rats by indomethacin, an inhibitor of prostaglandin biosynthesis, *Prostaglandins* 1:21, 1972.
3. Armstrong DT et al: Inhibition of ovulation in rabbits by intrafollicular injection of indomethacin and prostaglandin F antiserum, *Life Sci* 14:129, 1974.
4. Baker TG: Quantitative and cytological study of germ cells in human ovaries, *Proc R Soc Lond [Biol]* 158:417, 1963.
5. Bergland RM, Page RB: Pituitary secretion to the brain: anatomical evidence, *Endocrinology* 102:1025, 1978.
6. Bjersing L, Cajander S: Ovulation and the mechanism of follicle rupture, II: scanning electron microscopy of rabbit germinal epithelium prior to induced ovulation, *Cell Tissue Res* 149:301, 1974.
7. Bjersing L, Cajander S: Ovulation and the mechanism of follicle rupture, III: transmission electron microscopy of rabbit germinal epithelium prior to induced ovulation, *Cell Tissue Res* 149:313, 1974.
8. Bjersing L, Cajander S: Ovulation and the mechanism of follicle rupture, V: ultrastructure of tunica albuginea and theca externa of rabbit graafian follicles prior to induced ovulation, *Cell Tissue Res* 153:15, 1974.
9. Bruce NW et al: Rate of blood flow and growth of the corpora lutea of pregnancy and of previous cycles throughout pregnancy in the rat, *J Reprod Fertil* 71:445, 1984.
10. Canipari R, Strickland S: Studies on the hormonal regulation of plasminogen activator production in the rat ovary, *Endocrinology* 118:1652, 1986.
11. Diaz-Infante A et al: Effects of indomethacin and prostaglandin F$_{2\alpha}$ on ovulation and ovarian contractility in the rabbit, *Prostaglandins* 5:567, 1974.
12. Espey LL: Ovulation as an inflammatory reaction: a hypothesis, *Biol Reprod* 22:73, 1980.
13. Espey LL, Coons PJ: Factors which influence ovulatory degradation of rabbit ovarian follicles, *Biol Reprod* 14:233, 1976.
14. Espey LL, Lipner H: Enzyme-induced rupture of rabbit graafian follicles, *Am J Physiol* 208:208, 1965.
15. Epsey LL et al: Effect of various agents on ovarian plasminogen activator activity during ovulation in pregnant mare's serum gonadotropin-primed immature rats, *Biol Reprod* 32:1087, 1985.
16. Espey LL et al: Ovarian increase in kinin-generating capacity in the PMSG/hCG-primed immature rat, *Am J Physiol* 251 (suppl 3 pt 1):E362, 1986.
17. Fishman J: The catechol estrogens, *Neuroendocrinology* 4:363, 1976.
18. Filicori M et al: Characterization of the physiological pattern of episodic gonadotropin secretion throughout the human menstrual cycle, *J Clin Endocrinol Metab* 62:1136, 1986.
19. Filicori M et al: Ovulation induction with pulsatile gonadotropin-releasing hormone: technical modalities and clinical perspectives, *Fertil Steril* 56:1, 1991.
20. Fukumoto M et al: Collagenolytic enzyme activity in human ovary: an ovulatory enzyme system, *Fertil Steril* 36:746, 1981.
21. Gemzell CA et al: Clinical effect of human pituitary follicle stimulating hormone, *J Clin Endocrinol Metab* 18:1333, 1958.
22. Gilula NB et al: Cell-to-cell communication and ovulation: a study of the cumulus-oocyte complex, *J Cell Biol* 78:58, 1978.
23. Hamada Y et al: Inhibitory effect of prolactin on ovulation in the *in vitro* perfused rabbit ovary, *Nature* 285:15, 1980.
24. Hamilton JLA et al: Human synovial fibroblast plasminogen activator: modulation of enzyme activity by antiinflammatory steroids, *Arthritis Rheum* 24:1296, 1981.
25. Hodgen GD: The dominant ovarian follicle, *Fertil Steril* 38:281, 1982.
26. Ichikawa S et al: Blockage of ovulation in the explanted hamster ovary by a collagenase inhibitor, *J Reprod Fertil* 68:17, 1983.
27. Kelly AC, Jewelewicz R: Alternate regimens for ovulation induction in polycystic ovarian disease, *Fertil Steril* 54:195, 1990.
28. Kitai H et al: Microvasculature of preovulatory follicles: comparison of in situ and in vitro perfused rabbit ovaries following stimulation of ovulation, *Am J Obstet Gynecol* 152:889, 1985.
29. Kitai H et al: The relationship between prostaglandins and histamine in the ovulatory process as determined with the in vitro perfused rabbit ovary, *Fertil Steril* 43:646, 1985.
30. Knobil E: The neuroendocrine control of the menstrual cycle, *Recent Prog Horm Res* 36:53, 1980.
31. Larsen WJ, Wert SE, Brunner GD: A dramatic loss of cumulus cell gap junctions is correlated with germinal vesicle breakdown in rat oocytes, *Dev Biol* 113:517, 1986.
32. Laurent P, Bienvenu J: Acute inflammatory process. In Allen RC et al, editors: *Marker proteins in inflammation,* New York, 1982, Walter de Gruyter.
33. Lemaire WJ et al: Preovulatory changes in the concentration of prostaglandins in rabbit graafian follicles, *Prostaglandins* 3:367, 1973.
34. Lunenfeld B, Menzi A, Volet B: Clinical effects of human menopausal gonadotropin, *Acta Endocrinol Suppl* 51:587, 1960.
35. Martinat N, Combarnous Y: The release of plasminogen activator by rat granulosa cells is highly specific for FSH activity, *Endocrinology* 113:433, 1983.
36. McNatty K et al: The microenvironment of the human antral follicle: interrelationships among the steroid levels in antral fluid, the population of granulosa cells, and the status of the oocyte *in vivo* and *in vitro*, *J Clin Endocrinol Metab* 49:851, 1979.
37. Miyazaki T et al: The effect of intubation of oxygen free radicals on ovulation and progesterone production by the in vitro perfused rabbit ovary, *J Reprod Fertil* 91:207, 1991.
38. Motlik J, Fulka J, Flechon J-E: Changes in intercellular coupling between pig oocytes and cumulus cells during maturation in vivo and in vitro, *J Reprod Fertil* 76:31, 1986.
39. Navot D, Bergh PA, Laufer N: Ovarian hyperstimulation syndrome in novel reproductive technologies: prevention and treatment, *Fertil Steril* 58:249, 1992.
40. Okamura H et al: Ovarian smooth muscle in the human being, rabbit, and cat: histochemical and electron microscopic study, *Am J Obstet Gynecol* 112:183, 1972.
41. Oluda Y et al: An ultrastructural study of ovarian perifollicular capillaries in the indomethacin treated rabbit, *Fertil Steril* 39:85, 1983.
42. Orczyk GP, Behrman HR: Ovulation blockade by aspirin or indomethacin: in vivo evidence for a role of prostaglandins in gonadotropin secretion, *Prostaglandins* 1:3, 1972.

43. Osman P, Sullaart J: Intraovarian release of eggs in the rat after indomethacin treatment at pro-oestrus, *J Reprod Fertil* 47:101, 1976.

44. Page RB: Directional pituitary blood flow: a microcine photographic study, *Endocrinology* 112:157, 1983.

45. Pelletier G, Robert F, Hardy J: Identification of human anterior pituitary cells by immunoelectron microscopy, *J Clin Endocrinol Metab* 46:534, 1978.

46. Phifer RF, Midgley AR, Spicer SS: Immunohistologic and histologic evidence that follicle-stimulating hormone and luteinizing hormone are present in the same cell type in the human pars distalis, *J Clin Endocrinol Metab* 36:125, 1973.

47. Pincus F, Enzmann EV: The comparative behavior of mammalian eggs *in vivo* and *in vitro, J Exp Med* 62:665, 1935.

48. Reich R, Miskin R, Tsafriri A: Follicular plasminogen activator: involvement in ovulation, *Endocrinology* 116:516, 1985.

49. Reid RL et al: Effects on pituitary hormone secretion and disappearance rates of exogenous B-endorphin in normal human subjects, *J Clin Endocrinol Metab* 51:1179, 1981.

50. Rocereto T, Jacobowitz D, Wallach EE: Observations of spontaneous contractions of the cat ovary in vitro, *Endocrinology* 84:1336, 1969.

51. Rondell P: Biophysical aspects of ovulation, *Biol Reprod* 2 (suppl 2):64, 1970.

52. Schlaff S et al: Prostaglandin $F_{2\alpha}$, an ovulatory intermediate in the in vitro perfused rabbit ovary model, *Prostaglandins* 26:111, 1983.

53. Siebel MM et al: Ovulation induction in polycystic ovarian syndrome with urinary follicle-stimulating hormone or human menopausal gonadotropin, *Fertil Steril* 43:703, 1985.

54. Seifer DB, Collins RL: Current concepts of B-endorphin physiology in female reproductive dysfunction, *Fertil Steril* 54:757, 1990.

55. Smith C, Perks AM: The kinin system and ovulation: changes in plasma kininogens and in kinin-forming enzymes in the ovaries and blood of rats with 4-day estrous cycles, *Can J Physiol Pharmacol* 61:736, 1983.

56. Strickland S, Beers WH: Studies on the role of plasminogen activator in ovulation, *J Biol Chem* 251:5694, 1976.

57. Tsafriri A et al: Physiological role of prostaglandins in the induction of ovulation, *Prostaglandins* 2:1, 1972.

58. Vane JLR: Prostaglandins as mediators of inflammation, *Adv Prostaglandin Thromboxane Res* 2:791, 1976.

59. Virutamasen P, Wright KH, Wallach EE: Effects of catecholamine on ovarian contractility in the rabbit, *Obstet Gynecol* 39:225, 1972.

60. Wallach EE, Wright KH, Hamada Y: Investigation of mammalian ovulation with an in vitro perfused rabbit ovary preparation, *Am J Obstet Gynecol* 132:728, 1978.

61. Wallach EE et al: The effect of indomethacin on hMG-hCG induced ovulation in the rhesus monkey, *Prostaglandins* 9:645, 1976.

62. Wallach EE et al: Ultrastructure of ovarian follicles in in vitro perfused rabbit ovaries: response to human chorionic gonadotropin and comparison with in vivo observations, *Fertil Steril* 42:127, 1984.

63. Weiner S, Wright KH, Wallach EE: Lack of effect of ovarian denervation on ovulation and pregnancy in the rabbit, *Fertil Steril* 26:1083, 1975.

64. Weiner S, Wright KH, Wallach EE: Selective ovarian sympathectomy in the rabbit, *Fertil Steril* 26:253, 1975.

65. Willoughby DA, Sedgewick A, Edwards J: The inflammatory process. In Allen RC et al, editors: *Marker proteins in inflammation,* New York, 1982, Walter de Gruyter.

66. Yang NST, Marsh JM, LeMaire WJ: Prostaglandin changes induced by ovulatory stimuli in rabbit graafian follicles: the effect of indomethacin, *Prostaglandins* 4:395, 1973.

67. Yoshimura Y, Wallach EE: Studies of the mechanism(s) of mammalian ovulation, *Fertil Steril* 47:22, 1987.

68. Yoshimura Y et al: The effect of bradykinin on ovulation and prostaglandin production by the perfused rabbit ovary. Paper presented the 68th Annual Meeting of the Endocrine Society, Anaheim, Calif, 1986 (abstract no. 47).

69. Zacur HA: Ovulation induction with gonadotropin-releasing hormone, *Fertil Steril* 44:435, 1985.

70. Zamboni L: Fine morphology of the follicle wall and follicle cell-oocyte association, *Biol Reprod* 10:125, 1974.

Chapter 31

MONITORING OF OVULATION

Robert J. Stillman, MD
and Deborah I. Arbit, MD

WHY MONITOR OVULATION?

Spontaneous cycles

Spontaneous, natural ovulation may be monitored to predict its occurrence, to determine whether it has occurred, and to determine its adequacy. Clinical circumstance can determine the reasons for monitoring a spontaneous cycle and the type of monitoring used.

The prediction of when ovulation occurs may be useful in avoiding intercourse (e.g., for family planning) or in timing intercourse accurately (e.g., for resolution of infertility). However, basal body temperature (BBT) charts or progesterone determinations that may be used to document ovulation are generally poor predictors of the time of ovulation; determination of luteinizing hormone (LH) levels may better satisfy the sensitivity and specificity needed.

Documentation that ovulation has occurred, such as by BBT charts or serum progesterone levels, may be used as part of an infertility evaluation or as part of the work-up for an endocrine or anatomic abnormality (e.g., hypothyroidism or amenorrhea). Documentation of adequacy of ovulation in a spontaneous cycle generally is useful only as part of an infertility evaluation. Prolactin and thyroid function tests may be used to determine the cause of hormonally inadequate ovulation, but an endometrial biopsy is the classic test for assessing that adequacy itself.

Stimulated cycles

Stimulated ovulatory cycles generally are monitored to ensure efficacy and safety of therapy. Subsequent documentation of occurrence and adequacy of ovulation is an important goal within efficacy, but efficacy also entails the use of appropriate drug regimens designed to best ensure successful ovulation and conception (e.g., by individual dose adjustments for patients taking human menopausal gonadotropin (hMG). Safety includes the use of the most noninvasive monitoring techniques and the most risk-free therapy, as, for example, reducing the risk of ovarian hyperstimulation by monitoring estradiol levels.

PRINCIPLES OF MONITORING

Ideally, monitoring ovulation should fulfill a set of basic principles designed to bring about the greatest degree of accurate information most easily, a goal common to most medical procedures. These principles, often overlapping, at times competing, but clearly related, are discussed with illustrative examples. Ideally, ovulation monitoring needs to be efficacious, safe, cost effective, unintrusive, and noninvasive.

Efficacy

The critical goal of monitoring ovulation is to help ensure the greatest success in terms of optimal ovulation and conception. For example, ultrasound monitoring of follicular growth during high-dose clomiphene citrate therapy can be used to improve the efficacy of therapy by attempting to time the adjunctive human chorionic gonadotropin (hCG) injection. However, ultrasound assessment during low-dose clomiphene therapy when hCG will not be used may not improve success rates beyond those achieved with other methods to time ovulation that are more cost effective and less intrusive, such as urine LH testing kits.

Safety

Not all methods of monitoring ovulation are designed to maximize efficacy. Some are used to optimize safety and minimize risk; some may do both. For example, the use of ultrasound monitoring of follicular development during hMG therapy provides not only information on adequacy of stimulation but an important assessment of risk of subsequent multiple pregnancy, as might be indicated by the presence of multiple codominant follicles.

Cost effectiveness

The degree to which safety and efficacy can be enhanced in ovulation monitoring must be balanced with cost in a basic cost-benefit analysis. Little is to be gained by use of costly methods such as serial ultrasound measurements in spontaneous natural ovulation cycles when less-costly BBT charts or urine LH testing kits might do.

Unintrusiveness

Monitoring of ovulation can intrude into the daily lives of patients. It is worthwhile to explore means that offer less interference. For example, the first days of hMG therapy do not generally require monitoring, and thereafter days of monitoring occasionally can be skipped, depending on clinical responsiveness.

Noninvasiveness

Noninvasiveness in ovulation monitoring is the best means to ensure a safe outcome to the therapy that may be used. Another element involves the risk-benefit ratio of the methods themselves. For example, endometrial biopsy during the late luteal phase might not be worthwhile, given the potential risk of uterine injury/infection and the adverse influence on an implanted embryo.

Adherence to the principles of monitoring ovulation involves ideal goals, which can conflict with each other. However, efficacy and cost effectiveness do not have to be mutually exclusive; safety does not need to be forsaken to obtain some degree of unintrusive monitoring. A balance of all five ideal goals will provide a functional basis to monitoring. The right blend of efficacy, safety, cost effectiveness, unintrusiveness, and noninvasiveness is individualized by the physician's experience and skill and by the patient's clinical and personal needs into a functional monitoring regimen.

METHODS OF MONITORING
Spontaneous cycles

Direct demonstration of ovulation. Although ovulation theoretically can be visualized at the time of laparoscopy or laparotomy, generally the only direct demonstration that ovulation has occurred is pregnancy. All methods of monitoring ovulation are therefore indirect.

Indirect demonstration of ovulation. There are many windows into the normal spontaneous ovulatory cycle that provide indirect demonstration of ovulation. These include the patient's symptoms, BBT charts, cervical mucus, follicular development, endometrial development, hormonal changes, and electrical resistance (Fig. 31-1). Each indicator is a static test that monitors a dynamic event; hence each modality provides varying assurance that ovulation will occur (prediction)[9,15] or has occurred (detection). Each has advantages and disadvantages and each is considered in turn.

Prediction

Symptoms. In an idealized menstrual cycle of 28 days, ovulation generally occurs around day 14 of the cycle. However, even in regularly cycling women the cycle length can vary, so that cycle day alone is not a good predictor of ovulation.

Symptoms that can be associated with ovulation include abdominal pain (mittelschmerz), spotting, breast tenderness, cervical changes, and mood shifts. Cervical changes are associated with increased estrogen levels and include cervical softening, opening, and elevation in the vagina. Women can detect these symptoms to varying degrees, and hence their predictive value is variable.

Cervical mucus. First described by Billings in 1972, but long known to women, are changes in the mucous discharge from the vagina with the cyclic changes of the menstrual cycle. In response to increasing estrogen production during the follicular phase, the mucus, produced by the endocervical cells, changes in amount and characteristics (Fig. 31-1). These changes begin 5 days before ovulation and peak 12 to 24 hours before ovulation. By the time of follicular rupture, the cervical mucus score has decreased, concomitant with increasing progesterone production. Changes include translucency, from opaque early in the follicular phase to clear toward midcycle; amount, from scant to copious; spinnbarkeit, or stretchiness, from tacky and retractile to a length of more than 7 cm. Also, when placed on a glass slide and allowed to dry, midfollicular cervical mucus shows a ferning or arborization pattern, a consequence of its increasing salt content. Sperm penetration is maximal at the time of peak mucus production, along with maximal spinnbarkeit (8 to 9 cm) and maximal arborization.

Various scoring methods have been described to assess cervical mucus as a predictor of ovulation, as an adjunct to enhancing or preventing fertility. This method of predicting impending ovulation is simple and inexpensive. However, the day of peak mucus production can be known only in retrospect. In addition, cervical mucus production and quality may be adversely affected by medications (including fertility drugs and antihistamines), systemic illness, vaginal infection, previous cervical surgery, and in utero diethylstilbestrol (DES) exposure. These limit somewhat the applicability of this method.

Serum LH. Serum LH is secreted by the anterior pituitary gland and triggers ovulation. Ovulation occurs approximately 37 to 40 hours after the onset of the LH surge[34] and 15 to 20 hours after the LH peak (Fig. 31-1). Seasonal variations in the onset of the plasma LH surge have been

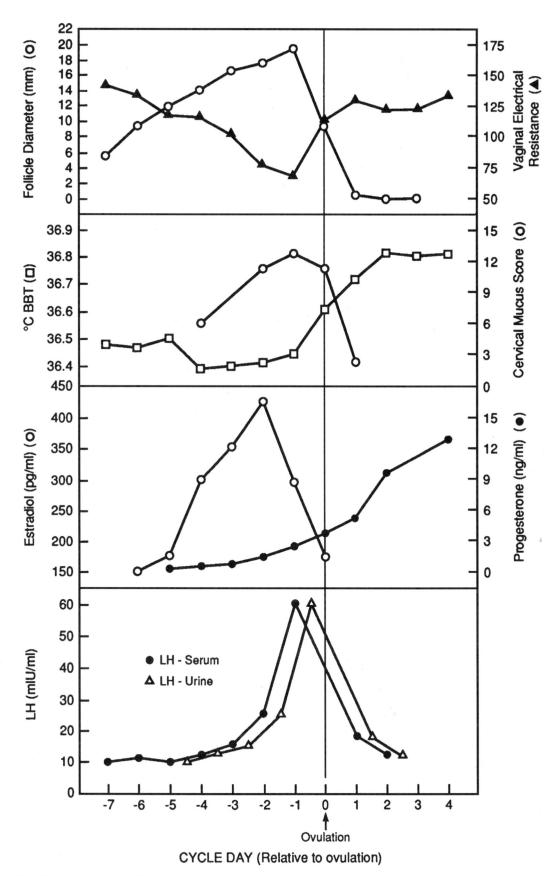

Fig. 31-1. A schematic illustration of the various monitoring methods in spontaneous cycles.

described.[35] In the spring, the LH surge onset occurred at 3 PM ± 1.5 hours in 28.6% of cycles, a statistically significant result. In autumn and winter, the LH surge onset began at 3 AM ± 1.5 hours in 42.5% of patients, also statistically significant. (Not enough patients were studied in summer months to include them in the analysis.) Therefore, ovulation occurs primarily in the morning during the spring, when 50% of women ovulate between midnight and 11 AM, and in the evening in autumn and winter, when 90% of women ovulate between 4 and 7 PM.[35]

Serum LH can be measured by radioimmunoassay (RIA) techniques. LH secretion from the pituitary is pulsatile, and in order to identify these pulses, blood samples need to be drawn every 10 minutes. However, less frequent sampling, once or twice daily, can identify general timing of the serum LH surge onset and peak. In one study, mean peak levels of LH were 64 ± 6 mIU/mL (Second International Reference Preparation).[37] A single value of greater than 40 mIU/mL was predictive of ovulation the following day in 86% of patients, the rest having increasing LH levels the following day with ovulation 1 day subsequently. Serum LH testing can accurately predict ovulation within 1 day in 86% of patients. However, since daily phlebotomy is required, this method has practical limitations in the clinical setting.

Urine LH. LH can be measured easily in urine via a semiquantatative assay using the enzyme-linked immunosorbent assay (ELISA) technique. The ELISA technique is exquisitely sensitive for detecting antigens and antibodies and is very economical in the use of reagents. It is widely used, since the test can be performed in a relatively short time, and has therefore been exploited for home urine ovulation predictor kits for measuring urinary LH. LH is detected in the urine simultaneously as in plasma in 33% of women.[5] In the rest, a delay of 3 to 21 hours has been noted. This is most likely due to renal function, the accumulation of urine in the bladder, and sampling frequency.

The ELISA technique "sandwiches" the LH molecule between two monoclonal antibodies, each specific for a different portion of the LH molecule (Fig. 31-2). Some kits use one antibody directed against the alpha subunit of the LH molecule with the other directed against the beta subunit, whereas others use two antibodies specific for different portions of the β-subunit. The first antibody is linked to the blotter, disc, or stick contained in the kit. If present, LH in the urine will attach to this antibody. Adding the second antibody causes a "sandwiching" of the LH molecule. Any unbound antibody is washed away. This second antibody is covalently coupled to an enzyme. When

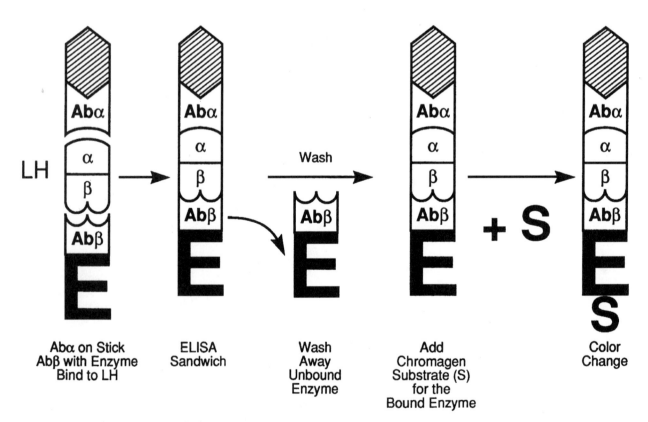

Fig. 31-2. ELISA technique—"sandwiching" of LH molecule between two monoclonal antibodies used in home urine LH testing kits.

a chromogen (a specific colorless substrate) is added, it is acted upon by the enzyme, and a colored end product results. The intensity of the color correlates with the amount of LH molecules in the given urine specimen. (See Chapter 62.)

There are many ovulation predictor kits available on the market, some of which are ingeniously named, such as Ovuquick, Clearplan Easy, First Response, and OvuGen, and they are constantly being refined. Ovuquick has one antibody against the α-subunit and one against the β-subunit of the LH molecule. First Response and OvuGen have both antibodies directed against the β-subunit. The detection of the LH surge is defined for each kit. Most predict ovulation 24 to 40 hours from a positive result. For example, with Ovuquick, the surge is the first color change above the test panel, and ovulation is said to occur the following day; with First Response, the surge is defined as the first significant color change above the previous day, and ovulation is said to occur on that same day. Most kits have a level of detection of 40 mIU/mL. This can be adjusted, depending on the amount of reagent used.

In practice, the kits are started usually beginning on day 10 to day 12 of a normal menstrual cycle. A urine specimen is collected and a specified number of drops are placed on the blotter. A buffer may be added, followed by the enzyme conjugate, the substrate, and then a stopping solution. The color is read by the patient within minutes, and reference spots are available for comparison. Kits come complete with directions and all supplies and have enough materials for testing from 5 to 10 days, depending on the brand. Most results may be stored, allowing a semipermanent record for later reference.

Studies (e.g., Whitehall Laboratories, 1989) claim 98% accuracy in detecting the LH surge compared with standard RIA. In studies of Ovuquick, 86% of those tested ovulated (by ultrasonographic criteria) the following day, and the remaining 14% ovulated 2 days after the surge, according to the kit.[37]

There is no consensus regarding the most desirable urine collection time for LH testing. Luciano et al.[19] note that the serum LH surge was more reliably reflected in the evening urine sample than in the morning urine sample when tested by RIA. OvuGen's literature states that first morning urine may contain high concentrations of LH, and therefore false-positive results may occur. Martinez et al.[23] state that the urine LH concentration may be diluted in the first voided urine specimen of the day. In addition, LH levels elevated above the reference range may persist for only 24 hours, so that the LH surge may occasionally be missed with once-daily testing. With more frequent testing, the sensitivity of the test improves.

Since the kits use an antibody to the β-subunit of LH, they are designed not to give false-positive results with follicle-stimulating hormone (FSH), thyroid-stimulating hormone (TSH), or hCG (which share a common α-subunit) at levels found in nonpregnant, normally cycling women. However, false-positive results of imminent ovulation can be obtained in any situation in which serum LH levels are elevated, such as menopause or chronic hyperandrogenic anovulation (polycystic ovary syndrome). Because the α-subunit of hCG and part of the β-subunit are identical with those of LH, a false-positive result can also be obtained in pregnancy. Medication containing LH or hCG, or compounds that may stimulate these hormones (e.g., gonadotropin-releasing hormone [GnRH]) may also cause false-positive results.

Home LH testing kits can predict ovulation accurately within 2 days of ovulation, are easily used by patients, and can be done in the privacy and convenience of home. Although they require some motivation by the patient, the kits enable the patient to be involved in monitoring her own physiologic events and have proven to be a widely used and important adjunct to daily practical infertility evaluation and treatment (Fig. 31-1).

Estrogen. Serum estrogen can be measured by RIA. Hackeloer et al.[11] demonstrated a linear correlation between plasma estradiol concentrations and mean follicular diameter from 5 days before the LH peak up to the LH peak (Fig. 31-3). Vermesh et al.[37] showed that peak estradiol levels were found before the LH peak in 97% of cycles, with a mean peak level of 463 ± 39 pg/mL. The variation in estrogen values limits their usefulness in predicting when ovulation will occur, as does the increased frequency of testing needed to detect an estrogen plateau or decrease that may precede the LH rise. Many of the same problems are true for urine estrogen assays.

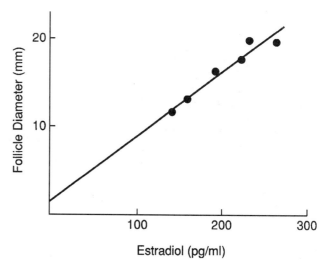

Fig. 31-3. Correlation between follicular diameter and mean serum estrogen beginning 5 days before LH peak. (Redrawn with permission from Hackeloer B et al: Correlation of ultrasonic and endocrinologic assessment of human follicular development, *Am J Obstet Gynecol* 135:1, 1979.)

Ultrasound. With serial ultrasonographic monitoring, the growth and subsequent rupture of the dominant follicle can be followed. (See Chapter 57.) An endovaginal ultrasound probe, with a 5.0-MHz transducer or greater, can readily enable visualization of the structures of the pelvis with minimal patient discomfort. The size, architecture, and location of the ovaries are easily noted.[16]

A baseline scan done early in the follicular phase can be used to identify any cystic structures that might later be confused with the growing follicle. By cycle day 5 to 7 the dominant follicle has been selected, and it can be identified ultrasonographically by cycle day 8 to 10. In the early follicular phase it is a cystic structure of 3 to 5 mm and progressively increases in size, usually progressing to ovulation.[14] Growth of the follicle is linear, approximately 1 to 4 mm/d. The follicle is sonolucent and is usually round or ovoid (Fig. 31-4A), but it can have various shapes resulting from compression by other follicles in the ovary, the ovarian capsule, or other pelvic structures or adhesions. In a normal ovulatory cycle, usually one dominant follicle is selected for subsequent ovulation, although not uncommonly a small secondary follicle develops.

The follicular diameter in spontaneous cycles before ovulation has been described in various texts as being from as small as 11 mm to as large as 32 mm. Some examiners have measured the single largest follicular diameter and others have calculated the mean diameter; this difference in measurement method may explain some of the wide diversity in reported follicle size before rupture. More accurate would be the uniform use of follicular volume, determined by the calculation for volume of a sphere or an ovoid sphere. The variability in follicle size at the time of rupture

limits use of this parameter alone in predicting when ovulation will occur. However, ultrasound evaluation of follicular growth in spontaneous cycles may occasionally have clinical utility, especially when it is important to know which ovary is developing a follicle in a particular cycle (e.g., when there is unilateral tubal occlusion or when donor insemination is planned).

Electrical impedance. Changes in the concentrations of electrolytes in the ionic state in vaginal fluids and saliva have led to development of instrumentation that measures electrical resistance. Changes in resistance have been correlated with the time of the cycle relative to ovulation. These probes measure electrical resistance at conductive electrodes connected to a current source.

Results of tabulated daily vaginal electrical resistance (VER) studies show a decrease at the time of the LH peak, followed by subsequent daily increase (Fig. 31-1). Salivary electrical resistance (SER) showed an increase 5 to 6 days before the LH peak; however, the results were not reproducible among individual women and were not shown to be statistically significant.

Although VER is a potential adjunct to predicting ovulation and can be accomplished in a home setting, further studies are needed to elucidate its role, if any, in actually predicting ovulation. To date the applications of VER appear limited compared with other methods.

Documentation

Symptoms. A history of regular cyclic menses, preceded or coincident with moliminal symptoms, is a reasonable way to document that ovulation has occurred. Molimina, a constellation of symptoms following the luteal withdrawal of progesterone, may include breast tenderness, bloating,

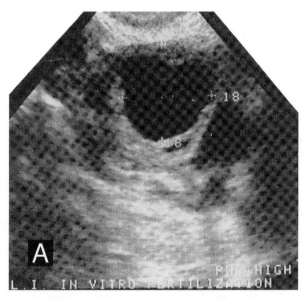 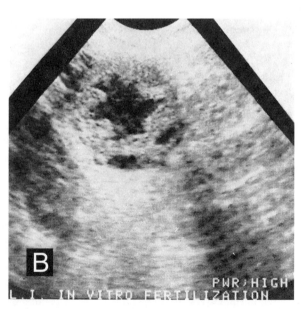

Fig. 31-4. Ultrasound evaluation of the ovary in the spontaneous cycle. **A,** Preovulatory follicle. **B,** Corpus luteum. (From Kenigsberg D: *Clin Obstet Gynecol* 32:533, 1989. With permission).

headache, irritability, fatigue, cramping, and others. The severity and number of these symptoms are generally stable and characteristic in an individual, but vary widely from woman to woman. They generally occur only in ovulatory cycles.

BBT charts. BBT is measured with an oral or rectal basal thermometer by the woman each morning upon awakening. BBT charting was first described by Van de Velde in 1904, and it has remained an inexpensive and easy method to document ovulatory cycles. A midcycle temperature rise is the result of progesterone, produced by the corpus luteum, which has a central effect on the hypothalamus, causing an increase in body temperature of 0.6°C in the luteal phase. A biphasic temperature chart is consistent with an ovulatory cycle, whereas a monophasic chart is consistent with anovulation. Daily variability of 0.1°C to 0.2°C is not atypical.

BBT charts are useful in documenting ovulation retrospectively, since the temperature rise is a consequence of postovulatory luteinization of the follicle. The thermogenic effect of progesterone does not take place until serum progesterone levels have reached 5 ng/mL.[19] BBT charts are classically described to have a dip or nadir before the rise; however, this has been an inconsistent finding. The nadir is defined as the lowest point in the curve, followed by at least two consecutive rises above the baseline. The nadir can be defined only after a persistent rise; therefore, BBTs can retrospectively define the periovulatory *period,* but they cannot prospectively predict the *day* of ovulation in any one cycle.

BBT charting is easily done, is inexpensive, and requires little training. Interpretation can be compromised by febrile episodes, daily lifestyle fluctuations, and missing measurements.

Ultrasound. There are three common ultrasonographic signs that ovulation has occurred: (1) follicular collapse, (2) fluid in the cul-de-sac, and (3) increased echogenicity of the follicle. The corpus luteum often has a stellate appearance, as seen in Fig. 31-4, *B,* with an irregular shape, thickened walls, and internal echoes. Also described by various ultrasonographers are echoes at the edge of the preovulatory follicle, thought to be the cumulus oophorus complex, and a double contour of the wall of the follicle a few hours before rupture.

Based on collapse or disappearance of the follicle, transvaginal ultrasonography can be an accurate method of detecting when ovulation has occurred. However, serial measurements are required.[41]

Initial data suggest that there may be correlations of ultrasound with other, more standard, assessments of luteal phase adequacy. This aspect is discussed later in this chapter.

Progesterone. Progesterone is secreted by the corpus luteum after ovulation. Investigators have therefore measured luteal phase progesterone levels to document ovula-

tion and to define the adequacy of the luteal phase. However, there are problems with each premise, especially the latter. Progesterone is secreted in a pulsatile fashion in the luteal phase, and therefore a single serum determination may be misleading. A high level of progesterone is reassuring regarding the occurrence of ovulation and perhaps the adequacy of the luteal phase; however, a lower value is more difficult to interpret. A serum progesterone level of at least 3 ng/mL is described as indicative of ovulation, and some evidence suggests that a serum concentration of 10 to 15 ng/mL may be indicative of adequate luteal function.[1] (See Chapter 24.) In nonconception cycles, peak progesterone levels are noted 7 days after ovulation, with a mean of 17.2 ± 1.7 ng/mL.[37] The initial rise of progesterone precedes ovulation (Fig. 31-1).

Search for alternate means to measure progesterone has led to measurements of urinary metabolites of progesterone, salivary progesterone, and peritoneal fluid progesterone. The urinary metabolite pregnanediol-3α-glucuronide (Pd-3G) has been shown to correlate well with serum levels in both 24-hour and first morning urine collections. Salivary progesterone has also been correlated with serum progesterone, but with varying ratios. Kruitwagen et al.[17] measured peritoneal fluid progesterone obtained by culdocentesis or laparoscopy concurrently with serum progesterone within 24 hours of ovulation as determined ultrasonographically by a decrease in the size of the follicle. They found markedly elevated levels of peritoneal fluid progesterone after ovulation. In three subjects with persistent cystic follicles after ovulation had occurred according to ultrasonographic criteria (reduction in the size of the follicle by at least 5 mm), no elevated peritoneal fluid progesterone level was noted. Kruitwagen et al.[17] postulated that after ovulation had occurred the stigmata had resealed, and hence the progesterone-rich fluid did not spill into the peritoneal cavity. Perhaps this phenomenon is consistent with the enigmatic luteinized unruptured follicle, wherein the hormonal profile is consistent with ovulation but ultrasonography shows persistence of the follicle.

Thus measurement of progesterone or its metabolites in serum or other body fluids can give assurance of the occurrence of ovulation. However, the adequacy of the ovulatory event is still not elucidated with this measurement alone. A more definitive assessment of the adequacy of ovulation is made with an endometrial biopsy.

Endometrial biopsy. The endometrium shows specific histologic changes in response to ovarian steroids, and these changes therefore provide a dynamic bioassay of the cyclic hormonal environment of the menstrual cycle. These changes enable definition of the periods of time in the hormonal cycle. In the proliferative phase, proliferative epithelial cells are seen, along with varying stages of coiling of glands, stromal edema, and mitoses that enable differentiation among early, mid-, and late proliferative stages. On the day of ovulation and 1 day after ovulation, the epithelium shows a mixture of secretory and proliferative cells and abundant mitoses, with less than 50% of the cells having subnucleolar vacuoles. This pattern may be seen in some anovulatory cycles, and hence is not sufficient to diagnose ovulation during this period. Beginning 2 days after ovulation, the endometrium shows specific changes that suggest, indirectly, that ovulation has taken place. In the secretory phase, vacuoles in the gland cells, stromal edema, and predecidual changes in the stromal cells to varying degrees are seen that enable definition of the postovulatory cycle day. By assessing the stroma and glands through the rest of the luteal phase, a determination can be made as to the hormonal adequacy of the ovulatory event and development of the corpus luteum.[24]

Traditionally, biopsy specimens have been dated by defining the onset of the next menstrual period as day 28, and subtracting the number of days from menses to the day that the biopsy was performed, to calculate the cycle day. This is compared with the histologic cycle day. A discrepancy of greater than 2 days is termed an out-of-phase biopsy, suggesting endometrial (implantation) inadequacy.[1] (See Chapter 24.) Recently, however, dating of the biopsy specimen using the next menstrual cycle has come under scrutiny, and investigators have determined that a more accurate assessment of the cycle day may be defined as the day remote from ovulation. Since the changes in the epithelium of the endometrium are a direct result of postovulatory progesterone secretion by the corpus luteum, this assessment makes both more intuitive and more scientific sense. Shoupe et al.[30] have compared endometrial biopsy dating using the next menstrual period as a reference versus ovulation as a reference (See Fig. 24-1.) They have shown that when ovulation was determined by daily transvaginal ultrasonographic disappearance of the follicle, 96.1% of the biopsies correlated with the histologically determined day, compared with 65% as determined by the next menses; 84.6% of the biopsies correlated with the histologically determined day when the day of ovulation was determined by daily serum LH peak. Unfortunately, Shoupe et al. did not quantify peak levels, differentiate between surge and peak, or indicate the length of time between the LH peak and ovulation.[30] Li et al.[18] noted that 90% of biopsies were in phase if the LH peak was used as an ovulatory reference point to determine dating, compared with 58% using the next menstrual period as a reference.

Although rarely used clinically, glycoprotein measurements in endometrial biopsy samples against which antibodies have been synthesized are also described to determine the occurrence of ovulation and warrant mention. Such an antibody against the D9B1 antigen, on a sialoglycoprotein in the endometrium, has been shown to be cycle dependent, with absent expression in the proliferative phase, maximal expression in the early secretory phase, and decreasing expression through the late secretory phase.[29]

Conclusion. It is possible to monitor different facets of the intricate physiologic responses of the human body during the menstrual cycle to predict or conclude that ovulation will occur or has taken place. Information from each method generally complements the other, with the best determinations made when combining different modalities. Increasing cervical mucus, midcycle symptoms, an enlarging follicle on ultrasonography, and particularly an LH surge give some prediction of ovulation. Collapse of the follicle ultrasonographically, an increased BBT, an elevated progesterone level, and a secretory endometrium may document that ovulation has indeed occurred. The combination of testing methods depends on the goal (i.e., to enhance or prevent pregnancy), the precision needed, and the time and monetary investments available.

Stimulated cycles

Ultrasound

Endometrium. The availability of reliable high-frequency transvaginal ultrasound transducers has opened a window to the endometrium. The state of preparation of the endometrium is one critical factor in the success of spontaneous and induced ovulatory cycles. Ultrasonographic evaluations of the endometrium to assess its thickness, its serial quantitative changes, and the qualitative changes in echogenicity patterns throughout the cycle have been described. Such evaluations have been performed in spontaneous cycles, during artificial estrogen/progesterone replacement therapies,[10] and in clomiphene-induced[26] and hMG-induced cycles.[3,7,38] These studies give promise to the use of endometrial ultrasound monitoring to predict positive and negative cycle outcomes. Color Doppler-flow ultrasound and higher-resolution vaginal ultrasound transducers may allow future study of this end-organ's responses.

Ultrasonographic monitoring of the endometrium in spontaneous and induced ovulation cycles began almost as a sidelight of the ovarian/follicular ultrasonographic studies. While scanning ovaries, the "winking" of bright lines of the endometrium in the miduterus was noted. Changes in these endometrial images were observed during serial measurements throughout the cycle. Observations brought correlations, and an important adjunct of ovulation monitoring was enjoined.

The method is easy, fast, reproducible, safe, noninvasive, and reasonably unintrusive. Only in correlation with other methods of monitoring (e.g., serum estradiol levels, follicular growth patterns, and endometrial biopsy) with the promise of efficacy and an analysis of cost benefit does the method invite scrutiny, especially in spontaneous cycles.

Two major areas of endometrial ultrasound evaluation and ovulation monitoring have so far emerged. The first is the *periovulatory* assessment of endometrial thickness and growth patterns. This may be either a static view, usually the day of or the day after the spontaneous LH surge/hCG injection, or a longitudinal view to assess changes in endometrial thickness or echo patterns from days before, up to, and through the LH/hCG surge. The second is the *luteal* assessment of endometrial reflective patterns. These represent morphologic changes in the endometrium associated with the hormonal impact of progesterone.[10]

Periovulatory. The endometrial ultrasound echo begins in the early proliferative phase as a narrow hyperechoic line in the miduterus (Fig. 31-5). In spontaneous cycles, endometrial thickness has been judged to increase significantly from a minimum of 6.1 mm 4 days before the LH surge to a maximum of 8.7 mm on the day of the LH surge onset.[27] This change in endometrial thickness correlates with the rise in serum estradiol level and an increase in the lead follicle's diameter. Aberrations of endometrial growth or reflectivity have so far not been studied in patients with unexplained infertility monitored in spontaneous cycles.

In clomiphene cycles,[7,8,26] the endometrial thickness also increased significantly from 4 days before the LH surge to the day of the LH surge. As with spontaneous cycles, there was a significant correlation among endometrial thickness, serum estradiol level, and follicle diameter. However, compared with spontaneous cycles, the thickness was significantly reduced (5.0 mm) when monitoring began and remained thinner until the day of the LH surge, despite a significantly greater serum estradiol concentration in the clomiphene cycles.

The aberration of clomiphene-induced endometrial growth correlates with clomiphene dose. The reduction in endometrial thickness on clomiphene may be an indication of its well-described antiestrogenic effect on the endometrium, especially in light of the greater serum estradiol concentrations in these cycles.

Data on endometrial growth have been gathered in stimulated cycles being monitored for ovum retrieval and subsequent in vitro fertilization (IVF), comparing patients who conceived and those who did not.[7,8] Gonen and co-workers evaluated the endometrium in clomiphene- and hMG-induced IVF cycles beginning on day 10 and continuing through the day after the hCG injection. Estradiol values on day 10, the change in estradiol levels from day 10 to the day after hCG injection, and the initial endometrial thickness on day 10 were not different. However, the endometrial thickness after hCG injection and the change in thickness from day 10 through the hCG injection were significantly greater in patients who subsequently successfully conceived in the IVF cycle being measured. Endometrial growth thus may be another predictive variable to achieving pregnancy[7,8] (Fig. 31-6). Importantly, this variable is known before oocyte retrieval. Thus, if appropriate confidence limits can be set on endometrial thickness, this variable may be utilized to abort a cycle by canceling oocyte retrieval until a more favorable endometrial pattern is observed. Smith et al.[32] reported on cycles in which there was failure to recover oocytes or recovery of immature oocytes led to low fertilization rates. These cycles were associated with an endometrial thickness of less than 5 mm.

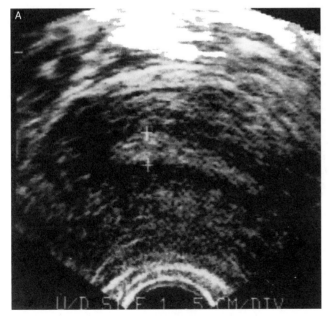

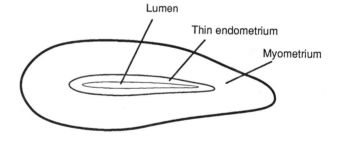

Fig. 31-5. Progression of endometrial patterns during the menstrual cycle as assessed by ultrasonography. (Modified from Grunfeld L et al: *Obstet Gynecol* 78:200, 1991, with permission of The American College of Obstetricians and Gynecologists.) **A,** Early proliferative phase: thin endometrial basalis surrounding the endometrial canal. (Ultrasound picture from Gonen Y, Casper R: *J In Vitro Fert Embryo Transfer* 7:146, 1990.)

Continued.

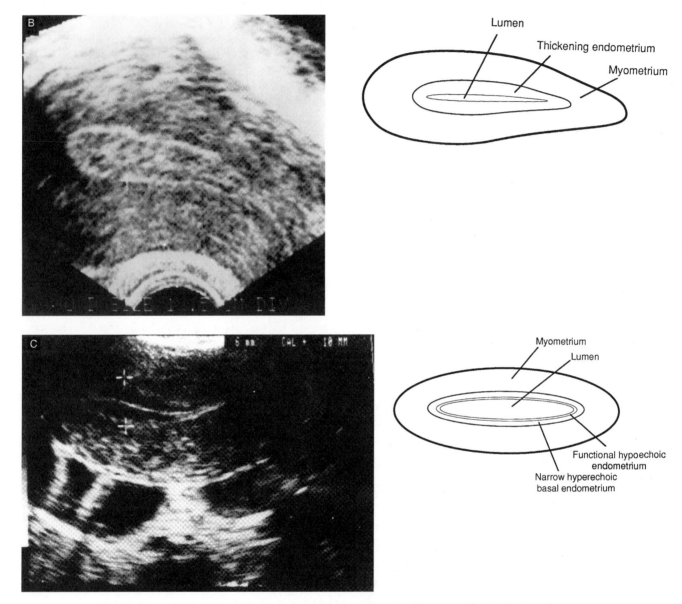

Fig. 31-5, cont'd B, Mid–proliferative phase. The inner functional layer proliferates but remains isoechoic with myometrium. The thinner surrounding basalis is relatively hyperechoic. (Ultrasound picture from Gonen Y, Casper R: *J In Vitro Fert Embryo Transfer* 7:146, 1990.) **C,** Late proliferative (preovulatory) phase. Triple-line sign is evident, composed of a hyperechoic basalis and a wide hypoechoic functional endometrium surrounding a hyperechoic central lumen. (Ultrasound picture from Gonen Y, Casper R: *J In Vitro Fert Embryo Transfer* 7:146, 1990.)

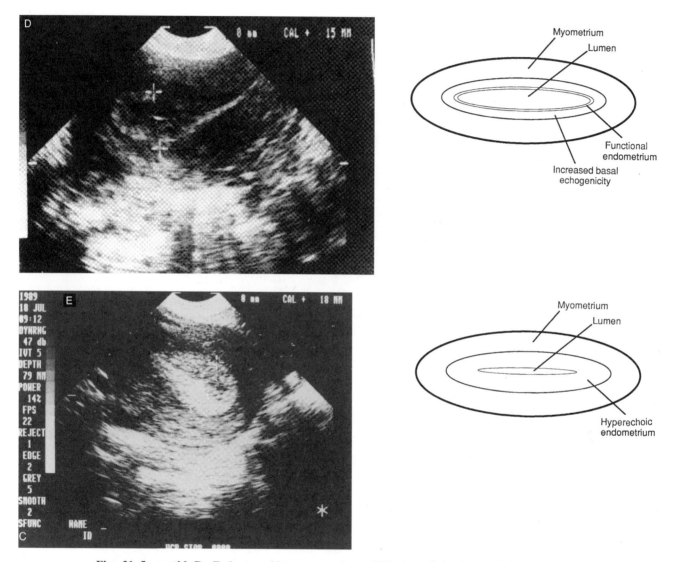

Fig. 31-5, cont'd D, Early to mid–secretory phase. Widening of the hyperechoic area as endometrial secretory activity presents echogenic interfaces to the ultrasound beam. (Ultrasound picture from Grunfeld L et al: *Obstet Gynecol* 78:200, 1991, with permission of The American College of Obstetricians and Gynecologists.) **E,** Mid- to late secretory phase: hyperechoic endometrium. (Ultrasound picture from Yee B, Rosen GF: *Infertil Reprod Med Clin North Am* 1:15, 1990.)

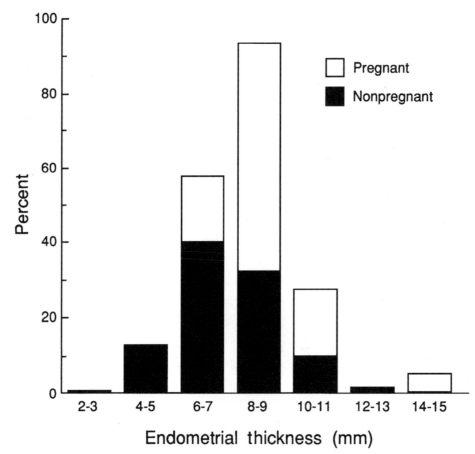

Fig. 31-6. The occurrence of clinical pregnancy related to endometrial thickness. Percentage, on the Y axis, refers to the percentage of each group that occurred at each level of endometrial thickness. (Redrawn from Gonen Y, Casper R: *J In Vitro Fert Embryo Transfer* 7:146, 1990.)

Welker et al.[38] found pregnancies only when the endometrial echo was 6 mm or more. Gonen et al.[8] report that endometrial thickness on the day after hCG of less than 6 mm carried with it a very poor prognosis for pregnancy. Glissant and co-workers[6] reported significantly greater conception rates correlated to greater endometrial thickness. The positive predictive value of endometrial thickness to conception is not as great as is the negative predictive value to failure to conceive.

Endometrial reflectivity patterns. In addition to endometrial thickness and growth rates, the reflectivity patterns of the echogenic endometrium have been described for spontaneous and stimulated cycles (see Fig. 31-5). Forrest et al.[4] described the dynamic endometrial pattern seen through spontaneous cycles. They also correlated these changes with histologic changes seen on endometrial biopsy done on the same day as the ultrasound scan. The development of proliferative endometrium was seen as a change from a thin, single-line endometrial cavity on cycle day 2 to a narrow, hypoechoic functional layer surrounding the canal on cycle day 8. This thin hypoechoic area

progressed to a wider hypoechoic area and formed the "triple-line sign." The wide hypoechoic area on either side of the central line of the endometrial cavity represents the functional proliferative endometrium. This is in turn surrounded by hyperechoic lines representing the barrier between the endometrial vessels and the myometrium. This effect produces a triple-line sign running longitudinally through the center of the uterus. How this triple-line sign, or its absence, may predict cycle outcome in spontaneous cycles has yet to be studied. Late proliferative endometrium and the endometrium seen during or shortly after the LH/hCG surge are characterized by (1) hypoechoism, (2) demonstration of little posterior acoustic enhancement (on abdominal ultrasound scanning), and (3) the well-defined triple-line sign. When all three characteristics were present, endometrial biopsy confirmed the histologic picture with a sensitivity of 100% and a specificity of 90%.

In stimulated cycles, a similar triple-line sign is seen on the day after hCG injection (Fig. 31-5). In IVF cycles, its absence correlates well with the failure of conception in that cycle, despite other similar cycle-monitoring parameters such as levels of estradiol and LH, number of follicles, number of oocytes, and number of embryos. The negative predictive value was 90.5% in cycles demonstrating an endometrial hyperechoic or isoechoic pattern, compared with the myometrium. Only the triple-line sign with its hypoechoic central area representing the developed functional endometrium was reassuring.[7] Welker et al.[38] recommend canceling oocyte retrieval or embryo replacement in cycles demonstrating a homogeneous hyperechoic pattern on the day after hCG. This is supported by Gonen and Casper.[7] Gonen and Casper, however, found that endometrial thickness might be even more important. Although most endometrium demonstrating a triple-line sign is also more than 6 mm thick, in rare cycles that had a good triple-line sign but an endometrial thickness of less than 6 mm, the cycle was highly likely to fail despite the triple-line sign. Conversely, cycles with a hyperechoic pattern and no triple-line sign, but an especially thickened endometrium (≥ 10 mm), occasionally led to conceptions. The best negative predictive value for cycle outcome combined the lack of a triple-line sign and lack of endometrial thickness. The best conception rates were found in patients demonstrating both a triple-line sign and an endometrial thickness greater than 6 mm.[7] Thus, clinically, if any pattern but a triple-line sign exists—especially if the endometrium is less than 6 mm thick—consideration should be given to withholding oocyte retrieval or to freezing embryos developed from oocytes in those cycles to permit subsequent embryo transfer into a more favorable endometrial environment.

Anecdotal reports have described a uterine cavity filled with 2 to 6 mm of fluid after hMG stimulation and hCG trigger.[20] This sequela has occurred in patients with known hydrosalpinges and obstruction, leading to speculation that fluid accumulation after stimulation in hydrosalpinges leads to fluid accumulation in the uterine cavity. Although one pregnancy in a report of six cases was recorded, it was recommended that the finding of fluid in the endometrial cavity on the day of oocyte recovery should lead to cryopreservation of all resultant embryos for later transfer into a more receptive endometrium.[20,38]

Much more work related to endometrial reflectivity patterns in the periovulatory period is needed in natural cycles and various stimulation protocols. Questions posed by Gonen and Casper[7] are appropriate: (1) Does an unfavorable pattern or thickness in the endometrium recur in the same patient? (2) Does the method of ovarian hyperstimulation contribute to the pattern and thickness of the endometrium (such as the differences between natural cycles and clomiphene cycles)? (3) Do favorable or unfavorable endometrial patterns or thicknesses occur in natural cycles? (4) Can an unfavorable endometrial pattern or thickness be improved by hormonal manipulation or alteration of stimulation protocols? These questions are worthy of continued investigation.

Luteal. Within approximately 48 hours of ovulation,

ultrasonographic changes indicating a transition from estrogen-stimulated, proliferative-stage endometrium to progesterone-stimulated, secretory-stage endometrium first become apparent (Fig. 31-5).[4] As the endometrium progresses from the periovulatory proliferative phase to the secretory phase, the functional layer of the endometrium undergoes a gradual transition from a hypoechoic to a hyperechoic texture. The hypoechoic appearance of the proliferative and periovulatory endometrium described has been related to its relative homogeneous histologic structure. The glands in the proliferative endometrium have a simple configuration, and therefore there are fewer enlarged vessels than in the secretory endometrium. The transition to a hyperechoic texture in the secretory endometrium has been related to the lengthening, coiling, and increased storage of echogenic mucus and glycogen in the endometrial glands. The spiral arteries supplying the functional layer lengthen and become more tortuous. The combination of glandular and vascular changes thus present more reflective interfaces to the incident ultrasound beam, resulting in the characteristic hyperechoic texture.

Grunfeld et al.[10] describe the gradual luteal transition from the periovulatory triple-line hypoechogenicity to the mid–luteal phase hyperechoic pattern. Gradual changes are seen in the early secretory phase, from a partial and increasingly thick hyperechoic pattern to greater than 50% of the endometrial thickness around the narrowing hypoechoic center above and below the endometrial lumen itself. The hyperechoic pattern increases from the basalis inward and continues through luteal phase day 7, when the whole pattern is hyperechoic. Grunfeld et al.[10] attempted to correlate these ultrasonographic features of endometrial luteal phase transition with morphologic assessment of endometrial biopsy. The model used was artificial replacement cycles in preparation for later transfer of donor oocytes (Estraderm patches containing 0.2 to 0.4 ng/mL given to reach a serum estradiol concentration of 200 to 400 pg/mL, to which is then added intramuscular progesterone in oil).[10] These cycles are meant to mimic physiologic cycles, and the serum estradiol and progesterone values found in these patients support this. The lack of current studies in the luteal phase of spontaneous ovulation cycles makes this the best available information about what may occur in the endometrium during the natural cycle. The first day of progesterone replacement was called luteal phase day 1 and was characterized by the triple-line sign. This mimic of the periovulatory period was correlated with biopsies of proliferative and very early luteal phase endometrium. Biopsy specimens were also assessed on luteal phase day 7 and compared with ultrasound evaluation. The finding of a uniform hyperechoic pattern in the endometrium at this time was correlated directly to an "in-phase" stromal endometrial maturation on biopsy. Ultrasound in this circumstance was 100% sensitive, providing reassurance of endometrial adequacy.

The finding of a partial hypoechoic area remaining in the

endometrium on luteal phase day 7 often correlated with endometrial luteal inadequacy on the biopsy specimen. However, some biopsy specimens at this time were interpreted as normal, despite the residual hypoechoism by ultrasound. The sensitivity of the ultrasound method for endometrial adequacy at this time in the cycle was only 62%. Thus, when luteal phase deficiency was detected by biopsy, endovaginal ultrasonography always detected the abnormal echogenic pattern in the endometrium. There were, however, cases in which a hyperechoic endometrium was not found (residual hypoechoism) but results of the endometrial biopsy were normal. Also, endovaginal ultrasound appears best at detecting stromal advancement, as some glandular abnormalities on biopsy were not detected on ultrasound. Because stromal adequacy has been linked to implantation potential, the normal ultrasound reflective pattern of the endometrium in the mid–luteal phase may be reassuring to adequate development of the secretory endometrium. Endometrial thickness alone was not helpful, since on luteal phase day 7 there was no difference in endometrial height from biopsy specimens found to be histologically normal (13 mm) versus those found to be abnormal (13.8 mm).[10]

Studies linking these endometrial luteal phase patterns to outcome in actual cycles of embryo replacement have not yet been performed. It may be useful to study spontaneous and induced ovulatory cycles detailing endometrial development correlated to both endometrial biopsies (as an assessment of functional endometrial adequacy) and subsequent cycle outcome. Studies also could evaluate the endometrium beyond luteal phase day 7 to determine the utility of ultrasound as a replacement or supplement to endometrial biopsy in natural and stimulated cycles. These results might yield a helpful advance in cycle monitoring, especially given the advantages of safety, noninvasiveness, and unintrusiveness that endovaginal ultrasonography holds over endometrial biopsy.

Follicles

Clomiphene cycles. Ultrasound follicular monitoring in clomiphene cycles can be used to assess the response to therapy and/or time the triggering hCG injection. At low doses of clomiphene, a patient's initial ovulatory response can most easily be assessed by LH kit, BBT, serum progesterone, biopsy, and/or conception. The need for ultrasound assessment of the developing follicle is minimal. Ultrasound studies that have serially followed follicular development in clomiphene cycles have found growth curves similar to those of spontaneous cycles,[27] but often with a lead follicle diameter significantly greater at the onset of monitoring and maintaining the significantly greater size throughout the follicular phase and at the time of the LH surge. This is especially true at higher clomiphene citrate doses.

Average follicle sizes on clomiphene citrate at the time of the LH surge are 27 mm (range of 16.5 to 32 mm).

Although these are generally larger than spontaneous cycles' follicle average of 21.6 mm (range 14 to 31 mm), there is considerable overlap. The wide range in clomiphene diameters at the time of the LH surge limit ultrasound follicle size for predicting the timing of ovulation.[27]

Ultrasound evaluation of clomiphene cycles has found many cycles to be multifollicular. Up to 25% of anovulatory women given 50 to 200 mg of clomiphene per day for 5 days demonstrate multifollicular development; the percentage increases to up to 95% of cycles on clomiphene 150 mg/d when given to otherwise ovulatory women.[27] With an overall twin conception rate of at least 8% with the use of clomiphene, patients who need ovulation induction, but in whom multiple gestation would be a significant problem (septate uterus, habitual abortion, in utero DES exposure), ultrasound assessment of follicle number may be an adjunct to therapy by recommending abstinence from intercourse if the LH surge occurs or by withholding hCG triggering of ovulation, since the increased rate of multiple gestation is due to multiple ovulation. Some sensitive patients and some patients who are otherwise ovulatory may develop many follicles, and for this reason special ultrasound assessment may be especially useful in them. However, the large majority of patients on clomiphene are at generally low risk, a risk that must be weighed against the cost and intrusiveness of ultrasound evaluation in these patients.

In the event of failure of conception in patients known to have multifollicular development or a history of cyst formation, ultrasound assessment before clomiphene citrate administration in the subsequent early follicular phase may be used to determine whether to withhold the clomiphene therapy for a cycle.

When a patient has failed to ovulate on low doses of clomiphene, consideration needs to be given to increasing the clomiphene dose or adding hCG to trigger ovulation. (See Chapter 32.) One paradigm to follow involves using ultrasound to segregate between these two choices. If ovulation has not been initiated after 100 mg daily for 5 days, as assessed by LH kit or BBTs, during the next cycle 150 mg daily is often tried. A transvaginal ultrasound assessment can be ordered for day 16 of the cycle. The patient is then followed for an LH surge, using a home urine LH kit. If this occurs, but conception is not initiated, clomiphene citrate 150 mg daily is continued without further monitoring in subsequent cycles. If no LH surge occurs, but follicular development by ultrasound did occur, hCG may be given in the next cycle in the same 150-mg dose, once the lead follicle reaches a mean diameter of 18 mm. The timing of ovulation—and therefore insemination/intercourse—follows as it does for an LH surge. Conversely, if little follicular development is seen on ultrasound, then a higher dose of clomiphene or other therapy is necessary because hCG alone will not provide benefit. O'Herlihy and co-workers[26] assessed 97 clomiphene/hCG cycles in 21 women; hCG was given when the lead follicle had a mean diameter greater than or equal to 18 mm. Ovulation occurred on cycle day 15 in 0%, on cycle day 16 in 41%, and on cycle day 17 in 33%. Given these rates, administering hCG without monitoring on day 16 or day 17 after clomiphene days 5 to 9 may appropriately trigger ovulation in a reasonable percentage of patients. However, individualizing the appropriate day for the hCG trigger may be more sensitively defined by ultrasound than by choosing any one day without monitoring.

Thus ultrasound monitoring of clomiphene cycles may have some utility by assessing an occasional patient with multifollicular development before ovulation, or persistent cyst formation from a previous cycle before starting the next course of therapy. It may also have benefit in evaluation of follicular development as a means to segregate therapy between hCG or a higher dose of clomiphene citrate in patients not ovulating on lower-dose therapies, and as a means by which to best time the hCG trigger.[33] However, the number of patients on clomiphene citrate in whom ultrasound monitoring is of use, as outlined above, is small. The routine or liberal use of ultrasound and low-dose clomiphene citrate—especially to predict ovulation or to detect the enigmatic luteinized unruptured follicle—must be looked at critically and compared with other, less expensive, less intrusive, monitoring methods.

GnRH pulsatile therapy. Follicular development during ovulation induction with pulsatile GnRH therapy is similar to that of development in spontaneous cycles once the therapeutic effect of the drug is initiated.[33] Most cycles have a dominant follicle whose growth characteristics and size resemble those seen with natural cycles. Multiple follicles (and subsequent multiple pregnancies that may ensue) are not common when using standard subcutaneous or even intravenous pulsatile regimens. Monitoring does provide an assessment of therapeutic response, and it allows alterations of drug dose should appropriate development fail to occur. Estrogen can be used alone or in conjunction with ultrasound follicle assessment, but ultrasound alone may provide enough information. This monitoring need be only occasional rather than daily. Patients other than those with Kallmann syndrome usually will mount a spontaneous LH surge in response to appropriate follicle development, and its detection can suffice for timing of intercourse/insemination and/or a switch to luteal phase support once the pump is discontinued, as is the most common protocol. Alternatively, somewhat closer ultrasound monitoring may be used to predict timing of the hCG trigger if required (e.g., mean follicle diameter ≥18 mm) instead of awaiting, if an LH surge will not occur.

Menotropins. Menotropin therapy bypasses the pituitary, which ordinarily provides feedback regulation to modify the degree of ovarian response in natural and clomiphene cycles. This direct effect on the ovary by menotropins provides the basis for their efficacy in many patients resistant to other forms of therapy, and in patients undergoing purposeful ovarian hyperstimulation for assisted reproduction. It also, of course, provides the setting for the major interrelated risks associated with this form of treatment, namely ovarian hyperstimulation syndrome, multiple gestation, and spontaneous abortion. Monitoring of ovulation during these therapies is clearly capable of enhancing efficacy and safety.[40] Ultrasound monitoring of follicular development has played a newer but increasingly central role in this monitoring. When combined with estrogen monitoring as the original staple of therapeutic assessment, a synergistic benefit can be appreciated. Monitoring should always be used judiciously. The potential risks of menotropin therapy warrant frequent monitoring to maximize success and minimize risk.[33]

In amenorrheic and anovulatory patients administered hMG, there is a significant correlation between ovarian follicular development (as assessed by ultrasound, based on either mean diameter of lead follicles or on total follicular volume) and estrogen secretion. Total follicular volume is derived by the addition of the volumes of each follicle ($v = 4/3 \times A^2B$, where A = long radius and B = short radius of each follicle ≥10 mm).[22] The size of the lead follicle develops progressively, as do the total follicular volumes. Individualized therapy to anovulatory patients often starts at two ampules of hMG daily. With this therapy, 77% of euestrogenic patients had two or more follicles of 16 mm or greater mean diameter at the time of hCG administration, but only 35% of hypoestrogenic patients under the same stimulation had two follicles of 16 mm or greater, and none had more than two follicles. This documents the variation in clinical response in patients presenting with different estrogen states underlying their anovulation and suggests that the monitoring may need to be more frequent (and dosing more cautious) in patients with euestrogenemic or hyperestrogenemic states than in patients with hypoestrogenemia (e.g., polycystic ovary disease versus hypothalamic amenorrhea).[22]

The hyperresponsiveness of patients with polycystic ovary disease and the panoply of regimens of ovulation induction designed to regulate these patients ("step-down" FSH, GnRH agonist + FSH, ovarian drilling, FSH + HMG, etc.) attest to the need for careful monitoring. Estradiol measurements also correlated with increases in total ovarian volume, total follicular volume, and the volume of each of the three largest follicles (although they correlated less well with this last important parameter) (Fig. 31-8).[12,22] With these correlations, it might seem appropriate to choose either estrogen or ultrasound for monitoring, but not both. In fact, if one were *required* to choose between estrogen and ultrasound for monitoring of menotropin therapies, ultrasound follicular development would be the choice. Ultrasound provides anatomic parameters that correlate better with follicle maturity and the number of

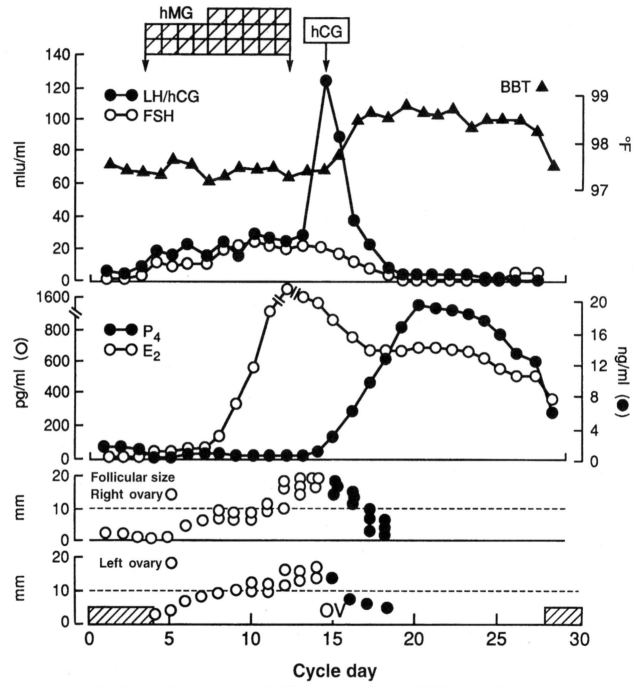

Fig. 31-7. Luteinizing hormone *(LH)*, follicle-stimulating hormone *(FSH)*, estradiol *(E₂)*, proges-terone *(P₄)*, follicular size, and basal body temperature *(BBT)* profiles in response to ovulation induction with human menopausal gonadotropin *(hMG)* and human chorionic gonadotropin *(hCG)*. (Redrawn from Stillman RJ: Ovulation induction. In DeCherney AH, editor: *Reproductive failure,* Churchill Livingstone, New York, 1986.)

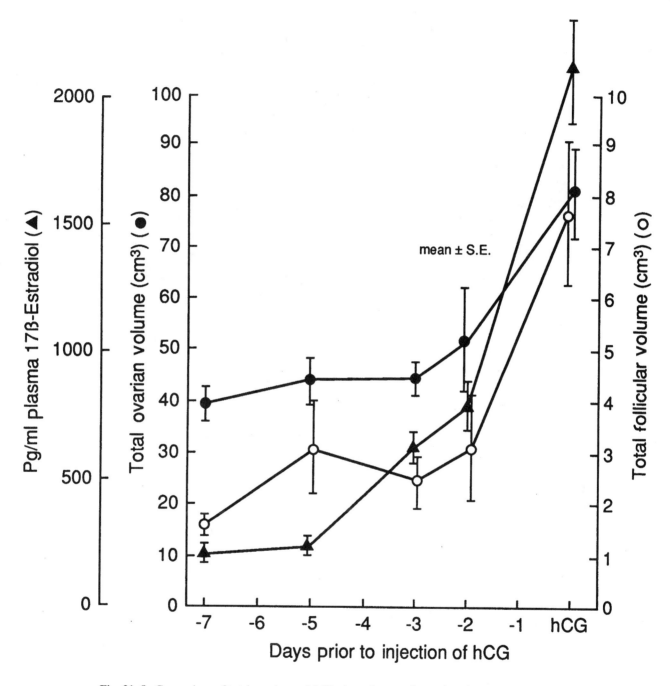

Fig. 31-8. Comparison of total ovarian and follicular volume and morning plasma 17 β-estradiol as a function of days before injection of hCG in cycles stimulated with hMG. (Redrawn from Haning R et al: *Fertil Steril* 37:627, 1982, with permission of the publisher, The American Fertility Society.)

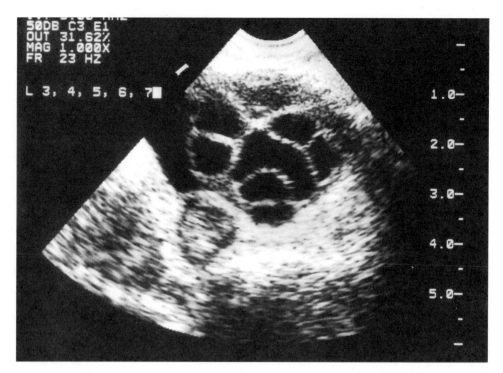

Fig. 31-9. Ultrasound of follicular development in menotropin-stimulated cycles.

mature follicles than does estrogen (Fig. 31-9). The poorer correlation of estrogen to size of the largest follicle or total follicular volumes results in poor predictive capability of estrogen for these important parameters. Multiple small follicles, each with its own relatively small estrogen production, can reproduce the estrogen levels that may also be associated with a single follicle or codominant mature follicles (e.g., an estradiol concentration of 1200 pg/mL may be seen with 10 follicles of 11 mm each or 3 follicles of 19 mm each). The difference with respect to the efficacy of the ovulation induction is great and can be differentiated by ultrasound. The likelihood of successful ovulation can be estimated, as can the number of fertilizable oocytes to be ovulated and, with it, the likelihood of multiple gestation.

Navot et al.[25] analyzed the risk factors and prognostic variables for multiple pregnancies during induction of ovulation with human menopausal gonadotropins. They examined 51 multiple pregnancy cycles and 51 consecutive control singleton pregnancy cycles. A statistically significant correlation was found between the occurrence of intermediate-sized follicles (15 to 17 mm) and multiple pregnancy. Also, the number of intermediate-sized follicles correlated directly with the number of fetuses. Since they tended to withhold hCG whenever more than two large follicles ($\geq$18 mm) were present, this tended to keep the large-sized follicle numbers similar in both groups.

In an important study, Silverberg and co-workers[31] assessed the follicle size of each follicle at the time of hCG administration and calculated its frequency of ovulation based on ultrasound criteria of collapse in each follicle in

Table 31-1. Predictor of the likelihood of a particular follicle ovulating by ultrasound criteria based on the size of that follicle at the time of hCG trigger in stimulated ovulation cycles

Follicle size (mm)	Ovulation (%)
<14	5/952 (0.5)
15–16	61/163 (37.4)
17–18	100/138 (72.5)
19–20	56/69 (81.2)
>20	21/22 (95.5)

From Silverberg KM, Olive DL, Schenken RS: Does follicular size at the time of hCG administration predict ovulation outcome? In The American Fertility Society Program Supplement, 46th Annual Meeting, Washington, DC, October 15–18, 1990. S12. Reproduced with permission of the publisher, The American Fertility Society.

122 treatment cycles in 48 patients (Table 31-1). The range was from 0.5% ovulation in follicles less than 14 mm to 95.5% in follicles greater than 20 mm. The frequency of multiple ovulation and therefore the risk of multiple gestation can be estimated from these data.

As is discussed in the section on estrogen monitoring, although ultrasound provides important measures entailed in menotropin monitoring, estrogen monitoring correlates best with the likelihood of ovarian hyperstimulation syndrome. Estrogens can help to modify hMG dose schedules when apparent ultrasound follicular development presents with low estrogen production. Thus the utilization of both estrogen and ultrasound provides the best current, mutually reinforcing, monitoring.[12]

Generally, menotropins are administered daily from day 3 of a cycle for 4 to 5 days at doses correlated to clinical indication for use. After the daily ultrasound and estradiol monitoring commences, results are available in the afternoon to individualize instruction for an evening dose or administration of an hCG trigger (or aborting of the cycle in cases of overstimulation). Steady growth on ultrasound (confirmed by estradiol rise) allows maintenance of dosing until at least one follicle is 16 to 17 mm or more in diameter. Based on growth rates rarely exceeding 1.5 mm mean diameter per day, days of monitoring occasionally may be omitted without decreasing the safety or efficacy. This sometimes results in decreased costs and less inconvenience for patients. Investigators report the triggering of ovulation after hMG with mean diameters of the largest follicles ranging from 14 to 25 mm, with most triggering at or around 16 mm or greater. Some of the timing as to when hCG is administered is arbitrarily chosen by the clinician in interrupting the cycle, as opposed to the physiologically prescribed timing of an LH surge. Since hMG therapy most often suppresses the spontaneous LH surge, it is unknown precisely when the follicle is actually "most" mature as opposed to when intervention occurs. Generally, however, it is believed that hMG-induced follicle(s) tend to be smaller at the time of hCG administration than are natural preovulatory follicles or clomiphene-induced follicles. The work of Silverberg et al.[31] has been mentioned regarding follicle sizes and likelihood of ovulation.

Regimens with fixed-dose schedules or with little monitoring, although successful in some patients, do not fulfill the principles of monitoring as frequently or for as many patients consistently as do individualized dose therapies based on frequent monitoring data.

The goal of ovulation induction with menotropins in anovulatory patients is the development of a single dominant, mature follicle in as physiologic a pattern as possible. Unfortunately, this is rarely possible without the hypothalamic and pituitary governors that are obviated by the direct stimulation of the ovaries by these therapies. Almost all hMG and FSH ovulation induction is associated with some degree of hyperstimulation. (See Chapter 33.) The goal is to use monitoring to control the hyperstimulation within a window that brings about ovulation but avoids ovarian hyperstimulation syndrome (OHSS) and its occasional concomitant multiple gestation. (See Chapter 35 for the classification of OHSS.) Aborting the cycle by withholding hCG ovulation induction (and intercourse) can be recommended in a risk-benefit consultation with the patient when the window is overshot.

Menotropins are widely utilized today for "purposeful" hyperstimulation—the attempt to induce multiple codominant follicles for assisted reproductive technologies (e.g., IVF, gamete intrafallopian transfer, and zygote intrafallo-

pian transfer) and derived procedures (e.g., intrauterine insemination). (See Chapter 30.) Their common denominator is the use of multiple extracorporeal or intracorporeal oocytes. The operative term here is *multiple* as a means to circumvent nature's human ovulatory cohort of one and thus hopefully increase cycle fecundity rates. Thus the window of therapeutic interest is much higher in these patients than in those with anovulation. What would often be an unacceptable degree of ovarian stimulation for the anovulatory patient is for assisted reproductive technologies the goal, and some degree of OHSS is uniform. Tolerance is higher often because follicular aspiration before ovulation that is associated with these programs appears to minimize the frequency or degree of OHSS, compared with that seen with the same number of follicles (and high estradiol levels) when follicular aspiration is not performed. Monitoring principles, especially the use of ultrasound to guide and adjust dose and determine the timing of hCG administration, are similar but cycles are less frequently aborted on the basis of monitoring except for low responses.

The daily growth of mean diameter of the largest follicle increases after hMG stimulation.[21] The mean diameter of the largest (of multiple) follicles at the time of hCG administration was 16.3 mm in patients with both ovaries and 18.5 mm in patients with one ovary. (The discrepancy in patients with one ovary may be due to the longer wait to obtain more developed follicles, since one ovary generally produces fewer follicles after hyperstimulation than do two ovaries.) According to Mantzavinos et al.,[21] high responders (estradiol > 600 pg/mL at the time of hCG injection) showed a somewhat larger mean follicular diameter (17.6 ± 1.5 mm) than did normal responders (estradiol 300 to 600 pg/mL), whose mean diameter was 16.9 ± 2.4 mm, and low responders (estradiol < 300 pg/mL), whose follicular diameter was 16.0 ± 1.1 mm. Similar growth dynamics of about 1.2 mm ± 0.3 mm per day were noted. There was no correlation between estradiol concentration and the diameter of the largest follicle on the day of hCG administration, but some correlation was noted with the total number of follicles developed.[21]

Serial, daily ultrasound monitoring of purposeful ovarian hyperstimulation with menotropins is an important staple in keeping the risks acceptable with these strategies. Adjunctive estradiol monitoring improves the opportunity to strike the therapeutic window that exists with both efficacy and manageable risk.

In conclusion, ultrasound evaluation of the endometrium may be able to take a rightful place beside follicle scanning as an important mainstay in monitoring ovulation induction. The expertise and training of an increasing number of practitioners in the area promises to increase ultrasound use for these patients. Ultrasound is of unquestioned value in menotropin therapy, especially those protocols designed to promote multifollicle development. More conservatism still should be exercised in the use of these monitoring techniques in nonstimulated spontaneous cycles and clomiphene-stimulated cycles.

Estrogen

Urine. Urinary levels of estradiol, estriol, and estrone were measured in initial experiments in ovulation induction. Retrospective data in early trials were translated into guidelines for prospective monitoring to minimize the risk of multiple gestation and hyperstimulation. There was no evidence that measurement of specific estrogens was at that time superior to determination of total urinary estrogens. The addition of semilog plots of total urinary estrogens versus days of treatment produced linear functions with an average increase of 53% per day. The straight line of the plot allowed prediction of the day on which total urinary estrogen might reach a given desired level. The urinary monitoring of estriol glucuronide by direct RIA simplified urinary assays by eliminating extraction steps previously required.[13]

Haning et al.[13] found that urinary estriol glucuronide correlated well with total ovarian volume, total follicular volume, and number of days of menotropin administration, and correlated especially well with coincident serum estradiol values. However, both estrogens correlated less well with volume of the largest follicle, making ultrasound the better anatomic parameter to monitor follicular maturation and number of mature follicles.[13] As mentioned in the section on ultrasound, multiple small follicles can produce the same urinary (or serum) estrogen pattern as a few large preovulatory follicles. Thus reliance on estrogen measurement without ultrasound is not a good monitoring protocol. In comparing serum estradiol with estriol glucuronide, Haning et al.[13] found that estradiol had a predictive value superior to estriol glucuronide in predicting OHSS. Importantly, they also found that estradiol had this superior predictive value for OHSS over ultrasound determination of number of follicles.[13]

Variation in patient body weight proved to be a source of error while attempting to predict OHSS using urinary estriol glucuronide. Thus the requirement of 24-hour urine collections; the variations in the completeness of the collections; the variations in output due to renal and enterohepatic circulation; the advent of easy, rapid, serum estradiol measurements; and the diminished predictive value of estriol glucuronide to OHSS have strictly limited urine estrogen monitoring.

A recent report of home urinary monitoring of estrone-3-glucuronide, the major urinary metabolite of 17β-estradiol, is encouraging.[36] The assay allowed the convenience and relative ease of patient home assay, lacked the need for 24-hour urine collections, and demonstrated a good correlation with serum values. The assay system uses overnight urine collection for a hapten-linked enzyme immunoassay. This requires a 45-minute assay (most of which time is spent in incubation steps) and a pocket-sized thermostatic rate colorimeter to measure the light transmis-

sion changes in the assay system relative to the concentration of estrone-3-glucuronide in the urine. The assay requires acquisition of some basic laboratory skills by the patient (e.g., measuring dilution steps) and some time (although less time than spent driving to the clinic for blood drawing), but its advantages in cost, convenience, increased patient involvement, and the ability to monitor patients distant from the clinic are all important to consider. The assay was used to determine when to initiate ultrasound monitoring (when estrone-3-glucuronide reached ≥ 200 nmol/24 hours). Thus ultrasound monitoring commenced after the urine estrogen monitoring reached a specific threshold. At this threshold, 80% of patients had at least a 16-mm lead follicle and were ready for the hCG trigger. The optimal range for estrone glucuronide turned out to be 200 to 750 nmol/24 hours on the day of the hCG trigger, with a 16% hyperstimulation rate between 500 and 750 nmol/24 hours, but only a 3% rate at levels less than 500 nmol/24 hours.

The assessment by Haning et al.[13] that the 24-hour estriol glucuronide assay had a poorer predictive value for OHSS than did serum estradiol invites more detailed comparison studies about the actual predictive value of home urinary monitoring using this estrone-3-glucuronide model. The use of this home monitoring as a threshold to initiate subsequent ultrasound and serum estradiol monitoring is one concept, but its ability to monitor further, later-stage ovulation induction is another. Nevertheless, further refinement and ease of urinary home monitoring, probably with the use of monoclonal ELISA assays similar to those now available for LH, will probably be an important adjunct to at least the initial stages of ovulation monitoring for menotropin cycles and perhaps for clomiphene-stimulated cycles, after which ultrasound and serum estradiol monitoring may be started.

Serum. As follicular development progresses there is a steady increase in estradiol level, a function of the increase in the number of granulosa cells; increased aromatase activity in granulosa cells; and gonadotropin stimulation in the early and mid–follicular phase. The rate of rise of estradiol, almost entirely from the dominant follicle after the early follicular phase, is essentially linear when the logarithm of the estradiol concentration is plotted against time in a semilog plot. Follicular volume and mean follicular size are closely correlated with the serum estradiol rise (Fig. 31-8).[12,28] However, the prediction of ovulation or determination of its occurrence by serum estradiol level is foiled by the range of values over which these events occur, clearly limiting the value of estradiol in monitoring spontaneous cycles.

Correlation of serum estradiol with the size of the largest follicle and especially to total follicular volume is also observed in ovulation induction for clomiphene citrate[2] and menotropin[22] cycles. Estimates have been made that clomiphene cycles generate estradiol concentrations of approxi-

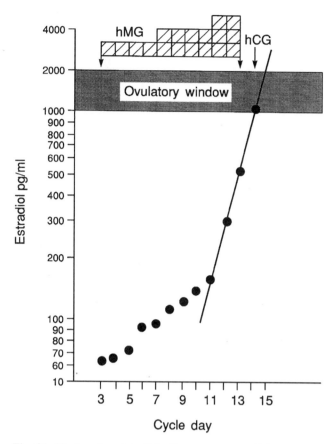

Fig. 31-10. Semilog plot of the 8 AM serum estradiol concentration in response to increasing 8 PM doses of hMG. In this example an ovulatory dose of hCG is administered on cycle day 14 when the estradiol concentration is between 1000 and 2000 pg/mL. (Redrawn from Stillman RJ: Ovulation induction. In DeCherney AH, editor: *Reproductive failure*, New York, 1986, Churchill-Livingstone.)

mately 300 to 460 pg/mL for each codominant large follicle and in hMG cycles approximately 250 to 350 pg/mL for each large follicle. Although these figures have been used occasionally to estimate follicular adequacy, the estrogen production from small follicles may throw this correlation off. As discussed previously, when monitoring is used ultrasound is important, because an estradiol concentration of 500 pg/mL can indicate one large follicle ready to ovulate or three small follicles destined to ovulate days subsequently. The difference with regard to outcome, of course, is important.

As for spontaneous cycles, the semilog plot[39] of serum estradiol during induced cycles is linear. This expression can predict an estradiol concentration days hence, but without evaluation of follicular size coincidentally, the time when ovulation should appropriately be triggered remains largely unknown (Fig. 31-10).

A monitoring program for serum estradiol in clomiphene-induced cycles has been discussed in the earlier

section on ultrasound. In low-dose clomiphene therapy, estrogen monitoring may have little clinical utility. In higher-dose therapy serum estradiol monitoring is an adjunct to ultrasound to determine whether an hCG ovulatory trigger can be effectively employed or whether a higher degree of follicular stimulatory growth is needed from more clomiphene or from menotropins.

The likelihood of ovulation, of conception, and of multiple pregnancy in cycles induced by hMG is best predicted by ultrasound. The alteration in dose based on ultrasound follicular growth parameters and the timing of hCG to maturing follicles optimizes ovulatory capacity. Conversely, hCG can be withheld and intercourse or insemination precluded when too many follicles are found. However, ultrasound parameters are not as effective as estradiol when predicting ovarian hyperstimulation.[13]

When follicular size is used as the parameter upon which to judge appropriate follicular growth, serum estradiol concentrations are generally higher than those reported in therapeutic regimens that used estradiol alone as an index of follicular growth (500 to 1000 pg/mL lower window and 1500 to 2000 pg/mL upper window).

Haning et al.[12] found that in cycles managed prospectively with ultrasound a 40% clinical pregnancy rate per cycle was obtained with at least one follicle of 14 mm or more. The plasma estradiol concentration in these cycles was less than 1000 pg/mL (their previous lower window) in 35% of patients; it was between 1000 and 3999 pg/mL in 48%, and more than 4000 pg/mL in 17%. The plasma estradiol level was above the previous upper window of 2000 pg/mL in almost half of the studied cycles. Pregnancy rates were correspondingly lower when the estradiol level was less than 1000 pg/mL (29%); there was a 44% pregnancy rate when estradiol was between 1000 and 3999 pg/mL and 50% when plasma estradiol was greater than 4000 pg/mL. No case of OHSS occurred in their series when plasma estradiol values were less than 1000 pg/mL and no severe ovarian hyperstimulation was found when the hCG was given as soon as the first follicle reached a diameter of 14 mm as long as the estradiol level was less than 4000 pg/mL. Haning et al. suggest that the ovulatory trigger of hCG should be withheld if the plasma estradiol concentration is greater than 4000 pg/mL. Many other practitioners remain more conservative and set a concentration lower than 4000 pg/mL as an upper therapeutic window. However, it is clear that conservative upper estradiol limits previously considered appropriate may need to be raised to allow time for appropriate follicular growth (as assessed by ultrasound) to ensure the best ovulation and pregnancy rates.[12]

It is important to emphasize that serum estradiol peaks approximately 8 to 10 hours after the injection of menotropin. Plasma estradiol values presented in the series by Haning et al.[12] relate to the schedule of 5:00 PM to 8:00 PM menotropin injection and 8:00 AM blood drawing (and ultrasound evaluation) the next morning. Some physicians still use an 8:00 AM menotropin injection based on results obtained from an 8:00 AM estrogen determination the previous day. Not only does this present a delay in the time of acting on the previous 24 hours of information, but the estrogen level may actually be lower than the peak value 12 to 14 hours earlier. Thus the timing of hMG injection and the timing of monitoring must be clearly understood in interpreting one's own monitoring results, pregnancy outcome data, and comparisons to the literature. Evening injection and morning monitoring is recommended. The data of Haning et al.[12] demonstrated the superiority of ultrasound over estrogen determination for the timing of hCG administration and demonstrated the value of estradiol monitoring for reducing the risk of severe ovarian hyperstimulation during ultrasound monitoring. A combination of ultrasound and plasma estrogen appeared to optimize induction of ovulation.[22]

CONCLUSION

Monitoring of ovulation has found an important role in the care rendered by gynecologists and reproductive endocrinologists, especially in the therapeutics—and economics—of infertility. A focus by the physician on the reasons for monitoring spontaneous or stimulated cycles and on the principles implied in undertaking monitoring (efficacy, safety, cost effectiveness, unintrusiveness, and noninvasiveness) will allow him or her to most effectively make use of the various methods available. In spontaneous cycles, this involves predicting the timing of ovulation and/or documenting its occurrence and adequacy. The area of greatest clinical need for more intensive ovulation monitoring, however, is clearly seen in stimulated cycles, especially those involving menotropins. Ultrasonographic depiction of follicular growth, supported by estrogen assays, allows as much efficacy and safety from these therapeutic interventions as can be mustered. The ultrasonographic evaluation of the endometrium and an increased number of sophisticated but simple methods of hormonal monitoring at home will serve to further the principles described, and therefore serve the patients who have entrusted us with their care.

REFERENCES

1. Cook C: Luteal-phase defect, *Clin Obstet Gynecol* 34:198, 1991.
2. DeCherney AH, Laufer N: The monitoring of ovulation induction using ultrasound and estrogen, *Clin Obstet Gynecol* 27:993, 1984.
3. Fleischer A et al: Sonographic depiction of endometrial changes occurring with ovulation induction, *J Ultrasound Med* 3:341, 1984.
4. Forrest T et al: Cyclic endometrial changes: US assessment with histologic correlation, *Radiology* 167:233, 1988.
5. Frydman R et al: Interrelationship of plasma and urinary luteinizing hormone preovulatory surge, *J Steroid Biochem* 20:617, 1984.
6. Glissant A, de Mouzon J, Frydman R: Ultrasound study of the endometrium during in vitro fertilization cycles, *Fertil Steril* 44:786, 1985.

7. Gonen Y, Casper R: Prediction of Implantation by the sonographic appearance of the endometrium during controlled ovarian stimulation for in vitro fertilization (IVF), *J In Vitro Fert Embryo Transfer* 7:146, 1990.
8. Gonen Y et al: Endometrial thickness and growth during ovarian stimulation: a possible predictor of implantation in in vitro fertilization, *Fertil Steril* 52:446, 1989.
9. Grinsted J et al: Prediction of ovulation, *Fertil Steril* 52:388, 1989.
10. Grunfeld L et al: High resolution endovaginal ultrasonography of the endometrium: a noninvasive test for endometrial adequacy, *Obstet Gynecol* 78:200, 1991.
11. Hackeloer B, Fleming R, Robinson H: Correlation of ultrasonic and endocrinologic assessment of human follicular development, *Am J Obstet Gynecol* 135:1, 1979.
12. Haning R et al: Ultrasound evaluation of estrogen monitoring for induction of ovulation with menotropins, *Fertil Steril* 37:627, 1982.
13. Haning R et al: Plasma estradiol is superior to ultrasound and urinary estriol glucuronide as a predictor of ovarian hyperstimulation during induction of ovulation with menotropins, *Fertil Steril* 40:31, 1983.
14. Hecht B, Hoffman D: The use of ultrasound in infertility, *Clin Obstet Gynecol* 32:541, 1989.
15. Jacobs M: Prediction of ovulation, *Infertil Reprod Med Clin North Am* 2:287, 1991.
16. Kenigsberg D: New tests for the prediction of ovulation, *Clin Obstet Gynecol* 32:533, 1989.
17. Kruitwagen R et al: Oestradiol-17 and progesterone level changes in peritoneal fluid around the time of ovulation, *Br J Obstet Gynaecol* 94:548, 1987.
18. Li T-C et al: A comparison between two methods of chronological dating of human endometrial biopsies during the luteal phase, and their correlation with histologic dating, *Fertil Steril* 46:6, 1987.
19. Luciano A et al: Temporal relationship and reliability of the clinic, hormonal and ultrasonographic indices of ovulation in infertile women, *Obstet Gynecol* 75:412, 1990.
20. Mansour R et al: Fluid accumulation of the uterine cavity before embryo transfer: a possible hindrance for implantation, *J In Vitro Fert Embryo Transfer* 8:157, 1991.
21. Mantzavinos T, Garcia J, Jones H: Ultrasound measurement of ovarian follicles stimulated by human gonadotropins for oocyte recovery and in vitro fertilization, *Fertil Steril* 40:461, 1983.
22. Marrs R, Vargyas J, March C: Correlation of ultrasonic and endocrinologic measurements in human menopausal gonadotropin therapy, *Am J Obstet Gynecol* 145:417, 1983.
23. Martinez A et al: Urinary luteinizing hormone testing and prediction of ovulation in spontaneous clomiphene citrate and human menopausal gonadotropin-stimulated cycles: a clinical evaluation, *Acta Endocrinol* 124:357, 1991.
24. Merrill J: The interpretation of endometrial biopsies, *Clin Obstet Gynecol* 34:211, 1991.
25. Navot D et al: Multiple pregnancies: risk factors and prognostic variables during induction of ovulation with human menopausal gonadotropins, *Hum Reprod* 6:1152, 1991.
26. O'Herlihy C, Pepperell R, Robinson H: Ultrasound timing of human chorionic gonadotropin administration in clomiphene stimulated cycles, *Obstet Gynecol* 59:40, 1982.
27. Randall J, Templeton A: Transvaginal sonographic assessment of follicular and endometrial growth in spontaneous and clomiphene citrate cycles, *Fertil Steril* 56:208, 1991.
28. Rogers P et al: Correlation of endometrial histology, morphometry and ultrasound appearance after different stimulation protocols for in vitro fertilization, *Fertil Steril* 55:583, 1991.
29. Seif M et al: A novel approach for monitoring the endometrial cycle and detecting ovulation, *Am J Obstet Gynecol* 160:357, 1989.
30. Shoupe D et al: Correlation of endometrial maturation with four methods of estimating day of ovulation, *Obstet Gynecol* 73:88, 1989.

31. Silverberg KM, Olive DL, Schenken RS: Does follicular size at the time of HCG administration predict ovulation outcome? Paper presented at the 46th annual meeting of The American Fertility Society, Washington, DC, October 15–18, 1990 (abstract).

32. Smith B et al: Ultrasonic assessment of endometrial changes in stimulated cycles in an in-vitro fertilization and embryo transfer program. *J In Vitro Fert Embryo Transfer* 1:233, 1984.

33. Stillman RJ: Ovulation induction. In DeCherney AH, editor: *Reproductive failure,* New York, 1986, Churchill Livingstone.

34. Testart J, Frydman R: Minimum time lapse between luteinizing hormone surge or human chorionic gonadotropin administration and follicular rupture, *Fertil Steril* 37:50, 1982.

35. Testart J, Frydman R, Roger M: Seasonal influence of diurnal rhythms in the onset of the plasma luteinizing hormone surge in women, *J Clin Endocrinol Metab* 55:374, 1982.

36. Thornton S, Pepperell R, Brown J: Home monitoring of gonadotropin ovulation induction using the ovarian monitor, *Fertil Steril* 54:1076, 1990.

37. Vermesh M et al: Monitoring techniques to predict and detect ovulation, *Fertil Steril* 47:259, 1987.

38. Welker B et al: Transvaginal sonography of the endometrium during ovum pickup in stimulated cycles for in vitro fertilization, *J Ultrasound Med* 8:549, 1989.

39. Wilson E, Jawad MJ, Hayden TL: Rates of exponential increase of serum estradiol concentrations in normal and human menopausal gonadotropin-induced cycles, *Fertil Steril* 37:46, 1982.

40. Yee B, Rosen GF: Monitoring stimulated cycles, *Infertil Reprod Med Clin North Am* 1:15, 1990.

41. Zandt-Stastny D et al: Inability of sonography to detect imminent ovulation, *AJR* 152:91, 1989.

Chapter 32

CLOMIPHENE CITRATE–INITIATED OVULATION

The State of the Art

Eli Y. Adashi, MD

The introduction of clomiphene citrate represented a major therapeutic breakthrough that literally revolutionized the practice of reproductive endocrinology. Having been in use for more than 20 years, clomiphene citrate is now often viewed as an established therapeutic agent, the workings of which are well characterized. However, such a conclusion represents a gross underestimation of the knowledge gap that still exists concerning many aspects of the action of clomiphene citrate. Numerous uncertainties remain regarding the mechanisms underlying the ability of clomiphene citrate to effect ovulation in women and the relative role of the various components of the reproductive axis in this connection. In addition, information on the circulatory pharmacodynamics of clomiphene citrate in humans and measurements of its circulating levels are extremely limited.

Nevertheless, the clinical utility of clomiphene citrate as an ovulation promoter is undisputed. The clinical use and abuse of clomiphene citrate have been delineated previously. This chapter provides a current account of the rationale underlying use of clomiphene citrate.

CONCEPT OF "CHEMICAL" INITIATION OF OVULATION

In effect, the use of clomiphene citrate represented the first widespread realization of the novel notion for the "chemical" (as opposed to "hormonal") initiation of ovulation.[13,38] Indeed, for the first time use was made of a chemically synthesized compound rather than a naturally occurring hormone (for example, human chorionic gonadotropin [hCG]) to effect ovulation in the human.

Synthesized in 1956 by Dr. Frank P. Palopoli,[74] then a chemist with the William S. Merrell Company, clomiphene citrate was first introduced for clinical trials in 1960. The first human studies were conducted by a relatively small group of investigators, including Dr. Robert Greenblatt (Medical College of Georgia), Dr. Robert Kistner (Harvard Medical School), and Dr. Charles Lloyd (then of the State University of New York). Many more investigators joined these efforts soon thereafter. This flurry of activity was followed shortly by the appearance of the first published report describing the successful use of clomiphene citrate in the induction of ovulation in women.[39] Still referred to by its code name MRL/41, clomiphene citrate was shown by Greenblatt and colleagues to effect ovulation in 28 of 36 chronic anovulators. Administration to normally cycling women resulted in a delay of menses and the extension of the usual 14-day postovulatory thermogenic shift to 20 to 25 days. Additional confirmatory reports followed soon.

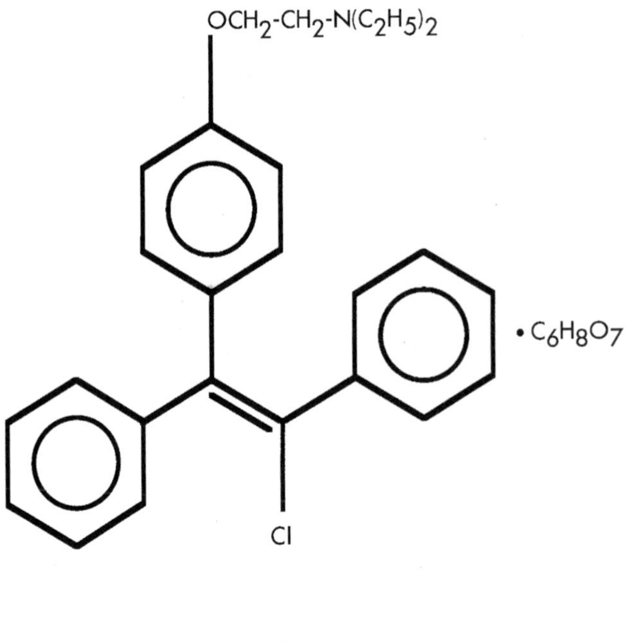

$$OCH_2-CH_2-N(C_2H_5)_2$$

$$\cdot C_6H_8O_7$$

Cl

2-[p-(2-chloro-1,2-diphenylvinyl) phenoxy] triethylamine dihydrogen citrate

Fig. 32-1. Structural formula of clomiphene citrate. (Redrawn from Adashi EY: *Semin Reprod Endocrinol* 4:255, 1980.)

An investigational new drug application was filed in 1962, and Food and Drug Administration approval for widespread clinical use was granted in 1967 with the stipulation that the total dose consumed per cycle not exceed 750 mg. Although current protocols may not always adhere to these upper dose limits, the original stipulation placing a cap on the total clomiphene citrate dosage still stands and continues to be listed in some, albeit not all, package inserts. The recent expiration of the original William S. Merrell Company patent rights resulted in the emergence of preparations listed under brand names other than Clomid, such as Serophene, a product of Serono Laboratories, Inc., Randolph, Mass. Although differences in the apparent efficacy of the various brands of clomiphene citrate have been considered, there appears to be no evidence supporting such concerns.[20]

CLINICAL PHARMACOLOGY

Structurally, clomiphene citrate is a triphenylethylene derivative. As such, it may be viewed as consisting of an ethylene (C=C) core, the four hydrogen atoms of which have been substituted with three phenyl rings and a chloride anion, respectively (Fig. 32-1). Only one of the three phenyl rings has been further modified by the addition of an aminoalkoxy ($OCH_2-CH_2-N[C_2H_5]_2$) side chain, the exact role of which in clomiphene citrate–initiated ovulation remains uncertain. The dihydrogen citrate moiety ($C_6H_8O_7$) simply denotes the fact that commercially available prepa-

rations as currently used represent the dihydrogen citrate salt form of clomiphene proper.

In clinical use, clomiphene citrate is provided as a racemic mixture of its two stereochemical isomers (Fig. 32-2). These were originally designated as the *trans*-isomer and the *cis*-isomer. By definition, the *trans*-isomer represents that molecule in which the two unsubstituted phenyl rings are found on opposite sides of a hypothetic plane dividing the clomiphene citrate molecule through its ethylene core. In contrast, the *cis*-isomer is defined as that molecule in which the two unsubstituted phenyl rings are found on the same side of the above-mentioned hypothetic plane. The *trans*- and *cis*-isomers were recently renamed as enclomiphene citrate and zuclomiphene citrate, respectively.[25] The racemic mixture administered to induce ovulation in women is generally made up of 38% zuclomiphene citrate and 62% enclomiphene citrate.

Clomiphene citrate, a nonsteroidal estrogen, is capable of interacting with estrogen receptor–binding proteins in a manner generally akin to that of native estrogens.[14] Several lines of evidence would seem to suggest, however, that the nature of the interaction of clomiphene citrate with estrogen receptor–binding proteins may nevertheless display qualitative differences vis-à-vis the naturally occurring ligand. Most important, clomiphene citrate, as well as a series of related triphenylethylene derivatives, is best characterized by the tendency to display prolonged nuclear receptor occupancy.[15] In fact, clomiphene citrate has been shown to

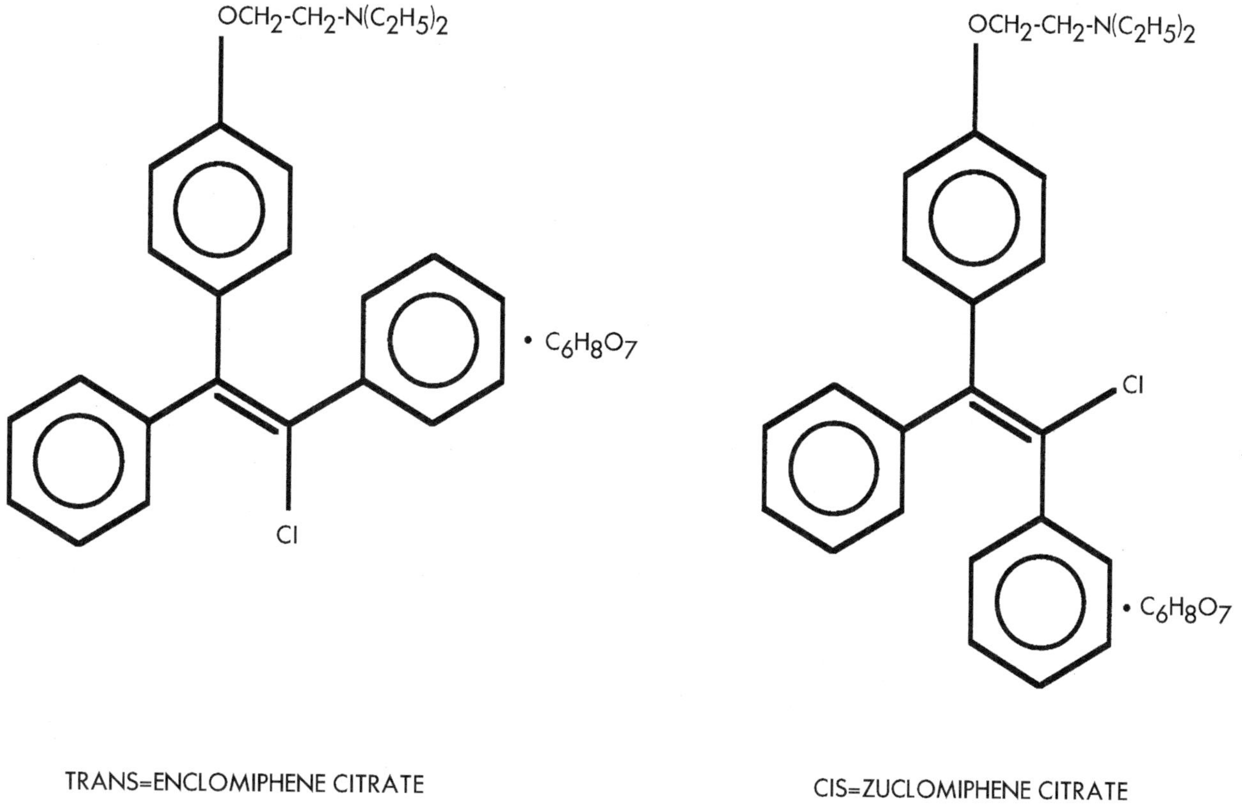

OCH$_2$-CH$_2$-N(C$_2$H$_5$)$_2$

• C$_6$H$_8$O$_7$

Cl

OCH$_2$-CH$_2$-N(C$_2$H$_5$)$_2$

Cl

• C$_6$H$_8$O$_7$

TRANS=ENCLOMIPHENE CITRATE

CIS=ZUCLOMIPHENE CITRATE

Fig. 32-2. Stereochemical isomers of clomiphene citrate. (Redrawn from Adashi EY: *Semin Reprod Endocrinol* 4:255, 1980.)

occupy nuclear receptor proteins for weeks on end, a phenomenon sharply contrasting with the rather brief interaction of native estrogens, which are known to clear the cell within 24 hours. Be that as it may, the relevance of these observations to the ability of clomiphene citrate to effect ovulation, to its possible progressive "nuclear" accumulation on repetitive administration, and to its possible lingering blastocytotoxic or teratogenic effects remains uncertain. It is noteworthy that triphenylethylenes and triphenylchloroethylenes have long been known as estrogen agonists of low potency but of unusually long duration of action in castrated or immature rodents. Moreover, these traits have been shown repeatedly to be augmented by an alkoxy substitution. Paradoxically, however, these early observations received relatively little attention until the "rediscovery" that clomiphene citrate may act as an estrogen, rather than an antiestrogen, in several species, including human. Clomiphene citrate has been shown to possess no progestational, corticotropic, androgenic, or antiandrogenic activities.

MECHANISMS AND SITES OF ACTION

It seems remarkable that despite intense basic and clinical investigation and a bibliography approaching 10,000 contributions, the mechanisms and sites of action of clomiphene citrate remain largely unknown. As currently

viewed, the ability of clomiphene citrate to initiate an ovulatory sequence is due primarily, and perhaps exclusively, to its ability to be recognized by and interact with estrogen receptors at the level of the hypothalamus. Acting in its capacity as an antiestrogen, clomiphene citrate is thought to displace endogenous estrogen from hypothalamic estrogen receptor sites, thereby alleviating the putative negative feedback effect exerted by endogenous estrogens. Alternatively, clomiphene citrate may be capable of inhibiting the positive cooperativeness triggered by the binding of estradiol to its receptor. The projected resultant alteration in the characteristics of pulsatile gonadotropin-releasing hormone (GnRH) released is assumed to "normalize" the release of pituitary gonadotropins, followed in rapid sequence by follicular recruitment, selection, assertion of dominance, and ultimately rupture. According to this view, the interaction of clomiphene citrate at the level of the hypothalamus is assigned a primary and essentially exclusive role, relegating other components of the reproductive axis to a secondary position (Fig. 32-3). Thus events occurring at either the pituitary or ovarian level are generally thought of as representing secondary phenomena contingent on the primary interaction of clomiphene citrate at the hypothalamic level.

Although evidence obtained in a variety of experimental models would suggest a hypothalamic site of action for

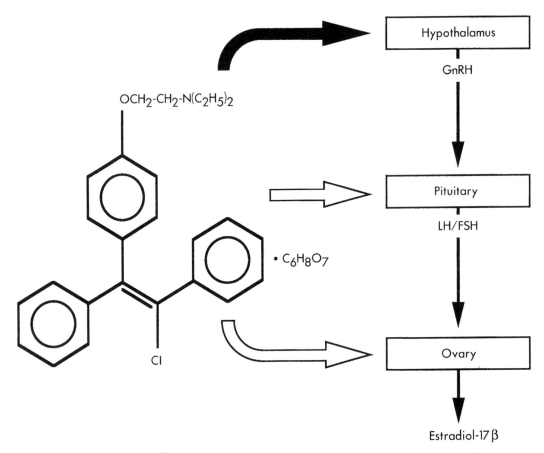

Fig. 32-3. Clomiphene citrate–initiated ovulation: current hypothesis as to presumed sites of action. (Redrawn from Adashi EY: Clomiphene citrate: mechanism(s) and site(s) of action—a hypothesis revisited, *Fertil Steril* 42:331, 1984.)

clomiphene citrate,[2] direct, unequivocal demonstration of such interaction in humans is not likely to be forthcoming. Indeed, definitive demonstration of a hypothalamic site of action would require direct measurements of the circulating levels of GnRH in the portal circulation so as to document a clomiphene citrate–induced alteration in the pattern of GnRH release. Given the obvious ethical difficulties associated with such an approach, evidence of a hypothalamic site of action for clomiphene citrate in humans necessarily remains indirect.

Along these lines, the recent study by Kerin and associates[52] is particularly noteworthy. In this investigation, gonadotropin pulse amplitude and frequency were evaluated in both normally cycling women (*n* = 5) and women treated with clomiphene citrate (150 mg/d on cycle days 2, 3, and 4). As expected, gonadotropin pulse frequency and amplitude remained unaltered in the placebo-treated control group for the duration of the 8-hour study period. In contrast, a significant increase in the pulse frequency of luteinizing hormone (LH) (from 3.3 ± 0.7 per 8 hours on day 2 to 6.8 ± 0.8 per 8 hours on day 5) was observed for the clomiphene citrate–treated group. Concurrently, the

pulse frequency of follicle-stimulating hormone (FSH) increased from 3.8 ± 0.6 to 5 ± 1.4 per 8 hours (Fig. 32-4). Significantly, clomiphene citrate therapy had little or no effect on the pulse amplitude of LH and FSH, or on the circulating levels of estradiol-17β or progesterone. Given that the pulsatile frequency of gonadotropin release is governed by hypothalamic mechanisms, these findings strongly suggest that the ovulation-initiating property of clomiphene citrate is exerted, at least in part, at the level of the hypothalamus and that an increase in GnRH pulse frequency may be involved.

Although the exact functional identity of clomiphene citrate as it interacts with the hypothalamic level is far from settled, the following observations suggest an antiestrogenic role, rather than an estrogenic role:

- Clomiphene citrate enhances GnRH release from estradiol-17β–exposed rat medial basal hypothalamus in vitro.[68]
- Clomiphene citrate antagonizes estrogen-stimulated medial basal hypothalamic tyrosine hydroxylase activity in vitro.[87]

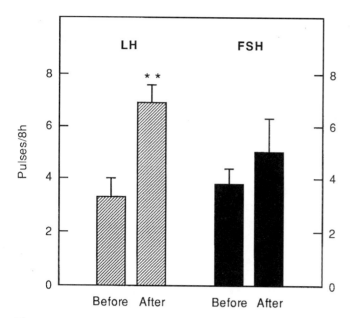

Fig. 32-4. Effect of clomiphene citrate on LH and FSH pulsatility. (Redrawn from Adashi EY: *Semin Reprod Endocrinol* 4:255, 1980.)

- Clomiphene citrate therapy is associated with the elicitation of hot flushes (a putative central nervous system phenomenon) in premenopausal women.[48]
- Clomiphene citrate antagonizes the beneficial aspect of estrogens on the occurrence of hot flushes in postmenopausal women.[51]
- Clomiphene citrate antagonizes the negative feedback effect of ethinyl estradiol (a hypothalamic phenomenon, as well as a pituitary phenomenon, by some accounts) in premenopausal women.[89]
- Clomiphene citrate is relatively inactive in initiating ovulation under estrogen-poor (hypogonadal) conditions.

Evidence has nonetheless recently been presented to suggest that consideration be given to the possibility that the pituitary and the ovary may not merely represent passive bystanders in the endocrine cascade initiated by clomiphene citrate, but that either organ, in its own right, may constitute a legitimate and active participant in the process.[2] It has therefore been proposed that the overall profertility effect of clomiphene citrate on the reproductive axis not only may reflect the consequences of its interaction with the hypothalamus but may represent the sum of its direct effects at the hypothalamic, pituitary, and ovarian levels.[2]

CLINICAL USE

Indications

The primary indication for the use of clomiphene citrate is infertility associated with normogonadotropic (or inap-

propriate), normoprolactinemic anovulation.[35,63,97] At the clinical level, the patients in question are likely to present with a chronic anovulatory disorder, commonly (but not always) dating back to puberty. Many patients are likely to report dysfunctional uterine bleeding, whereas others may be amenorrheic. Obesity and hirsutism may, but need not, be components of this overall clinical picture. Significantly, most women who respond to clomiphene citrate prove to be well estrogenized as judged by progestin-induced withdrawal bleeding, measurements of the circulating levels of estrone and/or estradiol-17β, and the occasional documentation of abnormal endometrial growth. Indeed, it is the euestrogenicity of responsive patients that prompted the suggestion that the ability of clomiphene citrate to initiate ovulation is due to its antiestrogenic property. Thus there is little doubt that an adequate estrogen milieu is most suitable for the initiation of ovulation with clomiphene citrate. Indeed, ovulation initiation is generally unsuccessful in hypogonadotropic (estrogen-poor) women.

Although an empirical trial of clomiphene citrate in a hypogonadotropic setting appears warranted, most such patients are not suitable candidates for this mode of ovulation initiation. In this connection it has been reported that hyperprolactinemic chronic anovulation may at times prove responsive to clomiphene citrate therapy. Whereas such an approach could be justified when no other therapeutic alternatives were available, the more appropriate approach to such patients at this time should include consideration of the use of bromocriptine. Needless to say, clomiphene citrate is of no use in the setting of hypergonadotropic chronic anovulation because of the obvious lack of ovarian function.

Although clomiphene citrate is primarily used to treat anovulatory infertility, this versatile drug has also been introduced as a component in management of luteal phase dysfunction,[21,24,75] oligoovulation, artificial insemination,[54] unexplained infertility,[28,34,65] and in vitro fertilization.[88] Under these circumstances, clomiphene citrate is used in an effort to promote the frequency of ovulation (as in the case of oligoovulation), to time ovulation better (as in the case of artificial insemination), or for its ability to effect "controlled hyperstimulation" of the ovarian cycle[31,59] (as in the cases of luteal phase dysfunction and in vitro fertilization). The latter effect was first and perhaps best demonstrated by Vandenberg and Yen,[90] whose findings indicate that the administration of clomiphene citrate in the early follicular phase to normally cycling women results in a substantial augmentation of all the hormonal variables evaluated. Specifically, the circulating levels of estradiol-17β in the course of the preovulatory surge reached levels approximating 1200 pg/mL, thereby suggesting the emergence of multiple follicles rather than a single dominant follicle (Fig. 32-5). As a corollary, luteal function in these patients was similarly "hyperstimulated," as evidenced by the substan-

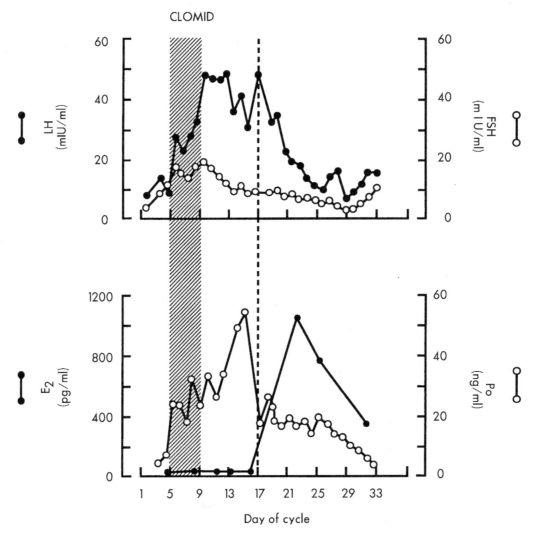

Fig. 32-5. Effect of clomiphene citrate on normally cycling women. (Redrawn from Adashi EY: *Semin Reprod Endocrinol* 4:255, 1980.)

tial elevation of the circulating levels of progesterone. Although a complete discussion of the secondary indications for the use of clomiphene citrate is beyond the scope of this chapter, there is little doubt that these more recent indications may in effect apply to larger numbers of patients than was originally predicted for the anovulatory patient pool.

Contraindications

The use of clomiphene citrate is governed by a relatively limited number of contraindications.

Ovarian cysts. Although the reasons generally are ill-defined, there appears to be general agreement as to the undesirability of administering clomiphene citrate in the face of a preexisting ovarian cyst or substantial post-treatment residual ovarian enlargement. Given the ability of clomiphene citrate to stimulate follicular growth, there is

the possibility of further enlargement of a preexisting ovarian cyst, resulting in potentially disastrous consequences.[77,78,81] Rare occurrences of massive ovarian enlargement have been reported.[84] Because the administration of clomiphene citrate is elective, there appears to be little reason to challenge this old dictum. It appears preferable that clomiphene citrate not be administered under such circumstances and that allowance be made for ovarian size normalization either spontaneously over time or by means of combination oral contraceptive–induced suppression of the reproductive axis. It is therefore generally accepted that, before the administration of clomiphene citrate, an effort be made to rule out the presence of ovarian cysts by means of a standard pelvic examination or pelvic ultrasound imaging. Similar maneuvers have been recommended for the intervals between treatment cycles before embarking on a new clomiphene citrate course, so as to rule out residual ovarian enlargement.

Concerns about the significance of residual ovarian enlargement are by no means universal, however. Indeed, "long-distance" (that is, over the telephone) initiation of ovulation with clomiphene citrate is not uncommonly practiced. Such an approach might be supported by the argument that the likelihood of hyperstimulation as a result of clomiphene citrate therapy appears to be relatively low. In addition, there is reason to believe that the earlier reports of the incidence of hyperstimulation may not be representative of contemporary practice and that current incidence rates may be substantially reduced. Aside from these considerations, the case of long-distance initiation of ovulation with clomiphene citrate is further bolstered by the argument that frequent office visits for pelvic examinations are inconvenient and impractical.

Thus whether or not compulsive monitoring for residual ovarian enlargement should constitute an absolute requirement or merely a highly desirable clinical requirement remains subject to individual clinical judgment. Clinical protocols used at the University of Maryland School of Medicine routinely call for the rigorous evaluation of ovarian size in connection with clomiphene citrate dose; no additional monitoring of ovarian size is undertaken. This clinical approach is based on the premise that ovarian responsiveness cannot be predicted with certainty while the treatment regimen is being adjusted. However, once a clomiphene citrate regimen has been established, ovarian responsiveness is expected to display a reasonable degree of predictability, thereby largely eliminating the need for intensive monitoring.

Pregnancy. Pregnancy is an obvious contraindication to clomiphene citrate therapy. The inadvertent administration of clomiphene citrate during pregnancy might occur if rigorous testing to rule out pregnancy has not been carried out. This is particularly likely under unmonitored circumstances when the lack of a menstrual period at the end of a clomiphene citrate cycle may be interpreted as an apparent treatment failure. In this connection, the old clinical dictum of "no period = no clomiphene citrate" appears to be as timely as it was when originally formulated. Awareness on the part of the physician, maintenance of a basal body temperature chart, and compulsive pregnancy testing should minimize the inadvertent administration of clomiphene citrate during early gestation. An additional advantage of the basal body temperature chart is that early post-treatment bleeding could be implantation bleeding rather than a true menstrual period. However, should the basal body temperature continue to be elevated under these circumstances, the inadvertent administration of clomiphene citrate during gestation might be avoided.

Needless to say, pregnancy testing should not take the form of a progestin challenge test, which, in the face of a potential early gestation, is equally undesirable. Instead, a standard urinary or serum determination of the concentrations of the beta subunit of hCG should be undertaken.

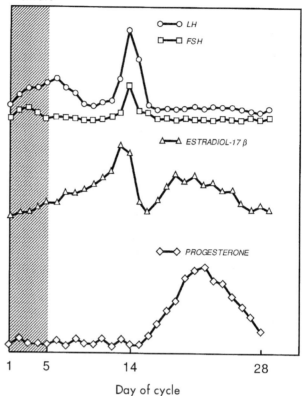

Fig. 32-6. Sequence of endocrine events in clomiphene citrate–initiated ovulation. (Redrawn from Adashi EY: *Semin Reprod Endocrinol* 4:255, 1980.)

Although the use of clomiphene citrate has not been associated with an increase in the incidence of congenital abnormalities, the impact of the administration of clomiphene citrate in the course of early gestation remains somewhat uncertain. A more complete discussion of the potential adverse effects of clomiphene citrate as regards early gestation and teratogenesis is found under Gestational Outcome.

Liver disease. The preexistence of liver disease or a history of liver dysfunction is generally construed as a contraindication to clomiphene citrate therapy. Given that clomiphene citrate is metabolized, at least in part, by the liver, its use in a patient with liver dysfunction is relatively unmanageable and potentially harmful.

Ovulation initiation

The sequence of endocrine events taking place in the course of a hypothetic, presumptively ovulatory, clomiphene citrate treatment cycle is illustrated in Fig. 32-6. The bar spanning days 1 through 5 of the cycle represents the period of administration of clomiphene citrate. The daily circulating levels of LH, FSH, estradiol-17β, and progesterone are expressed in relative terms and without unitage for the sake of generalization.

It is generally accepted that the first endocrine event attributable to the administration of clomiphene citrate is the concomitant citrate; or shortly thereafter, both gonadotropins gradually decline to a preovulatory nadir, only to surge again at mid cycle. At the same time, and presumably secondary to the rise in pituitary gonadotropins, a progressive and time-dependent increase in the circulating levels of estradiol-17β is observed, culminating in a preovulatory peak. The circulating levels of progesterone increase in the event of a "successful" ovulatory cycle, suggesting the formation of a functional corpus luteum.

The sequence of events just described is best referred to as clomiphene citrate–initiated ovulation, as opposed to clomiphene citrate–induced ovulation. This distinction is not merely one of semantics. Rather, such terminology denotes the temporal and causal relationship between the ovulation-producing agent and the actual event of ovulation. Whereas the administration of hCG is temporally as well as causally related to the ensuing (with 36 hours) rupture of the dominant follicle, clomiphene citrate therapy may be initiated as early as 14 days before the actual event of follicular rupture. Thus, rather than inducing ovulation, clomiphene citrate appears to set in motion (initiate) a series of endocrine events culminating in the generation of a preovulatory gonadotropin surge and hence follicular rupture. Consequently, it is proposed that the mechanisms whereby clomiphene citrate brings about ovulation be sought within the time frame of its administration.

Pretreatment work-up

Barring glaring infertility factors other than anovulation, it is generally agreed that a clomiphene citrate trial may be justified in the absence of a complete infertility work-up. This approach is based on the premise that clomiphene citrate trials are self-limited, discontinuation being relatively rapidly determined on the grounds of lack of suitability or efficacy. This policy markedly contrasts with that for pretreatment work-ups preceding ovulation induction with human menopausal gonadotropins (hMG). Under these circumstances, it is generally agreed that a complete (albeit individualized) infertility work-up may be in order because hMG therapy is generally complex, potentially hazardous, and rather costly. In contrast, before proceeding with clomiphene citrate administration, there is little harm in conducting an infertility work-up limited to relatively simple and noninvasive procedures, such as semen analysis or cervical cultures, thereby avoiding unnecessary time loss. An endometrial biopsy would appear to be a wise precaution given the possibility of abnormal endometrial growth. Before treatment, it also is advisable to rule out hyperprolactinemia, thyroid or adrenal dysfunction, a hepatic disorder, and pregnancy.

On the other hand, clomiphene citrate need not be administered indiscriminately in women with a known preexisting infertility factor. Indeed, there appears to be little point in embarking on clomiphene citrate–initiated ovulation in the face of tubal blockade or a significant male factor. Such circumstances clearly call for the clarification of infertility factors other than anovulation before embarking on a course of ovulation initiation.

Monitoring

Aside from monitoring for possible gestation and for residual ovarian enlargement, the use of clomiphene citrate is generally unencumbered by the intense monitoring requirements characteristic of the use of hMG. Nevertheless, the use of the basal body temperature chart as an adjunctive is strongly recommended for the obvious reasons of low cost, simplicity, and harmlessness. According to some clinicians, any additional monitoring in the course of clomiphene citrate therapy is largely redundant. For the most part, this recommendation is based on the pervasive feeling that clomiphene citrate constitutes a safe and effective drug, the empirical administration of which is often successful. Indeed, there is little doubt that monitoring may be redundant in patients who happen to be highly responsive to clomiphene citrate therapy. It is equally clear, however, that monitoring may be not only desirable but in effect essential in those patients often referred to as clomiphene citrate failures. A detailed discussion of the management of clomiphene citrate failure is given later; suffice it to say at this point that monitoring in this setting is crucial for the identification of those patients who may be candidates for hCG administration.

In the event that additional monitoring is desirable, several possibilities may be considered.

Circulating levels of estradiol-17β and progesterone: the "triple 7 regimen." This monitoring approach is based on the premise that the successful initiation of ovulation with clomiphene citrate is associated with characteristic alterations in the circulating levels of estradiol-17β and progesterone.[85] Specifically, this approach screens for the absence or presence of a typical preovulatory estradiol-17β surge and the subsequent rise of progesterone level, the hallmark of a presumptive luteal phase.[29,30]

In practical terms, the protocol used at the University of Maryland (the "triple 7 regimen") calls for a serum estradiol-17β determination 7 days after the last clomiphene citrate tablet has been consumed (Fig. 32-7). This places the monitoring for estradiol-17β well within the projected window of ovulation, which is predicted to occur any time between 5 and 10 days after the last oral dose of clomiphene citrate. Thus, pickup of a preovulatory estradiol-17β surge is almost always realized in the face of successful follicular recruitment, selection, and assertion of dominance.

Determination of the circulating levels of progesterone is generally carried out 7 days later, that is, 14 days after the

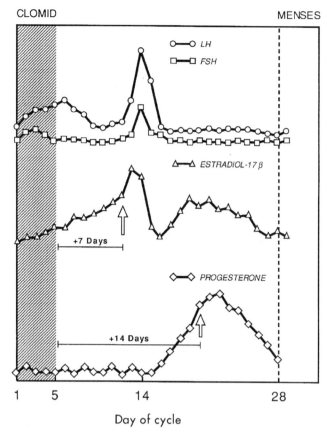

Fig. 32-7. Hormonal monitoring in clomiphene citrate–initiated ovulation: use of the "triple 7 regimen." (Redrawn from Adashi EY: *Semin Reprod Endocrinol* 4:255, 1980.)

last oral dose of clomiphene citrate. This test is thus timed favorably to pick up a possible luteal phase progesterone rise. Another office visit is scheduled 7 days after the progesterone determination, that is, 21 days after the last clomiphene citrate tablet.

This approach provides an efficient monitoring procedure, largely because of careful timing of the hormonal determinations. By timing the various hormonal determinations relative to the last oral dose of clomiphene citrate, the triple 7 regimen can be used regardless of whether clomiphene citrate is administered for 5, 7, or 10 days. Although this regimen calls for two hormonal determinations in the course of a cycle, we believe that this may be a price well worth paying in circumstances characterized by an apparent lack of response, in particular, in those instances in which the basal body temperature chart appears to be uninformative or in the face of an apparent treatment failure. When successful, this approach leads to unequivocal conclusions, given that the surging levels of estradiol-17β far exceed those observed under steady-state conditions in the chronic anovulatory state. Thus, given an appropriate baseline sample, there can generally be little doubt about the

detection of a clear-cut preovulatory estradiol-17β surge. Indeed, whereas the circulating levels of estradiol-17β under steady-state conditions are generally on the order of 50 pg/mL, preovulatory surge levels well in excess of 300 pg/mL are commonly encountered.[83] Similarly, given that the circulating baseline levels of progesterone are generally less than 1 mg/mL in the anovulatory state, a luteal rise of progesterone generally provides unequivocal, albeit presumptive, evidence of ovulation.

Follicular development by ultrasound. The widespread availability of ultrasound monitoring has led to the suggestion that monitoring of follicular maturation be employed independently of or in conjunction with hormonal determinations.[71] Although evidence of follicular responsiveness and of presumptive ovulation can be obtained by using this approach, the utility and cost effectiveness of this monitoring technique vis-à-vis the well-timed monitoring of the circulating levels of estradiol-17β and progesterone remain to be ascertained. Currently ultrasound monitoring of clomiphene citrate–initiated ovulation is not widely used. Nevertheless, ultrasound monitoring may turn out to be particularly useful in women who prove to be candidates for hCG administration.[72] In the absence of sonographic monitoring, the timing of hCG administration is commonly empirically determined (generally 6 to 7 days after the last oral dose of clomiphene citrate). However, in the future increasing reliance as to the timing of hCG administration may be placed on monitoring the diameter of the largest emerging follicles.

Clinical management

Clomiphene citrate is available only as scored 50-mg tablets, the recommended starting dose being 50 mg daily for a total of 5 days; lower doses may be particularly useful in patients displaying enhanced ovarian responsiveness. Therapy may be started at any time[96] if the patient has had no recent uterine bleeding. Indeed, uterine bleeding, be it spontaneous or induced, is not part of the process of ovulation initiation. Stated differently, given that the patients in question invariably demonstrate chronic anovulation, treatment can be started at any point in this steady-state condition. If, however, progestin-induced bleeding is intended or spontaneous dysfunctional uterine bleeding occurs, treatment should be started on or about day 5 of the cycle. In the most general terms, the clomiphene citrate dosage should be increased as soon as it becomes apparent that the current dosage is ineffective. Ideally, such a determination can and should be made within a single treatment cycle. The simplest protocols call for graded incremental therapy in which the dosage of clomiphene citrate is increased by 50 mg at a time.[23,79] For example, if ovulation does not occur after the first course of therapy, a second course of 100 mg daily for 5 days may be started. This course may begin as early as 30 days after the previous one. Lack of response at dose levels of 200 mg or 250 mg daily for 5 days should clearly signal a change of course as discussed.

Clinical experience indicates that more than 50% of patients destined to conceive will do so on the starting dose.[23] Increasing the dosage to 100 mg daily for 5 days will secure an additional increment in the conception rate of approximately 20% of the total observed. Thus more than 70% of clomiphene citrate–related conceptions occur at doses no higher than 100 mg daily for 5 days. Although higher dose levels provide additional, albeit minimal, increments in conception rates, their use generally can be obviated by prolonging the course of therapy at the lower dose levels or by other hormonal manipulations as discussed later. Originally approved for a total dose of up to 750 mg per cycle, clomiphene citrate use currently often exceeds this upper limit. Although a clear-cut relationship between dose level and multiple gestation has not been unequivocally established, it is reasonable to assume that such correlation exists. Consequently, it is recommended that one use the lowest dose of clomiphene citrate compatible with successful ovulation and conception[22] and that appropriate monitoring be used to avoid hyperstimulation.

When an ovulatory dose is reached, no additional modification of the dosage is required. When ovulation occurs at a given dose there is no advantage to increasing the dose in subsequent cycles of treatment. At that point a 4- to 6-month effort to conceive should be allowed to take place without any additional intervention. Indeed, as recently reviewed by Gysler and colleagues,[40] most clomiphene citrate–initiated conceptions are likely to occur within the first six ovulatory cycles. For optimal results, the patient is advised to have intercourse every other day for 1 week beginning 5 days after the last day of clomiphene citrate administration. Given the relatively high incidence of clomiphene citrate–associated luteal phase dysfunction,[32,49,92] a case can be made for screening all ovulatory patients for the presence of luteal phase dysfunction before attempting conception. A detailed discussion of the ovulatory patient who fails to conceive is offered later.

Although it would be highly desirable, there is at the present time no well-defined clinical or laboratory measure to predict clomiphene citrate responsiveness or dose requirements.[27,60] In this connection, the circulating concentrations of either androgens or estrogens did not show any correlation with the dose of clomiphene citrate that ultimately proved successful. On the other hand, there appears to be a significant correlation between body weight and the dose of clomiphene citrate required.[82] Despite this correlation, dose requirements in either obese or thin patients cannot be predicted prospectively; consequently, no definitive modifications of the treatment regimen can be anticipated on the basis of weight. Given that clomiphene citrate is not generally known to be stored in adipose tissue, the reasons underlying the apparent resistance of obese patients to clomiphene citrate remains uncertain. Several possibilities appear to warrant further consideration: (1) Given that obesity is associated with a decrease in the circulating levels of testosterone-estradiol–binding globulin and an increase in extraglandular aromatization, the consequent increase in the circulating levels of free estradiol-17β may be responsible for increased antagonism to clomiphene citrate action. (2) Given the decreased levels of testosterone-estradiol–binding globulin, the consequent increase in the circulating levels of free testosterone might interfere with the process of folliculogenesis. (3) Although ill-defined, it is possible that obesity may be associated with a hypothalamic dysfunction rendering clomiphene citrate relatively ineffective.

Clomiphene citrate failure

The term *clomiphene citrate failure* has been coined to designate in the most general terms the inability of clomiphene citrate to effect ovulation or conception, or both. It has been estimated that some 10% to 20% of women fail to conceive with peak clomiphene citrate doses even when supplemented with hCG. For the purpose of this discussion, a distinction is made between failure to ovulate and failure to conceive, each of which is discussed separately.

Failure to ovulate. In the broadest terms, clomiphene citrate ovulation failure may be defined as the inability to ovulate in the face of peak clomiphene citrate dosage. Although the determination of what constitutes peak clomiphene citrate dosage may be subject to interpretation, failure to ovulate in the face of a clomiphene citrate dosage of 200 mg daily for 5 days appears to constitute a satisfactory example.

Significantly, clomiphene citrate ovulation failure may be either partial or complete, thereby dictating major differences in the clinical response indicated.

Total lack of response. In this situation, rigorous monitoring has established a complete lack of response, that is, the absence of progressive folliculogenesis and the inevitable lack of ovulation. Under these circumstances, several therapeutic approaches may be considered.

Increasing duration of therapy. Increasing the duration of clomiphene citrate therapy has long been recognized by many clinicians as an effective means of overcoming apparent clomiphene citrate resistance.[1] The mechanisms underlying the increased efficacy of a prolonged clomiphene citrate course have nevertheless been poorly delineated. It is abundantly clear, however, that in some instances prolonged administration of relatively low doses of clomiphene citrate may succeed where shorter-term, high-dose regimens have failed. Indeed, there is no shortage of examples of patients resisting clomiphene citrate doses of 200 mg administered daily for 5 days only to respond to a 50-mg dose administered daily over a 10-day period.

By using this approach, Lobo and colleagues[62] recently compared the efficacy of an 8-day regimen of clomiphene citrate with that of an identical 5-day course (Fig. 32-8).

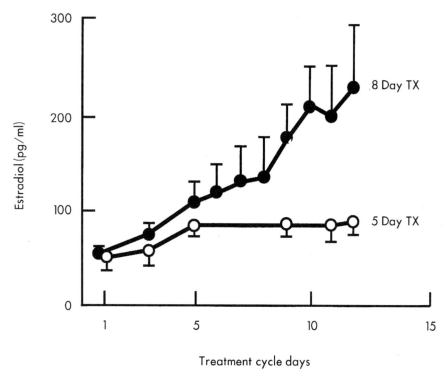

Fig. 32-8. Clomiphene citrate therapy administered for 5 or 8 days: impact on the circulating levels of estradiol. (Redrawn from Adashi EY: *Semin Reprod Endocrinol* 4:255, 1980.)

All 12 patients studied had failed to ovulate when treated with 250 mg of clomiphene citrate administered daily for 5 days. Extension of the duration of the clomiphene citrate course (to 8 days) resulted in ovulation in 8 of the 12 women studied. Hormonal monitoring suggested that the extended clomiphene citrate regimen resulted in higher circulating levels of estrogens, implying enhanced follicular maturation. Although the mechanisms underlying the phenomenon remain to be studied, it appears reasonable to speculate that the extended duration of clomiphene citrate therapy resulted in more persistent and seemingly more efficient increments in pituitary gonadotropin release and hence potent ovarian stimulation. It is therefore strongly recommended that consideration be given to increasing the duration of clomiphene citrate therapy in the event of an apparent total lack of response. Clinical experience suggests that as many as 50% of patients otherwise deemed "resistant" might achieve ovulation by using this approach.

A variation on the theme of increased duration of clomiphene citrate therapy has recently been reported by O'Herlihy and colleagues.[73] By using a complex therapeutic scheme involving alterations of both clomiphene citrate dose and duration, they were able to effect conception in 8 of 21 patients formerly considered resistant to conventional clomiphene citrate therapy. Although the protocol in question involves alteration of both dose and duration of therapy, it nevertheless provides additional evidence in

favor of attempts at increasing the duration of clomiphene citrate therapy in patients characterized by an apparent total lack of response.

Supplementation with dexamethasone. Although the mechanisms underlying the ability of dexamethasone to enhance the action of clomiphene citrate are not known, there is little doubt that these two agents may interact favorably to influence ovulation initiation. The ability of dexamethasone to increase the efficacy of clomiphene citrate is well recognized,* but only a few investigators have in effect documented this phenomenon. Check and co-workers[12] demonstrated that adding prednisone to the therapeutic regimen could induce ovulation in a hirsute woman who previously failed to ovulate with clomiphene citrate alone. According to Chang and Abraham,[11] nightly administration of dexamethasone (0.5 mg) diminished the circulating levels of dehydroepiandrosterone sulfate and testosterone, but not androstenedione. Although dexamethasone did not prove effective by itself, it nevertheless increased subsequent responsiveness to clomiphene citrate. Dexamethasone pretreatment also increased the circulating levels of estradiol-17β from undetectable to 40 to 70 pg/mL in a patient who previously did not experience withdrawal bleeding in response to a progesterone challenge test.

*References 11, 12, 18, 19, 45, 58, 61.

In a related study, Lobo and associates[61] compiled a study group of 12 women with polycystic ovary syndrome in whom ovulation could not be achieved despite the use of high-dose (250 mg/d) clomiphene citrate therapy. However, when a continuous nightly regimen of dexamethasone (0.5 mg/d) was superimposed, 6 of 12 patients ovulated, and 1 conceived. Two weeks after dexamethasone administration a significant decrease was noted in serum total testosterone, unbound testosterone, and dehydroepiandrosterone sulfate levels; no change was observed in LH, FSH, or prolactin levels. Moreover, women who ovulated were noted to have significantly higher pretreatment levels of dehydroepiandrosterone sulfate than those who did not ovulate.[46,61] In no case did the authors observe ovarian hyperstimulation. In addition, women who ovulated reproducibly continued to do so. Higher conception rates might have been expected, but the infertility work-up in the patients in question had not been completed at the time of study.

Daly and associates[18] reported a prospective, randomized, double-blind, crossover study of the use of dexamethasone in women undergoing ovulation initiation with clomiphene citrate. They compared 22 patients receiving clomiphene citrate alone with a group of 23 patients receiving combined therapy with both clomiphene citrate and dexamethasone and were able to demonstrate that the addition of dexamethasone (0.5 mg/d) resulted in higher ovulation and conception rates. Indeed, whereas all patients in the dexamethasone-supplemented group ovulated, only 14 of 22 did so in the clomiphene citrate–only group. Similarly, whereas 17 of 23 patients conceived in the dexamethasone treatment group, only 8 of 14 conceived in the absence of dexamethasone supplementation. Significantly, monitoring of dehydroepiandrosterone sulfate levels suggested that a beneficial effect for dexamethasone may be anticipated only at concentrations in excess of 200 μg/dL. Dexamethasone therapy should be discontinued as soon as a temperature rise is noted in the basal body temperature chart. If gradual tapering is considered necessary, the patient should be switched to hydrocortisone, thereby avoiding the use of dexamethasone during gestation.

It remains uncertain whether the dexamethasone effect is mediated via diminution in the circulating levels of adrenal androgens that might otherwise inhibit folliculogenesis or aromatase activity. In other words, it is possible that the dexamethasone-mediated decrease in adrenal androgens improves the microenvironment of the ovarian follicle and hence the responsiveness to pituitary gonadotropins. Alternatively, recent provocative data provided by Miyake and colleagues[69] suggest that glucocorticoids may synergize with clomiphene citrate at the level of the hypothalamus. Specifically, in vitro evidence was presented to the effect that hydrocortisone may participate in the generation of hypothalamic GnRH release.

Partial lack of response. As alluded to earlier, clomiphene citrate ovulation failure need not be complete. In-

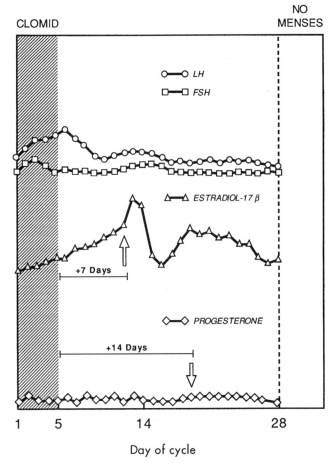

Fig. 32-9. Ovulation failure (partial lack of response) in clomiphene citrate–initiated ovulation. (Redrawn from Adashi EY: *Semin Reprod Endocrinol* 4:255, 1980.)

deed, in some instances clomiphene citrate is capable of causing follicular maturation associated with progressive increments in the circulating levels of estradiol-17β (Fig. 32-9). However, despite a seemingly adequate preovulatory estradiol-17β surge, ovulation fails to occur for reasons that are poorly understood. Although ovulation, and obviously conception, cannot be anticipated under these circumstances, the apparent lack of midcycle gonadotropin surge can be circumvented by the exogenous administration of hCG. Thus hormonal monitoring should allow the precise identification of those patients in whom clomiphene citrate was capable of effecting follicular maturation but not ovulation, and who are likely to benefit from hCG administration. In clinics in which hormonal monitoring is considered impractical or unnecessary, the detection of this type of apparent clomiphene citrate ovulation failure may not be possible. Instead, hCG-eligible patients can be "selected" only through the empirical administration of hCG. Although a given proportion of patients so managed are likely to benefit from this empirical approach, many other patients, ostensibly those displaying a total lack of response, will be subjected to an otherwise unnecessary therapeutic maneuver and a delay in the institution of alternative modes of therapy.

Failure to conceive. The straightforward designation of failure to conceive refers to the inability to conceive in the face of an apparent 4- to 6-month ovulatory pattern initiated by clomiphene citrate. Under these circumstances, a rather clear-cut clinical course can be charted. For one, it is generally agreed that the inability to conceive in the face of an apparently ovulatory pattern signals the need to rule out luteal phase dysfunction. Indeed, several studies have clearly demonstrated the association between clomiphene citrate–initiated ovulation and luteal phase dysfunction.[32,49,92] Although various figures have been provided for the incidence of luteal phase dysfunction in connection with clomiphene citrate–initiated ovulation, rates of 50% and more have been reported. This relatively high incidence of luteal phase dysfunction has prompted the suggestion that luteal phase dysfunction be ruled out as soon as ovulation is established, that is, well before the realization of an apparent conception failure. Once luteal phase dysfunction has been ruled out, the recognition of an apparent clomiphene citrate conception failure also signals the need for evaluation of other coexisting infertility factors (such as male factor or tuboperitoneal abnormalities) as possible contributors to the persistent sterility.

RESULTS

Although a wide range of figures has been reported, it can be stated that approximately 80% of well-selected patients can be expected to ovulate. In contrast, according to some studies, only about 40% of clomiphene citrate–treated patients ultimately achieve pregnancy.[43,95] This apparent discrepancy between ovulation and conception rates may be more apparent than real and may be due largely to other causes of infertility and loss to follow-up. Indeed, in the absence of other infertility factors, conception rates approaching 80% to 90% have been reported.[23,79] In addition, an earlier report by Lamb and associates[57] demonstrated that the conception rate per ovulatory cycle is the same in clomiphene citrate–initiated cycles as it is in spontaneous cycles. It is significant that these results were obtained by using life table analysis, thereby correcting for loss to follow-up. Moreover, the pregnancy rate in 70 patients ovulating for three cycles was 55.7%, the same pregnancy rate after 3 months of exposure in the general population.[37] Finally, a more recent report by Hammond and colleagues[42] further documented that in otherwise normal patients the monthly fecundity rate in clomiphene citrate–initiated cycles does not differ from that expected in women who discontinue diaphragm contraception. In fact, the pregnancy rate per ovulatory cycle in otherwise normal patients receiving clomiphene citrate proved to be 22%, remaining constant for at least 10 months. Taken together, these findings suggest that the pregnancy rate in clomi-

phene citrate–initiated ovulation may approach that of spontaneously occurring cycles, provided that therapy is sustained for the required duration.

ADVERSE EFFECTS
Hot flushes

Reportedly occurring in up to 11% of patients, the clomiphene citrate–associated hot flush superficially resembles its menopausal counterpart.[48] In contrast to the abundance of information now available regarding the menopausal hot flush, detailed contemporary hormonal and biophysical monitoring of the clomiphene citrate–associated hot flush is yet to be undertaken. The clomiphene citrate–associated hot flush is rarely severe and tends to disappear as soon as treatment is discontinued or completed. Although the mechanisms underlying this phenomenon remain to be carefully studied, it has generally been assumed to be due, at least in part, to the antiestrogenic properties of clomiphene citrate. According to this view, the clomiphene citrate–associated hot flush, like the menopausal hot flush, is causally related to net effective estrogenic deprivation. Whereas during menopause estrogenic deprivation is due to diminished estrogen biosynthesis, clomiphene citrate therapy produces an apparent state of estrogen deprivation consequent to clomiphene citrate, effecting an estrogen receptor blockade. Inasmuch as the menopausal hot flush is acceptable as a central neuroendocrine phenomenon, the clomiphene citrate–associated hot flush is likely to represent a similar, if not identical, occurrence.

Multiple gestation

A well-known corollary of clomiphene citrate ovulation initiation,[6,53] multiple gestation is likely due in large measure to the ability of clomiphene citrate to stimulate a pronounced rise in the circulating levels of pituitary gonadotropins. This phenomenon was highlighted by the mean early follicular FSH and LH levels, which are significantly higher than those of untreated control subjects. Representing primarily an increase in pulse frequency, this relatively acute burst of gonadotropins appears to be conducive to recruitment of several follicles. Inevitably, this increased follicular selection may result in the emergence of more than one follicle. Thus the relative increase in the incidence of multiple gestation associated with clomiphene citrate therapy is due virtually exclusively to multiple ovulation rather than to zygotic cleavage. Incidence rates established in earlier reports have ranged from 6.25% to 12.3%.[6] Particularly noteworthy is the large study conducted by Merrell National Laboratories analyzing the outcome of 2369 pregnancies.[6] When evaluated for multiple gestation incidence rates, the Merrell study revealed an overall figure of 7.9%, of which 6.9% were twins, 0.5% triplets, 0.3% quadruplets,[7] and 0.13% quintuplets. One set of sextuplets not included in the original series subsequently has been noted.[5] Thus, inasmuch as the spontaneous incidence of twinning is estimated at approximately 1%, these figures suggest a severalfold increase in the likelihood of twinning after clomiphene citrate therapy.

The aforementioned incidence rates have not, however, been reevaluated on a large scale recently. Moreover, there is reason to believe that the pattern of practice as regards the administration of clomiphene citrate has changed over the years. This is undoubtedly partly due to increased awareness by physicians of side effects, the increasing centralization of care in the hands of highly trained reproductive endocrinologists, the improved means of monitoring, and the availability of alternative methods for ovulation induction. Although ultrasound monitoring has clearly confirmed the ability of clomiphene citrate to promote the recruitment of multiple follicles, an incidence rate of 8% for multiple gestation may very well prove to be an overestimate.

Visual symptoms

Visual symptoms occasionally may occur with clomiphene citrate therapy; the incidence rate has been estimated at less than 2%.[6] Visual symptoms usually have been described as "blurring" or spots or flashes (scintillating scotomata) and have been correlated with increasing total dose. Symptoms often appear first during, or are accentuated upon, exposure to a more brightly lit environment. Although the mechanisms behind this phenomenon are entirely unknown (possibly intensification and/or prolongation of afterimages), this side effect is considered self-limited. Indeed, the symptoms tend to disappear within a few days or weeks after clomiphene citrate is discontinued. Although measured visual acuity generally has not been affected, severe diminution of visual acuity may occur in exceptional circumstances. Either way the phenomenon is reversible. As a matter of prudence, patients having any visual symptoms should discontinue treatment, and consideration should be given to other modes of ovulation initiation.

Cervical mucus abnormalities

Concerns regarding the apparent adverse effects of clomiphene citrate on cervical mucus generation constitute a persistent feature of the clomiphene citrate legacy.* Indeed, multiple reports appear to attest to the fact that the administration of clomiphene citrate may, in a certain percentage of cases, be associated with an unfavorable cervical mucus. Clearly, such a phenomenon, if common and true, could substantially influence the overall efficacy of clomiphene citrate therapy. The existence of reports to this effect notwithstanding, intuitive reasoning would strongly argue against such a possibility. Indeed, given the generation of a preovulatory estradiol urge capable of triggering a gonadotropin burst, it is difficult to rationalize why comparable efficacy cannot be expected at the level of the endocervical glands. Assuming midcycle levels of estradiol citrate in the 200 to 300 pg/mL range, effective mucus stimulation would seem predictable. If that in fact were not the case, one would have to invoke target-organ failure or else selective tissue sensitivity to the antiestrogenic potential of the drug. In this connection, consideration might also be given to the possibility that documentation of abnormal cervical mucus may in fact reflect poor timing and that midcycle cervical mucus may in fact be adequate. All told, this line of reasoning would argue against the use of estrogenic preparations designed presumably to overcome the adverse antiestrogenic action of clomiphene citrate at the cervical mucus level.

GESTATIONAL OUTCOME

Gestational outcome is a difficult area to assess. Most indications are that the use of clomiphene citrate is associated with an incidence rate of birth defects comparable to that observed in the population at large.* The reproductive impact of clomiphene citrate has therefore been the subject of numerous reports. Indeed, a computer-assisted literature search carried out in 1978 produced 445 relevant publications. Despite such apparent abundance, the disappointingly wide range of figures available virtually precludes the formulation of meaningful incidence rates for clomiphene citrate–related gestational outcome. This variability is best exemplified by evaluation of reported birth defect incidence rates, which have been observed to range from a "normal" 2% to a high of 12.7%.[6] It has been speculated that this highly variable outcome can be attributed in large measure to differences in sample size, lack of controls, and failure to recognize the potential impact of relevant "non–clomiphene citrate" variables on gestational outcome.

In a study of 2369 births, Merrell National Laboratories reported an incidence rate of birth defects of 2.4%, compared with a 2.7% incidence for the population at large.[6] Concerns about the possible teratogenicity of clomiphene citrate stem from a variety of experimental studies in which inordinately high doses resulted in a mild form of cataracts in offspring of pregnant rats, and gastroschisis, cranioschisis, stunted limbs, cleft palate, and hydrocephalus in offspring of pregnant rabbits. Multiple birth defects have also been observed in the offspring of pregnant rodents who received clomiphene citrate. Inhibition of uterine implantation, diminished fetal survival, and a blastocytotoxic effect have also been described. However, of 58 infants with birth defects reported to Merrell National Laboratories, 8 were born to 7 of 15 mothers who received an inadvertent course of clomiphene citrate during the first 6 weeks after conception.[6] Thus, aside from sporadic and otherwise inadvertent administration during pregnancy, the usual preconceptional

---

*References 8, 26, 55, 66, 86, 91.

*References 3, 4, 16, 36, 41, 44, 47, 50, 56.

administration of clomiphene citrate to women and its clearance kinetics would seem to make gestational exposure unlikely. However, recent evidence suggests that clomiphene citrate may be subject to delayed release by virtue of its long-term retention by nuclear receptor sites. Although gestational exposure of the fetus might be possible under such circumstances, the overall clinical experience and toxicologic studies in subhuman primates[17] thus far do not support such concerns. The incidence of spontaneous abortion after clomiphene citrate therapy has been widely reported to conform to that observed in the population at large. The possibility of clomiphene citrate–associated hydatidiform mole[10,70,80,93,94] and ectopic gestation[64] has been considered by several investigators. At the present time, however, final judgment on these possible associations must await further investigation.

Although a relatively limited body of literature supports the possibility that clomiphene citrate promotes the incidence of heterotopic pregnancies, several examples documenting such a possibility have been reported.[33,67,76] A report alleging superfetation secondary to ovulation with clomiphene citrate has also been published.[9] All told, the relatively small number of reports and the seemingly sporadic nature of the above occurrences argue against a cause-and-effect relationship between clomiphene citrate administration and the genesis of unusual gestational states.

CONCLUSION

It has been almost 40 years since the synthesis of clomiphene citrate. During that time it has firmly established its reputation as a dependable and versatile therapeutic agent. Although its mechanisms of action have not been entirely clarified, the original prediction of a hypothalamic site of action has recently received elegant and badly needed support. Recent years have also seen an expansion of the indications for the use of clomiphene citrate, which now include luteal phase dysfunctions, oligoovulation, and in vitro fertilization. Moreover, continued interest in the modification of clomiphene citrate regimens has contributed to further increases in its efficacy in the setting of anovulatory infertility. In this connection, increasing the duration of clomiphene citrate therapy and its supplementation with dexamethasone (and more recently with bromocriptine) have resulted in a substantial reduction in the number of cases originally deemed "resistant." If past performance is an indication, there is little doubt that clomiphene citrate will continue to play a major role in the practice of reproductive endocrinology in years to come.

REFERENCES

1. Adams R, Mishell DR Jr, Israel R: Treatment of refractory anovulation with increased dosage and prolonged duration of cyclic clomiphene citrate, *Obstet Gynecol* 39:562, 1972.
2. Adashi EY: Clomiphene citrate: mechanism(s) and site(s) of action—a hypothesis revisited, *Fertil Steril* 42:331, 1984.
3. Adashi EY et al: Gestational outcome of clomiphene-related conceptions, *Fertil Steril* 31:620, 1979.
4. Ahlgren M, Kallen B, Rannevik G: Outcome of pregnancy after Clomid therapy, *Acta Obstet Gynecol Scand* 53:371, 1976.
5. Aiken RA: An account of the "Birmingham sextuples," *J Obstet Gynaecol Br Commonw* 76:684, 1969.
6. Asch RH, Greenblatt RB: Update on the safety and efficacy of clomiphene citrate as a therapeutic agent, *J Reprod Med* 17:175, 1976.
7. Atlay RD, Pennington GW: The use of clomiphene citrate and pituitary gonadotropin in successive pregnancies: the Sheffield quadruplets, *Am J Obstet Gynecol* 109:402, 1971.
8. Bateman B, Nunley W, Kolp L: Exogenous estrogen therapy for treatment of clomiphene citrate-induced cervical mucus abnormalities: is it effective?, *Fertil Steril* 54:577, 1990.
9. Bsat FA: Superfetation secondary to ovulation induction with clomiphene citrate: a case report, *Fertil Fertil* 47:516, 1987.
10. Burke M: Ectopic pregnancy, hydatidiform mole and clomiphene, *Lancet* 1:41, 1976.
11. Chang RJ, Abraham GE: Effect of dexamethasone and clomiphene citrate on peripheral steroid levels and ovarian function in a hirsute amenorrheic patient, *Fertil Steril* 27:640, 1976.
12. Check JH, Rakoff AE, Roy BK: Induction of ovulation with combined glucocorticoid and clomiphene citrate therapy in a minimally hirsute woman, *J Reprod Med* 19:159, 1977.
13. Chemical induction of ovulation, *JAMA* 256:281, 1961 (editorial).
14. Clark JH, Markaverich BM: The agonistic-antagonistic properties of clomiphene: a review, *Pharmacol Ther* 15:467, 1982.
15. Clark JH, Peck EJ Jr: Oestrogen receptors and antagonism of steroid hormone action, *Nature* 251:446, 1974.
16. Correy IF, Marsden DE, Schokman FCM: The outcome of pregnancy resulting from clomiphene induced ovulation, *Aust N Z J Obstet Gynaecol* 22:18, 1982.
17. Courtney KD, Valerio DA: Teratology in *Macaca mulatta*, *Teratology* 1:1633, 1968.
18. Daly DC et al: A randomized study of dexamethasone in ovulation induction with clomiphene citrate, *Fertil Steril* 41:844, 1984.
19. Diamant YZ, Evron S: Induction of ovulation by combined clomiphene citrate and dexamethasone treatment in clomiphene citrate nonresponders, *Eur J Obstet Gynecol Reprod Biol* 11:335, 1981.
20. Diamond MP et al: Comparison of two brands of clomiphene citrate for stimulation of follicular development in a program for in vitro fertilization, *Fertil Steril* 45:522, 1986.
21. diZerega GS, Hodgen GD: Luteal phase dysfunction in fertility: a sequel to aberrant folliculogenesis, *Fertil Steril* 35:489, 1981.
22. Dodge ST, Strickler RC, Keller DW: Ovulation induction with low doses of clomiphene citrate, *Obstet Gynecol* 67:63S, 1986.
23. Drake TS, Tredway DR, Buchanan GC: Continued clinical experience with an increasing dosage regimen of clomiphene citrate administration, *Fertil Steril* 30:274, 1978.
24. Echt CR, Romberger FT, Goodman JA: Clomiphene citrate in the treatment of luteal phase defects, *Fertil Steril* 20:564, 1969.
25. Ernst S et al: Stereochemistry of geometric isomers of clomiphene: a correction of the literature and a reexamination of structure-activity relationships, *J Pharm Sci* 65:148, 1976.
26. Fedele L et al: Enhanced preovulatory progesterone levels in clomiphene citrate-induced cycles, *J Clin Endocrinol Metab* 69:681, 1989.
27. Feore JC, Taymor ML: The relationship between the pituitary response to luteinizing hormone-releasing hormone and the ovulatory response to clomiphene citrate, *Fertil Steril* 27:1240, 1976.
28. Fisch P et al: Unexplained infertility: evaluation of treatment with clomiphene citrate and human chorionic gonadotropin, *Fertil Steril* 51:828, 1989.
29. Fritz MA, Speroff L: The endocrinology of the menstrual cycle: the interaction of folliculogenesis and neuroendocrine mechanisms, *Fertil Steril* 38:509, 1982.
30. Fritz MA, Speroff L: Current concepts of the endocrine characteristics of normal menstrual function: the key to diagnosis and management of menstrual disorders, *Clin Obstet Gynecol* 26:647, 1983.

31. Gambrell RD, Greenblatt RB, Mahesh VB: Serum gonadotropins in a variety of ovulatory women treated with clomiphene citrate, *Int J Gynaecol Obstet* 11:90, 1973.

32. Garcia J, Jones SG, Wentz AC: The use of clomiphene citrate, *Fertil Steril* 28:707, 1977.

33. Glassner MJ, Araon E, Eskin BA: Ovulation induction with clomiphene and the rise in heterotopic pregnancies, *J Reprod Med* 35:175, 1990.

34. Glazener CMA et al: Clomiphene treatment for women with unexplained infertility: a placebo-controlled study of hormonal responses and conception rates, *Gynecol Endocrinol* 4:75, 1990.

35. Goldfarb AF, Crawford R: Polycystic ovarian disease, clomiphene and multiple pregnancies, *Obstet Gynecol* 34:307, 1969.

36. Goldfarb AF et al: Critical review of 160 clomiphene-related pregnancies, *Obstet Gynecol* 31:342, 1968.

37. Gorlitsky GA, Kase NG, Speroff L: Ovulation and pregnancy rates with clomiphene citrate, *Obstet Gynecol* 51:265, 1978.

38. Greenblatt RB: Chemical induction of ovulation, *Fertil Steril* 12:402, 1961.

39. Greenblatt RB et al: Induction of ovulation with MRL/41, *JAMA* 178:101, 1961.

40. Gysler M et al: A decade's experience with an individualized clomiphene treatment regimen including its effects on the postcoital test, *Fertil Steril* 37:161, 1982.

41. Hack M et al: Pregnancy after induced ovulation: follow-up of pregnancies and children born after clomiphene therapy, *JAMA* 220:1329, 1972.

42. Hammond MG, Halme IK, Talbert LM: Factors affecting the pregnancy rate in clomiphene citrate induction of ovulation, *Obstet Gynecol* 62:196, 1983.

43. Hancock KW, Oakey RE: The low incidence of pregnancy following clomiphene therapy, *Int J Fertil* 18:49, 1973.

44. Harlap S: Ovulation induction and congenital malformations, *Lancet* 2:961, 1976.

45. Higashiyama S et al: Ovulation induction with prednisolone-clomiphene therapy in clomiphene failure, *Jpn J Fertil Steril* 26:1, 1981.

46. Hoffman D, Lobo RA: Serum dehydroepiandrosterone sulfate and the use of clomiphene citrate in anovulatory women, *Fertil Steril* 43:196, 1985.

47. Insler V, Zakut H, Serr DM: Cycle pattern and pregnancy rate following clomiphene-estrogen therapy, *Obstet Gynecol* 41:602, 1973.

48. Jones GS, De Moraes-Reuhsen M: Induction of ovulation with human gonadotropins with clomiphene, *Fertil Steril* 16:461, 1965.

49. Jones GS et al: Pathophysiology of reproductive failure after clomiphene-induced ovulation, *Am J Obstet Gynecol* 108:847, 1970.

50. Karow WG, Payne SA: Pregnancy after clomiphene citrate treatment, *Fertil Steril* 19:351, 1968.

51. Kauppila J et al: Postmenopausal hormone replacement therapy with estrogen periodically supplemented with antiestrogen, *Am J Obstet Gynecol* 140:787, 1981.

52. Kerin JF et al: Evidence for a hypothalamic site of action of clomiphene citrate in women, *J Clin Endocrinol Metab* 61:265, 1985.

53. Kistner RW: The infertile woman, *Am J Nurs* 73:1937, 1973.

54. Klay LJ: Clomiphene regulated ovulation for donor insemination, *Fertil Steril* 27:383, 1976.

55. Kokia E et al: Addition of exogenous estrogens to improve cervical mucus following clomiphene citrate medication, *Acta Obstet Gynecol Scand* 69:139, 1990.

56. Kurachi K et al: Congenital malformations of newborn infants after clomiphene induced ovulation, *Fertil Steril* 40:187, 1983.

57. Lamb EL, Colliflower WW, Williams IW: Endometrial histology and conception rates after clomiphene, *Obstet Gynecol* 39:389, 1972.

58. Lisse K: Combined and clomiphene-dexamethasone therapy in cases with resistance to clomiphene, *Zentralbl Gynakol* 102:645, 1980.

59. Littman BA, Hodgen GD: A comprehensive dose-response study of clomiphene citrate for enhancement of the primate ovarian menstrual cycle, *Fertil Steril* 43:463, 1985.

60. Lobo RA et al: Clinical and laboratory predictors of clomiphene response, *Fertil Steril* 27:168, 1982.

61. Lobo RA et al: Clomiphene and dexamethasone in women unresponsive to clomiphene alone, *Obstet Gynecol* 60:497, 1982.

62. Lobo RA et al: An extended regimen of clomiphene citrate in women unresponsive to standard therapy, *Fertil Steril* 37:762, 1982.

63. Lunenfeld B, Insler V: Classification of amenorrhoeic states and their treatment by ovulation induction, *Clin Endocrinol* 3:233, 1974.

64. Marchbanks PA, Coulam CB, Annegers JF: An association between clomiphene citrate and ectopic pregnancy: a preliminary report, *Fertil Steril* 44:268, 1985.

65. Martinez AR et al: Intrauterine insemination dose and clomiphene citrate does not improve fecundity in couples with infertility due to male or idiopathic factors: a prospective, randomized, controlled study, *Fertil Steril* 53:847, 1990.

66. Maxson WS et al: Anti-estrogenic effect of clomiphene citrate: correlation with serum estradiol concentrations, *Fertil Steril* 42:356, 1984.

67. McLain PL, Kirkwood CR: Ovarian and intrauterine heterotopic pregnancy following clomiphene ovulation induction: report of a healthy live birth, *J Fam Pract* 24:76, 1987.

68. Miyake A et al: Clomiphene citrate induces luteinizing hormone release through hypothalamic luteinizing hormone-releasing hormone in vitro, *Acta Endocrinol* 103:289, 1983.

69. Miyake A et al: Hydrocortisone elicits the effect of clomiphene citrate on luteinizing hormone-releasing hormone in vitro, *Acta Endocrinol* 107:145, 1984.

70. Mor-Joseph S et al: Recurrent molar pregnancies associated with clomiphene citrate and human gonadotropins, *Am J Obstet Gynecol* 151:1085, 1985.

71. O'Herlihy C, de Crespigny LJCh, Robinson HP: Monitoring ovarian follicular development with real-time ultrasound, *Br J Obstet Gynaecol* 87:613, 1980.

72. O'Herlihy C, Pepperell RJ, Robinson HP: Ultrasound timing of human chorionic gonadotropin administration in clomiphene stimulated cycles, *Obstet Gynecol* 59:40, 1982.

73. O'Herlihy C et al: Incremental clomiphene therapy: a new method for treating persistent anovulation, *Obstet Gynecol* 58:535, 1981.

74. Palopoli FP et al: Substituted aminoalkoxytriarylhadoethylenes, *J Med Chem* 10:84, 1967.

75. Quagliarello J, Weiss G; Clomiphene citrate in the management of infertility associated with shortened luteal phases, *Fertil Steril* 31:373, 1979.

76. Raccuia J et al: Synchronous intrauterine and ectopic pregnancy associated with clomiphene citrate, *Surg Gynecol Obstet* 168:417, 1989.

77. Rojanasakul A: Massive ascites following induction of ovulation with clomiphene citrate: a case report, *J Med Assoc Thai* 71:86, 1988.

78. Roland M: Problems of ovulation induction with clomiphene citrate with report of a case of ovarian hyperstimulation, *Obstet Gynecol* 35:55, 1970.

79. Rust LA, Israel R, Mishell DR Jr: An individualized graduated therapeutic regimen for clomiphene citrate, *Am J Obstet Gynecol* 120:785, 1974.

80. Schneiderman CI, Waxman B: Clomid therapy and subsequent hydatidiform mole formation, *Obstet Gynecol* 39:787, 1982.

81. Scommegna A, Lash SR: Ovarian overstimulation, massive ascites and singleton pregnancy after clomiphene, *JAMA* 207:753, 1969.

82. Shepard MK, Balmaceda JP, Leiia CG: Relationship of weight to successful induction of ovulation with clomiphene citrate, *Fertil Steril* 32:641, 1979.

83. Shirai E, Lizuka R, Notake Y: Clomiphene citrate and its effects upon ovulation and estrogen, *Fertil Steril* 23:331, 1972.

84. Southam AL, Janovski NA: Massive ovarian hyperstimulation with clomiphene citrate, *JAMA* 181:443, 1962.

85. Swyer GIM, Radwanski E, McGarrigle HHG: Plasma oestradiol and progesterone estimation for the monitoring of induction of ovulation with clomiphene and chorionic gonadotropins, *Br J Obstet Gynaecol* 82:794, 1975.

86. Tepper R et al: The effect of clomiphene citrate and tamoxifen on the cervical mucus, *Acta Obstet Gynecol Scand* 67:311, 1988.

87. Tobias H, Carr LA, Voogt JL: Effect of estradiol benzoate and clomiphene on tyrosine hydroxylase activity and on luteinizing hormone and prolactin levels in ovariectomized rats, *Life Sci* 29:711, 1981.

88. Trounson AO et al: Pregnancies in humans by fertilization *in vitro* and embryo transfer in the controlled ovulatory cycle, *Science* 212:681, 1981.

89. Vaitukaitis JL et al: New evidence for an anti-estrogenic action of clomiphene citrate in women, *J Clin Endocrinol Metab* 32:503, 1971.

90. Vandenberg G, Yen SSC: Effect of anti-estrogenic action of clomiphene during the menstrual cycle: evidence for a change in feedback sensitivity, *J Clin Endocrinol Metab* 37:356, 1973.

91. Van der JV: The effect of clomiphene and conjugated estrogens on cervical mucus, *S Afr Med J* 60:347, 1981.

92. van Hall EV, Mastboom JL: Luteal phase insufficiency in patients treated with clomiphene, *Am J Obstet Gynecol* 103:165, 1969.

93. Wajntraub G, Kamar R, Pardo Y: Hydatidiform mole after treatment with clomiphene, *Fertil Steril* 25:904, 1974.

94. Weiss DB, Aboulafia Y: Ectopic gestation and hydatidiform mole in clomiphene-induced pregnancies, *Lancet* 2:1094, 1975.

95. Whitelaw ML, Kalman CG, Grams LR: The significance of the high ovulation rate versus the low pregnancy rate with Clomid, *Am J Obstet Gynecol* 107:865, 1970.

96. Wu CH, Winkel CA: The effect of therapy initiation day on clomiphene citrate therapy, *Fertil Steril* 52:564, 1989.

97. Yen SSC, Vela P, Ryan KJ: Effect of clomiphene citrate in polycystic ovary syndrome: relationship between serum gonadotropin and corpus luteum function, *J Clin Endocrinol* 31:7, 1970.

Chapter 33

HUMAN GONADOTROPINS

Bruno Lunenfeld, MD
and Vaclav Insler, MD

HISTORIC BACKGROUND

Probably the most far-reaching discovery in reproductive biology was made by Crowe et al.[29] in 1909 showing that the male and female reproductive systems are under the functional control of the anterior hypophysis. They demon-strated that partial hypophysectomy in adult dogs provoked atrophy of the reproductive organs, and prevented sexual development in juvenile animals. However, less than 20 years later Zondek and Ascheim[136] in Europe and Smith and Engle[118] in the United States discovered the gonadotropic hormones (follicle-stimulating hormone [FSH], luteinizing hormone [LH], and human chorionic gonadotropin [hCG]) and obtained firm evidence that the male and female reproductive systems were under the functional control of gonadotropins secreted by the pituitary gland. Zondek[134,135] demonstrated that implantation of the anterior pituitary caused a rapid development of sexual organs in immature animals. At approximately the same time, Smith[117] and Smith and Engle[118] showed that hypophysectomy resulted in a failure of sexual maturation in immature animals and in a rapid regression of sexual characteristics in adult animals. It took 30 more years to realize that the pituitary-ovarian axis was controlled by the hypothalamus and 20 additional years to identify the gonadotropin-releasing hormone (GnRH) and to recognize that its pulsatile release by the arcuate nucleus controlled gonadotropin secretion.

Sources of hormones

During the 1930s and 1940s gonadotropin extracts from different animal materials were prepared and applied for stimulation of ovarian function in humans. It was quickly realized, however, that these preparations were of very limited clinical value because nonprimate gonadotropins elicited in humans a rapid immunologic response that neutralized their therapeutic effect.[84] This discovery focused scientific and technologic efforts on extraction and purification of gonadotropins from human sources. In 1954 Borth et al.[16] were fortunate to demonstrate that kaolin extracts from pooled menopausal urine contained FSH and LH activity in comparable amounts. These extracts prevented Leydig cell atrophy and maintained complete spermatogenesis in hypophysectomized male rats and were capable of inducing follicular growth and promotion of multiple corpora lutea in hypophysectomized female rats.[17] On the basis of these observations we had predicted in 1954 that such extracts could open up interesting therapeutic possibilities.[16]

Table 33-1. Conception rates after gonadotropin therapy

Author	No. of patients	No. of cycles	Pregnancies		
			No.	% Cycles	% Patients
Australian Department of Health[4] (1981)	1056	4008	552	13.8	52.3
Bettendorf et al.[9] (1981)	756	1585	224	14.1	29.6
Butler[21] (1970)	134	438	31	7.1	23.1
Caspi et al.[25] (1974)	101	343	62	18.1	61.4
Ellis and Williamson[36] (1975)	77	332	43	13.3	55.8
Gemzell[45] (1970)	228	463	101	21.8	44.3
Goldfarb et al.[50] (1982)	442	1098	118	10.7	26.7
Healy et al.[57] (1980)	40	159	33	20.7	82.5
Kurachi[80] (1983)	2166	6096	523	8.6	24.2
Lunenfeld et al.[92] (1985)	1107	3646	424	11.6	38.3
Potashnik[105b] et al. (1986)	262	580	85	14.6	32.4
Spadoni et al.[119] (1974)	62	225	26	11.5	41.9
Thompson and Hansen[123] (1970)	1190	2798	334	11.9	28.1
Tsapoulis et al.[126] (1978)	320	?	163		50.9
Tuang[127] (1986)	95	320	72	22.5	75.8
CUMULATIVE	8036		2791		34.7

The recognition of the therapeutic potential of human gonadotropins stimulated the search for sources suitable for extraction of these hormones in amounts adequate for clinical use. Most investigators were purifying gonadotropins from urine of menopausal women (human menopausal gonadotropins [hMG]); however, the Stockholm group led by Gemzell[47] took the shorter route and obtained active gonadotropins by processing human pituitaries (human pituitary gonadotropin [hPG]). Gemzell and his co-workers reported the first successful induction of ovulation using hPG in 1958[47] and the first pregnancy in 1960.[48] Approximately at the same time Bettendorf et al.[8] succeeded in extracting a potent gonadotropic agent from human pituitaries and reported the first clinical experience with its use.

Of particular significance were the reports of Bettendorf[7] and Gemzell,[46] who were able to induce ovulation followed by pregnancy in hypophysectomized women. Lunenfeld and his group, working with hMG, achieved ovulations and pregnancies in anovulatory women. Their results were reported at various scientific and medical meetings beginning in 1959 and later published in 1963.[88] Because of the scarcity of postmortem pituitary glands, however, the possibility of their wide-scale use was limited. Thus attention of pharmaceutical companies (Serono Laboratories, Inc., Randolph, Mass., and Organon Inc., West Orange, N.J.) was directed toward preparation of purified extracts from menopausal urine.[34] Borth et al.[15] reported that this preparation was a potent ovarian stimulant in women, capable of promoting multiple follicular development.

Clinical studies

Large-scale clinical studies were then undertaken in numerous centers throughout the world and the results were reported in the literature. Induction of ovulation with human gonadotropins has been an integral part of the routine work of many fertility clinics for more than 15 years. During that time numerous reports describing in great detail all aspects of gonadotropin therapy have been published.[20,66,90,123] A survey of more than 22,000 gonadotropin treatments reported during the last several years (Table 33-1) indicates that this therapy has become universally accepted for induction of ovulation in anovulatory infertile women.[73,91]

The introduction of rapid and reliable hormone assays, and later the availability of ultrasound scanners enabling visualization and measurement of ovarian follicles, made monitoring of gonadotropin therapy accurate and objective and improved the results of treatment. In the 1980s the large-scale in vitro fertilization (IVF) programs used the principles developed for and the experience gained from induction of ovulation in infertile patients and added new important insights to the understanding of the mechanism of ovarian stimulation by gonadotropins.

The box on p. 613 describes briefly the most important milestones of the long and tedious way that led from the discovery of the gonadotropin principle to IVF. Experimental and clinical data obtained over the years also showed that FSH is capable of increasing the recruitment rate of new crops of small follicles, of maintaining the normal development of multiple follicles to the preovulatory stage, and, consequently, of enlarging the yield of fertilizable eggs. These findings prompted the use of gonadotropins as the preferred treatment modality in most IVF programs.

Conceptual protocols

With the use of gonadotropins for induction of superovulation in normally ovulating women, conceptual changes in the monitoring schemes had to be introduced. When

---

Milestones of developments leading to efficient treatment of female infertility

1926–1927	Discovery of the pituitary hormone controlling ovarian function
1955	Clinical use of urinary hormone assays (steroids and gonadotropins)
1959	Extraction and purification of gonadotropins from human pituitaries and menopausal urine
1961	Introduction of clomiphene citrate
1965	Wide-scale clinical use of gonadotropins and clomiphene
1968	Development of the first therapeutically oriented classification of anovulatory states
1970	Routine application of radioimmunoassays for estimation of hormone levels
1971	Isolation, determination of structure, and laboratory synthesis of GnRH
1972	Introduction of prolactin assays
1973–1976	Reports on pregnancies induced by GnRH therapy
1974	Development of prolactin-inhibiting drugs
1978	Discovery of pulsatile nature of GnRH secretion
1979	(a) Ultrasound imaging of ovarian follicles
	(b) Introduction of pulsatile GnRH therapy
	(c) Delivery of the first test-tube baby
1982	(a) Introduction of GnRH analogues for clinical use
	(b) Introduction of purified FSH for ovulation-inducing therapy
1984	Routine clinical use of IVF-ET and GIFT programs
1985	Application of combined pituitary suppression and ovarian stimulation therapy for the treatment of different types of fertility disturbances
1988–1990	Understanding of the interplay between endocrine, paracrine, and autocrine events in reproduction
1991	Introduction of recombinant gonadotropins

---

attempting to induce ovulation in anovulatory women, the principal aim is to achieve the development of a single dominant follicle. This approach has been directed at achieving ovulation and pregnancy in many patients while preventing multiple follicular growth, multiple pregnancies, and hyperstimulation in most of them. In contrast, the conceptual idea of IVF, gamete intrafallopian transfer (GIFT), or tubal embryo transfer (ET) programs is to use a superovulatory physiologic dosage in order to obtain a large number of fertilizable eggs. For this purpose many different protocols have emerged, each with its own merits and disadvantages and each using ultrasonographic scanning to estimate both the number and size of the growing follicles and estradiol assays to assess their functional integrity.

CHEMISTRY, PHARMACOKINETICS, AND ASSAY PROCEDURES

During the last 20 years the major elements of the mechanism of action, control, and regulation of secretion of gonadotropins has been elucidated, and more recently their structure has been determined.

Structure of gonadotropins

Gonadotropins have been found to be glycoproteins with a molecular weight of approximately 30,000d and containing about 20% carbohydrates. The carbohydrate moieties in their molecules are fucose, mannose, galactose, acetylglucosamine, and N-acetylneuraminic acid.[22] The sialic acid content varies widely among the glycoprotein hormones, from 20 residues in hCG and 5 in FSH to only 1 or 2 in LH. These differences are largely responsible for the variations in the isoelectric points of gonadotropins.

The carbohydrate moieties are complex. They may be branched or straight chains, and they contain sialic acid as important constituents, particularly at the end of the chains. The differing sialic acid content accounts for differences in molecular weight of the hormones isolated from various sources and in differences in biologic activity determined by in vivo assays. The higher the sialic acid content, the longer the biologic half-life. Thus the increased amount of the carbohydrate component in hCG is responsible for its significantly longer half-life than that of LH or FSH. Whereas the beta subunit of LH (β-LH) contains only one carbohydrate group, the beta subunit of hCG (β-hCG) contains six. The function of the carbohydrate is not fully known, except that removal of the terminal neuraminic acid (sialic acid) residues drastically shortens the half-lives of the circulating hormones in blood. For this reason desialized preparations of hLH, hCG, and hFSH show considerably reduced biologic activity in vivo but retain activity in vitro in biologic assays employing membrane receptors or isolated target cells. Hormone measurements by immunoassays or in vitro bioassay procedures do not therefore express the actual bioactivity of these hormones in vivo. Deglycosylated hormones can act in vitro as competitive antagonists of the actions of the intact hormone on the cyclic AMP production and to a lesser extent on steroid hormone biosynthesis.

The gonadotropic hormones consist of two hydrophobic, noncovalently associated α- and β-subunits. The three-dimensional structure of each subunit is maintained by internally cross-linked disulfide bonds. Gonadotropic hormones can be dissociated into the individual subunits by denaturing agents (10 M urea at pH 4.5 or 10 M propionic acid).[31] The subunits are practically without biologic activity, but the activity is regenerated by allowing the two subunits to recombine. All of the gonadotropins, as well as thyroid-stimulating hormone (TSH), share a common α-subunit of 92 amino acid residues in the same sequence, with five disulfide bonds and two carbohydrate moieties. The β-subunits (of FSH, LH, and hCG) are unique to each hormone and determine their biologic specificity. They have amino acid chains of variable lengths (116 to 147 amino acid residues) and contain six disulfide bonds. There is only one known gene that codes for the β chain of LH, whereas as many as six to eight genes or pseudogenes have been identified for the β chain of chorionic gonadotropin (CG).[13,122] (See Chapter 1.) It is not known how many of these CG genes are translated. Possibly some of the genes are expressed in the placenta, which would lead to the traditional, highly glycosylated CG and the differences we have encountered between pregnancy CG in urine and CG-like material that exists in the pituitary. Further studies, including carbohydrate and amino acid analyses, will help to determine the true nature of this CG-like material.

Metabolism of gonadotropins

Methodologies that have allowed analysis of genes and gene products have shown that the two subunits of the gonadotropic hormones are translated from separate messenger RNAs[41] and both are synthesized as precursors. The nascent polypeptide α- and β-subunits are then glycosylated in the Golgi apparatus by en bloc attachment of mannose-enriched oligosaccharide to two asparagine residues of each subunit. Excess mannose and glucose residues are trimmed from the intermediates. Monosaccharides, N-acetylglucosamine, galactose, and N-acetylneuraminic acid are then attached sequentially to complete the oligosaccharide structures.[65] The information regarding metabolism of gonadotropic hormones is scarce. It has been shown that purified preparations of hFSH, hLH, and hCG injected intravenously into humans had serum half-lives (as determined by bioassays) of 180 to 240 minutes, 38 to 60 minutes, and 6 to 8 hours, respectively. Although circulatory half-life estimates for pituitary LH ranged between 38 and 69 minutes, a separate analysis of the fast and slow compartments yielded values of 21 and 235 minutes, respectively. The half-life time of hCG as determined in women after intravenous administration ranged between 6 and 11 hours.[131] After intramuscular administration, as is usually used for therapeutic purposes, the differences between these two hormones are even more apparent.

The half-life of the α- and β-subunits of LH was found to be only 16 minutes. The higher carbohydrate content of hCG (10%) is responsible for its significantly longer half-life than that for hFSH (5%) and hLH (2%). Removal of the sialic acid of hCG reduces its half-life to minutes and a correspondingly low biologic activity in vivo, because of rapid hepatic uptake.

After the intramuscular administration of menotropins (Pergonal, containing FSH and LH derived from human menopausal urine) daily for 8 days, and testing blood levels twice daily, no increase in LH levels was observed.[33] However, after the intramuscular administration of hCG, peak serum levels of hCG were observed after 6 to 8 hours. Levels were reduced to about 50% after 36 hours, and hCG was still discernible after 6 days. Although this comparison is not totally adequate, since hCG was administered in a high dose (5000 IU) whereas LH was given in a low dose (150 IU), it can still be concluded that these differences are related to the half-lives of these hormones. FSH, which has an intermediate half-life longer than that of LH but shorter than that of hCG, even when given in a low dose (150 IU), accumulated in the plasma and was still elevated above the baseline level 3 days after the last injection.[33] Thus it is clear that hCG, when given as a substitute for LH, exerts a stronger and more prolonged biologic effect because of its significantly longer half-life. Also, the previously quoted differences between LH and hCG in animal studies[40] can be explained by this phenomenon, namely, that the differences are not of a qualitative nature but are quantitative expressions of a prolonged biologic effect. The mean metabolic clearance rate (MCR) of hFSH in women has been determined to be 14 mL/min and has not been determined in men. The MCR of hLH is 25 to 30 mL/min in women regardless of ovulatory state and is almost 50% higher in normal men. The disappearance curves for both hormones are multiexponential, indicating a distribution of these hormones in more than three mathematic compartments. In premenopausal women, daily production rates of hLH are 500 to 1000 IU, with a marked preovulatory rise; whereas daily production rates in postmenopausal women are 3000 to 4000 IU. These values indicate that the pituitary content of hLH (and probably of hFSH) is turned over once or twice daily and that rapid biosynthesis of gonadotropins must be necessary to maintain the normal levels of pituitary storage and secretion. Only 3% to 10% of the daily production of FSH and LH is excreted in the urine in a biologically active form, but nevertheless it reflects the rate of gonadotropin secretion in physiologic and pathologic conditions. The recovery of exogenous gonadotropins in the urine of fertile and infertile subjects is 10% to 20% of the administered dose. Urinary excretion of gonadotropins accounts for only 5% of the MCR. The MCR of hMG in hypogonadotropic subjects is 0.4 to 1.7 mL/min. The isoforms of FSH, with a more basic pH, clear faster from the circulation than do the acidic forms. It is now clearly established that the type of FSH secreted by the anterior pituitary gland changes during different endocrine states (Fig. 33-1). Thus the FSH activity within the pituitary appears to range between an extremely biopotent form of short half-life in the estrogenic milieu (due to a decrease in carbohydrate content) to a long-acting form with compromised bioactivity in a hypoestrogenic state. The microhet-

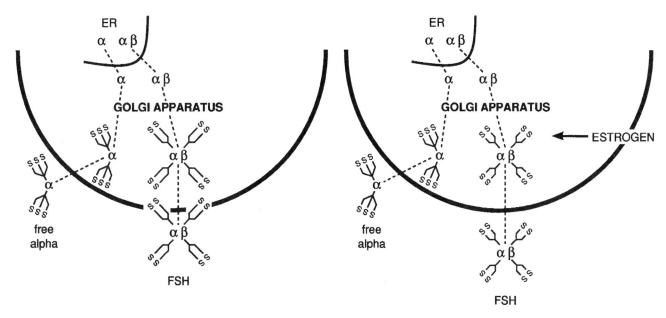

Fig. 33-1. Schematic presentation of FSH synthesis in the gonadotropin-producing cells. The two subunits of the gonadotropic hormones are translated from separate messenger RNAs, and both are synthesized as precursors in the endoplasmic reticulum (*ER*). The nascent polypeptide α- and β-subunits are then glycosylated in the Golgi apparatus. In a high-estrogenic environment the carbohydrate chains are shorter and the clearance of the hormone is more rapid. In a low-estrogenic environment the carbohydrate chains are longer and the clearance is slower.

erogeneity in the gonadotropic hormones is produced during post-translational events. The hormonal environment in various physiologic and pathologic conditions and during extraction or purification procedures may produce qualitative and/or quantitative changes in the carbohydrate or sialic acid content. To our knowledge heterogeneity due to structural changes in the amino acid sequence during the translational period has not been reported.

Assay procedures

The discussed structural differences in glycoprotein hormones must be taken into consideration when trying to interpret hormone assay results.

In vivo bioassays reflect the ability of the glycoprotein isohormones and their possible metabolites to exert their natural biologic actions in situ. In addition to measuring the bioactivity at target tissues, they also take into consideration the metabolic clearance rate of the hormone in the animal model used.

In an in vitro bioassay system the hormone-receptor interaction will depend on the β-subunit, although full biologic activity will be elicited only if this is combined with the α-subunit. These systems combine the assessment of binding and the measurements of a postreceptor response. The molecular heterogeneity of the gonadotropic molecules themselves may interfere with or augment binding at target cell receptors, leading to nonparallelism to standards. (See Chapter 62.)

In an immunoassay system the antibody may recognize the α chain, the β chain, or both. However, since these methods measure a composite of antigenic activity that is not necessarily related to the bioactivity of the hormone, the use of immunoassays for evaluating hormonal bioactivity is of limited value.

The carbohydrate component in gonadotropic hormone preparations may vary without significantly influencing the specific biologic reaction with an antiserum in immunoassay systems. However, the carbohydrate component will significantly influence the plasma half-life of the bioactivity of the glycoprotein hormone, as reflected in the response of the intact test animal or human recipient. Thus a biologic activity assessed by an in vitro system may in fact not equal its potency in vivo. For example, the biologic activity of hCG as measured by bioassays will be significantly reduced after desialization, whereas in in vitro assay systems it will retain most of its original activity. These differences have been clearly demonstrated by the fact that the decrease in biologic activity was correlated with the decrease of sialic acid and the disappearance rate from plasma of partially and fully desialized hCG preparations.[86]

Deglycosylation had no effect on the specificity of binding to its specific receptor. However, unlike receptor binding and immunologic activity, which were fully retained, the ability of the hormone to stimulate cAMP accumulation in vitro in rat interstitial cells was completely abolished.[94] Linda et al.[86] confirmed these findings by showing that, in the rat Leydig cell testosterone production assay in vitro, the maximal agonist activity of deglycosylated hCG was indistiguishable from that of intact hCG but its potency was reduced to 2.5% of that of intact hCG. Furthermore, both the deglycosylated and desialized hCG could elicit an initial testosterone increase when injected into the cynomolgus monkey. However, the duration of the testosterone response was significantly shorter than that produced by native hCG. The mean apparent plasma half-lives of the main components of the deglycosylated and desialized hCG were 23 minutes and 1.1 minutes, respectively, whereas the mean apparent plasma half-life of the main components of the native hCG was 275.4 minutes.

Differences were also found in potency estimations by in vitro bioassays, using granulosa cell aromatase bioassay or Sertoli cell aromatase bioassay compared with immunoassays, of serum samples containing FSH in various clinical situations.[105a] Similar potency differences were also described after certain purification procedures.

The differences between various assay methods may be of minor relevance in most routine diagnostic procedures, and probably will not significantly influence treatment or monitoring protocols. By knowing the limitation of each assay procedure and remembering the earlier mentioned principles, sensitive in vitro bioassays can be used in the control of purification procedures. However, to calibrate therapeutic preparations, in vitro procedures may either underestimate or overestimate potency and should therefore not be used. For these reasons, regulatory agencies demand in vivo bioassays for potency estimates of gonadotropic preparations.

The introduction of protein hormones produced by chemical synthesis, immunoabsorption, or recombinant DNA technology has provided detailed characterizations of the patterns of their properties in various biologic systems; this information is an essential element in the identification of such products and the assessment of their therapeutic value.

RATIONALE AND GOALS OF GONADOTROPIN THERAPY

The rationale of gonadotropin treatment is to provide gonadotropin levels of magnitude and timing similar to those observed in the normal ovulatory cycle and, consequently, to evoke recruitment of a follicular cohort, selection and full maturation of at least one dominant follicle, ovulation, and sustained corpus luteum function. Unfortunately, this goal has never been fully achieved. The FSH and LH levels and their ratios during gonadotropin-stimulated cycles are quite different from those of normal cycles.[56,132]

Estrogen levels and their daily rate of ascent, as well as progesterone values, are not identical to those observed in spontaneous cycles.[68] The follicular fluid levels of estradiol and progesterone are lower and the level of inhibin is higher in preovulatory gonadotropin-stimulated cycles than those in the dominant follicle of the natural cycle.[114] Moreover, the pregnancy rate in gonadotropin-induced cycles with steroid profiles closely resembling those found in spontaneous ovulations is dismally low.[67] Thus the theoretic rationale of gonadotropin therapy must be subordinated to its clinical aim, which is to achieve ovulation and pregnancy in all suitable cases while avoiding hyperstimulation.

Large-scale clinical experience indicates that this goal can be practically achieved. The unequivocal proof of the clinical efficacy of gonadotropin therapy is the thousands of babies born after gonadotropin-induced ovulations and conceptions.

SELECTION OF PATIENTS

Gonadotropin treatment is primarily a substitution therapy and as such should be applied in patients lacking appropriate gonadotropin stimulation but having target organs (gonads) capable of normal response. In daily practice, however, gonadotropins are also used in other groups of patients.

In 1968 Insler et al.[70] proposed a simple treatment-oriented classification of patients selected for gonadotropin therapy. This classification has been modified and adopted by the World Health Organization Scientific Group[127] and is still used in many centers today. According to this classification, gonadotropin treatment is applied in two main groups of women: *group I:* hypothalamic-pituitary failure—amenorrheic women with no evidence of endogenous estrogen production, nonelevated prolactin levels, normal or low FSH levels, and no detectable space-occupying lesion in the hypothalamic-pituitary region; *group II:* hypothalamic-pituitary dysfunction—women with a variety of menstrual cycle disturbances, including amenorrhea with evidence of endogenous estrogen production, and normal levels of prolactin and FSH. Theoretic considerations and clinical experience justify including women with polycystic ovary disease (PCOD) as a specific subgroup of patients belonging to group II. Regardless of the underlying pathophysiologic mechanism, when the ovarian disease reaches its structural and functional expression, the response to ovulation induction acquires distinctive characteristics. In group II, gonadotropins are usually applied after other types of ovulation-inducing therapy have failed.

It is theoretically plausible and clinically proven (Figs. 33-2 and 33-3) that the results of gonadotropin treatment are significantly better in group I than they are in group II.[93] Amenorrheic women of group I, however, represent a small and ever-diminishing proportion of the infertility clinic population.[9]

In recent years another group of patients, steadily growing in numbers, is being treated with human gonadotropins—women undergoing IVF. Obviously, these patients differ from both group I and group II in having

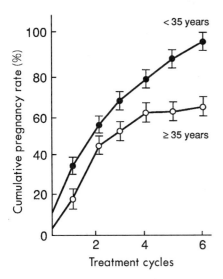

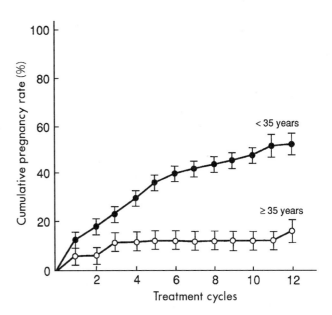

Fig. 33-2. Comparison of the cumulative pregnancy rates in amenorrheic women with hypothalamic-pituitary insufficiency (group I) above and below the age of 35 after ovulation induction with hMg/hCG.

Fig. 33-3. Cumulative pregnancy rates after ovulation induction with hMG/hCG in women with hypothalamic-pituitary dysfunction (group II) who did not responded to clomiphene treatment. Comparison is between women above and below the age of 35.

completely normal hormone levels and competent hypothalamic-pituitary-ovarian feedback mechanisms.

The general principles of gonadotropin therapy applied to these three groups of patients are similar, but the intensity of stimulation, course of treatment, and hormone patterns differ significantly. It may thus be summarized that, at present, four modes of gonadotropin treatment are used: (1) substitution therapy, given to patients of group I; (2) stimulation therapy, given to patients of group II; (3) regulatory therapy, given to patients of group II with PCOD and/or adrenogenital syndrome; and (4) superstimulation (controlled hyperstimulation) therapy, used in assisted reproduction programs.

PRINCIPLES OF GONADOTROPIN THERAPY

The basic principles of gonadotropin therapy were proposed by Insler and Lunenfeld[66,67] after observation of the course of treatment in several hundreds of patients. Ovarian response can be elicited only when a certain dose of FSH-like material has been applied. This amount of gonadotropins is called the *effective daily dose*. Administration of FSH at levels significantly below the effective daily dose does not evoke any measurable effect even when prolonged therapy is used (Fig. 33-4).

After the application of an effective daily dose of FSH a number of gonadotropin-dependent ovarian follicles are stimulated to begin growth and maturation. This period of gonadotropin therapy is called the *latent phase*. Since at this stage of follicular development appreciable amounts of estrogen are not yet secreted, the latent phase of therapy is clinically "mute" so far as secretion of sex steroids is

concerned. The recent introduction of high-resolution vaginal ultra-sonography will probably enable the detection of a newly recruited cohort of antral follicles measuring 2 to 3 mm. The latent phase begins with the application of the effective daily dose of gonadotropins and ends with the appearance of a measurable ovarian response, i.e., rising estrogen levels and increasing follicular diameter.

The second part of gonadotropin therapy, called the *active phase,* lasts from the initial estrogen rise until ovulation induction. It is characterized by an exponential rise of estrogen levels and steady growth of follicular diameter.

The duration of the latent phase is 3 to 7 days and is significantly longer in patients of group I than in women of group II. The length of the active phase is 4 to 6 days and is similar in all patients. The above principles, based on clinical observation and thorough analysis of patients' responses, received powerful theoretic support from the experimental work on primates by Hodgen and his group.[51,60,61] The introduction of ultrasound for monitoring of follicular size and the IVF programs allowing for direct laparoscopic observation of the size and appearance of ovarian follicles concomitant with the appreciation of the maturity of ova lend further support to the empirically developed principles of gonadotropin therapy. According to Hodgen's work in primates, the sequence of events leading to ovulation is as follows (Fig. 33-5):

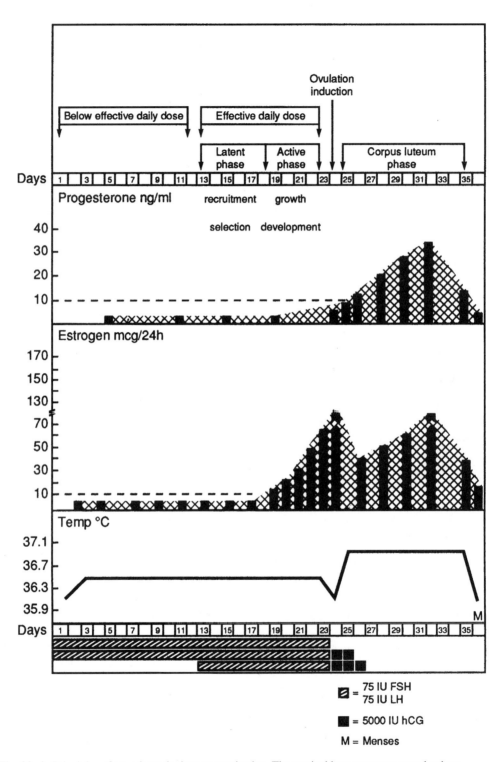

Fig. 33-4. Principles of gonadotropic therapy monitoring. The vertical bars represent actual values. The crosshatching represents the area under the curve.

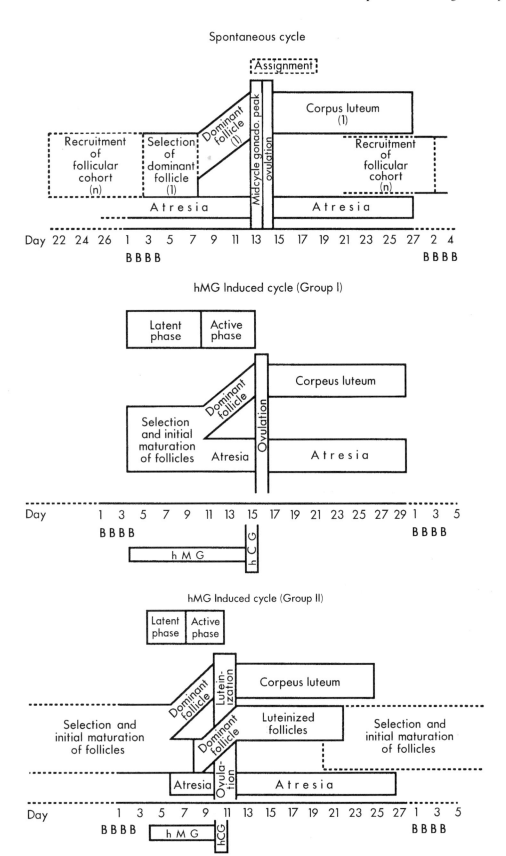

Fig. 33-5. Telescopic schematic presentation of different phases (selection, dominance, ovulation, and luteal phase) of spontaneous cycles and of stimulated cycles of amenorrheic women with hypothalamic-pituitary insufficiency (group I) and patients with hypothalamic-pituitary dysfunction (group II).

■ *Recruitment* (*rescue*) of a gonadotropin-dependent follicular cohort is brought about by a slight but significant FSH rise observed during the preceding late luteal phase. This process is usually completed by the third to fifth cycle day.

■ *Selection* of the dominant follicle is a process by which one follicle of the cohort is endowed with the ability to mature earlier and/or more quickly than all others. The exact mechanism of the selection process is not yet known. Our own theory is that the "assignment" of the follicle to be selected as the dominant one in the next cycle is brought about by the rescuing action of the midcycle FSH peak in the previous cycle, as well as by paracrine and autocrine events (growth factors, inhibin, activin, etc.). The process of selection of the dominant follicle is completed by the seventh cycle day.

■ *Dominance* is that part of the cycle when all the events, such as the exponential rise of estrogen, negative feedback action on the hypothalamus, modulation of pituitary secretion of gonadotropins, reduction of FSH secretion by inhibin, and positive feedback evoking the midcycle LH surge, are subordinated to the developmental rhythm of the dominant follicle. This controlling action of the dominant follicle lasts from the eighth cycle day until ovulation and persists also during the corpus luteum phase. The latent phase of gonadotropin therapy represents a "telescoped-in" version of the recruitment and selection phases of the spontaneous cycle. The active phase of therapy corresponds to the period of dominance.

The question of differences of response observed in patients of group I as compared with those of group II must now be briefly addressed. It is well known that in patients of group II the effective daily dose is smaller, the latent phase is shorter, and the response to treatment is less uniform.[90] It seems that these differences in response to stimulation with exogenous gonadotropins may be explained by the state of the ovary at the beginning of treatment.

In women of group I, at the initiation of each treatment course the ovaries are in a quiescent state with almost all follicles at a low stage of development. The pharmacologic dose of gonadotropins applied acts on a relatively uniform substrate. This is not so in patients of group II. In group II endogenous gonadotropins may cause a certain follicular development before or between treatments.

Gonadotropin therapy is thus applied to an ovary that already contains scores of follicles at various stages of development, provoking further growth of some of them, recruitment of additional ones, and atresia of others. No wonder that the response to treatment is less uniform and more prone to hyperstimulation. Gonadotropin therapy poses several interesting theoretic problems.

The exact size of the follicular cohort recruited in each cycle in women is not known. It is thus impossible to know whether gonadotropin therapy, using unphysiologic doses, provokes initial development of a larger cohort. Whatever the size of the initial cohort recruited, it seems that during the course of gonadotropin therapy additional follicles are stimulated and undergo partial or full maturation and others are rescued from atresia by the sustained high level of FSH. This process results in the development of several dominant follicles that reach full maturation hours or maybe even days apart one from the other. As indicated by the very low efficacy of single-dose or "trigger" schemes of therapy, to ensure follicular maturation during gonadotropin therapy relatively high FSH levels must be sustained throughout the treatment.

It is of interest to note that despite the somewhat high levels of estrogen occurring relatively early in the treatment, premature LH surges are rather rare.[44] This is true in patients with hypothalamic-pituitary failure (group I), but in patients with hypothalamic-pituitary dysfunction (group II) premature luteinization may occur in 25% of treatment cycles.[42] According to studies in primates,[112,118a] the hyperstimulated ovary may secrete a gonadotropin surge-inhibiting factor (different from inhibin), which blocks the LH surge triggered by the rising estrogen levels.

When using human gonadotropins for induction of ovulation one has to accept the fact that some features of spontaneous ovulatory cycles cannot be reproduced in gonadotropin-induced cycles. These features are as follows:

■ Premenstrual recruitment and initial selection of follicles
■ Feedback control of gonadotropin levels
■ Balanced effect of intraovarian sex steroids
■ Full maturation of one follicle only
■ Exact synchronization of structural, functional, and hormonal events throughout the entire genital system.

TREATMENT SCHEMES

A whole array of treatment schemes of gonadotropin therapy have been proposed and employed over the years. There are, however, only three essentially different types of therapy: (1) fixed-dose regimens, (2) individually adjusted schemes, and (3) combined therapy.

Fixed-dose regimen

In the fixed-dose regimens, a certain amount of hMG (or FSH) is administered on predetermined cycle days, followed by hCG given 1 day or more after the last injection of hMG or hPG. Although the dosages of gonadotropins and the days on which they were administered differed in various reports,[21,28,95] the general principles were identical. By using a fixed dose in each cycle, the patient's gonadotropin requirement (i.e., the effective daily dose) could be met only by successively increasing the dose in consecutive cycles.

Individually adjusted schemes

The individually adjusted treatment scheme[108] allows for successive increments of the gonadotropin dose according to the patient's response during the same cycle. It actually comprises the test course with the treatment course in one cycle, thus significantly increasing the efficiency of treatment (mean number of treatment courses per pregnancy). In some, particularly sensitive cases, the individually adjusted treatment scheme may avoid hyperstimulation that would have been brought about by using the fixed-dose schedule.

The problem of the size of initial dose of hMG (or FSH) and of its increments, as well as the ideal estrogen level to be arrived at before application of hCG, is still a matter of discussion. We usually start with two ampules of hMG per day in patients of group I and with one ampule in women belonging to group II. The successive dose increments are usually one ampule each, and hCG is administered when urinary estrogen reaches a level of 75 to 200 μg/24 hours or plasma estradiol attains a level of 300 to 900 pg/mL (Fig. 33-6).

It is interesting to note that with the advent of IVF programs, the whole circle of trial and error regarding the most efficient and safe treatment schemes of hMG was repeated. Different groups proposed fixed-dose schedules not much different from those that were tried and discarded years ago. Recently, however, more and more groups seem to adopt the individually adjusted treatment scheme, using some modifications suitable for the special purposes of an IVF program.[87,107]

For the sake of completeness, one additional mode of ovulation induction using human gonadotropins should be mentioned here. In 1983 Kemmann et al.[79] described their initial experience with a portable infusion pump delivering subdermally a constant amount of hMG over a period of 18 h/d. The authors claimed that with this method of delivery a better response was obtained than that obtained with the standard intramuscular injection of hMG.

Combined treatment

In the past most IVF programs used a combination of clomiphene citrate and hMG to stimulate a large-enough crop of follicles ready for ovum pickup. The claim was that this combination produced better, or at least more uniform, ovum maturation than did hMG alone. Proof for this claim, however, has not been established. Moreover, this mode of treatment is being abandoned because of the long half-life of clomiphene citrate and the high incidence of untimely LH surges.

It is well known that patients of group I respond better to gonadotropin therapy than do women of group II (Fig. 33-7). The efficiency of treatment (mean number of treatment courses per pregnancy) and the pregnancy rate are significantly better in the former group than in the latter group.[90] Some of the reasons for this discrepancy are obvious. First, patients of group II receive gonadotropin therapy only after they have failed to conceive when treated with other ovulation-inducing drugs. Second, the frequency of additional disturbances possibly affecting fertility, such as endometriosis, tubal factor, and polycystic ovaries, are much more frequent in group II.[90]

There are, however, differences in response to stimulation between patients of group I and those of group II that seem to be inherent to the functional characteristics of the hypothalamic-pituitary-ovarian axis. (See Principles of Gonadotropin Therapy.) In other words, with regard to gonadotropin therapy the presence of a functioning pituitary gland may be a disadvantage rather than an asset. To overcome the possible interference of untimely and/or unbalanced endogenous gonadotropin secretion, combined therapy using agents suppressing hypothalamic-pituitary function together with hMG or a purified FSH preparation was recommended.

Ben-Nun et al.[6] generated pharmacologic (drug-induced) hyperprolactinemia, causing a significant reduction of secretion and/or release of endogenous gonadotropins, and then stimulated the ovaries by exogenous hMG. They claimed that with this type of combined treatment ovulations and pregnancies could be obtained in several patients of group II who previously failed to conceive when treated with hMG/hCG alone. Laboratory synthesis of potent and/or long-acting analogues of GnRH makes it possible to efficiently reduce (down-regulate) the production and release of pituitary gonadotropins.[14,27,99,133] Treatment schemes combining pituitary suppression by GnRH analogues with ovarian stimulation by exogenous gonadotropins seemed therefore particularly attractive.

Even with the best protocols for inducing ovulation in anovulatory patients and superovulation in in vitro procedures, a number of patients may not ovulate. Of those who do ovulate, some produce poorly fertilizable eggs; in others, poor implantation may be observed. Some patients, even when given excessive amounts of gonadotropins, remain "poor" responders. Others (for example, those with PCOD) may be extremely sensitive to gonadotropins, responding to even very small amounts by producing multiple follicles whose growth is unsynchronized, culminating in various degrees of the ovarian hyperstimulation syndrome. During the last few years a number of new findings have emerged that may influence understanding of the ovarian cycle and ovulation-induction protocols. These include the following: (1) the effects of excessive LH in the follicular phase, (2) the effects of an untimely LH surge, (3) the role of growth factors in ovarian physiology and pathology, and (4) the role of growth factors and their binding proteins in regulating ovarian sensitivity and their possible connection with the pathogenesis of PCOD and the hyperstimulation syndrome.

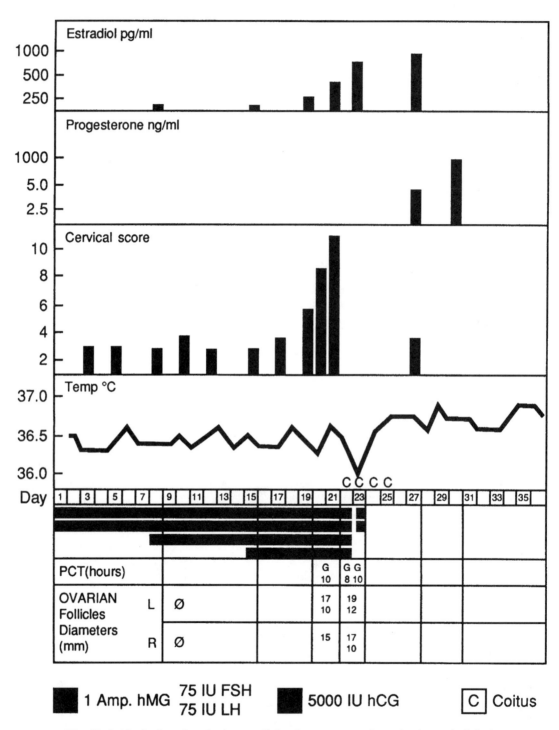

Fig. 33-6. Monitoring of cycles by estradiol and progesterone determination and clinical parameters (ultrasound and cervical score). Numbers at lower quadrant of figure represent hours postcoital (PCT) or the size of the follicles in mm.

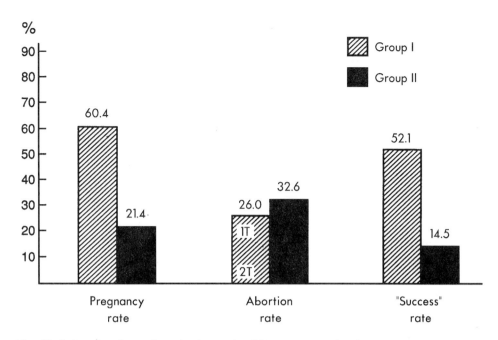

Fig. 33-7. Results of gonadotropin therapy in different groups of patients. *Pregnancy rate,* the percentage of patients who conceived during therapy; *1T,* first-trimester spontaneous abortions; *2T* second-trimester spontaneous abortions; *"success rate,"* the percentage of patients who took home at least one living child.

Effects of excessive luteinizing hormone in the follicular phase

Timely maturation of the oocyte is essential if fertilization and the development of an embryo are to occur. Before ovulation the chromosomes of the oocyte are arrested in the prophase stage of meiosis by an inhibiting factor that is itself inhibited by the action of LH at midcycle. This ensures the release of a mature egg at the appropriate time, that is, at ovulation.[125] Premature reactivation of meiosis caused by high basal concentrations of LH may lead to karyotypic abnormalities and death of the embryo and fetus.[109]

It has been suggested that a high concentration of LH through the follicular phase causes early maturation of the developing oocyte, producing at ovulation an egg that is physiologically aged.[62,63] These oocytes are unlikely to fertilize, but if conception is achieved early spontaneous abortion will result. Several investigators have reported that in IVF programs high concentrations of LH in the few days before oocytes are collected were associated with reduced rates of fertilization and conception.[64,96,106,120] McFaul et al.[96] suggested that exposure of the maturing oocyte to high levels of LH during follicular development is detrimental to fertilization and conception. These investigators[96] also demonstrated that, if conception is achieved in a cycle in which the oocyte is prematurely exposed to elevated LH levels there is a significantly higher probability that an early spontaneous abortion will result. According to McFaul et

al.,[96] this situation also occurs in patients diagnosed as having PCOD, in whom ovulation rates after ovulation induction are relatively high but pregnancy rates are low.

Johnson and Pearce[75] support this concept and conclude that pituitary suppression by GnRH analogues before induction of ovulation (reducing LH levels) reduces the risk of spontaneous abortion in women with PCOD and in patients with primary recurrent spontaneous abortion following induction of ovulation. Spontaneous abortion occurred in 11 of 20 women given clomiphene citrate, compared with only 2 of 20 who had pituitary suppression with buserelin followed by administration of pure FSH.

The reports just quoted permit the conclusion that an excessive endogenous LH environment may interfere with normal follicular development and might, by untimely inhibition of meiosis-inhibiting factors, provoke overaging of eggs with a significant reduction in their fertilization or implantation potential (Table 33-2). It has been shown that a definite correlation exists between mean LH levels in the follicular phase and the outcome of IVF.[64]

Infertile patients with pituitary or ovarian hypersensitivity (e.g., PCOD or PCOD-like patients) may benefit from ovulation-induction protocols using purified FSH preparations (e.g., Metrodin [Serono Laboratories]), which will decrease endogenous LH secretion and ensure a predominantly FSH environment during both the follicular recruitment and the follicular growth phase. The beneficial use of purified FSH, as expressed by pregnancy rate and by a

Table 33-2. Excessive LH in the follicular phase

May cause	Expression	Result
1. Excessive androgen production	Elevated intraovarian androgens	Abnormal follicular development
2. Excessive estrogen	Elevated intraovarian and serum estrogen	Negative influence on oocyte and embryo
		Negative influence on uterine receptivity
3. Premature luteinization	Elevation of progesterone prior to LH surge	Follicular luteinization
		Follicular atresia
		LUF* syndrome
4. Decrease of pituitary LH reserve	Diminished LH peak	Follicular luteinization
		Corpus luteum insufficiency
5. Inhibition of meiosis-inhibiting factor	Premature aging of oocyte	Unlikely to fertilize, implant, or survive

*LUF, Luteinized unruptured follicle.

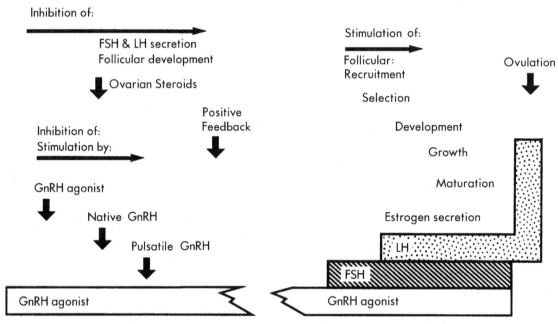

Fig. 33-8. The triphasic treatment scheme, comprising inhibition of the hypothalamic-pituitary-ovarian axis by GnRH agonist, stimulation of folliculogenesis by gonadotropins, and induction of ovulation by LH or hCG.

significant increase in the live birth rate, has also been adopted into the protocols for the induction of superovulation in IVF, GIFT, and intrauterine insemination (IUI).

Should this procedure not suffice, then desensitization of the pituitary with a GnRH agonist prior to follicular stimulation with gonadotropins may be necessary (Fig. 33-8). This will significantly inhibit the excessive LH production and normalize the endogenously induced abnormal hormonal environment. It will also inhibit the hypothalamic-pituitary-ovarian feedback system and prevent the occurrence of abnormal or premature LH surges. This, in turn, will permit stimulation of the ovary in tailor-made fashion, without hormonal interference from the patient's pituitary gland. If the ovaries of such patients are still capable of a normal response to gonadotropic stimulation, a correct and balanced FSH/hMG protocol will be adequate to recruit new crops of follicles, stimulate normal growth and development of the selected dominant follicles, and permit induction of ovulation of precisely matured follicles with hCG.

During the last few years many GnRH analogues became commercially available. Unfortunately, presently available analogues of GnRH are not deliverable orally. Nevertheless, progress has been made with alternatives to daily injection, first in the form of intranasal insufflation and then by potentially more compliance-compatible 1- to 3-month depot injectable formulations. However, not all patients respond to this triphasic regimen. In some of them

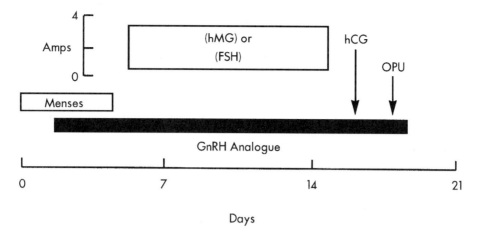

Fig. 33-9. Short protocol of GnRH analogue/hMG treatment. GnRH is started on day 2 to 4 after spontaneous or induced bleeding. The benefit of this treatment is economical because of the decreased gonadotropin dosage necessary for follicle stimulation. However, its disadvantages are an increased LH environment and an increased cancellation rate.

the ovaries are incapable of reacting normally to gonadotropic stimulation. The abnormal ovarian response to stimulation may result from any one (or a combination) of the following factors: abnormalities in the intraovarian compartment (e.g., overproduction of growth factors or lack of their binding proteins, imbalance of different P-450 enzymes), extragonadal influences (e.g., excessive adrenal androgens or decreased production of sex hormone-binding globulins [SHBG]) or metabolic disturbances due to obesity or hyperinsulinemia. A typical example of such a situation is PCOD. (See Chapter 11.)

Effects of an untimely luteinizing hormone surge

Premature luteinization is a specific category of anovulation. This entity frequently is unrecognized or is misdiagnosed as unexplained infertility or luteal phase defect. This situation can occur if an untimely LH surge occurs in response to rising estrogen levels at a time when the follicle is still immature. It can be diagnosed if an LH peak is detected in the presence of relatively small (<14 mm) follicles as demonstrated by ultrasonography.

It is possible that the etiology of this entity is an exaggerated sensitivity of the pituitary to estrogen. Rising, but relatively low estradiol (E_2) levels may evoke an LH surge. This assumption may explain the failure of clomiphene citrate or hMG to restore ovulation in such cases. Both agents cause multiple follicular development with an exaggerated estrogen rise, making the appearance of a premature LH peak even more likely. Therefore, the only rational therapy is to abolish the estrogen-evoked positive feedback mechanism. This can be effectively accomplished by the use of a potent GnRH agonist.[43,58,73] GnRH agonist is administered until the positive feedback is abolished. Although in about 75% of patients this will occur within 10

to 14 days, a short protocol should be avoided for the following reasons (Fig. 33-9): Although it will significantly reduce the amount of gonadotropins necessary for stimulation, due to the initial "flare up" effect, it will produce an exaggerated LH environment with an increase in ovarian androgens. These androgens may interfere with normal follicular development. Furthermore, it is estimated that with the short protocol in about 5% of cycles the premature LH peak is not prevented.

The long or intermediate protocol (Fig. 33-10) in which GnRH agonists are started in the midluteal phase 10 to 14 days before combined GnRH agonist/FSH/hMG administration is preferable, since in a progesterone-estrogen environment the initial stimulatory effect of the agonist will be reduced and thus the LH and resulting androgen environment will be diminished. With this protocol an endogenous premature LH peak is rare (occurring in less than 1% of cycles). The gonadotropin dosage necessary for ovulation or superovulation induction, however, is increased. FSH/hMG administration in conjunction with the agonist is continued until at least one follicle reaches maturation, as judged by ultrasonography and estrogen levels. hCG is then administered to induce ovulation.

A similar situation exists in ovulatory women with a normal pituitary-ovarian axis requiring IVF, GIFT, ZIFT, IUI, or artificial insemination by donor (AID). They receive pharmacologic doses of hMG/FSH to induce superovulation. The exaggerated E_2 levels in response to this therapy provoke in about 15% of treatment cycles an untimely spontaneous LH surge, leading to cancellation of ovum pickup or of the insemination procedure.

The possibility of desensitizing the pituitary gland with superactive GnRH analogues and thus inhibiting its capacity to respond to rising estradiol levels with an LH

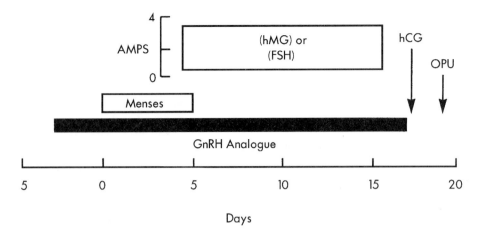

Fig. 33-10. Long (or intermediate) protocol of GnRH analogue/hMG treatment. GnRH is started during the luteal phase of the previous cycle, and hMG or FSH is started on day 2 to 5 after the beginning of bleeding. The benefit of this treatment is a decreased initial stimulation of the GnRH agonist, a decreased LH environment, and a decreased cancellation rate. The disadvantage of this protocol is the increased amount of medication necessary for follicular stimulation.

surge[43,116] has prompted many investigators to use GnRH analogues both prior to and in combination with FSH/hMG-hCG. The long protocol, starting with GnRH agonists 10 to 14 days before the FSH/hMG treatment regimen, has already proven its merits. By making logistics easier and by significantly reducing cancellation rates in IVF programs, it has increased the overall success rate. It allows the design of stimulation protocols creating a predominantly FSH environment during the recruitment phase and eliminating the interference of endogenous gonadotropins during the dominance and periovulatory phases. However, the temporary functional gonadotropin-specific hypophysectomy has introduced new challenges. Inhibition of endogenous gonadotropins following ovulation induced by hCG may, if not properly monitored, result in an inadequate luteal phase. This situation can usually be prevented by postovulatory periodic administration of hCG.

The choice of the GnRH analogue to be used should be based on a combination of factors, including its delivery system, its mode of administration, and its biologic half-life. All these criteria must be considered in designing the subsequent gonadotropin treatment protocol competent to stimulate follicular recruitment and development, timely ovulation induction, and adequate corpus luteum function.

Role of growth factors in ovarian physiology and pathology

Even with the best protocols for inducing ovulation in anovulatory patients or superovulion for in vitro procedures, some patients need excessive amounts of gonadotropins; despite this, some remain "poor" responders.

During the last few years the importance of intraovarian regulation via the potentiating effect of growth hormone (GH)-releasing factor (GRF), GH and growth factors, and insulin on both the thecal cell response to LH and the granulosa cell response to FSH has been demonstrated[1-3,30,37,74] (Fig. 33-11). These findings may have a significant impact on the understanding of ovulatory disorders such as PCOD, or on ovulation-inducing therapy and its main complication, the hyperstimulation syndrome.

Publications by Homberg et al.,[62,63] Volpe et al.,[128] and Barreca et al.[5] claimed that GH added to hMG protocols significantly reduces the hMG dose necessary for follicular stimulation. Ronnberg et al.,[111] however, could not confirm these findings in a study of ovulatory patients undergoing a randomized stimulation protocol for IVF. Based on our past and present studies, we believe that we can reconcile the discrepancy between these publications. We have shown that some patients with decreased levels of GH,[11] or anovulatory, normoprolactinemic, non–PCOD patients who are "bad responders" to gonadotropin stimulation and have a decreased level of GH reserve[100,101] may benefit from the addition of GH to gonadotropin stimulation protocols. The results of a prospective study demonstrated that patients who responded to clonidine or to arginine with elevation of GH responded normally to hMG therapy with a mean effective dose of 1.5 ampules per day (11.6 ampules mean total dose); patients who did not respond to clonidine with elevation of GH either needed excessive amounts of gonadotropins (mean effective dose of 3 ampules per day, mean total dose of 36.5 ampules) to obtain an acceptable response, or, despite higher doses of hMG, responded inadequately as expressed by either low serum E_2 levels or lack of sufficient follicular development, or both. The combined administration of GH and hMG to clonidine-negative patients resulted in a good ovarian response despite a significantly lower

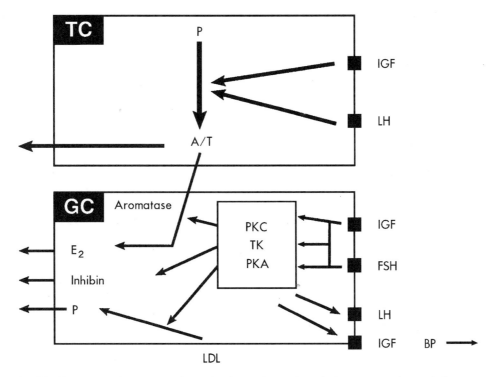

Fig. 33-11. Presumptive synergistic mechanisms of gonadotropic hormones and growth factors. Theca cells (*TC*): IGF-I enhances LH-induced androgen synthesis (*A/T*). Granulosa cells (*GC*): IGF-I and FSH enhance GC replication. IGF-I amplifies the following FSH effects: aromatase activity, LH receptor expression, progesterone (*P*) and estradiol (*E₂*) accumulation, and inhibin biosynthesis via cyclic AMP-dependent protein kinase (*PKA*), calcium–phospholipid-dependent protein kinase (*PKC*), and the tyrosine kinase (*TK*) systems. IGF-I binding protein (*IGF BP*) regulates IGF-I availability by competing for IGF-I binding sites. *LDL,* low-density lipoproteins.

dose of hMG. In clonidine-positive patients the addition of GH had no significant effect on response or hMG dosage (Fig. 33-12).

Role of growth factors and their binding proteins in regulating ovarian sensitivity

This study also demonstrated that the clonidine test might be a preliminary differentiating indicator of the relative sensitivity of patients to hMG. We think that it will help to select patients who might benefit from the concomitant GH-hMG therapy. One fact, however, should not be disregarded, namely, the connection between patients' body weight and their response to clonidine. Lean women have normal GH pulsatility and GH rise after application of clonidine. Obese patients may show negligible GH pulses and lack of response to clonidine, probably due to excess GH-binding protein (unpublished data). The usefulness of GH or GRF as adjunctive therapy with gonadotropins must not be overestimated, since insulin-like growth factor I (IGF-I) is not mandatory for normal ovarian response. It has been shown[35,82] that a Laron-type dwarf (an autosomal recessive syndrome characterized by elevated GH levels

concomitant with negligible serum IGF-I levels) can spontaneously ovulate, conceive, and deliver. This same patient, because of secondary infertility, was recently superovulated with gonadotropins for IVF, which permitted us to investigate her ovarian response in detail.[35] Despite undetectable GH-binding protein, negligible IGF-I, and elevated IGF-binding protein levels in her serum and follicular fluid, fertilizable eggs were obtained. This patient, who in effect provided an experiment of nature, together with IVF, permitted us to conclude that IGF-I is not obligatory for ovarian response but seems to play a permissive modulating role in ovarian physiology.

MONITORING OF THERAPY

Proper monitoring is crucial for the results of gonadotropin therapy, that is, for achieving a high rate of conceptions while avoiding hyperstimulation and reducing the incidence of multiple pregnancy to an acceptable minimum.

Rationale

Monitoring of the ovarian response to stimulation has four objectives:

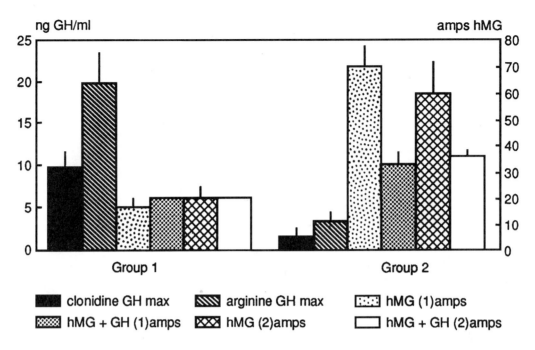

Fig. 33-12. Mean total dose ± SEM of hMG (number of ampules) in clondine- and/or arginine-positive and negative patients, with and without the addition of GH.

1. To determine the size of the effective daily dose of hMG
2. To determine the length of hMG application
3. To determine the suitability, size, and timing of administration of the ovulatory dose of hCG
4. To determine the occurrence and time of ovulation and to evaluate the corpus luteum function

Three different types of parameters are used in monitoring gonadotropin therapy: clinical, hormonal, and ultrasonic.

Clinical parameters include vaginal examination, basal body temperature (BBT) records, and cervical mucus evaluation expressed as a semiquantitative cervical score.[71,72] Hormone assays required for monitoring gonadotropin treatment consist of estrogen and progesterone estimations. The ultrasound examinations are aimed at determining the number and size of ovarian follicles and, if possible, also at observing their postovulatory transformation into corpora lutea.[23,53,110]

The latent phase of gonadotropin therapy is "mute" to hormonal monitoring. At that time neither the clinical nor the hormonal parameters can give an objective measure of the ovarian response to stimulation. The role of monitoring at this stage is to establish the size of the effective daily dose of hMG. This is done empirically by successively increasing the daily dose of hMG by one ampule every 5 to 7 days until a distinct ovarian response begins, as indicated by the initiation of steroidogenesis and by ultrasonically measurable follicular growth.

The main monitoring effort is centered at the active phase of treatment. The number of follicles developing and their growth rhythm must be established, and the time when at least one follicle is ready to receive the ovulatory LH stimulus must be determined as accurately as possible. The lessons learned from IVF indicate that in order to carry out this complicated task it is best to use all three monitoring parameters: clinical, ultrasonic, and hormonal. The number and diameter of follicles determined by ultrasound and the pattern of ascent of estrogen levels provide a good indication of the extent of follicular maturation. The clinical parameters (especially the cervical score), in addition to being an indirect indicator of estrogen levels, reflect the functional state of the genital tract with regard to sperm transport.

It has been shown repeatedly that both plasma 17β-estradiol and urinary total estrogen levels may be used for monitoring gonadotropin therapy with equal efficiency.[20,68,85] A steady exponential rise in urine or plasma estrogen is usually observed during the active phase of gonadotropin therapy. The ideal daily ascent rate is considered to be in the range of 40% to 100%. A slower ascent may reflect a suboptimal response, and a steeper daily increase is a warning sign of an exaggerated response, possibly heralding hyperstimulation.

For many years, the dominant follicle was considered to be the main source of estrogen, the contribution of smaller follicles being regarded as marginal. IVF and ultrasound proved that this is true in monofollicular cycles only. In cycles with multifollicular development, peripheral estrogen levels reflect the sum total of steroidogenic activity of several leading follicles as well as of a number of "runner-up" follicles. Nitschke-Dabelstein et al.[104] showed that an excellent correlation between the 17β-estradiol levels and the number and size of follicles observed on ultrasound examination could be found in monofollicular but not in multifollicular cycles. On the other hand, the follicular size as measured by ultrasound is inadequate as a sole parameter of follicular maturation, the functional integrity of the follicle probably being better expressed by its steroidogenic activity. This is the main reason for combining hormonal and ultrasonographic parameters in monitoring gonadotropin therapy. A steady daily increase in estrogen levels concomitant with a constant growth of follicular diameter on ultrasound assessment is the best indicator of successful ovarian stimulation, as well as a reasonably good predictor of hyperstimulation. Practical monitoring of gonadotropin treatment is carried out as follows.

Procedures

Patients are instructed to keep daily BBT records. Treatment is started between the third and fifth days of spontaneous or induced bleeding. If combined GnRH analogue-gonadotropin therapy is applied, the treatment is started when a sufficient pituitary-ovarian down-regulation has been obtained (i.e., plasma estrogen concentration does not exceed 30 pg/mL). The initial hMG dose is usually one ampule per day in patients of group II. In women of group I and in patients receiving the combined therapy, treatment is usually started with two ampules per day. If the patient had received gonadotropin therapy in the past, treatment is usually started at the level of the effective daily dose (EDD) of the previous course.

Before initiation of every course of treatment an ultrasonographic scan of the pelvic region is performed in order to rule out the presence of abnormal follicular structures or cysts. Since such structures may interfere with the ovarian response to stimulation, they should be punctured or the treatment should be delayed until their spontaneous disappearance.

Patients are examined every 1 to 3 days. This examination includes palpation of the ovaries, estimation of cervical score, postcoital tests when indicated, and a short interview with the patient regarding her general well-being. The dose of gonadotropins is adjusted according to the patient's response as indicated by estrogen levels, ultrasonography, and clinical findings.

If estrogen levels are low and are not rising, the initial dose of gonadotropins is continued for 5 to 7 days and then increased by one ampule. This procedure is repeated until the EDD (i.e., the dose that causes a significant and steady increase in estrogen level is achieved). In patients with low endogenous estrogens at initiation of therapy, cervical score estimations may replace estrogen assays for the estimation of EDD. From this day on the patient is examined daily or on alternate days. When estrogen levels reach or exceed 250 pg/mL, ultrasonography is performed. If estrogen levels increase too rapidly or the day-to-day difference exceeds the geometric rise, the dose is reduced by one ampule (75 IU of FSH) and treatment is continued at this reduced dosage. If the estrogen rise is steady and not excessive, the same dose is continued until a level of between 350 and 1200 pg/mL is reached.

Since the duration of the active phase is 4 to 6 days, this level should be reached within this time limit. At this stage of therapy the third ultrasonographic scan is performed. If, in both ovaries, the total number of measurable follicular structures does not exceed 10 and, 1 to 4 follicles have a diameter exceeding 17 mm, the ovulatory dose of hCG (10,000 IU) is administered. The patient is advised to have intercourse on 3 consecutive days starting on the day of hCG administration. After induction of ovulation the patient is examined 3 to 5 and 7 to 9 days after the hCG injection. Special care is taken not to overlook possible ovarian enlargement, abdominal pains, tenderness or distention, and weight gain exceeding 3 kg. At least one blood sample is drawn and sent for progesterone assay. The patient is instructed to report back to the clinic if abdominal pains, nausea, vomiting, or diarrhea appear. If a sustained high phase of BBT lasts for more than 14 days, hCG and progesterone assays should be performed.

No consensus has been reached with regard to exogenous hormonal support of the corpus luteum function after induction of ovulation. Some authors advise supporting the corpus luteum by administering progesterone by intramuscular injection or vaginal suppository. Others suggest two or three booster injections of 2500 to 5000 IU of hCG on days 5 and 7 after ovulation induction. This suggestion is based on two factors: the half-life of exogenous hCG is 6 to 8 hours and the endogenous hCG secreted by the trophoblast is detectable from day 7 to day 9 after ovulation. The additional hCG injections may be of special importance in patients of group I and after combined GnRH analogue-gonadotropin therapy.

Clinical research and experience have shown that in gonadotropin therapy multifollicular and multiluteal cycles are a rule rather than an exception.[68] However, only a small proportion of the multiluteal cycles results also in multiple clinical pregnancies. Brown[20] remarked that although multiple preovulatory follicles were seen by ultrasound in 50% of gonadotropin-induced cycles, the recorded multiple pregnancy rate was only 20%. O'Herlihy et al.[105] showed that multiple preovulatory follicles were found in 71% of clomiphene cycles, but the incidence of multiple pregnancy was only 14%. It is thus probable that in hMG-induced conception cycles a number of ova are usually released and possibly fertilized, but only one or two of them are destined to produce a fetus.

The IVF programs introduced a very important contribution to the management of gonadotropin therapy, particularly when multiple follicles are stimulated. Some of the excessive follicles may be punctured under ultrasound control, thus reducing the E_2 levels, leaving a smaller number of follicles to be luteinized by the hCG administration and diminishing the chance of clinical hyperstimulation.

COMPLICATIONS AND RESULTS OF GONADOTROPIN THERAPY

All complications of gonadotropin treatment are essentially due to ovarian stimulation, follicular development and luteinization, or ovulation. To the best of our knowledge direct side effects to the drug itself have not been reported. The main complications of gonadotropin treatment are (1) ovarian hyperstimulation syndrome (see Chapter 35), (2) high incidence of multiple pregnancy, and (3) spontaneous abortion rate higher than that in natural conceptions.

Hyperstimulation

Analysis of several large series encompassing 11,342 treatment cycles showed that the incidences of moderate and severe hyperstimulation were 3.4% and 0.84%, respectively (Table 33-3). It should be noted that all these series included cases treated without ultrasonographic monitoring. The influence of patient selection, treatment schedules, and monitoring methods on the relative risks of hyperstimulation have been discussed in previous sections. (See Selection of Patients, Treatment Schemes, and Monitoring of Therapy.) It is true that only some of the patients who received hCG, despite inappropriate increases or excessive levels of estrogen, developed ovarian hyperstimulation.[113] It is certain, however, that all women who did develop the syndrome had abnormally high preovulatory estrogen levels. Only future statistical analyses will demonstrate whether the additional use of ultrasonography will enable a further reduction in the rate of hyperstimulation or multiple births.

Multiple pregnancy

Multiple pregnancy is rather frequent after gonadotropin therapy. Brown[20] reviewed 1712 pregnancies resulting from ovulation induction by hPG or hMG and found that the average multiple pregnancy rate was 24.4%, fluctuating between 21% and 33%. As expected, small series showed a lower incidence of multiple gestations than did large series. The cause of multiple conceptions after induced cycles is very similar to that causing ovarian hyperstimulation, that is, the pharmacologic stimulation of multifollicular development. Thus the risk factors and the possibilities of avoiding (or at least reducing the incidence) of both complications are similar. (See Hyperstimulation.) Insler and Potashnik[68] reported that in 26% of gonadotropin-induced cycles three or more functional corpora lutea were produced and that mean plateau progesterone levels were

Table 33-3. The incidence of hyperstimulation after gonadotropin therapy

Authors	No. of treatment cycles	Mild hyperstimulation (%)	Severe hyperstimulation (%)
Australian Department of Health[4]	4008	3.7	0.9
Caspi et al.[25]	343	6.0	1.2
Ellis and Williamson[36]	322	5.0	0.6
Spadoni et al.[119]	225	4.4	1.8
Thompson and Hansen[123]	2798	?	1.3
Lunenfeld et al.[92]	3232	3.1	0.25
TOTAL	10928	3.4	0.84

higher in the conceptional cycles than in the nonconceptional cycles. Further analysis of the above data indicated that in hMG treatment cycles conception occurs in most cases in the presence of more than one corpus luteum and in one fourth of cases in the presence of three or more functioning corpora lutea. Since only around 25% of gonadotropin-induced pregnancies result in twins and only 5% produce three or more fetuses, and since the mean plateau progesterone levels are similar in single and multiple hMG-induced pregnancies, it could be speculated that in the majority of hMG conceptions a number of ova are released and fertilized but only one of them is destined to produce a living fetus. The others perish before reaching the uterine cavity or are absorbed or extruded before implantation. If, however, a quadruplet or quintuplet pregnancy reaches the gestational age of 7 to 8 weeks, its further development may represent a severe danger to the fetuses because of a very high probability of extreme prematurity, a considerable medical complication to the mother, and a pronounced psychologic social and financial burden to the family. A technique of fetal reduction under ultrasonographic control has been developed. Breckwoldt et al.[18] reported a gonadotropin-induced pregnancy with eight gestational sacs present in the uterus. Six of the fetuses were eliminated under ultrasonographic guidance. This technique, although medically simple and logical, is still controversial for ethical, legal, and religious reasons.

Spontaneous abortion

The spontaneous abortion rate in conceptions following gonadotropin therapy is approximately 21% (Table 33-4). Brown[20] compiled and reviewed a series of 1712 pregnancies and found that the combined spontaneous abortion and perinatal deaths rates fluctuated from 10% to 28% in different reports.

There was no significant difference in the spontaneous abortion rate in relation to diagnostic groups. The rate was 26% in patients of group I and 32.6% in women of group II,

Table 33-4. Spontaneous abortion rates in pregnancies after ovulation induction with hMG/hCG

Authors	Year	No. of patients	No. of pregnancies	Spontaneous abortions (%)
Bettendorf et al.[9]	1981	756	239 (9)	21.7
Australian Department of Health[4]	1981	1065	552	14.6
Caspi et al.[24]	1976	101	62	28
Ellis and Williamson[36]	1975	77	43	12
Spadoni et al.[119]	1974	62	26	31
Lunenfeld et al.[93]	1981	1107	424 (52)	25.2

Numbers in brackets are multiple pregnancies.

respectively.[10] However, the spontaneous abortion rate in the first conception cycle (28.8%) was significantly higher than that in the second or third gestation (12.8%). The main reasons for increased spontaneous abortion rates in conceptions resulting from induction of ovulation have been presumed to be (1) structural and functional inadequacy of the endometrium to ensure proper and timely nidation of the embryo; (2) functional incompetence of the corpus luteum, preventing it from proper reaction to the pregnancy signal (i.e., the initial increase in hCG level produced by the trophoblast); (3) multiple pregnancy; and (4) emotional factors. An in-depth analysis of the literature, however, seems to indicate that the dominant cause of early pregnancy wastage in conceptions resulting from ovarian stimulation is the poor quality of ova, which, in turn, depends on the nature of follicular environment during follicular maturation. This conclusion is also strongly supported by analysis of the fate of spontaneous pregnancies. According to Chard[25a] only 30% of natural conceptions produce a term pregnancy.

Conception rates

Conception rates after gonadotropin therapy are dependent on the following factors (in order of importance): (1) selection of patients, (2) type of monitoring, and (3) treatment scheme. In women with hypothalamic-pituitary failure (group I), substitution therapy with gonadotropins is very efficient in inducing ovulation and pregnancy. Gonadotropin treatment applied as stimulation therapy in patients having some, albeit deranged, hypothalamic-pituitary-gonadal function (group II) is by far more complicated and less efficient. (See Treatment Schemes.) Although in patients of group I pregnancy rates of up to 82% were achieved, in group II conception rates varied between 20% and 35%.[4,9,90,92] The same discrepancy was also seen when cumulative pregnancy rates were calculated by using the life-table analysis method. In group I, after six cycles of therapy, the cumulative pregnancy rate exceeded 90%. In contrast, patients of group II required 12 cycles of therapy in order to reach a cumulative conception rate of less than 60%.

Age of the patients also influences the outcome of treatment markedly. Women over 35 years of age had a significantly reduced conception rate regardless of the type of diagnosis and treatment.[69] The duration of amenorrhea, on the other hand, had no bearing on the results of gonadotropin therapy. The treatment was as efficient in women who had been amenorrheic for only 1 year as it was in those who had been amenorrheic for 10 years or more (unpublished data).

Table 33-1 shows the results of gonadotropin therapy as reported by 15 different groups working independently on four continents. This list does not purport to include all data on gonadotropin therapy published thus far. It shows, nevertheless, the overall dimension of this therapy and its importance in the therapeutic armamentarium of fertility clinics throughout the world. The list includes 22,000 treatment courses given to more than 8,000 women and nearly 3,000 conceptions. Since most entries deal with rather large groups of patients, this summary represents the results of gonadotropin treatment among unselected patients typical of busy fertility clinics. The pregnancy rates (per patient) ranged between 23.1% and 82.5%, with an average of 35.4%. Pregnancy rates per cycle ranged from 7.1% to 22.5%. The intensity of treatment (the mean number of treatment courses per patient) fluctuated from 2.0 to 4.2. By knowing the pregnancy rate per cycle specific to each clinic, one can easily calculate the overall prognosis and cost of this treatment.

Outcome of pregnancies. The course of gestation after induction of ovulation with hMG appeared to be normal. Analysis of the mode of delivery showed a high incidence of interventions, breech extraction, vacuum extraction, forceps delivery, and cesarean delivery. The high incidence of obstetric intervention may be explained by elevated multiple pregnancy rates, primiparity ratios, relatively high maternal age, and psychologic factors involved in delivering a "premium child" to patients with longstanding infertility.

Our 1987 study[89] showed that the sex ratio (M:F) of single births was 1.06 (54% boys) and of twins 0.72 (42% boys). The numbers of triplets were too small to analyze. In 1976 Caspi et al.[24] reported 32 males and 50 females among single births (39%) and a twin M:F ratio of 0.78. In the series reported by Bettendorf et al.,[9] the incidence of male children in single pregnancies was 51.8%. However,

Table 33-5. Congenital malformations after induction of ovulation with hMG/hCG

Authors	No. of births	No. of major malformations	No. of minor malformations
Kurachi[80a] (1985)	509	9	1
Hack and Lunenfeld[52] (1978)	209	4	4
Caspi et al.[24] (1976)	157	4	11
Harlap[54] (1976)	66	1	5
TOTAL	941	18 (1.91%)	21 (2.23%)
NORMAL POPULATION		1.27% (0.31%–2.25%)	7.24%

in that series the incidences of male children in twins and triplets were 53.8% and 66.7%, respectively. The normal secondary sex ratio at 28 weeks of gestation is considered to be 106 boys to 100 girls.[115,124] The sex ratio (M:F) for twins was found by Nicols[103] to be 1.043; for triplets, 1.007; and for quadruplets, 0.940. The high incidence of girls in our twin series and the high incidence of male children in twins and triplets in the series of Bettendorf et al.[9] are probably due to the rather small numbers involved. By combining all three series, one approaches the expected sex ratios, indicating clearly the importance of sufficiently large numbers in order to estimate similarities or divergencies in sex ratio.

Congenital malformations

Table 33-5 shows the rate of congenital malformations found in combined series of 941 babies born after induction of ovulation with hMG/hCG. The incidences were 22.3/1000 and 19.1/1000 of minor and major malformations, respectively. The incidence of congenital malformations in normal populations has been reported to be 12.7/1000 after 28 weeks of gestation, with a range of 3.1 to 22.5/1000.[98,121] There is a further rise to 23.1/1000 by the age of 5 years. Hendricks[59] reported a rate of 3% in the neonatal period, with twice as many malformations in twin births, mostly monozygotic twins. Shoham et al.[116a] reviewed a large number of reports dealing with congenital malformations in children born after induction of ovulation and concluded that clomiphene citrate, hMH/hCG, or the association of these drugs with IVF-ET and GIFT procedures do not carry an increased risk for congenital malformations as a whole, nor is there any specific malformation that has an increased incidence or is related in any way with the use of those drugs. It can thus be summarized that, at present, the clinical evidence does not indicate that babies born after hMG/hCG ovulation induction are at any greater risk of malformation than is the general population.

LONG-TERM SAFETY OF GONADOTROPIN THERAPY

Nulliparity has been a consistently reported risk factor for carcinoma of the breast and endometrium.[19,77,78,83,110a] With regard to cancer incidence among the 1438 functionally infertile patients in our 1987 series,[89] the rate of hormone-associated tumors was 1.5 times the expected rate. For carcinoma of the breast it was 1.4 and for endometrial cancer 8.0. In an attempt to assess whether risk factors could be linked to different etiologies within this heterogeneous group, these infertile patients were analyzed according to types: (1) amenorrheic patients with low endogenous estrogen and gonadotropin levels (141 women); (2) infertile patients having normal estrogen and postovulatory progesterone levels whose infertility was due to mechanical factors, male factor, or unexplained infertility (712 women); (3) amenorrheic or anovulatory patients displaying endogenous estrogens, but lacking or having less than normal postovulatory progesterone (992 women).

In the amenorrheic group of 141 patients with low endogenous estrogen and gonadotropins, the observed hormone-associated cancer rate was lower than the expected rate for all sites. Not a single case of breast, endometrial, or other hormone-associated cancer was detected (although 1.68 were expected) in patients of this group, independent of whether hMG/hCG therapy was followed by pregnancy or not.

In the 712 women with infertility due to mechanical or male factors and displaying both estrogen and postovulatory progesterone, no increased risk for hormone-associated cancer was observed.

In the 992 amenorrheic or anovulatory women who had fluctuating estrogen levels but lacked sufficient postovulatory progesterone, the observed rates of uterine and breast cancer were 10.3 and 1.8 times the expected rate. Of this group, 385 women were treated with hMG/hCG; 198 conceived and in 187 cases no record of conception exists.

In the former group not a single case of breast or uterine cancer was observed. On the other hand, in the 187 women who failed to conceive, the observed breast and uterine cancer rates were 2.83 and 28.57 times, respectively, higher than the expected rates.

These data indicate that hMG/hCG therapy does not increase the risk for cancer. Because the number of women receiving each specific treatment was small and the majority of patients has not yet reached the age of the maximal cancer risk, the statistical power to detect minor effects of treatment was low. However, a large cancer risk would certainly have been detected. It seems from the results presented that, among the infertile patients, only anovulatory women with unopposed estrogens are at increased risk for uterine and breast cancer. In these patients induction of ovulation with hMG/hCG followed by conception seems to reduce the risk.

In the last decades, a multitude of epidemiologic studies have been reported on the association of ovarian cancer with environmental factors, with hereditary factors, and with factors related to reproductive history. However, conclusive etiologic studies are scarce for the following reasons: (1) all examined associations appeared to be weak; (2) the etiology of ovarian cancer appeared to be multifactorial (this implies that considerable numbers of patients are needed to reach the threshold of statistical significance); and (3) based on the prevalence of ovarian carcinoma in the general population, it is difficult to find enough cases to undertake an epidemiologic study.

Several investigators have identified infertility as an independent risk factor in addition to the nulliparity effect. Whittemore et al.[129] called it "the ability to conceive," and found a significant correlation between the number of years of unprotected intercourse and the risk of ovarian cancer. Joly et al.,[76] like Nasca et al.[102] and McGowan et al.[97] calculated the pregnancy rates per 1000 woman-years at risk of pregnancy. All found significantly higher rates in control subjects than in infertile patients.

Hartge et al.[55] showed that infertile nulliparous women with a history of infertility had a 2.8 times higher risk than nulliparous women without such a history; Harlow[54a] estimated this figure to be much higher, a factor of 6. Booth[13a] concluded that the risk for ovarian cancer in nulligravid women with more than 10 years of unprotected intercourse is 6.5 times higher than in nulligravid women with less than 5 years of unprotected intercourse. Whittemore et al.[129] found a relative risk of 1.8 for the same risk factor in all women, regardless of parity.

The above findings are confirmed by the observations of Lais et al.,[81] who found 6 ovarian malignancies in 571 consecutive patients who underwent microsurgery for infertility. Five of the six patients were nulligravid. Of the five patients who had undergone laparoscopy some months previously, results in three had been negative; in two, small "trivial" lesions had been reported. This prevalence figure is grossly 10 times higher than the figure that was observed in general abdominal surgery or in pregnancy.[123a]

Hartge et al.[55] (296 cases and 343 controls) found a clear difference in cancer risk between unmarried nulliparous women (no risk increase) and married nulliparous women (70% risk increase). When they considered specifically nulliparous women who tried but failed to conceive, the risk ratio was 2.8. Hartke et al. thus demonstrated that infertility by itself is associated with an increased risk in addition to the effect of nulliparity.

Cramer et al.[26] (215 cases and 215 controls) did not find an effect of infertility only. They found a 2.5 times higher risk in nulliparous women. They also found an increased risk associated with postmenopausal estrogen replacement therapy.

Nasca et al.[102] (403 cases and 806 controls) concentrated on the infertility factor. They calculated the ratio of total pregnancies to the number of contraception-free years of marriage for each group. They found this ratio to be significantly lower in cancer patients (indicating an increasing risk with decreasing fertility). Their figures closely matched the findings of McGowan et al.[97] Nasca et al.[102] concluded that infertility played an important role in the relationship between gravidity/parity and ovarian cancer risk. Fertility drugs were not mentioned in this article. Joly et al.[76] did a case-control study of ovarian carcinoma and found a consistent risk increase linked with infertility. Their data were collected between 1957 and 1965, that is, before current use of fertility drugs.

In a recent publication Whittemore et al.,[130] using a large combined data set derived from case-control studies in the United States, interpreted their findings to show that an increased risk of ovarian cancer associated with infertility may be due in part to the use of fertility drugs.

The global study population of the three studies used by Whittemore et al.[130] in their analysis was 2278 women, of whom only 1723 were included in the analysis. The data related to infertility drugs were calculated from 20 never-married patients with invasive epithelial ovarian cancer treated with infertility drugs and 11 controls. This very small number of cases is responsible for the extremely wide 95% confidence interval of 2.3 to 315.6 with a mean risk of 27.0 for women who, despite receiving fertility drugs, did not conceive. Conception reduced this risk to levels of fertile controls. The study also found an increased relative risk for epithelial ovarian cancer of low malignant potential among women who had used fertility drugs. The mean relative risk for this group was 4.0 with 95% confidence limits of 1.1 to 13.9, based on four cases and nine controls.

If one translates the estimates of Whittemore et al.[130] into absolute figures, then the added risk of cancer possibility being attributable to fertility drugs would be approximately 8.3/100,000 (1 in 12,000/year) at ages 30 to 34 and

21.1/100,000 (1 in 5,000) for ages 40 to 44. This absolute risk would have to be balanced, however, against the benefit of achieving a birth.

Induction of ovulation with human gonadotropins is a well-established therapeutic modality. Its efficacy is unequivocal in women with hypothalamic-pituitary failure (group I). In patients with hypothalamic-pituitary dysfunction (group II), gonadotropin treatment, although less efficient than in group I, represents an additional therapeutic possibility, over and above that offered by other ovulation-inducing agents.

New insights provided by the introduction of ultrasonography and IVF and the constant search for better treatment schemes such as combined GnRH analogues-gonadotropin therapy constitute a firm basis for the prediction that, in the near future, gonadotropin therapy will become as efficient in group II as it now is in group I.

EPILOGUE

In the past gonadotropins were considered highly potent ovulation-inducing agents for first-line therapy in amenorheic patients with hypopituitary hypogonadism and as second-line therapy in anovulatory patients who failed to conceive with clomiphene citrate. Because of their potential to induce superovulation, their use since the early 1980s has expanded exponentially as the preferred drug in IVF, GIFT, and IUI programs.

In recent years it has been shown that an excess of LH during the early or late stages of folliculogenesis may have adverse effects on both the follicle and the oocyte, may interfere in conception, and may be a causal factor in early pregnancy loss. The possible adverse affects of LH are summarized in Table 33-3. These findings have prompted many investigators and clinicians to redesign protocols for ovulation and superovulation induction that safeguard against elevated LH levels. These protocols include administration of agents that reduce endogenous LH secretion and the use of predominantly FSH-containing preparations. The technical developments that have led to the production of highly purified FSH (Metrodin HP) and a deeper understanding of the pharmacodynamics and pharmacokinetics of these preparations have made it possible to redesign ovulation-inducing protocols (for example, low-dose regimens, low-dose increments, subcutaneous injection route). These new protocols may prove to be more efficient and may result in fewer multiple pregnancies, a lower spontaneous abortion rate, and an even lower risk of hyperstimulation.

With the use of a highly purified FSH preparation, a reevaluation of the role of estrogen as a marker of follicular development may be necessary. Now that highly purified urinary FSH preparations containing about 9000 IU of FSH per milligram of protein are becoming accessible, we are asking ourselves how we were able to use the earlier preparations containing 100 to 200 IU of FSH per milli-

gram of protein. These new and highly purified urinary preparations will surely replace both Pergonal and Metrodin within the next 2 years.

From figures published by the United Nations Population Division it can be estimated that during the last decade of this century in the developed world the population of women between the ages of 19 and 34 will be about 130 million. If we assume that at least 8% will be infertile, then the pool of the infertile population can be estimated to be above 10 million, with about 700,000 new patients entering this pool every year between the years 1990 and 1995. If for the purpose of this intellectual exercise we assume that gonadotropins represent a potential benefit for 5% of this infertile population as a first-line therapy, for 70% of the clomiphene failures, and for 45% of patients with infertility potentially treatable with IVF, GIFT, or IUI (due to mechanical factors or male partner problems), then the potential gonadotropin users theoretically could include nearly 7.5 million women with about half a million new patients every year.

The future of infertility therapy clearly relies on the capacity to produce pharmaceutical-grade gonadotropins in sufficient quantities to meet this ever-increasing worldwide demand. It has recently been shown that expression of a human FSH dimer could be achieved by transfecting Chinese hamster ovary cells with a genomic clone containing the complete β-FSH coding sequence together with the α-subunit minigene. The resulting recombinant FSH was more homogenous than the most purified pituitary FSH preparations, providing a basis for clinical use. The use of such recombinant FSH ovulation induction followed by pregnancies has been reported,[32,49] and the first set of healthy twins was born in the autumn of 1992.

With recombinant DNA technology and highly defined cell culture techniques using recombinant DNA, gonadotropins are now being prepared on an industrial scale. What would currently require 200 million liters of urine per year will ultimately be produced by genetically engineered cells in a chemically defined culture medium comprising only a small fraction of that volume. It is our hope that in the not-too-distant future DNA technology will provide an almost endless supply of human gonadotropins.

Moreover, recombinant DNA technology permits the design of potentially therapeutically active gonadotropin agonists and antagonists by altering key proteins and carbohydrate regions in the α- and β-subunits of FSH and LH.[12] FSH has a relatively short half-life and hCG a relatively long half-life. The long half-life of hCG is in part due to the presence of four serine O-linked oligosaccharides attached to an extended hydrophilic carboxy terminus. By using site-directed mutagenesis and gene transfer techniques it was possible to fuse the carboxy-terminal extension of β-hCG (CTP) to the 3′ end of the FSH coding sequence. The FSH-CTP fusion protein retained the same biologic activity as native FSH in vivo but had a prolonged circulating half-life. This resulted in a significant higher in vivo potency than native FSH and may represent an obvious candidate for a long-acting FSH agonist.[38,39]

Alternatively, deglycosylated mutants of this chimera can be engineered and, together with a deglycosylated α-subunit, could, by competitive binding to gonadotropin receptors, result in potent gonadotropin antagonists.[12]

When such recombinant FSH preparations reach the market, hMG and urinary FSH will have served their purpose, and the story of urinary gonadotropins will become history. If our modern society accepts the challenge of enabling every woman who desires it to experience the joy of motherhood, then industry will have to make the effort to solve the production problem, society will have to bear the cost, and the medical profession will have to provide the appropriate services.

REFERENCES

1. Adashi EY et al: Insulin-like growth factors as intraovarian regulators of granulosa cell growth and function, *Endocr Rev* 6:400, 1985.
2. Adashi EY et al: Somatomedin C synergizes with FSH in the acquisition of projection biosynthetic capacity by cultured rat granulosa cells, *Endocrinology* 116:2135, 1985.
3. Adashi EY et al: Somatomedin C enhances induction of LH receptors by FSH in cultured rat granulosa cells, *Endocrinology* 116:2369, 1985.
4. Australian Department of Health: Computer printout: the Human Pituitary Advisory Committee, courtesy of Prof R Shearman. Canberra, Australia, 1981, The Department.
5. Barreca A et al: Insulin like growth factor-I (IGF-I) and IGF-I binding protein in follicular fluids of growth hormone treated patients, *Clin Endocrinol* 32:497, 1990.
6. Ben-Nun I, Lunenfeld B, Ben-Aderet N: Prevention de la luteinisation premature du follicule par hyperprolactinemie iatrogene volontaire au cours des traitements par HMG hormons, *Reprod Med* 5:54, 1984.
7. Bettendorf G: Ovarian stimulation in hypophysectomized patients by human gonadotropins. In *Proceedings of the Fifth World Congress on Fertility and Sterility,* Amsterdam, 1966, Excerpta Medica, p 53.
8. Bettendorf G, Apostolakis M, Voigt KD: Darstellung hochaktiver gonadotropin fraktionen aus menschlichen hypophysen und deren anwendung beim menschen. In *Proceedings of the International Federation of Gynecologists and Obstetricians,* Vienna, 1961, p. 76.
9. Bettendorf G et al: Overall results of gonadotropin therapy. In Insler V, Bettendorf G, editors: *Advances in diagnosis and treatment of infertility,* New York, 1981, Elsevier/North-Holland.
10. Blankstein J, Mashiach S, Lunenfeld B: *Ovulation induction and in vitro fertilization,* Chicago, 1986, Year Book.
11. Blumenfeld Z, Lunenfeld B: The potential effect of growth hormone on follicle stimulation with human menopausal gonadotropin in a panhypopituitary patient, *Fertil Steril* 52:328, 1989.
12. Boime I et al: Expression of recombinant human FSH, LH, and CG in mammalian cells: a model for probing functional determinants. In Hunzicker-Dunn M, Schwarz NB, editors: *Follicle stimulating hormone: regulation of secretion and molecular mechanisms of action,* New York, 1990, Springer-Verlag.
13. Boorstein WR, Vamvakopoulos NK, Fiddes JC: Human chorionic gonadotropin beta subunit is encoded by at least eight genes arranged in tandem and inverted pairs, *Nature* 300:419, 1982.
13a. Booth M, Beral V, Smith P: Risk-factors for ovarian cancer: a case-control study, *Br J Cancer* 60:592, 1989.
14. Borgman V et al: Sustained suppression of testosterone production by the luteinizing hormone-releasing hormone agonist, buserelin, patients with advanced prostate carcinoma, *Lancet* 1:1097, 1982.
15. Borth R, Lunenfeld B, Menzi A: Pharmacologic and clinical effects of a gonadotropin preparation from human postmenopausal urine. In Albert A, Thomas MC, editors: *Human pituitary gonadotropins,* Springfield, Ill, 1961, Charles C Thomas.
16. Borth R, Lunenfeld B, de Watteville H: Activite gonadotrope d'un extrait d'urines de femmes en menopause, *Experientia* 10:266, 1954.
17. Borth R et al: Activite gonadotrope d'un extrait des femmes en menopause, *Experientia* 13:115, 1957.
18. Breckwoldt M et al: Induction of ovulation by combined GnRH-A/hMG/hCG treatment. Presented at the International Symposium on GnRH Analogues in Cancer and Human Reproduction, Geneva, Switzerland, 1988 (abstract 058).
19. Brinton LA, Hoover R, Fraumeni JF Jr: Reproductive factors in the aetiology of breast cancer, *Br J Cancer* 47:757, 1983.
20. Brown JB: Gonadotropins. In Insler V, Lunenfeld B, editors: *Infertility: male and female,* London, 1986, Churchill Livingstone.
21. Butler JK: Oestrone response patterns and clinical results following various Pergonal dosage schedules. In Butler JK, editor: *Developments in the pharmacology and clinical uses of human gonadotropins,* High Wycombe, UK, 1970, GD Searle.
22. Butt WR, Kennedy JF: Structure-activity relationships of protein and polypeptide hormones. In Margoulis M, Greenwood FC, editors: *Protein and polypeptide hormones,* Amsterdam, 1971, Excerpta Medica.
23. Cabau A, Bessis R: Monitoring of ovulation induction with human menopausal gonadotropin and human chorionic gonadotropin by ultrasound, *Fertil Steril* 36:178, 1981.
24. Caspi E, Ronen J, Schreyer P: Pregnancy and infant outcome after gonadotropin therapy, *Br J Obstet Gynaecol* 83:967, 1976.
25. Caspi E et al: Induction of pregnancy with human gonadotropins after clomiphene failure in menstruating ovulatory infertility patients, *Isr J Med Sci* 10:249, 1974.
25a. Chard T: Frequency of implantation failure and early pregnancy loss in natural cycles. *Baillieres Clin Obstet Gynaecol* 5:179, 1991.
26. Cramer DW et al: Determinants of ovarian cancer risk, I: reproductive experiences and family history, *J Natl Cancer Inst.* 71:711, 1983.
27. Crawley WF et al: Inhibition of serum androgen levels by chronic intranasal and subcutaneous administration of a potent luteinizing hormone-releasing hormone (LH-RH) agonist in adult men, *Fertil Steril* 37:1240, 1982.
28. Crooke AC: Comparison of the effect of Pergonal and pituitary follicle-stimulating hormone. In Butler JK, editor: *Developments in the pharmacology and clinical uses of human gonadotropins,* High Wycombe, UK, 1970, GD Searle.
29. Crowe SJ, Cushing H, Homans J: Cited by Lunenfeld B, Donini P: Historic aspects of gonadotropins. In Greenblatt RB, editor: *Ovulation,* Toronto, 1966, JB Lippincott.
30. Davoren JB, Hsueh AJW: Growth hormone increased ovarian levels of immunoreactive somatomedin C/insulin-like growth factor I in vivo, *Endocrinology,* 118:888, 1986.
31. De La Losa P, Jutisz M: Protein and polypeptide hormones. In Margoulis M, editor: Amsterdam, 1969, Excerpta Medica.
32. Devroe et al. Successful in vitro fertilisation and embryo transfer after treatment with recombinant human FSH, *Lancet* 339:1171, 1992.
33. Diczfalusy E, Harlin J: Clinical-pharmacological studies on human menopausal gonadotropin, *Hum Reprod* 3:21, 1988.
34. Donini P, Puzzuoli D, Montezemolo R: Purification of gonadotropin from human menopausal urine, *Acta Endocrinol* 45:329, 1964.
35. Dor J et al: Is insulin-like growth factor-I essential for the human graafian follicle development: observation in a Laron-type dwarf during in vitro fertilization, *J Clin Endocrinol Metab* 74:539, 1992.
36. Ellis JD, Williamson JG: Factors influencing the pregnancy and complication rates with human menopausal gonadotropin therapy, *Br J Obstet Gynaecol* 82:52, 1975.

37. Erickson GF, Garzo VG, Magoffin DA: Insulin-like growth factor-I regulates aromatase activity in human granulosa and granulosa luteal cells, *J Clin Endocrinol Metabol* 69:716, 1989.

38. Fares FAM et al: Design of a long-acting follitropin agonist by fusing the C-terminal sequence of the chorionic gonadotropin beta subunit to the follitropin beta subunit, *Proc Natl Acad Sci U S A* 89:4304, 1992.

39. Fares FAM et al: Design of a long-acting follitropin agonist using site-directed mutagenesis and gene fusion. Presented at the annual meeting of the Israel Endocrine Society, Jerusalem, 1993.

40. Farin CE et al: Effect of luteinizing hormone and human chorionic gonadotropin on cell populations in the ovine corpus luteum, *Biol Reprod* 38:413, 1988.

41. Fiddes JC, Goodman HM: Isolation, cloning and sequence analysis of the cDNA for the alpha-subunit of human chorionic gonadotropin, *Nature* 281:351, 1979.

42. Fleming R, Coutts JTR: Suppression of LH using a GnRH analog during induction of follicular growth blocks the pre-hCG progesterone rise suggesting that all peripheral estradiol derives from the theca cell layer. In the control of follicular development, ovarian and luteal function: lessons from in vitro fertilization, Serono Symposium, Paris, April, 1986.

43. Fleming R et al: Successful treatment of infertile women with oligomenorrhoea using a combination of an LHRH agonist and exogenous gonadotropins, *Br J Obstet Gynaecol* 92:369, 1985.

44. Garcia JE et al: Human menopausal gonadotropin/human chorionic gonadotropin in follicular maturation for oocyte aspiration: phase I, *Fertil Steril* 39:167, 1983.

45. Gemzell CA: Recent results of human gonadotropin therapy. In Bettendorf G, Insler V, editors: *Clinical application of human gonadotropins,* Stuttgart, 1970, Georg Thieme Verlag.

46. Gemzell CA: Induction of ovulation in patients following removal of pituitary adenoma, *Am J Obstet Gynecol* 117:955, 1973.

47. Gemzell CA, Diczfalusy E, Tillinger G: Clinical effect of human pituitary follicle stimulating hormone (FSH), *J Clin Endocrinol Metab* 18:1333, 1958.

48. Gemzell CA, Diczfalusy E, Tillinger G: Human pituitary follicle stimulating hormone, 1: clinical effect of a partly purified preparation, *Ciba Found Colloq Endocrinol* 13:191, 1960.

49. Germont et al: Successful in vitro fertilisation and embryo transfer after treatment with recombinant human FSH, *Lancet* 339:1170, 1992.

50. Goldfarb AF, Schlaff S, Mansi ML: A life-table analysis of pregnancy yield in fixed low-dose menotropin therapy for patients in whom clomiphene citrate failed to induce ovulation, *Fertil Steril* 37:629, 1982.

51. Goodman AL et al: Regulation of folliculogenesis in the rhesus monkey: selection of the dominant follicle, *Endocrinology* 100:155, 1977.

52. Hack M, Lunenfeld B: The influence of hormone induction of ovulation on the fetus and newborn, *Pediatr Adolesc Endocrinol* 5:191, 1978.

53. Hackeloer BJ: The role of ultrasound in female infertility management, *Ultrasound Med Biol* 10:35, 1984.

54. Harlap S: Ovulation induction and congenital malformations, *Lancet* 2:961, 1976.

54a. Harlow BL, Weiss NS, Roth CJ et al: Case-control study of borderline ovarian tumors: reproductive history; exposure to exogenous female hormones, *Cancer Res* 48:5949, 1988.

55. Hartge P et al: A case-control study of epithelial ovarian cancer, *Am J Obstet Gynecol* 161:10, 1989.

56. Healy DL, Burger HG: Serum FSH, LH and PRL during the induction of ovulation with exogenous gonadotropins, *J Clin Endocrinol Metab* 56:474, 1983.

57. Healy DL et al: A normal cumulative conception rate after human pituitary gonadotropin, *Fertil Steril* 34:341, 1980.

58. Hedon B et al: Agonist and gonadotropins for in vitro fertilization. In the control of follicular development, ovarian and luteal function: lessons from in vitro fertilization, Serono Symposium, Paris, April, 1986.

59. Hendricks CH: Twinning in relation to birth weight, mortality and congenital malformations, *Obstet Gynecol* 27:47, 1966.

60. Hodgen GD: The dominant follicle, *Fertil Steril* 38:281, 1982.

61. Hodgen GD et al: Selection of the dominant follicle and its ovum in the menstrual cycle. In Baier HM, Lindner HR, editors: *Fertilization of the human egg in vitro,* Berlin, 1983, Springer-Verlag.

62. Homberg R et al: Influence of serum luteinising hormone concentration on ovulation, conception and early pregnancy loss in polycystic ovary syndrome, *Br Med J* 297:1024, 1988.

63. Homberg R et al: Growth hormone facilitates ovulation induction by gonadotropins, *Clin Endocrinol* 29:113, 1988.

64. Howles CM et al: Effect of high tonic levels of luteinising hormone on outcome of in vitro fertilisation, *Lancet* 2:521, 1986.

65. Hussa RO: Biosynthesis of human chorionic gonadotropin, *Endocr Rev* 1:268, 1980.

66. Insler V, Lunenfeld B: Application of human gonadotropins for induction of ovulation. In Campos da Paz A et al, editors: *Human reproduction,* Tokyo, 1974, Igaku Shoin.

67. Insler V, Lunenfeld B: Human gonadotropins. In Philip EE, Barnes J, Newton M, editors: *Scientific foundation of obstetrics and gynaecology,* London, 1977, Heinemann.

68. Insler V, Potashnik G: Monitoring of follicular development in gonadotropin stimulated cycles. In Beier HM, Lindner HM, editors: *Fertilization of the human egg in vitro,* Berlin, 1983, Springer-Verlag.

69. Insler V, Potashnik G, Glassner M: Some epidemiological aspects of fertility evaluation. In Insler V, Bettendorf G, editors: *Advances in diagnosis and treatment of infertility,* New York, 1981, Elsevier/North-Holland.

70. Insler V et al: Functional classification of patients selected for gonadotropin therapy, *Obstet Gynecol* 32:620, 1968.

71. Insler V et al: Comparison of various methods used in monitoring of gonadotropic therapy. In Bettendorf G, Insler V, editors: *Clinical application of human gonadotropins,* Stuttgart, 1970, Georg Thieme Verlag.

72. Insler V et al: The cervical score: a simple semiquantitative method for monitoring the menstrual cycle, *Int J Gynecol Obstet* 10:223, 1972.

73. Insler V et al: The effect of different LHRH on the levels of immunoreactive gonadotropins, *Gynecol Endocrinol* 2:305, 1988.

74. Jia X Ch, Kalmijin J, Hsueh AJW: Growth hormone enhances FSH induced differentiation of cultured rat granulosa cells, *Endocrinology* 118:1401, 1986.

75. Johnson P, Pearce JM: Recurrent spontaneous abortion and polycystic ovarian disease: comparison of two regimens to induce ovulation, *Br Med J [Clin Res]* 300:154, 1990.

76. Joly DJ et al: An epidemiologic study of reproductive experience to cancer of the ovary, *Am J Epidemiol* 99:190, 1974.

77. Kelsey JL: A review of the epidemiology of human breast cancer, *Epidemiol Rev* 1:74, 1979.

78. Kelsey JL et al: A case-control study of endometrial cancer, *Am J Epidemiol* 116:333, 1982.

79. Kemmann E et al: The initial experience with the use of a portable infusion pump in the delivery of human menopausal gonadotropins, *Fertil Steril* 40:448, 1983.

80. Kurachi K: Problems concerning ovulation induction, *Nippon Sanka Fujinka Gakkai Zasshi* 35:1127, 1983.

80a. Kurachi K, Aono T, Suzuki M et al: Results of HMG (Humegon)-therapy in 6096 treatment cycles in 2166 Japanese women with ovulatory infertility, *Eur J Obstet Gynecol Reprod Biol* 19:43, 1983.

81. Lais CW, Williams TJ, Gaffey TA: Prevalence of ovarian cancer found at the time of infertility microsurgery, *Fertil Steril* 49:551, 1988.

82. Laron Z et al: Puberty in Laron type dwarfism. In Cacciari E, Prader A, editors: Serono Symposium No 36, New York, 1980, Academic Press.

83. LaVecchia C et al: Risk factors for endometrial cancer at different ages, *J Natl Cancer Inst* 3:667, 1984.

84. Leethem JH, Rakoff AE: Studies on antihormone specificity with particular reference to gonadotropic therapy in the female, *J Clin Endocrinol Metab* 8:262, 1948.

85. Lequin L et al: Oestrogens in urine or plasma to monitor ovarian response to exogenous gonadotropins. In the control of follicular development, ovarian and luteal function: lessons from in vitro fertilization, Serono Symposium, Paris, April, 1986.

86. Linda L et al: Stimulation of testosterone production in the cynomolgus monkey in vivo by deglycosylated and desialylated human choriogonadotropin, *Endocrinology* 124:175, 1989.

87. Lopata A et al: In vitro fertilization and embryo implantation. In Insler V, Lunenfeld B, editors: *Infertility: male and female,* London, 1986, Churchill Livingstone.

88. Lunenfeld B: Treatment of anovulation by human gonadotropins, *Int J Gynecol Obstet* 1:153, 1963.

89. Lunenfeld B, Blankenstein J, Ron E: Short and long term survey of patients treated with HMG/HCG and follow up of offspring. In Genazziani AR, Volpe A, Facchinetti F, editors: *Proceedings of the first international congress on gynecological endocrinology,* Parthenon Publishing.

90. Lunenfeld B, Insler V: *Diagnosis and treatment of functional infertility,* Berlin, 1978, Grosse Verlag.

91. Lunenfeld E, Lunenfeld B: Modern approaches to the diagnosis and management of anovulation, *Int J Fertil* 33:308, 1988.

92. Lunenfeld B, Mashiah S, Blankstein J: Induction of ovulation with gonadotropins. In Shearman R, editor: *Clinical reproductive endocrinology,* London, 1985, Churchill Livingstone.

93. Lunenfeld B et al: Therapy with gonadotropins: where are we today? In Insler V, Bettendorf G, editors: *Advances in diagnosis and treatment of infertility,* New York, 1981, Elsevier/North-Holland.

94. Manjunath WN, Sairam MR: Biochemical, biological and immunological properties of chemically deglycosylated human chorionic gonadotropin, *J Biol Chem* 257:7109, 1982.

95. Marshall JR, Jacobson A: A technique of dose selection in ovulation induction with HMG. In Butler JK, editor: *Developments in the pharmacology and clinical uses of human gonadotropins,* High Wycombe, UK, 1970, GD Searle.

96. McFaul PB, Traub AI, Thompson W: Premature luteinization and ovulation induction using human menopausal gonadotropin or pure follicle stimulating hormone in patients with polycystic ovary syndrome, *Acta Eur Fertil* 20:157, 1989.

97. McGowan L et al: The woman at risk for developing ovarian cancer, *Gynecol Oncol* 7:325, 1979.

98. McKeown J: Malformations in a population observed for five years. In *Foundations symposium on congenital malformations,* London, 1960, J&A Churchill.

99. Meldrum DR et al: Medical "oophorectomy" using a long-acting GnRH agonist: a possible new approach to treatment of endometriosis, *J Clin Endocrinol Metab* 54:1081, 1982.

100. Menashe Y et al: Can growth hormone increase, following clonidine administration, predict the dose of human menopausal hormone needed for induction of ovulation?, *Fertil Steril* 53:432, 1989.

101. Menashe Y et al: Effect of growth hormone on ovarian responsiveness, *Gynecol Endocrinol* 4:6, 1990.

102. Nasca PC et al: An epidemiologic case-control study of ovarian cancer and reproductive factors, *Am J Epidemiol* 119:705, 1984.

103. Nichols JB: Statistics of births in the USA, 1915–1948, *Am J Obstet Gynecol* 64:376, 1952.

104. Nitschke-Dabelstein S et al: Plasma 17beta-estradiol and plasma progesterone as indicators of cyclic changes in the follicle-bearing ovary. In Insler V, Bettendorf G, editors: *Advances in diagnosis and treatment of infertility,* New York, 1981, Elsevier/North-Holland.

105. O'Herlihy C et al: Incremental clomiphene therapy: a new method for treating persistent anovulation, *Obstet Gynecol* 58:535, 1981.

105a. Padmanabhan V, Chappel SC, Beiting IZ: An improved in vitro bioassay for follicle-stimulating hormone (FSH); suitable for measurement of FSH in unextracted human serum, *Endocrinology* 121:1088, 1987.

105b. Potashnik G, Glastner M, Holtberg G et al: Results of gonadotropin therapy. Personal communication based on unpublished data.

106. Punnonen et al: Spontaneous luteinizing hormone surge and cleavage of in vitro fertilized embryos, *Fertil Steril* 49:479, 1988.

107. Quigley MM: Selection of agents for enhanced follicular recruitment in an in vitro fertilization and embryo replacement treatment program, *Ann N Y Acad Sci* 442:96, 1985.

108. Rabau E, Lunenfeld B, Insler V: The treatment of fertility disturbances with special reference to the use of human gonadotropins. In Joel Ch A, editor: *Fertility disturbances in men and women,* Basel, 1971, S Karger.

109. Regan L, Owen EJ, Jacobs HS: Hypersecretion of LH, infertility and miscarriage, *Lancet* 336:1141, 1990.

110. Ritchie WGM: Ultrasound in the evaluation of normal and induced ovulation, *Fertil Steril* 43:167, 1985.

110a. Ron E, Lunenfeld B, Monczer J et al: Cancer incidence in a cohort of infertile women, *Am J Epidemiol* 2:516, 1980.

111. Ronnberg L, Martikainen H, Tapanainen J: Is there any benefit to use growth hormone in ovarian hyperstimulation? *Gynecol Endocrinol* 4:27, 1990.

112. Schenken RS, Hodgen GD: Follicle-stimulating hormone induced ovarian hyperstimulation in monkeys: blockade of the luteinizing hormone surge, *J Clin Endocrinol Metab* 57:50, 1983.

113. Schenker JG, Weinstein D: Ovarian hyperstimulation syndrome: a current survey, *Fertil Steril* 30:255, 1979.

114. Seegar-Jones GE et al: Specific effects of FSH and LH on follicular development and oocyte retrieval as determined by a program for in vitro fertilization, *Ann N Y Acad Sci* 442:119, 1985.

115. Serr DM, Ismajovich B: Determination of the primary sex ratio for human abortions, *Am J Obstet Gynecol* 87:63, 1963.

116. Shadmi AL et al: Abolishment of the positive feedback mechanism: a criterion for temporary medical hypophysectomy by LHRH agonist, *Gynecol Endocrinol* 1:1, 1987.

116a. Shohom Z, Zosmer A, Insler V, Early miscarriage and fetalmalformations after induction of ovulation by clomiphene citrate and/or human menopausal gonadotropins in in vitro fertilization and gamete interfallopian transfer, *Fertil Steril* 55:1, 1991.

117. Smith PE: Hastening of development of female genital system by daily hemoplastic pituitary transplants, *Proc Soc Exp Biol Med* 24:131, 1926.

118. Smith PE, Engle ET: Experimental evidence of the role of anterior pituitary in development and regulation of gonads, *Am J Anat* 40:159, 1927.

118a. Sopelak VM, Hodgen GD: Blockade of the estrogen induced luteinizing hormone surge in monkeys; a nonsteroid, antigenic factor in porcine follicular fluid, *Fertil Steril* 41:108, 1984.

119. Spadoni LR, Cox DW, Smith DC: Use of human menopausal gonadotropin for the induction of ovulation, *Am J Obstet Gynecol* 120:988, 1974.

120. Stanger JD, Yovitch JL: Reduced in vitro fertilisation of human oocytes from patients with raised basal luteinising hormone levels during the follicular phase, *Br J Obstet Gynaecol* 92:385, 1985.

121. Stevenson AC et al: Congenital malformations: a report of a study of a series of consecutive births in two centers, *Bull WHO* 34(9):1, 1966.

122. Talmadge K, Boorstein WR, Fiddes JC: The human genome contains seven genes for the beta sub-unit of chorionic gonadotropin but only one gene for the beta sub-unit of luteinizing hormone, *DNA* 2:279, 1983.

123. Thompson LR, Hansen LM: Pergonal (menotropin): a summary of clinical experience in the induction of ovulation and pregnancy, *Fertil Steril* 21:844, 1970.

123a. Thornton JG, Wells M: Ovarian cysts in pregnancy: does ultrasound make traditional management inappropriate? *Obstet Gynecol* 69:717, 1987.

124. Tricomi V, Serr DM, Solish G: The ratio of male and female embryos as determined by the sex chromatin, *Am J Obstet Gynecol* 75:504, 1960.

125. Tsafriri A, Pomeranz SH: Oocyte maturation inhibitor, *Clin Endocrinol* 15:157, 1986.

126. Tsapoulis AD, Zourlaz PA, Comninos AC: Observations on 320 infertile patients treated with human gonadotropins (human menopausal gonadotropin/human chorionic gonadotropin), *Fertil Steril* 29:492, 1978.

127. Tuang LC: Personal communication (1986) to B Lunenfeld: WHO scientific group report, *WHO Tech Rep Ser* 514, 1976.

128. Volpe A et al: Ovarian response to combined growth hormone-gonadotropin treatment in patients resistant to induction of superovulation, *Gynecol Endocrinol* 3:125, 1989.

129. Whittemore AS et al: Epithelial ovarian cancer and the ability to conceive, *Cancer Res* 49:4047, 1989.

130. Whittemore AS et al: Characteristics relating to ovarian cancer risk: collaborative analysis of 12 US case-control studies, II: invasive epithelial ovarian cancer in white women, *Am J Epidemiol* 136:1184, 1993.

131. Wide L et al: Metabolic clearance of human chorionic gonadotropin administered to non pregnant women, *Acta Endocrinol* 59:579, 1968.

132. Wu C: Plasma hormones in human gonadotropin induced ovulation, Obstet Gynecol 49:308, 1977.

133. Yen SSC: Clinical applications of gonadotropin-releasing hormone and gonadotropin-releasing hormone analogs, Fertil Steril 39:257, 1983.

134. Zondek B: Ueber die funktion des ovariums, *Dtsch Med Wochenschr* 18:343, 1926.

135. Zondek B: Ueber die funktion des ovariums, *Z Geburtshilfe Gynaekol* 90:327, 1926.

136. Zondek B, Ascheim S: Das Hormon des Hypohysenvorderlappens: Testobject zum Nachweis des Hormons, *Klin Wochenschr* 6:248, 1927.

Chapter 34

GONADOTROPIN-RELEASING HORMONE AND ANALOGUES IN OVULATION INDUCTION

**Howard A. Zacur, MD, PhD
and Yolanda R. Smith, MD**

The recent introduction of gonadotropin-releasing hormone (GnRH) and its analogues into clinical practice has had a significant impact on ovulation-induction protocols. A need for medical treatment of ovulatory disturbances may be required in 20-30% of infertile couples.[33, 89] Traditionally, this need has been fulfilled by prescribing one of the following medications: clomiphene citrate, bromocriptine, or human menopausal gonadotropins (hMG). Clomiphene citrate presumably acts by preventing the replenishment of estrogen receptors, possibly affecting the hypothalamic-pituitary-ovarian axis at many points,[1] and has usually been prescribed as an initial treatment to induce ovulation in women with chronic anovulation. Bromocriptine, a potent dopamine agonist, has been most effective in treating ovulatory dysfunction in women with hyperprolactinemia.[65] The use of hMG has been prescribed to directly stimulate the ovary.[47]

In 1971, research efforts by Schally[51,79] and Guillemin[10] led to the identification of a decapeptide, now known as GnRH, that stimulated luteinizing hormone (LH) and follicular-stimulating hormone (FSH) release from the pituitary gland. Evidence of the clinical utility of GnRH to induce ovulation prompted recent approval by the Food and Drug Administration (FDA) of intravenous pulsatile GnRH for ovulation induction in women with primary amenorrhea.[78] In addition, numerous agonist analogues have been developed and are used in ovulation induction protocols, either to suppress gonadotropins or to cause a flare in their secretion. It is the aim of this chapter to review the biochemistry of GnRH, its clinical application as an ovulation-inducing agent, and the usefulness of GnRH analogues to potentiate ovulation induction.

BIOCHEMISTRY OF GONADOTROPIN-RELEASING HORMONE

GnRH peptides, first isolated from porcine and ovine hypothalami, were found to have identical decapeptide sequences. These same 10 amino acids are now known to be the GnRH structure of all placental mammals that have been studied. Six forms of GnRH that are distinct from the mammalian sequence have also been identified. These distinct forms share 50% sequence identity and have been found in fish (jawless, cartilaginous, bony), amphibians (frogs), reptiles (alligators), chickens, and mammals[82] (Fig. 34-1). Actions of GnRH in other species include its well-known role in releasing pituitary LH and FSH, but also includes actions as a neurotransmitter, affecting sexual behavior.[66]

The GnRH gene is located on the short arm of chromosome 8[92] and consists of four exons (see Fig. 34-2). Exon I encodes a large 5′ untranslated region that is presumably important in regulating gene transcription. Exon II encodes the signal peptide, GnRH, and the first portion (AA1-11) of a 56 amino acid peptide called GnRH–associated peptide,

		1	2	3	4	5	6	7	8	9	10
Mammal	**(MGnRH)**	**pGLU–HIS–TRP–SER–TYR–GLY–LEU–ARG–PRO–GYL–NH$_2$**									
Chicken I	(cGnRH–I)	pGLu –HIS –TRP–SER–TYR–GLY–LEU GLN PRO–GLY–NH$_2$									
Catfish	(cfGnRH)	pGLu –HIS –TRP–SER–HIS GLY–LEU ASN PRO–GLY–NH$_2$									
Chicken II	(cGnRH–II)	pGLU –HIS –TRP–SER HIS GLY TRP–TYR PRO–GLY–NH$_2$									
Dogfish	(dfGnRH)	pGLU –HIS –TRP–SER HIS GLY TRP–LEU PRO–GLY–NH$_2$									
Salmon	(sGnRH)	pGLU –HIS –TRP–SER–TYR–GLY TRP–LEU PRO–GLY–NH$_2$									
Lamprey	(lGnRH)	pGLU –HIS –TYR SER LEU –GLU–TRP–LYS PrO–GLY–NH$_2$									

Fig. 34-1. Amino acid sequences of GnRH identified in mammals, birds, fish, and eels. (Modified From Sherwood NM, Lovejoy DA, Coe IR: *Endoc Rev* 14:241, 1993.)

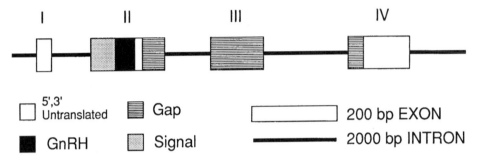

Fig. 34-2. Human GnRH gene consisting of four exons. Exon I encodes a 5′ untranslated region. Exon II encodes for GnRH and includes part of GAP. Exon III encodes GAP. Exon IV encodes the remainder of GAP and an untranslated region. (Modified from Sherwood NM, Lovejoy DA, Coe IR: *Endoc Rev* 14:241, 1993.)

or GAP. Exons III and IV encode the remaining amino acids for GAP, as well as an untranslated region.[81] GAP was initially thought to stimulate LH release and inhibit prolactin secretion from in vitro experiments,[62] but a significant in vivo effect has not been demonstrated.[94]

GnRH is synthesized by cell bodies located in the arcuate nucleus of the medial basal hypothalamus, released from axons into the hypothalamic-hypophyseal portal system, and transported to the anterior pituitary. GnRH concentrations, ranging from undetectable levels to 2000 pg/ml, have been reported in hypothalamic-hypophyseal portal blood obtained from rats,[18] monkeys,[11] and humans.[3] GnRH is released in a pulsatile fashion; however, the short half-life of GnRH makes it difficult to assess hypothalamic GnRH activity using peripheral serum measurements. Consequently, serum LH measurements have been used to infer hypothalamic GnRH physiology. To corroborate this indirect approach, similar studies have been performed in the ewe[55, 56] and the rhesus monkey.[91] These studies reveal a good correlation between hypothalamic GnRH pulses in portal blood and LH pulses in the peripheral circulation.

Events leading up to the release of LH and FSH from pituitary cells recently have been reviewed in detail.[14, 61] After GnRH binds to surface receptors located on pituitary gonadotropes, the bound receptors aggregate to open membrane channels, allowing the influx of extracellular calcium (Fig. 34-3). Bound GnRH receptors also activate G protein molecules, leading to activation of a phospholipase C enzyme. Phospholipase C cleaves inositol phospholipids into inositol triphosphate and diacylglycerol. Inositol triphosphate promotes accumulation of calcium in the cytosol by opening calcium channels in membranes and by releasing intracellular stores of calcium. Diacylglycerol activates calcium-dependent protein kinase C. These events trigger the release of preformed gonadotropins and stimulate gene transcription for additional gonadotropin synthesis. Occupancy of only 20% of the available GnRH binding sites is required to stimulate maximum LH release.[60] Following initial binding and internalization of the GnRH receptors, a loss of binding sites is observed (down-regulation), but this is soon followed by an increase in receptors, presumably due to increased synthesis (up-regulation).[21] Continuous exposure of GnRH receptors to GnRH leads not only to down-regulation, but also to a loss of sensitivity of vacant receptors to GnRH stimulation.[85]

Once released into the circulation, GnRH is rapidly degraded and has a half-life of only four minutes.[72] The peptide is attacked by endopeptidases between Tyr^5-Gly^6 and Gly^6-Leu^7 bonds,[43] as well as by a carboxamide peptidase at Pro^9, Gly-NH$_2$^{10} positions. Peptides that are not degraded bind to GnRH receptors. Amino acids at the amino and carboxyl terminals of the peptide appear to be most responsible for binding, with amino acids occupying the first three positions that are most responsible for causing LH and FSH release.[35]

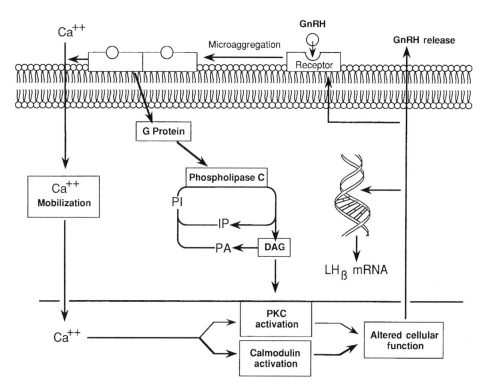

Fig. 34-3. Release of gonadotropin stimulated by GnRH. DAG denotes diacylglycerol; PKC is protein kinase C; PI is phosphatidylinositol; IP is inositol phosphate and PA is phosphatidic acid. (Modified from Conn PM, Crowley WF: *NEJM* 324:93-101, 1991.)

Knowledge of the chemical structure of the GnRH molecule, and of the importance of the various amino acids that determine biological activity and susceptibility to metabolism, has allowed analogues of the native molecule to be created with increased biological activity and a resistance to degradation. Substitutions at positions 6, 7, and 9, and/or deletion of the 10th amino acid, result in GnRH analogues with "agonistic activity." GnRH agonists currently produced are listed in Figure 34-6 on p. 645. These are all agonists because initial binding to the GnRH receptors causes a release in LH and FSH. Due to resistance in degradation of GnRH or to an increase in its binding affinity, pituitary gonadotropes exposed to GnRH agonists fail to release LH and FSH within two weeks. Thus, the biological consequence of GnRH agonist exposure is an initial release, or "flare," in gonadotropin levels, followed by persistent low levels of LH and FSH, similar to those seen in hypothalamic hypogonadism. The brief "flare" in gonadotropins, which lasts 4-7 days, may result in stimulation of follicle development, and may have potential clinical benefits in ovulation-induction protocols.

PATTERNS OF GONADOTROPIN HORMONE SECRETION

The pioneering efforts in the laboratory of Dr. Knobil, using the arcuate nucleus-lesioned monkey, led to the hypothesis that hourly pulsations in peripheral LH levels were the result of the hourly release of GnRH from the arcuate nucleus into the hypothalamic-hypophyseal portal blood.[58, 67] In arcuate-lesioned monkeys who were anovulatory, it was possible to administer GnRH at 90- to 120-minute intervals, eventually causing ovulation and the formation of a normal luteal phase.[41] If GnRH was administered at a lower frequency, ovulation did not occur and the basal LH to FSH ratio decreased.[90] Increasing the frequency of GnRH pulses resulted in a higher basal LH to FSH ratio, similar to that seen in chronically anovulatory women with hyperandrogenism.[71, 93] Thus, it was demonstrated that LH and FSH pulses follow GnRH pulses.

Although administration of GnRH at an unvarying frequency resulted in ovulation and a normal menstrual cycle in experimental monkeys,[41] this does not parallel events that occur in a normal human menstrual cycle. Peripheral measurements of LH pulses throughout the human menstrual cycle reveal changes in the frequency and amplitude of LH pulses,[69, 87] which infers that GnRH pulsatile secretion also must vary during the menstrual cycle. During the follicular phase of the human menstrual cycle, LH pulses are more frequent, but reduced in amplitude compared to the pulses seen during the luteal phase.[87]

It is currently believed that the GnRH pulse generator resides in the arcuate nucleus of the hypothalamus; the simplest hypothesis is that a single cell or cell group initiates each pulse.[42] It is also believed that in humans this

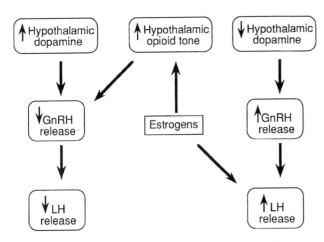

Fig. 34-4. Release of hypothalamic GnRH is influenced by many factors including steroids, opioids, and catecholamines.

pulse generator may be influenced by gonadal steroids, opiates, and catecholamines, as illustrated in Fig. 34-4. In brief, estradiol may alter pituitary LH release by altering hypothalamic GnRH release, stimulating pituitary cell synthesis and release of LH. Responses to estrogen may also be influenced by the dosage of steroid and the duration of exposure. Opiates and dopamine appear to inhibit hypothalamic release of GnRH. However, dopamine also appears to inhibit opiate release; thus, dopamine, depending upon dosage and the timing of administration, may either result in increased or diminished circulating LH levels.[34]

OVULATION INDUCTION WITH GONADOTROPIN-RELEASING HORMONE

The discovery of GnRH immediately raised expectations that this molecule could be used to induce ovulation in anovulatory women. In fact, this phenomenon occurred with a single injection of GnRH induced ovulation in a woman who had been receiving hMG.[36] When GnRH was given without hMG, as a single dose or single daily dose in other anovulatory women, ovulation either did not occur or occurred rarely.[2,8,39,59] Further use of GnRH as an ovulation-inducing drug was limited in the 1970s due to these failures. Improvement in the understanding of the physiology of GnRH–induced LH release later led to the development of clinical protocols that required GnRH to be given in doses once every 60-120 minutes. These new protocols consistently resulted in successful ovulation induction in anovulatory women.[95]

Patient selection

Anovulatory patients who presumably fail to release their own hypothalamic GnRH in the necessary amounts and intervals respond well to exogenous GnRH administration. These patients include those with primary GnRH administration. These patients include those with primary GnRH deficiency (e.g., Kallmann syndrome), as well as those with a secondary GnRH depression (e.g., "hypothalamic amenorrhea") resulting from stress.

Patients who are anovulatory because of hyperprolactinemia, premature ovarian failure, late-onset adrenal hyperplasia, and hyperandrogenic chronic anovulation syndrome (polycystic ovarian disease or syndrome) should be identified because they respond better to therapies other than GnRH. Anovulation in these patients results secondarily from other disturbances that may affect the pulse generator of GnRH, as well as other organs. Consequently, ovulation induction may prove difficult if only exogenous GnRH is given. Measurement of gonadotropins, prolactin, 17-hydroxyprogesterone, and testosterone should be sufficient to identify patients who would not respond well to GnRH ovulation induction.

Before considering GnRH therapy, consideration should be given to performing a semen analysis and demonstrating fallopian tube patency by hysterosalpingography. Identification of a male or tubal infertility factor permits corrective action prior to GnRH therapy, maximizing its efficacy.

Administration of GnRH as a "challenge" test prior to beginning GnRH ovulation induction has been recommended to identify patients with isolated pituitary deficiency of LH and FSH.[79] Because these patients are rare and the response to a single challenge of GnRH may not predict the pituitary's response to repeated exposure to GnRH,[26] GnRH challenge testing prior to attempting therapy is of limited benefit.

Route of administration, dosage, and frequency of GnRH for ovulation induction

GnRH may be absorbed following intravenous, subcutaneous, intramuscular, nasal, and sublingual administration.[2, 25, 39, 46] Pharmacokinetic studies reveal that, following intravenous administration of GnRH, LH rapidly rises and peaks within 30 minutes. The LH level then remains elevated for 2-3 hours.[25] Following subcutaneous or intramuscular GnRH administration, the time to reach the peak LH concentration is delayed, the peak concentration is lower, and the time to return to baseline is longer.[2, 25, 39]

Correlation exists between the administered dosage of GnRH and the peak LH response. Given intravenously, a GnRH dosage as low as 1 μg per bolus injection may induce ovulation,[15, 54] while dosages higher than 6 μg per bolus may cause supraphysiological stimulation of the pituitary-gonadal axis.[77] For intravenous administration, suitable bolus dosages for ovulation induction exist within the range of 26-100 ng/kg. Because some patients may require intravenous bolus dosages of 10-20 μg,[57] careful monitoring of the ovarian response to the bolus dosage is required. Excessively high dosages of GnRH may produce ovarian hyperstimulation and multiple gestation.[6] Furthermore, when administered to monkeys, higher GnRH dosages have resulted in declining levels of FSH,[73, 90] which could adversely affect follicular development. In summary, for intravenous administration, an initial dosage of 5 μg per bolus may be tried, with 5 μg dosage increments if there is no response in 10-14 days. Monitoring of patients receiving intravenous

GnRH may consist of serial plasma estradiol measurements and pelvic ultrasound imaging. This is discussed more fully in the chapter on monitoring of ovulation, Chapter 31.

GnRH may be administered subcutaneously to patients who are unable or unwilling to receive it intravenously. Required dosages for this route of administration are generally higher, ranging from 10-25 µg per bolus, with 15 µg usually being successful.[50] The subcutaneous route of administration may be less advantageous because the LH response to subcutaneously administered GnRH may be more variable than that observed following intravenous use. This may reflect varying absorption rates due to obesity. Consequently, gonadotropes may become "desensitized" to the somewhat "continuous" release of GnRH by the subcutaneous route, as opposed to the "intermittent" peak observed following intravenous treatment. Thus, administration of GnRH through the subcutaneous route may result in poor follicular development.

Most centers administer GnRH at a fixed rate of one bolus every 90 minutes. Administration of GnRH at rates more frequent than every 45 minutes,[16] or less frequent than every 120 minutes, impairs follicular development.[19] Although fixed rates of GnRH administration within a certain range results in ovulation, modification of GnRH dosage rates to more closely mimic the observed LH pulses during the human follicular phase of the menstrual cycle has been advocated. In particular, administration of GnRH at 60-minute intervals has been recommended to produce a more physiological reproduction of the endocrine features of a normal menstrual cycle.[20] Whether or not this improves pregnancy outcome rates remains to be seen.

Drug delivery systems

GnRH may be administered intravenously or subcutaneously by use of pulsatile pumps. FDA approval of intravenous GnRH has been granted for Lutrepulse (Ortho, Raritan, NJ), one of the two commercially available GnRH drugs. Factrel (Wyeth-Ayerst, Philadelphia, PA) is another GnRH drug that has been approved for diagnostic use.

Pumps available for drug administration include the AutoSyringe, Inc. model (Hooksett, NH), or the Pulsmat model from Ferring Laboratories, Inc. (Ridgewood, NJ). Although both pumps may be adjusted to vary the dosing interval, the drug volume may be altered only in the AutoSyringe, Inc., pump. Small needles (25-27 gauge) and catheters may be obtained for intravenous or subcutaneous use. The use of these pumps has been facilitated by the creation of home-care nursing programs affiliated with hospitals. These programs provide staff to restart IV lines on a 24-hour, seven-day-a-week basis.

Patient monitoring

Prior to initiating ovulation-induction therapy, a baseline estradiol level and pelvic sonogram should be obtained. These studies may alert the physician to underlying ovarian pathology, avoiding future confusion in trying to interpret the effect of therapy. After GnRH therapy has been started, plasma estradiol levels may be measured weekly. Some investigators recommend dosage adjustments if estradiol levels do not increase within one week,[76] while others have advised a dosage increase if evidence of a dominant follicle (greater than 12 mm) is not visible by pelvic ultrasound after 21 days of a particular intravenous GnRH dosage.[78]

Basal body temperature monitoring may be of use to detect the temperature shift that is expected following ovulation. A serum progesterone concentration that exceeds 3 ng/ml is confirmation that ovulation has occurred.

Luteal phase support

Once ovulation has been detected, continued therapy to support the luteal phase is necessary. Cessation of GnRH infusion during the early and midluteal phase in arcuate-lesioned monkeys resulted in premature menses.[32] Likewise, failure to continue GnRH following ovulation in humans has resulted in a luteal phase defect.[88] Furthermore, continuation of GnRH at a fixed dosage following ovulation in humans has resulted in luteal-phase deficiencies.[12, 63, 64] This outcome is not surprising because LH pulses during the normal human luteal phase are of greater amplitude and occur at a reduced frequency compared to those seen in the follicular phase, suggesting a physiological change in GnRH pulsatility that would not be possible in a fixed dosage regimen.

Support of the luteal phase may be provided by continuation of pulsatile GnRH administration at the same or slightly reduced dosage intervals (120-minute intervals). However, this form of luteal support increases discomfort and cost. Conversely, the GnRH infusion may be stopped after ovulation and human chorionic gonadotropin (hCG) may be given intramuscularly at 1000-2500 U doses every 3-4 days.[24, 30, 57, 70, 84] Alternatively, exogenous progesterone may be given as 50 mg vaginal suppositories twice daily.[5]

Response to treatment

When administered to women with hypothalamic hypogonadism, GnRH should be capable of successfully inducing ovulation once a satisfactory dosage has been determined. Braat et al. have shown with life table analysis that, when intravenous GnRH was given in 244 cycles to 48 hypogonadotropic women, the cumulative conception rate after 12 cycles was 93%. The mean conception rate per cycle was 22.5%.[7] These results are comparable to those expected following menotropin therapy. Rates of conception, spontaneous pregnancy loss, and multiple gestation were compared recently between women with hypogonadotropic amenorrhea who received either exogenous menotropins or intravenous pulsatile GnRH.[48] In this study, there were no significant differences in conception rates, pregnancy losses, or multiple gestations between the two groups.

In contrast to women with euprolactinemic hypothalamic hypogonadism given GnRH to induce ovulation,

GnRH has not proven to be as successful in inducing ovulation in women with hyperandrogenemic chronic ovulation syndrome, otherwise known as polycystic ovarian syndrome or disease (PCOD).[17] Given the fact that LH pulses are already increased in amplitude in patients with PCOD,[38] it is not surprising that GnRH treatment is less effective in inducing ovulation.

Side effects and risks

Mild ovarian hyperstimulation has been reported in patients induced to ovulate with GnRH,[83] and may reflect, in part, drug dosage.[45] Because moderate to severe ovarian hyperstimulation is unlikely, monitoring of patients receiving GnRH ovulation may be less intensive than those receiving hMG therapy.

Phlebitis during intravenous administration,[57] as well as infection at the site of subcutaneous needle placement,[31] have been reported. To prevent clot formation, intravenous GnRH solutions are usually prepared with low-dose heparin. Recent studies have demonstrated that systemic infections resulting from intravenous catheter use for GnRH–ovulation induction are rare, with a 2% incidence of positive blood cultures reported.[27] Consequently, patients with valve prostheses or mitral valve prolapse may be considered for alternative methods of ovulation induction.

The risk of developing antibodies to GnRH during therapy is also of concern. A 3% rate of GnRH antibody formation has been reported in 163 individuals (141 men, 22 women) who received GnRH for varying durations from 3 weeks to 9 months.[52] A separate study of 81 subjects found no antibody production against GnRH and offers some reassurance.[22] Interestingly, in both of these studies, the patients received GnRH subcutaneously.

GnRH AGONISTS AND OVULATION INDUCTION

Understanding the normal physiology of hypothalamic GnRH secretion has enabled physicians to be successful with inducing ovulation in amenorrheic women. The number of infertile women who might benefit from this therapy is minute compared to the number of women whose infertility is the result of another cause or is unexplained. Many of these women have been treated successfully using one of the new assisted reproductive technology procedures; for example, in vitro fertilization (IVF), intrauterine insemination (IUI), and gamete intrafallopian transfer (GIFT). These new procedures usually require hormonal induction of ovulation to produce sufficient numbers of oocytes and to improve the timing of the retrieval or insemination. A common ovulation-induction protocol (described in detail in Chapter 33) employs the use of hMG. Poor follicular maturation and/or premature luteinization of the follicles is observed sometimes in patients receiving hMG. Knowledge of the mechanism of desensitization of the pituitary gonadotropes, coupled with the development of GnRH analogues with agonist activity, has led to the use of these GnRH agonists in improved protocols.[68]

GnRH agonists are used in hMG protocols either to suppress pituitary secretion of LH and FSH, or to cause a brief flare in pituitary LH and FSH secretion, followed by suppression of gonadotropin secretion. The former is known as the luteal phase, or the late, long, or blocking protocol;[86] the latter is the follicular phase, or the short or "flare" protocol[28] (Fig. 34-5). In the luteal-phase protocol, GnRH agonists are administered in the midluteal phase (approximately day 21) with doses given twice daily or continuously. In this protocol, the GnRH agonist is continued alone until the plasma estradiol level is suppressed (generally less than 30 pg/ml) and no follicles greater than 15 mm are detected by sonography.[74] Once suppression has been achieved, menotropins are provided with the GnRH analogue until follicular development has proceeded to the point at which hCG may be administered.[53] When the dosage of the GnRH agonist is fixed at 1 mg/day, the duration of GnRH agonist administration prior to initiation of menotropins does not appear to alter ovarian responsiveness to exogenous gonadotropins.[80] Administration of a 1 mg dose per day for the first 10 days, followed by a 0.5 mg dose per day until hCG administration, has been advocated to decrease the number of ampules of menotropins required. A reduction in the number of hMG ampules required has also been one of the reasons given to support the short, or "flare," protocol for ovulation induction.

According to the "flare" protocol, GnRH agonists are administered between days one and three of the cycle. Menotropins and the GnRH agonist are administered to-

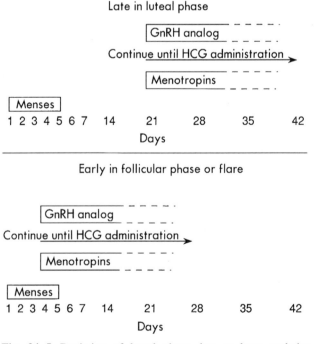

Fig. 34-5. Depiction of luteal phase, late or long ovulation induction protocols with GnRH agonists contrasted with follicular phase or short flare protocols.

gether until the day hCG is injected. This method has resulted in a higher rate of pregnancy success in one IVF program.[23]

It is unclear from the clinical data whether adjuvant use of a GnRH agonist in ovulation induction protocols significantly affects pregnancy rates. The clinical pregnancy rates for IVF cycles in which the GnRH agonist is started in the luteal phase have been reported to be significantly higher than when menotropins are used without a GnRH agonist (29% versus 12%).[13] However, a prospective randomized study of luteal or follicular phase administration of GnRH agonist with hMG, compared to hMG alone, found no differences in fertilization and implantation rates. With the GnRH agonist, though, cancellation rates were reduced and an increased number of oocytes were aspirated.[49] Similarly, comparing menotropins with early follicular or midluteal GnRH agonist administration, Ron-El et al. found no difference in pregnancy outcome.[75]

Improved pregnancy rates have been reported using the "flare" protocol in patients with a poor estradiol response to menotropins alone.[37] Unfortunately, using this protocol, an increased number of atretic follicles has also been reported.[9] Likewise, the number of mature oocytes in the preovulatory follicles of monkeys was found to be lower when a "flare" protocol was used.[44] These findings were also confirmed in a more recent, randomized prospective study.[40] Conversely, a recent meta-analysis of the literature concluded that the clinical pregnancy rate improved significantly after GnRH

analogue use in IVF.[29] It is clear that additional investigation is required to resolve this controversy.

Side effects

Side effects of GnRH analogues appear to be rare, usually minor, and generally due to those expected from a medically induced menopause (i.e., vaginal spotting, dryness, and hot flushes). Localized urticarial activity at the injection site of the GnRH analogue (wheal response) has been reported and is presumed to reflect the analogue's histamine-releasing capability. Mild, transient, neurological symptoms (paresthesia and numbness) have been reported recently in three women out of 536 receiving the D-Trp6 analogue of GnRH as part of their IVF ovulation induction protocol. A coincidental effect versus a direct neurological effect were discussed as possible causes.[4]

SUMMARY

Gonadotropin-releasing hormone and its analogues are now successful with inducing ovulation and assisting in ovulation induction with other medications (Fig. 34–6). Efficacious use of gonadotropin-releasing hormone for ovulation induction occurred only after the physiological role of gonadotropin-releasing hormone was understood. This validates the hypothesis that basic scientific investigation ultimately can provide important, clinically relevant information, even though the initial significance of the research may not be obvious.

Structure and relative potency of GnRH and GnRH agonist analogues.

Name	Relative Potency	Amino Acid Sequence									
		1 pyroGlu	2 His	3 Trp	4 Ser	5 Tyr	6 Gly	7 Leu	8 Arg	9 Pro	10 Gly–NH$_2$
GnRH	01										
	04										N–EtNH$_2$
	04						D–Ala				
	14						D–Ala				
Decapeptyl							D–Trp				
Leuprolide	15						D–Leu				N–EtNH$_2$
Buserelin	20						D–Ser (tBu)				N–EtNH$_2$
Nafarelin							D–Nal(2)				N–EtNH$_2$
Deslorelin	144						D–Trp				N–EtNH$_2$
Histrelin	210						D–His (ImBzl)				N–EtNH$_2$

Fig. 34-6. Analogs of GnRH formed by changing amino acids at positions 6 or 9 of the native hormone. Relative potencies of the analogs are indicated. (From Conn PM, Crowley WF: *NEJM* 324:93-101, 1991).

REFERENCES

1. Adashi EY: Clomiphene citrate: mechanism(s) and site(s) of action—a hypothesis revisited, *Fertil Steril* 331, 1984.

2. Akande EO, Bonnar J, Carr PJ, et al: Effect of synthetic gonadotropin-releasing hormone in secondary amenorrhea, *Lancet* 2:112, 1972.

3. Antunes JL, Carmel PW, Housepian EM, et al: Luteinizing hormone-releasing hormone in human pituitary blood, *J Neurosurg* 49:381, 1978.

4. Ashkenazi J, Goldman JA, Dicker D, et al: Adverse neurological symptoms after gonadotropin releasing hormone analog therapy for in vitro fertilization cycles, *Fertil Steril* 53:738, 1990.

5. Berger NG, Zacur HA: Exogenous progesterone for luteal support following gonadotropin-releasing hormone ovulation induction: case report, *Fertil Steril* 44:133, 1985.

6. Braat DDM, Ayalon D, Blunt SM, et al: Pregnancy outcome in luteinizing hormone releasing hormone induced cycles: a multicenter study, *Gynecol Endocrinol* 3:35, 1989.

7. Braat DD, Schoemaker R, Schoemaker J: Life-table analysis of fecundity in intravenously gonadotropin-releasing hormone treated patients with normogonadotropic and hypogonadotropic amenorrhea, *Fertil Steril* 55:266, 1991.

8. Breckwoldt M, Czygan PJ, Lehmann F, et al: Synthetic LH-RH as a therapeutic agent, *Acta Endocrinol (Copehn)* 75:209, 1974.

9. Brzyski RG, Muasher SJ, Droesh K, et al: Follicular atresia associated with concurrent initiation of gonadotropin-releasing hormone agonist and follicle-stimulating hormone for oocyte recruitment, *Fertil Steril* 50:917, 1988.

10. Burgus R, Butcher M, Amoss N, et al: Primary structure of the hypothalamic luteinizing hormone-releasing factor (LRF) of ovine origin, *Proc Natl Acad Sci USA* 69:278, 1972.

11. Carmel PW, Araki S, Ferin M: Pituitary stalk portal blood collection in rhesus monkeys: evidence for pulsatile release of gonadotropin releasing hormone (GnRH), *Endocrinology* 99:243, 1976.

12. Casas PRF, Badano AR, Aparicio N, et al: Luteinizing hormone-releasing hormone in the treatment of anovulatory infertility, *Fertil Steril* 26:549, 1975.

13. Chetkowski RJ, Druse LR, Nass TE: Improved pregnancy outcome with the addition of leuprolide acetate to gonadotropins for in vitro fertilization, *Fertil Steril* 52:250, 1989.

14. Conn PM, Crowley WF: Gonadotropin-releasing hormone and its analogues, *N Engl J Med* 324:93, 1991.

15. Crowley WF, McArthur JW: Simulation of the normal menstrual cycle in Kallmann's syndrome by pulsatile administration of luteinizing hormone-releasing hormone (LH-RH), *J Clin Endocrinol Metab* 51:173, 1980.

16. Crowley WF, Filicori M, Spratt DI, et al: The physiology of gonadotropin-releasing hormone secretion (GnRH) in men and women, *Recent Prog Horm Res* 41:473, 1985.

17. Eshel A, Abdulwahid NA, Armar NA, et al: Pulsatile luteinizing hormone releasing hormone therapy in women with polycystic ovarian syndrome, *Fertil Steril* 49:956, 1988.

18. Eskay RL, Mical RS, Porter JC: Relationship between luteinizing hormone releasing hormone concentration in hypophysial portal blood and luteinizing hormone release in intact, castrated and electrochemically stimulated rats, *Endocrinology* 100:263, 1977.

19. Filicori M, Flamigni C, Campaniello E, et al: Evidence for a specific role of GnRH pulse frequency in the control of the human menstrual cycle, *Am J Physiol* 257:E930, 1989.

20. Filicori M, Flamigni C, Merriggiola MC, et al: Ovulation induction with pulsatile gonadotropin-releasing hormone: technical modalities and clinical perspectives, *Fertil Steril* 56:1, 1991.

21. Frager MS, Pieper DR, Tonetta S, et al: Pituitary gonadotropin-releasing hormone (GnRH) receptors: effects of castration, steroid replacement and the role of GnRH in modulating receptors in the rat, *J Clin Invest* 67:615, 1981.

22. Fraser HM, Sandow J, Krauss B: Antibody production against an agonist analogue of luteinizing hormone-releasing hormone: evaluation of immunological and physiological consequences, *Acta Endocrinol (Copenh)* 103:151, 1983.

23. Garcia JE, Padilla SL, Boyati J, et al: Follicular phase gonadotropin-releasing hormone agonist and human gonadotropins: a better alternative for ovulation induction in in vitro fertilization, *Fertil Steril* 53:302, 1990.

24. Georzen J, Corenblum B, Wiseman DA, et al: Ovulation induction and pregnancy in hypothalamic amenorrhea using self-administered intravenous gonadotropin-releasing hormone, *Fertil Steril* 41:319, 1984.

25. Gonzalo-Barcena D, Kastin AJ, Schalch DS, et al: Synthetic LH-releasing hormone (LH-RH) administered to normal men by different routes, *J Clin Endocrinol Metab* 37:481, 1973.

26. Hashimoto T, Miyai K, Vozumi T, et al: Effect of prolonged LH-releasing hormone administration on gonadotropin response in patients with hypothalamic and pituitary tumors, *J Clin Endocrinol Metab* 41:721, 1975.

27. Hopkins CC, Hall JE, Santaro NF, et al: Closed intravenous administration of gonadotropin releasing hormone: safety of extended peripheral intravenous catheterization, *Obstet Gynecol* 74:267, 1989.

28. Howles CM, MacNamee MC, Edwards RG: Short-term use of an LH-RH agonist to treat poor respondents entering an in vitro fertilization program, *Hum Reprod* 2:655, 1987.

29. Hughes EG, Fedorkow DM, Saya S, et al: The routine use of gonadotropin releasing hormone agonists prior to in vitro fertilization and gamete intrafallopian transfer: a meta-analysis of randomized controlled trials, *Fertil Steril* 58:888, 1992.

30. Hurley DM, Brian RJ, Burger HG: Ovulation induction with subcutaneous pulsatile gonadotropin-releasing hormone singleton pregnancies in patients with previous multiple pregnancies after gonadotropin therapy, *Fertil Steril* 40:575, 1983.

31. Hurley DM, Brian R, Outch K, et al: Induction of ovulation and fertility in amenorrheic women by pulsatile low-dose gonadotropin releasing hormone, *N Engl J Med* 310:1069, 1984.

32. Hutchison JS, Zeleznik AJ: The rhesus monkey corpus luteum is dependent on pituitary gonadotropin secretion throughout the luteal phase of the menstrual cycle, *Endocrinology* 115:1780, 1984.

33. Jaffe SB, Jewelewic R: The basic infertility investigation, *Fertil Steril* 56:599, 1991.

34. Jaffe RB, Plosker S, Marshall L, et al: Neuromodulatory regulation of gonadotropin-releasing hormone pulsatile discharge in women, *Am J Obstet Gynecol* 163:1727, 1990.

35. Kalten MJ, Rivier JE: Gonadotropin releasing hormone analog design, structure function studies toward the development of agonists and antagonists: rationale and perspective, *Endocr Rev* 7:44, 1986.

36. Kastin AJ, Zarate A, Midgley AR, et al: Ovulation confirmed by pregnancy after infusion of porcine LH-RH, *J Clin Endocrinol Metab* 33:980, 1971.

37. Katayama KP, Roesler M, Gunnarson G, et al: Short-term use of gonadotropin-releasing hormone agonist (leuprolide) for in vitro fertilization, *J In Vitro Fert Embryo Transfer* 5:332, 1988.

38. Kazer RR, Kessel B, Yen SSC: Circulatory luteinizing hormone pulse frequency in women with polycystic ovary syndrome, *J Clin Endocrinol Metab* 65:233, 1987.

39. Keller PJ: Treatment of anovulation with synthetic luteinizing hormone-releasing hormone, *Am J Obstet Gynecol* 116:698, 1973.

40. Kingsland C, Tan SL, Bickertan N, et al: The routine use of gonadotropin-releasing hormone agonists for all patients undergoing in vitro fertilization. Is there any medical advantage? A prospective randomized study, *Fertil Steril* 57:804, 1992.

41. Knobil E, Plant TM, Wildt L, et al: Control of the Rhesus monkey menstrual cycle: permissive role of hypothalamic gonadotropin releasing hormone, *Science* 207:1371, 1980.

42. Knobil E: The GnRH pulse generator, *Am J Obstet Gynecol* 5:1721, 1990.

43. Koch Y, Baram T, Chobsieng P, et al: Enzymatic degradation of luteinizing hormone releasing hormone (LH-RH) by hypothalamic tissue, *Biochem Biophys Res Commun* 61:95, 1974.

44. Lefevre B, Gougeon A, Nome F, et al: Effect of a gonadotropin-releasing hormone agonist and gonadotropin on ovarian follicles in cynomolgus monkey: a model for human ovarian hyperstimulation, *Fertil Steril* 56:119, 1991.

45. Liu JH, Durfee R, Muse K, et al: Induction of multiple ovulation by pulsatile administration of gonadotropin-releasing hormone, *Fertil Steril* 40:18, 1983.

46. London DR, Butt WR, Lynch SS, et al: Hormonal responses to intranasal luteinizing hormone releasing hormone, *J Clin Endocrinol Metab* 37:829, 1973.

47. Lunenfeld B, Mashiach S, Blankstein: Induction of ovulation with gonadotropins. In Shearman RP, editor: *Clinical reproductive endocrinology*, New York, 1985, Churchill Livingstone.

48. Martin KA, Hall JE, Adams JM, et al: Comparison of exogenous gonadotropins and pulsatile gonadotropin-releasing hormone for induction of ovulation in hypogonadotropic amenorrhea, *J Clin Endocrinol Metab* 77:125, 1993.

49. Maroulis GB, Emery M, Verkauf B, et al: Prospective randomized study of human menotropin versus a follicular and luteal phase gonadotropin releasing hormone analog human menotropin stimulation protocols for in vitro fertilization, *Fertil Steril* 55:1157, 1991.

50. Mason P, Adams J, Morris DV, et al: Induction of ovulation with pulsatile luteinizing hormone-releasing hormone, *Br Med J* 288:181, 1984.

51. Matsuo H, Baba Y, Nair RMG, et al: Structure of the porcine LH and FSH releasing hormone I, the proposed amino acid sequence, *Biochem Biophys Res Commun* 43:1334, 1971.

52. Meakin JL, Keogh EJ, Martin CE: Human anti-luteinizing hormone-releasing hormone antibodies in patients treated with synthetic luteinizing hormone-releasing hormone, *Fertil Steril* 43:811, 1985.

53. Meldrum DR: Ovulation induction protocols, *Arch Pathol Lab Med* 116:406, 1992.

54. Miller DS, Reid Rr, Cetel NS, et al: Pulsatile administration of low-dose gonadotropin-releasing hormone, *JAMA* 250:2937, 1983.

55. Moenter SM, Caraty A, Karsch FJ: The estradiol induced surge of gonadotropin-releasing hormone in the ewe, *Endocrinology* 127:1375, 1990.

56. Moenter SM, Caraty A, Locatelli A, et al: Pattern of gonadotropin-releasing hormone (GnRH) secretion leading up to ovulation in the ewe: existence of a preovulatory GnRH surge, *Endocrinology* 129:1175, 1991.

57. Molloy BG, Hancock KW, Glass MR: Ovulation induction in clomiphene nonresponsive patients: the place of pulsatile gonadotropin-releasing hormone in clinical practice, *Fertil Steril* 43:26, 1985.

58. Nakai Y, Plant TM, Hess DL, et al: On the sites of negative and positive feedback actions of estradiol in the control of gonadotropin secretion in the Rhesus monkey, *Endocrinology* 102:1008, 1978.

59. Nakano R, Katayama K, Mizuno T, et al: Induction of ovulation with synthetic luteinizing hormone-releasing (FSH/LH-RH) in anovulatory sterility, *Fertil Steril* 25:160, 1974.

60. Naor Z, Clayton RN, Catt KJ: Characterization of GnRH receptors in cultured rat pituitary cells, *Endocrinology* 107:1144, 1980.

61. Naor Z: Signal transduction mechanisms of Cas2$^+$ mobilizing hormones: the case of gonadotropin-releasing hormone, *Endocr Rev* 11:326, 1990.

62. Nikolics K, Mason AJ, Szonyi E, et al: A prolactin-inhibiting factor within the precursor for human gonadotropin releasing hormone, *Nature* 316:511, 1985.

63. Nilius SJ, Fried H, Wide L: Successful induction of follicular maturation and ovulation by prolonged treatment with LH-releasing hormone in women with anorexia nervosa, *Am J Obstet Gynecol* 122:921, 1975.

64. Nilius SJ, Wide L: Gonadotropin-releasing hormone treatment for induction of follicular maturation and ovulation in amenorrheic women with anorexia nervosa, *Br Med J* 3:405, 1975.

65. Pepperell RJ: Prolactin and reproduction, *Fertil Steril* 35:267, 1981.

66. Pfaff DW: Luteinizing hormone-releasing factor potentiates lordosis behavior in hypophysectomized ovariectomized female rats, *Science* 182:1148, 1973.

67. Plant TM, Krey LC, Moossy J, et al: The arcuate nucleus and the control of gonadotropin and prolactin secretion in the female Rhesus monkey (*Macaca mulatta*), *Endocrinology* 102:52, 1978.

68. Porter RN, Smith W, Craft IL, et al: Induction of ovulation for in vitro fertilization using buserelin and gonadotropins, *Lancet* 2:1284, 1984.

69. Reame N, Sauder SE, Kelch RP, et al: Pulsatile gonadotropin secretion during the human menstrual cycle: evidence for altered frequency of gonadotropin-releasing hormone secretion, *J Clin Endocrinol Metab* 59:328, 1984.

70. Rebar R, Yen SSC, Vandenberg G: Gonadotropin responses to synthetic LRF: dose response relationship in men, *J Clin Endocrinol Metab* 36:10, 1973.

71. Rebar R, Judd HL, Yen SSC, et al: Characterization of the inappropriate gonadotropin secretion in polycystic ovary syndrome, *J Clin Invest* 57:1320, 1976.

72. Redding TW, Kastin AJ, Gonzalez-Barcena D, et al: The half-life, metabolism and excretion of tritiated luteinizing hormone releasing hormone (LH-RH) in man, *J Clin Endocrinol Metab* 37:626, 1973.

73. Reid RL, Sauerbrie E: Evaluation of techniques for induction of ovulation in outpatients employing pulsatile gonadotropin releasing hormone, *Am J Obstet Gynecol* 148:648, 1984.

74. Ron-El R, Golan A, Herman A, et al: Flexible menotropins initiation after long-acting gonadotropin releasing hormone analog, *Fertil Steril* 52:860, 1989.

75. Ron-El R, Herman A, Golan A, et al: The comparison of early follicular and midluteal administration of long-acting gonadotropin-releasing hormone agonist, *Fertil Steril* 54:233, 1990.

76. Rosen GF, Yee B: Inducing ovulation with gonadotropin releasing hormone and GnRH agonists, *Infert Reprod Med Clin North Am* 1:121, 1990.

77. Santoro N, Sierman ME, Filicori M, et al: Intravenous administration of pulsatile gonadotropin-releasing hormone in hypothalamic amenorrhea: effects of dosage, *J Clin Endocrinol Metab* 62:109, 1986.

78. Santoro N, Elzahn D: Pulsatile gonadotropin releasing hormone therapy for ovulatory disorders, *Clin Obstet Gynecol* 36:727, 1993.

79. Schally AV, Schally AMC, Kastin AJ: Present status of the use of LH-RH and its analogs in the diagnosis and therapy of infertility. In Beling CG, Wentz AC, editors: *The LH-releasing hormone*, New York, 1980, Masson.

80. Scott RT, Neal GS, Illions EH, et al: The duration of leuprolide acetate administration prior to ovulation induction does not impact ovarian responsiveness to exogenous gonadotropins, *Fertil Steril* 60:247, 1993.

81. Seeburg PH, Adelman JP: Characterization of CDNA for precursor of human luteinizing hormone releasing hormone, *Nature* 311:666, 1984.

82. Sherwood MN, Lovejoy DA, Cod DR: Origin of the mammalian gonadotropin-releasing hormones, *Endocr Rev* 14:241, 1993.

83. Skarin G, Millius SJ, Wide L: Pulsatile low-dose luteinizing hormone releasing hormone treatment for ovulation induction of follicular maturation and ovulation in women with amenorrhea, *Acta Endocrinol (Copenh)* 101:78, 1982.

84. Skarin G, Nilius SG, Wide L: Pulsatile subcutaneous low-dose gonadotropin-releasing hormone treatment of anovulatory infertility, *Fertil Steril* 40:454, 1983.

85. Smith MA, Vale WW: Desensitization to gonadotropin-releasing hormone observed in superfused pituitary cells on cytodex beads, *Endocrinology* 108:752, 1981.

86. Smitz J, Devroey P, Braechmans P, et al: Management of failed cycles in an IVF-GIFT programme with the combination of GnRH analogue and hMG, *Hum Reprod* 2:309, 1987.

87. Soules MR, Steiner RA, Clifton DK, et al: Progesterone modulation of pulsatile luteinizing hormone secretion in normal women, *J Clin Endocrinol Metab* 58:378, 1984.

88. Weinstein FG, Seibel MM, Taymore ML: Ovulation induction with subcutaneous pulsatile gonadotropin-releasing hormone: the role of supplemental human chorionic gonadotropin in the luteal phase, *Fertil Steril* 41:546, 1984.

89. Wilcox LS, Mosher WD: Use of infertility services in the United States, *Obstet Gynecol* 82:122, 1993.

90. Wildt L, Hausler A, Marshall G, et al: Frequency and amplitude of gonadotropin releasing hormone stimulation and gonadotropin secretion in the rhesus monkey, *Endocrinology* 109:376, 1981.

91. Xia L, VanVugt D, Alston EJ, et al: A surge of gonadotropin-releasing hormone accompanies the estradiol-induced gonadotropin surge in the rhesus monkey, *Endocrinology*, 131:2812, 1992.

92. Yang-Feng TL, Seeburg PH, Francke V: Human luteinizing hormone releasing hormone gene (LHRH) is located on the short arm of chromosome 8 (region 8p11, 2>p21), *Somat Cell Mol Genet* 12:95, 1986.

93. Yen SSC, Vela P, Rankin J: Inappropriate secretion of follicle stimulating hormone and luteinizing hormone in polycystic ovarian disease, *J Clin Endocrinol Metab* 30:435, 1970.

94. Yu WH, Seeburg PH, Nikolics K, et al: Gonadotropin-releasing hormone associated peptide exerts a prolactin inhibitory and weak gonadotropin-releasing activity in vivo, *Endocrinology* 123:390, 1988.

95. Zacur HA: Ovulation induction with gonadotropin-releasing hormone, *Fertil Steril* 44:435, 1985.

Chapter 35

OVARIAN HYPERSTIMULATION SYNDROME

Joseph G. Schenker, MD

Ovarian hyperstimulation syndrome (OHSS) is the least prevalent, albeit the most serious, complication of ovulation induction. OHSS is a syndrome in which induction of ovulation results in a wide spectrum of clinical and laboratory symptoms and signs. At one end of the spectrum there is only chemical evidence of ovarian hyperstimulation with an increased production of steroids; at the other end of the spectrum are massive ovarian enlargement, ascites, pleural effusion, hemoconcentration, oliguria, electrolyte imbalance, and hypercoagulability, a life-threatening derangement in hemostasis. This iatrogenic condition was first described toward the end of the 1930s with the use of gonadotropins extracted from pregnant mare serum (PMSG).[29] In all types of ovarian stimulation with different preparations (e.g., gonadotropins, clomiphene citrate, and gonadotropin-releasing hormone [GnRH] agonists) and different regimens of treatment, a nonphysiologic ovarian response may lead to the development of OHSS.

Induction of ovulation has become an acceptable and widespread medical therapy for anovulatory infertile women. The risk of severe OHSS varies between 0.5% and 1%.[159] In the last decade the development of assisted reproductive techniques expanded the use of ovulation-inducing agents in women with normal ovulatory cycles. A world collaborative report for 1989 revealed that infertile women participating in in vitro fertilization (IVF) and gamete intrafallopian transfer (GIFT) programs underwent 100,000 hyperstimulated treatment cycles.[188] Ovarian hyperstimulation after application of modern technologies is associated with incidences of moderate and severe OHSS in the range of 3% to 4% and 0.1% to 0.2%, respectively.[16,150]

Indications for controlled ovarian hyperstimulation are continuously expanding and are applied in cases of infertility other than anovulation, such as unexplained infertility, pelvic adhesions, endometriosis, luteal phase defect, and male infertility.[30,173] Even though the risk of severe OHSS with controlled ovarian hyperstimulation is below 1%, the absolute number of patients hospitalized for this iatrogenic syndrome will increase significantly.

Sporadic cases presenting with signs of OHSS due to increased endogenous secretion of gonadotropins have been reported.[13,154] They were associated with multiple pregnancies, hydatidiform mole, and the presence of lutein cysts.

The syndrome is explained by a sudden increase in

Table 35-1. Classification of OHSS

Degree	Symptoms and signs
Mild form	
Stage A	Chemical hyperstimulation; 17β-estradiol levels of 1000 to 1500 pg/mL
Stage B	Chemical hyperstimulation; ovaries up to 6 cm in diameter
Moderate form	
Stage A	17β-estradiol levels > 4000 pg/mL; ovaries 6 to 12 cm
Stage B	Ascites by ultrasound; findings as in stage A; vomiting, diarrhea
Severe form	
Stage A	17β-Estradiol > 6000 pg/mL; ovaries > 12 cm; ascites, liver dysfunction
Stage B	Tension ascites, ARDS, shock, renal failure, thromboembolism

capillary permeability, especially of the ovarian vessels, which results in a rapid fluid shift from the intravascular space to the third space, leading to acute hemodynamic changes and the wide-spectrum clinical picture.[129] Despite the cumulative knowledge of the pathogenesis of OHSS, there is still no reliable method for its prediction and complete prevention.

CLASSIFICATION OF OHSS

In 1967 Rabau et al.[134] classified OHSS into six categories. Based on clinical symptoms and signs and laboratory findings, Schenker and Weinstein[159] divided OHSS into three main categories (mild, moderate, and severe). Golan et al.[60] proposed a modified classification based on ultrasonographic findings that enables accurate definition of the size of the ovaries and the presence of ascites. With the practice of assisted reproductive technology in which normal ovulatory women are hyperstimulated, there is an increase in the incidence and severity of OHSS. We recently prepared a modified classification of OHSS based on clinical manifestations and laboratory and ultrasonographic findings (Table 35-1).

Mild form

In stage A there is chemical hyperstimulation with 17β-estradiol levels of 1500 to 2500 pg/mL. Estrogen levels in 24-hour urine are above 200 μg/mL. In stage B the laboratory findings as in stage A are present with enlargement of the ovaries up to 6 cm in diameter, based on clinical and ultrasonographic examinations.

Moderate form

In stage A 17β-estradiol levels are above 4000 pg/mL. The ovaries are enlarged to 6 to 12 cm in diameter, abdominal distention is present, and there is evidence of ascites on ultrasound examination. Stage B consists of the

criteria as in stage A, plus gastrointestinal symptoms of vomiting and/or diarrhea.

Severe form

In stage A, in addition to the findings in stage B of the moderate form, estradiol levels are above 6000 pg/mL; ovaries are enlarged to more than 12 cm in diameter; there is clinical evidence of ascites and/or hydrothorax; and/or there are clinical or laboratory findings of liver involvement. In stage B there is marked hemoconcentration (hematocrit ≥ 45%) with increased blood viscosity, which may result in coagulation abnormalities; tension ascites and/or adult respiratory distress syndrome (ARDS); and/or thromboembolic phenomena, and/or renal impairment, and/or hypovolemic shock.

CLINICAL SYMPTOMS AND SIGNS OF OHSS

Various clinical aspects of the different etiologies of OHSS have been described.[159] Several case reports have revealed unusual cases of severe OHSS.*

Mild hyperstimulation

Chemical hyperstimulation is a very common accompaniment of ovulation induction. Chemical hyperstimulation may follow administration of human chorionic gonadotropin (hCG); it may even occur with administration of clomiphene citrate, follicle-stimulating hormone (FSH), or human menopausal gonadotropin (hMG) alone. Superovulation in spontaneous ovulatory cycles within the framework of assisted reproductive programs leads to mild hyperstimulation in each case. Chemical hyperstimulation is of little clinical concern and usually resolves with the onset of menses. However, when conception occurs, the hCG produced by the syncytiotrophoblast maintains high levels of estradiol and progesterone for several weeks. Their actual levels depend on the number of gestational sacs.

The mild form of OHSS presents as a sensation of abdominal heaviness, tension, swelling, and pain. The physical findings are bilateral ovarian enlargement by multiple follicular and corpus luteum cysts; the ovaries may be up to 6 cm in diameter. In recent years mild hyperstimulation has become more common with induction of superovulation in ovulatory women participating in the various modalities of assisted reproductive programs. It is relatively more common than severe OHSS as a result of estradiol and ultrasonographic monitoring of ovulation induction in ovulatory patients. Occasionally the cyst may rupture or undergo torsion. The bloody contents of the ruptured follicles and corpus luteum cysts irritate the peritoneal cavity, and the patient experiences the symptoms of intraperitoneal hemorrhage. This often presents a difficult problem in the differential diagnosis between a ruptured cyst and an ectopic pregnancy. Endoscopic exploration may be

*References 4, 83, 88, 159, 161, 170.

necessary to establish an accurate diagnosis.

Twisting of an ovarian cyst may lead to infarction and thus present as an acute abdomen.

No therapy is necessary in the mild form of the syndrome, except for rest, observation, and medication for symptomatic relief. Pelvic examination or vaginal ultrasonographic examination should be performed carefully in order to prevent rupture of the cyst. It is advisable to avoid intercourse.

Moderate hyperstimulation

In cases of moderate hyperstimulation, the abdominal discomfort is more pronounced. The levels of 17β-estradiol are about 4000 to 5000 pg/mL. Gastrointestinal symptoms such as nausea, vomiting, and (less frequently) diarrhea are present. There is some weight gain and an increase in abdominal circumference. The ovaries are enlarged up to 12 cm in diameter, and some ascitic fluid is detected by ultrasonography. Most patients will have moderate OHSS within 10 days after hCG administration. In conception cycles the symptoms may appear later. OHSS is a self-limiting process. In nonconception cycles the symptoms disappear by the onset of menstruation, but regression of the ovarian cyst can take 2 to 4 weeks and sometimes even longer. Patients in this category require observation and should be hospitalized, since the condition may progress rapidly to the severe form, especially if conception occurs. It is therefore important to confirm conception as early as possible by estimation of β-hCG levels and ultrasonography.[159] In conception cycles, the symptom and signs of OHSS are often more protracted, lasting 14 to 30 days, and ovarian enlargement can persist for up to 8 to 12 weeks of gestation.[61,159,163]

The possibility of rupture of an ovarian cyst should always be considered. Pelvic and ultrasonographic examinations must be performed gently to minimize the likelihood of rupture, which may result in intraperitoneal hemorrhage and require surgical intervention. The ovarian cysts are large; therefore the incidence of torsion is limited.

During hospitalization the patients should be closely monitored by clinical symptoms, ultrasonography, and laboratory tests.

Severe hyperstimulation

Severe OHSS is a serious complication of ovulation induction in previously healthy women. The ovaries are greatly enlarged, more than 12 cm in diameter, and are easily palpated abdominally. Exceptional cases of severe manifestations of OHSS without ovarian enlargement have been reported.[83] The clinical manifestations may include a variable spectrum of symptoms and signs and abnormal laboratory findings, and include pleural effusion, pericardial effusion, hypovolemia, impairment of renal function, electrolyte imbalance, disturbance in liver function, thromboembolic phenomena, shock, tension ascites, ARDS, and

even death. Only two deaths following OHSS have been reported, both in Israel.[115,148] Since preparations for induction of ovulation are used extensively all over the world and cases of severe OHSS have been reported worldwide, it may be suggested that deaths occurring in other places have not been reported.

A patient with severe OHSS is critically ill and presents with many life-threatening problems that must be solved immediately with little margin for error. The clinician must understand the pathophysiology of this clinical iatrogenic syndrome, which may involve several organs and systems. The condition of a patient with severe OHSS improves within several days when she is correctly treated, when there are no complications, and when conception does not occur. The large ovarian cysts gradually subside after the abrupt appearance of clinical symptoms of hyperstimulation. In conception cycles recovery takes longer and complications are more frequent.

Specific complications of moderate and severe OHSS

The clinical symptoms and signs of 93 patients hospitalized in our institution with moderate and severe degrees of hyperstimulation are summarized in Figs. 35-1 and 35-2. The specific complications of tension ascites, thromboembolic phenomena, liver dysfunction, renal impairment, and ARDS are described below.

Tension ascites. The presence of ascites is a major sign of the capillary leak phenomenon present in OHSS. There is a direct connection between the intensity of capillary permeability and the severity of OHSS, as has been shown in an experimental model.[156] As this phenomenon continues, hypovolemia and oliguria are apparent. Administration of colloid solutions intravenously improves the hypovolemic state and increases the oncotic pressure, but the capillary leakage still exists and there will be sequestration of fluid in the third space. These dynamic changes in OHSS may cause the clinical picture of tension ascites, which is a severe, life-threatening condition. It has been demonstrated that the ascitic fluid is exudative, with a protein concentration of 4.8 g/dL.[122,181] In the presence of tension ascites the intraperitoneal pressure is increased. When the intraperitoneal pressure exceeds the normal intraluminal pressure of the abdominal vena cava, the inferior vena cava is compressed, and blood flow in the inferior vena cava is reduced. During these pathophysiologic changes there is reduced preload to the heart, leading to decreased cardiac output. The increased intraperitoneal pressure changes the balance between the abdominal and thoracic cavities. Problems of blood circulation and respiration arise as soon as the excursions of the diaphragm are decreased by a high intraabdominal pressure.

Pleural effusion, chiefly right-sided, commonly occurs in association with tension ascites. The hydrothorax is mainly a consequence of ascitic fluid seepage through diaphragmatic lymphatic vessels. In case of tension ascites there is

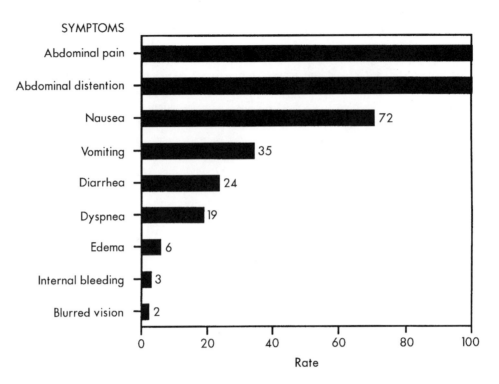

Fig. 35-1. Symptoms in 93 patients hospitalized with moderate and severe OHSS.

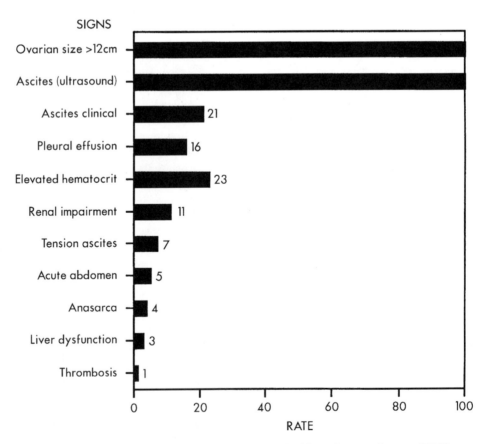

Fig. 35-2. Clinical signs in 93 patients hospitalized with moderate and severe OHSS.

also impairment of renal function. Therefore, in cases of OHSS with the presence of tension ascites, paracentesis guided by ultrasonography is indicated. By repeated paracenteses considerable amounts of proteins and electrolytes are lost, which may have serious consequences on fluid and electrolyte metabolism.[58,140]

Thromboembolic phenomena. Two severe cases of thromboembolic phenomena after hMG/hCG treatment have been reported from Israel; both patients died of carotid artery thrombosis.[115,148] The second case occurred in a 42-year-old woman.[148] Brachial vein thrombosis in one patient and deep vein thrombosis in another were observed after induction of ovulation with hMG/hCG.[31,55] A thromboembolic phenomenon resulting in a limb amputation was also recorded in Israel.[115] Recently a 30-year-old woman had a cerebrovascular accident with hemiplegia due to thrombosis of cerebral vessels after hyperstimulation for the GIFT procedure.[139] OHSS complicated by deep vein thrombosis in the absence of any signs of hemoconcentration has been reported in a patient who had low antithrombin III levels.[85] A case of internal jugular vein thrombosis and mediastinal thrombosis after ovulation induction with gonadotropins has also been reported.[46] The patient was successfully treated with heparin and had a normal, spontaneous delivery of healthy twins.

Evidence of hemoconcentration, with increased (6% to 10%) hematocrit values, has been observed. In most patients with evidence of hemoconcentration, coagulation parameters such as clotting time, bleeding time, platelet count, prothrombin time, and fibrinogen levels were within normal limits.[159] Phillips et al.[128] demonstrated abnormalities in coagulation factors in patients with OHSS. Arterial thrombosis in patients with OHSS possibly is caused by hemoconcentration resulting from increased hypovolemia due to an acute shift of fluids from the intravascular space to the third space. The high levels of estrogens in patients with moderate and severe OHSS also contribute to the incidence of thromboembolic phenomena, both arterial and venous. Ashkenazi et al.[6] observed mild, transient, neurologic symptoms after induction of ovulation with GnRH for IVF. The symptoms were numbness, headache, paresthesia, and paresis. The symptoms appeared abruptly and then disappeared, and might have been caused by transient cerebral ischemia.

Liver dysfunction. Recently abnormalities of liver function tests (LFT) in severe cases of OHSS were reported for the first time.[190] Additional reports[7,144,178] provide evidence for hepatic changes of both a hepatocellular and a cholestatic nature in cases of OHSS associated with and without conception. In two patients, elevated levels of serum aspartate aminotransferase (SGOT), alanine aminotransferase (SGPT), alkaline phosphatase, and bilirubin and a decreased concentration of albumin were observed. These results of LFT returned to normal within 1 month

while gestation was continuing uneventfully. Elevated levels of alkaline phosphatase, SGOT, SGPT, bilirubin, and creatine phosphokinase were found in cases reported by Sueldo et al.[178] Forman et al.[45] reported LFT abnormalities in three of eight patients with OHSS. Balasch et al.[7] reported a patient with jaundice and LFT abnormalities that subsided within 4 weeks.

Biopsy specimens of the liver demonstrated the following: Light microscopy disclosed a normal lobular pattern; there was no evidence of fibrosis; the vascular architecture was preserved; and fatty changes in some periportal areas and marked Kupffer cell hyperplasia were observed. Electron microscopy revealed paracrystalline inclusion in the mitochondria and some dilatation of the endoplasmic reticulum; no significant changes were found in the Golgi apparatus or glycogen granules.

One hypothesis is that the LFT abnormalities may be attributed to several factors: (1) the gestagen supportive treatment after preembryo transfer, (2) the increased vascular permeability observed in OHSS that, in turn, led to hepatic damage, and (3) the increased estrogen levels observed in OHSS.[190]

The ultrastructural changes found in liver specimens from women with OHSS have been described in specimens from women treated with sex hormones, estrogens, and gestagens, and from women taking contraceptive pills. The changes involving the mitochondria and endoplasmic reticulum may represent a morphologic compensation for the increased demand on the liver enzymes to metabolize the higher levels of sex hormones. The fact that LFT results returned to normal in all patients despite continuous progesterone support of the luteal phase negates the possibility that a gestagen may be involved in the etiology of LFT abnormalities.

Among various hormones known to be increased in OHSS, 17β-estradiol is the most prominent. Estradiol (E_2) administration to human subjects results in cholestatic changes, increased alkaline phosphatase concentrations, and impaired sulfobromophthalein excretion.[2] The correlation between estrogen levels and the appearance and disappearance of OHSS is well recognized. The E_2 levels reached in patients would explain, at least in part, the hepatic involvement in OHSS. Superovulation, usually induced in IVF programs, also leads to higher estrogen concentrations than those observed in induction of ovulation in anovulatory patients. This may be the reason that LFT abnormalities have been reported only recently in patients treated by assisted reproductive technology.

As for any patient showing abnormal liver function, several possible etiologies may have to be considered and excluded. The patient's medical history may exclude drug use, alcohol intake, gastrointestinal involvement, or exposure to toxins. Serologic tests may exclude the presence of viral infections such as hepatitis A and hepatitis B and the presence of cytomegalovirus, Epstein-Barr virus, and others. Hepatic imaging by ultrasonography can exclude biliary tract pathology.

If LFT abnormalities increase in severity, liver biopsy is indicated.

Renal impairment. Hypovolemia in severe cases of OHSS, due to a shift of fluid from the intravascular compartment to the third space, causes inadequate blood perfusion to the kidney and may lead to prerenal failure.[153] Oliguria is defined as the first stage of renal impairment, which may progress to anuria. Oliguria is a urinary output below 20 mL/h.[113] This condition leads to alteration of laboratory test results. Blood urea nitrogen (BUN) and creatinine levels are elevated, with a ratio of 20:1. Because of the low urinary flow, there is an increase in reabsorption of urea, leading to a rise in BUN to a greater degree than creatinine.[84] On the other hand, creatinine is not reabsorbed by the proximal tubule and therefore remains normal or only slightly elevated. Specific gravity is usually greater than 1.020, because the kidneys are stimulated to concentrate the urea. The urine sodium levels are less than 20 mEq/L. Urine osmolarity is above 480 mOsm/kg and is usually greater than plasma osmolarity. Therefore, in cases of renal impairment due to hypovolemia, it is of primary importance to observe changes in vital signs, to obtain accurate body weight measurements, and to record oral and intravenous fluid intake and urine output. When oliguria is diagnosed, the urinary output should be measured continuously by an indwelling catheter. Prerenal failure may lead to anuria, hyperkalemia, and uremia. Treatment of prerenal failure is aimed at restoring adequate circulation to the kidney. Correction of hypovolemia will improve the urine flow and reverse the signs of prerenal failure. Diuretics are contraindicated, since they may aggravate the hypovolemic state and even lead to shock.[159]

The first and best sign of recovery is an increase in urine output, especially with a severe complication such as tension ascites, ARDS, or shock.

Adult respiratory distress syndrome. ARDS is a rare but life-threatening manifestation of severe OHSS.[191] The main manifestations are respiratory failure and refractory hypoxemia that cannot be corrected by administration of 100% oxygen.[5] ARDS is caused by differing acute processes that directly or indirectly injure the lungs (e.g., sepsis, injury, shock, and fat embolism). The most frequent pathophysiologic change in ARDS is increased capillary permeability. OHSS is characterized by increased capillary leakage associated with increased prostaglandin production. In severe cases of OHSS the pulmonary capillary endothelium and alveolar epithelium are injured, leading to leakage of blood, plasma, and colloid solutions into the intestinal and intraalveolar spaces. Alveolar flooding and atelectasis result. The latter is due in part to reduced surfactant activity. An inflammatory process ensues within 2 to 3 days, leading later to fibrosis. The diagnosis of ARDS is

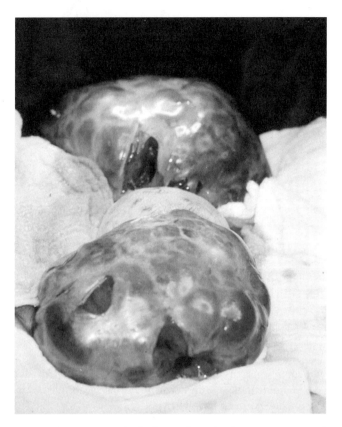

Fig. 35-3. Macroscopic findings of ovaries in a severe case of OHSS (rupture of follicular and corpus luteum cysts).

based on clinical manifestations and estimation of arterial blood gases, which discloses acute respiratory alkalosis. Chest x-rays usually show diffused bilateral alveolar infiltrates, as in acute pulmonary edema. The characteristic finding is low pulmonary arterial wedge pressure (below 15 mm Hg). If the severe hypoxemia of ARDS is not recognized and treated promptly, cardiorespiratory arrest occurs in 90% of patients. The survival rate of patients with severe ARDS is 50% with appropriate therapy.[127] Patients with OHSS complicated by ARDS should be treated in intensive respiratory units. The life-threatening hypoxemia should be treated as follows: The patient is intubated and ventilated with 100% oxygen, and a positive end-expiratory pressure (PEEP) is applied.[62] Intravenous fluid is administered, including blood plasma and colloid solutions to increase oncotic pressure and to restore peripheral perfusion, despite the presence of alveolar edema. Patients who respond to treatment and survive do not have residual pulmonary dysfunction.[93]

PATHOGENESIS OF OHSS

The main pathologic findings in severe OHSS are multiple ovarian cysts of more than 10 cm in diameter, follicular cysts, corpora lutea, and severe edema of the stroma[152] (Fig. 35-3). Massive enlargement of the ovaries is accompanied by different degrees of acute body fluid shifts with ascites formation, hydrothorax, and sometimes ana-sarca. The sudden body fluid shift seems to be caused by increased capillary permeability, especially of the ovarian vessels, as was demonstrated in experimental studies with the use of intravenous Evans blue and Pontamine sky-blue stains.[155] This experimental model of OHSS in the rabbit has been reproduced by Knox[91] and others, [57] who were able to block the manifestations of OHSS by the concomi-tant use of antihistamine preparations.

Evidence that increased capillary permeability is the pathogenetic mechanism of severe ovarian hyperstimula-tion is supported by the study by Tollan et al.[184] They demonstrated that during ovarian stimulation for IVF there is infiltration of fluids from the vascular space to the interstitial compartment 1 day before oocyte aspiration (1 day after hCG administration).

There is experimental evidence in the rat and in the rabbit that excessive estrogens may cause increased capil-lary permeability of the uterus and ovarian vessels.[34,125] It is well known that in cases of OHSS high levels of estrogen are found in the serum, urine, and follicular fluid. On the other hand, it is known that the administration of high doses of estrogens do not, by themselves, produce clinical hyper-stimulation; the syndrome could not be reproduced by administering huge doses of estrogen to female rabbits.[156]

Abnormally high serum levels of various steroids were detected in patients with OHSS after hMG/hCG treatment. As mentioned previously, it has been confirmed that the syndrome develops only after ovulation and corpus luteum formation.[159,181] In experimental animals the syndrome is not prevented by hysterectomy or by extraperitonealization of the ovaries. Moreover, OHSS cannot be induced in male animals or in men treated with large doses of hMG preparations.[152] Therefore it is assumed that the increased capillary permeability found in patients with OHSS is due to some excess of immediate metabolites secreted by the ovary after hMG/hCG stimulation.

Recent experiments set out to determine whether pros-taglandins are the "active substances" in the development of OHSS. It was demonstrated that indomethacin, a blocker of prostaglandin synthesis, can prevent the fluid shift associated with the ascites, pleural effusion, and hypo-volemia seen in this syndrome.[158] It may be that the excessive estrogen produced by the large numbers of developing follicles also stimulates increased production of prostaglandins, which in turn may be responsible for the increased capillary permeability observed in OHSS. In-domethacin has been used with good results by several investigators as a therapeutic measure in cases of severe OHSS.[40,87,157]

Histamine and OHSS

Gergely et al.[57] and Knox et al.[92] reproduced the animal model described earlier and showed that OHSS could be blocked in rabbits by administration of antihistaminic preparations. In animals treated with antihistamine regres-sion of the hyperstimulated ovaries was more rapid than in a control group. The difference in regression was found to be statistically significant. These investigators suggested that hyperstimulation can be prevented and treated by application of antihistaminic preparations.

Pride et al.,[132] using the rabbit model, studied the role of chlorpheniramine maleate, an H_1 receptor blockade in OHSS. H_1 receptor effectively blocked the ascites forma-tion but did not prevent the ovarian enlargement and augmentation of the intraovarian prostaglandin F (PGF) content. Pride et al. suggested that the protective effect of H_1 receptor blockade on ascites formation may be medi-ated, at least in part, by PGF. They also showed that steroidogenesis is not influenced by this preparation.

Renin-angiotensin system

Studies of plasma renin activity (PRA) and aldosterone in patients with ovarian hyperstimulation[119] have shown the following results: The pattern of PRA in hMG-hyperstimulated cycles is characterized by a mid–luteal phase peak that declines to normal in the late luteal phase in nonconception cycles, whereas a sustained elevation of PRA occurs in conception cycles. A direct correlation between the magnitude of PRA and the severity of OHSS was established. A significant correlation was demonstrated between PRA activity in the serum and levels of either progesterone or E_2. Elevated levels of plasma aldosterone were observed in cycles with OHSS, and especially in conception cycles with OHSS.

The demonstration of high levels of prorenin and the presence of angiotensin I, angiotensin-converting enzyme (ACE), and angiotensin II in human follicular fluid and the high plasma activity in cases of OHSS leads to the hypoth-esis that the renin-angiotensin system is involved in the pathogenesis of OHSS. Enlargement of the ovaries, caused by development of multiple follicular and corpus luteum cysts, requires extensive angiogenesis.[42,148]

Renin production has also been demonstrated in the human corpus luteum, and it is suggested that renin is involved in the extensive vascularization that occurs with formation of the corpus luteum. The renin-angiotensin system, in addition to its other actions (increased arterial vasoconstriction, arterial permeability, and synthesis of prostaglandins and aldosterone), also has angiogenic prop-erties. Follicular fluid and both nonluteal and luteal ovarian tissue contain factors that are capable of stimulating new vessel formation.[80]

The angiotensinogen concentration in follicular fluid is similar to that in plasma. Angiotensin I is split by a converting enzyme, dipeptidyl carboxypeptidase, forming angiotensin II. The converting enzyme is found mainly in the lungs and kidneys, but also in other organs. Angiotensin II is rapidly destroyed by angiotensinase. Its half-life in humans is 1 to 2 minutes. The product of angiotensin II

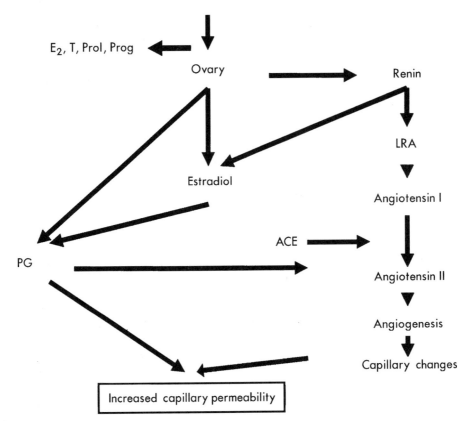

Fig. 35-4. Pathogenesis of OHSS. E_2, 17β-estradiol; T, testosterone; Prol, prolactin; Prog, progesterone; LRA, luteal phase renin activity; ACE, angiotensin converting enzyme; PG, prostaglandin.

destruction is angiotensin III, which has a lower biologic activity. It also increases vascular permeability, enlarging the pores through contraction of the endothelial cells by widening the gaps between cells.[126,141]

The presence of ACE activity, which converts angiotensin I to angiotensin II, was recently determined in human preovulatory follicular fluid. The ACE activity in follicular fluid was similar to that in plasma. Correlations were sought between follicular fluid ACE and both serum and follicular fluid E_2 and P_4. A highly significant correlation was found between ACE activity in follicular fluid and follicular fluid P_4. No linear correlation could be demonstrated between serum and follicular fluid ACE activity or between ACE activity and serum E_2 and P_4 or follicular fluid E_2.[148]

One concept of the pathogenesis of OHSS is that the increased capillary permeability present in OHSS is due to involvement of the renin-angiotensin system and synthesis of prostaglandins in the ovaries (Fig. 35-4). Enlargement of the ovaries and the increased capillary permeability, which leads to acute fluid shift, may explain the different clinical features observed in this syndrome (Fig. 35-5).

Rapid body fluid shifts in patients with ovarian hyperstimulation may lead to hypovolemia and hemoconcentration, as evidenced by increased hematocrit values and serum osmolarity.[131,159] When not corrected immediately, hypovolemia may lead to decreased renal perfusion, subsequently stimulating the proximal renal tubules to resorb salt and water, and resulting in clinical manifestations of oliguria, electrolyte imbalance, and azotemia. Urinary aldosterone levels were found to be markedly increased in several patients with OHSS.[84] High levels of aldosterone may prevent effective sodium diuresis once plasma volume and renal perfusion are restored after initial treatment.

With less sodium reaching the distal tubuli, there is a decrease in the exchange of hydrogen and potassium for sodium, resulting in hyperkalemic acidosis. A rise in the blood urea nitrogen concentration is due to decreased perfusion and increased urea absorption. Thus the patient is hypovolemic, azotemic, and hyperkalemic. The loss of fluid and protein into the peritoneal cavity accounts for the hypovolemia and hemoconcentration. This in turn results in low blood pressure and decreased central venous pressure.[159]

From a clinical point of view, the rapid body fluid shift may lead to hemoconcentration, increased blood viscosity and, finally, the thromboembolic phenomena that are associated with the syndrome. The dynamic fluid changes explain the clinical entities of tension ascites and ARDS, which are due to the vascular leak. Abnormal hormone

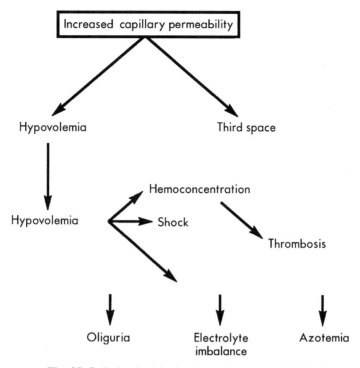

Fig. 35-5. Pathophysiologic changes in cases of OHSS.

levels may be the cause of liver dysfunction. The enlarged ovaries, composed of follicular and luteal cysts, may cause the intraperitoneal catastrophe bleeding, and torsion that require immediate surgical intervention.[79,159]

INCIDENCE AND SEVERITY OF OHSS

Factors affecting incidence and severity

The incidence and severity of OHSS vary with the different clinical conditions in which ovulation is induced in anovulatory patients or ovulatory patients hyperstimulated and treated by assisted reproductive technology. The incidence varies according to the types of pharmacologic preparations given and the doses and schedules of administration.

Careful monitoring of ovulation induction is the most important parameter affecting the incidence of OHSS. Data from the 1970s (Table 35-2), when induction of ovulation was monitored only by estrogen levels, showed mild hyperstimulation in 5% to 10% of cycles and severe hyperstimulation in 0.2% to 0.5%. More recent data on 3000 cycles of in vivo fertilization showed 1.1% moderate OHSS and 0.1% severe OHSS. The incidences in IVF cycles were 2.6% and 0.4%, respectively.

Pharmacologic preparations

Pregnant mare serum gonadotropin. Toward the end of 1930, PMSG was administered in clinical trials to stimulate the ovaries to ovulate, resulting in corpus luteum

Table 35-2. Incidence of OHSS

Years	No. of Cycles	Degree of OHSS	
		Moderate	Severe
1972–1980	865	30 (3.5%)	5 (0.5%)
1983–1985	1822	26 (1.4%)	10 (0.5%)
1986–1990 (In vivo fertilization)	3035	35 (1.1%)	3 (0.1%)
1986–1990 (In vitro fertilization)	1750	47 (2.6%)	8 (0.45%)

formation and pregnancy.[29] The results, however, were inconsistent and generally disappointing because of the formation of neutralizing antibodies to heterologous gonadotropins. Until 1962, 60 cases of OHSS, including two deaths, were reported in patients treated with PMSG.[41,43,117]

Human pituitary gonadotropin. In 1958 Gemzell et al.[54] first described the successful induction of ovulation and pregnancy in women utilizing human pituitary gonadotropin (hPG), derived from human pituitary glands removed at autopsy, in combination with hCG. During a 12-year period (1960–1971) 211 conceptions (36.8%) were achieved in 572 infertile women treated for 1045 cycles in Uppsala, Sweden. In 1963 Gemzell[52] reported that

OHSS had occurred in 4 of 22 treatment cycles. In later series the incidence of OHSS was about 2% of the treatment cycles as noted by monitoring estrogen levels. Among the OHSS cases was a case of right brachial vein thrombosis.

The incidence of OHSS with use of hPG has varied greatly.[56] Crooke et al.[31] recorded a case of deep vein thrombosis at 12 weeks of pregnancy. Several investigators have reported successful ovulation induction with potent gonadotropin extracts from human pituitary glands obtained post mortem. Data from the Australian Department of Health indicated that by the end of 1981 552 pregnancies occurred in 4008 treatment cycles.[102] The scarcity of human pituitary glands required for the production of hPG greatly restricted its global widespread use. Since the observation that Creutzfeldt-Jakob disease, a fatal slow viral disease of the central nervous system, had developed in patients who were treated with human growth hormone when they were children, the use of hPG has been restricted.

Clomiphene citrate. In 1961 Greenblatt and Barfield[65] introduced clomiphene citrate (CC) as a successful agent for ovulation induction. (See Chapter 32.) Its biologic action is to compete with estrogen for binding sites in the hypothalamus and possibly in the pituitary gland and ovary. During its administration there is a moderate increase in FSH and luteinizing hormone (LH) secretion, and a gradual increase in the estrogen production of the ovary. The therapy is individualized to patients with an intact hypothalamic-pituitary-ovarian axis. CC is therefore the drug of choice for induction of ovulation in patients belonging to group II of the World Health Organization classification, that is, anovulatory women having some spontaneous, albeit deranged, pituitary and ovarian activity. The rates of ovulation achieved are in the range of 80% to 90% for women with oligomenorrhea and 50% to 60% for women with amenorrhea, although the conception rate is relatively small (about 40% to 45%).

CC may be administered concomitantly with other agents such as hCG, GnRH, hMG, prednisone, and estrogen preparations. Combined therapy with CC/hMG/hCG may also result in OHSS.[72] One patient developed severe OHSS despite minimal doses of hMG and CC (without hCG) and careful monitoring. The administration of CC may trigger release of endogenous LH and, despite meticulous monitoring, a sudden LH surge may occur that in turn may lead to OHSS.

CC in different combinations is prescribed for superovulation of patients in IVF-embryo transfer (ET) programs. The regimens of CC/LH endogenous, CC/LH surge, and CC/hCG have been abandoned by most IVF programs because the number of oocytes obtained and the pregnancy rates are lower than those with other methods of follicular stimulation. The protocol of CC/hMG/hCG introduced by Lopata[99] was at one time accepted worldwide. In applying this protocol, almost all patients who respond develop mild OHSS.

The incidence of mild OHSS with CC therapy for induction of ovulation has been reported to be 13.5% in 8000 patients.[90] Gysler et al.[69] reported an incidence of 5.1% mild hyperstimulation during a decade of experience with individualized CC treatment regimens. Murray and Osmond-Clarke[118] encountered ovarian enlargement in only 2 of 328 patients treated with 100 to 200 mg of CC daily for 5 days. Rust et al.[143] reported an incidence of 9.6% of mild OHSS in patients receiving a high dose (up to 250 mg) of CC daily.

Severe OHSS with CC treatment is rare, but it has been reported. Southren and Janovsky[176] studied a patient with polycystic ovary (PCO) disease who developed massive ovarian enlargement, ascites, and pleural effusion after administration of CC for 14 days. A case of severe OHSS associated with conception similar to that observed in another patient[82] was reported by Scommegna and Lasch.[164]

Human menopausal gonadotropin. hMG—purified gonadotropin—is extracted from menopausal urine containing both FSH and LH in various proportions. It has been shown that administration of hMG can override the normal mechanism of ovarian follicle selection. Therefore hMG is a very active agent for stimulating the ovary to ovulate; with adequate therapy ovulation is achieved in 80% to 90% of cycles, although pregnancy can be expected in only 40% to 60%. Lunenfeld et al.[103] reported that 3120 (39.9%) conceptions were achieved in 8000 patients after 22,156 cycles of treatment.

With present methods of monitoring gonadotropin therapy, the incidence of OHSS has decreased. Taymor et al.[180] did not reduce the incidence of mild hyperstimulation (12% to 15%), but almost all severe cases were prevented. In that series an incidence of 0.25% severe OHSS was reported.

Experience with the use of gonadotropins for induction of ovulation in the last decade (Table 35-2) reveals the following data: From January 1983 to December 1985 ovulation was induced with hMG/hCG in 391 anovulatory patients during 1822 treatment cycles. The incidence of OHSS recorded was 3%. From January 1, 1986, through December 1990 there were 3035 cycles of induction of ovulation with hMG/hCG; 35 patients (1.1%) with moderate OHSS and 3 patients (0.14%) with severe OHSS were hospitalized. Among anovulatory patients who did not respond to CC, 211 responded to CC/hMG/hCG, resulting in 67 pregnancies (30.3%); 9% of these were complicated by ovarian hyperstimulation.

Data have shown that there is no difference in the incidence of OHSS when various combination regimens of hMG therapy are used (hMG/hCG, hMG/CC/hCG, hMG/dexamethasone/hCG, hMG/bromocriptine/hCG).[120] Usually smaller amounts of hMG were administered to patients who were treated by combined regimens and developed OHSS than were administered to the control group of patients induced by hMG/hCG who developed OHSS.

OHSS is more frequent in patients who conceive after induction of ovulation. Some forms of OHSS were observed in 50% of patients during the cycle in which conception resulted from ovulation induction.

In an IVF-ET program an aggressive stimulation regimen was applied during 1750 cycles to intervene with normal cycles. The protocol called for a high dose of hMG at the time of follicular recruitment and selection in order to obtain four to six large follicles. Fifty-five patients (3%) developed OHSS and were hospitalized; 47 (2.6%) had a moderate form and 8 (0.4%) had a severe form of OHSS (Table 35-2).

Follicle-stimulating hormone. FSH used in ovulation induction is a purified urinary extract. Purified FSH preparations are able to induce ovulation in anovulatory patients (group II of the WHO classification) when endogenous LH is available. Therefore it is indicated in patients with PCO disease in whom the hypothalamic-pituitary-ovarian axis is intact. Protocols of low-dose FSH administration without hCG resulted in low rates of ovulation and conception without the complication of OHSS.[15] When an intermediate dose of FSH (75 to 225 IU/d) was used without hCG administration, ovarian hyperstimulation was observed in cycles that were not carefully monitored.[49]

Stimulation of ovulation with FSH in a long protocol with additional triggering of ovulation with hCG may lead to OHSS. Preliminary results have shown that the incidence of OHSS will be lower if the cycles are well monitored by E_2 levels and ultrasonography.

Induction of ovulation by intermittent intravenous administration of purified FSH in eight patients with PCO disease resulted in 37% conception cycles and three patients with OHSS (one case of severe OHSS).[95] Evidence in support of pituitary FSH (pFSH) has been shown in the study by Raj et al.[137] who found a lower incidence of OHSS and of multiple pregnancies and a higher rate of pregnancies than with hMG. Check et al.[28] observed an incidence of OHSS of 23.7% in a series of 38 cycles of 18 women treated with urinary FSH. The incidence of severe OHSS in this series was 5.3%.

FSH alone and in combination with hMG are well-known regimens for superovulation of anovulatory patients in IVF programs. There are no conclusive data as to whether FSH alone has any advantages over hMG.

Gonadotropin-releasing hormone. GnRH is a decapeptidyl that is found in all mammalian species. It is released by the hypothalamus and transported to the anterior pituitary, where it stimulates release of LH and FSH. Normal menstrual cycles can be induced in GnRH-deficient women by pulsatile administration of GnRH. GnRH appears to be effective in the treatment of anovulation with isolated gonadotropin deficiency, chronic anovulation, and hypothalamic amenorrhea, with or without hyperprolactinemia. The dose, route, and frequency of GnRH pulses vary among the series reported in the literature.[98,169] OHSS has not been observed during low-dose GnRH stimulation. Use of higher pulsatile doses, mainly by the intravenous route, has led to multiple follicular development. Lunenfeld,[100] who reviewed the results of treated cycles in the literature, reported 10 cases (1.1%) of OHSS among 917 treatment cycles. The dose of GnRH in the cycles complicated by OHSS ranged between 10 and 20 µg per pulse. The rate of multiple pregnancy was 7.3%.

Gonadotropin-releasing hormone agonists (GnRHa). GnRHa are synthetic compounds similar to natural GnRH that have a high affinity for the pituitary receptor. The continuous stimulation of the GnRH receptor results in an initial increase in plasma gonadotropins followed by pituitary suppression—a medical hypophysectomy. GnRHa are routinely used in the medical management of a variety of endocrine conditions, including prostate cancer, PCO disease, endometriosis, uterine fibroids, and precocious puberty.[172]

Currently GnRHa with the gonadotropins hMG and FSH are used routinely for superovulation in assisted reproduction.[33,112,172]

GnRHa may be administered according to two different protocols, a short protocol and a long protocol. In the short protocol the GnRHa are administered by intramuscular or subcutaneous injection or by nasal spray. The short protocol of GnRHa utilizes the ability of the analogue to stimulate the pituitary on the first days of its administration. This effect is called the "flare-up" phenomenon. In the short protocol, GnRHa are administered daily starting on day 1 of the cycle, which results in an increased endogeneous secretion starting on day 1 to day 3 of the cycle. Continuous administration of the GnRHa establishes a hypogonadotropic state within 10 to 14 days. GnRHa and hMG are discontinued on the day of the hCG administration. In the long protocol GnRHa are administered by subcutaneous injection of slowly releasing microcapsules. In the long protocol GnRHa are started in the mid–luteal phase of the preceding cycle (day 21 of a 28-day cycle) and menotropin stimulation is started on day 3 to day 5 of the actual cycle, provided that medical hypophysectomy has been accomplished.[9] Under both protocols there is a luteal phase deficiency, and luteal function should be supported. The use of GnRH in superovulation in assisted reproduction increases the incidence of OHSS, especially its severe form. The data from the 1989 Registry of France showed an incidence of OHSS of 4.6% after application of both short and long protocols of GnRHa therapy.[16] Smitz et al.[175] reported 10 cases (0.6%) of severe OHSS in 1673 treatment cycles stimulated with buserelin and hMG. Some of the patients with OHSS had PCO disease. Caspi et al.[26] and Golan et al.[59] reported OHSS rates of 8.4% and 11%, respectively, in cycles treated with long-acting GnRHa. The

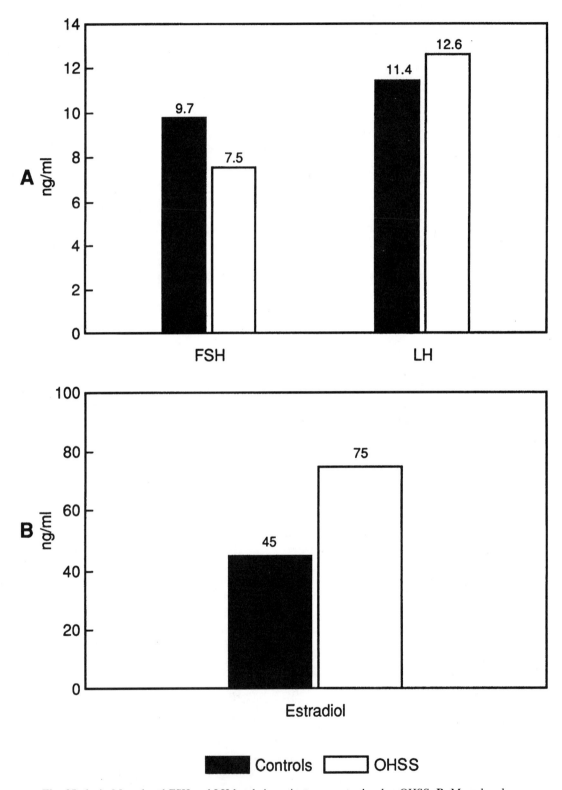

Fig. 35-6. A, Mean basal FSH and LH levels in patients prone to develop OHSS. **B,** Mean basal 17β-estradiol levels in patients prone to develop OHSS.

incidence of severe OHSS in such cycles ranges from 2% to 13.8%. Nine cases of severe OHSS were reported by an Egyptian group after the use of GnRHa.[1] The higher incidence of OHSS in GnRHa/hMG cycles may result from the large cohort of follicles recruited through the initial flare-up state of GnRH administration. This hypothesis is supported by experimental studies in primates and by clinical observation. It has been demonstrated that even subtherapeutic doses of GnRHa in women and monkeys can induce OHSS.[121]

Luteal phase supplementation with hCG can be an important factor in developing severe OHSS. Herman et al.[76] showed that OHSS occurred only in patients given hCG support through the luteal phase. The exacerbation was observed mainly in conception cycles. The severe symptoms occurred 12 to 20 days after oocyte aspiration, when the endogenous hCG levels from trophoblastic tissue began to rise.

Selection of patients

Experience of more than 25 years has shown that anovulatory patients who develop OHSS are younger and have a lower mean weight. Parameters such as height, duration of infertility, and type of infertility (primary or secondary) did not contribute to the development of OHSS.[120] The symptoms were observed more frequently in patients in group II than in patients in group I according to the WHO classification. Patients who develop OHSS have higher LH, prolactin, E_2, androstenedione, and testosterone levels[147] (Fig. 35-6, A and B). Patients belonging to group I require a higher dose of gonadotropins and a longer period of therapy. The incidences of mild and severe OHSS in 621 treated cycles of patients belonging to group I were 5% and 0.6%, respectively, compared with 10.1% and 1.2% in 784 treated cycles of patients in group II. The cumulative report by Thompson and Hansen[183] on 1286 patients who had received 3002 courses of hMG/hCG showed that in patients (257 treatment cycles) with primary amenorrhea (group I) no cases of OHSS were reported.

It has been noted that some women are hypersensitive to gonadotropin treatment and respond to it repeatedly with OHSS. Caspi et al.[25] reported an increased incidence of OHSS in menstruating, ovulatory, infertile patients (group II) treated with hMG/hCG. Greenblatt et al.[66] reported a large ovarian cyst after CC treatment of a patient with Stein-Leventhal syndrome. Southren and Janovsky[176] reported a case of severe OHSS among patients treated with CC. Patients with PCO frequently are sensitive to stimulation with hMG/hCG; therefore care must be taken to avoid the development of OHSS. These patients may ovulate spontaneously with an endogenous LH surge even if hCG is withheld. Therefore, it is of primary importance to withhold hCG from anovulatory patients when E_2 levels exceed 1500 pg/mL and more than four preovulatory follicles of 15 mm in diameter are detected. Administration of pituitary FSH in

low dose without hCG leads to ovulation and conception without OHSS. The use of urinary preparations of FSH does not confirm the results obtained with pituitary FSH, and cases of OHSS in patients with PCO disease have been reported.[50] Application of a long GnRHa protocol in patients with PCO disease induces follicular development, but there is a significant risk of OHSS.[27] On the other hand, the data of Thompson and Hansen[183] in 220 patients treated for 546 courses show that the incidence of OHSS in patients with PCO disease was similar to that in other diagnostic groups. Lunenfeld and Insler[101] reported that in 1405 cycles of treatment there was no significant difference in the incidence of OHSS, mild or severe, between patients of group I and II according to the WHO classification. Experience shows that there is a risk of OHSS in group II, and particular caution should be exercised before inducing ovulation in patients with PCO disease. Care must be taken to exclude endocrinopathies, especially syndromes associated with galactorrhea, that may be the cause of anovulation and for which specific therapy exists. To reduce the incidence of OHSS it is necessary initially to induce ovulation with CC in patients with PCO disease; only when conception has not been achieved after at least six treatment cycles, whether or not an adequate response was obtained, should gonadotropin therapy be considered despite the potential risk of OHSS.

It has been shown that postponement of hCG administration to patients with "imminent" OHSS may result in ovulation and conception without the development of OHSS.[135] Similar results may be obtained by selective follicular reduction.[136]

Patients who have undergone surgery for benign ovarian cysts and patients who have had unilateral oophorectomy are more prone to develop OHSS after induction of ovulation even with CC.[159] Thus, under these conditions, preparations for induction of ovulation should be administered with extreme caution, and the treatment should not be started before ultrasonographic examination to rule out the presence of an ovarian cyst.

Hormone levels in OHSS

Elevated levels of 17β-estradiol, progesterone, prolactin, and testosterone have been found in clinical studies of patients who had received hMG[159] (Fig. 35-7). In the experimental model of OHSS, increased levels of estradiol, progesterone, 17-hydroxyprogesterone, and testosterone were observed in peripheral and ovarian circulation.[162]

Patients with OHSS have increased serum levels of 17β-estradiol, estrone, progesterone, testosterone, and Δ^4 steroids. Abnormally high levels of urinary estrogens, pregnanediol, and 17-hydroxycorticosteroids have been found in patients with OHSS after hMG/hCG treatment.

Estrogens. The correlation between estrogen secretion and the appearance of OHSS is well recognized. The greater the number of follicles present at ovulation and the

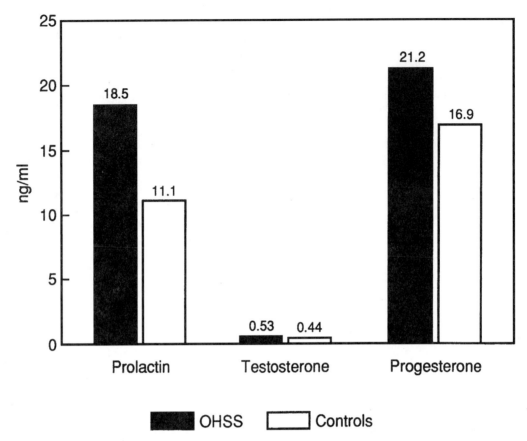

Fig. 35-7. Mean prolactin, testosterone, and progesterone levels on day 20 in cases of OHSS.

higher the E_2 level, the more likely it is that OHSS will occur. There is usually a correlation between the severity of OHSS and E_2 levels. On the other hand, cases of OHSS have been observed with urinary estrogen levels of less than 100 μg/mL amd serum E_2 levels of less than 750 pg/mL.

In our study series of 64 patients hospitalized for signs of moderate and severe OHSS, the E_2 levels on day 0 (before hCG administration) were as follows: In anovulatory patients treated with different modalities for induction of ovulation the E_2 levels ranged from 412 to 2680 pg/mL; in a group of ovulatory patients in the IVF program the range was 515 to 3315 pg/mL. Levels of E_2 above 6000 pg/mL of estradiol occurred in severe cases of OHSS. The high levels of estrogen in OHSS were not directly involved in the pathogenesis of OHSS. They may contribute to the development of the clinical features of thromboembolic phenomena and liver dysfunction.

Progesterone metabolites. High pregnanetriol levels reported in OHSS patients are not influenced by adrenal suppression.[106] Excessive stimulation of the ovaries by exogenous gonadotropin preparations increases ovarian steroidogenesis via the Δ^5 pathway.[67] A significant increase in serum testosterone levels has occasionally been noted with clinical evidence of virilization.[162]

High plasma levels of sulfate-conjugated androsterone and metabolites of progesterone, as well as a massive increase in urinary androsterone and pregnanediol, have been observed in cases of OHSS. Plasma concentrations of the metabolites of progesterone in overstimulated subjects have reached values of the order observed during the second and third trimesters of pregnancy.[104] In our experience, urine levels of hCG in patients with OHSS associated with conception of a single fetus were similar to those of normal single pregnancies at the same stage of gestation. Higher levels of hCG were observed in cases of OHSS associated with multiple pregnancy, as would be expected.

There has been controversy concerning the levels of steroid hormone concentration in pregnancies occurring after hMG therapy. Mishell et al.[114] have shown similarities of steroid hormone levels in hMG-treated patients without OHSS and during normal pregnancy. Patients who developed OHSS associated with pregnancy had markedly elevated levels of 17-hydroxyprogesterone and progesterone. High 17β-estradiol levels remained elevated for about 1 month, until multiple follicular enlargement subsided. Levels of 17-hydroxyprogesterone fell within 2 months to those of normal pregnancy at the same stage of gestation, whereas progesterone levels remained elevated. Rabau et al.[133] determined serial urinary steroids in patients with

OHSS associated with pregnancy. The high levels of 17-ketosteroids, 17-hydroxycorticosteroids, and pregnanetriol declined at the end of the first trimester of pregnancy (i.e., at the time when corpora lutea regress).

Prolactin. Ho Yuen et al.,[78] in addition to elevated steroid levels, have observed an increase in plasma prolactin values. They speculated that the hyperprolactinemia associated with elevated steroid levels may play a role in the pathogenesis of OHSS. Studies in rats show that prolactin may be involved in ascites formation in OHSS. Prolactin was shown to influence the permeability of guinea pig and human amniotic membranes.[107]

Hyperprolactinemia observed in patients with OHSS is due to the relatively high circulating estradiol levels present in OHSS. The hyperprolactinemia present in OHSS is transient and was first described in 1983.[12] The pattern of prolactin secretion in induced ovulatory cycles in anovulatory and ovulatory women is well documented in the literature. Prolactin levels during the early follicular phase of the cycle (days 2 to 5) are higher in patients with OHSS than in controls.

Ovarian renin-angiotensin system. There are sufficient data in the literature to indicate that the renin-angiotensin system is locally active in the human ovary. A ten-fold rise in prorenin concentration occurs in pregnancy. It reaches maximal levels 4 weeks after conception.[42] Prorenin measurements during the menstrual cycles show the following data: During the follicular phase there is no increase in the levels of prorenin. They increase about twofold at the time of the LH surge, and a second peak is observed during the mid–luteal phase.[81] Studies of primates have demonstrated that prorenin is secreted from the ovary.[123] Ovarian secretion of prorenin is stimulated after administration of hCG. In induction of ovulation the levels of plasma prorenin are directly related to the number of developing follicles in the ovaries. The concentration of prorenin in the follicular fluid is about 10 to 40 times higher than the concentration in the plasma.

A highly significant correlation exists between the plasma prorenin concentration during the luteal phase and the number of follicles. It was suggested that prorenin is secreted by the corpora lutea that were formed from the follicles.[119] Patients with OHSS who develop multiple follicular and corpus luteum cysts have increased levels of prorenin. The mechanism of prorenin conversion to active renin is not yet known. One possible mechanism is that the ascitic exudate present in OHSS contains proteases that are able to activate the conversion of prorenin to renin.

Elevated plasma renin concentrations have been observed in patients with OHSS. Renin is a proteolytic enzyme that is synthesized mainly by the juxtaglomerular apparatus of the kidney. Its inactive precursor is prorenin, a protein hormone with a molecular weight of approximately 60,000. Renin acts on angiotensinogen, releasing angiotensin I, which is a biologically inactive substance. Renin

production has also been demonstrated in human corpus luteum, and it is suggested that renin is involved in the extensive vascularization that occurs with the formation of corpus luteum. Levels of active renin, angiotensin I, and angiotensin II are higher in follicular fluid than in plasma.[148]

Angiotensin I appears to function solely as a precursor of angiotensin II and does not have any other established action. Angiotensin II is a potent vasoconstrictor. It produces arterial constriction and an increase in systolic and diastolic blood pressure. It acts directly on the adrenal cortex to increase the secretion of aldosterone. In primates, but not in humans, it affects the secretion of corticosteroids. Angiotensin II acts on peripheral adrenergic neurons to facilitate catecholamine synthesis and release; in this way it modulates sympathetic function. It increases permeability to high-molecular-weight material in large arteries, and stimulates the release of prostaglandins. Angiotensin II promotes angiogenesis. The newly formed capillaries show a greater permeability because of the increased pores present, since there is a widening of gaps between the endothelial cells. The presence of ACE activity has recently been shown in human preovulatory follicular fluid, which converts angiotensin I to angiotensin II.[148] One should emphasize, however, that in cases of OHSS hypertension has not been observed even with high activity of the renin-angiotensin system. The absence of hypertension may be due to other metabolites secreted by the ovary that prevent the hypertensive action of angiotensin II.

Aldosterone. Elevated plasma and urinary aldosterone levels are found in patients with OHSS.[39,73] Urinary excretion of aldosterone increases tenfold in OHSS, and it may reach about 2000 µg/24 hours. We have observed higher levels of plasma aldosterone in patients with OHSS, with a median level of 16 ng/dL (range 5.1 to 34 ng/dL). There was also a significant difference between plasma aldosterone levels in conception cycles with OHSS. There was no statistically significant correlation between plasma renin activity and aldosterone.[119] The lack of clinical manifestations of hyperaldosteronism may be due to the high progesterone levels in patients with OHSS, which may act as a competitive inhibitor of mineralocorticosteroids in distal renal tubules. In OHSS the contracted intravascular space may diminish the effect of aldosterone.

Increased plasma levels of antidiuretic hormone (ADH) have been reported.[73] Changes in levels of ADH are due to the hypovolemia present in OHSS.

Ultrasonographic findings in OHSS

Ultrasonic monitoring of follicular growth and ovulation has become an important method in the management of female infertility. The introduction of the transvaginal probe provided a simple and accurate tool to demonstrate follicular development, ovulation, and the presence of a corpus luteum during spontaneous and stimulated cycles.

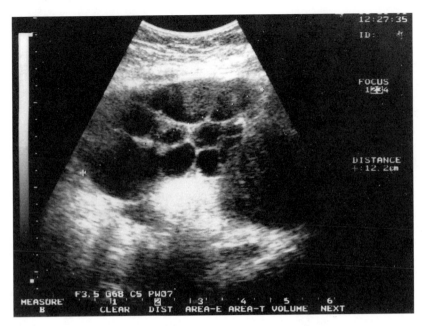

Fig. 35-8. Ultrasonographic findings in a patient with OHSS.

Ultrasound assessment of spontaneous cycles can detect abnormal follicular growth or disturbed ovulation in apparently normal cycles. The roles of ultrasonography in induced ovulation are to detect the number of developing follicles, adequacy of the follicular response, timing of hCG administration, and ovulation; to prevent the development of OHSS; and to diagnose OHSS and determine its severity as early as possible. OHSS is characterized by ovarian enlargement caused by multiple follicles and luteal cysts and by the presence of different degrees of ascitic fluid (Fig. 35-8). Ultrasonographic measurement of ovarian size is superior to clinical estimation, and enables better distinction between patients who will develop mild or moderate hyperstimulation. An abrupt increase in the amount of peritoneal fluid can be documented ultrasonographically before it is evident by physical examination.

Data from sequential ultrasonographic measurements of follicles during induction of ovulation show a strong positive correlation between the total number of follicles (all sizes) and the occurrence of OHSS.[160] Higher numbers of immature follicles (under 12 mm in diameter), small follicles (12 to 14 mm), and large follicles (more than 18 mm) were observed on the day of hCG administration in patients who developed OHSS[148] (Table 35-3). Blankstein et al.[18] demonstrated that estimation of the number of dominant follicles in ovulation induction was insufficient to prevent OHSS. In a series of 65 patients they found significantly more follicles in patients with OHSS at the time of hCG administration than in patients who did not develop OHSS. Mild OHSS was characterized by the presence of eight or

Table 35-3. Ultrasonographic findings in patients at risk to develop OHSS*

Follicle stage	Diameter (mm)
Immature	< 12
Small	12–14
Large	> 18

*There is a strong positive correlation between number of follicles and OHSS; there is a strong positive correlation between number of small follicles and OHSS.

nine follicles in 68% of cases. In moderate to severe OHSS, 95% of the preovultory follicles were less than 16 mm, and in 55% of cases the follicles were less than 9 mm in diameter.

Women with PCO disease are at increased risk of developing OHSS; therefore it is of primary importance to diagnose PCO disease before induction of ovulation. The ultrasonographic image of a polycystic ovary is typical in 75% of cases and seems to be pathognomonic—enlarged ovaries with many small follicles (3 to 5 mm in diameter) crowded on their surface, and the presence of abnormal ovarian stroma. Detection of an abnormal ovarian stroma is significantly improved by the use of vaginal ultrasonography.[47] It is important to obtain ultrasonographic evaluation of the ovaries before induction of ovulation, especially when ovulation was induced by GnRH in previous cycles. It has been noted that patients treated previously by GnRH

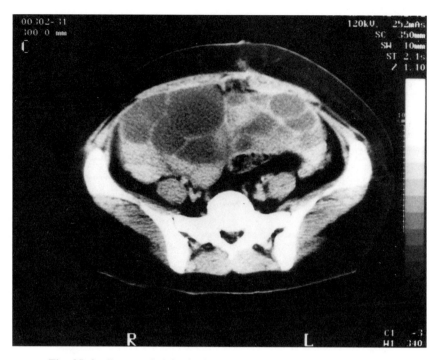

Fig. 35-9. Computed abdominal tomography in a severe case of OHSS.

have large ovarian cysts. These cysts should be aspirated before induction of ovulation.[171]

Pathologic changes in the ovaries and the presence of ascites may be demonstrated by computed tomography, which can be useful in differentiating OHSS from ovarian carcinoma (Fig. 35-9).

Blood flow measurements

The recent introduction of the new imaging technology, the transvaginal color Doppler, adds a novel approach to the noninvasive hemodynamic evaluation of ovaries in normal menstrual cycles, during induction of ovulation, and in OHSS. The technique is simple to perform and easy to interpret. It has been demonstrated by measurements of blood flow in the uterine arteries that perfusion increases in response to rising estrogen levels during the follicular phase, decreases in the preovulatory phase in response to the preovulatory estrogen decrease, and increases in the luteal phase in response to the combined effects of estrogen and progesterone.[63,94] Changes in the resistance index of the ovarian artery and volume flow during induction of ovulation have been shown.[182] Volume flow in the ovarian artery increases from 40 mL/min before treatment to 70 mL/min in midcycle and 90 to 100 mL/min in the late luteal phase. Within the treatment cycle of ovulation induction the ovarian flow more than doubles. The changing vessel resistance and flow volume throughout the treatment cycle demonstrate similar changes in the ovarian artery and the uterine artery and are associated with estrogen and, in particular, progesterone levels.

Blood flow measurements in patients with OHSS may provide additional information on the hemodynamic changes that occur in OHSS and may be an additional tool in evaluation of the severity of the syndrome and its clinical course.

TREATMENT OF OHSS

Mild and moderate forms of OHSS do not require any active therapy other than observation (Fig. 35-10). It is advisable to maintain hydration by frequent small amounts of hypotonic fluids, such as water, decarbonated ginger ale, cola, juice, or other soft drinks, especially in hot climates. Patients with moderate-grade OHSS require close observation (sometimes hospitalization), since they may rapidly progress to the severe form, especially if conception occurs. Patients with severe OHSS require hospitalization and prompt treatment.

On the premise that the basic physiologic change in the syndrome is an acute shift of fluids from the intravascular compartment to the third space, management should be conservative, consisting essentially of monitoring plasma volumes and correcting them[159] (see the box on p. 666). On hospitalization, fluid intake and output are assessed carefully. Fluids by mouth, as well as by regular diet, can be given. Vital signs are monitored and recorded, and an indwelling intravenous line is maintained. Urine output should be quantitated and recorded. Monitoring the trends in the patients' urine output provides an important guide to the accuracy of fluid resuscitation and the changing needs of the patient. A urine output in excess of 30 mL/h implies

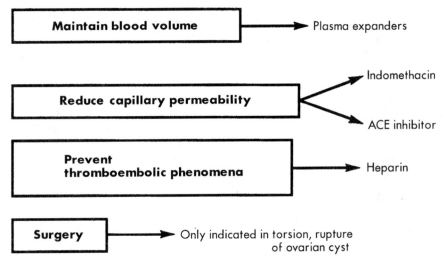

Fig. 35-10. Therapeutic approach in cases of OHSS.

Monitoring of patients with severe OHSS

Vital signs
Fluid balance
  Free intake, urinary output
  Daily weighing
  Daily waist measurement
  Hematocrit
  Hemoglobin
  Erythrocyte count
  Coagulation factors
  Electrolytes
    Serum
    Urine
  Central venous pressure
Blood tests
  Complete blood count
  Electrolytes
  Proteins
  Liver function tests
  Clotting parameters
  Osmolarity
  Acid base balance
  Blood gases
Urine tests
  Osmolarity
  Electrolytes
Imaging
  Ultrasonography
    Abdomen
    Chest
  Computed tomography
    Abdomen
    Chest

---

adequate perfusion to all vital organs and indicates that the patient is not hypovolemic. If urine output is less than 30 mL/h an in-dwelling urinary catheter should be introduced.

Basal blood studies, including complete blood count, urea, liver function tests, and clotting parameters, are obtained every day or every 2 to 3 days, depending on the clinical condition. Blood and urine electrolytes and osmolarity are measured.

Weight and waist measurements are recorded daily. In cases of severe hypovolemia, tension ascites, deterioration of respiration or renal function, or thromboembolic phenomena, central venous monitoring and evaluation of blood for acid-base balance are essential.

Abdominal ultrasonography is performed to assess ovarian size and the degree of ascites in cases of respiratory compromise. Chest X-ray will provide accurate assessment of the presence of pleural effusion and/or other signs of ARDS.

Maintenance of intravascular volume

To reverse the decrease of intravascular volume in a patient with severe OHSS one must understand the dynamic nature of fluid compartments and the use of specific fluids selectively. The relative merits of colloid solutions versus crystalloid solutions for fluid resuscitation continue to be controversial.[96,108]

Crystalloid solutions.

Normal saline. Normal saline is the preferred crystalloid solution, except in patients with hyperchloremic acidosis.

Ringer's lactate. Ringer's lactate has a slightly lower sodium concentration than normal saline; therefore less volume remains in the intravascular space. In addition,

Ringer's lactate contains more potassium, which is undesirable in patients with renal failure, oliguria, or hyperkalemia. Therefore Ringer's lactate should not be administered to patients with severe OHSS.

In cases of hypovolemia the crystalloids should be used in a relatively large volume and infused rapidly. Rapid infusion of crystalloid solutions will aggravate the capillary leak phenomenon in OHSS, with sequestration of fluid in the third space. One hour after infusion only 20% of the volume of administered isotonic crystalloid remains in the intravascular space. Therefore it is obligatory to monitor the patient's response closely by physical examination and measurement of central venous pressure or capillary wedge pressure.

Colloid solutions. Colloid solutions are more efficient and often more effective in expanding intravascular volume than are isotonic solutions. The vast majority of infused colloid remains in the intravascular space for many hours. However, colloid solutions are more expensive, carry an allergy risk, and are more difficult to store and to transport. Colloid solutions that may be used to restore intravascular volume include plasma, albumin, dextran, and hydroxyethyl starch (HES).

Fresh frozen plasma. Fresh frozen plasma provides a source for increased oncotic pressure. It contains all of the coagulation factors. Fresh frozen plasma carries a significant risk for allergic reaction and transmission of viral diseases, mainly hepatitis and acquired immunodeficiency syndrome (AIDS). The risk of transmission of viral diseases can be reduced by effective screening that can detect hepatitis B surface antigen and AIDS, but the risk remains for hepatitis of the non–A and non–B types and for AIDS in an early stage.

Albumin solutions. Albumin solutions are used as volume expanders. They are available in 5% isotonic or 25% hypertonic concentrations. The oncotic effect of 1g of albumin is to pull 18 g of water into the vascular space. Albumin leaks out of the intravascular space with a circulatory half-time of about 16 hours. Albumin is very expensive and carries the risk of allergic reaction. Its advantage over fresh frozen plasma is that it does not cause infections.

The advantages of albumin in treatment of OHSS patients are its tendency to increase colloid oncotic pressure, to remain in the vascular space, and to minimize intestinal edema.

Dextran. Dextran is a heterogenous mixture of polysaccharides available as 40,000 or 70,000 molecular weight solutions. Clearance of dextran occurs rapidly through renal filtration. Large molecules are taken up and metabolized by the reticuloendothelial system. A hyperoncotic solution of dextran produces an immediate and short-lived expansion of plasma volume. The effect of dextran on circulatory volume is relatively brief, with only 20% to 30% remaining in the intravascular space after 24 hours. One gram of dextran can bind about 25 g of water. A patient with OHSS receives an infusion of low-molecular-weight dextran (500 to 1000 mL/24 hours) with an appropriate electrolytic solution such as physiologic saline. In most cases the infusion is continued for 4 hours to 7 days, with good results.

The advantages of dextran in the treatment of patients with OHSS are as follows:

- Causes rapid plasma volume expansion, which increases venous return to the heart
- Increases arterial pressure, pulse pressure, cardiac output, and central venous pressure to restore normal circulatory dynamics
- Increases urinary output resulting from increased renal perfusion
- Prevents intravascular thrombus formation, decreases viscosity, and improves microcirculatory flow

Dextran also has several adverse effects:

- Reduces platelet adherence and is therefore contraindicated in cases of bleeding tendency; caution should be used when dextran is administered to OHSS patients with active hemorrhage
- Potentially causes renal failure secondary to tubular obstruction
- Rarely leads to a fatal anaphylactic reaction (we observed one case), but minor allergic reactions are observed in 5% of patients
- Interferes with several common laboratory tests and produces false elevations of serum plasma bilirubin and serum proteins

Hydroxyethyl starch. (HES) is a polysaccharide structurally similar to glycogen, supplied as a mixture of molecular weight fractions of 10,000 to 1,000,000. HES expands plasma volume in direct relationship to the amount infused. HES prolongs the partial thromboplastin time and causes a transient decrease in platelet count. Clotting abnormalities may be reversed with transfusion of fresh frozen plasma and platelets. Allergic reaction may occur in 1% of patients. Anaphylactic reaction is extremely rare. HES is cheaper than albumin but more expensive than dextran. Experience with the use of HES in the treatment of patients with OHSS is limited.

Continuous fluid replacement in cases of severe OHSS is performed as follows: after an initial dose of colloid solution, the additional amount administered is determined by the patient's urine output and the value of the central venous pressure (CVP). A urine output of less than 30 mL/h indicates that the patient is in a hypovolemic state and perfusion to vital organs is inadequate. CVP should be used as a guide for the rate and volume of fluid administration. CVP is usually monitored via a subclavian procedure. A low CVP generally indicates inadequate venous return to the heart (especially in cases of tension ascites). If venous return is inadequate, the cardiac chambers cannot distend to

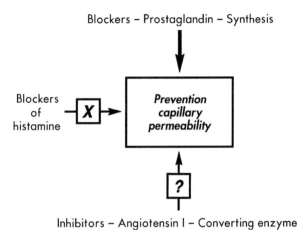

Fig. 35-11. Pharmacologic therapeutic approach in OHSS.

their normal filling capacity and cardiac output declines. If the level of CVP rises to 12 cm H_2O, fluid input should be reduced to a minimum.

Diuretics are ineffective in evacuating fluid from the third space (peritoneal and pleural cavities); moreover, they are contraindicated because a decrease in the volume of the already-contracted intravascular compartment may induce hypovolemic shock. We therefore do not share the view of Shapiro et al.,[167] who recommended severe sodium and fluid restriction as the only treatment. Thaler et al.[181] reported no change in patients' weight or abdominal circumference when sodium and water were restricted.

Pharmacologic preparations. On the basis of the concept of prostaglandin and the renin-angiotensin mechanism in OHSS, supported by the animal model referred to earlier [147, 158] and by clinical studies, pharmacologic preparations (Fig. 35-11) may be given to reduce capillary permeability and prevent fluid escape into the third space, a process occurring primarily in ovarian circulation.

Indomethacin. It has been demonstrated in an animal model that indomethacin blocks prostaglandin synthesis and can prevent the fluid shift associated with ascites, pleural effusion, and hypovolemia in OHSS without changing ovarian weight and estrogen secretion. On the basis of this concept 100 mg of indomethacin twice daily has been administered in severe cases of OHSS with good results.

Indomethacin is a potent nonsteroid drug with antiinflammatory, antipyretic, and analgesic properties. It should not be administered to patients with active gastrointestinal lesions. Indomethacin may aggravate psychiatric disturbances, epilepsy, and parkinsonism; it may depress bone marrow and may aggravate renal impairment; it is contraindicated in patients who are allergic to aspirin. Indomethacin is given in late pregnancy to prevent uterine contractions and preterm birth. In late pregnancy it may cause early closure of the ductus arteriosus.[168]

Katz et al.[87] reported 15 cases of OHSS treated with indomethacin for 3 to 8 days with good results. Eight of the patients were pregnant; no adverse effects on the fetuses were observed. In our series of pregnant patients no malformations were observed. Indomethacin may be contraindicated because of possible teratogenicity. Nevertheless, it is believed that indomethacin therapy is justified in severe OHSS even if the patient has conceived.[157]

Inhibitors of angiotensin-converting enzyme. There is evidence that the renin-angiotensin system is involved in the pathogenesis of OHSS. This may offer new possibilities for therapy with pharmacologic preparations that are specific competitive inhibitors of angiotensin I–converting enzyme.[153]

Captopril. Captopril, in tablets of 25 mg or 50 mg, is a highly competitive inhibitor of angiotensin I–converting enzyme, the enzyme responsible for conversion of angiotensin I to angiotensin II. The drug is indicated for treatment of hypertension or in cases of heart failure that have not responded adequately to or cannot be controlled by conventional diuretics and digitalis therapy. Captopril crosses the human placenta. There are no adequate, well-controlled studies in pregnant women. Embryocidal effects have been observed in rabbits.[166]

Analapril maleate. Analapril maleate, 5 mg or 20 mg, is a highly specific, long-acting, nonsulfydryl, ACE inhibitor. Its basic pharmacologic effects are vasodilatation, increased renal blood flow, and lowered blood pressure without a reflexive increase in sympathetic tone. Symptomatic hypotension is more likely to occur if the patient has been volume depleted, as in OHSS. It is contraindicated in patients with impaired renal function.

There are no adequate and well-controlled studies on the teratogenic effects of drugs that inhibit ACE. These drugs should be used during gestation only if the results justify the potential risk to the embryo. To our knowledge these preparations have not yet been used in cases of OHSS, but theoretically they may be used in severe cases.[153]

Antihistamines. Experimental studies in the rabbit demonstrated the role of histamines in the development of OHSS.[40,92] Chlorpheniramine maleate, an H_1 receptor blocker, has been used successfully in a case of severe OHSS. It enabled replacement fluid to remain in the intravascular compartment by stabilizing membrane permeability.[89]

Therapeutic approach to specific conditions associated with OHSS

Figure 35-12 indicates the therapeutic approach in liver impairment, ARDS, renal impairment, tension ascites, and thromboembolic phenomena.

Liver impairment. In most cases no special treatment is required. Dietary or activity restrictions are unnecessary and have no scientific basis. Most patients recover when the signs of OHSS disappear and results of liver tests return to normal.[178,190]

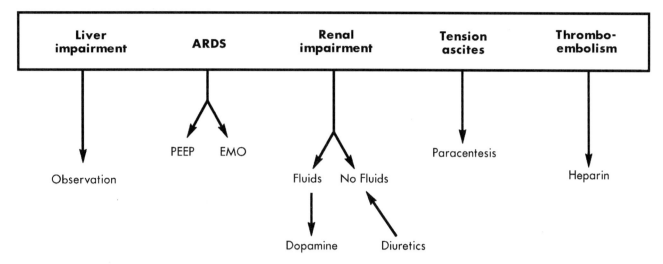

Fig. 35-12. Therapeutic approach to specific clinical conditions associated with OHSS.

Adult respiratory distress syndrome. No therapeutic modality exists at present that will halt or reverse the capillary leakage that exists in OHSS. Corticosteroids have theoretic benefit but have proven not to be efficacious. The first priority is to reverse the life-threatening hypoxemia. Positive end-expiratory pressure (PEEP) is the most effective supportive therapy.[75,191]

Further studies are needed to determine whether extracorporeal membrane oxygenation will help patients suffering from ARDS in cases of OHSS.[96]

Renal impairment. The deficit in intravascular volume observed in cases of OHSS decreases with an increase in renal function, stimulates the proximal renal tubuli to reabsorb salt and water, and is manifested clinically by oliguria and electrolyte imbalance.

Dopamine (DA) is a naturally occurring precursor of norepinephrine, whose effect varies with the dose administered.[77] At a low dose (2 to 5 μg/kg per minute) dopamine has primary β_1 effects. At such a dose DA independently stimulates renal DA receptors, increases renal blood flow, and promotes the filtration rate. Plasma volume should be restored before the administration of dopamine chloride (CVP of 10 to 12 cm H_2O or pulmonary wedge pressure of 14 to 18 mm Hg). DA may aggravate cardiac arrythmia and is thus contraindicated in thyrotoxicosis. There is no evidence of a teratogenic effect of dopamine hydrochloride.

DA in lower doses is used primarily to improve renal function. It may also increase urine flow in patients when output is within normal limits and thus may be of value in reducing the degree of preexisting fluid accumulation. At higher doses the adrenergic activity of DA becomes more prominent. In cases of shock in OHSS the use of DA can be justified even when the intravascular volume is depleted, since prolonged systemic hypotension does not provide adequate cerebral and coronary perfusion and may have a lethal consequence.

Tension ascites. Paracentesis is indicated in tension ascites, a life-threatening condition due to increased intraabdominal pressure, which prevents venous return to the right atrium. Several investigators[19,124] have observed dramatic clinical improvement after paracentesis, which improved circulatory function and renal perfusion. The procedure should be guided by ultrasonography to avoid puncture of large ovarian cysts, which can cause intraperitoneal hemorrhage. Drainage should be continuous. The presence of ascites is not an indication for drainage, as was proposed by several authors.[134] Pleural effusion should be drained in patients with respiratory disorders. In case of tension ascites there is immediate improvement in pleural effusion after paracentesis.[51]

Thromboembolic phenomena. Anticoagulant therapy is indicated only in cases in which there is clinical evidence of thromboembolic phenomena or laboratory findings of hypercoagulability.[159] One must check carefully for intraperitoneal bleeding due to rupture of a cyst when the patient is on anticoagulant therapy. A falling hematocrit without accompanying diuresis in a patient with OHSS is a good indicator of intraperitoneal bleeding.

Surgery

Surgical intervention should be avoided, the indications for surgery being limited to signs of intraperitoneal bleeding due to either rupture of an ovarian cyst or torsion of an ovarian cyst.[159]

The diagnosis of intraperitoneal hemorrhage sometimes may be difficult. The possibility of ovarian rupture should always be considered, and an examination should be done most gently to avoid iatrogenic rupture. Frequent monitoring of vital signs and hematocrit may help to confirm the diagnosis. A falling hematocrit without accompanying diuresis is a good indicator of intraperitoneal hemorrhage.

If surgery is necessary, as in patients with a ruptured

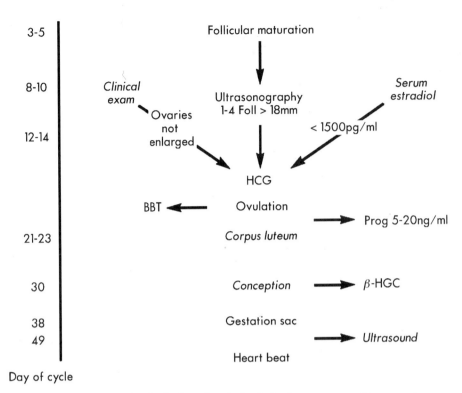

Fig. 35-13. Monitoring of ovulation induction as a preventive measure.

cyst, it should be conservative, and hemostatic measures should be undertaken in order to preserve gonadal tissue. Patients with acute abdomen have been subjected to laparotomy in which bilateral oophorectomy was performed.[8,68] Torsion of an ovarian cyst occurs more frequently in cases of mild OHSS, in which diameters of the cysts are smaller. The clinical symptoms are sudden severe pain and later peritoneal irritation that gives rise to abdominal muscle spasm and gastrointestinal symptoms. If the diagnosis is performed early, untwisting of the cyst can be performed by using endoscopic surgical techniques or laparotomy.[110]

PREVENTION OF OHSS

Theoretically OHSS can be prevented, provided the patient is monitored carefully and hCG is withheld whenever the physiologic range of ovarian response is exceeded. However, there are several reasons why, even with the most careful and painstaking preventive measures, OHSS cannot be completely eliminated. First, if the physiologic range is considered an adequate ovarian response, the efficiency of gonadotropin treatment is markedly reduced. The probable explanation for the difference between physiologic estrogen levels in spontaneous cycles and the higher minimally effective levels in stimulated cycles is the presence of multiple follicles, which reach a more advanced stage of maturation under both CC and gonadotropin induction of ovulation. Direct proof for this explanation is evident from studies in IVF. After CC stimulation the number of fertiliz-

able ova retrieved during follicular aspiration is usually two or three; after hMG stimulation the number may reach six or more. The overlap that exists between the minimally effective dose for conception and the dose that causes ovarian hyperstimulation is another reason for the inability to eliminate OHSS. However, the incidence of OHSS can be reduced significantly by clinical, biochemical, and bioelectronic methods used in monitoring ovulation induction.

Monitoring

In Fig. 35-13, the essentials of monitoring techniques in ovulation induction are illustrated. Since direct observation of follicular maturation is impossible, measurable parameters are followed that reflect more or less accurately the follicular maturation. Some parameters that indirectly reflect total estrogen activity are of academic interest (e.g., the karyopyknotic index [vaginal cytology]). Other clinical parameters are of great value both for backing up other laboratory evidence of follicular maturation and for semiquantitative estimations when adjunctive laboratory data are not available.

Estrogen levels. In our clinic, we have used the indirect method of assessment of estrogen activity by examination of the cervical score. Evaluation includes quantity of cervical mucus, crystallization of mucus (fern test), spinnbarkeit, and changes in the appearance of the external cervical os. Several investigators[44,64] have found that the gradual development of copious mucus with maximal ferning and changes in the external os are good indicators of follicular ripeness. During treatment, the cervical parameters must be estimated frequently enough to determine the expected day of follicular maturation. It usually takes 1 to 5 days from the initial cervical reaction until the follicle can respond to hCG by ovulation. A positive effect is found with estrogen values of 10 to 20 µg/24 h, whereas above 40 µg/24 h there may not be additional changes in the cervical score.

Individual responses of the endocervical glands may vary considerably; some patients will respond with high cervical scores when the estrogen levels are still very low; others will fail to respond at high estrogen levels.

CC, because of its antiestrogenic activity, may block altogether the response of the cervical glands to high levels of circulating estrogens. The sensitivity of an individual patient's endocervical glands may be determined by the administration of an estrogen preparation before gonadotropin therapy. In view of the disadvantages of cervical scoring, this method alone is considered unsatisfactory. Furthermore, the predictive value of impending ovarian hyperstimulation is poor, if it exists at all.[159]

Total urinary estrogen values and later serum estrogen values have established their effectiveness in monitoring induction of ovulation. Taymor et al.[180] were the first to report the correlation of high estrogen levels in urine with the appearance of OHSS. Experience has shown that this correlation is valid when a group of patients is considered, but in the individual case, there seems to be some disassociation between estrogen levels and the clinical findings. Subsequent reports have confirmed that estimations of estrogen levels in blood or urine have proved to be superior to indirect methods when monitoring ovulation induction to minimize, if not completely prevent, complications.[86,116,185]

Older methods of measuring total fractionated estrogens in urine permitted only assessment of the follicular response; thus OHSS resulted frequently. The introduction of rapid methods providing results of urinary estrogen measurement on the same day enables withholding the ovulatory dose of hCG or LH if the estrogenic response to menotropins is excessive, and thus minimizes the risk of OHSS.[21] Optimal preovulatory estrogen levels appear to be 75 to 150 µg/24 h, as judged by high pregnancy rates.

Rabau et al.[133] found that, when total estrogens were above 150 µg/24 h, the incidence of hyperstimulation was increased. Jewelewicz et al.[84] reported an incidence of hyperstimulation of 7.6% when the level of total estrogens measured was between 151 and 300 µg/24 h; when estrogen levels were above 800 µg/24 h, 90% of patients had hyperstimulation.

The development of sensitive, radiocompetitive binding techniques and radioimmunoassays for measuring plasma steroids has enabled more accurate assessment of ovarian response to treatment for induction of ovulation.

The experience of several investigators[111,153] has shown that monitoring of patients undergoing treatment by measurement of plasma estradiol may permit a direct and rapid assessment of follicular function. Although serum studies provide optimal control of therapy, practical difficulties are encountered because of the need for repeated blood sampling of patients and the requirement for greater laboratory expertise in serum determinations. Nevertheless, the advantage of measuring serum levels, which provide a measure of endogenous estradiol production on the day of hMG administration, over determining urinary estrogens, which represent the previous day's levels, is seen as sufficiently important to justify the use of serum estradiol monitoring. Moreover, the reliability of urinary estrogen determination is impaired by difficulties in urine collection and delivery to the laboratory.

Berquist et al.[14] reported that cases of severe hyperstimulation were completely avoided by serum E_2 determinations during 110 treatment courses with hMG. Mean preovulatory serum estradiol levels were 29% higher in the group in which OHSS was observed. Gemzell[53] summarized his experience with human gonadotropin therapy. He reported on 641 anovulatory women treated during 1365 courses. Comparisons were made before and after introduction of daily estrogen monitoring. Pregnancy rates were the same during the two periods of study (45% and 41%, respectively). The incidence of OHSS with clinical symptoms necessitating hospital care decreased from 2% to 0.5%.

The optimal dose of gonadotropins required to induce ovulation should produce a steroid pattern similar to that found during spontaneous, normal, ovulatory cycles. Attempts to reproduce the normal midcycle levels of plasma E_2 have not achieved an optimal pregnancy rate. Therefore higher levels of E_2 are reached in induced cycles. Haning et al.[74] have shown that the plasma E_2 level was the best predictor of the OHSS score. No cases of OHSS occurred in their series when plasma estradiol values were below 1000 pg/mL. In our series mean E_2 levels were 1041 ± 381 pg/mL on the day of hCG administration in cases of hyperstimulation, compared with control levels of 713 ± 333 pg/mL. On the other hand, we and others observed OHSS with peak levels of plasma E_2 below 1000 pg/mL. Therefore, in induction of ovulation in anovulatory patients, it is suggested that hCG be withheld when E_2 levels are above 1500 pg/mL. There is an additional warning sign—the slope of the rise of E_2 levels. A steep rise of E_2 levels during 2 or 3 consecutive days, when values are more than doubling, should be regarded as a serious warning sign, and hCG administration should be withheld. In induction of ovulation in ovulatory women participating in assisted reproductive programs, hCG administration should be withheld at E_2 levels above 2500 pg/mL.

Ultrasound. In the 1960s estrogen levels constituted the main parameters of monitoring ovulation induction.

Ultrasound monitoring has become a significant tool in the 1990s. Serial ultrasonographic measurements enable one to assess the number of follicles and their volume. Measurement of follicular size may reflect maturation of the follicles. At present, most centers employ ultrasonographic examination (most recently by the transvaginal route) for monitoring induction of ovulation. It has been shown that there is a linear correlation between follicular diameter and plasma E_2 levels in normal ovulatory cycles.[71,151] In induced cycles, generally more than one dominant follicle develops, and there are many follicles in various stages of maturation. In this condition, there is a poor statistical correlation between ovarian morphology, as determined by ultrasonography, and the concentration of plasma E_2 levels and/or total urinary estrogens.[109,142,165]

Cabau and Bessis[24] monitored by ultrasound and plasma E_2 levels 43 cycles of 27 patients. They found moderate hyperstimulation in four women of six who became pregnant. We compared two groups treated with hMG/hCG, the first under combined E_2 and ultrasonographic monitoring and the second under only E_2 monitoring. Ultrasonographic monitoring enabled shortening the duration of therapy, and pregnancy rates increased significantly. The incidence of OHSS was reduced from 5.4% to 2.9% by adjunctive use of ultrasonography. Bryce et al.[22] reported a case of OHSS despite close ultrasonographic monitoring in the absence of hormonal profiles, which retrospectively were found to be extremely high. Sallan et al.[146] suggested that ultrasonography may be used alone as a routine tool to monitor treatment of ovulation induction. Blankstein et al.[17,18] stressed the value of counting the number of follicles larger than 5 mm in diameter as a predictive score for OHSS. Mild OHSS and the time of hCG administration are characterized by the presence of more than eight follicles, of which 68% are of intermediate size (9 to 15 mm in diameter); moderate to severe OHSS is associated with 95% of preovulatory follicles that are less than 16 mm in diameter, of which 54% are less than 9 mm. A strong positive correlation has been shown between the total number of follicles (of all sizes) and the occurrence of OHSS. There were greater numbers of immature (<12 mm), small (12 to 16 mm), and large (>18 mm) follicles coexisting on the day of hCG administration. It was also found that the size of the ovaries on the day of hCG administration has a significant predictive value for the development of OHSS.

In cases of induction of ovulation in anovulatory patients, OHSS should be prevented in most cases by careful monitoring based on clinical, hormonal, and ultrasonographic parameters. If follicular stimulation is part of an assisted reproductive program, there is a need to define precise criteria that would enable clinicians to detect patients at risk for developing OHSS and a need for a system that permits manipulation in order to rescue the treatment cycle and prevent OHSS.

Manipulation and intervention during treatment cycles

Withholding hCG. Withholding hCG in treatment cycles has remained the most widely used and recommended measure for the prevention of OHSS.[159] By application of this approach there is almost no chance for conception. Discontinuation of hMG and withholding of hCG in cycles in which hormonal and ultrasonographic signs of imminent hyperstimulation are present bring about a decrease in hormone levels and the disappearance of ultrasonographic findings, and prevent the development of the clinical symptoms of OHSS.[135]

Rescue of overstimulated cycles. When an excessive response to induction of ovulation is observed (E_2 levels above 1500 pg/mL, leading follicles between 17 and 22 mm in diameter), hMG administration is withheld for several days and hCG is administered after a hiatus of several days. During the withholding period follicle growth continues, and ovulation and conception can be achieved. The longer the interval between hMG discontinuation and hCG administration, the lower the rates of ovulation and conception. In experience with this regimen all pregnancies occurred in patients who received hCG within 72 hours after the last dose of hMG. OHSS did not occur in any of the patients.

Aspiration of follicles. In 1987 it was reported that aspiration of the follicular contents in patients with laboratory signs of imminent OHSS may prevent the clinical symptoms and signs of this syndrome.[136] This observation may offer a possible explanation for the relatively low rates of OHSS in IVF stimulated cycles, despite multiple follicular development with high serum E_2 levels. Multiple follicular aspiration, which emptied most of the large, medium, and even small follicles of their follicular fluid and granulosa cells, prevented the development of OHSS. A significant decrease in serum levels of E_2 progesterone, and hCG was observed 1 hour after follicular aspiration. The remarkable decline in hormone levels after follicular aspiration may play a role in the prevention of OHSS. However, this approach does not offer complete protection against the development of OHSS.[48,59,105]

Reduction of follicles and cryopreservation. Belaisch-Allart et al.[10] induced ovulation with hMG/FSH/hCG in patients with PCO disease and advised the patients to have sexual intercourse 1 day after hCG administration. Thirty-five hours after hCG administration they aspirated all of the follicles except one. The retrieved oocytes were fertilized in vitro and cryopreserved. In the three reported cases two pregnancies were achieved without development of OHSS. This technique should be applied only in selected cases in order to avoid canceling the IVF cycles and prevent OHSS. It cannot replace proper monitoring of ovarian stimulation of E_2 assays and ultrasonography.

Amso et al.[3] suggested that in women who are at risk for developing OHSS, oocyte retrieval should be performed without preembryo replacement. The cryopreserved preembryos are transferred in future nonstimulated cycles.

Continuous application of GnRHa. It has been demonstrated that the combination of GnRHa and gonadotropins in IVF is associated with an increased incidence of severe OHSS. Charbonnel et al.[27] detected OHSS in all patients who were treated with GnRHa and hMG; 40% was moderate and 6% was severe. In patients with PCO disease the ovaries seem to respond even more intensely to this combined therapy. Salat-Baroux et al.[145] suggested that in a patient at risk for OHSS, when the E_2 level is about 2500 pg/mL, ovulation should not be induced but GnRHa should be continued to avoid a spontaneous peak of LH. They also induced ovulation in 33 patients with hCG, aspirated all follicles 36 hours later, cryopreserved the preembryos obtained, and continued the administration of agonist until complete ovarian inactivity was obtained. Only one case of severe OHSS was observed.

Since the introduction of clinical, laboratory, and ultrasonographic tools for monitoring ovulation induction, the incidence and the severity of OHSS have been reduced. The application of manipulative regimens and techniques for induction of ovulation in assisted reproductive methods contributes to the relatively low incidence of severe cases of OHSS. However, at present, it is doubtful that OHSS can be completely avoided because of the existence of a relatively small margin of safety between development of OHSS and the successful induction of ovulation and conception in anovulatory women and ovulatory women participating in assisted reproduction programs.

ADMINISTRATION OF HUMAN CHORIONIC GONADOTROPIN

Administration of hCG is critical for the development of hyperstimulation. It is well known that OHSS will not occur after the administration of the other gonadotropins alone, except in sporadic cases.[162] The dosage and timing of hCG administration vary from 1,000 to 25,000 IU or more and from one to several doses that can either overlap or not overlap the administration of the pharmacologic agents used for induction of ovulation. Ovulation rates were similar after hCG regardless of dose, but conception rates were higher after 5,000 to 15,000 IU. OHSS was less frequent in patients given 1000 to 5000 IU and more frequent in patients given higher dosages. hCG has been administered in a dosage of 10,000 IU, given in a single injection, 24 to 48 hours after the last injection of hMG. Occasionally the dosage was adjusted according to the patient's ovarian response based on clinical, hormonal, and ultrasonographic findings. The regimens in which hCG did not overlap hMG showed a significantly lower incidence of OHSS than the regimens in which hCG overlapped gonadotropin administration.[183] In highly responsive patients, therefore, withholding of hCG administration may prevent OHSS. The longer the delay between hMG discontinuation and hCG injection, the lower the rate of conception. Patients treated with different agents for induction of

ovulation show a continuous increase in hormone levels, especially serum E_2, after injection of hCG. The E_2 value on day 0, before administration of hCG, is critical and predictive for the development of OHSS and its severity.[153,159] The usual dose of hCG is between 5,000 and 15,000 U depending on the patient's risk of developing OHSS.

The recommendation is that hCG should be withheld whenever any of the following are found:

- The ovaries are enlarged more than 5 cm in the preovulatory phase.
- The total urinary estrogen level is more than 200 μg/24 h.
- The serum 17β-estradiol is more than 1500 pg/mL in cases of induction of ovulation in anovulatory patients, or more than 2500 pg/mL in superovulatory cycles of patients participating in assisted reproductive programs.
- The daily estradiol levels more than double in 24 hours.
- Enlarged ovaries (>5 cm) are detected by ultrasonography, with a predominance of many small follicles.

hCG administration for triggering ovulation can be substituted by purified human pituitary LH (hLH) given in repeated injections over a 24-hour period, mimicking the normal LH surge. No cases of severe OHSS were reported when hCG was substituted with hLH.[32] But it should be remembered that the availability of hLH for clinical use is very limited. hCG, however, differs biologically from human hLH: (1) hCG has a longer half-life (more than 1 day) than hLH (60 minutes)[177,189]; and (2) hCG has a higher affinity for ovarian receptors.

The biologic characteristics of hCG—longer half-life, higher affinity for and greater interreaction with ovarian receptor sites, and prolonged intracellular bioactivity—may contribute to the development of OHSS after administration of hCG to trigger ovulation, compared with the use of hLH.

It is possible to trigger ovulation in induced cycles by provoking an endogenous LH surge through the initial flare-up effect after administration of GnRHa. Recent reports show that if ovulation must be triggered in cycles at higher risk for OHSS, the release of endogenous LH through GnRHa may reduce the risk of the syndrome and the rate of multiple pregnancies, although the rate of conceptions per cycle is not reduced.[38]

LUTEAL PHASE SUPPORT

Several studies have demonstrated that induction of ovulation with different preparations is associated with a higher rate of luteal phase defect (LPD). LPD is found especially after superovulation in assisted reproduction.[11] The luteal phase may be supplemented with exogenous hCG/hLH, endogenous LH, or gestagenic preparations.[23] The use of 1000 to 2000 IU of hCG on alternate days increases the levels of E_2 and progesterone and prolongs the luteal phase, but does not increase pregnancy rates.

In recent years GnRHa have been used increasingly in superovulation in women undergoing IVF and GIFT. The hypogonadal state induced by those analogues is followed by better follicular recruitment, exogenous gonadotropins, and suppression of the LH surge, and has partially benefited women with PCO disease and other women who respond poorly to other treatment regimens.

The combined use of GnRHa and gonadotropins without luteal supplementation results in an inadequate luteal phase that may delay endometrial development, reduce subsequent implantation rates, and increase the chance of early preembryo loss. Several mechanisms have been suggested to explain the luteolytic action of GnRHa. Whatever the underlying mechanism may be, stimulated cycles employing GnRHa should be supported throughout the luteal phase by hCG or progesterone preparations. Luteal phase supplementation with hCG seems to be associated with the development of OHSS. The luteal phase can be supplemented by pusatile administration of GnRH. Weinstein et al.[187] have compared continuous GnRH administration in cases of luteal phase deficiency with supplementation of this phase with hCG. They found that it is advisable not to support the luteal phase with GnRH, since GnRH is not cost effective and is biologically inferior to hCG. Herman et al.[76] showed in their series that OHSS occurred only in patients supported with hCG through the luteal phase. Similar data were observed by others.[174]

The advantage of hCG over progesterone was demonstrated in a prospective, double-blind, randomized study of patients in IVF programs. It was shown that the ongoing pregnancy rate was significantly higher with hCG (1500 IU) administration on the day of embryo transfer and 4 days later than it was with progesterone supplementation (18.7% and 9.3%, respectively).[23]

To avoid hyperstimulation it may be advisable to refrain from hCG supplementation and administer intravaginal micronized progesterone. Recent data presented at the Seventh World Congress of IVF and Assisted Reproduction revealed that intravaginal micronized progesterone is superior to gestagen administrated by mouth or intramuscularly, and superior even to hCG.[36]

DOSAGES OF OVULATION-INDUCING AGENTS

Animal studies have revealed a direct relationship between the dose of hMG administered and the development of OHSS. It was found that the change in ovarian size, degree of capillary permeability, and severity of ascites and pleural effusion were related to the dose of gonadotropin administered.[158]

The incidence of mild OHSS in patients treated with CC is 13.8%. The incidence of ovarian enlargement was reduced to 5.5% in single-course therapy and to 7.8% in multiple-course therapy.[90] The incidence of severe OHSS is

very rare after CC administration. In induction of ovulation with CC the duration of therapy is probably a more important factor in developing OHSS than the dose used. A dosage up to 200 mg/d for 4 to 6 days is safe.

It has been demonstrated in clinical practice that the use of gonadotropin preparations results in a positive dose-response relationship with respect to ovulation and pregnancy rate. In addition, there is a direct positive association between the dose of gonadotropin and the probability of occurrence of OHSS. In the individual patient OHSS is a consequence of gonadotropin administration depending on the endogenous gonadotropin secretion and the state of follicular development at the beginning of stimulation, whereas in dealing with a group of patients we found no such correlation. The dosage of gonadotropin required to develop OHSS is usually related to the subgroup to which the patient belongs—high, normal, or low responders. There may be discrepancies in different dosages of gonadotropin in the same clinical group, and even in the individual patient the dose may vary from cycle to cycle.

Data show that patients who develop hyperstimulation use a fewer number of ampules of hMG than the controls. This tendency prevails in all subgroups of severity. Dosages of 14.8 ± 12.3, 13.1 ± 8, and 13 ± 8.9 ampules were administered to patients with severe, moderate, and mild OHSS, respectively, compared with 24 ± 17 ampules per cycle in the control group ($P > 0.005$).[120]

OHSS IN CONCEPTION CYCLES

OHSS is much more frequent and of a more severe grade in conception cycles. In cases of OHSS associated with pregnancy, the ovarian enlargement appears late in the luteal phase and the symptoms are aggravated with the increased endogenous hCG secretion. In conception cycles there is a prolongation of the active phase of the syndrome during the first trimester of gestation. In one series of OHSS, 40% of the cases occurred in conception cycles and 27.7% were of the severe form.[160] Tyler[186] reported that 50% of all patients who conceived had some degree of hyperstimulation. Rabau et al.[133] reported an incidence of 42.8% pregnancies in patients with OHSS.

The number of OHSS cases during conception cycles is increasing among women treated by IVF and GIFT, since the incidence of OHSS—particularly of the severe grade— is higher after application of these new technologies.

There are conflicting data on the association between OHSS and multiple pregnancies, despite the obvious common denominator of both entities, mainly the production of multiple follicles and multiple corpora lutea. Hack et al.[70] found a multiple pregnancy rate of 8.4% without any OHSS, whereas Drake et al.[37] observed OHSS in 6.6% of cases, none of which was complicated by multiple pregnancy. We have reported a quintuplet pregnancy that was associated with the severe form of OHSS after induction of ovulation with CC.

Multiple pregnancies and OHSS are observed more frequently in pregnancies induced by gonadotropin preparations. Recent protocols of induction of ovulation, combined preparations of GnRHa/hMG/hCG, especially in IVF and GIFT, induce a higher incidence of OHSS and a higher incidence of multiple pregnancies. In our series of hMG/hCG–treated patients, 18 of 73 women with moderate and severe OHSS had multiple pregnancies (2 quadruplets, 4 quintuplets, 4 triplets, and 8 sets of twins). Caspi et al.[26] reported an incidence of 66.6% of multiple births among patients with severe OHSS who conceived. Tulandi et al.[185] found a pregnancy rate of 34.6% among OHSS patients. Cases of high-order multiple pregnancies associated with OHSS have been reported. Pregnancies involving sextuplets, septuplets, octuplets, and even more fetuses have been reported.[160]

The frequency of multiple pregnancies, especially of high order, increased in the last decade after treatment of subfertility by new state-of-the-art reproductive technology. The rate of triplets and higher-order gestation achieved after IVF and GIFT is about 4%, compared with 1 in 8100 births in natural cycles.[149] Therefore a higher rate of multiple gestation associated with OHSS is expected. The management of OHSS associated with multiple pregnancies, especially of higher order, is based on the concept of the pathogenetic mechanism of the syndrome and selective embryo reduction.[20,97] An unusual case of severe OHSS with gestation after transfer of six preembryos has been reported[138]; the pregnancy was terminated in order to save the patient's life.

CONCLUSION

OHSS is an iatrogenic clinical condition associated with induction of ovulation that can be life-threatening. The syndrome is associated with a wide spectrum of clinical and laboratory findings. Patients with the severe form of the syndrome may suffer renal impairment, liver dysfunction, tension ascites, ARDS, thromboembolic phenomena, shock, and even death.

The incidences of the moderate form and the severe form are 1% to 2% and 0.2% to 0.5%, respectively. A higher rate of OHSS is expected in cycles resulting in gestation, especially in multiple gestation. Even though the incidence of severe OHSS is very low, the absolute number of cases is increasing as a result of induction of ovulation in assisted reproduction. Factors affecting the incidence and severity of this syndrome are the clinical condition for which induction of ovulation is performed, the pharmacologic agent used, the dosage, and the regimen of treatment. A new classification of OHSS is presented.

The main pathogenetic mechanism is considered to be increased capillary permeability, causing acute fluid shift from the intravascular space into the third compartment due to increased production of prostaglandins and ovarian contribution of the renin-angiotensin system.

There are no absolute criteria for identification of patients at risk to develop this syndrome. Preventive measures involve careful monitoring of ovulation induction and the ability to manipulate the treatment cycles. The syndrome cannot be absolutely prevented. Since it is a life-threatening condition in young healthy women treated only because of infertility, careful preventive measures should be provided to avoid OHSS. Therefore induction of ovulation should be administered only by qualified physicians.

REFERENCES

1. Aboulghar MA et al: The impact of follicular aspiration and luteal phase support on the incidence of ovarian hyperstimulation syndrome. Presented at the Seventh World Congress on IVF and Assisted Procreation, Paris, July 1991, *Hum Reprod* 6(suppl 1):174, 1991.
2. Adlercreutz X, Tenhunen R: Some aspects of the interactions between natural and synthetic female sex hormones and the liver, *Am J Med* 49:630, 1970.
3. Amso NN et al: The management of predicted ovarian hyperstimulation involving gonadotropin-releasing hormone analog with elective cryopreservation of all pre-embryos, *Fertil Steril* 53:1087, 1990.
4. Anderson K et al: Unilateral pleural effusion as the presenting feature of ovarian hyperstimulation syndrome, *Scott Med J* 33:338, 1988.
5. Ashbaugh IDG et al: Acute respiratory distress in adults, *Lancet* 2:319, 1967.
6. Ashkenazi J et al: Adverse neurological symptoms after gonadotropin-releasing hormone analog therapy for in vitro fertilization, *Fertil Steril* 53:738, 1990.
7. Balasch J et al: Acute prerenal failure and liver dysfunction in a patient with severe ovarian hyperstimulation syndrome, *Hum Reprod* 5:348, 1990.
8. Beclere C: Acute abdominal complications with massive luteinization of both ovaries caused by excessive doses of mare serum and chorionic gonadotropins, *C R Soc Fr Gynecol* 29:371, 1959.
9. Belaisch-Allart J: Interet de l'utilisation des agonistes de LHRH en protocole long, avec ou sans FSH, ou dans un protocole court dans un programme de FIV, *Contracep Fertil Sex* 16:32, 1988.
10. Belaisch-Allart J et al: Selective oocyte retrieval: a new approach to ovarian hyperstimulation, *Fertil Steril* 50:654, 1988.
11. Belaisch-Allart J et al: The effect of HCG supplementation after combined GnRH agonist/HMG treatment in IVF programme, *Hum Reprod* 5:163, 1990.
12. Ben-David M, Schenker JG: Transient hyperprolactinemia: a correctable cause for idiopathic female infertility, *J Clin Endocrinol Metab* 57:442, 1983.
13. Bergman P: Bilateral multiple lutein cyst of the ovary complicating normal pregnancy: report of a case, *Obstet Gynecol* 21:28, 1963.
14. Berquist C, Nillius SJ, Wide L: Human gonadotropin therapy, *Fertil Steril* 39:761, 1983.
15. Bettendorf G: Special preparations: pure FSH and desialo-hCG, *Baillieres Clin Obstet Gynaecol* 4:519, 1990.
16. Bilan: Responses aux stimulations de l'ovaulation dans les procreations medicalement assiste (PMA), *Contracep Fertil Sex* 18:592, 1989.
17. Blankstein J, Quigley MM: The anovulatory patient: an orderly approach to evaluation and treatment, *Postgrad Med* 83:97, 1988.
18. Blankstein J et al: Ovarian hyperstimulation syndrome prediction by number and size of preovulatory follicles, *Fertil Steril* 47:597, 1987.
19. Borenstein R et al: Ovarian hyperstimulation syndrome after different treatment schedules, *Int J Fertil* 26:279, 1981.
20. Breckwoldt M et al: Management of multiple conceptions after gonadotropin-releasing hormone analog/human menopausal

gonadotropin/human chorionic gonadotropin therapy, *Fertil Steril* 49:713, 1988.

21. Brown JG et al: A rapid method for estimating estrogens in urine using a semiautomated estimation, *J Endocrinol* 42:5, 1968.

22. Bryce RL et al: The value of ultrasound, gonadotropin, and estradiol measurements for precise ovulation prediction, *Fertil Steril* 37:42, 1982.

23. Buvat J et al: Luteal support after luteinizing hormone-releasing hormone agonist for in vitro fertilization: superiority of human chorionic gonadotropin over oral progesterone, *Fertil Steril* 53:490, 1990.

24. Cabau A, Bessis R: Monitoring of ovulation induction with human menopausal gonadotropin and human chorionic gonadotropin by ultrasound, *Fertil Steril* 36:178, 1981.

25. Caspi E et al: Induction of pregnancy with human gonadotropins after clomiphene failure in menstruating ovulatory infertile patients, *Isr J Med Sci* 10:249, 1974.

26. Caspi E et al., Results of in vitro fertilization and embryo transfer by combined long-acting gonadotropin-releasing hormone analog D-Trp-6-luteinizing hormone-releasing hormone and gonadotropins, *Fertil Steril* 51:95, 1989.

27. Charbonnel B et al: Induction of ovulation in polycystic ovary syndrome with a combination of a luteinizing-releasing hormone analog and exogenous gonadotropins, *Fertil Steril* 47:920, 1987.

28. Check JH et al: Severe ovarian hyperstimulation syndrome from treatment with urinary follicle-stimulating hormone: two cases, *Fertil Steril* 43:317, 1985.

29. Cole HH, Hart GH: The potency of blood serum of mares in progressive stages of pregnancy in effecting the sexual maturity of the immune rat, *Am J Physiol* 93:57, 1930.

30. Corsan GH, Kemman E: The role of superovulation with menotropins in ovulatory infertility: a review, *Fertil Steril* 55:468, 1991.

31. Crooke AC et al: Pregnancy in women with secondary amenorrhea treated with human gonadotropins, *Lancet* 1:184, 1964.

32. Crosignani PG Hormonal profiles in anovulatory patients treated with gonadotropins and synthetic luteinizing hormone releasing hormone, *Obstet Gynecol* 46:15, 1975.

33. Cummis JM, Yovich JM: Pituitary down-regulation using leuprolide for the intensive ovulation management of poor prognosis patients having in vitro fertilization, *J In Vitro Fert Embryo Transfer* 6:345, 1989.

34. Davis JS: Hormonal control of plasma and erythrocyte volume of rat uterus, *Am J Physiol* 199:841, 1960.

35. Demey H et al: Acute oligoanuria during ovarian hyperstimulation syndrome, *Acta Obstet Gynecol Scand* 66:741, 1987.

36. Devroey P et al: Micronized progesterone is the method of choice. Presented at the Seventh World Congress of IVF and Assisted Reproduction, Paris, July 1991, *Hum Reprod* 6(suppl 1):42, 1991.

37. Drake TS, Tredway DR, Buchanan GC: Continued clinical experience with an increasing dosage regimen of clomiphene citrate administration, *Fertil Steril* 30:274, 1978.

38. Emperaire JC, Ruffie A: Triggering ovulation with endogenous luteinizing hormone may prevent the ovarian hyperstimulation syndrome, *Hum Reprod* 6:506, 1991.

39. Engel T et al: Ovarian hyperstimulation syndrome: report of a case with notes on pathogenesis and treatment, *Am J Obstet Gynecol* 112:1052, 1972.

40. Erlik Y et al: Histamine levels in ovarian hyperstimulation syndrome, *Obstet Gynecol* 53:580, 1979.

41. Esteban-Altirriba J: Le syndrome d'hyperstimulation massive des ovaries, *Rev Fr Gynecol Obstet* 56:555, 1961.

42. Fernandez LA et al: Renin-like activity in ovarian follicular fluid, *Fertil Steril* 44:219, 1985.

43. Figueroa-Cases P: Reaccion ovarica monstruosa a las gonadotrofinas a proposito de un caso fatal, *Ann Chir* 23:116, 1958.

44. Flynn AM, Bertrand PV: The value of cervical score in the assessment of ovarian function, *J Obstet Gynaecol Br Commonw* 80:152, 1973.

45. Forman RG et al: Severe ovarian hyperstimulation syndrome using agonists of gonadotropin-releasing hormone for in vitro fertilization: a European series and a proposal for prevention, *Fertil Steril* 53:502, 1990.

46. Fournert N, Surrey E, Kerin J: Internal jugular vein thrombosis after ovulation induction with gonadotropin, *Fertil Steril* 56:354, 1991.

47. Franks S et al: Ovulatory disorders in women with polycystic ovary syndrome, *Clin Obstet Gynecol* 12:605, 1985.

48. Friedman CI et al: Severe ovarian hyperstimulation following follicular aspiration, *Am J Obstet Gynecol* 150:436, 1984.

49. Garcia N et al: Induction of ovulation with purified urinary follicle-stimulating hormone in patients with polycystic ovarian syndrome, *Am J Obstet Gynecol* 151:635, 1983.

50. Garcia N et al: Induction of ovulation with purified urinary follicle-stimulating hormone in patients with polycystic ovarian syndrome, *Am J Obstet Gynecol* 151:635, 1985.

51. Garcia-Compean D et al: Therapeutic paracentesis with albumin infusion for the treatment of tension ascites in cirrhotic patients, *Rev Gastroenterol Mex* 55:7, 1990.

52. Gemzell CA: The use of human gonadotropins in gynecological disorders. Keller RL, editor: *Modern trends in gynecology,* London, 1963, Butterworths.

53. Gemzell C: Induction of ovulation, *Acta Obstet Gynecol Scand Suppl* 47:1, 1976.

54. Gemzell CA, Diczfalusy E, Tillinger G: Clinical effect of human pituitary follicle-stimulating hormone (FSH), *J Clin Endocrinol Metab* 18:1333, 1958.

55. Gemzell CA, Roos P, Loeffler E: Follicle stimulating hormone. In Behrman SJ, Kistner RW, editors: *Progress in infertility,* Boston, 1975, Little, Brown.

56. Gemzell CA et al: Treatment of primary amenorrhea with human pituitary and chorionic gonadotropins, *J Obstet Gynaecol Br Commonw* 77:60, 1970.

57. Gergely RZ et al: Treatment of ovarian hyperstimulation syndrome by antihistamine, *Obstet Gynecol* 47:83, 1976.

58. Glickman RM, Isselbacker KS: Abdominal swelling and ascites. In Petersdorf RL, Adams RD, editors: *Harrison principles of internal medicine,* New York, 1983.

59. Golan A et al: Ovarian hyperstimulation syndrome following D-Trp-6 luteinizing hormone-releasing hormone microcapsules and menotropins for in vitro fertilization, *Fertil Steril* 50:912, 1988.

60. Golan A et al: Ovarian hyperstimulation syndrome: an update review, *Obstet Gynecol Surv* 44:430, 1989.

61. Goldfarb A, Rakoff A: Experience with the hyperstimulation syndrome during menotropin therapy. In Rosenberg E, editor: *Gonadotropin therapy in female infertility,* Amsterdam, 1973, Excerpta Medica.

62. Gong H: Positive pressure ventilation in ARDS, *Clin Chest Med* 3:69, 1982.

63. Goswamy RK: Doppler ultrasound in infertility. In Mashiach S et al, editors: *Advances in assisted reproductive technologies,* New York, 1990, Plenum Press.

64. Grant A, Robertson S: An evaluation of monitor tests for the induction of ovulation, *Aust N Z Obstet Gynaecol* 9:224, 1970.

65. Greenblatt RB, Barfield WE: Induction of ovulation with MRL/41, *JAMA* 178:101, 1961.

66. Greenblatt RB et al: Ovulation and pregnancy in the Chiari-Frommel syndrome: report of 10 cases, *Fertil Steril* 17:742, 1966.

67. Grodin JM et al: Functional studies of ovarian responsiveness to Pergonal. In Rosenberg E, editor: *Gonadotropin therapy in female infertility,* Amsterdam, 1973, Excerpta Medica.

68. Groot Wasnik C: Akutes abdomen nach gonadotrophin behandlung, *Zentralbl Gynakol* 92:449, 1970.

69. Gysler M et al: A decade's experience with an individualized clomiphene treatment regimen including its effect on the postcoital test, *Fertil Steril* 37:161, 1982.

70. Hack M et al: Outcome of pregnancy after induced ovulation: follow-up of pregnancies and children born after gonadotropin therapy, *JAMA* 211:791, 1970.

71. Hackeloer BJ et al: Ultrasonics of ovarian changes under gonadotrophine stimulation, *Geburtshilfe Frauenklin* 37:185, 1877.

72. Hammerstien J: Dangers of overstimulation in use of clomiphene and gonadotrophins, *Geburtshilfe Frauenklin* 27:1125, 1967.

73. Haning RV, Strawn EY, Nolten WE: Pathophysiology of the ovarian hyperstimulation syndrome, *Obstet Gynecol* 66:220, 1985.

74. Haning RV Jr et al: Diagnosis-specific serum 17 beta-estradiol (E_2) upper limits for treatment with menotropins using a 125I direct E_2 assay, *Fertil Steril* 42:882, 1984.

75. Hankins GD, Nolan TE: Adult respiratory distress in obstetrics, *Obstet Gynecol Clin North Am* 18:273, 1991.

76. Herman A et al: Pregnancy rate and ovarian hyperstimulation after luteal human chorionic gonadotropin in in vitro fertilization stimulated with gonadotropin-releasing hormone and menotropins, *Fertil Steril* 53:92, 1990.

77. Hoffman DB, Lebkowitz RJ: Catecholamines and sympathomimetic drugs. In Rall T, Nies AS, Taylor P, editors: *Goodman's and Gilman's pharmacological basis of therapeutics,* New York, 1990, Pergamon Press.

78. Ho Yuen B et al: Plasma prolactin, human chorionic gonadotropin, estradiol, testosterone and progesterone in the ovarian hyperstimulation syndrome, *Am J obstet Gynecol* 133:316, 1979.

79. Hurwitz A et al: Early unwinding of torsion of an ovarian cyst as result of hyperstimulation syndrome, *Fertil Steril* 40:393, 1983.

80. Itskovitz J, Sealey JE: The physiology of human ovarian prorenin-angiotensin system. In Mashiach S et al, editors: *Advances in assisted reproductive technologies,* New York, 1990, Plenum Press.

81. Itskovitz J et al: Plasma prorenin response to human chorionic gonadotropin in ovarian-hyperstimulated women: correlation with the number of ovarian follicles and steroid hormone concentrations, *Proc Natl Acad Sci U S A* 84:7285, 1987.

82. Jaffe H, Schenker JG: Severe OHSS due to combined treatment of HMG and clomiphene citrate and Pergonal therapy, *Infertility* 2:109, 1979.

83. Jewelewicz R, Vande Wiele RL: Acute hydrothorax as the only symptom of ovarian hyperstimulation syndrome, *Am J Obstet Gynecol* 121:1121, 1975.

84. Jewelewicz R et al: Ovarian overstimulation syndrome. In Rosenberg E, editor: *Gonadotropin therapy in female infertility,* Amsterdam, 1973, Excerpta Medica. p 235.

85. Kaaja R et al: Severe hyperstimulation syndrome and deep venous thrombosis, *Lancet* 2:1043, 1989.

86. Karam SK, Taymor ML, Berger MJ: Estrogen monitoring and prevention of ovarian hyperstimulation during gonadotropin therapy, *Am J Obstet Gynecol* 115:972, 1973.

87. Katz Z et al: Absence of teratogenicity of indomethacin in ovarian hyperstimulation syndrome, *Int J Fertil* 29:186, 1984.

88. Kingsland C et al: Ovarian hyperstimulation presenting as acute hydrothorax after in vitro fertilization, *Am J Obstet Gynecol* 161:381, 1989.

89. Kirshon B et al: Management of ovarian hyperstimulation syndrome with chlorpheniramine maleate, mannitol and invasive hemodynamic monitoring, *Obstet Gynecol* 71:485, 1988.

90. Kistner RW: Induction of ovulation with clomiphene citrate. In Behrman SJ, Kistner RW, editors: *Progress in infertility,* Boston, 1975, Little, Brown.

91. Knox GE: Antihistamine blockade of the ovarian hyperstimulation syndrome, *Am J Obstet Gynecol* 118:997, 1974.

92. Knox GE et al: Antihistamine blockade of the ovarian hyperstimulation syndrome, II: possible role of antigen-antibody complexes in the pathogenesis of the syndrome, *Fertil Steril* 26:418, 1975.

93. Koeninger EZ: Survivors of shock lung syndrome, *Lab Invest* 36:360, 1977.

94. Kurjak A, Zalud I: Transvaginal color doppler in the study of uterine perfusion. In Mashiach S et al, editors: *Advances in assisted reproductive technologies,* New York, 1990, Plenum Press.

95. Lanzone A et al: Induction of ovulation by intermittent intravenous purified follicle-stimulating hormone in polycystic ovary disease, *Fertil Steril* 48:105, 1987.

96. Layon AJ, Kirby RR: Fluids and electrolytes in the critically ill. In Civetta JM, Taylor RU, Kirby RR, editors: *Critical care* Philadelphia, 1988, JB Lippincott.

97. Le-Pors P et al: La 7e etait dans la trompe, *Rev Fr Gynecol Obstet* 83:167, 1988.

98. Leyendecker G, Struve T, Plotz EJ: Induction of ovulation with chronic intermittent (pulsatile) administration of LH-RH in women with hypothalamic and hyperprolactinemic amenorrhea, *Arch Gynecol* 229:177, 1980.

99. Lopata A: Concepts in human in vitro fertilization and embryo transfer, *Fertil Steril* 40:289, 1983.

100. Lunenfeld B: Ovulation induction and drugs efficiency. Paper presented at the ESCO meeting, Monto Carlo, 1984.

101. Lunenfeld B, Insler V: Classification of amenorrheic states and their treatment by ovulation induction, *Clin Endocrinol* 3:223, 1974.

102. Lunenfeld B, Mashiach S, Blanckstein J: Induction of ovulation with gonadotropins. In Sherman RP, editor: *Reproductive endocrinology,* Edinburgh, 1985, Churchill Livingston.

103. Lunenfeld B et al: Short and long term survey of treatment with hMG/hCG and follow-up of offsrping. In Genazzani A et al, editors: *Advances in gynecological endocrinology,* vol 1, Casterton-Hall, 1987, Parthenon.

104. Luukkainen T et al: Plasma and urinary steroids in hypophysectomized women during treatment with gonadotropins. In Bettendorf G, Insler V, editors: *Clinical Application of Human Gonadotropins,* edited Stuttgart, 1970, Georg Thieme Verlag.

105. Magnus O et al: Severe hyperstimulation syndrome: case reports, *Acta Eur Fertil* 19:89, 1988.

106. Mahesh VB, Greenblatt RB: Steroid secretion of the normal and polycystic ovary, *Recent Prog Horm Res* 20:341, 1964.

107. Manku MS, Mtabaji JP, Horrobin DF: Effect of cortisol, prolactin, and ADH on the amniotic membrane, *Nature* 258:78, 1975.

108. Marini JJ, Wheeler AP: Critical care medicine: the essentials, Baltimore, 1988, Williams & Wilkins.

109. Marrs RP, Vargyas JM, March CM: Correlation of ultrasonic and endocrinologic measurements in human menopausal gonadotropin therapy, *Am J Obstet Gynecol* 145:417, 1983.

110. Mashiach S et al: Adrenal torsion of hyperstimulated ovaries in pregnancies after gonadotropin therapy, *Fertil Steril* 53:76, 1990.

111. McGarrigle HH et al: The monitoring of gonadotropin therapy by plasma estradiol and progesterone determinations, *J Obstet Gynaecol Br Commonw* 81:651, 1974.

112. Meldrum DR et al: Routine pituitary suppression with leuprolide before ovarian stimulation for oocyte retrieval, *Fertil Steril* 51:1334, 1989.

113. *Merck manual of diagnosis and therapy,* ed 15, Rahway, NJ, 1957, Merck Sharpe & Dohme.

114. Mishell DR et al: Steroid and gonadotropin levels in normal pregnancies and pregnancies following HMG therapy. In Rosenberg E, editor: *Gonadotropin therapy in female infertility,* Amsterdam, 1973, Excerpta Medica.

115. Mozes M et al: Thromboembolic phenomena after ovarian stimulation with human menopausal gonadotropins, *Lancet* 2:1213, 1965.

116. Muechler EK, Kohler D, Huang KE: Monitoring of ovulation induction with HMG-HCG therapy by plasma estrogen and progesterone, *Int J Fertil* 26:273, 1981.

117. Muller P: In Beclere C, editor: *Gonadotrophines en gynecologie,* Paris, 1962, Masson et Cie.

118. Murray M, Osmond-Clarke F: Pregnancy results following treatment with clomiphene citrate, *J Obstet Gynaecol Br Commonw* 78:1108, 1971.

119. Navot D et al: Direct correlation between plasma renin activity and severity of ovarian hyperstimulation syndrome, *Fertil Steril* 48:57, 1987.

120. Navot D et al: Risk factors and prognostic variables in the ovarian hyperstimulation syndrome, *Am J Obstet Gynecol* 159:210, 1988.

121. Navot D et al: Gonadotropin-releasing hormone agonist induced ovarian hyperstimulation: low dose side effects in women and monkeys, *Fertil Steril* 55:1069, 1991.

122. Neuwirth R, Turksoy R, Vande wiele R: Acute Meigs' syndrome secondary to ovarian stimulation with human menopausal gonadotropins, *Am J obstet Gynecol* 91:977, 1965.

123. Ong ACM et al: The pathogenesis of the ovarian hyperstimulation syndrome (OHS): a possible role for ovarian renin, *Clin Endocrinol* 34:43, 1991.

124. Padilla SL et al: Abdominal paracentesis for the ovarian hyperstimulation syndrome with severe pulmonary compromise, *Fertil Steril* 53:365, 1990.

125. Pappan GD, Blanchette EJ: Transport of colloidal particles from small blood vessels correlated with cyclic changes in permeability, *Invest Ophthalmol* 4:1026, 1965.

126. Pessina AC, Hulme B, Peart WS: Renin-induced proteinuria and the effects of adrenalectomy, II: morphology in relation to function, *Proc R Soc Lond [Biol]* 180:61, 1972.

127. Petty TL: Adult respiratory distress syndrome: definition and historical perspective, *Clin Chest Med* 3:3, 1982.

128. Phillips LL, Glamstone W, Vande Wiele R: Studies of the coagulation and fibrinolytic systems in hyperstimulation syndrome after administration of human gonadotropins, *J Reprod Med* 14:138, 1975.

129. Polishuk WZ, Schenker JG: Ovarian overstimulation syndrome, *Fertil Steril* 20:443, 1969.

130. Porter R et al: Induction for ovulation for in vitro fertilization using buserelin and gonadotropins, *Lancet* 2:1284, 1984.

131. Pride J, Ho Y: The ovarian hyperstimulation syndrome, *Semin Reprod Endocrinol* 8:247, 1990.

132. Pride SM, Ho Yuen B, Moon YS: Clinical, endocrinological and intraovarian prostaglandin-F response to H-1 receptor blockade in the ovarian hyperstimulation syndrome, *Am J Obstet Gynecol* 148:670, 1984.

133. Rabau E, Lunenfeld B, Insler V: The treatment of fertility disturbances with special reference to the use of human gonadotropins. In *Fertility disturbances in men and women,* Basel, 1971, S Karger. p. 508.

134. Rabau E et al: Human menopausal gonadotropins for anovulation and sterility, *Am J Obstet Gynecol* 96:92, 1967.

135. Rabinovici J et al: Rescue of menotropin cycles prove to develop ovarian hyperstimulation, *Br J Obstet Gynaecol* 94:1098, 1987.

136. Rabinowitz R et al: Rate of ovarian hyperstimulation syndrome after high-dose HMG for induction of ovulation in IVF cycles. Presented at the Fifth Congress on IVF-ET, Norfolk, Va, April 5-10, 1987 (abstract 500).

137. Raj SG et al: The use of gonadotropins for the induction of ovulation in women with polycystic ovarian disease, *Fertil Steril* 28:1280, 1977.

138. Reed AP, Tausk H, Reynolds H: Anesthetic considerations for severe ovarian hyperstimulation syndrome, *Anesthesiology* 73:1275, 1990.

139. Rizk B, Meagher S, Fisher AM: Severe ovarian hyperstimulation syndrome and cerebrovascular accidents, *Hum Reprod* 5:697, 1990.

140. Robbins SL: *Pathologic basis of diseases,* ed 9, Philadelphia, 1974, WB Saunders.

141. Robertson AL, Khairallah PA: Effects of angiotensin II on the permeability of the vascular wall. In Page IH, Bumpus FM, editors: *Angiotensin,* Berlin, 1974, Springer-Verlag.

142. Robinson RD et al: Assessment of ovulation by ultrasound and plasma estradiol determinations, *Obstet Gynecol* 54:686, 1979.

143. Rust LA, Israel R, Michell DR: An individualized graduated therapeutic regimen for clomiphene citrate, *Am J Obstet Gynecol* 120:785, 1974.

144. Ryley NG et al: Liver abnormality in ovarian hyperstimulation syndrome, *Hum Reprod* 5:938, 1990.

145. Salat-Baroux J et al: Treatment of hyperstimulation during in vitro fertilization, *Hum Reprod* 5:36, 1990.

146. Sallan HN et al: Monitoring gonadotropin therapy by real time ultrasonic scanning of ovarian follicles, *Br J Obstet Gynaecol* 89:155, 1982.

147. Schenker JG: Pathogenesis of ovarian hyperstimulation syndrome: complications of induction of ovulation. In *Human reproduction: current status, future aspects,* Amsterdam, 1988, Excerpta Medica.

148. Schenker JG: Prevention and management of ovarian hyperstimulation syndrome. In Genazzani AR, Petraglia F, Volpe A, editors: *Progress in gynecology and obstetrics,* 1990, Parthenon.

149. Schenker JG: Outcome of high multiple pregnancies. Paper presented at the meeting the Fetus as a Patient, Bonn, August 1991.

150. Schenker JG: Unpublished data, 1991.

151. Schenker JG, Lewin A, Ben-David M: Principles of pathophysiology of infertility assessment and treatment. In Kurjak A, editor: *Ultrasound and infertility,* Boca Raton, Fla, 1989, CRC Press.

152. Schenker JG, Navot D: Complications of induction of ovulation. In Aravantinos DJ, editor: *Volume in honor of DB Kaskarelis,* Athens, 1985.

153. Schenker JG, Navot D: Complication of induction of ovulation. In Teoh E-S, Ratnam SS, Wong P-C, editors: *Ovulation and early pregnancy,* 1987, Parthenon.

154. Schenker JG, Polishuk WZ: Ascites in cases of twin pregnancy, *J Obstet Gynaecol Br Commonw* 74:451, 1967.

155. Schenker JG, Polishuk WZ: An experimental model of ovarian hyperstimulation syndrome. In Tichner M, Pilch J, editors: *Proceedings of the International Congress on Animal Reproduction,* vol 4, Krakow, Poland, 1976, Drukarnia Naukowa.

156. Schenker JG, Polishuk WZ: Ovarian hyperstimulation syndrome: clinical and experimental data. In *Excerpta Medica Int Congr Ser* No. 396, 1976.

157. Schenker JG, Polishuk WZ: Role of prostaglandins in ovarian hyperstimulation syndrome, *Obstet Gynecol Surv* 31:742, 1976.

158. Schenker JG, Polishuk WZ: The role of prostaglandins in ovarian hyperstimulation syndrome, *Eur J Obstet Gynecol Reprod Biol* 6:47, 1976.

159. Schenker JG, Weinstein D: Ovarian hyperstimulation syndrome: a current survey, *Fertil Steril* 30:255, 1978.

160. Schenker JG, Yarkoni S, Granat M: Multiple pregnancies following induction of ovulation, *Fertil Steril* 35:105, 1981.

161. Schenker JG et al: The ureters in ovarian overstimulation syndrome, *Int Surg* 53:286, 1970.

162. Schenker JG et al: Steroid pattern in experimental hyperstimulation syndrome and the response to indomethacin. Presented at the Second International Congress of Human Reproduction, Tel Aviv, October 1977.

163. Schwartz M, Jewelewicz R: The use of gonadotropins for induction of ovulation, *Fertil Steril* 35:3, 1981.

164. Scommegna A, Lasch SR: Ovarian overstimulation, massive ascites and singleton pregnancy after clomiphene, *JAMA* 207:753, 1969.

165. Seibel MM et al: The role of ultrasound in ovulation induction: a critical appraisal, *Fertil Steril* 36:573, 1981.

166. Setton I, Hirsh D: *Israel Drug Compendium,* Tel Aviv, 1986, Zmora-Bitan.

167. Shapiro AG, Thomas T, Epstein M: Management of hyperstimulation syndrome, *Fertil Steril* 28:237, 1977.

168. Sharpe GL, Larsson KS, Thalme B: Studies on closure of the ductus arteriosus, *Prostaglandins* 9:585, 1975.

169. Shoham Z, Homberg R, Jacobs HS: Induction of ovulation with pulsatile GnRH, *Baillieres Clin Obstet Gynaecol* 4:589, 1990.

170. Shulman D, Sherer D, Beilin B: Pulmonary edema in the ovarian hyperstimulation syndrome, *N Z Med J* 101:643, 1988.

171. Silverberg KM, Olive DL, Schenken RS: Ovarian cyst aspiration prior to initiating ovarian hyperstimulation for in vitro fertilization, *J In Vitro Fert Embryo Transfer* 7:153, 1990.

172. Simon A, Birkenfeld A, Schenker JG: Gonadotropin releasing hormone (GnRH): mode of action and clinical applications—a review, *Int J Fertil* 35:350, 1990.

173. Simon A et al: The value of menotropin treatment for unexplained infertility prior to an in-vitro fertilization attempt, *Hum Reprod* 6:222, 1991.

174. Smitz J et al: Luteal supplementation regimens after combined GnRH agonist HMG superovulation, *J Reprod Fertil Abstr Ser* 2:18, 1988.

175. Smitz J et al: Incidence of severe ovarian hyperstimulation syndrome after GnRH agonist/HMG superovulation for in vitro fertilsation, *Hum Reprod* 5:933, 1990.

176. Southren AL, Janovsky NA: Massive ovarian hyperstimulation with clomiphene citrate, *JAMA* 181:443, 1962.

177. Strickland TW, Puett D: Contribution of subunits to the function of luteinizing hormone/human chorionic gonadotropin recombinants, *Endocrinology* 109:1933, 1981.

178. Sueldo CE et al: Liver dysfunction in ovarian hyperstimulation syndrome: a case report, *J Reprod Med* 33:387, 1988.

179. Taymor ML: Gonadotropin therapy, *JAMA* 203:362, 1968.

180. Taymor ML, Karem S, Berger MJ: Estrogen monitoring and the prevention of ovarian overstimulation during gonadotropin therapy. In Rosenberg E, editor: *Gonadotropin therapy in female infertility,* Amsterdam, 1973, Excerpta Medica.

181. Thaler I et al: Treatment of ovarian hyperstimulation syndrome: the physiological basis for a modified approach, *Fertil Steril* 36:110, 1981.

182. Thaler I et al: In Mashiach S et al, editors: *Advances in assisted reproductive technologies,* New York, 1990, Plenum Press.

183. Thompson C, Hansen M: Pergonal: Summary of clinical experience in induction of ovulation and pregnancy, *Fertil Steril* 21:844, 1970.

184. Tollan A et al: Transcapillary fluid dynamic during ovarian stimulation for in vitro fertilization, *Am J Obstet Gynecol* 162:554, 1990.

185. Tulandi T, McInnes R, Arronet G: Ovarian hyperstimulation syndrome following ovulation induction with human menopausal gonadotropin, *Int J Fertil* 29:113, 1984.

186. Tyler E: Treatment of anovulation with menotropins, *JAMA* 205:16, 1968.

187. Weinstein DG, Seibel MM, Taymor ML: Ovulation induction with subcutaneous pulsatile gonadotropin-releasing hormone: the role of supplemental human chorionic gonadotropin in the luteal phase, *Fertil Steril* 41:546, 1984.

188. World collaborative report—1989. Presented at the Seventh World Congress on IVF and Assisted Reproduction, Paris, July 1991.

189. Yen SSC et al: Disappearance rate of endogenous luteinizing hormone and chorionic gonadotropin in man, *J Clin Endocrinol Metab* 28:1763, 1968.

190. Younis JS et al: Transient liver function test abnormalities in ovarian hyperstimulation syndrome, *Fertil Steril* 50:176, 1988.

191. Zosmer A et al: Adult respiratory distress syndrome complicating ovarian hyperstimulation syndrome, *Fertil Steril* 47:524, 1987.

Chapter 36

ADHESIONS IN REPRODUCTIVE SURGERY

Jacqueline Gutmann, MD,
Alan S. Penzias, MD,
and Michael P. Diamond, MD

Pathophysiology of adhesion formation
Surgical staging
Surgery versus assisted reproductive technology
Laparoscopy versus laparotomy
Surgical adhesiolysis
    Laser versus microelectrocautery
    Surgical adjuvants
    Mechanical separation

Intraabdominal adhesions are known to cause infertility, pain, and intestinal obstruction. These adhesions may be a result of earlier surgical intervention or inflammatory processes such as endometriosis, pelvic inflammatory disease, or appendicitis. The purpose of surgical adhesiolysis is to excise existing adhesions and prevent both the subsequent development of new adhesions and the re-formation of those already lysed. To achieve this goal, the pelvic surgeon has several tools available, including microsurgical technique, operative laparoscopy, the use of the carbon dioxide laser, and the use of surgical adjuvants. Despite these attempts, adhesions have been shown to re-form in 55% to 100% of women after reproductive pelvic surgery.[24] Perhaps even more sobering is the finding that approximately 50% of women undergoing laparotomy develop de novo adhesions.[27] This chapter reviews the pathogenesis of adhesion formation and reformation, surgical treatment of existing adhesions, surgical technique to minimize their formation and reformation, and the use of intraoperative and perioperative adjuvants.

PATHOPHYSIOLOGY OF ADHESION FORMATION

Adhesion formation represents the normal healing process gone awry. To understand how to prevent the formation of postsurgical adhesions, it is important to grasp the physiology of the normal healing process and the points in the process at which adhesions may develop (Figs. 36-1 to 36-8).

In response to peritoneal injury, an inflammatory response occurs with an increase in the permeability of blood vessels in the traumatized tissues secondary to release of histamine and vasoactive kinins.[34] This results in an outpouring of proteinaceous serosanguineous fluid, which generally coagulates within 3 hours. As a result, fibrinous bands, which have been infiltrated by monocytes, plasma cells, polymorphonuclear cells, and histiocytes, are formed between abutting surfaces. As a result of endogenous fibrinolytic activity, these adhesions are generally lysed within 72 hours after formation. Once these bands are lysed, metaplasia of the underlying mesenchymal connective tissue occurs and much of the healing is complete by 5 days. Because healing occurs from the base of the defect, large defects heal as quickly as the smaller lesions. If the fibrinous bands between abutting surfaces are not lysed by endogenous fibrinolysis, they become infiltrated by proliferating fibroblasts. Subsequently, vascular ingrowth occurs and an adhesion is created. Hence factors that disrupt this equilibrium, such as those that affect fibrinolytic activity or those that alter cell infiltration, may alter subsequent adhesion formation.[1,25,26,34,59] Although the exact etiology of pelvic adhesion formation is not completely understood, there are several well-known risk factors for their formation, including the following:

- Intraabdominal infection
- Tissue hypoxia
- Presence of a reactive foreign body
- Rough tissue handling at time of surgery
- Endometriosis
- Tissue drying
- Prior adhesions

681

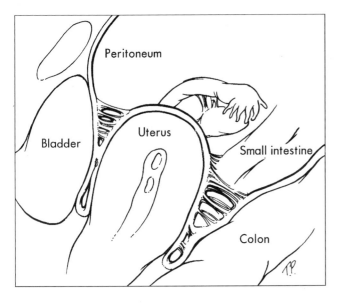

Fig. 36-1. Initial appearance with extensive pelvic adhesions.

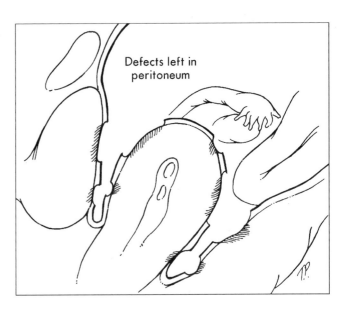

Fig. 36-2. After adhesiolysis with excision of all adhesions; many areas will look raw and oozing.

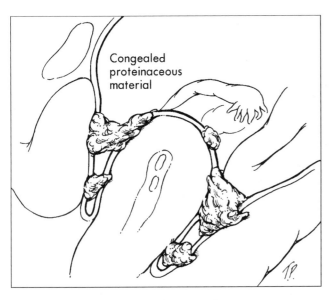

Fig. 36-3. Proteinaceous material congealing on many traumatized surfaces.

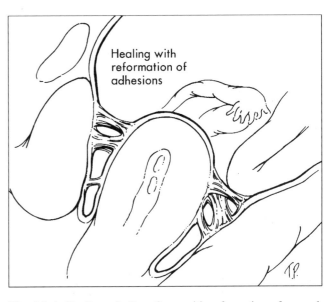

Fig. 36-4. Healing of all surfaces with reformation of several initial adhesions and a few new adhesions. This would be the appearance 7 to 10 days after surgery.

For example, a factor known to inhibit fibrinolysis, perhaps by inhibiting plasminogen activators, is tissue ischemia. Several investigators have shown that tissue ischemia, whether caused by handling, crushing, ligating, suturing, or stripping of the peritoneum, results in adhesion formation. In addition to diminished fibrinolytic activity, ischemia may induce adhesion formation by stimulating angiogenesis from a nonischemic site to one deprived of an adequate blood supply. Finally, ischemia of peritoneal tissue results in mesothelial cell desquamation, resulting in a raw basement membrane with fibrin deposition, thus also predisposing to adhesion formation.

Excessive formation of the fibrin mass also may result in the development of an adhesion. This is most commonly the result of a foreign body reaction. For example, talc from surgical gloves, when left in the field, is absorbed by peritoneal mesothelial cells. These cells subsequently undergo an inflammatory response resulting in death and desquamation. This then causes excessive fibrin deposition and predisposes to adhesion formation. Other foreign bodies commonly encountered during surgery include suture

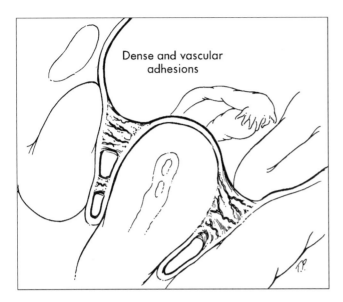

Fig. 36-5. Adhesions appear more dense and more vascular 1 to 2 years later, but there are no new adhesion locations.

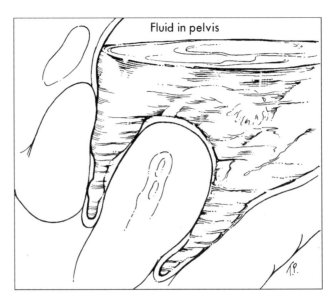

Fig. 36-6. With hydroflotation, the large amount of fluid in the pelvis causes separation of surfaces that previously were touching; i.e., the structures float in the fluid.

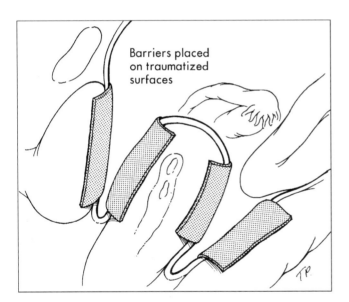

Fig. 36-7. Mechanical separation of traumatized structures.

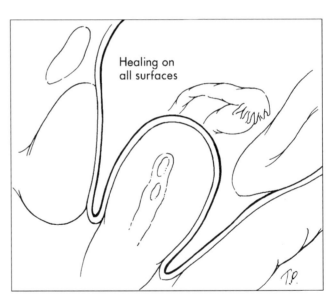

Fig. 36-8. Complete healing, with no adhesions.

material and lint from drapes, caps, gowns, masks, and laparotomy pads. Suture also acts to induce adhesion formation by causing tissue ischemia.[92] Interestingly, however, adhesion formation is less likely to occur in the presence of a foreign body if peritoneal injury has not occurred.[91]

The presence of intraabdominal blood has been suggested to induce adhesion formation, although its actual contribution is unclear. The volume of the blood instilled, the type of blood product used, and the presence or absence of serosal injury have been demonstrated to influence adhesion formation.

It is naively believed that the pathogenesis of adhesion reformation after lysis is the same as that for postoperative de novo adhesion formation. Despite this belief, investigators have demonstrated a greater propensity for adhesion reformation than formation in both animal models and clinical trials. This may be a result of a variation in the pathogenesis of adhesion reformation. Alternatively, previously damaged tissue may have a greater degree of ischemia and, consequently, have decreased fibrinolytic activity with a subsequent increase in adhesion development.

SURGICAL STAGING

It is clear that a common frame of reference is required to classify the extent of pelvic adhesive disease and allow a scientific comparison between methods of treatment. Classification also facilitates communication among surgeons and helps establish a commonality of understanding. Staging therefore serves a dual purpose: first, it allows a descriptive classification of patients on the quantitative or semiquantitative basis of organic disease present; second, it may afford a foundation for prognosis with or without therapy and before or after therapy.

Several such systems have emerged over time. In 1982 Hulka[65] published a prognostic classification system based on a 5-year retrospective survey of fertility surgery at his institution. Two primary factors emerged: the extent of ovarian involvement and the nature (filmy or dense) of the adhesions. With this system the poorest prognoses for achieving a spontaneous pregnancy were in those patients with less than 50% of the ovarian surface visible at laparoscopy and having adhesions that were classified as thick.

Currently the 1985 American Fertility Society classification of adnexal adhesions represents a forthright approach to classification. Despite some drawbacks, it nonetheless provides the critical element of quantitation that allows uniform reporting of results and comparisons among patients and therapies. (See Fig. 38-1.)

SURGERY VERSUS ASSISTED REPRODUCTIVE TECHNOLOGY

Surgical treatment of pelvic adhesions is usually performed in the context of assisting a couple achieve pregnancy. Historically this represented the only realistic option because the assisted reproductive technologies (ART) of today did not exist. However, the international experience with gamete intrafallopian transfer (GIFT), zygote intrafallopian transfer (ZIFT), tubal preembryo transfer (TPET), and in vitro fertilization and embryo transfer (IVF-ET) has risen exponentially in the 15 years since the birth of the first "test tube" baby, Louise Lesley Brown, in 1978. A clinical pregnancy rate of approximately 16% per retrieval for IVF-ET has been reported consistently over the past 4 years by the U.S. national IVF-ET registry.[86] This success rate modifies the treatment algorithm and calls for a more quantitative estimation of prognosis.

A number of studies have addressed the question of pregnancy rates after surgical treatment of pelvic adhesions. However, the lack of uniformity in etiology, staging, and follow-up make direct comparisons difficult. Reported pregnancy rates in these studies vary from 25% to 75%. Rock et al.[108] classified the extent of tubal disease with distal tubal obstruction and observed the patients' reproductive performance (Table 36-1). This study confirms the consensus in the literature; that is, mild disease is eminently treatable surgically whereas severe disease holds a poor

Table 36-1. Postoperative pregnancy rates after treatment of distal tubal occlusion of varying degrees of damage

Pregnancy	Tubal occlusion		
	Severe (%)	Moderate (%)	Mild (%)
Intrauterine	5	17	80
Ectopic	0	13	6

Modified from Rock JA et al: *Obstet Gynecol* 52:591, 1978.

prognosis for subsequent spontaneous pregnancy. The pregnancy rates reported after surgical treatment of moderate disease, however, and those after ART appear comparable. Another consideration is the rate of ectopic pregnancy. The 13% rate seen after surgical repair of moderate disease is nearly three times higher than the approximately 5% rate expected after IVF-ET. However, true comparisons of ART and surgical treatment of adhesions await the performance of properly designed and conducted studies.

The ultimate decision to choose either surgery or ART must take into account the patient's age, past reproductive performance, coexistent fertility factors (including a complete evaluation of semen parameters), and financial constraints.

LAPAROSCOPY VERSUS LAPAROTOMY

Diagnostic laparoscopy was first described in the 1930s but did not gain widespread popularity until the 1970s. Even then, the laparoscope was primarily used as a diagnostic tool. Not until the 1980s did American gynecologists join the pelviscopy procession led by innovative European surgeons. The early question was whether certain procedures could be done safely through the laparoscope. This led to a number of reports describing the safety of a variety of procedures ranging from the treatment of ectopic pregnancy to laparoscopically assisted vaginal hysterectomy. Many immediate benefits were obtained from a laparoscopic approach, including rapid recovery and decreased hospital stay, both of which provide the potential for dramatically decreased direct and attributable costs of the surgery. These forces quickly conspired against randomized clinical trials comparing laparoscopy and laparotomy. Therefore comparisons must be deduced from success rates reported in series of laparotomies and like treatments performed laparoscopically. The large body of literature supporting the laparoscopic treatment of ectopic pregnancy, for example, has established an admirable track record of treatment and follow-up. Clear end points have been established, including persistence, recurrence, and subsequent fertility. Other procedures, such as laparoscopic myomectomy, remain unproven in value.

The other source of comparative data is with animal studies. Luciano et al.[80] employed a rabbit model and demonstrated that de novo adhesion formation after laparoscopy in a normal pelvis was less than that found after a laparotomy. Also, adhesiolysis by laparoscopy was more successful at reducing adhesion score than the same procedure performed at laparotomy.

Unlike the treatment of ectopic pregnancy, for which clear end points have been established, the end points for surgical adhesiolysis are much more elusive. Restoration of normal anatomy is the surgical goal, but often subsequent pregnancy is the patient's desire. It is important to remember that even in well-documented cases of ectopic pregnancy, laparoscopy has equaled laparotomy only with regard to subsequent pregnancy rates. Laparoscopy in such cases is not superior to laparotomy. Likewise, there is no clear and convincing evidence that laparoscopic lysis of adhesions is superior to microsurgical adhesiolysis at laparotomy with regard to subsequent pregnancy.

The proliferation of laparoscopic equipment makes the laparoscopic approach to treatment a viable one for the general practitioner. Realistic self-assessment of surgical skills must take place before embarking on this form of treatment. Success rates reported by accomplished surgeons may not be attainable without significant advanced training.

SURGICAL ADHESIOLYSIS

Since adhesions do not generally correlate with clinical symptoms, it is difficult to assess the success of such surgery. Pregnancy is a deceptive measure of success, since confounding variables including patient age, desire for fertility, and coexistent fertility factors have an extraordinary effect on results. Another option is to reevaluate the pelvis laparoscopically, commonly referred to as second-look laparoscopy (SLL). Raj and Hulka[103] evaluated 60 women by SLL after microsurgical adhesiolysis at laparotomy. Sixty percent of their patients showed improvement in the degree of adnexal adhesions. They further determined that the optimal interval between primary surgery and SLL is 4 to 8 weeks, as newly formed or re-formed adhesions were most easily lysed at that time. Of the 40% of patients who showed no improvement at SLL, none became pregnant.

DeCherney and Mezer[21] compared the gross and histologic differences between adhesions found in early SLL, which they defined as 4 to 16 weeks after surgery, with laparoscopy after 18 months or more. The majority of adhesions seen at late laparoscopy were thicker and neovascularized, whereas early adhesions tended to be filmy and avascular. Trimbos-Kemper et al.[136] evaluated a large series of women 8 days after salpingostomy, fimbrioplasty, or adhesiolysis. More than 50% of the patients had some adhesion re-formation. These filmy adhesions were lysed and the patients were followed clinically. Those patients who did not conceive within 2 years were offered another laparoscopy. In this group, more than half did not have re-formation of adhesions. This study was followed by another series in which Diamond et al.[27] concluded that

reproductive pelvic surgery is complicated not only by adhesion re-formation but by de novo adhesion formation as well. This is the major justification for performing SLL. Additionally, the SLL helps define prognosis, allowing proper counseling of patients as to the success of their surgical procedure and possible referral for IVF or adoption. This invasive procedure may afford an early sign of ultimate prognosis and therefore not delay the pursuit of other avenues of treatment. Whether the risks and expense associated with SLL justify the benefit needs to be decided on an individual basis.

Unfortunately, postoperative adhesion development also occurs frequently after operative laparoscopy. Diamond et al.[32] reported that adhesion scores after operative laparoscopy significantly decreased, but that adhesion reformation occurred in the vast majority of patients (66 of 68 women, 97%).

Laser versus microelectrocautery

Much like laparoscopy, laser technology has proliferated over the past decade. The novel properties afforded by different laser sources have been adapted to the operating room. The modality most commonly used is the carbon dioxide laser, employed for its superficial site of action and variable spot size. Other lasers, including the neodymium:yttrium-aluminum-garnet (Nd:YAG), argon, and potassium-titanyl-phosphate (KTP), all penetrate beyond the surface—a principle that is most useful for ablative surgery but may be more detrimental than desirable in adhesiolysis.

Microelectrocautery is the alternative tool for adhesiolysis. At first glance, one might think it would cause more adjacent tissue damage than the carbon dioxide laser and therefore result in more postoperative adhesion reformation. However, a clinical study of the carbon dioxide laser and electrosurgery for adhesiolysis in 172 cases followed by early SLL[4] and experimental data in rabbits[81] revealed no difference in adhesion recurrence rates or histologic appearance of tissue between these modalities. The choice then is one of surgical convenience, since both sets of instrumentation have been adapted from hand-held units to laparoscopic use.

Surgical adjuvants

Various techniques have been used in an attempt to reduce postoperative adhesion formation and re-formation. As already reviewed, this includes avoidance of tissue trauma, meticulous attention to hemostasis, the use of minimally reactive or nonreactive suture material, and perhaps laparoscopic and laser surgery. In addition to these intraoperative interventions, pelvic surgeons have also used a wide variety of adjuvants to minimize adhesions.

These adjuvants act at one or more of the stages of adhesion formation; that is, they act to prevent the liberation of proteinaceous material from the site of peritoneal

Classes of adhesion-reduction adjuvants

Fibrinolytic agents	Mechanical separation
Urokinase	Intraabdominal
Hyaluronidase	Dextran
Chymotrypsin	Mineral oil
Trypsin	Silicone
Pepsin	Povidine
Plasminogen activators	Petroleum jelly
Anticoagulants	Crystalloid
Heparin	solutions
Citrates	Carboxymethyl-
Oxalates	cellulose
Antiinflammatory agents	Barrier separation
Corticosteroids	Endogenous tissue
Nonsteroidal	Omental grafts
antiinflammatory	Peritoneal grafts
agents	Bladder strips
Antihistamines	Fetal membranes
Progesterone	Exogenous material
Calcium-channel	Oxidized cellulose
blockers	Oxidized
Pentoxifylline	regenerated
Oxygen-derived free	cellulose
radical inhibitors	Polytetrafluoro-
Antibiotics	ethylene
Tetracyclines	Gelatin
Cephalosporins	Rubber sheets
	Metal foils
	Plastic hoods
	Polyglycolic acid
	Polaxamer 407
	Fibrin glue

Modified with permission from Diamond MP, DeCherney AH: *Microsurgery* 8:103, 1987.

injury, halt the generation of a coagulum from this material, stimulate fibrinolytic activity, keep peritoneal surfaces from abutting and reapproximating, and reduce the proliferative activity of fibroblasts (see the box).[25]

In a recent poll of the members of the Society of Reproductive Surgeons, it was found that the use of adjuvants is widespread.[62] This is the case despite conflicting results for many of these agents in the literature. Several explanations for the lack of uniformity in results exists. For example, there is great variability in experimental models; different animals are used; the means of inducing adhesion formation are not standard, nor are the locations of the adhesions induced; and the dosage and route of administration of the adjuvants are varied. Clinical studies are also affected by several of these variables. In addition, other factors such as obesity may play a role.[61] The following paragraphs review the literature examining surgical adjuvants in the reduction of postoperative pelvic adhesion development.

Antiinflammatory agents. Glucocorticoids act by reducing the initial inflammatory response to tissue injury. This is mediated by a reduction in vascular permeability, stabilization of lysosomes, and inhibition of the synthesis and release of histamines. Although older studies have demonstrated fibroblast inhibition with corticosteroid therapy,[58] more recent studies have failed to confirm this.[54,135]

Corticosteroids are commonly used in conjunction with an antihistamine, promethazine. In addition to its decreasing histamine release, promethazine may inhibit fibroblast proliferation. The efficacy of promethazine as a solo agent in inhibiting adhesion formation has not been evaluated.

Corticosteroids, administered before or immediately after surgery, have been demonstrated to decrease adhesion formation after peritoneal injury in small animals.[106,119] Because the dosages required are quite large, increased morbidity, such as infection and wound disruption, have been noted.[45,56] Most studies in nonhuman primates have failed to demonstrate a reduction in adhesion formation. Seitz and colleagues[117] evaluated adhesion reformation after adhesiolysis in monkeys receiving one of three therapies: normal saline, low-molecular-weight dextran, and dexamethasone/promethazine. Adhesion reformation was similar in each of the three groups. diZerega and Hodgen[35] also found perioperative dexamethasone and promethazine to be ineffective in preventing adhesion formation after trauma to the fallopian tube.

The widespread clinical use of corticosteroid therapy is perhaps based on the finding by Swolin[132] that intraperitoneal hydrocortisone decreased adhesion formation as found at SLL. Unfortunately, all patients receiving adjuvant therapy were operated on by Swolin, whereas those who did not receive glucocorticoids had other primary surgeons. There are few other clinical trials evaluating the use of corticosteroids, and the few that exist have failed to demonstrate its efficacy as an adhesion-reduction adjuvant.[66]

Prostaglandins have been shown to play a role in adhesion formation, and the intraperitoneal administration of prostaglandins has been shown to increase the formation of adhesions.[52] Hence it is postulated that by decreasing prostaglandin concentration with nonsteroidal antiinflammatory drugs (NSAIDs), adhesion formation may be reduced. Several possible mechanisms exist by which NSAIDs may reduce adhesion formation after peritoneal injury. They have been shown to inhibit platelet aggregation, leukocyte migration and phagocytosis, and lysosome release.[51] Others have suggested that tolmetin, an NSAID, acts to enhance macrophage function, thereby permitting more rapid clearance of tissue debris or fibrin through phagocytosis.[110] In addition, tolmetin and ibuprofen have been demonstrated to reduce the secretion of plasminogen-activator inhibitor activity. This results in increased plasminogen activator activity with an increase in plasmin and subsequent fibrinolysis.[109,110]

Intravenous administration of ibuprofen resulted in a reduction of peritoneal adhesions when given perioperatively in dosages of 7 to 10 mg/kg in a variety of rabbit models.[5,98,120] Intramuscular and intraperitoneal administration of ibuprofen in rat and rabbit models failed to produce a consistent reduction in peritoneal adhesions.[60,79] Perioperative administration of oxyphenbutazone has been reported to reduce postoperative adhesion formation in rats and monkeys,[68,69,73] as has administration of intraperitoneal indomethacin.[22] More recently, studies have demonstrated that intraperitoneal administration of tolmetin, either via a miniosmotic pump or in a series of micellar and vesicle preparations, significantly reduce adhesion formation.[110] Although there exists some evidence from animal models that suggests that NSAIDs may reduce adhesion formation, no clinical trials to date have been reported.

Progesterone has been shown to possess antiinflammatory and immunosuppressive properties. It has been demonstrated to impede the rejection of xenogenic tumor cells in hamsters,[94] inhibit leukocyte migration,[18] inhibit T-cell activation,[93] and reduce humoral antibody production.[16] Additionally, in rats, administration decreased vascular permeability and the resulting volume of transudate.[96] Initial interest in the use of progesterone for the prevention of postoperative adhesion formation resulted from the finding that adhesions were reduced after ovarian wedge resection if the traumatized ovary contained an active corpus luteum.[40] Subsequently, Maurer and Bonaventura[84] found that administration of intraperitoneal and intramuscular progesterone resulted in a decrease in adhesion development. Others have failed to confirm this and have, in fact, found an increase in adhesion formation after instillation of intraperitoneal progesterone.[6,8] In addition, intraperitoneal and intramuscular medroxyprogesterone acetate has also resulted in an increase in postoperative adhesion formation,[6,64] despite a significant reduction in antibody titers to peritoneum and myometrium.[60]

Colchicine, which has been shown to inhibit histamine secretion, mitotic activity, and collagen synthesis and secretion, has been demonstrated to reduce adhesion formation in two studies utilizing a rat model.[55,118] Despite these preliminary findings, little work has been performed in this area.

Pentoxifylline, a methylxanthine derivative, has several properties that make it a possible therapeutic candidate for adhesion prevention. It has been demonstrated to increase leukocyte membrane permeability,[114] enhance directed chemotaxis,[130] reduce neutrophil granulation, inhibit cytokine-induced granulocyte activation,[131] and inhibit tumor necrosis factor production by the macrophages.[129] Steinleitner and colleagues[128] have demonstrated a reduction in adhesion formation in a hamster uterine horn injury model with pentoxifylline therapy. In a follow-up study, this group also demonstrated its efficacy in inhibiting reformation of previously established adhesions after surgi-

cal resection.[126] Further work on this is required.

Oxygen-derived free radicals, which include superoxide anion (O_2) and hydrogen peroxide (H_2O_2), have been shown to be increased in tissue inflammatory reactions and may play a role in adhesion formation.[46] Superoxide dismutase (SOD) and catalase are compounds that are known to block the effects of oxygen free radicals and have been shown to reduce O_2- and H_2O_2-induced cellular injury in pulmonary tissue.[12,47,111] In a small study, intraperitoneal SOD and catalase administration showed a trend toward adhesion reduction in an endometriosis animal model.[101] It is of note that recent data suggest an increase in oxygen free radicals in the presence of endometriosis[143] and that this finding may not be applicable to other adhesion models.

Calcium is known to play a role in the regulation of the inflammatory response and regenerative process. This prompted the evaluation of calcium-channel blockers as surgical adjuvants in the prevention of postoperative adhesion formation. The mechanisms through which these medications act remain uncertain, although it is likely that they intervene at sequential loci of the adhesion-formation cascade.[127] Calcium antagonists may reduce tissue ischemia, which is known to play a role in adhesion formation. This has been demonstrated in both hepatic and cardiac tissue.[71,99] Administration of calcium-channel blockers has been shown to inhibit the release of vasoactive/inflammatory mediators such as histamine and prostaglandins E and F.[15] In addition, they have been shown to inhibit platelet aggregation,[87] protect against acute granulocyte-mediated tissue injury,[41] and inhibit fibroblast penetration into clot matrices.[3]

Several animal studies have investigated the use of calcium-channel blockers in the prevention of postoperative adhesions. Steinleitner and colleagues[123-125] have demonstrated reduction in primary post-traumatic pelvic adhesion formation in the hamster model with the use of subcutaneous verapamil, nifedipine, and diltiazem. In addition, therapy was well tolerated by all animals. To evaluate further the use of calcium-channel blockade in the prevention of adhesions, Steinleitner et al. extended their work to include a rabbit uterine horn model, which has previously predicted the outcome of adjuvant therapy in humans. They also sought to establish whether continuous intraperitoneal delivery offered any advantage over systemic administration. Intraperitoneal and subcutaneous verapamil were equally efficacious in the reduction of primary adhesion formation.[122,127]

Adhesion reformation is often more difficult to prevent than adhesion formation, and perhaps is also of greater clinical significance. Given this, Steinleitner and his colleagues sought to evaluate calcium-channel blockade in a reformation model. They demonstrated that intraperitoneal verapamil instillation resulted in a marked inhibition of adhesion reformation after lysis of peritoneal adhesions.[122]

Anticoagulants. As the development of a fibrinous

exudate is a necessary precursor to fibrinous organization and adhesion formation, prevention of fibrin deposition and enhanced fibrinolysis is likely to minimize adhesion formation. To this end, anticoagulants, primarily heparin, have been used. Encouraging reports were published in the 1940s on the use of high-dose intraperitoneal heparin.[76,83] Unfortunately, wound disruption and hemorrhage limited its use.[17,44] Recently Jansen[67] evaluated the use of low-dose heparin added to the irrigation solution. Jansen demonstrated that irrigation with a heparin solution (5000 IU/L) failed to reduce peritoneal adhesions when compared with Ringer's lactate solution, as assessed by early SLL.

As noted previously, peritoneal injury results in the release of a fibrin exudate into the peritoneal cavity. These resulting fine and fibrinous adhesions are either lysed by the fibrinolytic system or organized into permanent adhesions. Because it had been shown that suppression of fibrinolysis is associated with adhesion formation, it was believed that treatment with proteolytic enzymes such as streptokinase or urokinase would reduce postoperative adhesions. Unfortunately, when these agents were used in concentrations sufficient to reduce adhesions, hemorrhagic complications often occurred.[25]

Subsequently, investigators sought to evaluate tissue plasminogen activator (t-PA), which converts plasminogen to the active fibrinolytic enzyme, plasmin, as a surgical adjuvant. As activation of the plasmin occurs on the fibrin surface, the proteolytic activity is confined to the appropriate site and the potential for hemorrhagic complications is minimized. Further impetus to evaluate t-PA therapy is the finding that decreased t-PA activity has been associated with the development of pelvic adhesions.[13,14,39,134,139] Menzies and Ellis[88] demonstrated that the application of t-PA gel topically to a cecal injury resulted in reduction in primary adhesion formation and reformation when compared with vehicle. There was also no increase in complications, including wound healing, "colonic bursting pressure," or hemorrhage. In a rabbit uterine horn model, similar results were obtained; that is, a reduction in adhesion formation and reformation after adhesiolysis with the use of t-PA gel. It is of note that the degree of adhesion reduction was positively correlated with dosage, with a maximal effect seen at 25 mg of t-PA. No wound healing or hemorrhagic complications were found.[37] Others have confirmed this finding and have also demonstrated a positive effect of t-PA on sidewall adhesion formation.[39] Finally, intraperitoneal instillation of t-PA liquid also proved to be efficacious in the reduction of uterine horn adhesions after trauma.[38]

Antibiotics. Prophylactic systemic antibiotics are frequently used in reproductive pelvic surgery despite a paucity of literature delineating the specific benefits of such therapy. Whereas broad-spectrum cephalosporins were popular in the past, tetracyclines commonly are used now in order to protect adequately from chlamydia, a potentially

infectious organism in the female reproductive tract.[25] Unlike systemic antibiotic therapy, which is believed to be without significant potential for morbidity, the use of antibiotic peritoneal lavage has been demonstrated in some studies to cause peritoneal adhesions.[100,104]

Mechanical separation

Mechanical separation of pelvic structures, which can be accomplished with an instillate or a material barrier, has been used to reduce adhesion formation. It is postulated that mechanical separation of fibrinous-covered surfaces, while mesothelial healing occurs, will prevent these structures from becoming adherent. Many of the agents evaluated in the past resulted in an increase in adhesion formation secondary to severe foreign-body reactions.

Instillates. Crystalloid solutions, which are inert, have been used but have been proven ineffective because of rapid absorption. Because the rate of absorption of a substance from the peritoneal cavity is dependent on its physical properties and molecular weight, insoluble solutions such as dextran were evaluated. The length of time that dextran remains in the peritoneal cavity is dependent on the animal model used, the concentration of the solution, and the molecular weight of the solution.[36] diZerega and Hodgen[35] reported that in the monkey 32% dextran 70 in dextrose (Hyskon) remains in the peritoneal cavity for 5 days, but not 7 days.

Initially low-molecular-weight dextran (dextran 40) was used for adhesion prophylaxis. The results were variable, and its use was abandoned in favor of 32% dextran 70.[63]

In addition to the hydroflotation effect previously described (Fig. 36-6), 32% dextran 70 possesses other properties that are likely to play a role in its action. It is believed to have a "siliconizing effect" in coating raw serosal surfaces. Studies have also demonstrated that fibrin formed in the presence of low concentrations of 32% dextran 70 is structurally altered and is more susceptible to breakdown.[95,133] In addition, 32% dextran 70 inhibits lymphocyte proliferation and macrophage phagocytosis in vitro.[105] Supporting these additional actions of 32% dextran 70 is the finding that administration of dosages inadequate for hydroflotation was found effective in reducing adhesion formation.[95,133]

Most of the animal studies performed demonstrated a reduction in adhesion formation with the instillation of 32% dextran 70. Dosages varied from 2.5 mL/kg to 50 mL per rabbit.* Adhesion re-formation after lysis was reduced only when dosages of 5 to 10 mL/kg were used.[63,121] In women, this would require volumes greater than those currently regarded as safe. In fact, animal studies reported an increase in postoperative deaths when large volumes were used.[137]

*References 35, 63, 82, 97, 121, 137, 138.

Four large-scale clinical trials have been performed to evaluate the efficacy of 32% dextran 70 as a surgical adjuvant for adhesion reduction. Two reports demonstrated efficacy[2,113] and the other two failed to demonstrate adhesion reduction.[66,74] All trials were randomized and adhesion formation/reformation was evaluated by SLL. No significant side effects were encountered in the initial trials. Despite the conflicting nature of these studies, the use of 32% dextran 70 is widespread.[112]

Since then, case reports have appeared in the literature describing complications associated with the use of 32% dextran 70. These include labial edema, anaphylaxis, wound separation, disseminated intravascular coagulation, pleural effusion, and transient liver function abnormalities.[7,9,50,140] Although 32% dextran 70 has been demonstrated to be an excellent culture medium,[7] clinically this has not proven to be a problem. In fact, injection of several common "gynecologic" organisms into the peritoneal cavity of the mouse in the presence of 32% dextran 70 failed to increase mortality over that of control groups.[70]

Sodium carboxymethylcellulose (SCMC) is a high-molecular-weight polysaccharide that has undergone evaluation as a potential adjuvant. It is prepared by allowing sodium monochloroacetate to react with cellulose and may have a molecular weight as high as 350,000.[42,43] It acts by coating the intraperitoneal surfaces and also causes hydroflotation of the abdominoperitoneal structures. Several studies have found SCMC to be efficacious in inhibiting both adhesion formation and reformation.[29,42,48] In addition, Elkins et al.[43] found intraperitoneal SCMC to be significantly more efficacious than 32% dextran 70 in reducing adhesion reformation; SCMC was also found to be safe.[43,48] In a pony model, a transient elevation in blood glucose was noted but was thought to be secondary to a stress response rather than the medication.[90]

Endogenous barriers. Barrier agents act to reduce adhesion formation by preventing raw serosal surfaces from abutting. They have been used for more than half a century.[20] In 1917, free portions of omentum were used to decrease small bowel adhesions. Since that time, other natural materials have been tried—including fat, peritoneum, and amnion—without much success.[25] Recently trypsin-treated, gamma ray–irradiated human amniotic membranes were used to cover traumatized uterine horns. In this rabbit model, the investigators demonstrated a reduction in adhesions with use of an amniotic membrane.[142]

Exogenous barriers. In the past, other materials such as metal foils, plastic hoods, silk, and rubber sheets have been used in an attempt to reduce postoperative adhesions. Use of these substances has been abandoned because of lack of success,[116] and because they often required a second surgical procedure for removal.[25]

With advances in materials science, the use of exogenous materials as a barrier has become increasingly popular (Fig. 36-7). Silicone film placed over traumatized small-bowel serosa resulted in decreased adhesion formation, but unfortunately a second laparotomy was required for its removal.[19] Similarly, expanded polytetrafluoroethylene (PTFE, Gore-Tex), which is an inert membrane, also requires removal after placement. Initially used as a vascular graft, it was subsequently manufactured as a surgical membrane with a microporous structure that discouraged cellular penetration and tissue attachment.[11] Used as a pericardial patch, adhesion formation was shown to be minimized.[107] An initial study by Goldberg et al.,[53] however, failed to demonstrate efficacy of PTFE in reducing adhesion formation in a uterine horn model. Subsequently Boyers et al.[10] demonstrated that PTFE membrane was an effective barrier for reducing primary adhesions, as well as for reducing reformation of adhesions.[11] As noted by Boyers and co-workers,[10] the difference in results obtained in their study is likely to be secondary to study design. In the study by Goldberg et al.,[53] the control animals had a very low rate of adhesion formation. In addition, multiple sutures were used to hold the membrane in place, but sutures were not placed in the control defect.

Currently a clinical trial is in progress to evaluate the efficacy of the PTFE as a surgical adjuvant. Since animal studies found that the patch remained nonadherent to the pelvic sidewall,[11] its removal at SLL may not be difficult. Its use as an adjuvant may be limited by the fact that it is sutured in place, which may be cumbersome or difficult by laparoscopy.

The role of polyglycolic acid (PGA) mesh in the prevention of pelvic adhesions after radical pelvic surgery has been evaluated. Compared with controls, adhesions were found to be increased with the use of PGA after total abdominal hysterectomy, bilateral salpingo-oophorectomy, and intracolic omentectomy in dogs.[92] Although one cannot necessarily extrapolate these findings to infertility surgery, these results suggest that PGA is unlikely to be an effective surgical adjuvant.

Poloxamer 407, a copolymer of polyoxyethylene and polyoxypropylene, has been evaluated for use in adhesion prevention. Fluid at room temperature, it becomes a gel at body temperature. It is applied with an "applicating needle" as a fluid, but it gels within seconds at the site of application. In a rat uterine horn model, it was demonstrated to reduce effectively the formation of adhesions.[75] In addition, because it can be applied in the fluid phase, it is ideally suited for application through the laparoscope.

Fibrin glue is a compound made by combining a source of highly concentrated fibrinogen with thrombin, calcium, and factor VIII. The source of fibrinogen is either pooled, concentrated, human fibrinogen or single-donor human cryoprecipitate. Its role in adhesion prophylaxis has been evaluated. Although its mechanism of action is uncertain, it is postulated that fibrin glue acts by the separation of raw surfaces created by its rapid sealant effect. In a rat model, de Virgilio et al.[23] demonstrated a reduction in intraabdominal adhesion formation with the administration of fibrin glue with a high fibrinogen concentration (from cryoprecipitate) but not with the administration of fibrin glue with a low fibrinogen concentration (from fresh frozen plasma). Obviously, the use of human blood products to make the fibrin glue limits its attractiveness as a surgical adjuvant.

The role of blood in the formation of adhesions, as discussed earlier, is controversial. Recently, a number of procoagulant substances have been evaluated for their role as prophylaxis against adhesion formation. As already noted, fibrin glue appears to demonstrate antiadhesive properties. Other compounds, such as oxidized regenerated cellulose (ORC), also appear to have such properties. To assess whether their positive activity against adhesion formation represents a barrier or a hemostatic effect, McGaw and colleagues[85] compared a thrombin spray, which possesses only a procoagulant effect, with ORC in control animals. Overall, the ORC barrier appeared to reduce adhesion formation, whereas the thrombin failed to do so. This suggests that the barrier property of the ORC is an important component of its success as a surgical adjuvant.

Investigators evaluated ORC (Surgicel), which was initially designed as a hemostatic agent, for use in adhesion prevention because it was easy to apply and became a gel within hours after application.[89] Initial studies by Larsson et al.[72] and Rafferty[102] demonstrated the efficacy of ORC in the rat cecal trauma model. Others, however, did not find a decrease in adhesion formation in a similar model.[115] In a uterine horn model, most, but not all,[141] studies found ORC to be effective in preventing adhesion formation.[49]

The need for a more consistent reduction in adhesion formation and re-formation prompted the modification of the oxidation, porosity, knit, and weave of ORC to create Interceed (TC-7). Interceed becomes a gel approximately 8 hours after application to a peritoneal surface, and acts as a barrier between two otherwise opposing surfaces.[30] Macroscopically, the material appears to be almost entirely gone within 3 to 4 days. Microscopically, there is no evidence of a foreign-body reaction at the site of breakdown. Interceed is metabolized into glucose and glucoronic acid within a few days.[30]

Initial rabbit studies using a uterine horn model demonstrated a reduction in adhesion formation.[77] This was confirmed by Diamond et al.,[28] using both a sidewall and a uterine horn model. It is important to note that blood plus barrier (TC-4, which is similar to TC-7) failed to prevent adhesion formation in a rabbit uterine horn model.[78] Additionally, in this model, TC-4 alone did reduce adhesion formation. This underscores the need for careful hemostasis in order to ensure maximal effectiveness of this modified ORC. Furthermore, heparin, when added to the Interceed, appeared to act synergistically in the reduction of adhesion formation in the rabbit uterine horn model.[33] Yet, with use of a murine model, Interceed to a greater extent than

expanded PTFE (Gore-Tex surgical membrane) elicited a peritoneal inflammatory exudate.[57] Finally, in a randomized, multicenter clinical trial, Interceed was shown to reduce the incidence, extent, and severity of postsurgical pelvic adhesions as assessed at SLL.[31] Further clinical trials regarding the use of Interceed and heparin, and the laparoscopic placement of Interceed, are awaited.

REFERENCES

1. Abe H et al: The effect of intraperitoneal administration of sodium tolmetin-hyaluronic acid on the postsurgical cell infiltration in vivo, *J Surg Res* 49:322, 1990.
2. Adhesion Study Group: Reduction of postoperative pelvic adhesions with intraperitoneal 32% dextran 70: a prospective, randomized clinical trial, *Fertil Steril* 40:612, 1983.
3. Azzarone B et al: Modulation of fibroblast-induced clot retraction by calcium channel blocking drugs and the monoclonal antibody ALB6, *J Cell Physiol* 125:420, 1985.
4. Barbot J et al: A clinical study of the CO_2 laser and electrosurgery for adhesiolysis in 172 cases followed by early second-look laparoscopy, *Fertil Steril* 48:140, 1987.
5. Bateman BG, Nunley WC Jr, Kitchin JD III: Prevention of postoperative peritoneal adhesions: an assessment of ibuprofen, *Surg Forum* 32:603, 1981.
6. Beauchamp PJ, Quigley MM, Held B: Evaluation of progestogens for postoperative adhesion prevention, *Fertil Steril* 42:538, 1984.
7. Bernstein J et al: The potential for bacterial growth with dextran, *J Reprod Med* 27:77, 1982.
8. Blauer KL, Collins RL: The effect of intraperitoneal progesterone on postoperative adhesion formation in rabbits, *Fertil Steril* 49:144, 1988.
9. Borten M, Seibert CP, Taymor ML: Recurrent anaphylactic reaction to intraperitoneal dextran 75 used for prevention of postsurgical adhesions, *Obstet Gynecol* 61:755, 1983.
10. Boyers SP, Diamond MP, DeCherney AH: Reduction of postoperative pelvic adhesions in the rabbit Gore-Tex surgical membrane, *Fertil Steril* 49:1066, 1988.
11. Boyers SP, Jansen D: Gore-Tex surgical membrane. In diZerega GS et al, editors: *Treatment of postsurgical adhesions,* New York, 1990, Alan R Liss.
12. Britton L, Malinkovsk DP, Fridovich I: Superoxide dismutase and oxygen metabolism in *Streptococcus faecalis* and comparison with other organisms, *J Biol Chem* 245:4641, 1970.
13. Buckman RF et al: A physiologic basis for the adhesion-free healing of deperitonealized surfaces, *J Surg Res* 21:67, 1976.
14. Buckman RF et al: A unifying pathogenetic mechanism in the etiology of intraperitoneal adhesions, *J Surg Res* 20:1, 1976.
15. Chand N et al: Inhibition of allergic and non-allergic histamine secretion from rat peritoneal mast cells by calcium antagonists, *Br J Pharmacol* 83:899, 1984.
16. Clemens LE, Siiteri PK, Stites DP: Mechanism of immunosuppression of progesterone on maternal lymphocyte activation during pregnancy, *J Immunol* 122:1978, 1979.
17. Connolly JE, Smith JW: The prevention and treatment of intestinal adhesions, *Surg Gynecol Obstet* 110:417, 1960.
18. Contopoulos AN et al: Inhibition of leukocyte migration by progesterone in vivo and in vitro, *Soc Gynecol Invest* 8:110, 1977.
19. Cook GB: The silicone serosal interface, I: abatement of talc adhesions in dogs, *Surgery* 55:268, 1964.
20. Davis CB: Free transplantation of the omentum, *JAMA* 9:705, 1917.
21. DeCherney AH, Mezer HC: The nature of posttuboplasty pelvic adhesions as determined by early and late laparoscopy, *Fertil Steril* 41:643, 1984.
22. DeSimone JM et al: Indomethacin decreases carrageenan-induced peritoneal adhesions, *Surgery* 104:788, 1988.

23. de Virgilio C et al: Fibrin glue inhibits intra-abdominal adhesion formation, *Arch Surg* 125:1378, 1990.

24. Diamond MP: Surgical aspects of infertility. In Sciarra JJ, editor, *Gynecology and obstetrics,* Philadelphia, 1988, Harper and Row.

25. Diamond MP, DeCherney AH: Pathogenesis of adhesion formation/reformation: application to reproductive pelvic surgery, *Microsurgery* 8:103, 1987.

26. Diamond MP, Hershlag A: Adhesion formation/reformation. In diZerega GS et al, editors: *Treatment of postsurgical adhesions,* New York, 1990, Alan R Liss.

27. Diamond MP et al: Adhesion reformation and de novo adhesion formation following reproductive surgery, *Fertil Steril* 47:864, 1987.

28. Diamond MP et al: A model for sidewall adhesions in the rabbit: reduction by an absorbable barrier, *Microsurgery* 8:197, 1987.

29. Diamond MP et al: Assessment of carboxymethylcellulose and 32% dextran 70 for prevention of adhesions in a rabbit uterine horn model, *Int J Fertil* 33:278, 1988.

30. Diamond MP et al: Interceed (TC7) as an adjuvant for adhesion reduction: animal studies. In diZerega GS et al, editors: *Treatment of postsurgical adhesions,* New York, 1990, Alan R Liss.

31. Diamond MP et al: Reduction of adhesion reformation following adhesiolysis at laparotomy by INTERCEED[R] TC7. Abstract presented at the II Joint Meeting of ESCO-ESHRE, Milan, Italy, August 29–September 1, 1990.

32. Diamond MP et al: Postoperative adhesion development following operative laparoscopy: evaluation at early second-look procedures, *Fertil Steril* 55:700, 1991.

33. Diamond MP et al: Synergistic effects of Interceed (TC7) and heparin in reducing adhesion formation in the rabbit uterine horn model, *Fertil Steril* 55:389, 1991.

34. diZerega GS: The peritoneum and its response to surgical injury. In diZerega GS et al, editors: *Treatment of postsurgical adhesions,* New York, 1990, Alan R Liss.

35. diZerega GS, Hodgen GD: Prevention of postsurgical tubal adhesions: comparative study of commonly used agents, *Am J Obstet Gynecol* 136:173, 1980.

36. diZerega GS, Holtz G: The cause and prevention of postsurgical adhesions. In Osofsky H, editor: *Advances in clinical obstetrics and gynecology,* Baltimore, 1982, Williams & Wilkins.

37. Doody KJ, Dunn RC, Buttram VC: Recombinant tissue plasminogen activator reduces adhesion formation in a rabbit uterine horn model, *Fertil Steril* 51:509, 1989.

38. Dörr PJ et al: Prevention of postoperative adhesions by tissue-type plasminogen activator (t-PA) in the rabbit, *Eur J Obstet Gynecol Reprod Biol* 37:287, 1990.

39. Dunn RC, Buttram VC: Tissue-type plasminogen activator as an adjuvant for post surgical adhesions. In diZerega GS et al, editors: *Treatment of postsurgical adhesions,* New York, 1990, Alan R Liss.

40. Eddy CA, Asch RH, Balmaceda JP: Pelvic adhesion following microsurgical and macrosurgical wedge resection of the ovaries, *Fertil Steril* 33:557, 1980.

41. Elferink JGR, Deierkauf M: The effect of verapamil and other calcium antagonists on chemotaxis of polymorphonuclear leukocytes, *Biochem Pharmacol* 33:35, 1984.

42. Elkins TE et al: Adhesion prevention by solutions of sodium carboxymethylcellulose in the rat, I. *Fertil Steril* 41:926, 1984.

43. Elkins TE et al: Adhesion prevention by solutions of sodium carboxymethylcellulose in the rat, II. *Fertil Steril* 41:929, 1984.

44. Ellis H: The cause and prevention of postoperative intraperitoneal adhesions, *Surg Gynecol Obstet* 113:547, 1961.

45. Eskeland G: Prevention of experimental peritoneal adhesions in the rat by intraperitoneally administered corticosteroids, *Acta Chir Scand* 125:91, 1963.

46. Fantone JC, Ward PA: Role of oxygen-derived free radicals and metabolites in leukocyte-dependent inflammatory reactions, *Am J Pathol* 107:397, 1982.

47. Forman HF, York JL, Fisher AB: Mechanisms for the potentiation of oxygen toxicity of disulfuram, *J Pharmacol Exp Ther* 212:452, 1980.

48. Fredericks CM et al: Adhesion prevention in the rabbit with sodium carboxymethylcellulose solutions, *Am J Obstet Gynecol* 155:667, 1986.

49. Galan N et al: Adhesion prophylaxis in rabbits with Surgicel and two absorbable microsurgical sutures, *J Reprod Med* 28:662, 1983.

50. Gauwerky J, Heinrich D, Kubli F: Komplikationen und Nebenwirkungen des künstlichen Aszites zur Adhäsions-prophylaxe, *Geburtshilfe Frauenheilkd* 45:664, 1985.

51. Gernaat CM, Stubbs DF: Clinical brochure for investigators studying ibuprofen and myocardial infarction. Kalamazoo, Mich, 1980, Upjohn Co, 1980.

52. Golan A et al: Prostaglandins—a role in adhesion formation: an experimental study, *Acta Obstet Gynecol Scand* 69:339, 1990.

53. Goldberg JM, Toledo AA, Mitchell DE: An evaluation of the Gore-Tex surgical membrane for the prevention of postoperative peritoneal adhesions, *Obstet Gynecol* 70:846, 1987.

54. Granat M et al: Effects of dexamethasone on proliferation of autologous fibroblasts and on the immune profile in women undergoing pelvic surgery for infertility, *Fertil Steril* 39:180, 1983.

55. Granat M et al: Reduction of peritoneal adhesion formation by colchicine: a comparative study in the rat, *Fertil Steril* 40:369, 1983.

56. Grosfeld JL et al: Excessive morbidity resulting from the prevention of intestinal adhesions with steroids and antihistamines, *J Pediatr Surg* 8:221, 1973.

57. Haney AF, Doty E: Comparison of the peritoneal cells elicited by oxidized regenerated cellulose (Interceed) and expanded polytetrafluoroethylene (Gore-Tex surgical membrane) in a murine model, *Am J Obstet Gynecol* 166:1137, 1992.

58. Holden M, Adams LB: Inhibitory effects of cortisone acetate and hydrocortisone on growth of fibroblasts, *Proc Soc Exp Biol Med* 95:364, 1957.

59. Holtz G: Prevention of postoperative adhesions, *J Reprod Med* 24:141, 1980.

60. Holtz G: Failure of a nonsteroidal anti-inflammatory agent (ibuprofen) to inhibit peritoneal adhesion reformation after lysis, *Fertil Steril* 37:582, 1982.

61. Holtz G: Prevention and management of peritoneal adhesions, *Fertil Steril* 41:497, 1984.

62. Holtz G: Current use of ancillary modalities for adhesion prevention, *Fertil Steril* 44:174, 1985.

63. Holtz G, Baker E, Tsai C: Effect of thirty-two percent dextran 70 on peritoneal adhesion formation and reformation after lysis, *Fertil Steril* 33:660, 1980.

64. Holtz G et al: Effect of medroxyprogesterone acetate on peritoneal adhesion formation, *Fertil Steril* 40:542, 1983.

65. Hulka JF: Adnexal adhesions: a prognostic staging and classification system based on a five-year survey of fertility surgery results at Chapel Hill, North Carolina, *Am J Obstet Gynecol* 144:141, 1982.

66. Jansen RPS: Failure of intraperitoneal adjuncts to improve the outcome of pelvic operations in young women, *Am J Obstet Gynecol* 153:363, 1985.

67. Jansen RPS: Failure of peritoneal irrigation with heparin during pelvic operations upon young women to reduce adhesions, *Surg Obstet Gynecol* 166:154, 1988.

68. Kapur BML, Gulati SM, Talwar JF: Prevention of reformation of peritoneal adhesions: effect of oxyphenbutazone, proteolytic enzymes from carica papaya, and dextran 40, *Arch Surg* 98:301, 1969.

69. Kapur BML, Talwar JF, Gulati SM: Oxyphenbutazone: antiinflammatory agent in prevention of peritoneal adhesions, *Arch Surg* 105:761, 1972.

70. Kennedy EK, Rosenberg SM, Gebhart RJ: Effects of dextran-70 on bacteria-induced mortality in mice, *Infertility* 8:30, 1985.

71. Kloner RA, Braunwald E: Effects of calcium antagonists on infarcting myocardium, *Am J Cardiol* 59:84B, 1987.

72. Larsson B, Nisell H, Granberg I: Surgicel—an absorbable hemostatic material—in prevention of peritoneal adhesions in rats, *Acta Chir Scand* 144:375, 1978.

73. Larsson B, Svanberg SG, Swolin K: Oxyphenbutazone, an adjuvant to be used in prevention of adhesion in operations for fertility, *Fertil Steril* 28:807, 1977.

74. Larsson B et al: Effect of intraperitoneal instillation of 32% dextran 70 on post-operative adhesion formation after tubal surgery, *Acta Obstet Gynecol Scand* 64:437, 1985.

75. Leach RE, Henry RL: Reduction of postoperative adhesions in the rat uterine horn model with poloxamer 407, *Am J Obstet Gynecol* 162:1317, 1990.

76. Lehman E, Boys F: The prevention of peritoneal adhesions with heparin, *Ann Surg* 111:227, 1940.

77. Linsky CB et al: Adhesion reduction in the rabbit uterine horn model using an absorbable barrier, TC-7, *J Reprod Med* 32:17, 1987.

78. Linsky CB et al: Effect of blood on the efficacy of barrier adhesion reduction in the rabbit uterine horn model, *Infertility* 11:273, 1988.

79. Luciano AA, Hauser KS, Benda J: Evaluation of commonly used adjuvants in the prevention of postoperative adhesions, *Am J Obstet Gynecol* 146:88, 1983.

80. Luciano AA et al: A comparative study of postoperative adhesions following laser surgery by laparoscopy versus laparotomy in the rabbit model, *Obstet Gynecol* 74:220, 1989.

81. Luciano AA et al: A comparison of thermal injury, healing patterns, and postoperative adhesion formation following CO_2 laser and electromicrosurgery, *Fertil Steril* 48:1025, 1987.

82. Luengo J, van Hall EV: Prevention of peritoneal adhesions by the combined use of spongostan and 32% dextran 70: an experimental study in pigs, *Fertil Steril* 29:447, 1978.

83. Massie F: Heparin in the abdomen: a clinical report, *Ann Surg* 121:508, 1945.

84. Maurer JH, Bonaventura LM: The effect of aqueous progesterone on operative adhesion formation, *Fertil Steril* 39:485, 1983.

85. McGaw T et al: Assessment of intraperitoneal adhesion formation in a rat model: can a procoagulant substance prevent adhesions?, *Obstet Gynecol* 71:774, 1988.

86. Medical Research International and the Society of Assisted Reproductive Technology: In vitro fertilization/embryo transfer in the United States: 1987 results from the national IVF-ET registry, *Fertil Steril* 51:13, 1989.

87. Mehta J, Mehta P, Ostrowski N: Calcium blocker diltiazem inhibits platelet activation and stimulation of vascular prostacycline synthesis, *Am J Med Sci* 291:20, 1986.

88. Menzies D, Ellis H: The role of plasminogen activator in adhesion prevention, *Surgery* 172:362, 1991.

89. Meyer WR, DeCherney AH, Diamond MP: How good are the new adhesion-reduction adjuvants?, *Contemp Obstet Gynecol* 81, 1990.

90. Moll DH et al: Evaluation of sodium carboxymethylcellulose for prevention of experimentally induced abdominal adhesions in ponies, *Am J Vet Res* 52:88, 1991.

91. Montz FJ, Shimanuki T, diZerega GS: Postsurgical mesothelialepithelialization. In DeCherney AH, Polan ML, editors: *Reproductive surgery*, Chicago, 1987, Year Book.

92. Montz FJ, Wheeler JH, Lau LM: Inability of polyglycolic acid mesh to inhibit immediate post-radical pelvic surgery adhesions, *Gynecol Oncol* 38:230, 1990.

93. Mori T et al: Inhibitory effect of progesterone and 20 alpha hydoxypregn-4-en-3-one on the phytohemagglutinin-induced transformation of human lymphocytes, *Am J Obstet Gynecol* 127:151, 1977.

94. Moriyama I, Sugawa T: Progesterone facilitates implantation of xenogeneic culture cells in hamster uterus, *Nature* 236:150, 1972.

95. Muzaffar TZ, Youngson GG, Bryce WAJ: Studies on fibrin formation and effects of dextran, *Thromb Diath Haemorrh* 28:244, 1972.

96. Nakagawa H et al: Anti-inflammatory action of progesterone on carrageenin-induced inflammation in rats, *Jpn J Pharmacol* 29:509, 1979.

97. Neuwirth RS, Khalaf SM: Effect of thirty-two percent dextran on peritoneal adhesion formation, *Am J Obstet Gynecol* 121:420, 1975.

98. Nishimura K, Nakamura RM, diZerega GS: Biochemical evaluation of postsurgical wound repair: prevention of intraperitoneal adhesion formation with ibuprofen, *J Surg Res* 34:219, 1983.

99. Peck RC, Lefer AM: Protective effect of nifedipine in the hypoxic perfused cat liver, *Agents Actions* 11:421, 1981.

100. Phillips RKS, Dudley HAF: The effect of tetracycline lavage and trauma on visceral and parietal peritoneal ultrastructure and adhesion formation, *Br J Surg* 71:537, 1984.

101. Portz DM et al: Oxygen free radicals and pelvic adhesion formation, I: blocking oxygen free radical toxicity to prevent adhesion formation in an endometriosis model, *Int J Fertil* 36:39, 1991.

102. Rafferty AT: Absorbable haemostatic materials and intraperitoneal adhesion formation, *Br J Surg* 67:57, 1980.

103. Raj SG, Hulka JF: Second-look laparoscopy in infertility surgery: therapeutic and prognostic value, *Fertil Steril* 38:325, 1982.

104. Rappaport WD et al: Antibiotic irrigation and the formation of intraabdominal adhesions, *Am J Surg* 158:435, 1989.

105. Rein MS, Hill JA: 32% dextran 70 (Hyskon) inhibits lymphocyte and macrophage function in vitro: a potential new mechanism for adhesion prevention, *Fertil Steril* 52:953, 1989.

106. Replogle RL, Johnson R, Gross RE: Prevention of postoperative intestinal adhesions with combined promethazine and dexamethasone therapy, *Ann Surg* 163:580, 1966.

107. Revuelta JM et al: Expanded PTFE surgical membrane for pericardial closure, *J Thorac Cardiovasc Surg* 89:451, 1985.

108. Rock JA et al: Factors influencing the success of salpingostomy techniques for distal tubal fimbrial obstruction, *Obstet Gynecol* 52:591, 1978.

109. Rockwell WB, Ehrlich HP: An ibuprofen-antagonized plasmin inhibitor released by human endothelial cells, *Exp Mol Pathol* 54:1, 1991.

110. Rodgers KE: Nonsteroidal anti-inflammatory drugs (NSAIDs) in the treatment of postsurgical adhesion. In diZerega GS et al, editors: *Treatment of postsurgical adhesions*, New York, 1990, Alan R Liss.

111. Roos D et al: Protection of human neutrophils by endogenous catalase: studies with catalase deficient individuals, *J Clin Invest* 65:1515, 1980.

112. Rosenberg SM: Dextran 70—encouraging early clinical studies. In diZerega GS et al, editors: *Treatment of postsurgical adhesions*, New York, 1990, Alan R Liss.

113. Rosenberg SM, Board JA: High-molecular weight dextran in human infertility surgery, *Am J Obstet Gynecol* 148:380, 1984.

114. Schmalzer EA, Chien S: Filterability of subpopulations of neutrophils: effect of pentoxifylline, *Blood* 64:542, 1984.

115. Schroder M et al: Peritoneal adhesion formation after the use of oxidized cellulose (Surgicel) and gelatin sponge (Spongostan) in rats, *Acta Chir Scand* 148:595, 1982.

116. Seifer BD, Diamond MP, DeCherney AH: An appraisal of barrier agents in the reduction of adhesion formation following surgery, *J Gynecol Surg* 6:3, 1990.

117. Seitz HM Jr et al: Postoperative intraperitoneal adhesions: a double-blind assessment of their prevention in the monkey, *Fertil Steril* 24:935, 1973.

118. Shapiro I, Granat M, Sharf M: The effect of intraperitoneal colchicine on formation of peritoneal adhesion in the rat, *Arch Gynecol* 231:227, 1982.

119. Shikata Y, Yamaoka I: The role of topically applied dexamethasone in preventing peritoneal adhesions, *World J Surg* 1:389, 1977.

120. Siegler AM, Kontopoulos V, Wang CF: Prevention of postoperative adhesions in rabbits with ibuprofen, a non-steroid anti-inflammatory agent, *Fertil Steril* 34:46, 1980.

121. Soules MR et al: The prevention of postoperative adhesions: an

animal study comparing barrier methods with dextran 70, *Am J Obstet Gynecol* 143:829, 1982.

122. Steinleitner A, Kazensky C, Lambert H: Calcium channel blockade prevents postsurgical reformation of adnexal adhesions in rabbits, *Obstet Gynecol* 74:796, 1989.

123. Steinleitner A et al: Reduction of adhesion formation with perioperative verapamil treatment. Presented at the 36th Annual Meeting of the Pacific Coast Fertility Society, Palm Springs, Calif, April 1988.

124. Steinleitner A et al: The use of calcium channel blockade for the prevention of postoperative adhesion formation, *Fertil Steril* 50:818, 1988.

125. Steinleitner A et al: The use of diltiazem for prevention of postoperative adhesion formation, *J Reprod Med* 33:891, 1988.

126. Steinleitner A et al: Pentoxifylline, a methylxanthine derivative, prevents postsurgical adhesion reformation in rabbits, *Obstet Gynecol* 75:926, 1990.

127. Steinleitner A et al: Reduction of primary postoperative adhesion formation under calcium channel blockade in the rabbit, *J Surg Res* 48:42, 1990.

128. Steinleitner A et al: Use of pentoxifylline as an adjuvant to prevent postsurgical adhesion formation: preliminary investigations in a rodent model, *J Gynecol Surg* 5:367, 1989.

129. Strieter RM et al: Cellular and molecular regulation of tumor necrosis factor-alpha production by pentoxifylline, *Biochem Biophys Res Commun* 155:1230, 1988.

130. Sullivan GW et al: Enhancement of chemotaxis and protection of mice from infection, *Trans Assoc Am Physicians* 97:337, 1984.

131. Sullivan GW et al: Inhibition of inflammatory action of interleukin-1 and tumor necrosis factor (alpha) on neutrophil function by pentoxifylline, *Infect Immun* 56:1722, 1988.

132. Swolin K: Die Einwirkung von Grossen, intraperitonealen dusen Glukokortikoid auf die Bildung von postoperativen Adhäsionen, *Acta Obstet Gynecol Scand* 46:204, 1967.

133. Tangen O, Wik KO, Almquist IAM: Effects of dextran on the structure and plasmin-induced lysis of human fibrin, *Thromb Res* 1:487, 1972.

134. Thompson JN et al: Reduced human peritoneal plasminogen activating activity: possible mechanism of adhesion formation, *Br J Surg* 76:382, 1989.

135. Thrash CR, Cunningham DO: Stimulation of division of density inhibited fibroblasts by glucocorticoids, *Nature* 242:399, 1973.

136. Trimbos-Kemper TCM, Trimbos JB, van Hall EV: Adhesion formation after tubal surgery: results of the eighth-day laparoscopy in 188 patients, *Fertil Steril* 43:395, 1985.

137. Utian WH, Goldfarb JM, Starks GC: Role of dextran 70 in microtubal surgery, *Fertil Steril* 31:79, 1979.

138. Vemer M, Boeckx W, Brosens I: Use of dextrans for the prevention of postoperative peritubal adhesions in rabbits, *Br J Obstet Gynaecol* 89:473, 1982.

139. Vipond MN et al: Peritoneal fibrinolytic activity and intra-abdominal adhesions, *Lancet* 335:1120, 1990.

140. Weinans MJN et al: Transient liver function disturbances after the intraperitoneal use of 32% dextran 70 as adhesion prophylaxis in infertility surgery, *Fertil Steril* 53:159, 1990.

141. Yemini M et al: Prevention of reformation of pelvic adhesions by "barrier" methods, *Int J Fertil* 29:194, 1984.

142. Young RL et al: The use of an amniotic membrane graft to prevent postoperative adhesion, *Fertil Steril* 55:624, 1991.

143. Zeller JM et al: Enhancement of human monocyte and peritoneal macrophage chemiluminescence activities in women with endometriosis, *Am J Reprod Immunol Microbiol* 3:78, 1987.

Chapter 37

ENDOMETRIOSIS AND ITS MEDICAL MANAGEMENT

Jouko Halme, MD, PhD
and Dale Stovall, MD

BACKGROUND

Definition

Endometriosis is a common condition in women of reproductive age in which viable endometrial tissue is present outside the uterine cavity. Most commonly this tissue is found in the pelvis but occasionally in more distant areas of the body. Although ectopic endometrium is benign, it retains its responsiveness to physiologic fluctuations in sex steroids, which leads to changes in the ectopic tissue. These changes include proliferative, secretory, and inflammatory characteristics and are thought to be the basis of the symptoms of endometriosis: pain and infertility.

Epidemiology and risk factors

Endometriosis remains one of the most common and puzzling gynecologic disorders in women. The peak incidence is in the third and fourth decades of life, but endometriosis may be seen at any time in women of reproductive age. The accuracy of prevalence estimates is hampered by the fact that no reliable markers are available for endometriosis, and consequently a surgical procedure is always required for diagnosis. The indication for such a surgical procedure inevitably causes a bias in the estimate. Nevertheless, it is generally assumed that endometriosis probably is present in at least 1% of all women of reproductive age, is a principal contributing factor in 15% of infertile women, and can be found in 20% of women operated upon for pelvic pain.

The apparent perception that endometriosis is more commonly found in women of upper socioeconomic groups may result from detection bias, since these women may have better access to medical care and be more likely to be evaluated for their symptoms. Similarly, the impact of race remains unclear, although suggestive evidence exists that endometriosis is most common in Orientals, less common in whites, and least common in blacks. Probably many of these differences result from effects of confounding factors, such as variations in childbearing and birth control practices. Indeed, demographic changes in the population, such as delayed childbearing, may have contributed to the perceived growing incidence of endometriosis among contemporary women.

Many years of spontaneous menstrual cyclicity appear to predispose women for endometriosis. Also the fact that the disease has a tendency to regress during prolonged amenorrhea, as during pregnancy and menopause, points to the role of (retrograde) menstruation as a risk factor. Epidemiologic studies have, indeed, indicated that certain menstrual patterns such as early age of menarche, higher than average frequency of menses, and longer duration of flow are clearly associated with significantly increased risk for endometriosis.[22] Moreover, in teenaged females with severe endometriosis, defects in the outflow tract are very common. Hereditary factors confer a tendency for development of endometriosis, since a woman with a first-degree relative having the disease has a risk approximately seven times the normal risk of developing the disease.[107] The mechanisms by which genetic factors lead to this susceptibility have not been elucidated in detail, but recent studies have suggested that the immune system may be involved.

Pathogenesis

In the six decades since the term *endometriosis* was coined by Sampson,[104] a great deal of effort has gone to formulating hypotheses as to how this disease may develop. This is illustrated by the abundance of theories of histogenesis in the literature. However, less established are the theories, let alone evidence, for why endometriosis develops in some women and not in others.

Eleven major theories have been advanced to explain the mechanism(s) of how endometriosis develops, and these can be broadly divided into two categories: (1) those supporting transplantation or dissemination of shed endometrial cells or fragments and (2) those supporting the development of ectopic endometrium from other tissues by metaplasia.*

Six of the eleven theories of pathogenesis imply that endometrial tissue is derived from the endometrial cavity directly by extension; mechanically through the fallopian tubes, lymphatics, or vascular channels; or iatrogenically after surgery to the ectopic location. Many clinical situations support primarily one or more of these theories involving transplantation and so does the bulk of early experimental evidence. The pattern of endometriotic implants in the peritoneal cavity is consistent with the transplantation theory for the following reasons: The anatomic location is close to the entry of endometrial tissue into the pelvis and depends on gravity, since the uterine position influences the pattern of implants.[65] Furthermore, structures with inherent mobility, such as the tubes and bowel, are rarely sites of implantation. The most common site of endometriosis, the ovary, provides a fertile ground for implantation because of its active hormone production and frequent areas of surface breakdown at the sites of ovulation and rupture of functional cysts (Fig. 37-1). Thus the transplantation/implantation theory remains the most likely and widely supported concept.

The coelomic metaplasia theory is the earliest theory published to suggest that endometriosis may develop from the peritoneal lining by metaplastic transformation.[127] The concept is based on the common embryonic origin of müllerian ducts, surface epithelium and pelvic peritoneum from the epithelium of the coelomic wall. The basic tenet of this theory, that pelvic peritoneal cells have the potential to develop into active endometrium, has remained unsubstantiated by experimental or clinical evidence. The so-called induction theory[77] is an extension of this theory, suggesting that necrotic or denatured endometrium may contain substances that support or induce metaplastic change.

The metaplasia theory is attractive in that it would explain the occurrence of implants in any location of the body. However, the facts that men do not generally develop endometriosis and that endometriosis usually subsides after menopause are strong arguments against this concept, but they may just reflect the fact that the endometrium is a hormone-dependent tissue.

Whatever the tissue origin of ectopic implants in endometriosis, additional factors must play a role in determining who will develop the disease. In this regard attention has been focused on abnormal (retrograde) menstruation patterns, hormonal environment, and altered immune responses.

Numerous clinical reports have documented endometriosis in patients with reproductive outflow tract anomalies. Patients with müllerian anomalies have endometriosis generally if such anomalies include outflow obstruction.[91] In women with patent fallopian tubes, evidence for retrograde flow has been found in more than 90%.[50,78] However, since only 2% to 5% of healthy fertile women and some 25% to 35% of patients with longstanding infertility have endometriosis, it is reasonable to inquire as to whether the amount (or nature) of retrograde flow might differ from normal in those women. Epidemiologic evidence supports this concept indirectly. The risk of endometriosis is significantly increased with more frequent menses, longer duration, and heavy menstrual flow.[22] However, there is no clear evidence that women with endometriosis have more retrograde flow.[11] Uterine retrodisplacement does not appear to be important.[96,128] Neither is there any clear evidence that women with endometriosis have more retrograde flow.[11]

Even taking into account the role of retrograde flow and the need for estrogen in maintenance of endometriosis, the factors that determine who will develop the disease have remained elusive. It is clear that some other features of the host environment must contribute to the development of endometriosis either by influencing the probability of ectopic implantation or the sustained growth of such implants. Studies on steroid receptors of ectopic tissue have found significant variability, suggesting that the hormonal regulation of endometriotic tissue may be different at ectopic sites.* In addition to possible differences in the viability of the endometrial tissue itself, the hormonal and immunologic milieus may affect susceptibility to endometriosis.

There is no question that endometriotic implants are dependent on estrogen for their maintenance. Studies in experimental animals have indicated that estrogen and possibly also progestins have an impact on this mainte-

---

*References 24, 44, 61, 64, 77, 85, 92, 100, 105, 127.

*References 13, 43, 62, 68, 84, 89, 97, 126.

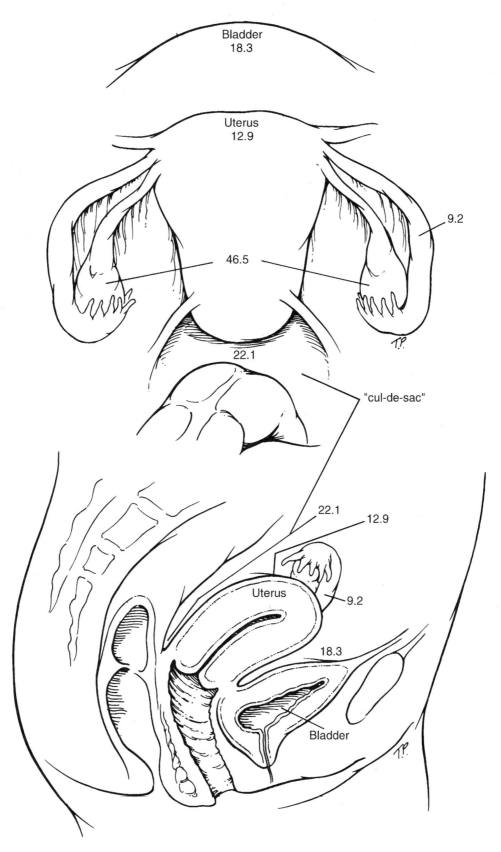

Fig. 37-1. The most common locations (percentages of cases) of pelvic endometriosis. (Modified from Scott RB et al: *Ann Surg* 131:706, 1950, and Jenkins S et al: *Obstet Gynecol* 67:336, 1986.)

nance.[29,106] The role of ovarian hormones in the etiology of endometriosis is less certain. The role of estrogenicity in development of endometriosis has recently won support from an epidemiologic study by Cramer et al.,[22] who found that smoking and heavy exercise, which are known to be inversely correlated with endogenous estrogen levels, significantly reduced the risk of endometriosis.

Changes in both cell-mediated and humoral immunity have been documented in women with endometriosis. Autoantibodies against endometrium and other reproductive tissues and phospholipids have been demonstrated in patients with endometriosis.[35,42,75,82] Furthermore, immunoglobulin G (IgG) and IgA deposits and complement component 3 have been detected in endometrium and endometriotic tissue, suggesting an immune activation.[4,60,129] Studies in monkeys and patients with severe endometriosis have revealed reduced reactivity to autologous endometrial antigens.[31,108]

The role of macrophages in the pathogenesis of endometriosis has been investigated extensively. These mononuclear phagocytes are essential in the host immune response. The macrophages digest and process peritoneal debris such as sperm and endometrial tissue and present antigens to the T cells. Several studies have indicated that endometriosis is associated with a significantly elevated number of macrophages in the peritoneal cavity.[45,48,52,114] In addition, the pelvic macrophage population has been shown to exhibit increased activational and maturational characteristics.[47,48,49] Endometriosis-associated peritoneal macrophages also have increased expression of human leukocyte antigen (HLA)-DR, competent cell-surface antigen modulation, and secretory activity, all of which may have important effects in the local peritoneal environment.[46] The competent antigen modulation as part of the antigen presentation may have relevance to the documented presence of autoantibodies in endometriosis. The activation of both the peripheral and the local monocyte/macrophage system via the secretion of cytokines or growth factors may facilitate the growth response of endometrial cells.[51,66] In summary, considerable information has accumulated to suggest that alterations in many facets of the hormonal and immune response are present in patients with endometriosis. Many of these alterations may be secondary features of the inflammatory process of endometriosis itself, but some may represent a more fundamental abnormality in these women.

ETIOLOGY AND PATHOGENESIS OF ASSOCIATED INFERTILITY

An association between endometriosis and infertility has been generally assumed, but most of the supporting evidence is indirect. The link appears stronger for advanced forms of endometriosis, whereas the association between minimal or mild stages of the disease and lower fecundity is much more tenuous.

Abnormalities in virtually every step in the female reproductive process have been suggested as the cause of infertility in endometriosis.[90,112] Marked anatomic alterations such as large endometriomas or tuboovarian adhesions in advanced disease clearly have the potential of distorting the delicate tuboovarian relationship and limiting fimbrial motility. Disturbances in the ovulatory process that have been suggested as possible mechanisms for infertility include occasional anovulation, abnormal prolactin secretion or follicular development, and luteal phase defects.[90,112] However, most recent studies have suggested that such abnormalities are present no more often in patients with endometriosis than in other infertile or fertile women. Although some earlier work had proposed a higher rate of clinical spontaneous abortion in endometriosis, studies with appropriate controls have not supported this mechanism.[93] However, since it has not been possible to investigate systematically the incidence of very early (e.g., preimplantation) pregnancy loss, this remains a possible mechanism. In fact, most of the proposed abnormalities dealing with altered immunity probably relate to this stage of development.

The role of endometriosis-associated inflammatory changes in the local peritoneal fluid environment has been receiving increasing attention.[115] Prostaglandins were initially proposed to be involved not only in pain symptoms but also in development of subfertility. The accumulated data on prostanoids in endometriosis remain hard to interpret, perhaps reflecting the short-lived nature of these compounds. Inflammatory cytokines, probably produced by activated macrophages such as interferon, interleukin-1, and tumor necrosis factor have also been implicated.[34,45,56,57] Whatever the mediating substance, the majority of studies that have tested the effects of endometriosis-associated peritoneal fluid on reproductive performance in vitro have noted impairment. Several reports (but not all) have demonstrated such effects on sperm motility and survival or sperm-oocyte interaction.[112] Peritoneal fluid has also been shown to affect adversely ovum pickup by the fimbria and to have toxic effects on early embryonic development in vitro.[56,111] It may be fair to say that the cause of infertility in patients with endometriosis appears to be multifactorial (Table 37-1).

DIAGNOSTIC APPROACH AND CLINICAL PRESENTATION

Presenting symptoms

Endometriosis should always be considered a possibility in patients with pelvic pain or infertility, particularly in the presence of a positive family history. The clinical diagnosis is based on characteristic symptoms and physical findings on pelvic examination. There is a great variability in the degree of symptoms in endometriosis. In patients presenting with infertility and found to have mild disease by laparoscopy, approximately 60% are asymptomatic. Pa-

Table 37-1. Support for the mechanisms of endometriosis-associated infertility

Mechanism	Stage of endometriosis	
	I–II	III–IV
Anatomic	−	++++
Ovulatory	+	++
Luteal	+	+
Ovum pickup	+	++
Gamete/embryo toxicity	++	++
Early pre- or postimplantation loss	+?	+?
Clinical pregnancy loss	±	−

tients with advanced endometriosis and large ovarian endometriomas may either be severely symptomatic or have no symptoms whatsoever. Because of this recognized variability it is essential that the diagnosis be verified by laparoscopy.

The most common symptoms of endometriosis are premenstrual pelvic pain and dysmenorrhea. Usually the pain has worsened progressively over the years. Some patients may always have had severe dysmenorrhea. The pain is usually lateral and deep in character, and often referred to the rectal area. In more advanced disease, the pain may be present throughout the month but intensifies during menses. Dyspareunia—pain during intercourse—is often associated with dysmenorrhea, seldom as an isolated symptom. Typically, pain is felt on deep penetration and can be somewhat alleviated by changing coital position. Uterine retroversion and tender uterosacral nodules are frequently observed in these patients.

Cyclic rectal pain and bowel urgency are common symptoms when endometriosis involves the bowel. Although the endometrial implants seldom penetrate to the mucosa, in situ bleeding in the muscularis or serosa results in such symptoms that sometimes include bloody stools at menses. With more advanced involvement of the bowel wall, peristaltic, crampy pain, typical of partial bowel obstruction, may be present.

Suprapubic pain that occurs during menstruation and is sometimes associated with dysuria and hematuria may be caused by the involvement of endometriosis with the bladder muscularis. Although endometriosis often involves the bladder serosa, this is seldom symptomatic. Deeper implants usually are associated with symptoms, and most commonly the dome of the bladder is involved.

Flank pain can be present in patients in whom endometriosis and associated scarring have led to ureteral obstruction and hydronephrosis. Febrile episodes and pyuria or hematuria can occur with intermittent ureteral obstruction.

Physical examination

There is no specific physical finding on pelvic examination that would allow a definitive diagnosis of endometriosis. However, bimanual palpation, including a bidigital rectovaginal examination, often gives valuable information on the extent of the disease.

More advanced disease may be manifested by pelvic induration with nodularity along the uterosacral ligaments or in the cul-de-sac, tender ovarian masses, or fixed retroversion of the uterus. The typical tender retrocervical nodules can be best felt with the rectal finger. Anterior palpation is sometimes helpful in identifying the involvement of bladder wall with endometriosis.

Tender adnexal masses commonly are found in patients with endometriosis. The mass almost always initially involves the ovary rather than the fallopian tube, although in more advanced disease adhesions may envelop both. Endometriotic cysts are bilateral in one third of cases. Fixed uterine retroversion is often present in advanced endometriosis, where posterior implants cause the obliteration of the cul-de-sac and adherence of the uterine fundus. However, a retroverted uterus is a common finding in healthy women and should not be a sole reason for suspecting endometriosis. Endometriotic nodules can sometimes be seen in the vagina, particularly in the posterior fornix, where they can be biopsied easily. This is the rare case in which a definitive, histologically verified diagnosis of pelvic endometriosis can be made without diagnostic laparoscopy. The diagnosis is of only limited value, however, since the extent of the disease still remains to be evaluated.

Diagnosis

Laparoscopy is the most important diagnostic method, but the search continues for identifying or developing a noninvasive means to diagnose endometriosis. A monoclonal antibody against an antigenic determinant in ovarian epithelium, called CA 125, has been used to develop an assay for this marker in serum. Serum CA 125 levels have been used as a tumor marker in the diagnosis and treatment of patients with ovarian epithelial carcinomas. However, numerous other physiologic and pathologic conditions (including menstruation, pregnancy, and pelvic inflammatory disease, and malignancies of the endometrium, breast, lung, and liver) are associated with elevated CA 125 levels. Levels of this marker have been shown to be elevated also in women with advanced stages of endometriosis.[10] Nevertheless, the low sensitivity and low specificity seen with CA 125 levels in the diagnosis of endometriosis limit its usefulness for diagnosis.[9] Other immunoassays attempting to detect the presence of antiendometrial antibodies in patients with endometriosis have so far not had enough sensitivity or accuracy to be useful as a diagnostic test. Imaging techniques that offer some potential for diagnosis of endometriosis include endovaginal ultrasound, computed tomography and magnetic resonance imaging.

Pelvic ultrasound, either transabdominal or endovaginal, is commonly used for evaluation of adnexal masses. Ultrasonographically, endometriomas often have a typical snowflake pattern or they may present a ground-glass appearance, but significant variability has been reported. The endometriosis-associated masses can be polycystic, mixed cystic and solid, or sonolucent or may exhibit complex patterns. Ultrasonography cannot reliably distinguish endometriosis from other ovarian cysts and tumors or tuboovarian abscesses. Endometriosis implants cannot be detected with this technique.

Computed tomography and magnetic resonance imaging have been so far found to be of little value and are seldom used in the diagnostic work-up of endometriosis.

Diagnostic laparoscopy

A definitive diagnosis of endometriosis can usually be made only by direct visualization of the pelvis. Diagnostic laparoscopy is the preferred procedure to confirm the diagnosis and to ascertain the extent of the disease. If the patient has a history of previous abdominal surgery, consideration should be given to performing a laparoscopy by an open technique in order to minimize the risk of perforating a hollow viscus. Laparotomy is indicated in the presence of a persistent large adnexal mass, bowel obstruction, or extensive abdominal wall adhesions, all of which render laparoscopy unsafe.

It is preferable to schedule the laparoscopy in the early follicular phase to minimize the chance that a hemorrhagic corpus luteum may be confused with an endometrioma. A thorough, systematic evaluation of the pelvis and upper abdomen is important. A second puncture instrument is usually needed for mobilization of pelvic organs to facilitate complete visualization. Adhesions may need to be lysed either with scissors or laser for the same purpose, particularly in patients who have had previous surgery. These adhesions are most commonly seen between the adnexa and the broad ligament or cul-de-sac and between the omentum and the abdominal wall.

Placing the patient in a 30-degree Trendelenburg position will help mobilization of bowel loops out of the pelvis and visualization of the cul-de-sac and its contents. Most patients with endometriosis have a tablespoonful or more of serosanguineous peritoneal fluid present at any time of the cycle, whereas this is seen in other patients usually during menses.[50] It is best to remove the fluid by aspiration in order to better see the deep cul-de-sac. By using a transcervical uterine manipulator such as the "Hulka tenaculum" (a combination of single-tooth tenaculum and uterine sound), the uterus is then tilted backward to allow inspection of the anterior cul-de-sac and bladder peritoneum. Next the uterus is tilted anteriorly and attention is focused on the adnexa. With the help of the second puncture instrument, either graspers or a probe, the tubes and ovaries are examined for evidence of endometriosis. The ovary is lifted and rolled over so that its lateral and inferior aspects can be seen. This is a common location of implants and occasionally "kissing lesions" are present on the ovary and the adjacent broad ligament. The posterior leaves of the broad ligament are carefully examined with particular attention to the ureters.

Uterosacral ligaments are then evaluated. A blunt probe is very helpful in assessment of the depth of lesions. Occasionally it is also useful to perform simultaneous digital rectovaginal palpation of the deeper lesions. The rectosigmoid colon and appendix are also inspected carefully. In cases of cul-de-sac obliteration a smooth, specially designed, rectal probe inside the bowel is very useful in establishing the extent of bowel involvement.

Findings should be recorded accurately by a careful description by dictation and sketching on appropriate forms to provide staging of the disease. Standardized criteria for this purpose have been published and should be followed. The American Fertility Society revised classification of endometriosis forms are available at cost from the American Fertility Society.* This form should be familiar to physicians treating patients with endometriosis. Classification is based on the presence and size of active implants and scarring in pelvic structures and divides the extent into stages I through IV. (See Fig. 38-1.) An optional videotape of the procedure is sometimes helpful but is time consuming to review. However, the development of routine editing of the tapes may make this kind of documentation more useful. Specially designed digital videoprinters recently have become available and have proved to be a very good method for documentation; the prints are easy to store in the patient's file and can be submitted to other physicians for review. In addition, this type of documentation of the extent of the disease has potential value in case of eventual litigation.

Endometriotic lesions

Macroscopic. Endometriotic implants in the ovary vary from small implants to large cysts. The cysts are usually dark brown to black, but sometimes thick-walled cysts are white or even yellow. When the cysts rupture, tarry chocolate-like material is released. In other areas of the pelvis cysts are rare. Endometriotic lesions have been found to be quite variable and to include both pigmented and nonpigmented types.[63,125] In patients with biopsy-proven endometriosis the most common lesions, in decreasing order, were found to be adhesions, scarred white lesions, peritoneal pockets, scarred black lesions, clear vesicles, polypoid red lesions, white vesicles, brown vesicles, flat or raised red lesions, fibrotic brown lesions, and black vesicles (Table 37-2).[81] In view of this wide array of lesions it is

---

*The American Fertility Society, 2140 Eleventh Avenue South, Suite 200, Birmingham, AL 35205-2800. Telephone (205)933-8494.

Table 37-2. The most common lesions observed in women with histologically confirmed endometriosis*

Type of lesion	Incidence (%)
Adhesions	91
Scarred white lesions	59
Peritoneal pockets	47
Scarred black lesions	46
Clear vesicles	30
Polypoid red lesions	26
White vesicles	25
Brown vesicles	24
Raised or flat red lesions	24
Fibrotic brown lesions	16
Black vesicles	7

*Based on data contained in Martin et al.[81]

possible to confuse them with nonendometriotic lesions such as hemangiomas, inflammatory cystic inclusions, residual ectopic trophoblastic tissue, or residual carbon from previous laser surgery.[81] Therefore, taking biopsy specimens of suspicious lesions is very important, especially if they have somewhat unusual characteristics. With experience and routinely performing careful biopsies one can increase the histologic confirmation of endometriosis in up to more than 90% of cases.[81] Reports exist of the presence of microscopic or nonvisible lesions in random biopsy specimens of the pelvic peritoneum in patients with and without endometriosis. The clinical significance of such lesions remains unknown.

Recent studies have indicated that the frequency of the typical pigmented lesions and endometriomas increases with age, whereas the subtle lesions are more commonly seen in younger women.[74,95] In addition, the deep infiltrating lesions are significantly more associated with pain than the superficial implants. Information from repeat laparoscopy studies suggests that, although there is a small but definite spontaneous regression rate of endometriotic implants, they generally have a significant tendency to progress and that treatment hinders progression in a majority of patients.[79,119,121]

Microscopic. The histology of ectopic endometriosis implants resembles that of eutopic endometrium but has certain specific features.[94] The implants, unlike endometrium, contain stromal hemorrhage and stromal fibrosis and may develop into cystic structures. Since the original description of endometriosis, the ectopic implants have been defined by the presence of endometrial glands and stroma, inflammatory cells (hemosiderin-laden macrophages), and scarring. The relative presence of each of these components varies with the type, age, biologic activity, and location of the lesion. Usually two of these components are required for making the histologic diagnosis. This requirement is too stringent to be the only basis for making a clinical diagnosis of endometriosis. As pointed out previously, adhesions were shown to be the most common macroscopic feature in patients with endometriosis. Since it is unlikely that old adhesions would always have others of these elements present, this may lead to underdiagnosing the disease.

Endometrial glands are more often irregular than in the normal endometrium. In early small lesions, the epithelial lining can be identified easily as endometrial, having columnar nonciliated epithelium without evidence of mucin production. Mitoses and pseudostratification can be seen in the late proliferative phase of the menstrual cycle. Secretion is sometimes evident with the presence of either subnuclear or supranuclear vacuoles or intraluminar secretion. There is considerable variability within the same implant and between different implants in the degree of recognizable secretory changes. In approximately one third of implants there is significant asynchrony as compared with eutopic endometrium.

During the menstrual phase the implants frequently exhibit glandular breakdown and stromal hemorrhage with the distinct presence of inflammatory cells emerging. The cystic structures enlarge and gradually will be enveloped by fibrotic connective tissue.

Hemorrhage in the interstitial space is a common feature of the implants. The blood accumulates when there is increased pressure and swelling within the cyst. Eventually the epithelium attenuates and disappears, and sometimes the cyst will rupture. Blood is gradually hemolyzed, and the degradation products form lipids and hemosiderin. Macrophages with lipid-containing foamy cytoplasm and yellowish hemosiderin are seen in these older lesions. The endometrial stroma is an important component of the ectopic implants. It consists of spindle-shaped cells with basophilic cytoplasm. The oval nuclei have finely granular chromatin and micronucleoli. Small arterioles are frequent. In older regressed implants the glandular elements may disappear completely, leaving only stroma. The stromal characteristics are quite typical, but they cannot be a basis of definite diagnosis since other spindle cells such as fibroblasts and ovarian stromal cells look similar. Scarring, accumulation of connective tissue, is the end result of repeated cyclic hemorrhagic changes in most endometriotic lesions.

In longstanding implants both collagen fibers and hemosiderin pigment are seen, but endometrial glands and stroma are sparse. It is important to look for them in many areas and several sections of the implant for confirmation of the diagnosis.

MEDICAL TREATMENT

The definitive diagnosis of endometriosis is made by either laparoscopy or laparotomy. Thus it seems logical to use a surgical approach as initial therapy for endometriosis and not use medical treatment in infertile patients, thereby causing a delay in attempts at pregnancy. However, in symptomatic patients after the diagnosis of the disease, medical management may be used postoperatively as an alternative to additional surgery or as a preoperative adjunct to surgical treatment. It is clearly indicated in the following:

- Suppression of active symptomatic disease
- Preoperative therapy in severe recurrent endometriosis to facilitate surgical excision (see Chapter 38)
- Postoperative therapy if excision is not complete or in the treatment of recurrent disease (see Chapter 38)
- Prevention of disease progression when conception must be delayed

Since the endometrium in ectopic implants should respond to steroid hormones in a fashion similar to that of the intrauterine endometrium, medical treatment of endometriosis has centered around the manipulation of steroid hormones. This accomplishes three goals: first, because of central suppression hormonal stimulation is removed from the existing implants; second, menstrual cyclicity is interrupted to prevent seeding of the disease during therapy; and third, the drugs may affect directly the growth and resolution of ectopic endometrium.

Medical therapy for endometriosis can be divided into four separate categories: (1) progestins and antiprogestins, (2) androgens/danazol, (3) synthetic gonadotropin-releasing hormone (GnRH) agonists, and (4) estrogen and progestin in combination. Each of these regimens is discussed with special attention to the mechanism of action, dosage and schedule, common side effects, and efficacy with regard to treatment of pelvic pain and infertility. Finally, comparison studies involving two or more medical treatment regimens are reviewed.

Progestins and antiprogestins

The use of progestational agents in the treatment of endometriosis is now entering its fourth decade.[72,73,122] The most widely studied progestational agents are norethindrone, levonorgestrel, and medroxyprogesterone acetate. Far fewer data and experience are available for some of the newer progestins and those not yet available in the United States, such as lynestrenol, gestrinone, desogestrel, and 3-ketodesogestrel. Norethindrone and levonorgestrel are 19-nortestosterone derivatives, and medroxyprogesterone acetate is a derivative of progesterone. Unlike the other compounds in this class, only gestrinone has antiprogestational effects, and it is discussed separately. It is theorized that each of the remaining agents affects ectopic endometrial tissue in a fashion similar to the way it affects the intrauterine endometrium. Therefore the ectopic implants would first decidualize, then slough, and eventually atrophy. These effects are mediated directly by cellular hormone receptors and are shown to include changes in estrogen metabolism in the endometrial tissue.[68] Levonorgestrel, gestrinone, desogestrel, and 3-ketodesogestrel were shown to inhibit 3β-hydroxysteroid dehydrogenase and 17,

20-lyase, and desogestrel was found to inhibit 17 α-hydroxylase in the rat ovary.[2] High doses of norethindrone and medroxyprogesterone acetate have been advocated. Doses of medroxyprogesterone acetate as high as 100 mg/d for 6 months have been used. In one prospective, double-blind, placebo-controlled study either total or partial resolution of peritoneal implants was observed in 63% of patients receiving medroxyprogesterone acetate 100 mg/d.[119] Only 18% of peritoneal lesions resolved in the group receiving placebo. Medroxyprogesterone acetate is more commonly given in a lower dosage (20 to 30 mg given orally in divided doses). It is also available in an injectable depot preparation. The dosage used for the depot preparation is 100 mg given intramuscularly each month. However, this regimen is less desirable because of its slower reversibility.

Although high-dose medroxyprogesterone acetate has proven efficacy in the reduction of peritoneal implants, its effects on the treatment of infertility associated with endometriosis are less clear. Hull et al.[58] found no significant differences in cumulative pregnancy rates as determined by life table analysis between 56 patients receiving no treatment and 36 patients receiving 30 mg of medroxyprogesterone acetate per day for 90 days. After 30 months of follow-up, 55% of controls conceived and 71% of patients receiving medroxyprogesterone acetate conceived.[58] Although this study focused on mild and minimal disease, it suggests that treatment with high-dose progesterone therapy may be inappropriate when treating infertility alone in patients with endometriosis.

Progestational agents, including norethindrone, medroxyprogesterone acetate, and lynestrenol, can produce numerous side effects. Breakthrough bleeding, fluid retention, and nausea are observed in as many as half of all patients. Also, depression may occur in as many as 10% of patients.[86,123] Fortunately, clinical trials report few dropouts related to intolerance of symptoms.

Unlike norethindrone, lynestrenol, and medroxyprogesterone acetate, gestrinone (ethylnorgestrien-one, R 2323) is a long-acting antiprogestational agent. Gestrinone has androgenic, antiprogestogenic, and antiestrogenic actions. It is commonly given at a dose of 2.5 mg twice weekly.[87] In a study of 50 patients with only 2 months of gestrinone therapy, a morphologic response was demonstrated in endometriosis implants. Included was a degree of cellular inactivation and degeneration of the endometriotic implants.[15,16] In a placebo-controlled study, Cooke and Thomas[20] demonstrated a significant improvement in endometriotic implants after treatment with 2.5 mg of gestrinone twice weekly.

Most studies evaluating pregnancy rates after the use of gestrinone have involved small numbers of patients. More importantly, few of these studies include a control group. Recently Fedele et al.[37] reported on 20 patients treated with gestrinone 2.5 mg twice weekly who had 18 months of follow-up after treatment. Their cumulative pregnancy rate was 33%.[37] Pregnancy rates as high as 59%[3] and 57%[21] have been reported. Since placebo controls were not used, the use of gestrinone for the treatment of infertility in patients with endometriosis is still in question. The data are more convincing for the use of gestrinone in the treatment of pelvic pain associated with endometriosis. Complete or partial relief of pelvic pain has been reported in 95%[21] to 97%[3] of patients. In the placebo-controlled study by Cooke and Thomas,[20] a significant improvement was documented in the volume of endometriosis implants when patients were treated with 2.5 mg of gestrinone twice weekly. The most common side effects experienced by patients taking gestrinone are seborrhea (71% to 81%), acne (65% to 79%), muscle cramps (35% to 45%), and breast hypotrophy (29% to 33%).[21]

Androgens/danazol

Danazol has been a commonly used treatment for endometriosis for the past 15 to 20 years.[7] It is an isoxazole derivative of 17α-ethinyl testosterone and could be best described as an attenuated androgen (Fig. 37-2). After absorption, danazol is metabolized into as many as 60 different compounds.[25] Two major metabolites of danazol, 17α-ethinyl testosterone and 2-hydroxymethyl ethisterone exhibit both progestational and androgenic activity. Thus the metabolic metabolites of danazol contribute to its efficacy and side effects. After an oral dose of 400 mg, peak blood levels of danazol are obtained in 2 hours and complete clearance by the liver occurs within 8 hours. The serum half-life of danazol is 4.5 hours. Barbieri et al.[8] have demonstrated danazol binding to androgen, estrogen, progesterone, and glucocorticoid receptors. They have also demonstrated the inhibition of numerous ovarian and adrenal enzymes by danazol,[9] and included are 21-hydroxylase, 11β-hydroxylase, 17β-hydroxysteroid dehydrogenase, 17α-hydroxylase, 17,20-lyase, and 3β-hydroxysteroid dehydrogenase isomerase. This complex pattern of enzyme inhibition serves to curtail estradiol synthesis.

Danazol or one of its metabolites, acting as a progesterone agonist, has been shown to suppress gonadotropin secretion in castrated animals.[28] In a prospective patient control study on eugonadal women with minimal en-

dometriosis, danazol administration resulted in an increase in the main luteinizing hormone (LH) pulse amplitude and a decrease in LH pulse frequency. The authors concluded that the changes in LH pulse amplitude represented a direct effect of danazol on the hypothalamic-pituitary axis.[80] Danazol has been shown to decrease follicle-stimulating hormone (FSH) and LH levels in postmenopausal women.[40] Although midcycle gonadotropin surges are eliminated by danazol, most clinical trials have shown no significant changes in basal serum gonadotropin levels. Danazol also displaces testosterone almost quantitatively from its binding globulin, and the endogenous androgen probably contributes to the effects of the drug. In a placebo-controlled, 6-month trial of danazol, with a dose of

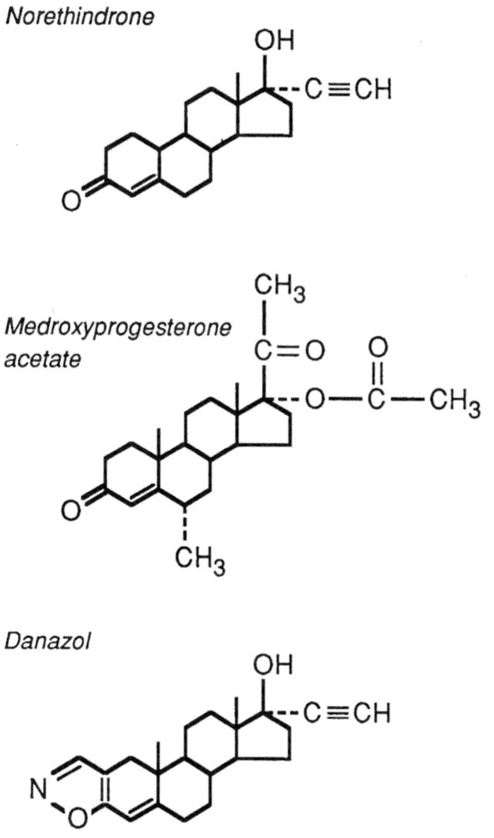

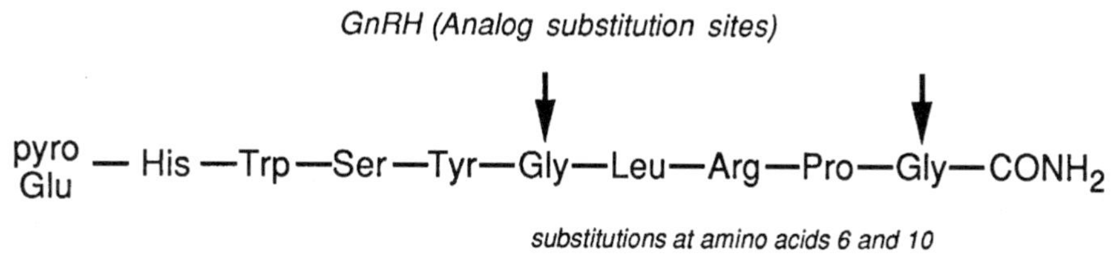

Norethindrone

Medroxyprogesterone acetate

Danazol

GnRH (Analog substitution sites)

substitutions at amino acids 6 and 10

Fig. 37-2. Medical treatment of endometriosis: molecular structures of basic compounds.

600 mg/d, Telimaa et al.[119] demonstrated a significant decrease in estrogen, progesterone, and sex hormone-binding globulin levels as compared with placebo. Therefore danazol induces a hypoestrogenic, hyperandrogenic state that suppresses ectopic endometrial growth. When patients given danazol for 6 months had endometrial biopsies, light, scanning, and transmission electron microscopy revealed progestational effects on the endometrial glands and stroma associated with a marked hypotrophy of the mucosa.[38] Danazol has also been shown to suppress growth of human endometrial cell cultures, suggesting a direct effect on endometrial tissue.[99]

The investigation of other tissue factors that may play a role in the proliferation of endometriotic implants has resulted in some interesting findings. Immunohistochemical staining for epidermal growth factor (EGF) receptors in endometriotic implants before and after treatment with danazol showed a decrease in the number of EGF receptors.[83] These data suggest that EGF may have a potential role in the maintenance of ectopic endometrial tissue. Danazol has also demonstrated an inhibition in the production of interleukin-1β and tumor necrosis factor production by stimulated monocytes in a dose-dependent fashion.[88] These findings suggest that danazol acts not only through inhibition of steroidogenesis but also by interfering with autocrine and paracrine functions.

Danazol is normally prescribed as 600 to 800 mg in divided doses per day; lower doses are not recommended because they may not suppress ovulation, and an accidental pregnancy while the patient is taking this potentially androgenizing drug is a risk. Vaginal or intrauterine administration has also been described.[59] The most common side effects are listed in Table 37-3. Unlike the side effects experienced with progestational agents, not all side effects of danazol are reversible after discontinuation of medication.[14] Although elevated liver enzymes have been reported in patients receiving danazol, the transaminases are most commonly affected and tend to normalize within 1 month of cessation of danazol therapy.[53] Many of the subjective side effects induced by danazol cause patient concerns, but it is not clear whether patient discontinuation of the drug occurs any more frequently than it does with progestins or GnRH agonists. Exercise has been shown to improve subjective acceptability of the drug.[19]

Over the past 5 years, numerous studies have been reported on the effects of cortical and trabecular bone mineral content after danazol therapy in patients with endometriosis.* Single- and dual-photon absorptiometry and quantitative computed tomography have been used to measure trabecular and/or cortical bone mineral content in the vertebral column, radius, and ulna. Baseline studies have revealed no differences between cortical and trabecu-

*References 27, 32, 110, 123, 130, 131.

Table 37-3. Medical treatment of endometriosis: common side effects

Medication and side effect	Patients affected (%)
Danazol	
Weight gain	85
Muscle cramps	52
Decreased breast size	48
Flushing	42
Oily skin	37
Acne	277
Hirsutism	21
Insomnia	10
Deepening of voice	7
GnRH analogues	
Hot flashes	80
Insomnia	75
Headache	52
Irregular vaginal bleeding	41
Decreased libido	38
Depression	38
Vaginal dryness	22
Arthralgias	14
Hair loss	8

lar bone mineral content in the lumbar spine between patients with endometriosis and age-matched controls.[27] Bone mineral content remained unchanged during and after 6 months of danazol therapy in all but one study. In that study a significant increase in bone mineral content of the spine was documented by single- and dual-photon absorptiometry.[130]

Because of the androgenic effects of danazol and many of its metabolites, one would expect an adverse effect on serum lipid profiles. Patients with endometriosis treated with danazol have consistently demonstrated such lipid profile effects.[17,23,55,120,124] Significant decreases in serum high-density lipoprotein (HDL), HDL₂, and apolipoprotein A-I levels have been demonstrated. In each of these studies, significant elevations in low-density lipoprotein (LDL) were found with no change in triglyceride levels. The significance of a 3- to 6-month adverse effect on the lipid profile is yet unknown in patients with familial hyperlipidemia, obesity, and/or hypertension; therefore it may be prudent to consider other treatments.

Danazol has proven efficacy in the treatment of peritoneal lesions. In two placebo-controlled trials, total or partial resolution of peritoneal implants was observed in 60% to 80% of patients.[55,119] Despite its desirable effects on peritoneal implants, danazol appears to have no effect on the regression of adhesions.[71] In patients with ovarian endometriomas, danazol is also less effective. Especially when cysts are greater than 3 cm in diameter, surgical therapy may be necessary.[103] Despite its lack of effect in decreasing existing pelvic adhesions, danazol is effective in the relief of pelvic pain associated with endometriosis. Danazol is effective in the treatment of dysmenorrhea, intermenstrual pelvic pain, and dyspareunia. Dysmenorrhea resolved in 100% of patients treated with danazol in one trial, only to recur in 92% of patients after 1 year.[36] Deep dyspareunia was minimally affected by treatment with danazol and had recurred in all patients 6 months after discontinuation of therapy. This high rate of recurrence is not unanticipated, since danazol is not a "cure" for endometriotic implants and has no effect on adhesions.

Endometriosis patients presenting with infertility as their only complaint do not appear to be good candidates for danazol therapy. In three placebo-controlled clinical trials, danazol treatment did not result in higher pregnancy rates when compared with placebo therapy. This was true not only for minimal and mild disease but also for moderate disease.[5,12,58] Not only is danazol ineffective in the treatment of infertility associated with endometriosis, but it has also been shown to delay pregnancy. Danazol has been demonstrated to delay pregnancy in treatment groups for 7 to 8 months over patients in the placebo group.[67,118]

Gonadotropin-releasing hormone agonists

Besides danazol, the only other medications that have received Food and Drug Administration approval for the treatment of endometriosis are some of the GnRH agonists. These compounds were first synthesized in the early 1970s, when it was discovered that substitutions in the amino acid sequence of GnRH led to changes in potency. Within the 10–amino acid sequence of GnRH, three peptidase cleavage sites are contained. These are found on either side of amino acid 6 and in between amino acids 9 and 10. Substitutions in the 6 and 10 position were found to increase not only the biologic half-life of GnRH but also its potency. The GnRH agonists' half-lives range from 80 to 480 minutes. Administration of these compounds can be accomplished by intranasal spray, subcutaneous injection, or intramuscular injection. GnRH analogues are also available in depot form.[33,109] After administration of a GnRH analogue, an agonistic phase with increased production of FSH, LH, and gonadal steroids is followed by desensitization and down-regulation of GnRH receptors with subsequent suppression of FSH, LH, and gonadol steroid synthesis and release. A hypogonadal, hypoestrogenic state is obtained. A variety of GnRH agonists with their amino acid substitutions and in vitro potencies are listed in Table 37-4.

The effects of GnRH analogues on endometriosis implants have been studied in experimental models and in clinical trials, especially in comparison with danazol. In an experimental model in which endometriosis was artificially induced in female rats, the GnRH agonist-treated group demonstrated significant reduction of endometriosis implants both grossly and histologically.[102] In clinical trials in which second-look laparoscopies were performed after GnRH agonist therapy, GnRH agonists were shown to be as

Table 37-4. Substitutions and relative potencies of some GnRH agonists

GnRH	Substitution	In vitro potency*	Half-life
Buserelin	D-Ser(tBu)^6 Pro^9	50	80 min
Decapeptyl	D-Trp^6	36	—
Goserelin	D-Ser(tBU), (Aza-Gly-NH$_2$)^{10}	75	6 h
Histrelin	imbzl-D-His^6-Pro^9	100	—
Leuprolide	D-Leu^6-Pro^9	15	3 h
Nafarelin	D-Nal(2)^6	100	4.3 h

*Relative to native GnRH (=1).
Modified from Barbieri RL, Friedman AI, editors: *Gonadotropin releasing hormone analogs: applications in gynecology.* New York, 1991, Elsevier Science Publishing.

effective as danazol in reduction of endometriotic implants.[38,55,71,98,123] Placebo-controlled studies, although few in number, suggest that GnRH agonists have similar effectiveness in reducing pelvic pain secondary to endometriosis as compared with danazol.[55,98] Surprisingly, there are no placebo-controlled studies that prove the effectiveness of GnRH agonists in the treatment of infertility. Comparisons of pregnancy rates between danazol and GnRH analogue treatment groups have shown no significant differences, yet the efficacy of either in the treatment of infertility associated with endometriosis is still in question.

Side effects of GnRH agonists are common. Because of the decrease in estrogen to menopausal levels, hot flashes occur in 80% to 100% of patients after the first 2 weeks of treatment. Occasionally, the lack of quality sleep due to the hot flashes can cause fatigue or difficulty with concentration or demanding mental tasks. It has been reported that adding progestin (e.g., 2.5 mg of oral norethindrone acetate) to the treatment regimen ameliorates these symptoms and maintains treatment efficacy.[112] Irregular vaginal bleeding or spotting occurs in 20% to 40% of patients.

Because of the hypogonadal state induced by GnRH agonists, one would expect possible changes in lipid profiles and/or bone density. Clinical trials measuring lipid profiles are commonly performed in comparison to danazol. Unlike danazol, the GnRH agonists produce little or no lipid effects. After 6 months of intranasal nafarelin acetate at a dose of 400 or 800 µg/d, HDL-cholesterol levels were shown to either increase by 10% to 20% or remain unchanged. LDL-cholesterol levels showed no significant changes.[17,23,54,124] However, an increase in total plasma cholesterol was demonstrated after 6 months of therapy in 12 patients receiving buserelin.[30] Still the bulk of evidence fails to demonstrate any significant adverse effects, although large, randomized, placebo-controlled studies with long-term follow-up are still needed.

Probably the most important untoward effect seen in

patients taking GnRH agonists is a change in bone mineral density. Because estradiol levels may be suppressed to the menopausal range, one would expect at least a minimal effect. Ylikorkala et al.[131] demonstrated a 50% rise in 24-hour urinary hydroxyproline output after 6 months of GnRH therapy. They also noted increases in serum osteocalcin and bone alkaline phosphatase activity by 80% to 120% and 34% to 40%, respectively. From these data they postulated that bone turnover is increased in patients taking GnRH analogues. Several studies using single- and dual-energy quantitative computed tomography have been used to measure spinal trabecular bone mineral content in endometriosis patients receiving GnRH analogues. Significant decreases in spinal trabecular bone mineral content have been documented after 6 months of therapy and range from 5.9% to 8.2%.[27,32,130] Both Dodin et al.[32] and Dawood et al.[27] have shown persistent, significant decreases in bone mineral content 6 months after stopping therapy. Conversely, in patients receiving supplemental oral calcium 1 g/d, there were no significant decreases in lumbar bone mineral density as evaluated by dual-photon absorptiometry.[123] In patients with normal bone mineral density the clinical significance of a temporary (and most likely reversible) bone loss is unknown. It has been recommended that before a 6-month course of agonist, especially in patients at risk for osteoporosis, the trabecular bone mineral density should be evaluated and GnRH agonist should be withheld in those with low values. In patients with normal bone mineral density, supplemental oral calcium (1 g/d) is also recommended during treatment. The addition of estrogen in an "add-back" fashion to a program of long-term GnRH analogue treatment appears to prevent loss of bone density while maintaining the ability of the analogue to treat effectively benign gynecologic conditions.[41,76] Although theoretically attractive, the concept of adding estrogen to medical suppression of endometriosis has not been clinically tested, and the maintenance of treatment efficacy remains a concern. However, adding norethindrone acetate to agonist therapy appears to offer the opportunity to reduce hot flashes and bone loss without limiting efficacy.[113]

Combination therapy

After successful treatment of pelvic pain associated with endometriosis with 3 to 6 months of medical therapy and in a patient who does not desire subsequent pregnancy, cyclic oral contraceptive treatment may be beneficial. A retrospective study suggested that patients treated with oral contraceptives had milder forms of endometriosis.[8] Continuous oral contraceptives containing both estrogen and progesterone, the so-named pseudopregnancy regimen, have been in use for more than 30 years.[73] This regimen induces a thin, pseudodecidualized endometrium, and this is its proposed mechanism of action on ectopic endometrial implants. In a study of 11 patients receiving 27 mg of cyproterone acetate

and 0.035 mg of ethinyl estradiol per day for 6 months,[36] follow-up laparoscopy showed partial regression of endometriotic lesions in all patients.

The use of danazol and a GnRH agonist in combination has been studied in endometriotic implants induced experimentally in female rats.[101] Histologic evaluation revealed a significantly greater increase in the atrophy of endometrial explants when danazol and leuprolide were used in combination, compared with either danazol or leuprolide alone. This regimen may be of some value to some severely symptomatic patients, but no clinical experience with it has been reported.

Monitoring treatment

Although the definitive diagnosis of endometriosis can be made only by laparoscopy, both serum CA 125 and antiendometrial antibody levels have been proposed as markers for the disease. Significant elevations of serum CA 125 levels have been demonstrated in patients with stage III and stage IV disease[10,26,69]; significant elevations have also been demonstrated in patients with minimal and mild endometriosis.[1] Most[6,26,116,117] but not all[39,69] studies have documented a correlation between CA 125 levels and the severity of the disease. The lack of postoperative suppression of serum CA 125 levels and persistent disease seem to be correlated, as do later elevations of CA 125 levels and disease recurrence. It is recommended that the baseline serum CA 125 level measured be upon initial diagnosis of endometriosis; if the level is elevated it can provide a guide for further management. In patients with improvement in endometriosis-associated symptoms and a decrease in serum CA 125 levels, rising levels with return of symptoms suggests recurrence of endometriosis. Another potential serum marker that may prove beneficial in the follow-up and treatment of patients with endometriosis is the level of antiendometrial autoantibodies. Kennedy et al.[70] studied 35 women with laparoscopy-proven endometriosis who were treated with either danazol or nafarelin; blood samples were drawn before and after treatment for measurement of antiendometrial antibody levels. Antiendometrial antibody levels were significantly elevated before treatment, compared with those of a control group. Significant suppression of antiendometrial autoantibodies was found in the group treated with GnRH agonist only.

The effects of danazol and GnRH agonist treatment on the production of autoantibodies was evaluated in a longitudinal, prospective, randomized study.[35] In that study only 50% of patients had significant elevations of their autoantibody levels before treatment. Significant reductions in autoantibodies (IgG, IgM, and IgA) were found only in the danazol-treated group. Again, further studies are necessary to assess accurately the role of antiendometrial and autoantibodies in the follow-up and treatment of patients with endometriosis.

INTERPRETATION OF TREATMENT RESULTS

Medical therapy has proven efficacy only in the treatment of pain associated with endometriosis. Medical therapy for endometriosis in the presence of infertility remains controversial because the exact nature of this association is unknown. In fact there is no conclusive evidence demonstrating an improvement in infertility associated with endometriosis with medical therapy. This is not surprising in view of the fact that the mechanisms involved in reproductive failure have not yet been elucidated to the extent that specific therapies would be available. Medical suppression of ovulation, menstruation, and ectopic implants, although effective in reducing symptoms, may not be specific enough to restore normal fecundity in most patients. Both danazol and the GnRH agonists are equally effective in the treatment of pain associated with endometriosis. Treatment with GnRH agonists has been reported to be associated with a different spectrum of side effects than that seen with treatment with danazol; however, in patients who are unable to tolerate therapy with GnRH agonists, it has been our experience that danazol often can be substituted with success. When treating patients with infertility associated with endometriosis, surgical therapy, usually at the time of initial diagnosis, seems most appropriate. (See Chapter 38.) Surgical therapy will not delay the couple's attempt at pregnancy as does medical therapy. In these patients, postoperative medical treatment should be reserved for patients with more extensive disease.

CONCLUSION

Endometriosis remains a challenging disease that prompts more questions about its etiology and biology the more that is learned about it. The recent recognition of the existence of the wide spectrum of peritoneal lesions and the possible variation in their biologic activity is very important but puzzling. The deep infiltrating lesions appear to be more associated with pain and the superficial peritoneal implants more with an inflammatory pelvic environment and subfertility. However, treatment of such lesions in patients with mild forms of the disease by any currently available method does not appear to improve pregnancy rates despite the documented decreases in implants and improvement in pain. Progress has been made in providing new treatment options for a great number of patients with symptomatic endometriosis. These new "tools" are helpful, albeit no one perfect treatment option has yet been developed. Pelvic pain tends to recur as early as 6 months after discontinuation of therapy.

Every physician who has had the opportunity to follow patients with endometriosis in the long term recognizes the chronic and progressive (fortunately slow in most cases) nature of the disease. This is still one of the biggest challenges in the modern management of endometriosis, since changing demographics and career opportunities have placed an ever-increasing emphasis on conservative approaches, trying to control the disease while preserving the best chances for immediate or future fertility. Even for the patient with debilitating pain we may need to find a way to provide chances for having a child. It is important to realize that a patient with endometriosis often will need several different treatment modalities, both surgical and medical, over the life span of the disease. Whenever feasible the modern long-term management should include an attempt to thwart progression of endometriosis by using low-dose progestin-dominant (monophasic) oral contraceptives if pregnancy is to be postponed or prevented.

Management of endometriosis should always be based on the individual needs of the patient and the recognition that no perfect cure yet exists. Selection of treatment and the long-term plan depend on the severity of symptoms, the extent of disease, the patient's age, and her reproductive desires.

REFERENCES

1. Acien P et al: CA-125 levels in endometriosis patients before, during, and after treatment with danazol or LH-RH agonists, *Eur J Obstet Gynecol Reprod Biol* 32:241, 1989.
2. Arakaw S et al: Inhibition of rat ovarian 3-β-hydroxysteroid dehydrogenase (3-β-HSD), 17-α-hydroxylase and 17, 20 -lyase by progestins and danazol. *Endocrinol Jpn* 36:87, 1989.
3. Azadian-Boulanger G et al: Hormonal activity profiles of drugs for endometriosis therapy. In Raynound J-P, Ojasso T, Mastini L, editors: *Medical management of endometriosis,* New York, 1984, Raven Press.
4. Badawy SZA et al: Autoimmune phenomena in infertile women with endometriosis, *Obstet Gynecol* 63:271, 1984.
5. Badawy SZ et al: Cumulative pregnancy rates in infertile women with endometriosis, *J Reprod Med* 33:757, 1988.
6. Barbieri RL: CA-125 in patients with endometriosis, *Fertil Steril* 45:767, 1986.
7. Barbieri RL, Evans S, Kistner RW: Danazol in the treatment of endometriosis: analysis of 100 cases with a 4-year follow-up, *Fertil Steril* 37:737, 1982.
8. Barbieri RL, Lee H, Ryan KJ: Danazol binding to rat androgen, glucocorticoid, progesterone and estrogen receptors: correlation with biologic activity, *Fertil Steril* 31:181, 1979.
9. Barbieri RL et al: Danazol inhibits human adrenal 21- and 11-beta-hydroxylation in vitro, *Steroids* 35:251, 1980.
10. Barbieri RL et al: Elevated serum concentrations of CA-125 in patients with advanced endometriosis, *Fertil Steril* 45:63, 1986.
11. Bartosik D, Jacobs S, Kelly LJ: Endometrial tissue in peritoneal fluid, *Fertil Steril* 46:796, 1986.
12. Bayer SR et al: The efficacy of danazol treatment for minimal endometriosis in an infertile population: a prospective randomized study, *J Reprod Med* 33:179, 1988.
13. Bergqvist A et al: Histochemical demonstration of estrogen and progesterone binding in endometriotic tissue and in uterine endometrium: a comparative study, *J Histochem Cytochem* 33:155, 1985.
14. Boothroyd CV, Lepre F: Permanent voice change resulting from danazol therapy, *Aust N Z J Obstet Gynaecol* 30:275, 1990.
15. Brosens IA: The rationale for endocrine therapy, *Acta Obstet Gynecol Scand Suppl* 150:21, 1989.
16. Brosens IA, Verleyen A, Cornillie F: The morphologic effects of short-term medical therapy of endometriosis, *Am J Obstet Gynecol* 157:1215, 1987.

17. Burry KA, Patton PE, Illingworth DR: Metabolic changes during medical treatment of endometriosis: nafarelin acetate versus danazol, *Am J Obstet Gynecol* 160:1454, 1989.

18. Buttram VC Jr: Cyclic use of combination oral contraceptives and the severity of endometriosis, *Fertil Steril* 31:347, 1979.

19. Carpenter SE, Markhan SM, Rock JA: Exercise may reduce side effects of danazol, *Infertility* 2:259, 1988.

20. Cooke ID, Thomas EJ: The medical treatment of mild endometriosis, *Acta Obstet Gynecol Scand Suppl* 150:227, 1989.

21. Coutinho EM, Husson JM, Azadian-Boulanger G: Treatment of endometriosis with gestrinone: 5 years experience. In Raynound J-P, Ojasso T, Mastini L, editors: *Medical management of endometriosis,* New York, 1984, Raven Press.

22. Cramer DW et al: The relation of endometriosis to menstrual characteristics, smoking and exercise, *JAMA* 255:1904, 1986.

23. Crook D et al: Zoladex versus danazol in the treatment of pelvic endometriosis: effects on plasma lipid risk factors, *Horm Res Suppl* 1:157, 1989.

24. Cullen TS: Adenomyoma of the round ligament, *Bull Johns Hopkins Hosp* 7:112, 1886.

25. Davison C, Banks W, Fritz A: The absorption, distribution, and metabolic rate of danazol in rats, monkeys, and human volunteers, *Arch Int Pharmacodyn Ther* 221:294, 1976.

26. Dawood MY, Khan-Dawood FS, Ramos J: Plasma and peritoneal fluid levels of CA-125 in women with endometriosis, *Am J Obstet Gynecol* 159:1526, 1988.

27. Dawood NY, Lewis V, Ramos J: Cortical and trabecular bone mineral content in women with endometriosis: effect of gonadotropin-releasing hormone agonist and danazol, *Fertil Steril* 52:21, 1989.

28. Desaulles PA, Krahenbuhl C: Comparison of the anti-fertility and sex hormone activities of sex hormones and derivatives, *Acta Endocrinol* 47:444, 1964.

29. DiZerega GS, Barber DL, Hodgen GD: Endometriosis: role of ovarian steroids in initiation, maintenance, and suppression, *Fertil Steril* 33:649, 1980.

30. Dlugi AM et al: A comparison of the effects of buserelin versus danazol on plasma lipoproteins during treatment of pelvic endometriosis, *Fertil Steril* 49:913, 1988.

31. Dmowski WP, Steele RW, Baker GF: Deficient cellular immunity in endometriosis, *Am J Obstet Gynecol* 141:377, 1981.

32. Dodin S et al: Bone mass in endometriosis patients treated with GnRH agonists implant or danazol, *Obstet Gynecol* 77:410, 1991.

33. Donnez J et al: Administration of nasal buserelin as compared with subcutaneous buserelin implant for endometriosis, *Fertil Steril* 52:27, 1989.

34. Eisermann J et al: Tumor necrosis factor in peritoneal fluid of women undergoing laparoscopic surgery, *Fertil Steril* 50:573, 1988.

35. El-Roeiy A et al: Danazol but not gonadotropin-releasing hormone agonists suppresses autoantibodies in endometriosis, *Fertil Steril* 50:864, 1988.

36. Fedele L et al: Comparison of cyproterone acetate and danazol in the treatment of pelvic pain associated with endometriosis, *Obstet Gynecol* 73:1000, 1989.

37. Fedele L et al: Gestrinone versus danazol in the treatment of endometriosis, *Fertil Steril* 51:781, 1989.

38. Fedele L et al: Endometrial patterns during danazol and buserelin therapy for endometriosis: comparative structural and ultrastructural study, *Obstet Gynecol* 76:79, 1990.

39. Fraser IS, McCarron G, Markham R: Serum Ca-125 levels in women with endometriosis, *Aust N Z J Obstet Gynaecol* 29:416, 1989.

40. Fraser IS, Thorburn GD: Effects of danazol on pituitary gonadotropins in postmenopausal women, *Aust N Z J Obstet Gynaecol* 18:247, 1978.

41. Friedman AJ: Treatment of leiomyomata uteri with short-term leu-prolide followed by leuprolide plus estrogen-progestin hormone replacement therapy for 2 years: a pilot study, *Fertil Steril* 51:526, 1989.

42. Gleicher N et al: Is endometriosis an autoimmune disease?, *Obstet Gynecol* 70:115, 1987.

43. Gould SF, Shannon JM, Cunha GR: Nuclear estrogen binding sites in human endometriosis, *Fertil Steril* 39:520, 1983.

44. Halban H: Hysteroadenosis metastatica: Die lymphogene Genese der sogenannte Adenofibromatosis heterotopica, *Arch Gynaekol* 124:457, 1925.

45. Halme J: Release of tumor necrosis factor by human peritoneal macrophages in vivo and in vitro, *Am J Obstet Gynecol* 161:1718, 1989.

46. Halme J, Becker S, Haskill S: Altered maturation and function of peritoneal macrophages: possible role in pathogenesis of endometriosis, *Am J Obstet Gynecol* 156:783, 1987.

47. Halme J, Becker S, Wing R: Accentuated cyclic activation of peritoneal macrophages in patients with endometriosis, *Am J Obstet Gynecol* 148:85, 1984.

48. Halme J et al: Pelvic macrophages in normal and infertile women: the role of patent tubes, *Am J Obstet Gynecol* 142:890, 1982.

49. Halme J et al: Increased activation of pelvic macrophages in infertile women with mild endometriosis, *Am J Obstet Gynecol* 145:333, 1983.

50. Halme J et al: Retrograde menstruation in healthy women and in patients with endometriosis, *Obstet Gynecol* 64:151, 1984.

51. Halme J et al: Peritoneal macrophages from patients with endometriosis release growth factor activity in vitro, *J Clin Endocrinol Metab* 66:1044, 1988.

52. Haney AF, Muscato JJ, Weinberg JB: Peritoneal fluid cell populations in infertility patients, *Fertil Steril* 35:696, 1981.

53. Heikkinen J et al: Serum bile acid concentrations as an indicator of liver dysfunction induced during danazol therapy, *Fertil Steril* 50:761, 1988.

54. Henzl MR, Kwei L: Efficacy and safety of nafarelin in the treatment of endometriosis, *Am J Obstet Gynecol* 162:570, 1990.

55. Henzl MR et al: Administration of nasal nafarelin as compared with oral danazol for endometriosis: a multicenter, double-blind, comparative clinical trial, *N Engl J Med* 318:485, 1988.

56. Hill JA, Haimovici F, Anderson DJ: Products of activated lymphocytes and macrophages inhibit mouse embryo development in vitro, *J Immunol* 139:2250, 1987.

57. Hu SK, Mitcho YL, Rath NC: Effect of estradiol on interleukin 1 synthesis by macrophages, *Int J Immunopharmacol* 10:247, 1988.

58. Hull ME et al: Comparison of different treatment modalities of endometriosis in infertile women, *Fertil Steril* 47:40, 1987.

59. Igarashi N: A new therapy for pelvic endometriosis and uterine adenomyosis: local effect of vaginal and intrauterine danazol application, *Asia Oceania J Obstet Gynaecol* 16:1, 1980.

60. Isaacson KB et al: Production and secretion of complement component 3 by endometriotic tissue, *J Clin Endocrinol Metab* 69:1003, 1989.

61. Iwanoff NS: Drusiges cysthaltiges Uterusfibromyom compliciert durch Sarcom und Carcinom (adenofibromyoma cysticum sarcomatodes carcinomatosum), *Monatsschr Geburtshilfe Gynaekol* 7:295, 1898.

62. Janne O et al: Estrogen and progestin receptors in endometriosis lesions: comparison with endometrial tissue, *Am J Obstet Gynecol* 141:562, 1981.

63. Jansen RPS, Russell P: Nonpigmented endometriosis: clinical, laparoscopic, and pathologic definition, *Am J Obstet Gynecol* 155:1154, 1986.

64. Javert CT: Pathogenesis of endometriosis based on endometrial homeoplasia, direct extension, exfoliation and implantation, lymphatic and hematogenous metastasis: including five case reports of endometrial tissue in pelvic lymph nodes, *Cancer* 2:399, 1949.

65. Jenkins S, Olive DL, Haney AF: Endometriosis: pathogenetic implications of the anatomic distribution, *Obstet Gynecol* 67:335, 1986.

66. Kauma S et al: Production of fibronectin by peritoneal macrophages and concentrations of fibronectin in peritoneal fluid from patients with and without endometriosis, *Obstet Gynecol* 72:13, 1988.

67. Kauppila AJ, Telimaa S, Ronnberg L: Steroidal drugs and endometriosis, *Acta Obstet Gynecol Scand Suppl* 150:7, 1989.

68. Kauppila A et al: Cytosol estrogen and progestin receptor concentrations and 17beta-hydroxysteroid dehydrogenase activities in the endometrium and endometriotic tissue: effects of hormonal treatment, *Acta Obstet Gynecol Scand Suppl* 123:45, 1984.

69. Kauppila A et al: Placebo-controlled study on serum concentrations of CA-125 before and after treatment of endometriosis with danazol or high dose medroxyprogesterone acetate alone or after surgery, *Fertil Steril* 491:37, 1990.

70. Kennedy SH et al: Antiendometrial antibodies in endometriosis measured by an enzyme-linked immunosorbent assay before and after treatment with danazol and nafarelin, *Obstet Gynecol* 75:914, 1990.

71. Kennedy SH et al: A comparison of nafarelin acetate and danazol in the treatment of endometriosis, *Fertil Steril* 53:998, 1990.

72. Kistner RW: The use of newer progestins in the treatment of endometriosis, *Am J Obstet Gynecol* 75:264, 1958.

73. Kistner RW: The treatment of endometriosis by inducing pseudopregnancy with ovarian hormones: a report of 58 cases, *Fertil Steril* 10:539, 1959.

74. Koninckx PR et al: Suggestive evidence that pelvic endometriosis is a progressive disease, whereas deeply infiltrating endometriosis is associated with pelvic pain, *Fertil Steril* 55:759, 1991.

75. Kreiner D et al: Endometrial immunofluorescence associated with endometriosis and pelvic inflammatory disease, *Fertil Steril* 46:243, 1986.

76. Leather AT et al: The prevention of bone loss in young women treated with GnRH analogues with "add-back" estrogen therapy, *Obstet Gynecol* 81:104, 1993.

77. Levander G, Normann P: The pathogenesis of endometriosis: an experimental study, *Acta Obstet Gynecol Scand* 34: 366, 1955.

78. Liu DTY, Hitchcock A: Endometriosis: its association with retrograde menstruation, dysmenorrhoea and tubal pathology, *Br J Obstet Gynaecol* 93:859, 1986.

79. Mahmood TA, Templeton A: The impact of treatment on the natural history of endometriosis, *Hum Reprod* 5:965, 1990.

80. Maouris P et al: The effect of danazol on pulsatile gonadotropin secretion in women with endometriosis, *Fertil Steril* 55:890, 1991.

81. Martin DC et al: Laparoscopic appearances of peritoneal endometriosis, *Fertil Steril* 51:63, 1989.

82. Mathur S et al: Autoimmunity to endometrium and ovary in endometriosis, *Clin Exp Immunol* 50:259, 1982.

83. Melega C et al: Tissue factors influencing growth and maintenance of endometriosis, *Ann N Y Acad Sci* 622:256, 1991.

84. Metzger DA, Haney AF: Etiology of endometriosis. In Rock JA, editor: Endometriosis, *Obstet Gynecol Clin North Am* 16(1): 1, 1989.

85. Meyer R: Uber den Stand der Frage der Adenomyositis und Adenomyome im Allgemeinen un ins Besondere uber Adenomyositis seroepithelialis und Adenomyometritis sarcomatosa, *Zentralbl Gynaekol* 36:745, 1919.

86. Moghissi KS, Boyce CRK: Management of endometriosis with oral medroxyprogesterone acetate, *Obstet Gynecol* 47:265, 1976.

87. Moguilewsky N, Philibert D: Dynamics of receptor interactions of danazol and gestrinone in the rat: correlations with biological activities. In Raynound J-P, Ojasso T, Mastini L, editors: *Medical management of endometriosis,* New York, 1984, Raven Press.

88. Mori H et al: Danazol suppresses the production of interleukin-1 beta and tumor necrosis factor by human monocytes, *Am J Reprod Immunol* 24:45, 1990.

89. Novak E, deLima OA: A correlative study of adenomyosis and pelvic endometriosis, with special reference to the hormonal reaction of ectopic endometrium. *Am J Obstet Gynecol* 56:634, 1948.

90. Olive DL, Hammond CB: Endometriosis: pathogenesis and mechanisms of infertility, *Postgrad Obstet Gynecol* 5:1, 1985.

91. Olive DL, Henderson DY: Endometriosis and müllerian anomalies, *Obstet Gynecol* 69:412, 1987.

92. Pick L: Ueber Neubildungen am Genitale, *Arch Gynaekol* 76:251, 1905.

93. Pittaway DE, Ellington CP, Klimek M: Preclinical abortions and endometriosis, *Fertil Steril* 49:221, 1988.

94. Ramzy I: Pathology. In Schenken RS, editor: *Endometriosis: contemporary concepts in clinical management,* Philadelphia, 1989, JB Lippincott.

95. Redwine DB: The distribution of endometriosis in the pelvis by age groups and fertility, *Fertil Steril* 47:173, 1987.

96. Reti LL, Bryne GA, Davoren RAN: The acute features of retrograde menstruation, *Aust N Z J Obstet Gynaecol* 23:51, 1983.

97. Roddick JW, Conkey G, Jacobs EJ: The hormonal response of endometrium in endometriotic implants and its relationship to symptomatology, *Am J Obstet Gynecol* 79:1173, 1960.

98. Rolland R, van-der-Heijden PF: Nafarelin versus danazol in the treatment of endometriosis, *Am J Obstet Gynecol* 162:586, 1990.

99. Rose GL et al: The inhibitory effects of danazol, danazol metabolites, gestrinone, and testosterone on the growth of human endometrial cells in culture, *Fertil Steril* 49:224, 1988.

100. Russell WW: Aberrant portions of the müllerian duct found in an ovary: ovarian cysts of müllerian origin, *Bull Johns Hopkins Hosp* 10:8, 1899.

101. Sakata N et al: Effects of danazol, gonadotropin-releasing hormone agonist, and a combination of danazol and gonadotropin-releasing hormone agonist on experimental endometriosis, *Am J Obstet Gynecol* 163:1679, 1990.

102. Sakura Y et al: Histological studies on the therapeutic effects of sustained-release microspheres of a potent LHRH agonist (luprorelin acetate) in an experimental endometriosis model in rats, *Endocrinol Jpn* 37:719, 1990.

103. Salat-Baroux J, Giacomini P, Antoine JM: Laparoscopic control of danazol therapy on pelvic endometriosis, *Hum Reprod* 3:197, 1988.

104. Sampson JA: Peritoneal endometriosis, due to menstrual dissemination of endometrial tissue into the peritoneal cavity, *Am J Obstet Gynecol* 14:422, 1927.

105. Schenken RS: Pathogenesis. In Schenken RS, editor: *Endometriosis: contemporary concepts in clinical management,* Philadelphia, 1989, JB Lippincott.

106. Scott RB, Wharton LR Jr: The effect of estrone and progesterone on the growth of experimental endometriosis in rhesus monkeys, *Am J Obstet Gynecol* 74:852, 1957.

107. Simpson JL et al: Heritable aspects of endometriosis, I: genetic studies, *Am J Obstet Gynecol* 137:327, 1980.

108. Steele RW, Dmowski WP, Marmer DJ: Immunologic aspects of human endometriosis, *Am J Reprod Immunol* 6:33, 1984.

109. Steingold KA et al: Treatment of endometriosis with a long-acting gonadotropin releasing hormone agonist, *Obstet Gynecol* 69:403, 1987.

110. Stevenson JC et al: A comparison of the skeletal effects of goserelin and danazol in premenopausal women with endometriosis, *Horm Res Suppl* 1:161, 1989.

111. Suginami H et al: A factor inhibiting ovum capture by the oviductal fimbriae present in endometriosis peritoneal fluid, *Fertil Steril* 46:1140, 1986.

112. Surrey ES, Halme J: Endometriosis as a cause of infertility, *Obstet Gynecol Clin North Am* 16:79, 1989.

113. Surrey ES, Judd HL: Reduction of vasomotor symptoms and bone mineral density loss with combined norethindrone and long-acting

gonadotropin-releasing hormone agonist therapy of symptomatic endometriosis: a prospective randomized trial, *J Clin Endocrinol Metab* 75:558, 1992.

114. Syrop CH, Halme J: Cyclic changes of peritoneal fluid parameters in normal and infertile patients, *Obstet Gynecol* 69:3, 1987.

115. Syrop CH, Halme J: Peritoneal fluid environment and infertility (Modern Trends), *Fertil Steril* 48:1, 1987.

116. Takahashi K et al: Prognostic potential of serum CA-125 levels in danazol-treated patients with external endometriosis: a preliminary study, *Int J Fertil* 35:226, 1990.

117. Takahashi K et al: Serum CA-125 and 17 beta-estradiol in patients with external endometriosis on danazol, *Gynecol Obstet Invest* 29:301, 1990.

118. Telimaa S: Danazol and medroxyprogesterone acetate ineffacicious in the treatment of infertility and endometriosis, *Fertil Steril* 15:872, 1988.

119. Telimaa S et al: Placebo-controlled comparison of danazol and high dose medroxyprogesterone acetate in the treatment of endometriosis, *Gynecol Endocrinol* 1:13, 1987.

120. Telimaa S et al: Circulating lipid and lipoprotein concentrations during danazol and high dose medroxyprogesterone acetate therapy of endometriosis, *Fertil Steril* 52:31, 1989.

121. Thomas EJ, Cooke ID: Successful treatment of asymptomatic endometriosis: does it benefit infertile women:, *Br Med J* 249:1117, 1987.

122. Timonen S, Johansson C-J: Endometriosis treated with lynestrenol, *Ann Chir Gynaecol Fenn* 57:144, 1968.

123. Tummon IS et al: Bone mineral density in women with endometriosis before and during ovarian suppression with gonadotropin-releasing hormone agonists or danazol, *Fertil Steril* 49:792, 1988.

124. Valimaki M et al: Comparison between the effects of nafarelin and danazol on serum lipids and lipoproteins in patients with endometriosis, *J Clin Endocrinol Metab* 69:1097, 1989.

125. Vernon MW et al: Classification of endometriotic implants by morphologic appearance and capacity to synthesize prostaglandin F, *Fertil Steril* 46:801, 1986.

126. Vierikko P et al: Steroidal regulation of endometriosis tissue: lack of induction of 17beta-hydroxysteroid dehydrogenase activity by progesterone, medroxyprogesterone acetate, or danazol, *Fertil Steril* 43:218, 1985.

127. Waldeyer: Eierstock und Ei, Leipzig, 1870. In Goodall JR, editor: *A study of endometriosis,* ed 2, Philadelphia, 1944, JB Lippincott.

128. Watkins RE: Uterine retrodisplacements, retrograde menstruation, and endometriosis, *West J Surg Obstet Gynecol* 46:480, 1938.

129. Weed JC, Arquembourg PC: Endometriosis: can it produce an autoimmune response resulting in infertility?, *Clin Obstet Gynecol* 23:885, 1980.

130. Whitehouse RW et al: The effects of nafarelin and danazol and vertebral trabecular bone mass in patients with endometriosis, *Clin Endocrinol* 33:365, 1990.

131. Ylikorkala O et al: Evidence of similar increases in bone turnover during nafarelin and danazol use in women with endometriosis, *Gynecol Endocrinol* 4:251, 1990.

Chapter 38

SURGICAL TREATMENT OF ENDOMETRIOSIS

**John A. Rock, MD
and Valerie S. Ratts, MD**

Surgery plays a key role in the diagnostic and therapeutic management of disease in patients with endometriosis. Although the diagnosis of endometriosis is suggested by a clinical presentation of infertility, dysmenorrhea, pelvic pain, and dyspareunia, surgical intervention is the only method that will accurately confirm the presence of endometriosis. Endometriosis is diagnosed by visualizing lesions at the time of operation or after finding the characteristic histologic appearance in resected or biopsied tissue. Surgery is useful not only for diagnosis, but also as an ideal therapeutic means to remove endometriosis and to restore normal pelvic anatomy that scarring from endometriosis may have altered. In patients with endometriosis, surgery may be used as a first-line therapy or as an alternative therapy when a course of medical therapy has failed. (See Chapter 37.)

DIAGNOSIS OF ENDOMETRIOSIS

The gynecologic surgeon must be well versed in recognizing endometriosis. Classic endometriosis appears as a pigmented lesion, usually puckered or raised, with a blue, brown, or black color due to tissue bleeding and hemosiderin deposition. Identifying typical implants of endometriosis with the characteristic pigmented, raised appearance is relatively straightforward. However, endometriosis may also present as lesions that are more difficult to recognize (refer to the box below). Atypical or nonpigmented lesions of endometriosis can have multiple appearances.[55,96] Thus endometriosis should be suspected when visualizing white, opacified, thickened areas of peritoneum with puckering from peritoneal scarring; raised, red, flamelike lesions; glandular lesions that resemble the mucosal lining of the endometrial cavity; yellow-brown patches that resemble café au lait plaques; circular peritoneal defects or "windows"; pink polyps; or clear translucent raised areas. The laparoscope is extremely helpful in diagnosing atypical lesions because it magnifies the tissue being examined. By using a working distance of 3 mm with the laparoscope, the peritoneum is magnified eight times. Small lesions signify-

---

Atypical appearances of endometriosis

White opacification
Red flame-like lesion
Glandular excrescences
Endometriosis in adhesions
Yellow-brown peritoneal patches
Peritoneal patches
Petechial peritoneum
Hypervascularization
Retroperitoneal disease

ing disease can be identified that may be missed with the naked eye.

Diagnosis requires a high index of suspicion, especially in patients with unexplained infertility. In one study of infertile patients undergoing laparoscopy by skilled, experienced surgeons, the diagnosis of endometriosis was missed in at least 6% of patients.[75] In another study, the reportedly "normal" appearing peritoneum in patients with documented endometriosis contained occult disease that was detected with scanning electron microscopy.[69] Microscopic endometriosis is often found in patients with pelvic adhesive disease. Thus a discovery of pelvic adhesions during surgery should alert the surgeon to search diligently for lesions of endometriosis.[67] Lesions suggestive of endometriosis can be confirmed by biopsy. Histologically, endometriosis is diagnosed when ectopic endometrial epithelium associated with endometrial stroma is seen.[22]

When endometriosis is diagnosed during laparoscopy or laparotomy, staging should also be performed. Staging of endometriosis requires a meticulous, systematic exploration of the entire pelvis for lesions. The extent of disease at each point of involvement is assessed, and the location, the number, and the size of endometriotic implants or endometriomas are noted. The pelvic structures involved with endometriosis are also documented. Specific attention is given to documenting involvement of the peritoneum, uterus, tubes, and/or ovaries. And finally, a thorough staging is complete only with documentation of the location and extent (filmy versus dense) of any adhesions.

Many systems for staging endometriosis have been introduced, including those of Acosta et al.,[1] Buttram,[12] Kistner et al.,[58] and the American Fertility Society (AFS)[4] and its revision (R-AFS).[5] The staging system currently in most common use is the R-AFS, which attempts to quantify the location and severity of endometriosis so that various therapies may be compared and evaluated. The point system devised for the R-AFS (Fig. 38-1) is heavily weighted toward ovarian involvement and adhesions as indicators of more severe disease.

Some surgeons advocate the use of laparoscopic ovarian puncture for accurate staging of endometriosis when the ovaries appear somewhat enlarged. A 16-gauge needle can be used to puncture the ovarian capsule. Aspiration of chocolate material is consistent with a previously undetected endometrioma, and may significantly alter the R-AFS staging. Quantification of the fluid can be used to assess the approximate size of the endometrioma.[17] Similarly, preoperative ultrasonograms in patients with endometriosis may be useful in screening for occult endometriomas.

Staging is useful in formulating a patient's prognosis, especially when infertility is an issue. Staging will also enable accurate comparisons between surgical procedures to be made, an important consideration when trying to follow the course of disease or when trying to determine whether there has been a response to previous therapy.

LAPAROSCOPIC THERAPY FOR ENDOMETRIOSIS

Operative laparoscopy offers the advantage of immediate diagnosis, and therapy for endometriosis should begin at the time of laparoscopic diagnosis. Initiation of treatment during an already in-progress surgery optimizes patient recovery and medical resources and decreases overall expense.

Laparoscopy is optimally performed during the follicular phase of the menstrual cycle. First, in the follicular phase the pelvic tissues are less hyperemic than in the luteal phase. When the tissue is less hyperemic, recognizing lesions of endometriosis is easier. Second, during the luteal phase the risk of damaging the corpus luteum, resulting in bleeding, is higher. Finally, operating during the follicular phase decreases the risk of interrupting an unrecognized early pregnancy. Ideally, diagnostic laparoscopy should not be performed during treatment with agents that suppress ovarian steroidogenesis, such as danazol or gonadotropin-releasing hormone (GnRH) analogues. Under suppression, endometriotic lesions are much more difficult to identify, and staging and assessment of disease therefore will be inaccurate.[36]

Because therapy for infertility patients usually begins at the time of laparoscopy, it is necessary that a complete evaluation of all infertility factors be performed before surgery. Many clinicians feel that the greatest fecundity rate occurs in the 6 to 18 months after ablation of endometriosis. An unrecognized male factor or ovulatory factor should be diagnosed and evaluated before surgery, because discovering it after surgery only delays the possibility of conception.

Laparoscopy may be used for all cases of endometriosis regardless of the stage of disease (Table 38-1). If there is difficulty in establishing tissue planes of dissection, or if a less-atraumatic technique is possible with the improved access of laparotomy, that should be the procedure of choice.[3,23]

Treatment of endometriotic implants through the laparoscope can be accomplished by a variety of techniques.[81] Small implants may be electrosurgically ablated with a unipolar or bipolar cautery. Cautery is applied until the lesion and surrounding tissue blanches. Bipolar cautery is usually safer. With this method, the implant is picked up between the two paddles and current is applied. Tissue necrosis is much more controlled, but implants deeper than 1 to 2 mm are difficult to remove. Unipolar cautery may be more beneficial in deeper lesions because of deeper penetration. However, it carries a greater risk of damaging adjacent structures such as ureter, bladder, bowel, or vessels by causing a greater area of thermal destruction.

Carbon dioxide (CO_2) laser ablation is a method of endometriosis ablation that allows great precision in removal of disease with minimal bleeding and minimal damage to surrounding tissue. One of the most appealing

Patient's name _____ Date _____

Stage I	(Minimal)	- 1-5
Stage II	(Mild)	- 6-15
Stage III	(Moderate)	- 16-40
Stage IV	(Severe)	- >40
Total _____		

Laparoscopy_____ Laparotomy_____ Photography_____

Recommended Treatment_____

_____

Prognosis_____

			<1cm	1-3cm	>3cm
Peritoneum	**Endometriosis**				
		Superficial	1	2	4
		Deep	2	4	6
Ovary	R	Superficial	1	2	4
		Deep	4	16	20
	L	Superficial	1	2	4
		Deep	4	16	20

		Partial		Complete	
Posterior culdesac obliteration		4		40	

			< 1/3 Enclosure	1/3-2/3 Enclosure	> 2/3 Enclosure
Ovary	**Adesions**				
	R	Filmy	1	2	4
		Dense	4	8	16
	L	Filmy	1	2	4
		Dense	4	8	16
Tube	R	Filmy	1	2	4
		Dense	4*	8*	16*
	L	Filmy	1	2	4
		Dense	4*	8*	16*

*If the fimbriated end of the fallopian tube is completely enclosed, change the point assignment to 16.

Additional endometriosis: _____   Associated pathology: _____

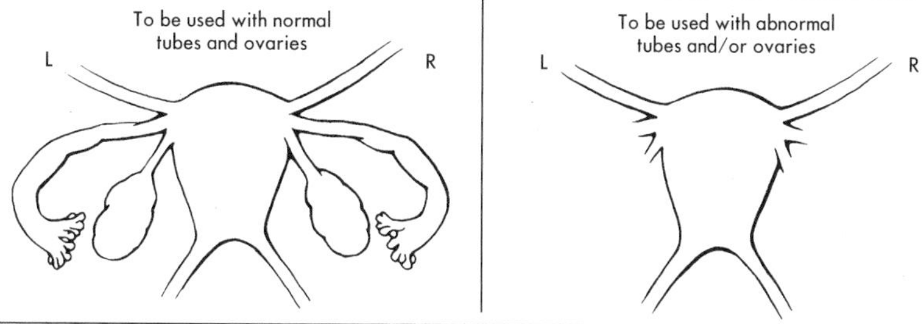

_____   _____

To be used with normal tubes and ovaries   To be used with abnormal tubes and/or ovaries

L   R   L   R

Fig. 38-1. Revised American Fertility Society staging for endometriosis. (From Revised American Fertility Society classification of endometriosis: 1985, *Fertil Steril* 43:351–352, 1985. Reproduced with permission of the publisher, The American Fertility Society.)

features of the CO_2 laser is that the energy does not penetrate much beyond the surface of the tissue being removed. Thermal damage is usually limited to 0.2 mm beyond visible damage. Therefore ablation by the CO_2 laser may be safer because of its greater accuracy. The zone of thermal necrosis for CO_2 laser vaporization is minimal, especially when in the superpulse mode. For implant ablation, the standard CO_2 laser laparoscope utilizes a focal point approximately 2 cm from the end of the delivery port. Depending on the area to be coagulated or vaporized, spot sizes vary from 0.5 to 2.5 mm. In the continuous firing mode, power densities of 2500 to 5000 W/cm^2 are used. Lesions that are close to vital structures may be ablated using single-pulse or superpulse modes of 0.05 to 0.1 second in order to limit the extent of tissue vaporization.[16] Endometrial implants should be vaporized completely. Copious irrigation should be used to remove carbon debris and

to expose the base of the lesion. Repeated vaporization may be necessary to eradicate the implant completely. Argon, potassium-titanyl-phosphate (KTP), and neodymium: yttrium-aluminum-garnet (Nd:YAG) fiber lasers are also being used for ablating endometriosis.

For larger lesions or atypical lesions, excision is available. With excision the lesion can be removed and sent for histologic confirmation of diagnosis (Fig. 38-2). The endometriotic focus is grasped, the peritoneum tented, and the lesion circumscribed. The edge of the lesion is then grasped and lifted so that the endometriotic implant can be excised. Care is taken to dissect the implant away from underlying healthy tissue and to identify underlying structures so that no inadvertent damage is done to adjacent tissue.[30,66,67]

Entering the retroperitoneal space is occasionally required for removal of endometriosis near the ureters or

Table 38-1. Algorithm for management of endometriosis

| Stage of disease | Desires childbearing | | Childbearing complete |
	Infertility*	Pelvic pain*	Pelvic pain*
Stages I and II	1. Expectant Rx 2. Laparoscopic Rx 2. Medical Rx 3. CSEL±PSN 3. IVF/ET	1. Laparoscopic Rx 2. Medical Rx 3. CSEL + PSN	1. Laparoscopic Rx 2. Medical Rx 3. TAH ± BSO 3. CSEL ± PSN
Stage III	1. Laparoscopic Rx 1. CSEL ± PSN 2. Medical Rx 3. IVF/ET	1. Laparoscopic Rx 2. CSEL + PSN 3. Medical Rx	1. Laparoscopic Rx 2. Medical Rx 3. TAH ± BSO 3. CSEL + PSN
Stage IV	1. CSEL + perioperative medical Rx 2. CSEL alone 3. Laparoscopic Rx + postoperative medical Rx 4. IVF/ET	1. CSEL + PSN + perioperative medical Rx 2. Medical Rx 3. Laparoscopic Rx + medical Rx	1. TAH ± BSO 1. CSEL + PSN + medical Rx 2. Laparoscopic Rx + medical Rx

Modified from Wheeler JM: Macro- and microsurgical treatment of endometriosis. In Thomas E, Rock JA, editors: *Modern approaches to endometriosis,* Boston, 1991, Kluwer Academic Publishers, with permission.
*Rx, Treatment; CSEL, conservative surgery for endometriosis at laparotomy; PSN, presacral neurectomy; TAH, total abdominal hysterectomy; BSO, bilateral salpingo-oophorectomy; IVF/ET, in vitro fertilization/embryo transfer; ±, adjunctive treatment option based on individual patient findings.

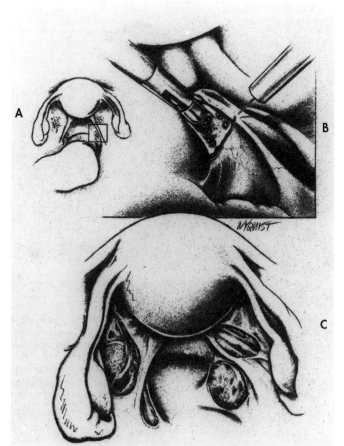

pelvic vessels. When laser laparoscopy is being used, aquadissection or hydrodissection is a useful technique[74] (Fig. 38-3). The tip of the irrigator is placed through a small incision in the peritoneum into the subperitoneal space. Fluid is delivered into the space to distend and elevate the peritoneum. The fluid provides a mechanical separation of the lesion to be excised from the surrounding structures. When the CO_2 laser is used, fluid also provides a thermal buffer, since the CO_2 laser beam does not penetrate water. Endometriosis of the peritoneum overlying crucial structures can be removed without fear of damaging adjacent structures. If aquadissection or hydrodissection is performed in the area of the broad ligaments or pelvic sidewall, the distending fluid may escape through the inguinal ring, resulting in edema of the external genitalia.

Adhesions associated with endometriosis may be removed through the laparoscope.[33] The surgical maxim to operate with minimal tissue trauma should be observed.

Fig. 38-2. Laparoscopic excision of peritoneal implant. **A,** Lesions of peritoneal endometriosis are identified. **B,** The endometriotic focus is grasped, the peritoneum is tented, and the lesion is circumscribed using the microelectrode as shown (or alternatively using the laser). **C,** The peritoneum is dissected free from underlying structures to excise the implant. (From Batt RE, Wheeler JM: Endometriosis: advanced diagnostic laparoscopy. In Hunt RB, editor: *Atlas of female infertility surgery*, Baltimore, 1992, Mosby.)

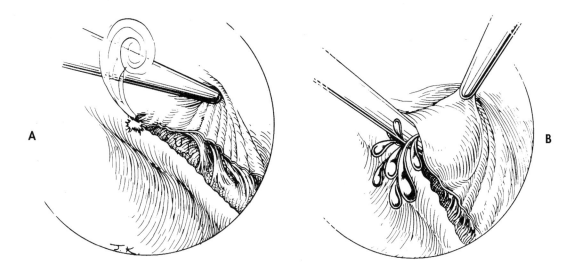

Fig. 38-3. Aquadissection. **A,** An incision is made in the peritoneum. **B,** The irrigator tip is inserted into the incision underneath the peritoneum. Fluid is injected into the space. (From Reich H, Hunt RB: Advanced laparoscopic surgery, In Hunt RB, editor: *Atlas of female infertility surgery,* Baltimore, 1992, Mosby.)

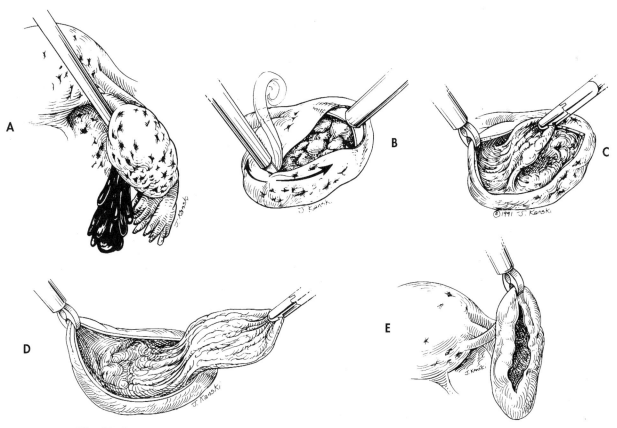

Fig. 38-4. Laparoscopic resection of an ovarian endometrioma. **A,** The ovary containing the endometrioma is mobilized. **B,** An incision is made in the cortex of the ovary over the most superficial area of the endometrioma. The endometrioma is lavaged and the cyst lining is inspected. **C,** The cyst wall is grasped. **D,** The cyst wall is stripped from the ovary. **E,** The defect may be closed with laparoscopic suturing or left to heal by secondary intention. (From Reich H, Hunt. RB: Advanced laparoscopic surgery, In Hunt RB, editor: *Atlas of female infertility surgery*, Baltimore, 1992, Mosby.)

Transparent, avascular adhesions may be excised with scissors, laser, or aquadissection. Dense adhesions will require a combination of blunt and sharp dissection. If bleeding is noted, hemostasis should be accomplished with a defocused laser beam or bipolar cautery. Adequate visualization is essential and can be accomplished with ancillary suprapubic instruments to orient the tissue planes. If exposure is not adequate, laparotomy should be considered.

Laparoscopic treatment of ovarian endometriomas has become an important technique[35,86] (Fig. 38-4) and can be as safe and effective as treatment at laparotomy.[2] It should generally be reserved for endometriomas less than 5 cm. Initially, the ovary must be adequately mobilized, which often requires lysis of adhesions. A careful inspection should then be performed in order to devise a planned approach. Superficial endometriosis of the ovary may be ablated by using any of the methods previously described for endometriotic implants. Note that sometimes the lesion that appears to be a small implant may in fact represent the superficial portion of a much larger endometrioma.

Removal of an ovarian endometrioma can be approached laparoscopically in one of two ways. In the first method, the endometriotic cyst is punctured, aspirated, opened, and lavaged. The cyst lining should be examined to confirm the diagnosis of an endometrioma; the lining should be smooth, without papillary excrescences. If the cyst is confirmed to be an endometrioma, the lining is ablated with electrocauterization or laser vaporization. Alternatively, the cyst wall can be removed by grasping the cyst lining and stripping it from the ovary with a corkscrew motion. Any portions of cyst lining left attached may then be ablated. The defect may be closed with laparoscopic suturing or left to heal by secondary intention. Experience suggests that minor adhesion formation will occur at the small ovarian defect.[18]

CONSERVATIVE THERAPY FOR ENDOMETRIOSIS AT LAPAROTOMY

Conservative therapy for endometriosis may require a laparotomy (see Table 38-1). The indications as described by Wheeler[102] for conservative surgery of endometriosis at laparotomy (CSEL) include the following:

- Persistence of symptoms or infertility in patients after a trial of expectant management, medical management, or laparoscopic treatment
- Severe disease exceeding the operative skill of the surgeon or availability of instrumentation
- Pathologic conditions that would be better approached through laparotomy (e.g., invasive bowel nodule or ureteral nodule)

Obtaining adequate exposure is absolutely necessary for resection of endometriosis. Usually a horizontal suprapubic incision is adequate unless other factors exist, such as a lesion suggestive of a neoplastic process, previous vertical incision, obesity, or need for better exposure for associated procedures such as presacral neurectomy. After opening the abdomen, the endometriosis should be staged. The next objective is to restore normal pelvic anatomy. Immobilizing adhesions are divided and can be excised later during the surgery. At this point, adnexal structures are raised from behind the uterus and placed on a Silastic platform for better visualization.

Conservative surgery with the intent of preserving or restoring reproductive function is based on the use of atraumatic microsurgical technique. The tissues should be handled gently with atraumatic instruments. Copious irrigation of the pelvic organs should be performed intermittently throughout the operation to prevent drying of tissues. We recommend use of Ringer's lactate with 5000 IU of heparin and 1 g of hydrocortisone added to each liter of solution. Adhesions should be removed with care not to damage or breach the underlying peritoneum. Since endometriosis can be diagnosed by histologic examination, adhesions should be excised and sent for pathologic review. Adhesions may contain microscopic foci of endometriosis. Any dissection should be performed with precision, whether by microelectrode cauterization, fine scissors, or laser. Meticulous hemostasis needs to be obtained, preferably with the use of a bipolar cautery. Finally, if suture materials are used they should be bioabsorbable and nonirritating.

The goal of conservative therapy for endometriosis is removal of all visible endometriosis. It is recognized that this surgery is probably more cytoreductive than ablative; multiple studies have shown endometriosis in visibly normal peritoneum.[69,75]

Endometrial implants are removed in a manner similar to that described for laparoscopy. Superficial implants may be ablated with bipolar coagulation or with the laser. Palpation is often useful for recognizing deeper lesions, which may not be visually apparent. Deeper implants should be excised rather than ablated, both to avoid extensive tissue damage by spread of thermal energy and to ensure complete resection. The endometriotic focus is grasped, the peritoneum is elevated, and the lesion is circumscribed. The tissue underneath is undercut, leaving a 2 to 4-mm margin. When removing implants, care should be taken in dissection so that underlying structures such as the uterine vessel and ureter are identified and not damaged. Some surgeons advocate hydrodissection, in which saline or lactated Ringer's solution is injected retroperitoneally to provide a barrier to the spread of laser energy. Others believe that hydrodissection actually distorts the anatomy, making identification of vital structures more difficult.

Deep nodules of endometriosis are not uncommon. In one study, 25% of patients with clinically recognized disease had lesions that penetrated deeper than 5 mm.[65] The pouch of Douglas and the uterosacral ligaments are two areas that need careful inspection and palpation for deeper implants of endometriosis. Deep infiltration (>5 mm) with active disease has been reported in 55% of patients with cul-de-sac involvement and in 34% of patients with uterosacral ligament involvement.[24] Endometriosis typically infiltrates until the level of the retroperitoneal fat is reached. Thus it is often necessary to dissect well into the retroperitoneal fat to remove adequately an entire endometriotic nodule. Deeply infiltrative lesions are rarely found in the ovarian fossae, where there is little retroperitoneal fat. Cornille et al.[24] reported that the very deep endometriotic lesions were most often confined to patients undergoing laparotomy for pelvic pain, whereas superficial implants were more commonly seen in patients undergoing surgery for infertility.

Once the implant is excised, if the defect in the peritoneum is hemostatic and small, it may be left open. Otherwise 5.0 polyglycolic acid suture may be used to loosely reapproximate the peritoneum. Sutures that are placed too tightly, producing tension on the peritoneum, may actually promote greater tissue necrosis and damage and increase the risk of adhesion formation.

Adhesiolysis is crucial to establishing normal pelvic and tuboovarian anatomy. Each individual adhesion should be isolated and removed with care not to damage or breach the adjacent peritoneum. This is most easily accomplished by fanning the adhesions out, using gentle traction with atraumatic forceps. A tapered Teflon-covered probe is useful if held behind an adhesion so that the adhesion can be tented away from the normal structures. Cutting the adhesion along the probe often makes excision more swift and more precise. When two structures are adherent to each other, attention must be paid to identify clearly the separate structures and establish a well-defined plane of dissection. Adequate distance must be present between the two structures for transection to be safely performed. The use of a needle or microelectrode is optimal for cutting. In addition, use of operating loupes (1.5 to 2.5×) will aid visualization so that excision will be exact.

Ovarian endometriosis

Removal of ovarian endometriosis is performed during laparotomy in a manner similar to that described for laparoscopy. Initially a careful inspection of the ovary is performed in order to identify all endometriotic lesions. Next, the ovary should be freed of any adhesions. Filmy adhesions of the ovary should be lifted and excised without cutting into the ovary. Note that 40% to 50% of subovarian adhesions contain endometriosis.[55] If the ovary is adherent to the ovarian fossa, great care should be used in the dissection so as not to damage an underlying ureter. Once the ovaries are mobilized, the use of a silastic platform behind the uterus aids in elevating the adnexal structures for better visualization. Superficial lesions of the ovary may be ablated with electrocautery, preferably bipolar or laser, using copious irrigation. The lesions should be elevated from the surrounding ovarian cortex before ablation so as

not to traumatize the surrounding normal ovarian surface.

Ovarian endometriomas are removed in a manner similar to that described for laparoscopy[8,43] (Fig. 38-5). An elliptical incision is made over the endometrioma with the longitudinal axis of the ellipse parallel to the line between the fimbria ovarica and the ovarian ligament. The electromicrosurgical needle is used to make the incision approximately 0.1 to 0.2 mm deep. Next, the capsule of the endometrioma is identified. A cleavage plane, using blunt curved scissors, is then developed to shell out the endometrioma. Ideally, the endometrioma is removed without rupturing the cyst wall. It is helpful to place a lint-free lap pack around the ovary containing the endometrioma so that if rupture with spillage of the contents occurs, the spread can be limited by the pack, which is immediately removed from the abdomen.

Once the endometrioma has been removed, hemostasis is achieved with the bipolar cautery and copious irrigation. Ovarian reconstruction is then performed. Mattress sutures of 5.0 nonreactive absorbable suture are used to close the deep portions of the ovary in layers, thereby eliminating dead space. The ovarian surface layer is closed with a subcortical layer of 6.0 delayed absorbable material (i.e., polyglycolic acid) to decrease exposure of suture material and thus decrease the incidence of adhesions. Adhesion barriers also may be placed across the suture line to decrease adhesion formation.[53] The advantage of laparotomy is that the ovary can be palpated so that smaller deep lesions can be appreciated. Larger endometriomas (greater than 10 cm) may actually be several smaller endometrial cysts in the involved ovary.

Previously, if disease was unilateral, the recommendation has been to remove the diseased adnexa. However, in this age of assisted reproductive technology, surgery should be as conservative as possible. Oocyte retrieval from small ovarian remnants has resulted in pregnancy.

Endometriosis of the fallopian tube

Endometriosis of the fallopian tubes usually results in peritubal adhesion formation and tubal damage, which causes infertility from mechanical factors. Adhesiolysis should be performed by using microsurgical techniques described previously with attention to establishing the normal anatomy of the tube and ovary. Tubal obstruction is usually the result of extensive adhesion formation rather than an obstructing nodule of endometriosis. Tubal reconstruction includes microsurgical techniques for ovariolysis, fimbrioplasty, and neosalpingostomy. Rarely, an endometriotic nodule can cause tubal occlusion. In this situation, diagnosis usually is made with a preoperative hysterosalpingogram combined with laparoscopic assessment. Sometimes medical management with danazol or GnRH analogues is helpful in shrinking the nodule so that tubal patency is reestablished. If medical management fails, tubal excision and anastomosis may be considered.

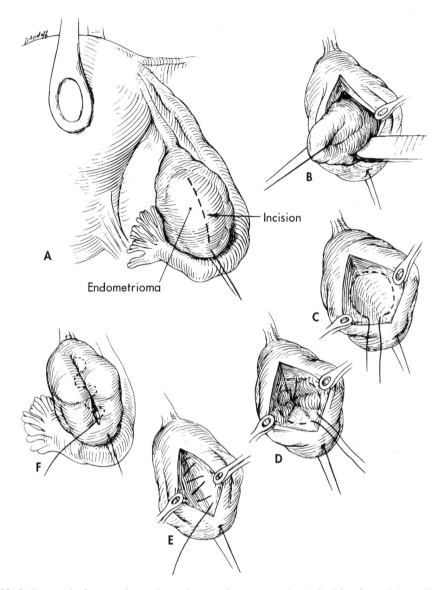

Fig. 38-5. Removal of an ovarian endometrioma at laparotomy. **A,** An incision is made over the endometrioma with the longitudinal axis of incision parallel to the line between the fimbria ovarica and the ovarian ligament. **B,** The capsule of the endometrioma is identified. A plane is developed to shell out the endometrioma. **C–E,** Deep portions of the ovary are closed using mattress sutures of a nonreactive absorbable suture. **F,** The ovarian surface layer is closed with a subcortical layer of 6.0 delayed absorbable material. (From Hesla JS, Rock JA: Endometriosis. In Rock JA, Murphy AA, Jones HW, editors: *Female reproductive surgery*, Baltimore, 1992, William & Wilkins.)

Retroperitoneal endometriosis

Retroperitoneal endometriosis usually causes severe pain, dysmenorrhea, and dyspareunia in patients. A typical examination will reveal tender nodules involving the cul-de-sac, uterosacral ligaments, rectosigmoid junction, and rectovaginal septum. Often the uterus is retroverted and fixed posteriorly.

Extensive retroperitoneal disease often is not easily accessible by the laparoscope. Removal of disease requires retroperitoneal dissection, which may be facilitated by placing a bougie in the rectum, sponge forceps in the vagina, and Foley catheter in the bladder (Fig. 38-6). The pararectal and paravaginal spaces may be exposed by applying traction in the appropriate direction. Careful dissection will allow complete excision of implants without damaging adjacent structures.

Endometriosis of the bowel

Endometriosis of the bowel is rare, but it occurs in up to 25% of women with endometriosis.[56] The treatment of such

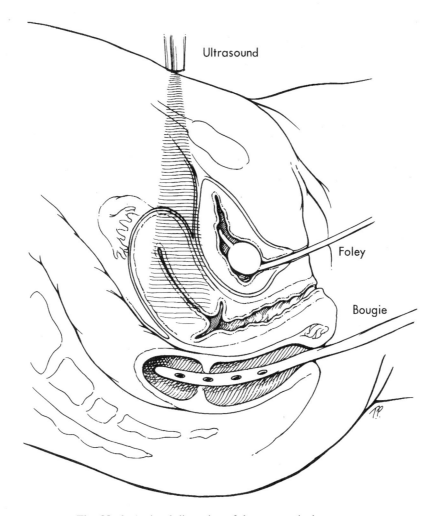

Ultrasound

Foley

Bougie

Fig. 38-6. Assisted dissection of the rectovaginal space.

patients must be individualized. Location of disease (rectosigmoid, large bowel, small bowel, or appendix) will determine the type of surgery necessary. Endometriosis of the gastrointestinal tract most commonly involves segments that are in close proximity to the uterus, fallopian tubes, and ovaries. In a study at the Mayo Clinic, 497 cases of bowel endometriosis were examined with the resulting distribution: 72.4% involved the sigmoid, rectosigmoid, or rectal areas; 13.5% involved the rectovaginal septum; 7% involved the small bowel; 3.6% involved the cecum; and 3% involved the appendix.[68] Results of a more recent study evaluating 163 cases of intestinal endometriosis were consistent with the previous findings. The distribution of disease revealed that 40% of lesions involved the descending colon; 20% involved the sigmoid; 10% involved the rectum; 20% involved the appendix; and the remaining 10% involved the ileum, cecum, or transverse colon.[101]

Before choosing the method of treatment of bowel endometriosis, the symptomatology of the patient should be assessed. A study by Coronado et al.[25] showed that patients with endometriosis of the intestinal tract will have symptoms suggestive of such involvement. Symptoms included

rectal pain (74%), dyspareunia (46%), constipation (49%), diarrhea (36%), and rectal bleeding (31%). Complete intestinal obstruction is rare, but when it occurs it is an absolute indication for laparotomy and resection of the involved portion of bowel.[80] If clinical symptoms are present before surgery, it is probably prudent to assess the bowel for evidence of involvement. Barium enema is most useful and will reveal a smooth (nonmalignant) crater if disease involves the mucosa. Endovaginal ultrasonography has been shown to be helpful in diagnosing disease of the anterior rectal wall.[44] Colonoscopy with biopsies will confirm endometriosis if there is mucosal involvement and will facilitate planning of the proper procedure.[7]

Before proceeding with laparotomy in patients with known or suspected bowel involvement, full mechanical and antibiotic bowel preparation is indicated. At laparotomy, superficial lesions of the bowel limited to the serosa may be excised, fulgurated, or laser vaporized. Lesions that extend more deeply are best treated with segmental bowel resection. If childbearing is complete, a total abdominal hysterectomy with bilateral salpingo-oophorectomy should be considered. Alternatively, ovarian preservation may be possible if the lesion can be resected completely.

Whether to perform an appendectomy during surgery for endometriosis is unclear. In one study of 926 patients who underwent laparotomy for bowel resection secondary to endometriosis, 126 patients (13.6%) underwent incidental appendectomy. Only two patients were shown to have microscopic involvement. Unless involvement of the appendix is evident, appendectomy is optional.[82]

The outcome for patients after bowel resection for endometriosis is quite good. Of the patients who attempted conception, 39% became pregnant. Improvement in pelvic pain was noted in 88% of patients.[25] However, if the deeply infiltrative endometriosis is not completely removed, bowel symptoms will recur.[65]

Endometriosis of the urinary tract

Urinary tract endometriosis is relatively rare, afflicting only 1.2% of women with endometriosis. Diagnosis begins with a high clinical index of suspicion. Symptoms of bladder involvement include frequency, dysuria, and hematuria. Cystoscopy is most useful for diagnosing vesicle endometriosis. Radiographic studies are most useful to assess accurately any ureteral involvement. An intravenous pyelogram is probably indicated for all patients undergoing surgery for extensive endometriosis. Ureteral involvement may be intrinsic or extrinsic; extrinsic disease is four times more common than intrinsic disease.

Treatment of urinary tract disease can begin with medical management with danazol or GnRH agonists, but close surveillance of renal function is necessary.[87] Endometriosis of the bladder that is superficial may be ablated or excised during laparoscopy or laparotomy. Extensive endometriosis of the bladder is treated with partial cystectomy.[94] Endometriosis of the ureter causing insidious ureteral obstruction and resulting in unrecognized severe loss of renal function has been described.[10,59] If ureteral obstruction occurs, surgery is absolutely indicated. The preferred treatment of ureteral obstruction is ureterolysis or resection of the involved segment accompanied with ureteroneocystostomy or ureteroureterostomy. Nephrostomy urinary diversion is considered when severe hydronephrosis is present and ureterolysis is not possible.[94]

Extrapelvic endometriosis

Extrapelvic endometriosis is rare, but it can cause clinically significant disease. Diagnosis needs to be confirmed by biopsy. The mainstay of therapy is excision of the lesion. If complete excision is not possible, hormonal suppression may be necessary. A staging system devised by Markham et al.[62] for extrapelvic endometriosis is presented in the box.

ADJUNCTIVE PROCEDURES FOR PAIN RELIEF

The dysmenorrhea and pelvic pain associated with endometriosis are most commonly treated with medical regimens such as hormonal suppressive therapy or nonsteroidal

---

Staging system for extrapelvic endometriosis

Classification of extrapelvic endometriosis

Class I: Endometriosis involving the intestinal tract
Class U: Endometriosis involving the urinary tract
Class L: Endometriosis involving the lung and thoracic cage
Class O: Endometriosis involving other sites outside the abdominal cavity

Staging of extrapelvic endometriosis

Stage I No organ defect
    1. Extrinsic: surface of organ (serosa, pleura)
       a. <1 cm lesion
       b. 1 to 4 cm lesion
       c. >4 cm lesion
    2. Intrinsic: mucosal, muscle, parenchyma
       a. <1 cm lesion
       b. 1 to 4 cm lesion
       c. >4 cm lesion
Stage II Organ defect*
    1. Extrinsic: surface of organ (serosa, pleura)
       a. <1 cm lesion
       b. 1 to 4 cm lesion
       c. >4 cm lesion
    2. Intrinsic: mucosal, muscle, parenchyma
       a. <1 cm lesion
       b. 1 to 4 cm lesion
       c. >4 cm lesion

From Markham SM, Carpenter SE, Rock JA: *Obstet Gynecol Clin North Am* 16:193, 1989, with permission of WB Saunders.

*Organ defect would depend on the organ of involvement and would include but not be limited to obstruction and partial obstruction of the urinary tract and the intestinal tract and hemothorax, hemoptysis, and pneumothorax resulting from pulmonary involvement.

---

antiinflammatory drugs. However, a significant portion of patients will receive no relief from pain with medical management. Surgery may be indicated in these patients.

Laparoscopic uterine nerve ablation

Laparoscopic uterine nerve ablation (LUNA) has been described for treatment of dysmenorrhea. In this procedure, interruption of the uterosacral ligament at the insertion into the cervix results in destroying a large number of sensory nerve fibers that innervate the cervix and lower uterine segment. LUNA can be performed with laser or electrocoagulation. Exposure of the uterosacral ligaments is key, usually achieved by flexing the uterus forward through manipulation of a uterine cannula. The course of the ureters should be noted before excision, to prevent damage. The CO_2 laser is used with a power density of 5,000 to 15,000 W/cm^2 to ablate a 2- to 5-cm segment of each uterosacral ligament immediately adjacent to the cervix to a depth of 1 cm. In addition, the area of the posterior cervix between the uterosacral ligaments may be superficially ablated to de-

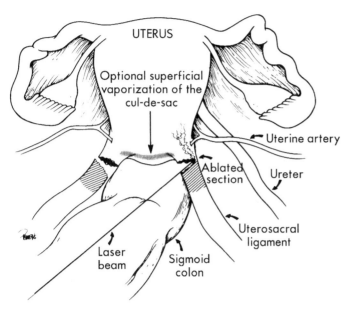

Fig. 38-7. Laparoscopic uterine nerve ablation (LUNA). (From Perry P, Azziz R: Laparoscopic uterine nerve ablation, presacral neurectomy, and appendectomy. In Azziz R, Murphy AA, editors: *Practical manual of operative laparoscopy and endoscopy*, New York, 1992. Springer-Verlag.)

stroy fibers that are crossing to innervate the contralateral side. Alternatively, bipolar cautery can be used. The uterosacral ligament is grasped with the bipolar forceps. Once the segment has been coagulated, laparoscopic scissors are used to transect the ligament. If bleeding is encountered, hemostasis is achieved by defocused laser beam or endocoagulation. The incision is carried no further because repeated bleeding may be extensive, making hemostatic control difficult (Fig. 38-7).

The usefulness of performing LUNA is mixed; the procedure can have significant morbidity and mortality. The degree of pain relief obtained after the procedure is quite varied. In a study by Lichten,[60] 10 of 20 patients with stage I endometriosis reported pain relief. Feste[39] reported that symptoms of dysmenorrhea and endometriosis-associated dysmenorrhea were improved in 71% of patients after LUNA. The most recent study, by Donnez,[34] has reported that 50% of 100 women experienced complete relief and 41% experienced mild to moderate relief.

Presacral neurectomy

Presacral neurectomy is an adjunctive procedure at laparotomy for treatment of dysmenorrhea due to endometriosis. Patient selection is an important factor in predicting the effectiveness of this procedure. Tjaden et al.[99] showed, in a small, randomized study, that in patients with *midline* pain, results were excellent after presacral neurectomy, but that in patients with adnexal pain symptoms the degree of relief was highly variable. Patients should also be reminded that presacral neurectomy does not increase pregnancy rates.

Presacral neurectomy should be performed through an incision that allows adequate exposure, such as either a vertical midline or a Maylard transverse incision. The intestines can then be easily displaced so that the bifurcation of the aorta is identified. Over the sacral promontory, the posterior parietal peritoneum is opened with Metzenbaum scissors for about 6 cm beginning caudally just below the bifurcation of the aorta and extending over the ventral surface of the sacrum (Fig. 38-8). The edges of the peritoneum are held outward by 3-0 silk stay sutures or Allis clamps.

Dissection begins with the right edge of the posterior peritoneum. With meticulous care, using fine-pointed scissors or a Kitner sponge, the areolar tissue containing nerve fibers is dissected off the posterior peritoneal flap. The blood vessels also lying in this area should not be disturbed. The right ureter is identified and retracted laterally. The common iliac artery lying immediately beneath the ureter is identified. Areolar tissue is bluntly freed from the ureter and artery. A right-angle clamp or probe is then inserted medially next to the promontory to dissect bluntly under the sheath until the glistening white of the sacral periosteum is reached. A window is made. Care should be taken to avoid the middle sacral vessels located on the surface of the promontory, because bleeding from these vessels can be significant and difficult to stop.

Similarly, beginning on the left peritoneal flap, areolar tissue is bluntly dissected off the posterior peritoneum. Dissection is carried down until the superior hemorrhoidal vessels are visualized. These vessels are left on the peritoneum, but the overlying areolar tissue is taken. Branch vessels to the iliac vein that are encountered should be ligated or clipped to avoid blood loss. The superior hypogastric nerve plexus is now isolated and may be elevated off the periosteum with blunt dissection. Two ties of 2-0 silk are placed proximally and distally around the nerve bundle, leaving approximately a 5- to 6-cm length of segment for excision. Once the nerve bundle is removed, the posterior peritoneum is then closed with a running suture.

The immediate complications of presacral neurectomy include damage to ureter and blood vessels. However, with meticulous surgical technique these risks are minimal. Side effects of constipation requiring laxative therapy, vaginal dryness, and bladder dysfunction have been described. As a rule these symptoms will resolve over several months.

POSTOPERATIVE ADHESION PREVENTION

The most reliable method for preventing postoperative adhesion formation is to follow meticulous surgical technique, thereby avoiding tissue trauma, anoxia, and ischemia. However, adhesions will form nevertheless and potentially can undo the reconstructive work performed after resection of endometriosis. Additional discussion of adhesion formation and prevention is found in Chapter 36.

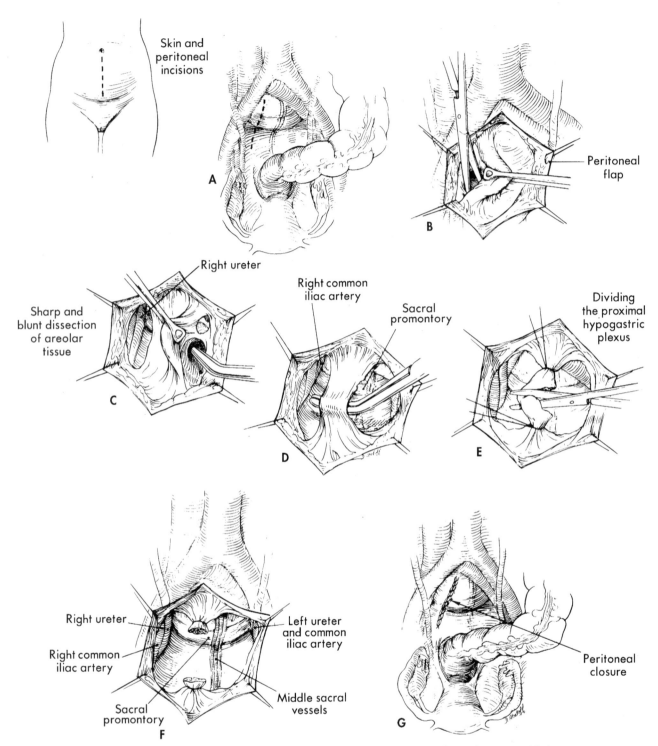

Fig. 38-8. Presacral neurectomy. (From Perry P, Azziz R: Laparoscopic uterine nerve ablation, presacral neurectomy, and appendectomy. In Azziz R, Murphy AA, editors: *Practical manual of operative laparoscopy and endoscopy*, New York, 1992. Springer-Verlag.) **A,** After the intestines are displaced, the aortic bifurcation is identified. The posterior parietal peritoneum is opened over the sacral promontory. **B,** The edges of the peritoneum are held outward with silk stay sutures. Areolar tissue containing nerve fibers is dissected off the posterior peritoneal flap. **C,** The right ureter should be identified and retracted laterally. Tissue is carefully dissected off the left peritoneal flap. **D,** The superior hypogastric nerve plexus is isolated. **E,** The hypogastric plexus is divided. **F,** The anatomy of the retroperitoneal space is seen and inspected for hemostasis. **G,** The peritoneum is closed.

Adjunctive agents

Multiple adjunctive agents have been used intraperitoneally and intravenously after resection of endometriosis to prevent adhesions, including dextran, nonsteroidal antiinflammatory agents, corticosteroids, promethazine, and heparin. Discussion of all of these agents exceeds the scope of this chapter but is presented in detail in Chapter 36. However, two mechanical adhesion barriers, oxidized regenerated cellulose (Interceed) and expanded polytetrafluoroethylene (PTFE) (Gore-Tex), deserve further attention. These products may be placed between the ovary and pelvic sidewall to try to prevent adhesion formation.

Oxidized regenerated cellulose designed in a knitted weave is known as TC-7. It is applied to a hemostatic peritoneal surface and will form a continuous gel covering within approximately 8 hours. This forms a mechanical barrier to prevent opposing raw surfaces from adhering to each other. Animal studies with rabbit uterine horns have shown that TC-7 significantly reduces adhesion formation.[32,61] The substance has been shown to be resorbed in 3 to 4 days. One multicenter, randomized, prospective human study[53] has shown TC-7 to be safe and efficacious in reducing adhesion formation. In this study, 74 women with bilateral adnexal adhesions served as their own controls. TC-7 was applied to the pelvic sidewall after adhesiolysis on one side. Second-look laparoscopy to assess adhesion formation was performed within 14 weeks of the original surgery. Adhesion formation was rated to be reduced on the sidewall where TC-7 had been placed. In contrast, animal studies have shown that oxidized, regenerated cellulose will actually elicit an acute peritoneal fluid inflammatory exudate in the mouse that may contribute to peritoneal injury and result in de novo adhesion formation in this model system.[47]

Another mechanical barrier, PTFE (Gore-Tex), is currently being evaluated. In one rabbit model study,[9] adhesions were statistically reduced. In a mouse model, PTFE was not associated with tissue injury despite a mild increase in the number of normal-appearing peritoneal fluid macrophages.[47] One disadvantage of this surgical membrane is that it is nonabsorbable and would require a second-look laparoscopy for removal. Human studies on the safety and efficacy of this barrier are pending.

Uterine suspension

Uterine suspension has been proposed as a method to reduce adhesion formation, especially when denuded peritoneal edges are located over the posterior uterus or in the cul-de-sac. In addition, theoretically the tubes and ovaries are elevated and thus will be at decreased risk for adherence to sites of previous adhesion excision or endometriosis resection. The procedure may be especially useful in patients with a retroflexed or retroverted uterus. The authors recommend the use of the modified Gilliam suspension in which the round ligament is shortened by pulling it through the internal ring and suturing it to the rectus sheath.

Second-look laparoscopy

Second-look laparoscopy is recommended by some investigators for patients with extensive endometriosis that has required extensive dissection. Patients whose ovaries were dissected from the cul-de-sac or posterior uterus are believed to benefit from this procedure. If laparoscopy is performed within 4 to 12 weeks after laparotomy, adhesions are usually thin and filmy and thus easy to remove. The effectiveness in improving pregnancy outcome has yet to be proven.

SEMICONSERVATIVE AND RADICAL SURGERY

Endometriosis can cause severe symptoms of pain due to extensive pelvic adhesive disease or recurrent endometriomas. For cases refractory to conservative management, when childbearing is no longer an issue, the last resort is to proceed with definitive abdominal surgery: total abdominal hysterectomy with or without bilateral salpingoophorectomy (see Table 38-1). The surgical dictum in this situation is to remove all visible endometriosis, thereby performing a complete cytoreduction.

Radical surgery requires careful counseling of the patient and significant preoperative preparation by the surgeon. Initial preoperative evaluation should include an imaging study of the pelvis to rule out the presence of other entities that can cause similar clinical presentations. A large endometrioma may present as a pelvic mass possibly consistent with an ovarian malignancy. In such situations, the pelvic mass should be treated as a malignancy until proven otherwise. Thus obtaining pelvic washings on entering the abdomen is essential. An intravenous pyelogram may be helpful if previous surgery or pelvic adhesions are suspected to have altered the course of the ureters and to rule out the presence of a double collecting system. A bowel preparation is an essential part of preoperative management in case large bowel mucosa is breached during extensive dissection. Bowel preparation will allow primary repair rather than the need for colostomy placement.

The protocol for bowel preparation used at Johns Hopkins begins with a clear liquid diet the day before scheduled surgery. Mechanical cleansing of the bowel begins the night before surgery with oral intake of 4 L of a polyethylene glycol 3350 and electrolyte solution preparation (i.e., Golytely, Colyte). This will induce diarrhea and mechanical bowel evacuation. To complete mechanical preparation, an enema is administered the night before surgery and the morning of surgery. In addition, antibiotic preparation of the bowel is performed by administering neomycin 500 mg orally every 2 hours for four doses and sulfasalazine 500 mg orally every 2 hours for four doses the night before surgery.

Once the decision has been made to proceed with a hysterectomy, the next problem that arises is whether or not the ovaries should be preserved. Whether to perform semiconservative surgery (thus preserving the ovaries) or to perform radical surgery (removing all ovarian tissue) re-

Table 38-2. Rates of recurrent symptoms or reoperation after hysterectomy with ovarian conservation in women with endometriosis

Author, year	No. of patients	No. of patients with recurrence* (%)	Comments
Cashman,[19] 1944	85	17 (20%)	3 patients died in postoperative period
Counsellor and Crenshaw,[26] 1951	517	23 (5%)	All received radiation therapy for recurrence of pain
Huffman,[51] 1951	155	9 (6%)	
Devereux,[31] 1963	22	0 (0%)	
Sheets et al.,[93] 1964	40	1 (3%)	Vaginal vault recurrence treated with radium
Ranney,[83] 1970	129	1 (1%)	
Gray,[45] 1973	42	14 (33%)	All cases had endometriosis involving the bowel
Andrews and Larsen,[6] 1974	130	3 (2%)	
Hammond et al.,[46] 1976	13	11 (85%)	
Williams and Pratt, 1977[105]	153	15 (10%)	10% were symptomatic; 6% had reoperation
Buttram and Betts,[14] 1979	14	1 (7%)	
TOTAL	1300	95 (7%)	

Modified from Walters MD: Definitive surgery. In Schenken RS, editor: *Endometriosis: contemporary concepts in clinical management,* Philadelphia, 1989, JB Lippincott.

*Defined as recurrent symptoms, reoperation, and/or radiotherapy.

mains controversial and requires a careful consideration of several factors: patient's age, severity of disease, and previous surgical history.

The risk of recurrence after ovarian conservation is thought to be low, although no randomized, prospective trials have been performed. Walters[100] reviewed several retrospective studies and calculated a risk of reoperation of 7% with a range of 1% to 85% (Table 38-2). In a review of patients at Johns Hopkins undergoing surgery for endometriosis with or without ovarian conservation, the incidence of recurrent symptoms after hysterectomy with ovarian conservation was significant (63%), although only half of the patients required reoperation. In this retrospective case review, women who underwent hysterectomy with bilateral oophorectomy also had a significant risk of recurrent symptoms (10%).[71]

Bilateral oophorectomy has the advantage of decreasing the risk of recurrent symptoms of endometriosis but the disadvantage of significant side effects, including severe menopausal symptoms and future risk of cardiovascular disease and osteoporosis. Although estrogen replacement therapy may address these risks, patient noncompliance reported with long-term use requires careful thought to the risk-benefit ratio of surgical castration.[95] Conservation of the ovaries at the time of hysterectomy performed for treatment of endometriosis is an option, provided the patient understands the risk of recurrent symptoms resulting in possible need for reoperation.

For most young women with severe disease, castration is the last resort. Ranney[84] has described several criteria that are indications for removal of the ovaries when hysterec-

tomy is being performed: (1) Resection of endometriosis results in damage to the hilar region of the ovary such that the blood supply is compromised or a sufficient portion of the ovary (at least one third) cannot be saved. When this situation occurs, the ovary is not expected to be hormonally functional and will only cause problems due to adhesions and postoperative pain. (2) Extensive deep endometriosis of the bowel or ureters is present that cannot be resected adequately. (3) Other pelvic pathology is present. (4) The patient is past or near menopause. (5) The patient desires oophorectomy after careful counseling. (6) Hemoperitoneum occurs that requires emergency surgery. In some patients repeated surgery for recurrent symptoms will be required until the last ovarian remnant is excised.[11, 50]

Once castration is completed, hormonal replacement therapy should be initiated. However, the difficult question of when to start estrogen replacement therapy remains unanswered. Although most studies show the incidence of recurrent symptoms to be minimal after hysterectomy with removal of the ovaries, whether or not estrogen replacement therapy can exacerbate disease by stimulating growth of microscopic or residual endometriotic implants remains a theoretic concern.

Despite theoretic concerns, many investigators support beginning estrogen replacement therapy immediately after surgery for endometriosis.[50, 98, 104] Henderson and Studd[49] advocated beginning estrogen replacement therapy immediately after surgery because they could not demonstrate any disease recurrence. One potential flaw with this study is that testosterone was included as a part of the hormonal replacement therapy. Although the dose of testosterone was low, androgen suppression of endometriotic implants may have biased these results. Successful use of estrogen add-back therapy with GnRH analogue in the treatment of endometriosis would support the contention that the amount of estrogen in replacement therapy is not enough to stimulate endometriosis.[40, 98]

COMBINATION THERAPY

A combined medical and surgical approach is often used for treatment of endometriosis. Preoperative and postoperative hormonal therapies have been proposed to enhance fertility rates. There is no "cure" for endometriosis, however, meaning that complete eradication of the disease has not been reported after any therapy, whether medical, surgical, or combination. Recurrence is the rule—probably because medical therapy only suppresses the disease, and surgical therapy removes only the visible implants, leaving multiple microscopic implants over the peritoneum that will grow in time.

The rationale behind preoperative medical therapy is that there will be less vascularity in the pelvis, requiring decreased operating time with less tissue manipulation and better hemostasis, and thus less adhesion formation. (See Chapter 37.) Theoretically, a better pregnancy rate will result. Furthermore, some surgeons prefer preoperative ovarian suppression, which allows ovarian reconstruction without the presence of a follicular cyst or corpus luteum.

The rationale for postoperative medical therapy is akin to the rationale for treatment of malignant mesothelial disease, that is, the disease is maximally cytoreduced. Any residual disease is then suppressed with "chemotherapy" (e.g., danazol, GnRH agonists).[104]

There are several objections to medical therapy in combination with surgery for treatment of endometriosis. One criticism with preoperative therapy is that one of the primary objectives of surgery is to remove disease. However, if the disease is shrunken and less visible after preoperative medical therapy, it will be difficult to recognize and therefore to remove. Another criticism is that the addition of a medical agent to surgical therapy will increase the cost of treatment. Finally, the time span required for treatment is increased when combination therapy is used. This is particularly important in patients with infertility, since couples must complete combination therapy before attempting to conceive. Many couples will be distressed at unnecessarily missing even one cycle of attempted conception. Preoperative therapy requires two surgical procedures: diagnostic laparoscopy and definitive surgical therapy. An interval of 3 to 6 months between the two procedures is needed to complete a course of medical therapy. In postoperative therapy, conception may be delayed for 3 to 6 months after surgery to complete a course of medical therapy. Many clinicians believe that the best chance for postsurgical conception is within the first 6 months after conservative surgery. Therefore, ideally, the infertility pa-

tient should be allowed to attempt pregnancy immediately after surgery for 6 months before postoperative medical therapy is started.[70, 72, 78] Alternatively, a short course of postoperative medical therapy (i.e., 3 months) may be used. With this option, attempts at conception are delayed only minimally.

In one study, preoperative danazol was shown to increase fecundity rates slightly, compared with surgical therapy alone. However, this study was flawed by the lack of randomization of patients.[15] In contrast to these data, based on the original AFS staging system,[4] Olive and Martin[78] compared monthly fecundity rates for patients with endometriosis who received surgery alone, preoperative danazol therapy, and postoperative danazol therapy. No significant differences were found in any of the treatment groups (Table 38-3). This was confirmed by a second study by Chong et al.[21] of 167 infertility patients with minimal pelvic endometriosis. Similar pregnancy rates were achieved regardless of therapy with laser (44.6%), danazol (48.9%), or combination of laser with danazol (51.4%).

The data on postoperative therapy also remains conflicting. Wheeler and Malinak[103] showed an improved pregnancy rate for patients with severe endometriosis who were treated with postoperative danazol. In contrast, Buttram et al.[15] reported that the fecundity rate for patients with severe disease was actually reduced with postoperative danazol in comparison to surgery alone. Thus the use of combination therapy utilizing danazol remains controversial for the treatment of endometriosis-related infertility. The use of GnRH analogues in combination therapy is currently being studied.

SUCCESS IN TREATMENT OF ENDOMETRIOSIS

The two measures used to assess the treatment of endometriosis are the resultant postoperative pregnancy rate and the degree of pain relief. One problem in assessing outcomes relates to the fact that there have been numerous classification systems, making comparisons among patients and studies over time difficult. To date there has been no comprehensive randomized clinical trial that compares all the different modalities of treatment available to the clinician, whether it be surgical therapy, medical therapy, or expectant management.

In a meta-analysis by Hughes et al.,[52] multiple modalities of therapy for treatment of endometriosis-associated infertility were evaluated, including ovulation suppression, laparoscopic ablation, and conservative laparotomy. The outcome measured was clinical pregnancy rate. Ovulation suppression was found to be an ineffective treatment for endometriosis-associated infertility. However, pooled data from the trials of laparoscopic surgery and laparotomy suggested treatment benefit. Potential flaws in this study existed because of the significant clinical and statistical heterogeneity present among the studies analyzed. Another study by Adamson et al.[3] reported a better pregnancy rate in

Table 38-3. Pregnancy rates after laparoscopic electrocoagulation of endometriosis

| Author | No. of pregnancies/No. treated | | | | | Length of follow-up (mo) |
	Minimal	Mild	Moderate	Severe	Combined	
Edward[37]	4/7 (57)[a]	10/18 (56)[b]	—	—	14/25 (56)	13
Hasson[48, c]	0/1 (0)	—	2/2 (100)	4/5 (80)	6/8 (75)	7
Sulewski et al.[97, d]	—	20/42 (48)	20/58 (35)	—	40/100 (40)	37
Daniell and Pittaway[28]	—	—	—	—	33/60 (55)	—
Reich and McGlynn[86]	—	—	—	—	15/23 (65)	18
Seiler et al.[92, e]	—	20/45 (44)	—	—	20/45 (44)	7
Nowroozi et al.[76, f]	—	42/69 (61)	—	—	42/69 (61)	8
Murphy et al.[70, f]	24/36 (67)	18/36 (50)	2/7 (29)	0/3 (0)	44/82 (54)	8
TOTAL	28/44 (64)	110/210 (52)	24/67 (36)	4/8 (50)	214/412 (52)	—

Modified from Cook AS, Rock JA: The role of laparoscopy in the treatment of endometriosis, *Fertil Steril* 55:663–680, 1991. Reproduced with the permission of the publisher, The American Fertility Society.
[a]Values in parentheses are percentages. Stage I by classification system of Mitchell and Farber.
[b]Stage II by classification system of Mitchell and Farber.
[c]Clinical judgment used to evaluate the extent of disease: 1, minimal; 2, moderate; 3, fairly extensive.
[d]Classification system not specified.
[e]Acosta classification system used.[1]
[f]The Revised American Fertility Society classification system used.[5]

Table 38-4. Pregnancy rates after laparoscopic CO_2 laser vaporization of endometriosis

| Author | No. of pregnancies/No. treated | | | | | Length of follow-up (mo) |
	Stage I	Stage II	Stage III	Stage IV	Combined	
Daniell and Brown[27]	—	—	—	—	3/10 (30)	5
Daniell and Pittaway[28]	—	—	—	—	3/15 (20)	6
Kelly and Roberts[57]	3/3 (100)[a]	3/7 (43)	—	—	6/10 (60)	6
Chong[20]	21/32 (66)[b]	—	—	—	21/32 (66)	12
Feste[39]	24/47 (51)	4/6 (66)	2/5 (40)	—	30/58 (52)	12
Martin[63]	7/27 (26)	3/19 (16)	1/4 (25)[c]	—	11/50 (22)	9
Martin[64]	25/56 (45)[d]	22/45 (49)[d]	9/14 (64)[c]	—	56/115 (49)	12
Davis[29, e]	20/31 (65)	—	15/26 (58)	2/7 (29)	37/64 (58)	15
Olive and Martin[78, f]	23/59 (39)	22/48 (46)	10/20 (50)	—	55/127 (43)	—
Donnez[33, g]	26/42 (62)	11/21 (52)	3/7 (43)	—	40/70 (57)	18
Paulson and Asmer[79, g]	109/140 (78)	60/88 (68)	—	—	169/228 (74)	8 to 32
Gast et al.[42, e]	36/70 (51)	12/33 (38)	9/19 (47)	—	50/122 (41)	10
Fayez et al.[38, c]	27/38 (71)	33/44 (75)	—	—	60/82 (73)	12
Nezhat et al.[73, g]	28/39 (72)	60/86 (70)	45/67 (67)	35/51 (69)	168/243 (69)	—
TOTAL	329/553 (59)	230/397 (58)	94/162 (58)	37/58 (64)	690/1170 (59)	—

Modified from Cook AS, Rock JA: The role of laparoscopy in the treatment of endometriosis, *Fertil Steril* 55:663–680, 1991. Reproduced with permission of the publisher, The American Fertility Society.

[a]Values in parentheses are percentages. The original American Fertility Society classification system is used unless noted.[4]
[b]Postop danazol for 132 days.
[c]Postop danazol for 6 months.
[d]3-month course of danazol for 6 to 18 months postop if not pregnant.
[e]Revised American Fertility Society classification system.[5]
[f]Patients treated with either a combination of laser laparoscopy only or a combination of laser laparoscopy and preop or postop danazol.
[g]Patients with factors other than endometriosis excluded from study.

patients treated by operative laparoscopy than in patients treated by expectant management, medical therapy, or laparotomy. These data would suggest operative laparoscopy as the treatment of choice for endometriosis-associated infertility unless severe tubal and/or fimbrial disease were present. Conservative surgery by laparotomy is probably not indicated in patients with minimal or mild disease with patent fallopian tubes. However, larger, randomized, controlled trials are needed to address this question.

Table 38-5. Monthly pregnancy rates with laser laparoscopy and adjunctive therapy

Disease severity and treatment	No. of patients	Monthly fecundity rate (%)	95% confidence limits
Stage I			
Laser only	44	3.5	1.8–4.9
Preoperative danazol	13	1.6	0–3.1
Postoperative danazol	2	3.5	0–10.2
Stage II			
Laser only	22	2.5	0.7–4.4
Preoperative danazol	21	4.4	2.0–6.8
Postoperative danazol	5	2.5	0–4.4
Stage III			
Laser only	12	5.6	1.5–10.1
Preoperative danazol	4	6.1	0–14.5
Postoperative danazol	4	1.5	0–4.4

Modified from Olive DL, Martin DC: Treatment of endometriosis-associated infertility with CO_2 laser laparoscopy: the use of one- and two-parameter exponential, *Fertil Steril* 48:18–23, 1987. Reproduced with the permission of the publisher, The American Fertility Society.

In a comprehensive review article by Cook and Rock,[23] multiple studies were compiled to evaluate pregnancy rates after laparoscopic electrocoagulation (Table 38-4) and laparoscopic CO_2 laser vaporization (Table 38-5). For laparoscopic electrocoagulation, the pregnancy rates were 64% for minimal disease, 52% for mild disease, 36% for moderate disease, and 50% for severe disease. For laparoscopic laser vaporization, the pregnancy rates were, respectively, 59%, 58%, 58%, and 64%. The difficulty in interpreting these data is that expectant management alone in patients with minimal endometriosis can yield pregnancy rates of 65% to 75%.[91] However, many patients are unwilling to wait without therapy. It does appear, however, that surgical therapy can shorten the interval to conception.[77] In reviewing the data, the majority of pregnancies after surgical therapy occur within the first 6 months of treatment.[70, 72]

In infertility patients with more severe endometriosis, there are data to suggest that conservative surgery yields a better pregnancy rate than does expectant management.[77] Mechanical factors from distorted anatomy interfering with ovum release and pickup are often offered as reasons that endometriosis causes infertility. These factors do not improve with observation. Surgery is required to reestablish the normal tuboovarian anatomy. However, the results of endoscopy appear to be as good as those obtained by laparotomy (Table 38-6 to 8) for advanced stages of endometriosis, suggesting that removal of disease may be more important than the particular approach to its removal.

Surgery results in more prompt and complete relief of pain symptoms than do the available medical regimens. Resection of endometriosis will reduce or eliminate pain in 80% of patients.[41] Combined with presacral neurectomy, conservative surgery can be quite effective. However, a significant portion of patients suffer recurrence of symp-

Table 38-6. Pregnancy rates after conservative surgery for mild endometriosis

Author, year*	No. pregnant/ No. treated	%	Cycle fecundity rate
Acosta et al.,[1] 1973	6/8	75%	
Hammond et al.,[46] 1976	2/3	67%	
Garcia and David,[41] 1977	2/3	67%	
Schenken and Malinak,[89a] 1978	11/34	32%	
Buttram,[13] 1979	61/88	69%	
Rock et al.,[88] 1981†	28/45	62%	0.022
Schenken and Malinak, 1982[90]	32/42	76%	
Rantala et al.,[85] 1983	26/44	59%	
Gordts et al.,[43] 1984†	8/20	40%	
Olive and Lee,[77] 1986	5/11	46%	0.039
TOTALS	181/298	61%	

Modified from Olive DL: Conservative surgery. In Schenken RS, editor: *Endometriosis: contemporary concepts in clinical management,* Philadelphia, 1989, JB Lippincott.

*All used staging system of Acosta et al.[1] except where indicated.
†AFS staging system.[4]

Table 38-7. Pregnancy rates after conservative surgery for moderate endometriosis

Author, year*	No. pregnant/ No. treated	%	Cycle fecundity rate
Acosta et al.,[1] 1973	30/60	50%	
Hammond et al.,[46] 1976	3/5	60%	
Garcia and David,[41] 1977	7/19	37%	
Sadigh et al.,[89] 1977	17/23	74%	
Schenken and Malinak,[89a] 1978	12/36	33%	
Buttram,[13] 1979	28/50	56%	
Rock et al.,[88] 1981†	48/88	55%	0.020
Rantala et al.,[85] 1983	22/39	56%	
Gordts et al.,[43] 1984†	42/99	42%	
Olive and Lee,[77] 1986	22/43	51%	0.039
TOTALS	231/462	50%	

Modified from Olive DL: Conservative surgery. In Schenken RS, editor: *Endometriosis: contemporary concepts in clinical management,* Philadelphia, 1989, JB Lippincott.

*All used staging system of Acosta et al.[1] except where indicated.

†AFS staging system.[4]

toms. The definitive surgery for pain related to endometriosis once childbearing is complete is a complete cytoreduction. Radical surgery including hysterectomy with or without adnexal removal should be considered. With this type of surgery only 3% of patients will develop recurrent pain symptoms.

Table 38-8. Pregnancy rates after conservative surgery for severe endometriosis

Author, year*	No. pregnant/ No. treated	%	Cycle fecundity rate
Acosta et al.,[1] 1973	13/39	33%	
Hammond et al.,[46] 1976	0/2	0%	
Garcia and David,[41] 1977	14/49	29%	
Sadigh et al.,[89] 1977	20/42	48%	
Schenken and Malinak, 1978[89a]	6/21	29%	
Buttram,[13] 1979	32/68	47%	
Rock et al.,[88] 1981†	39/81	48%	0.020
Rantala et al.,[85] 1983	18/46	39%	
Gordts et al.,[43] 1984†	20/57	35%	
Olive and Lee,[77] 1986	10/34	29%	0.039
TOTALS	127/439	39%	

Modified from Olive DL: Conservative surgery. In Schenken RS, editor: *Endometriosis: contemporary concepts in clinical management,* Philadelphia, 1989, JB Lippincott.

*All used staging system of Acosta et al.[1] except where indicated.

†AFS staging system.[4]

SUMMARY

Surgery plays a vital role in the management of endometriosis. Recognizing the disease at laparoscopy is key, because endometriosis may present with both typical and atypical lesions. An adequate assessment of the pelvis should be performed in order to stage the disease. Laparoscopy provides the ability to diagnose endometriosis and to begin surgical treatment immediately. Laparoscopy may be used to treat all stages of endometriosis. Laparotomy is necessary when appropriate visualization is not possible through the laparoscope or when the surgeon feels that his or her technique may be superior with a laparotomy. Regardless of the approach, the principles behind surgically treating endometriosis include removing all visible endometriosis and restoring normal pelvic anatomy. Adjunctive procedures for pain relief include presacral neurectomy and laparoscopic uterine nerve ablation. Radical surgical therapy should be reserved for the patient who has completed childbearing and for whom other more conservative therapy has not worked. The roles of second-look laparoscopy and combination therapy need further assessment. Finally, surgical management of endometriosis does not appear to improve pregnancy rates in patients with minimal disease regardless of the method of removal. However, surgery may play a role in decreasing the time to conception.

REFERENCES

1. Acosta AA et al: A proposed classification of pelvic endometriosis, *Obstet Gynecol* 42:19, 1973.
2. Adamson GD et al: Comparison of CO$_2$ laser laparoscopy with laparotomy for treatment of endometriomata, *Fertil Steril* 57:965, 1992.
3. Adamson GD et al: Laparoscopic endometriosis treatment: is it better?, *Fertil Steril* 59:35, 1993.
4. American Fertility Society: Classification of endometriosis, *Fertil Steril* 32:633, 1979.
5. American Fertility Society: Revised American Fertility Society classification of endometriosis, *Fertil Steril* 43:351, 1985.
6. Andrews WC, Larsen GD: Endometriosis: treatment with hormonal pseudopregnancy and/or operation, *Am J Obstet Gynecol* 118:643, 1974.
7. Badawy SZA et al: Diagnosis and management of intestinal endometriosis: a report of five cases, *J Reprod Med* 33:853, 1988.
8. Boeckx W, Brosens I: Microsurgery for endometriosis, *Contrib Gynecol Obstet* 16:286, 1987.
9. Boyers SP, Diamond MP, DeCherney AH: Reduction of postoperative pelvic adhesions in the rabbit with GoreTex surgical membrane, *Fertil Steril* 49:1066, 1988.
10. Bradford JA, Ireland EW, Giles WB: Ureteric endometriosis: 3 case reports and a review of the literature, *Aust N Z J Obstet Gynaecol* 29:421, 1989.
11. Brosens I, Boeckx W, Page G: Microsurgery of ovarian endometriosis, *Hum Reprod* 3:365, 1988.
12. Buttram VC Jr: An expanded classification of endometriosis, *Fertil Steril* 30:240, 1978.
13. Buttram VC Jr: Conservative surgery for endometriosis in the infertile female: a study of 206 patients with implications for both medical and surgical therapy, *Fertil Steril* 31:117, 1979.
14. Buttram VC Jr, Betts JW: Endometriosis, *Curr Probl Obstet Gynecol* 11:24, 1979.
15. Buttram VC, Reiter RC, Ward S: Treatment of endometriosis with danazol: a report of a 6 year prospective study, *Fertil Steril* 43:353, 1985.
16. Buyalos RP: Principles of endoscopic laser surgery. In Azziz R, Murphy AA, editors: *Practical manual of operative laparoscopy and hysteroscopy,* New York, 1992, Springer-Verlag.
17. Candiani GB, Vercellini P, Fedele L: Laparoscopic ovarian puncture for correct staging of endometriosis, *Fertil Steril* 53:994, 1990.
18. Canis M et al: Second-look laparoscopy after laparoscopic cystectomy of large ovarian endometriomas, *Fertil Steril* 58:617, 1992.
19. Cashman BZ: Hysterectomy with preservation of ovarian tissue in the treatment of endometriosis, *Am J Obstet Gynecol* 49:484, 1944.
20. Chong AP: Danazol versus carbon dioxide laser plus postoperative danazol: treatment of infertility due to mild pelvic endometriosis, *Lasers Surg Med* 5:571, 1985.
21. Chong AP, Keene ME, Thornton NL: Comparison of three modes of treatment for infertility patients with minimal pelvic endometriosis, *Fertil Steril* 53:407, 1990.
22. Clement PB: Endometriosis, lesions of the secondary mullerian system, and pelvic mesothelial proliferations. In Kurman RJ, editor: *Blaustein's pathology of the female genital tract,* New York, 1987, Springer-Verlag.
23. Cook, AS, Rock JA: The role of laparoscopy in the treatment of endometriosis, *Fertil Steril* 55:663, 1991.
24. Cornille FJ et al: Deeply infiltrating pelvic endometriosis: histology and clinical significance, *Fertil Steril* 53:978, 1990.
25. Coronado C et al: Surgical treatment of symptomatic colorectal endometriosis, *Fertil Steril* 53:411, 1990.
26. Counsellor VS, Crenshaw JL Jr: A clinical and surgical review of endometriosis, *Am J Obstet Gynecol* 65:930, 1951.
27. Daniell JF, Brown DH: Carbon dioxide laser laparoscopy: initial experience in experimental animals and humans, *Obstet Gynecol* 59:761, 1982.
28. Daniell JF, Pittaway DE: Use of the CO$_2$ laser in laparoscopic surgery: initial experience with the second puncture technique, *Infertility* 5:15, 1982.

29. Davis GD: Management of endometriosis and its associated adhesions with CO_2 laser laparoscope, *Obstet Gynecol* 68:422, 1986.

30. Davis GD, Brooks RA: Excision of pelvic endometriosis with the carbon dioxide laser laparoscope, *Obstet Gynecol* 72:816, 1988.

31. Devereux WP: Endometriosis: long-term observation, with particular reference to incidence of pregnancy, *Obstet Gynecol* 22:444, 1963.

32. Diamond MP et al: A model for sidewall adhesions in the rabbit: reduction by an absorbable barrier, *Microsurgery* 8:197, 1987.

33. Donnez J: CO_2 laser laparoscopy in infertile women with endometriosis and women with adnexal adhesions, *Fertil Steril* 48:390, 1987.

34. Donnez J: Carbon dioxide laser laparoscopy in pelvic pain and infertility. In Sutton C, editor: *Laparoscopic surgery,* London, 1989, Tindall.

35. Donnez J et al: CO_2 laser laparoscopy in peritoneal endometriosis and in ovarian endometrial cyst, *J Gynecol Surg* 5:361, 1989.

36. Evers JLH: The second look laparoscopy for evaluation of the results of medical treatment of endometriosis should not be performed during ovarian suppression, *Fertil Steril* 47:502, 1987.

37. Eward RD: Cauterization of stages I and II endometriosis and the resulting pregnancy rate. In Phillips JM, editor: *Endoscopy in gynecology,* Proceedings of the Third International Congress on Gynecologic Endoscopy, Downey, Calif, 1978, American Association of Gynecologic Laparoscopists.

38. Fayez JA, Collazo LM, Vernon C: Comparison of different modalities of treatment for minimal endometriosis, *Am J Obstet Gynecol* 159:927, 1988.

39. Feste JR: Laser laparoscopy: a new modality, *J Reprod Med* 30:413, 1985.

40. Friedman AJ, Hornstein MD: Gonadotropin-releasing hormone agonist plus estrogen-progestin "add-back" therapy for endometriosis-related pelvic pain, *Fertil Steril* 60:236, 1993.

41. Garcia C, David S: Pelvic endometriosis: infertility and pelvic pain, *Am J Obstet Gynecol* 129:740, 1977.

42. Gast MJ et al: Laser vaporization of endometriosis in an infertile population: the role of complicating factors, *Fertil Steril* 49:32, 1988.

43. Gordts S, Boeckx W, Brosens I: Microsurgery for endometriosis in infertile patients, *Fertil Steril* 42:520, 1984.

44. Gorell HA et al: Rectosigmoid endometriosis: diagnosis using endovaginal sonography, *J Ultrasound Med* 8:459, 1989.

45. Gray LA: Endometriosis of the bowel: role of bowel resection, superficial excision and oophorectomy in treatment, *Ann Surg* 177:580, 1973.

46. Hammond CB, Rock JA, Parker RT: Conservative treatment of endometriosis: the effects of limited surgery and hormonal pseudopregnancy, *Fertil Steril* 27:756, 1976.

47. Haney AF, Doty E: Comparison of the peritoneal cells elicited by oxidized regenerated cellulose (Interceed) and expanded polytetrafluoroethylene (Gore-Tex Surgical Membrane) in a murine model, *Am J Obstet Gynecol* 166:1137, 1992.

48. Hasson HM: Electrocoagulation of pelvic endometriotic lesions with laparoscopic control, *Am J Obstet Gynecol* 135:115, 1979.

49. Henderson AF, Studd JWW: The role of definitive surgery and hormone replacement therapy in the treatment of endometriosis. In Thomas E, Rock JA: *Modern approaches to endometriosis,* Boston, 1991, Kluwer Academic Publishers.

50. Henderson AF, Studd JWW, Watson N: A retrospective study of oestrogen replacement therapy following hysterectomy for endometriosis. In *Proceedings of the ICI conference on endometriosis,* Cambridge, Sept 1989, Cambridge, UK, 1990, Parthenon Press.

51. Huffman JW: External endometriosis, *Am J Obstet Gynecol* 62:1243, 1951.

52. Hughes EG, Fedorkow DM, Collins JA: A quantitative overview of controlled trials in endometriosis-associated infertility, *Fertil Steril* 59:963, 1993.

53. Interceed (TC-7) Adhesion Barrier Study Group: prevention of postsurgical adhesions by Interceed (TC-7), an absorbable adhesion barrier: a prospective randomized multicenter clinical study, *Fertil Steril* 51:933, 1989.

54. Jansen RPS: Early laparoscopy after pelvic operations to prevent adhesions: safety and efficacy, *Fertil Steril* 49:26, 1988.

55. Jansen RP, Russell P: Nonpigmented endometriosis: clinical, laparoscopic, and pathologic definition, *Am J Obstet Gynecol* 155:1154, 1986.

56. Jenkinson EL, Brown WH: Endometriosis: a study of 117 cases with special reference to constricting lesions of the rectum and sigmoid colon, *JAMA* 122:349, 1943.

57. Kelly RW, Roberts DK: CO_2 laser laparoscopy: a potential alternative to danazol in the treatment of stage I and II endometriosis, *J Reprod Med* 28:638, 1983.

58. Kistner RW, Siegler AM, Behrman SJ: Suggested classification for endometriosis: relationship to infertility, *Fertil Steril* 28:1108, 1977.

59. Koszczuk JC et al: Urinary tract endometriosis, *J Am Osteopath Assoc* 89:84, 1989.

60. Lichten E. Three years experience with LUNA: outpatient laser laparoscopic treatment of dysmenorrhea, *Am J Gynecol Health* 3:1, Sept/Oct 1989.

61. Linsky CB et al: Adhesion reduction in the rabbit uterine horn using an absorbable barrier TC-7, *J Reprod Med* 32:17, 1987.

62. Markham SM, Carpenter SE, Rock JA: Extrapelvic endometriosis, *Obstet Gynecol Clin North Am* 16:193, 1989.

63. Martin DC: CO_2 laser laparoscopy for the treatment of endometriosis associated with infertility, *J Reprod Med* 30:409, 1985.

64. Martin DC: CO_2 laser laparoscopy for endometriosis associated infertility with CO_2 laser laparoscopy: the use of one- and two-parameter exponential models, *Fertil Steril* 48:18, 1987.

65. Martin DC, Hubert GD, Levy B: Depth of infiltration of endometriosis, *J Gynecol Surg* 5:55, 1989.

66. Martin DC, Zwagg RV: Excisional techniques for endometriosis with the CO_2 laser laparoscope, *J Reprod Med* 32:753, 1987.

67. Martin DC et al: Laparoscopic appearance of peritoneal endometriosis, *Fertil Steril* 51:63, 1989.

68. Masson JC: President's address: present conception of endometriosis and its treatment, *Trans West Surg Assoc* 53:35, 1945.

69. Murphy AA et al: Unsuspected endometriosis documented by scanning electron microscopy in visually normal peritoneum, *Fertil Steril* 46:522, 1986.

70. Murphy AA et al: Laparoscopic cautery in the treatment of endometriosis-related infertility, *Fertil Steril* 55:246, 1991.

71. Namnoum AB et al: Incidence of symptom recurrence following hysterectomy for endometriosis. Paper presented at the American Fertility Society 49th annual meeting, Montreal, Oct 9–14, 1993.

72. Nezhat C, Crowgey SR, Garrison CP: Surgical treatment of endometriosis via laser laparoscopy, *Fertil Steril* 45:778, 1986.

73. Nezhat C, Crowgey S, Nezhat F: Videolaseroscopy for the treatment of endometriosis associated with infertility, *Fertil Steril* 51:237, 1989.

74. Nezhat C, Nezhat FR: Safe laser endoscopic excision or vaporization of peritoneal endometriosis, *Fertil Steril* 52:149, 1989.

75. Nisolle M et al: Histologic study of peritoneal endometriosis in infertile women, *Fertil Steril* 53:984, 1990.

76. Nowroozi K et al: The importance of laparoscopic coagulation of mild endometriosis in infertile women, *Int J Fertil* 32:442, 1987.

77. Olive DL, Lee KL: Analysis of sequential treatment protocols for endometriosis-associated infertility, *Am J Obstet Gynecol* 154:613, 1986.

78. Olive DL, Martin DC: Treatment of endometriosis-associated infertility with CO_2 laser laparoscopy: the use of one- and two-parameter exponential models, *Fertil Steril* 48:18, 1987.

79. Paulson JD, Asmar P: The use of CO_2 laser laparoscopy for treating endometriosis, *Int J Fertil* 32:237, 1987.

80. Perry EP, Peel ALG: The treatment of obstructing intestinal endometriosis, *J R Soc Med* 81:172, 1988.

81. Pouly JL et al: Laparoscopic treatment of endometriosis (laser excluded), *Contrib Gynecol Obstet* 16:280, 1987.

82. Prystowsky JB et al: Gastrointestinal endometriosis: incidence and indications for resection, *Arch Surg* 123:855, 1988.

83. Ranney B: Endometriosis, I: conservative operations, *Am J Obstet Gynecol* 107:743, 1970.

84. Ranney B: The prevention, inhibition, palliation, and treatment of endometriosis, *Am J Obstet Gynecol* 123:778, 1975.

85. Rantala AL et al: Fertility prognosis after surgical treatment of pelvic endometriosis, *Acta Obstet Gynecol Scand* 62:11, 1983.

86. Reich H, McGlynn F: Treatment of ovarian endometriosis using laparoscopic surgical techniques, *J Reprod Med* 31:577, 1986.

87. Rivlin ME et al: Leuprolide acetate in the management of ureteral obstruction caused by endometriosis, *Obstet Gynecol* 75:532, 1990.

88. Rock JA et al: The conservative surgical treatment of endometriosis: evaluation of pregnancy success with respect to the extent of disease as categorized using contemporary classification systems, *Fertil Steril* 35:131, 1981.

89. Sadigh H, Naples JD, Batt RE: Conservative surgery for endometriosis in the infertile couple, *Obstet Gynecol* 49:562, 1977.

89a. Schenken RS, Malinak LR: Reoperation after initial treatment of endometriosis with conservative surgery, *Amer J Obstet Gynecol* 131:426, 1978.

90. Schenken RS, Malinak LR: Conservative surgery versus expectant management for the infertile patient with mild endometriosis, *Fertil Steril* 37:183, 1982.

91. Seibel MM et al: The effectiveness of danazol on subsequent fertility in minimal endometriosis, *Fertil Steril* 37:183, 1982.

92. Seiler JC, Gidwani G, Ballard L: Laparoscopic cauterization of endometriosis for fertility: a controlled study, *Fertil Steril* 46:1098, 1986.

93. Sheets JL, Symmonds RE, Banner EA: Conservative surgical management of endometriosis, *Obstet Gynecol* 23:625, 1964.

94. Shock TE, Nyberg LM: Endometriosis of the urinary tract, *Urology* 31:1, 1988.

95. Speroff T et al: A risk-benefit analysis of elective bilateral oophorectomy: effect of changes in compliance with estrogen therapy on outcome, *Am J Obstet Gynecol* 164:165, 1991.

96. Stripling MC et al: Subtle appearance of pelvic endometriosis, *Fertil Steril* 49:427, 1988.

97. Sulewski JM et al: The treatment of endometriosis at laparoscopy for infertility, *Am J Obstet Gynecol* 138:128, 1980.

98. Thomas EJ: Combining medical and surgical treatment for endometriosis: the best of both worlds? *Br J Obstet Gynaecol* 99 (suppl 7):5, 1992.

99. Tjaden B et al: The efficacy of presacral neurectomy for the relief of midline dysmenorrhea, *Obstet Gynecol* 76:89, 1990.

100. Walters MD: Definitive surgery. In Schenken RS, editor: *Endometriosis: contemporary concepts in clinical management,* Philadelphia, 1989, JB Lippincott.

101. Weed JC, Ray JE: Endometriosis of the bowel, *Obstet Gynecol* 69:727, 1987.

102. Wheeler JM: Macro- and microsurgical treatment of endometriosis. In Thomas E, Rock JA, editors: *Modern approaches to endometriosis,* Boston, 1991, Kluwer Academic Publishers.

103. Wheeler JM, Malinak LR: Postoperative danazol therapy in infertility patients with severe endometriosis, *Fertil Steril* 36:460, 1981.

104. Wheeler JM, Malinak LR: Combined medical and surgical therapy for endometriosis, *Prog Clin Biol Res* 323:281, 1990.

105. Williams TJ, Pratt JH: Endometriosis in 1,000 consecutive celiotomies: incidence and management, *Am J Obstet Gynecol* 129:245, 1977.

Chapter 39

LEIOMYOMAS

Edward E. Wallach, MD

Uterine leiomyomas are the most common pelvic tumors in women. Traditionally they have been described as present in 20% of women over age 35 years, but their appearance at 50% of postmortem examinations of women suggests a much higher frequency. This neoplasm is variously referred to as leiomyoma, fibromyoma, myoma, leiomyofibroma, fibroleiomyoma, and fibroid. The term *myoma* is widely and acceptably used to describe these tumors, whereas *fibroid* is an inaccurate descriptor. The most acceptable term is *leiomyoma*, however, which more accurately describes its origin and predominant cellular composition. The high prevalence rate of leiomyomas suggests that they usually have a minor influence on ability to conceive but may exhibit a profound effect on pregnancy maintenance. A genetic basis for the presence and growth of uterine leiomyomas appears likely. For example, the incidence of leiomyomas among black women is significantly greater than that among white women. Nonetheless, the increased prevalence of leiomyomas with age, when viewed from the perspective of the current demographic trend toward postponing childbearing, justifies concern over the effects of these tumors on reproductive performance in future years.

PATHOLOGY

Malignant transformation of benign leiomyomas is extremely rare. The often-cited statistic that 0.5% of leiomyomas are malignant overstates the likelihood of malignant change. In view of the high frequency of leiomyomas, the large number of leiomyomas often found in a single uterus, and the rarity of metastases appearing after the removal of uteri containing multiple leiomyomas, the frequency of sarcomatous change is undoubtedly far less than 0.5%. In a review of 13,000 leiomyomas by Montague et al.[38] at Johns Hopkins, 38 (0.29%) cases demonstrated malignant change. Even this figure appears unduly elevated in light of the high prevalence of these benign tumors and the relative rarity of leiomyosarcoma. Corscaden and Singh[15] reported that malignant change developed in less than 0.13% of uterine leiomyomas; the true figure probably is in the order of 0.04%. Only a small percentage of uteri containing leiomyomas are ever surgically removed, thus yielding a much higher denominator than that based solely on surgical procedures performed in which uterine leiomyomas are found. Furthermore, not all of the leiomyomas contained in uteri removed at hysterectomy are sectioned and examined histologically. Also, unless pathologists use strict criteria for the determination of malignancy, cellular leiomyomas may be classified erroneously as leiomyosarcomas.

The microscopic diagnosis relies on the level of mitotic activity and degree of cellular atypism. The latter feature is based on presence of nuclear hyperchromatism and pleomorphism. Tumors with less than 5 mitotic figures per 10 high-power fields (HPF) and little if any cytologic atypia are classified as cellular leiomyomas; those with more than 10 mitotic figures per 10 HPF are considered malignant; those tumors with 5 to 10 mitotic figures per 10 HPF and no cellular atypia are referred to as "smooth muscle tumors of uncertain malignant potential," whereas those with this level of mitotic activity and cellular atypia are classified as leiomyosarcomas. From a prognostic standpoint, a poor outlook can be predicted when tumors display a high mitotic count and cytologic atypia. In contrast to leiomyosarcomas, leiomyomas are characterized microscopically by interlacing bundles of smooth muscle cells arranged in a whorl-like pattern. Nuclei are rod shaped and usually fairly uniform in both size and shape. The spindle shape of the cell is apparent when sectioned longitudinally, whereas in transverse sections the cell appears rounded or polyhedral. Smooth muscle cells are admixed with connective tissue elements to a varying degree.

The evolution of ultrasound as a routine diagnostic procedure during pregnancy over the past 10 to 15 years has increased our understanding of the behavior of leiomyomas in pregnancy. Prior to use of ultrasound, only large leiomyomas were detectable in pregnancy, and those were detected primarily by clinical examination. Aharoni et al.[2] followed 32 leiomyomas in 29 patients serially using ultrasound and found that an increase in size was apparent in only 7; 6 leiomyomas actually decreased in volume, and 19 changed in size by less than 10% of their initial volumes. Thus, in aggregate, 78% of the uterine leiomyomas followed by ultrasound examination actually failed to grow.

Although these data are reassuring, the rates of certain disturbances in reproductive performance—including infertility, spontaneous abortion, and preterm delivery—are increased when uterine leiomyomas are present. Degeneration of leiomyomas during pregnancy is not uncommon. Other complications associated with leiomyomas in pregnancy include preterm premature rupture of membranes, malpresentation, dysfunctional labor, increased abdominal delivery rate, retained placentas, postpartum hemorrhage, and puerperal uterine infections. In the series of Katz et al.,[30] 2% of pregnant women were found to have uterine leiomyomas, while 10% had complications related to leiomyomas per se. Acute red (carneous) degeneration is often accompanied by development of a heterogeneous pattern and anechoic or cystic spaces on ultrasonography.

The two changes in uterine leiomyomas discussed above—malignant change and degeneration—are the most significant. Other secondary changes with leiomyomas include hyaline degeneration, cyst formation, calcification, fatty change, infection, and necrosis not associated with pregnancy. As leiomyomas exhibit growth, they also risk diminution of blood supply, giving rise to a continuum of degenerative changes. The spectrum of manifestations of calcium deposition in leiomyomas ranges from a thin rim of calcium on the periphery, a diffuse honeycomb pattern, a series of concentric rings, or a solid calcific mass. All of these patterns can be appreciated radiographically. Infection or suppurative change most commonly occurs when a submucous leiomyoma protrudes through the cervix and into the vagina, as it ulcerates and becomes edematous. Infection of a submucous leiomyoma may accompany puerperal endometritis and advance to endomyometritis with or without abscess formation. Necrosis and cystic changes are also manifestations of compromised blood supply secondary to growth or to infarction accompanying torsion of a pedunculated leiomyoma. Fatty degeneration of a leiomyoma is relatively rare but may accompany hyalin-

ization of the tumor. More commonly, the yellow appearance observed macroscopically, which suggests deposition of fat, simply represents another stage of necrosis.

PATHOGENESIS OF GROWTH

Uterine leiomyomas are generally accepted as originating from smooth muscle cells of the uterus, although in certain instances an origin from the smooth muscle of uterine blood vessels is likely. Leiomyomas range in size from seedlings only millimeters in diameter to large uterine tumors that not only can fill the pelvis but can reach the costal margin. These tumors may be solitary or multiple. Excessive menstrual bleeding is often the only symptom produced by leiomyomas. Vascular alterations in the endometrium associated with leiomyomas have been correlated with hypermenorrhea. The obstructive effect on uterine vasculature produced by intramural tumors has been associated with the development of endometrial venule ectasia. As a consequence of this phenomenon, leiomyomas give rise to proximal congestion in the myometrium and endometrium. The engorged vessels in the thin atrophic endometrium that overlies submucous tumors contribute to excessive bleeding during cyclic sloughing of the endometrium. The increased size of the uterine cavity and the surface area of the endometrium are also contributing factors in increasing the quantity of menstrual flow. Hypermenorrhea associated with uterine leiomyomas may possibly be aggravated by the presence of endometritis, which is frequently observed histologically in the endometrium overlying submucous tumors.

The growth of uterine leiomyomas is clearly related to their exposure to circulating estrogen. These tumors are most prominent and demonstrate maximal growth during a woman's reproductive life, when ovarian estrogen secretion is maximal. They appear to exhibit a growth spurt just prior to menopause, a phenomenon that may relate to the frequency of anovulatory cycles and unopposed estrogen action, which prevail during the immediate premenopausal years. With the actual onset of menopause, leiomyomas characteristically tend to regress in volume. This regression is often counterbalanced by estrogen replacement therapy. Growth of leiomyomas in the absence of hormone treatment following menopause suggests an extraovarian source of estrogen or its elaboration from an enzymatically active ovarian stroma. Whenever leiomyomas undergo growth after menopause, the potential for malignancy must be seriously considered.

Leiomyoma growth is common during pregnancy and occurs less frequently during the cyclic use of estrogen-progestogen preparations, such as oral contraceptive pills. The increased size of leiomyomas during pregnancy may reflect their dependence on estrogen. In contrast to the influence of estrogens on leiomyomas, progesterone and progestational compounds tend to exert an antiestrogen effect; therefore, in view of this balance between estrogenic and progestational effects, gestational growth of leiomyomas must also represent enhancement of the uterine blood supply that accompanies pregnancy. The success of progesterone and synthetic progestogens in decreasing the size of uterine leiomyomas supports this concept. The relative infrequency of significant growth during oral contraceptive use may reflect, in part, the antiestrogenic properties of the progestogen and/or the low-dosage preparations in current use.

A higher concentration of estrogen receptors has been identified in uterine leiomyomas than in the adjacent myometrium itself and in normal uterine tissue. In addition, it has been reported that uterine leiomyomas bind approximately 20% more estradiol per milligram of cytoplasmic protein than does normal myometrium from the same uterus. Cramer et al.[17] demonstrated heterogeneity in growth potential of uterine leiomyomas when cells were cultured in the presence of hormones. During pregnancy, the rapid leiomyoma growth rate may exceed its blood supply and thereby lead to necrosis. The reduced circulation to these tumors can also result in thrombosis and extravasation of blood. The compromised tumors become dark and hemorrhagic, a characteristic finding in the red or carneous degeneration often associated with pregnancy.

CLINICAL MANIFESTATIONS AND DIAGNOSIS

Most patients with uterine leiomyomas are symptom free. When symptoms are produced they often relate to the location of the leiomyomas, their size, or concomitant degenerative changes. Pain is most often experienced in patients with a pedunculated leiomyoma as its pedicle undergoes torsion. Pain may also be attributed to cervical dilatation by a submucous leiomyoma protruding through the lower uterine segment, or to carneous degeneration associated with pregnancy. In each of these three conditions, pain is acute and requires immediate attention. Other pathologic conditions, including ectopic pregnancy, accident in an ovarian cyst, or acute pelvic inflammatory disease, must be considered in any patient who experiences acute abdominal pain and has identifiable leiomyomas.

Pressure and increased abdominal girth are more commonly encountered than pain, develop insidiously, are often less apparent, and are usually vaguely described by the patient. As leiomyomas grow, pressure is frequently exerted on adjacent viscera. Pressure on the urinary bladder usually provokes urinary frequency, especially when the leiomyoma is located in the subvesical region or when a large myomatous uterus fills the entire pelvis. When the leiomyoma is located adjacent to the urethra and bladder neck, acute urinary retention with overflow incontinence is likely to occur. An enlarging leiomyoma anatomically located just over the cervix may also cause protrusion of the base of the bladder and distention of the anterior vaginal wall, suggesting pelvic relaxation. Stress urinary incontinence may also reflect leiomyomas situated in the vicinity of the bladder

neck. Ureteral obstruction is one of the most serious consequences of chronic pressure on the urinary collecting system. This complication is usually silent and results from pressure of the myomatous uterus on the pelvic brim in the vicinity of the ureter. Unless the kidney has suffered parenchymal damage, this anatomic change is reversible once the pressure is alleviated. Chronic obstruction at the level of the bladder neck can also lead to hydroureter and hydronephrosis. Rectal pressure is rare unless the myomatous uterus is incarcerated in the cul-de-sac or contains a solitary large posterior wall leiomyoma. Constipation or tenesmus may also be associated with a posterior leiomyoma, representing pressure of the tumor on the rectosigmoid.

GROWTH PATTERNS

Since the incidence of malignancy in leiomyomas is relatively low, careful consideration must be paid to specific indications for surgery. A history of rapid growth, especially postmenopausal growth, should prompt removal even in the absence of associated symptoms. The most common reason for rapid growth of leiomyomas is pregnancy. Therefore, in younger patients in whom pregnancy has been ruled out and in older patients beyond menopause, rapid growth must raise the possibility of leiomyosarcoma. Small asymptomatic leiomyomas require only serial follow-up, initially at 1- to 2-month intervals to establish a growth curve pattern; if the growth pattern is stationary, pelvic examinations can be repeated at 3- to 4-month intervals. Leiomyomas often remain constant in size for many years. Since uterine size tends to vary with phase of the menstrual cycle and response to hormonal stimulation, selection of a uniform time in the cycle for each follow-up examination is appropriate. With larger asymptomatic tumors, expectant management may also be justified, provided the examiner has reason for confidence that the pelvic mass is a myomatous uterus and does not either represent an ovarian neoplasm or obscure the detection of such a tumor. If an adnexal neoplasm is suspected, further diagnostic studies are mandatory.

Exploratory laparotomy should be performed if diagnostic studies are not explicit in ruling out ovarian neoplasia. In any event, pelvic examination may be supplemented by ultrasonographic studies, which can provide objective information regarding the size of individual leiomyomas. Since a mass considered on pelvic examination to be a leiomyoma may in fact prove to be an ovarian tumor, an ultrasound study demonstrating normal-appearing ovaries clearly distinct from the uterus is an invaluable source of information. Ultrasound examination also assists in documenting growth of leiomyomas with a finer level of discrimination than that obtained by serial pelvic examination. The presence of hydronephrosis can also be determined through this noninvasive technique by visualizing kidney size and shape.

Conventional radiograms may also supplement pelvic examination. Characteristic radiographic findings of calcification are also reassuring. Intravenous pyelography is more precise than ultrasound in defining renal and ureteral characteristics. In specific cases computed tomography can supplement ultrasound and simple pelvic X-ray studies, although Tada et al.[46] have reported that 5% of patients diagnosed as having leiomyomas by computed tomography were subsequently found to have an ovarian tumor at the time of surgery. Magnetic resonance imaging (MRI) provides better definition of the source of a pelvic mass. Regardless of imaging procedures, in the event of diagnostic uncertainty, laparoscopy or laparotomy should be performed.

No standard size of an asymptomatic myomatous uterus has been invoked as an *absolute* indication for treatment. The presence of a large myomatous uterus in an asymptomatic patient in whom dimensions have not increased and malignancy is unlikely dictates that the patient's age, fertility status, and desire to retain the uterus or to avoid surgery be factored into any treatment decision. A size equivalent to a 12-week gestation had traditionally been the dividing point between surgery and a conservative approach in the asymptomatic patient, but at present, management tends to encompass more flexibility. The therapeutic options are reviewed in the next section of this chapter. In women approaching menopause, relatively large leiomyomas can often be observed serially by pelvic and ultrasound examinations with the confidence that they will diminish in size once ovarian function ceases. However, estrogen replacement therapy during menopause may offset the reduced growth that customarily accompanies cessation of ovarian function. Likewise, a conservative approach should be followed in the younger patient who wishes to preserve childbearing capacity or who desires to establish a pregnancy. Low-dose oral contraceptive tablets currently in use do not appear to exert a growth-promoting influence on leiomyomas. After menopause, asymptomatic small leiomyomas may generally be left undisturbed provided an ovarian neoplasm has been ruled out.

Careful observation is suitable management for most leiomyomas. The majority produce no symptoms, are confined to the pelvis, should not be confused with other pathologic conditions, and are rarely malignant, especially in the absence of rapid growth rate. The major indications for aggressive management of uterine leiomyomas are as follows:

- Abnormal uterine bleeding
- Rapid growth
- Growth after menopause
- Infertility
- Recurrent pregnancy loss
- Pain or pressure symptoms
- Urinary tract symptoms and/or obstruction
- Possibility of ovarian neoplasia

- Iron deficiency anemia secondary to chronic blood loss

THERAPEUTIC APPROACHES AND INDICATIONS

The therapeutic approaches and indications for uterine leiomyomas are conservative follow-up with observation by serial examination; hormone therapy, including use of progestins or gonadotropin-releasing hormone analogues; and surgical therapy, including myomectomy (sometimes in conjunction with hormone therapy) and hysterectomy.

Observation

If the conservative therapeutic approach is chosen for leiomyomas, serial follow-up should be carried out with precise and objective documentation of uterine size and configuration. Physical and ultrasound examinations performed initially and repeated in 6 weeks can provide the physician with a reasonable appreciation of whether the leiomyomas are enlarging and, if so, at what rate. (See Growth Patterns.) If the size appears stationary, serial examinations at 3- to 4-month intervals are reasonable. Temporizing is also appropriate if the patient is in the immediate premenopausal age range. Nevertheless, prediction of age at menopause in individual patients is often unreliable.

Hormone therapy

Progestins. Despite the fact that the endocrine alterations associated with pregnancy may favor the growth of uterine leiomyomas and be associated with profound alterations (enlargement, edema, and degeneration), progestational agents alone seem to have a salutary influence on leiomyoma growth. Progestational therapy has been successfully employed using norethindrone, medrogestone, and medroxyprogesterone acetate to achieve diminution in aggregate size of the myomatous uterus. These compounds produce a hypoestrogenic effect by inhibiting gonadotropin secretion and suppressing ovarian function. Progestational compounds may also exert a direct antiestrogenic effect at the cellular level.

Gonadotropin-releasing hormone analogues. More recently gonadotropin-releasing hormone analogues (GnRHa) have been used successfully to achieve hypoestrogenism in various estrogen-dependent conditions (e.g., endometriosis, precocious puberty, and uterine leiomyomas). Patients treated for uterine leiomyomas using this approach have experienced significant reduction in tumor size. This approach offers great promise as a primary means of conservative therapy or as an adjunct to surgical myomectomy.

The effects of either progestational therapy or GnRHa treatment are transient, and within several cycles after discontinuing administration, leiomyomas tend to return to their pretherapy size. Adjunctive therapy with a 3- to 4-month course of GnRHa should reduce leiomyoma size and render surgery easier, accompanied by less blood loss. This approach has special advantages in facilitating a hysteroscopic resection of a submucous leiomyoma, since the time consumed in the hysteroscopic resection itself is largely a function of tissue volume. An original concern that the tissue plane separating the leiomyoma from surrounding myometrium tends to be more fibrotic and less precise after GnRHa therapy has not been substantiated. Following a course of GnRHa, myomectomy is performed through a hypovascular myometrium, theoretically reducing blood loss.[1] Long-term treatment of young patients is neither practical nor desirable because of the possibility of bone loss as a consequence of hypoestrogenism during prolonged therapy with GnRHa. Pretreatment with GnRHa, however, not only facilitates the myomectomy itself but also provides an amenorrheic interval prior to surgery during which hemoglobin levels can be restored in the hypermenorrheic anemic patient, enabling presurgical blood donation for subsequent autotransfusion. The concern that presurgical shrinkage of small leiomyomas by GnRHa will render them undetectable at surgery and lead to early recurrence was not borne out by a randomized, double-blind study using placebo and leuprolide acetate.[23]

Since short-term use is desirable, GnRHa therapy may also be applied to perimenopausal women in whom reduction in leiomyoma volume may stabilize when menopause occurs shortly thereafter. In the study by Andreyko et al.,[4] a daily dose of 800 mg of nafarelin for 6 months caused a mean decrease in uterine volume of 57% in 10 patients followed by serial MRI. Maheux et al.[36] reported a mean decrease of 71% in leiomyoma size following treatment with intranasal buserelin in 9 patients. Schlaff et al.[44] used leuprolide in a double-blind, placebo-controlled study and demonstrated 42.7% and 30.4% declines in non–leiomyoma and leiomyoma volume, respectively, through serial MRI studies. The possibility of severe pelvic pain accompanying shrinkage of leiomyomas with GnRHa has been suggested by one report.[13] Results of clinical studies of GnRHa therapy for leiomyomas are variable, and at present accurate prediction of responders to GnRHa appear to be impossible.

Surgical therapy

Myomectomy

Indications. Myomectomy should be considered whenever preservation of the uterus is desired for its childbearing function and it is specifically requested. It is also the procedure of choice for a solitary pedunculated leiomyoma. Indications for myomectomy include interference with fertility or predisposition to repeated pregnancy loss due to the nature and/or location of the single leiomyoma or multiple leiomyomas. Infertility is rarely a consequence of uterine leiomyomas, but when a causal relationship is suspected, the location of leiomyomas is usually the significant element interfering with establishment or maintenance of

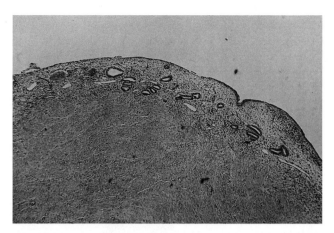

Fig. 39-1. Histologic section from a hysterectomy specimen with chronic endometritis in an atrophic endometrium overlying a submucous myoma.

pregnancy. Locations associated with difficulties in establishing pregnancy include the following: (1) directly under the endometrium, where leiomyomas may interfere with implantation and result in infertility or impair embryonic-fetal nutrition, giving rise to early pregnancy loss (Fig. 39-1) (in addition, chronic endometritis is common in the tissue overlying a submucous leiomyoma and may also adversely affect implantation); (2) impingement on the uterotubal junction, which may cause intramural obstruction of the fallopian tube; (3) a broad ligament site, where a leiomyoma can distort the anatomic relationship between the tubal ostium and the ovary; and (4) supracervical, where leiomyomas can alter the position of the cervix within the vagina, thereby interfering with the opportunity for the cervical os to be bathed in the ejaculate following coitus and thus prevent normal insemination. Indications for myomectomy are as follows:

- Pedunculated subserous leiomyomas
- Submucous leiomyomas with hypermenorrhea
- Rapidly enlarging leiomyomas
- Infertility secondary to leiomyomas
- Desire to retain fecundity
- Desire to retain uterus

Desire for uterine retention cannot be underestimated in our culture. Technology today even enables the uterus of a woman lacking ovaries to serve as a gestational vehicle through the processes of in vitro fertilization, endometrial preparation with exogenous hormone therapy, and ovum or embryo donation. Furthermore, publicity regarding unnecessary hysterectomy has sensitized women in the decision-making process regarding uterine retention in the presence of benign pathology. Wide dissemination of such attitudes may render myomectomy an even more prevalent procedure in the near future than it is today.

Preoperative evaluation. Once having arrived at a decision to perform myomectomy, the surgeon must carry out a

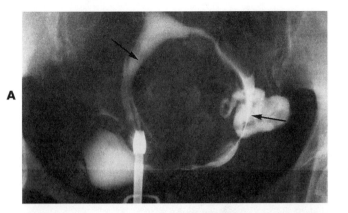

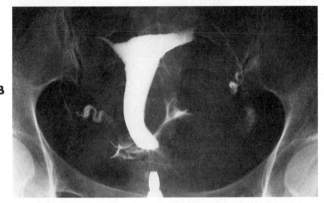

Fig. 39-2. A, Hysterosalpingogram illustrating an apparently normal uterine cavity. A left subserous broad ligament leiomyoma, located between the two arrows, is outlined by radiopaque material which has entered the peritoneal cavity from the patent left fallopian tube. **B,** Hysterosalpingogram illustrating an enlarged and asymmetrical uterine cavity, distorted by a left intramural leiomyoma.

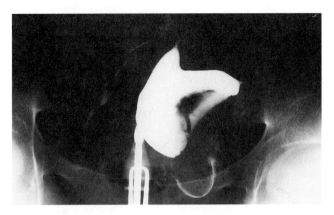

Fig. 39-3. Hysterosalpingogram in a patient with anemia secondary to cyclic episodes of hypermenorrhea. Despite a normal-sized uterus on pelvic examination, the hysterosalpingogram demonstrates a left-sided filling defect, representing a submucous leiomyoma.

careful preoperative appraisal. As with any gynecologic surgical procedure, evaluation of the cervix by Papanicolaou smear is mandatory. Use of imaging to evaluate the size and location of leiomyomas may be helpful, but it is not essential. Ultrasound examination alone may suffice to delineate the topography of the myomatous uterus. If adnexal neoplasia is a possibility, computed tomography or MRI is helpful to confirm whether adnexal pathology or normal ovarian tissue is present. Hypermenorrhea and other forms of abnormal bleeding merit evaluation of the endometrium prior to performing definitive surgery. In a younger patient, who is without significant risk of endometrial malignancy, office biopsy, aspiration, or curettage should suffice. In a patient over age 35 years, thorough curettage is warranted. In either event, a patient with leiomyomas and abnormal bleeding for whom myomectomy is contemplated should have a hysteroscopic examination to determine size, shape, and location of submucous leiomyomas, as well as the feasibility of hysteroscopic resection. At the time of hysteroscopy, a thorough endometrial sampling can be performed. Definitive surgery should be deferred until 4 to 6 weeks after hysteroscopy and

curettage to minimize the chance of disseminated infection through contamination of the endometrium.

A hysterogram is especially helpful before myomectomy because it provides a permanent record of the size and outline of the endometrial cavity (Figs. 39-2 and 39-3). This procedure also enables the surgeon to evaluate tubal patency and/or the proximity of submucous leiomyomas to the interstitial portion of the tubes or tubal ostia. Laparoscopic examination is indicated whenever the nature of the pelvic mass is unclear or adnexal neoplasia is a strong possibility. If the mass is larger than the equivalent of a 10-week gestation, laparoscopy may be technically difficult and is usually unnecessary. If there are sizable leiomyomas or broad ligament extension, intravenous pyelography provides information regarding location of the ureters and presence of obstruction to the renal outflow tract.

Hematologic status, especially when heavy or prolonged bleeding is present, should be appraised well in advance of surgery. The patient with a normal hemoglobin should have two units of her own blood obtained 2 weeks prior to surgery and stored, while she undergoes treatment with supplemental iron. If the patient is anemic, pretreatment with GnRHa or progestational agents can produce an amenorrheic state during which iron stores can be replenished. At the end of a hormonally induced 4- to 6-month interval of amenorrhea, the hemoglobin level should return to normal and permit preparations for phlebotomy and storage of blood for autotransfusion.

Since many patients use analgesics for pelvic pain, cramping, or pressure associated with leiomyomas, a history of drug use is important. If salicylates have been taken, they should be discontinued for a minimum of 2 weeks prior to elective surgery. Aspirin has an irreversible influence on platelet aggregation. Two weeks is ample time to reduce the likelihood of unnecessary blood loss related to medication, since a new population of unexposed platelets is normally generated within 9 days.

Even with stored autologous blood, typing and cross-matching additional units of blood provide protection against the hazards of significant blood loss during surgery.

Abdominal technique. Preoperative hysterography and hysteroscopy can be used to delineate the location and size of leiomyomas in preparation for their surgical removal. These parameters influence the site for the abdominal incision. A uterus with an aggregate size larger than the equivalent of a 12-week gestation or one containing prominent broad ligament leiomyomas usually merits a vertical abdominal incision to facilitate exposure. A transverse lower abdominal incision should be contemplated if the uterus is not of excessive size (greater than 18 to 20 weeks). No discussion of myomectomy is complete without paying homage to William Alexander,[3] who described the first multiple myomectomy; to Victor Bonney,[8] who felt that myomectomy is preferable to hysterectomy; and to I. C. Rubin,[43] who championed the procedure of multiple myomectomy. The general principles for myomectomy involve adequate exposure, hemostasis, and adhesion prevention.

Once the abdomen has been opened, the intraabdominal viscera should be explored, as during any abdominal operation. To optimize exposure, selection of an expedient abdominal incision, use of appropriate retractors, and elevation of the uterus in the pelvis/abdomen by preoperative insertion of a vaginal pack are helpful adjuncts.

To minimize blood loss and preserve the strength of the uterine musculature postoperatively, the site for the uterine incision should be carefully selected so as to facilitate removal of the maximal number of leiomyomas and to minimize the need for multiple uterine incisions. The

incision into the uterus should be made as close to the midline as possible (Fig. 39-4, **A**). A vertical incision made in the midline, although not always possible, can avoid incising vascular areas of the uterus and will help to reduce blood loss. A vertical midline incision also avoids injury to the interstitial portion of the fallopian tube. An anterior uterine incision has the advantage of minimizing the possibility of incorporating the adnexal structures in adhesions that may form postoperatively and usually adjacent to a posterior uterine incision. After selection of an anterior leiomyoma located close to the midline and in proximity to

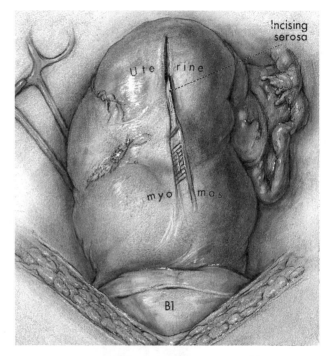

A

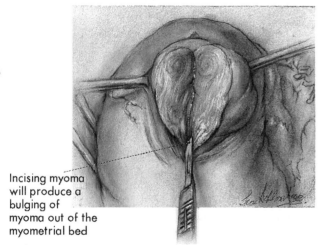

B

Incising myoma will produce a bulging of myoma out of the myometrial bed

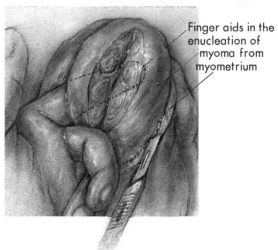

C

Finger aids in the enucleation of myoma from myometrium

Fig. 39-4. Technique of multiple myomectomy. **A,** A vertical incision is made over a leiomyoma on the anterior surface of the fundus as close to the midline as possible. Many leiomyomas can be removed through this single incision. **B,** The incision is extended into the substance of the leiomyoma. **C,** By progressively incising deeply into the leiomyoma, the plane between leiomyoma capsule and myometrium can be identified and bluntly dissected. *Continued.*

D

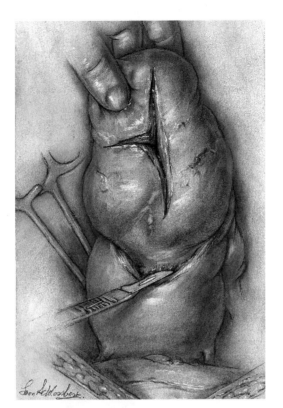

Multiple rows of
interrupted sutures
obliterate bed of
myoma

E

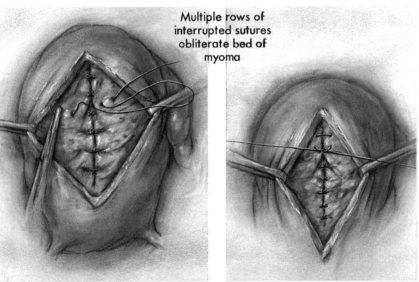

F

Fig. 39-4, cont'd D, Sharp dissection may be necessary to separate the leiomyoma from its capsule at its base. **E,** After the removal of as many leiomyomas as possible, the remaining cavity is obliterated and hemostasis secured. **F,** Multiple rows of nonreactive interrupted sutures of absorbable material are used to close the cavity. (From Wallach EE: Myomectomy. In TeLinde's *Operative Gynecology,* ed 7, Philadelphia, 1992, JB Lippincott Co.)

other leiomyomas, the incision is made in the serosa overlying the tumor and is then extended into the substance of the leiomyoma itself (Fig. 39-4, **B**). By progressively incising more deeply into the leiomyoma, the plane between the capsule of the tumor and the myometrium can usually be identified and dissected bluntly or with a knife (Fig. 39-4, **C** and **D**). Allis clamps or towel clips are then placed on each half of the bisected leiomyoma. While applying traction with the clamps, the base of the leiomyoma can be identified. Hemostasis is achieved once the leiomyoma is removed and when all other adjacent leiomyomas have been excised through the same uterine incision.

Prevention of blood loss. Many techniques have been used to lessen blood loss during myomectomy. An assistant may apply pressure to the edges of the uterine incision to

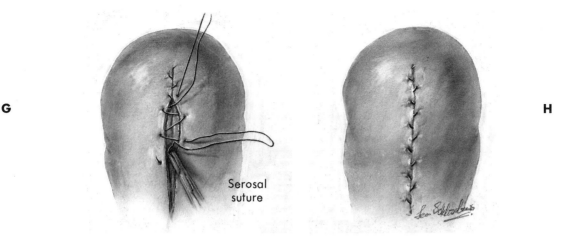

G

H

Serosal
suture

Fig. 39-4, cont'd G, When the dead space has been obliterated, the serosa is closed with a continuous "baseball-type" suture of 5-0 or 6-0 nonreactive absorbable material. **H,** This type of closure approximates the serosal edges. (From Wallach EE: Myomectomy. In TeLinde's *Operative Gynecology,* ed 7, Philadelphia, 1992, JB Lippincott Co.)

limit blood loss. A clamp designed by Bonney[8] encompasses and compresses both uterine arteries at the base of the broad ligament. Alternately, rubber-shod right-angle clamps can be used. Application of a hemostatic rubber tourniquet inserted through the broad ligament and encircling the uterine vessels has also been described. In this case the tourniquet is twisted and drawn taut (posterior to the uterus), grasped with a clamp, then loosened periodically to prevent uterine ischemia. Lock[35] suggested using ring forceps placed bilaterally across the infundibulopelvic ligament and lower portion of the broad ligament for hemostasis.

These approaches may help reduce blood loss from the myomectomy site yet preserve integrity of the blood supply to the remainder of the uterus. Operating with a Bonney clamp or tourniquet to grasp the uterine vessels is usually unnecessary, and these previously described maneuvers tend to be traumatic, especially in a procedure invoked for its conservatism. Rapid, but careful, surgery usually accomplishes the same objective without additional trauma to the uterus. Hemostatic agents such as epinephrine and vasopressin can be injected locally. Vasopressin (one ampule containing 20 units in 20 mL of lactated Ringer's solution or saline) may be injected into the myometrium to limit blood loss. Because of concerns over the possibility of delayed bleeding and a false sense of security with these agents, when this method is used the surgeon should pay careful attention to oozing from the sutured uterine surface prior to abdominal wall closure, which may signify hematoma formation in the myometrium. As previously mentioned, a preoperative course of GnRHa may diminish blood loss by creating a hypovascular myometrium.

Incisional closure. After the removal of as many leiomyomas as possible through a single uterine incision, the leiomyoma bed is closed in layers of interrupted sutures of nonreactive, absorbable material (Fig. 39-4, **E** and **F**). It is virtually impossible to identify discrete vessels throughout the myometrium, and a series of figure-of-eight or mattress sutures placed in the remaining defect is usually effective in controlling bleeding and in obliterating dead space. A pursestring suture may also be used to obliterate a deep cavity in the myometrium. When the dead space is obliterated and the serosal region is reached, a continuous suture is placed in the subserosal tissue using a "baseball-type" stitch (Fig. 39-4, **G** and **H**). This continuous suture traverses the inner aspect of the serosa prior to the superficial surface on each side throughout serosal closure. Alternatively, subserosal sutures of 5-0 or 6-0 nonreactive absorbable material may be used to approximate the serosal edges. If the uterus begins to engorge following serosal approximation, the surgeon should suspect continued bleeding into the leiomyoma bed secondary to inadequate hemostasis. In this case the sutures should be removed and the uterine defect reexamined and resutured to achieve hemostasis.

Prevention of adhesions. Adhesion prevention may be accomplished by careful packing of viscera using laparotomy pads contained in plastic bags. This step will reduce dissemination of lint throughout the abdomen. During the procedure irrigation is carried out using heparinized Ringer's lactate (5000 U of heparin per 1000 mL of Ringer's lactate). The irrigant can be delivered via syringe or through a hand-held apparatus attached to an intravenous fluid bottle and tubing.

As mentioned earlier, the anterior uterine incision is helpful in reducing the formation of adhesions, including those involving adnexal structures. This principle was described in 1898 by Alexander,[3] who stressed the concept of a single anterior uterine incision and removal of all tumors wherever they might be located. A posterior incision is more likely to lead to postoperative adhesions that incorporate the fallopian tubes and ovaries. An anterior

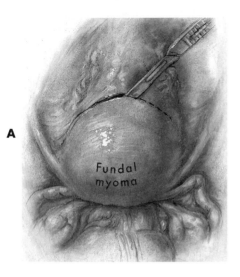

A

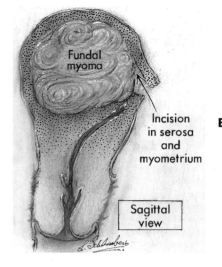

B

Fundal myoma

Incision in serosa and myometrium

Sagittal view

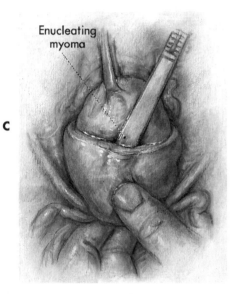

C

Enucleating myoma

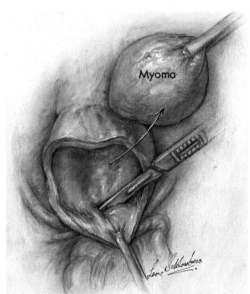

D

Myoma

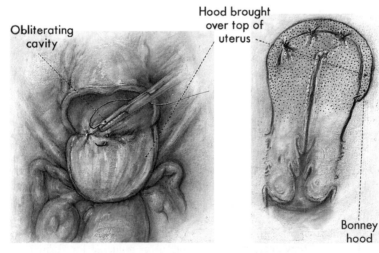

E

Obliterating cavity

Hood brought over top of uterus

F

Bonney hood

Fig. 39-5. Technique of myomectomy using an anterior hood type of incision as described by Bonney.[8] **A,** A transverse incision is made in the anterior fundal wall over the leiomyoma. **B,** Sagittal view of the location of the incision. **C,** Using blunt and sharp dissection, the leiomyoma is enucleated from its bed. **D,** Excess hypertrophied myometrium may be trimmed and removed. **E to G,** Posterior hood is folded over the anterior uterine wall. (From Wallach EE: Myomectomy. In TeLinde's *Operative Gynecology*, ed 7, Philadelphia, 1992, JB Lippincott Co.) *Continued.*

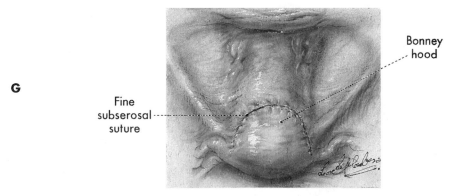

Fig. 39-5, cont'd **G,** Posterior hood is folded over the anterior uterine wall. (From Wallach EE: Myomectomy. In TeLinde's *Operative Gynecology,* ed 7, Philadelphia, 1992, JB Lippincott Co.)

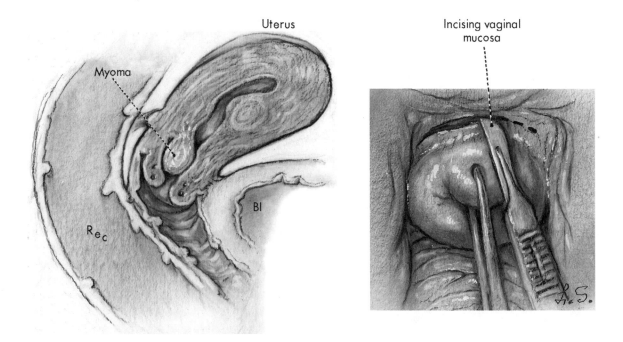

Fig. 39-6. Transvaginal removal of a pedunculated submucous leiomyoma that presents itself at the external cervical os. **A,** Sagittal view of uterus demonstrating the location of the leiomyoma originating on the posterior wall of the fundus just above the cervix. **B,** A transverse incision is made anteriorly through the vaginal mucosa at the cervicovaginal junction. *Continued.*

hood type of incision, as described by Bonney,[8] may be useful in avoiding a posterior fundal uterine incision when approaching posterior fundal leiomyomas (Fig. 39-5, **A** and **B**). This procedure can be accomplished by extending the myometrial incision overlying the leiomyoma to the fundal or posterior fundal region (Fig. 39-5, **C** and **D**), creating a posterior flap that is subsequently folded over the anterior uterine wall (Fig. 39-5, **E** to **G**). A posterior cervical leiomyoma usually cannot be reached through Bonney's hood approach. If the anterior incision is made low enough on the uterine corpus, the peritoneum of the bladder flap may be used to cover it. The uterus can be suspended by plication of the round ligaments, by attachment of the round ligaments to the anterior rectus sheath (Olshausen tech-

nique), or by a Gilliam technique using absorbable suture material such as chromic catgut, polyglycolic acid (Dexon), or polyglactin 910 (Vicryl).

Adjuvant antiadhesion medications should be considered as with reconstructive tubal surgery. Recently a material has been described that can be placed on traumatized tissues to separate raw edges and act as a barrier to the formation of adhesions in reconstructive tract surgery. Interceed (TC-7),[29] for example, a fabric composed of oxidized, regenerated cellulose, can be placed on the deperitonealized area of the pelvic sidewall prior to closure to reduce the extent of adhesion formation. Omental grafts should be avoided because of their adhesion-provoking tendency. In general, no regimen to prevent adhesion formation following recon-

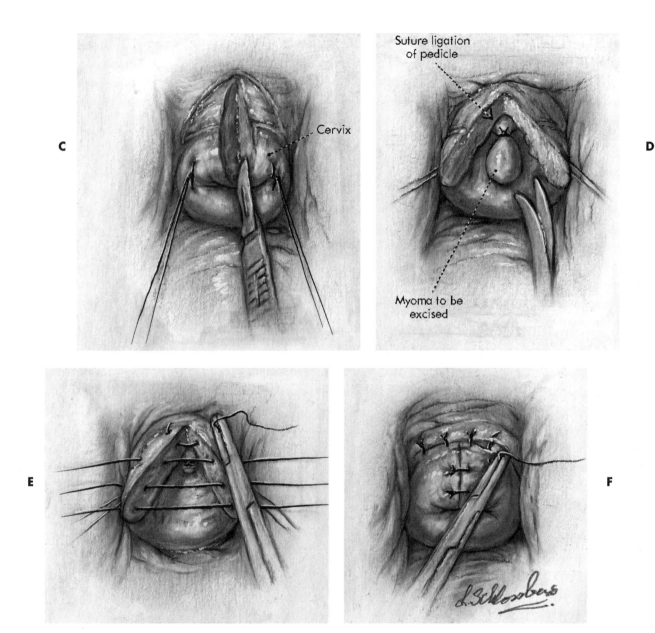

Fig. 39-6, cont'd C, After the bladder is advanced bluntly, the cervix is incised anteriorly in the midline. **D,** The leiomyoma and its pedicle are exposed and the pedicle is suture-ligated for hemostasis. **E,** After the leiomyoma is excised, the cervix is reapproximated with interrupted sutures of 0 absorbable, nonreactive material. **F,** The overlying vaginal mucosa is sutured with interrupted 3-0 absorbable sutures. (From Wallach EE: Myomectomy. In TeLinde's *Operative Gynecology,* ed 7, Philadelphia, 1992, JB Lippincott Co.)

structive surgery on the reproductive tract has been validated. Because of the heightened risk of infection with potential blood-filled spaces in the myometrium, preoperative antibiotics should be administered prophylactically and continued for at least 1 or 2 days after surgery.

Transvaginal technique. Submucous leiomyomas can be surgically removed using a vaginal approach in certain instances. A pedunculated submucous tumor occasionally presents itself at or through the cervix (Fig. 39-6, **A**). This type of tumor can be removed transvaginally through an already dilated cervix by advancing the bladder and making an anterior midline cervical incision (Fig. 39-6, **B** and **C**), or by vaginal hysterotomy. The pedicle of the leiomyoma is identified as high as possible, clamped close to its base, and transfixed (Fig. 39-6, **D**). If the cervix was vertically incised, it is reapproximated with interrupted sutures of 0 absorbable, nonreactive material and the overlying vaginal epithelium is reapproximated with interrupted 3-0 sutures (Fig. 39-6, **E** and **F**). Preoperative and perioperative antibiotic therapy is essential in this approach because of the

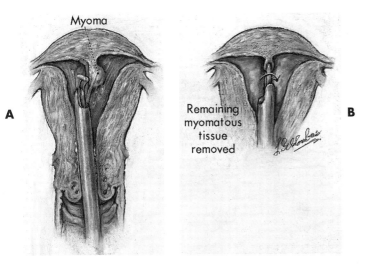

Fig. 39-7. Hysteroscopic removal of a submucous leiomyoma. **A,** After insertion of the resectoscope, the submucous leiomyoma is removed by a process of progressive shaving. The loop of the resectoscope is placed at the most distant portion of the leiomyoma and the current applied as the resectoscope is drawn toward the surgeon. Pressure is exerted by the loop against the leiomyoma with each stroke. **B,** A grasping forceps is used to twist off the remaining tissue once the size has been appreciably reduced. (From Wallach EE: Myomectomy. In TeLinde's *Operative Gynecology,* ed 7, Philadelphia, 1992, JB Lippincott Co.)

hazards of disseminating infection from the prolapsed, inflamed leiomyoma.

Hysteroscopic technique. Hysteroscopic resection of certain submucous leiomyomas avoids the need for an abdominal incision, eliminates the necessity for hysterotomy, and reduces the length of hospital stay. Technologic advances in fiberoptic light sources offer the opportunity to visualize the endometrial cavity directly, evaluate the extent of the leiomyomas, and identify bleeding sites. The development of instruments to resect tissue and electrosurgical means to secure hemostasis have also made hysteroscopic excision of submucous leiomyomas possible. A resectoscope or a cutting loop are adaptations of instruments used for transurethral prostatectomy. Delicate scissors can also be used to shave off portions of the leiomyoma. The medium for distending the uterus, 32% dextran 70, helps the surgeon visualize the tumor despite bleeding and washes away blood before cauterization. In most instances, laparoscopy should be done simultaneously to reduce the hazards of uterine perforation.

Although it is a useful technique, hysteroscopic resection of leiomyomas should not be undertaken by any surgeon unfamiliar and unskilled with either operative hysteroscopy or the specialized equipment needed to accomplish the procedure. Once the resectoscope or hysteroscope is introduced into the uterus, the submucous leiomyoma may be shaved and portions of the tumor removed (Fig. 39-7, **A**). The loop of the resectoscope is placed at the most distant reachable portion of the leiomyoma and drawn

toward the surgeon. In the process the operator exerts pressure similar to that exerted with a curette in performing a curettage. With repeated strokes of the loop, the excised slices of tissue float in the medium (32% dextran 70) and flow out from the uterine cavity as the resectoscope is periodically removed. A grasping forceps can be used to reduce the number of fragments of leiomyoma in the cavity. A forceps can also be used to twist off the residual leiomyoma from its pedicle (Fig. 39-7, **B**). Reinsertion of the telescope enables the surgeon to evaluate the extent of the resection. Rarely is it necessary to remove the entire leiomyoma. The remaining portion is usually passed through the cervix 2 to 3 weeks after the procedure. Most small pedunculated leiomyomas can be removed easily through the cervix.

The hysteroscopic approach is not applicable to all leiomyomas and should be reserved for submucous tumors that are simple, multiple yet not extensive, as well as pedunculated leiomyomas. Selection of patients should be focused on women who desire to retain childbearing capacity, women with a history of hypermenorrhea secondary to development of submucous leiomyomas, and those for whom laparotomy might be hazardous, for example, obese women. The patient and the operating team should also be prepared in each case for the possibility of laparotomy.

Pretreatment with GnRHa can facilitate hysteroscopic resection of leiomyomas by diminishing their size, thereby reducing operating time. Bleeding may be also lessened following a preliminary 2- to 3-month course of GnRHa. Postoperatively, hemostasis can also be achieved by insertion of a balloon catheter into the endometrial cavity. Inflation of the balloon tamponades the bleeding sites. The balloon can be deflated several hours after surgery and removed if bleeding has ceased. A gauze pack soaked in dilute vasopressin inserted into the uterus for less than an hour has been reported to reduce bleeding from the site of hysteroscopic resection of submucous leiomyomas.[47] (See Chapter 58.)

Laser vaporization. The carbon dioxide laser has also been used as a surgical adjunct for myomectomy. During laparotomy, small leiomyomas have been directly vaporized with the laser, and both medium and large leiomyomas were excised in McLaughlin's series.[37] This series cited improved hemostasis, greater precision enabling removal of only abnormal tissue, and ability to remove leiomyomas from previously inaccessible areas as definite advantages of laser vaporization, but acceptance of this technique must be borne out by long-term results through extended follow-up in a larger series of patients, as McLaughlin advises.

Baggish et al.[6] described treatment of submucous leiomyomas with the neodymium:yttrium-aluminum-garnet (Nd:YAG) laser. One approach involves multiple passes with the clear fiber into the substance of the leiomyoma. This maneuver devascularizes the leiomyoma, thereby destroying its blood supply. Alternatively, the base may be transected with the laser and the leiomyoma removed or left in the cavity to be expelled. Slicing the lesion plane by plane reduces the size of the leiomyoma. Elements of the leiomyoma can be removed with a sponge forceps or left to be passed spontaneously. As with the operating hysteroscope, concomitant laparoscopy is advisable.

Hysterectomy. With few exceptions removal of the uterus is the procedure of choice whenever surgery is indicated for leiomyomas and when childbearing has been completed. Hysterectomy is also the favored procedure whenever there is a reasonable likelihood of malignancy within a leiomyoma (e.g., as evidenced by rapid enlargement). If myomectomy is not technically feasible, hysterectomy should be carried out, especially in the presence of diffuse myomatosis of the uterus. Although it is unusual for myomectomy to be technically not possible, the procedure may be difficult, time consuming, and associated with a substantial complication rate. Therefore, to balance the risks of performing a difficult and potentially complicated myomectomy, sufficient indication for uterine preservation should be evident. Hysterectomy is usually a simpler procedure than multiple myomectomy, and it is the procedure to which most gynecologists are more accustomed.

COMPLICATIONS OF MYOMECTOMY

Multiple myomectomy is generally a more difficult and time-consuming procedure than hysterectomy. It is frequently accompanied by significant blood loss, a greater need for blood replacement, a higher frequency of postoperative anemia, paralytic ileus, and pain, as well as a longer hospital stay. Long-term complications must also be considered. The need for future uterine surgery to manage recurrence of leiomyomas is high. Roughly 20% to 25% of patients who have undergone myomectomy will ultimately require another surgical procedure—usually hysterectomy—for recurrences. The recurrence rate for patients with solitary leiomyomas is lower than that in women with multiple leiomyomas (26.8% versus 58.8%). Compared with women from whom a single leiomyoma was removed, the relative risk of recurrence was 1.2 in those with two or three and 2.1 with removal of four.[12]

With deep or multiple intramural myomectomy, cesarean delivery is usually advisable following establishment of pregnancy. Abdominal delivery is the procedure of choice whenever extensive dissection of the myometrium has been necessary. This rule of thumb should supercede the classic adage that cesarean delivery is indicated whenever the endometrial cavity has been entered. The incidence of late intestinal obstruction is higher after myomectomy than it is after hysterectomy, and pelvic adhesions are not uncommon, occasionally serving as a newly acquired factor in infertility. Anatomic impairment of the interstitial portion of the oviduct as a result of dissection in this location may represent an additional cause of postoperative infertility.

The patient contemplating myomectomy should be aware of the hazards of this "conservative" surgery as compared with those associated with hysterectomy for leiomyomas. She should also be advised of the possibility that hysterectomy may be required rather than the proposed myomectomy. Unusual cases of diffuse leiomyomatosis of the uterus discovered at the time of planned myomectomy have occasionally necessitated hysterectomy.[32] The reason for this note of caution is that myomectomy may not always be feasible. Unfortunately, the surgeon is not invariably able to predict the feasibility of uterine conservation, because unforeseen technical factors may accompany the excision of leiomyomas. Despite these drawbacks, most patients who wish to retain their childbearing function will select myomectomy over hysterectomy when given the option. For those who wish to conceive, a delay of 4 to 6 months before attempting pregnancy is advisable following the surgical procedure, since the myometrium is significantly disrupted during myomectomy.

OUTCOMES OF MYOMECTOMY

Evaluation of the outcome of myomectomy must be based on the specific indication for the surgery. Subsequent fertility, diminution of hypermenorrhea, achievement of a term pregnancy, alleviation of pain and/or pressure symptoms, and recurrence rate of leiomyomas can each individually serve as a useful index of successful outcome when keyed to the reason(s) for surgery. By and large, the removal of submucous leiomyomas should result in diminished menstrual blood loss in virtually all women in whom the bleeding has been related to their presence. Regression in size of the uterus is usually apparent immediately, but because of postoperative edema and absorption of blood from intercellular spaces, uterine size does not completely regress until approximately 12 weeks after surgery. The gynecologist may wish to reevaluate the uterine cavity by hysterography following myomectomy, but the procedure should be deferred until 4 to 6 months have elapsed from the time of surgery, when the shape of the endometrial cavity can be truly appreciated. Distortion of the cavity related to the surgical procedure itself persists for a long period of time and can be misleadingly troublesome when hysterography is performed within 1 to 2 months of myomectomy.

In the series of 139 myomectomy patients reported on by Ingersoll and Malone,[27,28] not all were married and desirous of childbearing when surgery was originally performed. The majority of patients under age 30 conceived, and 45% of those between age 31 and 35 established a pregnancy. None of those older than age 39 years at the time of surgery subsequently became pregnant. Of those conceiving, 70% did so within 2 years. In the series of Ranney and Frederick,[41] 28 of 34 married patients of reproductive age (82.4%) gave birth to a total of 48 babies following myomectomy. Berkeley et al.[7] reported that 25 of 50 patients in their series conceived a total of 36 pregnancies, resulting in 24 term and 3 premature viable infants. A striking finding, however, was that only 16% of women who underwent myomectomy for infertility with a myomatous uterus eventually conceived.

The above data are in contrast to those of Babaknia and co-workers,[5] who reported a term pregnancy rate of 38% among 34 patients with primary infertility who underwent myomectomy and of 50% in 12 patients with secondary infertility. None of the 6 women over age 35 conceived. The myomectomy-to-conception interval was short, with 73% conceiving within 1 year. The figures of Babaknia et al.[5] are in line with those of Lock,[35] who, after presenting his own experience and reviewing the literature, concluded that when multiple myomectomy is performed for primary infertility in the absence of other casual factors, between 40% and 50% of patients will subsequently become pregnant. Buttram and Reiter[11] reviewed 18 studies encompassing 1193 women in whom myomectomy was performed for infertility; 480 (40%) of these women conceived postoperatively. The same authors reviewed outcomes among 1941 myomectomy patients and compared preoperative and postoperative abortion rates. The reduction in abortion rate following myomectomy from 41% to 19% suggests improvement in reproductive salvage through the use of this procedure.

REFERENCES

1. Adamson GD: Treatment of uterine fibroids: current findings with gonadotropin-releasing hormone agonists, *Am J Obstet Gynecol* 166:746, 1992.
2. Aharoni A et al: Patterns of growth of uterine leiomyomas during pregnancy: a prospective longitudinal study, *Br J Obstet Gynaecol* 95:510, 1988.
3. Alexander W: Enucleation of uterine fibroids, *Br Gynaecol J* 14:47, 1898.
4. Andreyko J et al: Use of an agonistic analog of gonadotrophin-releasing hormone (nafarelin) to treat leiomyomas: assessment by magnetic resonance imaging, *Am J Obstet Gynecol* 158:903, 1988.
5. Babaknia A, Rock JA, Jones HW Jr: Pregnancy success following abdominal myomectomy for infertility, *Fertil Steril* 30:644, 1978.
6. Baggish MS, Sze EHM, Morgan G: Hysteroscopic treatment of symptomatic submucous myomata uteri with the Nd:YAG laser, *J Gynecol Surg* 5:27, 1989.
7. Berkeley A, DeCherney A, Polan M: Abdominal myomectomy and subsequent fertility, *Surg Gynecol Obstet* 156:319, 1983.
8. Bonney V: The technique and results of myomectomy, *Lancet* 1:171, 1931.
9. Briggs DW: Abdominal myomectomy in the treatment of uterine myomas, *Am J Obstet Gynecol* 93:769, 1966.
10. Brown AB, Chamberlain R, TeLinde RW: Myomectomy, *Am J Obstet Gynecol* 71:759, 1956.
11. Buttram VC Jr, Reiter RC: Uterine leiomyomata: etiology, symptomatology, and management, *Fertil Steril* 36:43, 1981.
12. Candiani GB et al: Risk of recurrence after myomectomy, *Br J Obstet Gynaecol* 98:385, 1991.
13. Chipato T et al: Pelvic pain complicating LHRH analogue treatment of fibroids, *Aust N Z J Obstet Gynaecol* 31:383, 1991.
14. Coddington C et al: Long-acting gonadotropin hormone-releasing hormone analog used to treat uteri, *Fertil Steril* 45:624, 1986.
15. Corscaden JF, Singh BP: Leiomyosarcoma of the uterus, *Am J Obstet Gynecol* 75:149, 1958.
16. Coutinho EM, Goncalves MT: Long-term treatment of leiomyomas with gestrinone, *Fertil Steril* 51:939, 1989.
17. Cramer S et al: Growth potential of human uterine leiomyomas: some in vitro observations and their implications, *Obstet Gynecol* 66:36, 1985.
18. Davids AM: Myomectomy: surgical treatment and results in a series of 1,150 cases, *Am J Obstet Gynecol* 63:592, 1952.
19. Dearnley G: The place of myomectomy in the treatment of primary infertility, *Proc R Soc Med* 49:252, 1956.
20. Donnez J et al: Treatment of uterine fibroids with implants of gonadotropin-releasing hormone agonists: assessment by hysterography, *Fertil Steril* 51:947, 1989.
21. Farber M et al: Estradiol binding by fibroid tumors and normal myometrium, *Obstet Gynecol* 40:479, 1972.
22. Farrer-Brown G, Beilby W, Tarbit M: Venous changes in the endometrium of myomatous uteri, *Obstet Gynecol* 38:743, 1971.
23. Friedman AJ et al: Recurrence of myomas after myomectomy in women pretreated with leuprolide acetate depot or placebo, *Fertil Steril* 58:205, 1992.
24. Fujii S: Leiomyomatosis peritonealis disseminata. In Williams CJ et al, editors: *Textbook of uncommon cancer,* New York, 1988, John Wiley & Sons.
25. Goldzieher J et al: Induction of degenerative changes in uterine leiomyomas by high-dosage progestin therapy, *Am J Obstet Gynecol* 96:1078, 1966.
26. Healy D, Fraser H, Lawson S: Shrinkage of a uterine fibroid after subcutaneous infusion of a LHRH agonist, *Br Med J* 289:1267, 1984.
27. Ingersoll F, Malone L: Fertility following myomectomy, *Fertil Steril* 14:596, 1963.
28. Ingersoll F, Malone L. Myomectomy: an alternative to hysterectomy, *Arch Surg* 100:557, 1970.
29. Interceed (TC7) Adhesion Barrier Study Group: Prevention of post-surgical adhesions by Interceed (TC7), an absorbable adhesion barrier: a prospective, randomized multicenter clinical study, *Fertil Steril* 51:933, 1989.
30. Katz VL, Dotters DJ, Droegemueller W: Complications of uterine leiomyomas in pregnancy, *Obstet Gynecol* 73:593, 1989.
31. Kelly HA, Cullen TS: *Myomata of the uterus,* Philadelphia, 1907, WB Saunders Co.
32. Lapan B, Solomon L: Diffuse leiomyomatosis of the uterus precluding myomectomy, *Obstet Gynecol* 53(suppl 3):82S, 1979.
33. Letterie GS et al: Efficacy of a gonadotropin-releasing hormone agonist in the treatment of uterine leiomyomata: long-term follow-up, *Fertil Steril* 51:951, 1989.
34. Lev-Toaff AS et al: Leiomyomas in pregnancy: sonographic study, *Radiology* 164:375, 1987.
35. Lock F: Multiple myomectomy, *Am J Obstet Gynecol* 104:642, 1969.
36. Maheux R, Lemay A, Merat P: Use of intranasal luteinizing hormone-releasing hormone agonist in uterine leiomyomas, *Fertil Steril* 47:229, 1987.
37. McLaughlin D: Micro-laser myomectomy technique to enhance reproductive potential: a preliminary report, *Lasers Surg Med* 2:107, 1982.
38. Montague A, Swartz A, Woodruff J: Sarcoma arising in a leiomyoma of the uterus, *Am J Obstet Gynecol* 92:421, 1965.
39. Neuwirth RS: Hysteroscopic management of symptomatic submucous fibroids, *Obstet Gynecol* 62:509, 1983.
40. Pfeffer WH: Adjuvants in tubal surgery, *Fertil Steril* 33:245, 1980.
41. Ranney B, Frederick I: The occasional need for myomectomy, *Obstet Gynecol* 53:437, 1979.
42. Replogle RL, Johnson R, Gross RE: Prevention of postoperative intestinal adhesions with combined promethazine and dexamethasone therapy, *Ann Surg* 163:580, 1966.
43. Rubin I: Progress in myomectomy, *Am J Obstet Gynecol* 44:196, 1942.

44. Schlaff WD et al: A placebo controlled trial of a depot GnRH analog (leuprolide) in the treatment of uterine leiomyomata, *Obstet Gynecol* 00:000, 199x.

45. Sutherland JA et al: Ultrastructure and steroid binding studies in leiomyomatosis peritonealis disseminata, *Am J Obstet Gynecol* 136:1992, 1980.

46. Tada S et al: Computed tomographic features of uterine myoma, *J Comput Assist Tomogr* 5:866, 1981.

47. Townsend DE: Vasopressin pack for treatment of bleeding after myoma resection, *Am J Obstet Gynecol* 165:1405, 1991.

48. Wallach EE: Evaluation and management of uterine causes of infertility, *Clin Obstet Gynecol* 22:43, 1979.

Chapter 40

SURGERY OF THE MALE REPRODUCTIVE TRACT

Abraham T. K. Cockett, MD

VARICOCELE PROCEDURE

Pathophysiology of varicocele

The varicocele, dilatation of the left spermatic vein due to venous insufficiency, has challenged andrologists and urologists for decades because of its role in male factor infertility. Many clinicians have noted that in an andrology clinic approximately 40% of husbands arriving for a complete evaluation for infertility have a left varicocele. Approximately 65% of this group also have a right varicocele, leading to a final diagnosis of bilateral varicoceles.

The pathophysiology of the varicocele has been recently summarized.[4] In the main, the male patient with a left varicocele or bilateral varicoceles may have an increased testicular core temperature, approximately 1.5°C higher than the scrotal temperature. The testicular volume is also significantly smaller on both sides, particularly in the presence of bilateral varicoceles, compared with a normal fertile male of similar height and weight.[5] For an average man who is 5 ft 9 in tall and weighs 165 to 170 lb the right testicle will have a volume of 24 mL ± 2 mL, and the left testicle will have a volume of 21 mL ± 1.5 mL. A man who is 6 ft tall and weighs 195 to 205 lb will have a right testicular volume of 32 to 34 mL and a left testicular volume of 28 to 30 mL.

A reduced sperm count (below 20 million/mL) will be reflected in a reduced testicular volume bilaterally even if only a left varicocele has been detected in the upright position.

Poor motility and a significantly higher percentage of immature spermatozoa or tapered forms (18% to 35%) are found in impressive numbers of patients with symptomatic varicoceles. Asymptomatic prostatic infection with *Ureaplasma urealyticum* or *Chlamydia trachomatis* organisms can also result in a very poor motility score, and such an asymptomatic infection needs antibiotic treatment.[6]

Over the past two decades at the University of Rochester Medical Center a right varicocele has been found to coexist with a left varicocele in most male patients (65%) with proven male infertility. The surgical approach is an extraperitoneal procedure that focuses on each spermatic vein, near or close to the point where the spermatic veins join their major emptying venous tributaries. On the left the spermatic vein empties into the left renal vein; on the right the spermatic vein empties into the vena cava. The spermatic venous, horizontal crossovers probably account for most of the right varicoceles found. These venous communications between the left and right spermatic veins occur at the level of L-2 (second lumbar vertebra), with the flow starting from the left spermatic vein and extending to the right spermatic vein because of pressure differences. It has also been confirmed that venous crossovers occur in the bony pelvic cavity, behind the symphysis pubis, and intrascrotally between the left and right spermatic veins.[3]

Serotonin levels have been reported to be elevated in spermatic vein blood in two groups of patients.[1] These increased concentrations might help to explain the poor motility and the increased numbers of tapered and immature spermatozoa in men with symptomatic varicoceles.

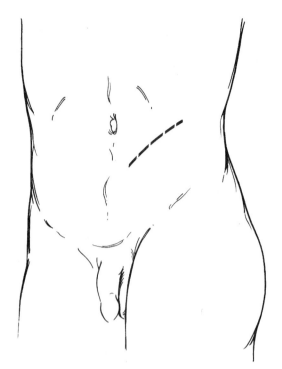

Fig. 40–1. Left-sided, slightly oblique line of incision for a bilateral approach. A similar incision is made on the opposite side. (Redrawn from Cockett ATK: *Manual of urologic surgery,* New York, 1979, Springer-Verlag.)

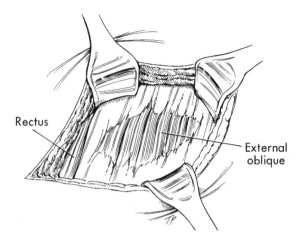

Fig. 40-2. The approach to the left spermatic vein is extraperitoneal. The muscles are separated between muscle fibers. In an obese patient only the external oblique muscle is incised along the horizontal plane. Added exposure can also be gained by incising the lateral left border of the rectus sheath. (Redrawn from Cockett ATK: *Manual of urologic surgery,* New York, 1979, Springer-Verlag.)

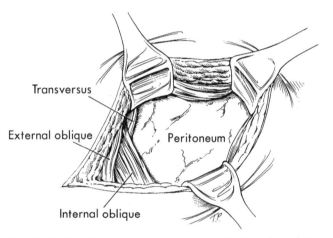

Fig. 40-3. The deeper muscles are separated. The edge of the rectus abdominis muscle can be seen on the medial aspect. The illustration includes the internal oblique and transversus abdominis muscles. By using narrow Deaver retractors medially, one can easily reach the floor of the cavity. (Redrawn from Cockett ATK: *Manual of urologic surgery,* New York, 1979, Springer-Verlag.)

Varicocelectomy

The surgical approach to varicocele repair is as follows: A left-sided, slightly oblique incision is made (Fig. 40-1). The abdominal muscles are then carefully and bluntly separated by forceps and finger dissection along the lines of the muscle fibers (Fig. 40-2). Next the peritoneal lining and its contents are carefully retracted medially to expose the psoas major muscle and the venous plexus (Fig. 40-3). Often the left spermatic vein and one or two secondary venous branches may be present. Each vein is dissected, doubly clamped, and divided in between (Fig. 40-4). The use of 2.0 silk provides permanent ligation of the veins. If the second vein is smaller, the use of 3.0 silk is recommended.

For a bilateral procedure a similar incision is made on the right side. Dissection is performed as described for a left varicocele. Unless the patient is obese, the bilateral varicocele operation can be completed in about 1 hour.

Results of surgery

The results of surgery at the University of Rochester are as follows: If only a left varicocele was present, the pregnancy rate after surgery is 71%. If bilateral varicocele surgery was performed, the pregnancy rate is 57%. The peak pregnancy rate occurs in the first 12 to 18 months after surgery.

PENILE AND SCROTAL PROCEDURES

Vasovasostomy

Microscopic vasovasostomy appears to be the most accurate way to reconstruct and repair both ends of the vas deferens in a patient who has previously undergone a bilateral partial vasectomy to achieve an infertile or sterile situation in his lifestyle. Microscopic vasovasostomy requires the use of a surgical operating microscope for anastomosis of both cleanly cut ends of the vas deferens. It is usually necessary to dilate the lumen of the proximal end,

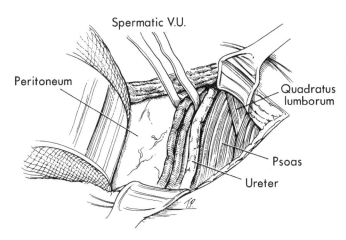

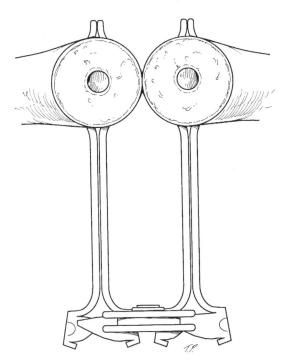

Fig. 40-4. By exposing the psoas major muscle medially, one comes upon the tranversalis fascia, which serves as an envelope around the spermatic vein. Careful dissection through the envelope will reveal at least one spermatic vein or, in most instances, two or more spermatic veins. After the veins are exposed they are doubly ligated and transected in between. The ureter is not exposed by carefully following this approach. In the illustration, however, the ureter is shown for orientation. The ureter is often slightly adherent to the posterior parietal peritoneum. (Redrawn from Cockett ATK: *Manual of urologic surgery,* New York, 1979, Springer-Verlag.)

Fig. 40-5. Diagram of both cut ends of the vas deferens in a vasovasostomy clamp, ready to start mucosal and seromuscular approximation. (Redrawn from Cos LR et al: *Urology* 22:567, 1983.)

which has not been under any pressure as a result of the previous bilateral partial vasectomy. The anastomosis is usually performed in two layers, having as a basic aim of the procedure an almost "perfect" mucosal approximation. Usually 9.0 absorbable suture is used, and the knots are exteriorized. For the most part stents are not routinely used. The procedure is as follows: After adequate hemostasis is obtained both cut ends of the vas deferens are carefully immobilized and placed in a special clamp (Fig. 40-5).

Placement of the first mucosal suture is illustrated in Fig. 40-6. Gentle spreading of the lumen using microsurgical forceps is emphasized. In Fig. 40-7 the first suture has been tied, clearly demonstrating the approximation of both edges of the mucosa. Several more sutures are placed in the posterior wall, allowing anastomosis of mucosal and muscular layers as shown in Fig. 40-8, which also shows placement of the anterior suture. In Fig. 40-9 the anastomosis is being completed with a second layer of sutures as demonstrated.[2]

It is now well known that antisperm antibodies develop in a man who has undergone a bilateral partial vasectomy. The highest antibody titers occur 3 to 5 years after surgery for sterilization, and it is usually appropriate to inform the man contemplating remarriage that the results of surgery—vasovasostomy—will be less successful in promoting a new pregnancy if the interval of sterilization is 5 years or more. High levels of the antisperm antibodies will diminish the likelihood of future pregnancies.

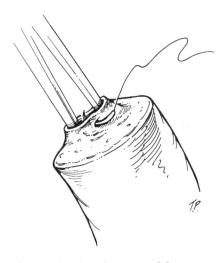

Fig. 40-6. Diagram showing placement of first mucosal suture; notice gentle spreading of the lumen, using microsurgical forceps. (Redrawn from Cos LR et al: *Urology* 22:567, 1983.)

Testicular biopsy

Testicular biopsy can be performed under local or regional anesthesia. A surgical incision 3 mm into the tunica albuginea will lead to expression outward of seminiferous tubules. (Use of a buffered solution to preserve the seminiferous tubules is important after biopsy.) After anchoring the tunica with 3-0 chromic catgut sutures, the tubules are sharply excised in a guillotine fashion with a

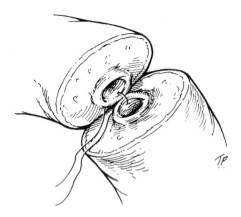

Fig. 40-7. First tied-down suture approximating both edges of the vas deferens mucosa. (Redrawn from Cos LR et al: *Urology* 22:567, 1983.)

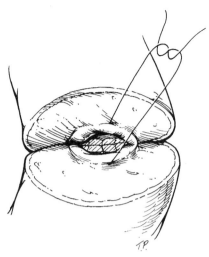

Fig. 40-8. Posterior wall anastomosis of the mucosal layer has been completed. Placement of anterior suture is shown. (Redrawn from Cos LR et al: *Urology* 22:567, 1983.)

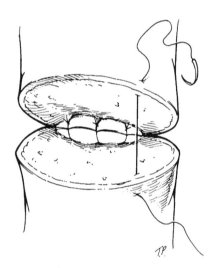

Fig. 40-9. Illustration showing anastomosis completed. (Redrawn from Cos LR et al: *Urology* 22:567, 1983.)

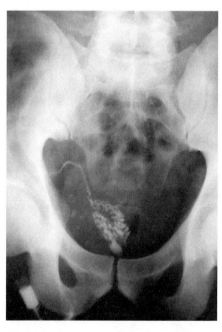

Fig. 40-10. Seminal vesiculogram performed by isolating the right vas deferens and cannulating the lumen with the pointed end directed proximally toward the verumontanum. Approximately 4 mL of diluted aqueous intravenous contrast medium was injected. The X-ray film reveals complete obstruction at the cap of the verumontanum.

small, sharp blade. Unilateral seminal vesiculography by carefully cannulating the lumen of the proximal vas deferens is often performed to rule out obstruction. This exposure is followed by a second incision over the vas deferens. Approximately 2.5 mL of a blue-tinged saline solution is then injected. Cystoscopy will confirm the presence of dye in the bladder (indigo carmine diluted in a syringe) and thus confirm the patency of the vas deferens, the ejaculatory duct, and the seminal vesicle.

Urethrotomy

Cystoscopy and urethroscopy are often necessary to rule out the presence of a urethral stricture or the rare presence of a blocked verumontanum (colliculus seminalis). If a stricture is encountered in the bulbous urethra, an internal urethrotomy is performed. The patient is treated before, during, and after this procedure with appropriate antibiotics. An indwelling urethral catheter is left in place for 2 to

5 days, depending on the character of the stricture and the ease of the urethrotomy.

PROSTATE (VERUMONTANUM) PROCEDURE
Case report

C. T., a 32-year-old white man, came to the andrology clinic for an infertility evaluation. He was active in sports, and had had knee surgery in 1978 and again in 1987. The remainder of his medical history was not remarkable. He was able to have erections and to perform sexually as a husband. A semen sample was analyzed, and it was noted that he had no sperm. The patient later came to our unit because of his infertility. We obtained a semen sample and confirmed the fact that he did not have any sperm, nor any seminal plasma. Blood was drawn for measurement of follicle-stimulating hormone, luteinizing hormone, and testosterone. All of the values were normal. We did see evidence for an asymptomatic infection (neutrophils in the semen); he and his wife were appropriately treated with doxycycline for 35 days to eradicate the asymptomatic infection. A transrectal ultrasound was thought to be indicated, which revealed enlarged ejaculatory ducts and seminal vesicles, pointing to an obstructive component. Seminal vesiculography subsequently was performed (Fig. 40-10). This study clearly showed obstruction at the utricle.

Outcome

The patient underwent two unroofing procedures of the verumontanum, but they did not result in any viable sperm.

However, from other reports involving younger patients, unroofing of the utricle has provided good spermatozoa and seminal plasma. Several reports indicate that pregnancies have occurred. A major emphasis of this report is that if complete azoospermia is seen without any ejaculum, transrectal ultrasound of the prostate and seminal vesicles is indicated; this should be performed at the second visit.

REFERENCES

1. Caldamone AA, Al-Juburi A, Cockett ATK: Varicoceles: elevated serotonin and infertility, *J Urol* 123:683, 1980.
2. Cos LR et al: Vasovasostomy: current state of the art, *Urology* 22:567, 1983.
3. Erturk E, Scheinfeld J, Cockett ATK: Case profile: male infertility due to communicating bilateral varicoceles, *Urology* 24:390, 1984.
4. Takihara H, Sakatoku J, Cockett ATK: The pathophysiology of varicocele in male infertility, *Fertil Steril* 55:861, 1991.
5. Takihara H et al: Significance of testicular size measurement in andrology, II: correlation of testicular size with testicular function, *J Urol* 137:416, 1987.
6. Valvo JR et al: Elevated seminal pH and *Ureaplasma urealyticum, J Androl* 3:144, 1982.

Part VI

ASSISTED REPRODUCTIVE TECHNOLOGIES

Chapter 41

HOMOLOGOUS ARTIFICIAL INSEMINATION

John S. Hesla, MD

Artificial insemination of women has been performed for centuries. However, it has only been over the past two decades that supracervical placement of a motile fraction of spermatozoa that has been separated from seminal plasma has gained widespread popularity as therapy for various etiologies of infertility. Unfortunately, the true efficacy of these techniques is still being determined, because few prospective, randomized, controlled clinical trials have been published that have been designed to provide definitive answers. This chapter attempts to provide the reader with a contemporary perspective regarding the evolving role of insemination with husband's sperm in clinical practice.

INTRACERVICAL INSEMINATION

Indications

Intracervical insemination (ICI) is appropriate therapy to enhance fecundity in only limited circumstances. These include conditions in which intravaginal intercourse with ejaculation in the pericervical area is not possible or, more commonly, when the use of donor sperm is planned.[131] Anatomic anomalies of the penis or vagina; organic, drug-related, or psychogenic impotence; and severe dyspareunia may prevent effective coitus. In cases of retrograde ejaculation, sperm may be recovered from urine after orgasm and placed in an intracervical or intrauterine location.[24] In addition, artificial insemination may be useful in an occasional case of severe hypospermia[125]; consistently low semen volume may lead to delayed conception.[108] Premature ejaculation, vaginismus, and psychologic impotence or dyspareunia are best approached through treatment by a sexual therapist, with artificial insemination reserved for refractory cases.[130] There are no substantive data to support the use of ICI for cases of infertility secondary to abnormalities of sperm density, motility, or morphology; immunologic or sperm-mucus hostility factors; and female infertility factors such as endometriosis, ovulation defects, and tubal disease (Tables 41-1 and 41-2).

Technique

Cervical mucus acts as both a filter and a reservoir for sperm during the periovulatory time period. The ability of sperm to penetrate the mucus is directly related to its motility.[124] Laboratory processing of sperm for insemination in the intracervical area is unnecessary, since normal cervical mucus provides this function naturally. No more than 0.5 mL of whole semen should be introduced into the cervical canal by use of an acorn-tip cannula or syringe when performing this procedure. Greater amounts may enter the endometrial cavity and cause severe cramping.[130]

Table 41-1. Intracervical insemination for oligospermia: cumulative pregnancy rates

	Year	Patients	Pregnant No.	%
Amelar and Hotchkiss*[12]	1965	10	4	40
Behrman and Sawada[17]	1966	4	1	25
Decker†[42]	1978	155	27	17
Eckerling[51]	1960	4	0	0
Harrison‡[72]	1978	20	0	0
Nunley et al.[133]	1978	17	4	23
Russell[148]	1960	34	2	6
Scott et al.[152]	1977	14	5	36
Speichinger and Mattox[162]	1976	13	1	8
Steiman and Taymor[163]	1977	22	5	23
Taymor and Idriss[170]	1978	7	1	14
Usherwood et al.[177]	1976	37	8	22
Whitelaw[183]	1976	82	10	12
TOTAL		419	68	16

From Nachtigall RD: Indications, techniques, and success rates for AIH. In *Seminars in Reproductive Endocrinology,* Volume 5, No. 1, New York, 1987, Thieme Medical Publishers, Inc. Reprinted by permission.
*Split ejaculate technique.
† Pooled frozen semen.
‡ Caffeine added to semen.

Excess semen is placed near the portio or deposited in a plastic cervical cap of appropriate diameter for application against the cervix. These cervical caps (oligospermia cup; Milex Products, Inc.) may help to maintain semen-mucus interaction and avoid the dilutional and spermicidal effects of acidic vaginal secretions. The cup is removed by the patient after 4 to 6 hours.

Results with ICI

The pregnancy outcome following ICI of whole semen for anatomic, impotence-related, or psychogenic conditions or as part of donor insemination is favorable provided that the fresh semen quality is good. The clinical pregnancy rate per treatment cycle has averaged 8% to 12%; at least 60% of couples should conceive within six treatment cycles.[96] The abortion rate, fetal malformation rate, and pregnancy outcome are comparable to natural conception.[131]

Use of the split ejaculate

If semen is collected so that the volume is split into two fractions, the first part of the ejaculate will contain approximately 80% of the sperm population and the most active forms.[73] Split ejaculate artificial insemination by husband has been advocated in the past as treatment of male infertility characterized by deficiencies in count and/or motility or in cases of a relatively high semen volume (greater than 5 mL) (Table 41-1).* In a 1979 review of six scientific papers that described the use of this technique in a total of 230 couples with oligospermia, the average

*References 12, 42, 133, 162, 163, 170.

Table 41-2. Intracervical insemination for poor postcoital test: cumulative pregnancy rates

	Year	Patients	Pregnant No.	%
Guttmacher[70]	1943	5	0	0
Harrison*[72]	1978	7	1	14
Mastroianni et al.[118]	1957	132	7	5
Russell[148]	1960	10	3	30
Steiman and Taymor[163]	1977	25	8	32
Usherwood et al.[177]	1976	13	4	31

From Nachtigall RD: Indications, techniques, and success rates for AIH. In *Seminars in Reproductive Endocrinology,* Volume 5, No. 1, New York, 1987, Thieme Medical Publishers, Inc. Reprinted by permission.
*Split ejaculate technique.

pregnancy rate was 18%.[131] This is not significantly different from the spontaneous rate of conception of 14% to 16% in an equivalent patient population. More promising results were achieved by Diamond et al.,[43] who reported an overall pregnancy rate of 53% in 61 couples with repeatedly poor postcoital tests and/or subnormal semen analyses who were treated by artificial insemination with cervical cap in the patient's home. Reasons proposed to explain these superior results with the cervical cap included minimal semen loss, protection of sperm from the vaginal environment, and the ability of the couple to control the timing and the procedure of insemination. However, this and similar studies have suffered in design because of lack of a control group. The general consensus in the literature is that other forms of assisted reproduction are more appropriate than homologous ICI for couples with infertility secondary to semen abnormalities or female factors.

INTRAUTERINE INSEMINATION
History

The first documented use of homologous artificial insemination occurred in London in the late eighteenth century. A man with severe hypospadias consulted John Hunter, who advised that the semen that escaped during coitus be collected in a warmed syringe and injected into the vagina.[151] A successful pregnancy ensued. In 1867 J. Marion Sims reported the first conception following therapeutic insemination for anatomic abnormalities of the cervix.[160] Homologous intrauterine insemination (IUI) using an aliquot of ejaculated semen was described 4 years later. Early trials of this therapeutic modality were associated with a high frequency of major side effects, including anaphylaxis, strong uterine contractions, and pelvic infection. Hence high seminal plasma concentrations of prostaglandins and bacterial contaminants limited the application of transcervical insemination for several decades.[169,185]

Medical interest in artificial insemination increased after the 1930s, when it became apparent that semen abnormalities were responsible for a significant proportion of infertility cases.[150] Nevertheless, the efficacy of therapeutic IUI was refuted by Mastroianni and colleagues[118] in the first published review of this procedure. Only one pregnancy was achieved by performing 69 IUI procedures in 29 patients. The authors concluded in this 1957 publication that the procedure should be abandoned unless further technologic advancements could be made to improve its success.

Various early attempts to concentrate the total amount of sperm by centrifugation and resuspension resulted in impaired sperm motility, although the use of the split ejaculate,[93] limitation of the volume of the inseminate,[182] and dilution and freezing of the specimen with egg yolk buffer[16] reduced the incidence of adverse reactions. Filtration methods utilizing albumin columns[46] and glass wool[139] were therefore devised to obtain a highly motile sperm fraction. However, it was only with the application of sperm separation techniques developed for in vitro fertilization (IVF) therapy that IUI could be performed with an acceptably low rate of side effects. These methods employ various media and gradient and/or column systems, all of which to varying extents select out the most fertile populations of sperm while limiting or eliminating the presence of abnormal morphologic forms, white blood cells, cellular debris, dead cells, and seminal plasma. The advances in semen processing and the advent of other assisted reproduction technologies have prompted a reassessment of what constitutes appropriate indications for homologous artificial insemination.

Prerequisites for IUI

Most couples seeking therapy for infertility do not have disorders that prohibit reproduction but rather have conditions that are associated with a relative diminution in the monthly likelihood of conception. Examples of these subfertile conditions include abnormalities in sperm concentration or motility, cervical factor infertility, endometriosis, minimal adnexal adhesions, luteal phase defect, and idiopathic infertility. An assessment of all major categories of infertility is necessary before initiation of artificial insemination in order to estimate the likelihood of response to therapy. Laparoscopic evaluation of the pelvis is desirable although not an absolute prerequisite to initiation of IUI provided that there are no risk factors, symptoms, or signs suggestive of pelvic adhesive disease or moderate to severe endometriosis. Cervical testing for chlamydia as well as bacteriologic culture for *Neisseria gonorrhoeae* should be performed.

Sperm penetration assay

The ability of sperm to capacitate, acrosome react, bind to, and penetrate the oocyte plasma membrane and to undergo nuclear decondensation can be assessed in the zona-free hamster egg penetration test, or sperm penetration assay (SPA).[57,147] Since the SPA provides an indirect evaluation of the functional capacity of a given ejaculate, it may be worthwhile to perform this test prior to consideration of proceeding with IUI therapy in cases of male factor or idiopathic infertility. There does appear to be a moderate degree of concordance between the results of the SPA and successful fertilization after human IVF procedures,[146] although the predictive value of the assay may be compromised by its high false-negative rate and the possible negative influence of female factors, if present, on conception and early development.[147] The ability of human spermatozoa to penetrate the human zona pellucida is not assessed by the SPA.

Whether IUI increases the pregnancy rate for a man with an abnormal penetration test is not known; however, several studies have noted a significantly lower fecundity rate after IUI for male factor infertility for those who demonstrated poor penetration in the zona-free hamster ova preparation, compared with men whose penetration results were normal.[32,103,111,184] Wiltbank et al.[184] reported that the combined results of the SPA and the postcoital test (PCT) predicted IUI success. For couples with poor PCTs, the pregnancy rates were 50% and 8% for those with SPA penetration values greater than 10% and less than 10%, respectively. If poor penetration of zona-free hamster ova is a consistent finding, a trial of IVF is recommended to determine whether sperm penetration and fertilization are also unsuccessful when tested against the female partner's ova.

Interpretation of IUI studies

To evaluate the efficacy of treatment of subfertility, it is necessary to perform controlled, randomized trials comparing pregnancy rates of treated and untreated subjects. Unfortunately, few such trials exist for homologous artificial insemination. Most studies are uncontrolled and describe heterogeneous groups of patients with dissimilar diagnostic entities, duration of infertility, prior therapy, and age. In addition, the techniques of semen processing, number and timing of inseminations per cycle, and method of ovulation prediction vary considerably. A key issue remains whether the beneficial outcome achieved is attributable to the technique of IUI as such or to close monitoring of the cycle and/or the use of ovulation-inducing agents.

The reliability of data from many series is compromised by small patient numbers. Many couples have more than one risk factor for infertility, which obviates assignment of utility based on etiology in such instances. Furthermore, the published cumulative pregnancy rates are usually for a relatively short treatment period; comparison of crude rates from a study involving few treatment cycles with those reporting 1- or 2-year cumulative pregnancy rates is not valid. Only recently have life table analyses of data been reported.[61,103]

An assumption that all pregnancies that occurred within a given treatment cycle can be attributed to IUI will lead to an overestimation of its efficacy. Many reports in the literature have failed to take into account the incidence of pregnancies among a treatment-independent control population that has been properly matched for similar infertility etiology. This "background" rate of spontaneous conception may be substantial. Collins et al.[29] examined the rate of treatment-independent pregnancy in 1145 infertile couples over a 2- to 7-year follow-up period and found that 35% of untreated couples achieved pregnancy, with the range varying from 14% to 44%, depending on the cause of infertility. These figures exclude patients with bilateral tubal disease or azoospermia. An additional 7% of the couples studied achieved pregnancies long after the cessation of therapy. Those with a normal infertility evaluation and secondary infertility have been shown to have a higher baseline fecundity than couples experiencing primary infertility.[104] Hence the heterogeneity of infertility necessitates the design and execution of well-controlled prospective studies to provide a true assessment of the value of IUI.

Indications for IUI

Sperm deposited in the vagina through coitus must penetrate cervical mucus and enter the endometrial cavity on their way to the usual site of fertilization, the tubal ampulla. Mortimer and Templeton[129] have shown that there is a reduction in sperm number of five to six orders of magnitude along the length of the female reproductive tract. Associated with this attrition is an increase in the percentage of rapidly motile sperm and a decrease in the percentage of morphologically abnormal sperm.[4] The sperm population present in the oviduct is directly proportional to the number of motile sperm deposited in the upper vagina.[155] Although there is evidence to suggest that sperm filtered out by the cervix are probably unfit to fertilize the oocyte,[124] placement of sperm directly into the uterine cavity may increase their numbers in the distal tube. Clinical data have been published that support this concept; Weathersbee et al.[180] noted that the rate of recovery of peritoneal sperm at laparoscopy was 25% higher after IUI than after ICI of unwashed semen in patients with a history of poor postcoital tests. General categories of fertility disorders that may respond to IUI include impaired semen quality, a failure of active sperm transport in the upper female genital tract, the presence of a local, hostile barrier at the intracervical level, and the possible existence of toxic substances in the peritoneal environment.

Female factors. An absence of quality cervical mucus during the periovulatory time period despite high circulating levels of estradiol is considered the primary rationale for IUI in couples with female factor infertility. Deficiencies in cervical mucus production may be due to loss of mucus-producing glands after cervical cauterization or conization, abnormal functional development of the cervical architecture secondary to diethylstilbestrol exposure in utero, and adverse effects of clomiphene citrate. In addition, a functional impairment in cervical mucus may arise from a biochemical defect of the endocervical glands, lack of normal hydration of mucus at midcycle as a consequence of cystic fibrosis, inflammatory processes of the cervix leading to changes in the normal physical properties or normal pH of the mucus, and antisperm antibody production.[96,99]

The primary test used to identify or rule out a cervical factor is the PCT, although the definition of what constitutes an abnormal study varies widely. Some authors have considered that a cervical factor was present only if there were no sperm in the PCT,[27] and others if there were less than 3, 5, 10, 15, or 20 motile sperm per high-power field.[84,142,158] Moreover, the validity of the PCT has been questioned because of the poor correlation of PCT results with successful conception. Jette and Glass[89] found similar pregnancy rates in patients with 0 to 20 sperm per high-power field and concluded that it is difficult to determine what constitutes an abnormal PCT. Many factors can influence the sperm findings, including the quality of cervical mucus. The frequent failure of authors to document diagnostic criteria compromises an objective evaluation of this indication for IUI.

Male factors. The generally accepted parameters of a "normal" semen analysis were established in 1951 by MacLeod and Gold.[107] They include a volume greater than 1 mL, a concentration greater than 20 million/mL and motility greater than 60%. At that time, only 5% of fertile men had a sperm count lower than 20 million/mL. However, in recent years the average sperm concentrations in the United States have declined such that currently 20% to 25% of proven fertile men have sperm counts below the "normal" range.[190]

A German investigation of 11,772 andrologic patients has revealed that fertility decreases substantially when the sperm count falls below 20×10^6/mL, and a second large drop occurs when the concentration is less than 10×10^6/mL.[69] In 1977 Zukerman et al.[190] compared the frequency distributions of sperm count in 4122 prevasectomy patients and 1000 infertile men. A significantly greater proportion of the infertile group had counts below 10×10^6/mL. No definitive studies have been published regarding the influence of other semen parameters in the process of natural fertilization.[3] IUI has been advised for couples with compromised semen quality under the premise that this therapy would increase the concentrations of competent sperm in the ampulla of the fallopian tube.

Sperm preparation

The semen specimen should be collected by masturbation or through use of a nonspermicidal condom after a 2- to 4-day abstinence period. There can be significant improvements in semen sample parameters in specimens obtained with semen-collection devices over samples obtained by masturbation from the same individual,[189] a factor that may be particularly important in the oligoasthenospermic patient. When sperm-directed antibodies have been detected in the seminal plasma, it is best to use a split ejaculate that has been diluted with culture medium immediately after collection.

Data derived from the use of the SPA have provided insight as to those factors that may influence the process of fertilization. The length of the abstinence period, exposure of sperm cells to seminal plasma for periods longer than 30 minutes, presence of leukocytes in concentrations equal to or exceeding 1 to 3 million/mL, individual differences in capacitation times, and the presence of dead cells all affect the results of this in vitro study.[91,147] Simple washing of sperm does not change the cellular components of an ejaculate, but it will reduce the bacterial count, because the sperm form a pellet at the bottom of the tube while the smaller bacteria stay in suspension.[102] Density gradient centrifugation with Percoll or a similar substance will filter motile sperm from bacteria, white blood cells, and debris.[22] Although the laboratory techniques of sperm processing usually improve sperm quality (such as by increasing the percentage with progressive motility), the fertility potential of the treated sperm is not necessarily increased.

Capacitation. Capacitation, a physiologic maturation of spermatozoa, is initiated by removal of sperm from inhibitory factors contained within the seminal plasma.[3] This process may occur in vivo during migration of sperm through cervical mucus to the tubal ampulla or as a consequence of laboratory semen separation techniques. The motility and oxygen uptake of a spermatozoon are increased by capacitation, a calcium-dependent process that is maintained by the cell for approximately 48 hours. Capacitation also results in alteration in the plasma membrane of the sperm so that the acrosome reaction can occur. The acrosome reaction requires a massive uptake of calcium, which in turn generates a high osmotic pressure, reduced negative surface charges, and partial or total release of the acrosome enzyme content. Fertility of the sample may be compromised if sperm processing promotes a premature acrosome response, because acrosome-reacted sperm will not bind and attach to the zona pellucida. This is rarely a problem when standard techniques of semen processing are employed.

Separation. The outcome of the sperm isolation procedure will be influenced by several factors, including the volume of the ejaculate, centrifugal force used for recovery, and total time employed for isolation. The percentage of sperm recovered by centrifugation and incubation may be increased by use of a higher centrifugal force, but the resultant sperm population has decreased motility.[96,128] Moreover, sperm longevity is reduced by repeated centrifugation and through centrifugation at speeds higher than 400*g*. Subtle changes in the plasma membrane of sperm can occur through this processing, including loss of integrity and fluidity; this iatrogenic damage may be mediated by reactive oxygen species.[6] Superoxide radicals cause peroxidation of sperm plasma membrane phospholipids and elevated superoxide production through a membrane-bound reduced form of nicotinamide-adenine dinucleotide phosphate (NADPH) oxidase system.[11] These alterations have been implicated in defective sperm function at the cellular level[5] and an impairment of their fertilizing ability in the zona-free hamster egg penetration test.[6] In extreme cases, notably men with already reduced sperm quality, the damage may prevent conception.[7]

The production of reactive oxygen species sufficient to cause sperm damage has been confirmed in almost one fourth of infertile patients.[86] Macrophages, neutrophils, and morphologically abnormal sperm—particularly those with a relatively high cytoplasmic volume—are the principal sources of oxygen free radical production in the centrifugal pelleting of human ejaculates.[6,11] Nevertheless, in the majority of semen specimens prepared for IUI, the above concern may not be critical, particularly if there is no baseline perturbation of sperm function that might otherwise impair or prevent fertilization. Normal samples from fertile men contain fewer leukocytes and residual cytoplasmic masses from round spermatids and a higher proportion of morphologically normal spermatozoa.

There is no particular culture medium or contemporary sperm separation technique that has been demonstrated to be clearly superior to another as based on sperm recovery or pregnancy rate per treatment cycle of IUI.[96] Sperm motility is influenced by ambient temperature and is dependent on media energy sources such as fructose, glucose, lactate, and pyruvate to support sperm metabolism.[165] HEPES-buffered media[143] are well suited for the IUI procedure because of their pH stability when exposed to air. Ham's F-10 and other bicarbonate-buffered media require an atmosphere containing 5% CO_2 to maintain a stable pH of around 7.4. Serum or albumin is frequently added to the culture medium to maintain sperm motility, decrease sperm agglutination, and support capacitation.[9] Serum-free medium may be used for short-term incubation of sperm, but for prolonged incubations under tissue culture conditions, a protein source is required, as well as sperm concentrations not exceeding 10^6/mL. Midcycle serum may be collected from the woman for use, although sperm motility may be better maintained if the blood sample is drawn in the early follicular phase.[9] Exposure of sperm to follicular fluid during semen processing may lead to enhanced capacitation or acrosome reaction.[20] Penicillin (6000 IU/dL) and streptomycin (12,000 IU/dL) are included in the culture medium used for dilution of the specimen. The IUI should be conducted within 30 minutes of completion of sperm processing.

Centrifugation-resuspension. A simple sperm wash is a satisfactory method of sperm preparation provided that the initial semen analysis reveals good motility and number of sperm, little debris, and minimal white blood cells, because all cell populations found in the ejaculate are present in the final specimen. The semen is diluted with buffered medium and centrifuged at low speed. The resultant sperm pellet is resuspended in medium and centrifuged once again. The sperm in the second pellet may be used for insemination or further processed by the swim-up technique or an additional wash prior to insemination. In order to decrease the chance of iatrogenic sperm membrane damage, 1 mL of ethiodol may be used to cushion the diluted ejaculate while it is undergoing centrifugation.[112] If the initial count or motility is low, the semen specimen should be processed as 0.5-mL aliquots. High-viscosity samples may require mechanical liquefaction.

The requirements for incubation of specimens under a CO_2 atmosphere with strict control of temperature and pH make IUI difficult to accomplish in the usual outpatient setting. The absolute need for such procedures was evaluated in a study by Baerthlein et al.[14] A simplified protocol that consisted of a double wash performed at room temperature using modified Ham's F-10 medium without protein supplementation yielded pregnancy rates equivalent to those achieved in the double-wash procedure when preovulatory serum was used, the pH was corrected, the medium was maintained at 37°C, and the final suspension was incubated at 37°C in a 5% CO_2 atmosphere for 30 to 45 minutes before insemination. Nevertheless, a compromised sperm population may be more sensitive to the alterations in the processing technique described above.

Swim-up technique (sperm migration). An alternative method of collecting a population of motile, morphologically normal sperm is through use of a "swim-up" technique. Protein-supplemented buffer (1 to 2 mL) is layered over the liquefied ejaculate or sperm pellet and incubated for 60 to 90 minutes at 37°C. In men with normal semen variables, a maximal number of spermatozoa will usually migrate into the overlying medium during the first 30 minutes of the incubation period.[112] The medium is aspirated and may be centrifuged at speeds not greater than 300g; the pellet is resuspended in 0.5 mL of medium for insemination. A variation of this approach involves lower centrifugation speeds that may reduce the incidence of damaged sperm, although a longer incubation time may be needed to recover adequate numbers of motile sperm through migration. Specimens prepared from swim-up migration without centrifugation escape the iatrogenic damage caused by pelleting of unselected sperm populations.[128] Nevertheless, the resultant samples are generally contained in a larger volume of medium that is subject to contamination by seminal plasma and nonmotile cells unless they are carefully aspirated.

The results of the SPA suggest that sperm recovered through direct swim up from semen may have better fertilizing potential than those processed by the simple wash method.[186] Kerin et al.[97] found that the sperm rise method of semen preparation resulted in an increase in motility 1.75 to 3.2 times that of the original, but the total number of motile sperm recovered was only 2% to 11% of the whole ejaculate. A wide variation in yields is possible that is dependent on the volumes of the semen aliquots used. Arny and Quagliarello[13] noted an average recovery rate of motile sperm of 25% using a 0.5-mL semen aliquot for the swim-up procedure. Studies reporting lower recoveries of sperm used fractions as large as 1 to 2 mL.[13]

Discontinuous gradient separation. Percoll is a suspension of colloidal silica particles conjugated to polyvinylpyrrolidone that exploits weight differences to filter debris and white blood cells from sperm cells.[140] Either continuous or discontinuous gradients can be used to accomplish the separation of a highly motile, morphologically normal spermatozoal population suitable for IUI.[150] Nycodenz, an iodinated, inert, nontoxic organic molecule dissolved in a tris(hydroxymethyl)aminomethane (TRIS) buffer, has also been used in a discontinuous gradient format to prepare motile sperm populations from oligospermic and asthenospermic patients.[63] Since soluble components released by leukocytes may influence sperm function, sperm processing using these filtering techniques may minimize damage from exposure to reactive oxygen species. In addition, the recovery rate of motile sperm is superior to that achieved with the swim-up procedure.[19] A layer of liquefied semen is placed over the top of the Percoll column and centrifuged at 300g for 20 to 30 minutes.[109] The layer of sperm is aspirated, rediluted in buffer, centrifuged, and resuspended in 0.3 to 0.5 mL of culture medium for insemination (Fig. 41-1).

Recent evidence has suggested that sperm separated on a Percoll column may have a greater fertilizing capacity than sperm separated by the swim-up technique.[168] An increase in overall penetration rates from 24.8% to 48.6% was reported by McClure et al.[109] using a two-step discontinuous Percoll gradient, with results being equal to or greater than those obtained with swim-up spermatozoa in 90% of 73 cases. Additional data supporting improved sperm functional capacity in infertile men after sperm preparation using density gradient centrifugation have been provided by Serafini et al.,[153] who reported hamster ova penetration rates of 16.3% ± 3.7% and 15.8% ± 3.3% for sperm populations prepared using Percoll and Nycodenz gradients respectively, compared with only 2.7% ± 1.7% for washed pellet swim-up spermatozoa.

It is theoretically possible that the silica particles of Percoll may cause an inflammatory reaction in the endometrium or peritoneum in much the same way as certain surgical glove powders have been shown to do. Nevertheless, Pickering et al.[140] failed to demonstrate any residual generalized peritoneal inflammatory response to Percoll 1 week after intraperitoneal injection, although a localized granulomatous response was seen at the presumed injection site. In addition, the washing procedure is efficient in removing residual particles from the spermatozoal preparation. Scanning electron microscopy has shown no evidence of alteration of sperm surface membrane morphology after exposure to Percoll.[140]

Other methods of sperm preparation include glass wool, rayon, and sterile cotton gauze filtration; albumin gradients;

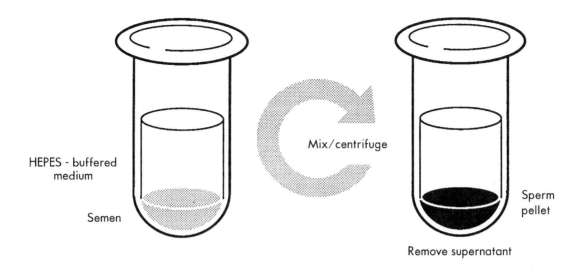

HEPES - buffered medium

Semen

Mix/centrifuge

Sperm pellet

Remove supernatant

A

Repeat medium addition, centrifugation, and supernatant removal

Overlay pellet and allow motile sperm to swim up into medium

Add medium and resuspend entire cellular pellet

Swim-up

Resuspension

Fig. 41-1. Semen processing for therapeutic insemination. **A,** Swim up or resuspension.

Continued.

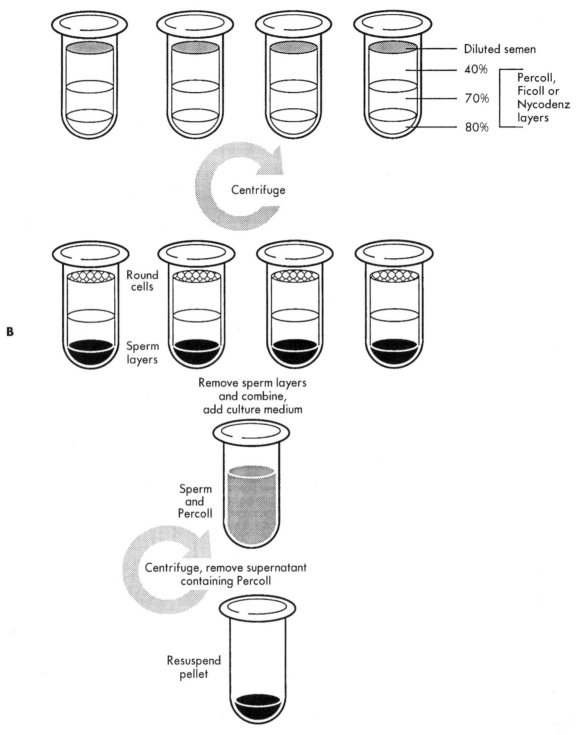

Fig. 41-1, cont'd. B, Discontinuous gradient centrifugation. (Modified from washed insemination symposium, *Contemp Ob/Gyn,* October 1990.)

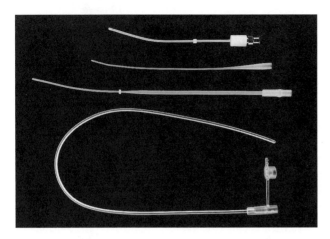

Fig. 41-2. A representative sample of catheters commonly used for intrauterine insemination. From top, Shepard catheter with stainless steel inner cannula, 5.4 Fr, Cook Ob/Gyn, Spencer, Indiana; Tom Cat catheter, 3.5 Fr, Sherwood Medical, St. Louis, Missouri; Tefcat intrauterine insemination catheter, 4 Fr, Cook Ob/Gyn, Spencer, Indiana; Accumark pediatric feeding catheter, 8 Fr, Concord Laboratories, Keene, New Hampshire.

and Sephadex and Ficoll columns. As noted previously, a potential disadvantage of these approaches is that foreign material may be washed into the specimen ultimately used for insemination. Another alternative for asthenospermic cases avoiding prior washing of the sperm is the "migration-sedimentation" method using liquefied semen in the special tubes described by Tea et al.[171]

The need for any type of laboratory processing of sperm before IUI in the treatment of male factor infertility was brought into question in a study by Cumming.[38] The author compared the use of whole semen derived from a split ejaculate to sperm collected after two washings in Ham's F-10 containing 10% human serum and found no difference in pregnancy rates between the patient populations. None of the 40 women in the group receiving unwashed sperm developed an infection, and the rate of mild cramping discomfort and/or spotting was no higher in the unwashed sperm group as compared with the washed sperm group. The cumulative pregnancy rate after six cycles of therapy was 20% in both groups. However, the study design did not include a nontreatment, control group. The weight of recent evidence suggests that use of sperm separated from seminal plasma is more appropriate for transcervical insemination, although no one technique of sperm processing has been proven to yield superior pregnancy rates.

Technique of IUI

IUI is performed with the patient in the lithotomy position after exposure of the cervix with a bivalve speculum. The cervix may be cleansed with sterile saline if significant debris is present in the region of the external os. The insemination device selected for use must be nonspermicidal and able to traverse the cervical canal and enter the superior aspect of the uterine cavity without traumatizing the cervical crypts or endometrium (Fig. 41-2). A tuberculin syringe fitted onto the end of the catheter is used to inject the sperm suspension. Since the endometrial cavity is a potential space, it is not physiologic to attempt to introduce a volume of greater than 0.5 mL. Insemination over a 30-to 60-second period minimizes the chance of retrograde flow. The catheter may be directed toward the uterotubal opening of the side in which ovulation will take place or the side of a unilaterally patent tube; experimental studies have suggested that IUI performed in this manner results in a direct flow of at least 20% of the fluid volume into the specified oviduct.[95]

Timing of IUI

Since the fertilizing life span of the ovum is estimated to be only 12 to 24 hours, the timing of artificial insemination procedures may critically influence success rates. This issue is particularly noteworthy in patients receiving transcervical insemination because, although a greater proportion of sperm should reach the tubal ampulla, there is less opportunity for sperm sequestration in the cervical crypts for slow release over time.[67] The uterine and tubal environment may be hostile to sperm longevity, particularly in cases of endometriosis, unexplained infertility, and antisperm antibody production. In addition, sperm from oligospermic men may be functionally compromised and have a decreased survival rate within the uterus.[95] Animal data confirm the importance of accurate timing of the insemination in maximizing therapeutic outcome. Mitchell et al.[123] showed that less than 10% of inseminated sperm were retained in the upper reproductive tract of the cow when studied 12 hours after IUI despite the use of small volumes of sperm suspension.

The majority of published series have documented the efficacy of one therapeutic insemination performed 36 to 40 hours after administration of human chorionic gonadotropin (hCG) in women undergoing controlled ovarian hyperstimulation. Nevertheless, a recent prospective, randomized trial by Silverberg et al.[159] described a significantly higher cycle fecundity with two IUIs timed 18 and 42 hours after hCG, as compared with one insemination procedure 34 hours after hCG. Codominant follicles that develop in response to menotropin therapy are never synchronous in their times of ovulation, resulting in a potentially greater time period in which sperm-oocyte fusion and fertilization may take place.

Ovulation in the natural menstrual cycle can be monitored by several means. Progressive follicular growth and collapse can be assessed ultrasonographically. The luteinizing hormone (LH) surge is detectable via rapid radioimmunoassay of the urine or serum, as well as by a monoclonal antibody urinary assay. The latter technique has gained widespread acceptance because of its reliability, availability, low cost, and patient convenience. Moreover, the urine forms a reservoir for LH and therefore is less likely to be influenced by the pulsatile release pattern of the gonadotropin. One recent study noted a significantly higher conception rate when IUI was performed on the day after the urinary LH surge rather than on the day of the LH rise.[95]

Less precise methods of timing of insemination in the natural menstrual cycle include reliance on basal body temperature or cervical mucus changes. In women with consistent cycle lengths, the IUI may be performed on the day of the nadir in temperature or approximately 14 days from the expected onset of menses; scheduling of insemination by this method yields pregnancy rates that are equivalent to that delivered by timing with urinary LH measurement for this patient population. A preovulatory increase in estrogen secretion stimulates the endocervical glands to produce a profuse, thin mucus high in glycogen, mucin, and salts. Measurement of spinnbarkeit, ferning, sodium chloride concentration, glucose concentration, and viscosity of the mucus are all methods that have been used to estimate follicular development.[10]

Response to therapy

Oligoasthenospermia. Traditional approaches to the treatment of oligospermia include varicocele ligation and hormonal stimulation of the male with clomiphene citrate, human menopausal gonadotropins (hMG), and hCG; however, unless hypothalamic hypogonadism is present, such treatments have not been shown to be more effective in achieving pregnancy than no therapy or placebo in prospective, controlled studies.[31] The poor results noted with these interventions have led to the recent focus on laboratory processing and insemination of selected populations of sperm. Assuming that the viability and fertilizing capacity of the sperm in the oligo/asthenospermic man are not greatly diminished, the placement of a few million sperm in the upper uterine cavity or fallopian tubes by IUI should theoretically increase the chances of fertilization and conception over intercourse or ICI.[76]

The interpretation of data derived from series of patients treated with IUI has been compromised by the wide variation in criteria used to define poor semen quality. Most reports concern sperm concentrations under 20 million/mL, but some have included maximal densities of 10 million/mL[64] or even 40 million/mL.[97,138] Furthermore, the presence of a male factor may be mentioned but not defined. In addition, there has been substantial disparity in parameters used to define normal morphology and motility.[84]

The spontaneous pregnancy rate among couples with previously diagnosed male factor infertility has been reported to range from 14% to 27%.[77,132,190] In a large study of 584 male factor couples, Aafjes et al.[1] found a 10.2% spontaneous pregnancy rate in patients with 2 to 4 years of infertility. The expectation of pregnancy was inversely related to the duration of infertility. Hence therapeutic insemination by husband must result in a cumulative pregnancy rate that is higher than approximately 20% in order

for this technique to be considered efficacious. Since many of the published trials of IUI for male infertility have not included an adequate control group, the results are often difficult to interpret.

Results with a natural cycle. There is a lack of consensus in the literature for the role of IUI in oligoasthenospermic couples. When strict criteria are used to diagnose male factor infertility, the efficiency of this method of treatment is very low. The average pregnancy rate with IUI using unprepared semen is approximately 18%.[131] Allen et al.[10] calculated an overall pregnancy rate of 25% for IUI-treated male factor infertility in their review of previously published data (range 7% to 66%).

Kerin and colleagues[95] described an 8.8% pregnancy rate per cycle following 296 cycles of LH-timed IUI as compared with a 2.8% pregnancy rate per cycle in 213 cycles of LH-timed intercourse in couples with male factor infertility. This difference in outcome among IUI and control cycles reached significance. Conception occurred in the first IUI treatment cycle in 13 of the 26 couples who were successful with this therapy. Although sperm number, motility, and morphology characteristics measured in either the fresh, whole semen or the washed sperm sample were similar in the pregnancy and nonpregnancy IUI cycles, the authors found that the conception rate for men with a severe semen defect was significantly improved through IUI (8.7% per cycle) as compared with timed intercourse (0%). There was no significant difference in outcome for patients with more moderate semen defects. Hence men with a severe impairment of semen quality (defined by inclusion of at least two of the following abnormalities: <10 million/mL count, <30% motility, <30% normal morphology) were unlikely to achieve conception from timed-intercourse cycles, but did benefit from semen washing and the deposition of these sperm high in the uterine cavity about the time of ovulation.

A later study from the same institution again revealed a marked improvement in conception rates through LH-timed IUI for couples in the severe semen defect group.[98] Patients were requested not to have intercourse for 3 days before the day of semen collection and insemination. Up to six cycles of IUI were alternated with timed intercourse in order to overcome one of the major limitations of some earlier studies, namely the absence of suitable controls to assess the spontaneous pregnancy rate in the same group of patients. Overall, IUI using motile sperm was significantly more effective than timed intercourse, with a pregnancy rate per cycle of 6.2% as compared with 3.4%. However, when success was characterized by category of abnormality, a statistically significant improvement in the pregnancy rate was found only for the severe semen defect group described previously and not for patients with a moderate semen defect, mucus hostility, or unexplained infertility. The pregnancy rates reported by other series are listed in Table 41-3. Fecundity is defined as percentage of treatment cycles in which pregnancy was achieved.

Table 41-3. IUI for male factor infertility

	Year	Patients	Pregnancies/cycle	Fecundity
Unstimulated cycles				
Byrd et al.[27]	1987	21	9/58	0.16
Chaffkin et al.[28]	1991	31	3/105	0.03
Confino et al.[30]	1986	27	0/108	0
Dmowski et al.[46]	1982	27	4/90	0.04
Francavilla et al.[58]	1990	68	15/335	0.05
Friedman et al.[61]	1991	81	18/276	0.07
Glass and Ericsson[65]	1978	19	0/67	0
Harris et al.[71]	1981	20	3/120	0.03
Hewitt et al.[74]	1985	18	1/32	0.03
Ho et al.[75]	1989	47	0/114	0
Hughes et al.[81]	1987	20	0/32	0
Hull et al.[82]	1986	8	0/20	0
Irianni et al.[84]	1990	NS	0/124	0
Kerin et al.[97]	1984	34	8/39	0.21
Kerin and Quinn[95]	1987	NS	26/296	0.09
Kirby et al.[98]	1991	188	10/331	0.03
Marrs et al.[115]	1983	4	0/12	0
te Velde et al.[172]	1989	30	3/112	0.03
Thomas et al.[174]	1986	8	0/24	0
Clomiphene citrate cycles				
Blumenfeld and Nahhas[20]	1989	13	5/43	0.12
Bolton et al.[22]	1986	29	5/158	0.03
Hewitt et al.[74]	1985	36	3/64	0.05
Irianni et al.[84]	1990	NS	3/23	0.13
Martinez et al.[116]	1990	NS	2/27	0.07
Menotropin cycles				
Blumenfeld and Nahhas[20]	1989	8	4/32	0.13
Chaffkin et al.[28]	1991	51	17/111	0.17
Cruz et al.[37]	1986	48	7/96	0.07
Dodson and Haney[47]	1991	39	13/85	0.15
Horvath et al.[79]	1989	39	6/175	0.03
Irianni et al.[84]	1990	NS	3/23	0.13
Sher et al.[158]	1984	4	1/4	0.25
Sunde et al.[166]	1988	40	8/56	0.14

Friedman et al.[61] reported 18 pregnancies among 81 male factor patients who underwent a total of 276 IUI cycles (6.5%/cycle). According to the life table analysis of these data, the success rate of IUI per treatment cycle reached a plateau after the fourth or fifth cycle. These results concur with other studies that have found that IUI is beneficial only in the first few cycles of treatment[30,37,76] and indicate that the continuation of IUI treatment beyond five or six cycles is unwarranted.

Several other controlled studies have failed to demonstrate any therapeutic benefit to IUI in cases of male factor infertility. Ho et al.[75] prospectively randomized 47 subfertile couples with oligospermia or asthenospermia to LH-timed IUI or LH-timed natural intercourse. No pregnancy occurred in 114 cycles of IUI with washed sperm, whereas one patient conceived during 1 of 124 natural intercourse cycles. The average sperm count after preparation by centrifugation and swim up was 3.16 ± 5.23 with 81% motility.

te Velde et al.[172] evaluated the efficacy of intrauterine insemination in couples with male factor infertility by randomly alternating IUI on the day after urinary LH rise and advising intercourse on the day of the LH rise and the following day. For male infertility not associated with an immunologic component, there was no difference in pregnancy rates of insemination and intercourse cycles. One patient conceived on the ninth and one on the eleventh IUI cycle. Hence, IUI in the natural menstrual cycle results in a marginal and perhaps insignificant enhancement of the fecundity of couples with compromised semen quality.

Prognostic characteristics of sperm.

Morphology. Most investigations have suggested that IUI may be of therapeutic value only if the cause of infertility is simple oligospermia without associated severe asthenospermia or teratospermia. Francavilla et al.[58] proposed that it is the presence of teratospermia, rather than oligospermia or asthenospermia per se, that limits the efficacy of IUI in the treatment of male subfertility. In their study, teratospermia affected the outcome of IUI when associated with moderate oligospermia and/or asthenospermia; the crude pregnancy rate per couple in such circumstances was 11.1%. The impairment was more profound when abnormal sperm morphology was associated with severe oligospermia and/or asthenospermia, because no pregnancies were achieved in such cases. In the absence of teratospermia, the cumulative success rates per couple both in severe and in moderate oligospermia and/or asthenospermia were quite similar, 33.3% versus 35.7%. These findings are consistent with the knowledge that sperm morphology is a strong discriminator of sperm fertilizing ability of human ova cultured in vitro.[101,106] Nevertheless, severe oligospermia and/or asthenospermia are usually associated with teratospermia as a consequence of a serious underlying disturbance of spermatogenesis.

Motility. Polansky and Lamb[141] found no difference in the treatment-independent, cumulative pregnancy rates among infertility patients with sperm motilities greater than 30% and motilities less than 30% over a 5-year period. Bostofte et al.[23] reported that the percentage of men with living children plummeted only when the sperm motility of the fresh ejaculate was less than 20%. Many studies analyzing outcome of IUI have failed to reveal any semen characteristic that differentiates conception from nonconception cycles. However, Arny and Quagliarello[13] noted that the percentage of motile sperm after swim up was of prognostic significance in couples undergoing IUI who had good semen quality and postcoital tests of less than or equal to 3 motile sperm per high-power field. Normal motility in this study was defined as greater than 30%. For patients with greater than 79% motility after swim up, discrimination provided by post–swim-up motility was enhanced by inclusion in the analysis of either the total number of motile sperm used for insemination or sperm concentration after swim up. The predictors of nonpregnancy and pregnancy were correct at rates of 93.3% and 70%, respectively.

This prognostic validity of sperm motility was supported by data of McGovern et al.,[110] who found that the only standard values of semen parameters that were useful in discriminating patients who conceived from those who did not through IUI performed in natural or clomiphene-stimulated cycles was a pre–swim-up motility of greater than or equal to 30% and a post–swim-up motility of greater than or equal to 70%. Patients with original sperm motilities consistently greater than or equal to 30% had a significantly higher cumulative pregnancy rate (62.9%) than patients with one or more semen samples with motility less than 30% (22%). In addition, patients with post–swim-up motilities consistently greater than or equal to 70% had a cumulative pregnancy rate of 51.2%, which was significantly greater than that for patients inconsistent for this parameter (15.6%). The findings were demonstrated in patients with negative infertility evaluations except for possible male factor, although all men included in the study had at least one semen sample with greater than or equal to 20 million sperm per milliliter.

Sperm numbers. Pregnancies have been achieved in patients with insemination of as few as 300,000 to 700,000 motile sperm.[27] Such success is infrequent; most centers recommend IVF when less than 1 million motile sperm are recovered after semen processing. Bohrer et al.[21] found no correlation between the number of sperm inseminated during IUI and the pregnancy rate per treatment cycle when the concentrations of sperm used were between 1 and 30 million. Others have reported no increase in pregnancy or multiple birth rates after the number of motile sperm surpassed 10 to 15 million in natural cycles.[78,96]

Results with a stimulated cycle. Although the success rate of therapeutic IUI by husband is poor when sperm concentrations are very low, recently published data suggest that the pregnancy rate per IUI cycle may be increased by ovarian stimulation with menotropins. The cycle fecundity rate for couples with male factor or cervical factor infertility was 0.14 when treatment consisted of hMG ovarian stimulation and IUI, as compared with a rate of 0.02 for IUI alone in one recent retrospective study.[28] Kemmann et al.[94] also showed that active ovulation management of women with male factor infertility or persistently abnormal postcoital tests significantly increased the monthly probability of pregnancy for IUI cycles. All patients in this series were initially treated with urinary LH-timed IUIs in spontaneous cycles that yielded a cycle fecundity of 0.022. When hMG was utilized and hCG was administered when the serum estradiol level reached between 400 and 1000 pg/mL, the cycle fecundity increased to 0.085.

Ovarian stimulation alone does not appear to lead to superior conception rates in couples with male factor infertility. Cruz et al.,[37] in a prospective, randomized, crossover study of 49 women with oligoasthenospermic husbands, reported that menotropin ovarian stimulation and IUI resulted in a cycle fecundity of 0.07, as compared with 0.01 in stimulated cycles with intracervical insemination. hCG was given when estradiol concentrations reached approximately 500 pg/mL. However, the confounding variable of the timing of insemination in the two treatment groups may have contributed to the difference in pregnancy rates, because IUI was performed 28 hours after midcycle hCG, whereas ICI was performed immediately after hCG. Another recent study also described a fecundity rate of 0.071 per IUI cycle when hMG was administered to achieve an equivalent number of large antral follicles.[117]

Dickey et al.[44] reported a clinical pregnancy rate of 12.5% per hMG-treated cycle when the partner's sperm count before preparation was 5 million/mL or more, as compared with 7.1% when the count was lower. Maximal pregnancy rates did not increase further when initial sperm concentrations were higher than 5 million/mL. The probability of conception remains essentially stable when greater than 1 million motile sperm are deposited transcervically in menotropin-stimulated cycles.[37,47,94] Multiple pregnancy rates may be increased in this patient population when the number of motile sperm inseminated exceeds 20 million.[48] Conflicting findings have been reported regarding the prognostic significance of sperm motility in menotropin-stimulated cycles.[33,44] Hence, although the data are limited, ovarian stimulation with gonadotropins appears to increase fecundity rates in male factor couples undergoing IUI, although the added medication expense and side effects of menotropins must be considered when counseling the couple regarding therapeutic options.

Retrograde ejaculation. Retrograde ejaculation is a condition in which semen is not expelled through the urethra at the time of orgasm but, because of an incompetent bladder neck, refluxes into the bladder. Etiologies for this condition include neurogenic disorders arising from diabetes or other chronic disease, neurologic trauma, or medication side effects.

The exposure of sperm to urine is detrimental to survival because of alterations in pH and osmolarity. Ingestion of sodium bicarbonate before ejaculation will alkalinize the urine to create a more favorable environment. If the urine pH is 7.6 to 8.1 and the osmolarity is between 300 and 500 mOsm/L, masturbation followed by immediate micturition permits successful recovery of fertile spermatozoa.[24] Urination is as effective as immediate bladder catheterization after orgasm to collect the sperm.[176] Laboratory processing of the specimen for IUI results in a relatively simple, cost-effective, and successful method of treating the infertility associated with this condition,[156] even when the total number of sperm isolated from the urine is less than 1 million and when the motility is as low as 30%.[156,176] Electroejaculation of paraplegic men also allows recovery of viable sperm that have been expelled in both an antegrade and retrograde fashion. IUI is preferred over standard cervical insemination because of the large volume of urine associated with the retrograde ejaculate obtained in this manner.[18]

Unexplained infertility. Ten to twenty percent of all cases of infertility are due to idiopathic causes. Considering that the cumulative conception rate after up to 5 years of follow-up fluctuates between 36.5% and 78.8% in patients whose infertility is unexplained, the real efficacy of any treatment modality may reside in accomplishing the pregnancy at an earlier time rather than increasing the total number of conceptions.[104]

Natural cycle. In the series of Kirby et al.[98] of patients with unexplained infertility treated with timed intercourse or IUI in the natural menstrual cycle, an overall pregnancy rate of 0.041 per cycle was noted, although the conception rate for the first cycle of therapy was 0.072 (Table 41-4). No pregnancies were achieved in 63 cycles of timed IUI and 39 control cycles of ICI among 21 couples with unexplained infertility in a study by Irvine et al.[85]

Table 41-4. IUI for idiopathic infertility

	Year	Patients	Pregnancies/ cycle	Fecundity
Unstimulated cycles				
Byrd et al.[27]	1987	14	6/48	0.13
Chaffkin et al.[28]	1991	3	0/11	0
Friedman et al.[61]	1991	59	14/224	0.06
Irianni et al.[84]	1990	NS	2/34	0.06
Irvine et al.[85]	1986	21	0/63	0
Kirby et al.[98]	1991	73	6/145	0.04
Martinez et al.[116]	1990	NS	1/35	0.03
Quagliarello and Arny[142]	1986	14	1/42	0.02
Serhal et al.[154]	1988	15	1/30	0.03
Clomiphene citrate cycles				
Blumenfeld and Nahhas[20]	1989	5	4/10	0.40
Deaton et al.[41]	1990	24	7/72	0.10
Hewitt et al.[74]	1985	9	1/12	0.08
Martinez et al.[116]	1990	NS	3/36	0.08
Menotropin cycles				
Blumenfeld and Nahhas[20]	1989	3	2/7	0.29
Chaffkin et al.[28]	1991	12	15/46	0.33
Dickey et al.[44]	1991	5	2/5	0.40
Dodson and Haney[47]	1991	57	17/116	0.15
Irianni et al.[84]	1990	NS	2/16	0.11
Moore et al.[126]	1987	NS	7/27	0.26
Serhal et al.[154]	1988	15	6/19	0.32
Sher et al.[158]	1984	5	2/5	0.40
Sunde et al.[166]	1988	11	1/15	0.07

In contrast to these poor results, Yovich and Matson showed a cycle fecundity of 0.08 in their series of 183 cycles of IUI for treatment of unexplained infertility, and Byrd et al.[27] reported a cycle fecundity of 0.13 in a series of 14 couples with the disorder. Friedman et al.[61] obtained a cycle fecundity of 0.063 in 59 idiopathic infertility patients following LH-timed IUI in 224 unstimulated menstrual cycles. Another recent prospective study by Martinez and colleagues[116] confirmed the existence of a statistically significant increase in conception rate with IUI over well-timed coitus in couples with longstanding idiopathic or male factor infertility.

Stimulated cycle. Subtle, unrecognized ovulatory or endocrine abnormalities may be important etiologic factors for unexplained infertility. Superovulation therapy appears to increase fecundity greatly compared with natural cycles in patients undergoing IUI; it is less clear that IUI benefits those infertility patients receiving empirical hMG therapy. The cycle fecundity rate with hMG stimulation and timed intercourse is approximately 0.10 for infertile couples when male factor, immunologic and mechanical factor infertility, is excluded.[154,181] Welner et al.[181] were able to achieve pregnancy with hMG treatment in 12.4% of couples with long-standing unexplained infertility who were awaiting an IVF cycle. Only 1% of patients in a nonrandomized control group conceived during the study period. Similarly, a recent randomized, double-blind multicenter study demonstrated that clomiphene citrate is more effective than placebo in inducing pregnancy in couples with unexplained infertility.[55] The authors suggested that the increased number of oocytes or the increase in gonadal steroids induced by clomiphene may be responsible for the beneficial effect of the medication in this patient population.

Large numbers of patients are necessary to demonstrate a statistically significant difference in cycle fecundity between timed intercourse and IUI in patients undergoing hMG therapy. One small series did suggest that IUI is helpful in improving cycle fecundity in women treated with menotropin protocols for unexplained infertility.[154] Serhal and colleagues[154] found that the combination of hMG superovulation and IUI was more effective in achieving pregnancy (cycle fecundity of 0.26) than IUI alone (0.03) or superovulation alone (0.06) in couples with unexplained infertility. All 22 women who conceived with IUI had failed to achieve pregnancy for a minimum of 4 years, despite a recognized spontaneous pregnancy rate of 20% per year in this category of infertility. Eight of nine women who conceived after combined therapy became pregnant during their first treatment cycle, and one conceived after two treatment cycles.

Dodson et al.[49] reported a cycle fecundity of 0.19 after hMG/IUI in a similar etiologic group. Other studies have shown favorable pregnancy rates for idiopathic infertility (8% to 19% per cycle) when ovarian stimulation was combined with IUI.[47] Among the idiopathic infertility patients of the Martinez et al.[117] 1991 hMG/IUI study, 8.7% of IUI cycles were conceptional. Whether the lower dosage schedule of hMG used in this study could account for a less favorable response remains a matter of speculation. In a more heterogeneous grouping of patients with male factor, cervical factor, endometriosis, and unexplained infertility, the overall cycle fecundity rate was 0.063 (15/238) for hMG therapy and 0.196 (70/357) for hMG/IUI treatment ($P < 0.0001$).[28]

Data generated from an animal model have suggested a mechanism for improved conception rates when these two therapies are combined. Ewes superovulated with follicle-stimulating hormone (FSH) or pregnant mare's serum gonadotropin had a lower density of motile sperm reaching the upper reproductive tract after intravaginal insemination as compared with inseminations performed during unstimulated estrous cycles.[53] The sperm density was restored to normal with IUI. Perhaps superovulation corrects aberrant folliculogenesis or ovulation and IUI is helpful in ensuring adequate sperm concentrations in the periovular region.

Cervical factor. Midcycle cervical mucus acts as a reservoir for sperm, both protecting the gametes from the hostile vaginal environment and slowly releasing them into the upper genital tract.[124] Patients who have persistently poor PCTs not specifically attributable to poor sperm quality are said to have cervical factor infertility, which encompasses between 5% and 10% of all cases of infertility. Two types of defective cervical mucus are recognized: quantitative insufficiencies, which are characterized by small volume; and qualitative insufficiencies, which are defined by an acid pH, inadequate penetration, and poor migration and survival of control sperm as well as husband's sperm. Despite these potential compromises to mucus quality, a negative postcoital test is usually indicative of male infertility rather than female infertility.[66]

Natural cycle. The success of IUI as treatment of cervical factor infertility is controversial. Although some studies have reported cycle fecundity approximating 0.20, others have noted intermediate or poor results (Table 41-5). Cumulative pregnancy rates have ranged from 14% to 68%.[103] In a review of six previously published papers, Nachtigall et al.[131] reported 39 pregnancies among 120 patients treated with IUI because of poor PCT results. This compares with a pregnancy rate of 12% in 192 women treated with cervical artificial insemination of husband's sperm in the same series. Although the analysis included heterogeneous patient populations and protocols, the overall success rate of 30% for IUI was encouraging. Friedman et al.[61] noted similar results, with 32 pregnancies achieved among 91 cervical factor infertility patients who underwent LH-timed IUI. Life table analysis demonstrated a pregnancy rate of 0.122 per cycle. te Velde et al.,[172] using a randomized crossover comparison of IUI with intercourse for couples with cervical factor infertility, showed a cycle fecundity of 0.16 after IUI and no pregnancies after inter-

Table 41-5. IUI for cervical factor infertility

	Year	Patients	Pregnancies/cycle	Fecundity
Unstimulated cycles				
Byrd et al.[27]	1987	29	10/112	0.09
Chaffkin et al.[28]	1991	20	3/58	0.05
Confino et al.[30]	1986	19	13/63	0.21
Friedman et al.[61]	1991	91	32/262	0.12
Hull et al.[82]	1986	19	3/65	0.05
Kirby et al.[98]	1991	24	7/58	0.12
Quagliarello and Arny[142]	1986	20	6/72	0.08
te Velde et al.[172]	1989	27	13/82	0.16
Clomiphene citrate cycles				
Hewitt et al.[74]	1985	30	2/59	0.07
Menotropin cycles				
Chaffkin et al.[28]	1991	35	24/91	0.26
Dodson et al.[49]	1987	4	2/7	0.29

course. Quagliarello and Arny[142] reported a 30% crude pregnancy rate in women with cervical factor treated by IUI as compared with no pregnancies in women with a cervical factor treated by ICI. Other large series have reported cumulative pregnancy rates per patient as high as 72.2%,[16] but some have achieved much less favorable results.[82,175] Therefore, even for this rather restricted indication, the literature does not provide a clear consensus of therapeutic efficacy, although the conception rates of the patient with a cervical factor are generally superior through transcervical insemination than through intravaginal insemination.

Stimulated cycle. Corson et al.[33] reported a statistically significant increase in cycle fecundity rate (from 5% to 11%) with hMG/IUI treatment as compared with IUI alone in patients who had cervical factor abnormalities. When a cervical factor was present in this series, IUI was helpful regardless of whether hMG was added, with high ratios noted versus no treatment. A study by Dodson et al.[49] found that the fecundity rate was 0.29 for cervical factor associated with normal seminal parameters when IUI and hMG were employed.

The etiology of poor cervical mucus production in women with cervical factor infertility is varied but may include aberrant follicular development in many cases. It is possible that the hMG improves conception rates in cervical factor infertility patients by correcting this abnormality. In addition, the increased cervical mucus production caused by supraphysiologic estradiol levels may serve as a reservoir for sperm. By using a low-dose hMG protocol, Soto-Albors et al.[161] were able to correct cervical mucus deficiency and achieve a viable cycle fecundity of 0.35 without IUI.

Immunologic infertility. An immunity to spermatozoa can be demonstrated in either partner in approximately one third of cases of cervical factor infertility.[26] Sperm antibodies of differing types may be bound to the sperm at the time of ejaculation, may be produced systemically in the female and diffuse into the reproductive tract, or they may be produced locally within the female reproductive tract. Mechanisms by which antisperm antibodies might interfere in vivo with reproduction include complement-mediated sperm cytotoxicity, enhanced phagocytosis of sperm by genital tract macrophages, restricted motion of spermatozoa within cervical mucus, interference with capacitation or the acrosome reaction, inhibition of sperm attachment to the zona pellucida or penetration of egg membranes, and interference with embryo implantation.[114] If cervical mucus antisperm antibodies act to impair sperm migration through the cervical canal, IUI may increase the cycle fecundity. Bypassing the cervix through IUI will not eliminate other sites of antigen-antibody reaction. Nevertheless, by increasing the number of sperm entering the uterus, the aggregate number of antigenic sites of the sperm might exceed the binding capacity of available female antisperm antibodies such that the total antibody burden is diminished.

Margalloth and colleagues[114] treated 91 women with longstanding infertility associated with the presence of humoral antisperm antibodies with intrauterine insemination in natural and stimulated cycles (Table 41-6). The pregnancy rate in unstimulated IUI cycles was 9/285 (3%), in clomiphene-stimulated IUI cycles was 6/86 (7%), and in hMG cycles was 11/102 (11%). The cumulative chance of conception with hMG stimulation was 40% in this patient population, with a 70% to 80% chance that the pregnancy would occur in the first two IUI cycles. Only 6/38 (16%) pregnancies resulted in abortion, suggesting that these women were not at an increased risk of this complication. However, the treatment assignments were not randomized and the results should be interpreted in light of similar pregnancy rates reported with no treatment. Other studies of the efficacy of IUI have reported pregnancy rates that ranged from 0% to 25% for male immune factor and from 17% to 40% for female immune factor.[103]

Apart from increasing the number of oocytes available for fertilization, it has been postulated that the high estro-

Table 41-6. IUI for immunologic infertility

	Year	Patients	Pregnancies/cycle	Fecundity
Unstimulated cycles				
Byrd et al.[27]	1987			
Male		4	0/17	0
Confino et al.[30]	1986			
Male		8	2/30	0.07
Female		10	4/38	0.11
Margalloth et al.[114]	1988			
Female		67	9/285	0.03
Clomiphene citrate cycles				
Margalloth et al.[114]	1988			
Female		20	6/86	0.07
Menotropin cycles				
Margalloth et al.[114]	1988			
Female		28	11/108	0.11

gen levels associated with multiple follicular development may lower antisperm antibody and complement concentrations in the female genital tract.[114,179] In addition, as sperm may have a shortened in vivo life span in the presence of antisperm antibodies, the better timing of insemination relative to ovulation after hMG-hCG treatment may contribute to the increased pregnancy rates in this group.

Although IUI overcomes the block to penetration of cervical mucus caused by head- or tail-directed antibodies, it cannot circumvent the impaired fertilizing ability of sperm caused by the binding of head-directed antibodies in the uterine and tubal fluids. Surface antisperm antibodies produced in the male genital tract may also interfere with the ability of the sperm to attach to the zona pellucida and have been shown to block or reduce penetration of zona-free hamster ova.[8] The hemizona binding assay may be helpful in differentiating between the populations of antibodies that will influence fertility and those that will not.[122] Nevertheless, when 100% of sperm are antibody bound, intrauterine insemination is not efficacious, regardless of the findings of other parameters of semen quality such as sperm motility.[59]

Sperm washing allows the removal of free or unbound antibodies present in the ejaculate. Unfortunately, because of the high affinity of antisperm antibodies for the sperm surface antigens, multiple washings and centrifugations fail to separate the bonds between them. Techniques required to remove the antibodies include washing with buffers of high ionic strength, which leads to loss of sperm function.[25] For treating seminal fluid antibodies that bind to sperm after ejaculation, immediate placement of the sperm into large diluting volumes or into solutions containing membrane fragments of freeze-thawed sperm as an immunoabsorbent may reduce the percentage of sperm that are antibody bound.[25] In most cases of refractory male immunologic infertility, IVF is the preferred method of therapy.

Endometriosis. Recent controlled studies have demonstrated no enhancement of fertility after medical therapy for endometriosis; cycle fecundity rates have ranged between 0.02 and 0.06 for both treated and expectantly managed groups.[136] IVF and gamete intrafallopian transfer (GIFT) have been successfully employed for this patient disease category. Because of the presence of apparently normal adnexal structures in most of these women, some investigators have suggested a role for alternative treatments such as superovulation with IUI in women with minimal or mild endometriosis (Table 41-7).

Kemmann et al.[94] noted that ovulatory stimulants improved the cycle fecundity of patients who had undergone laparoscopic CO_2 laser vaporization of minimal or mild endometriosis. Similarly, the data of Corson et al.[33] suggested that fecundity rates were higher in women with mild and minimal endometriosis undergoing IUI when hMG was added to the therapeutic program. IUI alone, however, was of no apparent help, and the authors concluded that the hMG was primarily responsible for the improved conception rate. In another recent retrospective study by Chaffkin et al.,[28] hMG alone was of minimal therapeutic benefit when compared with the cycle fecundity and cumulative pregnancy rates associated with combined menotropin/IUI therapy. Among couples who had failed to conceive despite laparoscopic laser surgery for endometriosis-associated infertility, the per-cycle pregnancy rates for hMG/coitus and hMG/IUI were 0.066 (5/76) and 0.128 (14/109), respectively. This increase in fecundity with the addition of homologous insemination approached, but did not meet, the criteria for statistical significance. In patients who had failed to conceive with prior hMG or IUI alone, the pregnancy rate per cycle following the introduction of hMG/IUI therapy equaled that of patients who received combined therapy from the onset. Considering the expense and risks involved with controlled hMG superovulation

Table 41-7. Clomiphene citrate and/or menotropin therapy with IUI for endometriosis-associated infertility

	Year	Patients	Pregnancies/ cycle	Fecundity
Clomiphene citrate cycles				
Deaton et al.*[41]	1990	27	7/76	0.09
Menotropin cycles				
Chaffkin et al.†[28]	1991	50	14/109	0.13
Dickey et al.[44]	1991			
All patients		NS	34/360	0.09
Minimal-mild		NS	28/246	0.11
Moderate-severe		NS	6/114	0.05
Dodson and Haney[47]	1991			
All patients		219	63/474	0.13
Minimal-mild		NS	54/409	0.13
Moderate-severe		NS	9/65	0.15

*24 of the 27 patients had minimal or mild stages of endometriosis that had been previously treated by laser laparoscopy.

†Patient population restricted to women who had previously received laparoscopic treatment of endometriosis.

therapy, it may be logical to maximize the benefits to the patient by the addition of IUI.

The cycle fecundity rates achieved through menotropin therapy and IUI in women with a history of endometriosis-associated infertility have approached those of GIFT and IVF in some assisted reproductive technology programs.[28,47] Hence controlled ovarian hyperstimulation, apart from oocyte retrieval and extracorporeal fertilization, may improve cycle fecundity in women with minimal or mild endometriosis.

Role of ovarian stimulation in IUI cycles

Clomiphene citrate. As with transcervical insemination in natural menstrual cycles, the overall efficacy of empirical clomiphene citrate administration to women undergoing IUI has been variable, with some studies reporting relatively good cycle fecundity[20] and others showing poor results.[22,74,94,114] Deaton and colleagues,[41] in a randomized prospective trial, compared clomiphene citrate and IUI with well-timed coitus in couples with either unexplained infertility or surgically corrected endometriosis. They found that the cycle fecundity rate in couples treated with clomiphene and IUI was 0.10, which compared with 0.033 for couples with well-timed intercourse. Using life table analysis and the log-rank test, the difference in fecundities was statistically significant. When comparing conception with nonconception cycles during treatment, no differences between the size of the lead follicle or the number of dominant follicles were detected.

Martinez et al.,[116] in a prospective, randomized, controlled study, found that IUI offered a definite advantage over timed intercourse in couples with idiopathic or male factor infertility, whereas the addition of clomiphene citrate did not improve fecundity. The pregnancy rate after IUI was 11.9% (8/67) per cycle or 20% (8/40) per couple. The

significantly higher number of follicles obtained in clomiphene-stimulated cycles did not substantially improve the pregnancy results either in IUI or timed intercourse cycles.

Similar findings in patients who received clomiphene were reported by Melis et al.[119]; however, these authors and others[20] have achieved significantly better results through IUI in polyovular cycles. Melis et al.[119] attributed this improvement to the higher number of developing follicles obtained with the addition of menotropins, although specific data on follicular recruitment were not presented in the publication. Hence the administration of clomiphene citrate may enhance fecundity rates, although it has yet to be established whether this response varies among infertility subgroups and through what mechanism this may occur.

Human menopausal gonadotropins. Correction of subtle ovulatory dysfunction has been the rationale for the use of agents such as clomiphene citrate, hMG, or both in combination in many categories of infertility. Abnormalities of folliculogenesis may include subnormal estradiol production, lower mean LH surges, and the luteinized unruptured follicle syndrome. Daly[40] found that dysfunctional ovulation as detected by ultrasound-determined follicular growth dynamics occurred in 12.2% of patients with unexplained infertility. The use of menotropin therapy in these women might overcome such deficiencies. Furthermore, the maturation of several oocytes per menstrual cycle should provide enhanced opportunity for fallopian tube capture, fertilization, and implantation. This may be particularly useful when the peritoneal environment is gametotoxic, such as has been ascribed to the infertile patient with endometriosis.[167] Multiple follicular development occurs in 5% to 10% of spontaneous cycles, as many as 35% to 60% of clomiphene-stimulated cycles, and is generally the rule in menotropin-induced cycles.[145]

The endometrium may provide a more favorable environment for implantation in some who receive hMG therapy. The combined use of hMG and luteal progesterone may treat patients with undiagnosed or borderline luteal phase deficiencies as well as those with clinically diagnosed luteal phase defects. Tubal motility and tubal and endometrial secretory products may be altered with hMG therapy and may play a role in conception rates. In addition, it is possible that couples with subtle, unrecognized defects in semen benefit from IUI. Asynchronous rupture of multiple follicles may lead to a widened time interval for fertilization to occur and a more optimal scheduling of the insemination procedure.

The weight of evidence suggests that for the categories of male factor, cervical factor, endometriosis, idiopathic, and possibly immunologic infertility, superovulation and IUI are additive in their enhancement of conception rates.[28,47,94,119,154] Kemmann et al.[94] reported that couples with male or cervical factor infertility had a cycle fecundity rate of 0.14 with superovulation and IUI, which compared with a rate of 0.02 for IUI in natural cycles. In a study comparing controlled ovarian hyperstimulation and IUI in women with unexplained infertility, Serhal et al.[154] noted that cycle fecundity increased from 0.06 with superovulation alone to 0.26 with combined menotropin/IUI therapy. Chaffkin and colleagues[28] determined that the mean cycle fecundity rate associated with hMG/IUI therapy (0.196) was significantly higher than either hMG or IUI therapy alone (0.063 and 0.034, respectively) in a heterogeneous group of 322 couples who underwent 751 cycles of therapy. In contrast to the decline in spontaneous pregnancy rates in untreated couples with increasing duration of infertility,[1] the success achieved with hMG/IUI may be independent of the duration of infertility.[47] Nevertheless, the above-cited findings are not universal; one recent controlled, prospective study of couples with male or idiopathic infertility receiving IUI therapy failed to confirm a beneficial effect of low-dose menotropin stimulation.[117]

Adjunctive gonadotropin-releasing hormone analogue therapy in controlled ovarian stimulation/IUI cycles. Several investigators have reported an increase in the number of collected oocytes, fertilization rate, length of the luteal phase, and pregnancy rate when a gonadotropin-releasing hormone (GnRH) analogue was included in the hMG stimulation protocol of IVF cycles.[62] Improvement of ovarian folliculogenesis, prevention of premature luteinization, homogenization of the cohort of oocytes, and enhancement of oocyte and embryo quality have all been proposed as possible mechanisms for this improved outcome.[173] Because of these results, Gagliari et al.[62] hypothesized that the addition of a GnRH analogue to the controlled ovarian hyperstimulation regimen followed by patients undergoing IUI would be beneficial in treating a population with multiple etiologies of infertility, including idiopathic, tubal factor, endometriosis, ovulatory dysfunctions, male factor,

luteal phase defect, and failed donor insemination. They achieved a significantly higher pregnancy rate per cycle when leuprolide was started in the midluteal phase of the menstrual cycle preceding hMG administration and continued until the day of hCG injection, as compared with that obtained in hMG only cycles (26.5% versus 16.0%; $P <$ 0.05). Sixty-three percent of both GnRH agonist-treated and nontreated women who achieved pregnancy did so during their first cycle of therapy. There was no increased rate of multiple gestations or fetal losses in the leuprolide-treated group. Thirteen of 28 patients who failed to conceive on hMG/IUI therapy conceived with GnRH analogue/hMG/IUI, and again the majority (69%) achieved pregnancy on their first cycle of such therapy.

Dodson et al.[50] recently assessed the use of leuprolide as adjunctive therapy in hMG/IUI cycles in a prospective study of 97 regularly ovulatory women with endometriosis, adnexal adhesions, idiopathic, and male factor infertility. An increase was noted in both the duration of stimulation and amount of menotropins required commensurate with the findings of Gagliardi et al.,[62] but a significant improvement in the cycle fecundity pregnancy rate was not obtained in leuprolide acetate/hMG/IUI cycles. The subjects in this report were regularly ovulating,[50] whereas 48% of the patients in the hMG group and 46% of the leuprolide/hMG group in the study by Gagliardi et al.[62] had some form of ovulatory dysfunction, luteal phase defect, or premature luteinization. Further trials will be necessary to establish the benefit of GnRH analogue administration to menotropin-stimulated patients undergoing IUI.

Superovulation parameters predictive of success. In the series by Dodson and Haney[47] describing the outcome of IUI in gonadotropin-stimulated patients, peak estradiol concentrations of greater than and less than 500 pg/mL were associated with cycle fecundities of 0.21 and 0.09, respectively. Nevertheless, there was no consistent correlation between the number of follicles measuring at least 17 mm in maximal diameter on the day of the initial hCG injection and the pregnancy rate per cycle. The age of the woman was inversely correlated with the rate of rise and peak estradiol and total number of follicles that developed. In addition, both the average serum estradiol concentration per follicle and cycle fecundity were inversely proportional to the age of the patient. Dickey et al.[44] also reported a significant correlation between estradiol and birth rate, which increased from 0.04 when estradiol was less than 500 pg/mL to 0.20 when estradiol was greater than or equal to 2500 pg/mL. The number of follicles greater than or equal to 17 mm at the time of hCG was correlated with fecundity and predicted all multiple births in this series of patients treated with gonadotropins and IUI. Other studies that restricted follicular response through a low-dose hMG regimen did not demonstrate a correlation between measures of multiple follicular development and cycle fecundity.[117]

Timing of conception

In accordance with the data of Friedman et al. and others regarding artificial insemination pregnancy rates in the natural menstrual cycle, it is appropriate to modify the approach to therapy of couples with cervical factor, male factor, and idiopathic infertility if conception has not occurred within four or five well-timed IUI cycles.[10,61,130] The same limitation of number of artificial insemination treatment cycles holds for patients who are undergoing controlled ovarian hyperstimulation, although a longer duration of therapy may be considered for the older woman. In the recently published series by Dodson and Haney,[47] no pregnancies were achieved with the fifth and sixth attempts, although few patients completed more than four courses who had not previously conceived with menotropin/IUI therapy. Life table analysis of the data of Chaffkin et al.[28] revealed that cycle fecundity declined significantly after three cycles of controlled superovulation with IUI. In addition, Remohi and colleagues[144] described a fecundity rate of 0.07 for the first four cycles of therapy and 0.03 for the fifth through 11th courses.

Risks of IUI in the natural or stimulated cycle

Spontaneous abortion. The rate of spontaneous abortion in patients treated with superovulation in conjunction with IUI has ranged from 20% to 29%.[47,79,103,157] This high incidence is comparable to those published statistics from IUI in natural cycles, 26%,[10] and through cervical insemination, 25%.[130] The increase in the observed rate of abortion in artificially inseminated patients over the 10% to 15% rate in the general population may be related to factors responsible for the infertility, such as sperm abnormalities, luteal phase defect, and genetic errors of the gametes. In addition, early detection of pregnancy in the subfertile population may lead to increased identification of early miscarriages.

Ectopic pregnancy. In patients with no history of pre-existing pelvic adhesive disease, the frequency of ectopic implantation of the conceptus after hMG administration and IUI is 4% to 5%.[47,79,157] However, in a series of patients with periovarian and peritubal adhesions treated in this manner, 18% of pregnancies were extrauterine.[2] These findings illustrate the fact that the incidence of ectopic pregnancies in an infertile population is significantly higher than the approximate 1% risk in the general population.[45]

Ovarian hyperstimulation syndrome. Ovarian hyperstimulation syndrome occurs in approximately 1 in 100 patients following hMG therapy. The syndrome is characterized by extreme ovarian enlargement, abdominal distention, ascites, pleural and occasional pericardial effusions, hemoconcentration, and electrolyte imbalance. Hyperstimulation may be particularly profound and prolonged with the occurrence of pregnancy. Risk factors associated with this condition include high serum estradiol levels and a large cohort of developing follicles. The full manifestations of ovarian hyperstimulation syndrome may be avoided in those patients identified to be at higher risk by withholding the injection of hCG. (See Chapter 35.)

Bleeding. Mild spotting will occur in 1% of patients after IUI, probably due to minor trauma inflicted by threading the insemination cannula through the external cervical os. The chance of establishing a pregnancy is reduced if the transfer causes intrauterine bleeding, for such trauma may induce the infiltration of phagocytic cells and initiate complement-mediated reactions, both of which may adversely affect the number and function of sperm in the upper genital tract.[96]

Pain. Transcervical insemination promotes uterine cramping in approximately 5% of treated patients. The mechanisms that may be responsible for this reaction include a reflex irritation caused by instrumentation of the cervical canal and stimulation by seminal prostaglandins that remain in the sample despite the usual laboratory processing procedures. In addition, disruption of the endometrium by the insemination cannula may initiate the prostaglandin cascade and stimulate the development of cramping 2 to 4 hours after completion of the procedure. A significant increase in baseline uterine activity and amplitude of contractions has been measured to last over 30 minutes when high concentrations of seminal plasma prostaglandins are present in the inseminate.[149] Diarrhea and nausea, prostaglandin-associated side effects, occur in 0.5% of all patients after IUI.[96]

Infection. Cervical mucus and semen may be colonized by a wide variety of aerobic and anaerobic bacteria, as well as by genital mycoplasma and *Chlamydia trachomatis.*[187] The cervical mucus and the cervical canal function as a physiologic barrier, allowing a preferential transport of sperm and inhibiting the passage of these microorganisms to the upper female genital tract, so that clinical infection rarely develops. By bypassing the protective filtration mechanism through IUI, the infectious risk may be increased because of the presence of microbes in the sperm suspension or through cervical contamination during catheterization. In vivo data lend credence to this concern. Stone et al.[164] demonstrated that peritoneal microorganisms could be isolated via laparoscopy from 56% of patients who underwent IUI, as compared with only 10% of cases of intracervical artificial insemination. Nevertheless, the reports of pelvic infection are extremely rare. Dodson and Haney[47] encountered one case of salpingitis after IUI in their series of over 800 inseminations, and Horvath et al.[79] reported a single occurrence of clinical salpingitis in 466 inseminations.

Sperm washing and swim-up techniques effectively reduce the microbial contamination of human semen.[187] This may occur through the bactericidal effect of penicillin and streptomycin present in the culture medium, separation of sperm and microorganisms during centrifugation, and the dilutional effect of the culture medium. Kuzan et al.[102]

compared the degree of bacterial contamination present by following three techniques of sperm separation. They found that a swimup over neat semen was superior to either a triple-wash technique or a combined wash and swim-up technique for separating bacteria from the final sperm suspension. Kaneko et al.[90] decreased bacterial density and numbers of species isolated using a double column, discontinuous Percoll density gradient. Similarly, Bolton et al.[22] found that a Percoll separation technique reduced the concentrations of skin and urethral bacteria that contaminated the semen. These laboratory results have not been correlated with relative clinical rates of infection.

Antisperm antibody formation. Injection of intact mouse sperm into the peritoneal cavities of mice has been shown to result in the production of antisperm antibodies.[52] Because with normal intercourse only tens of hundreds of sperm reach the peritoneal cavity, the greater antigenic load inherent with introduction of large numbers of sperm through intrauterine insemination may increase the risk of sensitization.[26] Fortunately, the findings of the majority of clinical trials have not justified this concern.

Preliminary data reported by Overstreet et al.[137] suggested that low pretreatment levels of antisperm antibodies in women may be significantly increased by IUI. Kremer[100] also found that the sperm agglutination titers of five women increased after IUI by two to four titer dilutions, but no sperm agglutination was measured in the serum of 15 previously negative women undergoing this therapy. In contrast, Goldberg et al.[68] measured only low, transient antisperm antibody titers in the serum and cervical mucus of women after four to six IUI cycles. These levels would not be expected to affect the prognosis for fertility. Moretti-Rojas et al.[127] tested the sera of 41 patients with agglutination and immobilization assays and the indirect immunobead assay before and after 1 to 15 cycles of IUI; two patients developed evidence of antisperm antibody formation. Neither higher total and motile sperm concentrations nor the presence of antisperm antibodies on the husband's sperm predisposed the patient to the development of antisperm antibodies. Furthermore, the level of antisperm antibody formation in menotropin-treated women has not been found to differ whether IUI or coitus is performed.[78] Hence the risk of inducing clinically significant antisperm antibody production is probably less than 3%.

Multiple gestation. Multiple gestations comprise 25% to 30% of all clinical pregnancies in women who receive hMG and IUI therapies.[48,157] Investigators have tried to identify risk factors associated with multiple gestation in this patient population, but a consensus has not been reached. Dodson et al.,[48] in a controlled study, found that no clinical parameter of semen quality or patient response to gonadotropin therapy was useful in predicting multiple gestation when ovulatory dysfunction was not present. The study controlled for age, parity, cause and duration of infertility, duration and amount of hMG used, serum estra-diol concentration on the day of hCG administration, number of preovulatory-sized follicles, and number of sperm used for insemination.

In a similarly designed study, Shelden and colleagues[157] found that insemination with greater than 20 million motile sperm significantly increased the risk of multiple gestation. The peak estradiol level, total dosage of hMG, and day of hCG administration were controlled for in analyzing the data, but not the number and size of preovulatory follicles.

In contrast to the results noted above, Gagliardi et al.[62] reported that a higher peak estradiol level and an increased number of follicles larger than 14 mm at the time of hCG administration after ovarian stimulation with leuprolide acetate and hMG were associated with a greater likelihood of multiple gestation. The peak estradiol level associated with singleton gestations was 1,046 pg/mL ± 82, whereas the peak estradiol concentration in multiple gestation cycles was 1,360 pg/mL ± 114. In addition, the mean follicle number associated with singleton gestations was 3.38 ± 0.38, whereas the mean follicle number leading to multiple gestations was 4.96 ± 0.23. Multiple gestations occurred with as few as 2.92×10^6 motile sperm in the insemination specimen. The patient population in this study had more diverse etiologies of infertility than that described by Shelden et al.,[157] who focused on couples treated with hMG/IUI for male or cervical factor infertility.

Unlike IVF and GIFT, hMG/IUI therapy provides no apparent mechanisms to control the occurrence of multiple pregnancies. Large numbers of preovulatory follicles may not be desirable in IUI cycles in order to limit this possibility. A sextuplet pregnancy has been reported in a patient undergoing hMG/IUI therapy despite the demonstration of only one follicle greater than 11 mm diameter.[60] For women who conceive with triplets or more, complete or selective pregnancy termination may be offered.

ALTERNATIVE THERAPIES

Gamete intrafallopian transfer

No comparative data have clearly shown IVF and GIFT to be superior to superovulation protocols in ovulatory women with normal pelvic anatomy. In one of the few published studies examining this issue, Kaplan et al.[92] retrospectively analyzed all GIFT and superovulation/IUI cycles at a single university center and found GIFT to be three times more efficient. However, as suggested by the authors, the inherent limitations of a nonrandomized, nonprospective study of this kind are obvious. Yovich and Matson,[188] in a nonrandomized study, compared the results achieved with IUI in couples with male factor, unexplained, and cervical factor infertility with those of a similar group of patients concurrently treated with GIFT. The overall cycle fecundity was 0.09 for IUI and 0.30 for GIFT; however, ovarian stimulation using clomiphene citrate or hMG was only applied to IUI patients with a history of disordered ovulatory cycles. IUI in canceled GIFT cycles has resulted in a cycle fecundity of 0.23, which compared with 0.40 in completed GIFT cycles.[39] Superovulation combined with IUI offers obvious benefits over other forms of assisted reproduction, for this treatment regimen costs substantially less than an IVF or GIFT cycle and has a lesser impact on the couple's lifestyle. Nevertheless, in couples with longstanding infertility, GIFT appears to offer a far greater chance of pregnancy than superovulation and IUI.[83]

Transuterine intratubal insemination

Transuterine intratubal insemination of capacitated sperm has been made possible by the development of catheters capable of being inserted through the uterus and placed in the ampulloisthmic region in an atraumatic fashion. This sonographically guided procedure has been suggested as a means to reduce the total number of motile sperm required for the insemination or decrease the need for superovulation in subfertile couples. Successful tubal catheterization in 46 of 50 cycles followed by insemination of frozen sperm samples resulted in six pregnancies.[87] Although the possibility of edema or blood clot formation in the proximal fallopian tube has been raised, there does not appear to be an increased rate of ectopic implantation in the few pregnancies that have been reported. Nevertheless, data from one study in which infertile patients were randomized to transuterotubal or IUI failed to demonstrate a significant difference in pregnancy rates between the two techniques.[135]

Direct intraperitoneal insemination

The technique of direct intraperitoneal insemination (DIPI) was initially described by Manhes and Hermabessiere in 1985.[113] Introduction of capacitated sperm to the peritoneal cavity around the time of ovulation may potentially bypass obstacles that inhibit fertilization and provide a useful treatment for certain categories of infertility such as cervical factor or male subfertility.[120] The indications, prerequisites, and exclusionary criteria for DIPI are very similar to those that exist for transcervical insemination. Menard et al.[121] have recommended the performance of an in vitro test of sperm survival and capacitation in peritoneal fluid and a control environment of buffered medium prior to consideration of direct intraperitoneal insemination.[134] In most cases, survival of sperm is higher in peritoneal fluid than in the reference environment, a result that is favorable for proceeding with therapy.

DIPI is usually performed in cycles of controlled ovarian hyperstimulation approximately 36 hours after administration of hCG, when the increased volume of peritoneal fluid and high local estrogen levels appear to favor the survival and capacitation of sperm.[54] After disinfecting the posterior vaginal fornix, a 19- or 21-gauge needle is inserted into the posterior cul de sac. Proper position of the needle is confirmed by identification of the free flow of peritoneal fluid. A 1- to 3-mL suspension of capacitated sperm is then injected. A second insemination may be performed on the following day if ultrasound study reveals a lack of follicular rupture.

In a large series of patients reported by Menard et al.,[121] DIPI resulted in a 19% pregnancy rate per couple and a 12% pregnancy rate per menstrual cycle. Two ectopic pregnancies occurred in patients with preexisting tubal lesions. These results contrast significantly with those of Jenkins and O'Donovan,[88] who noted only 1 pregnancy in 33 treatment cycles. An intermediate response was reported by Lesec et al.,[105] who achieved a pregnancy rate of 7% for male factor and unexplained infertility in a large study of 136 cases.

Crosignani and colleagues[36] reported on the outcome of 120 DIPI cycles in 77 couples with male subfertility and 44 DIPI cycles in 31 couples with unexplained infertility. Multiple follicular development was achieved with combined clomiphene-menotropin therapy. Twenty-three pregnancies were obtained, with fecundity rates of 0.227 per cycle and 0.322 per patient for unexplained infertility and 0.108 per cycle and 0.168 per patient for male subfertility. There were nine clinical abortions and one ectopic pregnancy among the conceptions. Two patients developed febrile pelvic infections after insemination; the authors subsequently introduced routine piperacillin antibiotic prophylaxis. Although pregnancies have been achieved with insemination of less than 1 million progressively motile spermatozoa, these cases are rare.[36,56,105]

Hovatta et al.[80] compared IUI versus DIPI in gonadotropin-stimulated women with unexplained, male factor, and endometriosis-associated infertility. The resultant pregnancy rates per treatment cycle were 8.6% for DIPI and 12.5% for IUI, values that were not statistically significant. The cumulative pregnancy rate per couple was 24% in the DIPI group and 31% in the IUI group. The pregnancy rates during the 326 control cycles of the same couples were markedly lower (1.1% and 0.6%, respectively). This equivalence in results has been confirmed in other series.[35] Since these data suggest that DIPI is not more effective than IUI, it may be more logical to select the more physiologic transcervical approach for the majority of inseminations, although some have suggested that embryo viability may be higher after DIPI.[15]

Besides the potential risk of introduction of bacteria directly into the peritoneal cavity, the intraperitoneal injection of larger numbers of washed sperm separated from seminal plasma may promote sperm immunization in women.[121] Although laboratory processing reduces the concentrations of seminal proteins that are antigenic to the female, it may remove the immunosuppressant properties of seminal plasma.[26] Critser et al.[34] found that eight of nine patients studied had positive antisperm antibody titers after two cycles of intraperitoneal insemination. Crosignani et al.,[36] on the other hand, found no antibody formation in 20 patients undergoing intraperitoneal insemination when evaluated 15 and 90 days after the procedure. Hence the relative risks and benefits of DIPI are still under investigation.

CONCLUSION

Although the valid indications for ICI are restricted to the use of donor sperm, extremes in semen volume, and certain conditions whereby intravaginal ejaculation is not possible, supracervical insemination appears to offer a broader range of applications in the treatment of subfertile conditions. Through use of semen separation techniques that minimize iatrogenic damage while ensuring sufficient recovery of a highly motile sperm fraction, well-timed IUI in the natural menstrual cycle may improve fecundity in certain cases of oligospermia, cervical factor infertility, and unexplained infertility. In addition, intracervical and intrauterine artificial insemination have been successfully used in men with retrograde ejaculation. There is increasing evidence that controlled ovarian hyperstimulation and IUI are additive in their enhancement of pregnancy rates for male factor, unexplained infertility, endometriosis, cervical factor, and possibly some forms of immunologic infertility.[28,31,47,94,154] This may occur through an increase in the number of gametes in the fallopian tube available for fertilization, a reduction in obstacles to sperm migration, correction of subtle defects of ovarian function through gonadotropin stimulation, or treatment of occult seminal abnormalities via laboratory processing. The relative merits of the more recently introduced techniques of transuterotubal insemination and direct intraperitoneal insemination have yet to be clearly established.

With the experience gained through controlled ovarian hyperstimulation in IVF centers, gonadotropin therapy has been extended to the ovulatory female, whereas previously these medications had been reserved for women with deficiencies in follicular development.[178] The emotional and financial expenses inherent with IVF and GIFT and the waiting period frequently required before commencing such therapy have provided added impetus to the application of gonadotropins for the empirical therapy of subfertile conditions. Nevertheless, the cost of superovulation is high, and this treatment carries with it the heightened risk of multiple pregnancy and possibly ectopic implantation. Effectiveness, expense, and safety must be carefully weighed before recommending this therapy to the individual couple.[178] Many questions remain to be answered by future controlled clinical trials of these techniques in assisted reproduction.

REFERENCES

1. Aafjes JH, van der Vijver JCM, Schenck PE: The duration of infertility: an important datum for the fertility prognosis of men with semen abnormalities, *Fertil Steril* 30:423, 1978.
2. Aboulghar MA, Mansour RT, Serour GI: Ovarian superstimulation in the treatment of infertility due to peritubal and periovarian adhesions, *Fertil Steril* 51:834, 1989.
3. Acosta AA et al: Assisted reproduction in the diagnosis and treatment of the male factor, *Obstet Gynecol Surv* 44:1, 1988.
4. Ahlgren M, Bostrom K, Malmquist R: Sperm transport and survival in women with special reference to the fallopian tube. In Hafez ESE, Thibault CG, editors: *The biology of spermatozoa,* Basel, Switzerland, 1975, S Karger.
5. Aitken RJ, Clarkson JS: Cellular basis of defective sperm function and its association with the genesis of reactive oxygen species by human spermatozoa, *J Reprod Fertil* 81:459, 1987.
6. Aitken RJ, Clarkson JS: Significance of reactive oxygen species and antioxidants in defining the efficacy of sperm preparation techniques, *J Androl* 9:367, 1988.
7. Aitken RJ et al: Analysis of the relationship between defective sperm function and the generation of reactive oxygen species in cases of oligozoospermia, *J Androl* 10:214, 1989.
8. Alexander NF: Antibodies to human spermatozoa impede sperm penetration of cervical mucus or hamster eggs, *Fertil Steril* 41:433, 1984.
9. Alexander NJ, Ackerman SB: Evaluation and preparation of spermatozoa for intrauterine insemination. In Acosta AA et al, editors: *Human spermatozoa in assisted reproduction,* Baltimore, 1990, Williams & Wilkins.
10. Allen NC et al: Intrauterine insemination: a critical review, *Fertil Steril* 44:569, 1985.
11. Alvarez JG et al: Spontaneous lipid peroxidation and production of hydrogen peroxide and superoxide in human spermatozoa: superoxide dismutase as major enzyme protectant against oxygen toxicity, *J Androl* 8:338, 1987.
12. Amelar RD, Hotchkiss RS: The split ejaculate: its use in the management of male infertility, *Fertil Steril* 16:46, 1965.
13. Arny M, Quagliarello J: Semen quality before and after processing by a swim-up method: relationship to outcome of intrauterine insemination, *Fertil Steril* 48:643, 1987.
14. Baerthlein WC, Muechler EK, Chaney K: Simplified sperm washing techniques and intrauterine insemination, *Obstet Gynecol* 71:277, 1988.
15. Barros A, Silva J, Maia J: Spontaneous abortions after intraperitoneal or intrauterine insemination, *Lancet* 337:302, 1991.
16. Barwin BW: Intrauterine insemination of husband's semen, *J Reprod Fertil* 36:101, 1974.
17. Behrman SJ, Sawada Y: Heterologous and homologous inseminations with human semen frozen and stored in a liquid nitrogen refrigerator, *Fertil Steril* 17:457, 1966.
18. Bennett CJ et al: Electroejaculation of paraplegic males followed by pregnancy, *Fertil Steril* 48:1070, 1987.
19. Berger T, Marrs RP, Moyer DL: Comparison of techniques for selection of motile spermatozoa, *Fertil Steril* 43:268, 1985.
20. Blumenfeld Z, Nahhas F: Pretreatment of sperm with human follicular fluid for borderline male infertility, *Fertil Steril* 51:863, 1989.
21. Bohrer M et al: The significance of the total number of motile sperm delivered with intrauterine insemination (IUI) in menotropin treated women. In Proceedings of the 42nd Annual Meeting of The American Fertility Society and the 18th Annual Meeting of the Canadian Fertility and Andrology Society, Toronto, Sept 27–Oct 2, 1986 (abstract).
22. Bolton VN, Warren RE, Braude PR: Removal of bacterial contaminants from semen for in vitro fertilization or artificial insemination by the use of buoyant density centrifugation, *Fertil Steril* 46:128, 1986.
23. Bostofte E, Serup J, Rebbe H: Relation between sperm count and semen volume, and pregnancies obtained during a twenty-year follow-up period, *Int J Androl* 5:267, 1982.
24. Brassesco M et al: Sperm recuperation and cervical insemination in retrograde ejaculation, *Fertil Steril* 49:923, 1988.
25. Bronson RA, Cooper GW, Rosenfeld D: Use of freeze-thawed sonicated human sperm as an in vitro immunoabsorbent, *Am J Reprod Immunol* 2:162, 1982.

26. Bronson R, Cooper G, Rosenfeld D: Sperm antibodies: their role in infertility, *Fertil Steril* 42:171, 1984.

27. Byrd W et al: Treatment of refractory infertility by transcervical intrauterine insemination of washed spermatozoa, *Fertil Steril* 48:921, 1987.

28. Chaffkin LM et al: A comparative analysis of the cycle fecundity rates associated with combined human menopausal gonadotropin (hMG) and intrauterine insemination (IUI) versus either hMG or IUI alone, *Fertil Steril* 55:252, 1991.

29. Collins JA et al: Treatment-independent pregnancy among infertile couples, *N Engl J Med* 309:1201, 1983.

30. Confino E et al: Intrauterine inseminations with washed human spermatozoa, *Fertil Steril* 46:55, 1986.

31. Corsan GH, Kemmann E: The role of superovulation with menotropins in ovulatory infertility: a review, *Fertil Steril* 55:468, 1991.

32. Corson SL et al: The human sperm-hamster egg penetration assay: prognostic value, *Fertil Steril* 49:328, 1988.

33. Corson SL et al: Intrauterine insemination and ovulation stimulation as treatment of infertility, *J Reprod Med* 34:397, 1989.

34. Critser JK et al: Sperm antibodies after intraperitoneal insemination of sperm. In Proceedings of the 6th World Congress of In Vitro Fertilization, Jerusalem, April 2–7, 1989 (abstract).

35. Crosignani PG, Walters DE, Solani A: The ESHRE multicentre trial on the treatment of unexplained infertility. In Proceedings of the 2nd Joint ESHRE ESCO Meeting, Milan, Italy, Aug 30, 1990, Oxford University Press (abstract).

36. Crosignani PG et al: Intraperitoneal insemination in the treatment of male and unexplained infertility, *Fertil Steril* 55:333, 1991.

37. Cruz RI et al: A prospective study of intrauterine insemination of processed sperm from men with oligoasthenospermia in superovulated women, *Fertil Steril* 46:673, 1986.

38. Cumming DC: Pregnancy rates following intrauterine insemination with washed or unwashed sperm, *Fertil Steril* 49:735, 1988.

39. Curole DN et al: Pregnancies in canceled gamete intrafallopian transfer cycles, *Fertil Steril* 51:363, 1989.

40. Daly D: Treatment validation of ultrasound-defined abnormal follicular dynamics as a cause of infertility, *Fertil Steril* 51:51, 1989.

41. Deaton JL et al: A randomized, controlled trial of clomiphene citrate and intrauterine insemination in couples with unexplained infertility or surgically corrected endometriosis, *Fertil Steril* 54:1083, 1990.

42. Decker WH: Pooled and frozen homologous (husband) semen for artificial insemination, *Infertility* 1:25, 1978.

43. Diamond MP et al: Pregnancy following use of the cervical cup for home artificial insemination utilizing homologous semen, *Fertil Steril* 39:480, 1983.

44. Dickey RP et al: Relationship of follicle number, serum estradiol, and other factors to birth rate and multiparity in human menopausal gonadotropin-induced intrauterine insemination cycles, *Fertil Steril* 56:89, 1991.

45. Dinsmoor M, Gibson M: Early recognition of ectopic pregnancy in an infertility population, *Obstet Gynecol* 68:859, 1986.

46. Dmowski WP et al: Artificial insemination homologous with oligospermic semen separated on albumin columns, *Fertil Steril* 31:58, 1982.

47. Dodson WC, Haney AF: Controlled ovarian hyperstimulation and intrauterine insemination for treatment of infertility, *Fertil Steril* 55:457, 1991.

48. Dodson WC, Hughes CL, Haney AF: Multiple pregnancies conceived with intrauterine insemination during superovulation: an evaluation of clinical characteristics and monitored parameters of conception cycles, *Am J Obstet Gynecol* 159:382, 1988.

49. Dodson WC et al: Superovulation with intrauterine insemination in the treatment of infertility: a possible alternative to gamete intrafallopian transfer and in vitro fertilization, *Fertil Steril* 48:441, 1987.

50. Dodson WC et al: Adjunctive leuprolide therapy does not improve cycle fecundity in controlled ovarian hyperstimulation and intrauterine insemination of subfertile women, *Obstet Gynecol* 78:187, 1991.

51. Eckerling B: Sterility due to oligospermia and hypokinesis of the sperm, *Fertil Steril* 11:475, 1960.

52. Edwards RG: Immunological control of fertility in female mice, *Nature* 201:582, 1964.

53. Evans G, Armstrong DT: Reduction of sperm transport in ewes by superovulation treatments, *J Reprod Fertil* 70:47, 1984.

54. Faundes A et al: Sperm migration of different stages of menstrual cycle, *Int J Gynaecol Obstet* 19:361, 1981.

55. Fisch P et al: Unexplained infertility: evaluation of treatment with clomiphene citrate and human chorionic gonadotropin, *Fertil Steril* 51:828, 1989.

56. Forrler A et al: Direct intraperitoneal insemination: first results confirmed, *Lancet* 1:1468, 1986.

57. Forster MS et al: Selection of human spermatozoa according to their relative motility and their interaction with zona-free hamster eggs, *Fertil Steril* 40:655, 1983.

58. Francavilla F et al: Effect of sperm morphology and motile sperm count on outcome of intrauterine insemination in oligozoospermia and/or asthenozoospermia, *Fertil Steril* 53:892, 1990.

59. Francavilla F et al: Failure of intrauterine insemination in male immunological infertility in cases in which all spermatozoa are antibody-coated, *Fertil Steril* 58:587, 1992.

60. Friedman AJ: Sextuplet pregnancy after human menopausal gonadotropin superovulation and intrauterine insemination, *J Reprod Med* 35:113, 1990.

61. Friedman AJ et al: Life table analysis of intrauterine insemination pregnancy rates for couples with cervical factor, male factor, and idiopathic infertility, *Fertil Steril* 55:1005, 1991.

62. Gagliardi CL et al: Gonadotropin-releasing hormone agonist improves the efficiency of controlled ovarian hyperstimulation/intrauterine insemination, *Fertil Steril* 55:939, 1991.

63. Gellert-Mortimer ST et al: Evaluation of Nycodenz and Percoll density gradients for the selection of motile human spermatozoa, *Fertil Steril* 49:335, 1988.

64. Gerris JM et al: The value of intrauterine insemination with washed husband's sperm in the treatment of infertility, *J Reprod* 2:315, 1987.

65. Glass RH, Ericsson RJ: Intrauterine insemination of isolated motile sperm, *Fertil Steril* 29:535, 1978.

66. Glazener CMA et al: The value of insemination with husband's semen in infertility due to failure of postcoital sperm mucus penetration: controlled trial of treatment, *Br J Obstet Gynaecol* 94:774, 1987.

67. Glezerman M, Bernstein D, Insler V: The cervical factor of infertility and intrauterine insemination, *Int J Fertil* 29:16, 1984.

68. Goldberg JM et al: Antisperm antibodies in women undergoing intrauterine insemination, *Am J Obstet Gynecol* 163:65, 1990.

69. Gunther VE, Radtke M, Schreiber G: Zur Korrelation von Spermaparametern und männlicher Fertilität, *Dermatol Monatsschr* 163:257, 1977.

70. Guttmacher AF: The role of artificial insemination in the treatment of human sterility, *Bull N Y Acad Med* 2nd Ser 19:573, 1943.

71. Harris SJ et al: Improved separation of motile sperm in asthenospermia and its application to artificial insemination homologous (AIH), *Fertil Steril* 36:219, 1981.

72. Harrison RF: Insemination of husband's semen with and without the addition of caffeine, *Fertil Steril* 29:532, 1978.

73. Harvey C, Jackson MJ: A method of concentrating spermatozoa in human semen, *J Clin Pathol* 8:341, 1955.

74. Hewitt J et al: Treatment of idiopathic infertility, cervical mucus hostility, and male infertility: artificial insemination with husband's semen or in vitro fertilization?, *Fertil Steril* 44:350, 1985.

75. Ho P-C, Poon IML, Chan SYW: Intrauterine insemination is not useful in oligoasthenospermia, *Fertil Steril* 51:682, 1989.

76. Hoing LM, Devroey P, Van Steirteghem AC: Treatment of infertility because of oligoasthenoteratospermia by transcervical intrauterine insemination of motile spermatozoa, *Fertil Steril* 45:388, 1986.

77. Homonnai ZT et al: Quality of semen obtained from 627 fertile men, *Int J Androl* 3:217, 1980.

78. Horvath PM et al: A prospective study on the lack of development of antisperm antibodies in women undergoing intrauterine insemination, *Am J Obstet Gynecol* 160:631, 1989.

79. Horvath PM et al: The relationship of sperm parameters to cycle fecundity in superovulated women undergoing intrauterine insemination, *Fertil Steril* 52:228, 1989.

80. Hovatta O et al: Direct intraperitoneal or intrauterine insemination and superovulation in infertility treatment: a randomized study, *Fertil Steril* 54:339, 1990.

81. Hughes EG, Collins JP, Garner PR: Homologous artificial insemination for oligoasthenospermia: a randomized controlled study comparing intracervical and intrauterine techniques, *Fertil Steril* 48:278, 1987.

82. Hull ME et al: Experience with intrauterine insemination for cervical factor and oligospermia, *Am J Obstet Gynecol* 154:1333, 1986.

83. Iffland CA et al: A within-patient comparison between superovulation with intrauterine artificial insemination using husband's washed spermatozoa and gamete intrafallopian transfer in unexplained infertility, *Eur J Obstet Gynecol Reprod Biol* 39:181, 1991.

84. Irianni FM et al: Therapeutic intrauterine insemination (TII): controversial treatment for infertility, *Arch Androl* 25:147, 1990.

85. Irvine DS et al: Failure of high intrauterine insemination of husband's semen, *Lancet* 2:972, 1986.

86. Iwasaki A, Gagnon C: Free radical formation in human semen: incidence and correlation with sperm motility. In Proceedings of the 35th Annual Meeting of the Canadian Fertility and Andrology Society, Vancouver, BC, Nov 8-11, 1989 (abstract).

87. Jansen RPS et al: Pregnancies after ultrasound-guided fallopian insemination with cryostored donor semen, *Fertil Steril* 49:920, 1988.

88. Jenkins DM, O'Donovan P: Direct intraperitoneal insemination, *Lancet* 1:655, 1988.

89. Jette NT, Glass RH: Prognostic value of the postcoital test, *Fertil Steril* 23:29, 1972.

90. Kaneko S et al: Continuous-step density gradient for the selective concentration of progressively motile sperm for insemination with husband's semen, *Arch Androl* 19:75, 1984.

91. Kanwar KC, Yanagimachi R, Lopata A: Effects of human seminal plasma on fertilizing capacity of human spermatozoa, *Fertil Steril* 31:321, 1979.

92. Kaplan CR et al: Gamete intrafallopian transfer versus superovulation with intrauterine insemination for the treatment of infertility, *J In Vitro Fert Embryo Transfer* 6:298, 1989.

93. Kaskarelis E, Comminos A: A critical evaluation of homologous artificial insemination, *Int J Fertil* 4:38, 1959.

94. Kemmann E et al: Active ovulation management increases the monthly probability of pregnancy occurrence in ovulatory women who receive intrauterine insemination, *Fertil Steril* 48:916, 1987.

95. Kerin JF, Quinn P: Washed intrauterine insemination in the treatment of oligospermic infertility, *Semin Reprod Endocrinol* 5:23, 1987.

96. Kerin JF, Quinn P: Supracervical placement of spermatozoa: utility of intrauterine and tubal insemination. In Soules MR, editor: *Controversies in reproductive endocrinology and infertility,* New York, 1989, Elsevier.

97. Kerin JF et al: Improved conception rate after intrauterine insemination of washed spermatozoa from men with poor quality semen, *Lancet* 1:533, 1984.

98. Kirby CA et al: A prospective trial of intrauterine insemination of motile spermatozoa versus timed intercourse, *Fertil Steril* 56:102, 1991.

99. Kredentser JV, Pokrant C, McCoshen JA: Intrauterine insemination for infertility due to cystic fibrosis, *Fertil Steril* 45:425, 1986.

100. Kremer J: A new technique for intrauterine insemination, *Int J Fertil* 24:53, 1979.

101. Kruger TF et al: Sperm morphologic features as a prognostic factor in IVF, *Fertil Steril* 46:1118, 1986.

102. Kuzan FB, Hillier SL, Zarutskie PW: Comparison of three wash techniques for the removal of microorganisms from semen, *Obstet Gynecol* 70:836, 1987.

103. Lalich RA et al: Life table analysis of intrauterine insemination pregnancy rates, *Am J Obstet Gynecol* 158:980, 1988.

104. Lenton EA, Weston GA, Cooke ID: Long-term follow-up of the apparently normal couple with a complaint of infertility, *Fertil Steril* 28:913, 1977.

105. Lesec G et al: In-vivo transperitoneal fertilization, *Hum Reprod* 4:521, 1989.

106. Liu DY et al: Human sperm-zona pellucida binding, sperm characteristics and in vitro fertilization, *Hum Reprod* 4:696, 1989.

107. MacLeod J, Gold RZ: The male factor in fertility and infertility, II: spermatozoon counts in 1000 cases of known fertility and in 1000 cases of infertile marriage, *J Urol* 66:436, 1951.

108. MacLeod J, Gold R, McLane CM: Correlation of the male and female factors in human infertility, *Fertil Steril* 6:112, 1955.

109. McClure RD, Nunes L, Tom R: Semen manipulation: improved sperm recovery and function with a two-layer Percoll gradient, *Fertil Steril* 51:874, 1989.

110. McGovern P, Quagliarello J, Arny M: Relationship of within-patient semen variability to outcome of intrauterine insemination, *Fertil Steril* 51:1019, 1989.

111. Makler A: Washed intrauterine insemination in the treatment of idiopathic infertility, *Semin Reprod Endocrinol* 5:35, 1987.

112. Makler A, Murillo O, Huszar A: Improved technique for separating motile spermatozoa from human semen, II: an atraumatic centrifugation method, *Int J Androl* 7:71, 1984.

113. Manhes H, Hermabessiere J: Fécondation intrapéritoneale: première grossesse obtenue sur indication masculine. In Proceedings of the Third International Forum on Andrology, Paris, June 18–19, 1985 (abstract).

114. Margalloth EJ et al: Intrauterine insemination as treatment for antisperm antibodies in the female, *Fertil Steril* 40:441, 1988.

115. Marrs RP et al: Clinical applications of techniques used in human in vitro fertilization research, *Am J Obstet Gynecol* 146:477, 1983.

116. Martinez AR et al: Intrauterine insemination does and clomiphene citrate does not improve fecundity in couples with infertility due to male or idiopathic factors: a prospective, randomized, controlled study, *Fertil Steril* 53:87, 1990.

117. Martinez AR et al: Pregnancy rates after timed intercourse or intrauterine insemination after human menopausal gonadotropin stimulation of normal ovulatory cycles: a controlled study, *Fertil Steril* 55:258, 1991.

118. Mastroianni L Jr, Laberge JL, Rock J: Appraisal of the efficacy of artificial insemination with husband's sperm and evaluation of insemination technic, *Fertil Steril* 8:260, 1957.

119. Melis GB et al: Pharmacologic induction of multiple follicular development improves the success rate of artificial insemination with husband's semen in couples with male-related or unexplained infertility, *Fertil Steril* 47:441, 1987.

120. Menard A: Liquide péritoneal et fertilité-insémination intrapéritonéale par culdocentèse, thèse, Paris, 1986,

121. Menard A et al: Evaluation and preparation of spermatozoa for direct intraperitoneal insemination. In Acosta AA et al, editors: *Human spermatozoa in assisted reproduction,* Baltimore, 1990, Williams & Wilkins.

122. Menge AC et al: The incidence and influence of antisperm antibodies in infertile human couples on sperm-cervical mucus interaction and subsequent fertility, *Fertil Steril* 38:439, 1982.

123. Mitchell JR, Senger PL, Rosenberger JL: Distribution and retention of spermatozoa with acrosomal and nuclear abnormalities in the cow genital tract, *J Anim Sci* 61:956, 1985.

124. Moghissi KS: The function of the cervix in human reproduction, *Curr Probl Obstet Gynecol* 7:1, 1984.

125. Moghissi KS et al: Homologous artificial insemination: a reappraisal, *Am J Obstet Gynecol* 129:909, 1977.

126. Moore DE et al: SOURCE; a nonsurgical alternative to IVF/GIFT. In Proceedings of the Pacific Coast Fertility Society Meeting, Palm Springs, Calif, May 6-10, 1987 (abstract).

127. Moretti-Rojas I et al: Intrauterine insemination with washed spermatozoa does not induce formation of antigen antibodies, *Fertil Steril* 53:180, 1990.

128. Mortimer D: Sperm preparation techniques and iatrogenic failures of in-vitro fertilization, *Hum Reprod* 6:173, 1991.

129. Mortimer D, Templeton AA: Sperm transport in the human female reproductive tract in relation to semen analysis characteristics and time of ovulation, *J Reprod Fertil* 64:401, 1982.

130. Nachtigall RD: Indications, techniques and success rates for AIH, *Semin Reprod Endocrinol* 5:5, 1987.

131. Nachtigall RD, Faure ND, Glass RH: Artificial insemination of husband's sperm, *Fertil Steril* 32:141, 1979.

132. Nelson CMK, Bung RG: Semen analysis: evidence for changing parameters of male fertility potential, *Fertil Steril* 251:503, 1974.

133. Nunley WC, Kitchin JD, Thiagarajah S: Homologous insemination, *Fertil Steril* 30:510, 1978.

134. Oak MK et al: Sperm survival studies in peritoneal fluid from infertile women with endometriosis and unexplained infertility, *Clin Reprod Fertil* 3:297, 1985.

135. Oei ML et al: A prospective, randomized study of pregnancy rates after transuterotubal and intrauterine insemination, *Fertil Steril* 58:167, 1992.

136. Olive DL, Haney AF: Endometriosis-associated infertility: a critical review of therapeutic approaches, *Obstet Gynecol Surv* 4:538, 1986.

137. Overstreet JW et al: Antisperm antibodies in women receiving intrauterine insemination. In Proceedings of the 35th Annual Meeting of the Society of Gynecologic Investigation, Baltimore, March 17–20, 1988 (abstract).

138. Pardo M et al: Spermatozoa selection in discontinuous Percoll density gradients for use in artificial insemination, *Fertil Steril* 49:505, 1988.

139. Paulson JD, Polakoski KI: The removal of extraneous material from the ejaculate, *Int J Androl Suppl* 1:163, 1978.

140. Pickering SH et al: Are human spermatozoa separated on a Percoll density gradient safe for therapeutic use?, *Fertil Steril* 51:1024, 1989.

141. Polansky FF, Lamb EJ: Do the results of semen analysis predict future fertility?: a survival analysis study, *Fertil Steril* 49:59, 1988.

142. Quagliarello J, Arny M: Intracervical versus intrauterine insemination: correlation of outcome with antecedent postcoital testing, *Fertil Steril* 46:870, 1986.

143. Quinn P, Warnes GM, Kerin JF: Improved pregnancy rate in human in vitro fertilization with the use of a medium based on the composition of human tubal fluid, *Fertil Steril* 44:493, 1985.

144. Remohi J et al: Intrauterine insemination and controlled ovarian hyperstimulation in cycles before GIFT, *Hum Reprod* 4:918, 1989.

145. Ritchie WGM: Ultrasound in the evaluation of normal and induced ovulation, *Fertil Steril* 43:167, 1985.

146. Rogers BJ: The usefulness of sperm penetration assay in predicting in vitro fertilization (IVF) success, *J In Vitro Fert Embryo Transfer* 33:209, 1986.

147. Rogers BJ et al: Variability in the human-hamster, in vitro assay for fertility evaluation, *Fertil Steril* 39:204, 1983.

148. Russell JK: Artificial insemination (husband) in the management of childlessness, *Lancet* 2:1223, 1960.

149. Sahmay S, Atasu T, Karacan I: The effect of intrauterine insemination on uterine activity, *Int J Fertil* 35:310, 1990.

150. Sato H et al: Improved semen qualities after continuous-step density gradient centrifugation: application to artificial insemination and pregnancy outcome, *Arch Androl* 24:87, 1990.

151. Schellen AMCM: *Artificial insemination in the human,* New York, 1957, Elsevier.

152. Scott JZ et al: The cervical factor in infertility: diagnosis and treatment, *Fertil Steril* 28:1289, 1977.

153. Serafini P et al: Enhanced penetration of zona-free hamster ova by sperm prepared by Nycodenz and Percoll gradient centrifugation, *Fertil Steril* 53:551, 1990.

154. Serhal PF et al: Unexplained infertility: the value of Pergonal superovulation combined with intrauterine insemination, *Fertil Steril* 49:602, 1988.

155. Settlage DS, Motoshima M, Tredway DR: Sperm transport from the external cervical os to the fallopian tubes in women: a time and quantitative study, *Fertil Steril* 24:655, 1973.

156. Shangold GA, Cantor B, Schreiber JR: Treatment of infertility due to retrograde ejaculation: a simple, cost-effective method, *Fertil Steril* 54:175, 1990.

157. Shelden R et al: Multiple gestation is associated with the use of high sperm numbers in the intrauterine insemination specimen in women undergoing gonadotropin stimulation, *Fertil Steril* 49:607, 1988.

158. Sher G et al: In vitro sperm capacitation and transcervical intrauterine insemination for the treatment of refractory infertility: phase I, *Fertil Steril* 41:260, 1984.

159. Silverberg KM et al: A prospective, randomized trial comparing two different intrauterine insemination regimens in controlled ovarian hyperstimulation cycles, *Fertil Steril* 57:357, 1992.

160. Sims JM: *Clinical notes on uterine surgery with special reference to the management of the sterile condition,* New York, 1871, William Wood and Co.

161. Soto-Albors C, Daly DC, Ying Y-K: Efficacy of human menopausal gonadotropins as therapy for abnormal cervical mucus, *Fertil Steril* 51:58, 1989.

162. Speichinger JP, Mattox JH: Homologous artificial insemination and oligospermia, *Fertil Steril* 27:135, 1976.

163. Steiman RP, Taymor ML: AIH and its role in the management of infertility, *Fertil Steril* 28:146, 1977.

164. Stone SC, de la Maza LM, Peterson EM: Recovery of microorganism from the pelvic cavity after intracervical or intrauterine artificial insemination, *Fertil Steril* 46:61, 1986.

165. Stumpf PG, Lloyd T: In vitro penetration of human sperm into bovine cervical mucus: effects of sperm washing and exposure to low temperatures, *Obstet Gynecol* 65:42, 1985.

166. Sunde A, Kahn J, Molne K: Intrauterine insemination, *Hum Reprod* 3:97, 1988.

167. Syrop CH, Halme J: Peritoneal fluid environment and infertility, *Fertil Steril* 48:1, 1987.

168. Tanphaichitr N et al: Egg penetration ability and structural properties of human sperm prepared by Percoll-gradient centrifugation, *Gamete Res* 20:67, 1988.

169. Taylor PL, Kelly RW: 19-OH E prostaglandins as the major prostaglandin of human semen, *Nature* 250:665, 1974.

170. Taymor ML, Idriss WK: The role of AIH in male subfertility. In Emperaire JC, Audebert A, editors: *First international symposium on artificial insemination homologous and male subfertility, Bordeaux, France, May 6-7, 1978,* Bordeaux, 1978, Institute Aquitain de Recherches sur la Reproduction Humaine.

171. Tea NT, Jondet M, Scholler R: A "migration-gravity sedimentation" method for collecting motile spermatozoa from human semen. In Harrison RF, Bonnar J, Thompson W, editors: *In vitro fertilization, embryo transfer and early pregnancy,* Lancaster, UK, 1984, MTP Press.

172. te Velde ER, van Kooy RJ, Waterreus JJH: Intrauterine insemination of washed husband's spermatozoa: a controlled study, *Fertil Steril* 51:182, 1989.

173. Thanki KH, Schmidt CL: Follicular development and oocyte maturation after stimulation with gonadotropins versus leuprolide acetate/gonadotropins during in vitro fertilization, *Fertil Steril* 54:656, 1990.

174. Thomas EJ et al: Failure of high intrauterine insemination of husband's semen, *Lancet* 2:693, 1986.

175. Toffle RC et al: Intrauterine insemination, the University of Minnesota experience, *Fertil Steril* 43:743, 1985.

176. Urry RL, Middleton RG, McGavin S: A simple and effective technique for increasing pregnancy rates in couples with retrograde ejaculation, *Fertil Steril* 46:1124, 1986.

177. Usherwood MMcD, Halim A, Evans PR: Artificial insemination (AIH) for sperm antibodies and oligospermia, *Br J Urol* 48:499, 1976.

178. Wallach EE: Gonadotropin treatment for the ovulatory patient: the pros and cons of empiric therapy for infertility, *Fertil Steril* 55:478, 1991.

179. Wang CF, Gemzell C: Pregnancy following treatment with human gonadotropins in primary unexplained infertility, *Acta Obstet Gynecol Scand* 58:141, 1979.

180. Weathersbee PS, Werlin LB, Stone SC: Peritoneal recovery of sperm after intrauterine insemination, *Fertil Steril* 42:322, 1984.

181. Welner S, DeCherney AH, Polan ML: Human menopausal gonadotropins: a justifiable therapy in ovulatory women with long-standing idiopathic infertility, *Am J Obstet Gynecol* 158:111, 1988.

182. White RM, Glass RH: Intrauterine insemination with husband's semen, *Obstet Gynecol* 47:119, 1976.

183. Whitelaw WJ: The cervical cap self-applied in the treatment of severe oligospermia, *Fertil Steril* 27:135, 1976.

184. Wiltbank MC, Kosasa TS, Rogers BJ: Treatment of infertile patients by intrauterine insemination of washed spermatozoa, *Andrologia* 17:22, 1984.

185. Witkin SS, Toth A: Relationship between genital tract infections, sperm antibodies in seminal fluid, and infertility, *Fertil Steril* 40:805, 1983.

186. Wolf DP, Sokoloski JE: Characterization of the sperm penetration bioassay, *J Androl* 3:445, 1982.

187. Wong PC et al: Sperm washing and swim-up technique using antibiotics removes microbes from human semen, *Fertil Steril* 45:97, 1986.

188. Yovich JL, Matson PL: Pregnancy rates after high intrauterine insemination of husband's spermatozoa or gamete intrafallopian transfer, *Lancet* 2:1287, 1986.

189. Zavos PM: Seminal parameters of ejaculates collected from oligospermic and normospermic patients via masturbation and at intercourse with use of Silastic seminal fluid collection device, *Fertil Steril* 44:517, 1985.

190. Zukerman Z et al: Frequency and distribution of sperm counts in fertile and infertile males, *Fertil Steril* 28:1310, 1977.

Chapter 42

THERAPEUTIC DONOR INSEMINATION

William D. Schlaff, MD

HISTORY

Although artificial insemination to many is a burgeoning practice of the twentieth century, the process was in fact contemplated as early as 300 B.C. by Talmudic scholars who pondered the possibility that a woman might conceive a child without any direct physical contact. This concern was further stimulated by an apocryphal story of a woman who conceived in a bath 24 hours after a male relative had used the same facility. While the purported events may not have been particularly accurate, these discussions clearly reflect both a theoretic and a practical appreciation for the possibility of artificial or donor insemination. In the Middle Ages, artificial insemination was reported to have been used in horses as well as fish. The first clearly recorded use of artificial insemination in the human was performed in 1799 by Dr. John Hunter, of Scotland. He obtained semen from his patient's husband, who had hypospadias, and deposited it in the patient's vagina with a resultant pregnancy. Interestingly, Lazaro Spallanzani had proved only 20 years previously that it was seminal fluid that was required to initiate pregnancy, and it was not until 25 years later that Prevost and Dumas proved that the sperm cells described by van Leeuwenhoek in the late seventeenth century were the component within the semen that was required for fertilization to occur. Subsequently, Girault in France in 1838 and J. Marion Sims in New York City in 1866 performed artificial insemination using husband's sperm on women believed to have anatomic abnormalities causing infertility. Interestingly, the specimen in most cases was inseminated directly into the uterine cavity. Seven of ten of Girault's patients conceived, and one of six patients of Dr. Sims became pregnant. Although these cases demonstrated the fact that artificial insemination could produce pregnancies, major concerns regarding timing, technique of insemination, and success rates arose even then.

The first recorded donor insemination success in the United States was performed in 1884 by Dr. William Pancoast, of the Jefferson Medical College in Philadelphia. A wealthy businessman, thought to be azoospermic after a bout of gonorrhea, requested help in establishing a pregnancy. Unbeknown to either husband or wife, the "best-looking member of the class" was solicited as a semen donor, and his specimen was injected into the wife's uterus while she was under anesthesia. Pregnancy resulted, and it was only after a significant delay and great ambivalence that Dr. Pancoast ultimately informed the husband of what had occurred. Fortunately, the husband was pleased, although all agreed that they would not discuss the incident further. Somewhat predictably, the secret ultimately was revealed by Dr. Addison Davis Hard, one of the medical students involved in the conspiracy, in an article published in 1909.[28] The facts in this case illustrate many of the dilemmas regarding informed consent, patient and donor screening, and record keeping that pertain even today. Only the increased scientific data and progressively open discussion of reproductive rights and donor insemination have resulted in the safer and better established standards and guidelines of the late twentieth century.

There have been various estimates of the number of children born through donor insemination in the United States. The generally accepted guess was about 1,000 per year through the 1940s, 1950s, and 1960s, increasing dramatically to the range of 5,000 to 10,000 or more per year in the 1970s and 1980s.[18,63] However, not until the Office of Technology Assessment of the U.S. Congress performed a national survey in 1987 was presumably more accurate information obtained; the survey showed that approximately 30,000 babies were born in the United States that year as a result of 170,000 women undergoing therapeutic donor insemination.[67] This number represents eight to ten times the number of successful pregnancies produced by all other forms of assisted reproduction combined. This chapter reviews the medical, legal, and social aspects of donor insemination as they pertain to the practice of contemporary reproductive medicine.

INDICATIONS

Poor quantity or quality of sperm

The indication for therapeutic donor insemination (TDI) is the absence of sperm sufficient in quantity and or quality to be likely to produce a pregnancy. Inherent in this description is a broad range of problems encompassing the man who is genetically or anatomically unable to produce any sperm to another who may have completely normal sperm but also have a genetic or psychologic reason compelling him and his partner to request donor insemination. At the other extreme may be the woman who has no sexual partner yet desires a child and seeks donor insemination. Thus the straightforward indications for TDI so commonly brought to mind are frequently clouded by other medical and social considerations. Furthermore, new assisted reproductive techniques can now provide some hope for many men who previously had been considered irreversibly subfertile. Therefore, before recommending donor insemination to any individual or couple, one must thoroughly understand the indications for the procedure, as well as the available alternatives.

The first step in this important process is to obtain a thorough history of the man's subfertility. Pertinent medical records frequently are available but not commonly brought to an initial consultation. In this case, a general discussion of donor insemination should be provided, but the physician should be discouraged from committing to a course of TDI without thoroughly reviewing the previous medical records. It is often striking that the couple's understanding of the nature of and reasons for pursuing donor insemination are unclear, and that the man's evaluation frequently is incomplete or suboptimal. Should the latter be true, it is most appropriate to defer any recommendation regarding TDI until a thorough evaluation has been completed and an accurate prognosis based on available reproductive techniques can be provided to the couple. An important part of this consultation is a discussion of alternatives. Although significant oligospermia or asthenospermia has heretofore been the most common indication for donor insemination, other techniques, including in vitro fertilization (IVF), may now be considered. Pregnancies through IVF have been accomplished with significantly fewer than 1 million motile sperm cells, and the possibilities using new microscopic techniques may expand this horizon even further. Admittedly, success rates for such procedures are likely to remain poor for some time, and expenses in the range of $8,000 to $10,000 per IVF cycle, compared with $150 to $350 per TDI cycle, may prompt the couple to eschew aggressive reproductive techniques. It is far more straightforward to recommend TDI when the husband has irreversible azoospermia, such as in gonadal failure. Yet it is still wise to discuss available alternatives (including adoption) even in this context.

Genetic problems

Abnormalities other than those directly related to sperm may be indications for donor insemination. These may include a specific genetic defect such as Huntington's chorea or multifactorial inherited problems such as early heart disease, cancer, or mental illness. The potential impact of these genetic problems, particularly when the inheritance pattern is less well defined, should be thoroughly reviewed with patients before initiating donor insemination. Psychologic difficulties prompting couples to seek donor insemination primarily include sexual dysfunction, but may also reflect marital discord. In all cases, counseling should be discussed thoroughly, and a decision regarding donor insemination should be deferred until the physician is confident that proceeding with insemination would be in the best interest of both the couple and the child likely to result.

Absence of a male partner

An important emerging indication for donor insemination is the absence of a male partner. Single women wishing to conceive but unwilling to have sexual relations with a known male partner in order to do so represent a significant body of patients now being considered for donor insemination. Many health professionals have biases regarding insemination of single women, particularly if they are also lesbians. There are few data examining the long-term outcome of these women and their children, and the existing data do not suggest any significant difference in outcome compared with married couples.[41,64] Insemination of single women should therefore be considered a legitimate indication for TDI, although practitioners often choose to reflect their own biases in their practice. Important legal issues relating to parental obligations are covered by laws in many states, as discussed later in this chapter. State statutes rarely address parental responsibilities of single women. These issues should be discussed with all single women before donor insemination is initiated.

SCREENING THE PATIENT

History and physical examination

Once the decision has been reached to proceed with donor insemination, a thorough patient history and physical examination should be performed. The purpose is to identify any factor that may reduce the fecundity of the woman and to identify potential risks for bearing an abnormal child. Therefore the history should include a detailed discussion of potential risk factors for subfertility. The history should also include a family history of genetic defects or reproductive failure, as well as a history of the woman's past reproductive performance. Regularity of menstrual cycles or any history of poor ovulatory performance should be elicited, and any past history of infertility, gynecologic infections, or abdominal or pelvic surgery should be discussed. A physical examination should similarly be directed at identifying any potential risk factor for subfertility or obstetric risk. A general physical examination should be performed, and the pelvic examination should include careful attention to potential vaginal or cervical factors or any abnormality of the uterus or adnexa. Obviously a pelvic mass or any finding on examination suggestive of endometriosis or adnexal adhesions should be investigated further.

Laboratory testing

Requisite laboratory testing should include any abnormality for which the patient or her offspring would be uniquely at risk of the basis of family or genetic history. Examples include screening for sickle cell disease in black patients or Tay-Sachs disease in eastern European Jewish women. All patients should be screened for transmissible diseases that might affect obstetric outcome. A Venereal Disease Research Laboratory (VDRL) test, rubella titer, cytomegalovirus (CMV) titer, hepatitis antigen status, and blood type should be obtained. Human immunodeficiency virus (HIV) antibody status should be assessed after informed consent is provided to the patient. Cervical cultures for gonorrhea and chlamydia are recommended at the time of the pelvic examination.[3] Blood typing should be performed, and documentation of the male partner's blood type should also be sought in order to identify an appropriate donor whose blood type is compatible with a natural liaison of the couple. On occasion, patients may report an incorrect blood type, and it is recommended that specific

documentation such as a Red Cross donation card be produced. As new screening tests emerge for diseases such as hepatitis C or cystic fibrosis, they too should be offered the patient considering TDI.

It is not recommended to screen all patients routinely with extensive fertility testing before initiating donor insemination. Assessment of ovulation is indicated in women who have irregular cycles or who are likely anovulatory, just as hysterosalpingography and laparoscopy are indicated in women with a history of gynecologic infection or a pelvic finding suggesting an anatomic abnormality. However, it is difficult to rationalize performance of these procedures in women with absolutely no risk factors unless they are coming to the end of their reproductive years and could be adversely affected by failure to diagnose an unsuspected problem on a timely basis.

DONOR SCREENING AND SELECTION

The former pattern of requesting semen specimens for donation from a convenient medical student, resident, or colleague is and should be considered a practice of the past that is unacceptable in contemporary treatment. Although insemination of specimens obtained from unscreened men fortunately resulted in few reported complications, including an infection rate of up to 7/1000 inseminations,[45,55] new guidelines reflect the conclusion that this type of practice is no longer consistent with medical standards. Fairly broad and nonspecific standards were established by the American Fertility Society's Ad Hoc Committee on Artificial Insemination in 1980.[2] In very brief form, these standards began to codify important issues such as family and medical history and very broadly began to address the issue of screening for infections. However, specific guidelines were largely lacking, reflecting the relatively nonrigorous view of TDI at the time. Many practitioners continued to obtain and use fresh semen specimens from donors who underwent only a brief interview, history, and physical examination. Retrospectively it is quite fortunate that the rate of significant complications proved to be so low.

Screening for human immunodeficiency virus

The emergence of the acquired immunodeficiency syndrome (AIDS) in the early to mid-1980s ultimately was responsible for a far more intense evaluation and codification of guidelines related to TDI. Before the emergence of AIDS as the most significant public health issue of the last decade, transmission of infections through TDI was feared primarily as an embarrassment or an inconvenience. However, with the new threat of HIV infection, TDI became a potentially life-threatening practice. This very real concern became compelling when four of eight women in Australia inseminated with semen from an infected, unscreened donor were reported to have become HIV positive in 1985.[62] The significant concerns related to HIV infection coupled with the increasingly common practice of TDI prompted a number of bodies to reconsider seriously the practice of TDI and to draft far more specific guidelines for screening. The American Fertility Society (AFS) published new guidelines in 1986 that addressed these issues in a variety of areas, most notably in donor screening, selection, and surveillance.[3] Ultimately, these guidelines, to a very great extent, ended the cavalier practice of enrolling occasional convenient donors and began the trend toward reliance on commercial banks that might have the resources and expertise to meet the new and more stringent guidelines.

Whether physicians enroll and screen their own donors or rely on a commercial sperm bank, the requirements and the responsibility of the physician are the same. That is to say, it behooves any physician who obtains semen from a commercial bank to be well aware of the screening criteria of that bank and to keep records reflecting ongoing confirmation that appropriate guidelines are being met. This critical issue may well require regular discussions with representatives of the bank to be updated about policies and procedures followed in the screening and specimen preparation.

History and physical examination

At the time of enrollment, potential donors should have a thorough medical, family, and genetic history taken. A sexual history should be obtained, and men who may be at high risk for AIDS (history of homosexual contact after 1978, intravenous drug user) or who have more than one sexual partner should be excluded. Men must be rejected if they have had evidence of a sexually transmitted disease within the previous 6 months, or any past history of genital herpes, genital warts, or chronic hepatitis. A physical examination is required, and the physician must be certain that there is no urethral discharge, genital warts, or genital ulcer. Additionally, urethral cultures for gonorrhea, chlamydia, and mycoplasma must be obtained. Serum antibody tests for hepatitis antigen and CMV should be obtained, as well as HIV antibody, VDRL, and blood type. Donors at risk for specific diseases because of their ethnic background (i.e., sickle cell disease, Tay-Sachs disease) should be screened for these diseases. Provided that they do not carry heritable factors, they can be enrolled as donors.[3,5] Ongoing monitoring of donor health status must also be performed. There is no universally accepted schedule for donor surveillance, although guidelines require that donors be rescreened for sexually transmitted diseases at least every 6 months. Furthermore, should a donor initiate a new sexual relationship, rescreening should take place even if it is earlier than scheduled.

Karyotyping

A number of reports have documented the occurrence of abnormal karyotypes in prospective donors, but all have found the likelihood to be quite low.[29,48,58] Certain donor programs and commercial banks may require karyotyping, but there are no data that show any clear benefit of this practice. Karyotyping is not mandated by current AFS guidelines. Present genetic screening guidelines also stipulate that the potential donor and his first-degree relatives (i.e., parents, offspring) must not have any nontrivial mendelian disorder (e.g., albinism) or malformation of complex cause (e.g., cleft lip or cleft palate). Furthermore, there must be no first-degree relative with major psychosis, epilepsy, juvenile diabetes mellitus, or early coronary disease. New guidelines recommend that the donor must be under age 40 years because of concern over an increased risk of chromosomal defects in offspring of older men.[4] Although the individual physician utilizing samples from a commercial bank will not interview the donor directly, he or she must be familiar with these criteria in order to be able to assure the recipient that all standards for genetic screening have been met.

Semen analysis

After the history and physical examination, and before proceeding with extensive laboratory evaluation, several semen analyses should be obtained. Minimum standards include a volume greater than 1 mL, greater than 60% of sperm moving actively in a purposeful direction, a concentration of 50 million motile sperm per milliliter or greater, and 60% or more normal oval forms. The presence of leukocytes in the semen should alert one to the possibility of infection or inflammation of the genital tract. Cultures should be obtained and specifically treated. Provided that a nonrecurring problem is identified and is appropriately treated, the man can be subsequently enrolled as a donor. While a number of authors and sperm banks have advocated the importance of post-thaw motility as a criterion for donor acceptability, the present guidelines require only that specimens must show the ability to survive freezing to allow the donor to be acceptable.[5] Most programs do not insist that donors have demonstrated prior fertility.

Use of fresh versus frozen semen

The guidelines published in 1986 specifically discussed the use of fresh versus frozen semen. The document addressed the risk of sexually transmitted diseases and noted that these diseases could occur with either fresh or frozen semen. The continued use of fresh semen was endorsed provided that scrupulous screening of donors was maintained. Data from insemination programs using fresh semen confirmed an exceedingly low rate of sexually transmitted diseases. However, with the increasing concern over HIV transmission and infection and increasing pressure from the Food and Drug Administration, the Centers for Disease Control and Prevention, and other bodies, guidelines of the AFS in early 1988 were revised to recommend exclusive use of frozen, quarantined semen specimens.[6] This modification required that all donors be screened before obtaining specimens, and that the specimens be frozen and quarantined for a minimum of 6 months, during which time the health status of the donor was to be monitored. HIV antibody tests were to be repeated, and only after at least 6 months of documented HIV-negative status was confirmed would the specimens be released for insemination. Although these recommendations have been described specifically as guidelines, they are widely accepted as standards for practice, and therefore one must conclude that the use of fresh semen for TDI, no matter how well the donor is known, must be considered inconsistent with present standards.

Limiting donors

There is a great deal of concern about limiting the use of donors so as to reduce the risk of consanguinity between the offspring of recipients of the same donor. This obviously could prove to be a problem in a small community in which a very limited supply of donors would likely be available to a practitioner. It is far less likely in an age of large commercial sperm banks that are geographically remote from the practitioner. Nevertheless, the present guidelines limit a donor to 10 pregnancies.[5] However, even in the contemporary practice of TDI, it is unlikely that this standard is universally observed. First, there is a widely held belief, whether accurate or not, that the relatively small number of pregnancies allowed per donor is inapplicable because commercial banks are providing specimens to practitioners throughout the entire country rather than to a local region. Second, and far more important, is the difficulty that many commercial sperm banks and other programs have in obtaining information regarding outcome of insemination. Generally, the feedback provided by practitioners to the commercial banks from which they obtain specimens is minimal. Informal estimates would suggest that only 20% to 30% of pregnancies produced through commercial specimens are ever reported to the sperm bank, and therefore the recommended limitation becomes a moot point. This deficiency is highly relevant, and aggressive attention should be paid to improving practitioner reporting of outcome to commercial banks. A difficult dilemma is produced for the director of the sperm bank in the case of an abnormal child born through TDI. The director would obviously have an obligation to investigate whether the defect was likely isolated or recurrent, and would therefore have to decide whether it would be prudent or ethical to continue to use specimens from that donor. Furthermore, the director would have an obligation to inform the donor himself should there be an increased risk of a transmissible defect to his own offspring. Again, in the absence of more stringent reporting mechanisms, these compelling obligations cannot be met.

Couple's selection of donor

The process by which the woman or the couple selects a donor is more difficult from a social standpoint than from a medical standpoint. The choice made by many couples may reflect their degree of comfort with each other and with their decision to undergo TDI, and may be a source of satisfaction on the one hand or conflict and disagreement on the other. The process of selection may therefore prove to be a subtle indicator of potential unease of either individual or of the couple as whole. Medical considerations demand that CMV-negative patients be inseminated by donors who are also CMV negative. Women who are CMV positive can be inseminated regardless of the CMV status of the donor. Furthermore, selecting a donor whose blood type is compatible with a natural child born of a couple is frequently a desirable goal. It is also wise to seek an RH-negative donor for an RH-negative woman. On occasion, it is difficult or impossible to find a donor with similar physical characteristics whose blood type would be compatible. In such a case, a thorough discussion of the advantages and disadvantages of the available choice should be undertaken with the couple. Most couples initially wish to try to match the physical characteristics of the husband. It is often helpful to the couple to reinforce the fact that any child would likely have some characteristics of each parent, and therefore a very specific match to the husband alone is not as crucial as it sometimes may seem. Most practitioners attempt to accommodate requests regarding the physical characteristics of the donor.

Some couples wish to have extensive information about educational and social characteristics of the donor. On occasion, the identification with the donor may even seem to be somewhat extreme. Interestingly, a recent study of 79 sperm donors suggested that 90% were willing to provide in-depth psychosocial information to the sperm bank, and 96% were willing to share this information in a nonidentifying manner with the recipient couple.[44] Even if anonymity could not be guaranteed, 36% said they would still participate as donors, and 60% said that they would be willing to meet or provide identifying information to the child at age 18. However, a similar study of 42 donors reported that anonymity was strongly desired by the majority of men and they did not favor disclosure of information.[54] In light of these and similarly conflicting observations, one can only conclude that there are presently no data to establish whether extensive social information should or should not be shared with couples, and it is ultimately the decision of the practitioner as to what should be supplied.

PATIENT MONITORING AND INSEMINATION

The goal of TDI is the establishment of a pregnancy as quickly and as inexpensively as possible. Therefore, the physician must strive to use the least-extensive monitoring techniques and the fewest inseminations required to produce optimal results. Although a plethora of new techniques and diagnostic adjuncts have been developed over recent years to monitor ovulatory cycles, a careful history alone continues to be extremely effective in timing insemination. Present data suggest that women with regular cycles who are inseminated 14 to 15 days before the expected menstrual period will have results equal to those observed when more extensive and expensive techniques are used. Basal body temperature charts may be helpful to some women, and they are certainly an inexpensive way of confirming ovulatory timing.[46] On the other hand, it is well known that these charts cannot be used specifically to identify the day of ovulation. Urinary luteinizing hormone (LH) testing has been used extensively, although it has not been demonstrated to increase cycle success rates in women who are very regular.[8,39] The use of ovulation indicators may well be quite helpful in women whose cycles are not strictly predictable.[25] More invasive monitoring, including ultrasound and hormonal assessments (sometimes in association with triggering of ovulation by human chorionic gonadotropin), should be reserved for women whose cycle irregularity makes simple timing or urinary LH monitoring inaccurate or undependable. The routine use of clomiphene citrate or any other ovulation-inducing agent should be strongly discouraged. Rather, such medications should be reserved only for women who have documented ovulatory dysfunction and in whom a thorough evaluation fails to identify a specific etiology for chronic, estrogenized anovulation.

Insemination techniques

Insemination techniques have evolved only slightly over the years. Vaginal placement of semen was proposed throughout the 1950s and 1960s, although insemination by intracervical injection or cervical cup was, and still is, much more widely performed. Intracervical insemination (ICI) is generally performed with gentle injection of the specimen, using a small syringe. A cervical cup or similar barrier is sometimes placed through the speculum to maintain the sperm at the cervical os. Alternately, the entire specimen can be placed in a cervical cup, which is then manually inserted over the os without the use of a speculum or any lubricant. The cup is left in place for 4 hours and can be removed easily by the patient. On some occasions, the patient will need to insert a finger vaginally to break the suction produced by placement of the cup to effect its removal. Another common technique of ICI is to inject a small amount of the specimen, generally 0.2 to 0.3 mL into the os and then to place the cup as described.

At least two recent articles have shown that intrauterine insemination (IUI) of frozen donor semen results in a higher rate of success than does ICI. In a prospective, randomized trial, Byrd and colleagues[13] found a pregnancy rate of 10% per cycle using IUI and only 4% using ICI. A subsequent study by Patton and his colleagues[47] showed a fecundity rate of only 5.1% with ICI and 23% by IUI. In both studies, a single insemination was performed on the day after detection of the LH surge by conventional urine kits. In both cases, semen samples for IUI were washed with either culture medium or human tubal fluid, and at least 20 million motile cells were inseminated. However, in the first study only 32 of 154 women conceived, and in the second only 23 of 69 conceived during the course of the study. The authors of both studies recognized that the many confounding factors such as number of inseminations per cycle, timing, length of follow-up, and total sperm used could have had an impact in the interpretation of their data. Nevertheless, the data from both studies suggest that IUI may well be associated with a higher fecundity rate than ICI. However, IUI generally costs 1.5 to 2 times more than ICI, and one must carefully consider the possibility that certain groups with a favorable prognosis may conceive quite effectively with ICI and not merit the additional cost.

There is significant controversy as to the optimal number of inseminations per cycle. The centers using LH surge monitors frequently choose to perform procedures on the day after the positive response if they wish to perform a single insemination, or on the day of the LH surge and the following day if they prefer two inseminations. In a well-designed, prospective trial, a two-inseminations-per-cycle approach was shown to result in a fecundity rate of 21%, compared with only 6% with one insemination per cycle.[14] However, the optimal number of inseminations and the mechanism of identifying the appropriate days continue to be subject to discussion and personal preference.

Admixture of husband and donor semen

A final controversial area relates to the admixture of semen from the oligospermic husband with that of the donor. There are a number of social issues related to this practice, but very little scientific direction. Many men wish to maintain the intellectual possibility that their own sperm may be successful in establishing a pregnancy. Therefore they request that their specimen be mixed with a donor sperm specimen for insemination of the wife. Obviously this is not a relevant concern for a couple whose husband is azoospermic. Although some practitioners may feel that the practice of admixture is desirable, others suggest that this request reflects failure on the part of the husband or wife to come to grips with the significantly reduced fertility. However, there are no data analyzing the social implications or successful adjustment in this area. The present guidelines recommend that the husband's semen should not be mixed with donor semen for TDI.[3] This recommendation is based on two poorly performed studies that showed a reduced pregnancy rate in those women in whom admixture with husband's sperm was performed.[49,50] The studies included only a small number of patients and had no control group. The authors speculated that the observed difference possibly was due to antibodies present in the husband's sperm.

However, the data to support this contention were fundamentally absent. A third study found no difference at all in pregnancy rates when husband and donor specimens were mixed.[31] In that study, the investigator added several drops of husband's semen to the donor specimen, thereby satisfying the husband's emotional desire for admixture without any real attempt to critically study the effect. In summary, there are no acceptable data at present that can direct the practitioner or the couple in the area of admixture of husband and donor semen. Presumably, this conclusion can also be applied to couples who wish to have intercourse after insemination for the same social reasons. Until a well-performed trial has been performed and reported, the ultimate decision of any practitioner may rest with his or her own bias as well as that of the couple in question.

LABORATORY METHODS

Cryopreservation of sperm

Cryopreservation of human sperm for insemination involves preparation, freezing, and thawing. There are a significant number of variables for each of these steps. Ultimately, the goal of all cryopreservation is to maintain viability of as many sperm as possible, and to provide a specimen of optimal fertilizing quality.

The freezing process in all cases makes use of a cryoprotectant, which prevents intracellular ice crystal formation during the cryopreservation procedure. According to a recent survey of semen bank facilities, the most common cryoprotectant used is glycerol, although a minority use a combination of glycerol and sucrose.[17] Dimethyl sulfoxide (DMSO), which is frequently used for cryopreservation of other cell types, is destructive to the acrosome and therefore is not used in sperm freezing. The glycerol concentration most frequently used ranges between 5% and 10%, and over half of the semen bank facilities use the cryoprotectant in association with some type of medium containing a citrate–egg yolk buffer. In general, the cryoprotectant is added at a 1:1 dilution in a dropwise manner. This procedure is usually performed at room temperature, after which the specimen is cooled in a stepwise fashion. Although programmable freezers commonly are used by commercial banks, a number of stepwise cooling and freezing methods are also used frequently. One-step cooling in liquid nitrogen vapor followed by plunging into liquid nitrogen for storage at −196°C is a common technique. A somewhat more involved process includes cooling in a refrigerator at 4°C, then placement into either liquid nitrogen vapor or a −70°C freezer, and finally insertion and storage in liquid nitrogen. Both glass ampules and plastic straws are frequently used for storage, although most commonly plastic vials containing a total of 0.5 to 2.0 mL of semen plus cryoprotectant are used. While a number of studies have addressed the optimal packaging, cryoprotectant, and freezing mechanism, there is as yet no compelling evidence to recommend one of these approaches over any other.[30,35,65] Similarly, a number of studies have looked at the effect of thawing rate and temperature on sperm viability. Thawing at room temperature appears to be just as effective as any other technique.

Cryopreservation is likely to cause injury to a varying proportion of sperm regardless of the technique chosen. Interestingly, specimens from a given donor tend to respond to freezing and thawing in a similar fashion most of the time.[36,52] That is to say, specimens of some donors freeze and thaw poorly with virtually every attempt despite normal semen parameters. For this reason, specimens from all donors should be checked periodically after thawing for adequacy based on percentage motility and morphology. Human specimens stored for more than 10 years have been demonstrated to produce pregnancies.[59] However, for obvious reasons, there are minimal long-term data on genetic integrity of sperm cryopreserved over many years. Many sperm banks have established a maximum storage time of 3 years, although data confirming significant risk in this regard do not exist.[19] A more detailed description of the principles and practice of cryopreservation of semen is covered in Chapter 43.

Preparation of sperm for insemination

If the specimen is to be inseminated intracervically, it is frequently helpful to bring up the total volume to approximately 2 mL by addition of culture medium at 37°C. This allows direct injection of 0.2 to 0.3 mL into the cervix, followed by placement of the cervical cup. If intrauterine insemination is anticipated, special preparation of the specimen must be performed to remove seminal fluid and reduce the likelihood of introducing bacteria into the uterus.[42,43] Most centers simply perform a standard sperm wash. This is done by centrifuging the specimen mixed with 5 to 7 mL of warm media at $200g$ to $300g$ for approximately 5 minutes to pellet the sperm and allow removal of unwanted supernatant. The pellet is then resuspended in 5 to 10 mL of warm media, gently mixed, and recentrifuged. The supernatant is again discarded and the pellet brought to a volume of 0.3 to 0.5 mL for insemination. Other methods include swim-up or various filtration columns. In the former technique, the initial specimen is centrifuged as described and then incubated at 37°C with approximately 0.5 mL of culture medium overlaid. Over the course of 1 hour, many of the active sperm will swim into the supernatant, which can then be aspirated for insemination. Various filtration methods, including use of a colloidal suspension of silica (Percoll) and cross-linked dextran beads (Sephadex), have also been used in an attempt to remove contaminants from the frozen-thawed specimen. Both of these latter techniques have been successful in producing clean-appearing specimens, but many viable sperm are lost in the preparation. In fact, a recent study demonstrated that only 5% to 7% of frozen-thawed sperm are retrieved for insemination after the swim-up procedure.[33] This loss of potentially excellent sperm ultimately may interfere with success rates. Therefore it is recommended that the sperm be evaluated microscopically before determining the best technique for preparation. Swim-up or column preparation should be performed only when the specimen is laden with debris or leukocytes.

The minimal number of sperm to be used for insemination is poorly established. The present guidelines recommend 30 to 50 million motile sperm per insemination, but do not specify whether this is recommended for ICI or IUI, or both.[5] Furthermore, the data on which this recommendation is based are not well established. For instance, the American Association of Tissue Banks recommends that ejaculates used for cryopreservation contain at least 75 million sperm per milliliter with 50% or greater motility after thawing.[1] This would result in approximately 20 million motile sperm per milliliter of insemination fluid. The guidelines of the French National Consortium results in insemination specimens containing about 15 million motile sperm per milliliter.[20] Published studies generally advocate using a total of 20 million motile cells or more; however, Brown and colleagues[12] recently showed that, in their hands, ICI using 125 million motile sperm per insemination produced a four-fold increase in fecundity compared with that observed using 25 to 75 million per insemination. There are even fewer available data addressing minimum sperm numbers required for IUI, although pregnancies using less than 5 million motile sperm are commonly established with IUI.[56] In the absence of better information, it is thus reasonable to require at least 20 million motile sperm for ICI and for the initial specimen (before preparation) for IUI, recognizing the possibility that future information may mandate modification of this guideline. This is clearly an area where further research is required.

SUCCESS RATES

Measurement

The success of TDI can best be measured by both cycle fecundity (pregnancy rate per cycle) and cumulative conception rates (number of women inseminated who ultimately conceive). In considering clinical outcome and making recommendations to patients, it is always important to distinguish between the two. A recent review summarized the numerous reports of success rates observed using fresh semen for TDI.[16] These studies generally show an overall pregnancy rate of 70% to 80%, with a mean of approximately three cycles needed to conceive. However, as noted, the use of fresh semen is no longer considered clinically acceptable. Therefore these quoted success rates are of little more than historic interest, particularly in light of the common observation that frozen-thawed semen used for TDI is less effective than fresh semen. In perhaps the best described study of this question, Richter and colleagues[51] showed that the fecundity rate using fresh semen was 0.18, whereas that observed using frozen semen was only 0.05. Other investigators, although almost universally showing better fecundity rates with fresh semen, have not shown the gap to be quite so large. The fecundity rate generally observed for TDI using frozen semen is approximately 10% per cycle (Table 42-1). The studies using frozen semen have suggested that 50% of women who will conceive will do so within approximately 6 months. This is in contrast to similar data using fresh semen showing a 50% success rate by month 3 to month 4. However, this observation should not discourage the couple from persisting past 6 months of insemination. Total cumulative success rates of 70% to 80% have been observed with 12 months of insemination. Interestingly, some data would suggest that cumulative conception rates using frozen semen compared to fresh will ultimately be almost equal, although the number of cycles required for conception with frozen specimens will be substantially (at least two times) longer.[61]

Effect of coexisting factors

The presence of coexisting factors interfering with fertility can clearly have an impact on fecundity. The data support the expectation that correction of complicating factors such as endometriosis or ovulatory disturbance will result in improved fecundity and crude pregnancy rates. The likelihood of pregnancy will approach that expected of a similar woman not undergoing TDI, although it may not be as good as that expected in a woman with no such complicating factors.[11,22,34] Similar observations can be applied to women based on the impact of age. Fecundity clearly decreases with age in the normal female population, and this decrease is paralleled by that observed in women undergoing TDI.[24] This consideration should be an important part of the counseling process for all women considering donor insemination.

Interestingly, the status of the husband may have significant implications for TDI success. A number of studies have convincingly demonstrated a higher fecundity rate in women whose husbands are azoospermic than in women whose husbands are oligospermic.[22,23,26,27,40] Presumably this finding reflects a form of selection bias in that many women of perfectly normal reproductive potential will conceive even with a severely oligospermic husband, whereas those whose potential is compromised by ovulatory or anatomic factors ultimately will seek medical therapy, often in the form of TDI. Wives of azoospermic men would not experience this selection process, and thus their fecundity rate would include women with both optimal and compromised reproductive potential.

In general, even for a woman with no infertility risk factors, a more aggressive diagnostic evaluation should be pursued if she has not conceived within 4 to 6 months. Such an evaluation should include assessment of anatomic factors by hysterography, evaluation of ovulation, evaluation of pertinent hormonal factors, and assessment of any other general medical problem that may be present. If the patient

Table 42-1. TDI success rates with frozen semen

Authors	No. of patients	Fecundity	Pregnancy rate (6 mo/12 mo)	Timing method*	Inseminations/ cycle	Route
Smith et al.,[61] 1981	238	0.08	NS/0.60*	Cx mucus	1-5	ICI
Trounson et al.,[66] 1981	1303	0.11	0.48/0.64	BBTC &/or NS LH	NS	ICI, IUI
Emperaire et al.,[23] 1982	131	0.09	NS	Cx mucus	1+	ICI
Richter et al.,[51] 1984	381	0.05	NS/0.45	Cx mucus	Every other day	ICI
Iddenden et al.,[37] 1985	40	0.09	NS/0.68	BBTC	1	ICI
		0.06	NS/0.58	BBTC	2	ICI
Bordson et al.,[10] 1986	120	0.10	NS	LH, hCG ℞	1-2	ICI, IUI
Hammond et al.,[34] 1986	226	0.10	0.50/0.65	BBTC	1-3	ICI
Brown et al.,[12] 1988	288	0.10	0.42/NS		2-3	ICI
Barratt et al.,[8] 1989	26	0.07	0.31/NS	BBTC	2	ICI
		0.04	0.23/NS	LH	2	ICI
Kossoy et al.,[39] 1989	54	0.12	NS	BBTC	1-2	ICI
		0.13	NS	LH	1-2	ICI
Silva et al.,[60] 1989	35	0.24	NS	LH, hCG ℞	NS	IUI
Wong et al.,[69] 1989	227	0.10	0.47/NS	BBTC	Multiple	ICI
DiMarzo et al.,[21] 1990	113	0.06	0.31/NS	LH	1-2	ICI
Centola et al.,[14] 1990	99	0.15	0.32/NS	LH	1	ICI
		0.21	0.78/NS	LH	2	ICI
Byrd et al.,[13] 1990	154	0.04	NS/0.38	LH	2	ICI
		0.10	NS/0.71	LH	2	IUI
Scott et al.,[57] 1990	81	0.15	0.52/NS	Cx mucus	1+	ICI
Odem et al.,[46] 1991	92	0.06	0.36/NS	LH	1	ICI
		0.13	0.65/NS	BBTC	2	ICI
Patton et al.,[47] 1992	69	0.05	NS	LH	1	ICI
		0.23	NS	LH	1	IUI

*NS, Not stated; Cx mucus, cervical mucus; ICI, intracervical insemination; IUI, intrauterine insemination; BBTC, basal body temperature chart; LH, LH monitoring; hCG ℞, human chorionic gonadotropin treatment.

has not conceived in more than 6 to 8 months, diagnostic laparoscopy should be strongly considered.

Anomalies

Many couples express concern over the potential risk that an abnormal child could result from donor insemination, particularly with the use of frozen semen. One could hypothesize that the freezing and thawing process might damage the genetic material contained within the sperm and therefore be associated with higher rates of abnormalities in the offspring. However, there is no experimental evidence for an increased rate of anomalies in pregnancies produced through TDI. As one would anticipate, there are numerous case reports of anomalies in offspring resulting from TDI, although no case-control study has ever been performed. However, a review of some 27 studies cataloguing anomalies seen in TDI offspring would suggest that the rate and nature of anomalies are similar to those seen in a comparable population of non–TDI pregnancies (1.8%).[68] In summary, in the absence of a well-performed cohort or case-control study, it is virtually impossible to conclude that there is no increased rate of anomalies associated with TDI pregnancies. However, it is nevertheless appropriate to inform couples that no such association has been demonstrated.

LEGAL CONSIDERATIONS

Both patients and practitioners frequently express concern over the legal status of the child born of TDI. In our contemporary society, it is difficult to suggest that all potential legal entanglements have been anticipated, although it is also fair to say that a substantial amount of legal guideline and precedent will serve to protect practitioner, patient, and child resulting from TDI. It is interesting to note that very few states have stipulations regarding the medical practice of donor insemination. Rather, the vast majority of statutory regulation is related to probate. That is to say, most laws are primarily directed at defining legitimacy, inheritance rights, and obligations of parents and donors to offspring rather than stipulating specific medical considerations. The majority of state laws that have been adopted are based on the Uniform Parentage Act (UPA) approved in 1973 by the National Conference of Commissioners on Uniform State Laws. Basically, the UPA stipulated that any child born by TDI with the consent of husband and wife is the legal child of the husband and the

Table 42-2. Legislated status of TDI

State	Relevant law	Who may perform	Written consent required	Reporting to state agency required	Comment
Alabama	Yes	Supervision*	Yes	Yes	UPA.†
Alaska	Yes	Physician‡	Yes		With written consent of couple, child is legitimate child of husband and wife.
Arizona	No				
Arkansas	Yes	Supervision	Yes		With written consent of couple, child is legitimate child of husband and wife. Section applies to married and unmarried women.
California	Yes	Supervision	Yes		UPA. Physician must retain consent in records.
Colorado	Yes	Supervision	Yes	Yes	UPA.
Connecticut	Yes	Physician	Yes	Yes	Child is legitimate if born to a married woman.
Delaware	Yes		Yes		UPA.
District of Columbia	No				
Florida	Yes		Yes		Child is irrefutably that of husband and wife.
Georgia	Yes	Physician	Yes		
Hawaii	No				
Idaho	Yes	Supervision	Yes	Yes	Must attempt to detect HIV or venereal disease in donor. If husband consents, child is his legitimate child.
Illinois	Yes	Supervision	Yes		Consent must be filed in patient medical record.
Indiana	Yes				Specimen must be quarantined for HIV.
Iowa	No				
Kansas	Yes		Yes	Yes	
Kentucky	No				
Louisiana	Yes				Husband cannot disavow paternity of TDI child if he signed permit.
Maine	No				
Maryland	Yes				Child conceived with consent of husband is legitimate child of both parents. Hospital and physician cannot be penalized for refusing to perform TDI.
Massachusetts	Yes		Yes		
Michigan	Yes		Yes		UPA.
Minnesota	Yes	Supervision	Yes		
Mississippi	No				
Missouri	Yes	Supervision	Yes	Yes	
Montana	Yes	Supervision	Yes	Yes	
Nebraska	No				
Nevada	Yes	Supervision	Yes	Yes	UPA.
New Hampshire	Yes	Supervision	No		Both donors and recipients must be medically evaluated and demonstrated to be medically acceptable.
New Jersey	Yes		Yes	Yes	UPA.
New Mexico	Yes	Supervision	Yes	Yes	UPA.

wife. The UPA further stipulated that the husband has all the rights and obligations of parentage, and the donor has neither. Other stipulations are included on a state-by-state basis.

Statutory requirements include those relating specifically to physicians, those relating to documentation, those relating to record keeping, and those relating to donor screening. Additionally, certain other stipulations may be included. These are summarized in Table 42-2. Although Table 42-2 is meant to be current, legal requirements are constantly changing, and the practitioner would be well advised to consult with legal counsel in his or her state of practice rather than relying on the guidelines outlined in this table.

The present practice of donor insemination does not require extensive medical training, but several states specify that only individuals certified to practice medicine are authorized to perform donor insemination. These states include Connecticut, Georgia, and Oklahoma. Many other states specify that only physicians or those acting under their supervision are authorized to perform donor insemination. Still others do not include any statement of who may perform donor insemination, thereby allowing virtually anyone to perform the procedure.

The vast majority of states that have legislated in the area of donor insemination have specified that a consent form is required. Most of these states direct that such a consent form be signed by both husband and wife. Oregon,

Table 42-2. Legislated status of TDI—Continued

State	Relevant law	Who may perform	Written consent required	Reporting to state agency required	Comment
New York	Yes	Physician	Yes		Child born to married woman with her husband's consent is legitimate child of both.
North Carolina	Yes		Yes		Child born with consent of husband and wife is the natural child of both.
North Dakota	Yes				UPA. Semen must be screened for AIDS.
Ohio	Yes	Supervision	Yes		UPA. Applies to married and unmarried women. A complete medical history of the donor is required. Semen and blood of donor must be tested as indicated.
Oklahoma	Yes	Physician	Yes	Yes	Applies to married and unmarried women. Child born with consent of husband and wife is legitimate child of both.
Oregon	Yes	Physician	Yes	Yes	Child born with consent of husband and wife is legitimate child of both.
Pennsylvania	No				
Rhode Island	Yes		Yes		UPA.
South Carolina	No				
South Dakota	No				
Tennessee	Yes		Yes		Child born with consent of husband and wife is legitimate child of both.
Texas	Yes		Yes		Child born with consent of husband and wife is legitimate child of both.
Utah	No				
Vermont	No				
Virginia	Yes		Yes		Child born with consent of husband and wife is legitimate child of both.
Washington	Yes	Supervision	Yes	Yes	UPA.
West Virginia	Yes		Yes		
Wisconsin	Yes	Supervision	Yes	Yes	Child born with consent of husband and wife is legitimate child of both.
Wyoming	Yes	Supervision	Yes		UPA.

*Insemination must be performed by or under the supervision of a physician.

†State has adopted the UPA stating that the child born of TDI is the legitimate child of husband and wife once consent is signed and that the donor has no rights or responsibilities of paternity.

‡Insemination must be performed by a licensed physician.

Arkansas, and Ohio also address the possibility that an unmarried woman may undergo donor insemination. Although one might infer that the single woman being inseminated assumes all rights and responsibilities for parenting the child, the state laws in the remainder of the states do not specifically address this potential problem. Therefore, the practitioner should consider developing a separate consent form for insemination of a single woman that specifies the acceptance of this responsibility in order to protect the donor and, possibly, the physician and his or her staff. Certain states also require that a copy of the consent form be kept on file in one or another state agency, such as the department of health, department of records, or probate court. Other states, such as California and Illinois, also require that the physician retain a copy of the consent form in the medical records of the patient. Finally, with the developing concern over transmissible disease in donor insemination, certain states specify the nature of screening of a potential donor. For instance, Indiana, Montana, and Michigan specify that a donor must be screened for HIV antibody.

Finally, legal precedent can be confusing and inconsistent in cases wherein a known donor rather than an anonymous donor is used. The vast majority of physicians clearly are unable to provide appropriate legal counsel when approached by couples wishing to use a known sperm donor. It is strongly recommended that the individuals seeking such an arrangement pursue independent legal counsel and establish a written document that defines the rights and obligations of each of the individuals involved.

Record keeping in TDI is fraught with uncertainty and inconsistencies. On the one hand, the practitioner wishes to have complete records on all donors, but at the same time usually fails to inform the sperm bank as to donor successes. Office records on the recipients are usually fairly accurate, but there is often profound ambivalence as to how long to hold them and what to release to other physicians, to insurance companies, or to other third parties. Hospital-based practices are often asked to provide copies of all outpatient notes to the hospital chart, almost certainly resulting in violation of the confidentiality many patients demand. Other potential conflicts that might possibly occur include the case wherein a child may wish to examine records pertaining to his or her conception with special interest in identifying the sperm donor. Obviously, many complicated confidences and legal issues are at stake in this area. Unfortunately, with rare exceptions, no statutory requirements or standards have been established. The sole AFS guideline stipulates that a permanent record designed to preserve confidentiality should be maintained. Thus, with the exception of clearly needing to maintain a copy of the signed consent, the practitioner has great latitude in structuring his or her record-keeping system. Ultimately, one can only recommend a well-organized and consistent approach that is shared with the couple before initiating TDI.

Aside from the legal concerns over parental rights and responsibilities, the patient should be thoroughly counseled regarding medical risks of donor insemination. These include sexually transmitted diseases and birth defects as previously noted. Emotional trauma is a rare complication of TDI, and adverse pregnancy outcome seems to occur at a rate comparable to that found in age-matched controls. Whether the practitioner prefers to include these risks as part of a formal permit or simply specifies that these concerns have been discussed is less important than clearly documenting in some form that these potential adverse events have been reviewed.

SOCIAL IMPLICATIONS

Perhaps the most common question asked of the practitioner is whether the patient should inform the child of the donor insemination. Although individuals and agencies may have their own biases in this matter, there are presently no firm data that clarify the best approach. This situation is representative of the common absence of prospective data to provide solid answers to most social questions. Therefore it is prudent to advise the couple to explore their own feelings thoroughly and to arrive at a conclusion with which they themselves will be comfortable over a long period of time. Counseling with a social worker, psychologist, or a member of the clergy frequently may be helpful in this regard. Counseling may also prove to be helpful in addressing many issues that are not immediately apparent to couples considering donor insemination. However, there are no data that clearly show that routine counseling before TDI will be helpful to the couple or will result in the exclusion of couples from treatment.

There are minimal data pertaining to the long-term outcome of TDI offspring or the family unit associated with TDI. A recent article describes the long-term outcome (up to 12 years) of 427 women who conceived more than 600 pregnancies through a TDI program.[7] This study was not prospective, but the large number of patients described does provide a reasonable basis on which to consider many of these questions. The authors found that 5.8% of the children demonstrated learning disabilities in school and that 10.5% were considered gifted. Neither of these figures appears to be different from those expected in the general population. Most of the couples (72%) had told their obstetrician that they had conceived through TDI, although only half had told any family member or friends. Sixty-one percent either did not plan to tell their child about TDI (47%) or probably did not plan to tell the child (14%). Almost identical observations have been reported by other investigators.[15,38,53] Unfortunately, there are no other scientific data that help couples to make a decision regarding informing their child of the donor insemination. Interestingly, the authors of the first study[7] found that the divorce rate among successful couples was only 7.2%, well below the national average. A lower rate of marital breakup has also been described for TDI couples in a Scandinavian study.[9] Interpretation of these data should take into consideration that a "self screening" process precedes the decision to embark on donor insemination. Thus the participants may represent an unusual group at the outset. Although patient satisfaction is difficult to analyze statistically, the observation that a significant number of patients, reported to be as high as 42%, return for a second, third, or even fourth child by TDI would clearly suggest that the process is felt to be a positive experience for the majority of patients.[32] While these data must be considered observational and are not derived from prospective, longitudinal studies, they nevertheless may be helpful in providing some direction that can be shared with couples considering donor insemination.

CONCLUSION

TDI has been shown to be a safe, cost-efficient, and overwhelmingly beneficial treatment for thousands of couples in the United States. It is the most successful infertility treatment available to practitioners. A thorough understanding of the clinical science and contemporary guidelines, as well as the legal and social implications of TDI, is required to provide this treatment safely and effectively. TDI should be initiated only after a thorough review of the indications and alternatives and a comprehensive discussion of donor screening and selection, medical risks, legal issues, and social implications.

REFERENCES

1. American Association of Tissue Banks: Guidelines for the banking of human semen, *AATB Newslett* 3:7, 1979.
2. American Fertility Society: Report of the Ad Hoc Committee on Artificial Insemination, Birmingham, Ala, 1980, The Society.
3. American Fertility Society: New guidelines for the use of semen donor insemination: 1986, *Fertil Steril* 46(suppl 2):95S, 1986.
4. American Fertility Society: Revised new guidelines for the use of semen donor insemination, *Fertil Steril* 49:211, 1988.
5. American Fertility Society: New guidelines for the use of semen donor insemination: 1990, *Fertil Steril* 53(suppl 1):1S, 1990.
6. American Fertility Society: Revised guidelines for the use of semen

donor insemination: 1991, *Fertil Steril* 56:396, 1991.

7. Amuzu B, Laxova R, Shapiro SS: Pregnancy outcome, health of children, and family adjustment after donor insemination, *Obstet Gynecol* 75:899, 1990.

8. Barratt CLR et al: A prospective randomized controlled trial comparing urinary luteinizing hormone dipsticks and basal body temperature charts with time donor insemination, *Fertil Steril* 52:394, 1989.

9. Bendvold E et al: Marital break-up among couples raising families by artificial insemination by donor, *Fertil Steril* 51:980, 1989.

10. Bordson BL et al: Comparison of fecundability with fresh and frozen semen in therapeutic donor insemination, *Fertil Steril* 46:466, 1986.

11. Bradshaw KD et al: Cumulative pregnancy rates for donor insemination according to ovulatory function and tubal status, *Fertil Steril* 48:1051, 1987.

12. Brown CA, Boone WR, Shapiro SS: Improved cryopreserved semen in an alternating fresh-frozen artificial insemination program, *Fertil Steril* 50:825, 1988.

13. Byrd W et al: A prospective randomized study of pregnancy rates following intrauterine and intracervical insemination using frozen donor sperm, *Fertil Steril* 53:521, 1990.

14. Centola GM, Mattox JM, Raubertas RF: Pregnancy rates after double vs single insemination with frozen donor semen, *Fertil Steril* 54:1089, 1990.

15. Clayton C, Kovacs G: AID offspring: initial follow-up study of 50 couples, *Med J Aust* 1:338, 1982.

16. Corson SL, Batzer FR: Indications, techniques, success rates, and pregnancy outcome: new directions with donor insemination, *Semin Reprod Endocrinol* 5:45, 1987.

17. Critser JK, Ruffing NA: Summary of a questionnaire completed by semen bank facilities. Presentation at the annual meeting of the American Society of Andrology, New Orleans, April 1989.

18. Curie-Cohen M, Luttrell L, Shapiro S: Current practice of artificial insemination by donor in the United States, *N Engl J Med* 300:585, 1979.

19. David G, Czyglik F: Limits of long term semen cryopreservation. In David G, Price W, editors: *Human artificial insemination and semen preservation,* New York, 1980, Plenum Press.

20. David G et al: The success of AID and semen characteristics: study on 1489 cycles and 192 ejaculates, *Int J Androl* 3:613, 1980.

21. DiMarzo SJ et al: Pregnancy rates with fresh versus computer-controlled cryopreserved semen for artificial insemination by donor in a private practice setting, *Am J Obstet Gynecol* 162:1483, 1990.

22. Edvinsson A et al: Factors in the infertile couple influencing the success of artificial insemination with donor semen, *Fertil Steril* 53:81, 1990.

23. Emperaire JC, Gauzere-Soumireu E, Audebert AJM: Female fertility and donor insemination, *Fertil Steril* 37:90, 1982.

24. Federation CECOS, Schwartz D, Mayhaux MJ: Female fecundity as a function of age, *N Engl J Med* 306:404, 1982.

25. Federman CA et al: Relative efficiency of therapeutic donor insemination using a luteinizing hormone monitor, *Fertil Steril* 54:489, 1990.

26. Formigli L, Formigli G, Gottardi L: Artificial insemination by donor results in relation to husband's semen, *Arch Androl* 14:209, 1985.

27. Foss GL, Hull MGR: Results of donor insemination related to specific male infertility and suspected female infertility, *Br J Obstet Gynaecol* 93:275, 1986.

28. Francoem T: *Utopian motherhood: new trends in human reproduction,* New York, 1970, Doubleday.

29. Fraser FC, Forse RA: On genetic screening of donors for artificial insemination, *Am J Med Genet* 10:399, 1981.

30. Friberg J: Survival of human spermatozoa after freezing with different techniques. In David G, Price W, editors: *Human artificial insemination and semen preservation,* New York, 1980, Plenum Press.

31. Friedman S: Artificial insemination with donor semen mixed with semen of the infertile husband, *Fertil Steril* 33:125, 1980.

32. Goss DA: Current status of artificial insemination with donor sperm, *Am J Obstet Gynecol* 122:246, 1975.

33. Graczykowski JW, Siegel MS: Motile sperm recovery from fresh and frozen-thawed ejaculates using a swim-up procedure, *Fertil Steril* 55:841, 1991.

34. Hammond MG, Jordan S, Sloan CS: Factors affecting pregnancy rates in a donor insemination program using frozen semen, *Am J Obstet Gynecol* 155:480, 1986.

35. Harrison RF, Sheppard BL: A comparative study in methods of cryoprotection for human semen, *Cryobiology* 17:25, 1980.

36. Heuchel V, Schwartz D, Price W: Within-subject variability and the importance of abstinence period for sperm count, semen volume and pre-freeze and post-thaw motility, *Andrologia* 13:479, 1981.

37. Iddenden DA, Sallan HN, Collins WP: A prospective randomized study comparing fresh semen and cryopreserved semen for artificial insemination by donor, *Int J Fertil* 30:54, 1985.

38. Klock SC, Maier D: Psychological factors related to donor insemination, *Fertil Steril* 56:489, 1991.

39. Kossoy LR et al: Luteinizing hormone and ovulation timing in a therapeutic donor insemination program using frozen semen, *Am J Obstet Gynecol* 160:1169, 1989.

40. Kovacs GT et al: The outcome of artificial insemination compared to the husband's fertility status, *Clin Reprod Fertil* 1:295, 1982.

41. Kritchevsky B: The unmarried woman's right to artificial insemination: a call for an expanded definition of family, *Harvard Women's Law Rev.* 4:1, 1981.

42. Kuzan FB, Hillier SL, Zarutskie PW: Comparison of three wash techniques for the removal of microorganisms from semen, *Obstet Gynecol* 70:836, 1987.

43. Leiva JL et al: Microorganisms in semen used for artificial insemination, *Obstet Gynecol* 65:669, 1985.

44. Mahlstedt PP, Probasco KA: Sperm donors: their attitudes toward providing medical and psychosocial information for recipient couples and donor offspring, *Fertil Steril* 56:747, 1991.

45. Mascola L, Guinan ME: Screening to reduce transmission of sexually transmitted diseases in semen used for artificial insemination, *N Engl J Med* 314:1354, 1986.

46. Odem RR et al: Therapeutic donor insemination: a prospective randomized study of scheduling methods, *Fertil Steril* 55:976, 1991.

47. Patton PE et al: Intrauterine insemination outperforms intracervical insemination in a randomized, controlled study with frozen, donor semen, *Fertil Steril* 57:559, 1992.

48. Perez MM, Marina S, Egozcue J: Karyotype screening of potential sperm donors for artificial insemination, *Hum Reprod* 5:282, 1990.

49. Quinlivan WLG, Sullivan H: The immunologic effects of husband's semen on donor spermatozoa during mixed insemination, *Fertil Steril* 28:448, 1977.

50. Quinlivan WGL, Sullivan H: Spermatozoal antibodies in human seminal plasma as a cause of failed artificial insemination, *Fertil Steril* 28:1082, 1977.

51. Richter MA, Haning RV, Shapiro SS: Artificial donor insemination: fresh vs. frozen semen: the patient as her own control, *Fertil Steril* 41:277, 1984.

52. Risum J et al: Evaluation of the quality variations of ejaculates from individual donors for establishing a quality control scheme, *Gynecol Obstet Invest* 17:149, 1984.

53. Rowland R: The social and psychological consequences of secrecy in artificial insemination by donor (AID) programmes, *Soc Sci Med* 21:391, 1985.

54. Sauer MV et al: Attitudinal survey of sperm donors to an artificial insemination clinic, *J Reprod Med* 34:362, 1989.

55. Schlaff WD: Transmission of disease during artificial insemination, *N Engl J Med* 315:1289, 1986 (letter).

56. Schlaff WD, Rock JA: Unpublished data, 1989.

57. Scott SG et al: Therapeutic donor insemination with frozen semen, *Can Med Assoc J* 153:273, 1990.

58. Selva J et al: Genetic screening for artificial insemination by donor (AID): results of a study on 676 semen donors, *Clin Genet* 29:389, 1986.

59. Sherman JK: Current status of clinical cryobanking of human semen. In Paulson JD et al, editors: *Andrology: male fertility and sterility,* Orlando, Fla, 1986, Academic Press.

60. Silva PD, Meisch J, Schauberger CW: Intrauterine insemination of cryopreserved donor semen, *Fertil Steril* 52:243, 1989.

61. Smith KD, Rodriguez-Rigau LJ, Steinberger E: The influence of ovulatory dysfunction and timing of insemination on the success of artificial insemination donor (AID) with fresh or cryopreserved semen, *Fertil Steril* 36:496, 1981.

62. Stewart GJ et al: Transmission of human T-cell lymphotropic virus type III (HTLV-III) by artificial insemination by donor, *Lancet* 2:581, 1985.

63. Stone S: Complications and pitfalls of artificial insemination, *Clin Obstet Gynecol* 23:667, 1980.

64. Strong C, Schinfeld JS: The single woman and artificial insemination by donor, *J Reprod Med* 29:293, 1984.

65. Thacil JV, Jewett AS: Preservation techniques for human semen, *Fertil Steril* 35:546, 1981.

66. Trounson AO et al: Artificial insemination by frozen donor semen: results of multicentre Australian experience, *Int J Androl* 4:227, 1981.

67. US Congress, Office of Technology Assessment: *Artificial insemination: practice in the United States: summary of a 1987 survey-background paper.* Pub No OTA-BB-BA-48, Washington, DC, 1988, US Government Printing Office.

68. Verp MS: Genetic issues in artificial insemination by donor, *Semin Reprod Endocrinol* 5:59, 1987.

69. Wong AWY et al: Factors affecting the success of artificial insemination by frozen donor semen, *Int J Fertil* 34:25, 1989.

Chapter 43

CRYOPRESERVATION OF SPERM

Don P. Wolf, PhD

BACKGROUND

The freezing of human sperm for use in therapeutic insemination (TI) is an established medical procedure with worldwide application. The procedure is safe if proper screening is employed to minimize the risk of infectious disease transmission, and semen samples can conveniently be maintained for prolonged time periods when stored at liquid nitrogen temperatures of −196°C, providing the flexibility required for most patient needs.

Sperm freezing has not always been an available option; moreover, the empirically derived recipes or protocols currently available for human semen, developed in large measure from experience with domestic animal sperm, do not often apply to the semen of other mammalian species.[42]

Following early observations by Spallanzini,[40] sperm survival after exposure to subzero temperatures was reported by Mantegazza[24] in 1866, who, recognizing the implications of the observation, suggested that frozen semen could be used for animal husbandry and clinically for the purpose of begetting a legitimate child after one's own death. Little progress toward these goals was made, apart from an 1897 report by Davenport[16] that human sperm could survive freezing at −17°C, until 1938, when Jahnel[19] found that some human sperm could be revived after freezing in glass tubes for 40 days at −79°C and for shorter periods at −196°C and −269°C. Shettles[39] in 1940 studied the low temperature tolerance of sperm in undiluted semen from 10 different donors and concluded that there is marked, donor-dependent variation in the sensitivity of human sperm that is temperature independent over the range of −79°C to −269°C. Although the motility recoveries were low (1% to 10%) in these experiments, the general conclusions drawn by Shettles concerning donor variability are still applicable to modern protocols using cryoprotectant and controlled rates of freezing. Shettles[39] also emphasized the importance of semen freshness; those samples stored for 5 or 10 hours before cryopreservation showed inferior survival, perhaps reflecting sperm damage or reduced cryoprotective action of seminal plasma secondary to proteolysis. These early experiments were usually conducted in glass capillary tubes; however, Parkes,[29] in 1945, concluded that freezing in bulk at −196°C or −79°C produced results superior to those obtained with films formed in capillary tubes. He also noted that the rate of freezing and thawing was not the primary factor in the survival of sperm exposed to low temperature.

The routine cryopreservation of human semen became feasible, on a theoretic basis, after the serendipitous discovery of the cryoprotective properties of glycerol by Polge and co-workers[32] in 1949. These workers studied the effects of glycerol, ethylene, and propylene glycol on rabbit, human, and fowl semen and reported success in

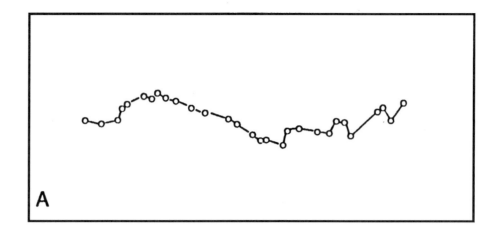

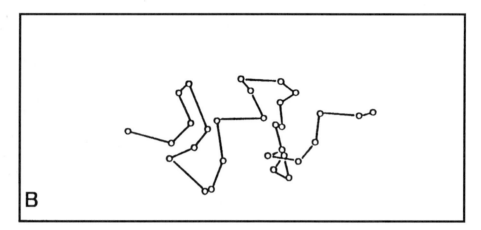

Fig. 43-1. Head trajectory of a nonhyperactivated (**A**) and a hyperactivated (**B**) human sperm cell.

protecting human and fowl sperm—but not rabbit sperm—against the effects of low temperature. With the discovery that sperm motility could be recovered after semen storage in glycerol, the question became, Do such motile cells retain fertilizing capacity? That is, does freezing affect the ability of sperm to fertilize the egg and induce normal embryonic development? This question was answered initially by Bunge and Sherman,[10] who described the establishment of three pregnancies in patients inseminated with sperm frozen and stored in dry ice (−78°C). In a subsequent report, Bunge and co-workers[9] described details of the pregnancies and the delivery of three normal infants, and reported a fourth pending pregnancy. Early success in the therapeutic use of frozen semen was also reported from Japan, as summarized by Sawada.[34] In 1963 Sherman[36] introduced the liquid nitrogen vapor technique for the freezing of human semen with subsequent storage at −196°C, a technique that is used with only minor modifications by many sperm banks today. An example of the protocol for this technique is presented in the chapter appendix.

These successes provided at least a superficial answer to the question, Do frozen-thawed sperm retain fertility and the ability to induce normal embryonic development? Additionally, they initiated an era of systematic studies of the optimal conditions for semen cryopreservation, for example, the use of dry ice versus liquid nitrogen (rate of cooling and storage temperature), the use of extenders, freezing in pellets, freezing in capillaries versus bulk, and the use of semen versus washed sperm. The major question now became the clinically relevant one: Is there DNA damage associated with cryopreservation such that congenital abnormalities or spontaneous abortion rates will be elevated in the offspring produced with frozen-thawed semen? After some 24,000 births worldwide, survey data summarized by Sherman[37] are reassuring—the incidence of abnormal progeny was cited as only about 1% and the incidence of spontaneous abortion was about 13%; both of these values are well within the range associated with the use of nonfrozen sperm. A recent, smaller but focused, study from the University of Wisconsin also concluded that children fathered by TI donors are at similar risk for congenital anomalies as are normally conceived children but, interestingly, they experience lower rates of family dissolution.[5]

Despite extensive interest and attention by a worldwide cadre of scientists and clinicians, no dramatic improvements have occurred in the cryopreservation of human semen since the early 1960s, the published results involving a multitude of studies notwithstanding.

This chapter reviews human sperm cryopreservation and management of a sperm bank as these activities stand in support of homologous (husband) or heterologous (donor) TI.

SPERM PHYSIOLOGY

Mammalian spermatozoa transport the paternal genetic contribution from the testis to the site of fertilization, the ampullary section of the oviduct or fallopian tube. Once at this site, sperm must find and recognize the egg, penetrate egg vestments, and fuse with the egg, inducing the latter's activation and the initiation of embryonic development. The number of sperm cells at the site of fertilization is imprecisely known in women; of the 100 million or so spermatozoa deposited at coitus, perhaps only as few as 100 reach the ampulla, reflecting the substantial sieving ability of the female reproductive tract. Since the liquid volume of the ampullary oviduct may be only 100 µL, sperm density at the fertilization site is approximately 1000/mL, substantially lower than the concentrations involved in in vitro fertilization.

Freshly ejaculated spermatozoa do not possess fertilizing capacity when in semen; rather, they must undergo a sequence of maturation events accomplished by "washing" in vitro or by exposure to the sieving effect of the female reproductive tract in vivo. After the removal of seminal plasma and the placement of washed cells in culture, sperm acquire fertilizing capacity, a process defined operationally—called capacitation—and discovered simultaneously but independently by Austin[6] and Chang[12] in 1951. The capacitation process is not well understood at the molecular level but undoubtedly involves cell surface changes that are reversible, since the addition of seminal plasma to once-capacitated spermatozoa results in decapacitation.[20] The second messengers, cyclic adenosine monophosphate and calcium, are undoubtedly involved in the capacitation process.[8]

Three of the unique features of capacitated spermatozoa are (1) their altered form of motility, called hyperactivation; (2) their ability to bind to the unfertilized egg's zona pellucida; and (3) their ability to undergo an acrosome reaction.

Hyperactivation

During capacitation, spermatozoa undergo a transition in motility from linear, progressive movement to a nonlinear, relatively nonprogressive motion that typifies hyperactivation (Fig. 43-1). With the availability of computer-assisted semen analyzers (CASA), the degree of hyperactivation can be quantitated rapidly in large numbers of cells. Specific characteristics that are associated with hyperactivation include increased curvilinear velocity and amplitude of lateral head displacement or flagellar beat amplitude and decreased linearity.[11,28,33] The degree of hyperactivation and the kinetics of its appearance in a washed population of human sperm may be donor dependent and thus of ultimate value in the diagnostic use of CASA.[22]

Binding to the zona pellucida

The capacitated cell is uniquely capable of binding, in a species-specific fashion, to the zona pellucida, a process mediated by a sperm receptor. This binding step is critical to sperm penetration of the egg, since it initiates the events that culminate in the induction of an acrosome reaction in the bound sperm. Binding is mediated by a specific glycoprotein called ZP3, which has been studied extensively in mice.[41] Evidence that ZP3 contains a sperm receptor is based on the following: (1) Receptor activity is found in the zona pellucida or purified ZP3 of unfertilized eggs but not fertilized eggs or embryos. (2) Binding of purified ZP3 occurs to the sperm head (not to the midpiece or tail) at nanomolar concentrations, which prevents sperm binding to eggs; the other major glycoproteins of the zona, ZP1 and ZP2, do not bind or influence sperm-zona binding. (3) Binding of purified ZP3 to sperm induces the acrosome reaction; purified ZP3 does not bind to cells that have undergone the acrosome reaction nor to a variety of other cells. (4) Finally, purified embryonic ZP3 does not possess any of these properties.

Acrosome reaction

The third characteristic of the capacitated cell is the ability to undergo an acrosome reaction (Fig. 43-2). This reaction exposes the enzymatic machinery, a trypsinlike protease called acrosin, required to digest the matrix of the zona pellucida and allow sperm passage, a process that involves secondary sperm receptors in ZP2.[41] Sperm penetration of the zona, then, is facilitated by both the mechanical forces generated by the hyperactivated sperm and the chemical forces represented by the acrosomal protease. Although species differences undoubtedly exist with regard to the details and sequence of these events in mammals, preliminary studies suggest that the human may be mechanistically similar to the mouse.[15]

A thorough understanding of human sperm physiology and the fertilization process should allow development of diagnostic approaches to the routine measurement of fertility or fertilizing ability. This information is important to any evaluation of cryodamage and the development of strategies to circumvent or avoid damage. Current knowledge levels and diagnostic approaches are far from ideal, as exemplified by the poor correlations that are now legendary among semen parameters, the sperm penetration assay or postcoital testing, and fertility status.

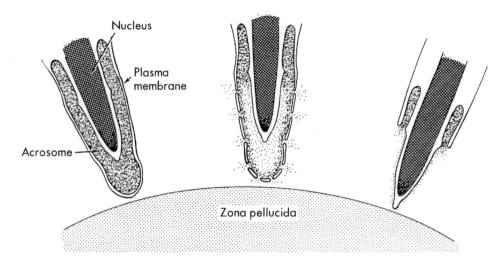

Fig. 43-2. Schematic representation of the acrosome reaction occurring in a capacitated cell attached to the outer margin of the zona pellucida.

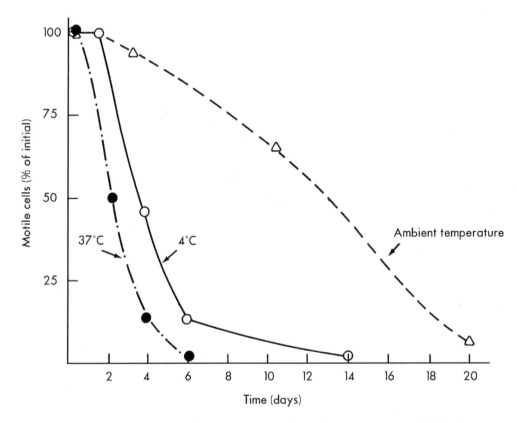

Fig. 43-3. Motility retention in washed human sperm stored at various temperatures. (Modified in part from Cohen et al.[13])

CRYOBIOLOGY

Cryobiology is the study of the effects of low temperature on cells. In mammalian systems, this includes temperatures below 37°C. It is, of course, possible to store human semen or washed sperm for limited time periods at temperatures below 37°C in the unfrozen state. This time is too short, however, to be of practical importance in the context of sperm banking. The relationship between motility survival and storage temperature for washed human sperm is illustrated in Fig. 43-3. Ambient temperature storage with motility retention is feasible, at best, for 1 or 2 weeks and for only 3 to 4 days at 4°C. Although exposure to 4°C is poorly tolerated by washed cells, noteworthy is the observation that human spermatozoa do not suffer from temperature shock, which has been so limiting in efforts to store domestic animal spermatozoa at low temperature.[35,42] Temperature shock, or damage that is induced when cells are cooled to suprafreezing temperatures, may reflect transition changes in membrane lipids that are critical to cell survival. From the considerations just discussed it should be obvious that long-term storage of human sperm requires low temperatures and freezing, freeze-drying, or vitrification, which leads to the unique set of problems discussed below.

Freezing is detrimental to most cells; cellular membranes are the principal targets of injury, and intracellular ice crystal formation is a primary mechanism along with cellular exposure to high solute concentrations and osmotic shock. The principal determinants in a cell's ability to survive freezing include size, shape, hydration state, and membrane permeability properties or ability to respond to osmotic challenges. Based largely on the pioneering studies of Mazur,[25] the response of cells can be predicted from considerations of the cell's permeability coefficient, its surface area, the osmotic gradient between outside and

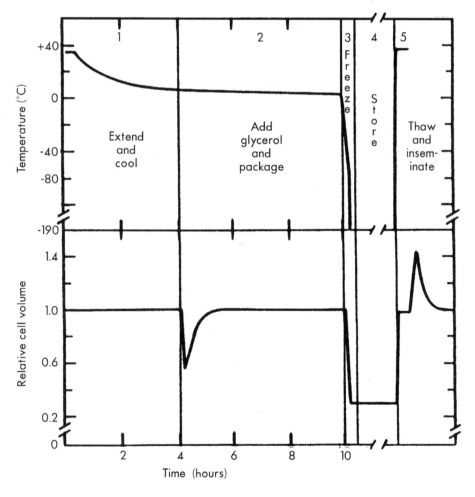

Fig. 43-4. Changes in temperature and cell volume associated with a cryoprocessing cycle for bull sperm. A time-event profile associated with a successful (but perhaps not optimum) cryopreservation process for bovine sperm is provided, with change in temperature plotted in the top panel and change in cell volume plotted in the bottom panel. (Reproduced with permission from Hammerstedt RH et al: *J Androl* 11:73, 1990.)

inside, and the temperature. The cryopreservation process per se involves selection and addition of the cryoprotectant, seeding the supercooled mixture (not normally done with sperm), determining the cooling rate and final holding temperature, setting the warming rate, and finally removing cryoprotectant(s). Human sperm are tolerant to a wide range of cooling ($0.5°C$ to $50°C$/minute) and warming rates and to the nature of cryoprotectants or extenders used as adjuncts to glycerol.[38] This may reflect their relatively low content of cytoplasm and thus of intracellular water. Additionally, the availability of large cell numbers means that only modest post-thaw survival is required to ensure fertility maintenance. On the other hand, acrosomal lability and susceptibility to cold shock has hampered efforts to apply this technology to sperm from a number of mammalian species.[42]

The cryopreservation process is characterized by dramatic changes in cellular volume. This relationship in bovine sperm is depicted in Fig. 43-4. Hammerstedt and co-workers[17] subdivided events into five distinct processing steps: (1) semen extension and cooling, (2) cryoprotectant addition and sample packaging, (3) freezing, (4) storage, and (5) thawing and insemination. Such time-temperature-volume relationships also apply for human semen, although semen extension and cryoprotectant addition normally are done at the same time and at ambient temperature for human specimens. As can be seen readily in Fig. 43-4, dramatic decreases in cell volume are associated with cryoprotectant addition and with the dehydration that occurs during cooling. Upon thawing, volume loss is reversed, with expansion beyond the original volume during cell removal from the freezing solution.

As mentioned earlier, cryoprotectants are used in the cryopreservation of human sperm. Their mechanism of action, which includes a lowering of the freezing point of the solution and cellular dehydration, is incompletely understood. Glycerol is much more effective in buffering the effects of low temperature on human sperm than are dimethyl sulfoxide and 1, 2-propanediol, yet the latter cryoprotectants also dehydrate and lower the solution freezing point. Parenthetically these latter two cryoprotectants are preferred in the cryopreservation of human one-cell to eight-cell embryos. Additionally, the ultrarapid cooling or vitrification protocols used successfully with embryos have not yet been examined with sperm, where a practical method for cryoprotectant removal must be developed.[21]

CRYOSURVIVAL

Although no entirely satisfactory laboratory method is available for measuring cryosurvival, the process is routinely assessed by post-thaw motility scores, determined in the presence of cryoprotectant. The premise, of course, is that the easily measured parameter of motility is reflective of fertility. A minimum standard of 50% survival of the initial motile sperm population is normally applied. Additionally, a stress test can be conducted wherein sperm are washed free of cryoprotectant and then incubated in an appropriate medium at $37°C$ for up to 24 hours. An example of the use of CASA to monitor changes induced by freeze-thawing in human sperm is illustrated in Table 43-1.[26] Semen was collected from four donors (eight ejaculates), and each specimen was divided equally into three portions for the nonfrozen control, cryoprotectant addition, and the frozen sample. Individual parameters of motility were measured on each aliquot at 1 and 3 hours after processing and expressed as mean values ± SD. As expected, addition and removal of cryoprotectant without freezing induced only minor changes in the percentage of motile cells and their averaged motility values (nonfrozen vs. cryocontrol). In contrast, freezing was associated with a dramatic decline in the percentage of motile cells, and declines were also seen in curvilinear velocity and in mean amplitude of lateral head displacement (nonfrozen or cryocontrol vs. frozen). On comparing the 1- and 3-hour time

Table 43.1. Influence of cryopreservation on human sperm

Time (after washing)	Parameter*	Results†		
		Nonfrozen	Cryocontrol	Frozen
1 Hour	% Motile	69 ± 6	66 ± 6	45 ± 13
	VCL_{30} (μm/s)	98 ± 12	90 ± 9	71 ± 13
	LIN	56 ± 7	59 ± 7	60 ± 2
	Mean ALD (μm)	4.3 ± 1.1	3.9 ± 0.7	3.0 ± 0.7
3 Hours	% Motile	68 ± 1	64 ± 4	42 ± 13
	VCL_{30} (μm/s)	94 ± 15	85 ± 10	68 ± 12
	LIN	56 ± 7	56 ± 6	60 ± 3
	Mean ALD (μm)	4.2 ± 10	3.4 ± 0.3	2.8 ± 0.5

*VCL_{30}, curvilinear velocity; LIN, linearity; ALD, amplitude of lateral head displacement.
†Mean values ± SD for eight samples from four different donors.

points, there was little suggestion of time-dependent loss of motility. However, by 24 hours the percentage of cryopreserved sperm that retained motility was so low (less than 10%) that CASA analysis was impractical.

With domestic animals, cryodamage is often monitored not only by motility measures but also by quantitative assessments of acrosomal status.[42] Since damage to the acrosome and the plasma membrane also occurs upon freezing human sperm,[23] acrosomal status should be considered as a potentially useful measure of cryodamage. Immunofluorescence assays for this purpose are readily available.[44] In a study of 23 sperm donors, Mahadevan and Trounson[23] saw the expected decline in motile sperm from 71.1% to 49.9% after freezing, well within the minimum standard of 50% survival described earlier. By using transmission electron microscopy, they noted that the mean percentages ± SD of cells with intact acrosomes were 51.2 ± 12.3, 40.5 ± 10.7, and 20.9 ± 8.1 for control, glycerol-exposed, and frozen-thawed samples, respectively, whereas the percentages with both intact acrosomes and plasma membranes were 31.8 ± 8.4, 21.7 ± 6.2, and 8.8 ± 3.5. These findings suggest that only a small percentage of the frozen-thawed sperm population is potentially fertile, since disrupted membranes are likely to compromise sperm fertility. The sperm penetration assay has been used by Critser and co-workers[14] to evaluate cryosurvival; however, this assay is cumbersome and impractical as a routine test for large sample numbers.

SCOPE OF THE SUBJECT

TI with either husband or donor sperm is a routine office procedure. For homologous TI, the principal indications are structural abnormalities of the vagina or cervix, abnormal postcoital testing, sexual dysfunction, immunologic infertility, abnormal semen parameters, and idiopathic infertility. For heterologous TI, indications include a severe male factor and genetic problems. The clinical uses for cryopreserved semen (as modified from Sherman[37]) are as follows:

1. Timed insemination with husband or donor semen even in the donor's temporary or permanent absence
2. Storage, pooling, and concentration of oligozoospermic samples
3. Preservation of semen before surgical, chemical, or radiologic cancer therapy or vasectomy
4. Backup for patients participating in the assisted reproductive technologies

The second application in the list remains a theoretic argument, since abnormal semen from patients does not usually survive freezing well. The fourth application has gained in importance with the increased usage of the assisted reproductive technologies in the treatment of infertility.[45] Detailed discussions of homologous TI and heterologous TI are found in Chapters 41 and 42, respectively.

DIAGNOSTIC APPLICATION

The ability of sperm to survive the freezing process is not used diagnostically as a measure of fertility potential despite the fact that male factor patients with presumed low fecundities are generally recognized to produce sperm that do not tolerate freezing well. On the other end of the spectrum, candidates for TI by a donor program with exceptional semen quality usually produce sperm that survive freezing (i.e., 50% retention of the motile population). As an example of the variation in this latter category, however, Beck and Silverstein[7] reported post-thaw motilities from 0% to 60% for random donors (potentially fertile) and 15% to 45% for pregnancy-proven donors. Another potential diagnostic application is cryosurvival based not on motility but on membrane integrity. Mahadevan and Trounson[23] described a positive correlation between TI donor fecundity and the degree of sperm acrosomal and plasma membrane intactness after freeze-thaw. Any future efforts to assign diagnostic significance to sperm cryosurvival might appropriately involve multiple measures, including— but by no means limited to—motility (retention before and after cryoprotectant removal and degree of hyperactivation), morphology (acrosomal and plasma membrane intactness and neck or tail abnormalities), and functional assessments (hemizona binding or sperm penetration assays).

SPERM BANK MANAGEMENT

Guidelines for the use of semen in TI have been established by the Centers for Disease Control and Prevention (CDC), the American Fertility Society (AFS), and the American Association of Tissue Banks (AATB). A detailed description of the management of a donor insemination program can be found in the article by Hummel and Talbert[18] and itemized in the sperm-freezing protocols of Sherman.[38] An overview of sperm banking, along with specific information from the program at the Oregon Health Services University (OHSU), is presented here.

Donor screening

Donors are usually recruited from the academic community by written advertisement in campus newspapers and must meet minimal educational requirements, such as 2 years of college or 14 years of formal education. They should be in good general health as determined by history and physical examination and in the age group from 21 to 40.[4] The results of a medical history that includes information on the health of family members (three generations) are reviewed by a medical geneticist and used to meet or exceed the exclusion criteria set by AATB and AFS. A sexual history is taken in an effort to identify members of groups at high risk for infectious diseases. In a recent retrospective review, approximately 8% of prospective donors at OHSU were rejected for medical reasons (Table 43-2).

Table 43-2. Screening prospective sperm donors ($n = 77$)

Screen	No. passed (% of original)
Medical history	71 (92.2)
Semen analysis	
Density minimum	55 (71.4)
Viscosity/motility minimum	52 (67.5)
Cryosurvival	48 (62.3)
Infectious disease	
Human immunodeficiency virus, chlamydia, gonorrhea, syphilis, hepatitis B surface antigen, *Mycoplasma hominis*	48 (62.3)
Cytomegalovirus, β-hemolytic streptococci, *Ureaplasma urealyticum, Gardnerella vaginalis*	31 (40.3)
Other	
Subsequent counts adequate	29 (37.7)
Continued interest	22 (28.6)
Active donor	21 (27.3)

Semen quality and cryosurvival

The concentration and motility of sperm in the initial semen sample is determined, with minimum levels set at 80 million/mL and 60%, respectively. Any additional deviations from the normal semen parameters established by the World Health Organization may also be the basis for exclusion.[43] Of 77 prospective donors characterized in the OHSU program from 1989 through 1990, 19 (26.8%) were disqualified because of inadequate initial semen parameters; most failed to meet the concentration minimum (Table 43-2). Trial freeze-thaws are also conducted on the initial sample, with the requirement that at least 50% of the motile sperm survive. Use of these criteria guarantees a post-thaw sample of 24 million or more motile sperm per milliliter. In our study, 7 of the 77 prospective donors (10%) failed to meet cryosurvival minimums.

Microbiologic screening

The human immunodeficiency virus (HIV) and the hepatitis C virus (HCV), along with a number of other infectious agents, can be transmitted heterosexually. The CDC reported that more than one fourth of those women in the United States acquiring HIV did so through heterosexual relations. Thus, with the possible exception of semen from a partner in a mutually monogamous relationship, fresh semen for TI carries a risk of virus transmission. Although Peterson et al.[31] do not describe any documented cases of acquired immunodeficiency syndrome (AIDS) transmission through TI in the United States, four of eight women in Australia who received semen from a seropositive donor subsequently seroconverted. Since morbidity and mortality in HIV-infected individuals is extremely high and effective treatment is unavailable, TI must be conducted with caution. The risk of virus transmission cannot be completely eliminated, because a "window" of 120 days or longer exists from initial infection or exposure to seroconversion and the appearance in the circulation of specific antibodies to the virus that can be detected by standard testing. In 1986,[1] use of fresh donor semen in TI was recommended as long as the donor was seronegative initially, did not belong to any of the high-risk groups, and was seronegative at 6-month intervals. However, in 1988[2] and again in 1990,[3] the AFS revised its guidelines to mandate the exclusive use of frozen semen that had been quarantined for 180 days. Thus, semen collected from a donor who was seronegative initially could not be released for TI until the sample had been held for at least 180 days and the donor had been retested and found to be seronegative for HIV. This recommendation revolutionized the TI process and, in the time frame of 1988 to 1990, many TI programs could not be sustained for lack of quarantined sperm.

A careful history of other sexually transmitted diseases must also be obtained; in fact, the testing outlined in Table 43-3[27] should be considered minimal, with the caveat that additional screens for infectious diseases will be added as they become available and/or necessary. Hummel and Talbert[18] provide additional details to consider in the microbiologic screening of prospective sperm donors. The incidence of positive screenings in our retrospective review was confined to CMV antibody (25%), β-hemolytic streptococci (14%), *Ureaplasma urealyticum* (9%), and *Gardnerella vaginalis* (5%).

Donor fecundity

A desirable screen that is not employed in current sperm bank management involves individual donor fecundity. It is recognized that even those donors who survive all of the screens discussed herein will display unique fecundities (pregnancies per insemination) ranging from 0 to over 0.5. Thus a mechanism should be developed for identifying donors at the low end of the fecundity range. This will entail a determination of the number of inseminations to be conducted before fecundity is established, presumably a number in the 25 to 50 range and an acceptable threshold fecundity, below which donors will be dropped.

Sperm banks

Quarantined donor semen may be purchased from a number of sperm banks, a listing of which is maintained by the AFS. The AATB also maintains a list of member banks. Policies vary between banks regarding (1) provision of samples to single versus married women, (2) shipping across state lines, (3) method of payment and fees, (4) the minimum number of motile sperm provided per insemination unit, (5) semen packaging (i.e., straws versus cryovials), (6) provision of samples directly to the recipient versus to the physician, (7) donor qualifications and screen-

Table 43-3. Infectious disease screen for potential semen donors

Organism or disease assessed	Test required			Basis for exclusion
	Serum	Semen	Urethral epithelium	
AIDS	Yes	No	No	Positive HIV antibody
Cytomegalovirus	Yes	No	No	Positive for antibody; antibody-positive donors may be accepted if periodic semen culture is negative
Hepatitis B	Yes	No	No	Positive for hepatitis B surface antigen or core antibody
Hepatitis C	Yes	No	No	Positive HCV antibody
Herpes simplex	No	No	No	History of herpes simplex lesion in donor or partner
Chlamydial infection	No	No	Yes	Positive by indirect immunofluorescence
N. gonorrhoeae	No	No	Yes	Positive culture
M. hominis	No	No	Yes	Positive culture
U. urealyticum	No	No	Yes	Positive culture
Streptococcal species	No	No	Yes	Positive culture
Trichomonas	No	Yes	No	Positive wet mount or culture
Warts (anal or genital)	No	No	No	History of warts (anal or genital)

ing, and (8) the release of nonidentifying donor characteristics.

Donor information that is usually provided by the bank includes physical characteristics such as height, weight, hair and eye color, and blood type. Racial and ethnic background information is also included and, occasionally, family medical history, educational attainment, intellectual quotient, religion, occupation, and interests or hobbies.

Donor-recipient matching can be based on the recipient's response to a questionnaire but will commonly include consideration of the physical characteristics listed above plus blood type, Rh factor, and race. Sperm from donors representing widely diverse backgrounds or characteristics can be accessed through the collective sperm banking activity in the United States. Samples may be shipped in liquid nitrogen transport tanks by overnight or 2-day delivery using one of several available express carriers. Dry ice transport is not considered as reliable and therefore is not recommended. Advance notice to sperm banks is judicious when timed inseminations are conducted and local liquid nitrogen storage is unavailable.

Patient semen

The major questions in homologous TI are when and how much semen to freeze. Variability in the success of the freezing process occurs between individuals as well as potentially between semen samples from the same individual; when male factors are present, cryosurvival expectations are low. The recommendation for an individual to proceed with cryopreservation is most appropriately made after determination of sperm count and motility before and after freeze-thawing, and the post-thaw numbers are the most significant. Based on this knowledge, conception rates by current technology, and individual needs and time

constraints, the patient, with the advice of his physician, can decide how many samples to freeze. In general, the recommendation is made that a minimum of 20×10^6 motile sperm be provided, post-thaw, per TI. Semen samples of average or better quality will yield this number per vial, three vials per ejaculate. Male factor patients will seldom produce these levels; however, TI should still be considered. Although in the United States cervical inseminations are often conducted with a minimum of 20 million motile sperm, markedly lower numbers have been used successfully in other countries, often involving multiple inseminations per cycle. If intrauterine insemination (IUI) is selected as the route of insemination, larger sperm numbers are required post-thaw, because sperm washing is only approximately 50% efficient. The recommended number of inseminations to perform per cycle is one or two, and the recommended route of insemination is intrauterine because of generally higher pregnancy rates.[30] Assuming that 12 vials, at 20×10^6 or more motile sperm per vial post-thaw, were frozen, 12 cycles of cervical insemination and four to six cycles of IUI at one insemination per cycle could be conducted with a high probability of establishing a pregnancy.

Sperm storage

The biochemical processes that occur in cells stored in liquid nitrogen are negligible; the major risk of storage damage is restricted to accumulated exposure to cosmic radiation. Hundreds of years may be required before the radiation damage becomes significant.[25] Nevertheless the evidence and/or bias persists that a decline in sperm survival occurs over time of storage, and the judicious recommendation would therefore be that storage time is limited, perhaps to 10 years.

SUMMARY

The ability to cryostore human semen, although not without significant limitations, as described above, provides a viable, cost-effective option for many couples attempting conception. This discussion of sperm cryopreservation with insights into the fundamentals of cryobiology, the physiology of sperm capacitation, the diagnosis of cryodamage, as well as the practical aspects of sperm banking, will hopefully encourage the reader to examine this important subject more thoroughly.

ACKNOWLEDGMENTS

The author acknowledges the secretarial and editorial skills of Patsy Kimzey. This work was supported in part by National Institutes of Health Grant RR00163. Publication No. 1894 of the Oregon Regional Primate Research Center.

REFERENCES

1. American Fertility Society: New guidelines for the use of semen donor insemination: 1986, *Fertil Steril* 46(suppl 2):95S, 1986.
2. American Fertility Society: Revised new guidelines for the use of semen donor insemination, *Fertil Steril* 49:211, 1988.
3. American Fertility Society: New guidelines for the use of semen donor insemination: 1990, *Fertil Steril* 53(suppl 1):1S, 1990.
4. American Fertility Society: Revised guidelines for the use of semen donor insemination: 1991, *Fertil Steril* 56:396, 1991.
5. Amuzu B, Laxova R, Shapiro SS: Pregnancy outcome, health of children, and family adjustment after donor insemination, *Obstet Gynecol* 75:899, 1990.
6. Austin CR: Observation on the penetration of the sperm into the mammalian egg, *Aust J Sci Res [B]*4:581, 1951.
7. Beck WW Jr, Silverstein I: Variable motility recovery of spermatozoa following freeze preservation, *Fertil Steril* 26:863, 1975.
8. Bedford JM, Hoskins DD: The mammalian spermatozoon: morphology, biochemistry and physiology. In Lamming GE, editor: *Marshall's physiology of reproduction,* vol 2, *Reproduction in the male,* ed 4, New York, 1990, Churchill Livingston.
9. Bunge RG, Keettel WC, Sherman JK: Clinical use of frozen semen, *Fertil Steril* 5:520, 1954.
10. Bunge RG, Sherman JK: Fertilizing capacity of frozen human spermatozoa, *Nature* 172:767, 1953.
11. Burkman LJ: Discrimination between nonhyperactivated and classical hyperactivated motility patterns in human spermatozoa using computerized analysis, *Fertil Steril* 55:363, 1991.
12. Chang MC: Fertilizing capacity of spermatozoa deposited into fallopian tubes, *Nature* 168:697, 1951.
13. Cohen J, Fehilly CB, Walters DE: Prolonged storage of human spermatozoa at room temperature or in a refrigerator, *Fertil Steril* 44:254, 1985.
14. Critser JK et al: Cryopreservation of human spermatozoa, I: effects of holding procedure and seeding on motility, fertilizability, and acrosome reaction, *Fertil Steril* 47:656, 1987.
15. Cross NL et al: Induction of acrosome reactions by the human zona pellucida, *Biol Reprod* 38:235, 1988.
16. Davenport CB: Experimental morphology: part I. In *Effect of chemical and physical agents upon protoplasm,* New York, 1897, Macmillan.
17. Hammerstedt RH, Graham JK, Nolan JP: Cryopreservation of mammalian sperm: what we ask them to survive, *J Androl* 11:73, 1990.
18. Hummel WP, Talbert LM: Current management of a donor insemination program, *Fertil Steril* 51:919, 1989.
19. Jahnel F: Über die widerstandsfähigkeit von menschlichen spermatozoen gegenüber starker kälte: wiederauftreten der beweglichkeit nach abkühlung auf − 196°C (flüssiger stickstoff) und −269.5°C etwa 3.7°

vom absoluten nullpunkt entfernt (flüssiges helium), *Klin Wochenschr* 17:1273, 1938.
20. Kanwar KC, Yanagimachi R, Lopata A: Effects of human seminal plasma on fertilizing capacity of human spermatozoa, *Fertil Steril* 31:321, 1979.
21. Kuzan FB, Quinn P: Cryopreservation of mammalian embryos. In Wolf DP, editor: *In vitro fertilization and embryo transfer: a manual of basic techniques,* New York, 1988, Plenum Press.
22. Mack SO, Tash JS, Wolf DP: Effect of measurement conditions on quantification of hyperactivated human sperm subpopulations by digital image analysis, *Biol Reprod* 40:1162, 1989.
23. Mahadevan MM, Trounson AO: Relationship of fine structure of sperm head to fertility of frozen human semen, *Fertil Steril* 41:287, 1984.
24. Mantegazza P: Sullo sperma umano, *Rend Reale Ist Lombardo* 3:183, 1866.
25. Mazur P: Freezing of living cells: mechanisms and implications, *Am J Physiol* 247:C125, 1984.
26. McClusky LL, Eaton DL, Wolf DP: Unpublished manuscript, 1993.
27. Mixon BA, Wolf DP: Unpublished manuscript, 1993.
28. Mortimer ST, Mortimer D: Kinematics of human spermatozoa incubated under capacitating conditions, *J Androl* 11:195, 1990.
29. Parkes AS: Preservation of human spermatozoa at low temperatures, *Br Med J* 2:212, 1945.
30. Patton PE et al: Intrauterine insemination outperforms intracervical insemination in a randomized, controlled study with frozen, donor semen, *Fertil Steril* 57:559, 1992.
31. Peterson EP, Alexander NJ, Moghissi KS: A.I.D. and AIDS—too close for comfort, *Fertil Steril* 49:209, 1988.
32. Polge C, Smith AU, Parkes AS: Revival of spermatozoa after vitrification and dehydration at low temperatures, *Nature* 164:666, 1949.
33. Robertson L, Wolf DP, Tash JS: Temporal changes in motility parameters related to acrosomal status: identification and characterization of populations of hyperactivated human sperm, *Biol Reprod* 39:797, 1988.
34. Sawada Y: The preservation of human semen by deep freezing, *Int J Fertil* 9:525, 1964.
35. Sherman JK: Temperature shock in human spermatozoa, *Proc Soc Exp Biol Med* 88:6, 1955.
36. Sherman JK: Improved methods of preservation of human spermatozoa by freezing and freeze-drying, *Fertil Steril* 14:49, 1963.
37. Sherman JK: Current status of clinical cryobanking of human semen. In Paulson JD et al, editors: *Andrology: male fertility and sterility,* Orlando, Fla, 1986, Academic Press.
38. Sherman JK: Cryopreservation of human semen. In Keel BA, Webster BW, editors: *CRC handbook of the laboratory diagnosis and treatment of infertility,* Boca Raton, Fla, 1990, CRC Press.
39. Shettles LB: The respiration of human spermatozoa and their response to various gases and low temperatures, *Am J Physiol* 128:408, 1940.
40. Spallanzini L: *Opuscoli di Fisica Animale, e Vegetabile,* 2 vols, Opuscolo II: *Osservazioni, e Sperienze intorno ai Vermicelli Spermatici dell' Uomo e degli Animali,* Modena, Italy, 1776, Presso la Societa' Tipographica.
41. Wassarman PM: Zona pellucida glycoproteins, *Annu Rev Biochem* 57:415, 1988.
42. Watson PF: Artificial insemination and the preservation of semen. In Lamming GE, editor: *Marshall's physiology of reproduction,* vol 2, *Reproduction in the male,* ed 4, New York, 1990, Churchill Livingstone.
43. *WHO laboratory manual for the examination of human semen and semen-cervical mucus interaction,* ed 2, New York, 1987, Cambridge University Press.
44. Wolf DP: Acrosomal status quantitation in human sperm, *Am J Reprod Immunol* 20:106, 1989.
45. Yavetz H et al: The efficiency of cryopreserved semen versus fresh semen for in vitro fertilization/embryo transfer, *J In Vitro Fert Embryo Transfer* 8:145, 1991.

Appendix

PROTOCOL FOR A GLYCEROL-BASED LIQUID NITROGEN VAPOR TECHNIQUE FOR THE FREEZING OF HUMAN SEMEN

PROCEDURE FOR FREEZING SEMEN

1. Make up TEST-MODIFIED cryoprotectant (giving 29.6% glycerol) just before use by adding 1.0 mL of glycerol (100%) to 4.0 mL of freezing medium-TEST yolk buffer with glycerol (12%: available commercially from Irvine Scientific, Santa Ana, California). Measure the glycerol carefully. After addition to extender, thoroughly wash the inside of the pipette by aspirating the glycerol-extender mixture in and out of the pipette. This mixture can be filter sterilized with a 0.45-µL filter. A 1:4 dilution of this stock will give a final glycerol concentration of 7.4%. At the Oregon Health Sciences University (OHSU), a semen dilution of three parts semen to one part cryoprotectant is used to increase sperm concentration and reduce storage volume.

2. Allow semen to liquefy for 30 minutes at 37°C. *Note:* Samples with high viscosity may require the additional step of repeated pipetting with a sterile Pasteur pipette or passage through an 18-gauge needle to reduce viscosity and to ensure thorough mixing.

3. After thorough mixing, transfer the entire sample, using a sterile serologic pipette, to a prelabeled, sterile, 15-mL conical tube. Measure and record volume.

4. Remove aliquots, using a positive displacement pipette (2×10 µL), for analysis. Determine count and motility. Note any abnormalities.

5. Determine amount of cryoprotectant to be added, using a ratio of three parts semen to one part cryoprotectant.

6. Add, at ambient temperature, the predetermined amount of cryoprotectant drop by drop, using a sterile serologic pipette. Mix well by gently pipetting up and down. Do not use a Vortex mixer or similar apparatus.

7. Label Nunc cryotubes or straws. At OHSU cryotubes are used as follows: Place the tube so that the screw top is to the left as you write in the label area. For DONOR sample, write donor (always four digits); under that, write donation number (three digits); below that, write vial number (two digits starting with 01, 02, etc.). For PATIENTS, write name, medical record number, and date on the Nunc cryotube, again having the screw cap to your left as you write in the label area.

8. Transfer the sample to prelabeled Nunc cryotubes. Fill the cryotube with no more than 90% of the tube's volume to permit ample expansion during freezing. Be sure the cryotube screw cap is tightened normally; overtightening will distort the seal and risk leakage. Be sure that the thread of the cryotube screw cap is completely dry before closing; liquid drops will impair the seal in liquid nitrogen. Always set up a vial to be thawed for test thaw results. This vial can be filled with only 0.5mL.

9. Place the cryotubes/vials at the top of the wand at the first clip located just below the labeling area. Use one wand for each vial. *Note:* Many programs skip steps 9 to 11.

10. Place the wands upside down and completely submerged in an ambient temperature bath. (A 600-mL plastic beaker can be used filled with 600 mL of water.)

11. Transfer bath (plastic beaker) containing the wands to a 4°C refrigerator for 1.5 hours to allow slow cooling of the sperm and cryoprotectant mixture (−0.2°/minute).

12. After the 4°C exposure, transfer the wands (right side up) to a Dewar flask or similar insulated jar containing enough liquid nitrogen so that the vials are 2 to 4 inches above the liquid nitrogen level. Leave the wands and vials suspended in the vapors for 30 to 45 minutes.

13. To avoid exposure to room temperature, work in the vapors of a wide-mouth Dewar flask containing liquid nitrogen. Transfer the vials from each donor or patient to prelabeled wands for permanent storage in a liquid nitrogen tank or freezer.

14. Place all vials in a preassigned liquid nitrogen tank/freezer for storage. Test vials can be thawed at a later time to determine the number of total motile sperm per vial.

15. Record the number of vials (excluding test vial) and their location in the storage container (the bucket or drawer number; the wand number or slot number in the drawer) on the appropriate donor or patient form and log this information into the computer.

QUALITY ASSURANCE

Trial thaw values for donors should contain a minimum of 30 million motile sperm per sample (sample size may vary but will usually be 1 mL). All sperm banking activities must be supported by extensive record keeping.

THAWING FROZEN SEMEN

1. Check the aluminum cane to make sure that you have the correct number of vials, and that the cane is marked with the correct patient name or donor ID number. *Important:* Never expose a frozen vial to room temperature until you are ready to thaw the vial, and never use an inadequately identified sample.

2. To thaw a vial, remove the cane with the desired vial from the tank, remove the vial from the cane, and simply let the vial stand at room temperature until thawing is complete, generally 10 to 20 minutes. Thawing may be hastened by holding the vial in hand or by exposure to warm (body temperature) water. Vials just removed from liquid nitrogen will be very cold and should not come in contact with bare skin.

3. When the vial is completely thawed, unscrew the cap and aspirate the contents into the insemination device, or into a pipette in the event the sample is to be processed before insemination. Check sperm motility under the microscope to ensure that sperm have survived the freezing process. Be sure the sample has warmed to ambient temperature before assessing motility, and also examine the motile sperm population for morphologic abnormalities. At least 30% of the cells should be progressively motile.

Chapter 44

GAMETE INTRAFALLOPIAN TRANSFER

Jose P. Balmaceda, MD,
Alejandro Manzur, MD,
and Ricardo H. Asch, MD

HISTORY AND PHYSIOLOGY BASES

The fallopian tubes play a fundamental role in human fertility, being responsible for picking up the mature oocyte once it has been released from the ovarian follicle, transporting it through its lumen while fertilization takes place (normally in the ampullary region), and, finally, allowing the entrance of the early embryo into the endometrial cavity just in time for proper implantation.

The contributions of Croxatto et al.[17,20] have helped us understand several aspects of human egg transport. They studied healthy, ovulatory, multiparous women undergoing elective surgical sterilization at different intervals after the luteinizing hormone (LH) peak. In their approach, both fallopian tubes were removed before segmental ligation into four compartments; the endometrial cavities were flushed through a transfundal approach, looking for the presence of an unfertilized ovum, and such presence was correlated with time after ovulation. They found that ovulation occurs approximately 17 hours after the LH peak, followed by rapid ovum pickup, since ova could be recovered from the fallopian tubes 24 hours after the LH peak. The oocyte remains in the ampullary portion for the next 72 hours, probably with back and forth movements, and travels for only a very brief time through the isthmus. Croxatto and co-workers found that the earliest an egg could be recovered from the human endometrial cavity was 96 hours after the LH peak (i.e., 80 hours postovulation) (Figs. 44-1 and 44-2).

On the other hand, Buster et al.,[12] while working with human embryo transfers, recovered embryos by flushing the endometrial cavity of donors and transferring them to synchronized recipients. They demonstrated that the great majority of pregnancies achieved by this technique were produced when an embryo of eight or more cells was recovered from the uterine cavity. These results suggested that the chronology of embryo entrance to the uterine cavity and probably the cellular stage of development are important variables in determining the chances of implantation.

These facts, combined with the indirect knowledge that human oocytes are fertilizable only within 24 hours after follicular extrusion, were fundamental physiologic considerations for developing gamete intrafallopian transfer (GIFT) as an alternative therapeutic technique for chronic infertility.

The GIFT procedure involves the direct placement of sperm and oocytes into the ampullary portion of the fallopian tubes, allowing in vivo fertilization to occur at the natural site. The assumption is that the embryos generated in this manner develop in the protective ambiance of the tube; by entering the uterus in a natural way, the chances of implantation should be increased.

The first tubal transfer-oriented study was reported in 1979 by Shettles,[40] who transferred a mature oocyte into

%
Recovery

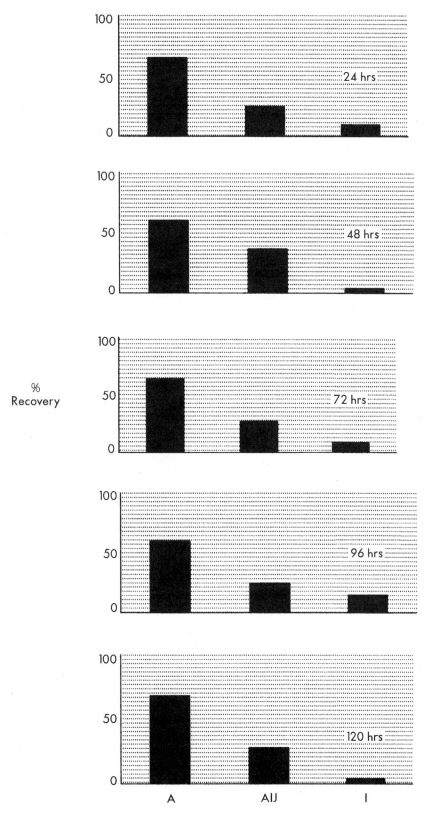

Fig. 44-1. Segmental distribution of ova recovered from the fallopian tube at different times after the LH peak. *A*, Ampulla; *AIJ*, ampulllary-isthmic junction; *I*, isthmus. (From Ortiz ME, Croxatto HB: 1988.)

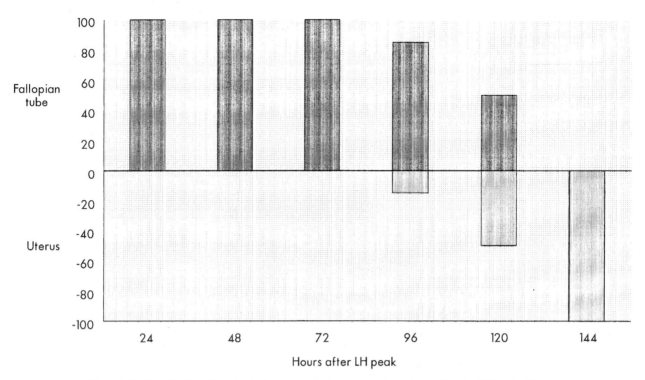

Fig. 44-2. Distribution of ova in the human genital tract at various times after the LH peak. (From Ortiz ME, Croxatto HB: 1988.)

the newly anostomosed fallopian tube of a 30-year-old patient who previously had undergone a tubal ligation. After successful in vivo fertilization, a normal infant was delivered at term. In 1980 Kreitman and Hodgen[33] published results achieved in primates with a technique termed low tubal ovum transfer. These investigators reported a 16% pregnancy rate in the animals after transferring sperm and oocytes to the isthmic portion of the fallopian tube. In 1983 Tesarik et al.[43] outlined the first successful attempt to develop a clinically useful technique of gamete tubal transfer that they called "oocyte in vitro insemination and tubal transfer." In a modification of Shettles' approach, they included ovarian stimulation, sperm capacitation in vitro, mixing of both gametes in vitro, and tubal transfer after tubal repair had been completed. Of four women treated, two achieved pregnancy, resulting in one spontaneous abortion 5 weeks after surgery and one normal term delivery.

In 1984 Asch et al.[5] reported the first pregnancy after translaparoscopic intrafallopian transfer of gametes in a woman with normal tubes. This procedure followed extensive research performed in primates by the authors, in which the concept proved to be efficient. That technique was recognized as GIFT and gained worldwide diffusion.[7] The patient was a 35-year-old woman with unexplained primary infertility of 7 years' duration, during which attempts with more conservative therapies, including intrauterine inseminations and controlled ovarian hyperstimula-

tion, had failed. She conceived a twin intrauterine gestation that progressed uneventfully to a vaginal term delivery.[6] Since then, mainly because of the reproducibility of the method and the consistency of its results, the number of patients treated with the GIFT procedure has grown rapidly. Approximately 4000 GIFT procedures are performed annually in the United States, and more than 130 infertility centers offer the procedure (national registry results 1990).[37]

The popularization of ultrasonographically guided transvaginal aspiration of follicles has enabled assessment of oocyte quality before subjecting patients to laparoscopy. Goals are now oriented to simplify the technique even more by performing tubal transfers through a transcervical approach by ultrasonically guided, blind transcervical, or hysteroscopic tubal catheterization.

No matter what changes have occurred in the technical aspects of the GIFT procedure during its 9 years of existence, its principles have remained the same, that is, to allow fertilization to occur in the protective natural tubal environment, with a more appropriate time of entry of the embryo into the uterine cavity and avoidance of undesirable endometrial trauma.

INDICATIONS

The GIFT technique was originally created for use in patients with unexplained infertility and patent tubes; however, as experience has accumulated, indications for GIFT have been extended to several other diagnoses of infertility and restricted to others, such as severe male factor and immunologic causes. It is still imperative that the patients undergoing a GIFT procedure have at least one functionally normal fallopian tube.

The main indications in management of the infertile couple include the following:

- Unexplained or idiopathic infertility
- Pelvic endometriosis
- Mild or moderate male factor
- Iatrogenic pelvic adhesions
- Failure of previous donor artificial insemination cycles
- Cervical factors
- Immunologic factors
- Premature ovarian failure with oocyte donation

Nevertheless, the diagnoses of unexplained infertility and mild endometriosis encompass the vast majority of patients.[4]

TECHNICAL ASPECTS

Several steps should be followed carefully in order to obtain the best results in a GIFT program. They are discussed in chronologic order.

Controlled ovarian hyperstimulation

As in other assisted reproductive technologies, the chances of achieving a pregnancy are increased by inducing multiple follicular development. Different hormonal therapeutic regimens are available to induce controlled ovarian hyperstimulation, but the most commonly used are the following:

Clomiphene citrate: 50 to 150 mg orally daily for 5 days, starting on day 3 to day 5 of the menstrual cycle.

Human menopausal gonadotropin (hMG): 75 to 450 IU intramuscularly daily, starting as early as day 2 of the menstrual cycle when used alone or as late as day 7 when combined with clomiphene citrate.

Pure follicle-stimulating hormone (FSH): 150 to 450 IU intramuscularly daily, starting on day 2 of the menstrual cycle. It can be used alone or combined with hMG.

Gonadotropin-releasing hormone (GnRH) analogues: The use of agonist analogues to down-regulate the anterior pituitary has led to significant progress in the schemata available for controlled ovarian stimulation.[27] Use of these drugs, combined with gonadotropins, has permitted the application of more aggressive regimens of stimulation that result in a larger number of mature oocytes recovered without the danger of premature ovulation. The agonistic analogues can be started during the luteal phase (day 21-25) of the preceding cycle (long protocol) or concomitant with gonadotropins on day 2 of the treatment cycles (flare-up). Our preference has been to use the long protocol.

Serial transvaginal ultrasonography is used to measure the number and size of follicular development. Usually an ultrasound assessment is required first before starting the hormonal therapeutic regimen, in order to rule out any preexisting ovarian cyst. Generally three or four other ultrasound examinations are done per cycle to monitor proper follicular growth and to choose the time of human chorionic gonadotropin (hCG) injection based on the diameter of the leading follicle. Recently we have incorporated ultrasonographic measurement of endometrial thickness as a reliable index of estrogenic activity. A triple layer pattern and an endometrial thickness of 8 mm or more at the time of oocyte retrieval has been clearly associated with a better chance of implantation.[21a] Although we continue to use serial serum estradiol (E_2) measurements to assist ultrasonographic follow-up of ovarian response, we have markedly reduced the frequency of this sampling since the incorporation of GnRH analogues. Today we consider obligatory the use of serum E_2 measurements in the following situations: presence of a cystic ovarian lesion at the time of initiation of gonadotropin stimulation; absence of ultrasonographic evidence of progress in ovarian response; and, most imperatively, to assess the risk of hyperstimulation in patients who have more than 15 follicles identified by ultrasound.

10,000 IU hCG intramuscularly is indicated in our protocol when the leading follicle has reached a diameter of 20 to 22 mm. In our experience, it has been extremely rare to cancel a cycle before hCG injection while using the long protocol of GnRH analogues. We have also been able to identify most of the potentially severe hyperstimulation cases in which preventive measures had been applied, such as lowering gonadotropin dosage or suspending it. These therapeutic modifications result in spontaneous follicular growth, with dramatic decreases in serum E_2 levels and apparently without compromising oocyte quality. The exact timing of hCG injection is controversial, but the latest reports in the literature seem to support the existence of a 3-day window period, once two or more follicles measure greater than or equal to 18 mm and the patient is under a GnRH agonist suppression protocol.[41]

Oocyte retrieval

As stated previously, follicular aspiration transvaginally with an ultrasonographically guided needle has become the routine form of oocyte retrieval in GIFT. This approach has allowed separation of the egg retrieval procedure from the actual surgical procedure chosen (laparoscopy or minilaparotomy) to replace the gametes into the fallopian tube. The laboratory team can thereby appropriately assess the quality of the oocytes before the patient is subjected to general anesthesia and surgery. Furthermore, transvaginal aspiration with ultrasound generally has facilitated oocyte recovery, as it identifies the follicle while being aspirated, and is more simple to perform than follicular aspiration by laparoscopy.

Once all of the follicles have been aspirated, the oocytes

retrieved are numbered and classified, and the most mature are selected to be transferred. As discussed later, the number of oocytes transferred and their maturity are critical variables affecting GIFT results. Supernumerary oocytes have been used for donation or fertilization, followed by freezing of resulting preembryos. Both of these alternatives are discussed in Results and Patient Selection.

Sperm preparation

Before acceptance of the couple for the GIFT procedure a semen sample is obtained and analyzed according to criteria of the World Health Organization to determine eligibility for the GIFT technique. In our institution, if 1.5 million or more total motile sperm with a progression of 2 to 3 or greater and at least 30% with normal morphology are not recovered, then GIFT is not performed due to poor pregnancy rate, and the couple is advised to have a procedure involving in vitro fertilization (IVF).

Two hours before a scheduled oocyte retrieval, the male partner produces a semen sample by masturbation, which is collected in a sterile container. After allowing time for liquefaction, the sample is examined for count, motility, and morphology; washed with culture medium in order to remove the seminal plasma; and, finally, the most motile fraction of the sperm is obtained by the swim-up technique[8] and used for the transfer. Usually 300,000 to 700,000 motile sperm are used for the GIFT procedure. The concentration of sperm is adjusted to allow the volume of fluid injected into the fallopian tube not to be in excess of 30 uL (usually between 20 and 30 uL). Volumes significantly higher than that would probably result in significant reflux from the ampullary portion, back to the peritoneal cavity.

Transfer of gametes

The sperm and oocytes are loaded into a special catheter that can be easily threaded through the fimbriated end of the tubes. The first one used by Asch et al.[5] was a modified cardiac catheterization catheter. Since then, several improved models have become available commercially. Basically they can be classified in two types: (1) a simple Teflon catheter and (2) a double-catheter system that allows manipulation and canalization of the tubes before the loaded catheter is brought into the surgical field. In our opinion, the type of catheter does not significantly affect the results; therefore surgeons should select the device according to their preferences. A visible graduation at the tip of the catheter facilitates determination of the degree of penetration. Ideally, the catheter should be inserted 3 cm before its contents are gently injected into the ampullary region.

Originally, gametes were loaded in the following order: aliquot of sperm, air space, oocytes, air space, aliquot of sperm, air space. The air spaces were used to avoid mixing gametes in vitro, although this is theoretical, because human fertilization requires hours and not minutes to be completed. This procedure is now maintained only for

those couples who request it because of religious or ethical beliefs; otherwise, both gametes are inserted together.

Once the contents of the catheter have been released, the catheter is removed and inspected in the laboratory to be sure that the gametes were transferred. The same procedure may be repeated for the contralateral tube.

The type of surgical transabdominal procedure used for the transfer has no apparent influence on the results. The main advantage of laparoscopic transfer is prompt postoperative recovery with minor discomfort; the advantage of minilaparotomy is the accuracy with which the gametes are introduced into the tubes. In that sense, if in a specific program the results with laparoscopic GIFT are significantly inferior to those reported in the literature, a change in the modality of transfer is justified before the technique is abandoned.

Patients are usually discharged 2 to 3 hours after the procedure, and minimal physical activity is recommended for the next 2 days.

Luteal phase support

Some form of luteal phase support has been used routinely in cases of GIFT, as in other assisted reproductive technology (ART) techniques. Although initially it was thought to be of questionable value, since the popularization of the use of GnRH analogues in controlled ovarian hyperstimulation protocols, we consider luteal phase support necessary. Not using it could be associated theoretically with luteal phase defect.

We have used injectable progesterone in oil (25 to 50 mg intramuscularly daily) starting 2 days after the transfer. Recently sublingual and vaginal suppositories of progesterone have also been employed. Our preliminary experience with hCG injections of 2000 IU given every 3 days has not shown significantly improved results, and such administration is clearly associated with a higher incidence of symptomatic ovarian hyperstimulation.[3a] We consider this latter therapeutic regimen only in patients with demonstrated progesterone intolerance or severe side effects in previous treatments.

The luteal phase support is continued until the β-hCG test is performed 2 weeks after the transfer. If the patient is pregnant, supplementation can be maintained for up to 8 weeks additionally, depending on the evolution of the pregnancy and the physician's criteria.

RESULTS AND PATIENT SELECTION

The procedure outcome is discussed first in general, and then each of the clinical variables that could affect it is analyzed.

GIFT outcome

The results of the 1987 first multinational collaborative study involving 2097 GIFT cases suggested immediately the technique to be reproducible.[4] Most of the clinics

Table 44-1. GIFT results in a multinational cooperative study: clinical pregnancies*

Etiology	No. of cases	No of pregnancies	% of pregnancies
Unknown	796	247	31
Endometriosis	413	132	32
Male factor	397	61	15
Tuboperitoneal factor	210	61	29
Failed donor insemination	160	66	41
Cervical factor	68	19	28
Oocyte donation	18	10	56
Immunologic factor	30	5	16
TOTAL	2092	601	28.7

*Data are from Asch et al.[4]

Table 44-2. GIFT results in a multinational cooperative study: pregnancy outcome*

Etiology	Spontaneous abortions (%)	Ectopic pregnancies (%)	Deliveries (%)
Unknown	16.1	2.4	81.5
Endometriosis	20.8	3.3	75.9
Male factor	12.7	3.9	83.4
Tuboperitoneal factor	16.3	11.0	72.7
Failed donor insemination	21.2	0.0	78.8
Cervical factor	15.8	21.0	63.2
Oocyte donation	10.0	0.0	90.0
Immunologic factor	20.0	0.0	80.0
TOTAL	16.8	3.9	79.3

*Data are from Asch et al.[4]

participating had similar outcomes, with an overall pregnancy rate of 28.7%, which was superior to IVF-embryo transfer (ET) results obtained during the same period of time. There was a significant difference depending on etiology, being as low as 15% or 16% for cases of male or immunologic factor and as high as 56% for those patients undergoing oocyte donation (Table 44-1). Once pregnancy had been achieved, approximately 80% progressed to third-trimester delivery, with a significant difference in oocyte donation patients (90%) compared with patients with other etiologies such as cervical factor (63.2%). The spontaneous abortion and ectopic pregnancy rates were 16.8% and 3.9%, respectively (Table 44-2).

Results of an international collaborative study of IVF-ET and GIFT for 1989[44] are shown in Table 44-3. The clinical pregnancy rate and take-home baby rate per puncture were significantly higher for GIFT than for IVF. The proportions of multiple pregnancies were similar for both procedures.

Other data presented by Cohen[14] in 1991 reporting statistics for the years 1987 through 1989 for the four main national registers (United States, Australia, United Kingdom, and France) also showed better results for GIFT, with clinical pregnancy rates that fluctuated between 20.8% and 27.5% (Table 44-4). In those same countries, the clinical

pregnancy rate per cycle was between 13% and 16.8% for IVF. The United States IVF registry for 1990[37] reports overall per-cycle take-home baby rates of 22% for GIFT and 14% for IVF.

Although in these multicenter reports the results achieved with GIFT appear to be superior to those achieved with IVF, one must remember that they represent two different populations that cannot be strictly compared because of the wide variation in IVF-ET results from clinic to clinic, as well as patient selection criteria. On the other hand, the value of comparing tubal and uterine transfers done by a single group of investigators, as opposed to national statistics, is that it decreases the interfering bias of differences between laboratories and operators; but the main disadvantage is that it may represent an effort to confirm a preconceived notion. Nevertheless, there are no large series in the literature to suggest that implantation rates of embryos vary strongly with the specific etiology of the couples' infertility.

The spontaneous abortion rate associated with GIFT is reported to be about 19%, which is comparable to IVF and

Table 44-3. Results of GIFT and IVF-ET in a world collaborative report*

Method	No. of centers	Clinical pregnancy rate	Take-home baby rate	Multiple pregnancy rate
GIFT	341	27.5	20.0	26.9
IVF-ET	500	16.4	11.9	25.7

*Data are from Asch et al.[4]

Table 44-4. National registry results achieved with GIFT*

Country	Year	No. of punctures	Clinical pregnancy rate (%)
United States	1988	3080	21.0
Australia	1988	2653	27.5
United Kingdom	1989	2840	20.8
France	1987-1989	2042	21.3
TOTAL		10615	22.6

*Data are from Cohen.[14]

ZIFT results and is not significantly different from the spontaneous abortion rate among natural conceptions within a fertile population.

The ectopic pregnancy rate for any ART procedure is higher than the spontaneous incidence in a normal population, and for GIFT it is reported to be approximately 5%. This higher rate of tubal pregnancy is probably the result of a combination of two factors: inevitable manipulation of the genital tract and undiagnosed tubal disease. Surprisingly, however, the incidence of ectopic pregnancy with GIFT is not higher than that with uterine transfer of embryos.

The incidence of chromosomal abnormalities and congenital malformations associated with GIFT does not differ from that reported with other ART procedures (2.1% and 3.1%, respectively).[37] Until now the interpretation of American statistics, corrected for patient age, is that this percentage of abnormalities does not represent a significant variation from the normal population. At the same time, according to the 1990 national registry statistics,[37] the premature delivery rate for GIFT is 18%. This elevated rate is obviously influenced by the higher number of multiple gestations.

As for other ART procedures it is not clear whether it is the influence of the GIFT technique itself or the selective population treated that explains the higher incidence of abnormalities (ectopic pregnancy and premature delivery) reported.

Oocyte quality

There is no doubt that certain variables can affect the outcome of the procedure, and quality of oocytes is maybe the most important one. This fact was originally demonstrated by Balmaceda et al.[10] in 1986, working with *Macaca fascicularis*. One group of animals underwent GIFT with immature oocytes and the others received only mature ones. Twenty-four hours after the transfer, they flushed the genital tracts of the animals and recovered the gametes and/or embryos. No embryos were recovered from any animal that had received immature oocytes, and the eggs retrieved showed advanced signs of degeneration and no signs of maturation. The group that had received mature oocytes had a fertilization rate of 37%, which is significantly lower than that obtained in vitro for the same quality of eggs.

The number of eggs transferred is not as crucial as the maturity of the oocytes, but it can definitely have an impact on the multiple pregnancy rate. There are several reports concluding that the clinical pregnancy rate is increased with the number of oocytes transferred when comparing the transfer of one, two, three, or four oocytes.[23,31,46] These figures are as low as 6.3% for one oocyte to as high as 41% for four oocytes transferred. Nevertheless, increasing the number of oocytes to five or more does not improve the pregnancy rate significantly, but it dramatically raises the multiple pregnancy rate (Table 44-5). The 1990 United

Table 44-5. Number of oocytes transferred and pregnancies with GIFT

Center	No. of oocytes	No. of cases	% Pregnancies
University of California, Irvine[23]	1	16	6.3
	2	48	20.8
	3	42	23.8
	4	89	39.3
Long Beach Memorial[46]	1	7	0
	2	32	18.8
	3	95	23.2
	4	112	42.9
Bourn Hall[16]	1-2	115	13.9
	3-4	263	24.7
	5-6	310	38.1
	7-8	243	42.8
	9-10	108	38.0
	>10	32	50.0

States IVF-ET registry reported an 11% clinical pregnancy rate when three or fewer oocytes were transferred and a 30% to 43% rate when four or more oocytes were transferred. In the same proportion, the delivery rates were 9% for the first group and 24% to 28% for the second group; but there was a marked difference in the multiple pregnancy rate, from only 1.4% when three or fewer oocytes were transferred, 8% when four were transferred, 8.5% when five or six were transferred, to 12.7% when more than six were transferred.

As described earlier, the new methods of controlled ovarian hyperstimulation result in a larger number of oocytes retrieved. The ability to cryopreserve supernumerary preembryos has allowed us to perform subsequent zygote intrafallopian transfer (ZIFT) or intrauterine frozen embryo transfer (FET) without requiring another ovarian hyperstimulation protocol. This possibility was originally demonstrated by Alam et al.,[1] who reported a 56.4% total cumulative pregnancy rate from one GIFT retrieval cycle, when cumulatively including all the consecutive frozen FETs to those patients who had a failed initial GIFT procedure. Although this is a theoretic mathematical calculation, based on our 17% pregnancy rate with frozen-thawed ET cycles, it clearly represents an increase of 8.9% in pregnancy rate per retrieval cycle (Fig. 44-3).

Sperm quality

The relevance of individual sperm parameters has also been accurately studied, and results obtained by Guzick et al.[23] in our center are shown in Table 44-6. Motility and morphology appeared to be the most important parameters, having an independent impact on the chances of pregnancy. In analyzing 218 GIFT cycles Guzick et al.[23] found a fivefold increase in pregnancy rate when normal morphol-

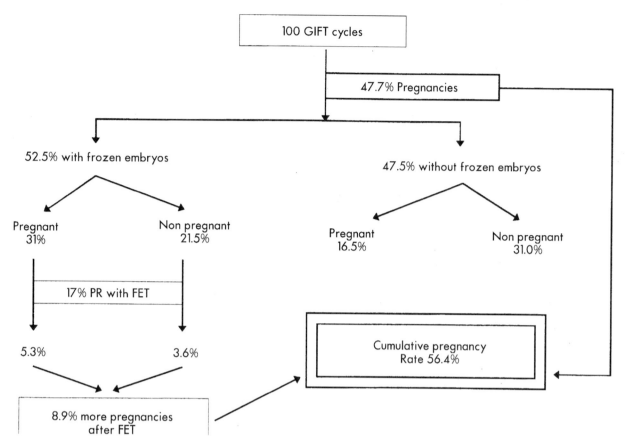

Fig. 44-3. Mathematical calculation of the cumulative pregnancy rate from 100 GIFT cycles and disposition of all remaining sibling preembryos. *PR,* Pregnancy rate; *FET,* frozen embryo transfer. (Data are from Alam et al.[1])

ogy was present in more than 50% of the ejaculate. If motility was more than 30% there was a threefold increase in the chances of pregnancy, but adding the total sperm count to this analysis had no significant effect. This last fact has a logical basis, as GIFT overcomes in part the numerical problems of a semen analysis by placing a high number of motile sperm directly into the ampulla (500,000 to 700,000 motile sperm). It cannot resolve a major functional problem in sperm parameters, such as very low motility or abnormal morphology, as demonstrated by Wiedemann et al.[45]

For this group of patients with a poor prognosis with GIFT because of a severe male factor, another technique is now available. It was first proposed by Devroey et al.[18] in 1986 and Yovich et al.[48] in 1987 and involves the transfer of embryos generated in vitro to the fallopian tubes. It receives the name of ZIFT, PROST (pronuclear stage transfer), or TET (tubal embryo transfer), depending on the stage of development of the embryos to be transferred. The advantage of this procedure over GIFT is that it documents fertilization before the transfer is performed; compared with IVF, it avoids the potential trauma related to direct

Table 44-6. Semen quality and pregnancies with GIFT

Study	Semen parameter	% Pregnancies
University of California, Irvine[23]		<20% 6.7
	Motility	
		>30% 31.9
		<50% 10.9
	Morphology	
		>50% 35.8
Wiedemann et al.[45]		<30% 23.3
	Motility and morphology	
		>30% 43.2

embryo transfer into the endometrial cavity. Theoretically the method conveys the same benefits as GIFT, in terms of allowing a chronologically appropriate entrance of the embryos to the uterus.

ZIFT results are generally less accurately reported in the literature, because the small number of centers that perform it often use different stages of embryo development. The

Table 44-7. Comparison of pregnancy rates achieved with GIFT, ZIFT, and IVF*

Study	Pregnancy rates with ART procedure (%)		
	GIFT	ZIFT	IVF
Yovich[47]	38.0	36.0	16.0
Hammitt et al.[25]	48.9	52.4	26.9
Bollen et al.[11]	19.4	38.5	28.4
Devroey et al.[19]	30.0	48.0	21.8
Tanbo et al.[42]	26.2	37.0	45.7

*Data are from Balmaceda et al.[9]

Table 44-8. Comparative results of GIFT and ZIFT for different age groups*

	GIFT/ZIFT		
Age group	Pregnancy rate (%)	Implantation rate (%)	Abortion rate (%)
<30	25/36	11/13	25/0
30-34	37/35	15/18	8/10
35-39	42/24	9/7	11/17
>40	46/6	10/1	50/66

*Data are from Balmaceda et al.[9]

outcome of this ART procedure seems to be comparable to that of GIFT and IVF, as shown in Table 44-7.[9] The United States IVF registry for ZIFT 1990 reported a 21% pregnancy rate and a 16% take-home baby rate.[37] For all the ART procedures, rates of spontaneous abortion, ectopic pregnancy, and heterotopic pregnancy are also similar, averaging 19%, 5% and less than 1%, respectively.[34]

Age of the patient

Age of the patient has a significant influence on the success of any ART procedure, and GIFT is not an exception. If we examine the fertility rate curve of a normal population, we find that there is a slight decrease when women reach the third decade of life. The decrease in fertility becomes more evident after age 35 years and is markedly apparent after age 40.

Defective oocytes may be responsible for this decrease in women's fertility, as has been clearly demonstrated by oocyte donation programs. We have obtained up to 50% pregnancy rates while working with poor responders or true ovarian failure recipients. Our success with this group implies that the problem is not endometrial but one of oocyte quality, which is probably related to the women's older age. Moreover, Cohen et al.[15] have postulated zona pellucida hardening as the main factor associated with defective oocytes in older women. These investigators published results of assisted zonal hatching performed in women with poor implantation rates despite normal fertilization, and found a significantly positive effect with this technique only in women over age 38 years. They concluded that assisted zonal hatching should be offered only to patients of that age group.

The relevance of age to the success of GIFT was reported by Craft and Brindsen.[16] These investigators reviewed 1071 GIFT procedures and found pregnancy rates between 33.5% and 40.2% in different age groups of patients, all under age 40, compared with only 19.2% in the group over age 40. Consequently, the incidence of multiple pregnancy was 29% in the group below age 40 and 16.2% in the group over age 40. They concluded that the chances of pregnancy and the risk of multiple pregnancies are

significantly lower in patients over age 40, even when 10 or more oocytes are transferred. Nevertheless, we believe, as do many other investigators,[23,31,46] that augmenting the number of oocytes transferred from four up to six or seven in this select age group increases the chances of pregnancy with GIFT. There is general acceptance that GIFT is the ART procedure that offers a better outcome for women above age 40, with an average pregnancy rate of 19% reported by several authors.[31,36,37] Results of IVF for this same age group of patients range around 10%. Table 44-8 presents data from our clinic collected during the years 1990 through 1991, and it compares results obtained by GIFT and ZIFT for women of different age groups. It clearly appears that GIFT has a better outcome than does ZIFT in patients over age 35 (42% versus 24% pregnancy rate). This difference becomes even more significant over age 40 years, with a pregnancy rate of 46% versus 6% and an implantation rate of 10% versus 1% for GIFT and ZIFT, respectively.

Table 44-9 also compares results achieved by GIFT and IVF according to women's ages and demonstrates higher figures for GIFT in the older age group.

Technical aspects

The use of one or both tubes to transfer the gamete does not seem to influence to the results. Yee et al.[46] found a 37.6% pregnancy rate when using both tubes and a 26.2% pregnancy rate when using only one. However, these figures are not statistically significant. Haines and O'Shea[24] reviewed 136 GIFT cycles and found a 57.1% pregnancy rate when one tube was used and 25.4% rate when both tubes were used. They concluded that the advantage of using only one tube was reduction in operating time and avoidance of any possible damage to the contralateral tube at the time of catheterization. In our center we perform single tubal transfers to the tube that appears healthier and easier to manipulate at the time of surgery.

The depth of entrance of the catheter into the tube was studied by Yee et al.,[46] who suggested that it should be at least 3 cm to maximize the chances of pregnancy. They reported a pregnancy rate of 32% when this condition was

Table 44-9. Comparative results of GIFT and IVF according to women's ages*

| Age group (y) | No. of transfers | GIFT/IVF | | | | |
		Clinical pregnancies (%)	Ectopic pregnancies (%)	Spontaneous abortions (%)	Deliveries (%)	Multiple deliveries (%)
<25	18/27	11.1/25.9	0/0	50/28.6	0/18.5	0/0
25-29	200/436	34/20.2	4.4/6.8	8.8/18.2	30/16.1	12.5/5.1
30-34	634/1331	36/23.7	5.7/7.6	15.8/15.9	28.9/19.3	10.1/5.6
35-39	532/1256	26.7/19.4	5.6/4.5	17.6/22.2	20.5/14.8	6.2/3.7
>40	214/350	16.8/10.9	2.8/7.9	38.9/28.9	8.9/6.6	1.4/1.7
TOTAL	1599/3405	29.8/20	5.3/6.3	17.2/19	23.2/16	7.8/4.4

*Data are from reference 37.

achieved, as opposed to only 16.7% when it was not. Results were independent of the total number of eggs transferred and whether one tube was used or both tubes were used. Our clinical experience confirms the data of Yee et al.[46] Furthermore, as previously discussed, we believe that the gametes should be inserted in a small volume to minimize chances of reflux to the peritoneal cavity.

The use of carbon dioxide (5% to 100%) to induce pneumoperitoneum apparently does not affect the results in terms of fertilization, cleavage, and pregnancy rates when doing laparoscopic GIFT.[32] Moreover, Pampiglione et al.[38] have prompted doing the GIFT procedure at the same time as diagnostic laparoscopy; they reported a 24% pregnancy rate (5 of 21 patients) using the combined procedures.[21] Later Gindoff et al.[21] and Johns[30] also reported similar results combining clomiphene citrate-induced ovulations for GIFT with diagnostic and operative laparoscopy.

Transcervical catheterization of the tubes, blindly, ultrasonically guided, or by hysteroscopy, may represent a simplified alternative to the classic transabdominal GIFT procedures. Although the first reports suggested that the results obtained were similar to those with the conventional method,[13,22,35] the consistency of these findings is under question today. In the literature describing the different transcervical methods utilized, a wide range of pregnancy rates is reported.[13,26,29,35] Some of the significant series published to date are summarized in Table 44-10. As can be seen in Table 44-10, the average pregnancy rate achieved is inferior to rates reported after transabdominal transfers. Furthermore, the ectopic pregnancy rate of 13% appears unacceptably high. On the other hand, the field of endoscopic surgery and the use of new fiberoptic technology may result in significant improvement of results achieved with transcervical tubal catheterization. New instruments are being proposed that may facilitate visualization of the ostium and the entrance to the tube without the need of uterine distention. This advance may represent a satisfactory alternative for patients presenting a difficult translaparoscopic approach because of pelvic adhesions or for patients with a high surgical risk, as this less-invasive technique does not require anesthesia or transabdominal surgery.

CONCLUSION

With the new regimens of ovarian hyperstimulation now available, we have reached limits that surpass the natural conception rate per cycle in normal couples. Furthermore, the capacity to cryopreserve preembryos increases the efficiency of the technique. For this last reason, we feel that GIFT should be performed mainly in centers that offer the complete array of ART procedures, which will allow for appropriate patient selection and permit full advantage of IVF technology.

At the present time there should not be any reason for

Table 44-10. Ultrasound-Guided GIFT

Authors	Year	Catheter	No. of cycles	No. of pregnancies (%)	No. of ectopic pregnancies
Bustillo et al.[13]	1989	K-JITS-1000	17	1 (5.9)	0
Hazout et al.[26]	1989	PRODIMED	18	1 (6.0)	0
Jansen and Anderson[28a]	1989	K-JITS-1000	1	1 (10.0)	0
Anderson and Jansen[28]	1989	K-JITS-2000	7	1 (14.0)	0
Lucena et al.[35]	1989	K-JITS-1000 and 1100	7	3 (42.8)	1
Anderson et al.[3]	1990	K-JITS	44	8 (18.2)	1
TOTAL			103	15 (14.6)	2 (13.3%)

excluding the GIFT technique from the therapeutic options that can be offered to a couple with patent fallopian tubes. We consider it a viable alternative to IVF, especially in women over age 40 years, who show consistently good and reproducible results.

Inclusion criteria for patient selection are fundamental for achieving the best results with GIFT. In general, couples with severe male factors and tubal abnormalities should be excluded.

The method of choice for transferring gametes is still laparoscopy. Simplifying techniques, such as transcervical catheterization of the fallopian tubes, will make GIFT even more attractive to physicians and patients.

Flexible protocols should be followed at the time of the transfer, considering variables such as the age of the patient, quality of the eggs, and characteristics of the sperm, instead of fixed formulas.

We are conscious that increased simplification and continuous improvement of the results achieved with IVF-ET may restrict the actual indication for GIFT. The decision of which therapeutic alternative to use must be made based mainly on individual results of the specific center.

REFERENCES

1. Alam V et al: Cumulative pregnancy rate from one gamete intrafallopian transfer (GIFT) cycle with cryopreservation of embryos: a practical mathematical calculation, *Human Reprod* 8(1):559, 1993.
2. See reference 28a.
3. Anderson JC et al: ultrasound-guided transvaginal catheterization of the fallopian tube for gamete or embryo transfer. 7th World Congress on In Vitro Fertilization and Assisted Procreation, Paris, 1991.
3a. Araujo E Jr et al: Luteal phase support for assisted reproductive technology: a prospective randomized study of human chorionic gonadotrophin versus intramuscular progesterone. The 41st Annual Meeting of the Pacific Coast Fertility Society, Indian Wells, California, April 1993.
4. Asch RH: GIFT: indications, results, problems, and perspectives. In Capitanio GL et al, editors: GIFT: from basics to clinics, Serono Symposia, Vol 63, New York, 1989, Raven Press.
5. Asch RH et al: Pregnancy following translaparoscopic gamete intrafallopian transfer (GIFT), *Lancet* 2:1034, 1984.
6. Asch RH et al: Birth following gamete intrafallopian transfer, *Lancet* 2:163, 1985 (letter).
7. Asch RH et al: Gamete intrafallopian transfer (GIFT): a new treatment for infertility, *Int J Fertil* 30:41, 1985.
8. Asch RH et al: Preliminary experiences with GIFT (gamete intrafallopian transfer), *Fertil Steril* 45:366, 1986.
9. Balmaceda JP, Gonzales J, Bernardini L: Gamete and zygote intrafallopian transfers and related techniques, *Curr Opin Obstet Gynecol* 4:743, 1992.
10. Balmaceda JP et al: In vivo versus in vitro oocyte maturation in a primate animal model. In Proceedings of the 42nd Annual Meeting of The American Fertility Society, Toronto, September 1986 (abstract).
11. Bollen N et al: The incidence of multiple pregnancy after in vitro fertilization and embryo transfer, gamete, or zygote intrafallopian transfer, *Fertil Steril* 55:314, 1991.
12. Buster JE et al: Biologic and morphologic development of donated human ova recovered by nonsurgical uterine lavage, *Am J Obstet Gynecol* 153:211, 1985.
13. Bustillo M et al: Transcervical ultrasound-guided intrafallopian placement of gametes, zygotes and embryos. In Proceedings of the Sixth World Congress of in Vitro Fertilization and Alternate Assisted Reproduction, Jerusalem, April 2-7, 1989.
14. Cohen J: The efficiency and efficacy of IVF and GIFT, *Hum Reprod* 6:613, 1991 (editorial).
15. Cohen J et al: Implantation enhancement by selective assisted hatching using zona drilling of human embryos with poor prognosis, *Hum Reprod* 7:685, 1992.
16. Craft I, Brindsen P: Alternatives to IVF: the outcome of 1071 first GIFT procedures, *Hum Reprod* 4:29, 1989.
17. Croxatto HB et al: Studies on the duration of egg transport by the human oviduct, II: ovum location at various intervals following luteinizing hormone peak, *Am J Obstet Gynecol* 132:629, 1978.
18. Devroey P et al: Pregnancy after translaparoscopic zygote intrafallopian transfer in a patient with sperm antibodies, *Lancet* 1:1329, 1986.
19. Devroey P et al: Zygote intrafallopian transfer as a successful treatment for unexplained infertility, *Fertil Steril* 52:246, 1989.
20. Diaz S, Ortiz ME, Croxatto HB: Studies on the duration of ovum transport by the human oviduct, III: time interval between the luteinizing peak and recovery of ova by transcervical flushing of the uterus in normal women, *Am J Obstet Gynecol* 137:116, 1980.
21. Gindoff PR et al: Efficacy of assisted reproductive technology during diagnostic and operative infertility laparoscopy, *Obstet Gynecol* 75:299, 1990.
21a. Gonen et al: Endometrial thickness and growth during ovarian stimulation: a possible predictor of implantation in in vitro fertilization cycles, *Fertil Steril* 52:446, 1989.
22. Guidetti R et al: Non-surgical tubal embryo transfer, *Hum Reprod* 5:221, 1990.
23. Guzik DS et al: The importance of egg and sperm factors in predicting the likelihood of pregnancy from gamete intrafallopian transfer, *Fertil Steril* 52:795, 1989.
24. Haines CJ, O'Shea RT: Unilateral gamete intrafallopian transfer: the preferred method?, *Fertil Steril* 51:518, 1989.
25. Hammitt DG et al: Comparison of concurrent pregnancy rates for in vitro fertilization: embryo transfer, pronuclear stage embryo transfer and gamete intrafallopian transfer, *Hum Reprod* 5:947, 1990.
26. Hazout A, Glissant A, Frydman R: Transvaginal ultrasound guided gamete intrafallopian transfer (GIFT). In Proceedings of the Sixth World Congress of in Vitro Fertilization and Alternate Assisted Reproduction, Jerusalem, Israel, April 2-7, 1989.
27. Hughes EG et al: The routine use of gonadotropin releasing hormone agonists prior to in vitro fertilization and gamete intrafallopian transfer: a meta-analysis of randomized controlled trials, *Fertil Steril* 58:888, 1992.
28. Jansen RPS, Anderson JC: Ultrasound-guided fallopian cannulation for gamete or embryo transfer. Paper presented at the 45th Annual Meeting of the American Fertility Society, San Francisco, November, 1989.
28a. Jansen RPS, Anderson JC: Ultrasound-guided gamete intra-fallopian transfer. Paper presented at the 6th World Congress on In Vitro Fertilization and Alternate Assisted Reproduction, Jerusalem, 1989.
29. Jansen RPS, Anderson JC, Sutherland PD: Nonoperative embryo transfer to the fallopian tube, *N Engl Med* 319:288, 1988.
30. Johns DA: Clomiphene citrate induced gamete intrafallopian transfer with diagnostic and operative laparoscopy, *Fertil Steril* 56:311, 1991.
31. Kerin J et al: The effect of maternal age on the pregnancy outcome of IVF and GIFT procedures. In Proceedings of the 44th Annual Meeting of The American Fertility Society, Atlanta, October 1988 (abstract).
32. Kham I et al: The effect of pneumoperitoneum gases on fertilization, cleavage and pregnancy in human in vitro fertilization and gamete intrafallopian transfer, *Hum Reprod* 4:323, 1989.
33. Kreitman O, Hodgen GD: Low tubal ovum transfer, an alternative to in vitro fertilization, *Fertil Steril* 34:374, 1980.
34. Li HP et al: Heterotopic pregnancy associated with gamete intrafallopian transfer, *Hum Reprod* 7:131, 1992.

35. Lucena E et al: Vaginal intratubal insemination (UITI) and vaginal GIFT, endosonographic technique: early experience, *Hum Reprod* 4:658, 1989.

36. Matson PL et al: The role of gamete intrafallopian transfer (GIFT) in the treatment of oligospermic infertility, *Fertil Steril* 48:608, 1987.

37. Medical Research International Society for Assisted Reproductive Technology (SART), The American Fertility Society: In vitro fertilization embryo transfer (IVF ET) in the United States, 1990: results from the IVF ET registry, *Fertil Steril* 57:15, 1992.

38. Pampiglione JS et al: Gamete intrafallopian transfer combined with diagnostic laparoscopy: a treatment for infertility in a district hospital, *Hum Reprod* 4:786, 1989.

39. Deleted in galleys.

40. Shettles LB: Ova harvest with in vivo fertilization, *Am J Obstet Gynecol* 133:845, 1979.

41. Tan SL et al: A prospective randomized study of the optimum timing of human chorionic gonadotrophin administration after pituitary desensitization in in vitro fertilization, *Fertil Steril* 57:1259, 1992.

42. Tanbo T, Dale PO, Abyholm T: Assisted fertilization in infertile women with patent fallopian tubes: a comparison of in vitro fertilization, gamete intrafallopian transfer and tubal embryo stage transfer, *Hum Reprod* 5:266, 1990.

43. Tesarik J et al: Oocyte recovery in in vitro insemination and transfer into the oviduct after its microsurgical repair at a single laparotomy, *Fertil Steril* 39:472, 1983.

44. Testart J et al: World collaborative report on IVF-ET and GIFT: 1989 results, *Hum Reprod* 7:362, 1992.

45. Wiedemann R, Noss U, Hepp M: Gamete intrafallopian transfer in male subfertility, *Hum Reprod* 4:408, 1989.

46. Yee B et al: Gamete intrafallopian transfer: the effect of the number of eggs used and the depth of gamete placement on pregnancy initiation, *Fertil Steril* 52:639, 1989.

47. Yovich J: Tubal transfers: PROST and TEST. In Asch RH et al, editors: *Gamete physiology,* Serono Symposia vol 273, New York, 1990, Raven Press.

48. Yovich JL et al: Pregnancies following pronuclear stage tubal transfer, *Fertil Steril* 48:851, 1987.

Chapter 45

MICROSCOPIC ASSESSMENT OF HUMAN OOCYTES, PREZYGOTES, AND PREEMBRYOS

Lucinda L. Veeck, MLT (ASCP), DSc (hon)

A program of in vitro fertilization (IVF) has been ongoing at the Jones Institute for Reproductive Medicine in Norfolk, Virginia, since 1980. During the first year of operation, treatment in only a few natural cycles was undertaken without success. Since 1981, in cycles utilizing gonadotro-

pins for ovarian stimulation, more than 49,000 oocytes have been harvested, evaluated, and handled in the laboratory as one part of a group effort to alleviate infertility in couples seeking assistance. The majority of oocytes have been healthy and seemingly capable of undergoing a normal fertilization process. Sixty-two percent of all oocytes harvested to date have been classified as mature, or nearly mature, without degenerative features. An additional 26% of the oocytes have been germinal vesicle-bearing, indicating a need for in vitro maturation before insemination, and 12% have been collected in a degenerative state, sometimes with damage to the oolemma or zona pellucida. To date, nearly 1300 babies have been born from this program, and many more are expected in the months to come. One advantage of working with such a large program is that the embryologist is given the opportunity to examine large numbers of oocytes and preembryos under the microscope and to learn, with experience, which nuclear and cytoplasmic features can be correlated with IVF success.

BACKGROUND, PHYSIOLOGY, AND SCOPE OF ASSESSMENT

Oocyte meiotic events

Each woman starts her life with about half a million germ cells as a result of mitotic proliferation of oogonia in the fetal ovary; more than 99% of these will degenerate over the woman's lifetime. Deoxyribonucleic acid (DNA) is replicated in germ cells in preparation for the first meiotic division. Prophase I of the first meiotic division is a complex stage during which homologous chromosomes exchange genetic material in a process known as crossing over. In the human ovary the transformation of oogonia to oocytes by entrance into prophase I begins from the third month of gestation. By birth, all germ cells are oocytes (with a tetraploid amount of DNA), and meiosis is arrested in prophase I at the dictyate (diplotene) stage; this arrest persists through infancy until just before ovulation.[1,2,5,17]

Before it can participate in the process of fertilization, the oocyte passes through a series of maturational steps. Still in meiosis I, the oocyte passes out of the dictyate stage (prophase I, PI). The nucleolus fades and the germinal vesicle (oocyte nucleus) membrane disappears. At metaphase of the first division, a spindle is formed, and chromosomes of recombined maternal and paternal genetic material line up randomly toward the poles (metaphase I, MI). At anaphase of the first division, whole members of homologous chromosome pairs separate randomly with their centromeres intact.

Because the germinal vesicle of the oocyte was tetraploid in respect to chromatids, each of the separated groups has a diploid amount of DNA (23 double-stranded chromosomes). At telophase of the first meiosis, division of the ooplasm occurs, and one of these chromosome groups is expelled in the first polar body and the other remains in the oocyte.

There is no true prophase of the second division; the cell passes directly to metaphase II without replication of DNA or formation of a nucleus. A spindle re-forms, and the 23 chromosomes of the oocyte, each with 2 chromatids, line up on the equatorial plate. Although there is only a haploid set of chromosomes, there is a diploid amount of DNA because the strands have not yet separated. Here the second meiotic arrest begins (metaphase II, MII); meiosis II is not resumed until the oocyte is activated by a penetrating spermatozoon or environmental forces. Once activated, final maturation occurs: at anaphase of the second division, chromatids split at the centromeres; at telophase of the second division, one set is extruded in the second polar body, leaving 23 single chromosomes to participate in the events of human fertilization.

These events occur naturally under gonadotropin stimulus in the natural or stimulated cycle. One must understand the fundamental maturation process in order to evaluate oocyte maturity fully at harvest.

Laboratory evaluation of the oocyte/preembryo

The following discussion encompasses morphologic features of the oocyte as evaluated at harvest, the sperm-penetrated oocyte (the prezygote), the fertilizing oocyte during syngamy (the zygote), and the preembryo from its first cytoplasmic division through the blastocyst stage of development. Nuclear, pronuclear, ooplasmic, and cytoplasmic aspects are covered and correlated to pregnancy potential. Other factors such as the effect of patient age and mode of ovarian stimulation, value of donor oocytes, and the developmental aspects of thawed preembryos are included.

Terminology

For clarification, the terminology used in the text is defined as follows:

Oocyte: The female gamete from inception of the first meiotic division until fertilization. In oogenesis, a cell that develops from an oogonium. *Metaphase II oocyte:* An oocyte with chromosomes at MII; characterized by the presence of a first polar body. A fully mature oocyte. A secondary oocyte. *Metaphase I oocyte:* An oocyte with chromosomes at MI; characterized by the absence of both a first polar body and a germinal vesicle. An oocyte at an intermediate stage of maturation. *Prophase I oocyte:* An oocyte with chromosomes at PI; characterized by a germinal vesicle.

Penetrated oocyte: An oocyte that has been penetrated by a spermatozoon; strictly defined, one in which gamete plasma membranes have become confluent. The stage before pronuclei are formed.

Prezygote: The penetrated oocyte that displays pronuclei and the second polar body; a pronuclear stage conceptus. The stage of development before syngamy. Some embryologists refer to this stage as an *ootid.* Pronuclei are commonly observed 10 to 20 hours after insemination.

Zygote: The one-cell stage after pronuclear membrane breakdown before first cleavage. This stage is characterized by maternal and paternal chromosomes that assume positions on the first cleavage spindle, thus the lack of a nucleus; commonly observed 18 to 24 hours after insemination. *Syngamy:* The union of two gametes in fertilization to form a zygote. The process of reorganization and pairing of maternal and paternal chromosomes in the zygote after pronuclear membrane breakdown.

Preembryo: The conceptus during early cleavage stages until development of the embryo. The preembryonic period ends at approximately 14 days after fertilization with development of the primitive streak. *Morula:* The 16-cell stage upward until blastocyst formation; the stage commonly observed between 72 and 96 hours postinsemination. Some embryologists believe that the term *morula* is inappropriate for mammals. *Blastocyst:* The conceptus in the post-morula stage possessing a fluid-filled cavity. Attached to the inner surface of the trophoblast is an inner cell mass from which the embryo develops.

Embryo: The stage of the organism after development of the primitive streak; persists until major organs are developed. Once the neural groove and the first somites are present, the embryo is considered formed. In women, the embryonic stage begins at approximately 14 days postfertilization and encompasses the period when organs and organ systems are coming into existence.

Conceptus: The derivatives of a fertilized oocyte at any stage of development from fertilization to birth; includes extraembryonic membranes and the preembryo, embryo, or fetus. The products of conception; all structures that develop from the zygote, both embryonic and extraembryonic. A term commonly interchanged with the term *preembryo* during IVF treatment.

DIAGNOSTIC APPROACH AND PRACTICE MANAGEMENT

Assessment of oocyte maturity and viability with bright-field microscopy

The accuracy and pace of microscopic work can depend in large part on the quality of the equipment used in the laboratory. The dissecting microscope, although invaluable to the embryology laboratory for oocyte handling and transfer, is simply not efficient for the precise evaluation of nuclear and cytoplasmic characteristics. An inverted microscope equipped with low-power and high-power objectives should be considered second in importance only to the quality and number of incubators in the laboratory. The oocytes and conceptuses described here were examined with one of several Nikon Diaphot microscopes purchased over a 10-year period. These microscopes have proven to be reliable and trouble free whether fitted with Hoffman optics, used for sensitive micromanipulative techniques, or attached to video time-lapse recorders for days on end. When fitted with special 2× long-working-distance objectives and 4×, 10×, 20×, and 40× objectives, the range of magnification has proved convenient for scanning follicular aspirates and necessary for the critical examination of oocyte, zona pellucida, and blastomere. Microscopic evaluation of oocytes at the time of harvest will determine when a semen sample should be delivered to the laboratory and at what approximate time the oocytes might be inseminated; the patient is counseled as to the expectation of fertilization success based on the laboratory's assessment of oocyte maturity and morphology. Because oocytes are inseminated only when they become fully mature, those that are individually evaluated at the time of collection tend to show slightly better fertilization outcomes than those that are not evaluated for maturational status; failure of fertilization does not occur because of inappropriate timing for sperm-oocyte interaction.

Embryology laboratories with poor fertilization rates should determine whether culture conditions need refining or whether poor oocyte assessment is leading simply to improper insemination times with subsequent fertilization failure. Experience has shown that waiting too long to inseminate a fully mature oocyte or placing an immature oocyte too quickly with spermatozoa will severely compromise the developmental potential of the gamete. Those inseminated before reaching metaphase II may be penetrated by spermatozoa and yet fail to initiate events leading to sperm chromatin decondensation; these oocytes ultimately lack functional male pronuclei.[34] Others may display three or more pronuclei when they are inseminated

in an immature or a postmature state; in immature oocytes the cortical granule numbers and response may be inadequate, whereas in postmature oocytes cortical granule release may be inhibited or the zona reaction may be poorly functional.[13] In addition to the confirmation of nuclear maturity, it is recognized that a brief period (at least 1 hour) may be needed after extrusion of the first polar body for the oocyte to gain full cytoplasmic competence.[42] If cytoplasmic maturation is significantly delayed after nuclear maturation is completed, a poor response to penetrating spermatozoa may follow, with failed oocyte activation or lack of sperm head decondensation. Therefore the practice of inseminating all oocytes at a set time, although most convenient for laboratory personnel, is not usually in the best interest of the patient unless sperm quality is exceptionally poor or large numbers of oocytes are collected after long-term cycle suppression with gonadotropin-releasing hormone agonists (GnRHa).

Better synchronization of oocyte maturity can be seen within a cohort of follicles after luteal phase suppression with GnRHa. The current practice at the Jones Institute is to assess directly the nuclear characteristics of all oocytes collected after standard gonadotropin stimulation of the ovary, and to perform only a gross visual evaluation on those with mature characteristics of the cumulus oophorus and corona radiata after luteal phase ovarian suppression with GnRHa. Because large numbers of fully mature oocytes generally are collected from younger patients after GnRHa suppression and exogenous ovarian stimulation (sometimes as many as 30 or more), this protocol has proven to be practical for the laboratory without affecting an individual patient's pregnancy outcome.

Assessment of oocyte maturity based on morphology of the cumulus oophorus and corona radiata. Evaluation of maturation generally has been based on the expansion and radiance of the cumulus-corona complex that surrounds the harvested gamete.[40,41] By studying this mucuslike mass, embryologists categorize specimens as mature when they possess an expanded, luteinized cumulus and a radiating layer of cells nearest the oocyte itself (Fig. 45-1, **A**). A less-expanded cumulus-corona complex denotes an intermediate stage of maturity (Fig. 45-1, **B**), and an unexpanded cumulus generally is associated with immaturity. While cellular luteinization often correlates well with oocyte maturity, it most significantly reflects the responses of other follicular cells to gonadotropin surges. In this regard, cellular evaluation may be imprecise; nuclear maturation of the oocyte and cellular maturation of the cumulus often show disparity.[22,41,45] If an oocyte is wrongly classified because of disparity, fertilization outcome may be compromised, ovulation induction protocols may not be suitably appraised, and male factor issues become difficult to interpret on the basis of fertilization results. Because correlation between cellular and nuclear events in sibling oocytes is particularly good with the use of GnRHa, a fixed insemina-

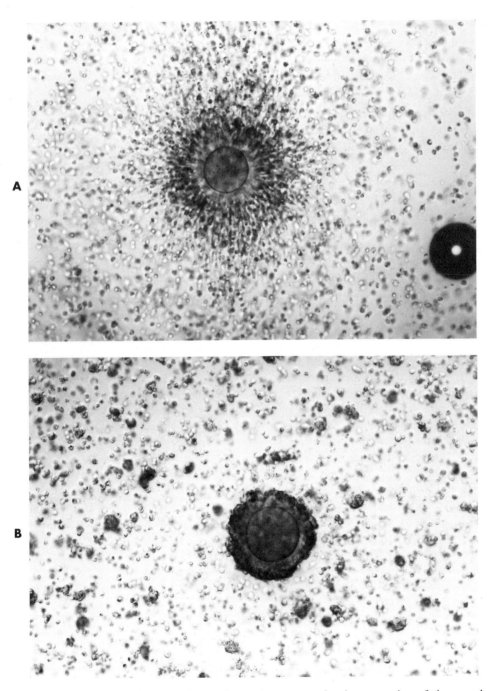

Fig. 45-1. A, Cellular characteristics of a mature oocyte showing expansion of the cumulus oophorus and corona radiata. **B,** Cellular characteristics of a less mature oocyte surrounded by compact layer of cells. (From Veeck LL: *Atlas of the human oocyte and early conceptus,* vol 2. © 1991, The Williams & Wilkins Co., Baltimore.)

tion time of 5 to 6 hours after harvest produces good results with this type of evaluation, especially with slightly longer intervals between administration of human chorionic gonadotropin (hCG) and collection. Oocytes very near maturity have adequate time in culture to complete their maturation process before meeting spermatozoa, and fully mature oocytes are not cultured past their optimal time for normal development.

Assessment of oocyte maturity and viability based on actual visualization of the oocyte and its associated structures. More exact methods may be used to assess accurately the meiotic status of the oocyte at harvest. With direct visualization of the ooplasm, perivitelline space, and zona pellucida, cumulus and corona cell radiance ceases to carry much importance in the evaluation of gamete maturity. Since late 1986 at the Jones Institute most oocytes have been evaluated for their exact meiotic status by means of a cumulus spreading technique. (See box).

With direct visualization, oocytes are classified as to the presence or absence of first polar bodies and germinal vesicles,[34,43] and are inseminated accordingly:

Metaphase II (MII): First polar body present, no germinal vesicle; inseminated 2 to 3 hours after collection (Fig. 45-2)

Metaphase I (MI): No first polar body, no germinal vesicle; examined for polar body every 2 to 3 hours after collection and inseminated 2 to 3 hours after verification that a metaphase II state has been reached (Fig. 45-3)

Prophase I (PI): Germinal vesicle present; incubated a full 24 hours before reassessing maturational status and inseminated after visualization of the first polar body (usually by 30 hours after collection) (Fig. 45-4)

The oocyte with chromosomes at metaphase II of maturation. By microscopic examination, the healthy MII oocyte is characterized by its round, even shape and ooplasm of a light color with homogeneous granularity. The first polar body is clearly visualized when the cumulus is flattened and may be situated to one side, above, or underneath the surface of the oocyte. The typical expanded,

---

Cumulus spreading to enable visualization of oocyte morphology

1. Place the oocyte-cumulus-corona complex in a droplet of culture medium or follicular fluid (approximately 50 μL) on the flat surface of a sterile Petri dish.
2. Jar the dish with the palm of the hand to flatten the cumulus for better visualization of the ooplasm and perivitelline space.
3. Examine the oocyte rapidly under an inverted microscope to identify physical characteristics.
4. Flush the oocyte immediately with equilibrated medium to restore pH and osmolality balance, transfer it to equilibrated culture medium, and incubate the specimen.

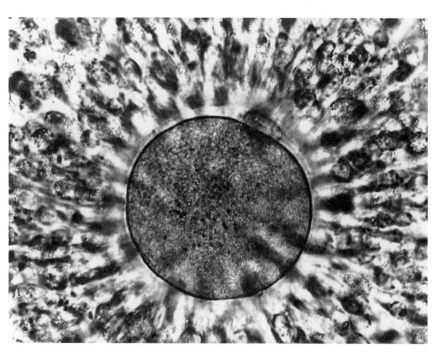

Fig. 45-2. Oocyte with chromosomes at metaphase II of maturation. Note the clear ooplasm and first polar body. (From Veeck LL: *Atlas of the human oocyte and early conceptus,* vol 2. © 1991, The Williams & Wilkins Co., Baltimore.)

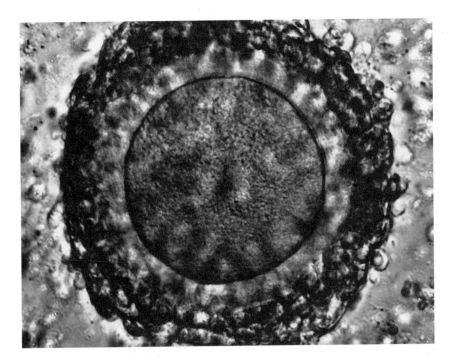

Fig. 45-3. Oocyte with chromosomes at metaphase I of maturation. Note the clear ooplasm and absence of a polar body and a germinal vesicle. (From Veeck LL: *Atlas of the human oocyte and early conceptus,* vol 2. © 1991, The Williams & Wilkins Co., Baltimore.)

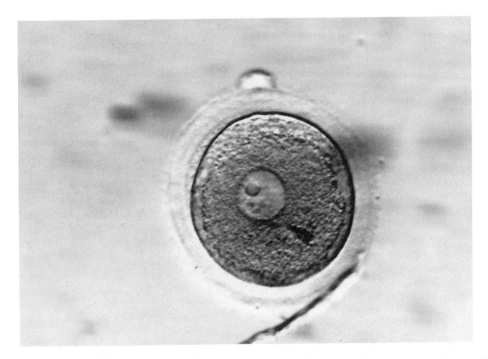

Fig. 45-4. Oocyte with chromosomes at prophase I of maturation. Note the darkened ooplasm and germinal vesicle. (From Veeck LL: *Atlas of the human oocyte and early conceptus,* vol 2. © 1991, The Williams & Wilkins Co., Baltimore.)

luteinized cumulus and radiating corona usually are associated with the fully mature gamete, but not always. Membrana granulosa cells harvested along with the MII oocyte are also luteinized and loosely aggregated, possessing features associated with adequate follicular response to hormone surges.[41,42,45,46]

This oocyte is at a resting stage of meiosis II after extrusion of the first polar body and passage to metaphase II. Chromosomes are divided between the oocyte and the polar body with $2n$ DNA from 23 chromosomes (46 chromatids) in each. For awhile, the first polar body remains connected to the oocyte by the meiotic spindle; generally a nucleus is not formed in the first polar body.[1,34] Although it is not possible to visualize most internal elements of the oocyte without special stains or electron microscopy, certain cytoplasmic structures are characteristic of the mature oocyte: One to three layers of cortical granules are uniformly distributed at the ooplasmic periphery, and the first polar body contains cortical granules because of its extrusion before sperm penetration and cortical granule release. Golgi complexes generally are absent in the mature oocyte; small aggregates of mitochondria and smooth endoplasmic reticulum are present.

Oocytes determined to be at metaphase II of maturation may be inseminated within the first 3 hours after collection. It is unknown exactly how long a mature, human oocyte remains capable of normal fertilization before postmaturity arises, but the window of time appears to be at least 12 hours and perhaps as long as 18 hours.

The oocyte with chromosomes at metaphase I of maturation. The MI oocyte may be nearly mature, several hours from full maturity, or just beyond the germinal vesicle stage. The oocyte has completed prophase of meiosis I; the germinal vesicle and its nucleolus have faded and disappeared, but as yet no first polar body has been extruded. During MI, a spindle forms and recombined maternal and paternal chromosomes line up randomly toward the poles. Later, at telophase, whole chromosomes sort independently to oocyte or first polar body.

Under the microscope, the MI oocyte is characterized by this absence of both nucleus and first polar body. A late (nearly mature) MI oocyte is round and even in form, with homogeneously granular and lightly colored ooplasm. Luteinized cumulus cells are usually associated with late stages. Early (less mature) MI oocytes may display minor central granularity and may be associated with unluteinized follicular cells.

An MI oocyte may require 1 hour or up to 24 hours in culture before reaching full maturity. Those needing less than 15 hours are considered to be nearly equivalent to MII oocytes in their fertilization performance and contribution to pregnancy, whereas those requiring more than 15 hours—although fewer in number—have not demonstrated the same fertilization potential, perhaps because of loss of sperm viability in vitro over the hours required for the

oocyte to reach maturity.[41-45] Because first polar body extrusion can occur at any time after harvest, it is necessary to examine the MI oocyte at regular intervals to determine the correct timing for insemination. As stated previously, if spermatozoa are placed with the oocyte before nuclear and cytoplasmic maturation are complete, they may fail to decondense within the ooplasm, or abnormal fertilization might occur. If insemination is delayed too long, in vitro aging may follow with similar undesired consequences.[34,42]

The oocyte with chromosomes at prophase I of maturation. The PI oocyte is often termed immature or unripened. It possesses a tetraploid amount of DNA because of the presence of 46 double-stranded chromosomes. This oocyte begins to mature in response to gonadotropin surges and reduction in follicular maturation inhibiting factors. The germinal vesicle, which persisted throughout earlier growth phases, begins its progression to germinal vesicle breakdown (GVBD), and the oocyte enlarges. Under the microscope, the PI oocyte is characterized by its distinct, spheric germinal vesicle, which contains a single, refractile, exocentric nucleolus. The germinal vesicle is centrally located within the ooplasm in early PI oocytes and in those that exhibit developmental arrest. It migrates to a more peripheral location in healthy oocytes before GVBD. As the oocyte continues toward maturation, defenses against polyspermy are established in the form of cortical granule accumulation and alignment at the oocyte periphery. These granules are sparse and discontinuous in immature oocytes.[34] The immature oocyte usually displays an irregular shape and centrally darkened, granular ooplasm. Attached cumulus cells may be compact and multilayered, or luteinized. Free follicular membrana granulosa cells within the immature follicle are usually small and appear in compact masses rather than possessing a luteinized expansion. PI oocytes with very mature characteristics (expanded cumulus and very radiant corona) generally represent arrested maturation and fail to undergo GVBD.[45]

Most PI oocytes collected for IVF are harvested from small antral follicles, have been stimulated to resume meiosis, and are in the final stages of the first meiotic prophase. GVBD may occur within minutes or require up to several hours after harvest; the length of time appears to depend on how far maturational events had progressed within the follicle before collection. Eighty-three percent (5743/6930) of PI oocytes collected at the Jones Institute since 1985 have succeeded in passing through metaphase I ultimately to reach full maturity under standard ovarian stimulation regimens with human menopausal gonadotropin (hMG) and/or pure follicle-stimulating hormone (FSH). If allowed to continue growth in culture after fertilization, our experience has been that 71% (286/405) will have arrested development before a 16-cell stage has been achieved, 12% (47/405) will have arrested development at a morula stage, and only 18% (72/405) will develop successfully into blastocysts. Preembryos developing from PI oocytes are capable of implanting in the uterus, but their overall potential for live birth is lower than that for preembryos developed from mature oocytes.[42-43] Occasionally an ongoing pregnancy has been realized after development and transfer of PI oocytes during IVF trials, and two live births have been achieved after the freezing and thawing of prezygotes developed from PI oocytes.

After maturation in vitro, morphologic features of oocytes maturing from PI oocytes are very comparable to those of MII oocytes at harvest, although some loss of cumulus and corona cells occurs during the culture period.

The zona pellucida. The zona pellucida is the prime controller of interspecific fertilization and, as such, forbids nonspecies spermatozoa from entering and contacting the oolemma. The human zona is a relatively thick (approximately 7 to 20 μm), transparent, acellular vestment that surrounds the oocyte and is separated from it by the perivitelline space.[34] During follicular growth the zona is deposited in patches between the surfaces of the oocyte and the surrounding cells. As the follicle grows, these patches enlarge, coalesce, and form a layer that separates most of the follicular cells from the oocyte surface. Whether the zona is formed from materials of the oocyte or the surrounding follicular cells is poorly understood.[15] Ultrastructural studies of zona morphology have demonstrated two types of surfaces: a smooth one and a meshlike one.[16] The smooth type is commonly associated with immature oocytes, whereas the meshlike one is typical of fertilizable oocytes. Spermatozoa are better able to bind to the meshlike zona, suggesting enhanced exposure or heightened development of binding sites. This observation is validated by the fact that, in the hemizona assay, spermatozoa bind to the zonae of mature oocytes in greater numbers than to those of immature or matured-in-vitro oocytes.[28] It is possible that during IVF trials, maturation of the zona has not occurred normally in some oocytes. This could result in poor exposure or a reduced number of binding sites with subsequent fertilization failure. Alternately, deterioration of zona material might contribute to penetration by multiple sperm.

An effective barrier to polyspermy is believed to be present in the inner zona; here the structure appears more compact and dense than the outer half.[34] After penetration by one spermatozoon, other spermatozoa are generally blocked from further penetration.

On about the sixth day after sperm penetration, the preembryo undergoes a hatching process whereby it expands and enlarges until it breaks free of the confining shell and becomes capable of implantation.

Under bright-field microscopy the healthy zona of an unfertilized oocyte appears to be clear and continuous, shows minor variation in its thickness, and usually displays some porosity and a slightly speckled aspect. Excessive porosity and breakup of the structure within a dispersed matrix of granular material can be associated with oocyte

aging and deterioration. As the period of in vitro culture passes, the zona often acquires increased porosity and additional variation in shape and thickness.[45]

Abnormal morphology of the human oocyte

Ooplasmic granularity. In our experience, approximately 8% of oocytes collected for IVF display a granular-appearing ooplasm at harvest (Fig. 45-5, **A**). Fertilization rates are similar for clear and granular oocytes (91% vs. 87%), although triploid fertilization is marginally higher in the granular group.[43,44] Pregnancy is often difficult to assess because many cycles have preembryos developing from both clear and granular oocytes. However, one study of 225 cycles produced the following results: Patients were matched for type of preembryo transferred (only cycles with preembryos developing from MII oocytes were considered), age (35.5 ± 4.0 years in the granular oocyte group vs. 35.1 ± 4.6 years in the mixed granularity group vs. 34.7 ± 4.1 years in the nongranular oocyte group), and time period of treatment (August 1990 to June 1991). Incidence of clinical pregnancy was 23.5% after 51 transfers in the granular group, 30.0% after 50 transfers in the mixed granularity group, and 32.3% after 124 transfers in the nongranular group. These percentages were not significantly different from one another because of the small number of transfers, but they showed a trend for better pregnancy rates after transfer of preembryos developing from oocytes with clear and light-colored ooplasm.

As opposed to a homogeneous type of ooplasmic granularity, oocytes displaying extremely darkened and granular centers with peripherally clear areas usually are associated with degeneration. When this situation is observed, fertilization often fails to occur and developmental potential is severely reduced. Nonetheless, the interpretation and significance of any type of ooplasmic granularity, homogeneous or central, is difficult to evaluate for two reasons: (1) assessment of granularity is quite subjective and prone to variability between observers; and (2) oocytes that are considered granular at harvest may possess clear blastomeres after cleavage, whereas others that are clear at harvest may develop into preembryos with excessively granular blastomeres.

The main organelles seen in oocytes are mitochondria, endoplasmic reticulum, and Golgi complexes. These organelles contain an array of enzymes and are involved in synthetic and metabolic activities.

Ooplasmic vacuoles. Ooplasmic vacuolization generally indicates a poor prognosis for optimal development of the oocyte. Vacuoles form by dilation and coalescence of vesicular elements of smooth endoplasmic reticulum, because of aggregation and fusion of preexisting smaller vacuoles, or may be the result of an aberrant endocytosis due to oolemma instability.[37] Under the light microscope, vacuoles are noticeably membrane bound and appear vacant or empty. Although very small vacuolar structures (<5 μm) are relatively common and may not affect overall

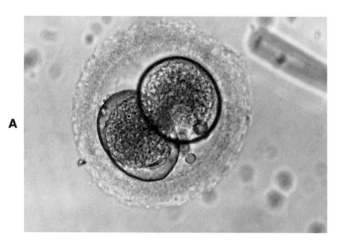

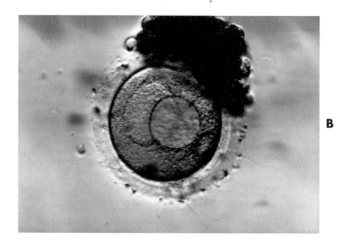

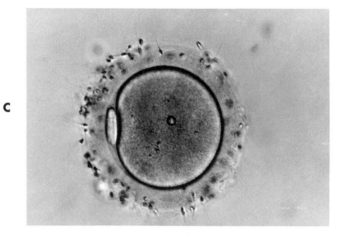

Fig. 45-5. Ooplasmic/cytoplasmic irregularities. **A,** Granularity in the blastomeres of a two-cell preembryo. **B,** Vacuolization. **C,** Refractile body.

developmental potential, large vacuoles (>25 µm) probably represent defects that interfere with subsequent growth (Fig. 45-5, **B**). In our experience, less than 20% of oocytes with large vacuoles display normal fertilization, and no pregnancy has been established with this type of oocyte.

Refractile body. Some inclusion bodies, such as the "refractile body" are associated with failure of fertilization. This structure, approximately 10 µm in diameter under bright-field microscopy, appears highly refractile because of its composition of lipid material and dense granules (Fig. 45-5, **C**). The evolution of this structure and its relationship to oocyte maturity and viability are not yet understood. Both mature and immature oocytes have demonstrated refractile bodies, and there is a strong tendency for recurrence in the same patient in repetitive treatment cycles. An association may exist with early stages of oocyte degeneration. In our experience, only 2% of oocytes with true refractile bodies are capable of undergoing a normal fertilization process. The correct identification of this structure is often difficult, and care must be taken to avoid confusing it with other small inclusions or very small vacuoles.[25,42,45]

Abnormal shapes and sizes of oocytes and polar bodies. Oocytes occasionally exhibit extraordinary shapes at the time of harvest from the ovary. Oval, comma, teardrop, and figure-of-eight contours have been noted, shapes that persist to preembryonic stages after sperm penetration. Amazingly, many of the oddest forms retain an ability to undergo monospermic fertilization and subsequent cleavage. Some of these unique shapes are thought to arise through mechanical stress at harvest, whereas others become malformed only later in their development. Overtly large and obviously small oocytes have also been seen; although the prognosis for normal fertilization is poor when oocytes are too large, very small oocytes quite often develop in a normal fashion.

Variation in the size of the first polar body (overly large or small) represents an unfavorable condition for the oocyte. Presumably, the factor determining the size of the polar body is the position of the meiotic spindle in relation

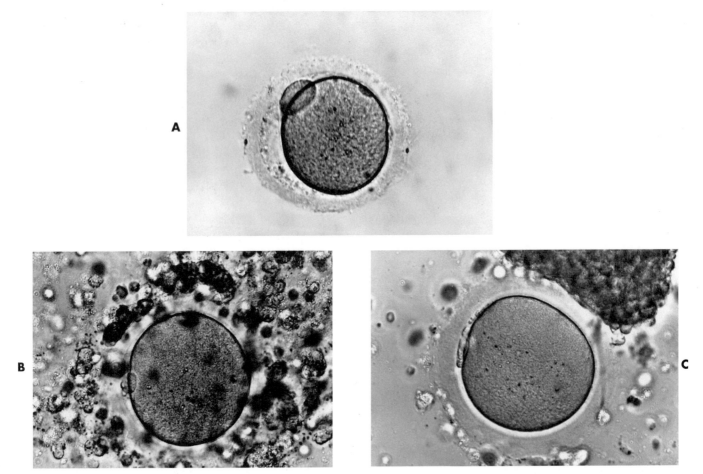

Fig. 45-6. Atypical polar bodies. **A,** Overly large. **B,** Very small. **C,** Fragmented.

to the surface of the oocyte. If this is true, inward displacement of the spindle would result in a polar body of atypically large size (Fig. 45-6, **A**). Aged oocytes are reported to extrude larger polar bodies in some instances.[1] In mice, one effect of oocyte aging is this migration of the second meiotic spindle to the center of the oocyte; when telophase occurs, the oocyte cleaves into two cells of similar size, one of which is the penetrated oocyte and the other of which is the second polar body. Some descriptions of immediate cleavage and parthenogenic division may be diagnosed incorrectly and merely be related to this type of unequal distribution of the ooplasm at the end of meiosis I. Truly enormous polar bodies are not commonly seen in human oocytes, and many described as such are in fact only large cytoplasmic fragments. On the other hand, oocytes with very small first polar bodies are more commonly observed and are associated with a reduced fertilization rate and increased incidence of triploidy (Fig. 45-6, **B**).[44] It may be postulated that in some instances chromosomes destined for the first polar body may remain entirely in the oocyte or be expelled incompletely, with subsequent triploid development of the prezygote after sperm penetration. Under these

conditions two pronuclei of maternal origin would be present. Oocytes with fragmented (Fig. 45-6, **C**) or completely detached first polar bodies also demonstrate a reduced potential for regular development in vitro. Oocyte postmaturity is often, but not always, the cause, and the incidence of triploid fertilization is high.[43]

Abnormalities of the zona pellucida

Breaks. The term *fractured zona* is commonly used to describe an oocyte with a breach in its zona pellucida and with a disrupted ooplasm (Fig. 45-7, **A**). The two most striking features of the fractured zona oocyte are the darkened ooplasm and the damaged zona pellucida. Degenerative changes in the oocyte and zona, brought on by atresia, likely predispose the structure to mechanical damage at harvest. Other oocytes with fractured zonae are clearly the result of excessive negative pressure during collection. Occasionally, minute breaks in the continuity of the zona allow the herniation of part of the ooplasm still surrounded by an intact oolemma.[45] Although these breaches are probably the result of excessive negative pressure at harvest, the damage may be aggravated by abnormalities of the zona pellucida. Depending on the

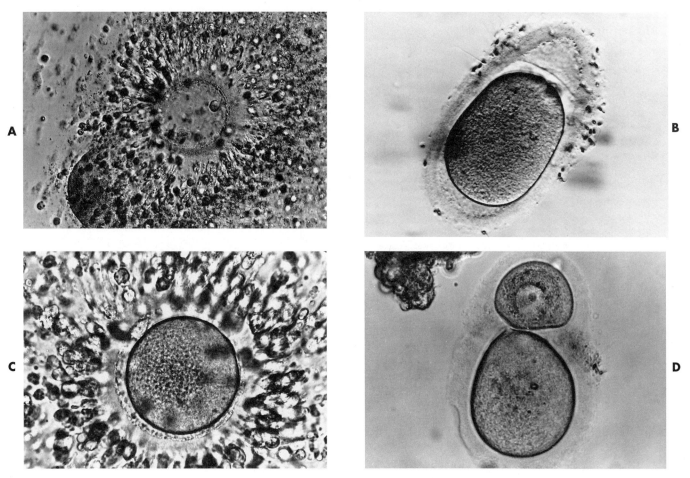

Fig. 45-7. Irregularities of the zona pellucida. **A,** Fractured zona. **B,** Degradation of zona material. **C,** Perivitelline debris. **D,** Binovular casing.

location of the meiotic spindle, either the intrazonal or extrazonal segment of cytoplasm may develop pronuclei after insemination. Because the effective block to polyspermy is altered, abnormal fertilization often occurs, especially in the extrazonal segment.

Abnormal color or thickness. A yellow-brown or dark brown tint to the typically speckled but clear zona pellucida is associated with reduced fertilization and poor development of the preembryo (personal observation). A zona thickness of greater than 30 μm is not generally demonstrated in fresh, unaged, and unfertilized oocytes; if observed, failure of fertilization is often seen.

Degradation of zona material. The zona may separate into distinct layers at one or more points in its continuity as it ages and deteriorates (Fig. 45-7, **B**). Again, increased rates of triploidy along with reduced potential of normal fertilization are associated with this type of degenerating zona pellucida.

Perivitelline debris. Deteriorating material may accumulate in the space between the oocyte and zona pellucida (Fig. 45-7, **C**). The debris-laden perivitelline space, when material is excessive, is associated with a poor fertilization

and pregnancy outcome (personal observation).

Binovular casing. More than one oocyte may be covered with a single zona pellucida, or two zonae may fuse together. Often, maturational stages of the two oocytes are disparate despite their identical follicular milieu. A primary, germinal vesicle–bearing oocyte or fully grown germinal vesicle–bearing oocyte is often seen to one side of a fully mature oocyte (Fig. 45-7, **D**).

Assessment of the sperm-penetrated oocyte with bright-field microscopy

The process of human fertilization involves the fusion of sperm and oocyte to produce a new genetic entity. (See box on p. 830). During the pronuclear phase, DNA synthesis is initiated.

Observed by light microscopy in a clinical setting, sperm tails and midpieces are not identifiable in human oocytes after sperm penetration. Neither can cortical granule release be evaluated without damaging the oocyte. Although these aspects are reliable indicators that sperm penetration has taken place, the embryologist must rely almost solely on the presence and number of pronuclei to determine whether or

The fertilization process

The spermatozoon, with a haploid number of chromosomes, penetrates the zona pellucida by digesting a path with acrosomal enzymes. The equatorial segment of the sperm head attaches to the plasma membrane of the oocyte, and sperm incorporation occurs through a process similar to phagocytosis.

Cortical granule exocytosis from the ooplasmic periphery invokes a chemical alteration of the zona pellucida that renders it impermeable to other spermatozoa. A slow or incomplete cortical granule exocytosis and zona reaction may be the most common cause of polyspermic fertilization.

The oocyte becomes *activated* by fusion with the spermatozoon and completes its second meiotic division.

Male and female pronuclei are formed from the sperm and oocyte chromatin. Pronuclei come in close contact, eventually lose their apposed pronuclear membranes, and enter into syngamy. This final event of the fertilization process involves the reorganization and pairing of maternal and paternal chromosomes and the formation of the zygote. There is a brief period of time in which the zygote remains single-celled until the first cleavage division.

not fertilization is in progress.[45] Practical criteria for the assessment of sperm penetration in living material are (1) observation of pronuclei at 10 to 20 hours postinsemination and (2) visualization of two polar bodies in the perivitelline space. Assessment of these two parameters is rapid and simple, involving a single observation. Unfortunately, the existence of two pronuclei is not proof of a normal fertilization process and cannot ensure that one pronucleus is of paternal origin and one is of maternal origin. Evaluating second polar bodies is also potentially misleading because of first polar body fragmentation and spontaneous second polar body extrusion. Although pronuclear and polar body determination is not ideal for the assessment of sperm penetration, it does provide the most useful and least threatening means of clinical evaluation. Because many triploid specimens demonstrate regular morphology after cleavage, failure to identify them could result in transferring an abnormal conceptus to the uterus. Monosomic and trisomic conditions cannot be recognized by any morphologic criteria used in the laboratory. Such conditions are the result of abnormal chromosome balance in gamete development or in grossly abnormal chromosome rearrangements during subsequent meiotic or mitotic divisions. These abnormalities would not be reflected in pronuclear number.

Evaluation of the prezygote should be done carefully. The number and size of pronuclei should be recorded, and the existence of nucleoli must be verified in each structure. Pseudopronuclei have been reported to confuse the evalua-

tion process and are presumably mistaken for pronuclei in a potentially alarming number of cases.[38] These structures are pronuclear-like vacuoles with the ability to move within the cytoplasm and become juxtaposed with true pronuclei. Use of a high-resolution inverted microscope and the consistent discipline of studying nucleoli should lessen the incidence of this error.

Normal fertilization. Male and female pronuclei usually are formed simultaneously; the male pronucleus forms near the site of sperm entry, and the female originates at the ooplasmic pole of the meiotic spindle.[50] The male pronucleus is somewhat larger in humans,[13] but the difference is not always easy to discern. (Fig. 45-8, **A**). Occasionally, when the oocyte is in a particular position, one pronucleus may entirely overlap another, giving the impression of a single pronucleus; in these instances, the double pronucleus structure appears much different from an individual pronucleus in that it displays a highly refractile quality.

Early in their formation, pronuclei may be seen at a distance from each other; later, they migrate together to the center of the cell. By 15 hours after insemination, pronuclei are most often observed lying close to one another; they may present a double-ring, figure-of-eight, or singular appearance if viewed in an overlapping position. Although they appear to contact or fuse, transmission electron microscopy has demonstrated that they remain separated by a narrow strip of ooplasm.[32,35,51] As male and female pronuclei become closely associated, adjacent areas of each appear to flatten out. During the same time, nucleoli move from random locations within each pronucleus to line up at the regions of juxtaposition. One to nine nucleoli can be observed in each structure, the smaller pronucleus often demonstrating a lower number. Pronuclei are surrounded by a dense aggregation of cellular organelles, which may appear granular or darkened under the light microscope. The female pronucleus often dismantles its envelope and undergoes membrane breakdown slightly ahead of the male.[33]

Abnormal fertilization. Prezygotes exhibiting aberrant numbers of pronuclei are not uncommon after IVF; the reported incidence of polyploidy ranges from 1% to 25%.* The development of a single pronucleus can also be observed. After the first division these abnormal specimens often demonstrate cleavage patterns indistinguishable from those of two-pronuclear origin. For this reason it is extremely important to assess the number of pronuclei before entrance into syngamy by viewing pronuclei from several different vantage points. The prezygote should be repositioned several times within its culturing vessel to view it from different angles and make a correct assessment. Although gross abnormalities in chromosome number generally predispose a conceptus to early death, implantation is possible; upward of 20% of aborted fetuses

*References 11, 14, 24, 26, 39, 49.

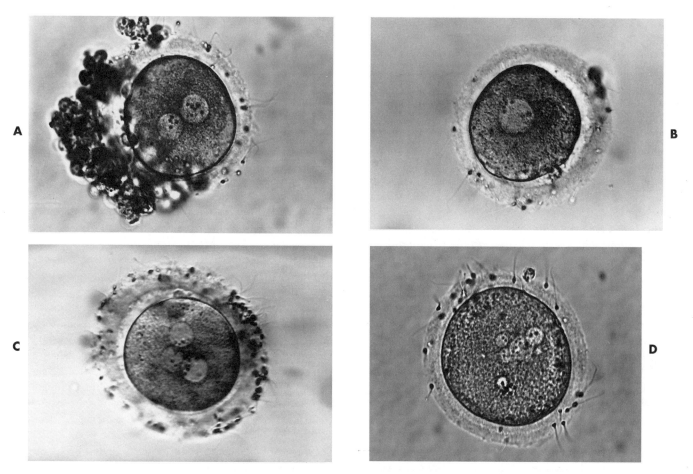

Fig. 45-8. Pronuclei. **A,** Two pronuclei. **B,** Single pronucleus. **C,** Three pronuclei. **D,** Pronuclear fragmentation.

are triploid.[13] Of special risk to the patient are the rare term delivery of a triploid child and the obstetric risk associated with early spontaneous abortion.

Single pronucleus. There are several theoretic causes for the development of a single pronucleus after IVF: (1) the oocyte may be accidentally activated by heat, cold, biochemical, osmotic, or mechanical means, which leads to extrusion of the first polar body and the development of a single haploid maternal pronucleus (the ability to activate oocytes is remarkably easy in some nonhuman species); (2) the maternal or paternal pronucleus may fail to develop during an otherwise routine process of fertilization, producing a haploid gynogenic or androgenic prezygote; or (3) a nuclear envelope may develop around the second metaphase chromosome group in an unpenetrated diploid oocyte, a condition common in some lower forms in which parthenogenesis occurs naturally, but is unreported in women.

The artificial activation of oocytes under experimental design produces haploid prezygotes capable of undergoing at least rudimentary cleavage.[7,18,19,21,27,36]

The single pronucleus observed after IVF in women may

be normally sized or larger than normal (Fig. 45-8, **B**). In some species, perhaps including human, haploid pronuclei of maternal origin can achieve roughly twice the nuclear and nucleolar volumes of the normal female pronucleus, despite the fact that they are derived from equivalent chromosomal material.[1] Diploid single pronuclei may also display larger volumes because of double amounts of DNA.[1] There is no certainty that human oocytes with single pronuclei, whether haploid or diploid, can give rise to preembryos capable of surviving to birth, but a rare cleavage to the blastocyst stage has been observed at the Jones Institute.

Polyploidy. Triploidy and, to a much lesser degree, tetraploidy, are not uncommonly observed in IVF laboratories. Polyploidy can arise through several different theoretic scenarios, many of which are well documented in the human: (1) the block to polyspermy may fail, resulting in a prezygote with excess male pronuclei; (2) a binucleate or diploid spermatozoon may penetrate an oocyte, resulting in a prezygote with one maternal and two paternal pronuclei; (3) a binucleate oocyte may be penetrated, resulting in a prezygote with one paternal and two maternal pronuclei; or

(4) an oocyte may retain either the first (rare) or second polar body chromosomes, resulting in a prezygote with one paternal and two maternal pronuclei, or retain both polar body chromosomes, resulting in one paternal and three maternal pronuclei.

Polyspermy (1) can be the result of failed or slow cortical granule exocytosis after insemination of an immature or postmature oocyte, may follow the insemination of an oocyte with a defective zona pellucida, or may occur through various other mechanisms. Some oocytes may be predisposed to polyspermic conditions despite low sperm numbers used for insemination. Experience has shown that the health and maturity level of the oocyte is the main determinant associated with normal fertilization. The number of inseminating sperm has shown little relationship to the incidence of abnormal fertilization. Sperm concentrations as low as 25,000/mL and as high as 1 million/mL have not differed in producing a rather constant rate of triploidy. On the other hand, various ovarian stimulation protocols produce higher rates of triploidy that can be correlated to extended high-dosage regimens and subsequent oocyte postmaturity.[12] Because of the obvious abnormal genetic constitution of these specimens, they are not replaced. Hydatidiform moles are thought to arise after two X-bearing paternal pronuclei enter syngamy; in such instances, all the genetic material of the molar conceptus is contributed by sperm.

Binucleate or diploid spermatozoa (2) account for up to 0.5% of spermatozoa observed in normal human semen populations.[6]

Binucleate oocytes (3) appear to occur rarely in nature, at least as judged by the incidence of oocytes recovered with two germinal vesicles at the Jones Institute. Only 5 such oocytes have been harvested among a population counting more than 8000 germinal vesicle-bearing oocytes over 10 years; how many are capable of maturing to metaphase II cannot be calculated.

Polar body retention (4), or retention of chromosomes from one or both polar bodies, may be fairly common, especially as involves the second polar body. Human oocytes display chromosomal aberrations at rates up to 30% or higher.[23,30,48]

It is often observed that triploid oocytes possess either two large and one small pronuclei, or two small and one large pronuclei (Fig. 45-8, **C**). It is assumed that these cases represent diandry and digyny, respectively. However, pronuclear size may be altered in the triploid or tetraploid specimen. It has been reported that the formation of multiple pronuclei results in an overall reduction in size for each.[1] If this concept is true for women, male and female pronuclei would be even more difficult to distinguish from one another, and the probable diagnosis of male versus female involvement would be more unreliable.

Preembryos developing from triploid prezygotes often appear to undergo more rapid cleavage than do diploid preembryos, but this is perhaps because most cleave abnormally at the first division. We have studied the first cleavage of triploid preembryos under time-lapse cinematography and have observed that the vast majority will divide directly into three blastomeres. Other investigators have observed the same situation; three patterns of cleavage have been documented for triploid prezygotes: (1) direct cleavage into three blastomeres with resulting variable and abnormal karyotypes displaying near-diploid complements (62%); (2) cleavage into two blastomeres with resulting uniform triploid karyotypes (24%); and (3) cleavage into two blastomeres plus a small extrusion mass with resulting diploid karyotypes in each blastomere and a probable haploid complement in the extrusion mass (14%).[20] With this information, a fascinating correlation is shown between the pattern of cleavage and the subsequent chromosomal complement of the preembryo. It furthermore indicates that some triploid preembryos might be capable of self-regulation and regular development. Nonetheless, because of the fear of molar pregnancy, triploid specimens are never replaced.

Pronuclear fragmentation. Pronuclei are capable of breaking up into multiple smaller structures called subnuclei, which contain scattered membrane-bound chromatin (Fig. 45-8, **D**). Similarly, unfertilized oocytes may develop subnuclei with chromatin that has disconnected from spindle microtubules during meiosis.[1,33] One would anticipate that chromosomes within these fragments would be unable to participate normally in meiotic or mitotic events, if they could do so at all. Aged oocytes appear to be more prone to develop these structures.

Assessment of the human preembryo with bright-field microscopy

Cleavage of the preembryo involves a series of mitotic divisions of the cytoplasm without any increase in its overall size.[1] Successive cell divisions occur approximately every 10 to 14 hours. Failure to proceed to the first cleavage after the development of two pronuclei is extremely rare.[37,45]

Normal morphology. A preembryo with a healthy appearance exhibits blastomeres of uniform size and shape without excessive granularity, distribution of color, or fragmentation. The actual events of cell division are well documented: As the first cleavage mitosis reaches telophase, the cytoplasm of the zygote elongates, and the surface contracts around the lesser circumference. This constriction continues until the zygote is divided into two blastomeres, and the process continues throughout subsequent cell divisions.[1] Individual blastomeres probably retain a totipotent capacity to develop independently into normal preembryos for several early cell divisions. For this reason the early conceptus surely possesses the ability to rid itself of defective cells while proceeding with growth and development of normal cell lines. Single blastomeres are

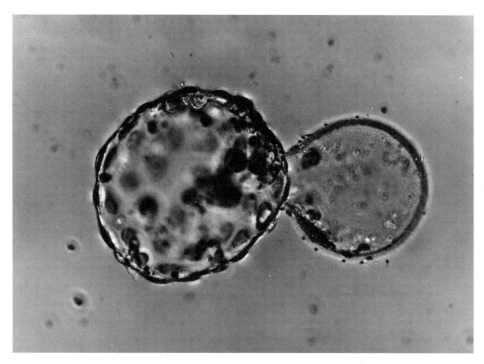

Fig. 45-9. Hatching blastocyst developed from a PI oocyte.

distinct until after the 8- to 16-cell stage, when changes occur in plasma membranes and cytoplasm; blastomeres become increasingly less distinct as they adhere more tightly to one another during the process of compaction.[13] A form of compaction occurs in the human morula when 16 to 32 cells are present, and the specimen often appears less healthy than the earlier-cleavage-stage conceptus. Twenty-four hours later, the preembryo enters the blastocyst stage, where a cavity is formed by coalescence of intercellular spaces and fluid accumulation. This occurs when the specimen has acquired as few as 32 cells, sometimes fewer, but usually more.[13] These cells are difficult, if not impossible, to count in a viable state under the light microscope. As the blastocyst accumulates fluid, it enlarges and the zona pellucida becomes thinner. The organism may exist in a fully expanded state for 24 hours or more before it hatches from the zona pellucida (Fig. 45-9).[9] Once free of its glycoprotein layer, it is able to implant in the uterine wall. The cells of the blastocyst form a spheric shell enclosing the cavity, with one pole distinguished by a thicker accumulation of cells. The outer layer is the trophoblast and will give rise to part of the placenta; the accumulation of cells inside the trophoblast is the inner cell mass, which gives rise to the embryo.

Abnormal morphology

Multinucleated blastomeres. Multinucleated blastomeres are commonly observed in cleaving preembryos.[34] Multinucleation may arise through complete or partial fragmentation of nuclei into subnuclei or from mitotic replication without cytoplasmic division (two complete nuclei). Although considered atypical, this situation has lost some of its impact as a pathologic condition, because it is often seen in preembryos associated with ongoing pregnancy.[37] It is not fully understood whether chromosomes of multinucleated blastomeres possess a corrective mechanism or whether these blastomeres degenerate, leaving others to establish cell lines.

Cytoplasmic fragmentation. It has long been observed that oocytes and preembryos are capable of undergoing a series of spontaneous and rapid cytoplasmic divisions, often in a manner that superficially resembles cleavage. Such divisions are, in fact, caused by a disorganized fragmentation of the cytoplasm. The fragments contain one or more subnuclei or—more likely—no nuclear material at all. Fragmentation is often associated with delayed insemination that predisposes an oocyte to postmaturity.[4,29]

Preembryo grading. Most preembryos have small cytoplasmic fragments and cellular debris in their perivitelline spaces, usually observable by light microscopy. Blastomeres constantly change shape, making and breaking cell contacts during cleavage, and in doing so can leave small fragments and debris.[34] This is particularly apparent if specimens are viewed under time-lapse cinematography, when constant pulsating, formation of blebs, and subsequent cytoplasmic restructure are noted. Cytoplasmic fragments generally are smaller than blastomeres, have the same complement of organelles, but lack nuclei. Acytoplasmic fragments can also be seen.

To determine the degree of fragmentation that is significant in terms of reduced conceptus viability, a morphologic grading system for early-stage preembryos has been developed. This system has shown to correlate reasonably well

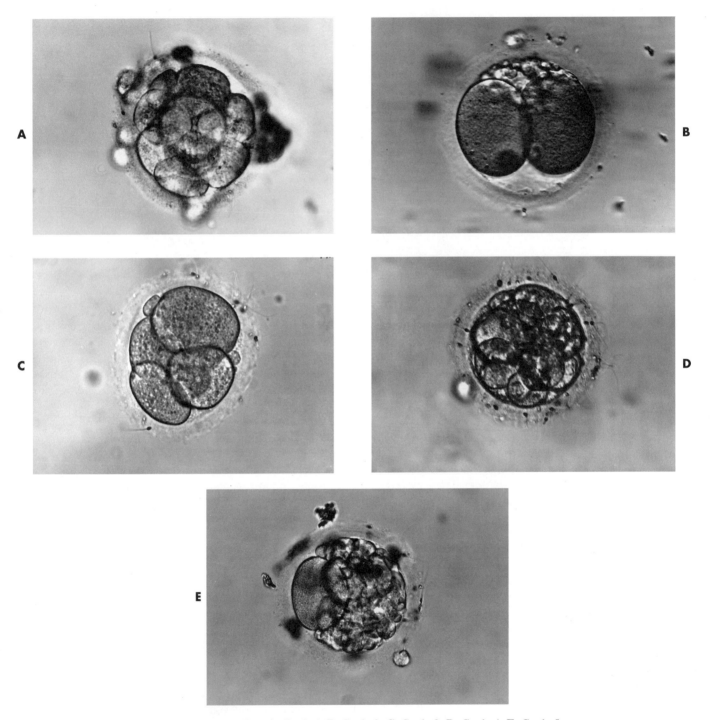

Fig. 45-10. Preembryo grading. **A,** Grade 1. **B,** Grade 2. **C,** Grade 3. **D,** Grade 4. **E,** Grade 5.

with IVF pregnancy rates. (See Interpretation of Results.) Under routine low-power light microscopy, the preembryo is graded according to its gross morphologic appearance (Fig. 45-10). This system has been used at the Jones Institute with two separate end points: (1) to grade the morphology of individual preembryos and (2) to classify transfers according to the highest score in the cohort of conceptuses being replaced. The grading system is as follows, with grade 1 representing perfect morphology:

Grade 1: Preembryo with blastomeres of equal size; no cytoplasmic fragments

Grade 2: Preembryo with blastomeres of equal size; minor cytoplasmic fragments or blebs

Grade 3: Preembryo with blastomeres of distinctly unequal size; few or no cytoplasmic fragments

Grade 4: Preembryo with blastomeres of equal or unequal size; significant cytoplasmic fragmentation

Grade 5: Preembryo with few blastomeres of any size; severe or complete fragmentation

Preembryo growth rate. Regularly cleaving two-cell conceptuses are observed any time after 22 hours of insemination, usually at around 24 hours, and may be seen for up to 44 hours postinsemination. Four-cell stages are routinely observed between 36 and 50 hours postinsemination. Eight-cell or greater stages are not commonly seen until after 48 hours but are usually noted before 72 hours. Three-, five-, and seven-cell stages commonly are interposed between these divisions, especially if examination is carried out during mitotic cell division. This asynchronous division persists throughout cleavage of the early conceptus, and any number of blastomeres can be noted in a given observation.[45] Morulae have been noted as early as 72 hours and are usually observed by 96 hours.[13,45] Blastocysts are not generally seen in the laboratory until after 120 hours.

An abnormally fertilized triploid specimen may cleave to the morula stage, but development usually is then arrested.[37,45] A rare triploid preembryo proceeds to the blastocyst stage. In normally fertilized specimens, slow cleavage has been suspected of indicating reduced viability, whereas rapid cleavage has been thought to be a reflection of a healthier conceptus. In reality, results from this center indicate that pregnancies can be established with slowly growing preembryos if morphology is good, and rapidity of growth cannot be correlated with better pregnancy rates.[44]

Preembryos have been evaluated at the Jones Institute for their growth rate in culture before intrauterine transfer. Conceptuses are classified as one of the following:

1. Rapidly cleaving with eight or more blastomeres at 36 to 48 hours after insemination
2. Cleaving at an average or normal rate, displaying two blastomeres by 24 hours postinsemination and four blastomeres by 40 hours postinsemination

3. Cleaving slowly, displaying only two blastomeres after 40 hours postinsemination

Morphology of thawed prezygotes and preembryos. As clinical pregnancy results continue to improve with human prezygote and preembryo freezing, established IVF centers are gaining the confidence to reduce the number of preembryos for fresh transfer and to increase the number for cryopreservation. This response, coupled with better methods of ovarian stimulation, contributes to a larger pool of cryopreserved material and creates great responsibility for the embryology laboratory. It is common practice to transfer three or four fresh preembryos and to cryopreserve the remaining ones for thaw during a later cycle. In selected cases replacement may be limited to one or two preembryos if multiple gestation is of particular obstetric concern.

By using a slow-freeze, slow-thaw protocol with 1,2-propanediol supplementation for cryoprotective purposes, approximately 70% of cryopreserved prezygotes survive the freezing and thawing process; survival after thawing is defined as the ability of the prezygote to enter syngamy and to proceed to at least the first cleavage.

Several investigators have reported that morphologically "good" (grades 1 and 2) preembryos survive freezing and thawing at rates similar to those of morphologically "poor" (grades 3, 4, and 5) specimens. Nevertheless, at least initially in most programs, preembryos with better morphology were transferred fresh and those with poor morphology were cryopreserved. As confidence in cryopreservation technology increased, groups began to opt for random selection to avoid possible bias when interpreting results. The morphologic condition after thaw appears to be better correlated with pregnancy than the morphologic status before freezing. At the Jones Institute random selection is performed for freezing without morphologic consideration. Prezygotes are usually photographed before and after the freezing and thawing procedure, and later after cleavage has occurred (Fig. 45-11). Interestingly, thawed specimens often present a better morphologic appearance on rehydration than they did before freezing. Cytoplasm may be clearer than before cryopreservation, and granularity may be lessened or more evenly distributed. Nucleoli usually are scattered within the pronuclei after thawing despite their alignment at pronuclear junctions before freezing. No correlation between this disruption of nucleolar order and reduced pregnancy rates has been noted. Distribution of morphologic grading groups among thawed specimens is strikingly similar to that of unfrozen controls from the same cycles.

INTERPRETATION OF RESULTS
Fertilization rate according to nuclear status at harvest

Oocytes were classified according to their nuclear maturity level at the time of harvest from the ovary (Table 45-1).

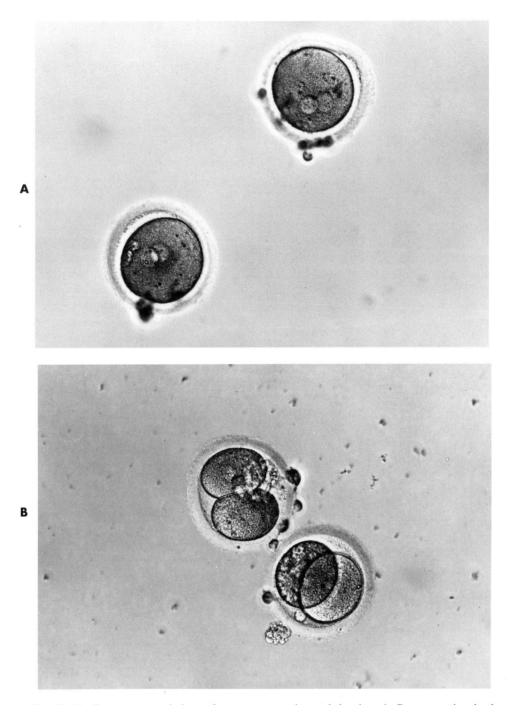

Fig. 45-11. Conceptus morphology after cryopreservation and thawing. **A,** Prezygotes involved with pregnancy and early miscarriage immediately after thawing. **B,** The same conceptuses after cleavage.

If nuclear maturation was not noted, but cumulus oophorus and corona radiata indicated probable maturity, the group was called unknown mature or unclassified; otherwise, oocytes were put into categories of MII, MI, or PI. MI were further divided between those that ultimately reached maturity within 15 hours and those that required more than 15 hours to achieve this level.

After analyzing the fertilization outcome of more than 21,000 oocytes, results indicate that fully mature oocytes (MII) demonstrate the greatest ability to become fertilized after insemination. Fertilization rates drop slightly with unclassified mature oocytes and MI oocytes requiring less than 15 hours in culture, and fertilization is markedly and significantly reduced when more than 15 hours are needed

Table 45-1. Fertilization performance of MII, MI, and PI oocytes*

Type of oocyte	No. inseminated	Total fertilized %†	No. normal %‡	No. abnormal %§
MII	10,849	10,207 (94.1%) a	9232 (85.1%) f	975 (9.0%) k
Unknown mature (mature cumulus)	1135	1023 (90.1%) b	897 (79.0%) g	126 (11.1%) l
MI (inseminated within 15 h)	5361	4592 (85.7%) c	4213 (78.6%) h	379 (7.1%) m
MI (inseminated after 15 h)	523	353 (67.5%) d	325 (62.1%) i	28 (5.4%) n
PI	3439	1780 (51.8%) e	1637 (47.6%) j	143 (4.2%) o

*Altogether 21,307 oocytes were collected over a 6½-year period.
†a > b > c > d > e; $P < .001$.
‡f > g > i > j; h > i; $P < .001$ (g = h).
§l > k > m > o; $P < .05$ (m = n, n = o).

to complete maturation. This drop in fertilizability is probably unassociated with oocyte maturity and more likely relates to degradation of sperm viability. When MII oocytes are harvested, semen samples are delivered within the hour; thus washed and capacitated sperm may be held for more than 24 hours before being placed with immature (PI) oocytes. Under these circumstances, the lower incidence of fertilization cannot be correlated solely with oocyte maturity because the reduction in sperm quality and motility is certainly also involved. A much better fertilization rate is always observed when fresh semen is collected on the second day for purposes of inseminating immature oocytes.[42] In this program, PI oocytes are often left uninseminated because of their reduced fertilizing ability and reduced contribution to pregnancy; if inseminated, they may be, with the patient's consent, part of the institutional review board–approved research protocols.

Abnormal fertilization (one pronucleus, three or more pronuclei) rates are significantly higher for MII, unclassified mature, and MI oocytes than those for PI oocytes that have matured in culture. Additionally, abnormal fertilization rates are significantly highest in the unclassified group, leaving a normally fertilized population equivalent to that found with late MI oocytes. Without inclusion of the unclassified group, abnormal fertilization rates drop with decreasing maturity levels at harvest.

Pregnancy rate according to nuclear status at harvest

Clinical pregnancy rates were evaluated in 3386 transfer cycles and correlated with original nuclear states of oocytes at harvest (Table 45-2). Of these transfers, 1566 can be placed into one of four "pure" transfer groups, groups denoting the transfer of one or more conceptuses of a single nuclear status at collection. For example, a pure MII group consists of transfer cycles in which only preembryos developed from metaphase II oocytes were transferred; a pure PI group had only the transfer of preembryos developing from prophase I oocytes. These pure groups would be opposed to "mixed" transfer groups in which more than one conceptus was transferred, the conceptuses were of different maturational origins, and identification of the preembryo responsible for pregnancy was therefore impossible.

Pure groups of metaphase II and unclassified mature conceptuses demonstrated similar pregnancy rates in younger patients (not significantly different), although a tendency was noted for better results with MII oocytes. MII transfers were significantly better than MI transfers in terms of pregnancy; these data show a larger difference between MII and MI transfers as compared to previous reports, perhaps because of the recent usage of GnRHa for ovarian suppression. GnRHa cycles that do not produce MII oocytes appear to result in poor pregnancy outcomes. As anticipated, preembryos developed from PI oocytes showed a significantly reduced ability to establish pregnancy, an observation that has been consistent in our laboratories over time.

Mixed transfer cycles represented a higher overall pregnancy rate, which could be attributed primarily to a larger number of preembryos transferred per cycle.

Older patients generally demonstrated lower pregnancy rates, although the differences were not significant because of the lower numbers of transfers. Pregnancy losses were similar in all groups.

Pregnancy rate according to number of preembryos transferred

Preembryos developing from MII, MI, or unclassified mature oocytes were evaluated for the effect of preembryo number on pregnancy rate in 3316 consecutive transfer cycles (Table 45-3). Results were as anticipated; it has long been observed that increasing the number of preembryos at transfer elevates the overall pregnancy rate and, unfortu-

Table 45-2. Analysis of 3386 consecutive transfers over a 6-year period: effect of oocyte maturity and patient age on pregnancy

Type of transfer	Patients under age 41 years (*n* = 3188 transfers)		Patients age 41+ years (*n* = 198 transfers)	
	Pregnancies/ transfers	%*	Pregnancies/ transfers	%†
Pure				
MII only	328/1065	31% a	21/87	24% e
Unknown mature only	24/100	24% b	3/11	27% f
MI only	43/218	20% c	0/15	0% g
PI only	3/67	4.5% d	0/3	0% h
Mixed				
MII + unknown mature	21/49	43%	—	—
MII + MI	323/1006	32%	7/41	17%
Unknown mature + MI	5/14	36%	0/1	0%
MII + unknown mature + MI	7/19	37%	—	—
All other combinations with PI oocytes	167/650	26%	11/40	28%

*a > c > d; b > d; *P* < .005 (a = b, b = c).
†Older patients: no significance between any group; younger patients vs. older patients: no significance.

Table 45-3. Analysis of 3316 consecutive transfers with mature oocytes over a 6-year period*: Effect of preembryo number on pregnancy

No. of preembryos transferred	Patients under age 41 years (*n* = 3121 transfers)		Patients age 41+ years (*n* = 195 transfers)	
	Pregnancies/ transfers	%†	Pregnancies/ transfers	%‡
1	63/449	14.0%a	6/44	13.6%e
2	158/652	24.2%b	9/43	20.9% f
3	192/683	28.1%c	11/46	23.9%g
4+	505/1337	37.8%d	16/62	25.8%h

*Seventy cycles with only prophase I oocytes were excluded.
†a < b = c < d; b < d; *P* < .001.
‡Older patients: no significance between any group; younger patients vs older patients: no significance.

nately, the multiple pregnancy rate. In this study, younger patients demonstrated significant increases in pregnancy with additional preembryos transferred, much more strikingly so as compared with older women. What has always been surprising is that the implantation rate per preembryo transferred consistently decreases as the number of preembryos transferred increases. Despite this, the number of multiple gestations observed at the Jones Institute is of great concern; more than 180 sets of twins, 25 sets of triplets, and 4 sets of quadruplets have already been delivered. Fortunately, triplet and quadruplet births have fared well, probably because of the strict prenatal care given to the mothers.

The incidence of multiple pregnancy according to num-ber of preembryos transferred is as follows: In younger patients, 15% when two were transferred, 22% when three were transferred, and 25% when four or more were transferred; in older patients, 11% when two were transferred, 18% when three were transferred, and 13% when four or more were transferred. Because the incidence of multiple pregnancy is higher in younger patients than in patients over age 40 years, guidelines are being established to limit preembryo number according to various factors, including age.

Effect of patient age on establishment of pregnancy

As shown in Tables 45-2 to 45-4, clinical pregnancy rates are generally higher in younger women undergoing

Table 45-4. Comparison of younger and older patients

Parameter	Patients under age 41 years	Patients age 41+ years
Average age (y)	34.5 ± 3.4	41.8 ± 1.2
Average no. of mature oocytes harvested	5.3 ± 4.4	4.0 ± 3.4
Average no. of mature oocytes transferred	3.0 ± 1.4	2.7 ± 1.3
Average no. of mature oocytes cryopreserved	1.0 ± 2.5	0.5 ± 1.9
Average no. cryopreserved/cycle with freezing	4.5 ± 3.8	4.3 ± 3.9
No. of total transfers/harvests (%)*	3188/3507 (91%) a	198/232 (85%) b
Pregnancies/transfers (%)†	918/3121 (29%) c	42/195 (22%) d
Term pregnancies/transfers (%)‡	643/3121 (21%) e	25/195 (13%) f

*a > b; $P < .01$.
†c > d; $P < .05$.
‡e > f; $P < .01$.

IVF treatment. Table 45-4 summarizes a general comparison between the younger and older populations described in Tables 45-2 and 45-3. These data reflect all patients treated over the past 6 ½ years regardless of male factor, etiology of infertility, resistance to ovarian stimulation, uterine anomalies, or other factors that might ordinarily exclude them from analysis. Surely within each of these groups, particularly in the over-age-40 group, there are patients who exhibit very poor prognoses because of multiple failed IVF cycles, elevated FSH levels, genetic anomalies in their oocyte population, and repeatedly poor preembryonic growth. In many of these cases, the element of poor oocyte quality would perhaps be benefited by acceptance of a donor oocyte.

Fate of donated oocytes

If it is determined that the oocytes of younger patients result in better opportunities for term pregnancy after transfer, it becomes interesting to evaluate whether this is an oocyte factor, an endometrial factor, or both. What rates of pregnancy are observed when young donors contribute oocytes that are placed in the uteri of older recipients? The oocyte donation program was evaluated during a 9-month period when the vast majority of donors (19 of 21) were not IVF patients but were young women donating for altruistic reasons or at the time of tubal ligation. Recipients were enrolled in the donation program after demonstrating ovarian failure, repeated failed ovarian stimulation during IVF trials, or repeatedly poor preembryo quality after IVF. Results are shown for this time period in Table 45-5. When donors were significantly younger and not of an infertile population, pregnancy rates were quite impressive (18 of 32 fresh transfers). Overall donor oocyte pregnancy rates have always been good when donors were under age 40, even when those same donors were part of the general IVF population; of 149 fresh transfers, 51 pregnancies have been established since November 1984 (34%), with an additional 21 pregnancies from cryopreserved and thawed

Table 45-5. Results of oocyte donation, November 1990 to June 1991

Parameter	Result
No. of different donors	21
No. of donation cycles	27
Average age of donor (y)	30.4 ± 3.9
No. of recipients	35
Average age of recipient (y)	39.7 ± 4.5
No. of fresh IVF transfers	32 (3 cycles had all prezygotes frozen)
No. of fresh IVF pregnancies	18 (56.3%)
No. of additional pregnancies from thaws	1
Total pregnancies/cycle with donation	19 (59.4%)
No. of grade 1 transfers (% pregnant)	9 (66.7%)
No. of grade 2 transfers (% pregnant)	17 (52.9%)
No. of grade 3 transfers (% pregnant)	1 (100%)
No. of grade 4 transfers (% pregnant)	5 (40.0%)
No. of grade 5 transfers (% pregnant)	None

prezygotes. This finding suggests that oocyte factors play an impressive role in the ability to produce pregnancy, perhaps more so than uterine factors in the older patient. Indeed, preembryo grading scores in recipient patients are skewed to higher grades, presumably as the result of receiving oocytes from young donors. Yet although the relationship to oocyte quality seems clear, one must consider other possibilities that may have played a role in preventing pregnancy in the recipient population, such as lethal genes shared by husband and wife that are avoided by a nonrelated oocyte, immunologic factors bypassed for the

Table 45-6. Preembryo grading versus IVF pregnancy over a 4-year period in patients under age 41 years

Preembryo grade	Pregnancies/ transfers	% Pregnant*	% Cycles with this grade
1	243/546	45% a	28.5%
2	226/714	32% b	37.3%
3	11/86	13% c	4.5%
4	97/422	23% d	22.1%
5	9/145	6.2% e	7.6%
TOTAL	586/1913	31% f	

*a > b > c; d > e; $P < .005$ (c = d, c = e).

Pregnancy rate according to preembryo grading

At the Jones Institute evaluations of preembryo grading schemes were initiated late in 1986. Although it is undoubtedly a subjective analysis, grading the extent of cytoplasmic fragmentation has proven to be remarkably repetitive between observers as demonstrated by blind scoring after photography. Our results indicate that transfers with at least one grade 1 or grade 2 preembryo demonstrate a significantly better chance for establishing a clinical pregnancy (Table 45-6). Although a higher score is favorable, pregnancy is possible even in cycles with grade 4 or grade 5 morphology demonstrating unequal-sized blastomeres and moderate to severe cytoplasmic fragmentation. Scores are remarkably repetitive for the same patient in succeeding cycles, and persistently poor scores have been recorded for some couples with idiopathic infertility. Grading information may be useful in counseling patients who fail to conceive after multiple attempts. Individuals who fail to conceive after repeated transfers of high-quality preembryos may require an aggressive evaluation of potential factors that could interfere with implantation. Those with repetitively poor scores might be counseled concerning possible gamete abnormalities, reduced potential for success, and justification for gamete donation. The impact of improving grading scores by virtue of altering ovarian stimulation regimens needs to be elucidated more thoroughly; at present, it appears that slight improvement is possible in patients with ovulation induction difficulties.

Pregnancy rate according to preembryo growth rate

Nearly 2000 transfers were analyzed for the effect of preembryo growth rate on the actual incidence of pregnancy (Table 45-6). Evaluation was made of the most rapidly growing preembryo in the cohort of conceptuses for replacement and transfers assigned to rapidly growing, normally growing, or slowly growing groups according to the criteria mentioned previously. Normal growth scores

accounted for the vast majority of transfers (85%) and presented the highest overall pregnancy rate. This means that 85% of the transfers done at the Jones Institute involve at least one preembryo that has two blastomeres by 24 hours and/or four blastomeres by 40 hours. No significant difference was seen between pregnancy rates achieved with rapidly and normally growing preembryos, but a significant drop in pregnancy rates was noted for slow growth. Six percent of cycles have been scored as rapidly growing (eight or more blastomeres by 36 to 48 hours postinsemination) and 9% have been classified as slowly developing (only two blastomeres after 40 hours postinsemination).

Pregnancy rate versus grading and growth rate

When cleavage rates were combined with preembryo grading data, several interesting observations were noted (Table 45-7). Although the slowly dividing preembryos scored low in their overall ability to establish pregnancy, their pregnancy potential equaled that of more rapidly developing conceptuses if they were of grade 1 quality (although numbers were low). Alternately, rapidly growing preembryos of grade 1 quality did not show an elevated pregnancy rate over normally growing ones of the same grade. In addition, the incidence of pregnancy was rather low for transfers scoring less than grade 2 in both rapidly and slowly cleaving groups, whereas preembryos dividing at average rates contributed to pregnancy even when grade 4 was associated with the transfer. Other investigators have observed this tendency for enhanced implantation with nonfragmented preembryos, particularly when cleavage rates fall within average or better limits.[3,8,10,31]

In vitro development of cryopreserved/thawed specimens

General results from our prezygote cryopreservation program are shown in Table 45-8. Prezygotes, including those with poor morphology, were randomly selected for freezing at approximately 12 to 19 hours postinsemination. All IVF cycles and prezygotes with freezing since the onset of the cryopreservation program were included in the analysis; many cycles had only a single prezygote frozen. Donor oocyte cycles are not included in Table 45-8 but represent an additional 16 pregnancies from 55 transfers (29%), a rate identical with that for IVF cycles. One might expect a higher pregnancy rate after thaw for recipients according to the results of fresh transfer in this group, but so far this is not the case, perhaps because of the higher fresh pregnancy rate and the lower number of recipients returning for thaw. Overall, the survival rate after thaw has been fairly consistent at 68% to 72% throughout 4 years, and the clinical pregnancy rate has been 29% to 30% after transfer. As seen in fresh transfer cycles, the number of preembryos replaced influences the opportunity for pregnancy.

Table 45-7. Combined grading and growth rates versus IVF pregnancy over a 4-year period in patients under age 41 years

Preembryo grade	Rapid growth rate*		Normal growth rate†		Slow growth rate‡	
	No. of transfers	% Pregnant	No. of transfers	% Pregnancy†	No. of transfers	% Pregnant
1	52	39%	488	45%	6	50%
2	44	27%	632	33%	38	13%
3	6	0%	63	17%	17	0%
4	17	6%	341	25%	64	19%
5	3	0%	93	6%	49	6%
TOTAL§	33/122	27%a	530/1617	33%b	23/174	13%c
% Cycles with this growth rate	6.4%		84.5%		9.1%	

* Eight or more blastomeres by 36 to 48 hours after insemination.
† Four blastomeres by 40 hours after insemination.
‡ Only two blastomeres by 40 hours after insemination.
§ a = b; a > c; $P < .005$; b > c; $P < .001$.

Table 45-8. Overall survival and pregnancy rates after cryopreservation and thaw: January 1987 to December 1990

Parameter	Result
No. of prezygotes frozen	2460
No. of prezygotes thawed	1248
No. of prezygotes surviving	875 (70%)
No. of prezygotes transferred	873
No. of implantations	112 (13%)
No. of cycles with freezing	582
No. of cycles with thawing	350
No. of cycles with survival	310
No. of cycles with transfer	308
No. of cycles with pregnancy	88 (29% Pregnancies/ transfer cycles)
No. of pregnancies/no. of cycles with 1 or 2 transferred	31/165 (19% Pregnancies/ transfer cycles)
No. of pregnancies/no. of cycles with 3 or 4 transferred	57/143 (40% Pregnancies/ transfer cycles)

Table 45-9. Preembryo grading versus pregnancy in thawed cycles: January 1987 to December 1990

Preembryo grade	Distribution of grade*		Thawed transfers	
	Fresh	Thaw	Pregnancies/ transfers	%†
1	29%	30%	38/92	41%a
2	42%	38%	38/118	32%b
3	4%	4%	2/11	18%c
4	16%	23%	9/71	13%d
5	8%	5%	1/16	6%e

*Distribution of grade: the percentage of cycles showing this grade of transfer.
†a > d; $P < .001$; a > e; $P < .05$; b > d; $P < .01$.

Table 45-9 shows that the distribution of preembryo grading scores is not different between fresh or thawed preembryos from the same harvest cycle; no negative effect on morphology was noted after thawing. In fresh IVF transfers, 71% of cycles were transferred with preembryos of either grade 1 or grade 2 morphology, compared with 68% in thawed transfers from the same cycles. Table 45-9 further demonstrates that a higher grading score predicts pregnancy in thawed transfers just as it does in fresh transfers, with grades 1 and 2 morphology resulting in a higher pregnancy rate.

Table 45-10 shows that actual and potential pregnancy rates are significantly elevated by virtue of the ability to cryopreserve and store excess prezygotes. In cycles with freezing, a fresh pregnancy rate of 36% has been observed. When additional pregnancies as a result of thawing are added to fresh pregnancies, the number of pregnancies divided by the number of cycles increases the actual pregnancy rate to 51%. When one predicts the pregnancy potential of prezygotes still in storage based on the current results with thawing and adds these to the calculation, the potential number of pregnancies divided by these same cycles reaches 63%. Table 45-10 further demonstrates that the use of GnRHa does not negatively affect the results of a cryopreservation program; cycles using GnRHa show the largest increase in actual and potential pregnancies, undoubtedly because of the greater number of prezygotes available for freezing.

SUMMARY

An attempt has been made to summarize the significance of morphologic and physiologic characteristics of oocytes,

Table 45-10. Real and projected pregnancy rates according to stimulation in cycles with freezing: January 1987 to December 1990

Stimulation	Fresh pregnancy rate		Actual augmented rate		Projected augmented rate	
	IVF pregnancies/ transfers	%	IVF + thaws to date	%	IVF + thaws to date + potential thaws with stored specimens	%
hMG	1/6	17%	1 + 1/6	33%	1 + 1 + 0/6	33%
FSH	25/75	33%	25 + 11/75	48%	25 + 11 + 5/75	55%
Combination	32/108	30%	32 + 17/108	45%	32 + 17 + 10/108	55%
GnRHa/hMG/FSH	149/393	38%	149 + 59/393	53%	149 + 59 + 54/393	67%
TOTAL*	207/582	36%a	207 + 88/582	51%b	207 + 88 + 69/582	63%c

* a < b < c; $P < .001$.

prezygotes, and preembryos. The role of nuclear maturation, cytoplasmic maturation, cytoplasmic inclusions, and associated miscellaneous factors has been correlated with actual pregnancy in a large IVF program. The effect of patient age, mode of treatment, preembryo number, grade, and growth rate has been related to actual results that reflect an overall potential for pregnancy. Certainly, chromosomal or genetic disorders may be present within preembryos and may represent disorders that are beyond the scope of recognition through simple bright-field microscopy. Unfertilized oocytes are reported to be chromosomally defective at rates reaching 30% to 50%,[23,30,48] and chromosomal aberrations have been observed in human preembryos in percentages as high as 36% of karyotyped specimens.[47] Without genetically healthy preembryos, success in establishing pregnancy is limited after IVF treatment, at least until scientists find means of a noninvasive, yet definitive, evaluation.

The ideal situation encountered during an IVF trial would proceed as follows: A patient under age 41 arrives at the center for treatment. Her hormones are suppressed with GnRHa starting in the luteal phase of her cycle (day 21), and ovarian stimulation with gonadotropins is begun on what will be called follicular cycle day 3. No severe male factor is present in the husband, and oocytes become fertilized at an expectedly good rate. She has intrauterine replacement of four preembryos, at least one of which is developed from an MII oocyte and classified as grade 1. She additionally has at least one prezygote frozen. Based on the actual analysis of 174 women with this precise profile, our patient would have an anticipated fresh pregnancy expectation of 51%. Her total expectation for at least one pregnancy after fresh transfer and subsequent thawing would be upward of 80%, with a more than 50% chance of actually taking home at least one healthy baby. Unfortunately, this optimistic profile fits only 7% of patients who have arrived at the Jones Institute for IVF treatment since 1987. With the more frequent use of GnRHa today, coupled with improvements in the laboratory, this patient will certainly represent a larger population in the near future. There still remain new frontiers in the world of in vitro fertilization.

REFERENCES

1. Austin CR: *The mammalian egg,* Oxford, UK, 1961, Blackwell Scientific Publications.
2. Beatty RA: The genetics of the mammalian gamete, *Biol Rev* 45:73, 1970.
3. Bolton VN et al: Development of spare human preimplantation embryos in vitro: an analysis of the correlations among gross morphology, cleavage rates, and development to the blastocyst, *J In Vitro Fert Embryo Transfer* 6:30, 1989.
4. Bomsel-Helmreich O: The ageing of gametes, heteroploidy, and embryonic death, *Int J Gynaecol Obstet* 14:98, 1976.
5. Byskov AG: Primordial germ cells and regulation of meiosis. In Austin CR, Short RV, editors: *Germ cells and fertilization,* vol 1, ed 2, Cambridge, UK, 1982, Cambridge University Press.
6. Carrothers AD, Beatty RA: The recognition and incidence of haploid and polyploid spermatozoa in man, rabbit, and mouse, *J Reprod Fertil* 44:487, 1975.
7. Chang MC: Development of parthenogenetic rabbit blastocysts induced by low temperature storage of unfertilized ova, *J Exp Zool* 125:127, 1954.
8. Claman P et al: The impact of embryo quality and quantity on implantation and the establishment of viable pregnancies, *J In Vitro Fert Embryo Transfer* 4:218, 1987.
9. Cohen J et al: Pregnancies following the frozen storage of expanding human blastocysts, *J In Vitro Fert Embryo Transfer* 2:59, 1985.
10. Cummins JM et al: A formula for scoring human embryo growth rates in in vitro fertilization: its value in predicting pregnancy and in comparison with visual estimates of embryo quality, *J In Vitro Fert Embryo Transfer* 3:284, 1986.
11. Dandekar PV, Martin MC, Glass RH: Polypronuclear embryos after in vitro fertilization, *Fertil Steril* 53:510, 1990.
12. Diamond MP et al: Polyspermy: effect of varying stimulation protocols and inseminating concentrations, *Fertil Steril* 43:777, 1985.
13. Edwards RG: *Conception in the human female,* New York, 1980, Academic Press.
14. Englert Y et al: Factors leading to tripronucleate eggs during human in vitro fertilization, *Hum Reprod* 1:117, 1986.
15. Familiari G, Sayoko M, Motta PM: The ovary and ovulation: a three-dimensional ultrastructural study. In Van Blerkom J, Motta PM, editors: *Ultrastructure of human gametogenesis and early embryogenesis,* Boston, 1989, Kluwer Academic Publishers.
16. Familiari G et al: The application of electron microscopy in the

evaluation of in vitro unfertilized human oocytes. In Spera G, de Kretser DM, editors: *Morphological basis of human reproductive function,* New York, 1987, Plenum Press.

17. Fowler RE, Edwards RG: The genetics of early human development, *Prog Med Genet* 9:49, 1973.

18. Fulton BP, Whittingham DG: Activation of mammalian oocytes by intracellular injection of calcium, *Nature* 273:149, 1978.

19. Kaufman MH, Surani MAH: The effect of osmolarity on mouse parthenogenesis, *J Embryol Exp Morphol* 31:513, 1974.

20. Kola I et al: Tripronuclear human oocytes: altered cleavage patterns and subsequent karyotypic analysis of embryos, *Biol Reprod* 37:395, 1987.

21. Komar A: Parthenogenetic development of mouse eggs activated by heat-shock, *J Reprod Fertil* 35:433, 1973.

22. Laufer N et al: Asynchrony between human cumulus-corona cell complex and oocyte maturation after human menopausal gonadotropin treatment for in vitro fertilization, *Fertil Steril* 42:366, 1984.

23. Martin RH et al: Chromosomal analysis of unfertilized human oocytes, *J Reprod Fertil* 78:673, 1986.

24. Michelmann HW, Bonhoff A, Mettler L: Chromosome analysis of polyploid human embryos, *Hum Reprod* 1:243, 1986.

25. Motta PM, Nesci E: The Call and Exner bodies of mammalian ovaries with reference to the problem of rosette formation, *Arch Anat Microsc Morphol Exp* 58:283, 1969.

26. Motta PM et al: Ultrastructure of human unfertilized oocytes and polyspermic embryos in an IVF-ET program, *Ann N Y Acad Sci* 541:367, 1988.

27. Muechler EK et al: Parthenogenesis of human oocytes as a function of vacuum pressure, *J In Vitro Fert Embryo Transfer* 6:335, 1989.

28. Oehninger S et al: Human preovulatory oocytes have a higher sperm binding ability than immature oocytes under hemizona (HZA) conditions: evidence supporting the concept of zona maturation, *Fertil Steril* 55:1165, 1991.

29. Peluso JJ, England-Charlesworth C, Hutz R: Effect of age and of follicular ageing on the preovulatory oocyte, *Biol Reprod* 22:999, 1980.

30. Plachot M et al: Chromosomal analysis of human oocytes and embryos in an in vitro fertilization program, *Ann N Y Acad Sci* 541:384, 1988.

31. Puissant F et al: Embryo scoring as a prognostic tool in IVF treatment, *Hum Reprod* 2:705, 1987.

32. Sathananthan AH: Ultrastructural morphology of fertilization and early cleavage in the human. In Trounson AO, Wood C, editors: *In vitro fertilization and embryo transfer,* London, 1984, Churchill Livingstone.

33. Sathananthan AH, Trounson AO: The human pronuclear ovum: fine structure of monospermic and polyspermic fertilization in vitro, *Gamete Res* 12:385, 1985.

34. Sathananthan AH, Trounson AO, Wood C: *Atlas of fine structure of human sperm penetration, eggs, and embryos cultured in vitro,* New York, 1986, Praeger Publishers.

35. Soupart P, Strong PA: Ultrastructural observations on human oocytes fertilized in vitro, *Fertil Steril* 25:11, 1974.

36. Uehara T, Yanagimachi R: Activation of hamster oocytes by pricking, *J Exp Zool* 199:269, 1977.

37. Van Blerkom J: Developmental failure in human reproduction associated with preovulatory oogenesis and preimplantation embryogenesis. In Van Blerkom J, Motta PM, editors: *Ultrastructure of human gametogenesis and early embryogenesis,* Boston, 1989, Kluwer Academic Publishers.

38. Van Blerkom J, Bell H, Henry G: The occurrence, recognition and developmental fate of pseudo-pronuclear eggs after in vitro fertilization of human oocytes, *Hum Reprod* 2:217, 1987.

39. Van der Ven HH et al: Polyspermy in in vitro fertilization of human oocytes: frequency and possible causes, *Ann N Y Acad Sci* 442:88, 1985.

40. Veeck LL: Extracorporeal maturation, *Ann N Y Acad Sci* 442:357, 1985.

41. Veeck LL: The morphologic estimation of mature oocytes and their preparation for insemination. In Jones HW Jr et al, editors: *In vitro fertilization—Norfolk,* Baltimore, 1986, Williams & Wilkins.

42. Veeck LL: Oocyte assessment and biological performance, *Ann N Y Acad Sci* 541:259, 1988.

43. Veeck LL: The morphological assessment of human oocytes and early conceptuses. In Keel BA, Webster BW, editors: *Laboratory diagnosis and treatment of infertility,* Boca Raton, Fla, 1990, CRC Press.

44. Veeck LL: Pregnancy rate and pregnancy outcome associated with laboratory evaluation of spermatozoa, oocytes, and preembryos. In Mashiach S et al, editors: *Advances in assisted reproductive technologies,* New York, 1990, Plenum Press.

45. Veeck LL: *Atlas of the human oocyte and early conceptus,* vol 2, Baltimore, 1991, Williams & Wilkins.

46. Veeck LL et al: Maturation and fertilization of morphologically immature human oocytes in a program of in vitro fertilization, *Fertil Steril* 39:594, 1983.

47. Wramsby H: Chromosomal analysis of preovulatory human oocytes and oocytes failing to cleave following insemination in vitro, *Ann N Y Acad Sci* 541:228, 1988.

48. Wramsby H, Fredga K, Liedholm P: Chromosomal analysis of human oocytes recovered from preovulatory follicles in stimulated cycles, *N Engl J Med* 316:121, 1987.

49. Wramsby H, Fredga K, Liedholm P: Ploidy in human cleavage stage embryos after in vitro fertilization, *Hum Reprod* 2:223, 1987.

50. Wright G et al: Observations on the morphology of pronuclei and nucleoli in human zygotes and implications for cryopreservation, *Hum Reprod* 5:109, 1990.

51. Zamboni L: *Fine morphology of mammalian fertilization,* New York, 1971, Harper & Row.

Chapter 46

IN VITRO FERTILIZATION AND ASSISTED REPRODUCTIVE TECHNOLOGIES

Marian D. Damewood, MD

ADVANCEMENTS OF IN VITRO FERTILIZATION

The first successful extracorporeal fertilization and cleavage of a human oocyte were performed by Rock and Menkin in 1944.[105] Thirty-four years later, the first successful in vitro fertilization (IVF) of a human oocyte with embryo transfer (IVF-ET) culminated in a live birth in the United Kingdom through the efforts of Edwards and Steptoe.[119] Before this procedure the extracorporeal fertilization of a human donor oocyte with cleavage to the blastocyst stage and transfer to a recipient's uterus was reported, but without establishment of pregnancy.[110] Since the first successful pregnancy by IVF in 1978, IVF technology has been associated with major ramifications in the field of human reproduction. Investigation of previously uncharted areas of human gamete function, fertilization events, and early embryonic development have been undertaken. Cryopreservation techniques for embryos, once limited to animal husbandry, have been successfully applied to the human conceptus. Alternate forms of reproduction such as gamete intrafallopian transfer (GIFT) have developed as corollary procedures of the IVF process. In addition, the scientific advances associated with human IVF have generated profound ethical issues associated with cryopreservation or micromanipulation of the fertilized human oocyte. The use of donor gametes, the use of a surrogate uterus, and the possibility of blastocyst manipulation and sperm microinjection have raised issues involving not only physicians and researchers but also scientific, clerical, and governmental leaders.[117]

The first human IVF-ET was performed by laparoscopic retrieval techniques in a natural cycle and resulted in the fertilization of one oocyte. Present-day technology includes control of the hypothalamic-pituitary axis with analogues of gonadotropin-releasing hormone (GnRHa) and induction of ovulation with human menopausal gonadotropins (hMG), resulting in the development of multiple follicles. Oocyte retrieval techniques have been modified to include an ultrasound-directed vaginal retrieval approach. Sperm microinjection techniques, as well as new cryopreservation techniques for embryos, sperm, and oocytes, are used in contemporary IVF laboratories.

Of utmost importance in the organization of successful IVF-ET programs is the team approach to these procedures: physicians, laboratory staff, nursing staff, anesthesiologists, and laboratory medicine specialists all contribute to successful outcomes. It is uncommon in medicine, with the exception of cardiac surgery teams or transplantation teams, to apply such a comprehensive team approach to a procedure—an approach that has contributed markedly to the innovative scientific advances and the role of this new technology in reproductive medicine.[29]

Table 46-1. Causes of infertility in patients in the Johns Hopkins IVF program

Major cause of infertility	Percent of total
Tubal disease	39.2
Endometriosis	25.8
Unexplained infertility	23.6
Oligospermia	6.2
Immunologic factors	3.1
Cervical factor	2.1

Modified from Damewood MD, editor: *The Johns Hopkins handbook of in vitro fertilization and assisted reproductive technologies,* Boston, 1990, Little, Brown.

SELECTION OF PATIENTS
General considerations

The major indication for IVF-ET is the failure of conventional medical or surgical therapy to result in establishment of pregnancy. The classic indication for IVF-ET, previous salpingectomy or salpingectomies for ectopic pregnancy, has been joined by other indications, including failed reconstructive tubal surgery, recurrent adhesions, or persistent cornual or distal tubal obstruction. Other diagnoses associated with infertility, such as endometriosis refractory to hormonal and surgical therapy, also have been treated successfully with the IVF procedure. Tubal factor infertility and endometriosis, along with the category of unexplained infertility, account for the majority of indications for IVF-ET. Additional indications include severe cervical factor, oligospermia, and immunologic factors such as sperm antibodies in the man or woman. An individual IVF candidate may have multiple causes of infertility, such as a combination of tubal disease and oligospermia. The causes of infertility and the IVF patients in the Johns Hopkins IVF program are summarized in Table 46-1.

The assessment of patients for IVF-ET includes consideration of infertility factors as well as general health, absence of contraindications to pregnancy, regularity of ovulation, luteal phase sufficiency, and absence of genital tract infections in husband and wife.[20,26] Each patient should be assessed individually, however, with emphasis on normal uterine function, ovulation, and semen parameters.[28] Accessibility of the ovaries for oocyte recovery by either laparoscopy or ultrasound retrieval, and other parameters including sperm count, motility, and morphology should be determined before initiation of the procedure. Laboratory screening for IVF couples may include a complete andrology survey for the man and a study of the woman's serum in a mouse embryo culture system. In addition, an interview with a psychologist to provide counseling for couples before the IVF attempt is arranged in specific instances.[46]

Indications for in vitro fertilization and embryo transfer

Before initiating a cycle of IVF-ET a complete infertility evaluation is mandatory, along with therapy by established and traditional techniques. Although the established and conventional infertility therapies are beyond the scope of this chapter, the major indications for the IVF-ET procedure and aspects of the traditional therapies are considered in an attempt to establish criteria for patient selection.

Tubal factors. In initial stages of IVF-ET technology, patients with intractable tubal disease or absence of the fallopian tubes were considered as primary candidates for the procedure. The use of microsurgical techniques in tubal surgery resulted in establishment of pregnancy in patients with tubal and peritoneal adhesive disease. However, large hydrosalpinges, absence of fimbriae, or severe adhesions are associated with a poor prognosis for full-term pregnancy. After tuboplasty the live birth rates are approximately 20% to 30% with an additional risk of ectopic pregnancy of 15% to 20%.[68,77] If a patient remains infertile for a period of 1 year to 18 months after a tuboplasty procedure, conception is unlikely to occur after a second tubal procedure.[78] The prognosis after a failed tubal anastomosis, although varying according to the sterilization procedure at the anastomosis site and the length of the tube, does not appear to improve after a repeated tubal surgical procedure. The risk of a third ectopic pregnancy after two conservative surgical procedures for ectopic pregnancy is considerable; only 30% of women with this diagnosis achieve an intrauterine pregnancy.[35] Thus repeated ectopic pregnancy is an indication for IVF-ET. Patients with tubal factor infertility may consider IVF-ET as an option when the expected pregnancy rate is at or below 20% after a failed surgical therapy, as well as patients for whom surgery is not an option.[76] Although patients with tubal disease or peritoneal adhesions may have reduced ovarian accessibility, the relatively recent development of ultrasound-directed vaginal oocyte retrieval has resulted in excellent oocyte retrieval rates comparable to those in women without pelvic factors. Patients with tubal factor infertility have been reported to have an 11.5% pregnancy rate per IVF-ET attempt when at least one embryo was transferred.[85]

Endometriosis. Stage I to stage IV endometriosis[3] has been increasingly considered as an indication for IVF-ET.[116] An IVF-ET attempt is usually recommended 1 to 2 years after previous unsuccessful medical or surgical therapy; the prognosis depends on the severity and extent of the endometriotic lesions as well as the patient's age and duration of infertility.[108] If pregnancy does not occur within 3 years of surgery the chances are poor that it will ever occur unless further intervention is undertaken using assisted reproductive technologies.[38] In moderate to severe endometriosis involving tubal obstruction, specifically when isthmic abnormalities are present or endometriotic cysts are present in the ovaries, IVF-ET is directly indicated within 1 year after failed reconstructive surgery.[109] When endometriosis was categorized with stage I to stage II disease and patent tubes, a 33.3% pregnancy rate per cycle was noted with at least one embryo transferred per cycle. Patients with stage III to stage IV disease and tubal blockage achieved only a 10% success rate per IVF-ET attempt. Thus severe disease with subsequent compromise of ovarian and tubal function appears to be associated with a deleterious effect on the outcome of a single IVF-ET attempt.[27] In the Norfolk program, patients with all categories of endometriosis achieved a pregnancy rate of 25.5% per cycle during a 3.5-year period.[74] Patients with a single diagnosis of endometriosis without other infertility factors had a 26.3% pregnancy rate per cycle, whereas patients with a secondary diagnosis (male factor, anovulation, cervical factor) achieved a 23.5% pregnancy rate.[23,71]

IVF-ET attempts in patients with a history of endometriosis without active disease, particularly those with mild to moderate disease, seemed to be associated with an 18.4% pregnancy rate per cycle and a 22.3% pregnancy rate per embryo transfer. Further evidence of compromise of reproductive function in patients with severe or extensive endometriosis was demonstrated by a lower IVF-ET pregnancy rate overall.[74] Factors responsible for this difference in severe disease may include an altered response to ovarian stimulation, a lower number of oocytes aspirated, the larger volumes of endometriosis present at the time of aspiration, and poor embryo quality at transfer. Although IVF is an alternative for patients with endometriosis, some investigations have shown evidence of lower fertilization rates in vitro.[125,136] These lower pregnancy rates have been attributed to poor oocyte quality in patients with stage III to stage IV endometriosis.

The possibility that GnRHa pretreatment can improve the outcome in these difficult cases has been considered.[34] Other investigators attribute the low pregnancy rate to poor-quality embryos or a defective luteal phase in patients with severe endometriosis.[23] Another study[125] also suggests impairment of oocyte fertilization parameters in patients with untreated endometriosis with persistent disease present at the time of an IVF attempt. One report addresses further surgical therapy in recurrent or persistent endometriosis in the IVF-ET setting with the use of operative laparoscopy. Although the IVF cycle was unsuccessful, pregnancy was established within a period of 10 months after operative laparoscopy in a significant number of patients with more than 5 years of primary infertility associated with endometriosis.[30] Cumulatively, IVF-ET in patients with stage I to stage IV endometriosis appears to yield pregnancy rates comparable to those of IVF patients with other factors. However, patients with mild disease appear to have better pregnancy rates than those with stage III or stage IV disease categories.[23,129]

Unexplained infertility. The term *unexplained* or *idiopathic* infertility is applied to couples who have failed to conceive after 2 to 5 years of regular intercourse and in whom no definitive abnormality or anomaly of the reproductive system or hormonal parameters can be elucidated. (See Chapter 25.) Unexplained infertility may be present in up to 15% of infertile couples.[92] The therapy of unexplained infertility is directed at improving cycle fecundity when expectant management has failed. Intrauterine insemination, superinduction of ovulation, or a combination of both techniques appears to increase pregnancy rates per cycle in unexplained infertility.[39,114] Unexplained infertility has been postulated to be related to subtle defects in ovulation, ovum or gamete transport, or tubal environment. An IVF attempt will also provide information as to whether fertilization has occurred. Observation of oocyte morphology as well as semen parameters in patients with unexplained infertility and fertilization failure will allow further insight into potential defects at the gamete level. Patients with unexplained infertility appear to have IVF results comparable to those of patients with tubal infertility and endometriosis, although couples with secondary unexplained infertility appear to be more likely to conceive.[83] Patients with idiopathic infertility were reported to have a 14.3% pregnancy rate per IVF attempt when at least one embryo was transferred.[85]

Cervical and other factors. Although cervical factor is not a primary indication for IVF-ET, it may be considered for couples with repeatedly poor postcoital tests in which cervical mucus cannot be improved medically and in whom intrauterine insemination is unsuccessful, particularly after an unsuccessful trial period of cervical bypass therapy.[2] However, IVF-ET is not usually indicated when these disorders are isolated conditions. In addition, IVF-ET may be efficacious in the therapy of refractory hypogonadotropic anovulation, oligoovulation, and luteal phase deficiency. In patients with luteinized unruptured follicle syndrome, IVF-ET or the GIFT procedure may be considered. In addition, donor oocyte technology in IVF has provided a means for achieving pregnancy in perimenopausal women or women with premature ovarian failure, oophorectomy, or gonadal dysgenesis.[21,50] In addition, for women with uterine factor such as müllerian agenesis, congenital uterine anomalies, or severe Asherman's syndrome refractory to surgical therapy, embryos developed through IVF-ET may be transferred to a surrogate uterus.[123] The legal and ethical issues for a surrogate uterus procedure are complex, and current guidelines are not completely outlined or effective with respect to the legalities involved.

Reproductive potential and age

Reproductive potential and the relationship to age is an important parameter in infertility therapy, particularly with consideration to assisted reproductive technologies.[113] Conflicting reports exist concerning the effect of the woman's age on reproductive potential. A study of women undergoing artificial insemination with frozen donor semen showed significant declines in fertility, fecundity rates, and cumulative pregnancy rates in the 36- to 40-year-old age group.[48] Some reports have noted IVF-ET pregnancy rates for women between ages 35 and 39 as generally acceptable.[129] Other investigators, however, demonstrated a decline in IVF-ET pregnancies with advancing patient age.[55] Women over age 35 years may demonstrate normal response to ovarian stimulation with gonadotropins but decreased receptivity of the endometrium or increased numbers of embryos with chromosomal abnormalities leading to a reduced rate of implantation.[113] Although oocytes produced by and retrieved from the women over age 35 in that study were as likely to be fertilized as those of younger patients, fewer fertilized oocytes cleaved into apparently normal embryos. Although patients older than age 40 are not completely excluded from IVF-ET procedures, additional reproductive difficulties may include poor follicular function as well as a high spontaneous abortion rate. Patients in the older age groups should be counseled about the risks and benefits of the procedure as well as maternal and fetal risks during pregnancy and the need for prenatal testing for chromosome disorders if pregnancy should occur.[76]

Male infertility

IVF-ET has provided new insights into the etiology and treatment of male infertility.[8] When considering male factor infertility, a complete evaluation of the man must be performed before an IVF-ET attempt, with associated infertility factors identified and treated accordingly. Since spermatozoa are placed in direct contact with oocytes, a relatively low concentration of sperm may be used for fertilization. With improving IVF techniques, fewer spermatozoa appear to be required to inseminate individual oocytes in vitro.[51] An important consideration is that the fertilizing potential of motile spermatozoa is not easily correlated with parameters of the original ejaculate used for infertility testing.[84]

IVF appears to be a logical alternative for oligospermic men. Fertilization rates, although lower for oligospermic men, are acceptable with sperm concentrations of 1.5×10^6/mL after a swim-up procedure.[124] Nonfertilizing sperm could not be distinguished from fertilizing sperm by conventional criteria but rather by the average concentration of motile spermatozoa in the swim-up fraction (12.5 ± 1.5 and $22.3 \pm 2.3 \times 10^6$/mL for a 0% and a 100% fertilization group, respectively).[51] The swim-up migration technique may serve as a predictive test for the in vitro fertilizing capacity of sperm. The minimum number of motile sperm required to fertilize human oocytes in vitro has not yet been determined, although fertilization has been achieved with only 10,000 motile sperm in culture media.[25,51] Optimal fertilization of an oocyte is achieved with the use of 0.5 to 2.0×10^5 motile sperm from oligospermic men.[131] Once fertilization occurs and embryos are transferred, pregnancy rates are comparable to or slightly lower than those for normospermic groups.[62] In general, oligospermic samples are less efficient in the fertilization of oocytes than normospermic samples.

Additional altered parameters such as lowered sperm motility, abnormal morphology, or other factors may be associated with reduced fertilizing ability.[66] The oligospermic sample may be unable to result in a minimum concentration of 1.5 million motile cells after swim-up.[132] Variability of fertilization rates in individual IVF-ET centers results in difficulty in establishing a minimum effective concentration of motile sperm for IVF-ET.[66] Additional variables in semen parameters, such as decreased motility (<40%), are associated with a marked decrease in fertilization rates.[132] Other studies have shown that fertilization rates did not decrease in samples with less than 20% motility unless the motile sperm count fell below 2×10^6/mL.[24] Although the establishment of acceptable motility criteria for IVF-ET programs is difficult, semen samples with sperm motility of less than 30% are associated with decreased fertilization rates.[66] Sperm morphology as a parameter is reported not to be associated with a statistically significant relationship with fertilization rates achieved in vitro.[62] However, other studies demonstrated delayed fertilization with morphology of more than 60% abnormal forms.[135] Standard World Health Organization criteria for abnormal morphology[133] may not be clinically useful in predicting IVF success. In general, severe abnormal morphology has compromised outcome and suitability of a semen sample for IVF-ET.

Although only 5% to 10% of men have autoimmunity to sperm,[60] in the presence of autoantibodies, fertilization rates are lower when immunoglobulin A (IgA) and IgG antibodies are present. Antisperm antibodies may interfere with sperm binding to the zona pellucida, cumulus dispersal, sperm penetration through the zona, or fertilization.[128] In other studies fertilization has been observed when 100% of motile sperm are bound by IgA and IgG antibodies.[85] Although combinations of factors such as oligospermia and sperm antibodies are associated with lower fertilization rates, statistically significant differences are difficult to demonstrate in patients with sperm antibodies alone as an isolated factor. Although fertilization rates may be lower, with male factor resulting in lower pregnancy rates, fertilization and cleavage has occurred in IVF cycles with establishment of pregnancy. The outcome of IVF-ET by infertility diagnosis in U.S. centers is shown in Table 46-2.[90]

Psychologic needs

Additional considerations for selection of patients include the evaluation and care for patients' psychologic

Table 46-2. Outcome by infertility diagnosis and treatment in IVF

Infertility diagnosis	Stimulation cycles	Canceled cycles*	Embryo transfers	Clinical pregnancies*	All deliveries*
Tubal disease/problem	3779	709 (19)	2348	468 (20)	333 (14)
Female unexplained	1042	207 (20)	247	58 (23)	50 (20)
Female immune	351	62 (18)	150	36 (24)	21 (14)
Endometriosis	2417	453 (19)	904	180 (20)	129 (14)
Male factor	2322	424 (18)	807	162 (20)	121 (15)

Modified from Medical Research International, Society for Assisted Reproductive Technology, The American Fertility Society: In vitro fertilization-embryo transfer (IVF-ET) in the United States: 1989 results from the IVF-ET registry, *Fertil Steril* 55:14-23, 1991, with permission of the publisher, The American Fertility Society, Birmingham, Ala.
*The numbers in parentheses are percentages.

needs. Frustration of the natural drive to procreate, involuntary childlessness, and abnormal biologic conditions often produce significant emotional distress in couples.[43,45,95] The infertile couple is thus at risk for emotional dysfunction, marital conflict, and sexual dysfunction.[46] The emotional and psychologic needs of participants in an IVF program should be considered by those performing the procedure as well as the members of the IVF team, of which a psychologist or counselor may be a member. Consideration of these factors is of importance before initiation of the medication in an IVF cycle. (See Chapter 26.)

PRINCIPLES OF IN VITRO FERTILIZATION

Induction of ovulation

The first successful IVF resulted from the fertilization of a single oocyte recovered from a dominant follicle in a natural cycle.[119] Further experience showed that pregnancy rates were improved by increasing the number of embryos available for transfer through controlled ovarian hyperstimulation.[127] Disadvantages associated with the use of the spontaneous menstrual cycles included frequent testing for the luteinizing hormone (LH) surge. The aims of ovarian stimulation in IVF are to promote the development of a relatively synchronous cohort of follicles. Close approximation of follicular size on ultrasound evaluation facilitates the appropriate timing of human chorionic gonadotropin (hCG) administration for timing of oocyte retrieval. In addition, the collection of multiple mature oocytes that have the capacity to fertilize and cleave is achieved with ovarian stimulation as well as the development of the proper endometrial environment for embryonic support. Newer protocols using GnRHa have minimized the premature LH surges with subsequent lower rates of cycle cancellations due to premature surges or poor parameters of follicular response.

Ovarian stimulation. The objective of ovarian stimulation is recruitment of a cohort of follicles in the time framework of the follicle-stimulating hormone (FSH) recruitment window that occurs between day 3 and day 5 in a 28-day cycle. Clinical monitoring parameters of follicular growth, such as serum estradiol assays and sequential real-time ultrasound measurements of follicular diameter, allow the determination of such critically timed steps such as the discontinuation of stimulatory agents, administration of hCG, and oocyte retrieval. Follicular induction regimens in current use include clomiphene citrate (CC), hMG, pure FSH, and GnRHa in combination with menotropins. In 1981 Trounson and colleagues[121] reported intrauterine pregnancies through transfer of multiple embryos in CC-stimulated IVF cycles. Regimens of CC alone and in combination with hCG as a substitute for the midcycle LH surge were used in the early years of IVF-ET technology to achieve the recruitment of more than one dominant follicle. Clomiphene citrate in doses of 50 to 150 mg/d was administered for 5 days, varying between days 3 and 7 of the cycle along with hCG given according to estrogen response and ultrasound measurement of the diameter of the dominant follicles. In 80% of CC cycles for IVF, oocytes were obtained (average of 1.6 to 2.1 retrieved per cycle). Pregnancy rates for CC cycles ranged from 11% to 20%, with a mean of 1.6 ± 0.2 embryos transferred.[28]

Because of the great variability of follicular response and a 30% to 50% frequency of spontaneous LH surges before hCG administration in patients stimulated by CC, other protocols were pursued.[73] An increase in the number of follicles recruited was seen with hMG supplementation of CC regimens. However, differences in ongoing pregnancy rates when the various treatments were compared were less marked. Investigators using a regimen of CC 100 mg/d on days 3 to 7 concurrent with one ampule of hMG per day described a 19% pregnancy rate per laparoscopic retrieval compared with a CC stimulation success rate of 11%.[134] A statistically significant increase in the total number of developing follicles, oocytes recovered, and embryos cleaving was achieved by administering CC with two ampules of hMG. However, no difference in pregnancy rates between this and single-agent therapy was reported.[37] More recently, reports of pregnancy rates per embryo transfer of 30.2% in patients treated with CC 100 mg/d from days 2 to 6 and hMG two or three ampules daily from day 4 onward were noted.[97] Continued trials of combination regimens suggested a general superiority of multiagent therapy over CC stimulation alone. In combination regimens the number of oocytes obtained was approximately 3 to 5.2 per cycle, with pregnancy rates ranging from 17% to 25% with 2.5 ± 0.3 embryos transferred.

Anticipating that the ovarian response may be more dependable than with CC alone and that the antiestrogenic effects of cervical mucus and the endometrium might be avoided, hMG/hCG treatment was instituted, with hMG administration in doses of one to four ampules per day beginning on day 3 of the cycle. The original two-cell theory for estradiol production described an equivalent activity of FSH and LH. Reflecting on this theory of gonadotropin action, urinary menotropin preparations were formulated at a 1:1 ratio of FSH to LH.[69] One ampule of hMG contains the equivalent of 75 IU of FSH and 75 IU of LH in the form of a lyophilized powder, which is reconstituted with normal saline for intramuscular injection.

Timing of initiation of therapy. The timing of initiation of gonadotropin therapy for controlled ovarian hyperstimulation in normally cycling women is critical for achieving optimal folliculogenesis.[97] The initiation of therapy on cycle day 3 appeared to provide favorable follicular recruitment. Menotropin administration in doses of one to four ampules per day beginning on cycle day 3 resulted in 3.6 to 5.1 oocytes per cycle with pregnancy rates of 20% to 26%. The mean number of embryos transferred was 2.3 ± 0.3. However, in evaluating results from world centers no significant difference was found in any of the stimulation regimens based on pregnancy rate alone.[31] In addition, higher hMG doses may lead to a greater percentage of atretic follicles or premature ovulation.[11] Very high estradiol values may also result in development of an endometrial environment that is hostile to nidation.[11]

Contemporary alterations in stimulation protocols attempted to enhance recruitment of follicles from the gonadotropin-sensitive pool by imitating the usual early follicular phase rise of FSH level in a spontaneous menstrual cycle without exposing the follicles to high concentrations of LH. Early in the cycle, the FSH contained within the hMG mixtures is the dominant component in stimulating folliculogenesis. In vitro studies suggest that the LH in hMG may impair oocyte development and successful implantation by altering theca androgen metabolism early in the cycle,[100] and exposure of the ovaries to a high level of LH during the first half of the follicular phase may be detrimental to IVF-ET success.[82] Gonadotropin preparations with a greater emphasis on pure FSH with minimally detectable LH present were then shown to be capable of stimulating ovarian estradiol secretion at a level not dissimilar to that obtained from the same dose of a urinary hMG preparation containing an equal ratio of FSH and LH.[16]

The elimination of the LH factor in the early portion of the follicular phase appeared to simulate more closely the natural cycle, thus allowing a more homogeneous follicular response and possibly producing oocytes of improved morphology than those produced with a mixed preparation of gonadotropins. The use of pure FSH in IVF-ET programs results in a larger number of oocytes retrieved (mean 5.8 to 8.1), perhaps reflecting events occurring in the FSH recruitment window. Although the addition of pure FSH offers theoretic advantages,[1] published reports have not shown consistently improved pregnancy rates.[12] Other investigators have determined that high-dose FSH stimulation at the onset of the menstrual cycle does not improve IVF-ET outcome in low-responder patients. In patients characterized as low responders,[75] follicular stimulation with FSH alone does not appear to offer a definite enhancement of oocyte quality,[79] particularly in patients with borderline to elevated serum FSH values when sampled in the follicular phase.[73]

Pretreatment with gonadotropin-releasing hormone agonists. Additional contemporary efforts to reduce the individual variability of follicular response to gonadotropin therapy include pretreatment with GnRHa. Administration of a GnRHa before initiation of menotropins maintains a relatively hypogonadotropic state with respect to endogenous gonadotropin secretion, resulting in increased homogeneity of ovarian estradiol secretion during therapy. With luteal phase GnRHa administration, reduction of the confounding problem of individual follicular variation with gonadotropin treatment is achieved, along with more uniform oocyte development. Suppression of endogenous gonadotropin secretion may be achieved by prolonged or short courses of GnRHa. Analogues of GnRH have a high affinity for the GnRH receptor and a decreased resistance to GnRH degradation, compared with the native releasing hormone. Initial exposure of a GnRHa at the pituitary level results in a prompt stimulation of LH and FSH secretion, or a "flare" effect associated with increased serum estradiol levels to a peak of two to four times the basal level. Repeated exposure of the pituitary to a GnRHa results in a reduction of available GnRH receptors, impairment of postreceptor mechanisms, and alternately unresponsiveness of the gonadotropin cells to GnRH. Basal and pulsatile secretions of FSH and LH diminish, and estrogen levels decline because of a lack of follicular stimulation.

Combined therapy with GnRHa and hMG. The combined use of GnRHa and hMG for superovulation in IVF has been advocated by many investigators.[101,127] Two major methods of utilizing GnRHa can be distinguished. In luteal phase suppression,[52] ovarian stimulation is initiated after at least 10 days of luteal phase administration of a GnRHa, continued until the day of hCG injection. Estradiol levels reach castration values of less than 25 pg/mL before the initiation of gonadotropins. The early follicular phase administration of GnRHa or "flare-up" approach,[22] takes advantage of the initial rise of serum gonadotropin levels on analogue administration to enhance follicular recruitment, with continuing administration until the day of hCG

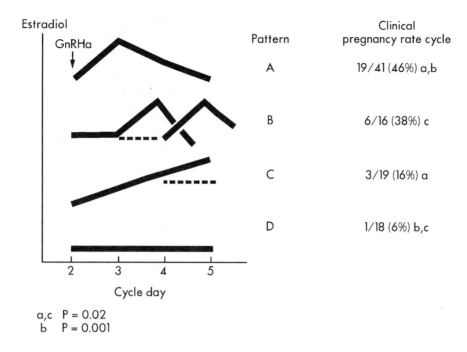

Pattern	Clinical pregnancy rate cycle
A	19/41 (46%) a,b
B	6/16 (38%) c
C	3/19 (16%) a
D	1/18 (6%) b,c

a,c P = 0.02
b   P = 0.001

Fig. 46-1. Pregnancy rates in women receiving follicular phase GnRHa. (Redrawn from Padilla SL et al: *Fertil Steril* 56:79, 1991.)

injection. The usefulness of GnRHa in IVF is associated with a reduction in variability of estradiol patterns in response to exogenous gonadotropin administration[94] and in prevention of premature LH surges. The suppression achieved results in the prevention of recruitment of follicles before exogenous stimulation, allowing a larger and more synchronous cohort of follicles to develop.[63]

In utilizing luteal suppression with GnRHa, patients require significantly more exogenous gonadotropin stimulation to achieve a desired logarithmic rise of circulating estradiol levels. As much as two or three times the total quantity of hMG is required in GnRHa/hMG cycles than in hMG cycles alone.[65] In addition, 2 or 3 extra days of stimulation are often necessary for adequate follicular development.[40] Presumably this prolongation of recruitment is due to absence of follicular response at the onset of hMG therapy. Several investigators have recommended decreasing the dose of analogue to one-half when menotropins are initiated after luteal phase initiation of GnRHa.[56] Other investigators have shown that in high-responder patients a combination of GnRHa and pure FSH results in lower estradiol levels during the stimulation cycle and a greater number of total mature oocytes retrieved and fertilized.[44] Other investigators have evaluated the length of administration of luteal phase suppression and showed no difference in the ovarian response to suppression by analogues for 12, 19, or greater than or equal to 26 days. With respect to numbers of oocytes, retrieval, and fertilization rates, women requiring extended GnRHa treatment responded comparably to those who suppressed quickly.[67]

An alternative technique in follicular stimulation takes advantage of the initial flare in pituitary gonadotropin secretion by introducing the GnRHa on cycle day 1 or 2.[107] Serum FSH values become elevated 1.5- to 6.0-fold over baseline, peaking on day 3 of agonist administration. Menotropin therapy is then usually initiated on cycle day 2 or 3. Some investigators suggest that the beneficial effects of this regimen are more likely to occur if the GnRHa is initiated on cycle day 3 rather than day 1.[14] In addition, some investigators have suggested that a significantly higher pregnancy rate is observed in patients receiving follicular phase GnRHa, compared with luteal phase administration,[54] particularly when patients were classified according to pattern of estradiol response during the first 4 days of leuprolide administration[96] (Fig. 46-1).

GnRHa do not appear to be associated with a measurable effect on fertilization, cleavage, or embryo growth rates. However, profound endocrinologic changes may occur in the luteal phase, such as short-term rescue of the corpus luteum, prevention of endogenous LH surge, and premature luteinization.[89] Improved implantation rates per embryo and a significantly higher ongoing pregnancy rate have been reported with the use of GnRHa/hMG treatment cycles, compared with other protocols.[80] Some investigators have described the flare approach as superior to luteal suppression,[54] whereas others have described the flare protocol as increasing oocyte atresia and reducing embryo quality, compared with stimulation cycles treated with luteal phase GnRHa.[18,82]

Other considerations. Many variables have been assessed with respect to predictive value for the outcome of any individual ovulation induction cycle for IVF. Assessment of follicular diameter and estradiol response patterns as well as evaluation of pretreatment pituitary gonadotropins have been considered. Studies have demonstrated better gonadotropin stimulation quality and pregnancy rates in IVF patients with low basal cycle day 3 FSH levels than in those with elevated FSH baseline values.[112] These laboratory parameters have been useful in counseling patients regarding the probability of achieving pregnancy through IVF and in determining optimal gonadotropin stimulation regimens.[95,111] Other approaches to IVF have included programmed cycles with oral contraceptives, which are reported to be useful in protocols in facilitating scheduling of cycles and prevention of spontaneous LH surges.[57] However, the ovary remains insensitive to gonadotropin stimulation in direct proportion to the time interval of steroid suppression. Prolongation of the latent phase of follicular development is more pronounced with contraceptive pill administration for more than 30 days.[87] Therefore few preovulatory follicles may be obtained after pretreatment with oral contraceptives. In general, GnRHa are the preferred agents for precycle regulation in IVF protocols.

Techniques of oocyte retrieval

Laparoscopic oocyte retrieval. In 1970 Steptoe and Edwards[118] first described the use of the laparoscope for oocyte aspiration, using a medium-gauge needle of 1.2 mm internal diameter placed in the left lower quadrant of the abdomen 7 cm from the midline. Oocyte recovery rate with this technique was 32%. Lopata,[81a] in 1974, using a 20-gauge aspirating needle with a 45° bevel on the end and a separate laparoscope, accessory trocar, and needle system, achieved an oocyte retrieval rate of 45%. These aspirations were performed at 200 mm Hg vacuum pressure. Other approaches include using a Teflon-lined needle system 23 cm long with an internal diameter of 1.6 mm and an external diameter of 2.1 mm resulting in an 80% to 100% egg recovery rate. With this system, 100 mm Hg negative pressure was adequate to obtain satisfactory aspirations.

Present-day IVF-ET laparoscopic aspiration methodology incudes a two-puncture system using an offset operating laparoscope containing an operating channel through which the operating needle is passed. A second puncture is performed for placement of a grasping forceps on the uteroovarian ligament. Oocyte aspiration is accomplished by a single-lumen needle (Teflon lined or without Teflon) ranging in size from 12- to 14-gauge with an internal diameter of 1.2 mm to 2.16 mm. In the Norfolk program a 12-gauge needle with a 2.16-mm internal diameter and a 45° bevel is used.[72] Of particular interest is the raised external band 5 mm from the most distal point of the needle tip that enables the operator to determine the depth of penetration of the needle into the follicle. Suction devices used once the needle is placed into the follicle are either a 50-mL syringe suction (which creates a negative pressure of approximately 200 mm Hg) or a wall suction system

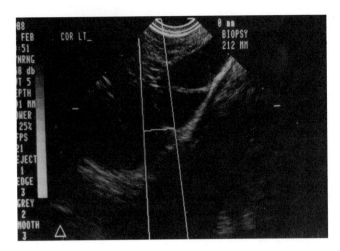

Fig. 46-2. Ultrasound-directed vaginal oocyte retrieval scanner views.

adjusted to approximately 100 mm Hg negative pressure. With the two-puncture system, an egg recovery rate of 89% to 94% has been achieved.

Other IVF teams use the operating laparoscope and a three-puncture technique; the operating channel of the laparoscope is used for lysis of adhesions and/or ovarian mobilization. Recovery rates are between 85% and 90% with this technique.[31] Lysis of adhesions, tubal and ovarian mobilization, and fulguration of ectopic endometrial tissue may be performed at the same time as the IVF-ET attempt, without adverse affects on IVF outcome. Investigators have examined the rate of treatment-independent pregnancies after IVF and reparative surgery, confirming the possibility that the rate of spontaneous conception may be increased, particularly with infertility associated with stage III or stage IV endometriosis.[30]

Ultrasound-directed follicular puncture. The major technique in use for IVF oocyte retrieval is ultrasound-directed follicular puncture, which is especially useful when the ovaries are inaccessible to the laparoscope because of severe adhesive distortion.[49,126] Real-time ultrasound and the modern sector scanner, adapted for use in oocyte retrievals, offer several advantages over laparoscopy, including use of local anesthesia and elimination of possible adverse effects on oocytes during the gas phase of carbon dioxide insufflation during laparoscopy.[81] In addition, patient acceptance of the technique is high, since ultrasound-guided retrieval does not require general anesthesia, possibly allowing additional attempts at IVF-ET. Ultrasound-guided retrieval may be performed through a transvesical approach or through a recently developed transvaginal approach.[36] A transvaginal sector scanner precisely locates follicles with an exact needle-guided puncture line. The viewing capacity of the transvaginal sector scanner is approximately at a 240° angle.[36] The needle guide is placed at an angle of 15° toward the scanner axis, and lines tracing the indicated direction of the needle in the sound field are fed into the scanner and are marked on the

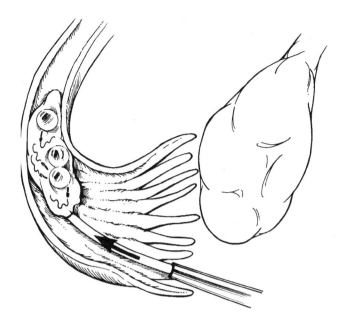

Fig. 46-3. GIFT procedure.[4]

Table 46-3. Outcome by infertility diagnosis and treatment in GIFT

Transfer cycles	Clinical pregnancies*	All deliveries*
335	82 (24)	58 (17)
378	126 (33)	99 (26)
81	28 (35)	19 (23)
704	229 (33)	177 (25)
578	180 (31)	146 (25)

Modified from Medical Research International, Society for Assisted Reproductive Technology, The American Fertility Society: In vitro fertilization-embryo transfer (IVF-ET) in the United States: 1989 results from the IVF-ET registry, *Fertil Steril* 55:14-23, 1991, with permission of the publisher, The American Fertility Society, Birmingham, Ala.
*The numbers in parentheses are percentages.

monitor by an electronic line (Fig. 46-2). Follicular puncture with the vaginal scanner may be carried out with an empty bladder and appears to carry less risk than a freehand technique. Several centers report oocyte retrieval rates between 85% and 95% per follicle with this method. The possibility of infection of the culture medium from a transvaginal route appears to be minimal.

GAMETE INTRAFALLOPIAN TRANSFER

The techniques of IVF-ET have led to a variety of alternative procedures associated with ovarian hyperstimulation and gamete retrieval. The ability of the fallopian tube to serve as the site of fertilization and sperm capacitation in women is the focus of an alternative procedure to IVF-ET, the GIFT procedure.[6,58] This approach involves the transfer of laparoscopically or ultrasonographically retrieved oocytes and washed sperm into the fallopian tube via laparoscopy (Fig. 46-3).[4] The first reported GIFT pregnancy and birth[4,5] occurred in a patient with unexplained infertility. Since that time, the GIFT procedure has been used for the treatment of infertility for many assumed or proven abnormalities in the transfer of sufficient numbers of normal gametes in the fallopian tube. GIFT has been used for patients with unexplained infertility, mild endometriosis, cervical factor, and male factor. Specific results in these diagnostic categories are described in Table 46-3.[90] Before performing a GIFT procedure the presence of at least one patent normal fallopian tube must be documented by laparoscopic examination or hysterosalpingography. An adequate response to superovulatory medications is similar to that obtained in the first step of IVF.

Theoretic advantages of GIFT over IVF-ET include the facts that fertilization occurs in the natural setting, gametes are minimally exposed to the in vitro environment, embryos are prevented from prematurely entering the endometrial cavity, and early embryo development does not occur in the laboratory, which may induce a lag in embryonic development. IVF-ET, however, has certain advantages over the GIFT procedure: documentation of fertilization, which is not possible with the GIFT procedure, and the ability to perform the procedure with ultrasound guidance completely, rather than with laparoscopy. Pregnancy rates with GIFT have been 20% to 23% per cycle; however, a randomized, controlled trial comparing GIFT and IVF-ET showed no significant differences in the pregnancy rates of couples presenting with idiopathic infertility.[79a] The overall success rate of the GIFT procedure may also be addressed in the context of patient selection.

LABORATORY MANAGEMENT OF IN VITRO FERTILIZATION

The success of any IVF program is highly correlated with careful attention to quality control procedures, maintenance of sterility, and attention to detail in the oocyte/embryo culture laboratory. Quality control standards are followed for the preparation of culture media and serum supplements used for follicular aspiration, semen preparation, oocyte culture, embryo culture, and embryo transfer.

Preparation of culture media

Standard culture media in widespread use in IVF laboratories include Ham's F-10 (GIBCO No. 430-1200) and Dulbecco's phosphate-buffered saline (GIBCO No. 3104287). Ham's F-10 is routinely used for oocyte culture, embryo culture, embryo transfer, and sperm washing. Dulbecco's phosphate-buffered saline is used at the time of oocyte retrieval for aspiration/needle flushing before and after follicular puncture. Before use in a human IVF procedure, each aliquot of medium is tested for embryo toxicity in the mouse embryo system and evaluated for its ability to enhance or promote the development of mouse embryos from the two-cell stage to the blastocyst stage. The blastocyst stage is observed after approximately 75 hours of culture. However, serum that inhibits embryo development can in most cases be identified after only 24 hours of culture.[115] Preparations of media that pass the mouse embryo test are used during the laboratory phase of IVF-ET. At the time of quality control testing, each medium is adjusted to an osmolarity of 280 mOsm/kg with sterile distilled water. Antibiotics such as 0.7 mL of a reconstituted penicillin-streptomycin (GIBCO No. 600-5145) may be added to each 100 mL of medium.

Culture medium for human IVF-ET has been supplemented with serum of various sources to improve culture conditions. Serum is also added to media used for preparation of sperm by the swim-up technique.[64] Serum has been obtained from various sources for human IVF-ET, including fetal cord serum, patient-specific serum, female donor serum, and pooled male serum. After centrifugation, serum is heat inactivated, filter sterilized, and frozen in separate lots at −20°C. Aliquots of each sample are tested for human immunodeficiency virus and hepatitis viruses. The use of serum supplements in human IVF-ET is prompted by the possibility that components present in serum may protect maturing oocytes from undergoing premature zona pellucida modification that would generate an egg of reduced fertilizability. Although controversial, studies have shown that IVF performed in the absence of serum[42] results in a 90% reduction in standard fertilization parameters in mouse eggs. The difficulties inherent with a serum system as described are that serum may be contaminated with viruses or other contagious organisms. Serum also may contain an unknown amount of antibodies or substances that interfere with fertilization or development.[41] Other substances, including inflammatory mediators released from platelets and white blood cells, are present in unknown and variable amounts.[59,70,106] In addition, serum from patients with minimal to mild endometriosis has been associated with an inhibition of early embryogenesis in a mouse embryo model, which may explain the decreased fertility rates observed in patients with nonobstructive endometriosis.[33]

Investigators have reported no significant differences in fertilization, cleavage, or implantation rates in serum-free culture media.[64] However, inclusion of a protein supplement in media used for oocyte maturation in an animal model system appears to improve IVF and development and has led many IVF-ET programs to include a protein supplement in oocyte maturation and fertilization media.[13] In addition, some laboratories omit serum and add a macromolecule such as bovine serum albumin to minimize variability in a culture system in which differences in fertilization and development may be attributed to the use of serum from different sources.[41] Oocytes that have undergone most or all of the maturation process before retrieval may not require serum to undergo fertilization, which could explain reports that the percentages of fertilization were similar in media containing either serum or bovine serum albumin.[7] Investigation to identify active inhibitory or promoting components in serum or follicular fluid will

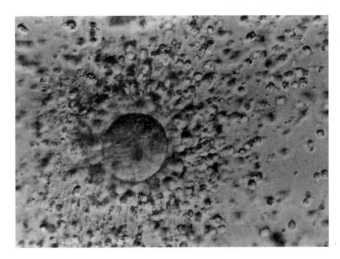

Fig. 46-4. Mature human oocyte approximately 15 minutes after aspiration.

allow further insight into protein and serum factor variables in IVF laboratory parameters.

Preparation of semen

Semen preparation for IVF-ET is of major importance. The sample is liquefied after collection for approximately 30 minutes in a 37°C warming oven. When the sperm concentration has been assessed, the sample is diluted and mixed with at least three times its original volume of insemination medium. Semen samples are centrifuged at 146g for 10 minutes, supernatants are discarded, and pellets are resuspended in fresh insemination medium and centrifuged again. The pellet is gently layered with 0.5 mL of insemination medium and incubated at 37°C for 1 hour, after which the top 0.4 mL of insemination medium containing the highly motile spermatozoa from each tube is combined and transferred. An aliquot of culture medium containing approximately 100,000 motile spermatozoa is added to each culture dish housing a mature oocyte. If a problem or combination of problems exist, such as low count, abnormal motility, or high percentage of abnormal morphology, additional manipulation such as use of a discontinuous colloidal suspension of silica (Percoll) gradient[15] may be necessary to enhance recovery of a population of highly motile and progressive spermatozoa.

Fertilization

Approximately 60% to 90% of human oocytes will fertilize after insemination in vitro (Fig. 46-4).[10] Approximately 15 to 18 hours after insemination, oocytes are examined for morphologic indications of fertilization, which include the formation and extrusion of the second polar body, the presence of two pronuclei, cytoplasm of the oocyte contracted away from the zona pellucida, or normal cleavage. If positive evidence of fertilization cannot be found, the oocytes are transferred to fresh insemination media. Of those oocytes that do not fertilize after initial insemination, 27% to 70% have been reported to fertilize after a fresh insemination with spermatozoa 24 hours later.[17,120] Pregnancy rates were significantly higher with transfers of embryos that cleaved after initial insemination (27% pregnancy rates) than those resulting solely from reinseminated oocytes (3% pregnancy rate). Only 1.3% of reinseminated embryos implanted, compared with a 12.9% implantation rate for those that fertilized and cleaved on initial fertilization.[98] Failure of the reimseminated embryo to produce a pregnancy may be due to abnormality. Failure of the initial insemination may be due to prematurely luteinized oocytes or abnormalities of sperm or oocyte function.[98] In addition, polyspermia may occur during the fertilization process, specifically when oocytes lose their block to polyspermic penetration, a suggestion that zona pellucida alteration has occurred. This may be due to aging of the oocyte[47] or previous sperm exposure.

The predictive value of factors associated with oocyte fertilization rates is difficult to assess. In a large study, grade of sperm motility was the only semen factor related to successful fertilization.[103] Fertilization did occur significantly more often in women with tubal infertility and in cases of secondary infertility, but the predictability of these variables was not reliable. Investigators have considered the first IVF cycle as a test fertilization "of oocyte and sperm," particularly in patients with unexplained infertility.[103]

Zygote monitoring

If fertilization is evident, the zygote or pronucleated oocyte is evaluated and transferred to growth medium for further development. Fertilized oocytes are placed back into a 5% carbon dioxide incubator under the same conditions used earlier during insemination. The fertilized oocyte is then observed for 38 to 40 hours after insemination for dividing cells of approximately equal size. After examination and evaluation the preembryos are placed back into the 5% carbon dioxide incubator. At this time embryo transfer is scheduled 43 to 48 hours after insemination.

Normally cleaving two-cell embryos may be observed any time after 22 hours postinsemination, usually at approximately 24 hours, and may be seen up to 44 hours post-insemination (Fig. 46-5). Four-cell stages are observed routinely between 36 and 50 hours postinsemination and the six- to eight-cell stages are seen after 48 hours. It is in a 48-hour and in some cases 72-hour period that embryo transfer is performed. Before embryo transfer the oocyte should have been fertilized normally, with blastomeres appearing healthy irrespective of size and fragmentation. If there are more than four or five normal embryos, excess embryos usually are cryopreserved, and thawed and replaced in a subsequent cycle if implantation failed to occur after the fresh embryo transfer.

Other methods of fertilization and culture

In the past decade IVF has undergone a number of

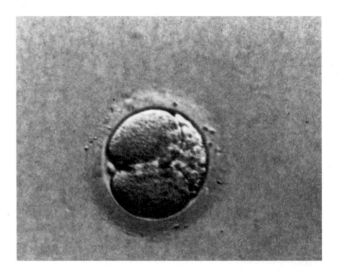

Fig. 46-5. Two-cell human embryo 38 hours postinsemination.

modifications both in ovulation induction and oocyte retrieval technology. Standard culture methodology has been described; however, other investigators have suggested simplified methods of fertilization such as intravaginal culture and microvolume straw. Intravaginal culture involves placing up to 10 oocytes into a 3-mL tube completely filled with culture medium with a concentration of 10,000 to 20,000 motile sperm per milliliter. The tube is hermetically sealed without either air or carbon dioxide, wrapped tightly in a Cryoflex envelope, placed into the vagina, and held in place with a diaphragm for approximately 44 to 50 hours. After removal of the tube the contents are poured into a Petri dish and examined for the presence of embryos.[104] A live birth rate of 13.5% has been reported with this technique. The intravaginal culture technique demonstrated that early embryo development can occur in the absence of either carbon dioxide or air. A 9-mL capillary tube is then used, and oocytes are aspirated in a microconcentration of 2000 to 4000 motile sperm. The straw is incubated at 37° C for 18 to 36 hours, and the contents are evaluated for fertilization. The straw technique yielded a 51.8% cleavage rate. These culture modifications represent a simplification of the laboratory steps currently necessary for IVF.[104]

EMBRYO TRANSFER AND THE LUTEAL PHASE

The technique of embryo transfer is usually accomplished with minimal difficulty. In the laboratory the embryos are loaded into an open-ended Teflon catheter with medium and air spaces in the following manner: 5 mL of medium, 5 mL of air, embryos, 5 mL of air, and 5 mL of medium. Before the procedure the patient is prepared for the embryo transfer on a suitable examining table with a sterile speculum placed in the vaginal canal. The cervix and vaginal vault are cleansed with warm Dulbecco's solution. The catheter is placed through the cervix into the uterine cavity, and the embryos are gently deposited with a slow

Table 46-4. Pregnancy rates versus number of embryos transferred

No. of embryos transferred	Pregnancy rate (%)
1	9–10
2	12–15
3	15–20
≥4	20–25

From Damewood MD, editor: *The Johns Hopkins handbook of in vitro fertilization and assisted reproductive technologies,* Boston, 1990, Little, Brown.

depression on the plunger of a 1-mL tuberculin syringe. Approximately 0.5 mL of air is required in the tuberculin syringe for complete depression of the plunger. The embryo transfer may be accomplished easily with placement of the catheter into the plane of the uterine axis that was predetermined at the time of oocyte retrieval.

Many instrument alternatives to Teflon catheters are available, particularly if a tortuous cervical canal is present. Although the embryo transfer is the simplest procedure associated with IVF, it is the procedure associated with the success rate of each individual cycle. An increasing number of embryos is associated with a higher pregnancy rate per transfer (Table 46-4).[29] However, endometrial receptivity may be the current rate-limiting step in the outcome of any IVF-ET individual cycle.[99] An asynchrony of the uterine endometrium, possibly induced by exogenous gonadotropins, has been investigated. Endometrium that has been altered by gonadotropin therapy may not be as receptive to implantation as endometrium during a natural cycle. This concept has been addressed in a study showing that clinical and ongoing pregnancy rates per cycle were higher in a group of patients who received embryos in a donor egg program but who did not receive the standard controlled ovarian hyperstimulation regimen given to the group of IVF patients.[99] A recent study reported that an artificial cycle mimicked the natural cycle, with endometrial biopsy results indistinguishable from those of natural cycles. Thus it is most likely that controlled ovarian hyperstimulation results in a hormonal environment that is inhibitory to embryo implantation.

Elevated estradiol secretion arising from multiple follicular stimulation may also have a detrimental effect on successful embryo implantation.[53] Additional studies have confirmed the existence of a shortened luteal phase and decreased progesterone production, reflected by urinary pregnanediol levels in gonadotropin-stimulated cycles.[91,102] Other investigations of the histology of the endometrium in IVF-ET patient cycles showed specimens having a normal in-phase histologic appearance but with an atypical pattern of protein secretion.[86] In addition, high luteal phase estrogen production may inhibit pituitary gonadotropin secretion and disrupt corpus luteum function.[88]

To promote an improved endometrial environment for nidation after ovarian stimulation, a protocol for luteal phase support has been used. A retrospective study evaluating luteal phase support using hCG and progesterone after embryo transfer in which the cycle included GnRHa pretreatment showed that clinical pregnancy rates and ongoing pregnancy rates were significantly higher in cycles with hCG luteal phase supplementation.[19] In other studies, cycles treated with GnRHa were associated with a significantly higher pregnancy rate with luteal phase hCG supplementation.[61] Progesterone administration initiated before either embryo transfer or ovulation is also employed as luteal phase support. In a study evaluating the efficacy of preovulatory progesterone administration on endometrial maturation and implantation rates, pregnancy rates per ET for patients who received progesterone supplementation initiated on the day of hCG administration were significantly higher than for those who did not receive the progesterone supplementation.[9] Other investigators have suggested that the addition of GnRHa pituitary suppression to the hMG ovarian stimulation improves the clinical IVF pregnancy rates by widening the implantation window from 7 days to 9 days after embryo transfer. This finding may in part explain the improved IVF-ET success rates with GnRHa/hMG stimulation protocols.[122] The time framework of administration of hCG should be considered when early pregnancy testing is performed after embryo transfer. Reports have shown the presence of hCG in the serum for as long as 10 to 14 days after injection of 10,000 IU.[32]

Asynchrony may also exist between embryo development in vitro and embryo development in vivo. Human embryos reach the blastocyst stage in vivo at approximately 100 hours, compared with 120 hours with in vitro incubation. This lag in embryo development may be associated with the percentage of successful implantation associated with any single IVF cycle. The receptivity of any one human cycle to the establishment of pregnancy may only be 20% to 25% per "cycle," since natural pregnancy rates appear to approach a similar statistical range of implantation per cycle according to life table analysis.

SUMMARY

In vitro fertilization and assisted reproductive technologies have provided the possibility of reproduction for those couples with infertility untreatable by contemporary methodology. Not only has in vitro fertilization provided the opportunity for insight into the workings of hypothalamic pituitary ovarian axis, but also has allowed observation of human gamete interaction in the laboratory. Investigations in the human in vitro fertilization laboratory have stimulated the development and refinement of assisted fertilization techniques. In addition, preimplantation diagnosis and genetic evaluation of blastomeres has also emanated from this technology and will be further refined in the 1990s. No recent procedure applicable to humans in the field of medicine has provided such insight in the short period of time since its inception and successful application in 1978.

REFERENCES

1. Abdalla HI et al: The effect of the dose of human chorionic gonadotropin and the type of gonadotropin stimulation on oocyte recovery rates in an in vitro fertilization program, *Fertil Steril* 48:958, 1987.
2. Allen NC et al: Intrauterine insemination: a critical review, *Fertil Steril* 44:569, 1986.
3. American Fertility Society: Revised American Fertility Society classification of endometriosis: 1985, *Fertil Steril* 43:351, 1985.
4. Asch RH et al: Pregnancy after translaparoscopic gamete intrafallopian transfer, *Lancet* 2:1034, 1984.
5. Asch RH et al: Birth following gamete intrafallopian transfer, *Lancet* 2:163, 1985.
6. Asch RH et al: Gamete intra-fallopian transfer (GIFT): a new treatment for infertility, *Int J Fertil* 30:41, 1985.
7. Ashwood-Smith MJ, Hollands P, Edwards RG: The use of Albuminar 5 (TM) as a medium supplement in clinical IVF, *Hum Reprod* 4:702, 1989.
8. Awadalla SG et al: In vitro fertilization and embryo transfer as a treatment for male factor infertility, *Fertil Steril* 47:807, 1987.
9. Ben-nun I et al: Effect of preovulatory progesterone administration on the endometrial maturation and implantation rate after in vitro fertilization and embryo transfer, *Fertil Steril* 53:276, 1990.
10. Ben-Rafael Z et al: Fertilization and cleavage after reinsemination of human oocytes in vitro, *Fertil Steril* 45:58, 1986.
11. Ben-Rafael Z et al: Dose of human menopausal gonadotropin influences the outcome of an in vitro fertilization program, *Fertil Steril* 48:964, 1987.
12. Benadiva CA et al: An increased initial follicle-stimulatory hormone/luteinizing hormone ratio does not affect ovarian responses and the outcome of in vitro fertilization, *Fertil Steril* 50:777, 1988.
13. Benadiva CA et al: Bovine serum albumin (BSA) can replace patient serum as a protein source in an in vitro fertilization (IVF) program, *J In Vitro Fert Embryo Transfer* 6:164, 1989.
14. Benadiva CA et al: Comparison of different regimens of a gonadotropin-releasing hormone analog during ovarian stimulation for in vitro fertilization, *Fertil Steril* 53:479, 1990.
15. Berger T, Marrs RP, Moyer DL: Comparison of techniques for selection of motile spermatozoa, *Fertil Steril* 43:268, 1985.
16. Bernardus RE et al: The significance of the ratio in follicle-stimulating hormone and luteinizing hormone in induction of multiple follicular growth, *Fertil Steril* 43:373, 1985.
17. Boldt J et al: The value of oocyte reinsemination in human in vitro fertilization, *Fertil Steril* 48:617, 1987.
18. Brzyski RG et al: Follicular atresia associated with concurrent initiation of gonadotropin-releasing hormone agonist and follicle-stimulating hormone for oocyte recruitment, *Fertil Steril* 50:917, 1988.
19. Buvat J et al: Luteal support after luteinizing hormone-releasing hormone agonist for in vitro fertilization: superiority of human chorionic gonadotropin over oral progesterone, *Fertil Steril* 53:490, 1990.
20. Campagnoli C et al: Patient selection for in vitro fertilization (IVF) and embryo transfer (ET), *Experientia* 41:1491, 1985.
21. Chan CLK et al: Oocyte donation and in vitro fertilization for hypergonadotropic hypergonadism: clinical state of the art, *Obstet Gynecol Surv* 42:350, 1987.
22. Charbonnel B et al: L'Association d'un analogue de la LHRH aux gonadotrophines améliorer le recrutement folliculaire et le taux de grossesse (fécondation in vitro), *Ann Endocrinol* 4:262, 1986.
23. Chillik CF et al: The role of in vitro fertilization in infertile patients with endometriosis, *Fertil Steril* 44:56, 1985.
24. Cohen J et al: In vitro fertilization: a treatment for male infertility, *Fertil Steril* 43:422, 1985.
25. Craft I et al: Sperm number and in vitro fertilization, *Lancet* 2:1165, 1981.
26. Daly DC: Advances in infertility therapy, *Compr Ther* 11:60, 1985.
27. Damewood MD: The role of the new reproductive technologies including IVF and GIFT in endometriosis, *Obstet Gynecol Clin North Am* 16:179, 1989.
28. Damewood MD: Current technology of in vitro fertilization and embryo transfer, *Md Med J* 39:331, 1990.
29. Damewood MD, editor: *The Johns Hopkins handbook of in vitro fertilization and assisted reproductive technologies,* Boston, 1990, Little, Brown.
30. Damewood MD, Rock JA: Treatment independent pregnancy with operative laparoscopy for endometriosis in an in vitro fertilization program, *Fertil Steril* 50:463, 1988.
31. Damewood MD, Wallach EE: IVF update, *Postgrad Obstet Gynecol* 6:1, 1986.
32. Damewood MD et al: Disappearance of exogenously administered human chorionic gonadotropin, *Fertil Steril* 51:398, 1989.
33. Damewood MD et al: Effect of serum from patients with minimal to mild endometriosis on mouse embryo development in vitro, *Fertil Steril* 54:917, 1990.
34. Damewood MD et al: Preparative GnRH agonist suppression and enhanced fertilization for stage III-IV endometriosis. Paper presented at the American Fertility Society 46th Annual Meeting, Washington, DC, Oct 13–18, 1990 (program supplement P-135 [S 121]).
35. DeCherney AH et al: Reproductive outcome following two ectopic pregnancies, *Fertil Steril* 43:82, 1985.
36. Dellenbach P et al: Transvaginal sonographically controlled follicle puncture for oocyte retrieval, *Fertil Steril* 44:656, 1985.
37. Diamond MP et al: Comparison of human menopausal gonadotropin, clomiphene citrate, and combined human menopausal gonadotropin-clomiphene citrate stimulation protocols for in vitro fertilization, *Fertil Steril* 46:1108, 1986.
38. Dmowski WP, Radwanska E: Endometriosis and infertility, *Acta Obstet Gynecol Scand Suppl* 123:73, 1984.
39. Dodson WC et al: Superovulation with intrauterine insemination in the treatment of infertility: a possible alternative to gamete intrafallopian transfer and in vitro fertilization, *Fertil Steril* 48:441, 1987.
40. Droesch K et al: Value of suppression with a gonadotropin releasing hormone agonist prior to gonadotropin stimulation for in vitro fertilization, *Fertil Steril* 51:292, 1989.
41. Ducibella T, Kopf GS, Schultz RM: Use of serum and timing of insemination for in vitro fertilization (IVF), *J In Vitro Fert Embryo Transfer* 7:121, 1990.
42. Ducibella T et al: Precocious loss of cortical granules during mouse oocyte meiotic maturation and correlation with an egg-induced modification of the zona pellucida, *Dev Biol* 137:46, 1990.
43. Edelmann RJ, Connolly KJ: Psychological aspects of infertility, *Br J Med Psychol* 59:209, 1986.
44. Edelstein MC et al: Ovarian stimulation for in vitro fertilization using pure follicle stimulating hormone with and without gonadotropin releasing hormone agonist in high responder patients, *J In Vitro Fert Embryo Transfer* 7:172, 1990.
45. Fagan PJ, Ponticas Y: Psychological issues in IVF: evaluation and care. In Damewood MD, editor: *The Johns Hopkins handbook of in vitro fertilization and assisted reproductive technologies,* Boston, 1990, Little, Brown.
46. Fagan PJ et al: Sexual functioning and psychologic evaluation of in vitro fertilization couples, *Fertil Steril* 46:668, 1986.
47. Familiari G et al: Is the sperm-binding capacity of the zona pellucida linked to its surface structure?: a scanning electron microscopic study of human in vitro fertilization, *J In Vitro Fert Embryo Transfer* 5:134, 1988.
48. Federation CECOS, Schwartz D, Mayaux MJ: Female fecundity as a function of age: results of artificial insemination in 2193 nulliparous

women with azoospermic husbands, *N Engl J Med* 306:404, 1982.

49. Feichtinger W, Kemeter P: Laparoscopic or ultrasonically guided follicle aspiration for in vitro fertilization?, *J In Vitro Fert Embryo Transfer* 1:244, 1984.

50. Feichtinger W, Kemeter P: Pregnancy after total ovariectomy achieved by ovum donation, *Lancet* 2:722, 1985.

51. Fisch B et al: The relationship between sperm parameters and fertilizing capacity in vitro: a predictive role for swim-up migration, *J In Vitro Fert Embryo Transfer* 7:38, 1990.

52. Fleming R, Coutts JRT: Induction of multiple follicular growth in normally menstruating women with endogenous gonadotropin suppression, *Fertil Steril* 45:226, 1986.

53. Forman R et al: Evidence for an adverse effect of elevated serum estradiol concentrations on embryo implantation, *Fertil Steril* 49:118, 1988.

54. Garcia JE et al: Follicular phase gonadotropin-releasing hormone agonist and human gonadotropins: a better alternative for ovulation induction in in vitro fertilization, *Fertil Steril* 53:302, 1990.

55. Gianaroli L et al: The role of the patient's age in the outcome of IVF cycles, *Hum Reprod* 3(suppl)1:83, 1988.

56. Gindoff PR, Hall JL, Stillman RJ: Ovarian suppression with leuprolide acetate: comparison of luteal, follicular, and flare-up administration in controlled ovarian hyperstimulation for oocyte retrieval, *J In Vitro Fert Embryo Transfer* 7:94, 1990.

57. Gonen Y, Jacobson W, Casper RF: Gonadotropin suppression with oral contraceptives before in vitro fertilization, *Fertil Steril* 53:282, 1990.

58. Guastella G, Comparetto G, Gullo D: Gamete intra-fallopian transfer (GIFT): a new technique for the treatment of unexplained infertility, *Acta Eur Fertil* 16:311, 1985.

59. Halliwell B, Gutteridge JMC, editors: *Free radicals in biology and medicine,* Oxford, UK, 1986, Clarendon Press.

60. Hargreave TB, Elton RA: Treatment with intermittent high dose methylprednisolone or intermittent betamethasone for antisperm antibodies: preliminary communication, *Fertil Steril* 38:586, 1982.

61. Herman A et al: Pregnancy rate and ovarian hyperstimulation after luteal human chorionic gonadotropin in in vitro fertilization stimulated with gonadotropin-releasing hormone analog and menotropins, *Fertil Steril* 53:92, 1990.

62. Hirsch I et al: In vitro fertilization in couples with male factor infertility, *Fertil Steril* 45:659, 1986.

63. Hodgen GD et al: Selection of the dominant ovarian follicle and hormonal enhancement of the natural cycle, *Ann N Y Acad Sci* 442:23, 1985.

64. Holst N et al: Optimization and simplification of culture conditions in human in vitro fertilization (IVF) and preembryo replacement by serum-free media, *J In Vitro Fert Embryo Transfer* 7:47, 1990.

65. Horvath PM et al: Exogenous gonadotropin requirements are increased in leuprolide suppressed women undergoing ovarian stimulation, *Fertil Steril* 49:159, 1988.

66. Hurst BS, Schlaff WD: Andrologic parameters for IVF-ET. In Damewood MD, editor: *The Johns Hopkins handbook of in vitro fertilization and assisted reproductive technologies,* Boston, 1990, Little, Brown.

67. Ibrahim ZH et al: Use of buserelin in an IVF programme for pituitary-ovarian suppression prior to ovarian stimulation with exogenous gonadotropins, *Hum Reprod* 5:258, 1990.

68. Jacobs LA et al: Primary microsurgery for post-inflammatory tubal infertility, *Fertil Steril* 50:855, 1988.

69. Jacobson A, Marshall JR: Ovulatory response rate with human menopausal gonadotropins of varying FSH/LH ratios, *Fertil Steril* 20:171, 1969.

70. Jinno M, Iida E, Iizuka R: A detrimental effect of platelets on mouse embryo development, *J Vitro Fert Embryo Transfer* 4:324, 1987.

71. Jones HW Jr: Impact of in vitro fertilization, *Int J Fertil* 31:108, 1986.

72. Jones HW Jr, Acosta AA, Garcia J: A technique for the aspiration of oocytes from human ovarian follicles, *Fertil Steril* 37:26, 1982.

73. Jones HW Jr et al: The importance of the follicular phase to success and failure in in vitro fertilization, *Fertil Steril* 40:317, 1983.

74. Jones HW Jr et al: Three years of in-vitro fertilization at Norfolk, *Fertil Steril* 42:826, 1984.

75. Karande VC et al: High-dose follicle-stimulating hormone stimulation at the onset of the menstrual cycle does not improve the in vitro fertilization outcome in low-responder patients, *Fertil Steril* 53:186, 1990.

76. Katz E, Hurst BS: Selection of patients for in vitro fertilization-embryo transfer. In Damewood MD, editor: *The Johns Hopkins handbook of in vitro fertilization and assisted reproductive technologies,* Boston, 1990, Little, Brown.

77. Laotikainen TJ et al: Factors influencing the success of microsurgery for distal tubal occlusion, *Arch Gynecol Obstet* 243:101, 1988.

78. Lauritzen JG et al: Results of repeated tuboplasties, *Fertil Steril* 37:68, 1982.

79. Lavy G et al: Ovarian stimulation for in vitro fertilization and embryo transfer, human menopausal gonadotropin versus pure human follicle stimulating hormone: a randomized prospective study, *Fertil Steril* 50:74, 1988.

79a. Leeton J et al: A controlled study between the use of gamete intrafallopian transfer (GIFT) and in vitro fertilization and embryo transfer in the management of idiopathic and male infertility. *Fertil Steril* 48:605, 1987.

80. Lejeune B, Barlow P, Puissant F: Use of buserelin acetate in an in vitro fertilization program: a comparison with classical clomiphene citrate-human menopausal gonadotropin treatment, *Fertil Steril* 54:475, 1990.

81. Lenz S, Lauritsen JG: Ultrasonically guided percutaneous aspiration of human follicles under local anesthesia: a new method of collecting oocytes for in vitro fertilization, *Fertil Steril* 38:673, 1982.

81a. Lopata A et al: Collection of human oocytes with laparoscopy and laparotomy, *Fertil Steril* 25:1030, 1974.

82. Loumaye E et al: Hormonal changes induced by short-term administration of a gonadotropin-releasing hormone agonist during ovarian hyperstimulation for in vitro fertilization and their consequences for embryo development, *Fertil Steril* 51:105, 1989.

83. Lutjen P et al: The establishment and maintenance of pregnancy using in vitro fertilization and embryo donation in a patient with primary ovarian failure, *Nature* 307:174, 1984.

84. Mahadevan MM, Trounson AO: The influence of seminal characteristics on the success rate of human in vitro fertilization, *Fertil Steril* 42:400, 1984.

85. Mahadevan MM, Trounson AO, Leeton JF: The relationship of tubal blockage, infertility of unknown cause, suspected male infertility, and endometriosis to success of in vitro fertilization and embryo transfer, *Fertil Steril* 40:755, 1983.

86. Manners CV: Endometrial assessment in a group of infertile women on stimulated cycles for IVF: immunohistochemical findings, *Hum Reprod* 5:128, 1990.

87. Marrs RP et al: The effect of the time of initiation of clomiphene citrate on multiple follicular development for human in vitro fertilization and embryo replacement procedures, *Fertil Steril* 42:682, 1984.

88. Martikainen H et al: Anterior pituitary dysfunction during the luteal phase following ovarian hyperstimulation, *Fertil Steril* 47:446, 1987.

89. Martikainen H et al: Endocrine responses to gonadotropins after LHRH agonist administration on cycle days 1-4: prevention of premature luteinization, *Hum Reprod* 5:246, 1990.

90. Medical Research International, Society for Assisted Reproductive Technology, The American Fertility Society: In vitro fertilization-embryo transfer (IVF-ET) in the United States: 1989 results from the IVF-ET Registry, *Fertil Steril* 55:14, 1991.

91. Messinis IE, Templeton A, Baird DT: Luteal phase after ovarian hyperstimulation, *Br J Obstet Gynaecol* 94:345, 1987.

92. Moghissi KS, Wallach EE: Unexplained infertility, *Fertil Steril* 39:5, 1983.

93. Morse CA, Van Hall EV: Psychosocial aspects of infertility: a review of current concepts, *J Psychosom Obstet Gynaecol* 6:157, 1987.

94. Muasher SJ: Stimulation protocols for patients with "atypical response," *Ann N Y Acad Sci* 541:82, 1988.

95. Muasher SJ et al: The value of basal and/or stimulated serum gonadotropin levels in prediction of stimulation response and in vitro fertilization outcome, *Fertil Steril* 50:298, 1988.

96. Padilla SL, Smith RD, Garcia JE: The Lupron screening test: tailoring the use of leuprolide acetate in ovarian stimulation for in vitro fertilization, *Fertil Steril* 56:79, 1991.

97. Pampiglione JS et al: The effect of cycle length on the outcome of in vitro fertilization, *Fertil Steril* 50:603, 1988.

98. Pampiglione JS et al: The clinical outcome of reinsemination of human oocytes fertilized in vitro, *Fertil Steril* 53:306, 1990.

99. Paulson RJ, Sauer MV, Lobo RA: Embryo implantation after human in vitro fertilization: importance of endometrial receptivity, *Fertil Steril* 53:870, 1990.

100. Polan ML: Ovulation induction with human menopausal gonadotropin compared to human urinary follicle-stimulating hormone results in a significant shift in follicular fluid androgen levels without discernible differences in granulosa-luteal cell function, *J Clin Endocrinol Metab* 63:1284, 1986.

101. Porter RN et al: Induction of ovulation for in vitro fertilization using buserelin and gonadotropins, *Lancet* 2:1284, 1984.

102. Quigley MM: Selection of agents for enhanced follicular recruitment in an in vitro fertilization and embryo replacement program, *Ann N Y Acad Sci* 442:96, 1985.

103. Ramsewak SS et al: Are factors that influence oocyte fertilization also predictive?: an assessment of 148 cycles of in vitro fertilization without gonadotropin stimulation, *Fertil Steril* 54:470, 1990.

104. Ranoux C, Seibel MM: New techniques in fertilization: intravaginal culture and microvolume straw, *J In Vitro Fert Embryo Transfer* 7:6, 1990.

105. Rock J, Menkin MF: In vitro fertilization and cleavage of human ovarian eggs, *Science* 100:105, 1944.

106. Ross R, Raines EW, Bowen-Pope DF: The biology of platelet-derived growth factor, *Cell* 46:155, 1986.

107. Sathanandan M et al: Adjuvant leuprolide in normal, abnormal and poor responders to controlled ovarian hyperstimulation for in vitro fertilization/gamete intrafallopian transfer, *Fertil Steril* 51:998, 1989.

108. Schmidt CL: Endometriosis: a reappraisal of pathogenesis and treatment, *Fertil Steril* 44:157, 1985.

109. Schoysman R: Tubal microsurgery versus in vitro fertilization, *Acta Eur Fertil* 15:5, 1984.

110. Schumacher GFB et al: In vitro fertilization of human ova and blastocyst transfer: an invitational symposium, *J Reprod Med* 11:192, 1973.

111. Scott RT et al: Follicle-stimulating hormone levels on cycle day 3 are predictive of in vitro fertilization outcome, *Fertil Steril* 51:651, 1989.

112. Scott RT et al: Intercycle variability of day 3 follicle-stimulating hormone levels and its effect on stimulation quality in in vitro fertilization, *Fertil Steril* 54:297, 1990.

113. Segal S, Casper RF: The response to ovarian hyperstimulation and in vitro fertilization in women older than 35 years, *Hum Reprod* 5:255, 1990.

114. Serhal PF et al: Unexplained infertility: the value of Pergonal superovulation combined with intrauterine insemination, *Fertil Steril* 49:602, 1988.

115. Shirley B et al: Effects of human serum and plasma on development of mouse embryos in culture media, *Fertil Steril* 43:129, 1985.

116. Steptoe P: The selection of couples for in vitro fertilization and embryo replacement, *Ann N Y Acad Sci* 442:187, 1985.

117. Steptoe P: Historical aspects of the ethics of in-vitro fertilization, *Ann N Y Acad Sci* 442:602, 1988.

118. Steptoe PC, Edwards RC: Laparoscopic recovery of preovulatory human oocytes after priming of ovaries with gonadotropins, *Lancet* 1:683, 1970.

119. Steptoe PC, Edwards RC: Birth after reimplantation of a human embryo, *Lancet* 2:366, 1978.

120. Trounson A, Webb J: Fertilization of human oocytes following reinsemination in vitro, *Fertil Steril* 41:816, 1984.

121. Trounson AO et al: Pregnancies in humans by fertilization in vitro and embryo transfer, *Science* 212:682, 1981.

122. Tur-Kaspa I et al: Ovarian stimulation protocol for in vitro fertilization with gonadotropin-releasing hormone agonist widens the implantation window, *Fertil Steril* 53:859, 1990.

123. Utian WH et al: Successful pregnancy after in vitro fertilization and embryo transfer from an infertile woman to a surrogate, *N Engl J Med* 313:1251, 1985.

124. Van Uem JFHM et al: Male factor evaluation in in vitro fertilization: Norfolk experience, *Fertil Steril* 44:375, 1985.

125. Wardle PG et al: Endometriosis and ovulatory disorders: reduced fertilization in vitro compared with tubal and unexplained infertility, *Lancet* 2:236, 1985.

126. Wikland M et al: Collection of human oocytes by the use of sonography, *Fertil Steril* 39:603, 1983.

127. Wildt L et al: Ovarian hyperstimulation for in vitro fertilization controlled by GnRH agonist administered in combination with human menopausal gonadotropins, *Hum Reprod* 1:15, 1986.

128. Wiley LM et al: Detection of antisperm antibodies: their localization to human antigens that are transferred to the surface of zona-free hamster oocytes during the sperm penetration assay, *Fertil Steril* 48:292, 1987.

129. Wilkes CA et al: Pregnancy related to infertility diagnosis, number of attempts, and age in a program of in vitro fertilization, *Obstet Gynecol* 66:350, 1985.

130. Williams RF, Hodgen GD: Disparate effects of human chorionic gonadotropin during the late follicular phase in monkeys: normal ovulation, follicular atresia, ovarian acyclicity, and hypersecretion of follicle stimulation hormone, *Fertil Steril* 33:64, 1980.

131. Wolf DO: Semen assessment in IVF, *J In Vitro Fert Embryo Transfer* 3:341, 1986.

132. Wolf DP et al: Sperm concentration and the fertilization of human eggs in vitro, *Biol Reprod* 31:837, 1984.

133. World Health Organization: *Laboratory manual for the examination of human semen and semen-cervical mucus interaction,* Cambridge, UK, 1987, Cambridge University Press.

134. Yee B, Vargyas JM: Multiple follicle development utilizing combinations of clomiphene citrate and human menopausal gonadotropins, *Clin Obstet Gynecol* 29:141, 1986.

135. Yovich JL, Stanger JD: The limitations of in vitro fertilization from males with severe oligospermia and abnormal sperm morphology, *J In Vitro Fert Embryo Transfer* 1:172, 1984.

136. Yovich JL et al: In vitro fertilization for endometriosis, *Lancet* 2:552, 1985.

Chapter 47

THE CRYOPRESERVATION OF HUMAN EGGS AND EMBRYOS

Alan Trounson, PhD
and Jillian Shaw, PhD

Cryopreservation of human embryos
    Cryopreservation by slow cooling techniques
    Results of freezing human embryos by slow cooling techniques
    Cryopreservation by rapid freezing and vitrification techniques
Cryopreservation of human oocytes
    Problems for the efficient cryopreservation of oocytes
    Cryopreservation of mature oocytes by slow cooling techniques
    Cryopreservation of oocytes by rapid freezing techniques

Table 47-1. Summary of methods used for cryopreservation of human embryos (pronuclear oocytes to four-cell embryos) in PROH

Step	Protocol*
Freezing solution	1.5 M PROH + 0.1 M sucrose in PBS + 20% human serum
Equilibration	15 min at RT in 1.5 M PROH; transfer to freezing solution and cool
Cooling rates	2°C/min to −7°C, seeding, then 0.3°C to −30°C
Rapid cooling and storage	50°C/min from −30°C to −190°C; store in LN
Thawing	In a 30°C water bath for 40 s
Removal of cryoprotectant	1.0 M PROH + 0.2 M sucrose for 10 min; 0.5 M PROH + 0.2 M sucrose for 5 min; culture medium for 10 min at RT

*Abbreviations: PBS, phosphate-buffered saline; RT, room temperature; LN, liquid nitrogen: PROH, 1, 2-propanediol.

The successful cryopreservation of mammalian embryos was first reported in 1972 by Whittingham et al.[78] and Wilmut.[83] These methods were based on the observations that long periods of slow cooling of mouse embryos in the presence of a cryoprotectant, in this case dimethyl sulfoxide (DMSO), enabled embryos to survive storage in liquid nitrogen providing that they were thawed slowly. Earlier workers had failed with embryo freezing mainly because they utilized cooling rates faster than 1°C/min, which does not allow adequate dehydration to occur. When cells surrounded by ice are slowly cooled, the intracellular water diffuses out of the cell and becomes incorporated into extracellular ice crystals. Embryos that are cooled faster than 1°C/min do not lose water fast enough, and ice can then form in the intracellular water. The rate of cooling that allows the loss of enough intracellular water to avoid intracellular ice formation during the whole cooling procedure can be calculated mathematically. The original freezing method of Whittingham, which utilized cooling rates of less than 1°C/min, approached the theoretic calculations for a cell's water content when it is in osmotic equilibrium with its surroundings.

The presence of a cryoprotectant in the cryopreservation solution is essential for embryo survival. Both dehydration and exposure to very high solute concentrations can damage cells because they cause, for example, irreversible conformational changes to proteins and membranes. Cryoprotectants interact with water and solutes in a way that reduces the damage to proteins and membranes. Very few compounds with cryoprotective properties, however, are sufficiently nontoxic to be useful for eggs or embryos. At the present time only three compounds, glycerol, DMSO, and 1,2-propanediol (PROH) are commonly used for embryo cryopreservation.

Slow cooling methods used to cryopreserve sheep[82] and cattle oocytes[67,81] are now used for human oocytes too. (Tables 47-1 to 47-3). Embryos of these species are usually cryopreserved at the late morula and blastocyst stages of

Table 47-2. Methods used to freeze human embryos (pronuclear oocytes to blastocysts) in DMSO

Step	Protocol*
Freezing solution	1.5 M DMSO in HEPES-buffered M 2 medium with either 20% human serum or 4 mg/mL human serum albumin
Equilibration	10 min in graded steps of 0.5, 1.0, and 1.5 M DMSO solutions at RT
Cooling rate	2°C/min to −7°C, ice nucleated
Rate and period of slow cooling	A. 0.3°C/min from −7°C to −36°C; store in LN *Thawing:* in a 35°C water bath until ice melts B. 0.3°C/min from −7°C to −45°C or below (to −80°C); store in LN *Thawing:* warm at 5°C to 15°C/min from −80°C to 0°C; warm rapidly to RT
Removal of cryoprotectant	10 min in graded steps of 1.5, 1.0, 0.5, and 0.25 M DMSO solutions; culture medium for 10 min at RT

*Abbreviations: HEPES, 4-(2-hydroxyethyl)-1-piperazineethanesulfonic acid; RT, room temperature; LN, liquid nitrogen; A and B protocols.

Table 47-3. Methods used to freeze human blastocysts in glycerol

Step	Protocol*
Freezing solution	1.0 M (8%) glycerol in PBS or HEPES-buffered culture medium + 20% human serum
Equilibration	10 min in 1, 2, 4, 6, and 8% glycerol solutions at RT
Cooling rate	Rapid cooling to −7°C; ice nucleate
Rate and period of slow cooling	0.3°C/min from −7°C to temperatures of −30°C to −36°C; transfer to LN
Thawing	In a 30°C to 37°C water bath until ice melts
Removal of cryoprotectant	10 min in 8, 6, 4, 2, and 1% glycerol solutions; culture medium for 10 min at RT

*Abbreviations: PBS, phosphate-buffered saline; HEPES, 4-(2-hydroxyethyl)-1-piperazineethanesulfonic acid; RT, room temperature; LT, liquid nitrogen.

development because they exhibit developmental-stage sensitivity to cooling and freezing.[36] It was noted by Willadsen[80] and confirmed by Whittingham et al.[79] that embryos could survive interruption of slow cooling at around −36°C to −40°C, instead of the lower temperatures of −60°C to −80°C used in the original methods (Tables 47-1 to 47-3). However, when slow cooling is interrupted at −36°C to −40°C, embryos need to be thawed rapidly to prevent the growth of small intracellular ice crystals, which probably form because of incomplete dehydration of cells. This interrupted slow cooling technique is often termed rapid freezing in publications on human embryo cryopreservation (Table 47-2, protocol A). Providing that the embryos are thawed slowly (5°C to 15°C/min) to prevent osmotic effects, which can also damage cells, the embryos will regain function and retain their full developmental potential.

For human embryos, Trounson and Mohr[64] used the original technique of slow cooling to −80°C with DMSO as the cryoprotectant to cryopreserve four- to eight-cell embryos. Pregnancies were established for infertile couples who had their supernumerary embryos cryopreserved by this technique.[17,37,64] Zeilmaker et al.[84] used the interrupted slow cooling method for the cryopreservation of early-cleavage-stage human embryos. They used DMSO as the cryoprotectant and interrupted the slow cooling at −40°C. Blastocyst-stage human embryos were also cryopreserved successfully by the interrupted slow cooling method developed for sheep and cattle blastocysts. Glycerol was used as the cryoprotectant, and slow cooling was interrupted at

−36°C.[11,12,15] The cryoprotectant PROH was also reported to be successful for cryopreservation of fertilized ova (pronuclear oocytes) and two- to eight-cell embryos.[33,58] In these procedures slow cooling was interrupted at −30°C. These reports formed the basis for the clinical use of cryopreservation in in vitro fertilization (IVF).

CRYOPRESERVATION OF HUMAN EMBRYOS

Human embryos can be cryopreserved throughout preimplantation development from the fertilized one-cell (pronuclear) ovum to the blastocyst stage. The post-thaw survival rate and the pregnancy rate per embryo transfer, however, is not the same for all developmental stages or for different freeze-thaw procedures. A literature review by Friedler et al.[18] showed that embryo survival rates ranged from 9% to 88%, and pregnancy rates ranged from 0 to 53%. In 1989 Fugger[19] reported from an analysis of clinical data in the United States that it required the transfer of an average of 11.5 cryopreserved pronuclear oocytes to establish a pregnancy, 16.0 early-cleavage-stage embryos, or 46.0 blastocysts. These data indicate that currently available cryopreservation procedures are most successful for one-cell fertilized oocytes and least suited to blastocyst-stage embryos.

Cryopreservation by slow cooling techniques

A range of compounds known as cryoprotectants enable cells to survive cooling to very low, subzero temperatures. The most widely used cryoprotectants are DMSO, PROH, glycerol, and ethylene glycol. These cryoprotectants are added to phosphate-buffered or 4-(2-hydroxyethyl)-1-piperazineethanesulfonic acid (HEPES)-buffered culture medium containing human serum (10% to 20%) or another protein supplement. Cryoprotectant solutions are generally made up on the day of use. It is not clear whether this gives the best results, since no large systematic studies comparing freshly prepared solutions with aged solutions have been carried out. The properties of solutions, however, may be influenced by the user. It is known that as water is incorporated into ice from a solution, other components of the solution (including gases, solutes, and ions) accumulate. This is particularly evident with advancing ice fronts, because gas bubbles form and grow as the concentration builds up in front of the advancing ice.[30] Gas bubbles are known to form in and around slowly cooled embryos. Thus it is possible that, as has already been demonstrated for cells, survival rates may be improved by using degassed cryoprotectant solutions. Kruuv et al.[31] observed increased survival rates of somatic cells frozen in serum and DMSO when the solution had been degassed in a vacuum of 25 mm Hg for 30 minutes. Degassing the medium may reduce the formation of gas bubbles during freezing and thawing. The appearance of gas bubbles within the embryo or in the vicinity can be an extremely damaging event for embryonic blastomeres.[2]

Embryos are normally cryopreserved at the pronuclear stage or after one or more cleavage divisions. When pronuclear-stage embryos are frozen, no selection based on embryo quality can be made, and the number of frozen embryos in storage may become quite large. Several larger IVF clinics prefer to freeze cleavage-stage embryos because it is then possible to establish the embryo quality before the transfer and freezing procedures are performed. Many groups choose to freeze only high-quality embryos, as these have better chances of surviving the freeze-thaw procedure.[4,60] Embryos with irregular-sized blastomeres, many anucleate fragments, and retarded cleavage are more likely to be damaged by freezing and rarely continue development to term after thawing and transfer to patients. Those embryos selected for cryopreservation are transferred to the freezing medium and allowed to equilibrate with the cryoprotectant. The procedures used for equilibration and freezing and thawing depend on the cryoprotectant chosen and are summarized in Tables 47-1 to 47-3. Pronuclear- and early-cleavage-stage (two- to four-cell) embryos are commonly frozen in 1.5 M PROH. Embryos of all cleavage stages may be frozen in 1.5 M DMSO, and blastocysts are most commonly frozen in 1.0 M glycerol solutions. The stepwise equilibration of embryos in cryoprotectant, described in Tables 47-1, 47-2, and 47-3, is necessary to allow water to pass out of the cells and for the cryoprotectant to pass in. During equilibration the cells contract rapidly in each solution as water leaves the cell and reexpand as the more slowly diffusing cryoprotectant enters the cell. Membrane permeability is temperature dependent, so that equilibration can be hastened by increasing the temperature or slowed by decreasing the temperature. Normally equilibration is carried out at room temperature

because the final cryoprotectant concentrations are generally well tolerated by the embryos at this temperature.

The equilibrated embryos may be frozen in a variety of containers ranging from glass ampules to plastic vials and insemination straws. Plastic containers are preferred to glass containers because they are safer for the embryologist and reduce the problems encountered with thermal fracture of ice,[48] which may cause severe damage to embryos. When the embryos are loaded into the container, they are cooled to approximately −7°C, which is a few degrees below the freezing point of the medium. Ice formation is initiated in the supercooled solution by touching the outside of the container, at some distance from the embryos, with a precooled object. Ice forms in the solution at the point of contact and then spreads through the whole solution. The container is kept at −7°C for a few minutes to ensure that ice formation has occurred. Ice will grow slowly from the point of seeding, forming large, rounded crystals, and the embryo will begin to dehydrate as the salt concentration rises in the surrounding solution. Slow cooling (less than 1°C/min) enables equilibrium conditions to be maintained as the intracellular water diffuses into the extracellular compartment and freezes.[35] Slow cooling to −30°C and below allows the majority of free water to leave the cell, with the remainder of the intracellular water vitrifying as the embryos are rapidly cooled to very low temperatures and stored in liquid nitrogen. The transition temperatures for the change from slow to rapid cooling are higher for PROH and glycerol than for DMSO; hence slow cooling can be terminated at approximately −30°C for PROH, but for DMSO slow cooling needs to continue until the temperature is −36°C or lower. When slow cooling is continued to temperatures of −45°C or lower, thawing must be slow. For slow thawing, the rates are usually between 5°C and 15°C/min from −80°C and 0°C to enable partial hydration and dilution of extracellular salts. If slow cooling is interrupted between −30°C and −40°C, thawing should be rapid to avoid the growth of intracellular ice crystals during warming (through devitrification and recrystallization).

The cryoprotectant can be removed by stepwise dilution in reducing concentrations (Tables 47-2 and 47-3) or can be removed in a sucrose solution without resorting to the gradual stepwise reduction of cryoprotectant. Sucrose maintains an extracellular osmotic gradient, preventing excessive water uptake of cells during removal of the cryoprotectant. When the cryoprotectant has diffused out of the cells, the embryos are placed in culture medium; in the absence of sucrose, water returns to the cells. This technique is commonly used to remove the cryoprotectant from human embryos (Table 47-1) and has been reduced to a one-step procedure by Freedman et al.[16] They incorporated the sucrose diluent in the freezing straw, mixing the embryos in the 1.5 M PROH freezing solution with the sucrose solution during thawing. However, it is doubtful whether this particular modification increases the survival rate of embryos because thawed embryos can simply be expelled into a sucrose solution.

Results of freezing human embryos by slow cooling techniques

Embryo freezing will increase the overall success of IVF and can be used in conjunction with gamete intrafallopian transfer (GIFT) by fertilizing supernumerary oocytes and cryopreserving the embryos that develop. In a review of published worldwide data, Friedler et al.[18] calculated that the overall survival rate of frozen embryos was 50% and the overall pregnancy rate with thawed embryos transferred to patients was 13%. Other large-scale studies have reported similar results. Mandelbaum et al.[34] reported that 62% of embryos frozen in PROH with 0.1 M sucrose had intact blastomeres after thawing, and transfer of these embryos resulted in a 19% pregnancy rate per transfer ($N = 228$). Van Steirteghem et al.[72] also reported a similar embryo survival rate (51%) of embryos frozen in PROH and DMSO but a higher pregnancy rate in patients receiving transferred embryos frozen in PROH (23%), compared with those frozen in DMSO (15%).

Data from our own IVF program (Table 47-4) in 1989-1990 using the slow cooling method in PROH show that about 70% of embryos should survive cryopreservation and about 20% of patients should become pregnant if one to three thawed embryos are transferred. In 1988-1989, 50% of embryos (150 embryos) survived cryopreservation by slow cooling in DMSO, and pregnancy was established in 17% of patients to whom thawed embryos were transferred (54 patients). Although it is not intended to compare these results because they cover quite different periods, it is generally considered that the results of freezing human embryos in PROH are better than results of freezing in DMSO. Camus et al.[4] reported very little difference in the pregnancy rate for patients transferred embryos frozen in DMSO (45 pregnancies from 311 transfers [14.5%]) and pronuclear zygotes frozen in PROH (20 pregnancies from 163 transfers [12.3%]). There is rather little interest in freezing blastocyst-stage embryos in glycerol because of the frequently reported low success rates.[19,70]

The overall benefit of cryopreservation for IVF can be difficult to compute because this will depend on the number of embryos transferred in the original cycle of IVF, the pregnancy success rate of fresh IVF, the number of patients having embryos frozen, and the success rate of cryopreservation. In a simple analysis of IVF pregnancies in the Monash IVF program in 1987,[61] 8% of the pregnancies were achieved with frozen-thawed embryos, but these pregnancies only increased the IVF success rate for patients entering the IVF program from 17% to 18%. There has been an increasing proportion of patients cryopreserving their supernumerary embryos and in the success rates for fresh and frozen embryo transfer since that time, but the benefits of cryopreservation for IVF patients entering clinical treatment should not be exaggerated. As more information from frozen cycles is becoming available it is now possible to address questions such as, does the pregnancy outcome depend more on embryo quality or uterine receptivity? In one such study Toner et al.[59] concluded that embryos collected in a cycle have similar pregnancy potential whether transferred in the fresh or frozen cycle.

Cryopreservation by rapid freezing and vitrification techniques

Embryos can be cryopreserved by direct transfer into liquid nitrogen. These techniques tend to use higher concentrations of cryoprotectants than do slow cooling procedures. Vitrification occurs if the cryoprotectant concentration exceeds 40%. A vitrified solution is in an amorphous state with the same molecular characteristics as the original solution and can be referred to as a glass. Concentrations of cryoprotectants that allow vitrification can be very toxic to cells; thus the time and temperature at which embryos are exposed to these solutions can determine their viability. The toxicity of these solutions is reduced at low temperatures, and embryos commonly are exposed to vitrification solutions at 0°C in preference to room temperature. Mouse embryos can be successfully vitrified in a range of solu-

Table 47-4. Survival of embryos and pregnancy rate in patients transferred embryos frozen by slow cooling in PROH (Monash IVF program, January 1989-June 1990)

Stage of embryo development	Time after insemination (h)	Embryos thawed		Pregnancies		
		N	% Surviving	No. of Transfers	N	%
Pronuclear zygote	16-26	70	74%	27	3	10%
2- to 4-cell	40-50	82	76%	31	9	29%
4- to 16-cell	64-74	240	69%	86	17	20%
TOTAL		392	71%	144	29	20%

tions,[47] and very high survival rates have been achieved for pronuclear- to morula-stage embryos.[26,38,40-42]

Solutions that contain less than 40% cryoprotectant do not vitrify completely; rather, ice crystals form at some stage during the cooling or warming procedure. When such solutions are used the procedure is referred to as rapid freezing rather than vitrification.

Mouse and human embryos have been rapidly frozen in solutions containing a range of concentrations of DMSO (1.5 to 4.5 M) and sucrose (0.25 M).[52,55,65,66,69] Solutions containing 1.5 to 3.0 M DMSO freeze fully or partially on cooling; solutions with more DMSO (e.g., 4.5 M) vitrify on cooling but freeze on warming. Very high survival rates can be achieved by exposing mouse embryos[52,55] briefly to solutions containing 4.5 M DMSO at room temperature or 0°C. The developmental capacity of these cryopreserved embryos in vitro or in vivo is not different from that of nonfrozen embryos, and the method can be used to cryopreserve the complete range of preimplantation development (pronuclear zygotes to blastocysts). Mouse embryos frozen in solutions containing low concentrations of DMSO (1.5 to 3.0 M) showed some chromosomal aberrations and reduced developmental capacity in vitro and in vivo; this damage appears to be correlated with ice formation in the cryoprotectant solution during the cooling step.[55] Cleavage-stage human embryos can also survive rapid freezing in 3.0 M DMSO and 0.25 M sucrose.[66,69] The embryos are transferred into a 0.25-mL clear plastic insemination straw containing the freezing solution, the straw is sealed, and after 3 minutes the straw is inserted into liquid nitrogen. Each straw is thawed in a 37°C water bath and the cryoprotectant is removed in a solution of 0.25 M sucrose (10 minutes). Using this technique Trounson[62] reported a survival rate of 73% to 75% of rapidly frozen human embryos and the establishment of four pregnancies (15%) in 27 patients to whom thawed embryos were transferred. However, one pregnancy was ectopic and three were aborted, two at 17 and 22 weeks of gestation. The two more advanced pregnancies were developmentally and chromosomally normal. These results were disappointing, but Gordts et al.[21] reported another five pregnancies with the use of 2.5 M DMSO and 0.25 M sucrose, exposing embryos to this solution for 2 to 2.5 minutes at room temperature. Their overall embryo survival rate was 69%. Four pregnancies were established from the transfer to 20 patients (20%). Again one pregnancy was ectopic and two were aborted, but one patient delivered twins. This patient conceived again with rapidly frozen embryos. Barg et al.[3] reported four pregnancies using a rapid freezing technique that involved a 3-minute exposure of embryos to 4.5 M DMSO and 0.3 M sucrose at 0°C before immersion in liquid nitrogen. They claimed an 86% embryo survival rate after thawing in a water bath at 37°C, and the four pregnancies were obtained by transfer of thawed embryos

to 38 patients (11%). Two patients delivered single babies and the other two were ongoing at the time of the report. Pregnancies have also been obtained by L. Gianaroli (personal communication) using a similar technique. These results are encouraging for the use of rapid freezing to cryopreserve human embryos, but large-scale trials are required to confirm the usefulness of this very simple and inexpensive technique.

CRYOPRESERVATION OF HUMAN OOCYTES

There are some particular advantages for the cryopreservation of gametes as distinct from embryos. Since embryos involve two parents there may be disagreement about their disposition and use during cryostorage. This situation does not occur if gametes are preserved. Mature preovulatory human oocytes have been successfully cryopreserved by using conventional slow cooling techniques[1,10,73]; however, the success rates have been low when compared with the cryopreservation of pronuclear zygotes or embryos[19,34] and there has been only a very limited interest in the clinical use of oocyte freezing in IVF and GIFT programs.

Oocytes are usually recovered from the preovulatory follicle at a mature stage (metaphase II) or they may complete maturation during a short period of incubation in culture.[68] Oocytes may also be recovered in an immature state (prophase or germinal vesicle stage) from superovulated patients[74] or from ovaries of unstimulated women.[9] There is interest in cryopreserving both mature and immature oocytes for patients involved in assisted conception technologies.

Problems for the efficient cryopreservation of oocytes

Mature metaphase II mouse oocytes can be successfully cryopreserved by slow cooling in 1.5 M DMSO,* but fertilization and developmental capacity are compromised in the frozen-thawed oocytes. It has been demonstrated that the reduction in fertilization is principally caused by zona hardening, since zona puncturing can restore the fertilization rate close to control values.[5] The zona is known to harden in response to DMSO, cooling, and dehydration.[63] DMSO has been shown to cause zona hardening in mouse oocytes by causing partial release of cortical granules.[75] Cooling of mouse oocytes from 25°C to 4°C also causes zona hardening.[25] DMSO has also been observed to cause progressive disassembly of the mouse metaphase II spindle, resulting in dispersal of chromosomes and polar pericentriolar material.[24] These observations raise concerns about the potential increase in chromosomal and developmental abnormalities in frozen-thawed metaphase II oocytes. Sathananthan et al.[50] also reported that cooling human oocytes from room temperature to 8°C and 0°C caused disorganization of the meiotic spindles and resulted in clumped and

*References 5, 6, 20, 44, 63, 77.

dislocated chromosomes. Effects on the cytoskeleton similar to those observed for DMSO were reported for PROH in rabbit oocytes, although barrel-shaped spindles were able to re-form after removal of PROH.[76] PROH has also been shown to be a potent activator of parthenogenetic development in mouse oocytes,[53] increasing the chromosomal abnormalities of ploidy in oocytes cryopreserved in PROH.[71] These problems require that mature oocytes be very carefully handled to minimize the risk of chromosomal and developmental abnormalities. Johnson[23] recommended that DMSO be added and removed from the mouse oocytes at 4°C and that a period of at least 1 hour is required at 37°C after removal of the cryoprotectant to enable re-formation of the meiotic spindle before insemination.

Mature human oocytes may be even more sensitive to cooling than mouse oocytes, and even short periods of 5 to 10 minutes of cooling to ambient temperatures may result in abnormalities of the meiotic spindle.[24,46] However, despite concerns about the normality of oocyte cytoskeletal structure and hardening of the zona pellucida to sperm penetration, it is possible that cryoprotectants and freezing techniques could be designed to minimize these effects. This may be best achieved by minimal exposure to cryoprotectants and rapid freezing and thawing.

Cryopreservation of mature oocytes by slow cooling techniques

Whittingham,[77] Glenister et al.,[20] Trounson and Kirby,[63] and Carroll et al.[5,6] reported similar results for the cryopreservation of mature mouse oocytes in 1.5 M DMSO. By equilibrating cumulus-intact oocytes in 1.5 M DMSO for 10 minutes in ice water and slow cooling (0.5°C/min) from the seeding temperature (−7°C) to low subzero temperatures (−40°C to −80°C) before rapid cooling and storage in liquid nitrogen, approximately 40% of slowly thawed (about 8°C/min) oocytes fertilized and developed to two cells in culture. This can be compared with 91% development to two cells by nonfrozen oocytes.[63] The surviving two-cell embryos may develop to fetuses at rates comparable to those of nonfrozen oocytes[77] or their developmental capacity may be significantly reduced (30% versus 64% for nonfrozen oocytes[63]). Using the same freezing technique, Schroeder et al.[51] obtained high survival rates after thawing (84%) and high fertilization and development rates to two cells (88% of those inseminated) and blastocysts (67% of two-cell embryos). The oocytes were frozen in 1.0 M DMSO after 30 minutes of equilibration on ice, and the medium contained 2.5% fetal calf serum. It is not known whether these minor modifications were responsible for the improved success rate of oocyte freezing reported in this study. It was certainly apparent that mouse oocytes should be equilibrated with DMSO on ice and that slow cooling should be continued to low subzero temperatures rather than interrupted at −36°C.[63] One recent study has investi-

gated whether glycerol could be used as a cryoprotectant for human or mouse oocytes.[22] The investigators found that when glycerol was used 8 of 19 solution control and 3 of 13 frozen-thawed human oocytes formed pronuclei, but the human oocytes exposed to glycerol did not cleave. By contrast, 67% of mouse oocytes frozen-thawed in glycerol fertilized and 50% formed hatching blastocysts.

It has been proposed that cryopreservation procedures should focus on immature (germinal vesicle stage) oocytes rather than mature oocytes because these may be less sensitive to the effects of cryoprotectants or cooling. Both rapid[85] and slow cooling[51] procedures have been used for germinal vesicle-stage oocytes. Schroeder et al.[51] compared the effects of cryopreservation on germinal vesicle-stage and in vitro-matured oocytes frozen after reaching metaphase II. They observed that, although 69% of germinal vesicle-stage oocytes survived freezing by slow cooling in DMSO, fertilization and development to two cells (9%) and blastocysts (0%) were severely compromised. By contrast, in vitro-matured, germinal vesicle-stage oocytes, matured with the addition of 1 μg of FSH per microliter to the maturation medium and cryopreserved at metaphase II, resulted in 55% fertilization and development to the two-cell stage and 77% development of two cells to blastocysts. These observations would indicate a preference for cryopreserving mature oocytes rather than immature oocytes, and that immature oocytes should be cultured to metaphase II before being frozen. Some research has also been carried out on freezing primary ovarian follicles of mice.[7,8] Freezing and thawing did not affect oocyte growth, and 61% of control and frozen oocytes resumed meiosis. Furthermore, 50% (5 of 10) of the frozen oocytes cleaved after insemination, and 2 of 4 that were transferred gave rise to live fetuses—a rate comparable to that of their nonfrozen controls (10 of 15 fertilized, 4 fetuses from 6 embryos transferred). Although these results represent only a very small proportion of all eggs that were collected, it is likely that improvements in culture conditions may allow better results to be obtained in the future.

Cryopreservation of oocytes by rapid freezing techniques

Mature mouse oocytes have been frozen by using a variety of rapid freezing procedures, but in most instances the survival, fertilization, and development rates have been lower than those that could be achieved with slow cooling procedures.[14,18,27-29] There has, however, been some progress in the field of rapid freezing of mature mouse oocytes. In 1989 Nakagata[39] modified the conventional vitrification procedure by reducing the equilibration time to 5 to 10 seconds. With this modification 87% of the oocytes had normal morphology after thawing; 78% of these formed two cells, and approximately 46% of these developed to live young. Similarly, Shaw et al.[54,56] showed that

Table 47-5. Proportion of mouse oocytes rapidly frozen in various cryoprotectant solutions forming two cells after IVF*

Solution	Nakagata[39]	VS1[47]	VS2[47]	VS3[47]	4.5 M DMSO	
Freezing method	no sucrose	no sucrose	no sucrose	no sucrose	0.25 M sucrose	0.5 M sucrose
Frozen after 10- to 15-s equilibration with cryoprotectant						
− cumulus	51†	44†	ND‡	ND	14†	80
+ cumulus	9†	53†	ND	ND	20†	55†
Frozen after 30-s equilibration with cryoprotectant						
− cumulus	33†	48†	3†	0†	80	67
+ cumulus	20†	54†	8†	0†	38†	94

*Data are expressed in percentages ([no. of 2-cell embryos formed/no. of oocytes frozen] × 100). Each group comprised a minimum of 40 frozen oocytes.
†Statistically different from control (73% − cumulus, $N = 394$; 86% + cumulus, $N = 81$).
‡ND, Not done.

although the original vitrification procedure resulted in only 24% blastocyst formation, a modified procedure increased this to 55%. Rubinsky et al.[49] found that the addition of 40 mg of antifreeze glycoproteins per milliliter to a vitrification solution containing 17.5% PROH, 2.5% glycerol, and 0.05 M sucrose increased the survival (percentage reaching metaphase II) of pig immature oocytes from 0% (0 of 47) to 24.5% (11 of 45). Although this percentage is lower than that for control oocytes (92%; 23 of 25), this approach may be worthy of fuller investigation.

The ultrarapid freezing procedure, although it achieves excellent results for mouse embryos,[52,55] proved to be poorly suited to unfertilized oocytes, with a maximum of approximately 30% blastocyst formation.[13,32,50,57] Our current research, however, does show that with appropriate modifications to the sucrose concentration in the cryoprotectant and the equilibration period, this procedure can also give excellent results for both cumulus-enclosed and cumulus-denuded mature oocytes (Table 47-5). Under optimal conditions we found no significant difference between the proportion of frozen-thawed and control oocytes reaching the blastocyst stage ($>70\%$) (unpublished results). The data for mice suggest that the rapid freezing procedures can achieve excellent results. The procedures for the mouse, however, are not necessarily successful for other species. Nakagata found that the vitrification procedure that gave excellent results for mouse oocytes[39,43] was not suited to hamster oocytes ($<5\%$ fertilization).[39] Research on rapid freezing procedures for human oocytes has started,[45] but it remains to be established how well the new vitrification and ultrarapid freezing protocols can be adapted to human oocytes.

REFERENCES

1. Al-Hasani S et al: Cryopreservation of human oocytes, *Hum Reprod* 2:695, 1987.
2. Ashwood-Smith MJ et al: Physical factors are involved in the destruction of embryos and oocytes during freezing and thawing procedures, *Hum Reprod* 3:795, 1988.
3. Barg PE, Barad DH, Feichtinger W: Ultrarapid freezing (URF) of mouse and human preembryos: a modified approach, *J In Vitro Fert Embryo Transfer* 7:355, 1990.
4. Camus M et al: Human embryo viability after freezing with dimethylsulfoxide as a cryoprotectant, *Fertil Steril* 51:460, 1989.
5. Carroll J, Depypere H, Matthews CD: Freeze-thaw-induced changes of the zona pellucida explains decreased rates of fertilization in frozen-thawed mouse oocytes, *J Reprod Fertil* 90:547, 1990.
6. Carroll J, Warnes GM, Matthews CD: Increase in digyny explains polyploidy after in-vitro fertilization of frozen thawed mouse oocytes, *J Reprod Fertil* 85:489, 1989.
7. Carroll J, Whittingham DG, Wood MJ: Growth *in vitro* and acquisition of meiotic competence after the cryopreservation of isolated mouse primary ovarian follicles, *Reprod Fertil Dev* 3:595, 1991.
8. Carroll J et al: Extra-ovarian production of mature viable mouse oocytes from frozen primary follicles, *J Reprod Fertil* 90:321, 1990.
9. Cha KY et al: Pregnancy after in vitro fertilization of human follicular oocytes collected from nonstimulated cycles, their culture in vitro and their transfer in a donor oocyte program, *Fertil Steril* 55:109, 1991.
10. Chen C: Pregnancy after human oocyte cryopreservation, *Lancet* 1:884, 1986.
11. Cohen J et al: Pregnancies following the frozen storage of expanding human blastocysts, *J In Vitro Fert Embryo Transfer* 2:59, 1985.
12. Cohen J et al: Factors affecting survival and implantation of cryopreserved human embryos, *J In Vitro Fert Embryo Transfer* 3:46, 1986.
13. Erasmus E et al: Comparative analysis of two cryopreservation techniques to freeze mouse oocytes, *Asstd Reprod Technol/Androl* 1:331, 1990.
14. Fahy GM: Vitrification. In McGrath JJ, Diller KR, editors: *Low temperature biotechnology: emerging applications and engineering contributions, BED* vol 10/*HTD* vol 98:113, 1989.
15. Fehilly CB et al: Cryopreservation of cleaving embryos and expanded blastocysts in the human: a comparative study, *Fertil Steril* 44:638, 1985.
16. Freedman M et al: Pregnancy resulting from cryopreserved human embryos using a one-step in situ dilution procedure, *Obstet Gynecol* 72:502, 1988.
17. Freeman L, Trounson A, Kirby C: Cryopreservation of human embryos: progress on the clinical use of the technique in human in vitro fertilization, *J In Vitro Fert Embryo Transfer* 3:53, 1986.
18. Friedler S, Giudice LC, Lamb EJ: Cryopreservation of embryos and ova, *Fertil Steril* 49:743, 1988.
19. Fugger EF: Clinical status of human embryo cryopreservation in the United States of America, *Fertil Steril* 52:986, 1989.
20. Glenister PH et al: The incidence of chromosome anomalies in

first-cleavage mouse embryos obtained from frozen-thawed oocytes fertilized in vitro, *Gamete Res* 16:205, 1987.

21. Gordts S et al: Survival and pregnancy outcome after ultrarapid freezing of human embryos, *Fertil Steril* 53:469, 1990.

22. Hunter JE et al: Fertilization and development of the human oocyte following exposure to cryoprotectants, low temperatures and cryopreservation: a comparison of two techniques, *Hum Reprod* 6:1460, 1991.

23. Johnson MH: The effect on fertilization of exposure of mouse oocytes to dimethyl sulfoxide: an optimal protocol, *J In Vitro Fert Embryo Transfer* 6:168, 1989.

24. Johnson MH, Pickering SJ: The effect of dimethylsulphoxide on the microtubular system of the mouse oocyte, *Development* 100:313, 1987.

25. Johnson MH, Pickering SJ, George MA: The influence of cooling on the properties of the zona pellucida of the mouse, *Hum Reprod* 3:383, 1988.

26. Kasai M et al: A simple method for mouse embryo cryopreservation in a low toxicity vitrification solution, without appreciable loss of viability, *J Reprod Fertil* 89:91, 1990.

27. Kola I et al: Vitrification of mouse oocytes results in aneuploid zygotes and malformed fetuses, *Teratology* 38:467, 1988.

28. Kono T, Kwon OY, Nakahara T: Development of vitrified mouse oocytes after in vitro fertilization, *Cryobiology* 28:50, 1990.

29. Kono T, Tsunoda Y: Ovicidal effects of vitrification solution and the vitrification-warming cycle and establishment of the proportion of toxic effects on nuclei and cytoplasm of mouse oocytes, *Cryobiology* 25:197, 1988.

30. Korber C, Rau G: Ice crystal growth in aqueous solutions. In Pegg DE, Karow AM Jr, editors: *The biophysics of organ cryopreservation*, NATO ASI series A: Life Sciences, vol 147, New York, 1987, Plenum Press.

31. Kruuv J et al: Effect of dissolved gasses on freeze-thaw survival of mammalian cells, *Cryo Lett* 7:233, 1985.

32. Lai AC-H, Ryan JP, Saunders DM: Ultrarapid cryopreservation of mouse oocytes and embryos: effect of cell stage and culture in vitro, *Asstd Reprod Technol/Androl* 1:320, 1990.

33. Lassalle B, Testart J, Renard J-P: Human embryo features that influence the success of cryopreservation with the use of 1,2-propanediol, *Fertil Steril* 44:645, 1985.

34. Mandelbaum J et al: Cryopreservation of human embryos and oocytes, *Hum Reprod* 3:117, 1988.

35. Mazur P: Equilibrium, quasi-equilibrium, and nonequilibrium freezing of mammalian embryos, *Cell Biophys* 17:53, 1990.

36. Mohr LR, Trounson A: Structural changes associated with freezing of bovine embryos, *Biol Reprod* 25:1009, 1981.

37. Mohr LR, Trounson A, Freemann L: Deep freezing and transfer of human embryos, *J In Vitro Fert Embryo Transfer* 2:1, 1985.

38. Nakagata N: High survival rate of pronuclear mouse oocytes derived from in vitro fertilization following ultrarapid freezing and thawing, *Jpn J Fertil Steril* 34:757, 1989.

39. Nakagata N: High survival rate of unfertilized mouse oocytes after vitrification, *J Reprod Fertil* 87:479, 1989.

40. Nakagata N: Survival of 4-cell mouse embryos derived from fertilization in vitro after ultrarapid freezing and thawing, *Jpn J Fertil Steril* 34:279, 1989.

41. Nakagata N: Survival of 2-cell mouse embryos derived from fertilization in vitro after ultrarapid freezing and thawing, *Jpn J Fertil Steril* 34:470, 1989.

42. Nakagata N: Cryopreservation of mouse strains by ultrarapid freezing, *Exp Anim* 39:299, 1990.

43. Nakagata N: Cryopreservation of unfertilized mouse oocytes from inbred strains by ultrarapid freezing, *Jikken Dobutsu* 39:303, 1990.

44. Parks JE, Ruffing NA: Factors affecting low temperature survival of mammalian oocytes, *Theriogenology* 37:59, 1992.

45. Pensis M, Loumaye E, Psalti I: Screening of conditions for rapid freezing of human oocytes: preliminary study toward their cryopreservation, *Fertil Steril* 52:787, 1989.

46. Pickering SJ et al: Transient cooling to room temperature can cause irreversible disruption of the meiotic spindle in the human oocyte, *Fertil Steril* 54:102, 1990.

47. Rall WF: Factors affecting the survival of mouse embryos cryopreserved by vitrification, *Cryobiology* 24:387, 1987.

48. Rall WF, Meyer TK: Zona fracture damage and its avoidance during the cryopreservation of mammalian embryos, *Theriogenology* 31:683, 1989.

49. Rubinsky B, Arav A, Devries AL: Cryopreservation of oocytes using directional cooling and antifreeze glycoproteins, *Cryo Lett* 12:93, 1991.

50. Sathananthan AH et al: The effects of ultrarapid freezing on meiotic and mitotic spindles of mouse oocytes and embryos, *Gamete Res* 21:385, 1988.

51. Schroeder AC et al: Developmental capacity of mouse oocytes cryopreserved before and after maturation in vitro, *J Reprod Fertil* 89:43, 1990.

52. Shaw JM, Diotallevi L, Trounson AO: A simple 4.5M dimethyl-sulfoxide freezing technique for the cryopreservation of one-cell to blastocyst stage preimplantation mouse embryos, *Reprod Fertil Dev* 3:621, 1991.

53. Shaw JM, Trounson AO: Parthenogenetic activation of unfertilized mouse oocytes by exposure to 1,2-propanediol is influenced by temperature, oocyte age and cumulus removal, *Gamete Res* 24:269, 1989.

54. Shaw JM et al: An association between chromosomal abnormalities in rapidly frozen 2-cell mouse embryos and the ice-forming properties of the cryoprotective solution, *J Reprod Fertil* 91:9, 1991.

55. Shaw PW et al: Morphological and functional changes in unfertilized mouse oocytes during a vitrification procedure, *Cryo Lett* 11:427, 1990.

56. Shaw PW et al: Vitrification of mouse oocytes: improved rates of survival, fertilization, and development to blastocysts, *Mol Reprod Dev* 29:373, 1991.

57. Surrey ES, Quinn PJ: Successful ultrarapid freezing of unfertilized oocytes, *J In Vitro Fert Embryo Transfer* 7:262, 1990.

58. Testart J et al: High pregnancy rate after early human embryo freezing, *Fertil Steril* 46:268, 1986.

59. Toner M et al: Cryomicroscopic analysis of intracellular ice formation during freezing of mouse oocytes without cryoadditives, *Cryobiology* 28:55, 1991.

60. Trounson A: Preservation of human eggs and embryos, *Fertil Steril* 46:1, 1986.

61. Trounson A: Embryo cryopreservation. In Wood C, Trounson A, editors: *Clinical in vitro fertilization,* Berlin, 1989, Springer-Verlag.

62. Trounson A: Cryopreservation, *Br Med Bull* 46:695, 1990.

63. Trounson A, Kirby C: Problems in the cryopreservation of unfertilized eggs by slow cooling in dimethyl sulfoxide, *Fertil Steril* 52:778, 1989.

64. Trounson A, Mohr L: Human pregnancy following cryopreservation, thawing and transfer of an eight-cell embryo, *Nature* 305:707, 1983.

65. Trounson A, Peura A, Kirby C: Ultrarapid freezing: a new low-cost and effective method of cryopreservation, *Fertil Steril* 48:843, 1987.

66. Trounson A, Sjoblom P: Cleavage and development of human embryos in vitro after ultrarapid freezing and thawing, *Fertil Steril* 50:373, 1988.

67. Trounson AO et al: Frozen storage and transfer of bovine embryos, *J Anim Sci* 46:677, 1978.

68. Trounson A et al: Effect of delayed insemination on in vitro fertilization, culture and transfer of human embryos, *J Reprod Fertil* 64:285, 1982.

69. Trounson A et al: Ultrarapid freezing of early cleavage stage human embryos and eight-cell mouse embryos, *Fertil Steril* 49:822, 1988.

70. Troup SA et al: Cryopreservation of human embryos at the pronucleate, early cleavage, or expanded blastocyst stages, *Eur J Obstet Gynecol Reprod Biol* 38:133, 1990.

71. Van der Elst J et al: Effect of 1,2-propanediol and dimethylsulfoxide on the meiotic spindle of the mouse oocyte, *Hum Reprod* 3:960, 1988.

72. Van Steirteghem AC et al: Cryopreservation of human embryos obtained after gamete intra-fallopian transfer and/or in vitro fertilization, *Hum Reprod* 2:593, 1987.

73. Van Uem JF et al: Birth after cryopreservation of unfertilized oocytes, *Lancet* 1:752, 1987.

74. Veeck LL et al: Maturation and fertilization of morphologically immature human oocytes, *Fertil Steril* 39:594, 1983.

75. Vincent C, Pickering SJ, Johnson MH: The hardening effect of dimethylsulfoxide on the mouse zona pellucida requires the presence of an oocyte and is associated with a reduction in the number of cortical granules present, *J Reprod Fertil* 89:253, 1990.

76. Vincent C et al: Solvent effects on cytoskeletal organization and in vivo survival after freezing of rabbit oocytes, *J Reprod Fertil* 87:809, 1989.

77. Whittingham DG: Fertilization in vitro and development to term of unfertilized mouse oocytes previously stored at −196° C, *J Reprod Fertil* 49:89, 1977.

78. Whittingham DG, Leibo SP, Mazur P: Survival of mouse embryos frozen to −196°C and −269°C, *Science* 178:411, 1972.

79. Whittingham DG et al: Survival of frozen mouse embryos after rapid thawing from −196° C, *J Reprod Fertil* 56:11, 1979.

80. Willadsen SM: Factors affecting the survival of sheep embryos during freezing and thawing. In Elliot K, Whelan J, editors: *The freezing of mammalian embryos,* CIBA Foundation Symposium 52, Amsterdam, 1977, Elsevier/North Holland.

81. Willadsen S, Polge C, Rowson LE: The viability of deep-frozen cow embryos, *J Reprod Fertil* 52:391, 1978.

82. Willadsen SM et al: Deep freezing of sheep embryos, *J Reprod Fertil* 46:151, 1976.

83. Wilmut I: The effect of cooling rate, warming rate, cryoprotective agent, and stage of development on survival of mouse embryos during freezing and thawing, *Life Sci* 11:1071, 1972.

84. Zeilmaker FH et al: Two pregnancies following transfer of intact frozen-thawed embryos, *Fertil Steril* 42:293, 1984.

85. Zhiming H, Jianchen W, Jufen Q: Ultrarapid freezing of follicular oocytes in mice, *Theriogenology* 33:365, 1990.

Chapter 48

DONOR OOCYTES IN ASSISTED REPRODUCTION

Owen K. Davis, MD
and Zev Rosenwaks, MD

The ready availability of donor sperm and the ease of artificial insemination have long enabled couples with refractory male factor infertility to achieve successful pregnancies. Before the development of in vitro fertilization (IVF) and related techniques, no similar option was available for women with premature ovarian failure, largely because of the inaccessibility of donor oocytes. With the advent of oocyte donation, this technology has proven useful in additional clinical contexts, including incipient ovarian failure/advanced maternal age, anatomically inaccessible ovaries, previous IVF failure resulting from poor oocyte quality, and hereditable genetic disorders.

This chapter provides an overview of oocyte donation both as a clinical tool and as a unique scientific model for investigation of the interplay among the conceptus, the endometrium, and the steroidal milieu.

HISTORIC BACKGROUND

Heape[14] reported successful donor embryo transfer in the rabbit more than a century ago. Experimentation was subsequently performed in a number of mammalian species, and this technology has gained wide application in the sheep and cattle industries.[39] Meyer and associates[21] were the first to perform successful donor embryo transfer in nonhuman primates.

The first human pregnancies after donor embryo transfer were reported by Buster et al.[3] in 1983. In these cases the donor embryos were obtained by transcervical uterine lavage of donor subjects 5 to 7 days after timed artificial insemination with sperm from the recipient's husband. The donor embryos were then transferred to the hormonally prepared recipient patients. This technique is both nonsurgical (and therefore relatively noninvasive) and cost effective, insofar as superovulation is not routinely used and virtually no laboratory phase is required. Application of this procedure is limited, however, by the availability of donors and by the risk of donor pregnancy due to retention of an embryo after failed uterine lavage,[35] as well as potential risk of introduction of a sexually transmitted disease (STD) transmission.

Subsequent to the original series of Buster et al.,[3] several early reports of successful human pregnancies after donor oocyte IVF appeared in the literature.[17, 34, 42] In this procedure the donor undergoes superovulation, as with conventional IVF, to effect multifollicular recruitment. Oocyte retrieval is performed, and the donor oocytes are inseminated in vitro with the recipient's partner's sperm. The fertilized ova are either transferred to the hormonally synchronized recipient in the same cycle or cryopreserved for transfer at a later date. Inevitably, other assisted reproductive techniques, including gamete intrafallopian transfer (GIFT) and zygote intrafallopian transfer (ZIFT), have been applied to oocyte donation, also with success.[1, 2]

Currently the use of donor oocytes in assisted reproduction is widespread. In the United States alone more than 500 donor embryo transfers had been performed by participating clinics, according to the 1990 U.S. IVF-ET Registry survey.[19]

DONOR OOCYTE RECIPIENTS

Indications and evaluation

Premature ovarian failure. Currently the major indication for oocyte donation is premature ovarian failure (POF), defined as hypergonadotropic hypogonadism occurring before the age of 40 years. It is estimated that POF afflicts approximately 1% of the female population.[6] The causes of POF are diverse, although a specific etiology frequently cannot be discerned. Iatrogenic causes of POF include gonadal extirpation, chemotherapy (particularly alkylating agents), and pelvic irradiation. Other causes and associations include X chromosome abnormalities (e.g., monosomy X), congenital thymic aplasia, hereditary galactosemia, and the "resistant ovary syndrome," which may result from a gonadotropin receptor or postreceptor defect.[30] (See also Chapter 54.)

Premature ovarian failure is frequently an autoimmune disorder; approximately 20% of karyotypically normal women with POF are found to have associated autoimmune processes.[5] Up to 17% of subjects with type I polyglandular autoimmune syndrome and 4% with the type II complex exhibit gonadal failure.[41] These patients often display elevated peripheral titers of antiovarian, antithyroid, and antiadrenal antibodies, and lymphocytic infiltration may be seen on ovarian biopsy specimens. A number of reports have demonstrated an associated elevation of Ia+ T cells in patients with endocrine disorders, including POF, Graves' disease, and idiopathic Addison's disease, suggesting that markers of cell-mediated autoimmunity should be sought.[9, 15, 28, 29]

Except in instances of surgical castration, previous antineoplastic chemotherapy, or pelvic irradiation, a thorough medical evaluation is indicated, particularly in women under the age of 35. The major purpose of this work-up is to exclude associated medical disorders, but it is also possible that a potentially correctable dysfunction may be discovered, thus avoiding the need for donor oocytes.

The medical history should elicit details of the timing and nature of secondary sexual maturation, menarche, and subsequent menstrual cycles; the onset of amenorrhea should be ascertained. The patient should be specifically questioned with regard to previous chemotherapy, radiation therapy, exposure to environmental toxins, and gonadal surgery (e.g., ovarian cystectomies). The review of systems should include documentation of coexisting medical conditions with an emphasis on possible endocrinopathies or autoimmune disorders.

The general physical examination should specifically include measurement of the patient's height, a survey of secondary sexual development, a pelvic examination, and a thorough search for stigmata of karyotypic disorders (e.g., features of Turner's syndrome) and endocrinopathies (e.g., thyromegaly, vitiligo). The basic laboratory evaluation should include documentation of hypergonadotropism (the hallmark of gonadal failure). It has been suggested that weekly assessment of follicle-stimulating hormone (FSH), luteinizing hormone (LH), and estradiol levels for 1 month may be useful; residual follicular activity is suggested if any one determination shows an estradiol concentration exceeding 50 pg/mL or an LH:FSH ratio greater than 1.[30] In these cases the prognosis for spontaneous ovulation or a response to ovulation induction might be slightly improved. A peripheral karyotype should be obtained in order to diagnose X chromosome abnormalities and, most significantly, to exclude the presence of a Y cell line. A streamlined endocrine evaluation should include thyroid functions, morning fasting blood glucose, serum calcium, and phosphorus levels; and an 8 AM serum cortisol level. Some clinicians advocate formal adrenocorticotropin-stimulation testing as a more sensitive screen for primary hypoadrenalism. The laboratory evaluation for autoimmunity should include a complete blood count (to screen for pernicious anemia) and antinuclear antibody titers. Although useful in a research setting, the clinical utility of routinely obtaining antiovarian, antithyroid, and antiadrenal antibody titers is questionable, since successful pregnancy after immunosuppressive therapy is, at best, a rare event. Ovarian biopsy generally should *not* be performed, because the prognosis for spontaneous or induced ovulation and pregnancy is uniformly poor even if the ovaries possess a near-normal complement of follicles (e.g., resistant ovary syndrome).

Incipient ovarian failure/advanced maternal age. It has long been appreciated that women over 40 years old have reduced fertility in general, and a poorer prognosis for success after IVF.[31] Most IVF programs have established age limits because of the reduced pregnancy rates and increased spontaneous abortion rates (60%) in these older patients. This striking decrease in fecundity is due primarily to oocyte senescence, rather than uterine aging, an issue that is explored more fully later in this chapter. This process of incipient ovarian failure is physiologic in the perimenopausal years, but it may also be seen in younger patients.

Ovarian reserve can be assessed by determining basal FSH and estradiol levels early in the follicular phase (day 3). An elevated FSH ($\geq$ 20 mIU/mL) and/or estradiol level may be indicative of incipient ovarian failure and a markedly diminished chance for success after therapy.[16, 37] It has been suggested that dynamic testing with clomiphene citrate can unmask occult ovarian failure if an exaggerated increase in the FSH level is seen.[22]

Increasingly, donor oocyte IVF is being applied to cases of incipient ovarian failure, both in younger patients and in women over 40 to 42 years of age, with success rates comparable to those seen in patients with POF.

Other indications for oocyte donation. Donor oocytes may be applied to cases of hereditable maternal genetic abnormalities (e.g., balanced translocations, autosomal dominant, or X-linked recessive disorders) to obviate the risk of transmission to the offspring. These patients currently comprise a small proportion of candidates for donor oocyte IVF, and this indication is likely to wane with the continued development of specific gene probes and the refinement of preimplantation genetic techniques such as embryo and polar body biopsy.

Women who have previously undergone multiple unsuccessful IVF attempts may also be candidates for donor oocytes, particularly when poor egg quality is suspected. Finally, the rare patient with ovaries that are physically inaccessible either transvaginally or laparoscopically is a potential candidate for oocyte donation. An example would be a patient with extensive abdominal and pelvic adhesions and ovaries fixed high in the pelvis.

Screening

Usually both the oocyte recipient and her partner should be healthy, and there should be no physical contraindications to pregnancy. The procedural aspects of donor oocyte IVF should be reviewed with the couple and should cover potential stresses, risks, and cost. Donor oocyte success rates for the individual center should be presented. In most programs, psychologic screening of the recipient couple is required in order to assess their emotional preparedness.

Physical examination of the female should include a pelvic examination to assess uterine size and position, at which time a uterine sounding may be performed with a trial embryo transfer catheter to determine uterine depth and ease of passage. A Papanicolaou smear and cervical cultures may also be obtained at this time. Screening for infectious diseases in the patient and her partner generally should include tests for human immunodeficiency virus (HIV), hepatitis, and syphilis.

Hysterosalpingography should be performed (or previous films reviewed) to evaluate for intrauterine abnormalities such as submucous leiomyomas, synechiae, polyps, or a congenital malformation that could compromise the chances for blastocyst implantation or increase the risk of pregnancy wastage. The male partner should have a semen analysis with a sperm wash and swimup in order to rule out a coexisting male factor.

OOCYTE DONORS

Donor availability

Perhaps the major difficulty in establishing a donor oocyte program is the limited availability of donor subjects. Donors can be anonymous or nonanonymous, the latter category including sisters and friends of the recipients.

Anonymous donors include other IVF patients who are willing to donate a portion of their oocytes, volunteers willing to undergo superovulation and oocyte retrieval solely for the purpose of ovum donation, and women scheduled for laparoscopic tubal sterilization who volunteer to undergo preoperative superovulation and monitoring, with oocyte harvest at the time of their surgery. The availability of embryo cryopreservation has diminished the pool of IVF patients willing to donate oocytes, as most

elect to freeze any "excess" embryos for possible future replacement. Paid anonymous volunteers and sisters therefore comprise the majority of donors at most centers. Complex social, ethical, and legal issues surround the recruitment and compensation of oocyte donors; a detailed discussion of this subject is beyond the scope of this chapter.

Women under the age of 35 years are sought as oocyte donors so as to maximize success rates and to reduce the risk of chromosomal abnormalities in the resulting pregnancies. Needless to say, in cases where the oocyte donor is older than 35 years, the recipient must be offered appropriate genetic counseling and prenatal testing (chorionic villus sampling or amniocentesis).

Screening

Prospective oocyte donors should undergo a rigorous and thorough screening process, including a detailed medical and genetic history, physical examination, and a formal psychologic assessment by an appropriately trained psychologist or psychiatrist. These women should be counseled regarding potential physical and emotional risks, including ovarian hyperstimulation syndrome and potential complications of oocyte retrieval such as pelvic infection and hemorrhage. The psychologic evaluation is intended to uncover any risk factors that may render a subject emotionally unsuitable for egg donation and to ensure that there is no element of coercion in her decision to donate oocytes (particularly in the case of nonanonymous donors).

Evaluation

The history and physical evaluation should exclude infectious diseases, significant hereditable disorders, and the possibility of reproductive dysfunction—including infertility or recurrent miscarriage. No contraindications to controlled ovarian hyperstimulation or oocyte recovery should exist. The laboratory evaluation should include a complete blood count and blood type to identify potential Rh incompatibility. In selected cases, hemoglobinopathies such as sickle cell trait should be ruled out. The screen for infectious disease should, at a minimum, include serology for HIV infection, hepatitis B and C, and syphilis.

Finally, written, informed consent must be obtained and must include a thorough review of all significant risks to the donor.

Given the relative scarcity of oocyte donors in the face of substantial numbers of potential recipients, other sources of donor eggs have been explored. Cha and associates[4] recently described the recovery of immature oocytes from unstimulated ovaries and ovarian biopsy specimens removed at the time of surgery, with subsequent in vitro maturation and fertilization. The transfer of five resulting embryos to a subject with POF resulted in a viable triplet pregnancy. Further investigation in this area is required to document the reproducibility of this technique, which may

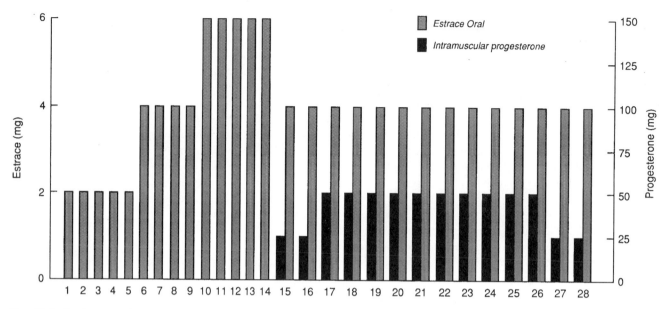

Fig. 48-1. Replacement protocol for ovarian failure using Estrace and progesterone injections.

have the potential to expand the pool of donor eggs, thus fulfilling the increasing clinical demand.

PREPARATION OF THE RECIPIENT

In the natural cycle, ovarian and endometrial function are intrinsically linked, allowing the orderly development of an endometrial milieu receptive to blastocyst implantation. Women with ovarian failure require exogenous hormonal replacement to simulate the natural cycle and to effect perinidatory uterine receptivity. Estrogen is required for endometrial proliferation and the induction of progesterone receptors. Although the importance of luteal phase estrogen in primates is unclear, progesterone is critical both for implantation and pregnancy maintenance.

A variety of steroid replacement regimens have been developed, all of which are designed to approximate the pattern of hormone secretion occurring in the natural menstrual cycle. Estrogen may be administered either orally or parenterally. Protocols have been described employing estradiol valerate; micronized estradiol-17β; estradiol-impregnated polysiloxane vaginal rings; and, more recently, transdermal estradiol patches.[11, 17, 32, 40] Progesterone is usually administered as intramuscular progesterone-in-oil or vaginal suppositories.[32] Replacement protocols typically result in late follicular and midluteal estradiol concentrations exceeding 200 pg/mL and 100 pg/mL, respectively, and midluteal progesterone levels of 20 ng/mL or greater.

A successful regimen employing micronized estradiol (Estrace) and intramuscular progesterone is depicted in Fig. 48-1. Currently we favor transdermal estradiol delivery,

which avoids the supraphysiologic serum estrone levels that follow oral administration (due to the "first pass" effect of hepatic metabolism) and results in relatively stable absorption kinetics.[11] In this protocol, estradiol transdermal patches (Estraderm; CIBA) are applied so as to deliver a dose of 0.1 mg on days 1 to 5, 0.2 mg on days 6 to 9, and 0.4 mg on days 10 to 13. Thereafter the dosage is decreased to 0.2 mg/d. Intramuscular progesterone-in-oil is started at a dose of 25 mg on day 15 and increased to 50 mg from day 16 on. Of note, with all replacement regimens, the length of the recipient's follicular phase may be adjusted to permit synchronization with the donor. The first day of progesterone administration is automatically designated as day 15. Synchronization is simplified when cryopreserved embryos are used, because transfer can be performed on the appropriate day in a future cycle without concern for the timing of oocyte retrieval.

At most centers, the recipient undergoes one or more preparatory cycles before the actual cycle of embryo transfer in order to ensure the adequacy of her response to the replacement regimen. Serial serum estradiol and progesterone determinations are performed, and a midluteal endometrial biopsy specimen is obtained on cycle day 21 to cycle day 23 and dated according to the histologic criteria of Noyes et al.[26] Replacement protocols frequently result in midluteal endometrium that displays glandular-stromal asynchrony, with glands lagging behind appropriately advanced stroma; when the stroma is in phase, pregnancy is not impeded.[32] If a late luteal phase biopsy is performed (day 25 or 26), it is generally found to be in phase and without evidence of asynchronous development. We do not routinely perform late luteal biopsies if the biopsy results for day 21 to 23 are normal.

Potential donor oocyte recipients who have intact ovarian function (e.g., women with genetic disorders or abnormal oocytes) are potentially problematic, as donor-recipient synchronization can be difficult to achieve if embryo transfer is planned for the natural cycle. The use of cryopreserved embryos can overcome this difficulty, but embryo cryosurvival is limited and, in many clinics, pregnancy rates are superior after the transfer of "fresh" embryos. An alternative approach, which has gained wide acceptance, is to render the recipient functionally agonadal with a gonadotropin-releasing hormone (GnRH) agonist, and then administer exogenous hormone replacement in the same fashion as described for patients with ovarian failure.[20]

DONOR SUPEROVULATION AND OOCYTE RETRIEVAL

A number of controlled ovarian hyperstimulation protocols have been developed; essentially all include the intramuscular administration of gonadotropins (human menopausal gonadotropin [hMG] or purified FSH), either alone or in conjunction with oral clomiphene citrate or a GnRH agonist. A detailed overview of these different regimens has been presented elsewhere.[33]

The basic approach to ovarian stimulation is a combined regimen of a GnRH agonist (leuprolide acetate), hMG, and purified FSH. Leuprolide is administered as a daily dose of 1 mg, commencing in the mid–luteal phase of the donor's previous cycle. Ovarian suppression is usually complete by the onset of menses, approximately 1 week later. A baseline ultrasonogram and estradiol level are obtained on the third day of the cycle to rule out ovarian cysts and to ensure adequate suppression, and the daily dose of leuprolide is then decreased to 0.5 mg. Gonadotropin therapy is initiated at a dosage of two ampules of hMG and two ampules of FSH (total, 300 IU) on days 3 and 4 of the cycle, and tapered to two ampules of hMG alone once follicular recruitment has occurred (generally by day 6 or 7). Endocrine and ultrasonographic surveillance is undertaken, and intramuscular human chorionic gonadotropin (hCG) is administered at a dose of 5,000 to 10,000 IU once appropriate follicular and hormonal criteria have been achieved, generally with the lead follicle(s) displaying a mean diameter of 16 mm or greater and the serum estradiol concentration exceeding 500 pg/mL. Oocyte retrieval is performed approximately 35 hours after the hCG injection. In cases of anonymous oocyte donation, the donors should be kept separate from the recipients during the daily office visits for monitoring in order to protect their anonymity.

Ultrasound-guided, transvaginal oocyte recovery is performed with intravenous sedation and analgesia. Laparoscopic oocyte harvest is undertaken in cases where the donor has been scheduled for tubal sterilization. The donor is advised to use barrier contraception during ovarian stimulation and after her oocyte retrieval, to reduce the risk of pregnancy.

After a preincubation interval of 2 to 8 hours, the donor oocytes are inseminated with the recipient's partner's sperm. The embryos that result are either cryopreserved or transferred to the synchronized recipient 48 to 72 hours after the retrieval. For donor oocyte GIFT, the eggs are mixed with the partner's sperm and transferred to the recipient via laparoscopic or transcervical tubal cannulation shortly after oocyte recovery.

SYNCHRONIZATION OF RECIPIENT AND DONOR

By definition, ovarian and endometrial events are dissociated in donor oocyte IVF cycles. Effective synchronization of embryonic and endometrial development is therefore key to the success of a donor egg program.

Clinical experience has indicated that a maximally efficient window of transfer exists. The transfer of embryos with four or more blastomeres into endometrium histologically developed to days 17 to 19 is most likely to result in implantation and pregnancy.[25, 32]

When cryopreserved donor embryos are used, synchronization is straightforward. The recipient is prepared with exogenous estrogen and progesterone as outlined earlier, with day 15 being the first day of progesterone administration. The frozen pronuclear embryos are thawed on day 16, allowed to cleave overnight, and transferred on day 17 at the two- to four-cell stage. Recipients possessing endogenous ovarian function either can be treated with an exogenous hormonal regimen, generally after suppression with a GnRH agonist, or may undergo frozen donated embryo transfer in the natural cycle. In the latter instance, luteal phase adequacy should be documented beforehand, and embryo thawing and subsequent transfer are timed according to the onset of the recipient's endogenous LH surge.

More commonly, fresh oocytes/embryos are used in donor egg cycles. Here, estrogen replacement of the recipient is initiated a few days before the donor's expected menses, because the donor's follicular phase may be significantly shortened by gonadotropin therapy. The length of the recipient's follicular phase is not critical and may be adjusted to accommodate the duration of the donor's stimulated follicular phase. Progesterone replacement is initiated the day before or the day of the donor's oocyte retrieval, thus permitting embryo transfer on cycle day 17 or 18 into a receptive endometrial milieu.

In donor oocyte GIFT cycles, the laparoscopic transfer of the oocytes and the sperm is generally performed on day 15, presumably allowing transport of any resulting embryo(s) to the recipient's endometrial cavity by cycle day 18 or 19.

EMBRYO TRANSFER AND POSTTRANSFER MANAGEMENT

After donor oocyte IVF, transcervical embryo transfer is performed in the routine manner, generally limiting the number of embryos to four or fewer. ZIFT and GIFT may also be applied to egg donation. The approach favored by a given center will be dictated by its particular method-specific success rates. After embryo replacement, the recipient is transferred to a holding area, where she remains at bed rest for an interval of 30 minutes or more before discharge. Normal activity may then be resumed, and the luteal estrogen/progesterone replacement is continued as in her earlier preparatory cycle(s). Serial measurement of the patient's luteal estradiol and progesterone levels documents the adequacy of the protocol, and a serum sample is assayed for the beta subunit of hCG (B-hCG) approximately 10 to 12 days after the embryo transfer. If pregnancy ensues, the hormonal replacement is continued. In a failed cycle, the medication is discontinued and withdrawal bleeding will then occur.

After a successful donor oocyte cycle, exogenous hormonal support is required during the interval preceding the luteoplacental shift. Monitoring of peripheral estradiol and progesterone concentrations is continued once pregnancy is documented. The onset of adequate placental steroidogenesis is marked by a significant rise in these steroid levels, at which point the dosage of the replacement hormone is halved. Estradiol and progesterone levels are reassessed in another week; if a continued rise is observed, hormonal therapy may be discontinued. Generally, hormonal replacement is unnecessary beyond the tenth week. Endovaginal ultrasonographic documentation of fetal heart activity is possible 4 to 5 weeks after embryo transfer. Early ultrasonographic assessment is useful for excluding an extrauterine gestation and in evaluation of a possible multifetal pregnancy.

RESULTS OF OOCYTE DONATION

Theoretically, success rates after ovum donation should exceed those with conventional IVF, as the oocytes are derived from young (<35 years old), normally fertile women. Furthermore, the resulting embryos are transferred to an endometrial bed primed by physiologic levels of estrogen and progesterone, unlike that priming in routine IVF, when ovarian hyperstimulation results in markedly supraphysiologic luteal phase sex steroid levels and, very likely, an increased incidence of abnormal endometrial histology.[13] These theoretic expectations have been confirmed by clinical experience. An analysis of the 1990 statistics of the U.S. IVF Registry revealed a 29% clinical pregnancy rate and a 22% delivery rate per transfer, resulting from a total of 547 donor oocyte cycles.[19] These statistics are clearly favorable when viewed in the context of overall per-transfer IVF clinical and viable pregnancy rates of 22% and 17%, respectively, reported in the same

Table 48-1. The Center for Reproductive Medicine and Infertility, Cornell University Medical College: Donor oocyte program, July 1990 to April 1992

Event	Result
No. of transfers	45
Clinical pregnancies	27
Ongoing pregnancies	24 (53.3%)
Implantation rate/embryo	28.3%

survey. Our recent cumulative donor oocyte data are presented in Table 48-1.

OOCYTE DONATION AS A SCIENTIFIC MODEL

This discussion has thus far focused on key aspects of clinical ovum donation. The remainder of this chapter explores some of the scientific insights afforded by this new technology. Because of the inherent dissociation of perinidatory embryonic and endometrial events in donor oocyte IVF, these two variables can be independently studied and manipulated, permitting a greater understanding of human reproductive physiology. In particular, oocyte donation has shed light on aspects of uterine receptivity, including the window of implantation, and on the time course of the luteoplacental shift.

Uterine receptivity

Conventional IVF and embryo transfer (ET) is of limited value as a scientific model for the characterization and definition of uterine receptivity. The efficiency of blastocyst implantation hinges on at least two variables: embryonic competence and endometrial receptivity. In routine IVF-ET, these variables cannot be isolated and individually controlled, because they are intrinsically linked in a given cycle. In theory, frozen embryo transfer permits dissociation of embryonic and endometrial development, but the relatively high attrition of thawed embryos and the possibility of reduced embryonic function due to the stresses of cryopreservation limit the usefulness of frozen embryo transfer as a physiologic model.

Furthermore, there is a large body of evidence suggesting that the processes of superovulation and, possibly, follicular aspiration result in unphysiologic endometrium in assisted reproduction cycles. This may be caused in part by supraphysiologic estradiol and progesterone levels in the luteal phase, and/or an increased estradiol-progesterone ratio. Graf and associates[13] obtained late luteal phase endometrial biopsy specimens in 25 stimulated patients not undergoing embryo transfer and found a 76% incidence of out-of-phase endometrium, defined as a histologic lag exceeding 2 days, a rate far exceeding the frequency of abnormal biopsy results reported in natural cycles of normal, fertile women.[10] Using scanning electron microscopy to evaluate the ultrastructure of uterine luminal epithelium,

Martel and colleagues[18] compared endometrial biopsies from spontaneous cycles in normal volunteers with those obtained from women treated with clomiphene citrate and hMG for IVF. In normal cycles, bulbous apical protrusions termed pinopods cover the luminal surface by the sixth postovulatory day (i.e., in the presumed window of implantation) in 78% of biopsy specimens studied. In contrast, only 15% of specimens obtained from IVF patients in stimulated cycles displayed similar morphologic changes on the sixth day after ovulation. These findings further suggest the unphysiologic nature of stimulated endometrium, although the importance of pinopods in the facilitation of embryo attachment has not been established. Finally, Paulson and associates[27] demonstrated higher per-embryo implantation rates in patients with POF receiving physiologic levels of hormone replacement than in patients undergoing standard superovulation/IVF, while controlling for age and embryonic morphology. These findings also support the contention that ovulation induction compromises endometrial receptivity.

Oocyte donation provides an elegant model for studying the temporal window of transfer, and, by inference, the window of implantation, as embryos of known cell number can be transferred to physiologic, histologically defined endometrium on different days of the luteal phase. Analysis of such data has shown that the transfer of embryos of two or more blastomeres to endometrium that is histologically developed to day 17 to day 19 of the idealized 28-day cycle permits implantation and viable pregnancies.[25, 32] Assuming that a 4- to 16-cell embryo develops to the blastocyst stage within 2 to 3 days after transfer, these results suggest that the window of endometrial receptivity in the woman does not extend beyond day 22 or 23. These and other studies indicate an implantation window width of approximately $3\frac{1}{2}$ days. At least one study has suggested a window of up to 7 days; Formigli and associates[12] obtained donor embryos by uterine lavage 5 days after ovulation and reported pregnancies after transfer anywhere from 4 days in front to 3 days behind the donor, including one transfer on day 22. This report has been faulted for potential sources of error, including imprecise delineation of ovulation, which was assessed only by ultrasonography, and the inability to exclude the possibility of spontaneous pregnancy in patients with ovarian function.

It must be stressed that conclusions about uterine receptivity that are derived from these data rely on assumptions regarding in vivo cleavage rates of embryos resulting from in vitro fertilized oocytes (i.e., the time required for the attainment of embryonic implantation competence). This problem may be obviated if advances in embryo culturing techniques evolve to permit the transfer of fresh blastocysts. Furthermore, although hormonal replacement protocols permit histologic definition of the endometrium, the inadequacy of currently available systems for grading embryos limits the ability to accurately define embryo quality/

normality. Acknowledging these limitations, oocyte donation has afforded a unique opportunity to investigate the temporal window of uterine receptivity.

Secretory endometrial receptivity is dependent on estrogen priming in the antecedent follicular/proliferative phase. The ability to manipulate endometrial maturation with exogenous hormones has enabled investigators to examine the impact of varying follicular phase length on the histology and histochemistry of the secretory endometrium which ensues. We have studied 12 women with ovarian failure, replacing gonadal steroids with oral micronized estradiol-17β and intramuscular progesterone-in-oil.[24] Using a standard 28-day replacement protocol as the control (see earlier), both short (6 days) and long (3 to 5 weeks) follicular phase protocols were studied. Day 20 and day 26 endometrial biopsy specimens were obtained in all groups and were histologically dated and histochemically characterized with respect to glycocalyx intensity and galactose residue content by periodic acid-Schiff staining and lectin (*Ricinus communis* I agglutinin) binding. All parameters compared favorably among the different groups, suggesting that a follicular phase of only 6 days is adequate preparation for normal secretory maturation, and, conversely, that a lengthened follicular phase is not deleterious. Donor embryo transfer was not performed in this study, precluding a direct appraisal of implantation and pregnancy outcome. As previously mentioned in the discussion of donor-recipient synchronization, these results do appear to confirm a substantial margin of safety in varying the length of the recipients' "follicular" phase to accommodate that of the donor.

Ovum donation has also proven a useful model in addressing a major controversy vis-à-vis the age-related decline in female fecundity, that is, the relative importance of uterine versus oocyte senescence. Success rates after conventional IVF decline significantly after the age of 40 years, and viable pregnancies are infrequent beyond the age of 42. Donor eggs permit dissociation of uterine and oocyte age. Sauer et al.[36] published a series of seven patients aged 40 to 44 years (mean age 41.4) who underwent appropriate hormone replacement and transfer of embryos derived from oocytes from donors under 35 years of age. They reported a per-embryo implantation rate of 35.7%, with an overall clinical pregnancy rate of 75%, which was not significantly different from success rates seen in donor egg recipients younger than age 40 years (mean age 31.8 years).

Although these results were derived from a small number of subjects, experience at other centers tends to be confirmatory, suggesting that the age-associated decline in both natural fecundity and assisted reproduction success rates is due principally to oocyte aging, and that the endometrium of women over the age of 40 retains normal receptivity to implantation of fertilized donor eggs, if adequately primed with exogenous steroids.

The luteoplacental shift

Donor oocyte IVF provides a unique human in vivo model for studying the luteoplacental shift, because recipient subjects with POF have no endogenous ovarian function. In the early 1970s, Csapo and colleagues[7, 8] estimated that placental "takeover" of steroidogenesis occurs during the eighth week of gestation, based on the study of luteectomized pregnant women. More recently, Navot and associates[23] used the donor oocyte model in an effort to demarcate the luteoplacental shift, but in this report the administration of pharmacologic doses of steroids led to supraphysiologic levels of estrogen and progesterone, consequently delaying the detection of significant placental steroidogenesis until the twelfth week of pregnancy.

We have recently studied a group of nine patients with ovarian failure who conceived after oocyte donation.[38] Hormone replacement consisted of oral or transdermal estradiol coadministered with intramuscular progesterone-in-oil, resulting in both constant and physiologic serum levels. Serum estradiol and progesterone concentrations were assayed serially, and statistically significant mean increases in these levels were noted by the fourth and fifth weeks after embryo transfer, respectively (sixth and seventh weeks of gestation by last menstrual period). Linear regression analysis of steroid concentrations versus gestational age was performed, and the intersection with basal levels was determined, suggesting onset of placental steroidogenesis during the third week after transfer. Although this model is imperfect, given the clinical necessity for exogenous sex steroid administration for early pregnancy maintenance, it nonetheless provides valuable insight into the time course of the development of placental steroidogenic competence.

CONCLUSION

The last decade has witnessed the emergence of donor oocyte IVF as a highly successful approach to the management of infertility caused by ovarian failure. The extension of this technology to women with poor oocyte quality, inaccessible ovaries, advanced age, and carriage of potentially transmissable genetic disorders has broadened both the indications and the demand for donor eggs. Indeed, the limited availability of oocyte donors appears to be the major limiting factor in the provision of this reproductive technology. Apart from its obvious clinical utility, oocyte donation has afforded investigators an unparalleled opportunity to study fundamental aspects of reproductive biology, including the window of implantation, uterine receptivity, and the placental "takeover" of steroidogenesis. Ongoing research undoubtedly will lead to further insight into these important aspects of human physiology.

REFERENCES

1. Abdalla HI, Leonard T: Cryopreserved zygote intrafallopian transfer for anonymous oocyte donation, *Lancet* 1:835, 1988.
2. Asch RH et al: Oocyte donation and gamete intrafallopian transfer in premature ovarian failure, *Fertil Steril* 49:263, 1988.
3. Buster JE et al: Non-surgical transfer of in vitro fertilized donated ova to five infertile women: report of two pregnancies, *Lancet* 2:223, 1983.
4. Cha KY et al: Pregnancy after in vitro fertilization of human follicular oocytes collected from nonstimulated cycles, their culture in vitro and their transfer in a donor oocyte program, *Fertil Steril* 55:109, 1991.
5. Coulam CB: Premature ovarian failure, *Fertil Steril* 38:645, 1982.
6. Coulam CB, Adamson SC, Annegers JF: Incidence of premature ovarian failure, *Obstet Gynecol* 67:604, 1986.
7. Csapo AI, Pulkkinen MO, Kaihola HL: The effect of estradiol replacement therapy on early pregnancy luteectomized patients, *Am J Obstet Gynecol* 117:987, 1974.
8. Csapo AI, Pulkkinen MO, Wiest WG: Effect of luteectomy and early progesterone replacement therapy in early pregnant patients, *Am J Obstet Gynecol* 115:759, 1973.
9. Davis OK, Ravnikar VA: Ovulation induction with clomiphene citrate in a woman with premature ovarian failure: a case report, *J Reprod Med* 33:559, 1988.
10. Davis OK et al: The incidence of luteal phase defect in normal, fertile women determined by serial endometrial biopsies, *Fertil Steril* 51:582, 1989.
11. Droesch K et al: Transdermal estrogen replacement in ovarian failure for ovum donation, *Fertil Steril* 50:931, 1988.
12. Formigli L, Formigli G, Roccio C: Donation of fertilized uterine ova to infertile women, *Fertil Steril* 47:162, 1987.
13. Graf MJ et al: Histologic evaluation of the luteal phase in women following follicle aspiration for oocyte retrieval, *Fertil Steril* 49:616, 1988.
14. Heape W: Preliminary note on the transplantation and growth of mammalian ova with a uterine foster mother, *Proc R Soc Lond* 48:457, 1890.
15. Jackson RA et al: Ia+ T cells in new onset Graves' disease, *J Clin Endocrinal Metab* 59:187, 1984.
16. Licciardi FL et al: Day 3 estradiol levels as prognosticators of pregnancy outcome in in vitro fertilization, both alone and in conjunction with day 3 FSH levels. Presented at the 38th annual meeting of the Society for Gynecologic Investigation, March 20–23, 1991 (abstracts handbook, p 169).
17. Lutjen P et al: The establishment and maintenance of pregnancy using in vitro fertilization and embryo donation in a patient with primary ovarian failure, *Nature* 307:174, 1984.
18. Martel D et al: Scanning electron microscopy of the uterine luminal epithelium as a marker of the implantation window. In Yoshinaga K, editor: *Blastocyst implantation,* Boston, 1989, Adams Publishing Group.
19. Medical Research International, Society for Assisted Reproductive Technology and The American Fertility Society: In vitro fertilization-embryo transfer in the United States: 1990 results from the IVF-ET Registry, *Fertil Steril* 57:15, 1992.
20. Meldrum DR et al: Artificial agonadism and hormone replacement for oocyte donation, *Fertil Steril* 52:509, 1989.
21. Meyer RK, Wolf RC, Arslan M: Implantation and maintenance of pregnancy in progesterone treated ovarectomized monkeys (Macaca mulatta). In Hofer H, editor: *Proceedings of the 2nd International Congress of Primatology,* vol 2, Atlanta, 1968.
22. Navot D, Rosenwaks Z, Margolioth EJ: Prognostic assessment of female fecundity, *Lancet* 2:645, 1987.
23. Navot D et al: Artificially induced endometrial cycles and establishment of pregnancies in the absence of ovaries, *N Engl J Med* 314:806, 1986.
24. Navot D et al: Hormonal manipulation of endometrial maturation, *J Clin Endocrinol Metab* 68:801, 1989.
25. Navot D et al: The window of embryo transfer and the efficiency of human conception in vitro, *Fertil Steril* 55:114, 1991.
26. Noyes RW, Hertig AT, Rock J: Dating the endometrial biopsy, *Fertil Steril* 1:3, 1950.
27. Paulson RJ, Sauer MV, Lobo RA: Embryo implantation after human

in vitro fertilization: importance of endometrial receptivity, *Fertil Steril* 53:870, 1989.

28. Rabinowe SL et al: Ia-positive T-lymphocytes in recently diagnosed idiopathic Addison's disease, *Am J Med* 77:597, 1984.

29. Rabinowe SL et al: Lymphocyte dysfunction in autoimmune oophoritis: resumption of menses with corticosteroids, *Am J Med* 81:347, 1986.

30. Rebar RW: Premature ovarian failure: a multifactorial disorder, *Contemp Ob/Gyn* 21:175, 1983.

31. Romeu A et al: Results of in vitro fertilization attempts in women 40 years of age and older: the Norfolk experience, *Fertil Steril* 47:130, 1987.

32. Rosenwaks Z: Donor eggs: their application in modern reproductive technologies, *Fertil Steril* 47:895, 1987.

33. Rosenwaks Z, Davis OK: In vitro fertilization and related techniques. In Scott JR et al, editors: *Danforth's obstetrics and gynecology,* Philadelphia, 1990, JB Lippincott.

34. Rosenwaks Z, Veeck LL, Liu H-C: Pregnancy following transfer of in vitro fertilized donated oocytes, *Fertil Steril* 45:417, 1986.

35. Sauer MV: Retained pregnancy complicating donor ovum transfer, *Int J Gynecol Obstet* 29:83, 1989.

36. Sauer MV, Paulson RJ, Lobo RA: A preliminary report on oocyte donation extending reproductive potential to women over 40, *N Engl J Med* 323:1157, 1990.

37. Scott RT et al: Follicle-stimulating hormone levels on cycle day 3 are predictive of in vitro fertilization outcome, *Fertil Steril* 51:651, 1989.

38. Scott R et al: A human in vivo model for the luteoplacental shift, *Fertil Steril* 56:481, 1991.

39. Seidel GEJ Jr: Super ovulation and embryo transfer in cattle, *Science* 211:351, 1981.

40. Stumpf PG et al: Development of a vaginal ring for achieving physiologic levels of 17 beta-estradiol in hypoestrogenic women, *J Clin Endocrinol Metab* 54:208-210, 1982.

41. Trence DL, Morley JE, Handwerger BS: Polyglandular autoimmune syndromes, *Am J Med* 77:107, 1984.

42. Trounson A et al: Pregnancy established in an infertile patient after transfer of a donated embryo fertilized in vitro, *Br Med J* 286:835, 1983.

Part VII

PROBLEMS WITH PREGNANCY

Chapter 49

REPEATED PREGNANCY LOSS

Howard A. Zacur, M.D., Ph.D.
and Sandra B. Goodman M.D.

Recurrent spontaneous abortion (RSA), defined as three or more consecutive pregnancy losses prior to the 20th gestational week, affects 0.5-1% of women.[88] Although the definition of RSA requires the occurrence of three or more pregnancy losses, an evaluation for RSA may be initiated following two miscarriages, depending upon the patient's prior history and desire. Diagnostic evaluation after two losses is appropriate in women more than 35 years of age and for individuals who have had no prior live births.

Reported frequency of pregnancy loss varies in the literature, depending upon the patient population being studied and the method used to diagnose pregnancy. In the general population, the risk of spontaneous abortion in women with the clinical diagnosis of pregnancy is 10-20%. However, the actual risk of abortion varies, depending upon the woman's age and past obstetrical history. In Denmark, Knudsen et al. reviewed the outcomes of 300,500 pregnancies and determined that the overall risk for a spontaneous

pregnancy loss was 11%, but increased to 16, 25, 45, and 54%, respectively, after one to four consecutive losses. For women older than 35, the risk of pregnancy loss was increased by 10%.[69] In the United Kingdom, Regan et al. prospectively studied 630 women planning to conceive, and found an overall incidence of pregnancy loss of 12% before 20 weeks of gestation. Nulligravida women and gravidas with prior successful pregnancy outcomes had a risk for spontaneous loss of 5% and 4%, respectively. Women whose sole previous pregnancy ended in a loss or who experienced losses in all previous pregnancies were at a 20% and 24% risk, respectively, of having another loss.[115] These reported risks pertained to losses of clinically diagnosed pregnancies. When sensitive urinary assays to measure human chorionic gonadotropin (hCG) are used, pregnancy may be diagnosed before a missed menstrual period. A loss rate of 22% of preclinically recognized pregnancies has been reported by Wilcox et al., using a sensitive urinary hCG assay.[159]

Knowledge of the various rates of RSA, coupled with the unique medical history of the patient, should determine when to begin an evaluation for repeated pregnancy loss. The purpose of this chapter is to review the known and proposed etiologies, evaluation, and current management for RSA.

ETIOLOGY

The causes of repeated pregnancy loss are multiple, but are identifiable in only 37-44% of cases.[141, 147] Identifiable causes may be categorized under genetic, endocrinological, anatomical, microbiological, and immunological headings. In the authors' recent study of 60 women with two consecutive early pregnancy losses, 50% were unexplained. Identifiable causes for the remainder are listed in Table 49-1.[162]

Genetics

Genetic material in the embryo's genome is provided by contributions from the mother's and father's genomes. If the parental genetic contribution is not assembled and processed properly, disordered embryo and fetal develop-

Table 49-1. Causes of repetitive pregnancy loss in 60 couples

Cause	%
Unidentified	50 %
Uterine abnormality	26.7%
Luteal-phase defect	10 %
Chromosome abnormality	1.6%
Positive cervical culture	1.6%
Endocrine	3.4%
Two or more combined causes	6.7%

ment may occur, resulting in pregnancy loss. Fetal chromosomal aberrations may occur at the time of fertilization or may result from the transmission of a parental chromosomal anomaly. Nondisjunction (failure to separate) of chromosomes during meiosis or mitosis may result in the presence of an extra chromosome, or in the loss of a chromosome in the fetus. Trisomies of all types (e.g., trisomy 16 or trisomy 21 [Down syndrome]) constitute the largest group of abnormal karyotypes analyzed from spontaneous abortuses. The most common single karyotypical abnormality is monosomy X (45X or Turner syndrome). Conditions suggested to predispose for fetal trisomy or monosomy include maternal[54] and paternal age,[80] seasonal variation at time of conception, sex of the fetus,[71] presence of maternal infection,[68] exposure to irradiation,[130] presence of maternal thyroid antibodies,[37] and delayed fertilization.[129] All of these factors, except seasonal variation, have been found to be associated with chromosomal aberrations. However, the mechanisms responsible for the resulting chromosomal abnormalities remain unknown.

Nuclear presence of three or more multiples of the haploid chromosome number is termed *polyploidy*. Triploidy (69 chromosomes) is more common than tetraploidy (92 chromosomes). Polyploidy may result from errors during meiotic division in oogenia or spermatogenia (e.g., cligyny, which results from a failure to extrude the second polar body) or from oocyte fertilization by more than one sperm (e.g., dispermy).

Although it has been stated traditionally that chromosomal abnormalities account for 50-60% of sporadic, early, spontaneous pregnancy losses,[9, 98, 136] some studies suggest that the prevalence of chromosomal anomalies may be as low as 8-22%.[16, 138]

Compared with the general population, couples who experience RSA have a higher incidence of structural chromosomal rearrangements in one partner. A rate of 6.2% was cited in a 1981 report,[131] whereas in 1990, 4.7% of 22,199 couples with repeated losses were found to have a cytogenetic abnormality in one partner,[10] compared with 1% in the general population. In this investigation, reciprocal translocations (exchange of chromosomal segments between chromosomes) were twice as frequent as Robert-

sonian translocations (fusion of two acrocentric chromosomes at or near the centromere with loss of the short arms). The chance of detecting a chromosomal translocation in couples may be increased to 20% if the couple's past history reveals repetitive losses with the delivery of a child with a fetal malformation.[147]

It has also become apparent that genetic causes for pregnancy loss may exist despite the presence of a normal karyotype in the abortus. For example, an alteration at a single gene site can produce a lethal mutation by disrupting synthesis of a protein critical for embryonic growth. Identification of such genetic errors may occur in the future through the use of restriction fragment length polymorphisms or gene knockout techniques (insertional mutagenesis).[81]

Recurrent euploid pregnancy losses can also result from genetic errors of "parental genetic imprinting." This recent scientific concept was developed based upon studies in mice that showed that germ cell genetic material may be marked or imprinted by either the maternal or paternal source. For example, embryos have been created using highly inbred strains of mice that possess both sets of chromosomes from either maternal or paternal origin. These embryos are constructed by replacing pronuclei from the oocyte following fertilization. When both chromosomal sets are paternally derived, the embryo is called an *androgenote*. When the chromosomes are all of maternal origin, the embryo is called a *gynogenote*. Although euploid, these genetically altered embryos do not develop normally or to term. Gynogenotes exhibit normal embryonal growth with poor placental development, whereas androgenotes exhibit poor embryonic development with good placental development[132, 133] (Fig. 49-1).

Medical and endocrinological causes of RSA

Poorly controlled diabetes mellitus has been associated with spontaneous abortion. Miodovnik et al. prospectively studied 43 pregnant, insulin-dependent diabetic women. Glycemic control was assessed by measuring hemoglobin A_{1C}. Women with spontaneous pregnancy losses had significantly higher hemoglobin A_{1C} levels than women without losses. Improvement in subsequent pregnancy outcome was attainable when the hemoglobin A_{1C} level was lowered.[87] Animal studies suggest a direct toxic effect of glucose on embryo growth and development.[21]

Hypothyroidism may cause infertility; however, its etiological role in RSA has been debated.[23, 44, 60] The biological mechanism(s) responsible for pregnancy loss during the hypothyroid state remains unknown. In fact, Montoro et al. have questioned whether hypothyroidism has any role in causing spontaneous abortion because none of the 11 pregnancies in their study population of nine hypothyroid women ended in abortion. However, in this study, only three out of nine patients did not receive thyroxine therapy.[90]

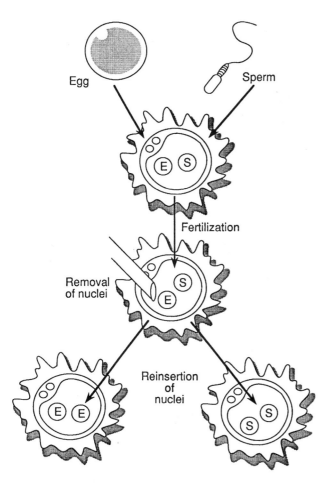

Fig. 49-1. Creation of a gynogenote (EE) or androgenote (SS). E represents the pronucleus from the egg and S represents the pronucleus from the sperm.

Existence of subclinical hypothyroidism has been suspected by some endocrinologists when antibodies to thyroglobulin and thyroid peroxidase (microsomal antigen) are detected in the serum. Stagnaro-Green et al. screened 552 women during the first trimester of pregnancy and found that women who tested positive for the thyroid autoantibody miscarried at a rate of 17%, compared with a rate of 8.4% for autoantibody-negative women.[135] A higher percentage of patients with RSA (31%) were found to have thyroid autoantibodies compared with controls (19%) in another study, although this difference did not reach statistical significance.[106] The presence of thyroid antibodies may reflect an underlying autoimmune problem that could be the cause of pregnancy loss rather than a result of the hypothyroid state.

Other medical illnesses associated with RSA include heart disease and systemic lupus erythematosus (SLE). Pregnancy loss rates of greater than 50% have been reported in women with congenital heart disease.[83] The risk of an adverse outcome depends upon the underlying cardiac anomaly. Cyanotic patients are more likely to be adversely affected than acyanotic patients.[127]

Women with SLE have fertility rates comparable to the general population, but are at a higher risk for pregnancy loss. The etiology for spontaneous loss in these patients may be attributable to the presence of circulating antiphospholipid antibodies (discussed later in this chapter). Diagnosis of SLE requires documentation of at least four of 11 signs or symptoms (see box below). The cause of this disorder remains unknown, but an immunological etiology is suspected.[137] Some RSA patients demonstrate a low positive antinuclear antibody titer, but do not have any other criteria of SLE.[162] This finding may reflect on underlying immune disturbance that is either the cause or consequence of pregnancy loss.

A deficiency in the luteal phase of the menstrual cycle was initially described by Jones in 1949.[57] Luteal-phase deficiency is defined as inadequate endometrial development, presumably due to insufficient progesterone secretion or activity. Diagnosis is made by endometrial biopsy obtained late in the luteal phase, 1-3 days prior to the anticipated onset of menstrual bleeding. The diagnosis is established if the calculated cycle date differs from the histological date by greater than two days during two cycles. (See box on p. 884.) More recently, Shoupe et al. have recommended that the histological date be correlated with a cycle date calculated from the time of ovulation.[128]

Other luteal-phase abnormalities have been described. These include a "short" luteal phase in which the onset of menses occurs earlier than 10 days following ovulation,[143] or an "inadequate" luteal phase in which progesterone levels are low.[1, 93] Luteal-phase deficiencies have been reported in 35-60% of couples who have experienced RSA.[43, 58] However, there is controversy over the existence of this entity[116] because the mechanism of pregnancy loss in patients diagnosed with a luteal-phase abnormality remains undetermined. Nonetheless, the importance of progesterone in maintaining early gestation is not contested,

---

Criteria for diagnosis of systemic lupus erythematosus

Malar rash
Discoid rash
Photosensitivity
Oral ulcers
Arthritis
Serositis
Renal disorder
Neurologic disorder
Hematologic disorder
Antinuclear antibody
Diagnosis of systemic lupus erythematosus requires any four or more of the above listed criteria.

Steinberg AD: Systemic Lupus Erythematosus. In Cecil *Textbook of Medicine.* Wyngaarden JD, Smith LH Bennet JC (eds). Philadelphia, 1992, WB Saunders.

Example: diagnosis of luteal-phase defect by biopsy

Endometrial biopsy taken
  March 1, 1994
First day of menses (defined by patient) occurs on March 3, 1994
March 3, 1994, is assigned as day 28 of the cycle. Determination of the day of ovulation is not needed.
The pathologist provides a histological date of the biopsy material. It should agree within two days of the day of menses (e.g., day 24-26 in the above example).
If the pathologist reads the biopsy as day 23, then the histological date would differ from the actual day of menses by greater than two days, consistent with an "out-of-phase" cycle.

---

especially in view of studies demonstrating induced pregnancy loss using the antiprogestin, RU-486.[4]

Infectious diseases and recurrent pregnancy loss

Reports have appeared periodically in medical literature implicating infectious organisms as a cause for RSA. Unfortunately, prospective, well-designed, controlled studies have not been performed to definitively answer the question of whether or not specific infections cause RSA.

Mycoplasmas are small bacteria that lack a cell wall. Although 64 types of mycoplasmas have been isolated,[146] only two of the T-strain mycoplasmas found in the human genital tract—*Mycoplasma hominis* and *Ureaplasma urealyticum*—have been implicated as causes of RSA. Cervical colonization by these organisms may occur following genital contact, but may also exist in the absence of prior sexual activity. Knudsen et al. were the first to report an association of genital tract *Ureaplasma urealyticum* with pregnancy loss.[67] Stray-Pedersen et al. noted a higher incidence of *Ureaplasma urealyticum* colonization in the cervix and endometrium in patients with three or more consecutive losses compared with control subjects. In this study, some of the RSA patients and their partners were treated with doxycycline (200 mg PO on day one, with 100 mg daily for the next 11 days). Treated patients had more successful pregnancy outcomes in gestation than untreated colonized patients.[140] Quinn et al. reported a higher rate of genital mycoplasma colonization in women with spontaneous abortion[108] and documented improved pregnancy outcome following antibiotic therapy.[109] Unfortunately, reported clinical trials have not been randomized, double-blind, or placebo-controlled. As a result, evidence linking mycoplasma colonization with recurrent pregnancy loss, as well as the role for antibiotic treatment, remains empirical.[144, 157]

Although other systemic and genital tract infections have been implicated as causes of sporadic spontaneous abortion, it is unlikely that they cause RSA. The parasite *Toxoplasma gondii,* acquired by eating raw, infested meat or inhaling oocytes from the feces of infected cats, may invade the placenta and embryo during an acute infection, resulting in fetal death. However, there is no evidence to suggest that this parasite plays a role in RSA[64] following initial infection. *Listeria monocytogenes* is a motile, gram-positive rod transmitted through the ingestion of contaminated dairy products.[38] Identification of the organism within the vagina is rare. Rabau and David found no evidence of *Listeria* infection among 554 patients who had experienced a spontaneous abortion, including 74 women with repeated pregnancy losses.[111] Conversely, Rappaport and Rabinovitz found *Listeria* in 25 of 34 women with recurrent abortions, while none of the 87 control patients who had not experienced a pregnancy loss tested positive for *Listeria.*[112] A subsequent ten-year prospective study of women with RSA failed to identify *Listeria monocytogenes* in the genital tract. The authors conclude that, although *Listeria monocytogenes* may contribute to fetal loss during acute infection, it is unlikely to be the causative agent on a recurrent basis.[79] *Salmonella typhi* and *Campylobacter* species (formerly known as *Vibrio fetus;* i.e., *C. jejuni, C. coli,* and *C. fetus*), as well as *Brucella* species (*B. abortus, B. melitensis,* and *B. suis*) may cause pregnancy loss during an acute infection, but are unlikely to result in RSA. Group B *β-hemolytic streptococci* (*Streptococcus agalactiae*), a gram-positive diplococcus frequently cultured from the genital tract of pregnant women,[2,3] has been associated with premature rupture of the membranes, preterm delivery, and neonatal infection.[114] However, there is no substantive evidence to date that links Group B *Streptococcus* vaginal colonization with RSA.

Viral infections also may cause spontaneous abortion, but do not appear to be responsible for repeated losses. Primary infections with rubella, cytomegalovirus, and herpes simplex virus during early pregnancy have been associated with severe congenital fetal anomalies and pregnancy loss. Immunity to the rubella virus is acquired following primary infection or immunization; thus, rubella is not a cause for RSA. Similarly, reactivation of cytomegalovirus, and secondary or recurrent herpes simplex infection, do not appear to be linked to abortion. Although the human immunodeficiency virus (HIV) may result in a 40-70% chance of maternal-to-fetal infection,[123, 124] precise risks for pregnancy loss or repeated losses in women infected with the HIV virus remain to be determined.

Chlamydia trachomatis is an obligate intracellular organism detected in some pregnant women. The effects of chlamydia infection on pregnancy outcome are controversial.[82] Quinn et al. reported an increased prevalence of immunoglobulin G antibodies to chlamydia in women with RSA compared with controls, although ongoing infection in these women was not present.[110] This raises the possibility that the existence of an antibody to chlamydia may result in pregnancy loss through mechanisms independent of active infection. Witkin and Ledger also found an increased incidence of elevated chlamydia antibody titer in women with RSA.[161] They speculated that prior chlamydial infection could induce an autoimmune response. The chlamydia organism has been shown to produce a 57 kd protein, which belongs to the 60 kd family of heat shock proteins.[91, 92] Developing mouse embryos have also been demonstrated to produce heat shock proteins.[6] Thus, antibodies initially generated in response to a chlamydia infection could potentially be directed against proteins produced by the developing embryo.

Uterine structural anomalies

The estimated frequency of müllerian duct anomalies in the general population is 0.1-0.5%. However, uterine anomalies are found at a rate of 10-14% in women with repeated pregnancy loss.[141, 147] Müllerian anomalies associated with RSA include unicornuate, didelphic, bicornuate, and septate uteri (see Fig 61-17, p. 1103). A septate uterus is indistinguishable from a bicornuate uterus on hysterosalpingography, but a notch in the uterine fundus may be seen in the bicornuate uterus at laparoscopy. The reasons for pregnancy loss in patients with müllerian anomalies remain hypothetical. Impaired blood supply to an embryo implanted onto a septum has been suggested. Fedele et al. determined with ultrasound the implantation site of 12 pregnancies in women with septate uteri and observed that all viable pregnancies were implanted into the lateral uterine walls. Of the eight pregnancies that ended in abortion, implantation in the septum was noted in six.[35]

Uterine anomalies resulting from diethylestilbesterol (DES) exposure in utero represent a special subset of patients who experience pregnancy loss. Studies attempting to determine if an increased risk for an unfavorable pregnancy outcome exists for women exposed to DES in utero have produced conflicting data. When ectopic pregnancy and preterm delivery are included with spontaneous abortion as outcome variables, it is clear that DES-exposed women are two to three times more likely than nonexposed women to experience an adverse outcome.[150] Whether or not DES exposure increases the risk for RSA is an important clinical question that has been difficult to answer due to the small number of women studied. It has been suggested, however, that the chance of having recurrent losses is twice as high for women exposed to DES.[49] The causes for pregnancy loss in DES-exposed women remain unknown. Recently, pregnancy outcome for women exposed to DES who underwent in vitro fertilization (IVF) was compared to that for women who were not exposed to DES with tubal disease who underwent in vitro fertilization. Term and ongoing pregnancy rates were lower in the DES-exposed group, although the pregnancy loss rates were not different from the group not exposed to DES. Perhaps hormonal manipulation associated with IVF prevented pregnancy loss

following implantation, but the results also suggest a reduced implantation rate for the uterus exposed to DES.[61]

Uterine synechiae

Intrauterine synechiae (adhesions within the uterine cavity) may be detected in 1.5% of patients undergoing hysterosalpingography.[31] Adhesions may form within the uterine cavity following traumatic endometrial curettage, myomectomy, cauterization of submucous fibroids or polyps, or infection. Curettage following pregnancy loss is the most common cause of adhesion formation,[121, 151] apparently resulting from a denudation of the endometrium, followed by fibrosis of the basalis layer.

Consequences of intrauterine adhesions include infertility, amenorrhea, hypomenorrhea, and pregnancy loss. Evaluation of over 2000 patients found to have intrauterine synechiae revealed that 43% complained of infertility, 37% were amenorrheic, 31% had hypomenorrhea, and 14% had repeated pregnancy losses.[121] A well-documented explanation for pregnancy loss in patients with intrauterine adhesions is lacking. Diminished uterine blood flow in areas of adhesion formation is a possible cause.[104] The importance of endometrial vascularization for successful embryonic growth was demonstrated in one study of chorionic villous vascularization of 40 patients with spontaneous, first-trimester abortion compared with 10 patients undergoing legal abortion. Deficient villous vascularization was found in cases of embryonic death and blighted ova. However, it could not be determined conclusively if the primary cause for the demise was embryonic in origin or secondary to poor endometrial vascularization.[84]

Leiomyomata

The effect of uterine leiomyomata on reproductive performance remains controversial. Submucous and intramural fibroids may result in pregnancy loss by disturbing endometrial development or by compromising the vascular supply to the implantation site. The association between leiomyomata and RSA remains tentative. Verkauf summarized the results from seven clinical studies published between 1983 and 1991 addressing the effect of myomectomy on fertility enhancement. Of 13 patients with RSA, nine successfully delivered following myomectomy, a success rate of 69.2%.[153] However, the studies were not prospective or controlled. Furthermore, a 69.2% successful pregnancy outcome is not significantly different from the 76% success rate reported prospectively by Regan, Braude, and Trembath for all women with RSA.[115] In a study of 1941 cases, Buttram and Reiter reported a reduction in the rate of spontaneous abortion from 41% preoperatively to 19% following myomectomy.[14] However, this was a retrospective study. A clear need exists for prospective, randomized investigations involving larger numbers of patients to assess the effect of leiomyomata on pregnancy outcome. Currently, myomectomy for RSA is recommended only after all other causes of pregnancy loss have been eliminated.

Environmental factors

A variety of environmental agents have been implicated as etiological factors in RSA. These include the use of prescription and illicit drugs, caffeine, tobacco, and alcohol, as well as exposure to radiation, pesticides, and other occupational toxins.

Despite early concerns, the use of oral-contraceptive pills prior to the time of conception is not associated with an increased risk of pregnancy loss.[47] Similarly, vaginal spermicides were initially implicated in pregnancy loss,[56] but follow-up studies found no evidence to suggest that spermicide exposure around the time of conception is harmful to the fetus.[85, 142]

Caffeine consumption has been reported to be associated with pregnancy loss.[8,134] However, in a recent report, moderate caffeine use was not associated with increased risk of pregnancy loss, particularly when other risk factors, such as smoking, were taken into account.[86]

Increased risk for adverse obstetrical outcome has been documented for women who use cocaine, alcohol, or tobacco during pregnancy. Cocaine use has been associated with an increased risk of pregnancy loss and congenital anomalies.[77] However, cocaine users also tend to abuse other drugs, suffer from poor nutrition, and have an increased incidence of sexually transmitted diseases, which could be responsible for their poor pregnancy outcomes.[13] Higher doses of alcohol consumption during pregnancy have been associated with congenital anomalies and increased risk of pregnancy loss.[20] Ingestion of more than two drinks per day, or one ounce of alcohol per week, increases the risk of a spontaneous loss to two times that of the general population.[46, 66] The cause of pregnancy loss associated with alcohol ingestion remains unknown, but the toxicity of alcohol itself and its metabolic product, acetaldehyde, may be causative.[45] Cigarette smoking has also been reported to be a risk factor for spontaneous abortion.[65] Women who smoke more than half a pack of cigarettes per day have been reported to have a 1.7 times increased rate of spontaneous abortion compared with nonsmokers. An adverse effect from passive smoke also has been reported.[160] It is believed that the adverse effects of smoking are mediated by its inducement of a hypoxic state.

High doses of ionizing radiation have been associated with congenital malformation and death in animals. Radiation exposure prior to implantation is likely to result in embryo death, whereas implantation exposure following implantation results in congenital malformation.[12] The effects of ionizing radiation are dose dependent. A dose response curve for human gestation has not been established.

Electromagnetic radiation from the use of video display terminals and electric blankets has also been suggested as a cause of pregnancy loss.[7, 158] However, a recent epidemiological study addressing the risk of spontaneous abortion associated with the use of video display terminals revealed no increase in abortifacient risk.[122]

Other environmental factors, including exposure to pesticides, heavy metals, and organic solvents, have been implicated in pregnancy loss. These potential environmental reproductive hazards have been addressed in several recent, excellent review articles.[41, 101, 103, 154]

Occupational exposure to antineoplastic drugs or nitrous oxide have been implicated in reproductive failure. Epidemiological studies have suggested adverse effects on fertility or pregnancy maintenance following occupational exposure to antineoplastic drugs[126] and nitrous oxide.[120] However, more work needs to be done to quantify exposure dose with the risk of infertility or pregnancy loss.

Immunological causes

Despite a thorough evaluation, the etiology for RSA remains undetermined in up to 60% of patients. Advances in the field of immunology have led to an increased understanding of the immune processes involved in normal pregnancy maintenance and pregnancy failure.[50, 51, 52] Immunological factors may be involved in more than 10% of pregnancy losses and in up to 80% of unexplained RSA. Thus, it is worthwhile to briefly review several salient features of the immune system and some of the hypotheses of how this system affects implantation and normal pregnancy maintenance.

Cells contain many surface antigens, including histocompatibility antigens, which are involved in cell recognition and immunity. The class I major histocompatibility complex (MHC) antigens, also called the *human leucocyte antigens* (HLA-A, -B, and -C), help cytotoxic T cells recognize foreign antigens. Class II MHC antigens, also called *HLA-DR, -DP and -DQ,* affect the ability of helper T lymphocytes to recognize foreign cell surface antigens. Thus, the MHC antigens participate in the immunological recognition and rejection of foreign tissue. When the immune system is stimulated by a foreign antigen, macrophages are activated, resulting in phagocytosis of the foreign substance and release of proteins called *cytokines.* Cytokines activate other cells of the immune system, including B lymphocytes, which release antibodies. Normally, the body's immune system recognizes its own cell surface antigens and attacks only tissue that is "foreign."

The immunological mechanisms invoked during gestation are unique because the products of conception contain paternal antigens that are foreign to the maternal host, yet are not rejected. Immunological sparing of the fetus may occur as a result of the production of immunosuppressive factors and blocking antibodies by the blastocyst, endometrium, or decidua that prevent fetal antigens from being detected by the maternal immune system.[117] (See Fig. 49-2.) Thus, it has been theorized that an inadequate production of these protective suppressor cells and blocking antibodies, or an exaggerated maternal immune response, could result in rejection of the conceptus and spontaneous abortion. The production of suppressor cells and blocking antibodies is hypothesized to be stimulated, in part, as a result of antigenic disparity between reproducing partners. It is presumed that when HLA antigenic sharing is present in partners, the conceptus could have an unusually high percentage of cell surface antigens, similar to those of the mother. The maternal immune system would be less likely to produce protective suppressor cells and blocking antibodies, leaving the products of conception vulnerable to immune attack.[5] Based upon this theory, couples with repeated pregnancy loss, identified as "sharing" HLA antigens, were treated by attempting to sensitize the maternal immune system to paternal cell antigens through paternal leucocyte immunotherapy.[94] However, recent studies demonstrated similar patterns of HLA sharing both in couples with RSA and in control couples,[34] and have not correlated HLA sharing with pregnancy failure. HLA sharing in couples with RSA may represent the sharing of a genetic marker for an HLA-linked gene defect, rather than being the cause of immunological intolerance.[42] Thus, these couples may possess a gene defect that is responsible for pregnancy losses.

A heightened maternal immune response to paternally derived antigens could result in rejection of the conceptus and spontaneous abortion. Hill et al. propose that leucocytes from some women with RSA produce cytokines, in response to reproductive antigenic stimulation, that are toxic to the conceptus and result in abortion.[53] Of the peripheral serum samples from 180 women with unexplained RSA in this study, 90% had production of embryo and/or trophoblast-toxic factors when challenged with sperm or trophoblast antigen in vitro. In contrast, none of the serum samples from 30 fertile control patients were toxic to embryo development or trophoblast growth following stimulation with sperm or trophoblast antigen. Thus, attenuation of the normal immunosuppressive response to pregnancy, or increased maternal immune response to reproductive antigens, represents potential immune mechanisms for pregnancy loss in women with otherwise unexplained RSA.

Another hypothesized immunological mechanism for RSA is that caused by maternal production of phospholipid antibodies,[33, 113] known as *antiphospholipid syndrome*. In this syndrome, IgG and IgM antibodies are attracted to phospholipid antigens, resulting in venous and arterial thrombosis, thrombocytopenia, and in some patients, recurrent reproductive failure. Two of the identified phospholipid antigens are cardiolipin and phosphatidylserine (Fig. 49-3). Circulating antibodies to these antigens can be measured. It is theorized that, because phospholipids are found on the surface of platelets and endothelial cells, antibodies binding to these antigens could result in platelet and/or endothelial

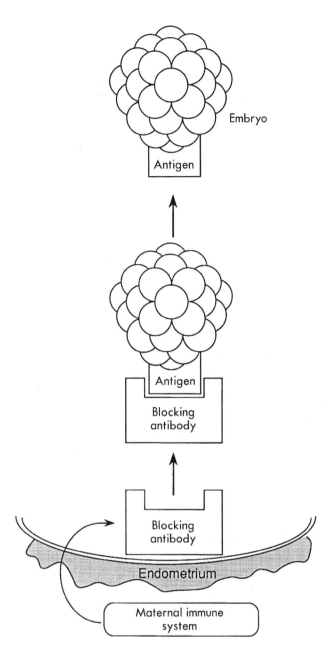

Fig. 49-2. Illustration of a maternally synthesized antibody that "blocks" or "masks" the presence of a "foreign" antigen on the cell surface of the embryo.

cell damage. This causes thrombosis and thrombocytopenia, which in turn may cause pregnancy loss. This proposed mechanism may not be correct because neither binding of immunoglobulin nor alterations in prostacyclin levels were observed when human umbilical vein endothelial cultures were incubated with sera from women who had high titers of phospholipid antibodies.[32] Alternatively, antiphospholipid antibodies may cause thrombosis by binding to protein C and inhibiting its activity. Protein C, activated by the thrombin-thrombomodulin complex, acts as an anticoagu-

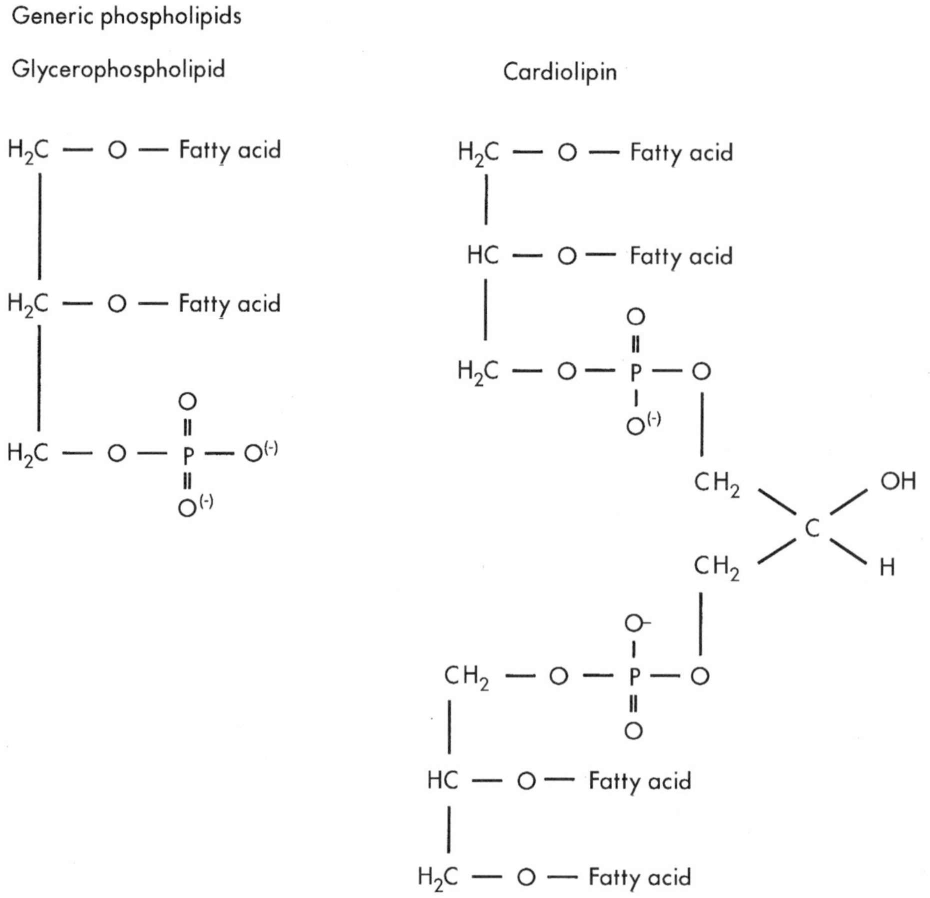

Generic phospholipids

Glycerophospholipid   Cardiolipin

Fig. 49-3. Examples of phospholipids. The general structure and the specific phospholipid cardiolipin.

lant by degrading coagulation factors VIII and V.[40, 155] It has been proposed that inactivation of protein C by phospholipid antibodies could result in enhancement of coagulation and thrombus formation.[39] The presence of antiphospholized antibodies in the maternal serum has been associated with adverse pregnancy outcome in both retrospective and prospective studies.[100]

One of the first phospholipid antibodies to be characterized was the lupus anticoagulant, identified in patients with SLE.[22] This antiphospholipid antibody affects the extrinsic activation of prothrombin in vitro, causing prolongation of the partial thromboplastin time.[148] In contrast, it is presumed that in vivo, the antibody binds to surface membranes, causing injury and eventually resulting in thrombosis.

Antibodies to cardiolipin may be detected by radioimmunoassay or enzyme-linked immunosorbent assay.[48] However, the definition of a positive cardiolipin antibody test remains controversial, because assays may require antibody titers to be greater than two to four standard deviations from the assay control mean to be labeled as positive.[74] Detection of the lupus anticoagulant phospholipid antibody is difficult because an immunoassay to measure an antibody titer for a specific phospholipid does not exist. Instead, the existence of this antibody is inferred by the ability of the patient's serum to interfere with in vitro coagulation tests. The most sensitive of these tests is Russell's viper venom time.[149] Russell's viper venom serves as a very potent extrinsic activator of the clotting system. Lupus anticoagulant evidently can bind to the venom and inhibit its activity, thus prolonging the in vitro clotting time.

PRECONCEPTION EVALUATION

An evaluation for RSA should be undertaken after two or three consecutive pregnancy losses. Couples who experience a pregnancy loss are frequently under intense emotional stress, particularly when an explanation for the pregnancy loss is not forthcoming. Suspicions about the effects of smoking even a single cigarette, drinking a single alcoholic beverage, or having had a pregnancy termination in the past may provoke intense guilt in the couple with a pregnancy loss. The physician should anticipate the possibility of these reactions and be prepared to recommend counseling when indicated.[72]

During the evaluation, a detailed history and complete physical examination are required. The history should include details about the patient's occupational exposures, use of prescribed or over-the-counter medications, cigarettes, alcohol, illicit drugs, in utero exposure to DES, and prior history of cervical or uterine manipulation. Physical examination may reveal evidence of an endocrinological disorder or a genital tract abnormality, such as a müllerian anomaly or leiomyomata.

Laboratory tests to evaluate thyroid, prolactin, and immune status should be obtained. Peripheral blood karyotype of both partners is recommended. Endocervical cultures for *Mycoplasma* and *Ureaplasma* may be obtained. Hysterosalpingography and/or hysteroscopy should be performed following cessation of the menstrual flow, but prior to ovulation, to exclude uterine anatomical defects. A timed endometrial biopsy is taken to evaluate the adequacy of the luteal phase (see Table 49-2).

Thyroid status may be evaluated using a sensitive thyroid-stimulating hormone (TSH) assay.[97] Measurement of thyroid antibodies may not be helpful; there is controversy about whether their existence is increased in patients with repeated pregnancy loss.[106] Even if these antibodies are present, it remains unclear how to treat affected patients.

A search for phospholipid antibodies is appropriate in view of their association with pregnancy loss. Currently, cardiolipin antibodies may be detected directly by immunoassay; the existence of lupus anticoagulant phospholipid antibodies is inferred by an alteration of standard clotting tests such as Russell's viper venom time.

Measurement of an ANA titer may identify individuals with an underlying connective tissue disease or potential immune disturbance.

The utility of additional assays to evaluate potential immune etiologies for RSA, including parental human leucocyte antigen profiles and mixed lymphocyte culture studies, remains controversial. The predictive value of these tests is unclear. In fact, the presence of cytotoxic antibodies and mixed lymphocyte culture inhibitors may be determined by the number and duration of prior pregnancies.

Although the prevalence of karyotypic anomalies is relatively low (3-5% of couples with repeated pregnancy losses) and the costs of performing a karyotype are high, a karyotype is recommended because an abnormal result provides couples with an explanation for their losses. Depending upon the karyotypic abnormality detected, the couple may be encouraged to conceive again or counseled to consider donor gametes or adoption.

Despite the controversy surrounding the effect of a mycoplasma infection on pregnancy maintenance, it is reasonable to treat a mycoplasma infection if no other cause for pregnancy loss is identified.

New diagnostic tests include measurement of chlamydial antibody titers. As previously mentioned, antibodies generated in response to a prior chlamydial infection may cross-react with embryo antigens. Further testing of this hypothesis, as well as formulating treatment protocols designed to reduce chlamydial antibody titers, are awaited.

The preconceptional evaluation of couples who have experienced repeated pregnancy losses affords the physician an opportunity to provide standard preconception advice. This includes the offer to obtain a rubella titer, with a recommendation for vaccination if the patient has not been immunized, and a baseline toxoplasmosis titer. Tay-Sachs and sickle-cell screening should be performed in genetically susceptible individuals. Couples can be counseled regarding the benefits of periconceptional folic acid supplementation (0.4 mg per day) to reduce the risk of neural tube defects.[27, 118] Additionally, patients should be counseled regarding the effects of passive smoke, as well as

Table 49-2. Diagnostic tests for patients undergoing evaluation for repeated pregnancy losses

Description	Purpose
Customary investigations	
Sensitive TSH assay	To identify hypothyroidism
Cardiolipin antibody titer	To identify phospholipid antibody
Russell's venom viper titer or comparable clotting assay	To identify lupus anticoagulant phospholipid antibody
Karyotype of paternal and maternal chromosomes	To identify anomalies
Hysterosalpingography and hysteroscopy	To identify uterine anomalies and adhesions
Endometrial biopsy	To identify luteal-phase dysfunction
Additional studies	
Cervical cultures	To detect *Mycoplasma nominis* and *Ureaplasma urealyticum*
Antinuclear antibody (ANA) titer	To screen for lupus erythematosus
Controversial investigations	
Determination of human leucocytic antigens in the couple	To detect an immunological cause of pregnancy loss
Mixed lymphocyte culture (MLC)	To detect an immunological cause of pregnancy loss
New diagnostic tests	
IgG antibody to *Chlamydia trachomatis*	Identification of an antibody that may cross-react with embryo antigen

the toxicity associated with maternal tobacco and alcohol use. Nutritional advice may be provided at this time. Benefits from preconceptional planning appear to be great, with minimal risk to the couple.[59]

TREATMENT

Assessing the response to any form of therapy is difficult because the rate of pregnancy maintenance is high, even in the absence of treatment.

Diagnosis of hypothyroidism is usually followed by treatment with exogenous thyroxine. Follow-up measurements of TSH are performed at 4-6-week intervals following each dosage adjustment. There is currently no evidence to suggest that euthyroid individuals with measurable thyroid antibodies and RSA benefit from "immune suppression." However, these patients should be monitored for the development of thyroid disease because patients with thyroid antibodies are at an increased risk for hypo-or hyperthyroidism secondary to autoimmune thyroiditis.

The recommended treatment for luteal phase deficiency is progesterone supplementation, administered either as a daily intramuscular injection of progesterone in oil (12.5 mg), or as vaginal suppositories (25 mg) given twice daily beginning on the third day of the basal body temperature rise. Treatment is continued until week 10-12 of gestation. Efficacy of progesterone treatment has been reported,[29] but doubts remain about its benefit.[78] Other methods used to treat luteal phase disturbances include clomiphene citrate and human menotropins. Such agents are presumed to work by improving follicular quality, resulting in increased estrogen stimulation of endometrial progesterone receptors, and by improved corpus luteum function following ovulation.

Following identification of a uterine anomaly, corrective surgical treatment may be recommended based upon the diagnosis. For a septate uterus, hysteroscopic resection, using scissors or wire loop cautery, has replaced the wedge metroplasty procedure performed previously through a laparotomy incision.[18] Septum resection has also been performed successfully under sonographic guidance.[107] Recently, hysteroscopic metroplasty was attempted to treat five DES-exposed patients with RSA. Three of these patients subsequently had viable pregnancies.[96] Spontaneous endometrial epithelial repair following hysteroscopic resection of a septum has been reported, suggesting that exogenous administration of estrogens after this procedure is not needed, and that pregnancy may be attempted as soon as two months after surgery.[15, 152] Pregnancy success following hysteroscopic metroplasty has been excellent; the percentage of live births following the procedure ranges from 73-87%.[36]

Suggested treatments for patients found to have antiphospholipid antibodies include the use of aspirin, prednisone, heparin, leucocyte immunization, and intravenous immunoglobulins. Lubbe et al. reported live births in five out of six women with RSA and positive lupus anticoagu-

lant who had been treated with aspirin and prednisone.[75, 76] Treatment is initiated at the time of the diagnosis of pregnancy. Aspirin is given at a dosage of 80 mg/day. Prednisone is given at a dosage of 40 mg/day until the activated prothrombin clotting time returns to normal. Higher prednisone dosages may be necessary. Upon normalization of the clotting time, the prednisone dosage may be gradually reduced to 10-15 mg/day, as long as the clotting time remains normal. Heparin therapy alone or with daily, low-dose aspirin (80 mg) has also been recommended to treat phospholipid antibody syndrome.[119] Different regimens of heparin therapy have been described, but usually 10,000-20,000 U of heparin/day is given subcutaneously in 2-3 divided doses as soon as a viable pregnancy is documented. Intravenous immunoglobulins have been used with some success in RSA patients found to be positive for antiphospholipid antibodies.[99, 125, 156] Rationale for this form of therapy remains speculative. Blocking of antibody binding to endothelial receptors has been cited as a potential reason.

Branch et al. noted that despite treatment with prednisone and aspirin, heparin and aspirin, prednisone, heparin, and aspirin, or immunoglobulins, pregnancy loss occurred. The overall rate of infant survival from all treatment groups reportedly averaged 63%.[11]

Risks of therapy to both mother and fetus following treatment have been investigated. Lockshin, Druzin, and Qamar reported that prednisone therapy did not improve pregnancy outcome in pregnant women with high antiphospholipid antibody titers. Results from this study, although not significant, indicated that untreated women did better than their treated cohorts.[73] This conclusion was in agreement with the findings by Out et al.[100] Cowchock et al. reported that, in a collaborative, randomized trial comparing prednisone with low-dose heparin therapy, heparin therapy was preferred because women given this treatment were less likely to deliver preterm or to develop preeclampsia.[25] Although children born to mothers treated for antiphospholipid syndrome tend to deliver prematurely, overall rates of minor to severe neonatal complications do not appear to be increased when compared with other prematurely delivered infants.[105] Maternal risks of prednisone therapy include poor wound healing, Cushingoid facies, osteoporosis, aseptic femoral head necrosis, and adrenal insufficiency. Heparin therapy has been associated with bleeding, thrombocytopenia, and fractures secondary to heparin-induced osteoporosis.[28] Combined therapy with prednisone and heparin appears to increase the risk for osteoporosis.

Patients sharing histocompatibility antigens or failing to mount a response in mixed lymphocyte cell cultures have been offered immunotherapy with paternal leucocytes.[145] Maternal immunization has usually been performed by subcutaneous administration of paternal or third-party leucocytes. Support for such therapy has depended upon the favorable results obtained from a randomized, controlled trial by Mowbray et al.[94] It is disappointing that other studies have failed to reproduce these results.[17, 55] Differences in results may be due to small numbers of patients and to heterogeneous patient populations.[24]

Reported complications from parental leucocyte immunization include anaphylactic reactions, transmission of infection, and elevation of anticardiolipin titers.[89] Because three follow-up studies have failed to corroborate the initial findings of Mowbray, it would seem that the risks of this therapy outweigh the benefits.[19, 30, 63] For example, a case of graft versus host disease (a potentially fatal illness in which transferred lymphocytes recognize and react against the host) has been reported in one recipient of paternal lymphocyte immunization.[62]

The ability to diagnose immunological disorders remains limited. For example, Cowchock and Smith recently studied the utility of tests for antinuclear antigens, cytotoxic antibodies to paternal lymphocytes, parental histocompatibility types, and blocking factors for maternal-paternal mixed lymphocyte reactions in predicting subsequent pregnancy outcome without immunological treatment. No significant correlation between immunological test results and pregnancy outcome could be found.[26] However, efforts to improve diagnostic capabilities for the detection of immunological disturbances are needed because favorable reproductive outcomes continue to be reported following treatment.[70] Intravenous immunoglobulin administration has been used not only for patients with antiphospholipid syndrome, but also for patients with unexplained RSA. Immunoglobulins, obtained from thousands of donors, may include immune factors such as blocking antibodies, potentially missing in the plasma of patients with unexplained pregnancy losses. Proof of this hypothesis has not been accomplished, but pregnancy success rates of 82-86% have been reported following immunoglobulin administration.[95]

CONCLUSION

Plouffe et al. compared the diagnosis and treatment outcomes for 100 couples evaluated between 1968 and 1977 with 131 couples seen between 1987 and 1991, and were unable to find a clear difference in pregnancy outcomes.[102] Thus, it appears that little progress has been made over the past 10 years in the ability to diagnose and successfully treat couples with RSA. With current advances in molecular biology, the potential for future breakthroughs in this area is promising. For example, a leukemia inhibitory factor has been identified that is expressed by the endometrium and is required for implantation of the embryo. In the absence of this factor, conception occurs, but the embryo cannot implant.[139] As more is learned about the role of the immune system in pregnancy maintenance, and more is understood about the mechanisms involved in implantation to a molecular level, a more optimistic outlook on the ability to diagnose and treat couples with RSA will be possible.

REFERENCES

1. Abraham GE, Maroulis GB, Marshall JR: Evaluation of ovulation and corpus luteum function using measurements of plasma progesterone, *Am J Obstet Gynecol* 44:522, 1974.
2. Anthony BF, Okada DM, Hobel CJ: Epidemiology of Group B *Streptococcus:* longitudinal observations during pregnancy, *J Infect Dis* 137:524, 1978.
3. Anthony BF, Okada DM, Obel C: Epidemiology of the Group B *Streptococcus:* maternal and nosocomial sources for infant acquisition, *J Pediatr* 95:431, 1979.
4. Baulieu EE: A novel approach to human fertility control and contragestation by the antiprogesterone RU-486, *Eur J Obstet Gynecol Reprod Biol* 28:125, 1988.
5. Beer AE, Quebberman JF, Ayers JWT, et al: Major histocompatibility complex antigens, maternal and paternal immune responses, and chronic habitual abortion in humans, *Am J Obstet Gynecol* 141:987, 1981.
6. Bensuade O, Babinet C, Morange M, et al: Heat shock proteins, first major products of zygotic gene activity in mouse embryo, *Nature* 305:331, 1983.
7. Blackwell R, Chang A: Video display terminals and pregnancy. A review, *Br J Obstet Gynaecol* 95:446, 1988.
8. Blugosz L, Bracken MB: Reproductive effects of caffeine: a review and theoretical analysis, *Epidemiol Rev* 14:83, 1992.
9. Boue J, Boue A, Lazar P: Retrospective and prospective epidemiologic studies of 1500 karyotyped spontaneous human abortions, *Teratology* 12:11, 1975.
10. Braekeleer MD, Dao TN: Cytogenetic studies in couples experiencing repeated pregnancy losses, *Hum Reprod* 5:519, 1990.
11. Branch DW, Silver RM, Blackwell JL, et al: Outcome of treated pregnancies in women with antiphospholipid syndrome: an update of the Utah experience, *Obstet Gynecol* 80:614, 1992.
12. Brent RL: Radiation teratogenesis: fetal risk and abortion, *Med Phys Monogr* 5:223, 1980.
13. Burkett G, Yasin S, Palen D: Perinatal implications of cocaine exposure, *J Reprod Med* 35:35, 1990.
14. Buttram VC, Reiter RC: Uterine leiomyomata: etiology, symptomatology and management, *Fertil Steril* 36:433, 1981.
15. Candiani GB, Vercellini P, Fedele L, et al: Repair of the uterine cavity after hysteroscopic septal incision, *Fertil Steril* 54:991, 1990.
16. Carr DH: Chromosome anomalies as a cause of spontaneous abortion, *Am J Obstet Gynecol* 97:283, 1967.
17. Cauchi MN, Lim D, Young DE, et al: Treatment of recurrent abortus by immunization with paternal cells—controlled trial, *Am J Reprod Immunol Microbiol* 25:16, 1991.
18. Chervenak FA, Neuwrith RS: Hysteroscopic incision of the septate uterus, *Am J Obstet Gynecol* 156:834, 1987.
19. Christiansen OB, Christiansen BS, Husth M, et al: Prospective study of anticardiolipin antibodies in immunized and untreated women with recurrent abortions, *Fertil Steril* 58:328, 1992.
20. Clarren SK, Smith DW: The fetal alcohol syndrome, *N Engl J Med* 298:1063, 1978.
21. Cockroff DL, Coppola PT: Teratogenic effects of excess glucose on head-fold rat embryos in culture, *Teratology* 16:141, 1977.
22. Conley CL, Hartman RC: A hemorrhagic disorder caused by circulating anticoagulant in patients with disseminated lupus erythematosus, *J Clin Invest* 31:621, 1952.
23. Corner GW: Endocrine factors in etiology of spontaneous abortion, *Clin Obstet Gynecol* 2:36, 1959.
24. Coulam CB, Clark DA: Report from the ethics committee for immunotherapy. American Society for the Immunology of Reproduction, *Am J Reprod Immunol Microbiol* 26:93, 1991.

25. Cowchock FS, Reece A, Balaban D, et al: Repeated pregnancy losses associated with antiphospholipid antibodies: a collaborative randomized trial comparing prednisone with low-dose heparin treatment, *Am J Obstet Gynecol* 166:1318, 1992.

26. Cowchock FS, Smith JB: Predictors for live birth after unexplained spontaneous abortions: correlations between immunologic test results, obstetric histories, and outcome of next pregnancy without treatment, *Am J Obstet Gynecol* 167:1208, 1992.

27. Czeizel AE, Dudas I: Prevention of the first occurrence of neural tube defects by periconceptional vitamin supplementation, *N Engl J Med* 327:1832, 1992.

28. Dahlman TC: Osteoporotic fractures and the recurrence of thromboembolism during pregnancy and the puerperium in 184 women undergoing thromboprophylaxis with heparin, *Am J Obstet Gynecol* 168:1265, 1993.

29. Daya S, Ward S, Burrows E: Progesterone profiles in luteal phase defect cycles and outcome of progesterone treatment in patients with recurrent spontaneous abortion, *Am J Obstet Gynecol* 158:225, 1988.

30. Doherty RA, Stubblefield P, Dostal-Johnson DA, et al: White blood cell immunization and anticardiolipin antibody levels in women with recurrent miscarriages, *Fertil Steril* 58:199, 1992.

31. Dmowski WP, Greenblatt FB: Asherman's syndrome and risk of placenta accreta, *Obstet Gynecol* 34:288, 1968.

32. Dudley DJ, Mitchell MD, Branch DW: Pathophysiology of antiphospholipid antibodies: absence of prostaglandin-mediated effects on cultured endothelium, *Am J Obstet Gynecol* 162:953, 1990.

33. Dudley DJ, Branch DW: Antiphospholipid syndrome: a model for autoimmune pregnancy loss, *Infertil Reprod Med Clin North Am* 2:149, 1991.

34. Eroghi G, Betz G, Torregano C: Impact of histocompatibility antigens on pregnancy outcome, *Am J Obstet Gynecol* 166:1364, 1992.

35. Fedele L, Dorta M, Brioschi D, et al: Pregnancies in septate uteri: outcome in relation to site of uterine implantation as determined by sonography, *Am J Roentgenol* 152:781, 1989.

36. Fedele L, Arcaini L, Parazzini F, et al: Reproductive prognosis after hysteroscopic metroplasty in 102 women: life-table analysis, *Fertil Steril* 59:768, 1993.

37. Fialkon PT: Thyroid antibodies, Down's syndrome and maternal age, *Nature* 214:1253, 1965.

38. Fleming DW, Cochi SL, MacDonald KL, et al: Pasteurized milk as a vehicle of infection in an outbreak of listeriosis, *N Engl J Med* 312:404, 1985.

39. Freyssinet JM, Wiesel ML, Cauchy J, et al: An IgM lupus anticoagulant that neutralizes the enhancing effect of phospholipid on purified endothelial thrombomodulin activity—a mechanism of thrombosis, *Thromb Haemost* 55:309, 1986.

40. Fulcher CA, Gardiner JE, Griffin JH, et al: Proteolytic inactivation of human factor VIII procoagulant protein by activated human protein C and its analogy with factor V, *Blood* 63:486, 1984.

41. Giacoia GP: Reproductive hazards in the workplace, *Obstet Gynecol Surv* 42:679, 1992.

42. Gill TJ: Invited editorial: influence of MHC and MHC-linked genes on reproduction, *Am J Hum Genet* 50:1, 1992.

43. Grant A, McBride WB, Moyes JM: Luteal phase defects in abortion, *Int J Fertil* 4:323, 1959.

44. Greenman GW, Gabrielson MO, Flanders JH, et al: Thyroid dysfunction in pregnancy, *N Engl J Med* 267:426, 1962.

45. Hadi HA, Hill JA, Castill RA: Alcohol and reproductive function: a review, *Obstet Gynecol Surv* 42:69, 1987.

46. Harlap S, Shiono PH: Alcohol, smoking and incidence of spontaneous abortions in the first and second trimester, *Lancet* 2:173, 1980.

47. Harlap S, Shiono PH, Ramcharan S: Spontaneous fetal losses in women using different contraceptives around the time of conception, *Int J Epidemiol* 9:49, 1980.

48. Harris EN, Gharavi AE, Patel SP, et al: Evaluation of the anticardiolipin antibody test: report of an international workshop help, *Clin Exp Immunol* 68:215, 1987.

49. Herbst AL, Senekjian EK, Fney KA: Abortion and pregnancy loss among diethylstilbestrol-exposed women, *Semin Reprod Endocrinol* 7:124, 1989.

50. Hill JA: Immunological mechanisms of pregnancy maintenance and failure: a critique of theories and therapy, *Am J Reprod Immunol Microbiol* 22:33, 1990.

51. Hill JA: Immunologic recurrent abortion, *Infertil Reprod Med Clin North Am* 2:137, 1991.

52. Hill JA: Cellular immune mechanisms of early reproductive failure, *Semin Perinatol* 15:225, 1991.

53. Hill JA, Polgar K, Harlow BL, et al: Evidence of embryo- and trophoblast-toxic cellular immune response(s) in women with recurrent spontaneous abortion, *Am J Obstet Gynecol* 166:1044, 1992.

54. Hook EB: Rates of chromosome abnormalities at different maternal ages, *Obstet Gynecol* 58:282, 1981.

55. Hwant JL, Ho H-N, Yang Y-S, et al: The role of blocking factors and antipaternal lymphocytotoxic antibodies in the success of pregnancy in patients with recurrent spontaneous abortion, *Fertil Steril* 58:691, 1992.

56. Jick H, Walker AM, Rothman KJ, et al: Vaginal spermicides and congenital disorders, *JAMA* 245:1329, 1981.

57. Jones GES: Some newer aspects of the management of infertility, *JAMA* 141:1123, 1949.

58. Jones GES, Delfs E: Endocrine patterns in term pregnancies following abortion, *JAMA* 146:1212, 1951.

59. Jones TB, Johnson MP, Burgon A, et al: Preconceptional planning, *Obstet Gynecol Clin North Am* 17:801, 1990.

60. Jones WS, Man E: Thyroid function in human pregnancy, *Am J Obstet Gynecol* 104:909, 1969.

61. Karende VC, Lester RC, Muasher SJ, et al: Are implantation and pregnancy outcome impaired in diethylstilbestrol exposed women after in vitro fertilization and embryo transfer? *Fertil Steril* 54:287, 1990.

62. Katz I, Fisch B, Amit S, et al: Cutaneous graft-versus-host-like reaction after paternal lymphocyte immunization for prevention of recurrent abortion, *Fertil Steril* 57:927, 1992.

63. Kilpatrick DC: Cardiolipin antibody levels are not influenced by leucocyte immunotherapy in patients experiencing recurrent spontaneous abortion, *Fertil Steril* 57:328, 1992.

64. Kimball AC, Ean BH, Fuchs F: The role of toxoplasmosis in abortion, *Am J Obstet Gynecol* 111:219, 1979.

65. Kline J, Stein ZA, Susser M, et al: Smoking: a risk factor for spontaneous abortion, *N Engl J Med* 297:793, 1977.

66. Kline J, Shrout P, Stein Z, et al: Drinking during pregnancy and spontaneous abortion, *Lancet* 2:176, 1980.

67. Knudsen RB, Driscoll SG, Ming PL: Strain of mycoplasma associated with human reproductive failure, *Science* 157:1573, 1967.

68. Knudsen RB, Ampola M, Streeter S, et al: Chromosomal aberrations induced by T-strain mycoplasms, *J Med Genet* 8:181, 1971.

69. Knudsen UB, Hansen V, Juul S, et al: Prognosis of a new pregnancy following previous spontaneous abortions, *Eur J Obstet Gynecol Reprod Biol* 39:31, 1991.

70. Kwak JUH, Gilman-Sachs A, Beaman KD, et al: Reproductive outcome in women with recurrent spontaneous abortions of alloimmune and autoimmune causes: preconception versus postconception treatment, *Am J Obstet Gynecol* 166:1787, 1992.

71. Lauritsen JG: Aetiology of spontaneous abortion: a cytogenetic and epidemiological study of 288 abortuses and their parents, *Acta Obstet Gynecol Scand* 52:3, 1976.

72. Leppert PC, Pahlka BS: Grieving characteristics after spontaneous abortion: a management approach, *Obstet Gynecol* 64:119, 1984.

73. Lockshin MD, Druzin ML, Qamar T: Prednisone does not prevent recurrent fetal death in women with antiphospholipid antibody, *Am J Obstet Gynecol* 160:439, 1989.

74. Lone PE, Santoro SA: Antiphospholipid antibodies: anticardiolipin and the lupus anticoagulant in systemic lupus erythematosus (SLE) and in non-SLE disorders, *Ann Intern Med* 112:682, 1990.

75. Lubbe WF, Butler WS, Palmer SJ, et al: Fetal survival after prednisone suppression of maternal lupus anticoagulant, *Lancet* 1:1361, 1983.

76. Lubbe WF, Liggins GC: Lupus anticoagulant and pregnancy, *Am J Obstet Gynecol* 153:322, 1985.

77. Lutiger B, Graham K, Einaison TR, et al: Relationship between gestational cocaine use and pregnancy outcome: a meta-analysis, *Teratology* 44(4):405, 1991.

78. MacDonald RR: Does treatment with progesterone prevent miscarriage? (Commentary), *Br J Obstet Gynaecol* 96:257, 1989.

79. Manganiello PD, Yearke RR: A 10-year prospective study of women with a history of recurrent fetal losses fails to identify *Listeria monocytogenes* in the genital tract, *Fertil Steril* 56:781, 1991.

80. Matsunaga E, Tonomura A, Oishi H, et al: Reexamination of paternal age effect in Down's syndrome, *Hum Genet* 40:259, 1978.

81. McDonough PG: The role of molecular mutation in recurrent euploidic abortion, *Semin Reprod Endocrinol* 6:155, 1988.

82. McGregor JA, French TI: *Chlamydia trachomatis* infection during pregnancy, *Am J Obstet Gynecol* 164:1782, 1991.

83. McNulty JH, Metcalfe T, Ueland K: Cardiovascular disease. In Burrown GN, Ferris TF, editors: *Medical complications during pregnancy,* Philadelphia, 1988, WB Saunders.

84. Meegdes BHLM, Ingenhoes R, Peeters LLA, et al: Early pregnancy wastage: relationship between chorionic vascularization and embryonic development, *Fertil Steril* 49:216, 1988.

85. Mills JL, Reed GF, Nugent RP, et al: Are there adverse effects of periconceptional spermicide use? *Fertil Steril* 43:442, 1985.

86. Mills JL, Holmes LB, Aarons JH, et al: Moderate caffeine use and the risk of spontaneous abortion and intrauterine growth retardation, *JAMA* 269(5):593, 1993.

87. Miodovnik M, Mimouni F, Siddiqi T, et al: Spontaneous abortions in repeat diabetic pregnancies: a relationship with glycemic control, *Obstet Gynecol* 75: 75, 1990.

88. Mishell DR, Recurrent abortion, *J Reprod Med* 38:250, 1993.

89. Moncayo A, Dupont O: Serum levels of anticardiolipin antibodies are pathologically increased after active immunization of patients with recurrent spontaneous abortion, *Fertil Steril* 54:619, 1990.

90. Montoro M, Collea JV, Frasier D, et al: Successful outcome of pregnancy in women with hypothyroidism, *Ann Intern Med* 94:31, 1981.

91. Morrison RP, Bellard RJ, Lyng K, et al: Chlamydial disease pathogenesis. The 57kd chlamydial hypersensitive antigen is a stress-response protein, *J Exp Med* 170:1271, 1984.

92. Morrison RP, Manning DS, Caldwell HD: Immunology of *Chlamydial trachomatis* infections: immunoprotective and immunopathogenetic mechanisms. In Gallin JI, Fauci AS, editors: *Advances in host defense mechanisms,* New York, 1991, Raven.

93. Moszkowski E, Woodruff JD, Jones GES: The inadequate luteal phase, *Am J Obstet Gynecol* 83:262, 1962.

94. Mowbray JF, Liddiee H, Underwood JL, et al: Controlled trial of treatment of recurrent spontaneous abortion by immunization with paternal cells, *Lancet* 1:941, 1985.

95. Mueller-Eckhardt G, Heine O, Neppert J, et al: Prevention of recurrent spontaneous abortion by intravenous immunoglobulin, *Vox Sang* 56:151, 1989.

96. Nael TC, Malo JW: Hysteroscopic metroplasty in the diethylstilbestrol-exposed uterus and similar nonfusion anomalies; effects on subsequent reproductive performance; a preliminary report, *Fertil Steril* 59:502, 1993.

97. Nicoloff TJ, Spencer CA: The use and misuse of the sensitive thyrotropin assays, *J Clin Endocrinol Metab* 71:553, 1990.

98. Ohno M, Maeda T, Matsunobu A: A cytogenetic study of spontaneous abortions with direct analysis of chorionic villi, *Obstet Gynecol* 77:394, 1991.

99. Orvieto R, Achiron A, Ben-Ratael Z, et al: Intravenous immunoglobulin treatment for recurrent abortions caused by antiphospholipid antibodies, *Fertil Steril* 56:1013, 1991.

100. Out HJ, Bruinse HW, Christiaens GCML, et al: A prospective, controlled multicenter study on the obstetric risks of pregnant women with antiphospholipid antibodies, *Am J Obstet Gynecol* 167:26, 1992.

101. Paul M, Himmelstein J: Reproductive hazards in the workplace: what the practitioner needs to know about chemical exposures, *Obstet Gynecol* 71:921, 1988.

102. Plouffe L, White EW, Tho SP, et al: Etiologic factors of recurrent abortion and subsequent reproductive performance of couples: have we made any progress in the past 10 years? *Am J Obstet Gynecol* 167:313, 1992.

103. Polifka JE, Friedman JM: Environmental toxins and recurrent pregnancy loss, *Infert Reprod Med Clin North Am* 2:195, 1991.

104. Polishuk WZ, Siew FP, Gordon R, et al: Vascular changes in traumatic amenorrhea and hypomenorrhea, *Int J Fertil* 22:189, 1977.

105. Pollard JK, Scott JR, Branch DW: Outcome of children born to women treated during pregnancy for the antiphospholipid syndrome, *Obstet Gynecol* 80:365, 1992.

106. Pratt D, Novotny M, Kaberlein G, et al: Antithyroid antibodies and the association with non-organ specific antibodies in recurrent pregnancy loss, *Am J Obstet Gynecol* 168:837, 1993.

107. Quenlen D, Brasme TL, Parmentier D: Ultrasound-guided transcervical metroplasty, *Fertil Steril* 54:995, 1990.

108. Quinn PA, Shewchuk AB, Shuber J, et al: Serologic evidence of ureaplasma urealyticum infection in women with spontaneous pregnancy loss, *Am J Obstet Gynecol* 145:245, 1983.

109. Quinn PA, Shewchuk AB, Shuber J, et al: Efficacy of antibiotic therapy in preventing spontaneous pregnancy loss among couples colonized with genital mycoplasmas, *Am J Obstet Gynecol* 1451;239, 1983.

110. Quinn PA, Petrie M, Barin M, et al: Prevalence of antibody to *Chlamydia trachomatis* in spontaneous abortion and infertility, *Am J Obstet Gynecol* 156:291, 1987.

111. Rabau E, David A: *Listeria monocytogenes* in abortion, *J Obstet Gynaecol Br Common W* 70:481, 1963.

112. Rappaport F, Rabinovitz M: Genital listeriosis as a cause of repeated abortion, *Lancet* 1:1273, 1960.

113. Reece EA, Gabrielli S, Cullen MT, et al: Recurrent adverse pregnancy outcome and antiphospholipid antibodies, *Am J Obstet Gynecol* 163:162, 1990.

114. Regan JA, Chao S, James LS: Premature rupture of membranes, preterm delivery and group B streptococcal colonization of mothers, *Am J Obstet Gynecol* 141:184, 1980.

115. Regan L, Braude PR, Trembath PL: Influence of past reproductive performance on risk of spontaneous abortion, *Br Med J* 299:541, 1989.

116. Rein MS: Luteal phase defect and recurrent pregnancy loss, *Infertil Reprod Med Clin North Am* 2:121, 1991.

117. Rocklin RE, Kitzmiller JL, Carpenter CB, et al: Maternal-fetal relation; absence of an immunologic blocking factor from the serum of women with chronic abortion, *N Engl J Med* 295:1290, 1976.

118. Rosenberg IH: Folic acid and neural tube defects—time for action. (Editorial), *N Engl J Med* 327:1875, 1992.

119. Rosove MH, Tabsh K, Wasserstrum N, et al: Heparin therapy for pregnancy in women with lupus anticoagulant or anticardiolipin antibodies, *Obstet Gynecol* 75:630, 1990.

120. Rowland AS, Baird DD, Weinberg CR, et al: Reduced fertility

among women employed as dental assistants exposed to high levels of nitrous oxide, *N Engl J Med* 327:993, 1992.

121. Schenker J, Margalioth E: Intrauterine adhesions: an updated approach, *Fertil Steril* 37:593, 1982.

122. Schnorr TM, Grajewksi BA, Hornung RW, et al: Video display terminals and the risk of spontaneous abortion, *N Engl J Med* 324:727, 1991.

123. Scott GB, Buck BE, Leterman JG, et al: Acquired immunodeficiency syndrome in infants, *N Engl J Med* 310:76, 1984.

124. Scott GB, Fischl MA, Klimas N, et al: Mothers of infants with the acquired immunodeficiency syndrome: evidence for both symptomatic and asymptomatic carriers, *JAMA* 253:363, 1985.

125. Scott JR, Branch DW, Kochenour NK, et al: Intravenous immunoglobulin treatment of pregnant patients with recurrent pregnancy loss caused by antiphospholipid antibodies and Rh immunization, *Am J Obstet Gynecol* 159:1055, 1988.

126. Selevan SG, Lindbohm ML, Pol-Sci C, et al: A study of occupational exposure to antineoplastic drugs and fetal loss in nurses, *N Engl J Med* 313:1173, 1985.

127. Shime J, Mocarski EJM, Hasting D, et al: Congenital heart disease in pregnancy: short- and long-term implications, *Am J Obstet Gynecol* 156:313, 1987.

128. Shoupe D, Mishell DR, Lacarra M, et al: Correlation of endometrial maturation with four methods of estimating day of ovulation, *Obstet Gynecol* 73:88, 1984.

129. Simpson JL: Genetic consequences of aging sperm or aging ova: animal studies and relevance to humans. In Sciarra JJ, Zatuchni GI, Speidel JJ, editors: *Risks, benefits and controversies in fertility control,* Hagerstown, MD, 1978, Harper and Row.

130. Simpson JL: What causes chromosome abnormalities and gene mutations? *Contemp Obstet Gynecol* 17:99, 1981.

131. Simpson JL: Repeated suboptimal pregnancy outcome, *Birth Defects* 17:113, 1981.

132. Solter D: Differential imprinting and expression of maternal and paternal genomes, *Ann Rev Gent* 22:127, 1988.

133. Sopienza C: Parental imprinting of genes, *Sci Am* 263:52, 1990.

134. Srisuphan W, Bracken MB: Caffeine consumption during pregnancy and association with late spontaneous abortion, *Am J Obstet Gynecol* 154:14, 1986.

135. Stagnaro-Green A, Roman SH, Cobin RH, et al: Detection of at-risk pregnancy by means of highly sensitive assays for thyroid autoantibodies, *JAMA* 264:1422, 1990.

136. Stein Z: Early fetal loss, *Birth Defects* 17:1, 1981.

137. Steinberg AD, et al: Systemic lupus erythematosis, *Ann Intern Med* 115:548, 1991.

138. Stevencher MA, Hempel JM, McIntyre MN: Cytogenetics of spontaneously aborted human fetuses, *Obstet Gynecol* 30:683, 1967.

139. Stewart CL, Kaspar P, Brunet LJ, et al: Blastocyst implantation depends on maternal expression of leukemia inhibitory factor, *Nature* 359:76, 1992.

140. Stray-Pedersen B, Eng J, Mannsaker-Reikvam T: Uterine T-mycoplasma colonization in reproductive failure, *Am J Obstet Gynecol* 130:307, 1978.

141. Stray-Pedersen B, Stray-Pedersen S: Etiologic factors and subsequent reproductive performance in 195 couples with a prior history of habitual abortion, *Am J Obstet Gynecol* 148:140, 1984.

142. Strobino B, Kline J, Lai A, et al: Vaginal spermicides and spontaneous abortion of known karyotype, *Am J Epidemiol* 123(3):431, 1986.

143. Strott CA, Cargille CM, Ross GT, et al: The short luteal phase, *J Clin Endocrinol Metab* 30:246, 1970.

144. Styler M, Shapiro SS: Mollicutes (mycoplasma) in infertility, *Fertil Steril* 44:1, 1985.

145. Taylor C, Faulk WP: Prevention of abortion with leucocyte transfusions, *Lancet* 2:68, 1981.

146. Taylor-Robinson D, McCormack WD: The genital mycoplasma, *N Engl J Med* 302:1003, 1980.

147. Tho PT, Byrd JR, McDonough PC: Etiologies and subsequent reproductive performance of 100 couples with recurrent abortion, *Fertil Steril* 32:389, 1979.

148. Thragarayan P, Shapiro SS, DeMarco L: Monoclonal immunoglobulin M coagulation inhibitor with phospholipid specificity-mechanism of a lupus anticoagulant, *J Clin Invest* 66: 397, 1980.

149. Thiagarajan P, Pengo V, Shapiro SS: The use of the dilute Russell's viper venom time for the diagnosis of lupus anticoagulants, *Blood* 68:869, 1986.

150. Tidey GF, Stillman RJ: In utero diethylstilbestrol exposure and pregnancy loss, *Infert Reprod Med Clin North Am* 2:105, 1991.

151. Valle RF, Sciarra JJ: Intrauterine adhesions: hysteroscopic diagnosis classification, treatment and reproductive outcome, *Am J Obstet Gynecol* 158:1459, 1988.

152. Vercellini P, Fedele L, Arcaini L, et al: Value of intrauterine device insertion and estrogen administration after hysteroscopic metroplasty, *J Reprod Med* 34:447, 1989.

153. Verkauf BS: Myomectomy for fertility enhancement and preservation, *Fertil Steril* 58:1, 1992.

154. Verp MS: Environmental causes of repetitive spontaneous abortion, *Semin Reprod Endocrinol* 7:188, 1989.

155. Walker FJ, Sexton PW, Esman CT: The inhibition of blood coagulation by activated protein C through the selective inactivation of activated factor V, *Biochem Biophys Acta* 571:333, 1979.

156. Wapner RJ, Cowchock FS, Shapiro SS: Successful treatment in two women with antiphospholipid antibodies and refractory pregnancy losses with intravenous immunoglobulin infusions, *Am J Obstet Gynecol* 161:1271, 1989.

157. Watts DH, Eschenbach DA: Reproductive tract infections as a cause of abortion and preterm bulk, *Semin Reprod Endocrinol* 6:203, 1983.

158. Wertheimer N, Leeper E: Possible effects of electric blankets and heated waterbeds on fetal development, *Bioelectromagnetics* 7:13, 1986.

159. Wilcox AJ, Weinberg Cr, O'Connor JF, et al: Incidence of early loss of pregnancy, *N Engl J Med* 319:189, 1988.

160. Windham GC, Swan SH, Fenster L: Parental cigarette smoking and the risk of spontaneous abortion, *Am J Epidemiol* 135:1394, 1992.

161. Witkin SS, Ledger WJ: Antibodies to *Chlamydia trachomatis* in sera of women with recurrent spontaneous abortions, *Am J Obstet Gynecol* 167:135, 1992.

162. Xu L, Chang V, Murphy A, et al: Antinuclear antibodies in sera of patients with recurrent pregnancy wastage, *Am J Obstet Gynecol* 163:1493, 1990.

Chapter 50

DEVELOPMENT OF FETAL STEROID-PRODUCING ORGANS DURING HUMAN PREGNANCY

Susan J. Spencer, MD,
Jaron Rabinovici, MD,
and Robert B. Jaffe, MD

Novel and unique mechanisms of steroid hormone formation and regulation, and the placental production of a wide array of peptide hormones and growth factors, characterize the endocrine milieu of the fetoplacental unit during pregnancy. In this chapter, we focus on the regulation of growth and differentiation of the human fetal adrenal gland and gonads, and the diverse peptide and steroid production of the human placenta.

HUMAN FETAL ADRENAL GLAND DEVELOPMENT

Embryogenesis

The fetal adrenal cortex comprises two histologically and functionally distinct zones, the inner, fetal zone and the outer, definitive zone. Both zones are derived from coelomic mesoderm. During weeks 4 to 6 of embryonic life, coelomic mesothelial cell proliferation occurs between the root of the mesentery and the developing gonad. These cells differentiate into a cluster of large, acidophilic cells to form the fetal zone of the cortex. At 10 weeks of gestation, another wave of mesothelial proliferation occurs and surrounds the original cell mass.[231] These smaller, basophilic cells form the definitive zone. The gland undergoes rapid growth, and by the end of the first trimester has attained a size equal to or greater than that of the fetal kidneys. By midgestation, the gland has increased more than seventy-fivefold in mass.[120] The bulk of fetal adrenal growth is attributable to the expansion of the fetal zone, which comprises 80% of the volume of the gland in midgestation.

As the cortex forms, beginning at around 7 weeks, neuroectoderm cells of sympathetic origin invade medially to establish a central cluster of chromaffin cells, which is the nascent adrenal medulla. As these primitive cells migrate toward the center of the gland they differentiate into either sympathetic ganglion cells or mature secretory chromaffin cells. This neuroectodermal cell migration continues through midtrimester, at which point a distinct medulla can be recognized.[231,468] Beginning at 14 weeks of gestation, two cell types can be recognized by morphology and by immunophenotype in the nascent adrenal medulla.[287] Nests of small, primitive-appearing cells that contain immunoreactive neurofilament protein and tyrosine hydroxylase are putative progenitors of ganglion cells. The large cell subpopulation, which contains immunoreactive chromogranin A and synaptophysin, as well as neurofilament protein and tyrosine hydroxylase, is postulated to be precursors of chromaffin cells of the mature medulla. Leu-enkephalin and the catecholamine-synthesizing enzymes, dopamine β-hydroxylase and phenylethanolamine *N*-methyltransferase, have been co-localized in the adrenal medulla at 24 weeks of gestation.[188,467]

Growth of the fetal adrenal cortex

Adrenocorticotropic hormone. Adrenocorticotropic hormone (ACTH) is a trophic factor for the developing adrenal. In animal models, hypophysectomy or stalk section causes progressive adrenal atrophy. In the rhesus monkey, dexamethasone-induced atrophy of the fetal cortex is reversed by the administration of ACTH to the fetus.[86] In the human, studies on the anencephalic fetus have provided insight into the regulation of human adrenal growth by ACTH. Evidence for a trophic role for ACTH is supported by the studies of Benirschke[35] and Gray and Abramovich,[152] which demonstrated that in the anencephalic fetus, adrenal fetal zone growth is normal until about 15 weeks. After this time, the fetal zone atrophies. Administration of ACTH to anencephalic fetuses restores the growth of the gland.[232] Thus ACTH is a critical adrenal trophic factor, at least after 15 weeks of gestation. Since ACTH does not cross the placenta, the ACTH that acts on the fetal adrenal must be of fetal origin.

Peptide growth factors. From more recent studies, evidence is accumulating for the intermediary role of peptide growth factors in the control of human fetal adrenal growth. The extent of expression of several of these factors is regulated by ACTH, and thus these growth factors may serve as autocrine or paracrine intermediates of ACTH action in modulating growth and function of the adrenal in utero.

The growth-promoting effects of epidermal growth factor (EGF) and related peptides have been demonstrated in a number of mammalian organ systems in development. EGF acts via a transmembrane receptor that contains tyrosine kinase activity. The primary biologic response to EGF in a variety of target cells in vitro and in vivo is increased cell proliferation. Crickard et al.[78] demonstrated the potent mitogenic effect of EGF on cultured midtrimester fetal adrenal cells. Furthermore, EGF receptors were identified on fetal zone and definitive zone adrenal cells. In vivo, EGF infusion causes hypertrophy of the adrenal in the ovine fetus.[438] In addition to its mitogenic action, EGF increases adrenal cortisol production in vitro.[108] Interestingly, EGF also has been shown to evoke ACTH secretion, as demonstrated in the chronically catheterized fetal lamb.[341] Thus EGF may prove to be a modulator of growth and function in the developing hypothalamic-pituitary-adrenal axis.

Basic fibroblast growth factor (bFGF) is a potent mitogen for a spectrum of mesoderm-derived cells.[148] Human fetal zone and definitive zone adrenal cells proliferate in response to bFGF.[78] Mesiano and colleagues[277] have demonstrated that expression of FGF messenger ribonucleic acid (mRNA) by midtrimester human fetal adrenal cells is stimulated by ACTH and by cyclic adenosine monophosphate (cAMP), the second messenger that mediates the actions of ACTH.

Another group of developmentally significant peptides, the insulin-like growth factors (IGFs), also are expressed by the human fetal adrenal.[276] IGF-II mRNA is expressed at high levels by the human fetal adrenal, and its expression is

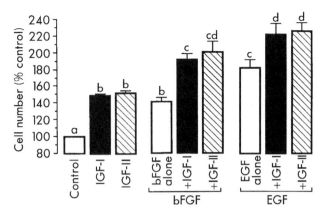

Fig. 50-1. Effects of insulin-like growth factor (IGF) I and IGF-II on fetal adrenal cell proliferation alone and in combination with basic fibroblast growth factor (bFGF) and epidermal growth factor (EGF). (From Mesiano S, Mellon SH, Jaffe RB: Mitogenic action, regulation and localization of insulin-like growth factors in the human fetal adrenal gland.[275])

enhanced by ACTH and cAMP. IGF-II can enhance fetal adrenal cell proliferation by itself and is additive with bFGF and EGF to further enhance adrenal cell growth (Fig. 50-1).[273] Furthermore, FGF is capable of up-regulating IGF receptors in vitro. The list of growth-promoting peptides has lengthened over the last two decades. However, the extent to which these mitogenic factors, under the influence of ACTH, leads to the preferential expansion of the fetal zone relative to the definitive zone during fetal life remains unclear.

Growth inhibitors also have been identified for the midgestation human fetal adrenal in vitro. Two members of the transforming growth factor (TGF) family of peptides, TGF-β and activin A, decrease fetal adrenal cell proliferation. TGF-β inhibits fetal adrenal cell proliferation in vitro without altering steroid production.[369] The TGF-β–related peptide, activin A, preferentially inhibits proliferation of fetal zone adrenal cells without altering the growth of definitive zone cells or adult cortical cells.[409] In addition, activin A enhances ACTH-induced cortisol production by fetal zone cells, but not definitive zone cells or adult adrenal cells (Fig. 50-2).[410] In this way, the pattern of steroidogenesis in the fetal zone is shifted to that more resembling the definitive zone in the adult, with predominant cortisol synthesis. The subunits of this peptide are synthesized by human fetal adrenals, and their expression is enhanced by ACTH in vitro.[410] By inhibiting proliferation and promoting the shift to the definitive, cortisol-producing phenotype, activin may prove to have a role in the postnatal remodeling of the human fetal zone. Further studies are needed to test this hypothesis.

Hypothalamic-pituitary-adrenal axis

The mechanisms for central control of adrenal function are established early in the second trimester. The hypothalamic-pituitary-adrenal axis is functional by 14 weeks of gestation,[41,386] and ACTH is able to increase dehydroepiandrosterone sulfate (DHEAS) and cortisol pro-

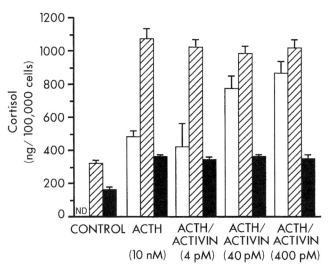

Fig. 50-2. Effects of increasing concentrations of recombinant human activin A on ACTH-stimulated cortisol production from cultured human fetal zone adrenocortical cells. Cortisol values are expressed as ng/ml per 10^5 cells per 48 h in conditioned medium from fetal zone (*white bars*), definitive zone (*hatched bars*), or adult (*black bars*) adrenal cell cultures. The data are means ± SE of triplicate experiments. (Redrawn from Spencer SJ et al: Activin and inhibin in the human adrenal gland: regulation and differential effects in fetal and adult cells.[410])

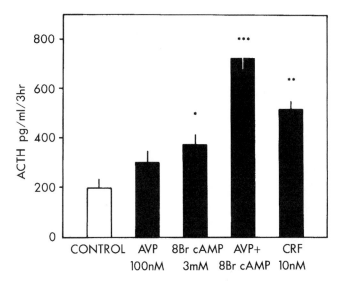

Fig. 50-3. Effects of arginine vasopressin (AVP), 8 bromo-cyclic adenosine monophosphate (8 Br cAMP) and corticotropin-releasing factor (CRF) on release of ACTH from human fetal pituitary cells. (From Blumenfeld Z, Jaffe RB: Hypophysiotropic and neuromodulatory regulation of ACTH in the human fetal pituitary gland, *J Clin Invest* 78:288, 1986.)

duction by human fetal adrenal cells at this time. Corticotropes are identifiable by 12 weeks of gestation, using immunocytochemical techniques.[21] From 14 weeks of gestation, the human fetal pituitary in vitro is able to secrete ACTH in response to corticotropin-releasing factor (CRF), arginine vasopressin (AVP), or 8-bromo-cAMP (Fig. 50-3).[41] Pretreatment with dexamethasone blunts the ACTH response to CRF. Fetal pituitary responsiveness to CRF and AVP, with negative feedback by glucocorticoids, is thus well established before midgestation.

Immunoreactive CRF also is present in syncytiotrophoblast and intermediate trophoblast, as well as in amnion, chorion, and decidua.[368,373] It has been suggested that the presence of immunoreactive CRF may indicate paracrine effects of placenta, fetal membranes, and decidua in the maturation of the hypothalamic-pituitary-adrenal axis.[368]

Steroidogenesis

There appears to be functional specialization of the fetal and definitive zones of the human fetal adrenal gland, as demonstrated by zone-separated superfusion studies.[387] The definitive zone produces primarily corticoids necessary for enzyme induction in a variety of fetal organs, as well as for maintenance of intrauterine homeostasis. In contrast, the fetal zone elaborates principally the placental estrogen precursor, DHEAS. The unique steroidogenic pattern of the fetal zone in utero is a consequence of the developmentally regulated pattern of steroidogenic enzyme gene expression. The distribution of enzyme activity in the adrenal is zone specific. 3β-Hydroxysteroid dehydrogenase (3β-HSD) ac-

tivity is present in the definitive zone but lacking in the fetal zone. This has been substantiated by molecular studies.[94,456] Voutilainen et al.[456] demonstrated a low level of expression of 3β-HSD in the human fetal adrenal as compared with adult adrenal. 3β-HSD expression is increased by ACTH and the phorbol ester tissue plasminogen activator (TPA) in vitro. Further 17α-hydroxylase/17,20-lyase (P-450c17) appears to be restricted principally to a narrow band between the fetal and definitive zones.[274]

Both fetal and definitive zone cells respond to the addition of ACTH with alteration of the steroidogenic patterns, and these changes have been examined in a number of studies.[78,118,257] There are several acute effects of ACTH. Upon binding to its receptor, ACTH increases the availability of adrenal free cholesterol by increasing the concentration of low-density lipoprotein receptors[60] and stimulating cholesterol esterase.[319] ACTH binding also facilitates transport of cholesterol into mitochondria and binding of cholesterol to the P-450 side-chain cleaving enzyme (P-450scc). In addition, ACTH acutely stimulates the release of newly synthesized steroid.[170] In contrast, the chronic action of ACTH is to increase accumulation of mRNAs for microsomal and mitochondrial steroidogenic enzymes. ACTH directly stimulates accumulation of mRNAs for P-450scc and P-450c17 in cultured human fetal adrenal cells.[89] The stimulatory effect of dibutyryl cAMP on P-450scc and P-450c17 mRNA accumulation is temporally similar to that of ACTH, indicating that the cAMP pathway probably mediates the long-term effects of ACTH on steroidogenic enzymes in the human fetal adrenal. P-450scc is the sole enzyme converting cholesterol to pregnenolone by catalyzing 20-hydroxylation, 22-

hydroxylation, and cholesterol side-chain cleavage on a single active site.[403] P450c17 is the single microsomal enzyme having both 17α-hydroxylase and 17,20-lyase activities.[296] Thus, after cholesterol is converted to pregnenolone by P-450scc, P-450c17 is the sole enzyme needed to produce DHEA, which, in its sulfurylated form (DHEAS), is the principal androgenic product of the human fetal adrenal gland. In addition to DHEAS, the principal steroid products of fetal zone cells stimulated by ACTH in vitro are pregnenolone, pregnenolone sulfate, and 17α-hydroxypregnenolone.[257]

As its name implies, the fetal zone is unique to intrauterine life. The fetal zone produces large amounts of DHEAS, which serves as the major precursor for placental aromatization to estrogens.[394] The fate of the majority of fetal zone DHEAS is 16α-hydroxylation by the fetal liver, followed by placental aromatization to estriol, which crosses freely into the maternal circulation. Circulating estriol may therefore reflect fetal adrenal function. Historically, urinary estriol was used as a marker for fetal well-being. A decline in DHEAS production has been associated with pregnancy loss.[222] Maternal serum estriol is also a reflection of the capacity of the fetal adrenal to synthesize adequate amounts of DHEAS.[114] As shown by Canick et al.,[56] midtrimester maternal serum estriol was significantly decreased in pregnancies affected by anencephaly as compared with normal pregnancies.

Fetal steroidogenesis is an interdependent process, requiring complementary enzyme activities of the adrenal, liver and placenta, or fetoplacental unit.[184] The human fetal adrenal is capable of synthesizing cholesterol from acetate; other sources of fetal corticoids include circulating low-density lipoprotein (LDL) cholesterol and placental pregnenolone and progesterone. The fetal gland is active in 17-hydroxylation of these latter precursors, which are then rapidly metabolized to DHEA. Sulfurylation of DHEA occurs extensively, as well as of pregnenolone and 17-hydroxypregnenolone.[186] Placental progesterone is utilized by the fetal cortex, particularly the definitive zone, to form Δ^4 compounds by 21-, 11β-, 17α-, and 18-hydroxylation to deoxycorticosterone, corticosterone, and cortisol.[88]

Fetal adrenal mineralocorticoid production has also been examined by incubation of fetal zone and definitive zone tissue with pregnenolone or corticosterone. Under basal and ACTH-stimulated conditions, aldosterone does not appear to be produced by the fetal adrenal in any significant quantity.[299,385]

The lymphokine tumor necrosis factor-alpha (TNF-α) is also produced by cultured fetal adrenal cells in response to ACTH.[374] In contrast to activin, TNF-α suppresses ACTH-stimulated cortisol and increases DHEAS synthesis.[183] Even in the absence of exogenous TNF-α, this pattern of predominantly DHEAS rather than cortisol production in response to ACTH is seen consistently with fetal zone cells in culture. Recent data[275] suggest that the interaction of

insulin-like growth factor-II (IGF-II) and estrogen also may drive steroidogenesis toward DHEAS production in the fetal adrenal gland.

The high androgen-corticoid ratio seen in the fetal adrenal relative to the adult is consistent with a developmentally regulated shift in the pattern of steroidogenic enzyme gene expression. The rise in fetal glucocorticoid levels that occurs in the third trimester is thought to stimulate fetal lung surfactant synthesis in preparation for extrauterine life. In addition to direct stimulation of fetal lung epithelium, the rise in glucocorticoid production may be required to counter the inhibitory effect of fetal androgens on surfactant synthesis by fetal lung seen in vitro.[439] Thus the balance of fetal adrenal steroids is critical for proper timing of lung development.

Although fetal glucocorticoid production is necessary for lung maturation, its role in parturition as elegantly demonstrated in the sheep studies of Liggins et al.,[242] has not been shown in the human. The pattern of human fetal ACTH secretion with parturition also has been investigated. Umbilical cord ACTH values were compared among groups of term neonates delivered vaginally or by cesarean section, with or without labor.[474] No significant differences in circulating ACTH were seen, suggesting that a rise in ACTH may not be essential for the initiation of labor in humans. The role of the increasing concentrations of placental corticotropin-releasing hormone (CRH) that occur at the end of pregnancy on the initiation of parturition currently is an active area of investigation.

Postnatal adrenal maturation

Fetal plasma DHEAS levels decline sharply in the postnatal period, within 96 hours of birth,[88] consistent with rapid involution of the fetal zone in the neonate. Postnatally the fetal zone disappears with the establishment of the adult cortical zonation pattern. It is not clear whether fetal zone involution also involves remodeling to contribute to this adult zonation. Based on morphologic studies, some investigators have proposed that the fetal zone may contribute to the nascent zona reticularis.[192] Sucheston and Cannon[416] suggested that the human fetal zone regresses as it is transformed into the zona fasciculata.

Studies in some subhuman primates suggest that this remodeling does not occur. In the baboon, the fetal zone undergoes postnatal involution, and within 2 weeks postpartum it occupies less than one third of the fetal cortex.[95] In this species, cell proliferation was observed in the definitive cortex, whereas areas of the fetal zone underwent necrosis. However, despite ultrastructural studies of the postnatal baboon adrenal, it is unclear whether definitive cortex or fetal zone remnant gives rise to the zona fasciculata of the adult gland. McNulty et al.[268] observed that the fetal zone of the rhesus monkey adrenal disappears slowly after birth without undergoing necrosis, and that this zone may contribute to the genesis of the nascent zona reticularis. Additional cytochemical data from the human postnatal adrenal are required to establish definitively the genesis of the adult cortical zones.

DEVELOPMENT OF HYPOTHALAMIC-PITUITARY-GONADAL FUNCTION IN THE HUMAN FETUS

Appropriate development of the hypothalamic-pituitary-gonadal axis during early fetal life provides the foundation for normal sexual prenatal and postnatal development, normal puberty, and adult reproductive function. Impairment in fetal gonadal function could result in loss of germ cells, endocrine function, and reproductive potential. Although our ability to correct such inadequate development currently is limited, understanding the mechanisms necessary for normal fetal gonadal development remains a prerequisite for the design of rational approaches to the diagnosis, prevention, and management of inadequate gonadal development.

Hypothalamus/pituitary

Early fetal development. The neuroendocrine axis develops early during fetal life, and recent evidence indicates that at least some of the autocrine/paracrine/endocrine factors that regulate this axis in the adult are already established in the fetus. The development of the brain is one of the earliest events in human fetal development. Although the classic view held that the pituitary develops from an epithelial evagination of Rathke's pouch, this has been questioned (for a more extensive discussion see reference 293). The emergence of the amine precursor uptake and decarboxylation (APUD) concept as signifying a common origin of certain peptide-secreting cells[318] suggests that the progenitors of the hormone-secreting cells originate in the ventral neural ridges of the primitive neural tube.[293] This region also gives rise in nonprimates to the diencephalon, which may suggest that the hypothalamus and anterior pituitary share a common embryonic origin.[429]

The pituitary increases in size and cell number from the sixth week of gestation[76] and at 8 weeks capillaries start to interdigitate the surrounding mesenchymal tissue about Rathke's pouch and the diencephalon.[76,106] Vascular casts demonstrated the presence of an intact hypothalamic-hypophysial vascular system in fetuses of 11.5 to 16.8 weeks of fetal age,[436] and it was suggested that during fetal life the hypothalamus and pituitary also could communicate through local diffusion of transmitters.[209]

During early fetal development the hypothalamus acquires the ability to secrete the decapeptide gonadotropin-releasing hormone (GnRH), and indirect evidence exists for the pulsatile release of GnRH during fetal life.[351,352] Secretion of GnRH begins early in fetal life. Hypothalamic GnRH can be detected around 8 to 10 weeks of gestational age in significant amounts.[136,209] From 10 to 22 weeks, the hypothalamic GnRH content increases significantly (from a range of 0.5 to 5 pg/mg at 8 to 10 weeks to 208 to 4300 pg/mg).[208,209,475] Immunologic studies of the fetal median eminence showed GnRH-containing neurons in the anterior hypothalamus, median eminence, and lamina terminalis.[51] Thus the hypothalamic nuclei and tracts,[349] as well as the hypophysiotropic factors (GnRH, thyrotropin-releasing hormone [TRH], and somatostatin)[209] are found at or before 14 to 16 weeks of gestation. In addition, high levels of dopamine are present in the fetal hypothalamus at 11 to 15 weeks,[181] and catecholamines are detected in cells of the hypothalamic arcuate nucleus that project to the median eminence.[305] In vitro studies demonstrated that human fetal hypothalami obtained from second-trimester human abortuses release GnRH in a pulsatile manner.[351,352] Furthermore, this calcium-dependent pulsatile release was inhibited by the addition of morphine, suggesting a functioning opiate receptor-mediated mechanism at this stage of fetal development.[352]

In addition to the evidence that the hypothalamus contains and secretes GnRH, the fetal pituitary probably also is able to react to this hypothalamic signal. Human fetal pituitary cells respond in vitro to the administration of GnRH with increased secretion of both luteinizing hormone (LH) and follicle-stimulating hormone (FSH).[96-98] In two in vivo studies in late gestational fetal rhesus monkeys, we also showed that serum LH levels increase after the pulsatile administration of LH[178] and that spontaneous LH secretion is pulsatile, presumably representing a pituitary response to pulsatile GnRH release.[252]

Human fetal pituitaries secrete intact LH in vitro as early as 5 to 7 weeks of gestational age,[156,399] and intact FSH and LH have been detected in fetal pituitaries and in fetal plasma by 10 weeks.[207] Pituitary gonadotropes were present by 10.5 to 13 weeks of gestation, and a rapid increase in gonadotrope cell number was seen by 25 weeks.[21] Pituitary levels of FSH reach a peak at 20 to 23 weeks of gestation, and levels in female fetal pituitaries are greater than in male pituitaries.[73,97,207] Studies performed during the 1970s indicated that circulating levels of FSH peak at 28 weeks and also are significantly higher in female fetuses than in males until the last 6 weeks of gestation.[73,207,427] Although pituitary LH levels also are greater in females than in males, plasma levels do not differ significantly.[73,207,427] Recently the introduction of cordocentesis permitted the determination of immunoreactive (I) FSH, LH, and bioactive FSH in cord blood of fetuses at gestational ages of 17 to 24 and 35 to 40 weeks.[28] A marked difference was found between male and female levels of I-FSH and I-LH and bioactive FSH during the second trimester but not the third trimester. In female fetuses, I-FSH and I-LH levels were as high as those recorded in normal postmenopausal women. In contrast, in male fetuses I-FSH and I-LH levels were within the low-normal adult male range. Furthermore, whereas female LH levels reached a peak during weeks 17 and 18, FSH levels increased gradually until week 24.[28] The sex differences in fetal pituitary and peripheral gonadotropin levels suggest that either a negative feedback loop operates in the male but not in the female fetus at this time in gestation or the testis secretes hormones that activate the feedback mechanism (androgens, inhibins) whereas the ovary does not.

In fetuses of both sexes, there is a marked excess of circulating free α-subunit, and levels in males and females are not significantly different.[28] The levels of the free alpha subunit are about 1000% to 1500% higher than expected on the basis of the molar concentrations of all glycoprotein hormones taken together.[28] The physiologic role of this augmented secretion of the free α-subunit and the contribution of placental secretion of free α-subunit to this excess are not fully understood.

Role of fetal pituitary and placental gonadotropins in the regulation of development of the fetal gonads. In the adult, gonadal function is regulated by pituitary gonadotropins. Receptors for FSH are present on testicular Sertoli cells and on ovarian granulosa cells. Activation of the LH/human chorionic gonadotropin (hCG) receptor by pituitary LH stimulates differentiation of testicular Leydig cells or ovarian theca and granulosa cells. However, the role of pituitary and/or placental gonadotropins in the control of fetal gonadal function is not fully understood. Human chorionic gonadotropin is detectable in the maternal circulation at about 9 to 13 days after conception.[65,185,225] Maternal hCG levels peak at around 10 weeks of gestation and decline thereafter to a nadir at 20 weeks.[250,453] Although the pattern of fetal hCG parallels that of the mother, immunoreactive hCG levels in fetal blood obtained by cordocentesis were about 1000 times lower than those recorded in the maternal circulation.[28] In the same study, fetal sex did not seem to influence maternal or fetal hCG levels at the gestational ages studied.[28] These findings are in contrast to previous observations that maternal hCG levels are higher in midgestational placentas[44] or at term in mothers of a female fetus.[49,306,466]

Anencephaly is a major congenital malformation caused by failure of the cranial vault to form during embryogenesis, resulting in extensive underdevelopment of the brain. This malformation results in the absence of the cerebrum and cerebellum, and the anterior pituitary is generally reduced in size.[26] The lack of hypothalamic releasing hormones (TRH, CRF, GnRH, growth hormone–releasing hormone [GHRH]) reduces or abolishes the secretion of anterior pituitary hormones (thyroid-stimulating hormone [TSH], ACTH, LH, FSH, and growth hormone [GH]) and causes a reduction in size of the target organs (thyroid, adrenal, gonads) of these hormones. However, primary (embryonic) sexual differentiation and early gonadal development in anencephalic fetuses is not impaired. Gonadal development of anencephalic male fetuses at different gestational ages is mainly characterized by a reduction in Leydig cell number, which is more pronounced with advancing gestation,[26,483] without significant morphologic changes of the seminiferous tubules.[26,68,483]

Female ovarian development is nearly identical in anencephalic and normal fetuses up to the seventh month of gestation, whereas after 32 weeks a more scattered distribution of primordial follicles is observed, with a lack of antral follicles.[26] At term, ovaries of anencephalic fetuses are of smaller size, and antral follicles are absent.[26] Signs of impaired fetal ovarian development in surgically hypophysectomized monkey fetuses include inadequate granulosa cell proliferation and differentiation.[162] After fetal hypophysectomy, a reduction in total germ cell number and an increase in atretic germ cells were seen.[162] Gonadal changes that were similar to those seen in anencephalic fetuses were reported after decapitation or hypophysectomy of fetal monkeys.[162,163,442] Baker and Scrimegeour[26] stressed that the proliferation of oogonia and their progression through meiosis until the development of primordial follicles was not inhibited in anencephalic females. Since granulosa cells are the presumed target cells for FSH in the fetal ovary and since FSH receptors appear only late in the primate ovary,[179] the timing of ovarian dependence on gonadotropins coincides well with the temporal appearance of FSH receptors in this tissue.[26]

Women carrying anencephalic fetuses have similar levels of placental hCG (cited in reference 26); therefore, the LH/hCG receptors of the testicular Leydig cells of anencephalics should be exposed to similar amounts of hCG. Some investigators have suggested that FSH might be needed for adequate hCG action.[26,77] Taken together, observations in anencephalics support the suggestion that extrapituitary factors, possibly of maternal and/or placental and/or gonadal origin, are able to control and promote gonadal development, at least in early gestation, and maintain some cell types throughout gestation. It is also possible that hCG of extraplacental origin, derived either from the fetal kidney or the fetal liver, may contribute to some extent to gonadal development in anencephalics.[262,263]

Placental hCG has long been regarded as the gonadotropic stimulus that induces testicular steroidogenesis in early pregnancy at a critical time for male genital development. This view has been based on several findings: (1) circulating fetal hCG concentrations reach a peak at 12 weeks of gestation, a time when testicular Leydig cell content is at its highest[324]; (2) in the second half of human pregnancy, when hCG and fetal testosterone levels fall, there also is a gradual regression in Leydig cells in the human fetal testis[74,132]; (3) fetal testes after 12 weeks of gestation contain binding sites for hCG.[175,288]

Several findings raise questions about the role attributed to hCG in regulating fetal testicular steroidogenesis. No data are available concerning whether hCG receptors are present and functional before 12 weeks of gestation, a time when hCG levels are peaking and testosterone levels are beginning to rise. In addition, discrepant results about the ability of hCG to stimulate fetal testicular testosterone secretion in vitro have been reported. Although increased testicular testosterone secretion in vitro in response to hCG stimulation and in response to concomitant perifusion of testis and placenta was described by several investigators,[1,4,175,177] recent studies failed to show hCG-dependent testosterone secretion from testes obtained at 15 to 18 weeks of gestation.[431,479] Word et al.[479] reported that in human fetal testes from late first-trimester and early second-trimester fetuses (weeks 10 to 18), testosterone synthesis as well as adenylate cyclase activity were independent of hCG stimulation. It is not clear which experimental differences caused these discrepancies. Because of the high circulating hCG levels at the gestational ages examined, hCG receptors of the freshly excised testes could have been fully occupied by endogenous hCG. Addition of exogenous hCG, therefore, might not have elicited an additional response in testosterone output. Thus the divergent results described could be explained by (1) maximal occupancy of the hCG receptors by endogenous hCG in some specimens with variable dissociation of the endogenous hCG occurring in the different studies; (2) failure of coupling of the immature binding sites to their second messenger (cAMP) in the younger testes; or (3) degradation of hCG binding sites during cell preparation. If coupling of the binding sites with the second messenger occurs only at a later time in development, then an intrinsic or extrinsic stimulator for the initiation of testicular testosterone secretion must be assumed. In the rabbit fetus, early testosterone synthesis occurs spontaneously, and only during later gestation is testosterone secretion dependent on gonadotropic stimulation.[125]

In addition to placental and pituitary gonadotropins, growth-promoting factors of placental origin may have an important role in fetal gonadal development. The human placenta produces many growth-promoting factors that are important for the development of different organ systems; some of these factors may play a role in the regulation of gonadal growth and differentiation. These putative regulatory factors include IGF-I[284] and IGF-II,[107] EGF,[151] TGF-α[414] and TGF-β,[116] and bFGF.[149] In addition, recently the mRNA of several growth factors and related peptides were localized to the fetal gonads.[345,459,481]

Human fetal gonadal development

Sexual development in human and subhuman primates, as in most mammals, can be divided into four stages: (1) pregonadal, (2) indifferent, (3) primary sex differentiation, and (4) secondary sex differentiation.[285] The pregonadal stage begins in the human embryo with the differentiation of primordial germ cells (PGCs) in 4.5-day-old blastocysts.[171] At this time the embryo lacks any specific gonadal structures, but the ultimate development of a female or male gonad is predetermined by its chromosomal sex.

The period of the indifferent gonad lasts in the human embryo about 7 to 10 days[191] and begins with the development of the gonadal or genital ridges.[132,202] The primate indifferent gonad forms by rapid proliferation and thickening of the genital ridge and its coelomic epithelium on the medioventral surface of the mesonephric fold to the root of the dorsal mesentery.[482] The PGCs start their ameboid migration from the entoderm of the yolk sac through the gut entoderm and into the mesoderm of the mesentery to the coelomic epithelium of the urogenital ridge.[119,477] The stimulus for the initiation and guidance of this migration has not been definitively established. An active cellular role of the coelomic epithelium has been suggested by some authors (for review see references 462 and 484).

In humans and other mammals, the development of a male gonad is specified by the presence of a Y chromosome or a critical fragment of the Y chromosome that contains the testis-determining gene(s) or factor(s) (TDF).[87,266] Several attempts to characterize this gene have been unsuccessful.[224,313,314,404] From microsurgical experiments it appears that the development of the gonad is not dependent on the presence or genetic expression of PGCs in the gonadal ridge.[260,272]

Appearance of Sertoli cells in the fetal male gonad signals the start of "primary sex differentiation."[200] In contrast, lack of differentiation of Sertoli cells at this critical time can be regarded as a sign of ovarian development. Chronologically, ovarian development in females occurs after the development of seminiferous tubules in the male gonad. If differentiation of Sertoli cells does not occur in chromosomal males, active ovarian differentiation is initiated.[198,199] During the "secondary sex differentiation" that follows, paracrine (müllerian inhibiting substance [MIS]) and endocrine (androgens) activity of the testis causes regression of the müllerian duct and stabilization of the wolffian duct and its derivatives in the male. Conversely, in the absence of the testicular hormones affecting these aspects of male development, and irrespective of the presence of a female gonad, the müllerian duct and the female genitalia form.

In the fetal testis, Sertoli cells aggregate to form testicular cords (43 to 50 days) that later enclose the germ cells.[191,462] The putative TDF gene is probably expressed at this time or shortly before and causes, presumably in combination with other autosomal gene products, the differentiation of the testicular cells into Sertoli cells and Leydig cells. The morphologic differentiation of the Sertoli cells is followed by the development of cellular junctions between adjacent Sertoli cells and formation of a basement membrane along the base of the tubules.[322] This is then followed by the secretion of MIS and the later cytologic differentiation of interstitial or Leydig cells.[201] The establishment of the peritubular disposition of myoid cells does not take place until the eighteenth week.[100] At present it is unknown which cells (Sertoli cells, peritubular cells) deposit the basement membrane, although in prepubertal rats there is evidence that both Sertoli cells and myoid cells cooperate in the deposition of the basal lamina.[406] After a period of rapid multiplication, Sertoli cells that surround the germ cells make up the majority of the testicular cord cells,[321] and they have important paracrine (MIS, activin [?]) and endocrine (estrogens, inhibin) functions during embryonic and fetal development. The developing testicular cords, which remain without lumina, grow in length, become circular, and anastomose during the fetal period.[323] They are enveloped by a discrete connective tissue investment (basal lamina) of three to five cell layers.[150] This basal lamina is detectable in the human fetus by 44 to 48 days.[452] The basement membrane and cellular investments of the testicular cords are remarkably similar to those in the adult.[150] Since myoid cells are found only later, it seems that at least the primary basement membrane is deposited by Sertoli cells. Whether the blood-testis barrier of the adult[99] is established during fetal life remains to be determined.

Fetal spermatogonia are found in the cords surrounded by Sertoli cells. Germ cells that are not enclosed by testicular cords degenerate rapidly. Some of the spermatogonia are found on the basal lamina at the end of the first trimester (days 87 to 97).[452] In contrast to the female, male germ cells do not start their meiotic division before puberty. This developmental pattern suggests that the fetal and prepubertal testis (possibly Sertoli cells) produces a meiosis-inhibiting factor. The spermatogonia in the periphery of the testicular tubules cease mitotic division at 18 to 20 weeks of gestation.[146] A large number of germ cells, particularly gonocytes, degenerate during fetal development. An increase in degeneration was seen between 16 and 20 weeks. The dead cells are removed by phagocytosis by neighboring Sertoli cells. These Sertoli cells are characterized by large phagosomes present in their cytoplasm.[146]

The first Leydig cells appear in the testis at a gestational age of 8 weeks.[324,452] They fill the area between the sex cords and are surrounded by mesenchymal cells and small capillaries.[150] The fetal Leydig cells have ultrastructural characteristics of steroid-secreting cells with extensive agranular endoplasmic reticulum.[324] Shortly after the time of their appearance, concentrations of androgens in testicular tissue, blood, and amniotic fluid start to rise and reach a maximum at 15 to 18 weeks.[90,363,395] This rise in androgens is accompanied by an increase in Leydig cell number, and ultimately Leydig cells fill the space between the testicular cords in the testis.[324] At 14 weeks, Leydig cells occupy 50% of the relative area of the human fetal testis and reach their maximal number.[172,303,452] Subsequently their number decreases, and only a few Leydig cells are seen in the fetal testis at term.[303,324] The life cycle of fetal Leydig cells in the human fetus parallels the rise, peak, and decline of fetal hCG levels during pregnancy, and the presence of hCG and hCG receptors in the testis [175,288] suggests a regulatory role

for this hormone.[176,324] (See also section on gonadotropic control of gonadal development.)

As outlined earlier, if differentiation of Sertoli cells does not occur in chromosomal males, active ovarian differentiation is initiated. In the human, as in other mammals, the indifferent gonadal stage persists longer in the female than in the male. Between 7 and 9 weeks, large ameboid-appearing primitive germ cells are scattered throughout the ovarian parenchyma and make up 8% to 10% of the ovarian cells.[228] Mesonephric cell cords occupy the medulla of the developing ovary before meiosis starts,[53] and at 3 months of gestation the ovarian cortex begins to thicken as a result of increased mitotic activity of the oogonia and the primitive granulosa cells.[337]

The two major patterns of ovarian differentiation are determined by whether the ovarian germ cells undergo "immediate" meiosis without prior steroidogenesis or "delayed" meiosis with ovarian steroidogenesis preceding the meiosis.[53] The human fetal ovary represents an intermediate example between these two types of development. In the human fetal ovary, meiosis begins shortly after ovarian differentiation, but despite the capacity for limited steroidogenesis few if any steroids are produced de novo in the fetal ovary during early gestation.[53] It seems that during normal fetal and postnatal development of the female, there is no apparent need of ovarian steroidogenetic function. However, adequate fetal and prepubertal ovarian development is necessary for normal puberty and reproductive life.

The stages of human intrauterine ovarian mitosis and meiosis are temporally regulated so that certain stages are initiated at certain times.* Oocytes of different developmental stages can be seen in the same ovary at a given time, suggesting that this regulation depends on two factors, one that induces the next developmental step to take place and another that selects which oocytes are "mature" enough to go to the next step. The large overlap in time between the different stages and the observation that oocytes of different degrees of maturation are located near each other indicate that some unknown intracellular mechanisms govern the individual maturational pace of each oocyte.

The peak number of germ cells is reached in the human fetal ovary at 16 to 20 weeks.[146] At this gestational age the number of germ cells increases to about 6 million then decreases subsequently to about 2 million cells at term.[146] The possible cause of the massive loss has been attributed to different factors. Some investigators have claimed that many oocytes regress during the early stages of meiosis if they are not enveloped by granulosa cells once they have entered the diplotene stage,[310] whereas others have observed that from early development of the ovary (weeks 7 to 12) until the postnatal period, germ cells in the cortical area have the ability to migrate toward the superficial coelomic layer covering the gonad.[290] As a result, oogonia and oocytes gradually become incorporated into the surface

*References 22-24, 43, 221, 228, 248, 309, 311, 407.

epithelium and are thereby eliminated from the ovary.[290] According to these authors, germ cells that are initially located deeper in ovarian tissue do not migrate and go on to become primary follicles.[290] Still others have attributed the increased germ cell atresia in the fetal ovary to meiotic pairing anomalies.[408]

Females with some chromosomal abnormalities (trisomy 21, trisomy 18, and 45,XO) experience inadequate ovarian development and excessive germ cell loss. Of these chromosomal defects, Turner syndrome (45,XO) is the most extensively studied.[62,370] In 45,XO fetuses, germ cells migrate to the gonadal ridge and undergo mitosis. However, oogonia do not undergo meiosis, and a more rapid degeneration occurs that leaves the ovaries at birth with either no or only few follicles. This suggests that both X chromosomes may be needed for meiosis and survival of oogonia in the human fetus.

During fetal development, primary oocytes become morphologically associated with the precursors of granulosa cells that originate either in the germinal epithelium or in the rete ovarii.[23] Follicular development occurs mainly between 16 and 21 weeks of gestation,[25,223] and primordial follicles can be seen around week 21.[223] At this stage, the most mature and developed primary follicles (in which flattened granulosa cells become cuboidal and begin to divide) are in the medullary portion of the ovary.[223] A translucent halo, the zona pellucida, appears around granulosa cell–engulfed oocytes[69] that consists of proteins synthesized by the oocyte.[241,463] Larger, preantral follicles, containing an enlarged oocyte with a zona pellucida, multiple layers of granulosa cells, and a theca cell layer that originates in the stroma, develop around the sixth month of gestation at the border between the cortex and the medulla.[326] Antral or graafian follicles with a fully developed oocyte, a fluid-filled cavity, multiple layers of granulosa cells, and a theca cell layer outside of the basement membrane, can be found in ovaries near term or in the neonate.[326,343] But these secondary and tertiary follicles are rare at term, constituting only 0.1% to 0.5% of all follicles.[228]

The fetal ovary also contains interstitial cells that possess typical ultrastructural characteristics of steroid-producing cells.[147,223] Their ultrastructure is reminiscent of fetal Leydig cells[147] and, similar to Leydig cells, they reach their maximal number at 18 weeks of gestation, followed by a gradual decline.[223] The different steroidogenic synthetic patterns observed in the fetal ovary when compared with later stages of life can be attributed to these interstitial cells. Theca cells with steroidogenic potential surrounding the developing follicles are found only during the latter third of pregnancy.[145,164]

Gonadal steroidogenesis and its regulation

Androgens are needed at different stages of mammalian intrauterine development for the adequate growth and differentiation of the internal and external genitalia[200] and, in some species, for imprinting of the brain along male lines.[111,355,357] The testes of all mammalian species studied to date are able to synthesize testosterone de novo from acetate,[364,388] and the interstitial Leydig cells are probably the site of this steroidogenesis. Changes in testicular steroidogenesis occur from the earliest appearance of Leydig cells until after puberty, and seem to depend on several factors, including changing sensitivity to gonadotropic hormones, levels of gonadotropins, number of steroid-producing Leydig cells, and progressive differentiation of these Leydig cells.

Human fetal testicular tissue can incorporate acetate into cholesterol.[61,258,399] However, testicular specimens obtained during the first and second trimesters can utilize acetate as well as LDL cholesterol as precursors for androgen formation.[61] Androgen formation from pregnenolone in the human fetal testis seems to proceed mainly through the Δ^5 (pregnenolone, 17α-hydroxypregnenolone, DHEA, and androstenediol) pathway.[174] Other studies have supported this observation,[2,182,258] although the Δ^4 (pregnenolone, progesterone, 17α-hydroxyprogesterone, androstenedione, and testosterone) pathway also may play a minor role in fetal testicular steroidogenesis.[432]

Shortly after the formation of the testicular cords and concomitant with the histologic differentiation of testicular Leydig cells (around week 8) testosterone synthesis begins in the human fetal testis.[395] Activation of 3β-HSD appears to play an important role in the increasing production of fetal androgens.[395] Testosterone synthesis reaches a maximum between 10 to 15 weeks and declines thereafter to low levels throughout the remainder of pregnancy.[90,395] Human fetal midgestational testes examined for mRNA levels of three steroid hormone enzymes, P450scc (cholesterol side-chain cleavage enzyme), P450c17 (17α-hydroxylase/17,20-lyase), and P450c21 (21-hydroxylase) showed highest abundance of P450scc and P450c17 mRNAs in the testes at 14 to 16 weeks.[457] These high mRNA levels diminished to 35% and 19% of their peak values, respectively, by 20 to 25.8 weeks.[457] All of these observations indicate that the gradual decline of Leydig cells is accompanied by a fall in testicular enzyme content and subsequently a decline of testicular androgen production. Serum testosterone levels during early gestation are significantly higher in umbilical cord blood of male fetuses (3.7 ± 0.9 ng/mL) than in maternal blood (1 ± 0.4 ng/mL), but at term both maternal and neonatal testosterone levels are comparably low (< 0.8 ng/mL).[90]

Several lines of evidence have highlighted the critical role of testosterone in the development of the male urogenital tract. Testosterone secretion begins immediately before the initiation of virilization of the urogenital tract in a variety of mammalian species.[395,472] The administration of androgens to female embryos at the appropriate time in development causes male development of internal and external genitalia.[380] Furthermore, the experimental administration of antiandrogenic agents during embryogenesis impairs adequate male development.[143,300] In addition, specific androgen receptors have been demonstrated in nongenital skin of human fetuses as early as 8 weeks, suggesting that these receptors appear very early in human development.[420] The role of testosterone in the virilization of the external genitalia of the male embryo that are not derived from the wolffian duct is probably exerted through its 5α-reduced derivative, dihydrotestosterone (DHT). In embryos of different species, including the human, 5α-reductase activity is maximal in the urogenital tubercle and in the urogenital sinus before virilization begins, whereas no activity can be detected in the wolffian duct derivatives until after their virilization has advanced.[395,471] The importance of DHT for the differentiation of the male genitalia that are not derived from the wolffian duct (i.e., urethra, prostate, and external genitalia) is further supported by studies of patients with 5α-reductase deficiency. Affected chromosomal males have female external genitalia, virilized wolffian duct derived–internal genitalia that terminate in a pseudovagina and bilateral testes.[327]

In the human, four single-gene defects in androgen synthesis ([1] cholesterol 20,22-desmolase deficiency; [2] 3β-HSD-isomerase deficiency; [3] 17α-hydroxylase/17,20-desmolase deficiency; and [4] 17β-HSD deficiency) can result in deficient testosterone synthesis, incomplete virilization of the male fetus, and an absence of müllerian ducts.[155,470] Depending on the severity of the enzymatic defect, affected males may exhibit characteristics ranging from mild developmental abnormalities of the external genitalia to a completely female phenotype.[155,470] The observation that müllerian duct–derived female genitalia are absent in these patients further reinforces the concept that regression of this ductal system is not dependent on adequate steroidogenic activity (see section on MIS). These "experiments of nature" are also supported by animal experiments: administration of androgens to female embryos at the appropriate time in development causes male development of internal and external genitalia.[380]

Gonadal steroids also exert endocrine effects that regulate the development and function of the fetal brain. The hypothalamus of the fetal primate brain contains receptors for androgens,[342] as well as aromatase and 5α-reductase activity.[70,190,356,378] Estrogen receptors can be demonstrated in hypothalamic and pituitary cytosolic extracts from midgestation fetuses,[85] and the midgestation hypothalamus can form catecholestrogens.[109] This suggests that gonadal steroids and their metabolites might act on the brain during embryogenesis and fetal life in a fashion similar to their actions in the adult.[280,353]

The establishment of negative feedback mechanisms that differentially influence gonadotropin levels in both sexes is further supported by gonadectomy studies that have shown that fetal orchidectomy in monkeys caused marked elevation of LH[103] and FSH,[360] whereas oophorectomy at the same time did not influence pituitary gonadotropin levels.

These results could explain the lower levels of gonadotropins found in male fetuses throughout the second half of pregnancy at a time when the fetal testis but not the fetal ovary is steroidogenically active. Furthermore, the recent study by Beck-Peccoz et al.[28] confirmed a negative correlation between fetal levels of free testosterone and of gonadotropin levels in both sexes, and the authors suggested that the negative feedback mechanism is operative from at least the seventeenth week to the end of gestation.

Although testosterone is quantitatively the major testicular androgen in fetal and postnatal life, several studies indicate that its role in virilization of the external genitalia of the male embryo that are not derived from the wolffian duct is exerted through its 5α-reduced derivative, DHT (see earlier discussion). Thus testosterone appears to be the principal steroid responsible for virilization of the internal genitalia.

In contrast to the male, ovarian steroid production is not essential for female phenotypic development. In primates, ovarian meiosis begins relatively early, but significant estradiol production does not start until follicular growth occurs late in fetal life.[316,434] However, some aromatizing activity could be found at 8 weeks of gestation, and this aromatizing ability of the ovaries (0 to 3 pmol/h/mg of protein) did not change with advancing gestational age.[124] These findings are supported by the presence of low levels of immunoassayable 17β-estradiol in human fetal ovaries[361] and the demonstration of aromatase mRNA in second-trimester fetal ovaries.[431] However, the aromatizing ability found in embryonic and fetal ovaries is minimal when compared to placental aromatization, which suggests that the fetal ovary is not a major contributor to circulating estrogens.[124] The fetal liver has half the capability per weight of the fetal ovary of forming estrogens from androgens, but because of its larger weight, its total aromatizing activity is greater than that of the ovary.[124]

In addition to its aromatizing ability, the human fetal ovary has other enzymatic activities that allow the partial conversion of steroidogenic intermediate hormones but are not sufficient for the conversion of acetate or cholesterol to C-19 or C-18 steroids. When homogenates of ovarian tissue from fetuses of 9 to 15 weeks of gestation were incubated with ^{14}C-progesterone, 20α-hydroxy-4-pregnene-3-one was the only metabolite detected.[40] In another study, fetal ovarian homogenates synthesized small amounts of progesterone and pregnenolone from radioactively labeled acetate,[40] with no evidence for androgen or estrogen production. Similarly, the fetal ovary was not able to synthesize testosterone de novo during the first half of pregnancy.[90,363,395]

The notion of incomplete steroidogenic activity of the fetal ovary is further supported by studies on the fetal ovarian mRNA content of steroid-metabolizing enzymes.[457] Cholesterol side-chain cleavage enzyme (P450scc) and 17α-hydroxylase/17,20-lyase mRNA were present in the ovary, but only at 6.2% and 1.8% of the maximal levels found in the testis.[457] Furthermore, these low levels did not vary throughout the second trimester (range of 14.9 to 21.5 gestational weeks).[457] Taken together, these findings suggest that the second-trimester fetal ovary is not able to synthesize C-18 steroids de novo from acetate, but certain steps, including cholesterol synthesis and metabolism of pregnenolone (sulfate) to androstenedione[316] are possible. This partial enzymatic activity and the low steroid content of primate fetal ovaries suggest that fetal human as well as rhesus monkey ovaries are steroidogenically relatively quiescent during gestation.[101,316] Furthermore, from studies of patients with steroidogenic enzyme deficiencies (e.g., 17α-hydroxylase deficiency), it can be concluded that absence of adequate steroidogenesis of gonadal androgens and estrogens does not have a major effect on female fetal gonadal and genital development.

Müllerian inhibiting substance. MIS is a dimeric glycoprotein (~140,000 d) produced in murine, bovine, and human fetal Sertoli cells at 7 weeks of gestational age.[92,93,336,441] In humans, the MIS gene is encoded on the short arm of chromosome 19.[64] MIS causes ipsilateral involution of the müllerian ducts—the embryologic precursors to the cervix, uterus, and fallopian tubes—in the male fetus. MIS was still detected by immunocytochemistry in Sertoli cells of human fetal testes at a gestational age of 22 weeks.[196] MIS mRNA was detectable and its levels were constant throughout the second trimester of pregnancy, a time when müllerian regression has already been completed.[458] The function of MIS during the latter stages of male fetal life is unknown. Since cryptorchid testes contained lower levels of MIS than normally developed testes, a role in the regulation of testicular descent was attributed to MIS.[92,180] Other investigators did not find differences in circulating serum levels between cryptorchid and normal boys.[197] Given the observation that MIS arrests the progression of the meiotic prophase in adult murine oocytes,[428] an analogous role for MIS in the regulation of human germ cell meiosis in fetal life has been proposed.[234a]

Human fetal ovaries between 14 and 22 weeks of gestation contain only small amounts of MIS mRNA (1.9% of the mean testicular MIS mRNA signal at this age), and these levels do not vary throughout the second trimester.[458] MIS mRNA was also demonstrated in adult cultured human granulosa cells and accumulated in these cells in response to physiologic concentrations of hCG.[458] In contrast to findings in male neonates, human female newborns did not have significant immunoassayable levels of MIS in serum.[283]

Inhibin/activin. Inhibin and activin are structurally related dimeric gonadal glycoproteins that were initially characterized by their ability to alter FSH secretion from the pituitary.[450] Inhibin selectively suppresses FSH secretion,[450] whereas activin stimulates pituitary FSH release in vitro and in vivo.[381] Inhibin is composed of one α-subunit

and one of two possible β-subunits (β_A, β_B). The three possible dimers consisting of the two β-subunits have been designated activin A (β_A/β_A), activin AB (β_A/β_B) and activin B (β_B/β_B).[243,382,449,450] Recent studies with these compounds have shown that both activin and inhibin modulate intragonadal processes, as well as functions in other organ systems. (For review see references 371 and 450.)

Several years ago, inhibin immunoreactivity was found in midtrimester human fetal testes at higher levels than in fetal ovaries.[391] We localized the subunits of inhibin and their mRNAs to Sertoli and Leydig cells of the human midtrimester fetus and (primarily) to the intratubular cells of the late-gestation rhesus monkey fetal testis (Fig. 50-4).[345] Our findings suggest a shift in the site of inhibin subunit production with advancing gestation. We have also demonstrated that the human fetal testis at midgestation is able to secrete inhibin in vitro and that inhibin secretion can be stimulated by both FSH and hCG.[345] Albers et al.[7] found bioactive inhibin in ovine testes during the last quarter of pregnancy (days 111 to 143), and the level of inhibin increased and testosterone secretion decreased after pulsatile FSH administration. It is unclear whether the decrease in testosterone was mediated by FSH or by the paracrine/autocrine action of inhibin within the testis.

Fetal human midtrimester ovaries contain only minimal amounts of immunoreactive inhibin/activin,[345,391] whereas inhibin/activin subunits can be detected in granulosa cells of numerous primary and secondary follicles in the late-gestation rhesus monkey ovary.[345] The paucity of immunoreactive inhibin/activin subunits in the fetal human midgestation ovary is in contrast to similar studies on human fetal testes of similar gestational age.[345] Thus the appearance of the inhibin/activin subunits in the fetal primate ovary occurs at a later gestational stage than in the testis.

Ample evidence exists that ovarian cells in adults synthesize and secrete inhibin/activin. Follicular fluid contains biologically active inhibin and activin.[450] Immunocytochemical and in situ hybridization studies have localized the subunits of inhibin/activin to granulosa and theca interna cells of follicles in murine, porcine, and primate ovaries.[279,382,440,478] The expression of the mRNA of these subunits was shown to undergo rapid changes throughout the stages of the menstrual cycle and to depend on the degree of development of the ovarian follicle.[74,382,440,478] We showed the presence of dimeric activin A in cells of human adult ovarian follicles and corpora lutea.[348]

Activin A has binding sites on rat granulosa cells and modulates both steroidogenesis and LH receptor accumulation in this species.[165,417,418] We recently reported that human recombinant activin A promotes proliferation[344] and inhibits some enzymatic steps of steroidogenesis[348] of human luteinized granulosa cells in vitro.

Circulating and pituitary levels of FSH decrease earlier in gestation in male fetuses than in females. These dissimi-

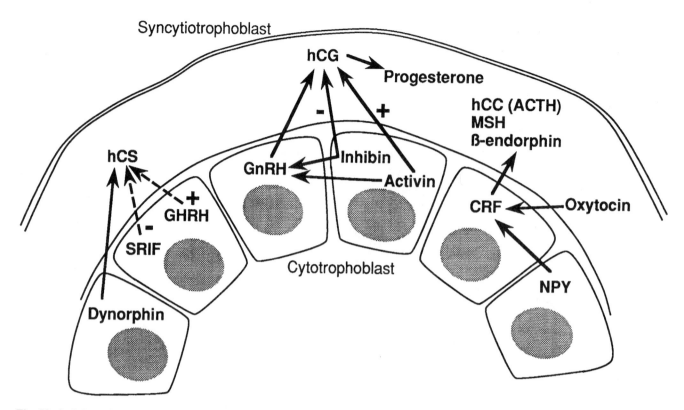

Fig. 50-4. Schematic representation of neurohormones and their potential interactions in the placenta. CRF, corticotropin-releasing factor; hCS, human chorionic somatomammotropin; hCC, human chorionic corticotropin; hCG, human chorionic gonadotropin; NPY, neuropeptide Y; ACTH, adrenocorticotropin; GHRH, growth hormone-releasing hormone; SRIF, somatostatin (somatotropin release-inhibiting factor); GnRH, gonadotropin-releasing hormone; MSH, melanocyte stimulating hormone. (Redrawn from Jaffe RB: Protein hormones of the placenta, decidua, and fetal membranes. In Yen SSC, Jaffe RB, editors: *Reproductive endocrinology,* ed 3, Philadelphia, 1992, WB Saunders.)

larities were attributed to either differences in maturation of the hypothalamic-pituitary axis or feedback of gonadal steroids (testicular testosterone). A comparison between the results obtained in fetuses of both sexes indicates that the differences observed (later appearance of all three subunits in the fetal ovary than testes) may contribute at least in part to the different sexual patterns of pituitary FSH secretion in the human and subhuman primate fetus (earlier decline in FSH in the male fetus). This possibility is further suggested by the demonstration of fetal pituitary sensitivity, that is, decrease in circulating FSH levels to parenteral administration of crude inhibin preparations,[8] which indicates that gonadal inhibin/activin-controlled pituitary feedback mechanisms may have their origins during intrauterine fetal life.

PROTEIN AND STEROID HORMONES OF THE PLACENTA

Placental glycoprotein and peptide hormones

It is now clear that, in addition to the pituitary trophic hormone-like proteins of the placenta (hCG, human chorionic somatomammotropin [hCS or hPL], and human chorionic corticotropin [hCC]), the placenta synthesizes an array

of hypothalamic-like hormones, as well as virtually all of the growth factors and their receptors, and the inhibin family of gonadal peptides.

Most intriguingly, production of placental protein hormones is no longer seen as autonomous; an increasing number of in vitro studies point to endogenous placental regulation of its hormonal products, simulating a miniature hypothalamic-pituitary-target hormone–regulated unit. In addition, substrates reaching the placental circulation may also regulate placental hormone production. If these in vitro studies are confirmed in vivo, the concept of autoregulation within the placenta will replace that of autonomous hormone production and constitute a new chapter in the understanding of placental biology. The site of origin and putative interactions of these placental hormones is presented schematically in Fig. 50-5. In addition to their actions within the placenta, it has been suggested that a number of these placental hormones exert effects on the fetus and/or the mother and thus participate in fetal and maternal homeostasis during pregnancy. Hormonal regulation within the placenta may be paracrine, autocrine, and/or endocrine.

Most, if not all, of the analogues of the hypothalamic

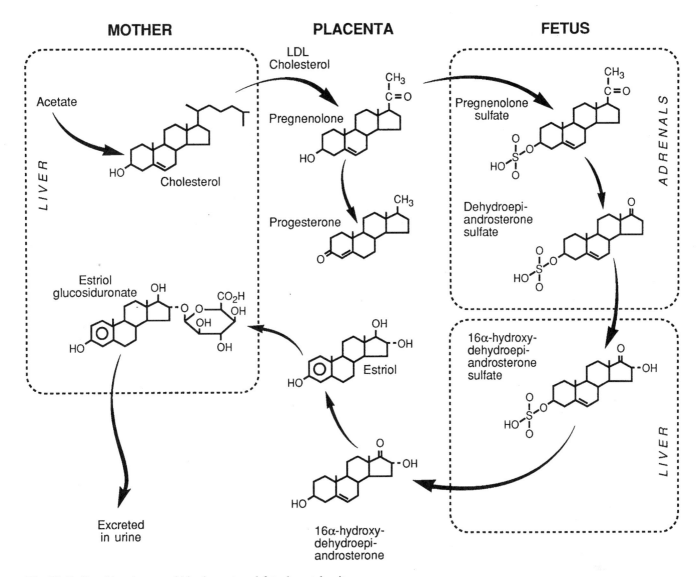

Fig. 50-5. Steroid pathways within the maternal-fetoplacental unit.

hormones are produced primarily in the cytotrophoblastic layer of the placenta. These include GnRH and its precursor GnRH-associated peptide (GAP), somatostatin (SRIF), corticotropin-releasing hormone (CRH or CRF), TRH, and the family of opioid peptides. Growth hormone–releasing hormone (GHRH or GRF) has been found in the rat placenta but has not yet been identified in the human.

Gonadotropin-releasing hormone. Gibbons and co-workers[127] reported in 1975 that GnRH is present in the human placenta. In addition, this material stimulated LH in vivo. Further support for this concept was provided by the studies of Khodr and Siler-Khodr.[127,216-218] These investigators demonstrated that placental tissue cultured in vitro demonstrated a marked increase in immunoreactive GnRH content[217] and enhanced hCG secretion.[216] They also demonstrated GnRH synthesis by placental tissue.[218] Furthermore, GnRH antagonists prevent the GnRH-induced increase in hCG release, as well as decreasing basal hCG

production.[400] The biochemical identity of this placental material was further established by Lee and colleagues,[234] using high-performance liquid chromatography. Subsequently, cloned genomic and complementary deoxyribonucleic acid (cDNA) sequences encoding the precursor form of GnRH in the human placenta were described,[383] further supporting the local synthesis of GnRH. Using immunohistochemical localization, the GnRH-like material was found to be localized principally in the cytotrophoblastic layer of the placental villus.[217]

As noted, the placental GnRH-like material enhances the secretion of hCG.[216] It stimulates the production of both the α- and β-subunits of hCG in placental explants. Interestingly GnRH-binding sites have been demonstrated in the human placenta,[81] raising the possibility that there is "autoregulation" of hCG production within the placenta. As is discussed subsequently, it also is possible that the hCG influences placental steroidogenesis, thus suggesting a complete placental internal regulatory system.

Cell membrane depolarization results in the release of placental GnRH by promoting the influx of calcium into the cells.[328] This is the same mechanism involved in the release of hypothalamic GnRH. Prostaglandins (PGE_2 and PGF_2) and epinephrine increase the release of GnRH from placental cells, probably acting via cAMP. Because propranolol (a β-adrenergic receptor antagonist) reverses the release of GnRH effected by epinephrine, and because isoproterenol (a β-adrenergic receptor agonist) mimics the effect of epinephrine on GnRH, it is possible that adrenergic receptors play a role in modulating placental GnRH release. Insulin and vasoactive intestinal peptide (VIP) can also stimulate placental GnRH in a dose-dependent manner.[335]

GnRH has been measured in the circulation of pregnant women.[397] Its concentration parallels that of placental GnRH concentrations, being highest in the first trimester. That there is a correlation between circulating GnRH and hCG[397] again suggests a possible role of GnRH in regulating hCG production.

Somatostatin. Immunoreactive somatostatin-like material has been demonstrated in human placental villi in early pregnancy.[227] Immunocytochemical localization studies demonstrated the presence of somatostatin in the cytotrophoblast but not in the syncytiotrophoblast.[227,464] With advancing gestational age, the amount of immunoreactive somatostatin decreased.[464] Since hCS increases as pregnancy progresses, the suggestion has been made that the placenta-derived somatostatin may exert an inhibitory influence on hCS,[464] and the diminution in somatostatin production by the cytotrophoblast may permit the progressive increase in hCS secretion by the syncytiotrophoblast. This, then, would be the parallel (albeit inhibitory rather than stimulatory) to the regulation of hCG production by placental GnRH.

Corticotropin-releasing hormone. In the pituitary gland, corticotropin-releasing hormone (factor) (CRH or CRF) of hypothalamic origin stimulates the release of the derivatives of pro-opiomelanocortin (POMC). These include ACTH, β-endorphin, β-lipotropin, and α-melanocyte–stimulating hormone (α-MSH). The human placenta synthesizes and secretes CRH, which is immunologically and biologically identical to hypothalamic CRH.[55,375,392,411,437] The CRH extracted from human placenta can stimulate the release of ACTH and β-endorphin from rat pituitary cells, as well as the ACTH-like material in the placenta.[249,331]

There is a remarkable increase in the mRNA for CRH of more than twentyfold in the last 5 weeks of pregnancy.[115] This parallels the increase in circulating maternal CRH levels and placental CRH content. The mRNA for CRH can be detected by the seventh week of human gestation. Interestingly, in contrast to the negative feedback effect of cortisol on hypothalamic CRH, glucocorticoids enhance CRH mRNA expression in the placenta.[372] CRH mRNA

can be found in both the cytotrophoblast and syncytiotrophoblast,[372] but Petraglia and associates,[331] using immunocytochemical techniques, demonstrated that CRH staining is more intense in the inner layer of the placental villi, that is, cytotrophoblast and intermediate trophoblast.

Petraglia and colleagues[329] also have demonstrated that prostaglandins, neurotransmitters and peptides can stimulate placental CRH release in vitro. They have shown that PGF_2 and PGE_2, norepinephrine, and acetylcholine all stimulate CRH release from cultured placental cells. In addition, the neuropeptides, arginine vasopressin and angiotensin II, along with oxytocin can stimulate CRH from placental cells, as they can from adult hypothalami. Furthermore, the cytokine, interleukin-1 (IL-1) can stimulate the release of CRH from cultured placental cells, whereas IL-2 does not.[329]

The marked increase in CRH expression at the end of gestation and the capacity of glucocorticoids to enhance this expression have led Robinson and colleagues[372] to propose a biologic role for CRH in the fetoplacental unit and in parturition. They suggest that the rise in placental CRH that precedes parturition could result from the rise of fetal glucocorticoids that occurs at this time. They suggest additionally that the increase in placental CRH may stimulate, via fetal ACTH, a further rise in fetal glucocorticoids, "completing a positive feedback loop that would be terminated by delivery." Since CRH of fetal hypothalamic origin may also stimulate fetal pituitary ACTH,[41,128,129,188] they postulate that environmental stresses may stimulate fetal hypothalamic, as well as placental, CRH production, leading to increases in fetal ACTH production. In addition, placental ACTH may stimulate the fetal adrenal directly.[246] Although these observations and hypotheses remain to be substantiated in vivo, they raise intriguing possibilities regarding the maintenance of fetal homeostasis and the initiation of parturition.

Thyrotropin-releasing hormone. A substance similar to the hypothalamic tripeptide TRH has been found in the human placenta.[127,390] It can stimulate pituitary TSH release in the rat both in vitro and in vivo.[127,390] Youngblood and colleagues[482a] have concluded that the material found in the placenta is not identical to hypothalamic TRH, although it has TSH-stimulating capacity. To date, a placental TSH has not been identified. Whether placental TRH plays a role in stimulating fetal or maternal pituitary TSH or prolactin remains to be ascertained. As is discussed subsequently, the thyroid-stimulating activity of the placenta has been ascribed to hCG.

Human chorionic gonadotropin. Human chorionic gonadotropin was the first placental protein hormone to be described. In 1927 Aschheim and Zondek[16] found a substance in the urine of pregnant women that they initially thought was produced by the anterior pituitary gland of the mother. Later studies indicated its production by the placenta.

Human chorionic gonadotropin, which has a molecular weight of 36,000 to 40,000 kd, is a glycoprotein hormone that is biologically and immunologically similar to LH from the pituitary. Details of its purification and chemical properties have been described by Bahl[20] and Carlsen et al.[59] The site of origin of hCG has been the subject of much controversy; immunocytochemical localization studies suggest that it is produced by the syncytiotrophoblastic layer of the placenta,[282] rather than the cytotrophoblast, as first believed.[126] It is elaborated by all types of trophoblastic tissue, including that from hydatidiform mole, chorioadenoma destruens, and choriocarcinoma. It also is produced by choriocarcinoma not following a pregnancy, as well as in the testes of men and the ovaries of women.

Like all glycoprotein hormones (LH, FSH, TSH), hCG is composed of two subunits, α and β. With very minor modifications, the α-subunit is common to all of the glycoprotein hormones and the β-subunit confers unique specificity to the hormone. Neither has activity by itself, and only the intact molecule exerts hormonal effects. The subunits can be recombined, and the α-subunits are interchangeable to a large degree. Several of the subunits have been characterized chemically. Antibodies have been developed to the β-subunits of several of the hormones. By utilizing an antibody to the β-subunit of hCG, a specific radioimmunoassay (RIA) has been developed.[445] This assay can distinguish hCG from pituitary LH, which most RIAs for the intact hormone are incapable of doing because of immunologic cross-reaction. Utilization of the β-subunit hCG RIA is useful clinically to follow the progress of trophoblastic disease, because LH will not interfere.

In normal pregnancy, the primitive trophoblast produces hCG very early. In a spontaneous pregnancy, we found that hCG is detectable 9 days after the midcycle LH peak, which is 8 days after ovulation and only 1 day after implantation.[185] Radioreceptor assays have been developed that also can detect the presence of early pregnancies.[230]

Concentrations of hCG rise to peak values by 60 to 90 days of gestation. In early pregnancy, there is an approximate doubling of hCG levels every 2 to 3 days. Thereafter there is a decrement in hCG levels to a plateau that is maintained during the remainder of the pregnancy. Maternal immunoassayable LH and FSH levels are virtually undetectable throughout pregnancy.[362,430] Recently bioactive FSH-like material has been found in the maternal circulation[312] perhaps secreted by the placenta. The half-life of hCG is approximately 32 to 37 hours,[281] appreciably longer than most other protein and steroid hormones, the half-lives of which often are measured in minutes.

Although much has been learned about the chemical nature, concentration, and site of production of hCG, information still is accumulating concerning its functional roles in pregnancy. It is known to play a luteotropic role in early pregnancy: it maintains the corpus luteum of the menstrual cycle, permitting its conversion to the corpus luteum of pregnancy, thus allowing the continued production of progesterone necessary for decidual development until the placenta takes over progesterone production. In addition, we have obtained data indicating that hCG may regulate steroid production in the fetus—both DHEAS by the fetal zone of the adrenal gland and testosterone by the testis.[175,187] These observations have been questioned by others.

Because of our interest in the role of hCG in the fetal gonad and adrenal, we quantified hCG in a variety of fetal tissues.[176] We found that hCG content was high not only in the fetal testis, in which we had demonstrated specific hCG binding and testosterone stimulation,[175] but also in other fetal tissues, including kidney, ovary, and thymus, as measured with an RIA for the β-subunit of hCG. These observations led to an investigation of the source of the hCG in these fetal tissues.[263] We speculated that hCG was being actively synthesized by these tissues rather than just being taken up from the fetal circulation. Therefore we compared human fetal kidney, liver, and lung with placenta in a tissue explant system, studying incorporation of ^{35}S-methionine. The data suggest that not only does the placenta produce hCG but the human fetal kidney actively synthesizes and secretes hCG as well. Preliminary studies suggest that the human fetal testis also has this capacity. Subsequently we demonstrated synthesis of α-subunit and the fact that the newly synthesized hCG was biologically active.[262] Immunocytochemical staining lent further support to these observations.[144] It is possible that the finding of chorionic gonadotropin in some adult, nontrophoblastic tumors represents an atavistic reversion to a fetal form of hormone synthesis. This also represented the first evidence that the genome of a human fetal tissue directs synthesis of what has been considered a placental hormone.

Two groups have shown that hCG has thyroid-stimulating activity and that much of the increased thyroid activity that occurs in pregnancy is a result of hCG.[215,304] Studies have shown that the hCG molecule contains the structural characteristics required for interaction with the human TSH receptor and activation of the membrane adenylate cyclase that regulates thyroid cell function. Highly purified hCG exhibits specific binding to human thyroid gland membranes.[58] In addition, hCG inhibits the binding of TSH,[12,58,320] and highly purified hCG stimulates adenylate cyclase in human thyroid gland membranes.[58] Furthermore, partial digestion of the hCG molecule with carboxypeptidase results in an increase in human thyroid adenylate cyclase–stimulating activity while retaining the ability to stimulate rat testicular adenylate cyclase activity.[57]

Finally, it is interesting to speculate whether hCG may have steroid regulatory effects within the placenta. Because hCG is produced in the syncytiotrophoblast and steroids also are produced within this cell layer, the intriguing possibility of "autoregulation" within the cell exists. The finding of hCG-specific adenyl cyclase stimulation in the placenta lends credence to this possibility.[271]

Human chorionic somatomammotropin. Another protein hormone, with immunologic and certain biologic similarities to pituitary growth hormone, was isolated from the human placenta by several groups of investigators in the early 1960s. Josimovich and MacLaren,[195] who found this material in peripheral maternal and retroplacental serum as well as in the placenta, designated it human placental lactogen (hPL) because it was found to be lactogenic in the pigeon crop sac assay and found to promote milk production by the mammary gland of the pseudopregnant rabbit.[195] However, whether it has lactogenic properties in women remains to be established. In addition to its effects in the lactational process, Josimovich and MacLaren[195] found that the hormone has luteotropic properties in the pseudopregnant, hypophysectomized rat.

Human placental lactogen or hCS is synthesized by the syncytiotrophoblastic layer of the placenta. It can be found in the serum and urine in both normal and molar pregnancies, and it disappears rapidly from the serum and urine after delivery of the placenta or evacuation of the uterus. After normal delivery, hCS cannot be detected in the serum after the first postpartum day. In addition to being found in normal and molar pregnancies, hCS has been found in the urine of patients harboring trophoblastic tumors and in men with choriocarcinoma of the testis.

In vitro biosynthesis of hCS has been accomplished.[421] Seeburg and co-workers[384] established the nucleotide sequence of part of the gene of hCS by a novel technique involving purification of DNA complementary to the predominant mRNA species. Human chorionic somatomammotropin is a single-chain polypeptide of 191 amino acids with two disulfide bridges and has a 96% homology with GH.[239,301] When circular dichroism is used, a marked similarity in secondary structure is also demonstrated.[36]

The somatotropic activity of hCS is 3% or less that of hGH, although the prolactin-like activity of the two hormones in animals is similar. Furthermore, hCS does have GH-like effects on tibial epiphyseal growth, body weight gain, and sulfate uptake by costal cartilage in the hypophysectomized rat, although the effective dose required is 100 to 200 times that of growth hormone.[158] In vitro, hCS stimulates thymidine incorporation into DNA and enhances the action of hGH and insulin.

In patients with idiopathic hypopituitarism, hCS has growth-promoting activity, as suggested by significant nitrogen and potassium retention and a decrease in blood urea nitrogen.[160] To demonstrate these changes, amounts of hCS were administered that achieved blood levels of 1 to 3 µ/mL, slightly below those of pregnant women in late gestation.

The effects of hCS on fat and carbohydrate metabolism are similar to those after treatment with hGH, including inhibition of peripheral glucose uptake and stimulation of insulin release. An increase in plasma free fatty acids occurs after administration of hCS or hGH to patients with hypopituitarism.[159]

Although hCS has potent mammotropic and lactogenic activity similar to that of hGH, prolactin-like activity was not demonstrable in a hypophysectomized woman treated with hCS.

Both RIAs and hemagglutination inhibition tests have been developed to quantify hCS. It is present in microgram-per-milliliter quantities in early pregnancy. Its concentration increases as pregnancy progresses, with peak levels being reached during the last 4 weeks. There may be a tenfold or greater increase in circulating levels of hCS from the first to the third trimester. Low levels of hCS (7 to 10 ng/mL) are present in the maternal circulation by 20 to 40 days of gestation. By the last 4 weeks of pregnancy, levels of 5.4 µg/mL are achieved.[160] Some investigators have found a significant relationship between placental weight and circulating hCS concentrations, although this has not been observed consistently. The concentration of hCS in maternal peripheral blood is about 300 times that in umbilical vein blood. Furthermore, the concentration of hCS in the blood leaving the gravid uterus is markedly greater than that in the peripheral circulation. The concentration of hCS is less in amniotic fluid than in maternal plasma but greater than that in fetal plasma.

As noted, there is a rapid disappearance of circulating hCS after removal of the placenta. Kaplan and colleagues[211] found multiexponential disappearance curves, with the half-life of the major component being 9 to 15 minutes. To maintain circulating concentrations, this would imply placental production of between 1 and 4 g of the hormone per day at term. Production of this hormone, therefore, must represent one of the major metabolic and biosynthetic activities of the syncytiotrophoblast.

A number of factors known to alter pituitary GH secretion are ineffective in altering hCS concentrations.[194] Prolonged fasting at midgestation[219] and insulin-induced hypoglycemia, however, were reported to raise hCS concentrations, and intraamniotic instillation of $PGF_{2\alpha}$ causes a marked reduction in hCS levels.

Grumbach and co-workers[158] proposed that hCS exerts its major metabolic effect on the mother to ensure the nutritional demands of the fetus. As pregnancy progresses, the fetus increases its substrate requirements, which leads to an increased functional role for this hormone in the second and third trimesters. Kaplan[204] suggests that hCS is the "growth hormone" of pregnancy. She notes that, during pregnancy, blood glucose is decreased and insulin secretion is increased with resistance to endogenous insulin. In addition, elevations in plasma free fatty acids occur. These GH-like and contrainsulin effects of hCS would lead to impaired glucose uptake and stimulation of free fatty acid release, with resultant decreased effective insulin.

Kaplan points out that, although free fatty acids cross the

placenta, the increased ketones induced by metabolism of free fatty acids are a more important energy source for the fetus. As a consequence of decreased effective insulin, muscle proteolysis and the formation of ketones may be enhanced. The decreased glucose utilization induced by hCS would ensure a steady supply of glucose for the fetus. In midgestation, hypoglycemia, which occurs with fasting, is related to fetal glucose consumption and not to an overall decrease in gluconeogenesis. In contrast, in the fed state, Kaplan suggests that the plasma insulin response to glucose would overcome the contrainsulin effects of hCS. This would allow restoration of hepatic glycogen and lipid stores. The increased insulin, acting in concert with hCS, would result in increased protein synthesis.

In this manner, maternal metabolism would be directed toward mobilization of maternal sources to furnish substrate for the fetus. There would be a steady source of various fuels for the fetus, of which glucose would be the major one. Insulin is seen as a fluctuating modifier of the effects of hCS on the mother. Feasting increases effective insulin and restores maternal substrates, whereas fasting results in decreased effective insulin and primary catabolic effects of hCS to ensure an adequate supply of metabolic nutrients for the fetus.

Human chorionic corticotropin. The production of ACTH-like material by the placenta has been suggested by several investigators. Liotta and colleagues[246] obtained data suggesting that the placenta may be the source of another pituitary-like hormone, hCC. They demonstrated both immunoassayable and bioassayable ACTH activity in extracts of extensively washed human placental tissue and dispersed viable trophoblasts. When the trophoblasts were incubated in tissue culture medium, the adrenal corticotropic content of both the cells and the medium was significantly greater than that during the preincubation level, suggesting its synthesis by trophoblastic cells. The physiologic role, if any, of hCC and its regulation remain to be elucidated. It has been suggested that it may be responsible for the relative resistance to negative feedback suppression of pituitary ACTH by glucocorticoids during pregnancy.[123,354] As noted earlier, however, because glucocorticoids stimulate expression of placental CRH, placental CRH may play a role in hCC production.

Other ACTH-related peptides. There is a common precursor glycoprotein in the pituitary gland, with a molecular weight of approximately 31,000 d, that gives rise to ACTH and a group of peptides, including β-lipotrophic hormone (β-LPH), β-endorphin, and α-MSH.[247] These substances are post-translationally derived from the parent hormone, variously referred to as pro-opiomelanocortin (POMC) or 31Kd ACTH/endorphin.

Both ACTH- and β-endorphin–like peptides have been demonstrated in human placental extracts by a variety of assay techniques.* Liotta and Krieger[245] demonstrated that

cultured human placental trophoblastic cells synthesize a high-molecular-weight glycoprotein with physicochemical similarities to those of pituitary POMC. ACTH(9-15)–like and β-endorphin(1-9)–like fragments were detected in a tryptic digests of this precursor. Subsequently this group showed that the β-endorphin–like peptide synthesized in placental cells is comparable to synthetic human β-endorphin.[244]

Thus the synthesis of both the 31Kd parent molecule and β-endorphin by the placenta furnishes yet another example of some of the similar biosynthetic capacities of placenta and pituitary. The biologic role, if any, of this placenta-derived β-endorphin awaits further study.

Immunoreactive β-endorphin in the maternal circulation remains relatively low throughout pregnancy, with mean levels of approximately 15 pg/mL.[141] Mean levels rise to approximately 70 pg/ml during late labor and rise further (mean 113 pg/mL) at delivery.[141] Similar concentrations of β-endorphin (mean 105 pg/mL) also are seen in umbilical cord plasma at term, suggesting secretion by the placenta and/or fetal pituitary. Many factors that cause an increase in pituitary ACTH also result in an increase in β-endorphin. Wardlaw and colleagues[460] have suggested that hypoxia and acidosis may cause an increase in β-endorphin (and β-LPH), as well as ACTH.

In addition to β-endorphin and β-LPH, which are derived from the parent POMC molecule, there are two other families of endogenous opioids—enkephalins and dynorphins. The former is derived from prepro-enkephalin A, the latter from prepro-enkephalin B. Immunoreactive methionine-enkephalin has been found in the human placenta that is chemically identical to the native molecule.[350] Circulating levels of met-enkephalin do not change appreciably throughout pregnancy.[350]

Three forms of dynorphin have been found in the human placenta.[236,451] Dynorphin binds to κ opiate receptors; these are abundant in human placenta,[34] and receptor number increases at term.[6] The placental content of dynorphin at term is of similar magnitude to that found in the pituitary gland and brain.[451] Relatively high concentrations of dynorphin have been found in amniotic fluid and umbilical cord venous plasma, and maternal plasma levels in the third trimester and at delivery are higher than those in nonpregnant women.[451] Because κ receptor agonists stimulate the release of hCS,[5] it is possible that dynorphin exerts local regulatory effects on hCS production.

Neuropeptide Y. Neuropeptide Y (NPY) is a 36–amino acid peptide that is found in the central and peripheral nervous systems and can exert effects centrally on such behavioral events as eating and satiety, as well as on neuroendocrine function.[9,154,433] Immunoreactive NPY has been found in extracts of term placenta, and its elution profile is similar to that of synthetic NPY.[333] In the placenta, NPY is found principally in the cytotrophoblast and intermediate trophoblast layers.[333] Additionally, bind-

*References 112, 244-247, 295, 307, 354.

ing sites for NPY recently have been found in the placenta.[333]

Maternal NPY levels are increased over those of nonpregnant women beginning early in gestation. They remain elevated until term and rise still further during labor, reaching their acme with cervical dilatation and parturition.[334] There is no significant change in NPY concentrations in the circulation of women undergoing cesarean section who are not in labor.[334] The levels of NPY fall rapidly after delivery, again suggesting a placental source of this neuropeptide. Elevated concentrations of NPY also are found in the amniotic fluid.[334]

Because NPY can stimulate CRH release from cultured placental cells, but not the release of GnRH, hCG, or hCS, NPY may play a role in the regulation of placental CRH release.

The inhibin family of peptides. As indicated earlier, several groups have succeeded in purifying the substances produced by the ovary and testis that inhibit pituitary FSH production, termed inhibin. Inhibins are glycoprotein hormones that are in the growth factor family that includes TGF-β, MIS, erythroid differentiation factor and the fly decapentaplegic gene complex. The major known sites of production of inhibin are the testes and ovary.

In addition to inhibin, which is a heterodimer, the homodimers (activins) β_A/β_A and β_A/β_B stimulate FSH production. The inhibin subunits have been found in the placenta, using both immunocytochemical and in situ hybridization techniques.[264,332,346] Placental inhibin has biologic activity,[264,332] and inhibin antibodies can block this activity. Using an antibody to a portion of the α-subunit of inhibin, Petraglia and associates[335] found immunoreactive cells in the cytotrophoblastic layer of human placental villi. Rabinovici and colleagues,[346] using immunocytochemistry, found all three subunits in the more central portions of the cytotrophoblast and the β_B-subunit in the syncytiotrophoblast. There were no observable changes in localization with advancing gestation. Meunier and co-workers[278] have identified the human β-subunit homodimer in RNA in the rat placenta, again suggesting the local synthesis of activin.

Cyclic adenosine monophosphate analogues and adenylate cyclase activators increase inhibin release from placental cells in culture, suggesting that cAMP may be the second messenger involved in the release of placental inhibin. This may also explain the increase in inhibin effected by hCG in placental cell cultures.[332] Furthermore, Petraglia and colleagues demonstrated that the neuropeptides VIP and NPY also increased inhibin release from the placenta in a dose-related manner.

A study of inhibin concentrations in patients with premature ovarian failure, who had undetectable circulating inhibin levels before becoming pregnant and high levels after in vitro fertilization and embryo transfer using donor ova,[278] again points to a placental source for the inhibin present in the maternal circulation. Levels of inhibin are high in both the maternal circulation and cord blood.

Addition of inhibin antiserum to placental cell cultures increases the production of hCG,[332] raising the possibility that inhibin plays an inhibitory role in regulating hCG release. Since inhibin antiserum also increases GnRH release in this system, it might also exert a local inhibitory action on placental GnRH and this may be the mechanism by which inhibin modulates hCG release.

In contrast, Petraglia and colleagues found that addition of activin to the placental cultures increased the concentrations of GnRH and progesterone and that these effects could be reversed by inhibin.[330] Since these authors also found that activin can augment the GnRH-induced release of hCG, the possibility exists of a local interaction of GnRH, hCG, and inhibin-related peptides.

Growth factors in the placenta. As indicated previously, inhibin is in the family of growth factors that includes TGF-β. Not only TGF-β[414] but also many other growth factors and their receptors have been found in the human placenta. These include insulin-like growth factors,[107] EGF,[229,256] platelet-derived growth factor,[151] and FGF.[149] Some or all of these may play a role in growth, development and differentiated function of the placenta, a fascinating biochemical factory.

Steroid hormone formation, metabolism, and function in pregnancy

In large measure, the integrated fetoplacental unit must control its destiny—its growth, development, and function, as well as the subsequent expulsion of the fetus and senescence of the placenta, and even its ability to survive in an alien environment.

From the endocrinologic point of view, these functions are subsumed by steroid hormone production by the fetal adrenal, gonad, and placenta; by neuropeptide and polypeptide hormone production by the fetal hypothalamo-pituitary unit and placenta; and by hormonal production by the fetal thyroid and pancreas. Contributing to this fetal and placental activity are the changes in maternal endocrine economy and the influence these have on the function of fetus and placenta.

In regard to steroid hormone formation in pregnancy, two aspects must be considered: (1) the integrated role and constant interaction of fetus, placenta, and mother in the formation of the large quantities of the sex steroids—estrogens and progesterone—extant during pregnancy; and (2) steroid hormone formation and regulation within the fetus itself, which we have considered in the previous sections.

Over the past three decades, the concept has evolved that the placenta is an incomplete steroid-producing organ, unlike the adult adrenal, testis, and ovary, and must rely on precursors reaching it from the fetal and maternal circulations. From the unique interdependence of fetus, placenta, and mother arose the concept of an integrated fetoplacental-maternal unit.

To understand this concept, the reader may find it useful to review the general biosynthetic pathways in steroid hormone formation. The individual adult steroid-producing glands are capable of the formation of progestins, androgens, and estrogens, but this is not true of the placenta. There is a constant interplay of fetus, placenta, and mother to form the bulk of the sex steroids in pregnancy. For estrogen formation by the placenta to occur, precursors must reach it from both the fetal and the maternal compartments, whereas placental progesterone formation is accomplished in large part from circulating maternal cholesterol.[167] In the placenta, cholesterol is converted first to pregnenolone and then rapidly and efficiently to progesterone.[338] Production of progesterone approximates 250 mg/d by the end of pregnancy, at which time circulating levels are in the order of 130 ng/mL.[193] To form estrogens, the placenta, which has an active aromatizing capacity, utilizes circulation androgens, primarily from the fetus but also from the mother. The major androgenic precursor in placental estrogen formation is DHEAS. This compound comes mainly from the fetal adrenal gland. Because the placenta has an abundance of the sulfatase (sulfate-cleaving) enzyme, DHEAS is converted to free (unconjugated) DHEA when it reaches the placenta, then to androstenedione, thereafter to testosterone, and, finally, to estrone and 17β-estradiol (see Fig. 50-5).

In human pregnancy, however, by far the major estrogen formed is neither estrone nor estradiol but another estrogen, estriol. Estriol is not secreted by the ovaries of nonpregnant women. It has an additional hydroxyl group in position 16 and constitutes more than 90% of the known estrogen in pregnancy urine, into which it is excreted as sulfate and glucuronide conjugates. Concentrations increase with advancing gestation and range from approximately 2 mg/24 hours at 26 weeks to 35 to 45 mg/24 hours at term.[114] Estriol also is found in high concentrations in amniotic fluid[379] and in the maternal circulation. At term, the concentration of estriol in the maternal circulation is between approximately 8 and 13 ng/dL.[140]

Estriol is formed by a unique biosynthetic process during pregnancy, which demonstrates the interdependence of fetus, placenta, and mother (Fig. 50-5). DHEAS quantitatively is the major steroid produced by the fetal adrenal gland; almost all of it is produced in the fetal zone.[387] When DHEAS of either fetal or maternal origin reaches the placenta, estrone and estradiol are formed. However, very little of either is converted to estriol by the placenta. Instead, some of the DHEAS undergoes 16α-hydroxylation, primarily in the fetal liver and, to a limited extent, in the fetal adrenal itself.[325] When the 16α-hydroxy-DHEAS (16α-OH-DHEAS) so formed reaches the placenta, the placental sulfatase enzyme acts to cleave the sulfate side chain, and the unconjugated 16α-OH-DHA is aromatized to form estriol. The estriol then is secreted into the maternal circulation. When it reaches the maternal liver, it is conjugated to form estriol sulfate, estriol glucosiduronate, and a mixed conjugate, estriol sulfoglucosiduronate, in which forms it is excreted by way of the maternal urine.[139]

With such relatively copious amounts of progesterone and estriol produced each day, the question of the function of these two steroids during pregnancy must be answered. In the case of progesterone, attention has focused on its effect in maintaining the uterine musculature—the myometrium—in a state of relative quiescence during much of the pregnancy.

Siiteri and colleagues[396] have proposed that progesterone produced by the placenta, the ovaries, or both is the essential hormone of mammalian pregnancy because of its ability to inhibit T lymphocyte cell-mediated responses involved in tissue rejection. On the basis of their experiments demonstrating the role of progesterone in prolonging xenogeneic grafts, preventing inflammation, and promoting the survival of human trophoblastic tissue in rodents, they have suggested that a high local (intrauterine) concentration of progesterone can effectively block cellular immune responses to foreign antigens. Siiteri et al. point out that progesterone has been aptly called the hormone of pregnancy because it appears to be essential for maintenance of pregnancy in all mammals examined, and its presence has been detected in species representing all classes of vertebrates and lower forms, such as molluscs. The essential nature of progesterone for pregnancy maintenance has been demonstrated by experiments in which abortion was induced after the administration either of drugs that inhibit progesterone synthesis or of progesterone antibodies. The specificity of the abortifacient effect was demonstrated by the concurrent administration of progesterone in these experiments. The studies of Moriyama and Sugawa[289] demonstrated that cultured xenogeneic cells injected into the estrogen-primed hamster uterus grow into solid, tumor-like masses during progesterone administration, suggesting that progesterone may be instrumental in conferring immunologic privilege to the uterus.

The functional role of estriol in pregnancy has caused a great deal of speculation. In many biologic systems, estriol is a weak estrogen, with approximately 0.01 the potency of estradiol and 0.1 the potency of estrone on a weight basis. However, there is one function for which estriol appears to be as effective as the other estrogens: its ability to increase uteroplacental blood flow. Therefore, Resnik and colleagues[359] have proposed that this may be the primary function of the large amounts of estriol produced each day. Its relatively weak estrogenic effects on other organ systems may make it an ideal candidate for this purpose. Resnik and Brink[358] demonstrated that estrogens exert their effect on blood flow by prostaglandin stimulation. Martucci and Fishman,[255] as well as Clark and associates,[71] have shown that although acute administration of estriol is ineffective as an estrogen and does not demonstrate extensive binding to estrogen receptors, prolonged exposure to estriol does produce estrogen effects, and binding occurs.

REFERENCES

1. Abramovich DR, Baker TG, Neal P: Effect of human chorionic gonadotrophin on testosterone secretion by the foetal human testis in organ culture, *J Endocrinol* 60:179, 1974.
2. Acevedo HF et al: Studies in fetal metabolism, II: metabolism of progesterone-4-(C^{14}) and pregnenolone-7α-(H^3) in human fetal testes, *J Clin Endocrinol Metab* 23:885, 1963.
3. Deleted in proofs.
4. Ahluwalia B, Williams J, Verma P: *In vitro* testosterone biosynthesis in the human fetal testis, II: stimulation by cyclic AMP and human chorionic gonadotropin (hCG), *Endocrinology* 95:1411, 1974.
5. Ahmed MS, Horst MA: Opioid receptors of human placental villi modulate acetylcholine release, *Life Sci* 39:535, 1986.
6. Ahmed MS, et al: Human placental opioid peptides: correlation to the route of delivery, *Am J Obstet Gynecol* 155:703, 1986.
7. Albers N et al: Hormone ontogeny in the ovine fetus, XXIII: pulsatile administration of follicle-stimulating hormone stimulates inhibin production and decreases testosterone synthesis in the ovine fetal gonad, *Endocrinology* 124:3089, 1989.
8. Albers N et al: Hormone ontogeny in the ovine fetus, XXIV: porcine follicular fluid "inhibins" selectively suppress plasma follicle-stimulating hormone in the ovine fetus, *Endocrinology* 125:675, 1989.
9. Allen JM, Bloom SR: Neuropeptide Y: a putative neurotransmitter, *Neurochem Int* 8:1, 1986.
10. Deleted in proofs.
11. Deleted in proofs.
12. Amir SM, Sullivan RC, Ingbar SH: *In vitro* responses to crude and purified hCG in human thyroid membranes, *J Clin Endocrinol Metab* 51:51, 1980.
13. Deleted in proofs.
14. Deleted in proofs.
15. Deleted in proofs.
16. Aschheim S, Zondek B: Anterior pituitary hormone and ovarian hormone in the urine of pregnant women, *Klin Wochenschr* 6:1322, 1927.
17. Deleted in proofs.
18. Deleted in proofs.
19. Deleted in proofs.
20. Bahl OP: Human chorionic gonadotropin, I: purification and physicochemical properties; II: nature of the carbohydrate units, *J Biol Chem* 244:575, 1969.
21. Baker BL, Jaffe RB: The genesis of cell types in the adenohypophysis of the human fetus as observed with immunocytochemistry, *Am J Anat* 143:137, 1975.
22. Baker TG: A quantitative and cytological study of germ cells in human ovaries, *Proc R Soc Lond [Biol]* 158:417, 1963.
23. Baker TG, Franchi LL: The fine structure of oogonia and oocytes in human ovaries, *J Cell Sci* 2:213, 1967.
24. Baker TG, Franchi LL: The fine structure of oogonia and oocytes in the rhesus monkey (Macaca mulatta), *Z Zellforsch Mikrosk Anat* 126:53, 1972.
25. Baker TG, Neal P: Oogenesis in human fetal ovaries maintained in organ culture, *J Anat* 117:591, 1974.
26. Baker TG, Scrimegeour JB: Development of the gonad in normal and anencephalic human fetuses, *J Reprod Fertil* 60:193, 1980.
27. Deleted in proofs.
28. Beck-Peccoz P et al: Maturation of hypothalamic-pituitary-gonadal function in normal human fetuses: circulating levels of gonadotropins, their common α-subunit and free testosterone, and discrepancy between immunological and biological activities of circulating follicle-stimulating hormone, *J Clin Endocrinol Metab* 73:525, 1991.
29. Deleted in proofs.
30. Deleted in proofs.
31. Deleted in proofs.
32. Deleted in proofs.
33. Deleted in proofs.
34. Belisle S et al: Functional opioid receptor sites in human placentas, *J Clin Endocrinol Metab* 66:283, 1988.
35. Benirschke K: Adrenals in anencephaly and hydrocephaly, *Obstet Gynecol* 8:412, 1956.
36. Bewley TA, Li CH: Circular dichroism studies on human pituitary growth hormone and ovine pituitary lactogenic hormone, *Biochemistry* 11:884, 1972.
37. Deleted in proofs.
38. Deleted in proofs.
39. Deleted in proofs.
40. Bloch E: Metabolism of 4-^{14}C-progesterone by human fetal testis and ovaries, *Endocrinology* 74:833, 1964.
41. Blumenfeld Z, Jaffe RB: Hypophysiotropic and neuromodulatory regulation of ACTH in the human fetal pituitary gland, *J Clin Invest* 78:288, 1986.
42. Blumenfeld Z et al: Partial loss of responsiveness of human fetal pituitary cells to GRF after chronic exposure, *Acta Endocrinol* 121:721, 1989.
43. Bojko M: Human meiosis, VIII: chromosome pairing and formation of the synaptonemal complex in oocytes, *Carlsberg Res Commun* 48:457, 1983.
44. Boroditsky RS et al: Serum human chorionic gonadotrophin and progesterone patterns in the last trimester of pregnancy: relationship to fetal sex, *Am J Obstet Gynecol* 121:238, 1975.
45. Deleted in proofs.
46. Deleted in proofs.
47. Deleted in proofs.
48. Deleted in proofs.
49. Brody S, Carlstrom G: Human chorionic gonadotrophin pattern in serum and its relation to the sex of the fetus, *J Clin Endocrinol Metab* 25:792, 1965.
50. Deleted in proofs.
51. Bugnon C, Bloch B, Fellman D: Cytoimmunological study of the ontogenesis of the gonadotropic hypothalamo-pituitary axis in the human fetus, *J Steroid Biochem* 8:565, 1977.
52. Bugnon C et al: Corticoliberin neurons: cytophysiology, phylogeny and ontogeny, *J Steroid Biochem* 20:183, 1984.
53. Byskov AG, Høyer PE: Embryology of mammalian gonads and ducts. In Knobil E, Neill J, editors: *The physiology of reproduction,* New York, 1988, Raven Press.
54. Deleted in proofs.
55. Campbell EA et al: Plasma corticotropin releasing hormone concentrations during pregnancy and parturition, *J Clin Endocrinol Metab* 64:1054, 1987.
56. Canick JA et al: Second-trimester levels of maternal serum unconjugated oestriol and human chorionic gonadotropin in pregnancies affected by fetal anencephaly and open spina bifida, *Prenat Diagn* 10:733, 1990.
57. Carayon P et al: Effect of carboxypeptidase digestion of the human choriogonadotropin molecule on its thyrotropic activity, *Endocrinology* 108:1891, 1981.
58. Carayon P, Lefort G, Nisula B: Interaction of human chorionic gonadotropin and human luteinizing hormone with human thyroid membranes, *Endocrinology* 106:1907, 1980.
59. Carlsen RB, Bahl OP, Swaminathan N: Human chorionic gonadotropin: linear amino acid sequence of the β subunit, *J Biol Chem* 248:6810, 1973.
60. Carr BR, Simpson ER: Lipoprotein utilization and cholesterol synthesis by the human fetal adrenal gland, *Endocr Rev* 2:306, 1981.
61. Carr BR et al: Regulation of human fetal testicular secretion of testosterone: low-density lipoprotein-cholesterol and cholesterol synthesized de novo as steroid precursor, *Am J Obstet Gynecol* 146:241, 1983.
62. Carr DH, Haggar RA, Hart AG: Germ cells in the ovaries of XO female infants, *Am J Clin Pathol* 19:521, 1968.

63. Deleted in proofs.

64. Cate RL et al: Isolation of the bovine and human genes for müllerian inhibiting substance and expression of the human gene in animal cells, *Cell* 45:685, 1986.

65. Catt KJ, Dufau ML, Vaitukaitis JL: Appearance of hCG in pregnancy plasma following the initiation of implantation of the blastocyst, *J Clin Endocrinol Metab* 40:537, 1975.

66. Deleted in proofs.

67. Deleted in proofs.

68. Ch'in KY: The endocrine glands of anencephalic foetuses, *Chin Med J Suppl* 2:63, 1938.

69. Chiquoine HD: The development of the zona pellucida of the mammalian ovum, *Am J Anat* 106:149, 1960.

70. Clark AS, MacLusky NJ, Goldman-Rakic PS: Androgen binding and metabolism in the cerebral cortex of the developing rhesus monkey, *Endocrinology* 123:9320, 1988.

71. Clark JH, Paszko Z, Peck EJ Jr: Nuclear binding and retention of the receptor estrogen complex: relation to the agonistic and antagonistic properties of estriol, *Endocrinology* 100:91, 1977.

72. Deleted in proofs.

73. Clements JA et al: Studies on human sexual development, III: fetal pituitary and serum and amniotic fluid concentrations of LH, CG, and FSH, *J Clin Endocrinol Metab* 42:9, 1976.

74. Codesal J et al: Involution of human fetal Leydig cells: an immunohistochemical, ultrastructural and quantitative study, *J Anat* 172:103, 1990.

75. Colenbrander B et al: Response of luteinizing hormone and follicle-stimulating hormone to luteinizing hormone releasing hormone in the fetal pig, *Biol Reprod* 27:556, 1982.

76. Conklin JL: The development of the human fetal adenohypophysis, *Anat Rec* 160:79, 1968.

77. Courot M: Effect of gonadotrophins on the seminiferous tubules of the immature testis. In Rosenberg E, Paulsen CA, editors: *The human testis,* New York, 1970, Plenum Press.

78. Crickard K, Ill C, Jaffe R: Control of proliferation of human fetal adrenal cells in vitro, *J Clin Endocrinol Metab* 53:790, 1981.

79. Deleted in proofs.

80. Deleted in proofs.

81. Currie AJ, Fraser HM, Sharpe RM: Human placental receptors for luteinizing hormone releasing hormone, *Biochem Biophys Res Commun* 99:332, 1981.

82. Deleted in proofs.

83. Deleted in proofs.

84. Deleted in proofs.

85. Davies JJ et al: A specific, high-affinity, limited-capacity estrogen binding component in the cytosol of human fetal pituitary and brain tissues, *J Clin Endocrinol Metab* 40:909, 1975.

86. Davies JJ et al: Dexamethasone and ACTH effects in the rhesus fetal adrenal, *Gynecol Invest* 8:83, 1977.

87. Davis RM: Localisation of male determining factors in man: a thorough review of structural anomalies of the Y chromosome, *J Med Genet* 18:161, 1981.

88. Dell'Acqua S et al: Adrenal function in the foetus. In James VHT et al, editors: *The endocrine function of the human adrenal cortex,* London, 1978, Academic Press.

89. DiBlasio AM et al: Hormonal regulation of messenger RNAs for P450scc (cholesterol side-chain cleavage enzyme) and P450c17 (17-hydroxylase/17,20-lyase) in cultured human fetal adrenal cells, *J Clin Endocrinol Metab* 65:170, 1987.

90. Diez d'Aux RC, Pearson Murphy BE: Androgens in the human fetus, *J Steroid Biochem* 5:207, 1974.

91. Deleted in proofs.

92. Donahoe PK et al: Müllerian inhibiting substance in human testes after birth, *J Pediatr Surg* 12:323, 1977.

93. Donahoe PK et al: Müllerian inhibiting substance activity in bovine fetal, newborn and prepubertal testes, *Biol Reprod* 16:238, 1977.

94. Doody KM et al: 3 Beta-hydroxysteroid dehydrogenase/isomerase in the fetal zone and neocortex of the human fetal adrenal gland, *Endocrinology* 126:2487, 1990.

95. Ducsay C et al: Endocrine and morphological maturation of the fetal and neonatal adrenal cortex in baboons, *J Clin Endocrinol Metab* 73:385, 1991.

96. Dumesic DA, Castillo RH, Bridson WE: Increase in follicle stimulating hormone content occurs in cultured human fetal pituitary cells exposed to gonadotropin-releasing hormone, *Life Sci* 48:1115, 1991.

97. Dumesic DA, Goldsmith PC, Jaffe RB: Estradiol sensitization of cultured human fetal pituitary cells to gonadotropin-releasing hormone, *J Clin Endocrinol Metab* 65:1147, 1987.

98. Dumesic DA et al: Increase in luteinizing hormone content occurs in cultured human fetal pituitary cells exposed to gonadotropin-releasing hormone, *J Clin Endocrinol Metab* 70:606, 1990.

99. Dym M, Fawcett DW: The blood-testis barrier in the rat and the physiological compartmentation of the seminiferous epithelium, *Biol Reprod* 3:308, 1970.

100. Elias W: Frühentwicklung des Samenkanälchen beim Menschen, *Verh Anat Ges* 68:123, 1974.

101. Ellinwood WE, Baughman WL, Resko JA: Control of pituitary gonadotropin secretion in fetal rhesus macaques. In Novy M, Resko J, editors: *Fetal endocrinology,* New York, 1981, Academic Press.

102. Deleted in proofs.

103. Ellinwood WE et al: Testosterone synthesis in rhesus fetal testes: comparison between middle and late gestation, *Biol Reprod* 22:955, 1980.

104. Deleted in proofs.

105. Deleted in proofs.

106. Falin LI: The development of human hypophysis and differentiation of cells of its anterior lobe during embryonic life, *Acta Anat* 44:188, 1961.

107. Fant M, Munro H, Moses AC: An autocrine/paracrine role for insulin-like growth factors in the regulation of human placental growth, *J Clin Endocrinol Metab* 63:499, 1986.

108. Fisher DA, Lakshmanan J: Metabolism and effects of epidermal growth factor and related growth factors in mammals, *Endocr Rev* 11:418, 1990.

109. Fishman J et al: Catechol estrogen formation by the human fetal brain and pituitary, *J Clin Endocrinol Metab* 42:177, 1976.

110. Deleted in proofs.

111. Forest M: Role of androgens in fetal and pubertal development, *Horm Res* 18:69, 1983.

112. Fraioli F, Genazzani AR: Human placental β-endorphin, *Gynecol Obstet Invest* 11:37, 1980.

113. Franchimont P, Pasteels JL: Secretion independante des hormones gonadotropes et de leurs sous-unites, *C R Acad Sci* [III] 275:1799, 1972.

114. Frandsen VA, Stakemann G: The clinical significance of oestriol determinations in late pregnancy, *Acta Endocrinol* 44:183, 1962.

115. Frim DM et al: Characterization and gestational regulation of corticotropin-releasing hormone messenger RNA in human placenta, *J Clin Invest* 82:287, 1988.

116. Frolik CA et al: Purification and initial characterization of a type β transforming growth factor from human placenta, *Proc Natl Acad Sci U S A* 80:3676, 1983.

117. Deleted in proofs.

118. Fujieda K et al: The control of steroidogenesis by human fetal adrenal cells in tissue culture, I: responses to adrenocorticotropin, *J Clin Endocrinol Metab* 53:34, 1981.

119. Fujimoto T, Miyayama Y, Fuyuta M: The origin of migration and fine morphology of human primordial germ cells, *Anat Rec* 188:315, 1977.

120. Gaillard DA et al: Fetal adrenal development during the second trimester of gestation, *Pediatr Pathol* 10:335, 1990.

121. Deleted in proofs.

122. Deleted in proofs.

123. Genazzani AR et al: Immunoreactive ACTH and cortisol plasma levels during pregnancy: detection and partial purification of corticotrophin-like placental hormone: the human chorionic corticotrophin (hCC), *Clin Endocrinol* 4:1, 1975.

124. George FW, Wilson JD: Conversion of androgen to estrogen by the human fetal ovary, *J Clin Endocrinol Metab* 47:550, 1978.

125. George FW et al: Studies on the regulation of the onset of steroid hormone biosynthesis in fetal rabbit gonads, *Endocrinology* 105:1100, 1979.

126. Gey GO, Jones GES, Hellman LM: The production of a gonadotropic substance (prolan) by placental cells in tissue culture, *Science* 88:306, 1938.

127. Gibbons JM, Mitnick M, Chieffo V: In vitro biosynthesis of TSH- and LH-releasing factors by the human placenta, *Am J Obstet Gynecol* 121:127, 1975.

128. Gibbs DM et al: Effects of synthetic corticotropin-releasing factor and dopamine on the release of immunoreactive β-endorphin/β-lipotropin and α-melanocyte-stimulating hormone from human fetal pituitaries in vitro, *J Clin Endocrinol Metab* 55:1149, 1982.

129. Gibbs DM et al: Synthetic corticotropin-releasing factor stimulates secretion of immunoreactive β-endorphin/β-lipotropin and ACTH by human fetal pituitaries in vitro, *Life Sci* 32:547, 1983.

130. Deleted in proofs.

131. Deleted in proofs.

132. Gillman J: The development of the gonads in man with a consideration of the fetal endocrines and the histogenesis of ovarian tumors, *Contrib Embryol Carnegie Inst* 32:81, 1948.

133. Deleted in proofs.

134. Deleted in proofs.

135. Gluckman PD: Maturation of hypothalamic-pituitary function in the ovine fetus and neonate, *Ciba Found Symp* 86:5, 1981.

136. Gluckman P, Grumbach M, Kaplan S: The human fetal hypothalamus and pituitary gland: the maturation of neuroendocrine mechanisms controlling the secretion of fetal pituitary growth hormone, prolactin, gonadotropin, and adrenocorticotropin-related peptides. In Tulchinsky D, Ryan K, editors: *Maternal-fetal endocrinology*, Philadelphia, 1980, WB Saunders.

137. Deleted in proofs.

138. Deleted in proofs.

139. Goebelsmann U, Jaffe RB: Oestriol metabolism in pregnant women, *Acta Endocrinol* 66:679, 1971.

140. Goebelsmann U et al: Plasma concentration and protein binding of oestriol and its conjugates in pregnancy, *Acta Endocrinol* 74:592, 1973.

141. Goland RS et al: Human plasma β-endorphin during pregnancy, labor, and delivery, *J Clin Endocrinol Metab* 52:74, 1981.

142. Deleted in proofs.

143. Goldman AS: Production of hypospadias in the rat by selective inhibition of fetal testicular 17α-hydroxylase and $C_{17,20}$-lyase, *Endocrinology* 88:527, 1971.

144. Goldsmith PC et al: Identification of cellular sites of chorionic gonadotropin synthesis in human fetal kidney and liver, *J Clin Endocrinol Metab* 57:654, 1983.

145. Gondos B, Bhiraleus P, Hobel CJ: Ultrastructural observations on germ cells in human fetal ovaries, *Am J Obstet Gynecol* 110:644, 1971.

146. Gondos B, Hobel C: Ultrastructure of germ cell development in the human fetal testis, *Z Zellforsch* 119:1, 1971.

147. Gondos B, Hobel CJ: Interstitial cells in the human fetal ovary, *Endocrinology* 93:736, 1973.

148. Gospodarowicz D, Neufeld G, Schweigerer L: Fibroblast growth factor: structural and biological properties, *J Cell Physiol Suppl* 5:15, 1987.

149. Gospodarowicz D et al: Fibroblast growth factor in the human placenta, *Biochem Biophys Res Commun* 128:554, 1985.

150. Gould SF, Bernstein MH: Fine structure of fetal human testis and epididymis, *Arch Androl* 2:939, 1979.

151. Goustin AS et al: Coexpression of the cis and myc proto-oncogenes in developing human placenta suggests autocrine control of trophoblast growth, *Cell* 41:301, 1985.

152. Gray ES, Abramovich DR: Morphologic features of the anencephalic adrenal gland in early pregnancy, *Am J Obstet Gynecol* 137:491, 1980.

153. Deleted in proofs.

154. Gray TS, Morley JE: Neuropeptide Y: anatomical distribution and possible function in mammalian nervous system, *Life Sci* 38:401, 1986.

155. Griffin J, Wilson J: Hereditary male pseudohermaphroditism, *Clin Obstet Gynecol* 5:457, 1978.

156. Groom C, Boyns A: Effect of hypothalamic releasing factors and steroids on release of gonadotropins by organ cultures of human fetal pituitaries, *J Endocrinol* 59:511, 1973.

157. Deleted in proofs.

158. Grumbach MM, Kaplan SL, Vinik AI: Human chorionic somatomammotropin (HCS). In Berson SA, Yalow RS, editors: *Methods in investigative and diagnostic endocrinology,* Amsterdam, 1973, Elsevier/North-Holland.

159. Grumbach MM et al: Plasma free fatty acid response to the administration of chorionic "growth hormone-prolactin," *J Clin Endocrinol Metab* 26:476, 1966.

160. Grumbach MM et al: Chorionic growth-hormone prolactin (CGP): secretion, disposition, biologic activity in man, and postulated function as the "growth hormone" of the second half of pregnancy, *Ann N Y Acad Sci* 148:501, 1968.

161. Deleted in proofs.

162. Gulyas BJ, Tullner WW, Hodgen GD: Fetal or maternal hypophysectomy in rhesus monkeys (Macaca mulatta): effects on the development of testes and other endocrine organs, *Biol Reprod* 17:650, 1977.

163. Gulyas B et al: Effects of fetal and maternal hypophysectomy on endocrine organs and body weight in infant rhesus monkeys (Macaca mulatta) with particular reference to oogenesis, *Biol Reprod* 16:216, 1977.

164. Guraya SS: Recent advances in the morphology, histochemistry, and biochemistry of the developing mammalian ovary, *Int Rev Cytol* 51:49, 1977.

165. Hasegawa Y et al: Induction of follicle stimulating hormone receptor by erythroid differentiation factor on rat granulosa cell, *Biochem Biophys Res Commun* 156:668, 1988.

166. Deleted in proofs.

167. Hellig HD et al: Steroid production from plasma cholesterol, I: conversion of plasma cholesterol to placental progesterone in humans, *J Clin Endocrinol Metab* 30:624, 1970.

168. Deleted in proofs.

169. Deleted in proofs.

170. Herrera J et al: Subcellular metabolic pools in the rat adrenal gland: in vivo effect of acute stimulation with ACTH on steroid biosynthesis, *J Steroid Biochem* 13:153, 1980.

171. Hertig AT et al: A description of 34 human ova within the first 17 days of development, *Am J Anat* 98:435, 1956.

172. Holstein AF, Wartenberg H, Vossmeyer J: Zur Cytologie der pränatalen Gonadenentwicklung beim Menschen, III: die Entwicklung der Leydigzellen im Hoden von Embryonen und Feten, *Z Anat Entwicklungsgesch* 135:43, 1971.

173. Deleted in proofs.

174. Huhtaniemi I: Studies on steroidogenesis and its regulation in human fetal adrenal and testis, *J Steroid Biochem* 8:491, 1977.

175. Huhtaniemi IT, Korenbrot CC, Jaffe RB: HCG binding and stimulation of testosterone biosynthesis in the human fetal testis, *J Clin Endocrinol Metab* 44:963, 1977.

176. Huhtaniemi IT, Korenbrot CC, Jaffe RB: Content of chorionic gonadotropin in human fetal tissues, *J Clin Endocrinol Metab*

46:994, 1978.

177. Huhtaniemi I, Lautala P: Stimulation of steroidogenesis in human fetal testes by the placenta during perifusion, *J Steroid Biochem* 10:109, 1979.

178. Huhtaniemi IT et al: Stimulation of pituitary-testicular function with gonadotropin-releasing hormone in fetal and infant monkeys, *Endocrinology* 105:109, 1979.

179. Huhtaniemi IT et al: Follicle-stimulating hormone receptors appear earlier in the primate fetal testis than in the ovary, *J Clin Endocrinol Metab* 65:1210, 1987.

180. Hutson JM, Donahoe PK: The control of testicular descent, *Endocr Rev* 7:270, 1986.

181. Hyppa M: Hypothalamic monoamines in human fetuses, *Neuroendocrinology* 9:257, 1972.

182. Ikonen M, Niemi J: Metabolism of progesterone and 17α-hydroxypregnenolone by the human testis *in vitro*, *Nature* 212:716, 1966.

183. Jaatela M et al: Regulation of ACTH-induced steroidogenesis in human fetal adrenals by rTNF-alpha, *Mol Cell Endocrinol* 68:R31, 1990.

184. Jaffe RB: Endocrine physiology of the fetus and fetoplacental unit. In Yen SSC, Jaffe RB, editors: *Reproductive endocrinology,* ed 2, Philadelphia, 1986, WB Saunders.

185. Jaffe RB, Lee PA, Midgley AR Jr: Serum gonadotropin before, at the inception of, and following human pregnancy, *J Clin Endocrinol Metab* 29:1281, 1969.

186. Jaffe RB, Payne AA: Gonadal steroid sulfates and sulfatase, IV: comparative studies on steroid sulfokinase in the human fetal testis and adrenals, *J Clin Endocrinol Metab* 33:592, 1971.

187. Jaffe RB et al: Regulation of the primate fetal adrenal gland and testes *in vitro* and *in vivo*, *J Steroid Biochem* 8:479, 1977.

188. Jaffe RB et al: Peptide regulation of pituitary and target tissue function and growth in the primate fetus, *Recent Prog Horm Res* 44:431, 1981.

189. Deleted in proofs.

190. Jenkins J, Hall C: Metabolism of [^{14}C] testosterone by human foetal and adult brain tissue, *J Endocrinol* 74:425, 1977.

191. Jirasek JE: Development of the genital system in human embryos and fetuses. In Cohen MM Jr, editor: *Development of the genital system and male pseudohermaphroditism,* Baltimore, 1971, John Hopkins University Press.

192. Jirasek JE: *Human fetal endocrines,* The Hague, 1980, Martinus Nijhof.

193. Johansson ENB: Plasma levels of progesterone in pregnancy measured by a rapid competitive protein binding technique, *Acta Endocrinol* 61:607, 1979.

194. Josimovich JB: Placental protein hormones in pregnancy, *Clin Obstet Gynecol* 16:46, 1973.

195. Josimovich JB, MacLaren JA: Presence in human placenta and term serum of highly lactogenic substance immunologically related to pituitary growth hormone, *Endocrinology* 71:209, 1962.

196. Josso N et al: Physiology of anti-müllerian hormone: in search of a new role for an old hormone. In Tsafriri A, Eshkol A, editors: *Development and function of reproductive organs,* New York, 1986, Raven Press.

197. Josso N et al: An enzyme linked immunoassay for anti-müllerian hormone: a new tool for the evaluation of testicular function in infants and children, *J Clin Endocrinol Metab* 70:23, 1990.

198. Jost A: Problems in fetal endocrinology: the gonadal and hypophyseal hormones, *Recent Prog Horm Res* 8:379, 1953.

199. Jost A: A new look at the mechanisms controlling sexual differentiation in mammals, *Johns Hopkins Med J* 130:38, 1972.

200. Jost A: Initial stages of gonadal development: theories and methods, *Arch Anat Microscop Morpholog Experiment* 74:39, 1985.

201. Jost A: Organogenesis and endocrine cytodifferentiation of the testis, *Arch Anat Microsc Morphol Exp* 74:101, 1985.

202. Jost A, Magre S, Agelopoulo R: Early stage of testicular differentiation in the rat, *Hum Genet* 58:59, 1981.

203. Deleted in proofs.

204. Kaplan S: Human chorionic somatomammotropin: secretion, biologic effects, and physiologic significance. In Jaffe RB, editor: *The endocrine milieu of pregnancy, puerperium and childhood,* Report of the Third Ross Conference on Obstetric Research, Columbus, Ohio, 1974, Ross Laboratories.

205. Deleted in proofs.

206. Deleted in proofs.

207. Kaplan SL, Grumbach MM: The ontogenesis of human foetal hormones, II: luteinizing hormone (LH) and follicle stimulating hormone (FSH), *Acta Endocrinol* 81:808, 1976.

208. Kaplan SL, Grumbach MM: Pituitary and placental gonadotrophins and sex steroids in the human and sub-human primate fetus, *J Clin Endocrinol Metab* 7:487, 1978.

209. Kaplan SL, Grumbach MM, Aubert ML: The ontogenesis of pituitary hormones and hypothalamic factors in the human fetus: maturation of central nervous system regulation of anterior pituitary function, *Recent Prog Horm Res* 32:161, 1976.

210. Deleted in proofs.

211. Kaplan SL et al: Metabolic clearance rate and production rate of chorionic growth hormone-prolactin in late pregnancy, *J Clin Endocrinol Metab* 28:1450, 1968.

212. Deleted in proofs.

213. Deleted in proofs.

214. Deleted in proofs.

215. Kenimer JG, Hershman JM, Higgins HP: The thyrotropin in hydatidiform moles is human chorionic gonadotropin, *J Clin Endocrinol Metab* 40:482, 1975.

216. Khodr GS, Siler-Khodr TM: The effect of luteinizing hormone releasing factor on human chorionic gonadotropin secretion, *Fertil Steril* 30:301, 1978.

217. Khodr GS, Siler-Khodr TM: Localization of luteinizing hormone-releasing factor in the human placenta, *Fertil Steril* 29:523, 1978.

218. Khodr GS, Siler-Khodr TM: Placental luteinizing hormone-releasing factor and its synthesis, *Science* 207:315, 1980.

219. Kim YJ, Felig P: Plasma chorionic somatomammotropin levels during starvation in midpregnancy, *J Clin Endocrinol Metab* 32:864, 1971.

220. Deleted in proofs.

221. Kindred JF: The chromosomes of the ovary of the human fetus, *Anat Res* 147:295, 1963.

222. Klopper AI, MacNaughton M: Hormones in recurrent abortion, *J Obstet Gynaecol Br Commonw* 72:1022, 1965.

223. Konishi I et al: Development of interstitial cells and ovigerous cords in the human fetal ovary: an ultrastructural study, *J Anat* 148:121, 1986.

224. Koopman P et al: Zfy gene expression patterns are not compatible with a primary role in mouse sex determination, *Nature* 342:940, 1989.

225. Kosasa TSA et al: Measurement of early chorionic activity with a radioimmunoassay specific for human chorionic gonadotropin following spontaneous and induced ovulation, *Fertil Steril* 25:211, 1974.

226. Deleted in proofs.

227. Kumasaka T et al: Demonstration of immunoreactive somatostatin-like substance in villi and decidua in early pregnancy, *Am J Obstet Gynecol* 134:39, 1979.

228. Kurilo LF: Oogenesis in antenatal development in man, *Hum Genet* 57:86, 1991.

229. Lai W, Guyda HJ: Characterization and regulation of epidermal growth factor receptors in human placental cell cultures, *J Clin Endocrinol Metab* 58:344, 1984.

230. Landesman R, Saxena BB: Radioreceptor assay of human chorionic gonadotropin as an aid in miniabortion, *Fertil Steril* 25:1022, 1974.

231. Langman J: *Medical embryology,* Baltimore, 1981, Williams & Wilkins.

232. Lanman JT: An interpretation of human foetal adrenal structure and function. In Currie AR, Symington J, Grant JK, editors: *The human adrenal cortex,* Edinburgh, 1962, E & S Livingstone.

233. Deleted in proofs.

234. Lee J-N, Seppala M, Chard T: Characterization of placental luteinizing hormone-releasing factor-like material, *Acta Endocrinol* 96:394, 1981.

234a. Lee MM, Donahoe PK: Müllerian inhibiting substance: a gonadal hormone with multiple functions, *Endocr Rev* 14:152, 1993.

235. Deleted in proofs.

236. Lemaire S et al: Purification and identification of multiple forms of dynorphin in human placenta, *Neuropeptides* 3:181, 1983.

237. Deleted in proofs.

238. Deleted in proofs.

239. Li CH, Dixon JS, Chung D: Primary structure of the human chorionic somatomammotropin (HCS) molecule, *Science* 173:56, 1971.

240. Deleted in proofs.

241. Liang LF, Chamow SM, Dean J: Oocyte-specific expression of mouse Zp-2: developmental regulation of the zona pellucida genes, *Mol Cell Biol* 10:1507, 1990.

242. Liggins GC, Kennedy PC, Holm L: Failure of initiation of parturition after electrocoagulation of the pituitary of the fetal lamb, *Am J Obstet Gynecol* 98:1080, 1967.

243. Ling N et al: A homodimer of the beta-subunits of inhibin A stimulates the secretion of pituitary follicle stimulating hormone, *Biochem Biophys Res Commun* 138:1129, 1986.

244. Liotta AS, Houghten R, Krieger DT: Identification of a β-endorphin-like peptide in cultured human placental cells, *Nature* 295:593, 1982.

245. Liotta AS, Krieger DT: In vitro biosynthesis and comparative post-translational processing of immunoreactive precursor corticotropin/β-endorphin by human placental and pituitary cells, *Endocrinology* 106:1504, 1980.

246. Liotta A et al: Presence of corticotropin in human placenta: demonstration of *in vitro* synthesis, *Endocrinology* 101:1551, 1977.

247. Mains RE, Eipper BA, Ling N: Common precursor to corticotropins and endorphins, *Proc Natl Acad Sci U S A* 74:3014, 1977.

248. Manotaya T, Potter EL: Oocytes in prophase of meiosis from squash preparations of human fetal ovaries, *Fertil Steril* 14:378, 1963.

249. Margioris AN et al: Corticotropin-releasing hormone and oxytocin stimulate the release of placental proopiomelanocortin peptides, *J Clin Endocrinol Metab* 66:922, 1988.

250. Marshall JR et al: Plasma and urinary chorionic gonadotropin during early human pregnancy, *Obstet Gynecol* 32:760, 1968.

251. Deleted in proofs.

252. Martin MC, Monroe SE, Jaffe RB: Pulsatile gonadotropin-releasing hormone secretion by the primate fetus *in utero.* Presented at the 34th annual meeting of the Society for Gynecologic Investigation, 1987 (abstract No 174).

253. Deleted in proofs.

254. Martin MC et al: Pulsatile luteinizing hormone secretion by the primate fetus in utero. Presented at the 37th annual meeting of the Society for Gynecologic Investigation, St. Louis, March 21–24, 1990 (abstract No 228).

255. Martucci C, Fishman J: Direction of estradiol metabolism as a control of its hormonal action—uterotrophic activity of estradiol metabolites, *Endocrinology* 101:1709, 1977.

256. Maruo T et al: Induction of differentiated trophoblast function by epidermal growth factor: relation of immunohistochemically detected cellular epidermal growth factor levels, *J Clin Endocrinol Metab* 64:744, 1987.

257. Mason JI, Hemsell PG, Korte K: Steroidogenesis in dispersed cells of the human fetal adrenal, *J Clin Endocrinol Metab* 56:1057, 1983.

258. Mathur RS, Wigvist N, Diczfalusy E: De novo synthesis of steroids and steroid sulphates by the testicles of the human foetus at midgestation, *Acta Endocrinol* 71:792, 1972.

259. Deleted in proofs.

260. McCarrey JR, Abbott UK: Chick gonadal differentiation following excision of primordial germ cells, *Dev Biol* 66:256, 1978.

261. Deleted in proofs.

262. McGregor WG, Kuhn RW, Jaffe RB: Biologically active chorionic gonadotropin: synthesis by the human fetus, *Science* 220:306, 1983.

263. McGregor WG et al: Fetal tissues can synthesize a placental hormone: evidence for chorionic gonadotropin beta-subunit synthesis by human fetal kidney, *J Clin Invest* 68:306, 1981.

264. McLachlan RI et al: The human placenta: a novel source of inhibin, *Biochem Biophys Res Commun* 140:485, 1986.

265. McLachlan RI et al: The maternal ovary is not the source of circulating inhibin levels during human pregnancy, *Clin Endocrinol* 27:663, 1987.

266. McLaren A: Sex determination in mammals, *Trends Genet* 4:153, 1988.

267. Deleted in proofs.

268. McNulty WP, Novy MJ, Walsh SW: Fetal and postnatal development of the adrenal glands in Macaca mulatta, *Biol Reprod* 25:1079, 1981.

269. Deleted in proofs.

270. Meijer JC et al: Development of pituitary gonadotropic cells in the pig fetus and the effect of luteinizing hormone-releasing hormone administration, *Biol Reprod* 32:137, 1985.

271. Menon KMJ, Jaffe RB: Chorionic gonadotropin-sensitive adenyl cyclase in human term placenta, *J Clin Endocrinol Metab* 36:1104, 1973.

272. Merchant H: Rat gonadal and ovarian organogenesis with and without germ cells: an ultrastructural study, *Dev Biol* 44:1, 1975.

273. Mesiano S, Jaffe RB: In the human fetal adrenal, interaction of estradiol (E_2) and insulin-like growth factor-II (IGF-II) directs fetal zone steroidogenesis toward dehydroepiandrosterone sulfate (DHAS). Presented at the 39th annual meeting of the Society for Gynecologic Investigation, San Antonio, March 18–21, 1992 (abstract No 259).

274. Mesiano S, Jaffe RB: The definitive zone of the human fetal adrenal does not express mRNAs for enzymes necessary for steroidogenesis. Presented at the 74th annual meeting of the Endocrine Society, San Antonio, June 24–26, 1992 (abstract No 1442).

275. Mesiano S, Mellon SH, Jaffe RB: Mitogenic action, regulation and localization of insulin-like growth factors in the human fetal adrenal gland, *J Clin Endocrinol Metab* 76:968, 1993.

276. Mesiano S et al: Both FGF and IGF-II expression are regulated by ACTH in the human fetal adrenal: a model for adrenal gland growth. Presented at the 72nd annual meeting of the Endocrine Society, Atlanta, June 20–23, 1990 (abstract No 21).

277. Mesiano S et al: Basic fibroblast growth factor expression is regulated by corticotropin in the human fetal adrenal: a model for adrenal growth regulation, *Proc Natl Acad Sci U S A* 88:5428, 1991.

278. Meunier H et al: Gonadal and extragonadal expression of inhibin alpha, beta A and beta B subunits in various tissues predicts diverse function, *Proc Natl Acad Sci U S A* 85:247, 1988.

279. Meunier H et al: Rapid changes in the expression of inhibin alpha-, beta A-, and beta B-subunits in ovarian cell types during the rat estrous cycle, *Mol Endocrinol* 2:1352, 1988.

280. Michael RP, Bonsall RW, Rees HD. Sites at which testosterone may act as an estrogen in the brain of the male primate, *Neuroendocrinology* 46:511, 1987.

281. Midgley AR Jr, Jaffe RB: Regulation of human gonadotropins, II: disappearance of human chorionic gonadotropin following delivery, *J Clin Endocrinol Metab* 28:1712, 1968.

282. Midgley AR Jr, Pierce GB Jr: Immunohistochemical localization of human chorionic gonadotropin, *J Exp Med* 115:289, 1962.

283. Miller WL: Immunoassays for human müllerian inhibitory factor (MIF): new insight into the physiology of MIF, *J Clin Endocrinol Metab* 70:8, 1990 (editorial).

284. Mills NC et al: Expression of insulin-like growth factors (somatomedins) in the human placenta. Presented at the 67th annual meeting of the Endocrine Society, 1985 (abstract No 1072).

285. Mittwoch U: Sex differentiation in mammals and tempo of growth: probabilities, *J Theor Biol* 137:445, 1989.

286. Miyakawa I, Ikeda I, Maeyama M: Transport of ACTH across human placenta, *J Clin Endocrinol Metab* 39:440, 1974.

287. Molenaar WM, Lee VM-Y, Trojanowski JQ: Early fetal acquisition of the chromaffin and neuronal immunophenotype by human adrenal medullary cells: an immunohistological study using monoclonal antibodies to chromagranin A, synaptophysin, tyrosine hydroxylase, and neuronal cytoskeletal proteins, *Exp Neurol* 108:1, 1990.

288. Molsberry RL et al: Human chorionic gonadotropin binding to human fetal testes as a function of gestational age, *J Clin Endocrinol Metab* 55:791, 1982.

289. Moriyama I, Sugawa T: Progesterone facilitates implantation of xenogeneic cultured cells in hamster uterus, *Nature New Biol* 236:150, 1972.

290. Motta PM, Makabe S: Germ cells in the ovarian surface during fetal development in humans: a three-dimensional microanatomical study by scanning and transmission electron microscopy, *J Submicrosc Cytol* 18:271, 1986.

291. Deleted in proofs.

292. Deleted in proofs.

293. Mulchahey JJ et al: Hormone production and peptide regulation of the human fetal pituitary gland, *Endocr Rev* 8:406, 1987.

294. Deleted in proofs.

295. Nakai Y et al: Presence of immunoreactive β-lipotropin and β-endorphin in human placenta, *Life Sci* 23:2013, 1978.

296. Nakajin S et al: Microsomal cytochrome P-450 activities (17α-hydroxylase and $c_{17,20}$-lyase) associated with one protein, *Biochemistry* 20:4037, 1981.

297. Deleted in proofs.

298. Deleted in proofs.

299. Nelson HP et al: Human fetal adrenal definitive and fetal zone metabolism of pregnenolone and corticosterone: alternate biosynthetic pathways and absence of detectable aldosterone synthesis, *J Clin Endocrinol Metab* 70:693, 1990.

300. Neumann F et al: Aspects of androgen-dependent events as studied by antiandrogens, *Recent Prog Horm Res* 26:337, 1970.

301. Deleted in proofs.

302. Deleted in proofs.

303. Niemi M, Ikonen M, Hervonen A: Histochemistry and fine structure of the interstitial tissue in the human foetal testis. In Wolstenholme G, O'Connor M, editors: *Endocrinology of the testis, Ciba Found Colloq Endocrinol* 1967.

304. Nisula BC, Ketlslegers JM: Thyroid-stimulating activity and chorionic gonadotropin, *J Clin Invest* 54:494, 1974.

305. Nobin A, Bjorkland A: Topography of the monoamine neuron systems in the human brain as revealed in fetuses, *Acta Physiol Scand Suppl* 388:1, 1973.

306. Obiekwe BC, Chard T: Human chorionic gonadotrophin levels in maternal blood in late pregnancy: relation to birthweight, sex and condition of the infant at birth, *Br J Obstet Gynaecol* 89:543, 1982.

307. Odagiri ED et al: Human placental immunoreactive corticotropin, lipotropin, and β-endorphin: evidence for a common precursor, *Proc Natl Acad Sci U S A* 76:2027, 1971.

308. Deleted in proofs.

309. Ohno S, Klinger HP, Atkin NB: Human oogenesis, *Cytogenetics* 1:42, 1962.

310. Ohno S, Smith JB: Role of fetal follicular cells in meiosis of mammalian oocytes, *Cytogenetics* 3:324, 1964.

311. Ohno S et al: Female germ cells of man, *Exp Cell Res* 24:106, 1961.

312. Padmanebhen V et al: Serum bioactive follicle-stimulating hormone-like activity increases during pregnancy, *J Clin Endocrinol Metab* 69:986, 1989.

313. Page DC et al: The sex-determining region of the human Y chromosome encodes a finger protein, *Cell* 51:1091, 1987.

314. Palmer MS et al: Genetic evidence that ZFY is not the testis-determining factor, *Nature* 342:937, 1989.

315. Pasteels JL, Brauman H, Brauman J: Etude comparee de la secretion d'hormone somatotrope par l'hypophyse humaine in vitro, et de son activite lactogenique, *C R Acad Sci Paris* 256:2031, 1963.

316. Payne AH, Jaffe RB: Androgen formation from pregnenolone sulfate by the human fetal ovary, *J Clin Endocrinol Metab* 39:300, 1974.

317. Peaker M, Philips JG, Wright A: The effect of prolactin on the secretory activity of the nasal salt gland of the domestic duck (Anas platyrhynchos), *J Endocrinol* 47:123, 1970.

318. Pearse AGE, Takor Takor T: Neuroendocrine embryology and the APUD concept, *Clin Endocrinol Suppl* 5:229, 1976.

319. Pederson RC, Brownie AC: Adrenocortical response to corticotropin is potentiated by part of the amino-terminal region of pro-corticotropin/endorphin, *Proc Natl Acad Sci U S A* 77:2239, 1980.

320. Pekonen F, Weintraub BD: Interaction of crude and pure chorionic gonadotropin with the thyrotropin receptor, *J Clin Endocrinol Metab* 50:280, 1980.

321. Pelliniemi LJ: Fine structure of germ cords in human fetal testis. In Horstmann E, Holstein A, editors: *Morphological aspects of andrology,* Berlin, 1970, Grosse Verlag.

322. Pelliniemi LJ: Development of sexual dimorphism of the embryonic gonad, *Hum Genet* 58:64, 1981.

323. Pelliniemi LJ, Dym M: The fetal gonad and sexual differentiation. In Tulchinsky D, Ryan K, editors: *Maternal-fetal endocrinology,* Philadelphia, 1980, WB Saunders.

324. Pelliniemi LJ, Niei M: Fine structure of the human foetal testis, I: the interstitial tissue, *Z Zellforsch Mikrosk Anat* 99:507, 1969.

325. Perez-Palacios G, Perez AE, Jaffe RB: Conversion of pregnenolone 7_α-^{3}H-sulfate to other Δ^5-3β-hydroxysteroid sulfates by the human fetal adrenal *in vitro*, *J Clin Endocrinol Metab* 28:19, 1968.

326. Peters H, Byskov AG, Grinsted J: Follicular growth in fetal and prepubertal ovaries of humans and other primates, *J Clin Endocrinol Metab* 7:469, 1978.

327. Peterson RE et al: Male pseudohermaphroditism due to steroid 5α-reductase deficiency, *Am J Med* 62:170, 1977.

328. Petraglia F, Lim ATW, Vale W: Adenosine 3',5'-monophosphate, prostaglandins, and epinephrine stimulate the secretion of immunoreactive gonadotropin-releasing hormone from cultured human placental cells, *J Clin Endocrinol Metab* 65:1020, 1987.

329. Petraglia F, Sutton S, Vale W: Neurotransmitters and peptides modulate the release of immunoreactive corticotropin-releasing factor from human cultured placental cells, *Am J Obstet Gynecol* 160:247, 1989.

330. Petraglia F, Vaughan J, Vale W: Inhibin and activin modulate the release of GnRH, hCG and progesterone from cultured human placental cells, *Proc Natl Acad Sci U S A* 86:5714, 1989.

331. Petraglia F et al: Evidence for local stimulation of ACTH secretion by corticotropin-releasing factor in human placenta, *Nature* 328:717, 1987.

332. Petraglia F et al: Localization, secretion, and action of inhibin in human placenta, *Science* 237:187, 1987.

333. Petraglia F et al: Identification of immunoreactive neuropeptide-Y in human placenta: localization, secretion, and binding sites, *Endocrinology* 124:2016, 1989.

334. Petraglia F et al: Plasma and amniotic fluid immunoreactive neuropeptide-Y levels changes during pregnancy, labor and at parturition, *J Clin Endocrinol Metab* 69:324, 1989.

335. Petraglia F et al: Neuroendocrinology of the human placental, *Front Neuroendocrinol* 11:6, 1990.

336. Picard JY et al: Cloning and expression of cDNA for anti-Müllerian hormone, *Proc Natl Acad Sci U S A* 83:5464, 1986.

337. Pinkerton JHM et al: Development of the human ovary—a study using histochemical technics, *Obstet Gynecol* 18:152, 1961.

338. Pion R et al: Studies on the metabolism of C-21 steroids in the human foeto-placental unit, I: formation of α,β-unsaturated 3-ketones in mid-term placentas perfused *in situ* with pregnenolone and 17α-hydroxypregnenolone, *Acta Endocrinol* 48:234, 1965.

339. Plant TM: A striking sex difference in the gonadotropin response to gonadectomy during infantile development in the rhesus monkey (Macaca mulatta), *Endocrinology* 119:539, 1986.

340. Plotsky PM: Hypophysiotropic regulation of adenohypophyseal adrenocorticotropic secretion, *Fed Proc* 44:207, 1985.

341. Polk D et al: Epidermal growth factor acts as a corticotropin releasing factor in chronically catheterized fetal lambs, *J Clin Invest* 79:984, 1987.

342. Pomerantz SM et al: Androgen and estrogen receptors in fetal rhesus monkey brain and anterior pituitary, *Endocrinology* 116:83, 1985.

343. Potter G: The ovary in infancy and childhood. In Grady H, Smith D, editors: *The ovary,* Baltimore, 1963, Williams & Wilkins.

344. Rabinovici J, Spencer SJ, Jaffe RB: Recombinant human activin-A promotes proliferation of human luteinized preovulatory granulosa cells *in vitro, J Clin Endocrinol Metab* 71:1396, 1990.

345. Rabinovici J et al: Localization and secretion of inhibin/activin subunits in the human and subhuman primate fetal gonads, *J Clin Endocrinol Metab* 73:1141, 1991.

346. Rabinovici J et al: Localization and regulation of the activin-A dimer in human placental cells, *J Clin Endocrinol Metab* 75:571, 1992.

347. Deleted in proofs.

348. Rabinovici J et al: Activin-A as an intraovarian modulator: actions, localization, and regulation of the intact dimer in human ovarian cells, *J Clin Invest* 89:1528, 1992.

349. Raiha N, Hjelt L: The correlation between the development of the hypophysial portal system and the onset of neurosecretory activity in the human fetus and infant, *Acta Paediatr Scand* 46:610, 1957.

350. Rama Sastry BV et al: Occurrence of methionine enkephalin in human placental villus, *Biochem Pharmacol* 29:475, 1980.

351. Rasmussen DD et al: Endogenous opioid regulation of gonadotropin-releasing hormone release from the human fetal hypothalamus *in vitro, J Clin Endocrinol Metab* 57:881, 1983.

352. Rasmussen DD et al: Pulsatile gonadotropin-releasing hormone release from the human mediobasal hypothalamus in vitro: opiate receptor-mediated suppression, *Neuroendocrinology* 49:150, 1989.

353. Rees HD, Bonsall RW, Michael RP: Estrogen binding and the actions of testosterone in the brain of the male rhesus monkey, *Brain Res* 14:28, 1988.

354. Rees LH et al: Possible placental origin of ACTH in normal human pregnancy, *Nature* 154:620, 1975.

355. Resko JA: Fetal hormones and development of the central nervous system in primates, *Adv Sex Horm Res* 3:139, 1977.

356. Resko JA, Connolly PB: C.E.R. Testosterone 5 alpha-reductase activity in neural tissue of fetal rhesus macaques, *J Steroid Biochem* 29:429, 1988.

357. Resko JA, Ellinwood WE: Negative feedback regulation of gonadotropin secretion by androgens in fetal rhesus macaques, *Biol Reprod* 33:346, 1985.

358. Resnik R, Brink GW: Modulating effects of prostaglandins on the uterine vascular bed, *Gynecol Invest* 8:10, 1977.

359. Resnik R et al: The stimulation of uterine blood flow by various estrogens, *Endocrinology* 94:1192, 1974.

360. Reyes, FI, Faiman C, Winter JSD: Development of the regulatory mechanisms of the hypothalamic-pituitary-gonadal system in the human fetus: the chorionic-hypothalamic-pituitary-gonadal axis. In Novy M, Resko J, editors: *Fetal endocrinology,* ORPRC Symposia on Primate Reproductive Biology, New York, 1981, Academic Press.

361. Reyes FI, Winter JS, Faiman C: Studies on human sexual development, I: fetal gonadal and adrenal sex steroids, *J Clin Endocrinol Metab* 37:74, 1973.

362. Reyes FI, Winter JSD, Faiman C: Pituitary gonadotropin function during human pregnancy: serum FSH and LH levels before and after LHRH administration, *J Clin Endocrinol Metab* 42:590, 1976.

363. Reyes FI et al: Studies on human sexual development, II: fetal and maternal serum gonadotropin and sex steroid concentration, *J Clin Endocrinol Metab* 38:612, 1974.

364. Rice BF, Johanson CA, Sternberg WH: Formation of steroid hormones from acetate-1-^{14}C by a human fetal testis preparation grown in organ culture, *Steroids* 7:79, 1966.

365. Riddick DH, Kusnik WF: Decidua: a possible source of amniotic fluid PRL, *Am J Obstet Gynecol* 127:187, 1977.

366. Riddick DH et al: De novo synthesis of prolactin by human decidua, *Life Sci* 23:1913, 1978.

367. Riddle O, Lahr EL, Bates RW: The role of hormones in the inhibition of maternal behavior in rats, *Am J Physiol* 137:299, 1942.

368. Riley S et al: The localization and distribution of corticotropin-releasing hormone in the human placenta and fetal membranes throughout gestation, *J Clin Endocrinol Metab* 72:1001, 1991.

369. Riopel L et al: Growth-inhibitory effect of TGF-β on human fetal adrenal cells in primary monolayer culture, *J Cell Physiol* 140:233, 1989.

370. Rivelis CF, Coco R, Bergada C: Ovarian differentiation in Turner's syndrome, *J Genet Hum* 26:69, 1978.

371. Robertson DM et al: Inhibin and inhibin-related proteins in the male. In Burger H, de Kretzer DM, editors: *The testis,* New York, 1989, Raven Press.

372. Robinson BG et al: Glucocorticoid stimulates expression of corticotropin-releasing hormone gene in human placenta, *Proc Natl Acad Sci U S A* 85:5244, 1988.

373. Saijonmaa O, Laatikainen T, Wahlstrom T: Corticotrophin-releasing factor in human placenta: localization, concentration and release in vitro, *Placenta* 9:373, 1988.

374. Saksela E, Jaatela M: Tumor necrosis factor in the human fetoplacentary unit, *Int J Dev Biol* 33:173, 1989.

375. Sasaki A et al: Isolation and characterization of a corticotropin-releasing hormone-like peptide from human placenta, *J Clin Endocrinol Metab* 67:768, 1988.

376. Sayers G, Portanova R: Secretion of ACTH by isolated pituitary cells: kinetics of stimulation by CRF and inhibition by corticosterone, *Endocrinology* 94:1723, 1974.

377. Schechter J: The cytodifferentiation of the rabbit pars distalis: an electron microscopic study, *Gen Comp Endocrinol* 16:1, 1974.

378. Schindler AE: Steroid metabolism in foetal tissue, IV: conversion of testosterone to 5α-dihydrotestosterone in human foetal brain, *J Steroid Biochem* 7:97, 1976.

379. Schindler AE, Siiteri PK: Isolation and quantitation of steroids from normal human amniotic fluid, *J Clin Endocrinol Metab* 28:1189, 1968.

380. Schultz FM, Wilson JD: Virilization of the wolffian duct in the rat fetus by various androgens, *Endocrinology* 94:979, 1974.

381. Schwall R et al: Multiple actions of recombinant activin-A in vivo, *Endocrinology* 125:1420, 1989.

382. Schwall R et al: Localization of inhibin/activin subunit mRNAs within the primate ovary, *Mol Endocrinol* 4:75, 1990.

383. Seeburg PH, Adelman JP: Characterization of cDNA for precursor of human luteinizing hormone releasing hormone, *Nature* 311:666, 1984.

384. Seeburg PH et al: Nucleotide sequence of part of the gene for human chorionic somatomammotropin: purification of DNA complementary to predominant mRNA species, *Cell* 12:157, 1977.

385. Serón-Ferré M, Jaffe RB: The fetal adrenal gland, *Annu Rev Physiol* 43:141, 1981.

386. Serón-Ferré M, Lawrence CC, Jaffe RB: Role of hCG in the regulation of the fetal zone of the human fetal adrenal gland, *J Clin Endocrinol Metab* 46:834, 1978.

387. Serón-Ferré M et al: Steroid production by the definitive and fetal zones of the human fetal adrenal gland, *J Clin Endocrinol Metab* 47:603, 1978.

388. Serra GB, Perez PG, Jaffe RB: De novo testosterone biosynthesis in the human fetal testis, *J Clin Endocrinol Metab* 30:141, 1970.

389. Shaaban MM et al: β-Endorphin and β-lipotropin concentrations in umbilical cord blood, *Am J Obstet Gynecol* 144:560, 1982.

390. Shambaugh G, Kubek M, Wilson JF: Thyrotropin-releasing hormone activity in the human placenta, *J Clin Endocrinol Metab* 48:483, 1979.

391. Sheth JJ, Sheth AR, Vin FK: Bioimmunoreactive inhibin-like substance in human fetal gonads, *Biol Res Pregnancy Perinatol* 4:110, 1983.

392. Shibaski T et al: Corticotropin-releasing factor-like activity in human placental extract, *J Clin Endocrinol Metab* 55:384, 1982.

393. Shiino M, Ishikawa H, Rennels EG: Specific subclones derived from a multipotential clone of rat anterior pituitary cells, *Am J Anat* 153:81, 1978.

394. Siiteri PK, MacDonald PC: The utilization of circulating dehydroisoandrosterone sulfate for estrogen synthesis during human pregnancy, *Steroids* 2:713, 1963.

395. Siiteri PK, Wilson JD: Testosterone formation and metabolism during male sexual differentiation in the human embryo, *J Clin Endocrinol Metab* 38:113, 1974.

396. Siiteri PK et al: Progesterone and maintenance of pregnancy: is progesterone nature's immunosuppressant?, *Ann N Y Acad Sci* 286:384, 1977.

397. Siler-Khodr TM, Khodr GS, Valenzuela G: Immunoreactive GnRH levels in maternal circulation throughout pregnancy, *Am J Obstet Gynecol* 150:376, 1984.

398. Siler-Khodr TM, Morgenstern LL, Greenwood FC: Hormone synthesis and release from human fetal adenohypophyses *in vitro*, *J Clin Endocrinol Metab* 39:891, 1974.

399. Deleted in proofs.

400. Siler-Khodr TM et al: Inhibition of hCG, α-hCG and progesterone release from human placenta tissue in vitro by a GnRH antagonist, *Life Sci* 32:2741, 1983.

401. Silman RE et al: Human pituitary peptides and parturition, *Nature* 260:716, 1976.

402. Simmer HH et al: On the regulation of estrogen production by cortisol and ACTH in human pregnancy at term, *Am J Obstet Gynecol* 119:283, 1974.

403. Simpson ER: Cholesterol side-chain cleavage, cytochrome P450, and the control of steroidogenesis, *Mol Cell Endocrinol* 13:213, 1979.

404. Sinclair AH et al: Sequences homologous to ZFY, a candidate human sex-determining gene, are autosomal in marsupials, *Nature* 336:780, 1988.

405. Skebel'skaya, YuB: Adrenocorticotropic activity of the human fetus hypophyses, *Probl Endokrinol* 4:77, 1965.

406. Skinner MK, Tung PS, Fritz IB: Cooperativity between Sertoli cells and testicular cells and testicular peritubular cells in the production and deposition of the extracellular matrix components, *J Cell Biol* 100:1941, 1985.

407. Speed RM: The prophase stages in human foetal oocytes studied by light and electron microscopy, *Hum Genet* 69:69, 1985.

408. Speed RM: The possible role of meiotic pairing anomalies in the atresia of human fetal oocytes, *Hum Genet* 78:260, 1988.

409. Spencer SJ, Rabinovici J, Jaffe RB: Human recombinant activin-A inhibits proliferation of human fetal adrenal cells in vitro, *J Clin Endocrinol Metab* 71:1678, 1990.

410. Spencer S et al: Activin and inhibin in the human adrenal gland: regulation and differential effects in fetal and adult cells, *J Clin Invest* 90:142, 1992.

411. Stalla GK et al: Human corticotropin-releasing hormone during pregnancy, *Gynecol Endocrinol* 3:1, 1989.

412. Stark RI, Frantz AG: ACTH-β-endorphin in pregnancy, *Clin Perinatol* 10:653, 1983.

413. Stark RI et al: Vasopressin secretion induced by hypoxia in sheep: developmental changes and relationship to β-endorphin release, *Am J Obstet Gynecol* 143:204, 1982.

414. Stromberg K et al: Human term placenta contains transforming growth factor, *Biochem Biophys Res Commun* 106:354, 1982.

415. Styne DM, Kaplan SL, Grumbach MM: Plasma glycoprotein hormone α-subunit in the neonate and in prepubertal and pubertal children: effects of luteinizing hormone-releasing hormone, *J Clin Endocrinol Metab* 50:450, 1980.

416. Sucheston ME, Cannon MS: Development of zonular patterns in the human adrenal gland, *J Morphol* 126:477, 1968.

417. Sugino H et al: Erythroid differentiation factor can modulate follicular granulosa cell functions, *Biochem Biophys Res Commun* 153:281, 1988.

418. Sugino H et al: Identification of a specific receptor for erythroid differentiation factor on follicular granulosa cell, *J Biol Chem* 263:15249, 1988.

419. Suh HK, Frantz AG: Size heterogeneity of human prolactin in plasma and pituitary extracts, *J Clin Endocrinol Metab* 39:928, 1974.

420. Sultan C et al: Androgen receptors and metabolism in cultured human fetal fibroblasts, *Pediatr Res* 14:67, 1980.

421. Suwa S, Friesen H: Biosynthesis of human placental proteins and human placental lactogen (HPL) *in vitro*, I: identification of ³H-labeled HPL, *Endocrinology* 85:1028, 1969.

422. Swaab DF, Boer GJ, Visser M: The fetal brain and intrauterine growth, *Postgrad Med J* 54 (Suppl 1):63, 1978.

423. Swaab DF, Honnebier WJ: The influence of removal of the fetal rat brain upon intrauterine growth of the fetus and the placenta and on gestation length, *J Obstet Gynaecol Br Commonw* 80:589, 1973.

424. Swaab DF, Honnebier WJ: The role of the fetal hypothalamus in development of the feto-placental unit and in parturition. In Swaab DF, Schade P, editors: *Integrative hypothalamic activity*, vol 7, *Prog Brain Res* 41:255, 1974.

425. Swaab DF, Martin JT: Functions of α-melanotropin and other opiomelanocortin peptides in labour, intrauterine growth and brain development, *Peptides* 81:196, 1981.

426. Swaab DF, Visser M, Tilders FJH: Stimulation of intrauterine growth in rat by α-MSH, *J Endocrinol* 70:445, 1976.

427. Takagi S et al: Sex differences in fetal gonadotropins and androgens, *J Steroid Biochem* 8:609, 1977.

428. Takahashi M, Koide SS, Donahoe PK: Müllerian inhibiting substance as oocyte meiosis inhibitor, *Mol Cell Endocrinol* 47:225, 1986.

429. Takor T, Pearse AGE: Neuroectodermal origin of avian hypothalamohypophyseal complex: the role of the ventral neural ridge, *J Embryol Exp Morphol* 34:311, 1975.

430. Talas M, Midgley AR Jr, Jaffe RB: Regulation of human gonadotropins, XIV: gel filtration and electrophoretic analysis of endogenous and extracted immunoreactive human follicle-stimulating hormone of pituitary, serum and urinary origin, *J Clin Endocrinol Metab* 36:817, 1973.

431. Tapanainen J, Voutilainen R, Jaffe RB: Low aromatase activity and gene expression in human fetal testes, *J Steroid Biochem* 33:7, 1989.

432. Tapanainen J et al: Age-related changes in endogenous steroids of human fetal testis during early and midpregnancy, *J Clin Endocrinol Metab* 52:98, 1981.

433. Tatemoto K: Neuropeptide Y: complete amino acid sequence of the brain peptide, *Proc Natl Acad Sci U S A* 79:5485, 1982.

434. Taylor T, Coutts JR, Macnaughton MC: Human foetal synthesis of testosterone from perfused progesterone, *J Endocrinol* 60:321, 1974.

435. Teasdale F et al: Human chorionic gonadotropin: inhibitory effect on mixed lymphocyte cultures, *Gynecol Invest* 4:263, 1973.

436. Thiveris JA, Currie RW: Observations on the hypothalamo-hypophyseal portal vasculature in the developing human fetus, *Am J Anat* 157:441, 1980.

437. Thomson M et al: Secretion of corticotropin releasing hormone by superfused human placental fragments, *Gynecol Endocrinol* 2:87, 1988.

438. Thorburn G et al: Epidermal growth factor: a critical factor in fetal maturation?, *Ciba Found Symp* 86:172, 1981.

439. Torday JS: Androgens delay human fetal lung maturation in vitro, *Endocrinology* 126:3240, 1990.

440. Torney AJ et al: Cellular localization of inhibin mRNA in the bovine ovary by in-situ hybridization, *J Reprod Fertil* 86:391, 1989.

441. Tran D, Meusy-Dessole N, Josso N: Anti-müllerian hormone is a functional marker of foetal Sertoli cells, *Nature* 269:411, 1977.

442. Tseng MT, Alexander NJ, Kittinger GW: Effect of fetal decapitation on the structure and function of Leydig cells in rhesus monkeys (*Macaca mulatta*), *Am J Anat* 143:349, 1975.

443. Tyson JE, Pinto H: Identification of the possible significance of prolactin in human reproduction, *Clin Obstet Gynaecol* 5:411, 1978.

444. Tyson JE et al: Studies of prolactin secretion in human pregnancy, *Am J Obstet Gynecol* 113:14, 1972.

445. Vaitukaitis JL, Braunstein GD, Ross GT: A radioimmunoassay which specifically measures human chorionic gonadotropin in the presence of human luteinizing hormone, *Am J Obstet Gynecol* 113:751, 1972.

446. Vale W, Rivier C: Substances modulating the secretion of ACTH by cultured anterior pituitary cells, *Fed Proc* 36:2094, 1977.

447. Vale W et al: Characterization of a 41-residue ovine hypothalamic peptide that stimulates secretion of corticotropin and β-endorphin, *Science* 212:1394, 1981.

448. Vale W et al: Effects of synthetic ovine corticotropin-releasing factor, catecholamines, neurohypophysial peptides and other substances on cultured corticotropic cells, *Endocrinology* 113:1121, 1983.

449. Vale W et al: Purification and characterization of an FSH releasing protein from porcine ovarian follicular fluid, *Nature* 321:776, 1986.

450. Vale W et al: Chemical and biological characterization of the inhibin family of protein hormones, *Recent Prog Horm Res* 44:1, 1988.

451. Valette AR et al: Immunoreactive dynorphin in maternal blood, umbilical vein and amniotic fluid, *Neuropeptides* 7:145, 1986.

452. van Wagenen G, Simpson ME: *Embryology of the ovary and testis in Homo sapiens and Macaca mulatta,* New Haven, Conn, 1965, Yale University Press.

453. Varma K, Larraga L, Serenkow HA: Radioimmunoassay of serum human chorionic gonadotropin during normal pregnancy, *Obstet Gynecol* 37:10, 1971.

454. Visser M, Swaab DF: Life span changes in the presence of β-melanocyte-stimulating hormone-containing cells in the human pituitary, *J Dev Physiol* 1:161, 1979.

455. Vlaskovska M, Hertting G, Knepel W: Adrenocorticotropin and β-endorphin release from rat adenohypophysis *in vitro:* inhibition by prostaglandin E$_2$ formed locally in response to vasopressin and corticotropin-releasing factor, *Endocrinology* 115:895, 1984.

456. Voutilainen R, Ilvesmaki V, Miettinen PJ: Low expression of 3 beta-hydroxy-5-ene steroid dehydrogenase gene in human fetal adrenals in vivo: adrenocorticotropin and protein kinase C-dependent regulation in adrenocortical cultures, *J Clin Endocrinol Metab* 72:761, 1991.

457. Voutilainen R, Miller WL: Developmental expression of genes for the steroidogenic enzymes P450scc (20,22-desmolase), P450c17 (17 alpha-hydroxylase/17,20-lyase), and P450c21 (21-hydroxylase) in the human fetus, *J Clin Endocrinol Metab* 63:1145, 1986.

458. Voutilainen R, Miller WL: Human müllerian inhibitory factor messenger ribonucleic acid is hormonally regulated in the fetal testis and in adult granulosa cells, *Mol Endocrinol* 1:604, 1987.

459. Voutilainen R, Miller WL: Developmental and hormonal regulation of mRNAs for insulin-like growth factor II and steroidogenic enzymes in human fetal adrenals and gonads, *DNA* 7:9, 1989.

460. Wardlaw SL et al: Plasma β-endorphin and β-lipoprotein in the human fetus at delivery: correlation with arterial pH and pO$_2$, *J Clin Endocrinol Metab* 79:888, 1979.

461. Wardlaw SL et al: Effects of hypoxia on β-endorphin and β-lipotropin release in the fetal, newborn and maternal sheep, *Endocrinology* 108:1710, 1981.

462. Wartenberg H: Differentiation and development of the testes. In Burger H, de Kretzer D, editors: *The testis,* New York, 1989, Raven Press.

463. Wassarman PM: Profile of a mammalian sperm receptor, *Development* 108:1, 1990.

464. Watkins WB, Yen SSC: Somatostatin in cytotrophoblast of the immature human placenta: localization by immunoperoxidase cytochemistry, *J Clin Endocrinol Metab* 50:969, 1980.

465. Weill J, Bernfeld J: Le syndrome hypothalamique. In *Libraires de l'Academie de Medicine,* Paris, 1954, Masson.

466. Wide L, Hobson B: Relationship between the sex of the fetus and the amount of human chorionic gonadotrophin in placentae from the 10th-20th weeks of pregnancy, *J Endocrinol* 61:75, 1974.

467. Wilburn L, Jaffe RB: Quantitative assessment of the ontogeny of met-enkephalin, norepinephrine and epinephrine in the human fetal medulla, *Acta Endocrinol* 118:453, 1988.

468. Williams RH: *Textbook of endocrinology,* Philadelphia, 1990, WB Saunders.

469. Williams JF et al: Receptor-binding activity of highly purified bovine luteinizing hormone and thyrotropin, and their subunits, *Endocrinology* 106:1353, 1980.

470. Wilson JD, Goldstein JL: Classification of hereditary disorders of sexual developments, *Birth Defects* 11:1, 1975.

471. Wilson JD, Lasnitzki I: Dihydrotestosterone formation in fetal tissues of the rabbit and rat, *Endocrinology* 89:659, 1971.

472. Wilson JD, Siiteri PK: Developmental pattern of testosterone synthesis in the fetal gonad of the rabbit, *Endocrinology* 92:1182, 1973.

473. Winter JS: Hypothalamic-pituitary function in the fetus and infant, *J Clin Endocrinol Metab* 11:41, 1982.

474. Winters A et al: Plasma ACTH levels in the human fetus and neonate as related to age and parturition, *J Clin Endocrinol Metab* 39:269, 1974.

475. Winters AJ, Eskay RL, Porter JC: Concentration and distribution of TRH and LRH in the human fetal brain, *J Clin Endocrinol Metabol* 39:960, 1974.

476. Witorsch RJ, Kitay JI: Pituitary hormones affecting adrenal 5α-reductase activity: ACTH, growth hormone and prolactin, *Endocrinology* 91:764, 1971.

477. Witschi E: Migration of the germ cells of human embryos from the yolksac to the primitive genital fold, *Contib Embryol* 32:67, 1948.

478. Woodruff TK et al: Dynamic changes in inhibin messenger RNAs in rat ovarian follicles during the reproductive cycle, *Science* 239:1296, 1988.

479. Word RA et al: Testosterone synthesis and adenylate cyclase activity in the early human fetal testis appear to be independent of human chorionic gonadotropin control, *J Clin Endocrinol Metab* 69:204, 1989.

480. Yates IE, Maran JW: Stimulation and inhibition of adrenocorticotropin release. In Knobil E, Sawyer WH, editors: *Handbook of physiology,* vol 4, sect 7, Washington, DC, 1974, American Physiological Society.

481. Yeh J, Osathanondh R, Villa-Komaroff L: Human first and second trimester fetal ovaries and uteruses express messenger RNA for basic fibroblast growth factor (bFGF) and the FGF receptor. Presented at the 47th Annual meeting of the American Fertility Society, Orlando, Fla, Oct 19–24, 1991 (abstract No 006).

482. Yoshinaga K et al: The development of the sexually indifferent gonad in the prosimian, Galago crassicaudatus crassicaudatus, *Am J Anat* 181:89, 1988.

482a. Youngblood WW, Humm J, Kizer JS: TRH-like immunoreactivity in rat pancreas and eye, bovine and sheep pineals, and human placenta: non-identify with synthetic Pyroglu-His-Pro-NH$_2$ (TRH), *Brain Research* 163:101, 1979.

483. Zondek LH, Zondek T: Observations on the testis in anencephaly with special reference to the Leydig cells, *Biol Neonate* 8:329, 1965.

484. Zuckerman S, Baker TG: The development of the ovary and the process of oogenesis. In Zuckerman S, Weir BJ, editors: *The ovary,* New York, 1977, Academic Press.

Chapter 51

ECTOPIC PREGNANCY

Alan S. Penzias, MD
and Alan H. DeCherney, MD

Ectopic pregnancy represents a serious aberration of the reproductive process. The consequences of this deviation range from the immediate loss of the present pregnancy to long-term compromise of fertility. Ectopic pregnancy is a life-threatening problem of epidemic proportions.

DEMOGRAPHICS

Between 1970 and 1985 the number of reported ectopic pregnancies in the United States quadrupled, increasing from 4.8 to 20.9 ectopic pregnancies per 1000 live births.[25] During this time period the number of hospitalizations for this condition tripled,[23] and it ranked among the top causes of maternal mortality[3] (Fig. 51-1). The most common cause of death from ectopic pregnancy is hemorrhage, occurring in 89% of these patients.[4] Although the absolute number of cases is on the rise, advances in diagnosis and therapy have significantly reduced the incidence of fatal outcome. A study of all deaths due to ectopic pregnancy occurring in 1979 and 1980 concluded that fully one third might have been prevented if the woman had notified or visited a physician more promptly after the onset of symptoms.[24]

Aside from the life-threatening nature of this disease, ectopic pregnancy has a major economic impact on the U.S. health care system. The total cost of ectopic pregnancy in 1990 was estimated to be nearly $1.1 billion, with a total direct cost per case of $9482.[81] Early diagnosis and intervention will prevent many fatalities, and appropriate use of cost-effective management approaches can reduce costs. Preventive measures that decrease the risk of ectopic pregnancy can save lives and lessen the financial burden of the disease.

ETIOLOGY

Ninety-seven percent of ectopic pregnancies are tubal, with another 2.5% located in the cornua. Other sites account for the remaining 0.5%. They occur with equal frequency in the left and right tubes, with some evidence that there is concordance with the side of the corpus luteum.[15] There is an abundance of descriptive data concerning the etiology of ectopic pregnancy. Quantitative estimates (Table 51-1) of risk factors for this disease have been published as well.[44]

Pelvic inflammatory disease

Pelvic inflammatory disease serves as the paradigm for understanding the etiology of ectopic pregnancy. Although *Neisseria gonorrhoeae* and *Chlamydia trachomatis* infections have been strongly identified with subsequent risk of ectopic pregnancy,[45,62,80,82] pelvic inflammatory disease is known to be of polymicrobial origin. Often the condition is diagnosed clinically without identification of a single causative organism. The sequelae of endotubal infection can include destruction of the fine and complex architecture of the tubal lumen. Hershlag and associates[35] examined fresh salpingectomy specimens by tuboscopy, light microscopy, and electron microscopy. They found that mild to moderate pathologic changes as documented by light microscopy and

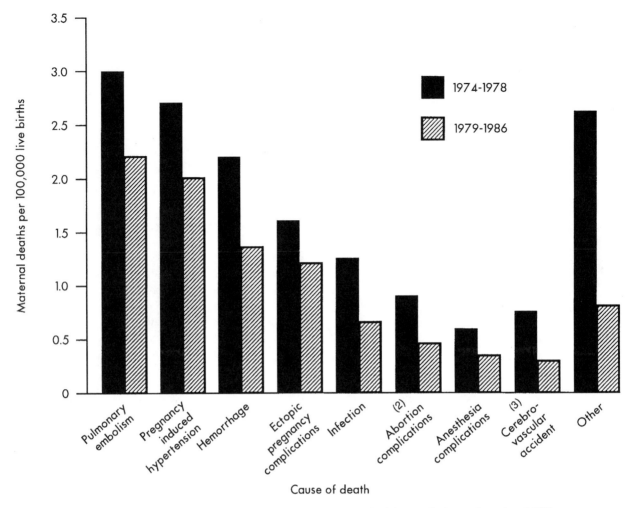

Fig. 51-1. Cause-specific maternal mortality rates in the United States. (Redrawn from Atrash HK et al: Maternal mortality in the United States, 1979–1986, *Obstet Gynecol* 76:1055-1060, 1990, with permission of The American College of Obstetricians and Gynecologists.)

Table 51-1. Risk factors for ectopic pregnancy*

Characteristic	Relative risk	95% Confidence interval
Current use of intrauterine device†	13.7	1.6-120.6
Tubal surgery†	4.5	1.5-13.9
Pelvic inflammatory disease†	3.3	1.6-6.6
History of infertility†	2.6	1.6-4.2
Abdominal/pelvic surgery	2.4	1.04-5.7
Acute appendicitis	4.0	2.2-7.2
Pelvic adhesions	5.6	2.3-13.8

*Based on data in reference 44.
†Strong, independent risk factor for ectopic pregnancy.

transmission electron microscopy were frequently not diagnosed, even with magnification, by tuboscopy. This finding implies that patients without visible evidence of previous pelvic infection might still have endotubal damage.

Salpingitis isthmica nodosa, a pathologic condition of the fallopian tubes caused by infection characterized by proximal tubal diverticula (Fig. 51-2), has also been associated with ectopic pregnancy.[36,43]

Previous therapeutic abortion

The relative risk of ectopic pregnancy after legal induced abortion in the United States is controversial. Levin et al.[39] reported a relative risk of 2.6 (95% confidence interval 0.9 to 7.4) in women with a history of two or more abortions; however, women with illegal abortions were not excluded from the final analysis. In contrast, Daling and associates[19] found that women with two or more legal abortions had a relative risk of 1.8 (95% confidence interval

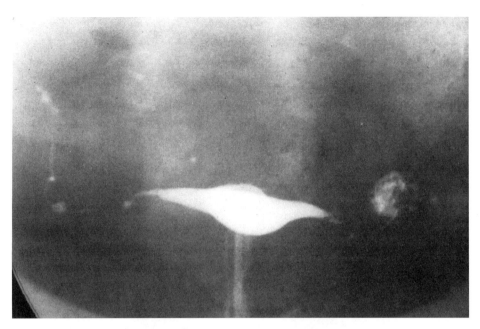

Fig. 51-2. Salpingitis isthmica nodosa (SIN). Hysterosalpingogram demonstrating a normal anteverted uterus and SIN in the right fallopian tube (left side of figure).

0.5 to 7.1) and concluded that this elevation could have been caused by chance (the 95% confidence interval crosses 1.0) (Table 51-2).

Reports from Japan[63,66] and Yugoslovia,[2] where therapeutic abortion is legal, reveal no association between induced abortion and risk of ectopic pregnancy. Panayotou et al.[55] reported that in Greece, where most abortions were illegal, there was a strong association (relative risk = 10) between pregnancy termination and ectopic pregnancy. In this case, postoperative infection may have contributed to the increased relative risk.

Larger studies are required to better define the potential association between therapeutic abortion and ectopic pregnancy.

Intrauterine device

A woman who conceives with an intrauterine device (IUD) in place is more likely to have an ectopic pregnancy than is a woman who conceives after failure of another contraceptive method. However, the *incidence* of ectopic pregnancy in women with an IUD in place is half that of women not using contraception.[31] This is due to the global efficiency of the IUD in preventing conception. It is not surprising, however, that the device is somewhat more effective at preventing intrauterine pregnancy than it is at preventing extrauterine pregnancy.

A growing body of data suggests that former IUD users, in the absence of infectious complications, are not at an increased risk of developing an ectopic pregnancy.[26,53,83]

Table 51-2. Standardized* relative risks of ectopic pregnancy according to selected risk factors

Characteristic	Relative risk	95% Confidence interval
History of 1 induced abortion	1.3	0.6-2.6
History of 2 induced abortions	1.8	0.5-7.1
Smoking status		
Current	2.6	1.4-4.8
Past	1.9	0.9-4.1
Dalkon Shield use	3.6	1.7-7.4
Age at first sexual intercourse		
≤ 17 y	1.0	—
18-20 y	1.6	0.9-3.1
21+ y	0.7	0.3-1.5
Condom use	0.4	0.2-1.0

From Daling JR et al: Ectopic pregnancy in relation to previous induced abortion, *JAMA* 253:1005-1008, 1985. Copyright 1985, American Medical Association. Reproduced with permission.
*Standardized for tabulated variables in addition to age, race, gravidity, and year of index pregnancy and whether the woman was using contraception at the time of conception, using a multiple logistic regression model.

Diethylstilbestrol

A number of reports suggest that the incidence of ectopic pregnancy is four to five times higher than that of the general population in women exposed to diethylstilbestrol (DES) in utero.[7,18,33,68,71] This dysfunctional outcome may be related to the grossly "withered" appearance of the fallopian tubes that has been described in women exposed to DES.[20]

As the cohort of women at risk of in utero DES exposure ages, the importance of this etiology will diminish.

Assisted reproductive technology

Infertility has been described as a risk factor for ectopic pregnancy.[15] Therefore it is not surprising that patients undergoing treatment of infertility by ovulation induction with both clomiphene citrate[15] and human menopausal gonadotropins[46] have a higher relative risk of ectopic pregnancy.

Patients who proceed to gamete intrafallopian transfer (GIFT) or in vitro fertilization and embryo transfer (IVF-ET) are also at risk for developing an ectopic pregnancy.[87] However, it would seem that this occurs almost exclusively in patients with a diagnosis of tubal factor infertility.[34]

Although the risk of combined intrauterine and tubal (heterotopic) pregnancy in the general population is generally reported to be 1/30,000, it has been reported as a complication of IVF-ET[88] with an incidence as high as 1/100 pregnancies.[48]

PATHOLOGY

Under normal circumstances, the trophoblast binds to the endometrial epithelium. This phenomenon is remarkable when one considers that this binding occurs between two polarized epithelial cells that are of disparate genetic and tissue derivation.[1] The embryo must penetrate this barrier in order to gain access to the maternal vasculature and establish placentation.[16] The highly invasive trophoblast can implant indiscriminately in a wide variety of ectopic sites regardless of host tissue, hormonal milieu, or timing.[38] Conversely, the only tissue in which this invasion does not occur indiscriminately is the endometrium.[48]

The vast majority of ectopic pregnancies are tubal. This is likely due to the fact that fertilization occurs predomi-

nantly in the tubal ampulla. Aberrations in mucosal epithelium or tubal motility secondary to scarring or hormonal conditions may then set the stage for anomalous implantation.

Chromosome analysis of ectopic and intrauterine pregnancies of comparable embryonic age show similar rates of chromosomal abnormalities.[28,60] This appears to exclude a genetic basis for ectopic pregnancy.

The anatomic position of the ectopic pregnancy along the fallopian tube can often yield a clue to its position in relation to the lumen. Cross-sectional studies of ampullary ectopic pregnancies reveal that in 75% of cases the trophoblast has invaded the mucosa and propagated in the extraluminal, subserosal space (Fig. 51-3). In contrast, isthmic pregnancies tend to propagate within the lumen[14,58] (Fig. 51-4). The importance of these observations lies in the fact that the tubal lumen frequently escapes destruction in the ampullary ectopic pregnancy, whereas luminal disruption is more common in the isthmus. These pathologic data based on anatomic siting may be useful when selecting a surgical approach to treatment.

DIAGNOSIS

Physicians have at their disposal a number of tests that aid in the diagnosis of ectopic pregnancy. These include culdocentesis, ultrasound, Doppler flow studies, and measurement of the hormones human chorionic gonadotropin (hCG) and progesterone. Before these tests were in routine use, nearly 80% of ectopic pregnancies were discovered only after they had ruptured.[11] When used alone or in combination, diagnostic tests enable timely diagnosis and treatment.

Signs and symptoms

The presenting symptoms vary greatly depending on (1) the location of the pregnancy, (2) the gestational age of the pregnancy, and (3) whether the ectopic pregnancy has bled or ruptured. Abdominal pain is the most frequent complaint. The presence of shoulder pain is an infrequent but ominous sign. Abnormal vaginal bleeding and amenor-

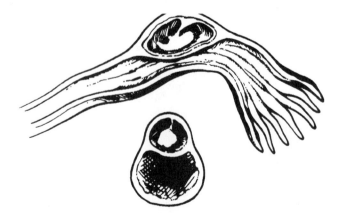

Fig. 51-3. Ampullary ectopic pregnancy. The trophoblast is shown propagating in the extraluminal, subserosal space.

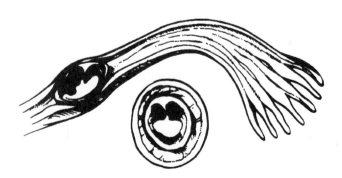

Fig. 51-4. Isthmic ectopic pregnancy. The trophoblast is shown propagating within the tubal lumen.

rhea are also common signs. A physical finding of a unilateral adnexal mass or tenderness is suggestive but not diagnostic.

The diagnosis of a catastrophic event requires only observation and physical examination. Premorbid diagnosis requires the combination of a raised index of suspicion and additional diagnostic studies.

Culdocentesis

Culdocentesis, although older and mildly invasive, can still provide excellent information. When it is used in combination with a positive pregnancy test, positive results strongly suggest the presence of an ectopic pregnancy. In a series of 158 patients with positive culdocentesis test results for whom the pregnancy test was not evaluated, Romero et al.[65] found that 86% had an ectopic pregnancy. When combined with a positive pregnancy test, the specificity for ectopic pregnancy rose to 99%. Although a positive culdocentesis often indicates the presence of an ectopic pregnancy, it does not mean that the pregnancy has ruptured. In fact, 65% of unruptured ectopic pregnancies will have a positive culdocentesis.

Human chorionic gonadotropin

The isolation and identification of the beta subunit of hCG revolutionized the diagnosis and management of early pregnancy. Early assays were confounded by a cross-reactivity with endogenous luteinizing hormone (LH) and sensitivity sacrificed so that a positive pregnancy test was not caused by an LH surge. The result was that only half of patients with an ectopic pregnancy had a positive pregnancy test. This assay was replaced by the radioreceptor assay with a sensitivity of 200 mIU/mL, followed by a radioimmunoassay with a sensitivity of 10 mIU/mL or less. Recently developed two-site "sandwich assays," including the immunofluorometric assay (IMFA) and the enzyme-linked immunosorbent assay (ELISA), have eliminated the requirement for environmentally hazardous radioactively labeled products while maintaining the high degree of sensitivity gained with the radioimmunoassay.

Isolated values of hCG can aid in the diagnosis of ectopic pregnancy only when used in combination with other diagnostic tests. However, the pattern of rise or fall of hCG can be extremely helpful. Normal intrauterine pregnancies show a mean doubling time ranging from 2.0 days during the fifth gestational week to 3.4 days in the seventh week.[59] When doubling time exceeds the 85th percentile, plateaus, or falls, the diagnosis of an abnormal gestation is almost certain. These patterns represent either an extrauterine gestation or an inevitable abortion of an intrauterine pregnancy.

Progesterone

Single values of progesterone have been reported to suggest the presence of an abnormal pregnancy. Yeko and

associates[85] showed that a progesterone level below 15 ng/mL strongly correlated with an abnormal gestation (Fig. 51-5). Buck et al.[13] found that a progesterone level below 20 ng/mL yielded a sensitivity of 92%, a specificity of 84%, a positive predictive value of 90%, and a negative predictive value of 87% for an abnormal gestation. Stovall and associates[74] reported that 81% of patients with an ectopic pregnancy had a serum progesterone level of less than 15 ng/mL, whereas 11% of patients with a normal pregnancy had a value below this level.

Ultrasound

Ultrasound evaluation is a noninvasive technique that utilizes transmitted and reflected sound waves to produce an image. The female pelvis is commonly imaged both transabdominally and transvaginally. The transvaginal route allows the transducer to be in closer proximity to the structures of interest. This, in turn, permits the use of high-frequency, high-resolution equipment.

Batzer et al.[8] described the ultrasonographic landmarks of the first 42 days of gestation. In all successful pregnancies, a gestational sac could be seen 28 days after ovulation. If no fetal heart motion was seen by 45 days or with a gestational sac of 30 mm or more, spontaneous abortion was likely. If no gestational sac was seen by 28 days

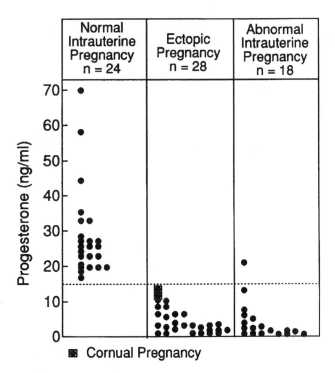

Fig. 51-5. Progesterone levels in early pregnancy, categorized by diagnostic group. (From Yeko TR, Gorrill MJ, Hughes LH, Rodi IA, Buster JE, Sauer MV: Timely diagnosis of early ectopic pregnancy using a single blood progesterone measurement, *Fertil Steril* 48:1048-1050, 1987. Reproduced with permission of the publisher, The American Fertility Society.)

postconception or with a β-hCG level of 7500 mIU/mL, ectopic pregnancy was suspected until proven otherwise.

The ultrasonographic appearance of the endometrium can also suggest whether the pregnancy is intrauterine or extrauterine. A developing intrauterine pregnancy will show the presence of a decidua capsularis and a decidua parietalis, the double sac sign (Fig. 51-6). In contrast, an extrauterine pregnancy will reveal only the decidualization of the empty endometrium, a pseudogestational sac[9,50] (Fig. 51-7).

The blood flow patterns in the inactive ovary, corpus luteum, and trophoblast can also be detected and characterized. The characteristic patterns of impedance to flow of each entity can help refine the interpretation of images seen by ultrasound.[22,77]

The combination of ultrasonography and hCG level is the mainstay of modern management of the suspected ectopic pregnancy. Romero and associates[64] concluded that a normal intrauterine gestational sac must be visualized by transabdominal ultrasound examination when the level of hCG reaches 6500 mIU/mL. The absence of a sac at this level has a sensitivity of 100% and a specificity of 96% for ectopic pregnancy.

The increasingly widespread use of transvaginal ultrasonography has led to a redefinition of the discriminatory zone. Shapiro et al.[70] reported on a series of 22 patients with proven ectopic pregnancy. Ninety-two percent of these patients had the ectopic pregnancy identified with titers below 3600 mIU/mL. Other reports suggest a discriminatory zone for transvaginal ultrasonography in the range of 1000 to 1500 mIU/mL.[30,51]

MANAGEMENT

Once the presence of an ectopic pregnancy is suspected or has been established, a therapeutic decision must be made. The choices include surgery, chemotherapy, and simple observation (Fig. 51-8). The selection of one approach over another is made with respect to the active clinical issues at the time of diagnosis.

Surgical management

There is active debate regarding the relative merits of laparoscopy and laparotomy in the treatment of ectopic

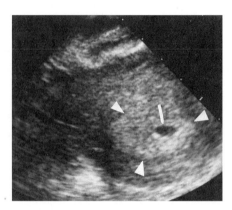

Fig. 51-6. The double sac sign of intrauterine pregnancy. The inner (*thin arrow*) and outer (*wide arrows*) sac margins are demonstrated. (Sonogram provided courtesy of Barbara Penzias.)

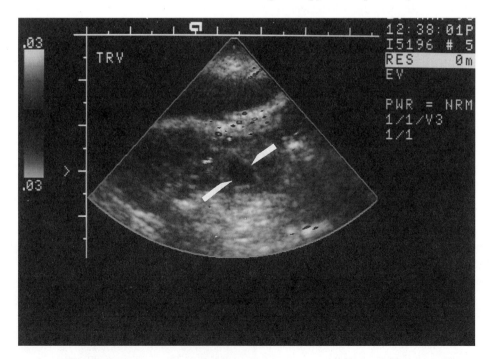

Fig. 51-7. Pseudogestational sac (*arrows*) of ectopic pregnancy. (Sonogram provided courtesy of Dr. Kenneth J. W. Taylor.)

pregnancy. To date, neither approach has proven superior to the other with regard to subsequent fertility. Laparoscopy has the advantage of fewer days in the hospital and more rapid recovery time. Contraindications to laparoscopy have been reported, only to be revised by the introduction of specialized instruments and the advancement of individual surgical skills.

The one remaining absolute contraindication to laparoscopy is hemodynamic instability. In such cases, the burden of a pneumoperitoneum could compromise both ventilatory capacity and venous return.

Salpingectomy. When a woman has finished her childbearing and is to be treated surgically for an ectopic pregnancy, salpingectomy is the procedure of choice. Whether performed laparoscopically or at laparotomy, salpingectomy generally avoids the intraoperative hemorrhage that can accompany more conservative procedures. In addition, the risk of a persistent ectopic pregnancy, which

also can complicate the conservative linear salpingostomy,[42,69] is virtually eliminated.

Guidelines for choosing salpingectomy in ectopic pregnancy can be proposed as follows:

- Childbearing completed
- Uncontrolled hemorrhage
- Recurrent ectopic pregnancy in the same tube
- Tubal destruction by the ectopic pregnancy

Intraoperative conditions should be considered in determining the procedure of choice. In performing a salpingectomy in a woman with a desire for future fertility, one must consider her reproductive potential. Oelsner[52] summarized reports on 1630 women who underwent salpingectomy for ectopic pregnancy and subsequently became pregnant. Forty-one percent achieved intrauterine gestation and 14% had another ectopic gestation (Table 51-3). Mitchell et al.[47] reported an intrauterine pregnancy rate of 61% in 39

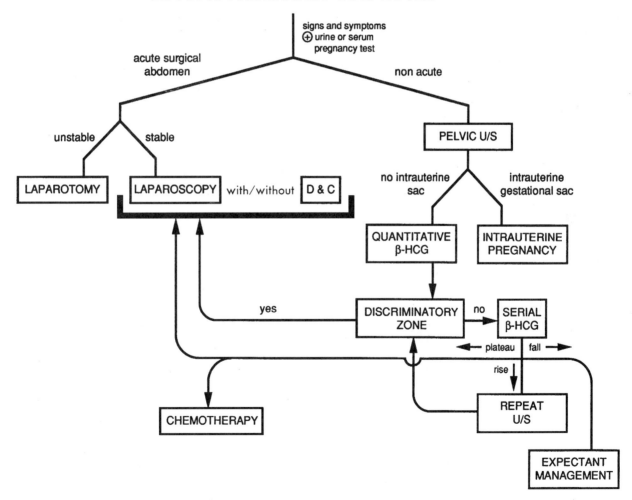

Fig. 51-8. Paradigm for management of suspected ectopic pregnancy. *U/S,* ultrasonography; *D&C,* dilation and curettage. The discriminatory zone is the quantitative β-HCG level above which an intrauterine pregnancy should be seen by ultrasound. *Yes* means the quantitative β-HCG is above the level of the discriminatory zone; *no* means it is below the level of the zone.

Table 51-3. Subsequent pregnancy outcome in women treated for an ectopic pregnancy

	Women desiring pregnancy	Women with intrauterine pregnancy (%)	Women with repeat extrauterine pregnancy (%)
Radical surgery	1630	667 (40.9)*	231 (14.2)*
Conservative surgery	442	201 (45.5)*	51 (41.5)*

From Oelsner G: Ectopic pregnancy in the sole remaining tube and management of the patient with multiple ectopic pregnancies, *Clin Obstet Gynecol* 30:225, 1987. Reproduced with permission.
*$P > 0.05$.

patients who attempted conception after salpingectomy.

Laparoscopic salpingectomy. Once the decision to perform a laparoscopic salpingectomy has been made, the surgeon has several choices. If the gestation is located in the ampulla, a prefabricated loop suture ligature can be placed proximal to the gestation (Fig. 51-9). A second loop is placed distally to retain control of the pedicle after the specimen is resected. This second loop allows the pedicle to be moved and inspected without fear of wrenching off the hemostatic suture. In choosing this procedure, care should be taken to avoid compromise to the ovarian blood supply. If hemostasis is not adequately achieved, unipolar or bipolar electrocautery can be selectively applied.

A theoretic concern in this situation is the migration of an embryo into the remaining proximal segment of fallo-

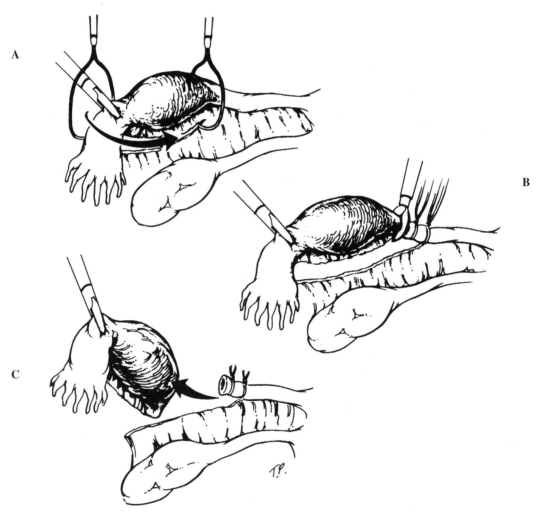

Fig. 51-9. Laparoscopic salpingectomy—suture loop excision. **A,** The forceps are passed through the open suture loop and the fallopian tube is grasped. **B,** The loop is slid over the ectopic pregnancy and tightened. **C,** A second loop is passed and tightened as the scissors resect the fallopian tube.

pian tube. This condition is rare in the natural state, but the patient is at some risk of an ectopic pregnancy after IVF-ET.

Alternatively, a salpingectomy can be performed by using serial electrocautery and transection (Fig. 51-10). Working from the proximal portion of the fallopian tube distally, the tissue is desiccated by the electrocautery and then transected with blunt-end scissors. A grasping forceps maintains gentle traction on the fallopian tube as it is freed. This facilitates exposure of the mesosalpinx as the surgery proceeds.

Segmental resection. Segmental resection is reserved for cases in which a small segment of the fallopian tube has been destroyed or hemostasis cannot be achieved. If what remains of the fallopian tube is unsuitable for immediate or later anastomosis, the newly created distal segment with its functional fimbria can be the site of a subsequent ectopic pregnancy. Under these circumstances, a salpingectomy should be considered. Of course, if the contralateral fallopian tube is occluded or absent, this risk is minimized.

Linear salpingostomy. Linear salpingostomy is the most conservative surgical procedure for treating an ectopic pregnancy (Figs. 51-11 and 51-12). Fallopian tubes treated in this way are potentially functional and can lead to subsequent intrauterine pregnancy. A literature review on the reproductive performance of women with a single fallopian tube who were treated for an ectopic pregnancy in that tube with linear salpingostomy[21] revealed that 61% subsequently achieved an intrauterine pregnancy and 17% had a recurrent ectopic pregnancy. This indicates that

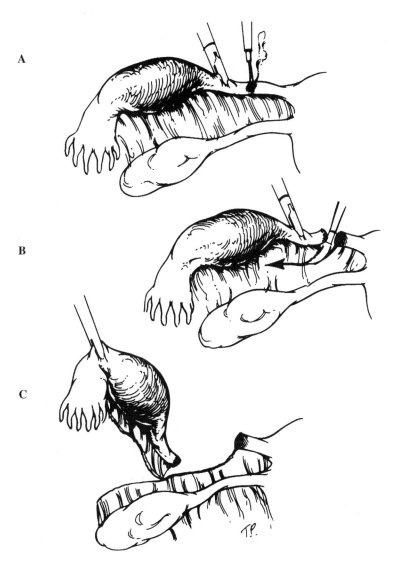

Fig. 51-10. Laparoscopic salpingectomy—electrocautery and excision. **A,** Grasping forceps stabilize the tube proximal to the ectopic pregnancy while coagulating current is applied. **B,** The coagulated area is transected. **C,** Serial cautery and transection free the specimen.

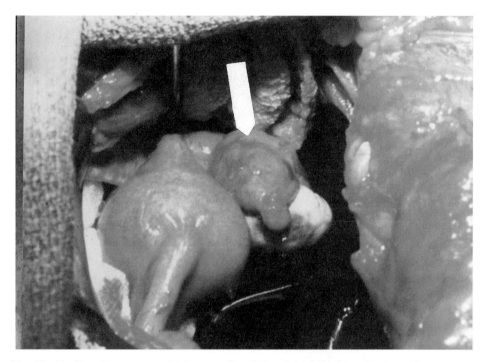

Fig. 51-11. Ectopic pregnancy in the ampulla of the right fallopian tube *(arrow)* as seen at laparotomy.

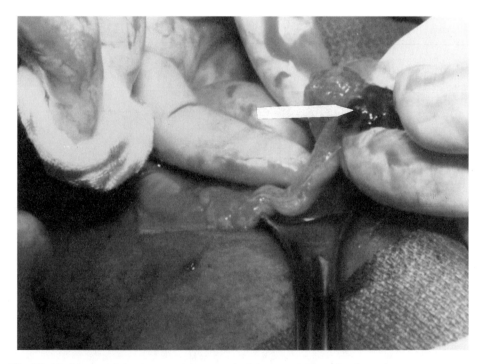

Fig. 51-12. Linear salpingostomy with removal of the ectopic gestation (arrow).

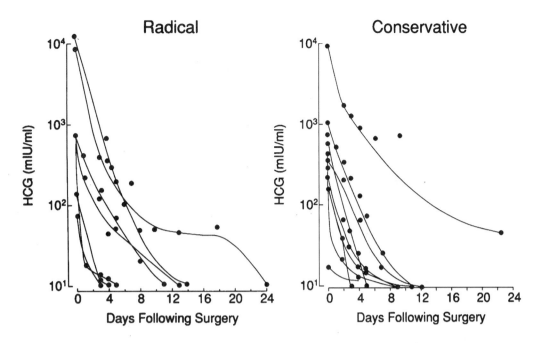

Fig. 51-13. β-hCG levels after radical (salpingectomy) and conservative (salpingostomy) surgery for ectopic pregnancy. (From Kamrava MM et al: Disappearance of human chorionic gonadotropin following removal of ectopic pregnancy, *Obstet Gynecol* 62:486-488, 1983. Reproduced with permission of The American College of Obstetricians and Gynecologists.)

subsequent intrauterine pregnancies in patients treated conservatively do not all occur through the contralateral tube. It also demonstrates that conservative surgery is successful in helping the patient achieve a pregnancy without increasing her risk of another ectopic pregnancy beyond that incurred by more radical treatment.

Patients who undergo linear salpingostomy are at risk of retaining active trophoblastic tissue. Under normal circumstances, β-hCG can be detected for as long as 12 days postoperatively[37] (Fig. 51-13). After this time period, the diagnosis of persistent ectopic pregnancy can be made and treatment options considered.

Laparoscopic linear salpingostomy. The performance of laparoscopic linear salpingostomy can be greatly enhanced by carefully stabilizing the fallopian tube both proximal and distal to the ectopic gestation (Fig. 51-14). An incision is made on the antimesenteric side of the tube at the point of maximal bulge. The trophoblast can then be gently teased from its implantation bed and irrigation applied to the site. Bleeding from the edge of the incision can be controlled with electrocautery. Bleeding from the base is often more difficult to control. Having two stabilizing graspers present in the abdomen, in addition to the operating port, allows the edges of the incision to be separated and the base more carefully inspected. A combination of careful localized electrocautery or simple pressure

with an atraumatic grasper at the site of hemorrhage in the implantation bed can often stop the bleeding.

Medical management

Methotrexate, a folic acid analogue used primarily in the treatment of gestational trophoblastic disease, was initially used for interstitial, cornual, and cervical ectopic pregnancies in which surgical therapy could lead to massive hemorrhage and result in a deformed uterus or even hysterectomy.[10,54,76,84] Primary medical treatment of ectopic pregnancy with the chemotherapeutic agent methotrexate is gaining in popularity. The medication can be given intramuscularly, orally,[57] or by direct injection into the ectopic gestation.[17,56,78]

Systemic therapy. Single- and multiple-dose regimens for systemic therapy have been proposed.[73,75] Commonly reported doses of methotrexate are (1) 50 mg/m² body surface area or (2) 1 mg/kg. The reported incidence of side effects with multiple-dose regimens ranges from 10% to 50%. These include nausea, elevated hepatic transaminase levels, leukopenia, and dermatitis. Reports of single-dose regimens indicate a lower incidence of these effects. Up to 20% of patients treated with methotrexate will ultimately require surgical intervention and therefore close follow-up is warranted.

After successful treatment, the hCG level declines and

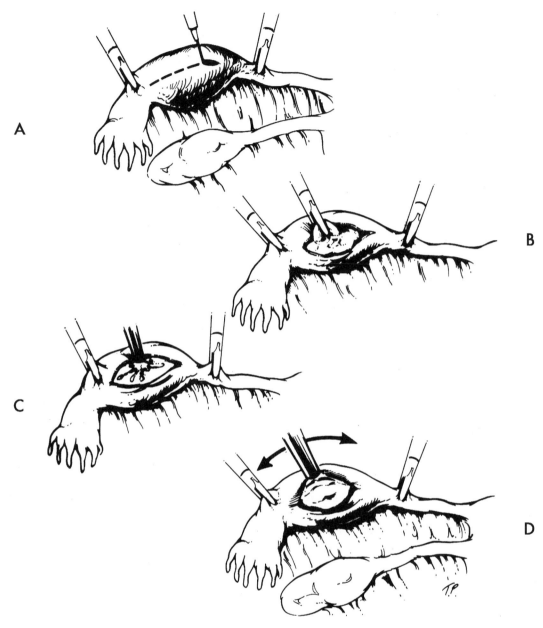

Fig. 51-14. Laparoscopic linear salpingostomy. **A,** The fallopian tube is stabilized proximal and distal to the ectopic pregnancy, pitressin is injected along the antimesenteric border at the point of maximal bulge, and the tube is incised in a linear fashion. **B,** The contents are gently removed. **C,** The bed is gently but copiously irrigated. **D,** The edges of the incision are grasped and the bed is examined with the laparoscope for residual tissue and hemostasis.

blood flow to the trophoblast declines (as indicated by a rising resistance to flow index); however, the intratubal mass remains (Fig. 51-15). It has been reported that the tubal mass may require as long as 3 months to resolve.[12] Stovall et al.[72] reported a post-treatment patency rate of 83% in 23 patients. Of these patients, 10 of 14 (71%) who attempted pregnancy achieved an intrauterine gestation.

Other agents that have been proposed for medical treatment of ectopic pregnancy include RU 486, actinomycin D, etoposide, and prostaglandins $F_{2\alpha}$ and E_2.

Direct injection. Whereas systemic medical therapy for ectopic pregnancy carries the risk of systemic side effects, injection of medication directly into the eccyesis has the theoretic appeal of avoiding these effects. Agents such as methotrexate, prostaglandin $F_{2\alpha}$, and hyperosmolar glucose have been used, with reports of success.[29,79] Local medical therapy can be administered at the time of diagnostic laparoscopy; however, advances in ultrasonographic technology have led advocates of local therapy toward ultrasonographically directed, transvaginal injection.

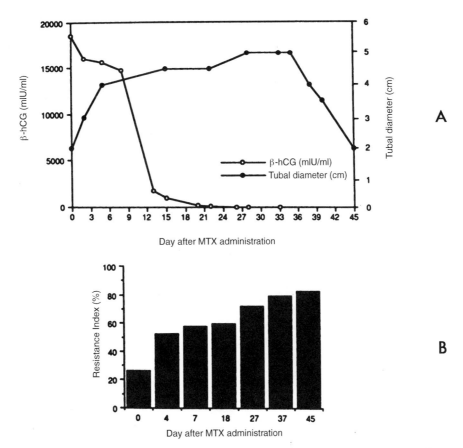

Fig. 51-15. A, Serum β-hCG levels and tubal diameter. **B,** Blood flow resistance index after methotrexate *(MTX)* administration in a patient with a tubal ectopic pregnancy. (From Tulandi T et al: Treatment of ectopic pregnancy by transvaginal intratubal methotrexate administration, *Obstet Gynecol* 77:627-630, 30, 1991. Reproduced with permission of The American College of Obstetricians and Gynecologists.)

The main advantage of transvaginal injection is that the patient avoids a laparoscopy. Variants of ultrasonographically directed transvaginal injection have been described and include transcervical cannulation of the fallopian tube.[61] The ultrasonographic appearance of a locally treated ectopic pregnancy can show enlargement with an increase in vascularity despite falling hCG levels. These changes might not indicate imminent rupture; on the contrary, they may reflect the healing process.[6]

Reproductive performance after local therapy has been reported to approximate that achieved with other forms of conservative treatment. One recent study reported an 86% tubal patency rate after therapy, with 70% achieving a subsequent pregnancy.[27] The presumption in direct injection therapy is that local therapy will decrease systemic exposure to significant levels of the treating agent. Furthermore, it is thought that there might be increased local concentration of the treating agent within the ectopic trophoblast. A recent study by Schiff et al.[67] compared the pharmacokinetics of methotrexate after local tubal administration by intramuscular (IM) injection. They found that after IM injection the peak level of methotrexate and the area under the curve were similar to the levels observed after intratubal injection. This finding challenges the purported advantages associated with local injection. Although early reports regarding local therapy were generally positive, Mottla et al.[49] recently attempted a randomized clinical trial comparing local methotrexate injection at laparoscopy with linear salpingostomy. They terminated the study prematurely because three of seven patients randomized to local methotrexate administration required reoperation and a fourth had a persistent ectopic pregnancy requiring a subsequent IM dose of methotrexate. These investigators propose an interesting hypothesis: if the methotrexate is not delivered directly to the trophoblast, it may be contained within a hematosalpinx and encapsulated in fibrinous material. The methotrexate may be unable to diffuse into local circulation and thus be inhibited from perfusing the trophoblastic tissue.

Although some evidence exists to recommend the use of laparoscopy in the treatment of ectopic pregnancy,[32] large-scale, randomized trials concerning minimally invasive methods such as local medical therapy are lacking, and the techniques should still be considered investigational.[40]

Expectant management

Although prompt surgical or medical treatment in cases of ectopic pregnancy have reduced the mortality of this disease, heightened awareness and better diagnostic tools may, in some cases, lead to premature intervention. The first prospective evaluation of expectant management was performed by Lund[41] in 1955. Group 1 consisted of 119 patients whose ectopic pregnancies were managed expectantly. These patients were compared with 85 patients who underwent immediate unilateral salpingectomy. Among those managed expectantly, 57% did not require surgery. Subsequent fertility in the two groups was not different, with 46% and 44% achieving an intrauterine pregnancy, respectively. More recently, Ylostalo et al.[86] followed 83 patients with decreasing levels of serum hCG in whom the diameter of the ectopic pregnancy was less than 4 cm and in whom there were no signs of rupture or acute bleeding by vaginal ultrasonography. In 57 patients (69%), spontaneous resolution occurred. Atri et al.[5] followed 13 patients with ectopic pregnancies ranging in size from 1 to 3.5 cm, with β-hCG levels less than 1000 IU/L. The serum β-hCG levels became undetectable within 3 to 45 days (mean 15.8 days). All ectopic pregnancies had completely resolved at follow-up transvaginal ultrasonography performed 10 to 63 days (mean 30 days) after initial examination. These investigators note that there was a detectable increase in the size of the ectopic pregnancy in 4 of the 13 patients and that an additional 4 ectopic pregnancies without detectable flow initially became mildly vascular during the course of resolution.

The difficulty with expectant management lies in selecting the proper patient. Certainly a patient with low, falling hCG titers should be considered; however, the ability to understand the risks involved and the ability to comply with instructions for follow-up are critical elements. Likewise, both patient and physician anxiety during the period of observation should be weighed against the potential risks associated with medical or surgical intervention. Finally, ultrasonographic changes such as enlargement of the ectopic pregnancy and an increase in vascularity do not appear to be good indicators of failed management, since these changes can be seen during the resolution phase. Although there have been no large-scale studies that examined subsequent tubal patency and conception rates, the collective experience seems to lean toward equivalence with conservative therapy.

CONCLUSION

Ectopic pregnancy is a common occurrence among women of reproductive age. The most important first step in diagnosis is suspecting that it may be present. Early suspicion combined with timely testing and appropriate intervention can effectively reduce the morbidity and mortality associated with the process.

REFERENCES

1. Anderson TL: Biomolecular markers for the window of uterine receptivity. In Yoshinaga K, editor: *Blastocyst implantation,* Serono Symposia USA, Boston, 1989, Adams Publishing Group.
2. Andolsek L, editor: *The Ljubljana abortion study 1971–1973,* Baltimore, 1974, National Institutes of Health Center for Population Research.
3. Atrash HK, Friede A, Hogue CJR: Ectopic pregnancy mortality in the United States, 1970–1983, *Obstet Gynecol* 70:817, 1987.
4. Atrash K et al: Maternal mortality in the United States, 1979–1986, *Obstet Gynecol* 76:1055, 1990.
5. Atri M, Bret PM, Tulandi T: Spontaneous resolution of ectopic pregnancy: initial appearance and evolution at transvaginal US, *Radiology* 186:83, 1993.
6. Atri M et al: Ectopic pregnancy: evolution after treatment with transvaginal methotrexate, *Radiology* 185:749, 1992.
7. Barnes AB et al: Fertility and outcome of pregnancy in women exposed in utero to diethylstilbestrol, *N Engl J Med* 302:609, 1980.
8. Batzer FR et al: Landmarks during the first forty-two days of gestation demonstrated by the β-subunit of human chorionic gonadotropin and ultrasound, *Am J Obstet Gynecol* 146:973, 1983.
9. Bradley WG, Fiske CE, Filly RA: The double sac sign of early intrauterine pregnancy: use in exclusion of ectopic pregnancy, *Radiology* 143:223, 1983.
10. Brandes MC et al: Treatment of cornual pregnancy with methotrexate: case report, *Am J Obstet Gynecol* 155:655, 1986.
11. Breen J: A 21 year survey of 654 ectopic pregnancies, *Am J Obstet Gynecol* 106:1004, 1986.
12. Brown DL et al: Serial endovaginal sonography of ectopic pregnancies treated with methotrexate, *Obstet Gynecol* 77:406, 1991.
13. Buck RH, Joubert SM, Norman RJ: Serum progesterone in the diagnosis of ectopic pregnancy: a valuable diagnostic test?, *Fertil Steril* 50:752, 1988.
14. Budowick M et al: Histopathology of the developing tubal ectopic pregnancy, *Fertil Steril* 34:169, 1980.
15. Cacciatore B et al: Suspected ectopic pregnancy: ultrasound findings and hCG levels assessed by an immunofluorometric assay, *Br J Obstet Gynaecol* 95:497, 1988.
16. Chlafke S, Enders AC: Cellular basis of interaction between trophoblast and uterus at implantation, *Biol Reprod* 12:41, 1975.
17. Clark L et al: Treatment of ectopic pregnancy with intraamniotic methotrexate: a case report, *Aust N Z J Obstet Gynaecol* 29:84-85, 1989.
18. Cousins L et al: Reproductive outcome of women exposed to diethylstilbestrol in utero, *Obstet Gynecol* 56:70, 1980.
19. Daling JR et al: Ectopic pregnancy in relation to previous induced abortion, *JAMA* 253:1005, 1985.
20. DeCherney AH, Cholst I, Naftolin F: Structure and function of the fallopian tubes following exposure to diethylstilbestrol (DES) during gestation, *Fertil Steril* 36:741, 1981.
21. DeCherney AH, Maheaux R, Naftolin F: Salpingostomy for ectopic pregnancy in the sole patent oviduct: reproductive outcome, *Fertil Steril* 37:619, 1982.
22. Dillon IH, Feyock A, Taylor KJ: Pseudogestational sacs: doppler US differentiation from normal or abnormal intrauterine pregnancies, *Radiology* 176:359, 1990.
23. Dorfman SF: Epidemiology of ectopic pregnancy, *Clin Obstet Gynecol* 30:173, 1987.
24. Dorfman SF et al: Ectopic pregnancy mortality, United States, 1979 to 1980: clinical aspects, *Obstet Gynecol* 64:386, 1984.
25. Ectopic Pregnancy—United States, 1984 and 1985, *MMWR* 37:637, 1988.

26. Edelman DA, Porter CW: The intrauterine device and ectopic pregnancy, *Adv Contracept* 2:55, 1986.

27. Egarter C et al: Reproductive performance after local and systemic prostaglandin for ectopic pregnancy, *Arch Gynecol Obstet* 252:45, 1992.

28. Elias S et al: Chromosome analysis of ectopic human conceptuses, *Am J Obstet Gynecol* 141:698, 1981.

29. Feichtinger W, Kemeter P: Conservative treatment of ectopic pregnancy by transvaginal aspiration under sonographic control and injection of methotrexate, *Lancet* 1:381, 1987.

30. Fossum GT, Davajan V, Kletzky O: Early detection of pregnancy with transvaginal ultrasound, *Fertil Steril* 49:788, 1988.

31. Franks AL et al: Contraception and ectopic pregnancy risk, *Am J Obstet Gynecol* 163:1120, 1990.

32. Grimes DA: Frontiers of operative laparoscopy: a review and critique of the evidence, *Am J Obstet Gynecol,* 166:1062, 1992.

33. Herbst AL et al: A comparison of pregnancy experience in DES-exposed and DES-unexposed daughters, *J Reprod Med* 24:62, 1980.

34. Herman A et al: The role of tubal pathology and other parameters in ectopic pregnancies occurring in in vitro fertilization and embryo transfer, *Fertil Steril* 54:864, 1990.

35. Hershlag A et al: Salpingoscopy: light microscopic and electron microscopic correlations, *Obstet Gynecol* 77:399, 1991.

36. Homm RJ, Holtz G, Garvin AJ: Isthmic ectopic pregnancy and salpingitis isthmica nodosa, *Fertil Steril* 48:756, 1987.

37. Kamrava MM et al: Disappearance of human chorionic gonadotropin following removal of ectopic pregnancy, *Obstet Gynecol* 62:486, 1983.

38. Kirby DRS: The transplantation of mouse eggs and trophoblast to extrauterine sites. In Daniel JC, editor: *Methods in mammalian embryology,* San Francisco, 1965 WH Freeman.

39. Levin AA et al: Ectopic pregnancy and prior induced abortion, *Am J Public Health* 72:263, 1982.

40. Lindblom B. Ectopic pregnancy: laparoscopic and medical treatment, *Curr Opin Obstet Gynecol* 4:400, 1992.

41. Lund JJ: Early ectopic pregnancy treated nonsurgically, *J Obstet Gynaecol Br Emp* 62:70, 1955.

42. Lundorff P et al: Persistent trophoblast after conservative treatment of tubal pregnancy: prediction and detection, *Obstet Gynecol* 77:129, 1991.

43. Majmudar B, Henderson PH III, Semple E: Salpingitis isthmica nodosa: a high-risk factor for tubal pregnancy, *Obstet Gynecol* 62:73, 1983.

44. Marchbanks PA et al: Risk factors for ectopic pregnancy: a population based study, *JAMA* 259:1823, 1988.

45. Mardh PA et al: *Chlamydia trachomatis* infections in patients with salpingitis, *N Engl J Med* 296:1377, 1977.

46. McBain JC et al: An unexpectedly high rate of ectopic pregnancy following the induction of ovulation with human pituitary and chorionic gonadotrophin, *Br J Obstet Gynaecol* 87:5, 1980.

47. Mitchell DE, McSwain HF, Peterson HB: Fertility after ectopic pregnancy, *Am J Obstet Gynecol* 161:576, 1989.

48. Molloy D et al: Multiple-sited (heterotopic) pregnancy after in vitro fertilization and gamete intrafallopian transfer, *Fertil Steril* 53:1068, 1990.

49. Mottla GL, Rulin MC, Guzick DS: Lack of resolution of ectopic pregnancy by intratubal injection of methotrexate, *Fertil Steril* 57:685, 1992.

50. Nyberg DA et al: Ultrasonographic differentiation of the gestational sac of early intrauterine pregnancy from the pseudogestational sac of ectopic pregnancy, *Radiology* 146:755, 1983.

51. Nyberg DA et al: Early pregnancy complications: endovaginal sonographic findings correlated with human chorionic gonadotropin levels, *Radiology* 167:619, 1988.

52. Oelsner G: Ectopic pregnancy in the sole remaining tube and the management of the patient with multiple ectopic pregnancies, *Clin Obstet Gynecol* 30:225, 1987.

53. Ory HW and the Women's Health Study: Ectopic pregnancy and intrauterine contraceptive devices: new perspectives, *Obstet Gynecol* 57:137, 1981.

54. Palti Z et al: Successful treatment of a viable cervical pregnancy with methotrexate, *Am J Obstet Gynecol* 161:1147, 1989.

55. Panayotou PP et al: Induced abortion and ectopic pregnancy, *Am J Obstet Gynecol* 114:507, 1972.

56. Pansky M et al: Local methotrexate injection: a nonsurgical treatment of ectopic pregnancy, *Am J Obstet Gynecol* 161:393, 1989.

57. Patsner B, Kenigsberg D: Successful treatment of persistent ectopic pregnancy with oral methotrexate therapy, *Fertil Steril* 50:982, 1988.

58. Pauerstein CJ et al: Anatomy and pathology of tubal pregnancy, *Obstet Gynecol* 67:301, 1986.

59. Pittaway DE, Wentz AC: Evaluation of early pregnancy by serial chorionic gonadotropin determinations: a comparison of methods by receiver operating characteristic curve analysis, *Fertil Steril* 43:529, 1985.

60. Poland BJ, Dill FJ, Styblo C: Embryonic development in ectopic human pregnancy, *Teratology* 14:315, 1976.

61. Risquez F et al: Transcervical cannulation of the fallopian tube for the management of ectopic pregnancy: prospective multicenter study, *Fertil Steril* 58:1131, 1992.

62. Robertson JN, Hogdton P, Ward ME: Gonococcal and chlamydial antibodies in ectopic and intrauterine pregnancy, *Br J Obstet Gynaecol* 95:711, 1988.

63. Roht LH, Aoyama H: Induced abortion and its sequelae: Prevalence and associations with outcome of pregnancy, *Int J Epidemiol* 2:103, 1973.

64. Romero R et al: Diagnosis in ectopic pregnancy: value of the discriminatory human chorionic gonadotropin zone, *Obstet Gynecol* 66:357, 1985.

65. Romero R et al: Value of culdocentesis in the diagnosis of ectopic pregnancy, *Obstet Gynecol* 65:519, 1985.

66. Sawazaki C, Tanaka S: The relationship between artificial abortion and extrauterine pregnancy. In *Harmful effects of induced abortion,* Tokyo, 1966, Family Planning Federation of Japan.

67. Schiff E et al: Pharmacokinetics of methotrexate after local tubal injection for conservative treatment of ectopic pregnancy, *Fertil Steril* 57:688, 1992.

68. Schmidt G et al: Reproductive history of women exposed to diethylstilbestrol in utero, *Fertil Steril* 33:21, 1980.

69. Seifer DB et al: Persistent ectopic pregnancy following laparoscopic linear salpingostomy, *Obstet Gynecol* 76:1121, 1990.

70. Shapiro BS et al: Transvaginal ultrasonography for the diagnosis of ectopic pregnancy, *Fertil Steril* 50:425, 1988.

71. Siegler AM, Wang CF, Friberg J: Fertility of the diethylstilbestrol-exposed offspring, *Fertil Steril* 31:601, 1979.

72. Stovall TG, Ling FW, Buster JE: Reproductive performance after methotrexate treatment of ectopic pregnancy, *Am J Obstet Gynecol* 162:1620, 1990.

73. Stovall TG, Ling FW, Gray LA: Single-dose methotrexate for treatment of ectopic pregnancy, *Obstet Gynecol* 77:754, 1991.

74. Stovall TG et al: Preventing ruptured ectopic pregnancy with a single serum progesterone, *Am J Obstet Gynecol* 160:1425, 1989.

75. Stovall TG et al: Methotrexate treatment of unruptured ectopic pregnancy: a report of 100 cases, *Obstet Gynecol* 77:749, 1991.

76. Tanaka T et al: Treatment of interstitial pregnancy with methotrexate: report of a successful case, *Fertil Steril* 37:851, 1982.

77. Taylor K et al: Ectopic pregnancy: duplex doppler evaluation, *Radiology* 173:93, 1989.

78. Tulandi T et al: Treatment of ectopic pregnancy by transvaginal intratubal methotrexate administration, *Obstet Gynecol* 77:627, 1991.

79. Tulandi T et al: Transvaginal intratubal methotrexate treatment of ectopic pregnancy, *Fertil Steril* 58:98, 1992.

80. Walters MD et al: Antibodies to *Chlamydia trachomatis* and risk for tubal pregnancy, *Am J Obstet Gynecol* 159:942, 1988.

81. Washington AE, Katz P: Ectopic pregnancy in the United States:

economic consequences and payment source trends, *Obstet Gynecol* 81:287, 1993.

82. Westrom L, Bengtsson LP, Mardh PA: Incidence, trends and risks of ectopic pregnancy in a population of women, *Br Med J* 252:15, 1981.

83. Wilson JC: A prospective New Zealand study of fertility after removal of copper intrauterine contraceptive devices for conception and because of complications: a four year study, *Am J Obstet Gynecol* 160:391, 1989.

84. Yankowitz J et al: Cervical ectopic pregnancy: review of the literature and report of a case treated by single-dose methotrexate therapy, *Obstet Gynecol Surv* 45:405, 1990.

85. Yeko TR et al: Timely diagnosis of early ectopic pregnancy using a single blood progesterone measurement, *Fertil Steril* 48:1048, 1987.

86. Ylostalo P et al: Expectant management of ectopic pregnancy, *Obstet Gynecol* 80:345, 1992.

87. Yovich JL, Turner SR, Murphy AJ: Embryo transfer technique as a cause of ectopic pregnancies in in vitro fertilization, *Fertil Steril* 44:318, 1985.

88. Yovich JL et al: Heterotopic pregnancy from in vitro fertilization, *J In Vitro Fert Embryo Transfer* 2:146, 1985.

Chapter 52

PHYSIOLOGY OF LACTATION AND BREASTFEEDING

John E. Tyson, MD

The human breast is viewed consistently as an accessory sex organ contributing to the completion of the mammalian reproductive cycle through the provision of nutrition to the neonate. Subjected as it is to the enormous fluctuations in maternal hormone secretion, both in intrauterine life and thereafter, the mammary gland should be redefined as a major organ responsible for preservation of the species,[105] for it not only facilitates maternal-fetal bonding,[59] but provides essential immunobiological components that have been elucidated over the past decade and that provide for the survival of the newborn until it achieves immunological competence. The rejection and/or abandonment of breastfeeding enhances the risk of infant mortality.[5,73]

Harmonious gestational metabolic interactions between the maternal and fetal compartments are a prerequisite, not only to intrauterine fetal growth and development, but to the creation of a maternal reserve energy for the future nutritional and immunological support of the neonate.[94]

During the first trimester of pregnancy, enhanced maternal lipid storage is facilitated by increased sensitivity to circulating insulin concentrations. Hepatic glycogen storage is also increased, and more efficient protein metabolism is present. Although most authors account for maternal weight gain by citing an inventory of organ-system weight gain, increased deposition of adipose tissue anticipates neonatal caloric needs that are available and distributed through breastfeeding.

The breasts' ability to lactate is acquired early in gestation. Breast secretions arise in unsuppressed postabortal women as early as the 16th week of gestation. However, little has been reported on the composition of such secretions, or whether or not immunological protection is afforded a neonate if such "milk" were ingested.

INTRAUTERINE BREAST DEVELOPMENT

Because puerperal lactational performance relies on a competent endocrinologically prepared mammary gland, the development of the primordial breast during embryogenesis serves as an important benchmark against which future abnormalities of breast development and function may be measured. A comprehensive review is provided by Vorherr.[125] Beginning in the fifth week of gestation, a 2-4 cell streak of ectodermal tissue becomes a galactic band, doubling in size by the sixth week. At this time, the thoracic mammary ridge becomes apparent, while an involution of any remaining tissue occurs. However, if subinvolution of the mammary streak is apparent, there may be subsequent supernumerary mammary tissue, whether complete or incomplete. In the adult this is seen as pigmented nipples along the milk line.

At the seventh gestational week, the round ectodermal mammary ridge migrates immediately to invaginate and form the disc stage, where the cells are seen as a globular protrusion in the overlying skin. This globular stage is characterized by multidirectional invasion of the mesenchyme. At eight weeks, a conical invagination of the epithelial anlage occurs from the globular configuration previously seen. Complete between the 12th and 16th weeks of gestation, the overlying skin becomes indented, while mesenchymal cells differentiate to form smooth muscle cells in both the nipple and the areola.

Differentiation of the duct tissue occurs between the 15th and 25th weeks of intrauterine life, giving rise to the secondary mammary anlage, which ultimately evolves into the surrounding sebaceous and sweat glands of the areola. The mammary gland adopts special apocrine and holocrine functions thereafter. Such functions are divided between the areolar sebaceous glandular tissue and the areolar tissue of the breast.

Beyond the sixth month of gestation, 15-25 mammary ducts merge with sebaceous glands at the epidermal surface to form the fetal mammary gland. Thus, it is possible to date a gestation based upon pathological evaluation of such fetal tissue.[122] Throughout the remainder of gestation, increasing canalization with vascular fibers of fatty tissue occurs and the mammary gland increases four-fold in size, assuming the capability of producing colostrum between the 32nd and 34th weeks of gestation. Circular elliptical structures of smooth muscle are in place and the areola, which is gland- and hair-free, indents to become pigmented, while the mammary ducts converge into a central duct with an exterior ostium. Under the influence of maternal estrogen, the epidermis of the areola mammae is thickened, and squamous epithelial components extend into the infundibular part of the milk duct to produce sebaceous discharge.

Subcutaneous connective tissue serves as a supporting structure for the glandular elements and divides into three layers in the latter part of gestation. A superficial layer, consisting of connective tissues, attaches to overlying corium and surrounds the primary mammary anlage. An intermediate zone surrounds the ducts and extends into the peripheral connective tissue, while an interconnective tissue layer is highly vascular and contains the longitudinal capillaries that ultimately serve the alveoli. Even in intrauterine life, mammary tissue is found to contain hematological cellular components, including red cells, lymphocytelike cells, mass cells, histiocytes, and leucocytes. The differentiation of the vascular system during this time can be used to confirm fetal age (please refer to the box below).[122]

Cellular differentiation of the mammary-vascular system

Gestational weeks

7	Erythroblast and premature blood vessels
9 - 10	Vessel budding
12	Capillary formation and connective tissue
13	Vascular network divided into three zones

Because of the influence of maternal hormones in late gestation, features of mammary growth and development, principally lobular growth, may be increased, leading to postnatal mammary secretion. However, the breast does not regress after delivery, and studies of tissue from the breasts of infants succumbing to sudden infant death syndrome (SIDS) between three months and two years of age show no sex difference in the tissue.[122] Well-formed ducts and apocrine secretions within these ducts are associated with adult-type fat. Myoepithelial cells are preserved, but premature red and white blood cells suggest that extramedullary erythroypoiesis occurs. Thus, these studies show that postpartum neonatal mammary involution takes many months, and the role of elevated prolactin concentrations suggests that both estradiol, and possibly testosterone, play a role in breast development.[76,77]

PUBERTAL DEVELOPMEENT

Moving from a stage of relative quiescence, the mammary gland begins to develop through its second developmental stage at the time of puberty.

Thelarche is marked by the further branching of the ductal system, maturation of the alveolar network, and the acquisition of cellular precursors that make lactation possible.[26]

The pubertal surge in gonadotropin-releasing hormone (GnRH), and the subsequent increase in peripheral concentrations of follicle-stimulating hormone (FSH) promote excitation of steroidogenic function of ovarian tissue. However, six months prior to the onset of menstruation, mammary growth is clearly detected, where estrogen, principally estradiol, stimulates the growth in allometric elongation of the mammary ducts with reduplication of the lining. Tissue sprouts and lobular buds for future breast lobules are observed. The volume and elasticity of periductal connective tissue increases, along with vascularization and fat deposition. These changes are the first major increase in the preadolescent breast.[82]

At the time of puberty, ductal and periductal growth is under the control of the cyclic concentrations of both estradiol and progesterone. However, it should be emphasized that earlier, between the approximate ages of eight and 10, breast bud growth and fat deposition begin as a precursor matrix for subsequent parenchyma.

Beyond puberty, visible and often symptomatic changes occur premenstrually in the breast, including lobular edema with epithelial basement membrane thickening and increased alveolar diameter and secretory activity.

Fluctuations in breast size can be noted as regression of endocrine support in the luteal phase of the menstrual cycle, leading to reduced lobular alveolar size and a degeneration of the glandular cells. However, it is important to note that the mammary ductal proliferation and alveolar branching that occurs during estrogen stimulation never really de-

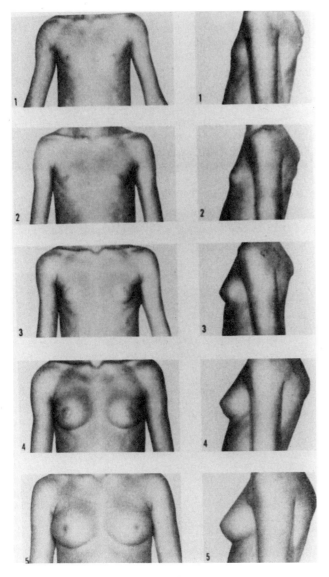

Fig. 52-1. Phases of breast growth

PHASE 1	Preadolescent evaluation of the mammilla (nipple only)
PHASE 2	Mammillary growth and sprouting of subnuclear ductule breast tissue with the formation and protrusion of nipple and increased diameter of the areola (age 10-12)
PHASE 3	Nipple growth, budding of breast tissues with contours remaining the same (age 12-14)
PHASE 4	An areola elevation with increased growth of subareolar tissue. Globular shape to the breast (age 14-15)
PHASE 5	Development of mature breast in response to cyclic estradiol and progesterone stimulation. Mammillary protrusion associated with isometric growth and proportionate to body size (age 15 and beyond)

(From Tanner JM: *Wachstrum und reifung des Menschen.* Stuttgart, Thieme.)

clines to premenstrual dimensions. Thus, cyclic hormone-dependent increases in breast tissue continue up to the age of 35. There is no longstanding augmentation of breast size that occurs as a result of pregnancy, whereas the accumulation of fat tissue during pregnancy is rapidly lost in the first few months of postpartum breastfeeding.

Phases of breast growth are shown in Fig. 52-1. When Phase IV of breast development is reached, enhanced peripubertal growth of the breast can be achieved if pregnancy occurs, especially in early adolescence. The effect of this growth on the mammary gland may be sufficient to provide some maternal protection from the subsequent development of breast cancer as claimed from recent epidemiological studies.[58,68,83] Although some attribute this protection to prolonged ovarian quiescence and decreased hormonal stimulation of the breast by estrogen and progesterone,[89] nursing-induced migration of lymphocytes, immunoglobulins, and antimitogenic agents may offer protection locally against viral oncogens.

LYMPHATIC NEURAL AND VASCULAR CONSIDERATIONS

The lymphatic, neural, and vascular anatomy of the breasts is shown in Fig. 52-2. Supplied with a generous network of lymphatics, the breasts are drained by two systems, consistent with a cutaneous areolar and a glandular network. Most somatic sensory and autonomic motor nerves innervate the breast. Somatic sensory innervation of the nipple and the areolar is abundant, and postganglionic unmyelinated sympathetic fibers from the thoracic paravertebral bodies follow the mammary vessels because there is no known direct innervation of mammary epithelial cells.

Sympathetic nervous stimulation of the mammary gland is displayed as concentrations within the smooth muscle both of the nipple and the areola. The release of norepinephrine induces stimulation of myoepithelial β-adrenergic receptors, causing muscular relaxation.[126] Similarly, lactiferous ducts are innervated by sensory fibers. The neuroafferent reflex component induces the adequate release of both prolactin and oxytocin,[1a,2,20] and, as described below, the separation of both the stimulation of milk synthesis and its subsequent secretion can be identified.

The major sensory cutaneous innervation of the areola and nipple is from the fourth and sixth intercostal nerves, which carry autonomic motor fibers to the smooth muscle of both the areola and the nipple. The sensory innervation of the areola and nipple elicits responses to temperature change, touch, and pain. These fibers run radially to the glandular body. Sympathetic postganglionic fibers from the second to the sixth intercostal and supraclavicular nerves innervate the smooth muscles of the areola, the nipple, and the mammary blood vessels. The dynamic interaction between neural afferent stimulation, vascular, and lymphatic responses to such stimulation emphasizes the

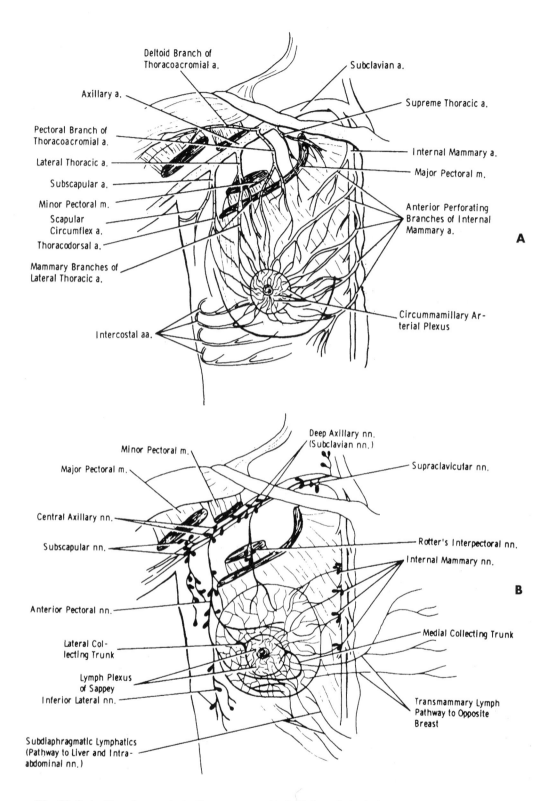

Fig. 52-2. A, Vascular supply to the mammary gland; **B,** Lymphatc drainage;

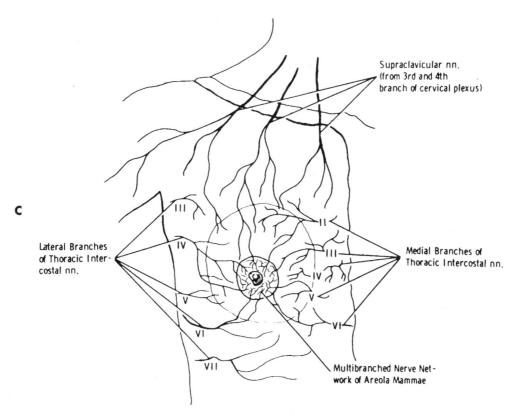

Fig. 52-2. C, Mammary nervous innervation (From Vorherr H: *The breast; morphology, physiology and lactation,* New York, 1974, Academic Press.)

importance of an anatomically intact mammary gland for breastfeeding.

EPIDEMIOLOGY OF BREASTFEEDING

The acceptability and adoption of breastfeeding as a biological necessity of infant nutrition in the first months of life has varied worldwide over the last 40 years.[52] Cultural and socioeconomic differences have led to various approaches in support of breastfeeding.[22,23] Where adequate adult nutrition is unavailable due to scarce food supplies, breastfeeding has proven the only economical way of managing the newborn infant.[74] In such cases, adequate maternal caloric intake serves two individuals. Continuous effort, however, is required by government agencies to maintain public support for breastfeeding.

During the 1970s, in some developing countries, breastfeeding was discouraged.[29] The provision of free or subsidized artificial nutritional sources for the newborn was considered politically appropriate as it implied advanced social status. Women were informed that breastfeeding represented poor socioeconomic standing. To be able to afford or to receive gratuitous infant formula became a symbol of success.[92] Unfortunately, infant mortality rates rose and were eventually linked to the widespread nonmaternal infant food supply. In the late 1970s and the early 1980s, resurgence in both the interest in and practice of breastfeeding occurred.

The simplification of infant formula preparations, product pricing, and the assumption of prosperity when women breastfeed has now increased a global move toward lactation suppression.[92] However, despite all presumed physiological benefits to both mother and child, breastfeeding has once again experienced a decline as sophisticated socialization takes place.[29]

An increasing number of women entering the workplace by necessity has created a definite sign of increasing gender parity. However, the perceived economic gains from women entering the workplace mitigates against such women remaining at home for long periods. As a result, not only is age at the time of first childbearing advancing, the requirement to return to work has forced more and more mothers to reduce the period of peripheral lactation. In anthropological studies, Margaret Mead observed that "ladies" stopped breastfeeding because they were not animals and had wet nurses.[79] The introduction of bottle-feeding became a marvelous, labor-saving device for all concerned.

Now employers and governments are adopting policies that include spousal benefits associated with pregnancy and childbearing that may benefit breastfeeding mothers up to 29 weeks. Specialists in reproductive medicine, therefore, must consider breastfeeding as a positive influence,[84] not only for the initial neonatal benefits to behavior and nutrition, but more important, for the potential benefits to continued maternal health and disease prevention, including prevention of breast, ovarian, and uterine malignancy.

The implementation of breastfeeding reduces the incidence of neonatal upper respiratory tract infections,[3,55] and decreases infant mortality due to intestinal bacteria.[51] Necrotizing enterocolitis and diarrheal diseases are also notably reduced.[70] Sudden infant death assigned to overwhelming systemic infection may also be reduced. Combined, the reduction in infant mortality due to breastfeeding is reportedly 4:100,000 of all births, and among the diseases felt to be delayed in onset or averted by breastfeeding are regional ileitis, celiac disease, lymphoma, atopic dermatitis, and autoimmune thyroiditis.[7] The extrapolation of the benefits of breastfeeding up to the first six months of life clearly outweigh the disadvantages of time and effort expended.

The definition of breastfeeding should be taken into consideration by caregivers involved in evaluating lactation. Breastfeeding may be defined as *full,* meaning *without any substitution,* or *partial,* where *variable nutritional supplements,* usually fruit, are supplied. Bottle-feeding leads to the increased risk of neonatal infection, depending on the local water supply. Thus, obstetricians who remain neutral in the decisions of women to breastfeed might appear, by default, to encourage formula feeding.[84] Modifiers to the acceptance of breastfeeding as a promoter of disease include maternal age; birth order of the proband;

the social, economic, and educative status of the mother; and the standards of infant care that are available in a given jurisdiction, including the availability of daycare.[23]

Industrialization has had a negative impact on breastfeeding. Although the traditional hunter-gatherer society utilized prolonged breastfeeding exclusively and provided infant spacing of up to 24 months,[62] this was accompanied by culturally sanctioned abstinence for similar periods. Industrialization critically curtailed the duration of breastfeeding with a resulting increase in the need for alternative interventions directed at child spacing. Introduction of infant formulas had an adverse effect on infant survival in the first year of life, and also increased the risk of pregnancy by reducing the period of natural infertility that normally follows parturition.[52,119]

With the introduction of clinical/mechanical means of contraception, breastfeeding once again declined, and with it, the benefits to the neonate.[9] Fig. 52-3 presents a schematic of three evolutionary periods related to declines in breastfeeding and child spacing.

GESTATIONAL CHANGES IN MAMMARY ARCHITECTURE

A specific and ordered cascade of pregnancy-specific maternal endocrine events induces further mammary growth and development. These include ductal growth, extension of the lobular differentiation and proliferation, alveolar growth, and secretory activity.[117]

The first trimester of pregnancy is marked by ductal

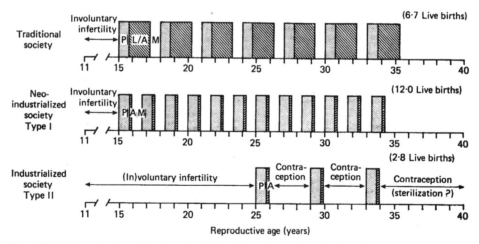

Fig. 52-3. Reproductive behavior is depicted in three theoretical settings. In a traditional aboriginal society, menarche was followed by a period of sexual abstinence based on cultural norms. This was followed by pregnancy (P), a prolonged period of lactational amenorrhea (L/A), and anovulation followed by a brief period of menses (M). Infant mortality might remove as many as two children from the family, regardless of lactation.

Better sanitation, housing, and nutrition, along with industrialization and urbanization, reduced the period of L/A and resulted in a population explosion.

In today's industrialized and technologically advanced society, contraception has reduced by L/A and P rates. Western societies now turn to advanced reproductive technologies to overcome increasing infertility in males and females.[17] (From Tyson JE: Neuroendocrine control of lactational infertility. In Fertility regulation during human lactation, *J Biosoc Sci Suppl* 4:23, 1977.)

sprouting and lobular formation; by eight weeks, the enlarged breast shows dilated veins and increased turgor. Nipple and alveolar pigmentation are also exaggerated. In midpregnancy, the early formation of colostrum is concealed by a lack of specific secretion from the nipple; however, at midpregnancy, epithelial proliferation is decreased while acinar activity is increased. Lactation may occur as early as 14-16 weeks with the acute interruption of pregnancy, as in elective abortion. Secretion at this time is colostrum-like; however; true colostrum is not apparent until the third trimester of pregnancy.[24]

PROLACTIN (PRL) AND LACTATION

From the initial studies of Erdheim and Stumme, investigators have proven a gestationally dependent increase in pituitary size and volume, related principally to hypertrophy and hyperplasia with prolactin-secreting cells of the pituitary gland.[30] These cells, which contain large nuclei and an increased cytoplasmic fraction, increase in size due to the unopposed stimulation of the lactotrope by increasing circulating concentrations of estradiol. Increased pituitary weight up to 1.5 µg/mg of wet weight has been identified.[110] However, this weight increase is not associated with an increase in the volume or size of peripheral pituitary cells, including growth hormone-secreting cells. Somatotrope cells remain relatively dormant through pregnancy, as reflected in the suppression of peripheral growth hormone concentrations observed beyond the 12th week of gestation, following the administration of an arginine infusion, or insulin-induced hyperglycemia.[114,116]

Likewise, the release of PRL into the medium by monkey pituitary cells is increased when such cells are obtained from the pituitaries of pregnant animals.

The role of PRL on mammary growth and development throughout gestation remains speculative, although there is some evidence to support the regulatory role of PRL on salt and water balance across the alveolar membrane. The role of insulin, cortisol, growth hormone, estradiol, progesterone, and PRL during gestation is well documented in the animal model. During gestation, peripheral PRL concentrations rise from 5-20 mg/ml to as high as 300 mg/ml at term. (Fig. 52-4). There is a multiphasic pattern of PRL release during labor and delivery,[75] the mechanisms of which may be related to alterations in central dopamine turnover.[97] PRL secretion during the third trimester of pregnancy has been tested both through the administration of thyrotropin releasing hormone (TRH) and with direct nipple stimulation.[4,118] The release of PRL in this stage of gestation is equally blunted with the administration of dopamine agonists.[124] The gradually increasing secretion of PRL is noted following the intravenous administration of TRH in various stages of pregnancy. However, corrected for blood volume, PRL response in late gestation is four to five times that of earlier gestation, related perhaps to the high circulating concentrations of estradiol, mentioned previously. No engorgement or milk let-down is noted in response to such secretion, due once again to the negative effects high peripheral concentrations of progesterone have on mammary cell enzymes that induce milk production.

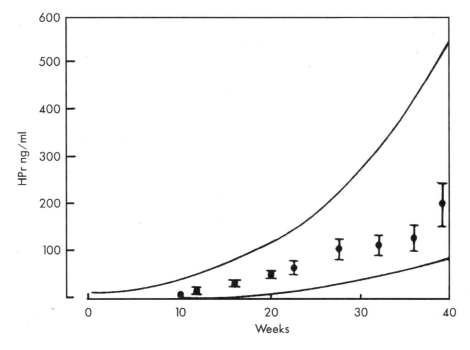

Fig. 52-4. Mean basal PRL serum levels in normal women during gestation. (From Tyson JE, et al: Studies of prolactin secretion in human pregnancy, *Am J Obstet Gynecol* 113:14, 1972.)

At delivery, the removal of the principal steroid-hormone producing organ, the placenta, creates an accelerated decline in the peripheral concentration of estradiol and progesterone. During gestation, the actions of PRL on the mammary gland are blunted in two ways. First, by estrogen at the PRL receptor; second, by progesterone, which is known to attenuate or inhibit the activation of N-acetyllactosamine synthetase, which is responsible for the production of lactose.

Studies in the authors' laboratory have shown the total absence of growth hormone is no impairment to the production of milk in the immediate puerperium.[112] Indeed, physiological suppression of growth hormone secretion in the normal individual is noted in postpartum studies using insulin-induced hyperglycemia or arginine infusion.[67,116]

Differences also appear in the secretion of growth hormone (hGH) and PRL between lactating and nonlactating women, suggesting a potential reciprocal relationship that may be mediated more by neurotransmitter secretion than by peripheral estrogen concentrations. In breastfeeding, PRL levels are elevated and hGH response to provocative stimuli is low. In nonbreastfeeding women, hGH secretion has returned to prepregnancy levels by the 28th postpartum day.

The profile of postpartum PRL secretion is based upon the temporal relationship of the stimulus to delivery, and the duration of the stimulus. PRL release can be provoked within the first 72 hours postpartum and thereafter by direct nipple stimulation. Oophorectomy, on the other hand, has no effect on lactation. Although the initiation of lactation is known to be PRL dependent, its maintenance may depend more upon an elevated basal concentration of PRL than

acute increments observed after varying periods of nursing. Fig. 52-5 presents the normal incremental differences in PRL secretion in response to fixed periods of suckling in healthy postpartum lactating women. Pituitary responsiveness to neural excitation at the level of the nipple appears to depend on intensity of sucking in that the application of stimulation to both nipples simultaneously, as in the case of suckling twins, can as much as triple the output of PRL; milk yield and composition may also be affected.[101,121] However, the destruction of a direct connection between somatic sensory nerves and the nipple, as in the case of breast augmentation or reduction with nipple removal and reimplantation, removes a woman's ability to nurse, as well as the provoking effect of suckling on the release of PRL. Likewise, anesthetizing the nipples of healthy, postpartum nursing mothers reduces and, in some instances, completely ablates the peripheral PRL response. Notably, under such circumstances there is a reduction in the overall volume of milk produced.[119]

The release of PRL during a 15-minute nursing interval may not be responsible for activating either a let-down or production of milk during that feeding. Rather, subsequent milk production is predicated on the frequency, duration, and intensity of the suckling stimulus. These factors not only define the yield of milk, but in many instances, its composition and subsequent volume.[118,120] However, milk volume often is directly related to the state of maternal hydration, as well as to the nutritional and fluid needs of the nursing infant.

A quantitative measure of both the frequency and duration of nursing is possible, as can be seen in Fig. 52-6. However, the variable of intensity is much more difficult to

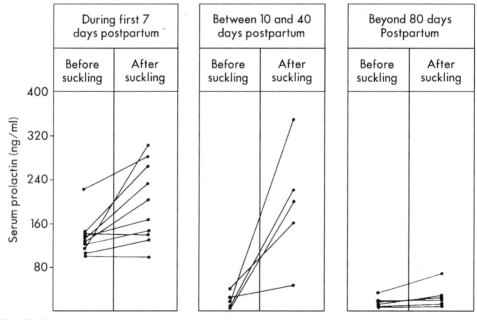

Fig. 52-5. Serum PRL responses to nipple stimulation during nursing at the time of the first morning breastfeed. (From Tyson JE, Friesen HG, Anderson MS: Human lactational and ovarian response to endogenous prolactin release, *Science* 177:897, 1972.)

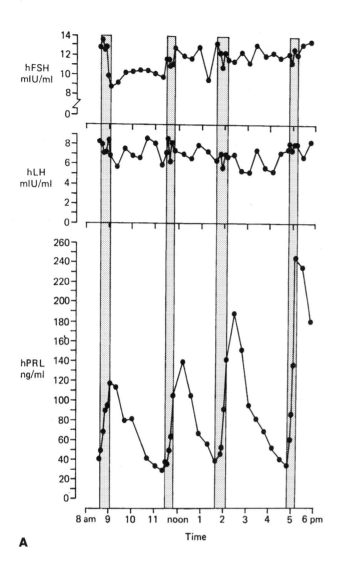

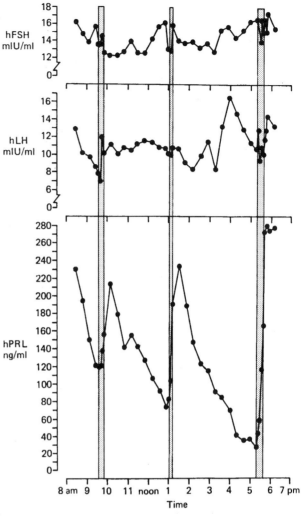

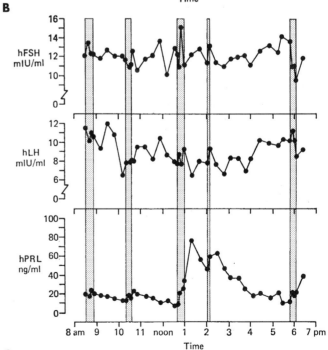

Fig. 52-6. Three examples of PRL secretion in response to variable frequencies and durations of nipple stimulation by nursing infants (hatched areas indicate nursing interval).

(A)   Frequent, scheduled, demand feedings, each of 15 minutes duration. Gradual increase in PRL increments. -39 days postpartum.

(B)   Nursing of infrequent and short duration in immediate puerperium. Pituitary excitability is marked. -41 days postpartum.

(C)   Frequent, demand feeding beyond the third postpartum month. Note low to absent PRL response. -56 days postpartum.

(From Tyson JE: Neuroendocrine control of lactational infertility. In Fertility regulation during human lactation, *J Biosoc Sci Suppl* 4:23, 1977.)

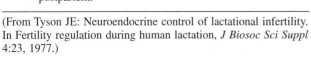

quantitate because it depends on the negative pressure of the infant's sucking. Indeed, after the 18th postpartum month, women who continue to breastfeed frequently are noted to have no significant increase in peripheral PRL concentration.

Breast milk can be synthesized and stored up to 48 hours without material changes in the rate of milk synthesis. However, breast engorgement and involuntary milk let-down occurs in some instances. PRL secretion is measurably related to the frequency, duration, and intensity of nipple stimulation, as can be shown when twins are applied to the same breasts consecutively, or to both breasts concurrently, in a lactating woman.

OXYTOCIN AND HUMAN LACTATION

The nonopeptide, oxytocin, is synthesized in cells of the paraventricular and supraoptic nuclei of the brain. Stimulating the nipple sends impulses via efferent somatosensory fibers via the spinal column and ipsolateral dorsolateral funiculus to the lateral cervical nucleus. Oxytocin is then released and moves from an average basal concentration of 0.7 ± 0.1 μU/ml[53] to as high as 5.9 ± 0.5 μU/ml within three minutes. Such an elevation is still evident approximately 15 minutes after the elicited stimulus.[71] The mean cumulative oxytocin concentration in the peripheral plasma of women who are nursing is significantly higher in breastfeeding on demand. The mean stimulated oxytocin concentration is elevated in response to suckling in a consistent fashion between the fourth and 11th postnatal weeks.[78]

The suckling-induced increase in oxytocin has been shown to be blocked by drugs that disrupt the α-noradrenergic transmission, including synthesis inhibition and α-adrenergic receptor blockade.[14] Escalation of the oxytocin response by an α-adrenergic stimulus is perhaps equal to the physiological component of milk ejection; however, dopamine receptors are involved in the secretion of oxytocin, and dopamine has been shown to be excitatory to the release of oxytocin through the D_1 receptor, where positive coupling to adenylate cyclase occurs. The hormone, however, is negatively coupled to the D_2 dopamine agonist. D_2DA agonists inhibit oxytocin release indirectly via PRL, which is inhibited by the D_2DA agonist, but stimulated by D_2 receptor agonists parallel with oxytocin. With a half-life of 1.5 minutes, the turnover rate of oxytocin is exceedingly high. However, its action at the level of the mammary myoepithelial cell brings about a contraction of the ducts, which in turn shorten, widen, and then eject the milk by toxic contraction.[38, 39, 126]

Studies on milk ejection suggest that oxytocin release is selective for nipple stimulation, except for osmoregulatory homeostasis. Oxytocin release also increases in response to pain, cold, heat, and immobilization stress in laboratory animals. An increase in osmolarity associated with hypovolemia may also be associated with changes in oxytocin secretion.[6] Neural outbursts of oxytocin have been reported

to occur in response to nipple stimulation, the amplitude and frequency of which are synchronized with the release of oxytocin from pituitary explants.[21] However, continuous nipple stimulation does not change the frequency of such bursts. If the maternal organism is dehydrated, as might occur postpartum, oxytocin firing increases and the amplitude of each burst is increased.[6] Because oxytocin and vasopressin neurons are interwoven, selected stimulation and firing occurs.[56] Magnicellular neurons of the supraoptic nucleus and paraventricular nucleus have membranous apposition, which might explain the dual response.

Further understanding of the role of oxytocin in milk let-down has been observed in the use of the oxytocin contraction test.[44,50,100] Peripheral oxytocin concentrations were increased in association with up to 30 minutes of nipple stimulation. The release also occurred in pulses, and more important, can provoke uterine contractions. The oxytocin release under these circumstances, however, is much less than that seen in the postpartum period.[13] Oxytocin release does not affect the levels of adrenocorticotropic hormone (ACTH), cortisol, or growth hormone[86] Corticotropin releasing hormone- (CRH) induced release of ACTH, however, is inhibited by oxytocin; secretion of PRL and growth hormone are not.[17] Oxytocin and PRL can be released in the nonpuerperal state and increases in peripheral oxytocin concentration have been noted after TRH-induced PRL secretion during the menstrual cycle.[16] It is clear, though, that oxytocin release is cyclic and, under most circumstances, is designed to bring about contractions of paraductal smooth muscle normally found in the mammary gland.[126]

MILK YIELD DURING PHYSIOLOGICAL FULL LACTATION

In the last 6-8 weeks of gestation, a dramatic rise in peripheral PRL concentration is observed, coincident with the onset of colostrum production. Colostrum's composition is identified under normal circumstances between birth and the third postpartum day.[18] Transitional milk is identified between the third and seventh day, when concentrations of lactose and fat begin to rise. Although transitional milk is rich in immunoglobulins, true milk has a consistent composition of lactose, fat, and protein beyond the seventh day; components vary, depending upon the intensity and frequency of each nursing stimulus. Peripheral elevations in the concentration of oxytocin and PRL are observed beginning at the fourth postpartum day, and continues up to third or fourth month.[44] Thereafter, little if any change is seen in response to suckling. Studies have shown that PRL stimulates nuclear ribonucleic acid (RNA) polymerase activity, which in turn gives rise to the synthesis of messenger RNA within the alveolar and syncytial cells of the breast. In suckling, PRL rises, the alveolar and acinar tissues collapse, there is a decrease in intraductal pressure, the glandular cells are flattened, and milk is extruded. However, milk yield is not correlated with oxytocin or peripheral PRL concentrations. Levels of oxytocin do not correlate well with the duration of lactation; PRL concentrations do.

The average daily milk yield in a woman participating in full lactation is 700-800 ml. By weight, 0.84 to 2.16 kg of weight is lost per 24 hours in the form of milk. Milk yield is proportionate to suckling, but is in no way correlated with either peripheral oxytocin or PRL concentrations.[101] Daily water turnover in lactating women, including insensible loss, is approximately 2 L greater than that of nonbreastfeeding controls, or 6.4 L per 24 hours. Nutritional deprivation in the mother gives rise to changes in milk osmolarity, including changes in sodium, urea, and creatinine.[91] However, compensatory methods are in play in women who consume 25% more fluid 26-140% during breastfeeding in order to effect a stable production of milk. Although fasting causes changes in milk osmolarity, fluid deprivation appears to have no effect on milk production or composition.[27]

SUPPRESSION OF LACTATION

Although the ideal source of neonatal nutrition remains human milk, lactation suppression developed for reasons stated elsewhere in this chapter. However, the use of hormonal medications such as testosterone and estrogen was empiric and ultimately shown to block the action of PRL at the ductoalveolar level. This blockade in the absence of nipple stimulation suffices until pituitary PRL secretion falls to prepregnancy basal levels, usually by day 7 postpartum. It is presumed that the absence of afferent neural stimulation of the nipple and areola impedes both PRL and oxytocin release, thus representing a natural, noninvasive means of lactation suppression. The most effective approach to lactation suppression remains breast binders. Cloth binders effectively provide counterpressure against the breast and block tactile stimulation of the nipples. The most common, and second least-invasive methodology for treating breast engorgement in cases of failed natural suppression, is the use of ice packs and analgesics. Both methods result in a reduction of mammary sympathetic activity and lactation inhibition. Suppression of lactation is predominantly based upon clinical observation of effect, rather than on sound scientific inquiry and discovery. Thus, combinations of injectable androgens and estrogens were used to produce lactation suppression. However, as has been shown from intraductal samples of milk, levels of testosterone in such samples reach adult male levels[66] at 24 hours following injection, and may remain as much as five times the normal female range five weeks after the injection.

More ominous, perhaps, was the use of diethylstilbestrol, with a potency measured to be 5 to 10 times that of naturally occurring estrogen, which was given in dosages of 5-20 mg daily for up to 10 days. The effect was a dose-dependent reduction in milk production. Although small doses produced mammary secretion, larger doses had an inhibitory effect. Another synthetic, nonsteroidal, estrogenlike substance also has captured the imagination of obstetricians. Chlorotrianisene was used postpartum in various dosage regimens with results similar to those obtained with diethylstilbestrol. Pyridoxine (vitamin B_6), in dosages of 200 mg, three times a day for six days, has also been used for the suppression of lactation, presumably through the suppression of PRL, as a secondary response to an increase in dopamine decarboxylase. The inhibition of the mammary response to PRL appears to be the mode of action of these drugs, thus blocking the initiation of lactation in the first 24 postpartum hours. The mechanism of action of these steroids at the end-organ was seen in studies where PRL secretion was stimulated in response to nipple manipulation in puerperal women who had received estradiol and testosterone preparations. Increments in PRL following such stimulation were similar to those seen in breastfeeding women who had not received steroid suppression.[117]

Since 1972, specific inhibitors of PRL secretion have been available. Orally active, 2-bromo-α-ergocryptine has been used extensively with good results.[124] Modifications to the original oral regimen have now been reported, including the use of long-acting oral and depot-injectable analogues.[63] The use of the medication has been followed by side effects in a small, seemingly stratified, group of women. These postpartum women exhibited hypertension vascular spasm. Cerebral vascular actions have also been reported with the use of the medication. Occasional reports have implicated bromocriptine in the onset of acute myocardial infarction. Unfortunately due to additional reports of adverse vascular side effects of parladel, this medication was withdrawn by the FDA for use in postpartum lactation suppression in September of 1994. Newer, nonergotamine-derived dopamine agonists, such as CV 205-502, appear to be promising alternatives because of fewer side effects.[93,123] The administration of high doses of estrogen, progesterone, or testosterone, however, must be weighed against the potential adverse side effects known to occur, including thromboembolism, liver dysfunction, and endometrial hyperplasia with bleeding.

BREASTFEEDING AND MATERNAL/INFANT BEHAVIOR

Maternal and emotional deprivation of the neonate often creates altered personality and behavior.[43,107] Directed by pheromones or other chemical attractants, skin-to-skin thermal contact regulates bouts of nursing; water conservation in the dehydrated maternal rat may be achieved by ingesting fetal urine.[41] Instinctively, coital behavior drops with lactation and it has been shown in humans that maternal sexual behavior may decrease coital frequency to 1.25 times/week for 6-9 months.[108] This may be due to a partial ovarian quiescence, which gives rise to low estradiol concentrations and subsequent low libido with dry vagina and decreased pheromone production. However, maternal-fetal bonding, as outlined by Kennell, Joos, and Klaus[59] indicates that maternal adaptive behavior is subject to expression by fetal signals. In anxiety states, increased sympathetic tone impairs lactation by reducing let-down, thus impairing oxytocin-related milk ejection.[45] Limbic structures of the brain are involved in mediating these actions, but it is important not to underestimate the multisensory control of maternal behavior associated with sights, sounds, and tactile sensations obtained from the newborn infant. An individual genome may be available for maternal behavioral expression, but as described above, this may be voluntarily suppressed for societal reasons. Maternal-infant bonding represents a symbiotic relationship between mother and child with potential long-term expression.

LACTATION AND EXERCISE

Aerobic exercise contributes not only to cardiovascular fitness, but, depending upon the motivation to exercise and the body habitus of the woman, may promote acute alterations in hormonal secretions.[42] Shangold, Gatz, and Thysen recorded significant increases in plasma PRL concentrations of women during acute exercise.[104] Changes were also noted in testosterone secretion in these women. Previous studies in the authors' laboratory identified an adaptive reaction in normally menstruating women who regularly exercise aerobically. That is, acute alterations in both plasma PRL and cortisol secretion during the first two weeks of aerobic exercise were blunted thereafter, and were essentially absent as exercise performance improved. Similar responses to such exercise were identified by Brisson et al. and were related to specific sporting habits of the individual;[10] Coiro et al. found oxytocin blocked exercise-induced ACTH and cortisol in men.

During the initial phases of lactation, caloric energy expenditure on aerobic exercise may induce acute increments in PRL. Though considered beneficial to increasing milk volume or composition, these increments may be offset by the competition for calories between mother and child. However, this is not detrimental to breastfeeding.[25] It has been shown that vigorous aerobic exercise between the sixth and 12th postpartum week fails to have an adverse effect on lactation or milk composition.[69] Caloric expenditure during this time increases to greater than 400 kilocalories per day; this is compensated for with increased caloric intake.

A 13% increase in caloric intake was noticed in breastfeeding mothers who exercised, compared to sedentary breastfeeding controls.[25] Physiological declines in milk-protein concentration were similar. Although basal PRL responses remain slightly elevated in nursing women by the fifth postpartum month, no statistically significant difference could be found in such women who actively exercised.

Exercise by nursing mothers is not contraindicated and hormonal paremeters associated with breastfeeding remain stable, even in the presence of significant maternal weight loss.

LACTATION AND MATERNAL DRUG INGESTION

Hazards to the neonate exist from maternally ingested drugs during the lactation interval.[98] Such hazards have been studied extensively, but no unifying consensus has been put forth about the individual risk to the infant. Because 90% of all infants receive breast milk during the first 3-6 postpartum weeks, concern must be focused on what medications pose the greatest risk to the neonate. The potential for transcellular transport of maternally ingested drugs is determined by the status of the drug in the maternal circulation. Because a carrier state exists with maternally ingested drugs, and because only the free or non–protein-bound portion of a medication enters breast milk, binding affinity of drugs in the maternal circulation must be determined. In addition, those compounds that are lipid soluble have a greater chance of traversing the blood-alveolar barrier.[96] Molecular size impairs transport from the maternal circulation to the breast; however, events in the transfer of maternally ingested compounds to the breastfeeding neonate follow the pattern shown in Fig. 52-7. Variations in the concentration of drugs in human milk also depend on the temporal relationship that exists between maternal ingestion, peak maternal plasma concentration, metabolic clearance rate, and equally important, the interval

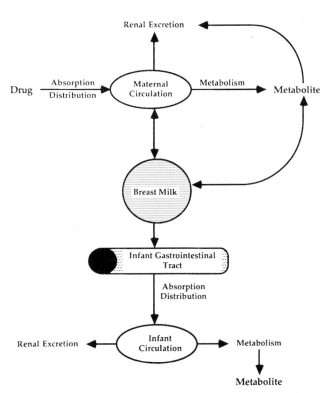

Fig. 52-7. Events during drug transfer from lactating mothers to infants. (From Reider MJ: Prescribing for the lactating woman, *Med North Am* 38:6913, 1989.)

between maternal ingestion and subsequent infant feeding. Depending upon the time of feeding, the pH of milk also is important to the activity of the compound.

Prophylactic antibiotics are used increasingly in women who experience premature labor.[87] Antibiotics are used as frequently in women who have suffered premature rupture of the membranes, although clinical opinion varies on the efficacy of such treatment.[87,99] However, the widespread use of antibiotics may enhance the risk of postpartum transfer of such agents into milk, increasing the risk of altered neonatal intestinal bacterial colonization, thereby increasing the chance of necrotizing enterocolitis.[70]

Many drugs may be used safely during lactation because studies have failed to identify significant transmembrane transport of the medication. Some of these medications obviously enhance PRL secretion, including benzodiazepines and tricyclic antidepressants. Maternal drowsiness has been reported with the use of these medications because of the influence on dopaminergic neural function. Protracted use of such medications, including chlorpromazine, prochlorperazine, and thioridazine, at the time of weaning may lead to persistent galactorrhea and a delay in the resumption of cyclic postovulatory menstruation.[96] Some of these medications have been tried as stimulants to milk production.[118,129]

There is no contraindication to the *prescribed* use of nonsteroidal antiinflammatory drugs, acetaminophen, or acetylsalicylic acid. It is generally appropriate to establish an inventory of maternal medications prior to labor and delivery and, where possible, to restrict or reduce the dosage of medication in anticipation of breastfeeding.

Drug dependency in pregnant and postpartum women is a growing problem worldwide. The fact that such dependence may frustrate physiological lactation is superseded only by the risks of neonatal drug addiction, which may preclude nursing.[127] It is beyond the scope of this chapter to review the many social, moral, and ethical issues raised by this reality.

IMMUNOLOGY OF COLOSTRUM AND LACTATION

The aqueous form of human milk is isosmotic compared with plasma and contains both lactose and electrolytes. Sodium and chloride, however, may be lower in milk than in maternal plasma.[34,36] Transcellular diffusion may account for the extrusion of lactose, water, and electrolytes, the latter occurring by electrochemical gradients. The major osmol in milk is lactose and, because of the measurement of electrical potential gradients between blood and milk, active transport mechanisms must be involved in creating this substance. Mammary blood flow influences milk secretion. It is decreased in stress and in fasting, and stasis can be identified by increased sodium and chloride, and decreased concentrations of lactose and potassium. The initial

product of mammary synthesis and secretion occurs during the latter part of the third trimester, when a lipid-rich solution called *colostrum* is produced. With an average protein content of 10g%, colostrum is rich in globulins. The principal immunoglobulin in colostrum is IgA.[102,106,128] The postnatal transfer of passive immunization and the absorption of these immunoglobulins by the neonatal intestinal tract occurs as a result of mucosal pinocytosis, whereby immunoglobulins are transferred to the neonatal lymphatics and venous system.[8] This provides passive immunity for up to three months.

Mammary glands contain immune substances associated with both respiratory and gut immune mechanisms.[90,106] Classical anatomical immune systems include lymphocytes, monocytes, and polymorphonuclear leucocytes, derived from primary or central sites (e.g., bone marrow and the thymus).[12] Secondary tissues include lymph nodes, the mucosal immune system, as well as the gut-associated lymphoid tissue (GALT). These tissues include Peyer's patches, mesentery lymph nodes, and the appendix. Linkage is also noted between the lacrimal and salivary glands, and the bronchus and tonsils. The IgA class of proteins are immunoprotective of the gut, and exist preferentially in external secretions (Fig. 52-8). sIgA is a secretory IgA, and is 90% of the immunoglobulin found in milk. It is produced by plasma cells, 37% of which are in mammary tissue and are transported by endocytosis from the basal lateral surface of the mucosal membrane.[57] Although sIgA is not bactericidal, it blocks the adhesion of pathogens to mucosal epithelial surfaces.[3] The maternal serum component of IgA is IgA_1; the secretory component is IgA_2. Specific patterns of lymphocyte migration are regulated by the antigen to which they are sensitized. GALT-derived, antigen-sensitized lymphocytes migrate to the antigen-free mammary gland. In colostrum, up to 20% of cells are lymphocytes, in which T and B cells decrease in the first week following delivery. Sensitized IgA-containing B-cells move to home in on the mammary gland, where terminal maturation occurs in plasma cells, producing IgA against both respiratory and gastrointestinal pathogens.

Because the breast is part of the mucosal immune system,[106] the lactational transmission of cellular immunity becomes extremely important when considering breastfeeding for all infants, including those who are born prematurely.[49,109] Preterm infants who were allowed breast milk thrived better than those who were not give colostrum.[109] Breastfeeding reduced mortality rates in low-birth-weight infants.[5] In addition to reduced mortality rates, PRL concentrations were higher in preterm infants and related positively to successful future outcome and lower morbidity. When PRL concentrations were low, as in the case of infants who were not breastfed, the outcome was more precarious.

The overwhelming use of cow's milk in infant feeding

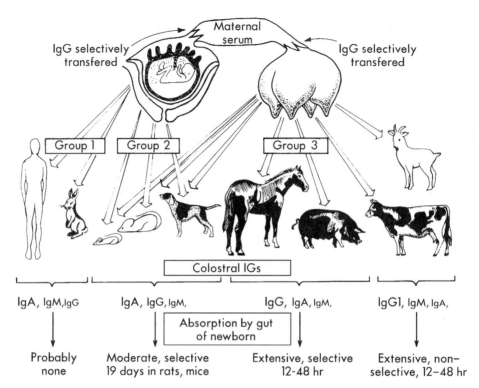

Fig 52-8. Partitioning and migration of maternally derived immunoglobulins in various animal species, including humans. (From Butler JE: Immunoglobulins of the mammary secretions. In Larson BL, Smith BR, editors: Lactation: a comprehensive treatise, vol 3, Nutrition and biochemistry of milk maintenance, New York, 1974, Academic Press.)

has been associated with claims of allergies that are influenced more by family history than by the early introduction of cow's milk.[72] However, recent studies have suggested that cow's milk is a possible trigger of the autoimmune response that destroys pancreatic β-cells in genetically susceptible hosts, resulting in diabetes. The isolation of an albumin peptide containing 17 amino acids is now considered to be a reactive epitope. Studies suggest that patients with insulin-dependent diabetes mellitus have an immunity to cow's-milk albumin, with antibodies to an albumin peptide, that may be capable of reacting with the β-cell–specific surface protein and subsequent islet cell dysfunction.[54]

Such evidence suggests a protective effect of maternally derived immunoglobulins as they occur in breastmilk. The differential absorption of immunoglobulins has been studied in the cow, where colostrum maintains its potency over a number of hours. Studies at one, six, and 12 months indicate that immunoglobulins reach a peak in the blood at 12-18 hours after ingestion. IgA is absorbed most; IgM is absorbed least. Subcategories of IgG are also absorbed with varying frequencies.[61] In the feline, IgG1, IgA, and IgM are transferred with some irregularity with half-lives of 2-4 days. Endogenous IgM and IgG production, however, occurs in the later postpartum period.[64] In humans, IgA$_1$ and IgA$_2$ are found in human milk. Colostral milk proteins, in

effect, can suppress T-lymphocyte proliferation.[80] The modulation of the effect on T cells, however, is dosage dependent and may be responsible for an exaggerated fetal response. It has also been reported that colostrum can inhibit proliferation of T cells activated by coenzyme A.[48] Interleukin-1 (IL-1) and interleukin-2 (IL-2) are found in human milk; interleukin-6 (IL-6) is closely associated with the production of IgA. In the calf, colostral lymphocytes traverse the intestinal wall and seem to regulate a blastogenic response, increasing the formation of antibodies dependent on T-helper cells.[95]

Perhaps most important to the immunoprotective effect of colostrum on the newborn infant is the half-life of immunoglobulins. With a half-life of 20-25 days, IgG is present in much higher concentrations than IgA (with a half-life of 14-20 days) and IgM (with a half-life of 8-10 days).[128] Secretory IgA inhibits the adherence of enteropathic bacteria to HEP-2 cells, and monocytes are found in similar concentrations in both early and late milk, along with increasing concentrations of ILg and IgA.[19]

T-cells infected with human T-cell leukemia/lymphoma virus (HTLV) were not found in the cord blood of mothers with HIV II, but cells were found in infants after breast-feeding.[46]

The sIgA antibodies measured in the saliva of newborns were lower in allergic infants who were fed breast milk than in those fed cow's milk.[72] Class-specific antibodies exist in human milk for a variety of pathogens, which probably makes this the most important aspect of natural feeding.[55] Immunoglobulins IgG and IgA have been found against *Hemophilus* influenza B, pertussis, shigellosis,[15] *Streptococcus pneumoniae,*[3,65] *Giardia lamblia,*[35,103] as well as *Neisseria meningitidis,* schistosomiasis,[28] and coliforms. Isaacs et al. suggest that both antiviral and antibacterial lipids are produced by the neonatal gut as a result of stimulation by maternally derived immunoglobulins and T cells.[51]

The homing of lymphocytes to the mammary gland is regulated by lactogenic hormones. Fetal (newborn) mucosal immunity is low, with activation and maturation soon after birth. Milk increases the sIgA mucosal membrane production in the fetus; thus, the synergy is established between maternal and fetal immune systems. Memory T cells (antigen primed) are an expression of antibodies to surface antigens by colostrum T cells and supports the fact that the infant benefits from the mother's previous immune experience.[85]

ABNORMAL LACTATION

Breast development may be induced under pseudophysiological circumstances, such as the administration of exogenous steroid hormones, specifically estrogen and its derivatives. This development occurs with the use of estrogenlike substances to induce premature epiphyseal closure in prepubertal girls deemed too tall for esthetic reasons. Such treatment promoted an arrest of linear femoral growth, and breast development characterized by areolar pigmentation, ductal and alveolar development was noted. Similarly, estrogen administration to posthypophysectomized women results in normal breast development. Breast development is absent, however, in women suffering from Turner syndrome. Ovulation induction with menopausal gonadotropins in hypophysectomized women with intact ovaries finally induces terminal development of the mammary alveolar tissue.

The classic nomenclature commonly used for abnormal lactation arose from the sporadic identification, classification, and reporting of breast secretions unrelated to the puerperium as noted elsewhere in this text. The report by Forbes et al., of the Forbes-Albright syndrome, includes both amenorrhea and galactorrhea, as well as the presence of pituitary adenomata.[32] In short, galactorrhea, the persistent discharge of milklike secretion six months beyond the post-partum period in nonpregnant women, is pathological. By far, the most common type of galactorrhea is associated with the abnormal secretion of PRL, now perceived to be a disorder of hypothalamic neurotransmitter turnover, specifically, the elaboration and turnover of dopamine.[130] The resulting chronic depletion of dopamine sometimes leads to hyperprolactinemia with or without pituitary tumor, for

which the most successful treatment is chemotherapy.[11,31,81,123]

Many studies have continued to support the existence of a distinct prolactin-inhibiting factor (PIF) based upon studies involving extracts of porcine median eminence. The preponderance of evidence, however, favors dopamine as the principle PIF, being totally responsible for the control of PRL secretion. Thus, disturbances or distribution of the tuberoinfundibular axis disrupts the direct action of dopamine at the level of the pituitary lactotrope, resulting in abnormally elevated PRL secretion and subsequent galactorrhea.

HYPOGALACTIA

Inadequate lactation has serious ramifications for both mother and infant. However, the precise diagnosis of hypogalactia remains elusive because it involves so many factors in its diagnosis. Prior to pregnancy, surgical augmentation of the breast or breast reduction operations may result in transection of the neural innervation of the nipple and areola. Thus, in spite of adequate endocrine priming throughout pregnancy, milk letdown is impossible due to both the loss of ductal continuity and nipple and areolar neural integrity. [117]

Hygogalactia may also result from acute postpartum pituitary necrosis. The Sheehan syndrome in its complete form leads to a loss of dopaminergic pathways between the hypothalamus and the pituitary gland. This leads to the absence of PRL synthesis and release.

Skopichev and Gaidukov suggest that impending hypogalactia may be diagnosed objectively during the first 24 hours postpartum. Using a cytologic evaluation of leukocyte aggregation in colostrum, the authors have noted maximum leukocytic infiltration in the first 18-24 hours. The lack of leukocytic aggregation suggests, to the authors, adequate prenatal and prelactational breast preparation. They also conclude that the measurement of alkaline phosphatase and other leukocytic enzymes aid in the diagnosis of this condition.[105a]

Impaired dietary intake of micronutrients occurring in women during pregnancy in developing countries is a leading cause of hypogalactia.[1, 41a] These conclusions have been drawn from the Nutrition Collaborative Research Support Program (CRSP). Using data from Egypt, Kenya, and Mexico, the CRSP concluded that beyond maternal age, weight gain in pregnancy, and fat deposition, all of which determine fetal birth weight, the absence of adequate dietary supplies and the bioavailability of Vitamins B12, B6, zinc, and iron contribute to hypogalactia and ultimately to fetal demise.[82a]

Of equal importance to the development of hypogalactia is the presence of puerperal mastitis and breast abscess, which usually reduces milk production while antibiotic and analgesic therapy is administered to the patient. Just as acute auditory and visual stimuli can evoke milk letdown, chronic stress may also inhibit lactation. Kolodina and Lipovskii manipulated both tryptophan and thyroxine intake in lactating rats who were under chronic stress conditions and concluded that hypogalactia was indeed due to an enhanced catecholaminergic activity and decreased serotonergic tone, leading to decreased milk production.[61a]

Adequate prenatal nutrition is obviously necessary for the avoidance of postpartum vascular collapse, which could promote pituitary hemorrhage or infarction. Treatment of hypogalactia must also be predicated on the knowledge that a mother has received adequate prenatal instructions regarding the application of the infant to the postpartum breast. The patient must also be aware of the frequency, intensity, and duration of infant sucking, which serves as the principle means of stimulating adequate milk production and milk flow.

Chemical therapy for hypogalactia has included attempts to augment milk production with thyrotropin-releasing hormone[115a], as well as chlorpromazine and metaclopramide. Acupuncture has also been considered.[30a] None of these treatments appear to be successful. The incidence of true hypogalactia, however, is extremely rare.

THE POSTMENOPAUSAL BREAST

Postmenopausally, the breast undergoes involution where a dramatic and quantitative decrease in the number and size of alveolar cells occurs. This progressive hypoplasia and atrophy, the result of the absence of estrogen and progesterone, is also associated with an increase in adipose and stromal tissue replacing glandular elements.

The sequential administration of estrogen and/or progesterone results in increased breast tissue turgor and fat deposition, simulating the breast of the premenopausal woman. However, alveolar and acinar redevelopment is absent.[60]

Fluid secretion from the breast, itself a modified apocrine gland, takes several forms. The simplest and most benign form is the release of desquamated cells from the terminal ducts. The examiner should exert caution in determining if breast secretion exists, and more important, the procedure of nipple aspiration should be standardized using a breast pump, single duct aspirator, or gentle massage.

Breast secretion is defined as the appearance or collection of 20-30 microliters of fluid from the breast. Without spontaneous discharge, there is nevertheless duct secretion, known as *nipple aspirate fluid* (NAF). The volume of NAF varies little from woman to woman, regardless of race. However, there appears to be a positive correlation between the availability of breast secretions and genetically determined earwax.[88]

More important, perhaps, are the correlations that may exist between the presence of breast secretions and duct pathology. Spontaneous nipple discharge occurs in only 3-6% of women who seek specialty breast services.[60] However, spontaneous nipple discharge has been reported in 10-15% of women who are subsequently found to have benign breast disease, including duct ectasia and duct papillomata. The latter are usually solitary and found in the terminal duct near the nipple. NAFs are various colors and concentrations and may be cloudy, purulent, or bloody. Bloody fluid is associated with a duct papilloma or other benign disease in 38% of cases. However, carcinoma is found in 69% of women with this complaint. Nipple discharge of any kind is not necessarily associated with carcinoma, especially in cases of galactorrhea in a woman of child-bearing age. However, the correlation between palpable breast masses and carcinoma is even more difficult to make.

EVALUATION OF NIPPLE DISCHARGE

Evaluation may vary significantly, depending upon the volume, color, consistency, and timing of a nipple discharge. Should the discharge occur spontaneously, a history of the timing of the discharge, its frequency, and the events surrounding the observation are equally important. For example, Frantz noted galactorrhea in circumstances such as sexual intercourse, and in the presence of visual or auditory stress.[33] It should be emphasized that, in the acquisition of a sample of breast secretion, unnecessary compression of the breast should be avoided because such compression leads to the transudation of tissue fluids, as well as to displacement of damaged endothelial cells that will cause misdiagnosis.

In most instances, a spontaneous breast discharge can be expressed onto a glass cytology slide, then fixed with either 95% ethanol or ether. Plated and examined under a microscope, the cellular elements of the discharge can be identified.[47] However, it should be noted that the quality and number of cells in the secretion may differ, depending upon whether the aspirate is obtained from the fore or the after portion of the breast duct. Samples may be collected by a suction cup device. A negative pressure of approximately 100 mm of mercury over 15 seconds should be sufficient to obtain a suitable aspirate.

Commonly, the composition of nipple aspirate includes lactose, lipids, cholesterol, alphalactalbumin, and immunoglobulins. As a secretory product, nipple aspirate has been shown to contain concentrations of estradiol far above those found in peripheral plasma, while cholesterol and its oxidation products, β-epoxides, are found in the ductal discharge. Attempts should be made to correlate the color of breast secretions with the composition. The darker the color, the more likely it is that the sample has high cholesterol and epoxides. However, the oxidation of lipids in contact with air may account for color changes that occur after the sample has been obtained.[40]

CYTOLOGICAL COMPONENTS OF BREAST FLUID

Identifying the normal stratification of cell types and breast secretion involves knowing the precise age of the menstrual cycle at which the secretions are obtained. It is important to note that the cell content of breast secretion changes with age, as epithelial cells become more prominent in the sample. Studied microscopically, breast secretions contain epithelial cells, occasional erythrocytes, lymphocytes, and foam cells. Histocytes compose 14-15% of cells; foam cells account for nearly 69% of all cells. Foam cells may be referred to as *colostrum bodies* and are found to have increased nuclear vacuolation, especially in pregnant women.[47]

SUMMARY

Goldman and Garza summarize the issues related to future research into breast milk.[37] The rapidly emerging role of breastfeeding gains importance in the initiation and development of the neonatal immune system. Breastfeeding may provide immunity against certain factors that promote breast cancer. However, such protection may be specific for the age of the woman at which the first pregnancy is delivered.

The goal of future research may be directed at seeking the etiological factors that predispose women to breast disease and which, when identified, may be modified to reduce the risk of disease.[90]

Several conclusions may be drawn from the diverse pattern of research that has been conducted in the last two decades. The first is the clear relationship between PRL and lymphocytic migration. The second is the stimulatory effect that nursing has on hormone secretion and immunoglobulin production and transport. And last, the implicit understanding that the avoidance of nursing and the suppression of puerperal lactation is one of the most unphysiological and unscientific maneuvers to beset contemporary women.

REFERENCES

1. Allen LH: The Nutrition CRSP: What is marginal malnutrition and does it affect human function? *Nutr Rev* 51:255, 1993.
1a. Amico JA, Seif SM, Robinson AG: Oxytocin in human plasma: correlation with neurophysin and stimulation with estrogen, *J Clin Endocrinol Metab* 52:988, 1981.
2. Amico JA, Finley BE: Breast stimulation in cycling women, pregnant women and a woman with induced lactation: pattern of release of oxytocin, prolactin and luteinizing hormone, *Clin Endocrinol* 25:97, 1986.
3. Anderson B, et al: Inhibition of attachment of *Streptococcus pneumoniae* and *Haemophilus influenzae* by human milk and receptor oligosaccharides, *J Infect Dis* 153:232, 1986.
4. Anderson B, Huth J, Tyson JE: Plasma thyrotropin releasing hormone, prolactin TSH and T concentrations following the intravenous or oral administration of TRH[4], *Am J Obstet Gynececol* 135:737, 1979.
5. Awasthi S, Malik GK, Misra PK: Mortality patterns in breast versus artificially fed term babies in early infancy: a longitudinal study, *Indian Pediatr* 28(3):243, 1991.
6. Balment RJ, Brimble MJ, Forsling ML: Release of oxytocin induced by salt loading and its influence on renal secretion in the male rat, *J Physiol (Lond)* 308:439, 1980.
7. Bauchner H, Leventhal JM, Shapiro ED: Studies of breastfeeding and infections: how good is the evidence? *JAMA* 256:887, 1988.

8. Bertotto A, et al: Human breast milk T lymphocytes display the phenotype and functional characteristics of memory T cells, *Eur J Immunol* 20:1877, 1990.
9. Briend A, Fauveau V, Chakraborty J: Contraceptive use and breastfeeding duration in rural Bangladesh, *Eur J Clin Nutr* 45(7):341, 1991.
10. Brisson GR, et al: Exercise-induced dissociation of the blood prolactin response in young women according to their sports habits, *Horm Metab Res* 12:201, 1980.
11. Brue T, et al: Effects of the dopamine agonist CV 205-502 in human prolactinomas resistant to bromocriptine, *J Clin Endocrinal Metab* 74:577, 1992.
12. Butler JE: Immunoglobulins of the mammary secretions. In Larson BL, Smith BR, editors: *Lactation: a comprehensive treatise, vol 3, Nutrition and biochemistry of milk maintenance*, New York, 1974, Academic Press.
13. Christensson K, et al: Effect of nipple stimulation on uterine activity and on plasma levels of oxytocin in full term, healthy, pregnant women, *Acta Obstet Gynec Scand* 68:205, 1989.
14. Clarke G, Lincoln DW, Merrick LP: Dopaminergic control of oxytocin release in lactating rats, *J Endocrinol* 83:409, 1979.
15. Cleary TG, et al: Human milk secretory immunoglobulin A to *Shigella* virulence plasmid-coded antigens, *J Pediatr* 119:34, 1991.
16. Coiro V, et al: Oxytocin enhances thyrotropin-releasing hormone-induced prolactin release in normal menstruating women, *Fertil & Steril* 47:565, 1987.
17. Coiro V, et al: Oxytocin reduces exercise-induced ACTH and cortisol rise in man, *Acta Endocrinol* 119:405, 1988.
18. Cowie AT, Tindal JS: *The physiology of lactation,* London, 1971, Arnold Edward.
19. Cravioto A, et al: Inhibition of localized adhesion of enteropathogenic *Escherichia coli* to HEp-2 cells by immunoglobulin and oligosaccharide fractions of human colostrum and breast milk, *J Infect Dis* 163(6):1247, 1991.
20. Crowley WR, Armstrong WE: Neurochemical regulation of oxytocin secretion in lactation, *Endocr Rev* 13:33, 1992.
21. Crowley WR, et al: Evidence for stimulatory noradrenergic and inhibitory dopaminergic regulation of oxytocin release in the lactating rat, *Endocrinology* 121:14, 1987.
22. Cunningham AS: Breast-feeding and morbidity in industrialized countries: an update. In Jelliffe DB, Jelliffe EFP, editors: *Advances in international maternal and child health,* New York 1981, Oxford University.
23. Cunningham AS, Jelliffe DB, Jelliffe EFP: Breast-feeding and health in the 1980s: a global epidemiologic review, *J Pediatr* 118(5):659, 1991.
24. Dabelow A: Die Milchdruse. In Bergmann W, Mollendorf W, editors: *Handbuch der mikroskopischen anatomie des menschen,* Berlin, 1957, Springer-Verlag.
25. Dewey KG, et al: A randomized study of the effects of aerobic exercise by lactating women on breast milk volume and composition, *N Engl J Med* 330:449, 1994.
26. Drife JO: Breast development in puberty, *Ann N Y Acad Sci* 464:58, 1986.
27. Dusdieker LB, et al: Effect of supplemental fluids on human milk production, *J Pediatr* 106:207, 1985.
28. Eissa AM, et al: Transmission of lymphocyte responsiveness to schistosomal antigens by breast feeding, *Trop Geogr Med* 41:208, 1989.
29. Emery JL, Scholey S, Taylor EM: Decline in breastfeeding, *Arch Dis Child* 65:369, 1990.
30. Erdheim J, Stumme E: Über die schwanger schaftsver änderung in der hypophyse, *Beitr Pathol Anat* 46:1, 1909.
30a. Fava A, Bongiovanni A, Frassoldati P: Acupuncture therapy of hypogalactia, *Minerva Med* 22:71, 1980.
31. Ferrari C, et al: Cabergoline: long-acting oral treatment of hyperprolactinemic disorders, *J Clin Endocrinol Metab* 68:1201, 1989.

32. Forbes AP, et al: Syndrome characterized by galactorrhea, amenorrhea and low urinary FSH: comparison with acromegaly and normal lactation, *J Clin Endocrinol Metab* 14:265, 1954.

33. Frantz AG: Prolactin, *N Eng J Med* 298:201, 1978.

34. Garza C, et al: Special properties of human milk, *Clin Perinatol* 14:11, 1987.

35. Gillin FD: *Giardia lamblia:* the role of conjugated and unconjugated bile salts in killing by human milk, *Exp Parasitol* 63:74, 1987.

36. Goldman AS, Goldblum RM: Human milk: immunologic-nutritional relationships, *Ann N Y Acad Sci* 587:236, 1990.

37. Goldman AS, Garza C: Future research in human milk, *Pediatr Res* 22(5):493, 1987.

38. Grosvenor CE, Mena F: Neural and hormonal control of milk secretion and milk ejection. In Larson BL, Smith BR, editors: *Lactation: a comprehensive treatise: the mammary gland/development and maintenance,* New York, 1974, Academic Press.

39. Grosvenor CE, Mena F: Regulating mechanisms for oxytocin and prolactin secretion during lactation. In Muller EE, MacLeod RM, editors: *Neuroendocrine perspectives,* New York, 1982, Elsevier Biomedical.

40. Gruenke LD, et al: Breast fluid, cholesterol and cholesterol epoxides. Relationship to breast cancer risks and other characteristcs, *Cancer Res* 47:5483, 1987.

41. Gubernick DJ, Alberts JR: Maternal licking of young: resource exchange and proximate controls, *Physiol Behav* 31:593, 1983.

41a. Guilarte TR: Vitamin B_6 and cognitive development: recent research findings from animal and human studies, *Nutr Rev* 51:193, 1993.

42. Hale RW, et al: A marathon: the immediate effect on female runners' luteinizing hormone, follicle-stimulating hormone, prolactin, testosterone, and cortisol levels, *Am J Obstet Gynececol* 146:550, 1983.

43. Harlow HR, Zimmerman RR: Affectional responses in the infant monkey, *Science* 130:421, 1959.

44. Hatjis CG, et al: Oxytocin, vasopressin, and prolactin responses associated with nipple stimulation, *South Med J* 82:193, 1989.

45. Herrenkohl LR, Rosenberg PA: Exteroceptive stimulation of maternal behavior in the naive rat, *Physiol Behav* 8:595, 1972.

46. Hino S: Milk-borne transmission of HTLV-l as a major route in the endemic cycle, *Acta Paediat J Overseas Ed* 31:428, 1989.

47. Holmquist DG, Papanicolaou GN: The exfoliative cytology of the mammary gland during pregnancy and lactation, *Ann N Y Acad Sci* 63:1422, 1956.

48. Hooton JW, et al: Human colostrum contains an activity that inhibits the production of IL-2, *Clin Exp Immunol* 86:(3):520, 1991.

49. Howie PW, et al: Protective effect of breastfeeding against infection, *Br Med J* 300:11, 1990.

50 Huddlestone JF, Sutcliff G, Robinson D: Contraction stress test by intermittent nipple stimulation, *Obstet Gynecol* 63:699, 1984.

51. Isaacs CE, et al: Antiviral and antibacterial lipids in human milk and infant formula feeds, *Arch Dis Child* 65:861, 1990.

52. Jelliffe DB, Jelliffe EFP: *Human milk in the modern world,* Oxford, 1978, Oxford University.

53. Johnston JM, Amico JA: A prospective longitudinal study of the release of oxytocin and prolactin in response to infant suckling in long-term lactation, *J Clin Endocrinol Metab* 62:653, 1986.

54. Karjalaiaen J, et al: A bovine albumin peptide as a possible trigger of insulin-dependent diabetes mellitus, *N Eng J Med* 327:302, 1992.

55. Kassim OO, et al: Class-specific antibodies to *Bordetella pertussis, Haemophilus influenzae* type b, *Streptococcus pneumoniae* and *Neisseria meningitidis* in human breast-milk and maternal-infant sera, *Ann Trop Paediatr* 9:226, 1989.

56. Kasting NW: Simultaneous and independent release of vasopressin and oxytocin in the rat, *Can J Physiol Pharmacol* 66:22, 1988.

57. Keller MA, et al: IgG4 in human colostrum and human milk: continued local production or selective transport from serum, *Acta Paediatr Scand* 77(1):24, 1988.

58. Kelsey J: Breast cancer epidemiology: summary and future directions, *Epidemiol Rev* 15:256, 1993.

59. Kennell JH, Voos DK, Klaus MH: Parent-infant bonding. In Osofsky JD, editor: *Handbook of infant development,* New York, 1979, John Wiley & Sons.

60. King EB, Goodson WH: Discharges and secretions of the nipple, In Bland KI, Copeland EM, editors: *The breast: comprehensive management of benign and malignant disease,* 1991, WB Saunders.

61. Klobasa F, Butler JE, Habe F: Maternal-neonatal immunoregulation: suppression of de novo synthesis of IgG and IgA, but not IgM, in neonatal pigs by bovine colostrum, is lost upon storage, *Am J Vet Res* 51(9):1407, 1990.

61a. Kolodina LN, Lipovskii SM: Dynamics of the serotonin content in the blood of puerperae with normal lactation and in hypogalactia, *Akush Ginekol (Mosk)* 2:18, 1980.

62. Konner M, Worthman C: Nursing frequency, gonadal function, and birth spacing among !Kung hunter-gathers, *Science* 207:788, 1980.

63. Kremer JA, et al: Postpartum return of pituitary and ovarian activity during lactation inhibition with the new dopamine agonist CV 205-502 and during normal lactation, *Acta Endocrinol* 122(6):759, 1990.

64. Ladjeva I, Peterman JH, Mestecky J: IgA subclasses of human colostral antibodies specific for microbial and food antigens, *Clin Exp Immunol* 78(1):85, 1989.

65. Lämmler C, Frede C, Blobel H: Interactions of streptococci with human colostral immunoglobulin A, *Comp Immunol Microbiol Infect Dis* 11(2):115, 1988.

66. Lev-Gur M, et al: Serum hormone changes in parturients given steroid preparations to suppress lactation, *Int J Fertil* 35(2):95, 1990.

67. Liu J, Rebar RW, Yen SS: Neuroendocrine control of the postpartum period, *Clin Perinatol* 10:723, 1983.

68. London SJ, et al: Lactation and risk of breast cancer in a cohort of U.S. women, *Am J Epidemiol* 132:17, 1983.

69. Lovelady CA, Lonnerdal B, Dewey KG: Lactation performance of exercising women, *Am J Clin Nutr* 52:103, 1990.

70. Lucas A, Cole TJ: Breast milk and neonatal necrotizing enterocolitis, *Lancet* 336:1519, 1990.

71. Lucas A, Drewett RB, Mitchell MD: Breast feeding and plasma oxytocin concentrations, *Br Med J* 281:834, 1980.

72. Lucas A, et al: Early diet of preterm infants and development of allergic or atopic disease: randomised prospective study, *Br Med J* 31:300(6728):837, 1990.

73. Macedo CG: Infant mortality in the Americas, *PAHO Bull* 22:303, 1988.

74. Majumder AK: Breast-feeding, birth interval and child mortality in Bangladesh, *J Biosoc Science* 23(3):297, 1991.

75. McCoshen JA, Bose R, Embree JE: Uterine prolactin and labor: modulation by human chorionic gonadotropin affects prostaglandin (PG) E_2 and PGF_2 a production, *Semin Reprod Endocrinol* 10:294, 1992.

76. McKiernan J: Postnatal breast development of preterm infants, *Arch Dis Child* 59:1090, 1984.

77. McKiernan J, Coyne J, Cahalane S: Histology of breast development in early life, *Arch Dis Child* 63:136, 1988.

78. McNeilly AS, et al: Release of oxytocin and prolactin in response to suckling, *Br Med J* 286:257, 1983.

79. Mead M: Family contexts of breastfeeding. In Raphael D, editor: *Breastfeeding and food policy in a hungry world,* New York, 1979, Academic.

80. Mincheva-Nilsson L, et al: Human milk contains proteins that stimulate and suppress T lymphocyte proliferation, *Clin Exp Immunol* 79(3):463, 1990.

81. Molitch Me, et al: Bromocriptine as primary therapy for prolactin-secreting macroadenomas: results of a prospective multicenter study, *J Clin Endocrinol Metab* 60:698, 1985.

82. Monaghan P, et al: Peripubertal human breast development, *Anat Rec* 226:501, 1990.

82a. Neumann CG, Harrison GG: Onset and evolution of stunting in infants and children. Examples from The Human Nutrition Collaborative Research Support Program, Kenya and Africa studies, *Eur J Clin Nutr* 48 (Suppl 1): 590, 1994.

83. Newcomb PA, et al: Lactation and a reduced risk of premenopausal breast cancer, *N Engl J Med* 330:81, 1994.

84. Newman J: Encouraging, supporting, and maintaining breastfeeding: the obstetrician's role, *J Soc Obstet Gynecol Canada* 13:15, 1991.

85. Nikolova E, et al: Interleukin production by human colostral cells after in vitro mitogen stimulation, *Am J Reprod Immunol Microbiol* 23(4): 104, 1990.

86. Nussey SS, et al: The effect of oxytocin infusion on adenohypophysial and adrenal cortical responses to insulin-induced hypoglycaemia, *Clin Endocrinol (Oxf)* 29:257, 1988.

87. Owen J, Groome LJ, Hauth JC: Randomized trial of prophylactic antibiotic therapy after preterm amnion rupture, *Am J Obstet Gynecol* 169:976, 1994.

88. Petrakis NL: Cerumen genetics and human breast cancer, *Science* 173:347, 1971.

89. Pike MC, et al: Estrogens, progestogens, normal breast cell proliferation and breast cancer risk, *Endomiol Rev* 15:17, 1993.

90. Pittard WB III: Breast milk immunology: a frontier of human nutrition, *Am J Dis Child* 133:83, 1979.

91. Prentice AM, et al: The effect of water abstention on milk synthesis in lactating women, *Clin Sci* 66:291, 1984.

92. Raphael D: Social myths and economic realities about breastfeeding. In Raphael D, editor: *Breastfeeding and food policy in a humgry world,* New York, 1979, Academic Press.

93. Rasmussen C, et al: Long-term treatment with a new non-ergot long-acting dopamine agonist, CV 205-502, in women with hyperprolactinemia, *Clin Endocrinol (Oxf)* 29:271, 1988.

94. Report of the task force on the assessment of the scientific evidence relating to infant-feeding practices and infant health, *Pediatr* 74:579, 1984.

95. Riedel-Caspari G, Schmidt FW: The influence of colostral leukocytes on the immune system of the neonatal calf. I. Effects on lymphocyte responses, *Deutsche Tierarztliche Wochenschrift* 98(3):102, 1991.

96. Rieder MJ: Prescribing for the lactating woman, *Med North Am* 38:6913, 1989.

97. Rigg LA, Yen SS: Multiphasic prolactin secretion during parturition in human subjects, *Am J Obstet Gynececol* 128:215, 1977.

98. Rivera-Cabimbim L: The significance of drugs in breast milk, *Clin Perinatol* 14:51, 1987.

99. Romero R et al: Antibiotic treatment of preterm labour with intact membranes: a multi-centred randomized double blinding placebo controlled trial, *Am J Obstet Gynecol* 169:764, 1994.

100. Rosenzweig BA, et al: Comparison of the nipple stimulation and exogenous oxytocin contraction stress tests. A randomized, prospective study, *J Reprod Med* 34:950, 1989.

101. Saint L, Maggiore P, Hartmann PE: Yield and nutrient content of milk in eight women breast-feeding twins and one woman breast-feeding triplets, *B J Nutr* 56:49, 1986.

102. Saito S, et al: Detection of IL-6 in human milk and its involvement in lgA production, *J Reprod Immunol* 20(3):267, 1991.

103. Samra HK, Ganguly NK, Mahajan RC: Human milk containing specific secretory IgA inhibits binding of *Giardia lamblia* to nylon and glass surfaces, *J Diarrhoeal Dis Res* 9:100, 1991.

104. Shangold MM, Gatz ML, Thysen B: Acute effects of exercise on plasma concentrations of prolactin and testosterone in recreational women runners, *Fertil Steril* 35:699, 1981.

105. Short R: Breast feeding, *Sci Am* 250:35, 1984.

105a. Skopichev VG, Gaidukov SN: A physiological validation for the early diagnosis of hypogalactia in women, *Fiziol Zh SSSR Im I M Sechenova* 77:(5):92, May 1991.

106. Slade HB, Schwartz SA: Mucosal immunity: the immunology of breast milk, *J Allergy Clin Immunol* 80:348, 1987.

107. Stern JM: Licking, touching and suckling: contact stimulation and maternal psychobiology in rats and women, *Ann N Y Acad Sci* 95, 1986.

108. Stern JM, Leiblum S: Postpartum sexual behaviour of American women as a function of absence or frequency of breast feeding: a preliminary communication. In Else J, Lee P, editors; *Primate ontogeny, cognition and social behavior, proceedings of the international primatological society,* Cambridge, England, 1980, Cambridge University.

109. Stine MJ: Breastfeeding the premature newborn: a protocol without bottles, *Hum Lactation* 6(4):167, 1990.

110. Sulman FG: Hypothalamus-pituitary axis b)prolactin-inhibiting factor. In Gross F, Labhart A, Mann T, et al, editors: *Hypothalamic control of lactation,* Germany, 1970, William Heinemann.

111. Tanner JM: *Wachstrum und reifung des Menschen,* Thieme, Stuttgart.

112. Tyson JE, et al: Isolated growth hormone deficiency: studies in pregnancy, *J Clin Endocrinol Metab* 31:147, 1970.

113. Tyson JE, et al: Patterns of insulin, hGH and hPL release after protein and glucose-protein ingestion in pregnancy, *Am J Obstet Gynecol* 110:934, 1971.

114. Tyson JE, et al: Studies of prolactin secretion in human pregnancy, *Am J Obstet Gynecol* 113:14, 1972.

115. Tyson JE, Friesen HG, Anderson MS: Human lactational and ovarian response to endogenous prolactin release, *Science* 177:897, 1972.

115a. Tyson JE, Friesen HG, Anderson MS: Human milk secretion after TRH-induced prolactin release in hypothalamic hypophysiotropic hormones. In Gual C, Rosenberg E, editors: *Physiological and Clinical Studies,* Excerpta Medica, 1973.

116. Tyson JE, Friesen HG: Factors influencing the secretion of human prolactin and growth hormone in menstrual and gestational women, *Am J Obstet Gynecol* 116:377, 1973.

117. Tyson JE, Khojandi M, Huth J, et al: The influence of prolactin secretion on human lactation, *J Clin Endocrinol Metab* 40:764, 1975.

118. Tyson JE, Perez A, Zanartu J: Human lactational response to oral thyrotropin releasing hormone, *J Clin Endocrinol Metab* 43:760, 1976.

119. Tyson JE: Neuroendocrine control of lactational infertility. In Infertility regulation during human lactation, *J Biosoc Sci Suppl* 4:23, 1977.

120. Tyson JE, et al: Nursing medicated prolactin and luteinizing hormone secretion during puerperal laction, *Fertil Steril* 30:154, 1978.

121. Uvnäs-Moberg K, et al: Oxytocin and prolactin levels in breast-feeding women. Correlation with milk yield and duration of breast-feeding, *Acta Obstet Gynecol Scand* 69:301, 1990.

122. Valdes-Dapena MD: *Histology of the fetus and the newborn,* Philadelphia, 1979, WB Saunders.

123. Vance ML, et al: CV 205-502 treatment of hyperprolactinemia, *J Clin Endocrinol Metab* 68:336, 1989.

124. Varga L, et al: Suppression of puerperal lactation with an ergot alkaloid: a double-blind study, *Br Med J* 2:743, 1972.

125. Vorherr H: The breast; morphology, physiology and lactation, New York, 1974, Academic Press.

126. Wakerley JB, Clarke G, Summerlee AJS: Milk ejection and its control. In Knobil E, Neill J, editors: *The physiology of reproduction,* New York, 1988, Raven.

127. Wilton JM: Breastfeeding and the chemically dependent woman, *Clin Iss Perimat Womens Health Nurs* 3(4):667, 1992.

128. Yamada T, Nagai Y, Matsuda M: Changes in serum immunoglobulin values in kittens after ingestion of colostrum, *Am J Vet Res* 52(3):393, 1991.

129. Ylikorkala O, et al: Treatment of inadequate lactation with oral sulpiride and buccal oxytocin, *Obstet Gynecol* 63:57, 1984.

130. Zacur HA, Foster GV, Tyson JE: Multifactorial regulation of prolactin secretion, *Lancet* 1:410, 1976.

Part VIII

MENOPAUSE

Chapter 53

MENOPAUSE OVERVIEW

Nicole Fournet, MD
and Howard L. Judd, MD

Pathophysiology of menopause
    Premenopause and the transitional period
    Hormonal changes associated with menopause
    The menopausal hot flash
    Urogenital atrophy
    Skin changes
    Psychologic changes
Treatment of menopause
    Complications
    Contraindications and precautions
    Management of hormone replacement therapy

Menopause is the permanent cessation of menstruation resulting from the loss of ovarian activity. No specific alteration can be identified at the time of the last menses and, consequently, the onset of menopause can be determined only retrospectively.

The mean age at menopause is approximately 50 years and has shown a remarkable stability throughout the centuries. Because of increasing longevity, one third of women currently are postmenopausal in the United States. It is estimated that 350 million women will be age 60 or older worldwide by the year 2000. The steady expansion of the aging population is having a tremendous impact on health care resources. Loss of ovarian function contributes to this impact, since it is associated with the development of morbid conditions such as osteoporosis and heart disease. This chapter reviews the hormonal changes associated with menopause, the pathophysiologic mechanisms responsible for climacteric symptoms, and the current strategies used for hormone replacement.

PATHOPHYSIOLOGY OF MENOPAUSE
Premenopause and the transitional period

Epidemiologic studies of female reproduction have shown that the fecundability rate declines rapidly after age 35 years.[119] The mean age at the birth of the last child is 40 years, which is approximately 10 years before menopause. These data suggest that the biologic potential of the ovary is compromised a decade or more before complete cessation of menses. The decline of reproductive function seems to correlate with subtle alterations of menstrual and hormonal patterns that become more pronounced as menopause approaches.

A gradual decrease in the mean cycle length after the age of 26 years has been reported.[136] The shortest cycles (25.5 days) occurred between 3 and 9 years before menopause and were followed by the onset of menstrual irregularities characteristic of the transitional period. A decrease in the length of the follicular phase accounted for these shortened menstrual cycles (Fig. 53-1).[120] The mean midcycle serum estradiol (E_2) peak (192 pg/mL) and the mean E_2 concentration throughout the cycle (92 pg/mL) were lower than those of younger women. The preovulatory luteinizing hormone (LH) surge tended to occur earlier in the cycle, but the peak level was not statistically different. Serum follicle-stimulating hormone (FSH) levels were found to be increased throughout the cycle, the concentrations being strikingly elevated in the early follicular phase and falling gradually as E_2 concentrations increased.[121] Urinary gonadotropin studies in women over the age of 40 have confirmed that the FSH elevation was most pronounced during and before menstruation.[93]

This early rise of FSH concentration appears to have a substantial impact on the reproductive capacity of older women. It is suggested that the increased concentrations of FSH reflect a reduction in the functional residual ovarian follicles.[94] FSH priming in the late luteal phase results in the precocious recruitment and hurried development of the remaining follicles, which, in turn, seem to have a diminished ability to secrete estrogens. The ovulatory potential of these women, however, is maintained, as shown by the presence of a normal midcycle LH peak.[93,121] Luteal phase length and corpus luteum progesterone secretion also are similar to those of younger women.[120]

The onset of irregular menses announces the climacteric transition and is associated with more striking hormonal disturbances. Long menstrual intervals alternate with un-

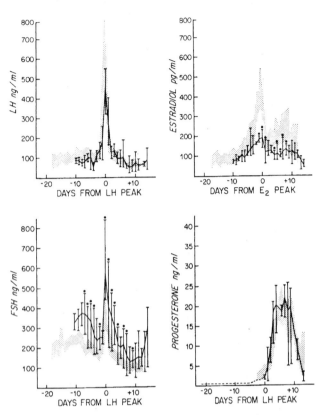

Fig. 53-1. Mean and range of serum LH, FSH, estradiol, and progesterone levels in women over age 45 with regular cycles. By comparison, the shaded area represents mean ± 2 SE in cycles of women aged 18 to 30. (From Sherman BM, Korenman SG: Hormonal characteristics of the human menstrual cycle throughout reproductive life. Reproduced from the *Journal of Clinical Investigation,* 1975, 55:699, by copyright permission of the American Society of Clinical Investigation.)

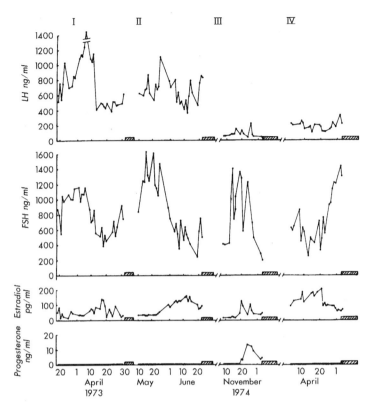

Fig. 53-2. Daily serum LH, FSH, estradiol, and progesterone levels during four cycles in one perimenopausal woman experiencing irregular menses. Shaded bars indicate menstruation. (From Sherman BM, West JH, Korenman SG: The menopausal transition: analysis of LH, FSH, estradiol and progesterone concentrations during menstrual cycles of older women, *J Clin Endocrinol Metab* 42:629, 1976, © by The Endocrine Society.)

usually short cycles, probably because of the erratic maturation of residual ovarian follicles.[136] In short cycles, serum E_2 levels remain typically low (<75 pg/mL) but display a definite increase at midcycle.[120] The peak of E_2 is followed by evidence of progesterone secretion. Progesterone levels, however, are typically decreased (<10 ng/mL) and most likely reflect inadequate corpus luteum function. In longer cycles, vaginal bleeding is often preceded by a rise and fall in E_2 levels without evidence of progesterone secretion. Consequently, it is probable that these cycles are anovulatory. In the transitional period, FSH and, often but less consistently, LH serum levels are elevated within the postmenopausal range.[121] Midcycle peak E_2 levels correlate with a proportional decrease of both FSH and LH levels, but FSH soon escapes and rises again sharply in the late luteal phase, as E_2 levels decline (Fig. 53-2). Interestingly, LH levels seem to be less sensitive and fail to show a significant variation at that time. Thus it appears that E_2 secretion is maintained during the transitional period despite the presence of postmenopausal gonadotropin levels. Indeed, a spontaneous rise in E_2 (100 to 250 pg/mL) has

even been observed sporadically after the establishment of menopause and probably results from the stimulation of the remaining follicles by high FSH levels.[24]

Most intriguing is the dissociation of the responses of FSH and LH. The role of hypothalamic gonadotropin-releasing hormone (GnRH) in the control of LH secretion is now well established.[67] The regulation of FSH release is less well understood. To date, the etiology of FSH elevation in premenopause remains unclear. Steroid feedback cannot entirely account for it, since E_2 levels are usually within the normal range for menstruating women. There is increasing evidence that inhibin, another ovarian follicular product, regulates pituitary FSH. It is suggested that the increasing follicular depletion in the later reproductive years may result in diminished inhibin production and the escape of FSH from its negative regulatory control.[108] In a group of infertile patients with incipient ovarian failure, as shown by their persistently elevated FSH levels, inhibin levels remained low throughout the cycle as compared with those of normal women (Fig. 53-3).[19] FSH levels were inversely correlated with those of inhibin.

Another alternative is that neuroendocrine events are responsible for increased FSH secretion perimenopausally.

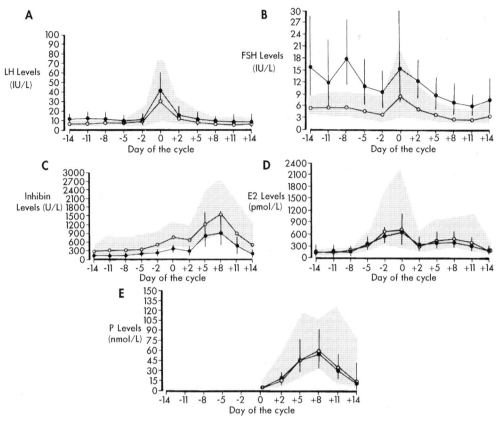

Fig. 53-3. LH (**A**), FSH (**B**), inhibin (**C**), estradiol (**D**), and progesterone (**E**) levels in incipient ovarian failure cycles (•). The geometric mean and 67% confidence limits are shown. The geometric mean (○) and the 95% confidence limits of the normal control group are shown in the shaded area. All data are log transformed. (From Buckler HM et al: Gonadotropin, steroid, and inhibin levels in women with incipient ovarian failure during anovulatory and ovulatory rebound cycles, *J Clin Endocrinol Metab* 72:116, 1991, © by The Endocrine Society.)

The evidence of enhanced pituitary responsiveness of FSH to GnRH administration in postmenopausal women supports this hypothesis.[112] Although age-related changes in neurotransmitters such as catecholamines have been documented in rodents,[152] a similar mechanism remains speculative in humans.

Hormonal changes associated with menopause

Androgens. In normally cycling women, androstenedione (Δ^4) is the major ovarian androgen and circulates at mean levels of approximately 1500 pg/mL (150 ng/dL).[73] Levels of Δ^4 do not show significant fluctuation except for a 15% increase at midcycle. After spontaneous menopause, the Δ^4 concentration is reduced by approximately 50% to a level of 800 to 900 pg/mL, a level comparable to that observed in premenopausal women after oophorectomy[71] (Fig. 53-4).

The metabolic clearance rate (MCR) of Δ^4, approximately 1800 L/h, is not affected by menopause or oophorectomy.[74] This high metabolic rate is explained by the fact that Δ^4 is minimally bound to sex hormone–binding globulin (SHBG) and loosely bound to albumin.[109] In postmenopausal women, the production rate (serum concentration multiplied by MCR) of Δ^4 is approximately 1.6 mg/24 h.

Oophorectomy after menopause further reduces Δ^4 levels by 20% (mean decrease 180 pg/mL). Because peripheral conversion of precursor steroids to Δ^4 is minimal,[2] the nonovarian fraction of Δ^4 reflects the adrenal secretion of this hormone. Ovarian secretion of Δ^4 is maintained but to a much lesser magnitude than in the reproductive years. Consequently, the adrenal gland is the primary source of circulating Δ^4 in postmenopausal women.

In normally cycling women, circulating testosterone (T) levels are lower than Δ^4 levels (mean 325 pg/mL), and a 20% increase is observed at midcycle.[73] The postmenopausal T concentration, approximately 250 pg/mL, is only minimally lower than that observed in younger women.[71] Because of its greater affinity for SHBG, T has a slower rate of clearance (mean 600 L/24 h),[74] resulting in a T production rate of approximately 200 μg/24 h. Since menopause does not influence the MCR_T,[21] T production rate is

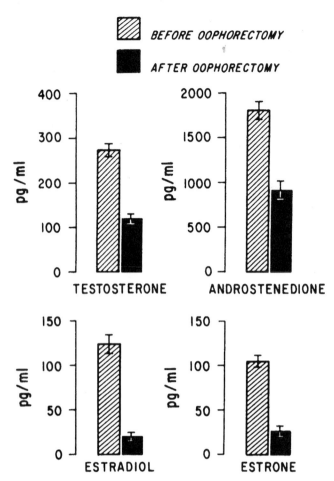

Fig. 53-4. Mean ± SE serum androgen and estrogen levels in five premenopausal women with endometrial cancer before and 6 to 8 weeks after oophorectomy. (From Judd HL: Hormonal dynamics associated with the menopause, *Clin Obstet Gynecol* 19:775, 1976.)

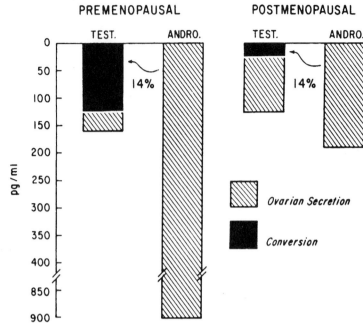

Fig. 53-5. Net fall of serum testosterone and androstenedione levels in premenopausal and postmenopausal women following oophorectomy. The theoretic amounts of hormone that are the result of peripheral conversion are shown in black. (From Judd HL: Hormonal dynamics associated with the menopause, *Clin Obstet Gynecol* 19:775, 1976.)

approximately 150 μg/24 h in postmenopausal subjects.

The source of circulating T is difficult to identify for the following reasons: First, 14% of circulating Δ^4 is peripherally converted to T; this conversion accounts for at least 50% of circulating T.[64] (Fig. 53-5) Second, oophorectomy decreases MCR_T in premenopausal women.[2] Therefore, serum T concentrations may not completely reflect alterations of T production in these subjects.

The ovary is a major source of T, as shown by the significant reduction of this hormone after oophorectomy in both premenopausal and postmenopausal women[71] (Fig. 53-5). Because the ovarian contribution to circulating Δ^4 levels is small after menopause[71] and only 14% of Δ^4 is converted to T, it is likely that peripheral conversion of Δ^4 accounts for only a minimal amount of the relatively high T concentrations observed in older subjects. Therefore, circulating T levels result mainly from direct secretion by the postmenopausal ovary. This view is substantiated by the larger step-up of T found in the ovarian veins of postmenopausal as compared with premenopausal subjects[75] (Fig. 53-6). This finding supports the hypothesis that postmeno-

pausal ovaries secrete directly more T than the premenopausal gonad. A potential explanation for this increased ovarian T production is the stimulation of androgen-secreting cells, such as hilus cells or stromal theca cells, by the elevated gonadotropins of older women. This relative hyperandrogenism coupled with postmenopausal estrogen depletion may explain in part the development of symptoms of defeminization, hirsutism, and even virilism observed in some older women.

Dehydroepiandrosterone (DH) and its sulfate (DHS) are mainly produced by the adrenal gland after menopause.[3] It is now well established that these two weak androgens steadily decline with age.[85,90] By the seventh decade, DH and DHS mean concentrations are 1.8 ng/mL and 0.3 μg/mL, respectively.[85] The decrease in Δ^5 androgens appears to be selective, since a similar change is not observed for androstenedione.[90] It has been hypothesized that an age-related decrease of adrenal 17,20-desmolase activity could account for this disparity.

Whether the decline of adrenal androgens is an aging phenomenon or is related to ovarian failure is unclear. Current data tend to support the latter hypothesis. Investigators have reported an increase in DHS in postmenopausal women receiving conjugated estrogens and have postulated that ovarian estrogens may stimulate adrenal DHS production.[3] The finding of DHS levels in normally menstruating women higher than in those who are postmenopausal or with premature ovarian failure supports this view.[28] However, long-term estrogen replacement failed to increase

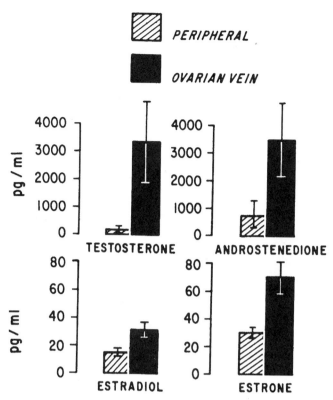

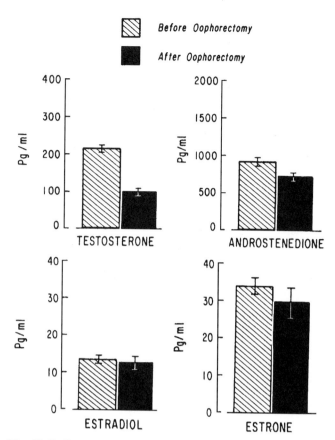

Fig. 53-6. Mean ± SE peripheral and ovarian vein androgen and estrogen levels in 10 postmenopausal women. (From Judd HL et al: Endocrine function of the postmenopausal ovary: concentrations of androgens and estrogens in ovarian and peripheral vein blood, *J Clin Endocrinol Metab* 39:1020, 1974, © by The Endocrine Society.)

Fig. 53-7. Serum androgen and estrogen levels in 16 postmenopausal women before and after oophorectomy. (From Judd HL: Hormonal dynamics associated with the menopause, *Clin Obstet Gynecol* 19:775, 1976.)

DHS levels. Taken together, these data suggest that ovarian factors other than estrogens exert a regulatory effect on adrenal production of DHS.

Estrogens. The most prominent hormonal change associated with menopause is a dramatic reduction in circulating E_2 levels. The mean peripheral concentration is approximately 13 pg/mL, and is comparable to the level seen in premenopausal women after oophorectomy[3,75] (Fig. 53-4). The MCR_{E_2} is decreased by 3.0% in postmenopausal women to approximately 900 L/24 h.[83] This results in a mean production rate of 12 µg/24 h. E_2 is bound to both SHBG and albumin, but more loosely than T. Studies have shown that the E_2 fraction bound to SHBG exits the circulation in vivo and is probably available to most tissues.[103]

In postmenopausal women, the majority of circulating E_2 is derived from the peripheral conversion of estrone (E_1), which in turn is the product of the peripheral aromatization of adrenal Δ^4.[76] Adrenal gland hormonal production plays a central role in menopause, as shown by the profound decrease in circulating sex steroids observed in older women with Addison's disease or adrenalectomy.[141] The conversion of precursor androgens such as Δ^4 and T

appears to contribute minimally to the circulating E_2 pool. Direct secretion of E_2 by the ovary is not significant either, since its circulating levels are similar before and after oophorectomy[72] (Fig. 53-7). Furthermore, only a small E_2 step-up is found in the ovarian veins of postmenopausal subjects.[75]

In contrast with the reproductive years, the circulating level of E_1 is higher than that of E_2 after menopause, the mean E_1 level being approximately 30 pg/mL.[72,75] Its MCR is more rapid than that of E_2. After menopause, MCR_{E_1} is reduced by 20% to approximately 1600 L/24 h. In postmenopausal women, most of the circulating E_1 results from the peripheral aromatization of Δ^4 of adrenal origin.[124] Direct glandular secretion of E_1 by either the ovary or the adrenal gland appears to be minimal. The rate of conversion of Δ^4 to E_1, as well as circulating estrogen levels, strongly correlates with obesity and excess fat and has been implicated in the genesis of endometrial cancer.[75,142] Whether age influences peripheral aromatization and estrogen levels remains a matter of debate.[24]

Progestins. Progesterone (P_4) secretion is the hallmark of corpus luteum function. In the normal menstrual cycle, serum P_4 levels increase steadily from the day of the LH surge and reach a plateau of 10 to 20 ng/mL at the midlutal phase (day 5 to day 10 after the LH peak).[4] After luteal phase day 10, P_4 levels decline sharply concomitant with corpus luteum demise to reach a level of 0.8 ng/mL on the first day of menses. During the follicular phase, circulating P_4 levels remain very low (0.3 to 0.8 ng/mL).

Early in the perimenopausal period, there is evidence of a dissociation in the corpus luteum capacity for E_2 and P_4 secretion, with reduced E_2 concentrations but normal luteal phase P_4 levels.[121] As menopause approaches, further disruption of the menstrual cycle results in lower P_4 levels consistent with luteal phase inadequacy and, finally, anovulation.

After menopause, low peripheral P_4 levels of 0.1 to 0.4 ng/mL have been measured. In the hands of different investigators, these values are similar to or lower than those observed in the follicular phase of premenopausal controls.[85,140] No further change in circulating P_4 levels has been noted with advancing age.[90]

In the absence of data concerning the ovarian vein concentration of P_4, the origin of postmenopausal P_4 secretion remains unclear. Indirect data on using the dexamethasone suppression test are conflicting. The ovarian origin of postmenopausal P_4 is suggested by one study showing no change in P_4 levels after administration of dexamethasone for 7 days.[85] In that study, however, P_4 secretion was still maintained after dexamethasone suppression in two subjects who had undergone bilateral oophorectomy. The ovarian theory is further supported by the observation that both hilus and stromal cells from postmenopausal ovaries secrete P_4 in vitro.[30,31] P_4 production is further enhanced by the addition of human chorionic gonadotropin (hCG) to the culture media.

Another investigator showed complete suppression of P_4 secretion after administration of a similar dose of dexamethasone for 5 days and concluded that postmenopausal P_4 was predominantly of adrenal origin.[140] Sustained P_4 levels in postmenopausal women who have undergone oophorectomy support this hypothesis. In addition, adrenocorticotropic hormone (ACTH) stimulation increased P_4 levels by 500%, whereas hCG stimulation did not significantly alter P_4 levels.

A peripheral 17-hydroxyprogesterone (17-OHP) level of approximately 0.4 ng/mL has been found in postmenopausal women.[85,140] This value is significantly lower than 17-OHP levels measured in the follicular phase of premenopausal subjects. Although both the ovary and the adrenal gland have been shown to contribute to 17-OHP secretion, the role of the latter seems to be predominant based on the following findings[140]: (1) postmenopausal 17-OHP levels are similar before and after oophorectomy; (2) ACTH stimulation increases 17-OHP levels by 500%; (3) dexamethasone suppresses 17-OHP levels by half.

Circulating levels of 17-hydroxypregnenolone of adrenal origin decrease significantly after menopause, whereas pregnenolone concentration remains unaffected.[1] No age-related changes in concentrations of 17-OHP, 17-hydroxypregnenolone, or pregnenolone have been substantiated.[90]

Gonadotropins. Circulating FSH and LH levels are consistently elevated in postmenopausal women, with FSH usually being higher than LH. These elevations reflect the increased pituitary production due to the removal of inhibitory gonadal steroid feedback. The slower clearance of FSH is in part responsible for the higher FSH levels.

The pulsatile pattern of gonadotropin secretion is exaggerated after menopause. As in the follicular phase of cycling women, pulsatile release of the gonadotropins occurs at 60 to 90-minute intervals, but the amplitude of the pulses is much greater in older subjects.[153] This increased amplitude reflects the increased responsiveness of the pituitary gland to GnRH secretion from the hypothalamus.[112] GnRH secretion also is increased after cessation of ovarian function.

The menopausal hot flush

The most characteristic symptom of the climacteric is an episodic disturbance consisting of sudden flushing and perspiration, referred to as the hot flash or flush. This phenomenon has been observed in 65% to 76% of women who experience a natural or surgical menopause.[55,68,88,98,134] Of those, 82% will experience the disturbance for more than 1 year and 24% to 50% will complain of the symptom for more than 5 years.[98,135]

Subjectively, a hot flush begins with a sensation of increasing pressure in the head followed by a feeling of heat in the head, neck, upper chest, and back that can spread to the entire body.[98] It is followed immediately by an outbreak of perspiration in the affected areas.[55] Patients often complain of insomnia, and there is a close temporal relationship between the occurrence of hot flushes and waking episodes. The mean duration of a whole episode is 3.3 minutes but can vary from 5 seconds to 60 minutes.[137] The frequency of these episodes varies greatly among subjects and can be as frequent as one every 20 minutes.[89] Mean frequency in women with severe complaints is approximately once per hour. Hot flushes are not affected by age at menopause, socioeconomic status, parity, or racial background.[96,135] In contrast to other menopausal symptoms such as urogenital atrophy or osteoporosis, vasomotor symptoms improve with advancing age.

There are measurable changes in physiologic function that accompany hot flushes. Cutaneous vasodilatation occurs, is generalized, and results in measurable increases in the skin temperature of the fingers and toes that last for 30 to 40 minutes.[89,95,134] The next sign is a decrease in skin resistance, a measurement of perspiration. This reaches its maximum in about 4 minutes and returns to baseline in 18 minutes (Fig. 53-8). As heat is lost from the body by cutaneous vasodilatation and perspiration, there is a drop in

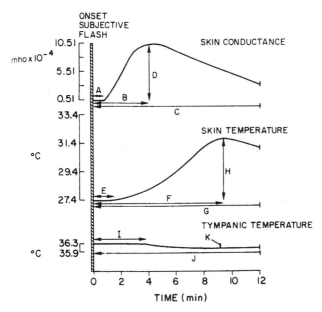

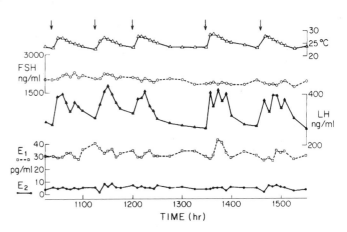

Fig. 53-9. Serial measurements of finger skin temperature and serum FSH, LH, E_1, and E_2 in a postmenopausal patient. Arrows mark the onset of the subjective flushes as expressed by the patient (From Meldrum et al: Gonadotropins, estrogens, and adrenal steroids during the menopausal hot flash, *J Clin Endocrinol Metab* 50:685, 1980, © by The Endocrine Society.)

Fig. 53-8. Characteristics of the changes in chest skin conductance, finger skin temperature, and tympanic membrane temperature based on recordings of 25 menopausal hot flushes. (From Tataryn et al: Postmenopausal hot flushes: a disorder of thermoregulation, *Maturitas* 2:101, 1980.)

core temperature beginning at about 4 minutes after the onset of the subjective flush and lasting for about 30 minutes.[89,134] Since the subjective symptoms last for an average of 4 minutes,[89] it is obvious that objectively recorded changes continue many minutes after disappearance of the symptomatic flush.

The pathophysiologic mechanism responsible for the occurrence of hot flushes remains to be fully elucidated. Since the phenomenon occurs after surgical or spontaneous loss of ovarian function, it has been postulated that estrogen withdrawal plays a central role. The observation that flushes occur simultaneously with the pulsatile release of LH but not FSH from the pituitary was the key finding that suggested a neuroendocrine mechanism[133] (Fig. 53-9). Although LH release is associated with hot flushes, it is unlikely that this hormone itself triggers these aberrant thermoregulatory events. This conclusion is supported by the observation that hot flushes are observed in women with surgically induced pituitary insufficiency with low, nonpulsatile LH release.[91] In addition, administration of GnRH agonist to premenopausal women results in the suppression of pulsatile LH release and induces vasomotor symptoms.[23] Taken together, these data suggest that the neuroendocrine mechanism responsible for the pulsatile release of LH must also influence the thermoregulatory centers (Fig. 53-10). LH secretion is mediated by the release of GnRH from the hypothalamus into the portal vein. Patients with isolated gonadotropin deficiency, due to a defect in hypothalamic GnRH secretion, have typical menopausal hot flushes after

estrogen withdrawal.[43] Thus it is unlikely that GnRH itself is responsible for vasomotor symptoms.

Patients with hypothalamic amenorrhea are thought to have a neurotransmitter disorder of the hypothalamus resulting in decreased GnRH secretion and consequently hypogonadism. Despite postmenopausal levels of estrogens, these patients rarely if ever experience hot flushes.[43] It is therefore hypothesized that the same neuroendocrine event that causes hypothalamic amenorrhea is responsible for the absence of hot flushes. This theory is supported by the observation that GnRH neurons are in close proximity to the thermoregulatory centers in the preoptic anterior hypothalamus.[82] Furthermore, brain norepinephrine and endorphins play a role in both thermoregulation and GnRH release.[69] The decrease in hot flush frequency after administration of clonidine, an α_2-adrenergic receptor agonist, supports the role of catecholamines in vasomotor symptoms.[80] Infusion with Naloxone, an opioid antagonist, elicits rises of LH levels in ovulatory but not postmenopausal women. Estrogen and progestin administration to older women will lower LH levels that can be reversed by this opiate antagonist[29] (Fig. 53-11). Based on these observations, the following hypothesis is proposed: Loss of ovarian function with its accompanying reduction of hypothalamic opioid tone results in thermoregulatory instability and the triggering of hot flushes. E_2 administration, through enhancement of hypothalamic opioid activity, lowers gonadotropin levels and relieves hot flushes.

This hypothesis is further supported by a recent study using veralipride, a dopamine antagonist.[92] Because this drug both reduces vasomotor symptoms and decreases circulating LH levels, it has been hypothesized that it exerts its activity by increasing endogenous opioid tone in postmenopausal women.

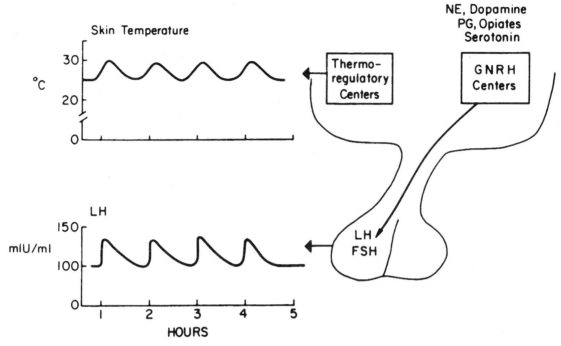

Fig. 53-10. A proposed neuroendocrine mechanism of menopausal hot flushes. (From Judd HL: The basis of menopausal vasomotor symptoms. In Mastroianni L Jr, Paulsen CA, editors: *Aging, reproduction and the climacteric,* New York, 1986, Plenum Press.)

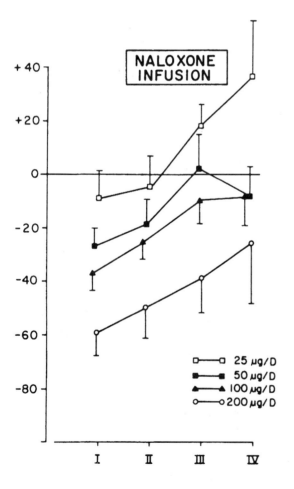

Urogenital atrophy

Postmenopausal urogenital atrophy is a relatively late manifestation of estrogen deficiency. The epithelia of the vagina, urethra, and bladder trigone have a common origin in the urogenital sinus and exhibit estrogen receptors.[65] These cells are sensitive to estrogens and develop similar atrophic changes with its withdrawal. Lower genital tract atrophy occurs in all postmenopausal women, but the degree of epithelial change varies greatly from one subject to another. Some women will maintain a healthy vaginal cytology and good function for many years, whereas others will rapidly develop epithelial atrophy and marked discomfort with sexual relations. In this latter group, distressing symptoms such as vaginal dryness, burning, pruritus, dyspareunia, dysuria, and urinary frequency may develop. Although approximately half of postmenopausal women experience some degree of lower genital tract disorder,[66]

Fig. 53-11. The mean ± SE percentage change in LH levels from values observed before naloxone infusion in the pretreatment study (before estrogen administration) in postmenopausal women. The data are divided into zone I (prenaloxone), zone II (first 2 hours of naloxone), zone III (last 2 hours of naloxone), and zone IV (postnaloxone). Naloxone infusions were performed on day 27 of 28-day treatment period for each E_2 dosage. (From D'Amico JF et al: Induction of hypothalamic opioid activity with transdermal estradiol administration in postmenopausal women, *Fertil Steril* 55:754, 1991. Reproduced with permission of the publisher, The American Fertility Society.)

most of them are reluctant to bring up this issue spontaneously. Physicians should therefore inquire about these problems, particularly since estrogen replacement therapy provides relief from most of these symptoms.[143]

Atrophic vaginitis and cervical changes. With the decline of estrogen, the vagina loses elasticity and subepithelial connective tissue increases.[100] This results in progressive shortening and narrowing of the vagina and loss of rugae. The vaginal epithelium becomes attenuated, pale, or erythematous with fine petechial hemorrhages. The atrophic epithelium is easily traumatized, leading to ulcerations and bleeding. It can account for 15% of postmenopausal bleeding.[18] Estrogen withdrawal results in the loss of cellular glycogen, increased vaginal pH, and the replacement of lactobacilli by other bacteria causing vaginal infections. The decrease in vaginal fluid and reduced vaginal lubrication during coitus result in dyspareunia and diminished interest in sexual relations.[116] Although estrogen therapy is the treatment of choice for these complaints, there is evidence that regular sexual activity per se prevents excessive shrinkage of the vagina and allows maintenance of better coital function.[18]

Cytologic examination of vaginal cells can be used as an indicator of hormonal exposure. The maturation index measures the relation of superficial, intermediate, and parabasal cells (S/I/P).[10] Estrogen deprivation results in the loss of maturation of the vaginal epithelium, which leads to the disappearance of superficial cells and the increase in intermediate and parabasal cells. However, superficial cells have still been identified in 25% of women over the age of 75.[100] Nonhormonal medications such as digitalis and tetracycline promote the maturation of vaginal cells and may mislead the physician. The maturation index is therefore of limited value in clinical practice. Because it does not appear to correlate with either circulating estrogen levels or menopausal symptoms, the maturation index should not be used to determine the need for estrogen replacement therapy.[130]

The cervix undergoes similar atrophic changes. Some of the fibromuscular stroma is lost and the cervix shrinks. Eventually, its vaginal portion no longer projects into the vagina, and the external os becomes flush with the vaginal vault.[100] The cervical epithelium thins and may bleed easily during pelvic examination. The endocervical glands undergo atrophy and the cervical mucus is scant, contributing to vaginal dryness. The external and internal ossa may be stenotic, and the squamocolumnar junction migrates up into the cervical canal. This may hinder obtaining an adequate sample for a Papanicolaou test, or the colposcopic evaluation of cervical lesions.

Urodynamic changes. The urethral epithelium is sensitive to estrogens and exhibits cytologic changes throughout the menstrual cycle similar to those seen in vaginal epithelial cells.[18] The urethra is composed of transitional cells proximally and squamous cells distally. In the reproductive years, the squamous epithelium extends upward toward the urethrovesical junction and increases the thickness of the urethral epithelium. After menopause, the squamous epithelium regresses and becomes thin and friable. Inflammatory changes may be observed. The maturation index of the urethral mucosa reveals predominantly parabasal cells.[9]

Atrophic changes of the urethra and the bladder trigone are responsible for the development of the so-called senile urethral syndrome.[115] Affected subjects experience urgency, frequency, dysuria, and suprapubic pain in the absence of a urinary tract infection.

The thinning of the urethral epithelium and the sclerosis of periurethral connective tissues are responsible for a 30% drop in urethral pressure.[107] Postmenopausal women experience an increased incidence of recurrent lower urinary tract infections[66] and urinary incontinence.[138] This latter phenomenon is often exacerbated by some degree of pelvic relaxation. After menopause, pelvic muscles and ligaments lose their tone and elasticity.[18] The changes are usually more pronounced in multiparous women. The descent of pelvic structures removes the urethrovesical junction from its intraabdominal location. Thus an increase in the abdominal pressure is transmitted to the bladder only, without urethral compensation, and results in the loss of urine.

Vulva. Postmenopausal vulvar changes are more a consequence of the aging process than of hypoestrogenism. Hair distribution becomes more sparse over the labia majora and the mons pubis. The labia majora appear wrinkled because of the loss of elastic tissue and subcutaneous fat.[78] The labia minora become more prominent. Like the vaginal epithelium, the vulvar skin thins. It is easily traumatized, and ulcerations and fissures may be present. During sexual arousal, labial swelling is diminished and mucus secretion from the Bartholin gland is reduced. Most of the time, vulvar atrophy is asymptomatic and should be considered "physiologic."[100] In some instances, excessive shrinkage of the paravaginal tissues results in severe constrictions of the introitus, which renders intercourse virtually impossible.[18] As in most vulvar atrophic changes, these alterations are not directly attributable to estrogen deficiency.[78]

Skin changes

Skin alterations such as atrophy, loss of elasticity, dryness, and impaired wound healing occur with advanced age. These are usually more pronounced in sun-exposed areas. It has become increasingly evident, however, that alterations in skin quality cannot be ascribed to the aging process alone. Data have accumulated to show that the decline in sex steroids at the time of menopause has a major impact on skin changes. Multiple studies have now suggested that estrogen replacement therapy not only helps maintain skin resilience but also reverses some of the changes observed in older women.

Epidermal changes. The epidermis is a thin layer composed primarily of keratinocytes. As these cells mature, they become cornified and form the outermost layer of the epidermis, providing a barrier against the external environment. With aging, the keratinocytes undergo a reduction in vertical height, an increase in surface area, a decrease in adhesions, and an increase in cytoarchitectural disruption.[11] There is an associated flattening of the dermoepidermal junction. These changes account for the dryness, increased fragility, and easy bruising of aging skin.

The epidermis contains estrogen target cells. The nuclei of basal keratinocytes of ovariectomized mice incorporate tritiated E_2.[132] Estrogen receptors have also been isolated from human skin.[57] Early studies in rodents showed a thinning of the epidermis after administration of estrogens.[38,63] A subsequent study noted initial epidermal thickening, followed later by thinning.[20] Data on the effect of estrogen on the epidermis have been somewhat confusing. In women, epidermal biopsy specimens measured by planimetry showed that the longer the time after castration the thinner the epidermis became.[106] The difference in thickness was statistically significant 7 months after oophorectomy, compared with preoperative biopsy specimens. After 3 months of treatment with either estriol succinate or estradiol valerate, increases in epidermal thickness and epidermal mitotic activity were noted. However, 24% of the patients taking estradiol valerate exhibited a thinning of the epidermis at 6 months of treatment. This biphasic effect, somewhat comparable to the results of rodent experiments, might be attributed to an inhibitory effect of estrogens at pharmacologic rather than physiologic doses. This hypothesis is further supported by findings that showed that high concentrations of E_1 significantly reduced mitotic activity of human epidermis in vitro.[118]

Dermal changes. The dermis is a connective tissue that forms the bulk of skin. Its major component is collagen, which accounts for 97.5% of dermal fibers; elastin fibers (2.5%) make up the rest.[14] The stroma contains fibroblasts, blood vessels, nerve fibers, and immunocompetent cells. The dermis also surrounds important skin appendages such as hair follicles and sebaceous glands.

The rate of dermal collagen synthesis declines with age, leading to dermal atrophy and impaired wound healing.[11] Dermal collagen fibers, however, remain structurally stable and do not exhibit age-related morphologic changes. In contrast, dermal elastic fibers show progressive structural and functional degenerative changes after age 30 years.[123] With electron microscopy, formation of cysts and splitting and fragmentation of the fibers are observed with increasing frequency with aging. The decrease in sebaceous gland secretion further contributes to skin dryness.

In laboratory animals, estrogen receptors have been identified on dermal fibroblasts.[132] Fibroblasts are responsible for the production of dermal collagen, elastin, and mucopolysaccharides. Although it has little morphologic effect on fibroblasts, estrogen has been shown to enhance the synthesis of hyaluronic acid and, as a result, increase the water content of the mouse dermis.[51]

Extensive studies have been performed on the effect of estrogens on dermal collagen content and skin thickness of postmenopausal women. Women treated with both estrogen and testosterone implants for 2 to 10 years were compared with an untreated, aged-matched group.[15] Both forearm skin thickness and thigh skin collagen content were significantly greater in the treated group (Fig. 53-12). In untreated postmenopausal subjects, a gradual depletion of collagen

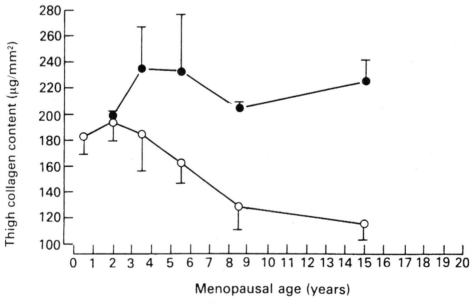

Fig. 53-12. Relation between thigh skin collagen content and menopausal age in women treated with sex steroid implants (•) and in untreated patients (o). (From Brincat et al: Long-term effects of the menopause and sex hormones on skin thickness, *Br J Obstet Gynaecol* 92:256, 1985.)

content of 2% per year was noted.[17] The role of sex steroids was further stressed by the finding that the decline in skin collagen correlated with the number of postmenopausal years but not with chronologic age.[15] Skin collagen content and skin thickness were improved with administration of estrogen only or a combination of estrogen and testosterone.[16] However, women with the lowest collagen values benefited most from the treatment, with little additional action being noted in subjects who started with a high skin collagen content. This observation seems to indicate that in women with reduced skin thickness and collagen content, estrogen replacement may be therapeutic as well as prophylactic, whereas in women with high values it can only prevent loss.

Although these studies are of great interest, they are flawed by the lack of a placebo-controlled randomized study design. Until this is accomplished, these drug trials cannot be considered conclusive.

Psychologic changes

Menopause has been associated with an array of affective symptoms such as nervousness, irritability, anxiety, and depression. Other neuropsychologic disturbances include insomnia, disruption of concentration, and impairment of memory.[33] The precise role of endocrine changes in the development of these symptoms has been difficult to define because of the lack of control for other interfering factors. For example, the aging process alone could account for these changes. In fact, two studies have suggested that insomnia was related to advanced age rather than menopause.[34] Some reports have shown that stressful life events, such as the departure of children from the home, an ailing husband, the lack of suitable confidants, and professional dissatisfaction, may have substantial psychologic implications during the climacteric.[32] Finally, cross-cultural differences seem to play an important role. Several epidemiologic studies have identified fewer climacteric complaints in women who belong to cultures in which aging is associated with an improvement of their social condition.[34]

Although numerous studies have now reported that minor psychologic disturbances occur with greater frequency in the transitional period,[32] others have failed to show this association.[88,99] These inconsistencies probably reflect methodologic problems, including the use of unstandardized questionnaires, the reliance on cross-sectional designs, and the confusion between chronologic age and menopausal status. There is, however, good evidence that menopause is not associated with an increase in major psychiatric disorders. The early psychiatric literature referred to a disease known as involutional melancholia. It was characterized by the late onset of depression, anxiety, and hypochondriacal symptoms in individuals without previous history of psychiatric illness, and was thought to be confined to the involutional period. In the 1970s, the concept of involutional melancholia was challenged after multiple studies failed to support the existence of such a distinct entity.[146] As a result, involutional melancholia was removed from the American Psychiatric Association's *Diagnostic and Statistical Manual* (DSM-III). Further studies have failed to show an increase in major depressive illnesses in middle-aged women.[154] The peak of mental disorders in women is between the ages of 35 and 44 years and declines thereafter.[146]

More consistent results have been observed with drug trials of estrogen replacement therapy. In a 4-month double-blind, crossover trial, estrogen was found to be significantly more effective than placebo in relieving 12 symptoms, including hot flushes, insomnia, irritability, poor memory, anxiety, worry about age, headaches, worry about self, and optimism.[22] It was noted, however, that women who had previously experienced severe hot flushes were relieved of a greater number of symptoms with estrogen, compared with women without vasomotor instability. It was hypothesized that the disappearance of hot flushes resulted in a "domino effect," with decreased insomnia and consequently less irritability. It was also stressed that placebo alone improved psychologic symptoms, suggesting that medical attention per se may have been responsible for these improvements.

In another large, well-controlled study, patients who had undergone surgical menopause were treated with ethinyl estradiol and levonorgestrel, separately or in combination, or placebo.[35] Ethinyl estradiol elicited the greatest benefit on the psychologic profile as measured by Hamilton Score and ordinal ratings of general well-being, depression, fatigue, anxiety, irritability, and insomnia. The impact of vaginal atrophy on sexual function is well recognized. Whether the loss of ovarian function plays a role in other aspects of female sexuality remains controversial.[34] Again, the influence of hormonal replacement on sexual function is better established. Investigators have found that ethinyl estradiol improved sexual desire, enjoyment, vaginal lubrication, and orgasmic frequency in postmenopausal women, where as administration of conjugated estrogens was associated with increased coital satisfaction.[22,36]

The impact of exogenous androgens on sexual function remains to be defined. In an uncontrolled study, significant improvement of sexual function was reported in patients treated with both estradiol (50 mg) and testosterone (100 mg) implants.[131] In one of the few double-blind, randomized trials, women failed to show additional benefit of testosterone over estradiol alone.[37] Estradiol or a combination of estradiol and testosterone improved sexual interest and responsiveness. In a recent double-blind, crossover study, testosterone was reported to increase sexual desire and arousal significantly but did not influence coital frequency.[122] Clearly, a major problem with studies on postmenopausal sexual activity has been the questionable validity of the rating scales used, the lack of information on the availability of a suitable sexual partner, and the limited number of double-blind trials.

In summary, menopause increases minor psychologic complaints but not major psychiatric disorders. In addition to the endocrine changes of menopause, stressful life events, sociocultural factors, and individual vulnerability can contribute to the psychologic distress of middle-aged women and need to be addressed by health care providers. Hormone replacement therapy appears to be beneficial in some women in relieving affective, cognitive, and sexual complaints and therefore should be offered. Care must be exercised in administering larger than usual doses of hormones for this indication because of the likely occurrence of placebo effects.

TREATMENT OF MENOPAUSE

As long as ovarian function is sufficient to maintain some uterine bleeding, replacement therapy usually is not required. As the menstrual pattern alters and symptoms appear, patients begin to seek help; the need for medical intervention must then be addressed.

Every woman with climacteric symptoms deserves an adequate explanation of the physiologic event she is experiencing in order to dispel her fears and minimize symptoms such as anxiety, depression, and sleep disturbances. Specific reassurance about continued sexual activity is important.

Estrogen replacement is the hallmark of treatment of menopause. Before administering this form of therapy, a discussion of the advantages, as well as the complications and contraindications, should be held with each patient.

Complications

Hyperplasia and endometrial cancer. Continuous and unopposed stimulation of endometrial cells by estrogens results in transformation from atrophic to proliferative to hyperplastic.[45] Cystic and adenomatous hyperplasia can progress further to atypical adenomatous hyperplasia, a well-recognized precancerous lesion that, in turn, may lead to endometrial adenocarcinoma.[52]

In the mid-1970s, epidemiologic studies reported an alarming increase in the incidence of endometrial carcinoma, which seemed to coincide with a rise in the sales of estrogens in the United States.[50,145] These findings were later supported by several case-control studies that showed convincing evidence of an association between exogenous estrogens and endometrial cancer.[49,84,125,155]

Postmenopausal women receiving unopposed estrogens have a threefold to fifteenfold increased risk of developing endometrial cancer. The risk appears to correlate with both the dose[49,84] and the duration[6,49,84,155] of estrogen exposure. Administration of estrogens in a cyclic fashion provides little or no protection.[6,114] Although the risk declines after discontinuation of estrogen use, the precise interval that is sufficient to eliminate excessive risk has not been determined. Some studies have suggested that a significant risk persists for up to 6 to 10 years after cessation of

treatment.[110,117] It is important, however, to put this risk clearly in perspective. The absolute risk of developing endometrial cancer is increased from 1/1000 in unexposed women to 2.7/1000 per year in estrogen users.[104] Thus the risk remains small. There is also good evidence suggesting that estrogen-linked endometrial cancer has a good prognosis. In a study of 363 women with endometrial cancer, estrogen users (>1 year) tended to have localized disease (stage 0 or I) and well-differentiated tumors.[26] The degree of myometrial invasion was significantly lower compared with the nonuser group. Women with tumors who were treated with estrogen have a significantly higher survival rate at 5 years, 94%, compared with 81% in nontreated patients (Fig. 53-13).[39] These reassuring findings may explain why there has been no demonstrable increase in mortality from endometrial cancer despite increased estrogen usage.

It has been suggested that the addition of a progestin reduces the risk of estrogen-induced endometrial carcinoma.[44,53,97] Administration of 10 mg of medroxyprogesterone acetate for 10 days each month has been shown to be protective. Duration as well as dosage of progestin therapy is critical.

It has been reported that the combination estrogen-progestin not only protects the endometrium from the influence of unopposed estrogens but may also decrease the incidence of endometrial cancer below that of women using no hormones.[44] This latter finding and the increasing evidence of long-term advantages of estrogen therapy suggest that postmenopausal women with previously cured endometrial cancer may benefit from estrogen replacement. Indeed, a nonrandomized study has shown that former endometrial cancer patients treated with estrogens had a better survival rate than the non–estrogen-treated group.[27] Until additional studies confirm these findings, the administration of exogenous estrogens to former endometrial cancer patients should be limited to carefully selected subjects.

Breast cancer. There is substantial evidence to support the role of sex hormones, particularly estrogens, in the genesis of breast cancer. Experimental data have shown that estrogens act as promotors of breast cancer in rodents. Factors that are associated with prolonged estrogenic exposure, such as low parity, first childbirth after age 30, obesity, anovulatory infertility, early menarche, and late menopause, increase the relative risk of breast cancer.[59] Based on these findings, exogenous estrogens have long been suspected to increase the risk of breast cancer. However, it has been surprisingly difficult to substantiate this risk. Since the mid 1970s, more than 20 well-designed cohort and case-control studies have yielded inconsistent results, creating confusion among physicians and patients.

To summarize the findings of these epidemiologic studies, nearly all have shown no statistically significant increase in the overall risk of breast cancer with estrogen

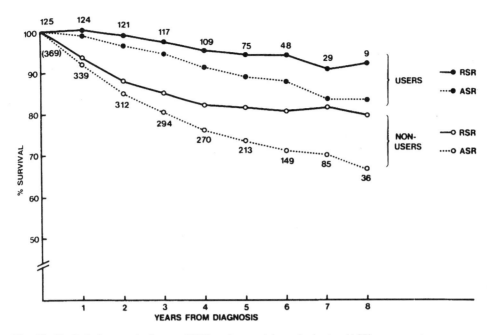

Fig. 53-13. Relative survival rates (*RSR*) and actuarial survival rates (*ASR*) among estrogen users and estrogen nonusers. Numbers indicate how many women were under observation at each year interval. (From Elwood JM, Boyes DA: Clinical and pathological features and survival of endometrial cancer patients in relation to prior use of estrogens, *Gynecol Oncol* 10:173, 1980.)

replacement. Some have reported enhanced risks in subsets of women, such as those exposed to estrogen for longer durations or in larger doses, those with intact ovaries, those who underwent premenopausal oophorectomy, those with benign breast disease, or those who used injectable estrogens. In nearly all cases, subsequent reports have been published that have not confirmed these findings. The one finding that has been supported by a majority of studies is an increased risk with long-term usage. Recently investigators reviewed 15 of the most pertinent studies and used a summary dose-response slope to calculate the proportional increase in breast cancer for each year of estrogen use[128] (Table 53-1). They concluded that estrogen use did not result in increased risk of breast cancer for the first 5 years but rose slightly thereafter to reach a 30% increase at 15 years. The risk was also increased in women with a family history of breast cancer. The authors stressed, however, that the results of three European studies negatively influenced the total results.[8,41,81] These studies may have somewhat distinctive features. All of them reported predominantly synthetic estrogen usage, whereas American studies reported primarily conjugated equine estrogen administration; more premenopausal and perimenopausal women were included in the data analysis; progestins were more commonly used in association with estrogens. Finally, geographic factors may play a role in the risk distribution.

The impact of progestins on the risk of breast cancer remains controversial. Progestins counteract the effect of estrogen on endometrial proliferation, thereby preventing the development of endometrial cancer. There is, however, evidence to suggest that the effects of progestins on the breast are different from those on the endometrium.[60] First, the breast epithelial cell division rate peaks in the luteal phase, on day 23 to day 25, at the time of maximal progesterone levels.[79] In contrast, maximal endometrial mitotic activity occurs in the follicular phase. Second, extensive case-control and cohort studies have shown that long-term use of oral contraceptives (OCs) is associated with a marked reduction in risk of endometrial cancer, whereas there is no evidence of a protective effect on breast cancer. It has actually been suggested that prolonged early use of OCs may enhance risk of breast cancer in premenopausal women.[60] Finally, the data on menopausal combined estrogen-progestin therapy have been inconclusive. Some have shown protection,[46,97] others have reported no effect, and the remainder have suggested enhanced risk.[8,41]

In conclusion, there is no consistent evidence currently that postmenopausal administration of estrogens increases the incidence of breast cancer. Very prolonged use (>15 years), particularly of synthetic estrogens, may increase risk. However, it must be remembered that none of these studies was randomized. This design flaw raises serious questions about whether the women who were treated or not treated were of equal risk for this disease with the exception of estrogen usage. The possibility of differences in risk besides use of estrogens may explain the lack of consistency of findings and raises questions about the reality of the small increase of risk with long-term use.

Table 53-1. Effect of estrogen replacement therapy on breast cancer risk in women: data from 15 case-control studies stratified and pooled by high, moderate, and low quality scores, 1977 through 1989.

Reference, y	Quality score	Proportional increase in risk for each year of estrogen use	Mean proportional increase in risk for each year of estrogen use by quality score (95% confidence interval)*
		HIGH QUALITY SCORE: 71-83	
Wingo et al,[151a] 1987	83	0.008	
Bergkvist et al,[8] 1989	82	0.006	
Ross et al,[109a] 1980	75	0.060	
Hoover et al,[63a] 1981	72	0.066	
Hiatt et al,[61a] 1984	71	0.053	
	77 (66-88)†		0.040 (0.030-0.050)
		MODERATE QUALITY SCORE: 40-57	
Nomura et al,[99a] 1986	57	−0.002	
Brinton et al,[17a] 1986	51	0.001	
Kaufman et al,[77a] 1984	45	−0.007	
LaVecchia et al,[81] 1986	43	0.308	
Kelsey et al,[78a] 1981	40	−0.091	
	47 (33-61)†		−0.008 (−0.0017−0.000)
		LOW QUALITY SCORE: 15-38	
Hulka et al,[64a] 1982	38	0.068	
Jick et al,[68a] 1988	38	0.007	
Ravinhar et al,[106a] 1979	26	−0.016	
Wynder et al,[152a] 1978	25	−0.203	
Sartwell et al,[111a] 1977	15	−0.084	
	28 (9-47)†		0.006 (0.000−0.012)

From Steinberg KK et al: *JAMA* 265:1985, 1991.
*Results obtained by combining dose-response slopes across studies for each quality score category, then converting the results to mean proportional increase in risk per year of estrogen use.
†Mean quality score (95% confidence interval).

Because the effect of progestins on the breast is controversial, their use in women without a uterus is not recommended. Although there is continued evidence that the beneficial effects of estrogen replacement therapy outweigh its risks, physicians should consider the risk-benefit ratio for each patient on an individual basis. Screening for breast disease should be performed regularly in accordance with established guidelines.

Hypertension. The association of OC use with blood pressure elevation has been documented. Large population studies, such as the Kaiser-Permanente Contraceptive Drug Study, have reported that elevated blood pressure occurs more frequently in OC users than in controls.[42] The mean increment of blood pressure was statistically significant, although small (5 mm Hg systolic and 1 mm Hg diastolic).

Based on these results, attempts have been made to identify a causal relationship between estrogen replacement and hypertension. At least seven case-control studies have been published between 1976 and 1988, with five showing no association.[58,86] In the two studies that found an increase in blood pressure, the temporal relationship between hormone use and hypertension either was not determined or, when assessed, it was discovered that most of the hypertensive women had elevated blood pressure before therapy was initiated. At least five prospective drug trials have also been conducted, of which three were randomized.[58] None found a significant increase in blood pressure, whereas a small but consistent lowering of both systolic and diastolic blood pressures was reported with estrogen use.

In summary, the available data do not support the role of estrogen replacement in the development of hypertension. Although isolated cases have been documented, they probably represent idiosyncratic reactions to hormone administration.

Thromboembolic disease. The administration of oral contraceptives increases the risk of overt venous thromboembolic disease and the occurrence of subclinical thrombosis that is extensive enough to be detected by laboratory procedures, such as ^{125}I-labeled fibrinogen uptake[111] and plasma fibrinogen chromatography.[5] Thrombophlebitis has been reported with estrogen replacement therapy in an uncontrolled study, whereas this association has not been present in controlled trials.[13,53,97]

Theoretically, estrogens may promote clotting mechanisms by acting at three different sites: the vascular endothelium, platelets, and coagulation mechanism. Estrogens have been associated with endothelial cell proliferation and reductions of venous blood flow.[77] The available data on endothelial prostaglandin production are inconclusive. Administration of estrogen to laboratory animals tends to reduce prostacyclin production, whereas synthetic estrogen seems to increase the activity of this vasodilating compound in postmenopausal women.[101] The role of progestins needs further clarification.

Platelet aggregation is usually not affected by estrogens, although one study demonstrated an increase.[105] The mild decrement in platelet count observed after administration of sex steroids does not appear to be clinically important.

Both procoagulant and anticoagulant factors are present in blood to maintain its fluidity while allowing hemostasis with vascular injury. Like other hepatic proteins, fibrinogen and factors II, VII, IX, X, and XII are increased with use of estrogens.[101] The degree of increment is related to the potency of the estrogen and is more pronounced with synthetic estrogens such as ethinyl estradiol. Nonoral estrogens do not influence the production of clotting factors.[25] These findings should be placed in perspective since elevation of blood coagulation factors do not directly correlate with a clinically hypercoagulable state.

Estrogen replacement therapy can also lower anticoagulant factors such as antithrombin III and anti-Xa. Numerous studies have shown that OCs can decrease antithrombin III activity.[147] Deficiency of antithrombin III is associated with an increased incidence of venous thrombosis. A reduction of antithrombin III activity by 50% is believed to increase substantially the risk of overt venous thrombosis. A reduction of 20% or more has been found to be highly predictive of the occurrence of subclinical venous thromboembolic disease that is extensive enough to be detected by ^{125}I-labeled fibrinogen uptake.[77] Postmenopausal administration of a synthetic estrogen, mestranol, has resulted in a 10% decrease in antithrombin III activity.[12] Although a similar decrease has been documented with a natural estrogen, 17β-estradiol,[126] the doses tested of estradiol valerate[12] and conjugated estrogens[7,12] did not appear to affect antithrombin III activity.

Estrogens also exert an anticlotting effect by stimulating the fibrinolytic system. Fibrinolysis is activated by the release of plasminogen activators from the vascular endothelium. Plasminogen is converted into plasmin, an enzyme that degrades fibrin and fibrinogen. Hepatic synthesis of plasminogen increases with administration of sex hormones. Conjugated estrogens significantly increased plasminogen activity in oophorectomized women.[102]

Review of these data indicates that the role of estrogen on coagulation mechanisms is not fully understood. Caution should therefore be exercised in administering hormone replacement to women who have recently experienced a vascular thrombosis or embolism.

Hepatic function. Estrogens have an impact on both protein and lipid metabolism by hepatocytes. These effects are particularly prominent with oral preparations, which are delivered in large concentrations through the portal circulation, and exert a bolus effect on the liver. As a result, oral estrogens induce a pharmacologic elevation of renin substrate and carrier globulins at dosages that are insufficient to relieve hot flushes, correct vaginal atrophy, or prevent osteoporosis.[70]

Alteration of hepatic lipid metabolism by estrogen leads to an increase of saturation of bile with cholesterol.[61] Because bile saturation of cholesterol is between 75% and 90%, small increases are associated with precipitation and stone formation. This pathophysiologic mechanism has been proposed to explain the increased incidence of gallbladder disease observed with oral estrogens.[13] A recent study has shown that transdermal administration of estradiol did not increase bile lithogenicity, suggesting that the nonoral route may be less detrimental.[139] This finding awaits further confirmation. The effects of hormones on other lipoproteins is reviewed in Chapter 15.

Contraindications and precautions

Contraindications to estrogen replacement therapy include undiagnosed vaginal bleeding, acute liver disease, chronic impaired liver function, a recent history of thromboembolism or thrombophlebitis, and suspected breast or endometrial carcinoma or a past history of these tumors. Estrogens may have adverse effects with preexisting hypertension, benign disease of the breast, uterine leiomyoma, familial hyperlipidemia, migraine headaches, chronic thrombophlebitis, endometriosis, and gallbladder disease.

A past history of breast or endometrial cancer used to be considered an absolute contraindication to estrogen replacement, but this concept has recently been challenged. There is increasing evidence that in some patients who have a good prognosis and long disease-free intervals, relief of severe postmenopausal symptoms with estrogens may be an appropriate alternative.[27,151] Until further data are available, however, such a treatment should be limited to highly selected patients.

Management of hormone replacement therapy

General guidelines of hormone replacement for all postmenopausal patients cannot be outlined. The risk-benefit ratio of estrogen administration needs to be determined for each woman individually as a function of her symptoms and risk factors. Before the institution of estrogen replacement therapy, a complete and thorough evaluation of the patient should take place. This examination includes: (1) a history, with specific reference to contraindications and precautions; and (2) a physical examination, including blood pressure, breast and pelvic examinations, and a Pap smear. A baseline mammogram should also be performed to rule out a subclinical breast cancer. After prescription of the treatment, the patient should be reevaluated in 3 months. Subsequent visits should be scheduled at 6- to 12-month intervals.

Principles of estrogen therapy. Current recommendations for hormone replacement are aimed toward the relief of disruptive climacteric symptoms such as hot flushes and urogenital atrophy. The prevention of osteoporosis is another major indication for long-term therapy and is reviewed in Chapter 55. Several studies have indicated that estrogens may be beneficial in the prevention of cardiovascular disease and the relief of postmenopausal psychologic symptoms, but hormonal treatment has yet to be approved by the U.S. Food and Drug Administration for such indications.

Estrogen therapy can be given in a cyclic or continuous fashion. Because the available data indicate that there is little or no benefit to interrupted schedules,[114] we generally recommend continuous administration. Continuous administration is less confusing to the patient and avoids the return of symptoms during the medication-free interval. It is also good practice to prescribe the lowest dosage compatible with effective treatment of the symptom.

For hot flushes, estrogen replacement should be considered when the symptom causes discomfort. Transdermal estradiol by skin patch at a dose of 0.05 mg reduces objectively measured hot flushes by 50% (Fig. 53-14).[129] It is a clinical impression that conjugated equine estrogens at a dose of 0.625 mg elicit a similar suppression. Thus higher doses of estrogens are required in the remainder of the patients in order to alleviate the complaint. Rarely, as much as 0.3 mg of transdermal estradiol or 2.5 mg of conjugated estrogens may be necessary. Before prescribing such a high estrogen dosage, the physician should make every attempt to confirm the accuracy of the diagnosis. As soon as clinically feasible, the medication should be decreased gradually to the standard dosage. Because hot flushes usually improve with time, the treatment should be discontinued and reevaluated at periodic intervals.

If the patient cannot take estrogens because of contraindications, a progestin may be administered. Medroxyprogesterone acetate at a dose of 10 to 20 mg[113] or megestrol acetate at a dose of 20 to 80 mg[40] provides substantial relief of the symptom.

Alpha-adrenergic antagonists and agonists, such as clonidine (0.1 to 0.4 mg twice daily)[80] or α-methyldopa (375 to 1125 mg/d at bedtime),[54] partially suppress hot flushes but have unpleasant side effects. A new dopamine antagonist, veralipride (100 mg/d), has shown promising results in a controlled, randomized study and may become in the future a better alternative when sex steroids are contraindicated.[92]

For urogenital atrophy, all routes of estrogen administration can be effective. Oral conjugated estrogens at a dosage of 0.625 to 1.25 mg[47] and transdermal estradiol at dosages of 0.05 to 0.1 mg[25] have been shown to revert the vaginal epithelium to maturation indexes that are indistinguishable from those of premenopausal women (Fig. 53-15). Similar effects are achieved with the daily administration of 0.5 g of vaginal cream (0.3 mg of conjugated estrogens). Since this dosage is difficult to administer, we usually prescribe use of 1 g every other day or less frequently. Although the package insert recommends use of 2 to 4 g of cream daily, this amount is almost never required. Silastic vaginal rings for continuous low-dose release of E_2 may become available in the United States in the future.[62] The ease of

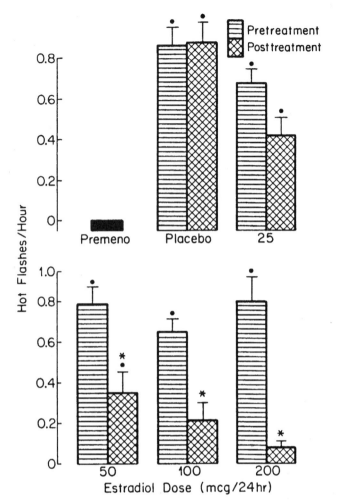

Fig. 53-14. Mean ± SE rate of occurrence of hot flushes in postmenopausal women treated with various doses of transdermal estradiol. *Premeno* indicates the premenopausal control group. (From Steingold KA et al: Treatment of hot flashes with transdermal estradiol administration, *J Clin Endocrinol Metab* 61:627, 1985, © by The Endocrine Society.)

application and long-term drug delivery offer an advantage for older patients.

Progestin regimens: administration and monitoring. Because administration of unopposed estrogens has been shown clearly to increase the incidence of hyperplasia and endometrial carcinoma,[49,125] the addition of a progestin should be offered to all women undergoing estrogen replacement therapy, unless they have had a hysterectomy. Progestins protect the endometrium from estrogen-induced hyperstimulation by decreasing endometrial DNA synthesis and nuclear estradiol-receptor content.[150] Progestins also induce various enzymes, such as 17β-estradiol and isocitric dehydrogenases. These changes correlate histologically with secretory transformation of the endometrium. Progestins unfortunately are associated with adverse metabolic effects and unpleasant symptoms such as headache, depression, abdominal bloating, and weight gain. For these

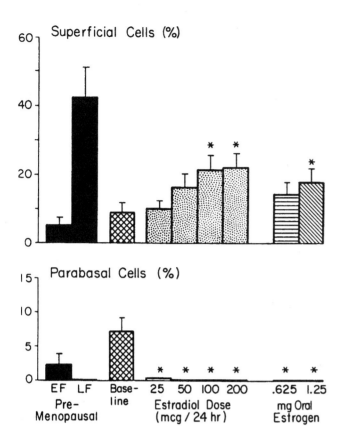

Fig. 53-15. Mean ± SE percentages of vaginal superficial and parabasal cells in premenopausal women during the early (*EF*) and late (*LF*) follicular phases, and in postmenopausal women before and during the administration of transdermal estradiol and oral conjugated estrogens. (From Chetkowski RJ et al: Biologic effects of transdermal estradiol. Reprinted by permission of *New England Journal of Medicine,* vol 314, p 1615, 1986.)

reasons, use of the lowest progestin dosage associated with a protective effect on the endometrium is recommended. This dosage, however, remains to be determined. Duration of usage is also critical. From a biochemical standpoint, maximal progestin suppression of DNA synthesis and nuclear estradiol receptor expression is not achieved until the sixth day of progestin administration.[150] Use of progestins for 7 days decreased the incidence of endometrial hyperplasia from approximately 30% with estrogen only to 4%.[148] When the progestin was given for durations of 10 and 12 days, the incidence of hyperplasia further decreased to 2% and 0%, respectively. On the basis of these findings, we advocate the administration of sequential progestins for 12 to 13 days each month.

A 10- to 12-day schedule of medroxyprogesterone 10 mg, norethindrone 0.7 to 1.0 mg, norgestrel 0.15 mg, and micronized oral progesterone 300 mg/d has been shown to provide adequate endometrial protection when added to standard estrogen regimens equivalent to 0.625 mg and 1.25 mg of conjugated estrogens.[149] In an attempt to decrease the dose of progestins, studies have evaluated the antiestrogenic effects of sequential administration of medroxyprogesterone acetate 2.5 mg, 5 mg, and 10 mg for 11 days.[48] Although all of these dosages reduced estrogen receptor concentrations to pretreatment values when added to 0.625 mg of conjugated estrogens, the dose of 2.5 mg resulted in insufficient suppression with 1.25 mg. Furthermore, the 10-mg dose was the only one producing a homogeneous, secretory pattern within the endometrium. One of the major problems when studying low-dose progestins is the great interpatient variation in absorption, metabolism, and endometrial sensitivity to the administered steroid.[149] Medroxyprogesterone acetate 5 mg for 12 to 13 days monthly is sufficient to be protective in most patients. However, a small percentage will develop hyperplasia. Thus routine endometrial sampling of these women is recommended.

More recently investigators have concentrated on the development of low-dose continuous progestin regimens. The rationale for such a schedule is to minimize metabolic side effects and symptoms, simplify administration, and induce amenorrhea. The last goal is particularly important for older women, who usually find vaginal bleeding most inconvenient. It should be emphasized that the variety of study designs and progestin regimens used makes their interpretation difficult, and thus the findings presented here should be considered preliminary. Norethindrone at a daily dose of 0.35 to 2.0 mg has been shown to induce endometrial atrophy when added to oral micronized estradiol or conjugated estrogens.[87,127] Additional studies reported similar findings with administration of 200 to 300 mg of oral micronized progesterone[56] and 2.5 mg of medroxyprogesterone acetate daily.[144] Although amenorrhea was achieved with most of the patients, up to 30% of them still experienced vaginal bleeding after 1 year of use.[149] In general, the bleeding pattern was unpredictable and therefore more disruptive than with sequential progestin use. A review of the current data indicates that the incidence of vaginal bleeding was particularly high within the first 3 months of treatment[149] and among perimenopausal women.[87,127] These bleeding problems have accounted for a high rate of discontinuation of therapy. These regimens do not seem to antagonize the beneficial effects of estrogens on liver metabolism and menopausal symptoms. Most investigators have reported well-known progestin side effects such as depression, bloating, drowsiness, and weight gain as a cause for dropout, suggesting that even very low doses do not entirely eliminate these disconcerting side effects.

The use of low-dosage vaginal creams does not usually result in serum estrogen levels sufficient to stimulate the endometrium. In this group of patients, we administer a course of medroxyprogesterone acetate, 10 mg for 12 days once a year. In the rare occurrence of withdrawal bleeding, the progestin should be given on a monthly basis. As previously mentioned, we do not recommend progestin administration to women who have undergone a hysterectomy.

Monitoring sequential administration of progestin is usually easy, because scheduled withdrawal bleeding is expected. If the patient has not complained of vaginal bleeding or does not have an enlarged uterus, it is our opinion that endometrial biopsy is not required before institution of estrogen replacement therapy. Patients with endometrial pathology will usually declare themselves with irregular bleeding once the hormone treatment is initiated. If breakthrough bleeding occurs during drug therapy, an endometrial biopsy should be performed to exclude the presence of abnormal histology. Currently we use the Pipelle or Mylex biopsy instruments. The timing of further biopsies, if needed, is a clinical decision based on the results of the histologic examination of the endometrium obtained. The presence of endometrial hyperplasia dictates more prolonged use of the progestin or discontinuation of hormone replacement.

Continuous administration of the progestin is more difficult to follow because all bleeding is breakthrough bleeding. Unless the irregular spotting is prolonged, heavy, or frequent, usually an endometrial biopsy is not performed. In patients who wish to remain on this regimen and have persistent bleeding episodes, several biopsies may be necessary. If results of all are normal, the need for continued endometrial evaluation is reduced.

For postmenopausal women who do not accept or tolerate progestins, unopposed estrogen therapy may be prescribed, as long as the influence of estrogen on the genesis of endometrial carcinoma is discussed with the patient. We recommend both pretreatment and annual endometrial biopsies in this group of women. If hyperplasia is present, a progestin should be administered or the estrogen therapy discontinued.

If these guidelines are followed, the occurrence of serious problems will be reduced. It must be understood that all women cannot tolerate hormone replacement. No matter what strategy is used or how much reassurance is provided, there are women who cannot continue treatment. When possible, substitutional regimens can be prescribed, but patient satisfaction is problematic. Continuous efforts are being exerted to define better, safer, and less disruptive forms of hormone replacement. These efforts can only be applauded.

REFERENCES

1. Abraham GE: Radioimmunoassay of plasma pregnenolone, 17-hydroxypregnenolone and dehydroepiandrosterone under various physiological conditions, *J Clin Endocrinol Metab* 37:140, 1973.
2. Abraham GE, Lobotsky J, Lloyd CW: Metabolism of testosterone and androstenedione in normal and ovariectomized women, *J Clin Invest* 48:696, 1969.
3. Abraham GE, Maroulis GB: Effects of exogenous estrogen on serum pregnenolone, cortisol, and androgens in postmenopausal women, *Obstet Gynecol* 45:271, 1975.
4. Abraham GE et al: Simultaneous radioimmunoassay of plasma FSH, LH, progesterone, 17-hydroxyprogesterone, and estradiol-17β during the menstrual cycle, *J Clin Endocrinol* 34:312, 1972.
5. Alkjaersig N, Fletcher A, Burstein R: Association between oral contraceptive use and thromboembolism: a new approach to its investigation based on plasma fibrinogen chromatography, *Am J Obstet Gynecol* 122:199, 1975.
6. Antunes CMF et al: Endometrial cancer and estrogen use, *N Engl J Med* 303:485, 1980.
7. Astedt B: Does estrogen replacement therapy predispose to thrombosis?, *Acta Obstet Gynecol Scand Suppl* 130:71, 1985.
8. Bergkvist L et al: The risk of breast cancer after estrogen and estrogen-progestin replacement, *N Engl J Med* 321:293, 1989.
9. Bergman A, Brenner PF: Alterations in the urogenital system. In Mishell DR Jr, editor: *Menopause: physiology and pharmacology,* Chicago, 1987, Year Book.
10. Blaustein RL: Cytology of the female genital tract. In Kurman RJ, editor: *Pathology of the female genital tract,* New York, 1987, Springer-Verlag.
11. Bolognia J: Aging skin, epidermal and dermal changes, *Prog Clin Biol Res* 320:121, 1989.
12. Bonnar J et al: Coagulation system changes in postmenopausal women receiving estrogen preparations, *Postgrad Med J* 56(suppl 6):30, 1976.
13. Boston Collaborative Drug Surveillance Program: Surgically confirmed gallbladder disease, venous thromboembolism, and breast tumors in relation to postmenopausal estrogen therapy, *N Engl J Med* 290:15, 1974.
14. Brincat M, Studd J: Skin and the menopause. In Mishell DR Jr, editor: *Menopause: physiology and pharmacology,* Chicago, 1987, Year Book.
15. Brincat M et al: Long-term effects of the menopause and sex hormones on skin thickness, *Br J Obstet Gynaecol* 92:256, 1985.
16. Brincat M et al: Skin collagen changes in postmenopausal women receiving different regimens of estrogen therapy, *Obstet Gynecol* 70:123, 1987.
17. Brincat M et al: A study of the decrease of skin collagen content, skin thickness, and bone mass in the postmenopausal woman, *Obstet Gynecol* 70:840, 1987.
17a. Brinton LA, Hoover R, Fraumeni JF Jr: Menopausal estrogens and breast cancer risk: an expanded case-control study. Br J Cancer 54:825, 1986.
18. Brown KH, Hammond CB: Urogenital atrophy, *Obstet Gynecol Clin North Am* 15:13, 1982.
19. Buckler HM et al: Gonadotropin, steroid, and inhibin levels in women with incipient ovarian failure during anovulatory and ovulatory rebound cycles, *J Clin Endocrinol Metab* 72:116, 1991.
20. Bullough HF: Epidermal thickness following oestrone injections in the mouse, *Nature,* 159:101, 1947.
21. Calanog A et al: Testosterone metabolism in ovarian cancer, *Am J Obstet Gynecol* 124:60, 1976.
22. Cambell S, Whitehead M: Oestrogen therapy and the menopausal syndrome, *Clin Obstet Gynecol* 4:31, 1977.
23. Casper RF, Yen SSC: Menopausal flushes: effect of pituitary gonadotropin desensitization by a potent luteinizing hormone-releasing factor agonist, *J Clin Endocrinol Metab* 53:1056, 1981.
24. Chang RJ, Judd HL: The ovary after menopause, *Clin Obstet Gynecol* 24:181, 1981.
25. Chetkowski RJ et al: Biologic effects of transdermal estradiol, *N Engl J Med* 314:1615, 1986.
26. Chu J, Schneid AI, Weiss NJ: Survival among women with endometrial cancer: a comparison of estrogen users and nonusers, *Am J Obstet Gynecol* 143:569, 1982.
27. Creasman WT: Estrogen replacement therapy: is previously treated cancer a contraindication?, *Obstet Gynecol* 77:308, 1991.
28. Cumming DC et al: Evidence for an influence of the ovary on circulating dehydroepiandrosterone sulfate levels, *J Clin Endocrinol Metab* 54:1069, 1982.

29. D'Amico JF et al: Induction of hypothalamic opioid activity with transdermal estradiol administration in postmenopausal women, *Fertil Steril* 55:754, 1991.

30. Dennefors BL: Hilus cells from human postmenopausal ovaries: gonadotrophin sensitivity, steroid and cyclic AMP production, *Acta Obstet Gynecol Scand* 61:413, 1982.

31. Dennefors BL et al: Steroid production and responsiveness to gonadotropin in isolated stromal tissue of human postmenopausal ovaries, *Am J Obstet Gynecol* 136:997, 1980.

32. Dennerstein L: Depression in the menopause, *Obstet Gynecol Clin North Am* 4:33, 1987.

33. Dennerstein L: Psychologic changes. In Mishell DR Jr, editor: *Menopause: physiology and pharmacology,* Chicago, 1987, Year Book.

34. Dennerstein L: Psychologic and sexual effects. In Mishell DR Jr, editor: *Menopause: physiology and pharmacology,* Chicago, 1987, Year Book.

35. Dennerstein L et al: Hormone therapy and affect, *Maturitas* 1:247, 1979.

36. Dennerstein L et al: Hormones and sexuality: effect of estrogen and progestogen, *Obstet Gynecol* 56:316, 1980.

37. Dow MGT, Hart DM: Hormonal treatments of sexual unresponsiveness in postmenopausal women: a comparative study, *Br J Obstet Gynaecol* 90:361, 1983.

38. Ebling FJ: Some effects of oestrogen on epidermis, *J Endocrinol* 9:xxxi, 1953.

39. Elwood JM, Boyes DA: Clinical and pathological features and survival of endometrial cancer patients in relation to prior use of estrogens, *Gynecol Oncol* 10:173, 1980.

40. Erlik J et al: Effect of megestrol acetate on flushing and bone metabolism in postmenopausal women, *Maturitas* 3:167, 1981.

41. Ewertz M: Influence on noncontraceptive exogenous and endogenous sex hormones on breast cancer risk in Denmark, *Int J Cancer* 42:832, 1988.

42. Fisch LR, Freedman SH, Myatt AV: Oral contraceptives, pregnancy and blood pressure, *JAMA* 222:1507, 1972.

43. Gambone J et al: Further delineation of hypothalamic dysfunction responsible for menopausal hot flashes, *J Clin Endocrinol Metab* 59:1097, 1985.

44. Gambrell RD Jr: The menopause: benefits and risks of estrogen-progestogen replacement therapy, *Fertil Steril* 37:457, 1982.

45. Gambrell RD Jr: Clinical use of progestins in the menopausal patient, *J Reprod Med* 27:531, 1982.

46. Gambrell RD Jr, Maier RC, Sanders BI: Decreased incidence of breast cancer in postmenopausal estrogen-progestogen users, *Obstet Gynecol* 62:435, 1983.

47. Geola FL et al: Biological effects of various doses of conjugated equine estrogens in postmenopausal women, *J Clin Endocrinol Metab* 51:620, 1980.

48. Gibbons WE et al: Biochemical and biological effects of sequential estrogen/progestin therapy on the endometrium of postmenopausal women, *Am J Obstet Gynecol* 154:456, 1986.

49. Gray LA Sr, Christopherson W, Hoover RN: Estrogens and endometrial carcinoma, *Obstet Gynecol* 49:385, 1977.

50. Greenwald P, Caputo TA, Wolfgang PE: Endometrial cancer after menopausal use of estrogens, *Obstet Gynecol* 50:239, 1977.

51. Grosman N: Studies on the hyaluronic acid protein complex, the molecular size of hyaluronic acid and the exchangeability of chloride in skin of mice before and after oestrogen treatment, *Acta Pharmacol Toxicol Scand* 33:201, 1973.

52. Gusberg SB: The individual at high risk for endometrial carcinoma, *Am J Obstet Gynecol* 126:535, 1976.

53. Hammond CB et al: Effects of long-term estrogen replacement therapy, II: neoplasia, *Am J Obstet Gynecol* 133:537, 1979.

54. Hammond MG, Hatley L, Talbert LM: A double blind study to

55. Hannan JH: *The flushing of the menopause,* London, 1927, Bailliere, Tindall & Cox.

56. Hargrove JT et al: Menopausal hormone replacement therapy with continuous daily oral micronized estradiol and progesterone, *Obstet Gynecol* 73:606, 1989.

57. Hasselquist MB et al: Isolation and characterization of the estrogen receptor in human skin, *J Clin Endocrinol Metab* 50:76, 1980.

58. Hazzard WR: Estrogen replacement and cardiovascular disease: serum lipids and blood pressure effects, *Am J Obstet Gynecol* 161:1847, 1989.

59. Henderson BE, Ross RK, Pike MC: Breast neoplasia. In Mishell DR Jr, editor: *Menopause: physiology and pharmacology,* Chicago, 1987, Year Book.

60. Henderson BE et al: Re-evaluating the role of progestogen therapy after the menopause, *Fertil Steril* 49(suppl):9S, 1988.

61. Heuman R et al: Effects of postmenopausal ethinyl estradiol treatment on gallbladder bile, *Maturitas* 2:69, 1979.

61a. Hiatt RA, Bawol R, Friedman GD et al: Exogenous estrogen and breast cancer after bilateral oophorectomy, *Cancer* 4:139, 1984.

62. Holmgren PA, Lindskog M, von Shoulz B: Vaginal rings for continuous low-dose release of estradiol in the treatment of urogenital atrophy, *Maturitas* 11:55, 1989.

63. Hooker CW, Pfeiffer CA: Effect of sex hormones upon body growth, skin, hair and sebaceous glands in the rat, *Endocrinology* 32:69, 1943.

63a. Hoover R, Glass A, Finkle WD et al: Conjugated estrogens and breast cancer risk in women, *J Natl Cancer Inst* 67:815, 1981.

64. Horton R, Tait JF: Androstenedione production and interconversion rates measured in peripheral blood and studies on the possible site of its conversion to testosterone, *J Clin Invest* 45:301, 1966.

64a. Hulka BS, Chambless LE, Duebner DC et al: Breast cancer and estrogen replacement therapy, II: neoplasia, *Am J Obstet Gynecol* 133:537, 1979.

65. Ingelman-Sundberg A et al: Cytosol oestrogen receptors in the urogenital tissues in stress incontinent women, *Acta Obstet Gynecol Scand* 60:585, 1981.

66. Iosif CS, Bekassy Z: Prevalence of genito-urinary symptoms in the late menopause, *Acta Obstet Gynecol Scand* 63:257, 1984.

67. Jaffe RB et al: Neuromodulatory regulation of gonadotropin-releasing hormone pulsatile discharge in women, *Am J Obstet Gynecol* 163:1727, 1990.

68. Jaszmann L, Van Lith ND, Zaat JCA: The perimenausal symptoms, *Med Gynaecol Sociol,* 4:268, 1969.

68a. Jick H, Walker AM, Watkins RN et al: Replacement estrogens and breast cancer, *Am J Epidemiol* 112:586, 1988.

69. Judd HL: The basis of menopausal vasomotor symptoms. In Mastroianni L Jr, Paulsen CA, editors: *Aging, reproduction and the climacteric,* New York, 1986, Plenum Press.

70. Judd HL: Effects of estrogen replacement on hepatic function. In Mishell DR Jr, editor: *Menopause: physiology and pharmacology,* Chicago, 1987, Year Book.

71. Judd HL, Lucas WE, Yen SSC: Effect of oophorectomy on circulating testosterone and androstenedione levels in patients with endometrial cancer, *Am J Obstet Gynecol* 118:793, 1974.

72. Judd HL, Lucas WE, Yen SSC: Serum 17β-estradiol and estrone levels in postmenopausal women with and without endometrial cancer, *J Clin Endocrinol Metab* 43:272, 1976.

73. Judd HL, Yen SSC: Serum androstenedione and testosterone levels during the menstrual cycle, *J Clin Endocrinol Metab* 36:475, 1973.

74. Judd HL et al: Androgen and gonadotropin dynamics in testicular feminization syndrome, *J Clin Endocrinol Metab* 34:229, 1972.

75. Judd HL et al: Endocrine function of the postmenopausal ovary: concentrations of androgens and estrogens in ovarian and peripheral vein blood, *J Clin Endocrinol Metab* 39:1020, 1974.

76. Judd HL et al: Origin of serum estradiol in postmenopausal women, *Obstet Gynecol* 59:680, 1982.

77. Judd HL et al: Estrogen replacement therapy: indications and complications, *Ann Intern Med* 98:195, 1983.

77a. Kaufman DW, Miller DR, Rosenberg L et al: Noncontraceptive estrogen use and risk of breast cancer, *JAMA* 252:63, 1984.

78. Kaufmann RH: *Atrophic, desquamative, and postradiation vulvovaginitis,* Chicago, Year Book.

78a. Kelsey JL, Fischer DB, Holford TR et al: Exogenous estrogens and other factors in the epidemiology of breast cancer, *J Natl Cancer Inst* 67:327, 1981.

79. Key TJA, Pike MC: The role of oestrogens and progestagens in the epidemiology and prevention of breast cancer, *Eur J Cancer Clin Oncol* 24:29, 1988.

80. Laufer LR et al: Effect of clonidine on hot flashes in postmenopausal women, *Obstet Gynecol* 60:583, 1982.

81. LaVecchia C et al: Noncontraceptive oestrogens and the risk of breast cancer in women, *Int J Cancer* 38:853, 1986.

82. Lomax P, Knox GV: The sites and mechanisms of action of drugs affecting thermoregulation. In Schonbaum E, Lomax P, editors: *The pharmacology of thermoregulation,* Basel, 1973, S Karger.

83. Longcope C: Metabolic clearance and blood production rates of estrogens in postmenopausal women, *Am J Obstet Gynecol* 111:778, 1971.

84. Mack TM et al: Estrogens and endometrial cancer in a retirement community, *N Engl J Med* 294:1262, 1976.

85. Maroulis GB, Abraham GE: Ovarian and adrenal contributions to peripheral steroid levels in postmenopausal women, *Obstet Gynecol* 48:150, 1976.

86. Mashchak CA, Lobo RA: Estrogen replacement therapy and hypertension, *J Reprod Med* 30(suppl 10):805, 1985.

87. Mattsson LA, Cullberg G, Samsioe G: Evaluation of a continuous oestrogen-progesterone regimen for climacteric complaints, *Maturitas* 4:95, 1982.

88. McKinlay S, Jefferys M: The menopausal syndrome, *Br J Prev Soc Med* 28:108, 1974.

89. Meldrum DR et al: Elevation in skin temperature of the finger as an objective index of postmenopausal hot flashes: standardization of the technique, *Am J Obstet Gynecol* 135:713, 1979.

90. Meldrum DR et al: Changes in circulating steroids with aging in postmenopausal women, *Obstet Gynecol* 57:624, 1981.

91. Meldrum DR et al: Objectively recorded hot flushes in patients with pituitary insufficiency, *J Clin Endocrinol Metab* 52:684, 1981.

92. Melis GB et al: Effects of the dopamine antagonist veralipride on hot flushes and luteinizing hormone secretion in postmenopausal women, *Obstet Gynecol* 72:688, 1988.

93. Metcalf MG, Livesey JH: Gonadotrophin excretion in fertile women: effect of age and the onset of the menopausal transition, *J Endocrinol* 105:357, 1985.

94. Metcalf MG, Livesey JH: Gonadotrophin excretion in fertile women: effect of age and the onset of the menopausal transition, *Obstet Gynecol Surv* 41:101, 1986.

95. Molnar GW: Body temperatures during menopausal hot flashes, *J Appl Physiol* 38:499, 1975.

96. Moore B: Climacteric symptoms in an African community, *Maturitas* 3:25, 1981.

97. Nachtigall LE et al: Estrogen replacement therapy, II: a prospective study in the relationship to carcinoma and cardiovascular and metabolic problems, *Obstet Gynecol* 54:74, 1979.

98. Neugarten BL, Kraines RJ: Menopausal symptoms in women of various ages, *Psychosom Med* 27:266, 1965.

99. Neugarten BL, Wood V, Kraites RJ: Women's attitudes toward the menopause. In Neugarten BL, editor: *Middle age and aging,* Chicago, 1968, University of Chicago Press.

99a. Nomura AMY, Kolonel LN, Hirohata T et al: The association of replacement estrogens with breast cancer, *Int J Cancer* 37:49, 1986.

100. Notelovitz M: Gynecologic problems of menopausal women, I: changes in genital tissues, *Geriatrics* 33:24, 1978.

101. Notelovitz M: Estrogen replacement therapy: indications, contraindications, and agent selection, *Am J Obstet Gynecol* 161:1832, 1989.

102. Notelovitz M, Kitchens CS, Ware MD: Coagulation and fibrinolysis in estrogen-treated surgically menopausal women, *Obstet Gynecol* 63:596, 1983.

103. Pardridge WM, Meitus LJ: Transport of steroid hormones through the rat blood-brain barrier: primary role of albumin-bound hormone, *J Clin Invest* 64:145, 1979.

104. Peterson HB, Lee NC, Rubin GL: Genital neoplasia. In Mishell DR Jr, editor: *Menopause: physiology and pharmacology,* Chicago, 1987, Year Book.

105. Poller L, Thompson JM, Thomas W: Conjugated equine oestrogens and blood clotting: a follow-up report, *Br Med J* 1:935, 1977.

106. Punnonen R: Effect of castration and peroral estrogen therapy on the skin, *Acta Obstet Gynecol Scand Suppl* 21:1, 1972.

106a. Ravinhar BA, Seigel DG, Lindtner J: An epidemiologic study of breast cancer and benign breast neoplasias in relation to the oral contraceptive and estrogen use, *Eur J Cancer* 15:395, 1979.

107. Reed T: Urethral pressure profile in continent women from childhood to old age, *Acta Obstet Gynecol Scand* 59:331, 1980.

108. Richardson SJ, Senikas V, Nelson JF: Follicular depletion during the menopausal transition: evidence for accelerated loss and ultimate exhaustion, *J Clin Endocrinol Metab* 65:1231, 1987.

109. Rosner W: Interaction of adrenal and gonadal steroids with proteins in human plasma, *N Engl J Med* 281:658, 1969.

109a. Ross RK, Paganini-Hill A, Gerkins VR et al: A case-control study of menopausal estrogen therapy and breast cancer, *JAMA* 243:1635, 1980.

110. Rubin GL et al: Estrogen replacement therapy and the risk of endometrial cancer: remaining controversies, *Am J Obstet Gynecol* 162:148, 1990.

111. Sajar S et al: Oral contraceptives, antithrombin III activity, and postoperative deep-vein thrombosis, *Lancet* 1:509, 1976.

111a. Sartwell PE, Arthes FG, Tonascia JA: Exogenous hormones, reproductive history, and breast cancer in women with natural menopause, *J Natl Cancer Inst* 56:839, 1976.

112. Scaglin H et al: Pituitary LH and FSH secretion and responsiveness in women of old age, *Acta Endocrinol* 81:673, 1976.

113. Schiff I, Tulchinsky D, Cramer D: Oral medroxyprogesterone in the treatment of postmenopausal symptoms, *JAMA* 244:1443, 1980.

114. Schiff I et al: Endometrial hyperplasia in women on cyclic or continuous estrogen regimens, *Fertil Steril* 37:79, 1982.

115. Scotti RJ, Ostergard DR: The urethral syndrome, *Clin Obstet Gynecol* 27:515, 1984.

116. Semmens JP, Wagner G: Estrogen deprivation and vaginal function in postmenopausal women, *JAMA* 248:445, 1982.

117. Shapiro S et al: Recent and past use of conjugated estrogens in relation to adenocarcinoma of the endometrium, *N Engl J Med* 303:485, 1980.

118. Shahrad P, Marks R: A pharmacological effect of oestrone on human epidermis, *Br J Dermatol* 97:383, 1977.

119. Sherman BM: Endocrinologic and menstrual alterations. In Mishell DR Jr, editor: *Menopause: physiology and pharmacology,* Chicago, 1987, Year Book.

120. Sherman BM, Korenman SG: Hormonal characteristics of the human menstrual cycle throughout reproductive life, *J Clin Invest* 55:699, 1975.

121. Sherman BM, West JH, Korenman SG: The menopausal transition: analysis of LH, FSH, estradiol and progesterone concentrations during menstrual cycles of older women, *J Clin Endocrinol Metab* 42:629, 1976.

122. Sherwin BB, Gelfand MM: Differential symptoms response to parenteral estrogen and/or androgen administration in the surgical menopause, *Am J Obstet Gynecol* 151:152, 1985.

123. Shuster J, Black MM, McVitie E: The influence of age and sex on skin thickness, skin collagen and density, *Br J Dermatol* 93:693, 1975.

124. Siiteri PK, MacDonald PC: Role of extraglandular estrogen in human endocrinology. In Greep RO, Astwood E, editors: *Handbook of physiology,* vol 2 pt 1, *Endocrinology,* Washington, DC, 1973, American Physiological Society.

125. Smith DC et al: Association of exogenous estrogen and endometrial carcinoma, *N Engl J Med* 293:1164, 1975.

126. Sporrong T et al: Haemostatic changes during continuous oestradiol-progestogen treatment of postmenopausal women, *Br J Obstet Gynaecol* 97:939, 1990.

127. Staland B: Continuous treatment with natural oestrogens and progestogens: a method to avoid endometrial stimulation, *Maturitas* 3:134, 1981.

128. Steinberg KK et al: A meta-analysis of the effect of estrogen replacement therapy on the risk of breast cancer, *JAMA* 265:1985, 1991.

129. Steingold KA et al: Treatment of hot flashes with transdermal estradiol administration, *J Clin Endocrinol Metab* 61:627, 1985.

130. Stone SC, Mickal A, Rye PH: Postmenopausal symptomatology, maturation index, and plasma estrogen levels, *Obstet Gynecol* 45:625, 1975.

131. Studd JWW, Parsons A: Sexual dysfunction: the climacteric, *Br J Sex Med* vol 4, p 11, Dec 1977.

132. Stumpf WE, Madhabananda S, Joshi SG: Estrogen target cells in the skin, *Experientia* 30:196, 1974.

133. Tataryn IV et al: LH, FSH and skin temperature during the menopausal hot flash, *J Clin Endocrinol Metab* 49:152, 1979.

134. Tataryn IV et al: Postmenopausal hot flushes: a disorder of thermoregulation, *Maturitas* 2:101, 1980.

135. Thompson B, Hart SA, Durno D: Menopausal age and symptomatology in general practice, *J Biol Sci* 5:71, 1973.

136. Treloar AE et al: Variation of the human menstrual cycle through reproductive life, *Int J Fertil* 12:77, 1967.

137. Tulandi T, Samarthji L: Menopausal hot flush, *Obstet Gynecol Surv* 40:553, 1985.

138. Ulmsten V, Henriksson L, Iosif S: The unstable female urethra, *Am J Obstet Gynecol* 144:93, 1982.

139. Van Erpecum KJ et al: Different hepatobiliary effects of oral and transdermal estradiol in postmenopausal women, *Gastroenterology* 100:482, 1991.

140. Vermeulen A: The hormonal activity of the postmenopausal ovary, *J Clin Endocrinol Metab* 42:247, 1976.

141. Vermeulen A: Sex hormone status of the postmenopausal woman, *Maturitas* 2:81, 1980.

142. Vermeulen A, Verdonck L: Sex hormone concentrations in postmenopausal women, *Clin Endocrinol* 9:59, 1978.

143. Walter S et al: Urinary incontinence in postmenopausal women treated with estrogens, *Urol Int* 33:135, 1978.

144. Weinstein L, Bewtra C, Gallagher JC: Evaluation of a continuous combined low dose regimen of estrogen-progestin for treatment of the menopausal patient, *Am J Obstet Gynecol* 162:1534, 1990.

145. Weiss NS, Szekely DR, Austin DF: Increasing incidence of endometrial cancer in the United States, *N Engl J Med* 294:1259, 1976.

146. Weissman MM: The myth of involutional melancholia, *JAMA* 242:742, 1979.

147. Wessler S et al: Estrogen-containing oral contraceptive agents: a basis for their thrombogenicity, *JAMA* 236:2179, 1976.

148. Whitehead MI, Fraser D: Controversies concerning safety of estrogen replacement therapy, *Am J Obstet Gynecol* 156:1313, 1987.

149. Whitehead MI, Hillard TC, Crook D: The role and use of progestogens, *Obstet Gynecol* 75(suppl):59S, 1990.

150. Whitehead MI et al: Effects of various types and dosages of progestogens on the postmenopausal endometrium, *J Reprod Med* 27(suppl):539, 1982.

151. Wile AG, DiSaia RJ: Hormones and breast cancer, *Am J Surg* 159:438, 1989.

151a. Wingo PA, Layde PM, Lee NC et al: The risk of breast cancer in postmenopausal women who have used estrogen replacement therapy, *JAMA* 257:209, 1987.

152. Wise PM et al: Contribution of changing rhythmicity of hypothalamic neurotransmitter function to female reproductive aging, *Ann N Y Acad Sci* 592:31, 1990.

152a. Wynder EL, MacCornack FA, Stellman SD: The epidemiology of breast cancer in 785 United States Caucasian women, *Cancer* 41:2341, 1978.

153. Yen SSC et al: Pulsatile pattern of gonadotropin release in subjects with and without ovarian function, *J Clin Endocrinol Metab* 34:671, 1972.

154. Young DD: Some misconceptions concerning the menopause, *Obstet Gynecol* 75:881, 1990.

155. Ziel KH, Finkle WD: Increased risk of endometrial carcinoma among users of conjugated estrogens, *N Engl J Med* 293:1167, 1975.

Chapter 54

PREMATURE OVARIAN FAILURE AND HYPERGONADOTROPIC AMENORRHEA

Robert W. Rebar, MD

Incidence
Clinical features
Etiology
    Genetic causes
    Enzymatic defects
    Physical insults
    Immune disturbances
    Defects in gonadotropin structure or action
    Idiopathic
    Myth of a distinct resistant ovary syndrome
Evaluation
Therapy

Concepts regarding premature ovarian failure have changed considerably since the disorder was first defined as consisting of the triad of amenorrhea, hypergonadotropinism, and hypoestrogenism in women under the age of 40 years by de Moraes and Jones[27] in 1967. With the report of Goldenberg and colleagues[30] documenting that ovarian follicles were absent in all amenorrheic women with serum FSH concentrations greater than 40 mIU/mL (Second International Reference Preparation of human menopausal gonadotropins), the definition was refined to specify that follicle-stimulating hormone (FSH) levels should be greater than that level. With the first appearance in the literature of isolated cases documenting the initiation or resumption of cyclic menses and/or pregnancy,[45,55,89] questions about the permanence of the ovarian "failure" were first raised. The potential "reversibility" of this condition was confirmed subsequently by several large series noting spontaneous pregnancies in well-documented cases.[1,36,68,77,78] Moreover, these series served to underscore the heterogeneity of the women presenting with presumptive premature ovarian failure. Thus it is perhaps most appropriate in this chapter to consider the clinical spectrum of individuals presenting with hypergonadotropic amenorrhea, many of whom in fact may suffer from permanent ovarian failure.

INCIDENCE

The incidence of women with hypergonadotropic amenorrhea and diminished secretion of estrogen is not well established but has been estimated to be 0.9% (with a 95% confidence interval of 0.3% to 1.5%) for women under the age of 40.[21] Other groups have suggested that its incidence among women with primary or secondary amenorrhea approximates 2% to 10%.[5,95]

CLINICAL FEATURES

In an effort to describe the varied clinical characteristics of women with hypergonadotropic amenorrhea, the findings in 128 sequential patients seen with this disorder between 1978 and 1989 have been tabulated.[82] Inclusion criteria were (1) amenorrhea of 3 or more months' duration, (2) age under 40 years at onset of amenorrhea, and (3) circulating FSH concentrations of greater than 40 mIU/mL on two or more occasions.

Of the 128 women with hypergonadotropic amenorrhea, 18 (14.1%) had never had a single menstrual period and had a mean age of 22.7 years at the time of diagnosis. The remaining 110 patients (85.9%) with secondary amenorrhea averaged 27.9 years in age at the time the amenorrhea began. As outlined in Table 54-1, several distinctions exist

Table 54-1. Women with hypergonadotropic amenorrhea presenting with primary or secondary amenorrhea

	Primary amenorrhea		Secondary amenorrhea		Significance (x^2 test)
Total number of patients (%)	18	(14.1%)	110	(85.9%)	
Symptoms of estrogen deficiency	4	(22.2%)	91	(82.7%)	$P < 0.001$
Incomplete sexual development	16	(88.9%)	8	(7.3%)	$P < 0.001$
Chromosomal abnormalities	10	(55.6%)	6/49	tested (12.2%)	$P < 0.01$
Immune abnormalities*	4	(22.2%)	21	(19.1%)	NS‡
Spinal bone density < 90% of controls	3/4	(75%)	16/33	(48.5%)	NS
Withdrawal bleeding after progestin	2/9	(22.2%)	41/75	(54.7%)	NS
Pregnancies before diagnosis	0		41	(37.3%)	$P < 0.025$
Evidence of ovulation after diagnosis	0		27	(24.5%)	$P < 0.05$
Pregnancies after diagnosis	0		9	(8.2%)	NS

Updated data from Rebar and Connolly[76]; from Rebar et al.[82] with permission.
*Not including any test for antiovarian antibodies.
†NS, Not significant.

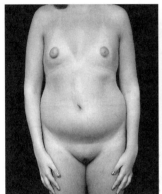 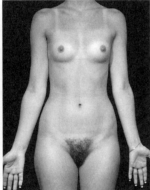

Fig. 54-1. Diverse appearances of two women with hypergonadotropic amenorrhea and incomplete sexual development. Other patients may show complete sexual development. Based on sequential determinations of circulating gonadotropins and estradiol levels, neither had evidence of remaining functional follicles. *Left,* A 16-year-old with primary amenorrhea who noted some breast development and pubic hair growth at age 11. Karyotype was 46,XX and laparoscopic ovarian biopsy showed stroma only. *Right,* A 23-year-old who had one episode of spotting at age 17 before being given oral contraceptive agents. Note that breast development is really only Tanner stage 3 and pubic hair, stage 4. Her pubic hair does not extend onto the inner aspects of her thighs.

between those patients with primary and those with secondary hypergonadotropic amenorrhea.

In just under 75% of the women evaluated, symptoms of estrogen deficiency, most commonly hot flushes and dyspareunia, were present. Such complaints were far more common in the women with secondary amenorrhea. In contrast, incomplete development of secondary sexual characteristics and chromosomal abnormalities were much more common in women with primary amenorrhea (Fig. 54-1). Chromosomal abnormalities were identified in more than half of the women with primary amenorrhea who were karyotyped. Moreover, the individuals with primary amenorrhea more often had deletions of some or all of one X

Table 54-2. Women with hypergonadotropic amenorrhea with various immune abnormalities

Immune abnormalities*	Primary amenorrhea 4	Secondary amenorrhea 21
Thyroid disturbances	3	10
Addison's disease		1
Hypoparathyroidism		1
Vitiligo		1
Diabetes mellitus	1	
Polymyositis		1
Antinuclear antibody	1	5
Rheumatoid factor		2

Updated data from Rebar and Connolly[76]; from Rebar et al.[82] with permission.
*More than one abnormality per individual possible.

chromosome, whereas those with secondary amenorrhea were more likely to have additional X chromosomes.

Immune disturbances were noted in over 20% of patients tested. As demonstrated by a solid-phase enzyme-linked immunosorbent assay (ELISA), 5 of the 22 (22.7%) karyotypically normal women with secondary hypergonadotropic amenorrhea tested had antibodies to ovarian tissue.[49] In all, 25 of the 128 women had documented immune abnormalities aside from antiovarian antibodies (Table 54-2). Abnormalities involving thyroid function were most commonly associated with hypergonadotropic amenorrhea.

A variety of other disorders were also found in association with hypergonadotropic amenorrhea. Seven patients with secondary amenorrhea had received chemotherapy with alkylating agents and, in some cases, radiation therapy, as well, before becoming amenorrheic. Four patients developed amenorrhea immediately after an infectious disease: one with chickenpox, one with severe shigellosis, one with malaria, and one with an undefined viral syndrome. Four individuals with normal karyotypes had a family history of menopause before age 40.

Nineteen of the 37 women (over 50%) undergoing dual-photon absorptiometry of the lumbar spine had bone densities that were less than 90% of the mean value observed in age-matched controls. Surprisingly, withdrawal bleeding in response to progestin occurred in more than 50% of the women tested. Withdrawal bleeding even occurred in two of the nine individuals with primary amenorrhea who were tested. Interestingly, withdrawal bleeding did not predict the possibility of subsequent ovulation.

Although none of the women with primary amenorrhea obviously had conceived before diagnosis, more than one-third of those with secondary amenorrhea had had pregnancies. Similarly, evidence of ovulation was not detected after diagnosis in any women with primary amenorrhea but was found in almost one fourth of the women with secondary amenorrhea. Because none of the patients resumed regular monthly menses after diagnosis, it must be presumed that ovulation occurred only occasionally. One ninth of the patients with secondary amenorrhea (8.2%) later conceived.

Basal FSH and luteinizing hormone (LH) concentrations were markedly increased in all patients, with mean FSH levels of 107.9 mIU/mL ± 8.5 (SEM) and mean LH levels of 90.0 ± 5.9 mIU/mL. In contrast, concentrations of both estrone and estradiol were low, similar to those observed in the early follicular phase of the normal menstrual cycle.

Twenty-seven patients with secondary amenorrhea were given clomiphene citrate in an effort to induce ovulation, but only four (14.8%) ovulated. Because the four women who ovulated all had evidence of spontaneous episodic ovulation before therapy, it is unclear whether the clomiphene therapy actually induced ovulation or whether there was a temporal association only.

Nineteen women had serum gonadotropin levels suppressed for 1 to 3 months with either exogenous estrogen (and progestin) or a gonadotropin-releasing hormone agonist. Ovulation induction was then attempted with human menopausal gonadotropins. Only two of the patients (of the five suppressed with the agonist) ovulated, and only one conceived. In contrast with this lack of success, two of the four patients in this series who received donor oocytes delivered normal infants.

Fourteen of the women with secondary amenorrhea had ovarian biopsies, with apparently viable oocytes and follicles noted in nine of the specimens. Yet two of the nine pregnancies involving their own oocytes in this group of women occurred in women with no observable follicles on biopsy specimens. Seven of these nine pregnancies occurred while the patients were taking exogenous estrogen; the other two pregnancies occurred, as noted, after ovulation induction. Only three of the patients with primary amenorrhea underwent gonadal biopsy. The two with 46,XY karyotypes proved to have dysgerminomas. One other patient had only fibrous streaks.

From this large series of affected women, it is apparent

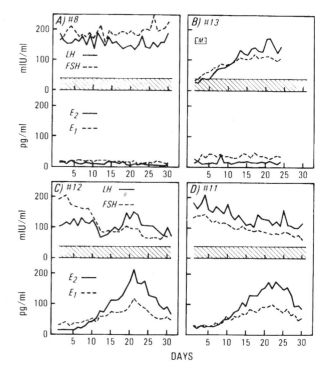

Fig. 54-2. Representative patterns of concentrations of circulating LH, FSH, estrone (E_1), and estradiol (E_2) in daily samples collected from women with hypergonadotropic amenorrhea. Progesterone levels (not shown) were always less than 1.0 μg/mL. The shaded areas indicate concentrations of less than 40 mIU/mL, the level above which ovarian failure has been considered to exist. The patient depicted in **B** had her first menstrual period (*M*) in more than 1 year at the time the sampling began; at that time gonadotropin levels were less than 40 mIU/mL. The changing ratio of LH to FSH and the increasing concentrations of E_2 in **B**, **C**, and **D** strongly suggest the presence of remaining functional follicles. (From Rebar et al.,[78] with permission.)

that individuals with hypergonadotropinism who present with primary and secondary amenorrhea have quite distinct features. Hypergonadotropic amenorrhea is clearly heterogeneous. Use of the term *premature ovarian failure* to describe all young women with hypergonadotropic amenorrhea is inappropriate because some of these women will ovulate and conceive after elevated gonadotropin levels are identified. Recommendations for diagnosis, evaluation, and therapy also follow from the findings in this series and are considered subsequently.

These conclusions are supported by an earlier, more detailed evaluation of circulating hormone concentrations in a subset of these same patients.[78] Blood samples were obtained daily for 1 month from 18 women for measurement of gonadotropins and gonadal steroids. In nine of the women, estradiol levels were very low and FSH and LH levels were very high (Fig. 54-2 A). This pattern of hormone secretion is typical of postmenopausal and oophorectomized women and indicates that there is no follicular activity. However, in nine of the women, evidence

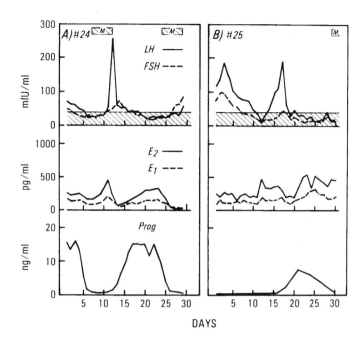

Fig. 54-3. Patterns of daily concentrations of circulating LH, FSH, E_1, E_2, and progesterone (*Prog*) in women with hypergonadotropic amenorrhea and evidence of ovulation during sample collection. The shaded areas indicate concentrations of less than 40 mIU/mL. In one patient (**A**) the follicular phase apparently was very short, with an LH surge occurring just after the cessation of menstrual bleeding (*M*). This patient had documented thyroiditis. In another patient (**B**) falling gonadotropin levels preceded the follicular phase increase in E_2. This individual had four cyclic menses followed again by hypergonadotropic amenorrhea. (From Rebar et al.,[78] with permission.)

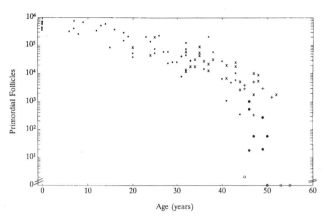

Fig. 54-4. The relationship between age and primordial follicle number in normal adult women, using data from four separate studies (hence the different symbols), as summarized by Richardson and Nelson.[83] The rapid fall in follicle number that occurs just before menopause is apparent. If this same rapid decrease in follicle number occurs in women who develop premature ovarian failure, irregular and sporadic ovulations may occur just before follicle depletion. (From Richardson and Nelson,[83] with permission.)

of follicular function, as based on increased circulating estradiol concentrations, was present (Fig. 54-2 C and D). In fact, two of the women studied had presumptive evidence of ovulation, with elevated serum progesterone levels during the sampling period (Fig. 54-3). These findings certainly are in concert with reports that pregnancies occasionally occur spontaneously in women with hypergonadotropic amenorrhea.

ETIOLOGY

de Moraes-Ruehsen and Jones[27] suggested three possible explanations for the early completion of atresia that they presumed existed in women with hypergonadotropic amenorrhea and premature ovarian failure: (1) decreased germ cell endowment, (2) accelerated loss of oocytes (atresia), and (3) postnatal germ cell destruction. These reasonable possibilities, however, cannot apply in those circumstances where considerable numbers of oocytes still remain, suggesting that a block to gonadotropin action in ovarian follicles can also exist.

Given older information that even postmenopausal women may have a few remaining follicles[20,39] and more recent information that follicle number decreases rapidly in the last several months before menopause,[83,84] occasional

ovulations and rare pregnancies may occur in women with this disorder who are in reality "perimenopausal" (Fig. 54-4). Among the various causes of hypergonadotropic amenorrhea, some cannot occur in women with any viable follicles and others have the potential for spontaneous pregnancy (see the box on p. 4).

Genetic causes

Familial inheritance. Several reports[23,60,95] have described "familial" premature ovarian failure with vertical transmission of the trait, implying autosomal dominant, sex-linked inheritance. In such families, premature depletion of oocytes might result from failure of all available germ cells to migrate to the genital ridges, from a reduced germ cell complement, or from accelerated atresia arising on a genetic basis. It is well recognized that the number of oocytes differs widely among various strains of mice.[46] In addition, both mice[46] and humans[7,8,11,12] show marked individual variability in the rates of follicular atresia. Although the etiology of the premature ovarian failure that may coexist with the neurologic disorder myotonia dystrophica[37] is unknown, it may be due to a genetically endowed decrease in germ cell number or to accelerated atresia.

Gonadal dysgenesis. Individuals with the various forms of gonadal dysgenesis typically present with hypergonadotropic amenorrhea, regardless of the extent of pubertal development and the presence or absence of associated anomalies or stigmata. It is well recognized that cytogenetic abnormalities of the X chromosome can impair ovarian development and function. Studies of 46,X individuals and those with various X chromosomal depletions have confirmed that two intact X chromosomes are necessary for maintenance of oocytes.[92] The gonads of 45,X fetuses

---

Tentative classification of hypergonadotropic amenorrhea

I. Genetic and cytogenetic etiologies

    A. Reduced germ cell number
    B. Accelerated atresia (?)
    C. Structural alterations or absence of an X chromosome
    D. Trisomy X with or without mosaicism
    E. In association with myotonia dystrophica

II. Enzymatic defects

    A. 17α-Hydroxylase deficiency
    B. Galactosemia

III. Environmental insults

    A. Ionizing radiation
    B. Chemotherapeutic agents
    C. Viral infection
    D. Cigarette smoking
    E. Surgical extirpation

IV. Defective gonadotropin secretion or action (?)

    A. Secretion of biologically inactive gonadotropin
    B. α- or β-Subunit defects
    C. Gonadotropin receptor or postreceptor defects

V. Immune disturbances

    A. In association with other autoimmune disorders
    B. Isolated
    C. Congenital thymic aplasia

VI. Idiopathic

From Rebar et al.[82] with permission.

contain the normal complement of oocytes at 20 to 24 weeks of fetal age, but these rapidly undergo atresia so that none are present at birth.[94] Primary and secondary amenorrhea typically occur in women with deletions in either the short or the long arm of one X chromosome.[92] Structural abnormalities of the X chromosome also can have a negative impact on ovarian function and are present in some women with premature ovarian failure.[1,50,77] Relatively recent investigation of a family in which three women had premature ovarian failure documented submicroscopic deletions of Xq26-27,[52] suggesting that perhaps other affected individuals may have similarly subtle molecular defects in chromosomal structure.

It is important to remember that, although individuals with Turner syndrome are generally evident on inspection,[99] patients with pure and mixed gonadal dysgenesis may be difficult to identify on physical examination alone. Women with pure gonadal dysgenesis, who generally present with primary amenorrhea and sexual infantilism, are of normal height and do not have the somatic abnormalities associated with Turner syndrome.[29,93] Such indi-

viduals have either a 46,XX or a 46,XY karyotype. In the extremely rare disorder of mixed gonadal dysgenesis, a germ cell tumor or a testis accounts for one gonad, with an undifferentiated streak, rudimentary, or no gonad accounting for the other.[25] Such individuals are generally mosaic, with the 45,X/46,XY karyotype being the most frequent, but with several other chromosomal patterns reported. Almost all affected individuals are raised as females, with mild to moderate virilization occurring at puberty. Abnormal genitalia may be noted at birth. Because of the malignant potential of intraabdominal gonads in individuals with a Y chromosomal component,[59,87,88] the gonads should be removed.

Trisomy X with or without mosaicism. It is now apparent that an excess of X chromosomes also may be associated with decreased germ cell number of accelerated atresia.[26,32,101] In most of these individuals normal ovarian function is generally present for several years before the onset of premature ovarian failure. Yet even here a few individuals with sexual infantilism have been reported.

Enzymatic defects

17α-Hydroxylase deficiency. Individuals with the rare disorder of 17α-hydroxylase deficiency are easily identified because of the constellation of findings, including primary amenorrhea, sexual infantilism, hypergonadotropinism, hypertension, hypokalemic alkalosis, and increased circulating levels of deoxycorticosterone and progesterone, found in girls who survive into their teenaged years.[10,31,58] Ovarian biopsies of a few affected individuals have shown the presence of numerous large cysts and follicular cysts, with complete failure of orderly follicular maturation.[58]

Galactosemia. Women with galactosemia develop amenorrhea with elevated gonadotropin levels, even when treatment with a galactose-restricted diet begins at an early age.[41,48] The precise etiology of the premature ovarian failure in galactosemia is unknown. It is very tempting to suggest that the carbohydrate moieties on gonadotropin molecules are altered, thus rendering them biologically inactive or changing their metabolism. Yet a direct effect of galactose on the oocyte is suggested by the experimental finding that pregnant rats fed a 50% galactose diet delivered pups with significantly reduced numbers of oocytes, apparently as a result of decreased germ cell migration to the genital ridges.[18]

Physical insults

Destruction of oocytes by various environmental insults is one potential cause of ovarian failure.[100] Conditions that have been implicated include ionizing radiation, various chemotherapeutic agents, certain viral infections, and cigarette smoking.

Ionizing radiation. Of the patients irradiated for Hodgkin disease who receive 400 to 500 rads to the ovaries over 4 to 6 weeks, permanent hypergonadotropic amenorrhea results in approximately 50%.[3,6,74] In general, for any given dose of radiation, the older the woman, the greater the likelihood of her developing amenorrhea, presumably because the number of viable oocytes remaining is smaller. It appears that a total of 800 rads is sufficient to lead to permanent sterility in all women.[3,6,74] That the amenorrhea following radiation therapy might not always be permanent was first noted by Jacox[43] in 1939. This observation suggests that many follicles may be damaged but not destroyed by relatively low doses of radiation. It has been suggested that the ovaries be transposed surgically outside of the field of irradiation before radiation therapy begins to prevent ovarian failure,[6,74] but how fertile such women are after successful curative therapy has not been examined in detail.

Chemotherapeutic agents. As the prognoses for young women with various malignancies, particularly Hodgkin disease, acute forms of leukemia, and breast cancer, have improved after appropriate radiation and chemotherapy, it has become apparent that the chemotherapeutic agents, in addition to the ionizing radiation, may produce either temporary or permanent ovarian failure.* The alkylating agents, especially cyclophosphamide, have been studied most extensively and appear particularly prone to affect reproductive function. In general, the younger the individual patient at the time of therapy, the more likely it is that ovarian function will not be compromised by the chemotherapeutic agents.* As noted in considering the effects of radiation therapy, it may well be that the number of oocytes in the ovaries at the time of therapy is important in determining whether ovarian function will persist after therapy. In a recent study, Green and his associates[33] examined the effect of chemotherapy beginning before age 20 on the outcome of subsequent pregnancies. The frequency of congenital anomalies was 8.1% (5 of 62) among the liveborn children of the women, not greater than that observed in the general population. No relationship between the mother's age at diagnosis or the length of time from completion of therapy to pregnancy and the presence of congenital anomalies was identified. The results of the study suggest, however, that one particular chemotherapeutic agent, dactinomycin, may be associated with an increased risk of a specific type of anomaly, congenital structural cardiac anomalies, and indicate the need for future studies.

Viral and other agents. Although viruses have been thought to have the potential to cause ovarian destruction for many years, it has been difficult to document the involvement of these agents. Morrison and his colleagues[65] reported three presumptive cases in which mumps oophoritis preceded "premature menopause," including cases in a mother and her daughter in which the mother had documented mumps parotiditis and abdominal pain during preg-

*References 24, 42, 51, 95, 97, 104.

Table 54-3. Reported cases of autoimmune diseases associated with premature ovarian failure

Thyroid	26
Adrenal	8
Polyendocrinopathy (type I)	20
Polyendocrinopathy (type II)	19
Diabetes mellitus	3
Multiple endocrinopathy	6
Myasthenia gravis	9
Pernicious anemia	2
Idiopathic thrombocytopenia	1
Glomerulonephritis	1
Rheumatoid arthritis	1
Crohn disease	1
Vitiligo	1
Systemic lupus erythematosus	2
Asthma	1
Ovarian lymphocytic infiltrate	3
Unspecified	15
TOTAL	119 out of 380 cases

Data tabulated from LaBarbera et al.[53] and from Rebar et al.[82] with permission.

nancy just before delivery of the daughter. Finally, Jick and co-workers[44] have reported that cigarette smokers experience menopause at an earlier age than do nonsmokers.

Immune disturbances

Several autoimmune disturbances and diseases associated with altered immunity—both endocrine and nonendocrine—are known to be associated with hypergonadotropic amenorrhea (Table 54-3).[53,82] As is true for autoimmune disorders in general, the ovarian "failure" in affected individuals often waxes and wanes, and pregnancies may occur at least early in the disease process in affected women.

Isolated cases first were reported in the early 1950s in which hypergonadotropic amenorrhea preceded, followed, or occurred together with the onset of other autoimmune illnesses. In fact, Guinet and Pommatau[34] first reported a case in which premature menopause and myxedema preceded development of Addison disease. In a recent review of 119 cases from the literature,[53] 17.5% had an autoimmune disorder associated with ovarian failure. Further evidence for an autoimmune etiology in some cases of hypergonadotropic amenorrhea is provided by sporadic reports confirming return of ovarian function after either immunosuppressive therapy or recovery from an autoimmune disease.[9,22,55] Also supporting an autoimmune etiology for ovarian failure are some cases in which lymphocytic infiltrates have been observed in ovarian tissue.[72,90]

It is tempting to suggest that an antigen-specific suppressor cell defect, possibly to an ovarian antigen such as the FSH receptor, might permit a "forbidden" clone of helper T cells to stimulate production of antibodies to this ovarian antigen by sensitized B lymphocytes (plasma cells). Antibodies to ovarian cell antigens might cause cytotoxicity directly through complement fixation or indirectly by activating killer (K) cells. K cells have surface receptors to the Fc region of immunoglobulin G. Thus antibody-dependent cytotoxicity can result if high titers of antiovarian antibodies bound to the target tissue in turn bind to K cells and induce cell damage. Mechanisms similar to that just described have been proposed for autoimmune thyroiditis.[102] It is true that cases documenting any leukocytic infiltration of the ovary are rare, whereas such cases are common in thyroiditis. However, these differences may merely reflect differences in the target tissue rather than in the disease process and/or the difficulty in obtaining ovarian tissue during acute episodes. Moreover, ovarian biopsies sample only a small portion of the ovary and may not include areas containing follicles showing leukocytic infiltrates.

A number of other immune alterations have been documented in some cases. Enhanced release of leukocyte migration inhibition factor (MIF) by peripheral lymphocytes after exposure of the lymphocytes to crude ovarian proteins has been reported.[28,70] The release of MIF in response to organ-specific antigens provides evidence of activation of cell-mediated immunity. Alterations in the proportions of the various types of lymphocytes also have been noted.[40,73] Further supporting an autoimmune basis for premature ovarian failure in some patients is the report of a significant association with HLA-DR3.[103] Associations between autoimmune endocrinopathies and HLA antigens are well known and indicate a genetic susceptibility to autoimmunity in some individuals. In addition, McNatty and co-workers[57] noted both antibodies to corpus luteum and complement-dependent cytotoxic effects on cultured granulosa cells, as documented by inhibition of progesterone production and cell lysis, in sera from 9 of 23 patients with hypergonadotropic amenorrhea and Addison disease. Indirect immunofluorescence of ovarian biopsy specimens also reveals antibodies reacting with various ovarian components in some patients.[66] Circulating immunoglobulins to ovarian proteins have been detected by immunocytochemical techniques by several investigators.[53] Utilizing a solid-phase ELISA, antibodies to ovarian tissue have been detected in 22% of karyotypically normal women with premature ovarian failure.[49] The most convincing study to the present time remains that by Chiauzzi and co-workers,[19] who demonstrated that two patients with ovarian failure had circulating immunoglobulin G that blocked binding of FSH to its receptor. It is important to realize that ovarian autoantibodies may not be the cause of ovarian failure. The ovarian failure may result from cell-mediated autoimmunity, and autoantibodies may appear only because of the resultant cell death.

Although the importance of the thymus gland to immunologic function has been known for many years, only relatively recently has any relationship between the thymus and reproductive function become evident. This is true despite the documentation by Miller and Chatten[63] in 1967 that congenitally athymic girls who died before puberty had ovaries that contained no oocytes on autopsy.

Data now suggest that the thymus gland is essential early in development for normal gonadotropin secretion. Congenitally athymic mice, known to develop premature ovarian failure,[54] actually have lower gonadotropin concentrations prepubertally than their normal heterozygous littermates.[80] Moreover, these hormonal aberrations and the accelerated loss of oocytes[71,85] can be prevented by thymic transplantation into the thymus gland at birth.[79] In comparing ovarian development in the rodent with that in the primate, it is important to realize that development occurring during the first few weeks of extrauterine life in the mouse occurred in utero in the human female. Thus extirpation of the thymus in rhesus monkeys in utero is associated with a marked reduction in oocyte numbers at birth.[38] A possible explanation for this association of thymic aplasia and ovarian failure may be found in the observation that peptides produced in the thymus can stimulate release of gonadotropin-releasing hormone (GnRH) and consequently LH.[81]

Determining which patients have an autoimmune basis for their hypergonadotropic amenorrhea is important because affected patients might be effectively treated early in the disease process. Sequential studies of one teenaged patient in whom gonadotropin levels decreased and pubertal development ensued only when corticosteroids administered for adrenal insufficiency were taken regularly suggest this possibility.[55] In other reports, ovulation temporarily returned after plasmapheresis in a woman with myasthenia gravis[9] and with glucocorticoid therapy in a woman with a perifollicular lymphocytic infiltrate.[22]

Defects in gonadotropin structure or action

At present the possibility that defects in gonadotropin structure or function can cause hypergonadotropic amenorrhea is only theoretic. This is, however, a tempting speculation. Abnormal molecular forms of gonadotropin, especially FSH, with reduced biologic activity might lead to accelerated follicular atresia early in development and premature ovarian failure. Support for the need for normal levels of gonadotropins early in development is provided by the observation that fetal removal of the pituitary gland in rhesus monkeys leads to the newborns' having ovaries containing no oocytes.[35] In addition, cases of male pseudohermaphroditism with immunologically active but biologically inactive LH are well documented.[4,69] Moreover, altered forms of immunoreactive LH and FSH have been noted in urinary extracts from women with premature ovarian failure compared with those from oophorectomized and postmenopausal women,[91] suggesting that metabolism and/or excretion of gonadotropins and possibly their subunits are altered in some cases of this disorder. Because individuals who still have viable oocytes in their ovaries at the time of diagnosis should ovulate in response to normal exogenous gonadotropins, it would be important to identify such individuals so that therapy can be instituted.

It is also possible that receptors for LH, FSH, or some other gonadotropic factor might be absent or defective. Postreceptor cellular systems that mediate hormone action could be absent or defective as well.

Idiopathic

At present the diagnosis of "idiopathic" premature ovarian failure must be considered a diagnosis of exclusion. However, it is true that no apparent cause for hypergonadotropic amenorrhea is found in the majority of cases. It is also likely that other causes for hypergonadotropic amenorrhea will become apparent as more is learned about this enigmatic disorder.

Myth of a distinct resistant ovary syndrome

As originally defined, the resistant ovary or Savage syndrome is a disorder in young amenorrheic women consisting of (1) elevated peripheral gonadotropin levels, (2) the presence of normal but immature follicles in the ovaries, (3) a 46,XX karyotype, (4) complete development of secondary sexual characteristics, and (5) diminished sensitivity to stimulation with exogenous gonadotropins.[47] From the previous discussions it is clear that this syndrome is itself heterogeneous and a part of the spectrum of hypergonadotropic amenorrhea, overlapping with several of the various causes outlined. Findings such as these may occur relatively early in the disease process, in the "perimenopausal" period prior to destruction of all remaining oocytes. Affected individuals also might have an autoimmune basis for their ovarian failure or a gonadotropin receptor or postreceptor defect. It would seem inappropriate to separate this category of women from others who present with hypergonadotropic amenorrhea.

EVALUATION

The purposes for evaluating young women with hypergonadotropic amenorrhea are to identify (1) specific, potentially treatable causes and (2) other potentially dangerous associated disorders. A thorough history and physical examination are always warranted. A maturation index and evaluation of the cervical mucus may help determine whether any endogenous estrogen is present.

Several simple laboratory tests should be performed to rule out thyroid disease, hypoparathyroidism, hypoadrenalism, diabetes mellitus, and other evidence of autoimmune dysfunction. How extensive such testing should be, however, is unsettled at present, and suggested appropriate tests are listed in the box at right. In addition to the clinical evaluation of estrogen status, measurement of circulating LH, FSH, and estradiol concentrations on more than one occasion may help determine whether any functional follicles are present. If the estradiol concentration is greater

---

Evaluation of hypergonadotropic amenorrhea in young women

1. Complete history and physical examination
2. Maturation index
3. Karyotype (? limited to patients with onset before age 30)
4. Complete blood count with differential, sedimentation rate, total serum protein and albumin-globulin ratio, rheumatoid factor, antinuclear antibody
5. Fasting blood sugar, serum calcium and phosphorus, evaluation of adrenal status
6. Thyroxine, thyrotropin, anti-thyroglobulin, and antimicrosomal antibodies
7. LH, FSH, and estradiol on at least two occasions
8. Evaluation of bone density
9. Evaluation of sella turcica

Adapted from Rebar et al.[77]

---

than 50 pg/mL or if the LH level is greater than the FSH level (in terms of milli-international units per milliliter) in any sample, then at least a few viable oocytes are still present. Irregular uterine bleeding, indicative of continuing estrogen production, also suggests the presence of remaining functional oocytes. It has been suggested recently that the presence of follicles on transvaginal ultrasonography also can be used to identify women with remaining oocytes,[61] but this possibility remains to be explored in more detail, especially because follicles sometimes can be identified even in the ovaries of postmenopausal women.

If available, testing of the patient's serum for antibodies to endocrine tissues, including ovary, may be of some value. The difficulty with this recommendation is the fact that no test for antibodies to any specific antigen, except for one to the LH receptor,[64] has been developed. In addition, as noted previously, antibodies may develop because of cytotoxicity in the ovary and may not cause ovarian failure.

It is also unclear in which patients chromosomal studies should be conducted. It would seem prudent to obtain a karyotype in women with the onset of hypergonadotropic amenorrhea before age 30 to identify those with various forms of gonadal dysgenesis, individuals with mosaicism, those with trisomy X, and those with a portion of a Y chromosome. If a Y chromosome is present, gonadal extirpation is warranted because of the increased risk of malignancy.[59,87,88] Chromosomal evaluation also may be warranted in women who develop hypergonadotropic amenorrhea after the birth of a girl or girls who may suffer later from the same inherited malady.

Although controversial, it does not appear that ovarian biopsy is warranted in women with hypergonadotropic amenorrhea and a normal karyotype. It is not clear how the results would alter therapy. Aiman and Smentek[1] reported that one of their two patients who eventually conceived had no oocytes present on biopsy. Similarly, Rebar and Connolly[76] noted that two of eight subsequent pregnancies among 97 women with secondary hypergonadotropic amenorrhea occurred in women with no follicles present in ovarian tissue obtained by laparotomy. As noted by Aiman and Smentek,[1] if five sections of an ovarian biopsy sample are examined and each is 6 μm thick, then the presence of follicles is sought from a sample representing less than 0.15% of a 2- by 3- by 4-cm ovary. Thus the absence of follicles on biopsy may not be indicative of the remainder of the ovary. Moreover, affected individuals almost always require estrogen replacement regardless of the results of the biopsy.

Evaluation of bone density appears warranted in women with hypergonadotropic amenorrhea because of the high incidence of osteopenia.[62,82] Periodic assessment may be warranted, regardless of therapy, to assess the rapidity of bone loss. Similarly, monitoring patients for the development of autoimmune endocrinopathies may be warranted even if all tests are normal when the patient is first evaluated; development of other disorders after diagnosis of hypergonadotropic amenorrhea does occur.[76]

Almost all reported FSH-secreting pituitary adenomas are found in elderly men. It seems prudent, however, to rule out existence of a large adenoma by radiographic evaluation of the sella turcica. Given the very low probability of identifying any lesion, a lateral skull film would seem sufficient.

THERAPY

It is reasonable to suggest that all young women with hypergonadotropic amenorrhea should be treated with exogenous estrogen whether or not they are interested in childbearing. The accelerated bone loss frequently accompanying this disorder may well be prevented by administration of exogenous estrogens.[62] In addition, almost all spontaneous pregnancies in this disorder occur during or after estrogen administration.[2,76,96] However, even with exogenous estrogens, the possibility of spontaneous pregnancy appears to be less than 10% even though, as noted, perhaps 25% of women have evidence of ovulation after the diagnosis of hypergonadotropic amenorrhea. Because of this possibility of pregnancy, women taking exogenous estrogens in any form, even as part of oral contraceptive agents, should be advised to contact their physician if they develop any signs or symptoms of pregnancy or do not have withdrawal bleeding. Although it may not be necessary to advise the use of barrier forms of contraception, the possibility of pregnancy must be discussed. Either oral contraceptives or sequential estrogen-progestin therapy may be utilized, but sequential therapy is more physiologic. It is important to remember that these young women may require twice as much estrogen as do menopausal women to alleviate their signs and symptoms of hypoestrogenism.

Several isolated case reports have suggested that ovarian suppression with estrogen or a GnRH agonist followed by stimulation with human menopausal gonadotropin may be efficacious in inducing ovulation and allowing conception.[14,17] Most of these reports emanate from one group. Larger series suggest that the possibility of successful ovulation induction and pregnancy is small indeed and may be no greater than what occurs spontaneously in these patients.[67,76]

A brighter hope for women with hypergonadotropic amenorrhea rests with in vitro fertilization involving oocyte donation. The first successful case of oocyte donation in humans was reported in 1984. A young woman with ovarian failure was given oral estradiol valerate and progesterone pessaries to prepare the endometrium for transfer of a single donated oocyte after fertilization with her husband's sperm.[56] Critical to the development of programs utilizing oocyte donation have been (1) improvements in transvaginal ultrasonography, allowing follicular aspiration and oocyte collection without surgery; (2) improvements in success with embryo cryopreservation and subsequent embryo transfer to the donor; and (3) improved ability to synchronize the artificial cycles in the recipient with the hyperstimulation cycles in the donor, generally by use of GnRH agonists.[13,75,86] A number of replacement protocols have been developed for the donor with hypergonadotropic amenorrhea, including use of oral, transvaginal, and transdermal administration of estradiol and oral, transvaginal, and intramuscular administration of progesterone. Should pregnancy develop from the transferred embryo, given the absence of functional gonads in the recipient, exogenous supplementation with estradiol and progesterone must be continued until placental production of progesterone is well established. Success rates generally have exceeded those observed in standard in vitro fertilization programs.[13,86] Thus oocyte donation provides the possibility of pregnancy to all women with premature ovarian failure so long as a normal uterus is present.

REFERENCES

1. Aiman J, Smentek C: Premature ovarian failure, *Obstet Gynecol* 66:9, 1985.
2. Alper MM, Jolly EE, Garner PB: Pregnancies after premature ovarian failure, *Obstet Gynecol* 67:595, 1986.
3. Ash P: The influence of radiation on fertility in man, *Br J Radiol* 53:271, 1980.
4. Axelrod L, Neer RM, Kliman B: Hypogonadism in a male with immunologically active, biologically inactive luteinizing hormone: an exception to a venerable rule, *J Clin Endocrinol Metab* 48:279, 1979.
5. Bachmann GA, Kemmann E: Prevalence of oligomenorrhea and amenorrhea in a college population, *Am J Obstet Gynecol* 144:98, 1982.
6. Baker JW et al: Preservation of ovarian function in patients requiring radiotherapy for para-aortic and pelvic Hodgkin's disease, *Lancet* 1:1307, 1972.
7. Baker TG: A quantitative and cytological study of germ cells in human ovaries, *Proc R Soc Lond* [Biol] 158:417, 1963.
8. Baker TG: Primordial germ cells. In Austin CR, Short RV, editors:

Reproduction in mammals, vol 1, *Germ cells and fertilization,* London, 1972, Cambridge University Press.

9. Bateman BG, Nunley WC, Kitchin JD III: Reversal of apparent premature ovarian failure in a patient with myasthenia gravis, *Fertil Steril* 39:108, 1983.

10. Bigleri EG, Herron MA, Brust N: 17-Hydroxylation deficiency in man, *J Clin Invest* 45:1946, 1966.

11. Block E: Quantitative morphological investigations of the follicular system in women: variations at different ages, *Acta Anat* 14:108, 1952.

12. Block E: A quantitative morphological investigation of the follicular system in newborn female infants, *Acta Anat* 17:201, 1953.

13. Chan CLK et al.: Oocyte donation and *in vitro* fertilization for hypergonadotropic hypogonadism: clinical state of the art, *Obstet Gynecol Surv* 42:350, 1987.

14. Check JH, Chase JS: Ovulation induction in hypergonadotropic amenorrhea with estrogen and human menopausal gonadotropin therapy, *Fertil Steril* 42:919, 1984.

15. Check JH, Chase JS, Spence M: Pregnancy in premature ovarian failure after therapy with oral contraceptives despite resistance to previous human menopausal gonadotropin therapy, *Am J Obstet Gynecol* 160:114, 1989.

16. Check JH et al: Ovulation induction and pregnancy with an estrogen-gonadotropin stimulation technique in a menopausal woman with marked hypoplastic ovaries, *Am J Obstet Gynecol* 160:405, 1989.

17. Check JH, Wu CH, Check M: The effect of leuprolide acetate in aiding induction of ovulation in hypergonadotropic hypogonadism: a case report, *Fertil Steril* 49:542, 1988.

18. Chen Y-T et al: Reduction in oocyte number following prenatal exposure to a diet high in galactose, *Science* 214:1145, 1981.

19. Chiauzzi V et al: Inhibition of follicle-stimulating hormone receptor binding by circulating immunoglobulins, *J Clin Endocrinol Metab* 54:1221, 1982.

20. Costoff A, Mahesh VB: Primordial follicles with normal oocytes in the ovaries of postmenopausal women, *J Am Geriatr Soc* 23:193, 1975.

21. Coulam CB, Adamson SC, Annegers JF: Incidence of premature ovarian failure, *Obstet Gynecol* 67:604, 1986.

22. Coulam CB, Kempers RD, Randall RV: Premature ovarian failure: evidence for the autoimmune mechanism, *Fertil Steril* 36:238, 1981.

23. Coulam CB, Stringfellow SS, Hoefnagel D: Evidence for a genetic factor in the etiology of premature ovarian failure, *Fertil Steril* 40:693, 1983.

24. Damewood MD, Grochow LB: Prospects for fertility after chemotherapy or radiation for neoplastic disease, *Fertil Steril* 45:443, 1986.

25. Davidoff F, Federman DD: Mixed gonadal dysgenesis, *Pediatrics* 52:725, 1973.

26. Day RW, Larson W, Wright SW: Clinical and cytogenetic studies on a group of females with XXX sex chromosome complements, *J Pediatr* 64:24, 1964.

27. de Moraes-Ruehsen M, Jones GS: Premature ovarian failure, *Fertil Steril* 18:440, 1967.

28. Edmonds M et al: Autoimmune thyroiditis, adrenalitis, and oophoritis, *Am J Med* 54:782, 1973.

29. Espiner EA et al: Syndrome of streak gonads and normal male karyotype in phenotypic females, *N Engl J Med* 283:6, 1970.

30. Goldenberg RL et al: Gonadotropins in women with amenorrhea, *Am J Obstet Gynecol* 116:1003, 1973.

31. Goldsmith O, Solomon DH, Horton R: Hypogonadism and mineralocorticoid excess, the 17-hydroxylase deficiency syndrome, *N Engl J Med* 277:673, 1967.

32. Gordon DL, Paulsen CA: Premature menopause in XO/XX/XXX/XXXX mosaicism, *Am J Obstet Gynecol* 97:85, 1967.

33. Green DM et al: Congenital anomalies in children of patients who received chemotherapy for cancer in childhood and adolescence, *N Engl J Med* 325:141, 1991.

34. Guinet P, Pommatau E: Le pseudo-panhypopituitarisme par insuffisiences associées ovarienne, thyroidienne, et semenale, *Ann Endocrinol* 15:327, 1954.

35. Gulyas BJ et al: Effects of fetal or maternal hypophysectomy on endocrine organs and body weight in infant rhesus monkeys (Macaca mulatta): with particular emphasis on oogenesis, *Biol Reprod* 16:216, 1977.

36. Hague WM et al: Hypergonadotropic amenorrhea—etiology and outcome in 93 young women, *Int J Gynaecol Obstet* 25:121, 1987.

37. Harper PS, Dyken PR: Early onset dystrophica myotonia, *Lancet* 2:53, 1972.

38. Healy DL, Bacher J, Hodgen GD: Thymic regulation of primate fetal ovarian-adrenal differentiation, *Biol Reprod* 32:1127, 1985.

38. Hertig AT: The aging ovary—a preliminary note, *J Clin Endocrinol Metab* 4:581, 1944.

40. Ho PC et al: Immunologic studies in patients with premature ovarian failure, *Obstet Gynecol* 71:622, 1988.

41. Hoefnagel D, Wurster-Hili D, Child EL: Ovarian failure in galactosaemia, *Lancet* 2:1197, 1979.

42. Horning SJ et al: Female reproductive potential after treatment for Hodgkin's disease, *N Engl J Med* 304:1377, 1981.

43. Jacox HW: Recovery following human ovarian irradiation, *Radiology* 32:538, 1939.

44. Jick H, Porter J, Morrison AS: Relation between smoking and age of natural menopause, *Lancet* 1:1354, 1977.

45. Johnson TR Jr, Peterson EP: Gonadotropin-induced pregnancy following "premature ovarian failure," *Fertil Steril* 31:351, 1979.

46. Jones EC, Krohn PL: The relationship between age, numbers of oocytes and fertility in virgin and multiparous mice, *J Endocrinol* 21:469, 1961.

47. Jones GS, de Moraes-Ruehsen M: A new syndrome of amenorrhea in association with hypergonadotropism and apparently normal ovarian follicular apparatus, *Am J Obstet Gynecol* 104:597, 1969.

48. Kaufman FR et al: Hypergonadotropic hypogonadism in female patients with galactosemia, *N Engl J Med* 304:994, 1981.

49. Kim JG et al: Determination by ELISA of antiovarian antibodies in premature ovarian failure. In Program of the 45th Annual Meeting of the American Fertility Society, San Francisco, Nov 13–16, 1989 (abstract).

50. Kinch RAH et al: Primary ovarian failure: a clinicopathological and cytogenetic study, *Am J Obstet Gynecol* 91:630, 1965.

51. Koyama H et al: Cyclophosphamide-induced ovarian failure and its therapeutic significance in patients with breast cancer, *Cancer* 39:1403, 1977.

52. Krauss CM et al: Familial premature ovarian failure due to an interstitial deletion of the long arm of the X chromosome, *N Engl J Med* 317:125, 1987.

53. LaBarbera AR et al: Autoimmune etiology in premature ovarian failure, *Am J Reprod Immunol Microbiol* 16:115, 1988.

54. Lintern-Moore S, Pantelouris EM: Ovarian development in athymic nude mice, I: the size and composition of the follicle population, *Mech Ageing Dev* 4:385, 1975.

55. Lucky AW et al: Pubertal progression in the presence of elevated serum gonadotropins in girls with multiple endocrine deficiencies, *J Clin Endocrinol Metab* 45:673, 1977.

56. Lutjen P et al: The establishment and maintenance of pregnancy using *in vitro* fertilization and embryo donation in a patient with primary ovarian failure, *Nature* 307:174, 1984.

57. McNatty KP et al: The cytotoxic effect of serum from patients with Addison's disease and autoimmune ovarian failure on human granulosa cells in culture, *Clin Exp Immunol* 22:378, 1975.

58. Mallin SR: Congenital adrenal hyperplasia secondary to 17-hydroxylase deficiency: two sisters with amenorrhea, hypokalemia, hypertension, and cystic ovaries, *Ann Intern Med* 70:69, 1969.

59. Manuel M. Katayama KP, Jones HW Jr: The age of occurrence of gonadal tumors in intersex patients with a Y chromosome, *Am J*

Obstet Gynecol 124:293, 1976.

60. Mattison DR et al: Familial premature ovarian failure, *Am J Hum Genet* 36:1341, 1984.

61. Mehta AE et al: Noninvasive diagnosis of resistant ovary syndrome by ultrasonography, *Fertil Steril* 57:56, 1992.

62. Metka M et al: Hypergonadotropic hypogonadic amenorrhea (World Health Organization III) and osteopenia, *Fertil Steril* 57:37, 1992.

63. Miller ME, Chatten J: Ovarian changes in ataxia telangiectasia, *Acta Paediatr Scand* 56:559, 1967.

64. Moncayo H et al: Ovarian failure and autoimmunity: detection of autoantibodies directed against both the unoccupied luteinizing hormone/human chorionic gonadotropin receptor and the hormone-receptor complex of a bovine corpus luteum, *J Clin Invest* 84:1857, 1989.

65. Morrison JC et al: Mumps oophoritis: a cause of premature menopause, *Fertil Steril* 26:655, 1975.

66. Muechler EK, Huang K-E, Schenk E: Autoimmunity in premature ovarian failure, *Int J Fertil* 36:99, 1991.

67. Nelson LM et al: Gonadotropin suppression for the treatment of karyotypically normal spontaneous premature ovarian failure: a controlled trial, *Fertil Steril* 57:50, 1992.

68. O'Herlihy C, Pepperell RJ, Evans JH: The significance of FSH elevation in young women with disorders of ovulation, *Br Med J* 281:1447, 1980.

69. Park IJ et al: A case of male pseudohermaphroditism associated with elevated LH, normal FSH and low testosterone possibly due to the secretion of an abnormal LH molecule, *Acta Endocrinol* 83:173, 1976.

70. Pekonen F et al: Immunological disturbances in patients with premature ovarian failure, *Clin Endocrinol* 25:1, 1986.

71. Pierpaoli W, Besedovsky HO: Role of the thymus in programming of neuroendocrine functions, *Clin Exp Immunol* 20:323, 1975.

72. Rabinowe SL et al: Lymphocyte dysfunction in autoimmune oophoritis: resumption of menses with corticosteroids, *Am J Obstet Gynecol* 81:348, 1986.

73. Rabinowe SL et al: Monoclonal antibody defined T lymphocyte abnormalities and anti-ovarian antibodies in premature menopause, *Endocrinology* 118(suppl 1):24, 1986.

74. Ray GR et al: Oophoropexy: a means of preserving ovarian function following pelvic megavoltage radiotherapy for Hodgkin's disease, *Radiology* 96:175, 1970.

75. Rebar RW, Cedars MI: Hypergonadotropic forms of amenorrhea in young women, *Endocrinol Metab Clin North Am* 21:173, 1992.

76. Rebar RW, Connolly HV: Clinical features of young women with hypergonadotropic amenorrhea, *Fertil Steril* 53:804, 1990.

77. Rebar RW, Erickson GF, Coulam CB: Premature ovarian failure. In Gondos B, Riddick D, editors: *Pathology of infertility,* New York, 1987, Thieme Medical Publishers.

78. Rebar RW, Erickson GF, Yen SSC: Idiopathic premature ovarian failure: clinical and endocrine characteristics, *Fertil Steril* 37:35, 1982.

79. Rebar RW et al: Reduced gonadotropins in athymic mice: prevention by thymic transplantation, *Endocrinology* 107:2130, 1980.

80. Rebar RW et al: The hormonal basis of reproductive defects in athymic mice, I: diminished gonadotropin concentrations in prepubertal females, *Endocrinology* 108:120, 1981.

81. Rebar RW et al: Thymosin stimulates secretion of luteinizing hormone-releasing factor, *Science* 214:669, 1981.

82. Rebar RW et al: Hypergonadotropic forms of amenorrhea. In Hunzicker-Dunn M, Schwartz NB, editors: *Follicle stimulating hormone: regulation of secretion and molecular mechanisms of action,* New York, 1992, Springer-Verlag.

83. Richardson SJ, Nelson JF: Follicular depletion during the menopausal transition, *Ann N Y Acad Sci* 592:13, 1990.

84. Richardson SJ, Senikas V, Nelson JF: Follicular depletion during the menopausal transition: evidence for accelerated loss and ultimate exhaustion, *J Clin Endocrinol Metab* 65:1231, 1987.

85. Sakakura T, Nishizuka Y: Thymic control mechanism in ovarian development: reconstitution of ovarian dysgenesis in thymectomized mice by replacement with thymic and other lymphoid tissues, *Endocrinology* 90:431, 1972.

86. Sauer MS, Paulson RJ: Oocyte donation for women who have ovarian failure, *Contemp Obstet Gynecol* 125, November 1989.

87. Schellhas HF: Malignant potential of the dysgenetic gonad, part I, *Obstet Gynecol* 44:298, 1974.

88. Schellhas HF: Malignant potential of the dysgenetic gonad, part II, *Obstet Gynecol* 44:455, 1974.

89. Schreiber JR, Davajan V, Kletzky OA: A case of intermittent ovarian failure, *Am J Obstet Gynecol* 132:698, 1978.

90. Sedmak DD, Hart WR, Tubbs RR: Autoimmune oophoritis: A histopathologic study of involved ovaries with immunologic characterization of the nononuclear cell infiltrate, *Int J Gynecol Pathol* 6:73, 1987.

91. Silva de Sa MF, Matthews MJ, Rebar RW: Altered forms of immunoreactive urinary FSH and LH in premature ovarian failure, *Infertility* 11:1, 1988.

92. Simpson JL: Phenotypic-karyotypic correlations of gonadal determinants: current status and relationship to molecular studies. In Vogel F, Sperling K, editors: *Proceedings of the International Congress of Human Genetics.* Heidelberg, 1987, Springer-Verlag.

93. Simpson JL et al: Gonadal dysgenesis in individuals with apparently normal chromosomal complements: tabulation of cases and compilation of genetic data, *Birth Defects* 7:215, 1971.

94. Singh RP, Carr DH: The anatomy and histology of XO human embryos and fetuses, *Anat Rec* 155:369, 1966.

95. Siris ES, Leventhal BG, Vaitukaitis JL: Effects of childhood leukemia and chemotherapy on puberty and reproductive function in girls, *N Engl J Med* 294:1143, 1976.

96. Starup J, Philip J, Sele V: Oestrogen treatment and subsequent pregnancy in two patients with severe hypergonadotropic ovarian failure, *Acta Endocrinol* 89:149, 1978.

97. Stillmann RJ, Schiff I, Schinfeld J: Reproductive and gonadal function in the female after therapy for childhood malignancy, *Obstet Gynecol Surv* 37:385, 1982.

98. Surrey ES, Cedars MI: The effect of gonadotropin suppression on induction of ovulation in premature ovarian failure patients, *Fertil Steril* 52:36, 1989.

99. Turner HH: A syndrome of infantilism, congenital webbed neck and cubitus valgus, *Endocrinology* 23:566, 1938.

100. Verp MS: Environmental causes of ovarian failure, *Semin Reprod Endocrinol* 1:101, 1983.

101. Villanueva AL, Rebar RW: Triple-X syndrome and premature ovarian failure, *Obstet Gynecol* 62:705, 1983.

102. Volpé R: Autoimmune thyroid disease. In Volpé R, editor: *Autoimmunity and endocrine disease,* New York, 1985, Marcel Dekker.

103. Walfish PG et al: Association of premature ovarian failure with HLA antigens, *Tissue Antigens* 21:168, 1983.

104. Whitehead E et al: The effect of combination chemotherapy on ovarian function in women treated for Hodgkin's disease, *Cancer* 52:988, 1983.

Chapter 55

OSTEOPOROSIS IN THE POSTMENOPAUSAL WOMAN

Robert Lindsay, MD, PhD

Osteoporosis is a disease characterized by low bone mass and microarchitectural deterioration of bone tissue, leading to enhanced bone fragility and a consequent increase in fracture risk.[1] Intrinsic to this definition is the realization that this is a skeletal disease in which the only important clinical outcome is fracture. However, the skeletal changes that precede fracture can take many years to develop, and are asymptomatic. Osteoporosis affects primarily postmenopausal women, and is causally related to the failure of ovarian function. Important secondary causes of osteoporosis exist, including glucocorticoid excess, the long-term use of heparin, the use of methotrexate, dilantin, and excessive thyroid-hormone replacement. In such instances, the effect of the secondary agent is enhanced in the already-at-risk postmenopausal population. Osteoporosis also affects males, but less frequently than females. Important causes among men include testosterone deficiency and alcoholism. An aggressive, rare, idiopathic type can afflict men in their middle years. In the context of this volume, only the postmenopausal variety of the disease is considered in detail.

EPIDEMIOLOGY

The incidence of fractures is greatest among the very young and the very old.[2,3] Fractures associated with osteoporosis occur most frequently among the elderly. Classically, only fractures of the femoral neck, spine (vertebral crush fractures), and Colles fractures were considered osteoporotic. However, the incidence of fractures increases with age at many other skeletal sites (Fig. 55-1). Therefore, the majority (if not all) of the fracture syndromes among the elderly can be considered osteoporotic fractures.[4] The degree to which the reduction in bone mass contributes to each fracture clearly varies among anatomical sites, and trauma exerts an equally variable influence that is also site specific. Other important fractures include fractures of the pelvis, proximal humerus, tibial table, and ribs (especially with glucocorticoid-induced disease).

The impact of these fractures upon the health of many countries is now recognized, and osteoporosis has been classified as a major problem in public health for much of the Western world.[5] The prevalence of osteoporotic fractures is increasing in many areas of the world, including the Asian countries. In the United States, there are currently at least 1.5 million osteoporotic fractures each year.[2] Deformities of the vertebral bodies, often recognized on radio-

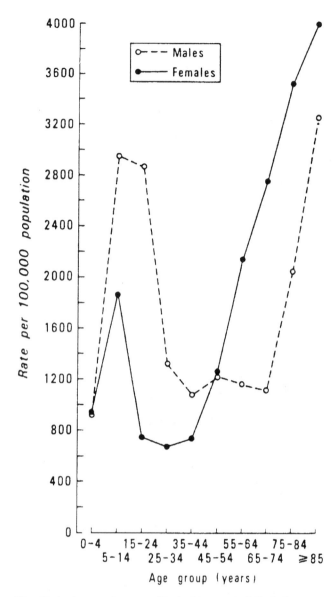

Fig. 55-1. Age- and sex-specific incidence of all limb fractures among the residents of Rochester, Minnesota, 1969-1971. (From Garraway WM, Stauffer RN, Kurland LT, et al: Limb fractures in a defined community. 1. Frequency and distribution, *Mayo Clin Proc* 54:701, 1979.)

graphs, are the most prevalent and may be among the most frequent, but reliable data on the incidence of crush fractures are lacking. However, fractures of the proximal femur clearly have the greatest impact in terms of cost, morbidity, and mortality. Almost 300,000 fractures of the hip (femoral neck and intertrochanteric fractures) occur each year in the United States (Fig. 55-2). These fractures most often affect the population over the age of 70 years, and are 2-3 times more common among women than men.[2,3] (Because women live longer than men, the actual number of fractures among women represents about 80% of the clinical load.) The cost of these fractures is estimated to be in excess of

$10 billion annually. Because the elderly are the most rapidly increasing segment of society, it is not surprising that the number of fractures is also increasing, thus, the cost also is expected to increase. By the year 2025, the cost of osteoporotic fractures may exceed $100 billion.[6] The populations of Asian countries is increasing, particularly among the elderly, at a faster rate than in other countries, so the impact of osteoporosis in these countries will be especially great in the early part of the next century.[7]

Bone loss with age occurs at all skeletal sites, so it is not surprising that common clinical experience dictates that, once a patient has presented with one osteoporotic fracture, she is more likely to incur another. Patients with hip fractures often have evidence of vertebral deformity and are twice as likely to have had a Colles fracture.[2,8] However, many individuals who experience a fracture once never have a recurrent fracture, and osteoporosis exhibits significant clinical heterogeneity in its expression. This often makes it difficult to design authoritative clinical and epidemiological studies in this field.

Hip fracture

Fractures of the femur increase with age in both men and women. Typically, hip fractures occur after a fall, although they occasionally occur before a fall. The exponential increase in fracture with age results in a lifetime fracture risk of 15-17% in Caucasian women, about 6% for African-American women, and correspondingly lower risks for males (5% and 3% for Caucasian and African-American males, respectively).[9]

Hip fracture usually results in hospital admission and a semiemergent surgical procedure to stabilize the fracture or replace the hip. The consequence of this treatment is significant mortality and high morbidity. The combination of advanced age and frailty of the patients, coupled with the greater risks associated with surgery on the hip, cause a peri- and postoperative mortality of 5-20%, in excess of that expected for age and sex.[2,3,10,11] Ten to 20% of patients become dependent and may require long-term care after the acute hospital stay.[12]

There is considerable geographical variability in the incidence of hip fracture. Fracture rates are generally high in Northern Europe and the United States, although there is considerable variability within both regions[9,13-15] (Fig. 55-3). In the United States, fracture rates apparently are inversely related to average social status in any community.[9] The lowest recorded incidence is in the Bantu,[16] although fracture rates are generally higher among whites than nonwhites in all societies.[2] The generality that fracture rates increase with increasing latitude does not appear to hold true within the United States,[13] and perhaps is not true when examined more critically in other countries. In most societies, hip-fracture rates are higher among women than men[17,18] of the same age, with the rate in men lagging 5-10 years.

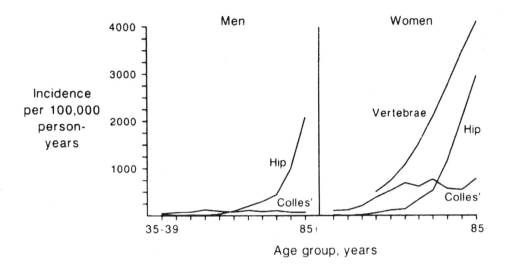

Fig. 55-2. Incidence of osteoporotic fractures as a function of age in men (left) and women (right). (From Melton III LJ: Epidemiology of fractures. In Riggs BL, Melton LJI, editors: *Osteoporosis: etiology, diagnosis and management,* New York, 1988, Raven Press.)

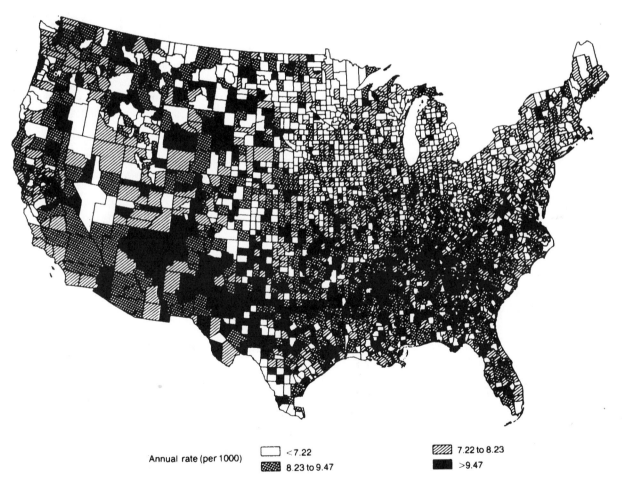

Fig. 55-3. Age-adjusted annual incidence of hip fracture among white women aged 65 years and older by county of residence, 1984 through 1987. (From Jacobsen SJ, Goldberg J, Miles TP, et al: Regional variation in the incidence of hip fracture: US white women aged 65 and older, *J Am Med Assoc,* 264:500, 1990.)

Hip fracture generally requires some degree of trauma, although all clinicians who see such patients report anecdotal experiences of patients who apparently suffer a spontaneous fracture before falling.[19] For most patients, the predisposing trauma is a fall from a standing height. The incidence of falls increases with age, and falls may occur more frequently among women, at least up to the age of 75 years[20] (Fig. 55-4). The occurrence of a fall predisposes to recurrence, and frequent fallers among the elderly can be identified. Falls are most common among the very elderly and infirm, and frequency of falls increases with the number of medical diagnoses present. Only a small fraction of falls result in hip fracture, probably about 1% or less. Whether the fraction of falls that results in hip fracture increases with age is not known; however, as age increases and gait slows, the likelihood of a lateral fall directly on the hip increases.[19,21] As age advances, the capability of individuals to protect themselves from injury declines (with declining strength and speed of reflexes).[22] The increased use of alcohol, sedatives, and other medications[23] among the elderly also contributes to the risk of falling and injury, as does the presence of confusion. The combination of these factors increases the chances of a direct injury to the hip in circumstances in which the energy of the fall cannot be diverted from the femoral neck, in individuals in whom the femoral neck is already prejudiced by loss of mass.[24] The femoral neck, unlike other tubular bones, does not compensate for declining mass by increasing width, a feature that is particularly true among women. The resulting application of a force across the neck is clearly sufficient to produce a fracture in an already weakened bone. Recent evidence suggests that the length of the femoral neck (from the head to the trochanter) correlates with fracture risk, and that the lower fracture incidence in some populations might be related to the geometry of the femoral neck, in addition to the mass of bone present.[25]

Vertebral fracture

Although fractures of the proximal femur are considered to contribute most to the public-health cost of osteoporosis, fractures of the vertebrae are those most feared by the younger female population, who view the height loss and change in body shape among their aging relatives with considerable concern. The epidemiology of vertebral fracture is not well understood, and prevalence rates among the older population appear to vary from 15-75%.[2,26] In part, this variability results from a lack of consensus about the definition of a vertebral fracture. Most abnormalities seen on radiographs are of the anterior-wedge type and are not associated with specific instances of back pain (at least of the type that can be remembered by the patient). These probably occur gradually, and perhaps should not be classified as fractures, but rather as shape changes induced by modeling of the vertebral body. However, these deformities add to the morbidity of the primary disorder, and are likely to occur more frequently in patients with an initial kyphosis secondary to a true crush fracture event.[27] Thus, irrespective of the mechanism by which multiple anterior wedges occur, by their addition to the morbidity they must be considered part of the osteoporotic syndrome. Vertebral fractures are often asymptomatic and found on routine radiographs.[2] In such instances, the use of bone-mass measurement to determine the presence of osteoporosis is useful in making a correct diagnosis[28] (vertebral fractures can be traumatic). When symptomatic, the common presenting symptom is acute back pain.

Colles fracture

Fractures of the distal radius constitute the third most common osteoporotic fracture.[2] These are precipitated by a fall on the outstretched hand. The incidence of distal forearm fractures increases with age in women from the fourth decade until the sixth, but not after that.[2,3] Several reasons have been proposed for the plateau in fracture frequency after age 65, the most appealing being a change in the direction of falling with age that increases the chance of a direct fall on the hip, but reduces the chance of a forward fall onto the outstretched hand.[22] The natural age-related reduction in gait could conceivably produce such an effect (Fig. 55-2). Fractures are painful, and require reduction and fixation. Often, return of function is incomplete, and occasionally reflex-sympathetic dystrophy occurs. Colles fractures, however, are not fatal and are not as serious a problem as other osteoporotic fractures. Colles fractures seem, in the author's practice, to rarely be recognized as osteoporotic in nature, and patients are rarely referred for evaluation of skeletal status.

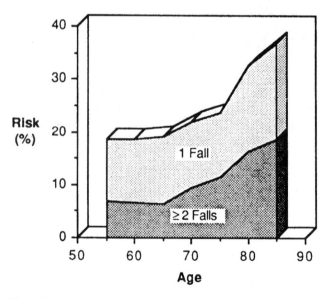

Fig. 55-4. Annual risk of falling among older women. (From Cummings SR, Nevitt MC: *Epidemiology of hip fractures and falls.* In Kleerekoper M, Krane S, editors: *Clinical disorders of bone and mineral metabolism,* New York, 1989, Mary Ann Liebert.)

Other fractures among the elderly are likely to be osteoporotic in nature. A recent, large study of fractures among Caucasian women over 65 years of age in the United States found that fractures of the pelvis, humerus, tibial table, and other skeletal sites are related to a decline in bone mineral density.[4] Thus, such fractures, which are not normally considered part of the spectrum of osteoporotic fractures, need to be considered when evaluating the cost of osteoporosis. The consequence is that the cost of osteoporosis to society is significantly greater than is usually stated in estimates that include only fractures of the hip, spine, and distal radius. The full extent of the cost of osteoporotic fractures is presently unknown.

CLINICAL CHARACTERISTICS

Most patients with osteoporosis are asymptomatic, and many patients present with questions about their personal risk for the disease, rather than with the symptoms of fracture. The most common symptomatic expression is back pain. Osteoporosis causes back pain for two reasons. First, acute collapse of a vertebral body may result in sudden severe back pain, centering around the site of fracture. The pain is usually described as sharp, often episodic, and characteristically radiates around the dermatome anteriorly. It is exacerbated by coughing and sneezing, and relieved by rest. The pain of an acute fracture lasts one to several weeks and gradually subsides with rest and analgesics. Occasionally, muscle spasms in the paravertebral muscles are sufficiently severe to require the use of an antispasmodic. With lumbar vertebral collapse, the pain may radiate into the pelvis or follow sciatic distribution. Constipation may be a problem in such patients, presumably secondary to the loss of intestinal mobility. In the acute phase, tenderness may be elicited over the affected vertebra.

In contrast to the acute presentation, most vertebral collapses appear to occur without symptoms and may gradually progress, rather than suddenly collapse. Most patients of this type present with kyphosis, loss of height, or a dull, chronic, lower back pain. Radiographs often confirm the presence of several vertebral fractures, although if the primary fracture occurs at the level of T 7-8, a gibbus deformity may develop with only one fracture and modest height loss. Such deformities may be highly symptomatic in some patients; others have remarkably few symptoms.

Many patients are referred when vertebral fractures are identified on routine radiographs. Other patients seek care when loss of height or kyphosis becomes noticeable. Increasingly, however, physicians are faced with asymptomatic individuals who are concerned about their risk of osteoporotic fracture. Often these are perimenopausal women who have had a parent or other relative with a fracture of the hip. Others may have read about the disease in one of the many articles about osteoporosis that are published in the popular press. Rarely, patients with a recent Colles fracture present for evaluation of osteoporosis, suggesting that it remains widely unappreciated that a Colles fracture may be an early sign of osteoporosis.

Physical examination is helpful in patients with an acute fracture, but apart from the signs of height loss and kyphosis that may be present, is largely unhelpful in most patients. A complete examination of the back is useful and should be performed to elicit symmetry, mobility, tenderness, and the presence of kyphosis or loss of lumbar lordosis. Height loss can be estimated by measuring pubis to crown and pubis to heel. Each should approximate one-half the arm span and, if the former is reduced, height loss has occurred. The presence of some loss of height is not pathognomonic for osteoporosis. Some loss occurs naturally with age (probably not more than 1 inch), and other disorders can also cause loss of height. Progressive, multiple, vertebral fractures can cause remarkable height loss of several inches (8-9 inches in height loss has been seen in some osteoporotic patients). Eventually, height loss ceases when the ribs abut on the anterior superior iliac crests, and the rib cage assumes the weight of the upper body. Back pain may be reduced at this stage, but may be replaced by rib pain where the ribs rub on the ilium. Such advanced cases of osteoporosis are associated with marked deformity, and anterior abdominal protrusion is a common complaint (often confused with obesity by the patient). The anatomical change in abdominal contents that occurs can produce serious constipation. There is often a forward pelvic tilt and pseudospondylolisthetic abnormalities. The hips are kept flexed and the feet pronated. The consequence is a shuffling gait, easily observed by asking the patient to walk across the room.

DIFFERENTIAL DIAGNOSIS

Back pain is a common presenting symptom of many disorders, and osteoporosis is only one of many differential diagnoses that must be kept in mind. Kyphosis can also be caused by a wide variety of conditions, including trauma, tumors, osteomalacia, skeletal dysplasias, and in younger patients (particularly females), Scheuermann disease. Asymptomatic vertebral fractures can be the presenting sign of malignancy, and every patient should be screened for multiple myeloma, although intractable pain is more common with this latter diagnosis.

In addition to nonosteoporotic conditions, secondary causes of osteoporosis must be considered in every patient. The clinical stigmata of Cushing syndrome may be evidence of steroid therapy or endogenous excess glucocorticoid production. Thyrotoxicosis, gastrointestinal disease or surgery, alcoholism, renal disease, liver disease, and osteomalacia must all be considered. A complete drug history is an important aspect of the history and falls into the category of secondary causes of osteoporosis that have been reviewed elsewhere.[29]

LABORATORY AND RADIOLOGICAL INVESTIGATION

Laboratory tests are within the normal range in uncomplicated postmenopausal osteoporosis, and are performed to exclude other diagnoses and secondary forms of osteoporosis. Baseline investigations include a complete blood count (CBC) and automated biochemistry. In older individuals, thyroid function (TSH) and protein electrophoresis in serum and urine are performed. If clinical evaluation suggests Cushing syndrome, it is appropriate to measure serum cortisol and, if necessary, urinary free cortisol, or to perform a formal dexamethasone suppression test. A serum 25-hydroxyvitamin D level is the best estimate of vitamin D status, and parathyroid hormone (PTH) levels rule out hyperparathyroidism in all but a few individuals. If serum alkaline phosphatase is elevated, malignancy, Paget disease, renal and liver disease, osteomalacia, hyperparathyroidism, hypercortisolism, polymyalgia rheumatica, and multiple fractures must be considered as causes. Alkaline phosphatase is elevated also in chronic heart failure, osteomyelitis, and with the use of a wide range of therapeutic agents.

An increasing number of tests are becoming available that allow evaluation of bone turnover.[30,31] These include skeletal alkaline phosphatase and osteocalcin, which are associated with bone formation; tartrate-resistant acid phosphatase; urinary excretion of hydroxyproline; and a variety of immunoassayable, collagen-degradation products, including cross-linking molecules particular to type 1 collagen (deoxypyridinoline), which are associated with bone resorption. Measurement of urinary calcium (24-hour) is useful as an indicator of calcium intake and bone resorption, but is reduced in osteomalacia and hypocalciuric hypercalcemia. The use of these markers of bone turnover is being evaluated and these tests remain investigational. Potentially, these measurements could assist in predicting the rate of bone loss[32] or the response to therapy.

The assessment of fractures in patients with osteoporosis is performed by radiological evaluation. The number and severity of vertebral fractures is evaluated by properly positioned lateral radiographs of the dorsal and lumbar spine. Early osteoporotic changes include loss of horizontal trabeculae, creating an appearance of greater prominence of the vertical trabeculae, vertebral biconcavity, and anterior wedging. Schmorl nodes, an invagination of the disc into the body of the vertebrae, is a common finding, but is not pathognomonic of osteoporosis because these can be found in other bone diseases, including osteomalacia, and can be found also in myeloma.[33] Complete crush fractures include collapse of both anterior and posterior segments of the vertebral bodies. Posterior collapse alone is suggestive of other causes, including malignancy. The commonly stated term *osteopenic* is misleading when applied subjectively to radiographs. If this term is used, it should be ignored, especially in the absence of other signs. For determination of bone mass, radiographs are not useful unless peripheral radiographic techniques are used with computer assessment.[34] The Singh index[35] is another semiquantitative technique that is used to evaluate the trabecular pattern of the femoral neck and to classify skeletal status according to the remaining trabecular pattern. The index does not correlate particularly well with bone-mass measurement, and is only a rough guide to the status of the skeleton.[36]

PATHOGENESIS OF OSTEOPOROSIS

Peak bone mass

The pathogenesis of osteoporotic fracture can be described in a fairly simple model[37] (Fig. 55-5). The disease is important clinically only because of fractures, which are its complication. As far as is known, the changes in the skeleton are asymptomatic and, in the absence of fracture symptoms (e.g., back pain), should probably not be ascribed to osteoporosis. The strength of the skeleton is related to its mass, anatomy, and architecture. In the young adult, the amount of bone in the skeleton—so-called peak skeletal mass—is primarily under genetic control.[38,39,40] A recent study conducted in Australia suggests that there is a relationship between the genetics of the vitamin D receptor and bone mass.[41] In this study, originally conducted among twins, the presence of the BB genotype was associated with higher bone mass than the bb genotype. A similar relationship was found among nonrelated adults. This exciting finding requires confirmation, but suggests that it is possible to identify those most at risk for osteoporosis by examining their vitamin D receptor genetics, something that potentially would require only a blood sample.

Environmental influences during growth can also have an impact upon the capacity to reach peak bone mass. These include chronic illness, disuse, and poor nutrition. The potential magnitude of the effects of these environmental influences is best observed in the skeletal development of children, paralyzed since birth, whose skeletons are grossly inadequate to withstand the stresses placed upon bone during normal ambulation, but are sufficient for a bed-bound existence. However, within the confines of normal growth and development, the impact of any environmental factor is still unclear. A recent evaluation of the effects of calcium supplementation performed in a cohort of identical twins suggests that increased calcium intake is associated with increased accretion of bone mass.[42] The effects were most evident in prepubertal children, but after discontinuing supplementation, the effects were lost.[43] In cross-sectional studies, calcium intake and physical activity both influenced peak bone mass[44,45,46] and it seems likely that environmental factors may affect as much as 10-20% of the variance in peak bone mass.[47] In effect, this means that adoption of a reasonable program of physical activity and a good diet during growth may maximize peak bone mass. This has yet to be confirmed with longitudinal data. Low peak bone mass is also associated with amenorrhea,

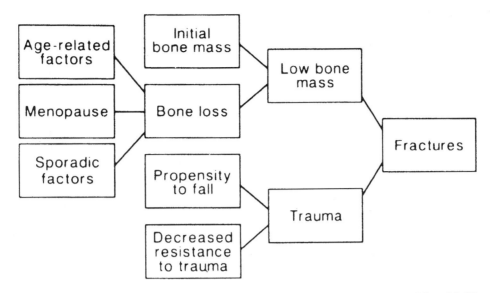

Fig. 55-5. Model of risk factors for osteoporotic bone loss and fractures. (From Melton LJ, III: Epidemiology of fractures. In Riggs BL, Melton LJI, editors: *Osteoporosis: etiology, diagnosis, and management*, New York, 1988, Raven Press.)

independent of the pathogenesis. Thus, hypothalamic amenorrhea, hyperprolactinemia, and anorexia nervosa all can reduce bone mass by inhibition of ovarian function.[48-56] Bone mass is also low in Turner syndrome and Klinefelter syndrome.[57,58] Other abnormalities associated with a reduction in bone mass in the young adult years (i.e., prior to menopause) include thalassemia[59] and pseudohypoparathyroidism.[60] Peak bone mass is low among Eskimos and is higher in the African-American population.[61-65] A family history of osteoporosis may also confer a risk by resulting in low peak bone mass, presumably through genetic influences.[66,67]

Young adults with lower bone mass tend to have a higher frequency of fracture, but those are of the traumatic type, generally affecting peripheral bones; typical osteoporotic fractures are rarely seen in young individuals.[68] Osteoporosis occurs sporadically in children and young adults, and its cause in these situations remains obscure.

Bone loss

Bone mass is relatively stable among premenopausal women.[69] In most cross-sectional studies, and in the few longitudinal studies currently available, there is almost no bone loss in vertebral bone, at least until the age of 40 years, but there may be some bone loss at the femoral neck.[61,70-72] The discrepant behavior of these sites raises the intriguing possibility that different parts of the skeleton may respond to different stimuli. This has been assumed under some circumstances for cancellous and cortical bone, but it has not been examined critically for differing anatomical sites. Further evaluation of this is clearly required. Bone loss occurs ubiquitously among postmenopausal

women, independent of race or social class.[73-76] In all populations studied, bone loss follows cessation of ovarian function.[61] In those without other risk factors, the factors controlling the rate and duration of bone loss are inadequately understood. The data clearly suggest that loss of ovarian estrogen is the dominant factor in initiating bone loss. The relationship between loss of ovarian function and osteoporosis was originally suggested by Albright who, in an elegant series of clinical studies, showed that osteoporosis occurred more frequently among oophorectomized women and those who had undergone premature menopause. Albright[77-78] also demonstrated that estrogens can be used in the treatment of the disease.[79] In a follow-up study of Albright's original patients, Henneman and Wallach[80] showed that further height loss does not occur in osteoporotic patients treated with estrogen.

Noninvasive measurement of bone mass made possible the detection of bone loss among asymptomatic, postmenopausal women.[81] It became evident that bone loss occurs universally after loss of ovarian function, but the rate of loss is considerably variable among individuals. The acceleration of bone loss immediately after menopause or oophorectomy may last five years or more, but this too may be somewhat variable among skeletal sites and individuals.

The alterations in skeletal homeostasis that must occur to cause bone loss can be measured by the biochemical changes that are evidence of the increased skeletal turnover, occurring with loss of ovarian function.[82] Serum and urine markers of bone formation and resorption increase by approximately 50% or more through menopause (Fig. 55-6). There is increased alkaline, acid phosphatase, and osteocalcin in serum, and increased urinary excretion of

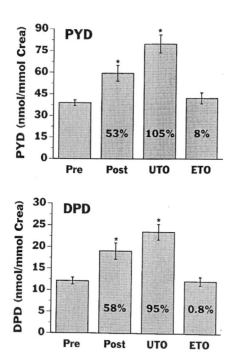

Fig. 55-6. Mean urinary concentrations of the hydroxypiridinium cross-links pyridinoline (PYD) and deoxypyridinolene (DPD) in postmenopausal (POST) healthy women, and untreated (UTO) and estrogen-treated (ETO) women with postmenopausal osteoporosis compared to premenopausal (PRE) healthy women. Column inserts denote percentage change of mean value compared to normal premenopausal controls (PRE). Bars represent standard error of mean (SEM). Asterisks indicate p values < 0.01. UTO levels of both PYD and DPD were higher than post (p < 0.01). (From Seibel M, Cosman F, Shen V, et al: Urinary hydroxypyridinium cross-links of collagen as markers of bone resorption and estrogen efficacy in post-menopausal osteoporosis, *J Bone Miner Res* 8:881, 1993.)

calcium, hydroxyproline, and the cross-linking molecules of collagen deoxypyridinoline and pyridinoline. Modest alterations in circulating PTH and vitamin D metabolites have been observed sometimes[83] and, to detect changes in this endocrine axis, dynamic tests are required.[84,85] The alterations in the calcium homeostatic systems that have been observed suggest that the primary disturbance is in the skeleton, and that these are simply secondary perturbations.[86] However, there is some evidence from dynamic investigation of the axis that estrogen deficiency may affect the set point, relating calcium in serum to PTH secretion. It may also affect the synthesis of 1,25-dihydroxyvitamin D by the kidney, a finding that may account for the reduction in the efficiency of intestinal calcium absorption seen in postmenopausal women.[87]

Bone loss appears to follow loss of ovarian function at any age, independently of the cause. Thus, situations such as athletic amenorrhea, hyperprolactinemia, anorexia, and the use of GnRH superagonists are followed by bone loss.[50-56,88] In each case, it appears to require suppression

of ovarian function to disrupt skeletal metabolism. However, in anorexia, the dietary indiscretions undoubtedly exacerbate the problem. The possibility that more subtle alterations in the pituitary ovarian axis can affect skeletal homeostasis, as has been suggested in one study,[89] remains an open question and requires further evaluation.[90] The modest declines in bone mass seen in some studies of premenopausal women may result from the gradual failing of ovarian function that precedes overt signs of menopause.

Pathophysiology of bone loss. To understand the process of the loss of bone mass, and the architectural alterations that are seen in cancellous bone, it is important to understand something of the process of bone remodeling. In adults, remodeling is a process of repair in which older bone tissue is removed (resorption) and replaced with new tissue[91-94] (Fig. 55-7). Remodeling occurs in small units, discrete from time and space.

The overall rate of remodeling (i.e., the number of these units at work in the skeleton at any point in time) is

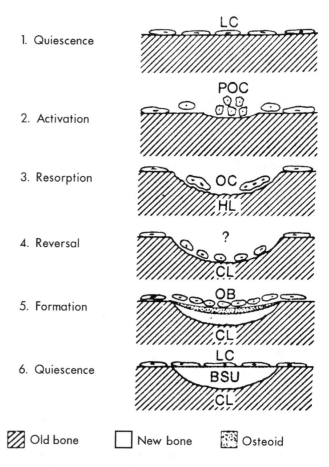

Fig. 55-7. Normal bone remodeling. LC, lining cell; POC, preosteoclast (mononuclear); OC, osteoclast (multinucleated); HL, Howship's lacuna; CL, cement line (reversal line); OB, osteoblast; BSU, bone structure unit. (From Parfitt AM: Bone remodeling: relationship to the amount of bone and structure of bone, and the pathogenesis and prevention of fractures. In Riggs BL, Melton LJI, editors: *Osteoporosis: etiology, diagnosis, and management,* New York, 1988, Raven Press.)

dependent upon a number of factors, the most important of which may be a variety of endocrine factors (e.g., thyroid, parathyroid, and sex steroids).[95,96,97] Control of the function of each remodeling unit, and the cells that constitute its work force, is provided locally with the probable input of a variety of paracrine and autocrine factors; of these, there are a myriad within marrow (e.g., TGFs interleukins, IGFs, tumor necrosis factors [TNFs] and prostaglandins).[98,99] Superimposed upon these factors is endocrine control. Strains produced within the skeleton by physical activity are also factors that can influence the behavior of remodeling units, but the mechanism of action remains obscure.[100] The result is an almost incomprehensible array of potential controlling factors, the interplay of which is not well understood. In vitro studies, the most common method used to evaluate the effects of a single factor or of two factors on the behavior of single-cell systems, or organ culture preparations, usually of fetal bone, cannot replicate the complex behavior surrounding remodeling processes in vivo. No reliable system for evaluation of a remodeling cycle exists in vitro, and only inferences can be drawn from these types of experiments. In vivo experiments with bone have been difficult to perform. Animal models are mostly inadequate unless primates are used, although recently it has been realized that significantly useful data may be generated using rodent models of bone loss.[101]

Two separate alterations in the functioning of remodeling have been proposed for the loss of ovarian function.[102-105] First there is an increase in the activation of new remodeling cycles.[91] Because resorption of old bone is the first function of the remodeling unit, it follows that increased activation temporarily causes removal of some bone tissue. This tissue (often called the *remodeling space*) would be replaced under normal situations as each cycle proceeds to new bone formation. The total amount of tissue in the remodeling space at any one time is dependent upon the frequency of activation of the woman's cycles. Thus, if activation were to slow again, a temporary increase in bone mass would be observed as the remodeling space contracts. Therefore, to produce permanent bone loss, other changes must occur in remodeling with sex-steroid deficiency.[106] One proposed mechanism relies on excessive recruitment or activity of the osteoclast population, the cells responsible for bone resorption.[91] In this hypothesis, the osteoclasts either become more aggressive with sex-steroid deficiency, or there is a larger number of osteoclasts recruited to a remodeling site. Consequently, in either instance, the resorption cavity created by each team of osteoclasts is larger. In order for actual loss of tissue to occur, the osteoblasts recruited to the resorbed area would not be able to detect the enhanced size of the cavity, but would simply deposit a predetermined amount of osteoid, which would subsequently be mineralized. The amount of new bone therefore would be less than the amount resorbed and thus, insufficient to completely repair the deficit, creating a negative

balance at each remodeling unit. That process would result in a permanent deficit in bone, at least until remodeling was initiated at the same site, where it might (at least potentially) be reversed. A second hypothesis (and the two are not mutually exclusive) entails the failure of the message that recruits osteoblasts to the resorption site.[107] In this hypothesis, resorption would occur normally and, at the end of the resorption process, activity within the cavity would cease; that is, there would be no new bone formation, leaving the resorption cavity unfilled.

Either of these mechanisms could result in rapid loss of bone, and both mechanisms may occur in cancellous bone. Perhaps more important is that both mechanisms would account for the increased penetration of trabeculae by osteoclasts that occurs after menopause, a process by which entire trabecular structures are gradually eliminated.[108] It is this loss of trabeculae that influences the pattern of fractures.[109] For example, the horizontal trabeculae in vertebral bodies are preferentially lost, creating a scaffolding without cross-struts, and consequently, a weakened structure liable to collapse.[110]

Loss of cortical bone tissue also occurs with declines in ovarian-steroid production.[92] Indeed, in the early studies in which bone mass was measured after oophorectomy, the measurements were made at sites of predominantly cortical bone, such as the midshaft of the radius or the metacarpal bones.[76] The mechanisms of loss of cortical bone have been inadequately studied, but it appears that tissue loss is produced by excessive remodeling at the inner corticotrabecular junction.[111] This process is probably no more than a variant of the mechanisms by which cancellous bone is removed. Excessively active or aggressive osteoclast teams tunnel into the cortex from the corticotrabecular junction and the defect is inadequately repaired by osteoblasts or, by virtue of recruitment failure, no osteoblasts appear within the resorption site to fill in the defect. The consequence, an apparent outward migration of the endocortex, is called *trabecularization of the cortex*. Because most long bones continue to expand with new bone formation on the outer surface of the cortex, the inner damage produces less impact upon the mechanical strength of the bone than might occur otherwise. However, cortical thinning is an important contributor to the mechanical instability of the skeleton among elderly women.[112]

Superimposed upon the loss of bone related to disruption of ovarian function are a wide variety of factors that can influence the skeleton of the aging individual.[19] These can be divided into age-related and sporadic factors. Age-related (and menopause-related) declines in intestinal calcium absorption,[113-115] coupled with a decline in calcium intake, form the major nutritional factor influencing the skeleton.[116] Calcium deficiency clearly causes osteoporosis in both animals and humans.[117-120] The problem for the clinician is that calcium deficiency is difficult to detect. Unlike iron, there is no serum ferritin for calcium. Thus, recommendations for calcium intake are somewhat arbitrary, but designed to ensure that the vast majority of individuals can achieve an adequate intake without side effects.

It is clear also that insufficient physical activity is detrimental to the skeleton,[121-127] as is exposure to zero gravity.[128,129] However, the best (and most achievable) program for good skeletal health is not known.[130] Again, the clinician is forced into generalities. Melding advice about cardiovascular health and skeletal health seems logical, and in counseling patients, we often simply use the guidelines of the American Heart Association. Whether this has much effect on the skeleton of normal healthy adults has not been rigorously tested.

Excessive alcohol intake is also harmful to the skeleton, increasing urinary calcium losses and inhibiting bone formation.[131-133] However, moderate alcohol intake may be less harmful, and may show a positive relation with bone mass.[134] Cigarette use also appears harmful to the skeleton.[135,136] The mechanism of the tobacco effect is not entirely clear, but there is an interaction with low body weight, and perhaps also a negative effect upon estrogen metabolism.[137] Other factors are probably minor; for example, protein intake, zinc, and boron.[19]

A wide variety of medications can affect the skeleton. The most severe is the pharmacological use of glucocorticoids. Reviews of the effects of steroids on bone recently have been published.[29,138,139] The use of excess thyroid hormone also is thought to be detrimental to skeletal health by increasing activation of remodeling.[140,141] If this is correct, then the postmenopausal population is most at risk. Methotrexate, heparin (long-term, high dosage), dilantin, and loop diuretics have all been incriminated as potentially harmful to the skeleton.[29]

EVALUATION OF THE ASYMPTOMATIC WOMAN

Increasing numbers of women are requesting an evaluation of their risk for osteoporosis. The situation is analogous to the evaluation of asymptomatic individuals for the risk of heart disease or stroke. Because osteoporosis is more easily prevented than treated, as are heart disease and stroke, this approach has considerable clinical usefulness. Although it is acceptable to provide general advice to patients of any age, particular concern must be given to perimenopausal patients, for these women are at the start of the accelerated phase of bone loss. This population therefore should be targeted for intervention. These patients, entering this period of their lives with reduced bone mass, are most likely to be at risk for osteoporosis in later life.[142] There is no simple method the physician can use for clinical detection of the status of the skeleton. Risk-factor analysis (e.g., family history, nutrition, and life-style) is insufficiently sensitive to be used as a determination of the skeletal status of individual patients.[143,144] This is not to say that risk assessment should not be performed. Several of the factors epidemiologically associated with osteoporo-

sis are likely to increase the rate or duration of bone loss. These include insufficient dietary calcium, excess alcohol and caffeine intake, and perhaps, cigarette consumption.[19] In addition, many of the secondary causes of osteoporosis are likely to exacerbate the bone loss that occurs as a consequence of the loss of ovarian function.[29] Thus, risk assessment is useful to alter the behavior of patients and to reevaluate the use of medications.

Determining skeletal mass, however, requires the use of one of the noninvasive techniques that allow accurate and precise quantification of the skeleton.[145-147] There is a close relationship between skeletal mass and strength; consequently, a measurement of mass allows an estimate of strength.[148] Bone-mass measurement has been demonstrated to be predictive of the risk of future fractures.[149-153] The power to predict fracture is at least as good as the prediction for cholesterol (or any lipoprotein) and heart disease. For each standard deviation decline in bone mass, there is an approximate doubling of the risk for fracture.[151] Thus, bone-mass measurement has become a clinical tool that can be used to determine those most at risk for osteoporosis, allowing the physician to treat only those most likely to suffer from fracture.

Several methods are available for bone-mass measurement. The most commonly used is dual-energy x-ray absorptiometry (DXA), which allows measurement of the lumbar spine and femoral neck, as well as the total body and forearm.[145] Because bone mass at all sites predicts the risk of all fractures, the site of measurement is not crucial to risk prediction. Thus, other techniques that cannot be used to measure the sites of important osteoporotic fractures can be used, including computed tomography (CT); which measures the spine; single-energy x-ray, which measures the wrist and hand; and radiographic absorptiometry. As would be expected, there is some specificity of site when prediction of individual fractures is the goal; thus, measurements of the hip predict hip fractures somewhat better than measurements at other sites.[156] Guidelines for the clinical use of bone-mass measurements have been published.[28]

In addition to the use of bone-mass measurement, it has been suggested that measurement of bone turnover, using the biochemical indices of bone remodeling, might be a useful method of determining the rate of loss of bone mass.[30] This seems intrinsically logical, but has yet to be evaluated in a rigorous fashion. The precise biochemistry that would give the most accurate prediction of skeletal change is not known; thus, the routine use of these investigations as an aid to predict fracture risk cannot be recommended.

PREVENTION

The initial approach to the prevention of osteoporosis is similar to that for heart disease; that is, the elimination of risk factors. For osteoporosis, this requires altering nutrition and life-style, and eliminating any therapeutic agent that might exacerbate bone loss, where possible. The factors that are most commonly considered include calcium nutrition and physical activity. However, it is also important to eliminate cigarette consumption and to reduce alcohol intake. More modest risk factors to consider include the intake of caffeine and protein, though the effects of modifying these is not known.

Calcium

Data generated over the past several years have established the average intake of calcium among adults in the United States to be approximately 500 mg/day, with almost one-third of adult women obtaining less than 400 mg/day.[155] As noted above, there are inherent difficulties in determining the adequacy of calcium intake for any individual patient. There is no test of sufficiency, and there is considerable variability in the physiology of handling calcium in the population.[156-158] Although there is doubt about the precise calcium intake required for an individual, an impressive body of data indicates that the vast majority of adults would be in the range of sufficiency if calcium intake were increased to 1000-1500 mg/day.[156,159] Because intakes of this magnitude are generally safe, it seems reasonable to recommend these levels for the population at large. Indeed, this was the recommendation of a consensus development conference held under the auspices of the National Institutes of Health in 1984.[160] This was reemphasized at a further concensus conference in 1994.

The debate has continued since then. However, both epidemiological and observational data indicate that modest increases in calcium intake can reduce the risk of fractures among the aging population.[161-164] Whether or not such intake should be lifelong is not finally established. Recent controlled studies in older individuals showed that calcium supplementation reduced the rate of bone loss in women well past menopause,[163] although the effect was most evident only in those whose calcium intake was less than 400 mg/day. Therefore, it seems prudent to suggest intakes of 1000 mg/day for all adults, with increases to 1500 mg/day for those with osteoporosis, pregnant and lactating women, and for teenagers through the growth period.

Such intakes are achievable by dietary modification. In the United States this usually means increasing dairy intakes, to which many are resistant due to a fear of calories or cholesterol, or because of lactase insufficiency or other intolerances for milk. Consequently, dietary supplementation has become usual to achieve intakes of 1000-1500 mg of calcium. For most individuals, a supplement of 500-1000 mg easily achieves this result. Calcium supplements in the United States are regulated as food supplements (distinct from drugs) and consequently, the rigor of quality assurance for tablet preparation is somewhat less than that usually required for pharmaceuticals. The result has been concern about the bioavailability of some preparations.[165] In general, calcium from any reputable manufacturer is well formulated. If patients have doubts about the calcium preparation they have purchased, simply testing the tablet dissolution in 8 ounces of vinegar (in which it would disintegrate within 45 minutes) provides a rough guide to bioavailability. The authors generally use chewable calcium tablets to ensure bioavailability, adding a 200-500 mg tablet to the end of each meal. Taken this way, the calcium salt provided (with these preparations it is carbonate) is less important. Where there is evidence of achlorhydria, calcium citrate may be used as an alternative preparation because this salt does not rely on gastric acid for availability.[166]

Side effects of calcium in these dosages are unusual. Among the elderly, constipation may be a problem, with consequent intestinal complaints. Calcium carbonate is also an antacid and its use will produce CO_2 in the presence of gastric acid. This occasionally results in complaints of eructation. In those who do not have an active history of renal stones, there is no evidence that calcium intakes of this amount increase the risk of stone formation. If renal stones are a problem, full investigation of the pathophysiology is required before calcium is used.

Exercise

Because disuse is an established cause of osteoporosis, it is logical to recommend increased physical activity to prevent skeletal atrophy. Within the confines of normal activity, it is far from clear if increasing activity has much effect on bone mass. It is difficult to conduct adequately controlled clinical trials in this arena, which, at least in part, contributes to the problem. However, the overall health benefits of exercise are sufficiently well documented and understood so that it seems only prudent to add an activity regimen to both prevention and treatment of osteoporosis.

There are no accepted standardized guidelines for exercise prescription for osteoporosis. In the authors' practice, the guidelines for exercise developed for cardiovascular health are used, and 30 minutes of aerobic activity, at least three times per week, is recommended. Patients starting a program for the first time (or after a significant inactive time) should have a physical examination, should be counseled about beginning carefully, and should be instructed to gradually increase the strenuousness of the activity. In general, it is better if the activities are fun (and social) to encourage ongoing compliance with what is often seen by the patient to be an imposition on life-style.

ESTROGEN INTERVENTION

Since Albright originally demonstrated that estrogens could be useful in the treatment of osteoporosis,[79] a large body of evidence has appeared in the scientific literature to support the concept.[80,167-186] As techniques for bone mass became available, cross-sectional data suggested that bone mass (or density) was greater among postmenopausal women treated with estrogens.[177,187] The first controlled clinical studies appeared in the early 1970s demonstrating—initially in short-term,[172] but later in long-term studies[167,168]—that estrogen intervention reduced the rate of bone loss in both oophorectomized and postmenopausal women.(Fig. 55-8). Controlled studies have also demonstrated that 0.625 mg conjugated equine estrogen (or its equivalent) is, for most individuals, an effective dose.[169] Data over the past several years have demonstrated that estradiol (either micronized or esterified), estrone, and synthetic estrogen are effective[188-190] (Fig. 55-9). Estriol might also be effective if it could be given several times daily in high doses.[191] The route of administration appears to be irrelevant to the effect on bone, and data have been obtained with estrogens given orally, transdermally, percutaneously, subcutaneously, and per vaginam.[173,185,192-195]

For estrogen efficacy in prevention of bone loss among postmenopausal women, the important issue appears to be the dosage administered. Oral estrogens are metabolized in both the intestinal wall and the liver before appearing in circulation. Consequently, the relationship between a particular estrogen in serum and the biological effect is somewhat difficult to establish. The delivery of estradiol across the skin facilitates the evaluation of the relationship. In the studies that have been conducted, it appears that the attainment of physiological circulating concentrations of estradiol are associated with reduction in bone turnover and prevention of the loss of mass.[192,193] Effects on bone have been observed with circulating estradiol levels of 50-100 pg/ml within the early to mid follicular phase levels seen in premenopausal women.[193]

Mechanism of action

The mechanism by which estrogens produce their effect on the skeleton is as inadequately understood as the alteration in skeletal homeostasis through menopause.[173] It has been established that cells derived from osteoblasts have functional estrogen receptors;[196,197] however, the net effect of estrogen administration is exactly the converse of the changes in skeletal metabolism that occur through menopause.[82] The activation of new remodeling cycles is reduced, and there is apparent correction in the defect in osteoclast function.[97] Biochemically, these changes in cell function in the skeleton cause a return of the indicators of bone remodeling to approximately their premenopausal levels[82] (see Fig. 55-6). The understanding of the mechanism by which these changes occur is as indistinct as the understanding of bone remodeling. It is tempting to speculate that the presence of specific receptors within osteoblasts indicates a central role for that cell type in estrogen action, but the issue is open to debate. In several cell systems derived from osteoblasts, estrogens have been shown to stimulate growth, inhibit growth, alter the secretion of a variety of cytokines, or mediate no changes in cell physiology.[198-200] In one series of experiments, it was proposed that estrogen effects on osteoclast function in vitro could be observed only when significant numbers of

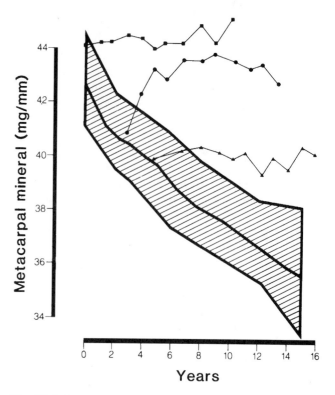

Fig. 55-8. Long-term prevention of bone loss by estrogen. The hatched areas represent the placebo using (mean ± SD) a prospective controlled study in oophorectomized women. The three lines show the mean values only for three estrogen-treated groups; treatment initiated at the time of oophorectomy (squares), 3 years after (circles), or 6 years after (triangles). Bone loss is prevented in all three situations. However, the earlier treatment is begun, the better the outcome, in terms of bone mass, after 10 years of therapy.

osteoblasts were cocultured in the system.[201] These are not universal findings, and the recent suggestion that osteoclasts themselves may have estrogen receptors allows a postulate for a direct action.[202] However, in vitro, estrogens in concentrations close to physiological do not reduce bone resorption by osteoclasts.[203]

Although it seems most likely that at least some of the effects of estrogen on bone are mediated by bone cells, there are alternative explanations. Other cells within bone marrow could be the specific targets for sex-steroid effects,[204] or perhaps the vitamin D PTH system could be regulated by sex-steroid status.[205-208] It has been suggested that the secretion of interleukin-1 (IL-1) by mononuclear cells in circulation is under the control of estrogens.[209] The synthesis of IL-1 is increased among postmenopausal women, and this increment is reversed by estrogen.[210] In a rat model of osteoporosis, an IL-1 receptor antagonist was shown to reduce bone loss after ovariectomy.[35] If similar alterations in IL-1 secretion occur in marrow, and because IL-1 can be a potent stimulator of bone resorption, IL-1 could be an important modulator of osteoclast activity among postmenopausal women.[211] It has also recently been

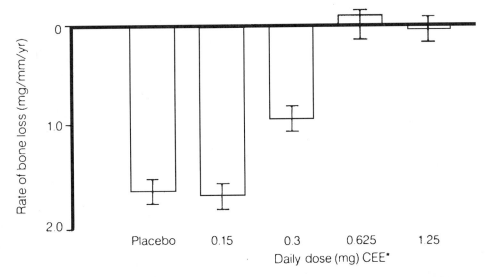

Fig. 55-9. The effects of various doses of conjugated equine estrogen on bone loss. Allocation to treatment program was done randomly using placebo and 0.15, 0.30, 0.625, and 1.25 mg doses of conjugated estrogens. Rate of loss was calculated for each individual patient over a 2-year period. (From Lindsay R, Hart DM, Clark DM: The minimum effective dose of estrogen for prevention of postmenopausal bone loss, *Obstet Gynecol* 61:759, 1984.)

demonstrated with a mouse model that IL-6 secretion is increased after oophorectomy[212] and that blocking antibodies prevent the bone loss that occurs after oophorectomy.[213] In a rodent model system, it has been suggested that prostaglandin production locally could be influenced by oophorectomy and mediate osteoclast activity.[214] Estrogens also can affect other cytokines that play potentially important roles in bone remodeling.[215] Estrogens in vitro can modify the action of TGF-β, and potentially its secretion into bone.[211] TGF-β appears to play a role in bone formation, including osteoblast recruitment, and perhaps in the inhibition of bone resorption. It is one candidate for the so-called coupling factor, linking resorption and formation in the remodeling cycle.[211] Finally, estrogens stimulate the production of IGFs, especially IGF-1, which has also been implicated in bone formation.[216-220] Thus, estrogens within marrow, on skeletal cells, and on peripheral cells exert myriad effects that could potentially interact to modulate the bone remodeling process. Integrating these in vitro and in vivo effects of estrogen has not been easy. It is perhaps best to view the in vitro effects, especially those on single-cell systems, as least representative of the mediators in vivo (although there are undoubtedly clear effects in vitro, these are often confusing and conflicting). Unfortunately, the in vivo data are far from providing a comprehensive view of estrogen effects, in part because of the sketchy understanding of bone remodeling.

Estrogens also modulate calcium homeostasis,[205-208] although the effects are somewhat more subtle than the effects upon bone.[208] Estrogen administration to postmenopausal women results in a small fall in serum calcium and phosphate and a significant reduction in urinary calcium, but an increase in urinary phosphate (or more correctly, a decrease in the tubular maximum for phosphate resorption [TmPO₄/ GFR]).[167,172] These biochemical changes are compatible with an increase in parathyroid hormone activity, although this has been difficult to document.[208] In addition, increments in 1,25(OH)$_2$D have been reported.[221,222] The majority of studies performed have been with oral estrogens, so this increase, in part, is related to enhanced hepatic production of vitamin D-binding protein; increased serum levels for 1,25(OH)$_2$D simply reflect an increase in serum concentrations of vitamin D-binding protein. However, it has been shown that concentrations of the free steroid are elevated with estrogen use.[221] The consequence appears to be enhanced intestinal calcium absorption.[158,222,223] In view of the difficulty in evaluating alterations in the calcium homeostatic systems, the authors recently undertook a series of investigations, electing to stress the system using dynamic tests of a nature similar to those used in other areas of endocrinology.[206,207] It was demonstrated that there is increased renal response of the 1α-hydroxylase, suggesting that estrogens do stimulate 1,25(OH)$_2$D production. The authors also showed that there is skeletal resistance to the effects of PTH in the presence of estrogen, and that there may well be increased PTH activity at other end-organs (notably the kidney). Thus, the effects of estrogen on the skeleton and calcium metabolism are complex, and require further unraveling. Finally, estrogen administration may result in an increase in circulating levels of calcitonin.[205,224-226] It has been suggested that at least some of the effects of estrogen on bone turnover are mediated by calcitonin. The data are conflicting on this issue and all are not in agreement with this as an action of estrogens.[227]

Fracture prevention. The effects of estrogen on bone mass have been clearly demonstrated in prospective, double-blind, controlled studies. However, fractures occur many years after the process of bone loss begins at menopause. Thus, data evaluating fracture prevention with estrogens have been obtained most often using an epidemiological approach.

There are now several epidemiological studies that have examined the relationship between estrogen and hip fractures.[228-236] In general, all of the published data support the concept that estrogen use is associated with a reduction in the risk of hip fracture (Table 55-1). The consensus from the published data suggests a reduction of approximately 50% in the risk of hip fracture with the long-term use of estrogen. The current data do not allow definition of the precise period of estrogen use that results in such a risk reduction. However, most agree that at least 5-10 years of therapy is probably necessary, although the duration may need to be longest with those whose therapy is initiated at the earliest age.[237] In situations where the issue was examined, it originally appeared that the beneficial effects are greatest for those whose treatment began closest to menopause,[233] a finding that is consistent with the bone-density data.

Nonetheless, bone loss begins again when estrogen therapy is discontinued.[238-240] The rate of bone loss is approximately parallel to that which occurs after oophorectomy; indeed, cessation of estrogen therapy can be regarded as a form of medical oophorectomy. The more years that pass from the last use of estrogen, the closer the bone mass or density of an estrogen-treated woman will be to the population who have never used estrogen postmenopausally.[237] It would not be surprising, therefore, if the estrogen effects on fracture waned from the last exposure. That may be the case, but there does seem to be some reduction of the risk for fracture conferred by exposure to estrogen for 1 or more years at any time after menopause.[233] This raises several questions, but perhaps the two most frequently asked in relation to this are:

1. What is the optimum duration of estrogen therapy for maximum fracture protection?
2. What is the age range at which estrogens should be initiated for protection against hip fracture?

Neither question can be answered definitively with the current state of knowledge. From the most recent data on the evaluation of bone mass in women previously on estrogen,[237] the continued, almost lifetime use of estrogen appears to be required to maintain skeletal status. However, as noted above, some fracture prevention appears to continue after estrogens are stopped. This dichotomy could result because of biases in the epidemiological data, i.e., only healthy women get estrogen[241], estrogen affecting fracture risk through non–bone-mass mechanisms, or early demise of individuals with low bone mass.[242] Because these questions cannot be answered at present, the duration of therapy for maximum efficacy is unknown.

The second question is equally difficult to answer. Most of the bone-mass studies have evaluated effects of estrogen when initiated shortly after menopause.[173] Risk reduction may occur even when estrogens are initiated at a late age.[193] Thus, while estrogen initiation at menopause may be required for symptoms[243] or for cardiovascular effects,[244,245] a later start could give a greater benefit-to-cost ratio for osteoporosis prevention.

Fewer data are available regarding the effects of estrogen on vertebral fracture risk. However, one prospective study, based upon alterations in vertebral configuration on lateral radiographs, suggests that long-term estrogen use results in an approximately 80% reduction in vertebral fractures[168] (Table 55-2). The only study of an epidemiological nature published thus far supports that conclusion.[178] The data for fractures of the distal radius are similar to those for hip fractures, with the epidemiological studies suggesting a risk reduction of approximately 50%. No data have been published examining the effects of estrogen intervention on other fractures in the elderly.

Table 55-1. Studies indicating a reduction in fractures with estrogen use

Author	Journal	Year	Fracture	Relative risk
Hutchinson	*Lancet*	1979	H, C	0.17[a]
Johnson	*Am J Public Health*	1981	H	0.67[a]
Kreiger	*Am J Epidemiol*	1982	H	0.5[a]
Paganini-Hill	*Ann Intern Med*	1981	H	0.42[a]
Weiss	*N Engl J Med*	1980	H, C	0.46[a]
Williams	*Obstet Gynecol*	1982	H, C	variable
Kiel	*N Engl J Med*	1987	H	0.65[a]
Ettinger	*Ann Intern Med*	1985	All	—
Lindsay	*Lancet*	1980	V	—
Naessen	*Ann Intern Med*	1990	H	0.79[a]

[a]p < 0.05.
H, Hip; C, Colles; and V, vertebral

Table 55-2. Radiographic changes following estrogen or placebo treatment for 10 years

Treatment	Spine score*	Percentage positive scores	Crush fractures
Estrogen	0.35	27.6	1
Placebo	1.65	66	5
	p < 0.01	p < 0.01	

*Spine score was obtained by reviewing all vertebrae from T1 to L5 and scoring 1 for wedge and 2 for "crush" fractures. (From Lindsay R, Hart DM, Lindsay R, Hart DM, Forrest C, et al: Prevention of spinal osteoporosis in oophorectomized women, *Lancet* 2:1151, 1980.)

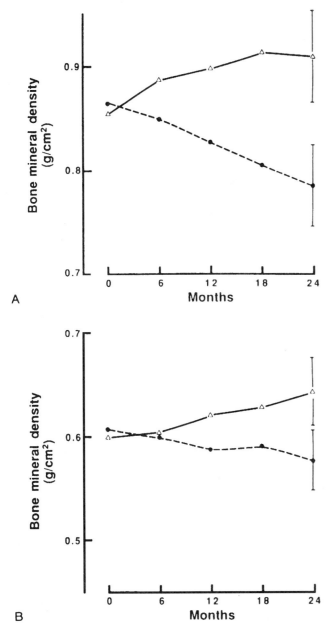

Fig. 55-10. Mean changes in bone mineral density of the lumbar spine (A) and the femoral neck (B) during 2 years of therapy with estrogen and calcium (triangles) or calcium (circles). At the end of 2 years, the mean bone mineral density of the lumbar spine was significantly greater in the calcium- and estrogen-treated group than at the initiation of the study (P <0.01), and than the final mean for the calcium-treated group (P <0.01). (From Lindsay R, Tohme J: Estrogen treatment of patients with established postmenopausal osteoporosis, *Obstet Gynecol* 76:1, 1990.)

Estrogens and established osteoporosis. In the United States, only estrogens and salmon calcitonin are approved by the FDA for use in osteoporosis. However, many clinicians believe that estrogens are of value only in prevention. This is not the case.[173] Estrogen intervention in patients with osteoporosis and in the older population (at least up to the age of 75 years) reduces bone turnover, stabilizes bone mass, and thereby prevents worsening of the disease.[180,181,193,246,247] Several studies have shown a small, but significant, increment in bone mass[119] (Fig. 55-10). This increase, which is generally greatest in the spine, occurs gradually over the first 12-18 months of therapy. It is presumed that this transient increase is caused by initial suppression of the activation of new remodeling sites, and a consequent reduction in resorption. Those remodeling units still active at the start of therapy continue their progress. Thus, bone formation is affected little during the early phase of therapy, while resorption is reduced, resulting in a positive bone balance.[97] This phenomenon is the reverse of that seen during phases of rapid bone loss, such as in the early years after menopause.

The majority of data showing that estrogens reduce fracture risk were obtained when estrogens were used for prevention, but recent controlled data show that a reduction in recurrent fractures can be seen with estrogen therapy in patients with osteoporotic crush fractures.[193] Intervention with estrogen therapy is therefore beneficial even in fairly late stages of the disease.

Other effects of estrogens. Estrogens are clearly potent steroids with effects on multiple organ systems. Estrogen therapy clearly reduces menopausal symptoms and the genitourinary atrophy that follows menopause. In addition, estrogens may reduce the risk of coronary artery disease, and perhaps stroke, among the aging female population. On the other side remains the increased risk of endometrial malignancy, largely offset by provision of a progestin, and the potential for an increase in the risk of breast cancer, which continues to be debated. The reader is referred to the appropriate chapters of this volume for in-depth discussions of these issues.

Estrogen prescription in osteoporosis. As noted above, the skeleton is extremely sensitive to estrogens;[169] thus, a skeletal response is usually obtained at standard dosages of estrogen even when estrogens are used for other indications, such as for the suppression of menopausal symptoms. The dosages of estrogen recommended specifically for osteoporosis are shown in Table 55-3. Estrogen can be given by any route of administration, and generally, the authors provide estrogens on a continuous basis. For patients with a uterus, progestin is added for 12-14 days per month; in older individuals, a continuous progestin is tried. The dominant effect of estrogen on the skeleton is not negatively affected by the addition of the progestin.[248] Indeed, there are data indicating that certain progestins are skeletally active and can prevent bone loss.[170,249-251] One publication suggests that norethindrone acetate can enhance the effect of estrogen on bone by uncoupling formation and resorption.[247,252] This requires confirmation.

In addition, all patients are given the recommendation to

Table 55-3. Estrogens: effective daily doses

Estrogens	Doses
Conjugated equine estrogens	0.625
Micronized estradiol	0.5 - 1 mg
Piperazine estrone sulphate	1.25 mg
Estradiol valerate	1 - 2 mg
Transdermal estradiol	50 - 100 mcg
Ethinylestradiol*	20 mcg

The doses of estrogen noted above are some average values for patients seen by the author. Readers are referred to their own regulatory agencies or manufacturers for doses recommended in their country.

*For reference only

increase their calcium intake to 1000-1500 mg/day and to reduce the impact of other risk factors. This includes reducing alcohol and caffeine intake, eliminating cigarette use, and increasing physical activity. For patients with established osteoporosis, the implementation of a program of physical therapy is a useful method of reducing pain, increasing mobility, and providing specific instruction on activities that strengthen the back and limit the chance of injury.

ALTERNATIVES TO ESTROGEN

As mentioned previously, the only FDA-approved therapeutic agents for the treatment of osteoporosis are estrogens and salmon calcitonin. Other therapeutic agents are being developed, and clearly are needed as alternatives. Presently in the United States, salmon calcitonin must be given by subcutaneous injection, and thus remains a poor alternative for patients who cannot or should not take estrogen therapy. Potential therapeutic agents are listed in the box in column 2, and a brief discussion of those for which there is at least some clinical data follows.

Calcitonin

The major biological action of the 32 amino acid peptide, calcitonin, is inhibition of osteoclastic bone resorption. Thus, calcitonin has been used in situations of excessive bone resorption, such as Paget disease and hypercalcemia of malignancy.[253] The use of calcitonin in osteoporosis was first described by Chesnut et al.[254] The net effect of pharmacological calcitonin administration is the reduction in bone remodeling, similar to that seen with estrogens[255-265] (Fig. 55-11). It has been assumed that the effect is due to inhibition of resorption by a direct effect on osteoclasts.[254] In in vitro experiments, osteoclasts from both rodent and human species do not create resorption cavities in inert bone in the presence of calcitonin.[266] In experiments in which patients were treated with calcitonin in therapeutic dosages, and subdivided into those with high remodeling states and those whose remodeling status was normal (often described as low turnover), the effects of

Pharmacological agents for osteoporosis

"Anti-resorptive" agents
  Sex steroids
    Estrogens
    Progestins
    "Anti-estrogens" (estrogen analogues)
    Testosterone (and anabolic agents)
  Bisphosphonates
  Calcitonins
  Calcium
Formation stimulators
  Fluoride
  Parathyroid hormone (and analogues)
Action not known
  Vitamin D and analogues
  Thiazides
Potential agents*
  Growth hormone
  Growth factors (IGFs)
  Interleukin inhibitors
  Integrins
  Proton pump inhibitors
  Bone morphometric proteins

*Agents not known to be in clinical development

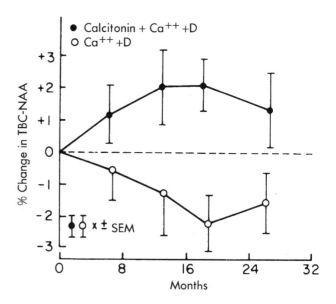

Fig. 55-11. Effect of synthetic salmon calcitonin (100 U/day), calcium, and vitamin D on total body calcium measured by neutron activation analysis (TBC-NAA) in 24 osteoporotic women (●). Twenty-one control osteoporotic women (○) received only 400 U of vitamin D and 1200 mg of calcium as calcium carbonate during the study. Iliac crest bone biopsies revealed a significantly greater percentage of total bone in calcitonin-treated patients, compared with control patients after 2 years of treatment. (From Gruber HE, Ivey JL, Baylink DJ, et al: Long-term calcitonin therapy in postmenopausal osteoporosis, *Metabolism* 33:295, 1984.)

calcitonin on bone mass in the spine was most marked in the patients with high turnover.[267] No differences were seen in the femoral diaphysis, where calcitonin appeared to have little effect. When calcitonin is compared with estrogen, the net effects on bone mass are somewhat similar, although estrogen may have the edge because the effects on femoral neck bone density were slightly better with estrogen.[268]

There is currently no consensus about the dosage, regimen, or duration of calcitonin required for prevention or treatment of osteoporosis. Dosages of 50-100 U/day, delivered subcutaneously, appear to be effective. Some data suggest that intermittent therapy (e.g., 3 months on; 3 months off) is more effective than continuous, daily, or alternate-day administration.[253] The fact that calcitonin is delivered by injection virtually limits its use to the treatment of patients with fractures.

Limitations on the use of calcitonin, especially in cultures where injectable agents are not widely used (e.g., the United States), have resulted in the development of intranasal sprays. The effect of calcitonin delivered in this fashion has been studied in postmenopausal and oophorectomized women, but the results have been mixed. Studies of one group[263] suggest that dosages as low as 50 U of calcitonin by the nasal route prevent bone loss in the immediate postmenopausal period. Others have found that the required dosage is much higher, as much as 400 U/day.[264] Dosages of 200 U/day may be effective as treatment for established osteoporosis. This preparation is not currently available in the United States.

Perhaps the most attractive claim for calcitonin has been that it can relieve the pain associated with vertebral crush fractures, obviating or reducing the requirement for narcotic analgesics.[269-272] Controlled data have confirmed calcitonin's analgesic effect.[272] The authors' clinical experience suggests that such an effect does exist, but only in some patients. The reason for the variability in response is not clear. In patients with acute vertebral fractures and significant pain, calcitonin is a useful adjunct to management of acute pain (Fig. 55-12). Evidence that there is no reduction in pain associated with calcitonin within 10 days prompts consideration of discontinuing therapy, unless the patient is willing to use the injectable agent for a longer period for maintenance of skeletal mass.

Bisphosphonates

The development of bisphosphonates for the prevention and treatment of osteoporosis might have been predicted many years ago, but has been slow in coming. These agents, analogues of pyrophosphate, inhibit bone resorption and increase calcium content of bones in growing rodents.[273] Their actions in animals and in a variety of human situations have been well reviewed recently.[274] Nearly all bisphosphonates that have been evaluated have been shown to effectively prevent bone loss. The first-generation bisphosphonate, etidronate, has been studied in two controlled clinical trials in osteoporotic patients. Etidronate causes a small increment in bone mass, compatible with reduction in activation frequency, with some suggestion of a reduction in fracture recurrence (Fig. 55-13).[275,276] However, the effect on fractures is not convincing for several reasons, and etidronate, at close to therapeutic dosages, is associated with inhibition of mineralization, limiting its use in osteoporosis.[274] Successors to etidronate include alendronate, tiludronate, and risedronate. The former two compounds

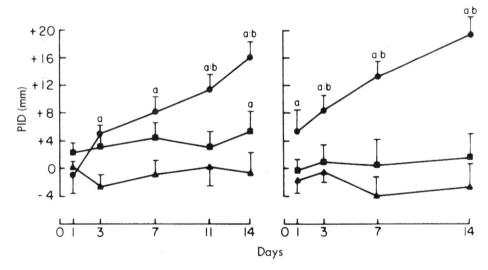

Fig. 55-12. Time-course of pain intensity difference (PID) (mean ± SEM) as scored by patients with malignancy and bone pain (left panel) and physician (right panel) during treatment with placebo (▲, n=10); human calcitonin (■, n=11). "a" = Statistically significant versus placebo; "b" statistically significant versus human calcitonin. Note that salmon calcitonin (●) was more effective in reducing bone pain than either human calcitonin or placebo. (From Gennari C, Chierichetti SM, Bigazzi S, et al: *Calcif Tissue Int* 38:3, 1986.)

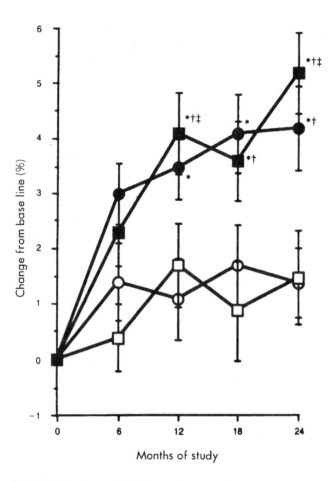

Fig. 55-13. Mean (±SE) changes in bone mineral density of the spine (as measured by dual-photon absorptiometry) in group 1 (placebo and placebo; open circles) group 2 (phosphate and placebo; open squares), group 3 (placebo and etidronate; solid circles), and group 4 (phosphate and etidronate; solid squares). The asterisk indicates a significant change from base line (P <0.017); the dagger, a significant change compared with group 1 (P <0.01); and the double dagger, a significant difference as compared with group 2 (P <0.01). (From Watts NB, Harris ST, Genant HK, et al: *N Engl J Med* 323:73, 1990.)

have effects on bone mass in controlled studies, but as yet there are no fracture data.[277-279] The latter has yet to be rigorously evaluated in humans.[274]

No bisphosphonate is currently approved for use in osteoporosis in the United States, but some are approved in other countries. When used in osteoporosis, etidronate is given for two weeks every three months at a daily dose of 400 mg. There is no good reason this regimen is required, and lower doses, given continuously, would probably be as effective. Most other bisphosphonates are being evaluated clinically on a continuous regimen. Bisphosphonates must be given on an empty stomach to facilitate absorption, and can be associated with gastrointestinal irritation, but appear to have few other side effects. The long residence of these compounds in bone[274] emphasizes the importance of ensuring that long-term safety data are obtained.

Anabolic agents

As noted, osteoporosis results in women primarily because of the loss of the ovarian secretion of estrogen. However, other changes could contribute to bone loss with age in women. Reductions in the weak steroids, androstenedione and dehydroepiandrosterone, occur with age, and there has been some suggestion that bone loss in later life may be related to the remaining circulating concentrations of androgens.[280,281] Consequently, anabolic or androgenic agents have been tested for their effects in osteoporosis. The results are generally similar to those observed with estrogen. Anabolic agents reduce bone turnover and prevent loss of bone.[282-288] The effects may be blurred by the increase in lean mass that occurs; consequently, these agents may be somewhat less effective than estrogens.[289] Because these agents generally are poorly tolerated among postmenopausal women and have detrimental effects on lipids, their use in osteoporosis will remain limited. There may be some advantage to their effects on skeletal muscle in the treatment of the frail elderly, but no rigorous controlled trial has been completed.

Calcitriol

The malabsorption of calcium seen in osteoporotic patients,[290] and improvement with administration of calcitriol, has suggested a role for this active metabolite of vitamin D in therapy of osteoporosis.[245] Several controlled studies have been performed using calcitriol.[291-297] Although some of the data are conflicting, calcitriol seems to reduce bone loss, and two studies have found evidence for prevention of fracture recurrence.[297,298] Part of the variability in the data could be explained by geographical differences in the importance of one or more pathogenetic factors, principally calcium deficiency and true vitamin D deficiency. Calcitriol

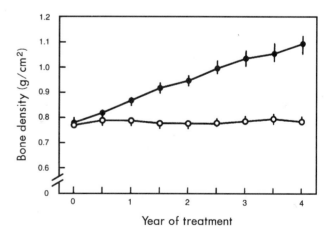

Fig. 55-14. Mean (±SE) bone density of the lumbar spine in the fluoride group (solid circles) and the placebo group (open circles). (From Riggs BL, Hodgson SF, O'Fallon WM, et al: *N Engl J Med* 302:802, 1990.)

Table 55-5. Nonvertebral fractures during a study in women with osteoporosis in fluoride and placebo groups*

Site	Incomplete fractures		Complete fractures		Total fractures	
	Fluoride	Placebo	Fluoride	Placebo	Fluoride	Placebo
Radius (Colles fracture)	0(0)	0(0)	1(1)	4(4)	1(1)	4(4)
Humerus	0(0)	0(0)	5(6)	1(1)	5(6)	1(1)
Rib	1(1)	0(0)	10(13)	8(8)	11(14)	8(8)
Pelvis	3(4)	0(0)	3(3)	1(1)	6(7)	1(1)
Proximal femur	4(5)	1(1)	7(8)	3(3)	11(13)	4(4)
Tibia	10(11)	0(0)	2(2)	0(0)	12(13)	0(0)
Metatarsus or calcaneus	7(10)	1(1)	2(2)	2(2)	9(12)	3(3)
Other†	1(1)	0(0)	5(5)	3(3)	6(6)	3(3)
All sites	7(10)	1(1)	2(2)	2(2)	9(12)	3(3)
Relative risk (95% confidence interval)‡	16.8 (3.9-71.7)		1.9 (1.1 -3.4)		3.2 (1.8-5.6)	

*No. of patients (no. of fractures).

†Other fractures involved the clavicle (two), the shaft or distal femur (two), and the small bones of the wrist or foot (two) in the fluoride group, and the ulna, fibula, and hand in the placebo group.

‡The fluoride group had 310 person-years of follow-up and the placebo group had 325 person-years of follow-up. Patients were evaluated every six months for nonvertebral fractures.

(From Riggs BL, Hodgson SF, O'Fallon WM, et al: N Engl J Med 302:802, 1990.)

appears more effective in Japan and New Zealand than in the United States. Calcitriol is not approved for use in osteoporosis in the United States, and remains an investigative agent. The therapeutic window is narrow, and calcitriol must be used with caution to avoid hypercalciuria and hypercalcemia.

Fluoride

Fluoride has been recommended for use in the treatment of osteoporosis for many years.[299] It became clear from patients with fluorosis and from experiences when patients were treated with high doses of sodium fluoride that there was an increase in the mineral content of the spine and other areas in the axial skeleton.[300-304] However, clinical trials were recently initiated to determine if this effect results in a reduction in fracture recurrence[305,306] (Fig. 55-14). These two studies in the United States suggested a reduction of vertebral fracture, but this was not significant. One study suggested an increased risk of peripheral fractures in the fluoride-treated group,[305] and others have raised the question that fluoride increases the risk of fractures of the hip[307,308] (Table 55-5). Other preparations of fluoride currently are being evaluated.[309]

Estrogen agonists

Several years ago, the authors observed that postmenopausal patients with breast cancer who were being treated with tamoxifen were not losing bone mass.[310] This has been confirmed in a controlled clinical trial and in subsequent experiments in oophorectomized animals.[311-313] Tamoxifen appears to function much like a weak estrogen in postmenopausal women, and indeed, can cause endometrial stimulation.[314] Consequently, there has been interest in alternative compounds that function like tamoxifen on bone, without endometrial stimulation. One compound,

raloxifene, is now in clinical trial. In short-term studies, this compound appeared to be capable of reducing bone remodeling in a fashion similar to estrogens, but did not cause similar endometrial growth.[315] Similar results have been obtained in rodents.[316-318] Preliminary data also suggest that the changes that occur in lipoproteins may be similar to those produced by estrogen, thus raising the possibility that raloxifene could produce similar effects on cardiovascular disease. Finally, raloxifene was developed as an analogue to tamoxifen and might also reduce the risk of breast cancer.[319] Many further studies are required before this compound can be recommended, but it provides an approach toward what might be called the "perfect estrogen." Only time will tell if it will succeed.

One other compound that is marketed in several parts of the world is OD14 or Livial. This is a hybrid compound related to norethindrone. It appears to have potent bone-sparing effects in postmenopausal women,[320,321] without much endometrial stimulation. This compound provides an alternative to estrogen, although its effects on other target tissues, such as the heart and breast, are not known.

Parathyroid hormone

It has been known for many years that PTH not only stimulates bone remodeling, but also can be anabolic to the skeleton.[322] The anabolic effects of PTH have been reviewed in detail recently.[323] PTH clearly causes an increase in bone mass in human and animal experiments,[324-326] and might be a promising therapy, especially because the increments in bone mass seen in animal experiments resulted in increased bone strength.[326] PTH presently requires administration on a daily basis by injection, clearly limiting its use. In addition, the effects on bone mass appear to be limited to the axial skeleton, and there is apparently little, if any, effect on the femoral neck.

CONCLUSIONS

Osteoporosis is a serious public-health problem for the postmenopausal population. It is defined as a reduction in bone mass or density, accompanied by microarchitectural deterioration of bone tissue that results in an increase in the risk of fractures. Fractures that occur include those of the spine, hip, and wrist, but other fractures are also part of the disease. Estrogen deficiency after menopause is the major reason that these fractures are more common among women than men. Estrogen deficiency (irrespective of cause) increases bone turnover and remodeling, and results in the loss of bone mass. Intervention with estrogen reduces turnover to premenopausal levels and prevents loss of bone. Long-term estrogen intervention results in a reduced risk for fractures—as much as 50% for hip fractures and perhaps a considerably greater reduction in vertebral crush fractures. Although estrogens have been classically used in the immediate postmenopausal period, intervention much later in life may be equally beneficial in the prevention of osteoporosis. Estrogen intervention is also effective in the treatment of the established disease, even after fractures have occurred. The route of administration for estrogens is unimportant, but dosage is critical.

Other therapeutic agents are available, or are being evaluated, for osteoporosis in this postmenopausal population. These include bisphosphonates, calcitonin, vitamin D and its analogues, fluoride anabolic agents, and parathyroid hormone. Most recently, it was demonstrated that weak estrogen agonists, similar to tamoxifen, might also be of benefit in osteoporosis. This has resulted in the development of compounds that are analogues of tamoxifen. This class of compound provides a potentially exciting mode of therapy for the future.

1. Consensus Development Conference: Osteoporosis, *Am J Med* 90:107, 1991.
2. Melton III LJ: Epidemiology of fractures. In Riggs BL, Melton LJI, editors: *Osteoporosis: etiology, diagnosis, and management,* New York, 1988, Raven Press.
3. Cummings SR, Kelsey JL, Nevitt MC, et al: Epidemiology of osteoporosis and osteoporotic fractures, *Epidemiol Rev* 7:178, 1985.
4. Seeling DG, Browner WS, Nevitt MC, et al: Which fractures are associated with low appendicular bone mass in elderly women, *Ann Intern Med* 115:837, 1991.
5. Kelsey JL, White, AA, Tastives H, et al: The impact of musculoskeletal disorders in the population of the Unites States, *JBJS* 61A:959, 1979.
6. Cummings SR, Rubin SM, Black D: The future of hip fractures in the United States, *Clin Orthop Rel Res* 252:163, 1990.
7. Cooper C, Campion G, Melton III LJ: Hip fractures in the elderly: a world-wide projection, *Osteo Int* 2:285-289, 1992.
8. Pogrund H, Makin M, Robin G, et al: Osteoporosis in patients with fractured femoral neck in Jerusalem, *Clin Orthop* 124:165, 1977.
9. Cummings SR, Black DM, Rubin SM: Lifetime risks of hip, Colles', or vertebral fracture and coronary heart disease among white postmenopausal women, *Arch Intern Med* 149:2445, 1989.
10. Cummings SR: Osteoporotic fractures: the magnitude of the problem. In Christiansen C, Johansen JS, Riis BJ, editors: *Osteoporosis 1987,* ed 2, Copenhagen, 1987, Osteopress.
11. Melton III LJ, Riggs BL: Epidemiology of age-related fractures. In Avioli LV, editor: *The osteoporotic syndrome,* New York, 1983, Grune & Stratton.
12. Fitzgerald JF, Moore PS, Dittus RS: The care of elderly patients with hip fracture: changes since implementation of the prospective payment system, *N Engl J Med* 319:1392, 1988.
13. Jacobsen SJ, Goldberg J, Miles TP, et al: Regional variation in the incidence of hip fracture: US white women aged 65 and older, *J Am Med Assoc* 264:500, 1990.
14. Farmer ME, White LR, Brody JA: Race and sex differences in hip fracture incidence, *Am J Public Health* 74:1374, 1984.
15. Elffors L, Allander E, Kanis JA, et al: The variable incidence of hip fracture in southern Europe: the MEDOS study, *Osteopor Int* 4:in press, 1994.
16. Solomon L: Osteoporosis and fracture of the femoral neck in the S.A. Bantu, *J Bone Joint Surg* 50B:2, 1968.
17. Stott S, Gray DH: The incidence of femoral neck fractures in New Zealand, *NZ Med J* 91:6, 1980.
18. Wong PCN: Femoral neck fractures among the major racial groups in Singapore. Incidence patterns compared with non-Asian communities, *Singapore Med J* 5:150, 1964.
19. Lindsay R, Cosman F: Primary osteoporosis. In Coe F, Favus M, editors: *Disorders of bone and mineral metabolism,* New York, 1992, Raven Press.
20. Campbell AJ, Reinken J, Allan BC, et al: Falls in old age: a study of frequency and related clinical factors, *Age Ageing* 10:264, 1981.
21. Frankel VH, Pugh JW: Biomechanics of the hip. In Frankel VH, editor: *Basic biomechanics of the skeletal system,* Philadelphia, 1980, Lea & Febiger.
22. Cummings SR, Nevitt MC: Epidemiology of hip fractures and falls. In Kleerekoper M, Krane S, editors: *Clinical disorders of bone and mineral metabolism,* New York, 1989, Mary Ann Liebert.
23. Ray WA, Griffin MR, Schaffner W, et al: Psychotropic drug use and the risk of hip fracture, *N Engl J Med* 316:363, 1987.
24. Mastens M, VanAudekarcke R, Delport P, et al: The mechanical characteristics of cancellous bone at the upper femoral region, *J Biomech* 16:971, 1983.
25. Nakamura T, Yoshikawa T, Mizuno Y, et al: Do geometric properties of the femoral neck explain Japanese-American differences in hip fracture incidence? *J Bone Miner Res (suppl)* 8:133, 1993.
26. Melton III LJ, Kan SH, Frye MA, et al: Epidemiology of vertebral fractures in women, *Am J Epidemiol* 129:1000, 1989.
27. Wasnich RD, Davis JW, Ross PD: Spine fracture risk is predicted by non-spine fractures, *Osteopor Int* 4:1, 1994.
28. Johnston CC, Melton III LJ, Lindsay R, et al: Clinical indications for bone mass measurement, *J Bone Miner Res, (suppl)* 4:1, 1989.
29. Marcus R: Secondary forms of osteoporosis. In Coe F, Favus M, editors: *Disorders of bone and mineral metabolism,* New York, 1992, Raven Press.
30. Delmas PD: Biochemical markers of bone turnover in osteoporosis. In Riggs BL, Melton LJI, editors: *Osteoporosis: etiology, diagnosis and management,* New York, 1990, Raven Press.
31. Lindsay R, Mellish R, Cosman F, et al: Biochemical markers of bone remodeling. In Nordin BEC, editor: *Osteoporosis: contributions to modern management,* London, 1990, Parthenon.
32. Christiansen C, Riis BJ, Rodbro P: Prediction of rapid bone loss in postmenopausal women, *Lancet* 1:1105, 1987.
33. Genarri HK: The radiology of osteoporosis. In Riggs BL, Melton LJI, editors: *Osteoporosis: etiology, diagnosis and management,* New York, 1988, Raven Press.
34. Lindsay R, Cosman F, Herrington BS, et al: Radiographic absorptiometry: a simple technique for determination of low bone mass, *Osteoporo Int* 2:34, 1991.
35. Singh M, Nagrath AR, Maini PS: Changes in trabecular pattern of the upper end of the femur as an index of osteoporosis, *J Bone Joint Surg* 52A:457, 1970.

36. Bohr H, Schaadt O: Bone mineral content of femoral bone and the lumbar spine measured in women with fracture of the femoral neck by dual photon absorptiometry, *Clin Orthop* 179:240, 1983.

37. Riggs BL, Melton III LJ: Involutional osteoporosis, *N Engl J Med* 314:1676, 1986.

38. Maller M, Horsman A, Harvald B, et al: Metacarpal morphometry in monozygotic and dizygotic elderly twins, *Calcif Tissue Res* 25:197, 1975.

39. Pocock NA, Eisman JA, Hopper JL, et al: Genetic determinants of bone mass in adults, *J Clin Invest* 80:706, 1987.

40. Smith DM, Nance WE, Kang K, et al: Genetic factors in determining bone mass, *J Clin Invest* 52:2800, 1973.

41. Morrison NA, Cheng QL J, Tokita A, et al: Prediction of bone density from vitamin D receptor alleles, *Nature* 367:284, 1994.

42. Johnston CCJ, Miller JZ, Slemenda CW, et al: Calcium supplementation and increases in bone mineral density in children, *N Engl J Med* 327:82, 1992.

43. Slemenda CW, Reister TK, Peacock M, et al: Bone growth in children following the cessation of calcium supplementation, *J Bone Miner Res, (suppl)* 8:154, 1993.

44. Kanis JA, Passmore R: Calcium supplementation of the diet I, *Br Med J* 298:137, 1989.

45. Kanders B, Dempster DW, Lindsay R: Interaction of calcium nutrition and physical activity on bone mass in young women, *J Bone Miner Res* 3:145, 1988.

46. Pocock NA, Eisman JA, Gwinn T, et al: Muscle strength, physical fitness but not age predict femoral neck bone mass, *J Bone Miner Res* 4:441, 1989.

47. Kelly PJ, Eisman JA, Sambrook PN: Interaction of genetic and environmental influences on peak bone density, *Osteopor Int* 1:56, 1990.

48. Lindberg JS, Fears WB, Hunt MM: Exercised induced amenorrhea and bone density, *Ann Intern Med* 101:747, 1984.

49. Linnel SL, Stager MM, Blue PW: Bone mineral content and menstrual regularity in female runners, *Med Sci Sports Exec* 16:343, 1989.

50. Marcus R, Cann C, Madvig D: Menstrual function and bone mass in elite women distance runners, *Ann Intern Med* 102:158, 1985.

51. Klibanski A, Neer RM, Beitins IZ, et al: Decreased bone density in hyperprolactinemic women, *N Engl J Med* 303:1511, 1980.

52. Sanborn CF, Martin BJ, Wagner WW: Is athletic amenorrhea specific to runners? *Am J Obstet Gynecol* 143:859, 1982.

53. Cann CE, Martin MC, Genant HK: Decreased spinal mineral content in amenorrheic women, *J Am Med Assoc* 251:626, 1984.

54. Drinkwater BD, Nilson KL, Chesnut CHI: Bone mineral content of amenorrheic and eumenorrheic athletes, *N Engl J Med* 311:277, 1984.

55. Nystrom E, Leman J, Lundberg PA, et al: Bone mineral content in normally menstruating women with hyperprolactinaemia, *Horm Res* 29:214, 1988.

56. Rigotti NA, Nussbaum SR, Herzog DB, et al: Osteoporosis in women with anorexia nervosa, *N Engl J Med* 311:1601, 1984.

57. Beals RK: Orthopedic aspects of the XO (Turner's) syndrome, *Clin Orthop* 97:19, 1973.

58. Smith DAS, Walker MS: Changes in plasma steroids and bone density in Klinefelter's syndrome, *Calcif Tissue Res* 22:225, 1976.

59. DeVernejoul MC, Girot R, Gueris J, et al: Calcium phosphate metabolism and bone disease in patients with homozygous thalassemia, *J Clin Endocrinol Metab* 54:276, 1982.

60. Avioli LV: Hyperparathyroidism, hypoparathyroidism, pseudohypoparathyroidism, and pseudopseudohypoparathyroidism. In Goldensohn ES, Appel SH, editors: *Scientific approaches to clinical neurology*, vol 2, Philadelphia, 1977, Lea & Febiger.

61. Looker AC, Johnston CCJ, Wahner HW, et al: Women at risk for hip fracture in the U.S. population: prevalence of low femur bone density from NHANES III, *J Am Med Assoc* (in press), 1994.

62. Trotter M: Densities of bones of white and Negro skeletons, *J Bone Joint Surg* 42A:50, 1960.

63. Smith Jr RW, Frame B: Concurrent axial and appendicular osteoporosis: its relation to calcium consumption, *N Engl J Med* 273:73, 1965.

64. Mazess RB, Barden HS, Christiansen C, et al: Bone mineral and vitamin D in Aleutian Islanders, *Am J Clin Nutr* 42:143, 1985.

65. Solomon L: Bone density in aging Caucasian and African populations, *Lancet* 1:1326, 1979.

66. Seeman E, Hopper JL, Bach LA, et al: Reduced bone mass in daughters of women with osteoporosis, *N Engl J Med* 320:554, 1989.

67. Evans R, Marel GM, Lancaster EK, et al: Bone mass is low in relatives of osteoporotic patients, *Ann Intern Med* 1:870, 1988.

68. Boden SD, Labroupoulos PA, Saunders R: Hip fractures in young patients: is this early osteoporosis? *Calfic Tissue Int* 46:65, 1990.

69. Lindsay R: Bone mass measurement for premenopausal women, *Osteopor Int (suppl)* 4: (in press), 1994.

70. Lindsay R, Nieves J, Golden A, et al: Bone mass among premenopausal women, *Int J Fertil (suppl)* 38:83, 1993.

71. Sowers MFR, Wallace RB, Lemke JH: Correlates of mid-radius bone density among premenopausal women: a community study, *Prev Med* 14:585, 1985.

72. Sowers MFR, Clark MK, Hollis B, et al: Radial bone mineral density in pre- and perimenopausal women: a prospective study of rates and risk factors for loss, *J Bone Miner Res* 7:647, 1992.

73. Christiansen C, Lindsay R: Estrogens, bone loss and preservation, *Osteo Int* 1:7, 1991.

74. Johnston CC, Hui SL, Witt RM, et al: Early menopausal changes in bone mass and sex steroids, *J Clin Endocrinol Metab* 61:905, 1985.

75. Lindsay R, Coutts JRT, Sweeney A, et al: Endogenous estrogen and bone loss following oophorectomy, *Calcif Tissue Res* 22:213, 1984.

76. Aitken JM, Hart DM, Anderson JB, et al: Osteoporosis after oophorectomy for non-malignant disease, *Br Med J* 1:325, 1973.

77. Albright F, Bloomberg F, Smith PH: Postmenopausal osteoporosis, *Trans Assoc Am Physicians* 55:298, 1940.

78. Albright F, Smith PH, Richardson AM: Postmenopausal osteoporosis, *J Am Med Assoc* 116:2465, 1941.

79. Albright F: The effect of hormones on osteogenesis in man, *Recent Prog Horm Res* 1:293, 1947.

80. Henneman PH, Wallach S: A review of the prolonged use of estrogens and androgens in postmenopausal and senile osteoporosis, *Arch Intern Med* 100:705, 1957.

81. Genant HK, Steiger P, Glueer CC: New developments in bone densitometry, *Postgrad Med* 18-22:33, 1989.

82. Seibel M, Cosman F, Shen V, et al: Urinary hydroxypyridinium crosslinks of collagen as markers of bone resorption and estrogen efficacy in postmenopausal osteoporosis, *J Bone Miner Res* 8:881, 1993.

83. Stock JL, Coderre JA, Mallette E: Effects of a short course of estrogen on mineral metabolism in postmenopausal women, *J Clin Endocrinol Metab* 595 1985.

84. Cosman F, Shen V, Xie F, et al: A mechanism of estrogen action on the skeleton: protection against the resorbing effects of (1-34)hPTH infusion as assessed by biochemical markers, *Ann Intern Med* 118:337, 1992.

85. Cosman F, Shen V, Herrington BS, et al: Response of the parathyroid gland to infusion of (1-34)hPTH: demonstration of suppression of endogenous secretion using IRMA intact (1-84)PTH assay, *J Clin Endocrinol Metab* 73:1345, 1991.

86. Avioli LV, Lindsay R: The osteoporoses. In Krane S, Avioli LV, editors: *Metabolic bone disease*, Philadelphia, 1990, WB Saunders.

87. Cannigia A, Gennari C, Borella G, et al: Intestinal absorption of calcium-47 after treatment with oral estrogen and gestagen in senile osteoporosis, *Br Med J* 3:30, 1970.

88. Riis BJ, Christiansen C, Johansen JS, et al: Is it possible to prevent bone loss in young women treated with luteinizing hormone-releasing hormone agonists? *J Clin Endocrinol Metab* 70:920, 1990.

89. Prior JC, Vigna YM, Schecter MT, et al: Spinal bone loss and ovulatory disturbances, *N Engl J Med* 323:1221, 1990.

90. Drinkwater BL, Bruemner B, Chesnut CHI: Menstrual history as a determinant of current bone density in young athletes, *J Am Med Assoc* 263:545, 1990.

91. Parfitt AM: Bone remodeling: relationship to the amount and structure of bone, and the pathogenesis and prevention of fractures. In Riggs BL, Melton LJI, editors: *Osteoporosis: etiology, diagnosis, and management,* New York, 1988, Raven Press.

92. Dempster DW, Lindsay R: Pathogenesis of osteoporosis, *Lancet* 34:797, 1993.

93. Parfitt AM: Quantum concept of bone remodeling and turnover implications for the pathogenesis of osteoporosis, *Calcif Tissue Int* 28:1, 1979.

94. Dempster DW: Bone remodeling: implications for the pathogenesis, prevention and treatment of osteoporosis. In Riggs BL, Melton LJI, editors: *Osteoporosis: etiology, diagnosis and management,* ed 2 (in press), New York, 1994, Raven Press.

95. Parfitt AM: *Accelerated cortical bone loss: primary and secondary hyperparathyroidism,* Berlin, 1986, Springer-Verlag.

96. Parfitt AM: The physiological and clinical significance of bone histomorphometric data. In Recker R, editor: *Bone histomorphometry. techniques and interpretation,* Boca Raton, 1983, CRC.

97. Steiniche T, Hasling C, Charles P, et al: A randomized study of the effects of estrogen/gestagen or high-dose oral calcium on trabecular bone remodeling in postmenopausal osteoporosis, *Bone* 10:313, 1989.

98. Mundy GR: Local control of osteoclast function, *Osteopor Int (suppl),* 3:126, 1993.

99. Raisz LG: Local and systemic factors in the pathogenesis of osteoporosis, *N Engl J Med* 318:818, 1988.

100. Lanyon LE: Functional strain as a determinant for bone remodeling, *Calcif Tissue Int* 36:556, 1984.

101. Kalu DN: The ovariectomized rat model of postmenopausal bone loss, *Bone Miner* 15:175, 1991.

102. Recker RR, Kimmel DB, Parfitt AM: Static and tetracycline-based bone histomorphometric data from 34 normal postmenopausal females, *J Bone Miner Res* 3:133, 1988.

103. Vedi S, Compston JE, Webb A: Histomorphometric analysis of bone biopsies from the iliac crest of normal British subjects, *Metab Bone Dis Rel Res* 4:231, 1982.

104. Vedi S, Compston JE, Webb A, et al: Histomorphometric analysis of dynamic parameters of trabecular bone formation in the iliac crest of normal British subjects, *Metab Bone Dis Rel Res* 5:69, 1983.

105. Melsen F, Mosekilde L: Tetracycline double-labeling of iliac trabecular bone in 41 normal adults, *Calcif Tissue Res* 26:88, 1978.

106. Eriksen EF: Normal and pathological remodeling of human trabecular bone: three-dimensional reconstruction of the remodeling sequence in normals and in metabolic bone disease, *Endocr Rev* 7:379, 1986.

107. Riggs BL, Melton III LJ, Wahner HW: Heterogeneity of involutional osteoporosis: evidence for two distinct osteoporotic syndromes. In Frame B, Potts JTJ, editors: *Clinical disorders of bone and mineral metabolism,* Amsterdam, 1983, Excerpta Medica.

108. Dempster DW, Shane E, Horbert W, et al: A simple method for correlative light and scanning electron microscopy of human iliac crest bone biopsies: qualitative observations in normal and osteoporotic subjects, *J Bone Miner Res* 1:15, 1986.

109. Parfitt AM: Trabecular bone architecture in the pathogenesis and prevention of fracture, *Am J Med* 82:68, 1987.

110. Kleerekoper M, Villanueva AR, Stanciu J, et al: The role of three-dimensional trabecular microstructure in the pathogenesis of vertebral compression fractures, *Calcif Tissue Int* 37:594, 1985.

111. Parfitt AM: Surface specific bone remodeling in health and disease. In Kleerekoper M, editor: *Clinical disorders of bone and mineral metabolism,* New York, 1989, Mary Ann Liebert.

112. Mazess RB: Fracture risk: a role for compact bone, *Calcif Tissue Int* 47:191, 1990.

113. Gallagher JC, Riggs BL, Eisman JA, et al: Intestinal calcium absorption and serum vitamin D metabolites in normal subjects and osteoporotic patients, *J Clin Invest* 64:729, 1979.

114. Alevizaki CC, Ikkos DG, Singhelakis P: Progressive decrease of true intestinal calcium absorption with age in normal man, *J Nucl Med* 14:760, 1973.

115. Bullamore JR, et al: Effect of age on calcium absorption, *Lancet* 2:535,

116. Abraham S, Carrol MD, Dresser CM, et al: *U.S. dietary intake findings,* 1971-1974, HEW Publication No.:77-1647, National Center for Health Statistics, 1974.

117. Bauer W, Aub JC, Albright F: Studies of calcium phosphorous metabolisms: study of bone trabeculae as readily available reserve supply of calcium, *J Exp Med* 49:145, 1929.

118. Jaffe HL, Bodansky A, Chandler JP: Ammondium chloride decalcification as modified by calcium intake: the relation between generalized osteoporosis and osteitic fibrosa, *J Exp Med* 56:823, 1932.

119. Jowsey J, Gershon-Cohen J: Effect of dietary calcium levels on production and reversal of experimental osteoporosis in cats, *Proc Soc Exp Biol Med* 116:437, 1964.

120. Heaney RP: Calcium, bone health and osteoporosis. In Peck WA, editor: *Bone and mineral research 4,* New York, 1986, Elsevier.

121. Whedon GD: The influence of activity on calcium metabolism, *J Nutr Sci Vitaminol (Tokyo)* 31:41, 1991.

122. Issekutz B, Blizzard JJ, Burkhead NC, et al: Effect of prolonged bed rest on urinary calcium output, *J Appl Physiol* 21:1013, 1966.

123. Gieser M, Trueta J: Muscle action, bone rarefaction and bone formation, *J Bone Joint Surg* 40B:282, 1958.

124. Dietrick JE, Whedon GD, Sherr E: Effects of immobilization upon various metabolic and physiologic functions of normal men, *Am J Med* 47:3, 1948.

125. Mazess RB, Whedon GD: Immobilization and bone, *Calcif Tissue Int* 35:265, 1983.

126. Uhthoff HK, Jowarski ZF: Bone loss in response to long-term immobilization, *J Bone Joint Surg* 60B:420, 1978.

127. Young DR, Niklowitz WJ, Brown RJ, et al: Immobilization-associated osteoporosis in primates, *Bone* 7:109, 1986.

128. Smith MC, Rambout PC, Vogel JM, et al: Bone mineral measurement in experiment M078 in biomedical records from Skylab, *NASA Pub* 183, 1977.

129. Mack PB, LaChance PA, Vose GP, et al: Bone demineralization of foot and hand of Gemini-Titan IV, V, and VII astronauts during orbital flight, *Am J Roentg* 100:503, 1967.

130. Smith Jr EL, Smith PE, Ensign CJ, et al: Bone involution decrease in exercising middle-aged women, *Calcif Tissue Int* 36:S129, 1984.

131. Nilsson BE, Westlin NE: Changes in bone mass in alcoholics, *Clin Orthop* 90:229, 1973.

132. Baran DT, Teitelbaum SL, Bergfeld MA, et al: Effect of alcohol ingestion on bone and mineral metabolism in rats, *Am J Physiol* 223837:507, 1980.

133. Farley JR, Fitzsimmons R, Taylor AK, et al: Direct effects of ethanol on bone resorption and formation in vitro, *Arch Biochem Biophys* 237:305, 1985.

134. Bikle DD: Effects of alcohol abuse on bone, *Compr Ther* 14:16, 1988.

135. Daniell HW: Osteoporosis of the slender smoker, *Arch Intern Med* 136:298, 1976.

136. Daniell HW: Postmenopausal tooth loss. Contributions to edentulism by osteoporosis and cigarette smoking, *Arch Intern Med* 143:1678, 1983.

137. Haarbo J, Hassager C, Schlemmer A, et al: Influence of smoking, body fat distribution and alcohol consumption on serum lipids, lipoproteins, and apolipoproteins in early postmenopausal women, *Atherosclerosis* 84:239, 1990.

138. Dempster DW: Bone histomorphometry in glucocorticoid-induced osteoporosis, *J Bone Miner Res* 4:137, 1989.

139. Lukert BP, Raisz LG: Glucocorticoid-induced osteoporosis: pathogenesis and management, *Ann Intern Med* 112:352, 1990.

140. Melsen F, Mosekilde L: Morphometric and dynamic studies of bone changes in hyperthyroidism, *Acta Pathol Microbiol Scand* 85:141, 1977.

141. Meunier PJ, Bressot C: Endocrine influences on bone cells and bone remodeling evaluated by clinical histomorphometry. In Parsons JA, editor: *Endocrinology of calcium metabolism,* New York, 1982, Raven Press.

142. Cummings SR, Black DM, Nevitt MC, et al: Appendicular bone density and age predict hip fracture in women, the study of osteoporotic fractures research group, *J Am Med Assoc* 263:665, 1990.

143. Slemenda CW, Hui SL, Longcope C, et al: Predictors of bone mass in perimenopausal women. A prospective study of clinical data using photon absorptiometry, *Ann Intern Med* 112:96, 1990.

144. Lindsay R, Dempster DW, Clemens TL, et al: Incidence, cost, and risk factors of fracture of the proximal femur in the U.S.A. Proceedings of the international symposium on osteoporosis, *Osteoporosis* 1:311, 1984.

145. Chesnut III CH: The imaging and quantitation of bone by radiographic and scanning methodologies. In Coe FL, Favus MJ, editors: *Disorders of bone and mineral metabolism,* New York, 1992, Raven.

146. Chesnut III CH: Noninvasive methods for bone mass measurement. In Avioli LV, editor: *The osteoporotic syndrome,* ed 3, New York, Wiley Liss.

147. Mazess RB, Barden HS, Bisek JP, et al: Dual-energy x-ray absorptiometry for total-body and regional bone-mineral and soft-tissue composition, *Am J Clin Nutr* 51:1106, 1990.

148. Hansson T, Roos B, Nachemson A: The bone mineral content and ultimate compression strength of lumbar vertebrae, *Spine* 5:46, 1980.

149. Hui SL, Slemenda CW, Johnston CC: Age and bone mass as predictors of fracture in a prospective study, *J Clin Invest* 81:1804, 1988.

150. Ross PD, Wasnich RD, Vogel JM: Detection of prefracture spinal osteoporosis using bone mineral absorptiometry, *J Bone Miner Res* 3:1, 1988.

151. Cummings SR, Black DM, Nevitt MC, et al: Bone density at various sites for prediction of hip fractures, *Lancet* 341:72, 1993.

152. Hui SL, Slemenda CW, Johnston CCJ: Baseline measurement of bone mass predicts fracture in white women, *Ann Intern Med* 111:355, 1989.

153. Gardsell P, Johnell O, Nilsson BE: Predicting fractures in women by using forearm bone densitometry, *Calcif Tissue Int* 44:235, 1989.

154. Wahner HW, Fogelman I: *The evaluation of osteoporosis: dual-energy x-ray absorptiometry in clinical practice,* London, 1994, Martin Dunitz.

155. Abraham S, Carrol MD, Dresser CM, et al: Dietary intake findings, U.S. 1971-1974, *HEW Publication 2975* 77:1647, 1974.

156. Heaney RP, Recker RR, Saville PD: Calcium balance and calcium requirements in middle-aged women, *Am J Clin Nutr* 30:1603, 1990.

157. Heaney RP, Recker RR: Distribution of calcium absorption in middle-aged women, *Am J Clin Nutr* 43:299, 1986.

158. Heaney RP, Recker RR, Saville PD: Menopausal changes in calcium balance performance, *J Lab Clin Med* 92:953, 1978.

159. Lindsay R, Nieves J: Milk and bones, *Br Med J* 308:930, 1994.

160. Consensus Development Conference on Osteoporosis, *J Am Med Assoc* 252:799, 1984.

161. Nordin BEC, Horsman A, Crilly RG, et al: Treatment of spinal osteoporosis in postmenopausal women, *Br Med J* 16:451, 1980.

162. Riggs BL, Seeman E, Hodgson SF, et al: Effect of the fluoride/calcium regimen on vertebral fracture occurrence in postmenopausal osteoporosis, *N Engl J Med* 306:446, 1982.

163. Dawson-Hughes B, Dallal GE, Krall GE, et al: A controlled trial of the effect of calcium supplementation on bone density in postmenopausal women, *N Engl J Med* 323:878, 1990.

164. Holbrook TL, Barrett-Connor E, Wingard DL: Dietary calcium and risk of hip fracture: 14-year prospective population study, *Lancet* 2:1046, 1988.

165. Carr CJ, Shangraw RF: Nutritional and pharmaceutical aspects of calcium supplementation, *Am Pharm* NS27:149, 1987.

166. Recker RR: Calcium absorption and achlorhydria, *N Engl J Med* 333:70, 1985.

167. Lindsay R, Aitken JM, Anderson JB, et al: Long-term prevention of postmenopausal osteoporosis by oestrogen, *Lancet* 1:1038, 1976.

168. Lindsay R, Hart DM, Forrest C, et al: Prevention of spinal osteoporosis in oophorectomized women, *Lancet* 2:1151, 1980.

169. Lindsay R, Hart DM, Clark DM: The minimum effective dose of estrogen for prevention of postmenopausal bone loss, *Obstet Gynecol* 63:759, 1984.

170. Lindsay R, Hart DM, Purdie P, et al: Comparative effects of oestrogen and a progestogen on bone loss in postmenopausal women, *Clin Sci* 54:193, 1978.

171. Abdalla HI, Hart DM, Lindsay R: Differential bone loss and effects of long-term estrogen therapy according to time of introduction of therapy after oophorectomy. In Christiansen C, Arnaud C, Nordin BEC, et al, editors: *Osteoporosis II,* Glostrup, 1984, Aalborg Stiftsbogtrykkeri.

172. Aitken JM, Hart DM, Lindsay R: Oestrogen replacement therapy for prevention of osteoporosis after oophorectomy, *Br Med J* 3:515, 1973.

173. Lindsay R: Sex steroids in the pathogenesis and prevention of osteoporosis. In Riggs BL, editor: *Osteoporosis: etiology, diagnosis and management,* New York, 1988, Raven Press.

174. Christiansen C, Riis BJ: Five years with continuous combined oestrogen/progestogen therapy. Effects on calcium metabolism, lipoproteins, and bleeding pattern, *Br J Obstet Gynaecol* 97:1087, 1990.

175. Christiansen C, Christiansen MS, McNair P: Prevention of early postmenopausal bone loss: conducted 2 years study in 315 normal females, *Eur J Clin Invest* 10:273, 1980.

176. Civitelli R, Agnusdei D, Nardi P, et al: Effects of one-year treatment with estrogens on bone mass, intestinal calcium absorption, and 25-hydroxyvitamin D-1-hydroxylase reserve in postmenopausal osteoporosis, *Calcif Tissue Int* 42:76, 1988.

177. Davis ME, Lanzl LH, Cox AB: Detection, prevention and retardation of postmenopausal osteoporosis, *Obstet Gynecol* 36:187, 1970.

178. Ettinger B, Genant HK, Cann CE: Long-term estrogen therapy prevents bone loss and fracture, *Ann Intern Med* 102:319, 1985.

179. Horsman A, Gallagher JC, Simpson M, et al: Prospective trial of estrogen and calcium in postmenopausal women, *Br Med J* 2:789, 1977.

180. Nachtigall LE, Nachtigall RH, Nachtigall RD: Estrogen replacement therapy I: a 10-year prospective study in the relationship to osteoporosis, *Obstet Gynecol* 53:277, 1979.

181. Quigley MET, Martin BL, Burnier AM, et al: Estrogen therapy arrests bone loss in elderly women, *Am J Obstet Gynecol* 156:1516, 1987.

182. Recker RR, Saville PD, Heaney RP: The effect of estrogens and calcium carbonate on bone loss in postmenopausal women, *Ann Intern Med* 87:649, 1977.

183. Riggs BL, Jowsey J, Goldsmith RS, et al: Short- and long-term effects of estrogen and synthetic anabolic hormones in postmenopausal osteoporosis, *J Clin Invest* 5159:1659, 1972.

184. Meema S, Bunker ML, Meema HE: Preventive effect of estrogen on postmenopausal bone loss, *Arch Intern Med* 135:1436, 1975.

185. Riis BJ, Thomsen K, Strom V, et al: The effect of percutaneous estradiol and natural progesterone on postmenopausal bone loss, *Am J Obstet Gynecol* 156:61, 1987.

186. Jensen GF, Christiansen C, Transbol I: Treatment of postmenopausal osteoporosis: a controlled therapeutic trial comparing oestrogen/gestagen, 1,25-dihydroxyvitamin D3 and calcium, *Clin Endocrinol* 16:515, 1982.

187. Al-Azzawi F, Hart DM, Lindsay R: Long-term effect of oestrogen replacement therapy on bone mass as measured by dual photon absorptiometry, *Br Med J* 294:1261, 1987.

188. Christiansen C, Lindsay R: Estrogens, bone loss and preservation, *Osteoporosis Intern* 1:7, 1991.

189. Harris ST, Genant HK, Baylink DJ, et al: The effects of estrogen (Ogen) on spinal bone density of postmenopausal women, *Arch Intern Med* 151:1980, .

190. Horsman A, James M, Francis R: The effect of estrogen dose on postmenopausal bone loss, *N Engl J Med* 309:1405, 1983.

191. Lindsay R, Hart DM, MacLean A, et al: Bone loss during oestrial therapy in postmenopausal women, *Maturitas* 1:279, 1979.

192. Stevenson JC, Cust MP, Gangar KF, et al: Effects of transdermal versus oral hormone replacement therapy on bone density in spine and proximal femur in postmenopausal women, *Lancet* 336:265, 1990.

193. Lufkin EG, Wahner HW, O'Fallon WM, et al: Treatment of postmenopausal osteoporosis with transdermal estrogen, *Ann Intern Med* 117:1, 1992.

194. Garnett T, Studd J, Watson N, et al: A cross-sectional study of the effects of long-term percutaneous hormone replacement therapy on bone density, *Obstet Gynecol* 78:1002, 1991.

195. Farish E, Hart DM, Jackanicz TM, et al: Hormone replacement therapy by vaginal ring pessaries: effects on biomechanical indices of bone metabolism. Proceedings of the international symposium on osteoporosis, 1984, Copenhagen, Denmark.

196. Komm BS, Terpening CM, Benz DJ: Estrogen binding, receptor mRNA, and biologic response in osteoblast-like osteosarcoma cells, *Science* 241:81, 1988.

197. Erikssen EF, Colvard DS, Berg NJ: Evidence of estrogen receptors in normal human osteoblast-like cells, *Science* 241:84, 1988.

198. Ernst MC, Schmid C, Frankenfoldt ER, et al: Estradiol stimulation of osteoblast proliferation in vitro: mediator roles for TGFB, PFE2, IGF1, *Calcif Tissue Int (suppl)* 42:117, 1988.

199. Keeting PE, Scott RE, Colvard DS, et al: Lack of a direct effect of estrogen on proliferation and differentiation of normal human osteoblast-like cells, *J Bone Miner Res* 6:297, 1991.

200. Rickard DJ, Gowen M, MacDonald BR: Proliferative responses to estradiol, IL-1 and TGFB by cells expressing alkaline phosphatase in human osteoblast-like cell cultures, *Calcif Tissue Int* 52:227, 1993.

201. McSheehy PHJ, Chambers TJ: Osteoblastic cells mediate osteoclastic responsiveness to parathyroid hormone, *Endocrinology* 118:824, 1986.

202. Oursler MJ, Osdoby P, Pyfferoen J, et al: Avian osteoclasts as estrogen target cells, *Proc Natl Acad Sci USA* 88:6613, 1991: PNAS 1991 88; 6613-6617.

203. Arnett TR, Lindsay R, Dempster DW: Effect of estrogens and anti-estrogens on osteoclast activity in vitro, *J Bone Miner Res* 1:99, 1986.

204. Kalu DN, Salerno E, Liu C-C, et al: Ovariectomy-induced bone loss and the hematopoietic system, *Bone Miner* 23:145, 1993.

205. Stevenson JC, Abeyasekera G, Hillyard CJ: Regulation of calcium-regulating hormones by exogenous sex steroids in early postmeno-pause, *Eur J Clin Invest* 13:481, 1983.

206. Cosman F, Shen V, Herrington BS, et al: Mechanism of estrogen action in osteoporosis treatment as assessed by human (1-34)PTH infusion. In Christiansen C, Overgaard K, editors: *Osteoporosis III,* Copenhagen, 1990, Osteopress.

207. Cosman F, Nieves J, Horton J, et al: Effects of estrogen on response to EDTA infusion in postmenopausal osteoporotic women, *J Clin Endocrinol Metab* (in press), 1994.

208. Stock JL, Coderre JA, Mallette E: Effects of a short course of estrogen on mineral metabolism in postmenopausal women, *J Clin Endocrinol Metab* 61:595, 1985.

209. Pacifici R, Brown C, Puscheck E, et al: Effect of surgical menopause and estrogen replacement on cytokine release from human blood mononuclear cells, *Proc Natl Acad Sci U S A* 88:5134, 1991.

210. Pacifici R, Rifas L, Vered I, et al: Interleukin-1 secretion from human blood monocytes in normal and osteoporotic women: effect of menopause and estrogen/progesterone treatment, *J Bone Miner Res* 3A:541, 1988.

211. Gowen M: Cytokines and celluar interactions in the control of bone remodeling, *Bone Miner* 6:77, 1994.

212. Jilka RL, Hangoc G, Girasole G, et al: Increased osteoclast development after estrogen loss: mediation by Interleukin-6, *Science* 257:88, 1992.

213. Girasole G, Jilka RL, Passeri G, et al: 17-beta estradiol inhibits interleukin-6 production by bone marrow-derived stromal cells and osteoblasts in vitro: a potent mechanism for the anti-osteoporotic effects of estrogens, *J Clin Invest* 89:893, 1992.

214. Clinical applications of TGE-β, Ciba Foundation Symposium 157, Chichester, 1991, Wiley.

215. Raisz LG: Local and systemic factors in the pathogenesis of osteoporosis, *N Engl J Med* 318:818, 1988.

216. Ernst M, Rodan GA: Estradiol regulation of insulin-like growth factor-1 expression in osteoblastic cells: evidence for transriptional control, *Mol Endocrinol* 5:1081, 1991.

217. Ernst M, Heath JK, Rodan GA: Estradiol effects on proliferation, messenger ribonucleic acid for collagen and insulin-like growth factor-I, and parathyroid hormone-stimulated adenylate cyclase activity in osteoblastic cells from calvariae and long bones, *Endocrinology* 125:825, 1989.

218. Hock JM, Canalis E, Centrella M: Transforming growth factor-b stimulates bone matrix apposition and bone cell replication in cultured fetal rat calvariae, *Endocrinology* 126:421, 1990.

219. McCarthy TL, Centrella M, Canalis E: Regulatory effects of insulin-like growth factor I and II on bone collagen synthesis in rat calvarial cultures, *Endocrinology* 124:301, 1989.

220. Canalis E, Centrella M, Burch W, et al: Insulin-like growth factor I mediates selective anabolic effects of parathyroid hormone in bone cultures, *J Clin Invest* 83:60, 1989.

221. Cheema C, Grant BF, Marcus R: Effects of estrogen on circulating "free" and total 1,25-dihydroxyvitamin D on the parathyroid-vitamin D axis in postmenopausal women, *J Clin Invest* 83:537, 1989.

222. Gallagher JC, Riggs BL, DeLuca HF: Effect of estrogen on calcium absorption and serum vitamin D metabolites in postmenopausal osteoporosis, *J Clin Endocrinol Metab* 51:1359, 1980.

223. Cannigia A, Gennasi C, Borella G, et al: Intestinal absorption of calcium 47 after treatment with oral estrogen and gestagen in senile osteoporosis, *Br Med J* 4:30, 1970.

224. Stevenson JC, White MC, Joplin GF, et al: Osteoporosis and calcitonin deficiency, *Br Med J* 285:1010, 1982.

225. Stevenson JC, Hillyard CJ, MacIntyre I, et al: A physiological role for calcitonin in protection of the maternal skeleton, *Lancet* 2:767, 1979.

226. Stevenson JC, Abeyasekera G, Hillyard CJ: Deficient calcitonin response to calcium infusion in postmenopausal osteoporosis, *Lancet* 1:693, 1982.

227. Body JJ, Heath HHI: Effects of age, sex, calcium and total thyroidectomy on circulating monomeric calcitonin concentrations, *Calcif Tissue Res* 35#6:A45, 1983.

228. Gordan GS, Picchi J, Roof BS: Antifracture efficacy of long-term estrogens for osteoporosis, *Trans Assoc Am Physicians* 86:326, 1973.

229. Hutchinson TA, Polansky JM, Feinstein AR: Postmenopausal oestrogens protect against fracture of hip and distal radius, *Lancet* 2:705, 1979.

230. Kiel DP, Felson DT, Anderson JJ: Hip fracture and the use of estrogens in postmenopausal women, *N Engl J Med* 317:1169, 1987.

231. Kreiger N, Kelsey JL, Holford TR: An epidemiological study of hip fracture in postmenopausal women, *Am J Epidemiol* 116:141, 1982.

232. Paganini-Hill A, Ross RK, Gerkins VR, et al: Menopausal estrogen therapy and hip fractures, *Ann Intern Med* 95:28, 1981.

233. Weiss NS, Ure CL, Ballard JH: Decreased risk of fractures of the hip

and lower forearm with postmenopausal use of oestrogen, *N Engl J Med* 303:1195, 1980.

234. Naessen T, Persson I, Adami HO, et al: Hormone replacement therapy and the risk for first hip fracture. A prospective, population-based cohort study, *Ann Intern Med* 113:95, 1990.
235. Williams AR, Weiss NS, Ure C, et al: Effect of weight, smoking, and estrogen use on the risk of hip and forearm fractures in postmenopausal women, *Obstet Gynecol* 60:695, 1982.
236. Johnson BE, Lucasey B, Robinson RG, et al: Contributing diagnoses in osteoporosis, *Arch Intern Med* 149:1069, 1989.
237. Felson DT, Zhang Y, Hannan MT, et al: The effect of postmenopausal estrogen therapy on bone density in elderly women, *N Engl J Med* 329:1141, 1993.
238. Lindsay R: Osteoporosis: an updated approach to prevention and management, *Geriatrics* 44:45, 1989.
239. Christiansen C, Christiansen MS, Transbol I: Bone mass in postmenopausal women after withdrawal of estrogen/gestagen replacement therapy, *Lancet* 1:459, 1981.
240. Horsman A, Nordin BE, Crilly RG: Effect on bone of withdrawal of oestrogen therapy, *Lancet* 2:33, 1979.
241. Barrett-Connor E: Postmenopausal estrogens and prevention bias, *Ann Intern Med* 115:455, 1991.
242. Reference deleted.
243. Reference deleted.
244. Mishell Jr DR: Estrogen replacement therapy: measuring benefit vs. cardiovascular risk, *J Reprod Med* 30:795, 1985.
245. Barrett-Connor E, Bush TL: Estrogen and coronary heart disease in women, *J Am Med Assoc* 265:1861, 1991.
246. Lindsay R, Tohme J: Estrogen treatment of patients with established postmenopausal osteoporosis, *Obstet Gynecol* 76:1, 1990.
247. Christiansen C, Riis BJ: Beta-estradiol and continuous norethisterone: a unique treatment for established osteoporosis in elderly women, *J Clin Endocrinol Metab* 71:836, 1990.
248. Abbasi R, Hodgen GD: Predicting the predisposition to osteoporosis. Gonadotropin-releasing hormone antagonist for acute estrogen deficiency test, *J Am Med Assoc* 255:1600, 1986.
250. Stevenson JC: Pathogenesis, prevention, and treatment of osteoporosis, *Obstet Gynecol* 75:36, 1990.
251. Gallagher JC, Kable WT, Goldgar D: Effect of progestin therapy on cortical and trabecular bone: comparison with estrogen, *Am J Med* 90:171, 1991.
252. Christiansen C, Riis BT, Nilas L, et al: Uncoupling of bone formation and resorption by combined oestrogen and progestogen therapy in postmenopausal osteoporosis, *Lancet* 2:800, 1985.
253. Martin TJ, Moseley JM: Calcitonin. In Avioli LV, Krane S, editors: *Metabolic bone disease*, ed 2, Avioli.
254. Gruber HE, Ivey JL, Baylink DJ, et al: Long-term calcitonin therapy in postmenopausal osteoporosis, *Metabolism* 33:295, 1984.
255. Gonzalez D, Ghiringhelli G, Mautalen C: Acute antiosteoclastic effect of salmon calcitonin in osteoporotic women, *Calcif Tissue Int* 38:71, 1986.
256. McDermott MT, Kidd GS: The role of calcitonin in the development and treatment of osteoporosis, *Endocr Rev* 8:377, 1987.
257. Caniggia A, Gennari C, Bencini M, et al: Calcium metabolism and 47 calcium kinetics before and after long-term thyrocalcitonin treatment in senile osteoporosis, *Clin Sci* 38:397, 1970.
258. Maresca V: Human calcitonin in the management of osteoporosis: a multicentre study. *J Int Med Res* 13:311, 1985.
259. Gennari C, Chierichetti SM, Bigazzi S, et al: Comparative effects on bone mineral content of calcium and calcium plus salmon calcitonin given in two different regimens in postmenopausal osteoporosis, *Curr Ther Res* 38:455, 1985.
260. Mazzouli GF, Passeri M, Gennari C, et al: Effects of salmon calcitonin in postmenopausal osteoporosis: a controlled double-blind clinical study, *Calcif Tissue Int* 38:3, 1986.
261. Wallach S, Cohn SH, Ellis KJ, et al: Effect of salmon calcitonin on skeletal mass in osteoporosis, *Curr Ther Res* 22:556, 1977.

262. Polatti F, Montrasio MG, Caprotti M, et al: Bone mineral content after oophorectomy: effects of salmon calcitonin and oral calcium, *Min Metab Res* 5:159, 1984.
263. Reginster JY, Albert A, Lecart MP, et al: 1-year controlled randomized trial of prevention of early postmenopausal bone loss by intranasal calcitonin, *Lancet* 2:1481, 1987.
264. Christiansen C, Baastrup PC, Transbol I: Development of 'primary' hyperparathyroidism during lithium therapy: longitudinal study, *Neuropsychobiology* 6:280, 1980.
265. Stancer H, Forbath N: Hyperparathyroidism, hypothyroidism, and impaired renal function after 10 to 20 years of lithium treatment, *Arch Intern Med* 149:1042, 1989.
266. Murrills RJ, Shane E, Lindsay R, et al: Bone resorption by isolated human osteoclasts in vitro: effects of calcitonin, *J Bone Miner Res* 4:259, 1989.
267. Civitelli R, Gonnelli S, Zaccher F, et al: Bone turnover in postmenopausal osteoporosis. Effect of calcitonin treatment, *J Clin Invest* 82:1268, 1988.
268. Cosman F, Nieves J, Walliser J, et al: Current therapies for postmenopausal osteoporosis: a comparison of three anti-resorptive agents, *J Women's Health* (in press), 1994.
269. Schiraldi GF, Scoccia S, Soresi E: Analgesic activity of high doses of salmon calcitonin in lung cancer, *Curr Ther Res* 38:592, 1985.
270. Fiore CE, Castorina F, Malatino LS, et al: Antalgic activity of calcitonin: efffectiveness of the epidural and subarachnoid routes in man, *Int J Clin Pharmacol Res* 3:257, 1983.
271. Gennari C, et al: Effects of calcitonin treatment on bone pain and bone turnover in Paget's disease of bone, *Miner Metab Res It* 2:109, 1981.
272. Gennari C, Chierichetti SM, Bigazzi S, et al: Comparative effects on bone mineral content of calcium and calcium plus salmon calcitonin given in two different regimens in postmenopausal osteoporosis, *Curr Ther Res* 38:455, 1985.
273. Schenk R, Merz WA, Muhlbauer R, et al: Effect of ethane-1-hydroxy-1,1-disphosphonate (EHDP) and dichloromethylene bisphosphonate (C1 2 MDP) on the calcification and resorption of cartilage and bone in the tibial epiphysis and metaphysis of rats, *Calc Tissue Res* 11:196, 1973.
274. Reference deleted.
275. Watts NB, Harris ST, Genant HK, et al: Intermittent cyclical etidronate treatment of postmenopausal osteoporosis, *N Engl J Med* 323:73, 1990.
276. Storm T, Thamsborg G, Steiniche T, et al: Effects of intermittent cyclical etidronate therapy on bone mass and fracture rate in women with postmenopausal osteoporosis, *N Engl J Med* 322:1265, 1990.
277. Reginster JY, Lecart MP, Deroisy R, et al: Prevention of postmenopausal bone loss by tiludronate, *Lancet* 2:1469, 1989.
278. Santora AC, Bell NH, Chesnut CH, et al: Oral alendronate treatment of bone loss in postmenopausal osteopenic women, *J Bone Miner Res (suppl)* S131, 1993.
279. Passeri M, Baroni MC, Pedrazzoni M, et al: Intermittent treatment with intravenous 4-amino-1-hydroxybutylidene-1,1-bisphosphonate (AHBuBP) in the therapy of postmenopausal osteoporosis, *Bone Miner* 15:237, 1991.
280. Marshall DH, Crilly RC, Nordin BEC: Plasma androstenedione and oesetrone levels in normal and osteoporotic postmenopausal women, *J Am Med Assoc* 171:1637, 1959.
281. Taelman P, Kaufman JM, Janssen X, et al: Persistence of increased bone resorption and possible role of dehydroepiandrosterone as a bone metabolism determinant in osteoporotic women in late postmenopause, *Maturitas* 11:65, 1989.
282. Chesnut III CH, Ivey JL, Gruger HE, et al: Stanozolol in postmenopausal osteoporosis: therapeutic efficacy and possible mechanisms of action, *Metabolism* 32:577, 1983.

283. Chesnut CHI, Nelp WB, Baylink DJ, et al: Effect of methandrostanoline on postmenopausal bone wasting as assessed by changes in total bone mineral mass, *Metabolism* 26:267, 1977.

284. Dequeker J, Geusens P: Anabolic steroids and osteoporosis, *Acta Endocrinol (suppl),* 271:45, 1985.

285. Johansen JS, Hassager C, Podenphant J, et al: Treatment of postmenopausal osteoporosis: is the anabolic steroid nandrolone decanoate a candidate? *Bone Miner* 6:77, 1989.

286. Aloia JF, Kapoer A, Vaswani A, et al: Changes in body composition following therapy of osteoporosis with methandrostaenolene, *Metabolism* 6:1076, 1989.

287. Need AG, Horowitz M, Bridges A, et al: Effects of nandrolone decanoate and antiresorptive therapy on vertebral density in osteoporotic postmenopausal women, *Arch Intern Med* 149:57, 1989.

288. Need AG, Challerton BE, Walker CJ, et al: Comparison of calcium, calcitriol, ovarian hormones and nandrolone in the treatment of osteoporosis, *Maturitas* 8:275, 1986.

289. Reference deleted.

290. Frances RM, Peacock M, Taylor GA, et al: Calcium malabsorption in elderly women with vertebral fracture: evidence for resistance to the action of vitamin D metabolites on the bowel, *Clin Sci* 66:103, 1984.

291. Gallagher JC, Riggs BL, Recker RR, et al: The effect of calcitriol on patients with postmenopausal osteoporosis with special reference to fracture frequency, *Proc Soc Exp Biol Med* 191:287, 1989.

292. Caniggia A, Nuti R, Lore F, et al: Long-term treatment with calcitriol in postmenopausal osteoporosis, *Metabolism* 39:43, 1990.

293. Arthur RS, Piraino B, Candib D, et al: Effect of low-dose calcitriol and calcium therapy on bone histomorphometry and urinary calcium excretion in osteopenic women, *Miner Electrolyte Metab* 16:385, 1990.

294. Gallagher JC, Jerpbak CM, Jee WSS, et al: 1,25-dihydroxyvitamin D3 in patients with postmenopausal osteoporosis, *Proc Natl Acad Sci U S A* 79:3325, 1982.

295. Aloia JF, Vaswani A, Yeh JK, et al: Calcitriol in the treatment of postmenopausal osteoporosis, *Am J Med* 84:401, 1988.

296. Ott SM, Chesnut CHI: Calcitriol treatment is not effective in postmenopausal osteoporosis, *Ann Intern Med* 110:267, 1989.

297. Orimo H, Shiraki M, Hayashi T, et al: Reduced occurrence of vertebral crush fractures in senile osteoporosis treated with 1-alpha(OH)-vitamin D3, *Bone Miner* 3:47, 1987.

298. Tilyard M: Lose-dose calcitriol versus calcium in established postmenopausal osteoporosis, *Metabolism* 39:50, 1990.

299. Riggs BL: Treatment of osteoporosis with sodium fluoride: an appraisal. In Peck WA, editor: *Bone and mineral research,* New York, Elsevier.

300. Jowsey J, Riggs BL, Kelly PJ, et al: Effect of combined therapy with sodium fluoride, vitamin D and calcium in osteoporosis, *Am J Med* 53:43, 1972.

301. Briancon D, Meunier PJ: Treatment of osteoporosis with fluoride, calcium, and vitamin D, *Orthop Clin North Am* 12:629, 1981.

302. Harrison JE, Bayley TA, Josse RG, et al: The relationship between fluoride effects on bone histology and on bone mass in patients with postmenopausal osteoporosis, *Bone Miner* 1:321, 1986.

303. Davies MC, Hall ML, Jacobs HS: Bone mineral loss in young women with amenorrhea, *Br Med J* 301:790, 1990.

304. Hodsman AB, Drost DJ: The response of vertebral bone mineral density during the treatment of osteoporosis with sodium fluoride, *J Clin Endocrinol Metab* 69:932, 1989.

305. Kleerekoper M, Peterson EL, Nelson DA, et al: A randomized trial of sodium fluoride as a treatment for postmenopausal osteoporosis, *Osteo Int* 1:155, 1991.

306. Riggs BL, Hodgson SF, O'Fallon WM, et al: Effect of fluoride treatment on the fracture rate in postmenopausal women with osteoporosis, *N Engl J Med* 322:802, 1990.

307. Hedlund LR, Gallagher JC: Increased incidence of hip fracture in osteoporotic women treated with sodium fluoride, *J Bone Miner Res* 4:223, 1989.

308. Gutteridge DH, Price RI, Nicholson GC, et al: Fluoride in osteoporosis—vertebral but not femoral fracture protection, *Calcif Tissue Int* 36:481, 1984.

309. Pak CYC, Sakhaee K, Zerwekh JE, et al: Safe and effective treatment of osteoporosis with intermittent slow release sodium fluoride: augmentation of vertebral bone mass and inhibition of fractures, *J Clin Endocrinol Metab* 68:150, 1989.

310. Turken S, Siris E, Seldin D, et al: Effects of tamoxifen on spinal bone density, *J Natl Cancer Inst* 81:1086, 1989.

312. Turner RT, Wakley GK, Hannon KS, et al: Tamoxifen inhibits osteoclast-mediated resorption of trabecular bone in ovarian hormone-deficient rats, *Endocrinology* 122:1146, 1988.

313. Reference deleted.

314. Reference deleted.

315. Draper MW, Flowers DE, Huster WJ, et al: Effects of raloxifene (LY 139481 HC1) on biochemical markers of bone and lipid metabolism in healthy postmenopausal women. In Christiansen C, Riis, editors: *Proceedings of the fourth international symposium on osteoporosis,* Neuropsychobiology 6:280, 1980.

316. Black LJ, Sato M, Rowley ER, et al: Raloxifene (LY 139481 HC1) prevents bone loss and reduces serum cholesterol without causing uterine hypertrophy in ovariectomized rats, *J Clin Invest* (in press), 1983.

317. Bryant HU, Black LJ, Rowley ER, et al: Raloxifene (LY 139481 HC1): bone, lipid and uterine effects in the ovariectomized rat model, *J Bone Miner Res (suppl),* 8:123, 1993.

318. Sato M, McClintock C, Kim J, et al: DEXA analysis of raloxifene effects on the lumbar vertebrae and femora of ovariectomized rats, *J Bone Miner Res* (in press), 1994.

319. Clemens JA, Bennett DR, Black LJ, et al: Effects of new antiestrogen keoxifene LY 156758 on growth of carcinogen-induced mammary tumors and on LH and prolactin levels, *Life Sci* 32:2869, 1983.

320. Lindsay R, Hart DM, Kraszewski A: Prospective double-blind trial of a synthetic steroid (Org OD14) for prevention of postmenopausal osteoporosis, *Br Med J* 1:1207, 1980.

321. Geusens P, Dequeker J, Gielen J, et al: Non-linear increase in vertebral density induced by a synthetic steroid (ORG OD 14) in women with established osteoporosis, *Maturitas* 13:155, 1991.

322. Bauer W, Aub JC, Albright F: Studies of calcium phosphorous metabolism: study of bone trabeculae as ready available reserve supply of calcium, *J Exp Med* 49:145, 1929.

323. Dempster DW, Cosman F, Parisien M, et al: Anabolic actions of parathyroid hormone on bone, *Endocr Rev* 14:690, 1993.

324. Liu CC, Kalu DN: Human parathyroid hormone (1-34) prevents bone loss, augments bone formation in sexually mature ovariectomized rats, *J Bone Miner Res* 5:973, 1990.

325. Slovik DM, Rosenthal DI, Doppelt JH, et al: Restoration of spinal bone in osteoporotic men by treatment with human parathyroid hormone (1-34) and 1,25-dihydroxyvitamin D, *J Bone Miner Res* 1:377, 1986.

326. Shen V, Dempster DW, Birchman R, et al: Loss of cancellous bone mass and connectivity in ovariectomized rats can be restored by combined treatment with parathyroid hormone and estradiol, *J Clin Invest* 91:2479, 1993.

Chapter 56

MENOPAUSE, HORMONE THERAPY, AND THE PREVENTION OF CARDIOVASCULAR DISEASES

An epidemiologic perspective

Trudy L. Bush, PhD
and Susan R. Miller, ScD

Menopause is a very profound physiologic transition in a woman's life. It is viewed not only as a progression from a reproductive to a nonreproductive state, but also as a time of accelerated biologic aging. Premenopausally, the occurrence of serious medical conditions and diseases are rare; however, in the postmenopausal period, a time both of increased age and reduction of endogenous ovarian hormones, many health problems—including cardiovascular

disease and osteoporosis—become more common. The role of endogenous hormones in the pathogenesis of many diseases, including cardiovascular disease, has not been well defined, although it is commonly believed that premenopausal women are protected from developing atherosclerosis because of high levels of circulating estrogens.

Cardiovascular disease, including coronary heart disease and stroke, is unquestionably the major cause of death among women in the United States, accounting for more than two thirds of all deaths that occur in women.[39] In the United States each year, for example, more than twice as many women die of cardiovascular disease than die of all cancers combined. Heart disease and stroke are also associated with serious morbidity in women, thus influencing not only the quantity but also the quality of life. Finally, cardiovascular disease in women, as well as in men, accounts for a tremendously high percentage of health care costs.

Despite these statistics, both women and the physicians who treat them are often unaware of the magnitude of the impact of cardiovascular disease in postmenopausal women, and may believe that breast or uterine cancer or even osteoporosis is more common than coronary disease and stroke. Fig. 56-1 presents in graphic form the relative annual impact of each of these conditions in 2000 healthy women over age 50 years. As seen in Fig. 56-1, each year 20 of the 2000 women will develop cardiovascular disease, and 12 of those 20 will die. Eleven of these women will experience a bone fracture each year, and one will succumb to her hip fracture. In contrast, six women will develop breast cancer (two of whom will die) and three will develop endometrial cancer (one of whom will die). Clearly, in terms of morbidity and particularly mortality, cardiovascu-

AMONG 2,000 POST-MENOPAUSAL WOMEN IN ONE YEAR:

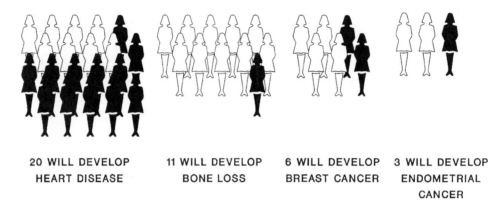

| 20 WILL DEVELOP HEART DISEASE | 11 WILL DEVELOP BONE LOSS | 6 WILL DEVELOP BREAST CANCER | 3 WILL DEVELOP ENDOMETRIAL CANCER |

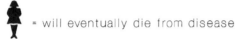 = will eventually die from disease

Fig. 56-1. Illness and death in postmenopausal women.

lar disease, which is a preventable condition, has the greatest impact on the lives and well-being of postmenopausal women.

The association between postmenopausal hormone use and cardiovascular disease in women is perceived by many as being inconsistent. This chapter reviews the epidemiologic studies that have examined the effect of hormone therapy on the risk of heart disease in women, assesses whether the evidence from the epidemiologic studies on hormone use and cardiovascular disease meets the epidemiologic criteria for a causal association, and briefly explores the overall risks and benefits of hormonal use in postmenopausal women.

EPIDEMIOLOGIC STUDIES

The studies reviewed in this chapter are presented separately by study type, since some study formats are more likely to produce biased results than others (e.g., prospective cohort studies are likely to be less biased than case-control studies). Therefore the degree of confidence in the results of any study is a function of both study type and procedural integrity, and overview approaches (including meta-analyses of results from a variety of studies) need to take these factors into account.

During the last 25 years there have been a sizable number of epidemiologic studies that have assessed whether estrogen use in women is associated with a decreased risk of heart disease and stroke. Although it is difficult to summarize the results of these often-disparate reports, it is nonetheless important to assess these studies qualitatively and to provide a quantitative approach to the

measurement of the risk of cardiovascular disease seen with estrogen use. Reports included in this chapter were selected based on the following criteria: studies were selected from published medical literature if they (1) included menopausal women who were at risk of heart disease; (2) inquired about noncontraceptive estrogen use; (3) had a major cardiovascular disease as an outcome; and (4) had risk estimates unadjusted or age adjusted only. A total of 28 published studies were found that met these criteria and are included here.

Study type

There are two basic types of epidemiologic studies: experimental and observational.

Experimental. Experimental studies include clinical trials in which assignment to the therapeutic regimen is done randomly and patients are followed prospectively for predefined outcomes. Clinical trials inspire the highest confidence level, since there is an unbiased selection to active therapy, patients are followed prospectively, and outcomes are determined by investigators who are unaware of the treatment status of the participant. However, clinical trials are very costly in both time and dollars. Thus the number of clinical trials in human populations is generally limited, since large numbers of patients must be followed for long periods of time to answer the hypothesis.

Observational. There are four major subtypes of observational studies: prospective or cohort studies, clinical cross-sectional studies, case-control studies, and population-controlled studies. Of these four subtypes, prospective studies tend to inspire the most confidence, since exposure (in this

Table 56-1. Observational studies: prospective approach

Reference	No. of women	% Users	Follow-up (mean y)	Recency of use*	End points†	Risk estimate
Lafferty and Helmuth[30]	124	49%	8.6	C	MI	0.16‡
Stampfer et al.[47]	32,317	58%	4.0	C	All CVD	0.30‡
Hammond et al.[22]	610	49%	5.0	C	All CVD	0.33‡
Bush et al.[13]	2,270	26%	8.5	C	CVD death	0.34‡
Potocki[41]	198	47%	10.0	C	CHD	0.47
Henderson et al.[23]	8,807	56%	4.5	E	MI	0.54‡
Petitti et al.[40]	6,093	43%	11.5	C	CVD death	0.60
Wolf et al.[56]	1,944	27%	16.0	C	CVD death	0.66
van der Giezen et al.[53]	13,740	6%	10.0	E	CVD death	0.67
Boysen et al.[9]	5,602	22%	5.0	E	Stroke	0.81
Criqui et al.[16]	1,868	39%	12.0	E	CVD death	0.81
Wilson et al.[54,55]	1,234	24%	10.0	E	All CVD	1.94

*C, Current user; E, ever user.
†MI, Myocardial infarction; CVD, cardiovascular disease.
‡$P < 0.05$.

case exogenous hormones) is assessed before the outcome; that is, estrogen users and nonusers are first identified as such and then followed prospectively to the end of the study period. Prospective studies differ from clinical trial in only one important area: assignment to therapy is by self-selection, instead of by random selection.

Clinical cross-sectional studies are similar to case-control studies, inasmuch as individuals are defined as diseased or nondiseased (cases or controls) by virtue of a medical examination. The exposure of interest is then assessed concurrently with the diagnosis. Thus patients are asked to recall their use of hormones. An example of this type of study would be an angiographic study, wherein women referred to this procedure would be divided into two groups: those with serious coronary artery occlusion and those with no disease. These two groups of women would then be asked about their use of hormones. Clinical cross-sectional studies are robust, since disease is defined anatomically and the cases and controls come from the same population (women referred for angiography). The major limitation is that the exposure is assessed after the medical intervention, and can be influenced by incorrect patient recall.

Case-control studies, in which estrogen use in women who have clinical heart disease (i.e., women with myocardial infarction) is compared with that seen in women who have not had infarctions (controls), provide useful information. However, these studies may be biased because women are already ill when the exposure is assessed, and those who are sick may be more or less likely to recall an exposure than those who are well. Furthermore, the possibility of including nonrepresentative cases and controls can seriously bias the risk estimate. Because of these limitations, case-control studies are often viewed as less reliable than prospective approaches.

Population-controlled studies are those in which the experience of a group of patients is compared with the experience of the population in general. For example, the death rate of estrogen users in one large clinical practice would be compared with the death rate of all the women in the state. This study design, while providing us with some information, may be the least well controlled and thus the least reliable of all the study designs.

Overview of studies

Although estrogens have been used clinically in the United States for more than 50 years, there is only one randomized prospective clinical trial of hormone use in women with cardiovascular disease (myocardial infarction) as the end point.[37] In this small study, 84 pairs of women, matched for age and medical condition, were randomly assigned to hormone therapy or placebo. These patients were long-term residents of a chronic disease hospital in New York City and were followed after randomization for 10 years. Because this trial was small, the results were not statistically significant; however, the risk estimate for estrogen users compared with nonusers for myocardial infarction was 0.3, essentially a 70% reduction of myocardial infarction in estrogen users. This trial is one of the few studies in which progestins were concurrently added to an estrogen regimen.

There are 12 prospective studies, ranging in size from very small[30] to the very large Nurses' Health Study,[47] and they are ranked in Table 56-1 according to the magnitude of their risk estimates. Six of the 12 prospective studies have risk estimates below 0.6, and five of these estimates are statistically significant. Only one prospective study, the Framingham study, shows an increased risk of cardiovascular disease of about 20% among estrogen users, but this was not statistically significant.[54,55] Another report from Framingham (not included in Table 56-1), however, showed a slight decrease in coronary disease occurrence in estrogen users.[18]

Clinical cross-sectional studies are presented in Table 56-2. As can be seen here, when atherosclerosis is defined

Table 56-2. Observational studies: clinical cross-sectional approach

Reference	No. of diseased/nondiseased women	Current use	End point	Risk estimate
Gruchow et al.[21]	154/779	Yes	Severe occlusion	0.37*
Sullivan et al.[49]	1444/744	Yes	> 70% occlusion	0.44*
McFarland et al.[35]	137/208	Yes	> 70% occlusion	0.50*
Manolio et al.[33]	2955	Yes	Carotid thickness	†

*$P < 0.05$.
†Estrogen users had significantly thinner carotid walls.

Table 56-3. Observational studies: case-control approach

Reference	No. of cases/controls	Type of control	Current use	End point	Risk estimate
Talbott et al.[52]	64/64	Community	Yes	Sudden death	0.34
Rosenberg et al.[42]	336/6730	Hospital	Yes	MI	0.47
Beard et al.[6]	86/150	Community	No	MI and sudden death	0.55
Avila et al.[3]	103/721	Community	Yes	MI	0.70
Adam et al.[1]	76/151	Community	Yes	MI	0.79
Szklo et al.[51]	36/39	Hospital	No	MI	0.83
Rosenberg et al.[43]	105/303	Hospital	Yes	MI	1.05
La Vecchia et al.[31]	116/160	Hospital	Yes	MI	1.62
Jick et al.[28]	17/34	Hospital	Yes	MI	7.50*

*$P < 0.05$.

Table 56-4. Observational studies: population-controlled approach

Reference	No. of women	Follow-up (y)	End point*	Risk estimate
MacMahon[32]	1891 users	12.0	ASHD death	0.30†
Burch et al.[10]	737 users	13.3	CHD death	0.43†
Hunt et al.[26]	4544	10.1	CVD death	0.37†

*ASHD, Arteriosclerotic heart disease; CHD, coronary heart disease; CVD, cardiovascular disease.
†$P < 0.05$.

anatomically all of the studies show significantly less coronary artery disease in estrogen users as compared with nonusers. Furthermore, the magnitude of the reduction in coronary lesions ranges from 50% to 63% among hormone users.

Overall, there have been nine published case-control studies that have examined the association of hormone use with cardiovascular disease in women (Table 56-3), and these range in size from very small (17 cases in reference 28) to relatively large (336 cases in reference 42). Although the majority of these studies report a 20% or greater reduction in the risk of cardiovascular disease and death in women using hormones postmenopausally, none of these results is statistically significant. Furthermore, two reports[28,31] found an increase in risk of myocardial infarction (MI) among women taking hormones.

The three published population controlled studies are presented in Table 56-4, and all show statistically significant reductions in the risk of heart disease ranging from 50% to 70%. Two of these studies are from the United States[10,32] and one is from Great Britain.[26]

If the risk estimates in these 28 published studies are weighted for study type (clinical trials > prospective studies > clinical cross-sectional studies > case-control studies > population-controlled studies) and study size (larger studies > smaller studies), an overall summary risk estimate can be calculated. This is a simple but direct way to summarize a large amount of information while taking into account the quality of the study (study type) as well as the stability of the estimates (study size). When this is done, the summary risk estimate is 0.5, suggesting a 50% reduction in the risk of cardiovascular disease in women using hormones postmenopausally. This degree of reduction (approximately 50%) has also been reported with more sophisticated statistical approaches.[20,46]

EPIDEMIOLOGIC CRITERIA FOR CAUSALITY

Although many believe that a causal association between an exposure and an outcome cannot be demonstrated in the absence of a clinical trial, it is difficult, expensive, and sometimes unethical to conduct a randomized, double-blind, clinical trial to assess the effect of a given exposure.

Because of this problem, a set of criteria has been developed that, if met, would provide sufficient evidence of a causal association in lieu of clinical trial (experimental) data.[34] One example of this approach, which uses epidemiologic reasoning, is the association between lung cancer and cigarette smoking in humans. Given the quality, quantity, and biologic plausibility of data on smoking and lung cancer risk, nearly all scientists conclude that smoking causes lung cancer. However, this conclusion is based on implicit reasoning, using these epidemiologic criteria for causality rather than on any clinical trial evidence. This same logical process can be used to assess the relationship of postmenopausal estrogen use and heart disease in women. Six criteria for causality include the following:

1. Consistency of the association
2. Proper time sequence demonstrated
3. Dose-response demonstrated
4. Strength of association meaningful
5. Change in risk with change in exposure
6. Biologic plausibility

Consistency of the association

Consistency of the association requires that the data be consistent, and one way to assess consistency is to examine the association over time, across different geographic areas, or with different methods or different populations. Regarding the hormone use–cardiovascular disease association, some degree of reduction in heart disease in women using estrogen has been reported in the 1960s, the 1970s, the 1980s, and the 1990s. Furthermore, a reduction in risk is seen with a variety of end points, including nonfatal and fatal myocardial infarction, stroke, coronary stenosis, fatal heart disease, sudden death, and all cardiovascular disease. Reductions in cardiovascular disease risk among estrogen users also is seen in disparate geographic areas, including Poland, England, New Zealand, Israel, Germany, Canada, and in various states in the United States. There is also consistency across different age groups, since hormone users in their sixth, seventh, eighth, and even ninth decade had reductions in cardiovascular disease.[23,33] Based on these findings, it can be concluded that the association between postmenopausal hormone use and cardiovascular disease meets the first criterion for causality.

Proper time sequence

Demonstration of proper time sequence requires that the exposure occurred before the outcome event. In the one clinical trial and in all of the prospective and population-controlled studies, hormone use preceded the occurrence of cardiovascular disease.

Dose-response

Very few of these studies addressed the issue of whether the dose of estrogen taken was associated with a differential risk of disease. Only four reports assessed a dose-response, and three found no association between increasing dose of estrogen and protection against heart disease. However, one, the Leisure World study,[23] found that a dose of 1.25 mg of conjugated estrogen was superior to a dose of 0.625 mg. Given the limited information available, it cannot be determined whether a dose-response relationship exists. Furthermore, this criterion may not be entirely appropriate for evaluating the hormone–cardiovascular disease association, since high doses of estrogen may produce a hypercoagulable state in selected women, leading to an increased risk of adverse events, including thromboembolic disease.

Strength of the association

To fulfill this criterion, the strength of the association between exposure and outcome must be substantial and meaningful. About two thirds of all the studies reviewed in this chapter have estimated that the risk of cardiovascular disease in estrogen users is less than 0.5. A 50% reduction in the risk of the most important cause of morbidity and mortality in women represents a very strong effect.

Change in risk with change in exposure

This is a very important criterion, since if a change in risk occurs with a change in exposure (i.e., smoking cessation leads to a reduction in risk of lung cancer) it is unlikely to be the result of other factors. Three of the studies have assessed whether current estrogen users had lower risks of cardiovascular disease than women who had ever taken estrogen (some women had stopped using estrogen previously). The results of all three studies show that current users have a lower risk of cardiovascular disease than ever users.

Biologic plausibility

Oral estrogens have long been known to alter plasma lipids in a generally favorable manner, and moderate doses of both natural and synthetic estrogens decrease low-density lipoprotein (LDL) cholesterol by about the same amount as dietary restrictions, and increase high-density lipoprotein (HDL) cholesterol about the same amount as moderate alcohol consumption. As reported by Barnes et al.,[5] a dose of 0.625 mg of oral conjugated estrogen reduces total cholesterol approximately 4% to 6%, reduces LDL cholesterol about 15%, and increases HDL cholesterol by approximately 15%. These beneficial changes in lipoprotein levels have been hypothesized to account for 30% to 50% of the observed reduction in cardiovascular risk (Table 56-5).[13,21]

More recently scientists in the United States and elsewhere have been investigating nonlipid, cardioprotective effects of estrogen on the vascular system in an attempt to explain the remaining 50% to 70% reduction in risk. Current data suggest that estrogens have direct salutary effects on the vascular wall, can increase cardiac output and coronary flow, and can decrease peripheral systemic resistance.

Table 56-5. Cox model results from the Lipid Research Clinics Program follow-up study. Risk of cardiovascular death by selected factors.

Factors	β	SE*	p†	OR‡
Five year increase in age	.805	.024	.000	2.24
Five mm Hg increase in SBPss	.680	.006	.018	1.97
Cigarette smoking	.416	.012	.000	1.52
Non-use of estrogen	-.981	.448	.010	2.70

*SE, standard error
†p, probability
‡OR, odds ratio
ssSBP, systolic blood pressure.

Table 56-6. Studies of secondary prevention

Reference	End point	% Reduction
Nachtigall et al.[38]	CVD death	74
Bush[11]	CVD death	82
Henderson et al.[24]	CHD death	66
Cooperative Study Group[2]	Death, stroke, or retinal infarction	82
Sullivan et al.[50]	Death	90

With one exception (i.e., dose-response), the estrogen–cardiovascular disease association appears to meet the epidemiologic criteria for causality. The hypothesis that estrogens cause a reduction in the risk of cardiovascular disease must now be seriously considered. To summarize this chapter at this point, the quantitative evaluations of the published studies on this association suggest that estrogen use is associated with approximately a 50% reduction in cardiovascular disease occurrence, and a qualitative evaluation suggests that estrogen use is causally associated with the reduction of cardiovascular disease.

HORMONES AND THE SECONDARY PREVENTION OF CARDIOVASCULAR DISEASE

Although most of the studies that evaluated the effect of estrogen use on cardiovascular disease are studies of primary prevention, there are actually five reports in the literature that have assessed the effect of estrogen use on the occurrence of cardiovascular death and further events in women who already have frank cardiovascular disease.[2,11,24,38,50] In comparison to those studies of primary prevention, these five studies all show that hormone use in women with established disease reduces the risk of death and further events by approximately 70% to 90% (Table 56-6). This degree of reduction in risk is marked and has rarely been seen with any pharmacologic treatment. It also suggests that estrogens influence the risk of subsequent cardiovascular disease via a powerful nonlipid mechanism.

This mechanism probably results in a stabilized vascular system resistant to spasm. This hypothesis is plausible, given that estrogens have long been used very effectively to treat perimenopausal and postmenopausal hot flashes and flushes (vasomotor instability). These results further suggest that much of the primary prevention of cardiovascular disease seen with estrogen use may be effected by lipoprotein changes, whereas the secondary prevention of cardiovascular disease seen with estrogen use may be mediated via a stabilized vascular system.

ESTROGEN/PROGESTIN USE AND CARDIOVASCULAR DISEASE

Many women now use a combined estrogen/progestin regimen for treatment of menopausal symptoms and prevention of osteoporosis and heart disease. However, the effect of progestins on risk of these conditions is not well studied. Although some investigators have suggested that this combination of hormone therapy is superior to estrogen only,[57] others are less sanguine. Because progestins may negate or overwhelm the effect of estrogen on many biologic systems, and because these hormones may have adverse effects not mediated through estrogen receptors, the full impact of their use is not known. Future studies, including the postmenopausal estrogen and progestin intervention (PEPI) trial, may shed some much-needed light on this issue.

The issue concerning progestins is an important one. All progestins have androgenic effects, which decrease HDL cholesterol, increase LDL cholesterol, and increase glucose intolerance. These alterations should result in a worse cardiovascular profile. There is little information on cardiovascular risks in postmenopausal women using estrogen/progestin compounds, but there is evidence from women using oral contraceptives that the rate of arterial disease increases with the increase in progestin content of oral contraceptives.[29] This increase in disease is paralleled by a reduction in HDL cholesterol, which is also dose-dependent.

ESTROGEN THERAPY: BENEFITS VERSUS RISKS

Concern remains as to whether the benefits of estrogen therapy outweigh the known risks, and this concern is emphasized because some investigators do not agree that estrogen use is causally associated with a reduction in coronary risk. Instead, it is argued that selection bias to estrogen use, rather than estrogen use per se, accounts for much of the protective effect seen in the studies of cardiovascular disease. That is, healthier women are more likely to take estrogen than less healthy women; therefore estrogen users are protected not because of the estrogens but because they were healthier initially.

In all of the observational epidemiologic studies, selection bias cannot be ruled out. That is, women who take estrogen may do better because of some factors associated with their taking the drug rather than the drug itself. Although a clinical trial is considered necessary to address this issue fully, subgroup analysis can provide insights into whether selection bias exists and, if so, how much of the effect may be due to it. Several studies described below suggest that selection bias for hormone use does not markedly influence the magnitude of the protection afforded estrogen users.

The Lipid Research Clinics Program follow-up study included 2270 white women between the ages of 40 and 69 years at entry who were followed for an average of 15 years.[11,13] The study found a 70% decreased risk of cardiovascular death in estrogen users compared with women who were not using estrogen at entry into the study. A strong protective effect of estrogen was seen across a broad age span, in hypertensive and in normotensive women, in better educated and in less educated women, and in nonsmokers as well as in those currently smoking. As seen in Table 56-5, non-use of estrogen remained a strong significant predictor of cardiovascular death after adjusting for the other risk factors. Although selection bias for estrogen use may be real, it does not appear to explain much of the protective effect in this population.

Another study provides further evidence that the issue of selection bias may be inflated. Using angiographically defined end points, Sullivan et al.[49] found that estrogen was protective regardless of cholesterol level at baseline or smoking habits. Patients who were nonsmokers with a cholesterol level less than 235/dL had a 69% decrease in risk, whereas those with a cholesterol level greater than 235 mg/dL had an 88% decrease. Among smokers, those with low cholesterol had a 33% decrease in risk and those with high cholesterol had a 71% decrease in actual coronary lesions.

There are questions, however, regarding the effect of route of administration on cardioprotection. There are no data on the effects of non–oral estrogens on cardiovascular disease per se. Furthermore, compared with oral agents, lipid and lipoprotein changes with non–oral estrogens are either absent or diminished.[12,27] Thus it cannot be assumed that the cardioprotective and other metabolic effects will be similar to those seen with oral estrogen.

There are two important risks associated with use of unopposed estrogen therapy: the documented increased risk of uterine cancer and a perceived increased risk of breast cancer. Uterine cancer occurs in 2/1000 postmenopausal women per year.[36] After 2 to 4 years of unopposed estrogen use, that rate is increased three to five times; furthermore, the risk is also dose and duration dependent, and it persists for several years after therapy is halted.[45]

Estrogen-associated endometrial cancer, however, tends to be small, low-grade, and an early-stage disease, which is treatable and has a high cure rate. Collins et al.[14] compared the survivorship of women with endometrial cancer using estrogens with those who had never used estrogen. After 10 years, women who used estrogen and developed endometrial cancer had better survival rates than women who did not use estrogen and did not get cancer. The 10-year survivorship was about 75% for nonusers who did not develop cancer, compared with 90% for estrogen users who did develop endometrial cancers.

The evidence regarding hormone therapy and breast cancer risk is equivocal at best. There are good reasons to hypothesize an association between estrogen and breast cancer, because estrogen stimulates mitoses in breast cells and has been shown to promote breast tumors in rats. (This may not be true in humans.) Estrogen, as a major endocrine product of the ovary, also is associated with a variety of risk factors for development of breast cancer, including early menarche, late age at first birth, late age at menopause, and early oophorectomy. However, it should be noted that postmenopausal ovarian products, specifically dehydroepiandrosterone, have also been linked to the development of breast cancer.[19]

There have been several meta-analyses published that have attempted to examine the estrogen–breast cancer association.[17,20,48] Overall, these summary reports suggest a very small increase in breast cancer incidence among women who have ever used estrogens (relative risk = 1.1). However, survivorship after diagnosis of breast cancer in women who have used estrogens is markedly improved compared with that of women who have never used estrogens,[7,8,16,24] a situation similar to that seen in endometrial cancer. One conclusion that may be derived from these results is that breast cancer may be promoted but not initiated by estrogen use. A second possibility is that women using estrogens are more likely to have their breast tumors diagnosed earlier, since they are under the care of a physician. Nonetheless, these data should be relatively reassuring in that the risk of breast cancer does not appear to be markedly increased among estrogen users. In fact, given that investigators have been looking for an estrogen–breast cancer link for decades, the lack of significant findings should be very reassuring.

ESTROGEN USE IN WOMEN WITH CANCER

One of the most pressing clinical questions today is whether the use of postmenopausal hormonal therapy is safe in women who have or who have had cancer.[4,15] Many women are now being diagnosed with small, noninvasive lesions within their breasts found on screening mammography. These women by and large survive their breast cancers only to remain at risk for developing menopausal symptoms and the other conditions associated with estrogen, that is, heart disease and osteoporosis.[44] This same question regarding safely also is true for women who have had endometrial cancer.

Answers to these questions will be forthcoming, because women with breast and uterine cancer seek treatment with these hormones to preserve quality of life and to protect themselves against osteoporosis and heart disease. Several observation studies under way in both the United States and Australia are following women with breast cancer treated with postmenopausal hormonal therapy to determine whether they experience a different survivorship than that of untreated women.

SUMMARY

A net-benefit equation for estimated changes in mortality with estrogen therapy has been calculated by Henderson et al.[25] Even assuming a twofold increase in the risk of breast cancer with estrogen use, there is a 41% decrease in all-cause mortality in women who receive estrogen therapy, because of the magnitude of beneficial effects on osteoporotic fracture and heart disease incidence. Since cardiovascular disease is the major cause of morbidity and mortality in postmenopausal women, and since the beneficial effects of estrogen outweigh the documented and perceived risk of estrogen use, estrogen ought to be considered as prophylactic therapy, particularly in women at high risk of heart disease.

REFERENCES

1. Adam S, Williams V, Vessey MP: Cardiovascular disease and hormone replacement treatment: a pilot case-control study, *Br Med J* 282:122, 1981.
2. American-Canadian Cooperative Study Group: Persantine aspirin trial in cerebral ischemia, III: risk factors for stroke, *Stroke* 17:12, 1986.
3. Avila MH, Walker AM, Jick H: Use of replacement estrogens and the risk of myocardial infarction, *Epidemiology* 1:128, 1990.
4. Baker DP: Estrogen replacement therapy in patients with previous endometrial carcinoma, *Compr Ther* 16(1):28, 1990.
5. Barnes RB, Roy S, Lobo RA: Comparison of lipid and androgen levels after conjugated estrogen or depo-medroxyprogesterone acetate treatment in postmenopausal women, *Obstet Gynecol* 66:216, 1985.
6. Beard CM et al: The Rochester Coronary Heart Disease project: effect of cigarette smoking, hypertension, diabetes, and steroidal estrogen use on coronary heart disease among 40- to 59-year-old women, 1960–1982, *Mayo Clin Proc* 64:1471, 1989.
7. Bergkvist L et al: Prognosis after breast cancer diagnosis in women exposed to estrogen and estrogen-progesterone replacement therapy, *Am J Epidermiol* 130:221, 1989.
8. Bergkvist L et al: The risk of breast cancer after estrogen and estrogen-progestin replacement, *N Engl J Med* 321:293, 1989.
9. Boysen G et al: Stroke incidence and risk factors for stroke in Copenhagen, Denmark, *Stroke* 19:1345, 1988.
10. Burch JC, Byrd BF Jr, Vaughn WK: The effects of long-term estrogen on hysterectomized women, *Am J Obstet Gynecol* 118:778, 1974.
11. Bush TL: Long-term effect of estrogen use on cardiovascular death in women: results from the Lipid Research Clinics' (LRC) Follow-Up Study. American Heart Association 31st Annual Conference on Cardiovascular Disease Epidemiology, March 1991, Orlando, Florida.
12. Bush TL, Miller V: Effects of pharmacologic agents used during menopause: impact on lipids and lipoproteins. In Mishell D, editor: *Menopause, physiology and pharmacology,* Chicago, 1987, Year Book.
13. Bush TL et al: Cardiovascular mortality and noncontraceptive estrogen use in women: results from the Lipid Research Clinics Program follow-up study, *Circulation* 75:1102, 1987.
14. Collins J et al: Oestrogen use and survival in endometrial cancer, *Lancet* 2:961, 1980.
15. Creasman WT: Recommendations regarding estrogen replacement therapy after treatment of endometrial cancer, *Oncology* 6:23, 1992.
16. Criqui MH et al: Postmenopausal estrogen use and mortality, *Am J Epidemiol* 128:606, 1988.
17. Dupont WD, Page DL: Menopausal estrogen replacement therapy and breast cancer, *Arch Intern Med* 151:67, 1991.
18. Eaker ED, Castelli WP: Coronary heart disease and its risk factors among women in the Framingham study. In Eaker ED et al, editors: *Coronary heart disease in women,* New York, 1987, Haymarket Doyma.
19. Gordon G et al: Relationship of serum levels of dehydroepiandrosterone and dehydroepiandrosterone sulfate to the risk of developing postmenopausal breast cancer, *Cancer Res* 59:3859, 1990.
20. Grady D et al: Hormone therapy to prevent disease and prolong life in postmenopausal women, *Ann Intern Med* 117:1016, 1992.
21. Gruchow HW et al: Postmenopausal use of estrogen and occlusion of coronary arteries, *Am Heart J* 115:954, 1988.
22. Hammond CB et al: Effects of long-term estrogen replacement therapy, I: metabolic effects, *Am J Obstet Gynecol* 133:525, 1979.
23. Henderson BE, Paganini-Hill A, Ross RK: Estrogen replacement therapy and protection from acute myocardial infarction, *Am J Obstet Gynecol* 159:312, 1988.
24. Henderson BE, Paganini-Hill A, Ross RK: Decreased mortality in users of estrogen replacement therapy, *Arch Intern Med* 151:75, 1991.
25. Henderson BE, Ross RK, Paganini-Hill A: Estrogen use and cardiovascular disease, *J Reprod Med* 30:814, 1985.
26. Hunt K, Vessey M, McPherson K: Mortality in a cohort of long-term users of hormone replacement therapy: an updated analysis, *Br J Obstet Gynaecol* 97:1080, 1990.
27. Jensen J, Riis BJ, Strom V: Long-term effects of percutaneous estrogens and oral progesterone on serum lipoproteins in postmenopausal women, *Am J Obstet Gynecol* 156:66, 1987.
28. Jick H, Dinan B, Rothman K: Noncontraceptive estrogens and nonfatal myocardial infarction, *JAMA* 239:1407, 1978.
29. Kay C: Progestogens and arterial disease, evidence from the Royal College of General Practitioners study, *Am J Obstet Gynecol* 142:762, 1982.
30. Lafferty FW, Helmuth DO: Post-menopausal estrogen replacement: the prevention of osteoporosis and systemic effects, *Maturitas* 7:147, 1985.
31. La Vecchia C et al: Risk factors for myocardial infarction in young women, *Am J Epidemiol* 125:832, 1987.
32. MacMahon B: Cardiovascular disease and non-contraceptive oestrogen therapy. In Oliver MF, editor: *Coronary heart disease in young women,* Edinburgh, 1978, Churchill Livingstone.
33. Manolio T et al: Associations of postmenopausal estrogen use with cardiovascular disease and its risk factors in older women, *Circulation* 88:2163, 1993.
34. Mausner JS, Kramer S: *Epidemiology: an introductory text,* Philadelphia, 1985, WB Saunders.
35. McFarland KF et al: Risk factors and noncontraceptive estrogen use in women with and without coronary disease, *Am Heart J* 117:1209, 1989.
36. Miller BA et al, editors: *Cancer statistics review: 1973–1989,* NIH Pub No 92-2789, Bethesda, Md, 1992, National Cancer Institute.
37. Nachtigall LE et al: Estrogen replacement therapy, II: a prospective study in the relationship to carcinoma and cardiovascular and metabolic problems, *Obstet Gynecol* 54:74, 1979.
38. Nachtigall M et al: Incidence of breast cancer in a 22-year study of women receiving estrogen-progestin replacement therapy, *Obstet Gynecol* 80:827, 1992.
39. National Center for Health Statistics: *Vital statistics of the United States, 1986,* vol II, *Mortality,* part A, DHHS Pub No 88-1122, Public Health Service, Washington, DC, 1988, US Government Printing Office.
40. Petitti DB, Perlman JA, Sidney S: Noncontraceptive estrogens and mortality: long-term follow-up of women in the Walnut Creek Study, *Obstet Gynecol* 70:289, 1987.

41. Potocki J: Wplyw leczenia estrogenami na niewydolnose wiencowa u kobiet po menopauzie, *J Pol Tyg Lek* 216:1812, 1971.

42. Rosenberg L, Armstrong B, Jick H: Myocardial infarction and estrogen therapy in post-menopausal women, *N Engl J Med* 294:1256, 1976.

43. Rosenberg L et al: Noncontraceptive estrogens and myocardial infarction in young women, *JAMA* 244:399, 1980.

44. Satariano WA, Ragheb NE, Dupuis MH: Comorbidity in older women with breast cancer: an epidemiologic approach. In Yancik R, Yates R, editors: *Cancer in the elderly: approaches to early diagnosis and treatment,* New York, 1989, Springer Publishing.

45. Shapiro S, Kelly JP, Rosenberg L: Risk of localized and widespread endometrial cancer in relation to recent and discontinued use of conjugated estrogens, *N Engl J Med* 313:969, 1985.

46. Stampfer MJ, Colditz GA: Estrogen replacement therapy and coronary heart disease: a quantitative assessment of the epidemiologic evidence, *Prev Med* 20:47, 1991.

47. Stampfer MJ et al: A prospective study of postmenopausal estrogen therapy and coronary heart disease, *N Engl J Med* 313:1044, 1986.

48. Steinberg KK, Thacker SB, Smith JC: A meta-analysis of the effect of estrogen replacement therapy on the risk of breast cancer, *JAMA* 265:1985, 1991.

49. Sullivan JM et al: Postmenopausal estrogen use and coronary atherosclerosis, *Ann Intern Med* 108:358, 1988.

50. Sullivan JM et al: Estrogen replacement and coronary artery disease: effect on survival in postmenopausal women, *Arch Intern Med* 150:2557, 1990.

51. Szklo M et al: Estrogen use and myocardial infarction risk: a case-control study, *Prev Med* 13:510, 1984.

52. Talbott E et al: Biologic and psychosocial risk factors of sudden death from coronary disease in white women, *Am J Cardiol* 39:858, 1977.

53. van der Giezen AM et al: Systolic blood pressure and cardiovascular mortality among 13,740 Dutch women, *Prev Med* 19:456, 1990.

54. Wilson PWF, Garrison RJ, Castelli WP: Postmenopausal estrogen use, cigarette smoking, and cardiovascular morbidity in women over 50: the Framingham Study, *N Engl J Med* 313:1038, 1985.

55. Wilson PWF, Garrison RJ, Castelli WP: Postmenopausal estrogen use and heart disease, *N Engl J Med* 315:135, 1986 (letter).

56. Wolf PH et al: Reduction of cardiovascular disease-related mortality among postmenopausal women who use hormones: evidence from a national cohort, *Am J Obstet Gynecol* 164:489, 1991.

57. Wood H, Wang-Cheng R, Nattinger AB: Postmenopausal hormone replacement: are two hormones better than one?, *J Gen Intern Med* 8:451, 1993.

Part IX

SPECIALIZED PROCEDURES

Chapter 57

THE ROLE OF ULTRASOUND IN THE MANAGEMENT OF INFERTILITY

Roger C. Sanders, MD

Conception is an intricate and complex event. Some of the most important aspects of the process of union of the sperm and the oocyte occur on such a microscopic scale that visualization with ultrasound is not feasible. Some portions of the conception route are obscured by intestinal gas or bone. Nevertheless, high-frequency ultrasound can be used to look at the testes, epididymides, prostate gland, seminal vesicles, some portions of the vasa deferentia, the ovaries, the fallopian tubes, and the uterus. The only portion of the pathway that is not well visualized is most of the course of the vas deferens and the intimate details of the fallopian tube anatomy. Real-time ultrasound is cinematic and is, so far as is known, harmless; thus repeated studies can be performed and dynamic events such as ovulation can be imaged. Ultrasound therefore has become an invaluable tool in the investigation and treatment of infertility.

MALE INFERTILITY

The testes and epididymides are exquisitely seen with ultrasound because they are so superficial. High-frequency transducers (e.g., 7.5 and 10 MHz) can be used with or without a standoff pad.

Infertility problems in the scrotum

The normal adult testis is approximately $3.5 \times 4 \times 2.5$ cm. Smaller testes may be seen in hypofertile individuals. Normally the epididymis is seen as a tubular echopenic structure on the posterior aspect of the testis. Its relationship to the testis is most variable; sometimes it lies laterally, sometimes posteriorly. The appendix epididymis is a relatively large cranial portion of the epididymis that is well visualized if a hydrocele is present (Fig. 57-1). Otherwise it tends to blend in with the surrounding peritesticular tissue.

Undescended testes. Sperm production by undescended testes commonly is diminished. Visualization of undescended testes with ultrasound is satisfactory as long as they lie at or below the inguinal ligament. If they are intraabdominal, they cannot be seen with ultrasound. Undescended testes are of the same size and ovoid shape as descended testes and of the same acoustic texture (Fig. 57-2).

Varicocele. The most common cause of infertility seen in the scrotum is a varicocele. Varicoceles are associated with low sperm count and sperm hypomotility. The typical varicocele is visible in the left scrotal wall as a series of dilated veins that lie lateral and superior to the testis (Fig. 57-3). Venous structures in this area are considered to constitute a varicocele if one or more veins measure at least 3 mm when maximally distended. A tortuous configuration of the venous drainage of the scrotum, however, is suggestive of varicocele even though the caliber of the largest vein is smaller than 3 mm. Although many varicoceles can be palpated, some can be seen only with ultrasound and cannot be felt.[49] There is a difference between the diameter of the vein at rest, in the supine position, and when venous pressure is increased by straining or by the erect position.[64] Varicoceles may also occur on the right. If a right varico-

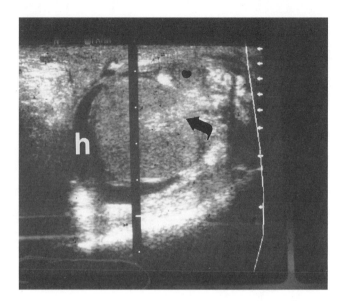
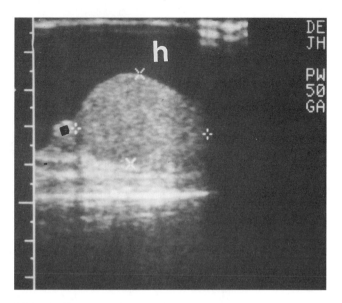

Fig. 57-1. A, Transverse view of the testis and the epididymis. The mediastinum testis (*arrow*), the site where the tubules leave the testis, can be seen adjacent to the epididymis (*black dot*). There is a small hydrocele (*h*) present. **B,** Longitudinal view. The appendix epidydymis (*black square*) lies superior to the testis. There is a large hydrocele (*h*) present.

cele is larger than the left or an abnormality is present only on the right, a renal mass may be occluding the testicular vein. With large left varicoceles it is also worthwhile to look in the left renal fossa to ensure that no renal mass is present. Venous flow can be seen within the dilated veins with high-quality real-time systems. Doppler can be used to confirm venous flow. Color flow may also be used, although the amount of flow is so small that color flow does not add much information.[59]

Ischemia and torsion. With acute infection of the epididymis or the testis (e.g., mumps) the vascular supply of the testis is compressed and infarction may occur. Testicular torsion may also result in infarction. Torsion has a predisposition to be bilateral in a testis with a "bell clapper" deformity. Bilateral torsion will result in infertility. After infarction the testis becomes atrophic and small. It is usually echogenic (Fig. 57-4).

Seminal vesicles and vasa deferentia

Unfortunately, the vasa deferentia cannot be visualized between the region superior to the scrotum and posterior to the bladder, but they can be seen in the area immediately superior to the seminal vesicles and the prostate gland and posterior to the bladder. To visualize the vasa deferentia and seminal vesicles transrectal ultrasonography is performed. The seminal vesicle lies lateral to the vas deferens, but the two organs are easily confused because the textures of both are very similar (Fig. 57-5). The ejaculatory ducts lead through the prostate gland to the seminal vesicles (Fig. 57-6). Congenital absence of the seminal vesicles or vasa

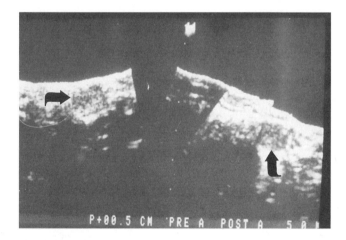

Fig. 57-2. Transverse B-scan view of both groins. Undescended testes (*arrows*) can be seen on both sides as ovoid echopenic masses.

deferentia (vasal aplasia) can be seen readily with ultrasound (Fig. 57-7). It occurs in 1% to 6% of series of infertile men and accounts for 4.4% to 17% of cases of azoospermia.[15, 57] In a series of 85 patients with azoospermia with a low volume of ejaculate, transrectal ultrasound showed bilateral absence in 12 and unilateral absence in 18.[69] In most instances both the seminal vesicles and vasa deferentia are absent, but this is not always the case. If the vasa deferentia are absent or narrowed, cysts may be seen superior to the area of blockage posterior to the bladder at the termination of the vasa deferentia. It is possible that aspiration of such cysts might yield spermatozoa that could

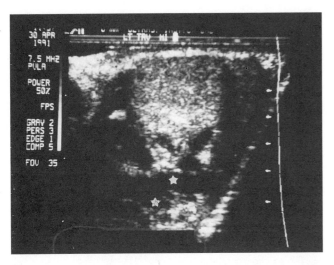
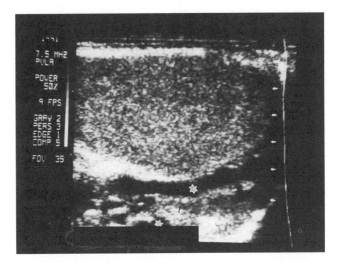

Fig. 57-3. Varicocele. **A,** Transverse view. **B,** Longitudinal view. Posterior to the left testis large venous tubular structures (*asterisks*) can be seen that showed flow when color flow was used.

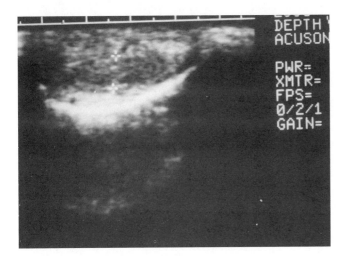

Fig. 57-4. Atrophic testis. The testis (*between asterisks*) is much smaller than usual and has a more echogenic structure.

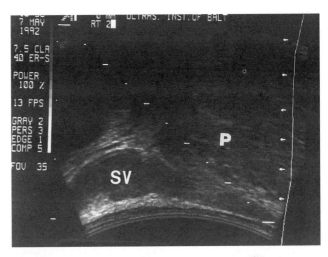

Fig. 57-5. Normal seminal vesicle and prostate gland. Longitudinal view. The seminal vesicle (*SV*) can be seen posterior to the bladder. *P,* Prostate.

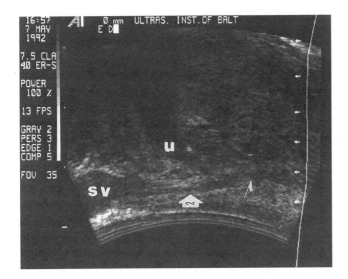

Fig. 57-6. Longitudinal view. The ejaculatory duct (*arrowhead*) can be tracked to the verumontanum (*small arrow*). The urethra can be seen (*u*). *SV,* Seminal vesicle.

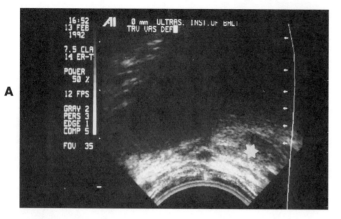

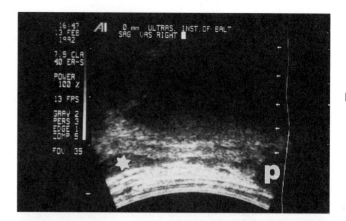

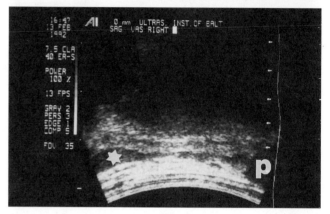

Fig. 57-7. A, Absence of right vas deferens and seminal vesicle. Transverse view. A seminal vesicle (*asterisk*) is seen only on the left. **B,** Partial absence of left seminal vesicle. Sagittal view on the left. No seminal vesicle can be seen. *p,* Prostate gland. **C,** Sagittal view on the right. An attenuated seminal vesicle can be seen between the normal seminal vesicle portion (*asterisk*) and the prostate gland (*p*).

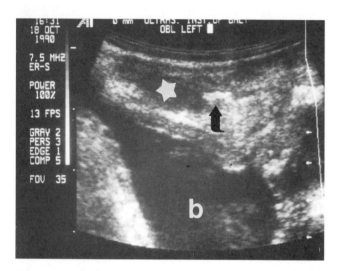

Fig. 57-8. Ejaculatory duct blockage. The ejaculatory duct is dilated (*star*) because of the presence of a calcification (*arrow*) within the ejaculatory duct. *b,* Bladder.

then be inseminated into the partner's uterus, but this has proved unsuccessful thus far.

Ejaculatory duct blockage may sometimes be seen with ultrasound (Fig. 57-8). Blockage is usually unilateral, but bilateral ejaculatory duct blockage due to calculi may occur.[57] Calculi develop close to the verumontanum at the narrowest point of the ejaculatory duct. The ducts become dilated proximal to the calculi. Isolated absence of the ejaculatory ducts may occur. In this situation the seminal vesicles are dilated and full of spermatozoa. In one patient, injection of contrast medium into the seminal vesicles under ultrasound control with subsequent roentgenography showed absence of the ejaculatory ducts and the presence of a cystic müllerian duct that both seminal vesicles joined. A new channel from the müllerian duct cyst to the veru-

montanum was created with a neodymium:yttrium-aluminum-garnet (Nd:YAG) laser with subsequent normal semen analysis.[23]

FEMALE INFERTILITY

Follicle production takes place within the ovaries. The ovaries can be seen throughout life with transabdominal ultrasound, but visualization is poor in small children and menopausal women, at which time only the transabdominal approach can be used. The vaginal probe permits much greater detail,[2,55] and, fortunately, this technique is usable during the ages when infertility is being assessed. Occasionally patients with high ovaries can be investigated only by the transabdominal approach. The seminal studies by Hackeloer[29] showed that follicular development could be followed with ultrasound.

Ovaries

The ovaries are located in the broad ligament, and on transabdominal ultrasonography the usual location of the ovaries is at the same level as the uterine horns; this site is often adjacent to the echogenic focus in the iliopsoas muscle that represents the sciatic nerve. When using the endovaginal probe fewer anatomic landmarks are available, but the ovaries usually lie close to the uterus alongside the iliac vessels (Fig. 57-9). If there is any free fluid present the fallopian tube may be outlined; the ovaries will be seen

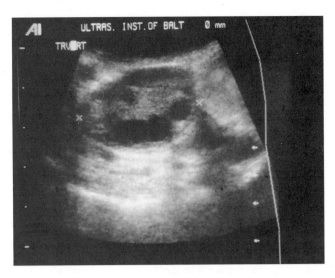

Fig. 57-9. Normal ovary. There are three small follicles within the ovary, which is in the follicular phase of the cycle; none of the follicles has yet become a dominant follicle.

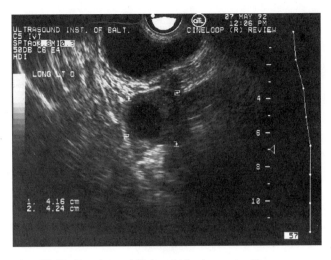

Fig. 57-10. Dominant follicle within the ovary (*between measurement marks*). The patient is at day 14 of the cycle. The follicle is 2.3 cm in diameter and about to ovulate.

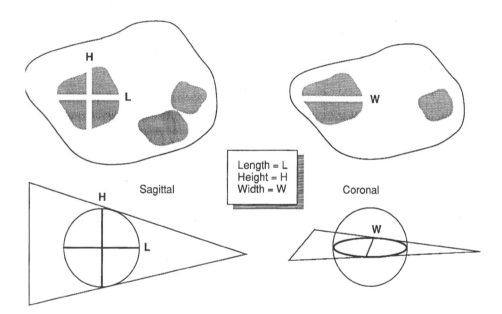

Length = L
Height = H
Width = W

Fig. 57-11. Diagram showing appropriate measurement technique to measure the follicle in all three dimensions. Follicles are measured in both the sagittal and coronal plane so that volume can be calculated. (Redrawn with permission from *Clinical sonography: a practical guide*, ed. 2.)

adjacent to the fimbriated end of the fallopian tube. The normal menarcheal ovary is approximately 3 × 2 × 2 cm.

Ovulation usually alternates from the left ovary to the right ovary (some dispute this)[7]; the dominant follicle becomes larger than other waiting follicles at about the eighth day of the cycle and thereafter gradually increases in size[16,30] (Fig. 57-10). The dominant follicle grows from about 8 mm to at least 15 mm in size. Follicular rupture takes place when the follicle is between 1.5 and 2.7 cm in size.[44,48,65] In most women other, smaller, follicles (less than 8 mm in diameter) are visible dispersed throughout the

ovary. Endovaginal ultrasonic measurements of follicle size have been shown repeatedly to be more accurate than measurements derived from the transabdominal approach.[4] Measurements are best made in three dimensions; the volume is then calculated by using the formula for a prolate ellipse (length × width × height × 0.5233) for each follicle (Fig. 57-11). The follicle should be named in the same fashion as a fetus; that is, the presenting follicle should be termed follicle A, the next follicle B, the next follicle C, and so forth, and day-to-day consistency in naming should be maintained so that the same follicle is measured on consecutive days—providing the same follicle can be recognized. Although this is a simple task when using a transabdominal probe, orientation with the endovaginal probe is not as easy. Nabothian cysts in the cervix have been mistaken for intraovarian follicles, so it is important to look at both the uterus and ovaries.

At birth there are approximately 2,000,000 primary oocytes in each ovary. When menarche occurs there are approximately 400,000 follicles per ovary remaining. Most primary oocytes become atrophic or do not develop. Maturation of the oocytes and follicles depends primarily on changes in levels of follicle-stimulating hormone (FSH), luteinizing hormone (LH), and circulating estrogen. Impending ovulation is associated with (1) the development of internal echoes in the dominant follicle and (2) the appearance of crenation or wall irregularity and wall thickening.[38]

Although size at ovulation varies, it is relatively consistent in a given individual. Some investigators have suggested that impending ovulation can be recognized by visualization of the cumulus oophorus. The following ultrasonic signs of the cumulus oophorus have been described: (1) an echogenic area projecting into the lumen[8]; (2) a linear, poorly defined, echogenic focus[51]; and (3) a zone of decreased echogenicity around the follicle.[60] The cumulus oophorus complex is approximately 1 mm in diameter, so it is not surprising that it is difficult to see with ultrasound.[79] There is no consensus on whether one can see the cumulus oophorus with ultrasound.[60] Some consider the visualization of a septum or a small clump of echoes within the follicle as evidence that the cumulus oophorus has been seen and that ovulation is imminent. In any event, the visualization of a cumulus oophorus does not appear to be sufficiently consistent to allow it to be used as a marker for when human chorionic gonadotropin (hCG) should be administered or for the timing of intercourse (if the patient is trying to time intercourse to coincide with ovulation). Most investigators consider ultrasound measurements of follicle size not to be helpful in predicting ovulation because follicle size at ovulation is so variable,[44,67] and suggest that the maximal diameters of the ovarian follicles and the peak plasma estradiol determination are equally effective in predicting ovulation time. Others use LS assays and ultrasound to predict ovulation.

Successful ovulation can be recognized by (1) complete disappearance of the follicle; (2) loss of the circular shape of the follicle; (3) thickening of the follicle wall; (4) replacement of the clear follicle by an irregular echogenic area; (5) the development of fluid in the cul-de-sac[31, 61]; and (6) an increase in maximal Doppler velocity[10] (Fig. 57-12). The secretory phase is characterized by a high diastolic and systolic flow, whereas the flow is low in diastole during the proliferative phase.[10] Follicles start on the pathway to ovulation some months before ovulation occurs. Often two follicles develop side by side, but only one actually progresses to become the dominant follicle and the other

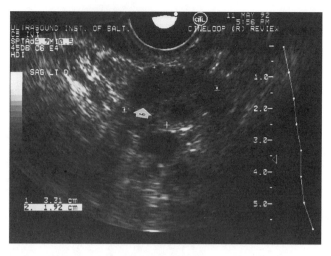

Fig. 57-12. Postovulation image. An echopenic area representing the corpus luteum is visible (*arrowhead*).

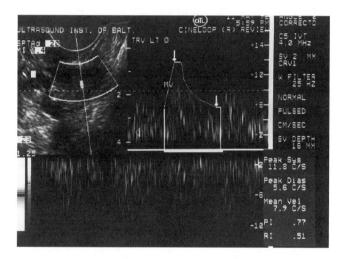

Fig. 57-13. Doppler study showing the normal Doppler pattern in the secretory phase with a high diastolic flow related to the corpus luteum.

regresses when it reaches a size of approximately 10 mm. Occasionally two dominant follicles develop. If ovulation is not imminent no dominant follicle will be seen. The midcycle LH surge initiates completion of the first meiotic division of the oocyte, and ovulation typically occurs within 36 hours of the LH surge. Pulse Doppler and color-flow Doppler have been used to follow the normal ovary over the course of the menstrual cycle. It has been shown that there is increased flow associated with the development of the corpus luteum[21] (Fig. 57-13). The significance of the flow variation seen with Doppler in the management of infertility is as yet uncertain. It may be that one will be able to detect defective follicular growth by the Doppler pattern.

After ovulation a corpus luteum develops at the site of the ruptured dominant follicle.[11,54] A corpus luteum may be seen as a cyst with internal echoes and irregular walls, or an

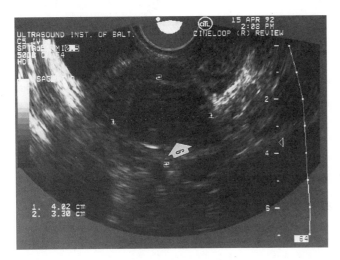

Fig. 57-14. Echopenic mass related to hemorrhage into a corpus luteum (*arrowhead*). This mass has an appearance similar to endometriosis.

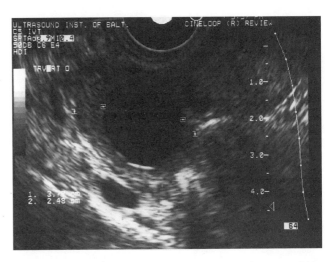

Fig. 57-15. Follicular cyst. There is a large echo-free cyst within the ovary with no internal structure. These cysts can be any diameter between 3 and 10 cm and will disappear over the next few weeks.

actual hematoma may develop at the site of the dominant follicle (Fig. 57-14). This hematoma can be larger than the dominant follicle and may contain even, low-level echoes consistent with hemorrhage. It usually is not possible to distinguish between a corpus luteum with hemorrhage and an endometrioma on a single examination.

Defective follicular growth. Various types of unsatisfactory follicular growth can be seen. Ovulation failure is the cause of infertility in about 20% of women.

Premature ovarian failure. Ovarian failure is characterized by an absence of follicles. Premature menopause (ovarian failure in a woman aged less than 40) is not treatable by ovulation induction. Ovaries in this syndrome are measurably smaller than those of normally ovulating women of this age group.

Resistant ovary syndrome. In the resistant ovary syndrome, primordial or immature follicles are present.[50] A dominant follicle may fail to develop (anovular cycle) or a dominant follicle may develop but it may never rupture. The latter situation is known as the luteinized unruptured follicle syndrome. Luteinization is recognized by wall thickening with persistent temperature elevation.[9] The luteinized unruptured follicle can achieve a large size (Fig. 57-15). Although such cysts may reach 3.5 to 6 cm in diameter, larger cysts (e.g., 8 cm) have been reported. The unruptured follicle, otherwise known as a follicular retention cyst or a follicular cyst, disappears over the next 4 weeks. A second ultrasound study approximately 1 month later is generally arranged when a single ovarian cyst is seen by ultrasound in a menstruating woman. This unimportant follicular cyst is distinguished from a pathologic process since it will spontaneously disappear rapidly. At the site where a follicle is expelled a small opening (a stigma) develops on the ovarian surface. This is not visible with ultrasound. If no aperture is apparent but signs of luteiniza-

tion exist (i.e., an elevated basal body temperature, increased serum progesterone level, and presence of secretory endometrium), the luteinized unruptured follicle syndrome can be diagnosed.[39] In cycles in which the follicle shrinks after the LH surge but impregnation is unsuccessful, the presence of the corpus luteum cyst is sometimes associated with lower progesterone levels than anticipated.[32]

In other individuals a dominant follicle develops but discontinues growth and starts to atrophy 1 or 2 days before the LH surge occurs. In another group there is normal follicular phase growth, but a poor estradiol surge occurs and there is failure to rupture with continuing growth subsequent to the LH peak; no efficient luteinization is observed.

Hypoplastic ovary. Infertility may be due to defective ovarian development. This most frequently occurs in Turner's syndrome. (See Chapter 2.) Streak ovaries may be present. On ultrasound a thin ovary is visible that does not contain follicles.[46]

Polycystic ovary syndrome. Polycystic ovary (PCO) syndrome is common and is seen in 5% of the female population.[3] From an ultrasonographic point of view in the PCO syndrome, both ovaries are enlarged and rounder than usual and there is more stromal tissue within the ovary than normal (Fig. 57-16). Small cysts surround the periphery of the ovary, which are presumed to represent small follicles but may be dysplastic cysts. These cysts are approximately 5 mm in diameter. As many as 18 to 20 cysts can be seen around the border of the ovary on any given ultrasonographic section. The ultrasonographic pattern of the PCO syndrome can be seen in women who are menstruating and ovulating normally; on the other hand, not all individuals with biochemical evidence of PCO syndrome have the typical ultrasonographic appearance. The PCO syndrome is

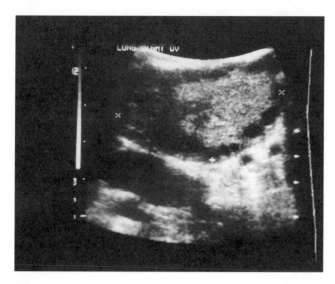

Fig. 57-16. Polycystic ovary. Using the endovaginal probe, numerous small, peripherally placed cysts can be seen located around the periphery within the ovary (*between markers*). There is increased central stromal tissue.

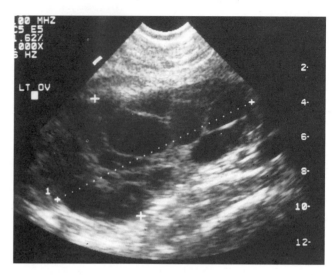

Fig. 57-17. Hyperstimulation. Numerous large cysts can be seen within a markedly enlarged ovary (7 cm). This is mild hyperstimulation.

associated with obesity and hirsutism, although these clinical findings may not be seen. (See Chapter 11.) Transvaginal ultrasound-guided follicular aspiration of polycystic ovaries has been performed in an attempt to induce ovulation and pregnancy. A 50% pregnancy rate was achieved after cyst aspiration.[52]

Ovulation induction

Clomiphene citrate. Clomiphene citrate (Clomid, Serophene) is a nonsteroidal synthetic estrogen antagonist that binds to estrogen receptors in the pituitary gland and the hypothalamus. Follicular development during clomiphene administration is different on ultrasonography from that in a spontaneous cycle. Individual follicles develop but at an accelerated rate, or the rate may be slowed down so that the largest follicle on a given day may not be the largest 2 days later. Since there are several follicles present, they tend to compress each other with the result that follicular shape may be distorted and irregular (Fig. 57-17). Clomiphene also affects the endometrial cavity. Endometrial cavity echo thickness is diminished when clomiphene is given.[62]

Human menopausal gonadotropins. FSH and LH are glycoprotein hormones that can be extracted from the urine of postmenopausal women. In this form, they are marketed under the generic name of menotropins or human menopausal gonadotropins (hMG) (Pergonal). These compounds do not require an intact pituitary gland or hypothalamus. If follicular activity is observed and is visible on the ultrasound study usually less hMG is required and there is rapid development of follicles that exhibit different growth rates. There is a significant risk of hyperstimulation, so ultrasonographic monitoring is important to time hCG administration. Clomiphene is capable of inducing ovulation in many

women with PCO disease and women with hypothalamic amenorrhea. Induction of ovulation with hMG and hCG is generally reserved for women in whom clomiphene has failed. (See Chapters 30, 32, 33, and 35.) Ovulation induction with all drugs will fail in women with ovarian failure whose ovaries lack primordial follicles (e.g., Turner's syndrome). Ovulation usually occurs within 48 hours of hCG administration. In infertile women when the follicle reaches 15 mm in diameter hCG is given.

Preinduction studies. Progestogen withdrawal bleeding may be induced before beginning ovulation induction to normalize the endometrium. At the same time a baseline ultrasound study is performed before hMG administration so that a preexisting ovarian cyst is not confused with a follicle. Several different schemes exist for the use of ultrasound in monitoring the menstrual cycle. In one approach a study is performed on baseline day 5 to rule out a preexisting condition hindering fertility, such as endometriosis or the presence of leiomyomas. Some limit subsequent ultrasound studies to the day of the LH surge to document the presence of satisfactory follicular activity. In this approach another study is performed the following day to determine whether ovulation has occurred. A subsequent study is performed 4 days after the LH surge to assess the uterine lining on the day of implantation, and another study is conducted on days 7 and 11 to determine whether the uterine lining is continuing to develop. Others perform more frequent ultrasonographic studies so that they can observe the dominant follicle as it grows, and administer hCG when the follicle reaches 15 mm in diameter to induce ovulation. With clomiphene and hMG stimulation, corpus luteum development may be inhibited and follicles may persist.[17] It has been suggested that ovulation induction can

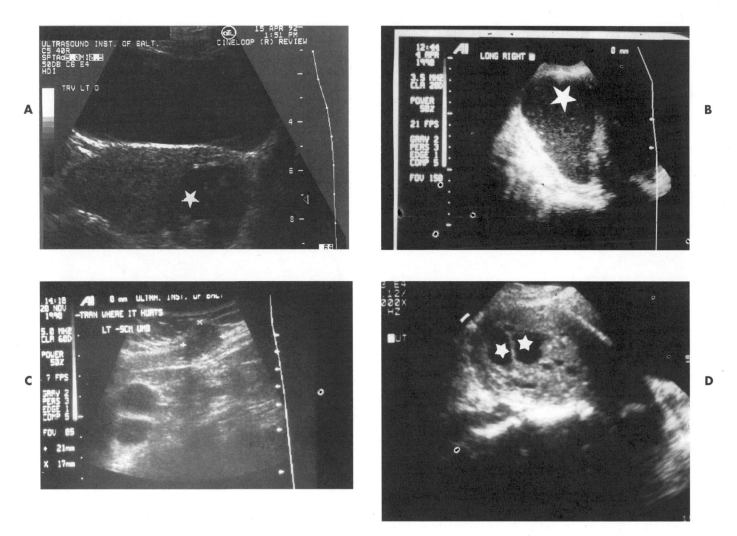

Fig. 57-18. A, Endometriosis. Large mass with mixed acoustic pattern in the left ovary representing an endometrioma (*star*). **B,** Extraovarian mass with low-level echoes (*star*), which is an endometrioma. **C,** Endometriosis of the abdominal wall at the site of an operative incision site (*between markers*). **D,** Adenomyosis. Sonolucent spaces within the uterus represent foci of endometriosis (*stars*).

be successfully monitored by ultrasound alone without estradiol estimation.[70]

Hyperstimulation syndrome. In individuals who are overdosed with follicle-stimulating therapy, an ovarian hyperstimulation syndrome (OHSS) may develop. (See Chapter 35.) hMG induces hyperstimulation much more often than clomiphene. The follicles within the ovary become very large and numerous, with the formation of bilateral multilocular intraovarian cysts. The syndrome begins to develop about 3 days after hCG administration. Fluid retention may occur, with the development of ascites or even pleural effusions. Severe OHSS is a serious condition with potential mortality (2%). A mild degree of ovarian hyperstimulation (Fig. 57-17) may be appropriate (10% to 20%) and may be required for successful conception (an ovarian size of about 5 cm is acceptable). Steering a pathway between mild and major hyperstimulation may require continuous ultrasonographic monitoring. OHSS is characterized by cysts of greater than 10-cm diameter, ascites, and hemoconcentration.[48] In moderate hyperstimulation the ovaries reach a size of up to 10 × 10 cm; there may be a small amount of ascites.[33]

Endometriosis. Endometriosis is a common cause of infertility. The abnormal endometrial tissue is deposited at many sites in the pelvis, including within or alongside the ovary, and within or alongside the fallopian tube. (See Chapter 37.) At these two sites infertility is caused either by the presence of adhesions and fibrosis or by blockage of sperm transport. Endometriomas arise when the ectopic endometrial tissue desquamates and results in the creation of a hematoma (Fig. 57-18). Such hematomas are indistinguishable from blood-filled structures such as a hemorrhagic corpus luteum. Since a fresh hematoma is created with each menstrual cycle, these hematomas persist and

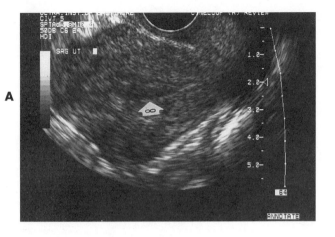

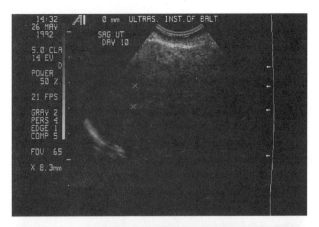

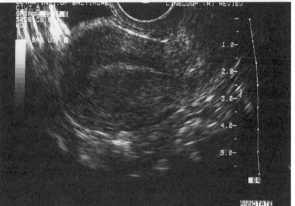

Fig. 57-19. Endometrial cavity in proliferative and secretory phases. **A,** In the proliferative phase of the cycle, the endometrial cavity is thin and there is a single line with a subtle echopenic area on either side (*arrowhead*). **B,** At the time of ovulation, three lines are seen (*between markers*). This finding can be of value in determining ovulation time. **C,** In the secretory phase the central echogenic area is markedly thickened.

enlarge, whereas hematomas related to corpus luteum formation disappear after a month or so. A repeated study in a few weeks' time is usually helpful in distinguishing these two entities. A similar appearance in both ovaries is most unlikely to relate to a corpus luteum hemorrhage. Endometrial implants have not been visualized consistently with ultrasound, although some ultrasonographers have claimed that there is increased echogenicity in the region where abnormal endometrial deposits exist. Since the hematoma related to an endometrioma is of varied age, an endometrioma may have areas of different echnogenicity within a single mass. Septa are common, but the most typical appearance is that of an even, low-level echogenicity (Fig. 57-18, **B**). Endometriomas can be very large and are often bilateral. They are locally tender when the endovaginal probe is used on some occasions. When they are located within the ovary, distinction between a single endometrioma and a corpus luteum with hemorrhage may not be possible on a single examination.

If an endometrioma in the fallopian tube causes blockage, blood may be seen within the tube. This structure has a more complex appearance than the echo-free fluids seen with a hydrosalpinx; blood typically has even, low-level echoes. However, it may not be possible to distinguish a hematosalpinx from a pyosalpinx related to pelvic inflammatory disease.

Uterus

Over the course of the menstrual cycle a small change occurs in uterine size, but a great change occurs in the appearance of the endometrial cavity (Fig. 57-19). In the proliferative phase immediately after menstruation the en-

dometrial echoes are thin. There is a hypoechoic area around the endometrial cavity, with a hyperechoic perimeter. At the time of ovulation the hypoechoic area starts to become echogenic, and during the secretory phase the endometrial cavity echoes thicken and can reach a width of approximately 16 to 22 mm.[18] A small hypoechoic area around the thick echogenic endometrial stripe remains visible. Echoes become thinner during menstruation, and a small amount of fluid may accumulate within the endometrial cavity. Ultrasound can therefore be used as a means of assessing whether or not the endometrium is in the secretory or proliferative phase and whether the change from the proliferative phase to the secretory phase is taking place in a normal fashion during the menstrual cycle.[22,27]

A multilayered appearance has correlated with successful implantation in in vitro fertilization (IVF) patients who were suppressed with a gonadotropin-releasing hormone agonist and then stimulated with hMG,[21,25] and patients with a thin cavity more often had a poor response to IVF.[5] A thin endometrial cavity echo correlated with poor results in stimulated patients.[25] Efforts to use the thickness of the endometrial cavity as an index of whether or not intrauterine fertilized ovum placement will be successful have not been helpful.[20] Welker et al.[77] suggest that a pattern that correlates with a successful implantation is one in which there is an outer hyperechoic layer and an inner hypoechoic layer. Uniform cavity echogenicity or fluid within the cavity did not correlate with success.[77]

Clomiphene citrate and hMG have the potential to stimulate the endocervical glands. The degree of mucus production can be quite large and can be detected as an anechoic cervical region in about 5% of patients.[35]

Uterine perfusion has been assessed with doppler ultrasound. The normal uterine artery has a diastolic component. It has been suggested that if the uterine arterial flow shows complete or partial absence of diastolic components, treatment with progesterone and estradiol for a 3-month period will increase fertility.[26]

In women with premature ovarian failure there is usually a variable endometrial response to standard hormone replacement therapy. Endometrial cavity thickness fails to thicken in women with Turner's syndrome and in other women with a poor response to hormone therapy.[42]

Pregnancy detection. Ultrasound is used to follow infertility therapy, and pregnancy detection by ultrasound is possible 23 to 24 days after hCG administration.[58] A small intrauterine gestational sac will be seen. In 3% of stimulated pregnancies an ectopic pregnancy will be found. No intrauterine gestational sac will be seen, although a decidual cast may be visible. Instead, in about 35% of ectopic pregnancies it will be possible to see a gestational sac outside the uterus and ovary, alongside the fallopian tube. One may see only the hematoma associated with ectopic development or fluid in the cul-de-sac, which represents blood that has leaked from the ectopic pregnancy.

Multiple pregnancy is a complication that occurs in about 10% of stimulated pregnancies. Ultrasound is used to monitor such pregnancies and to establish how many fetuses are present.

Structural abnormalities. Foreign bodies, such as fragments of a previously aborted fetus or a retained intrauterine device, may prevent implantation. These are very easily identified with ultrasound.

Several congenital anomalies of the uterus are associated with infertility. Uterine abnormality as a cause of fertility occurs in 0.1% to 0.5% of instances of infertility. (See Chapter 61.) In most instances the uterine abnormality is uterine hypoplasia or an absent uterus (66%); however, double uterus and unicornuate uterus have also been associated with infertility.[24,45] In a study of 13,470 infertile persons, 8.6% of female infertility was due to congenital uterine anomalies. The ultrasonographic appearances are characteristic (Fig. 57-20 A, B). (See Fig. 61-17 for a diagrammatic presentation of different types of uterine anomalies.) Examination should be performed in the secretory phase of the menstrual cycle because the endometrial cavity is so well seen. In a uterus subseptus (bicornuate uterus) two endometrial cavities will be seen within the uterine outline.[53] In uterus didelphys two separate uteri are seen at about a 45-degree angle to each other. In a unicornuate uterus

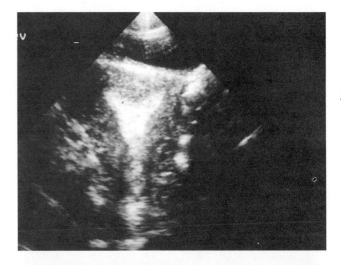

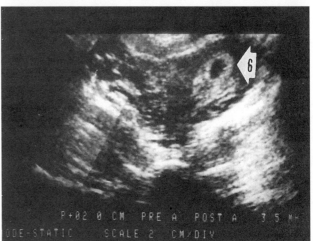

Fig. 57-20. A, Normal uterine coronal view with ultrasonography. **B,** Bicornuate uterus with pregnancy in left horn (*arrowhead*).

the uterus will slope toward the side with a formed horn. In severely bicornuate uteri two endometrial cavities are seen at the fundus only. It should be remembered that renal malformations such as renal agenesis are associated with all of the various types of uterine anomalies.[1]

Diethylstilbestrol (DES) is known to be associated with infertility. It causes a T-shaped uterus with a boxlike contour and a shortened cervix; this abnormality can be suspected on ultrasound because of the small size of the uterus. Fundal expansion is absent.[75] Such uteri have half the normal volume. Cervical incompetence is common in patients with DES changes but may be an isolated finding. It occurs in 0.2/1000 pregnancies. Cervical incompetence can be detected with ultrasound when the pregnancy reaches approximately the 12- or 13-week stage. The cervix is shortened (less than 3.5 cm) and there may be evidence of fluid in the cervical canal.

Leiomyomas. Leiomyomas that relate to the endometrial cavity are known to influence normal fertility adversely in a number of ways. (See Chapter 39.) The endovaginal probe allows the recognition of a number of leiomyomas that were invisible by using the transabdominal approach alone. Leiomyomas can be categorized by location. They may be pedunculated, subserosal, or intramural. None of these locations affects conception. Those that are in a submucosal or intracavitary position are of more consequence. A submucosal leiomyoma distorts the endometrial cavity and lies alongside the endometrial cavity (Fig. 57-21). When a leiomyoma is intracavitary the endometrial cavity echoes can be seen surrounding, or almost surrounding, the intracavitary mass. It may be difficult to distinguish between an endometrial cavity polyp and an intracavitary leiomyoma with ultrasound.

Ultrasound can be used as an aid in the planning of a myomectomy. An endovaginal probe is used to measure the size and extent of the leiomyoma and the size and extent of impingement on the endometrial cavity.

Asherman's syndrome. Preexisting infection or instrumentation may result in synechiae within the endometrial cavity. Such synechiae can prevent implantation. They may be visible by using hysteroscopy but can be missed. Ultrasound performed with fluid injected into the endometrial cavity may reveal such synechiae.

Fallopian tubes

Obstruction. Impediments to normal sperm transport may prevent fertilization and have already been described. Fallopian tube problems also prevent follicle transport. Previous tubal reanastomosis or endometriosis may obstruct the tubes and be associated with a hydrosalpinx.[63] Fluid is normally secreted within the fallopian tube. Obstruction at the fimbriated end may lead to the accumulation of fluid in the tube and the development of a hydrosalpinx. A hydrosalpinx has a characteristic ultrasonographic appearance (Fig. 57-22). The ampullary end of the tube is much more easily distensible than the proximal (interstitial) end of the tube; typically the distal end bends medially and posteriorly, whereas the less dilated central portion of the tube lies more anteriorly within the broad ligament. The fallopian tube makes a right-angle bend when it is significantly dilated. Since the condition is usually bilateral, the two dilated tubes may end up adjacent to each other posterior to the uterus. Depending on the severity of the infection that caused the hydrosalpinx, the wall of the tube may be variably thickened. Making a diagnosis of hydrosalpinx hinges on distinguishing an intraovarian from a periovarian cystic process. The presence of hydrosalpinx may confuse the process of IVF, since portions of the dilated tube may be mistaken for follicles. Aspiration of bilateral hydrosalpinges before IVF has been found helpful.[68]

Patency. Recently it has become possible to diagnose hydrosalpinx by using ultrasonographically guided injection into the tubes. Fluid such as normal saline or ultrasonographic contrast medium is injected into the uterus by a

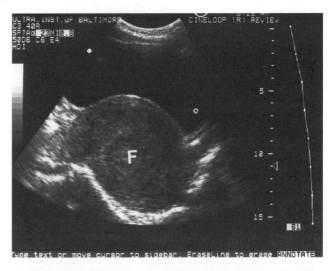

A

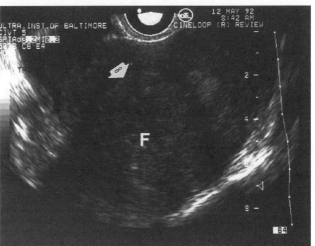

B

Fig. 57-21. Submucosal leiomyoma. **A,** There is a large leiomyoma within the uterus on the transabdominal views, but its relationship to the endometrial cavity cannot be seen. **B,** Endovaginal views show that the endometrial cavity is bowed anteriorly (*arrowhead*) and lies alongside the leiomyoma (*F*).

transcervical approach, and real time with color-flow and pulse doppler is used to determine whether the saline passes through the fimbriated end of the tube. Exit of contrast medium from the tube establishes tubal patency.[13] At the time of the intrafallopian tube catheterization, an attempt at relieving the hydrosalpinx has been made. In this technique the fimbriated end is perforated by the catheterization device, which may relieve the hydrosalpinx.[43,71] Ultrasound has also been used as a means of testing tubal patency. Saline is injected at the time of an ultrasound study and can be seen to flow out of the ampullary end of the tube. A catheter is placed under ultrasound control in the cornu of the uterus; smaller catheters are then introduced in a coaxial approach into the fallopian tube. A 45% success rate of fallopian tube catheterization[6] has been reported using this approach.

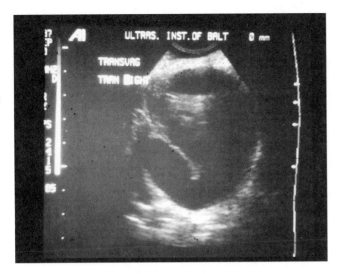

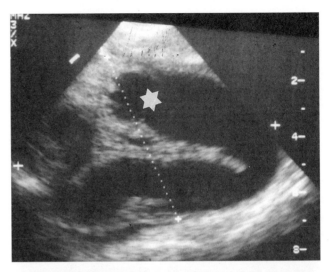

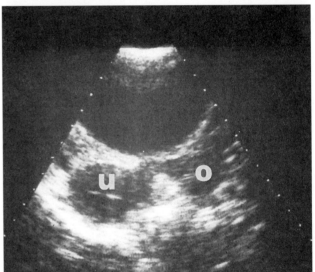

Fig. 57-22. A, Hydrosalpinx. The dilated tube forms a Z shape, with the ampullary end markedly larger than the remainder of the dilated tube. **B,** Chronic hydrosalpinx. A dilated fimbriated end (*asterisk*) with markedly thickened walls can be seen. **C,** Thickened tube related to chronic inflammation. The tube can be seen between the ovary (*o*) and the uterus (*u*).

ULTRASOUND IN ASSISTED REPRODUCTIVE TECHNIQUES

Monitoring

Patients undergoing IVF, gamete intrafollicular transfer (GIFT), or zygote intrafallopian transfer (ZIFT) procedures are monitored with ultrasound. During the initial phase, when clomiphene is used to stimulate follicle production, ultrasound studies are performed on a daily basis to determine the number of follicles that are being recruited and to determine whether growth is taking place at a normal rate. Sufficient doses of clomiphene are given to cause the development of approximately six large follicles per ovary. Timing of hCG administration is again controlled with ultrasound. Ultrasound is also used to monitor for evidence of hyperstimulation. (See Hyperstimulation Syndrome.)

Guidance of follicular aspiration

Four methods of guidance of follicular aspiration have been proposed (Fig. 57-23, **A, B,** and **C**). At one time laparoscopic follicular aspiration was used exclusively. This was followed by a phase when needle insertion was performed through the vagina alongside the cervix, with monitoring of the performance of the needle placement by a transabdominal transducer.[12,19] Transurethral aspiration was next introduced, again with transabdominal monitoring of the procedure.[56] A third procedure involved the transabdominal puncture of the follicle under transabdominal ultrasonographic monitoring. A percutaneous transvesical route to follicular aspiration was also used, but was ultimately discarded because it was both painful and difficult.

Currently in almost all centers the approach used is that of needle insertion through a guidance tube placed alongside the vaginal transducer. A template appears on the screen that directs the course of the needle into the center of the follicle (Fig. 23, **C**). The needle is pushed against the edge of the follicle and then inserted swiftly to enable aspiration of the follicle contents. The follicle is then flushed with normal saline. The flushing procedure, which may yield the oocyte, has been shown to be without hazard[41] and to increase oocyte yield.[76] This technique was originally described by Feichtinger et al.[18] in 1984, and numerous groups have since shown that it is less traumatic than other procedures.[78] Oocyte yield per retrieval attempt is greater by using this approach than when a laparoscopic or transvesical approach is used.[14] Doppler can be used to assess the success rate. If the flow pattern changes at ovulation induction from a high-resistance to a low-resistance finding with an increase in systolic velocity, the success rate is higher.[72] Once the follicles have been

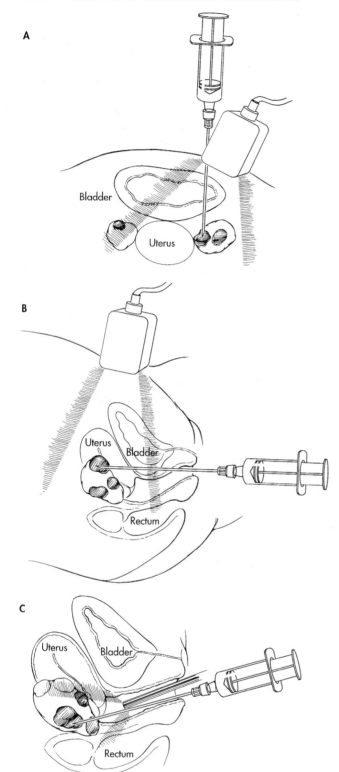

aspirated they are fertilized in vitro and replaced. Despite the fact that the ultrasonographic method of oocyte retrieval may well involve penetration of the intestinal tract, reported complications are increasingly rare. Pelvic infection has occurred, however, requiring antibiotic treatment.[36]

Techniques for replacing the fertilized eggs within the patient have undergone change in recent years. Initially blind reinsertion into the uterine cavity was performed. Later, ultrasound was used as a guidance technique and the fertilized gametes were placed at the fundus within the uterine cavity.[37] An increased pregnancy rate was achieved. In some instances clinicians had not appreciated that the insertion tube had coiled within the uterine cavity until ultrasound was used. The GIFT and ZIFT procedures initially required laparoscopic insertion into the fallopian tube; now ultrasonographically guided fallopian tube catheterization with gamete placement has been developed. In the first instance an endovaginal ultrasonographic guidance technique was used, but more recently transabdominal guidance with a full bladder was found to be more successful.[74] As with stimulated pregnancy, ectopic pregnancy may occur after IVF, ZIFT, and GIFT[28]; 90% of such ectopic pregnancies can be seen with ultrasound. Heterotopic pregnancy may occur after IVF if the fertilized eggs are placed in the uterus.[66] Seventeen cases were reported among 1648 pregnancies; it is a relatively common complication.[66]

CONCLUSION

The use of ultrasound has revolutionized the ability to observe various aspects of the reproductive process. It is particularly valuable in monitoring ovulation on a daily basis. Its use in men in infertility management has been much less explored but is very promising. Various obstructing processes in both men and women can be visualized.

Fig. 57-23. Diagram showing the techniques for obtaining follicles by using a needle under ultrasound guidance. **A,** Follicle puncture is shown under transabdominal ultrasound guidance. The needle is passed through the bladder. **B,** Follicular aspiration using the needle inserted through the vagina but with guidance performed with a transducer placed on the abdomen, viewing the area through the bladder. **C,** Follicular aspiration performed with both the transducer and the needle inserted into the vagina. (Modified with permission from *Clinical sonography: a practical guide,* ed 2.)

REFERENCES

1. Acien P et al: Renal agenesis in association with malformation of the female genital tract, *Am J Obstet Gynecol* 165:1368, 1991.
2. Andreotti RF et al: Endovaginal and transabdominal sonography of ovarian follicles, *J Ultrasound Med* 8:555, 1989.
3. Barbieri RL: Polycystic ovarian disease, *Annu Rev Med* 42:199-204, 1991.
4. Belaisch-Allart J et al: Comparison of transvaginal and transabdominal ultrasound for monitoring follicular development in an in-vitro fertilization programme, *Hum Reprod* 6:688-689, 1991.
5. Brandt TD et al: Endometrial echo and its significance in female infertility, *Radiology* 157:225, 1985.
6. Breckenridge JW, Schinfeld JS: Technique for US-guided fallopian tube catheterization, *Radiology* 180:569, 1991.
7. Check JH, Dietterich C, Houck MA: Ipsilateral versus contralateral ovary selection of dominant follicle in succeeding cycle, *Obstet Gynecol* 77:247, 1991.
8. Coulam CB, Hill LM, Breckle R: Ultrasonic assessment of subsequent unexplained infertility after ovulation induction, *Br J Obstet Gynaecol* 90:460, 1983.
9. Coulam CB, Moore SB, O'Fallon W: Investigating unexplained fertility, *Am J Obstet Gynecol* 158:1374, 1988.
10. Crade M, Solis D: Intrafollicular blood flow during human ovulation, *Ultrasound Obstet Gynecol* 1:220, 1991.

11. deCrespigny LC, O'Herlihy C, Robinson HP: Ultrasonic observation of the mechanism of human ovulation, *Am J Obstet Gynecol* 139:636, 1981.

12. deCrespigny LC et al: Pregnancy after percutaneous transvesical ultrasound-guided follicle aspiration for in-vitro fertilization, *Med J Aust* 140:31, 1984.

13. Deichert U et al: Transvaginal hysterosalpingo-contrast sonography for the assessment of tubal patency with gray scale imaging and additional use of pulsed wave Doppler, *Fertil Steril* 57:62, 1992.

14. Deutinger J et al: Follicular aspiration for in vitro fertilization: sonographically guided transvaginal versus laparoscopic approach, *Eur J Obstet Gynecol Reprod Biol* 26:127, 1987.

15. Dominguez C et al: Agenesis of seminal vesicles in infertile males: ultrasonic diagnosis, *Eur Urol* 20:129, 1991.

16. Dornbluth NC et al: Assessment of follicular development by ultrasonography and total serum estrogen in human menopausal gonadotropin-stimulated cycles, *J Ultrasound Med* 2:407, 1983.

17. Eissa MK et al: Characteristics and incidence of dysfunctional ovulation patterns detected by ultrasound, *Fertil Steril* 47:603, 1987.

18. Feichtinger W, Kemeter P: Ultrasonic and hormonal evaluation of luteal phases and early ongoing pregnancies after in vitro fertilization and embryo replacement, *Ann N Y Acad Sci* 424:445, 1984.

19. Feldberg D et al: Transvaginal oocyte retrieval controlled by vaginal probe for in vitro fertilization: a comparative study, *J Ultrasound Med* 7:339, 1988.

20. Fleischer AC et al: Sonography of the endometrium during conception and nonconception cycles of in vitro fertilization and embryo transfer, *Fertil Steril* 46:442, 1986.

21. Fleischer AC et al: Transvaginal sonography of the endometrium during induced cycles, *J Ultrasound Med* 10:93, 1991.

22. Forrest TS et al: Cyclic endometrial changes: US assessment with histologic correlation, *Radiology* 167:233, 1988.

23. Gaboardi F et al: The neodymium:YAG laser recanalization in a patient with azoospermia due to ejaculatory duct agenesis, *J Urol* 146:1120-1122, 1991.

24. Golan A, Caspi E: Congenital anomalies of the mullerian tract, *Contemp Ob Gyn* p 39, Feb 1992.

25. Gonen Y et al: The impact of sonographic assessment of the endometrium and meticulous hormonal monitoring during natural cycles in patients with failed donor artificial insemination, *Ultrasound Obstet Gynecol* 1:122, 1991.

26. Goswamy RK, Steptoe PC: Doppler ultrasound studies of the uterine artery in spontaneous ovarian cycles, *Hum Reprod* 3:721, 1988.

27. Grunfeld L et al: High-resolution endovaginal ultrasonography of the endometrium: a noninvasive test for endometrial adequacy, *Obstet Gynecol* 78:200, 1991.

28. Guirgis RR, Craft IL: Ectopic pregnancy resulting from gamete intrafallopian transfer and in vitro fertilization, *J Reprod Med* 36:793, 1991.

29. Hackeloer BJ: The role of ultrasound in female infertility management, *Ultrasound Med Biol* 10:35, 1984.

30. Hackeloer BJ et al: Correlation of ultrasonic and endocrinologic assessment of human follicular development, *Am J Obstet Gynecol* 135:122, 1979.

31. Hall DA et al: Sonographic morphology of the normal menstrual cycle, *Radiology* 133:185, 1979.

32. Hamilton MPR et al: Luteal cysts and unexplained infertility: biochemical and ultrasonic evaluation, *Fertil Steril* 54:32, 1990.

33. Haning RV, Zwiebel WJ: Update on ultrasound in clinical management of infertility, *Semin Ultrasound CT MR* 6:337, 1985.

34. Hann LE et al: Sonographic demonstration, *JAMA* 245:2731, 1979.

35. Hill LM et al: Sonographic evaluation of the cervix during ovulation induction, *Am J Obstet Gynecol* 157:1170, 1987.

36. Howe RS et al: Pelvic infection after transvaginal ultrasound-guided ovum retrieval, *Fertil Steril* 49:726, 1988.

37. Hurley VA et al: Ultrasound-guided embryo transfer: a controlled trial, *Fertil Steril* 55:559, 1991.

38. Jaffe R, Aderet NB: Ultrasonic screening in predicting the time of ovulation, *Gynecol Obstet Invest* 18:303, 1984.

39. Katz E: Why study luteinized unruptured follicle syndrome?, *Contemp Ob Gyn* 00:97, 1987.

40. Kaufman D: The sons of DES: the complete story, *Voice* 2:82, 1989.

41. Lenz S et al: Are ultrasonic guided follicular aspiration and flushing safe for the oocyte?, *J In vitro Fert Embryo Transfer* 4:159, 1987.

42. Li TC et al: The variation of endometrial response to a standard hormone replacement therapy in women with premature ovarian failure: an ultrasonographic and histological study, *Br J Obstet Gynaecol* 98:656, 1991.

43. Liss K, Sydow P: Fallopian tube catheterization and recanalization under ultrasonic observation: a simplified technique to evaluate tubal patency and open proximally obstructed tubes, *Fertil Steril* 56:198, 1991.

44. Luciano AA et al: Temporal relationship and reliability of the clinical, hormonal, and ultrasonographic indices of ovulation in infertile women, *Obstet Gynecol* 75:412, 1990.

45. Maneschi M, Maneschi F, Fuca G: Reproductive impairment of womb with unicornuate uterus, *Acta Eur Fertil* 19:273, 1988.

46. Massarano AA et al: Ovarian ultrasound appearances in Turner syndrome, *J Pediatr* 114:568, 1989.

47. McArdle CR: Ovulatory response vs follicular maturity, *AJR* 145:195, 1985.

48. McArdle CR et al: Induction of ovulation monitored by ultrasound, *Radiology* 148:809, 1983.

49. McClure RD et al: Subclinical varicocele: the effectiveness of varicocelectomy, *J Urol* 145:789, 1991.

50. Mehta AE et al: Noninvasive diagnosis of resistant ovary syndrome by ultrasonography, *Fertil Steril* 57:56, 1992.

51. Mendelsohn EB et al: The role of imaging in infertility management, *AJR* 144:415, 1985.

52. Mio Y et al: Transvaginal ultrasound-guided follicular aspiration in the management of anovulatory infertility associated with polycystic ovaries, *Fertil Steril* 56:1060, 1991.

53. Nasri MN, Setchell ME, Chard T: Transvaginal ultrasound for the diagnosis of uterine malfunctions, *Br J Obstet Gynaecol* 97:1043, 1990.

54. Nitschke-Dabelstein S, Hackeloer BJ, Sturm G: Ovulation and corpus luteum formation observed by ultrasonography, *Ultrasound Med Biol* 7:33, 1981.

55. Orsini LF et al: Ultrasound monitoring of ovarian follicular development: a comparison of real-time and static scanning techniques, *J Clin Ultrasound* 11:207, 1983.

56. Parsons J et al: Oocyte retrieval for in-vitro fertilisation by ultrasonically guided needle aspiration via the urethra, *Lancet* I:1076, 1985.

57. Patterson L, Jarow JP: Transrectal ultrasonography in the evaluation of the infertile man: a report of 3 cases, *J Urol* 144:1469, 1990.

58. Pellicer A et al: Comparison of implantation and early development of human embryos fertilized in vitro versus in vivo using transvaginal ultrasound, *J Ultrasound Med* 10:31, 1991.

59. Petros JA et al: Correlation of testicular color doppler ultrasonography, physical examination and venography in the detection of left varicoceles in men with infertility, *J Urol* 145:785, 1991.

60. Picker RH et al: Ultrasonic signs of imminent ovulation, *J Clin Ultrasound* 11:1, 1983.

61. Pupols AZ, Wilson SR: Ultrasonographic interpretation of physiological changes in the female pelvis, *J Assoc Can Radiol* 35:34, 1984.

62. Randall JM, Templeton A: Transvaginal sonographic assessment of follicular and endometrial growth in spontaneous and clomiphene citrate cycles, *Fertil Steril* 56:208, 1991.

63. Reuter K, Cohen S, Daly D: Ultrasonic presentation of giant hydrosalpinges in asymptomatic patients, *J Clin Ultrasound* 15:45, 1987.

64. Rifkin MD et al: The role of diagnostic ultrasonography in varicocele evaluation, *J Ultrasound Med* 2:271, 1983.

65. Ritchie WGM: Sonographic evaluation of normal and induced ovulation, *Radiology* 161:1, 1986.

66. Rizk B et al: Heterotopic pregnancies after in vitro fertilization and embryo transfer, *Am J Obstet Gynecol* 164:161, 1991.

67. Robertson RD et al: Assessment of ovulation by ultrasound and plasma estradiol determinations, *Obstet Gynecol* 54:686, 1979.

68. Russell JB, Rodriguez Z, Komins JI: The use of transvaginal ultrasound to aspirate bilateral hydrosalpinges prior to in vitro fertilization: a case report, *J In Vitro Fert Embryo Transfer* 8:213, 1991.

69. Shinohara K, Carter S, Lipshultz L: Transrectal ultrasonography for disorders of seminal vesicles and ejaculatory ducts, *Urol Clin North Am* 16:773, 1989.

70. Shoham Z et al: Is it possible to run a successful ovulation induction program based solely on ultrasound monitoring?: the importance of endometrial measurements, *Fertil Steril* 56:836, 1991.

71. Stern JJ, Peters AJ, Coulam CB: Transcervical tuboplasty under ultrasonographic guidance: a pilot study, *Fertil Steril* 56:359, 1991.

72. Strohmer H et al: Prognostic appraisal of success and failure in an in vitro fertilization program by transvaginal Doppler ultrasound at the time of ovulation induction, *Ultrasound Obstet Gynecol* 1:272, 1991.

73. Tessler FN et al: *Handbook of endovaginal sonography,* New York, 1992, Thieme Medical Publishers.

74. Thurmond AS: US-guided fallopian tube catheterization, *Radiology* 180:571, 1991.

75. Viscomi GN, Gonzalez R, Taylor KJW: Ultrasound detection of uterine abnormalities after diethystilbestrol (DES) exposure, *Radiology* 136:733, 1980.

76. Waterstone JJ, Parsons JH: A prospective study to investigate the value of flushing follicles during transvaginal ultrasound-directed follicle aspiration, *Fertil Steril* 57:221, 1992.

77. Welker BG et al: Transvaginal sonography of the endometrium during ovum pickup in stimulated cycles for in vitro fertilization, *J Ultrasound Med* 8:549, 1989.

78. Wikland M et al: Use of a vaginal transducer for oocyte retrieval in an IVF/ET program, *J Clin Ultrasound* 15:245, 1987.

79. Winfield AC, Fleischer AC, Moore DE: Diagnostic imaging of fertility disorders, *Curr Probl Diagn Radiol* 19:6, 1990.

Chapter 58

HYSTEROSCOPY AND ENDOMETRIAL ABLATION

Robert S. Neuwirth, MD

Hysteroscopy is a technique first attempted 120 years ago that was virtually abandoned by 1960. However, in the past 20 years the technique has been reborn and refined, and is replacing in part the classic techniques of curettage, metroplasty, myomectomy, and hysterectomy in the management of a variety of reproductive and gynecologic, diagnostic, and therapeutic problems. Hysteroscopy has become linked to other technologies to derive new methods that are quite specialized, such as tubal manipulation with fine balloon catheters and flexible endoscopes, in vivo cervical cytologic diagnosis, and laser and electrosurgical techniques. These marriages of technology and new techniques have offered women more precise diagnoses and more options for therapy. Several of the recent applications of hysteroscopy are still undergoing evaluation for effectiveness, as well as for risk, and are not yet fully accepted. Nonetheless, many hysteroscopic techniques have been clearly established and are replacing older, classic, surgical methods.

This chapter reviews the basic principles of hysteroscopy, the techniques, and the diagnostic and surgical applications and summarizes the state of the art, including endometrial ablation. Hysteroscopic endometrial ablation is one of the most promising and far-reaching applications of hysteroscopy. It deserves special attention because of the role it can play in new managements of menorrhagia, an old and very common clinical problem.

HISTORY OF HYSTEROSCOPY

The earliest hysteroscopic examination was reported in 1869 by Pantaleoni,[22] who used an endoscope of Desormeux. The instrument was essentially a tube with a proximal flame for illumination through which the surgeon could see into hollow organs such as the bladder. A major advance was made in 1879 by Nitze,[20] who developed a tubular instrument with lenses, an internal illumination system using a heated platinum wire, and a cooling and distending system of circulating water. The incandescent lamp of Edison soon replaced the platinum wire. This gave more satisfactory illumination for cystoscopy, but a distal bulb remained a problem in a uterine cavity that was smaller. Although the development of cystoscopy with the Nitze instrumentation moved in the direction of a circulating liquid to fill and flush the bladder, early hysteroscopy was performed without distention until Rubin[26] tried carbon dioxide with a cystoscope in 1925 and reported modest results. The use of liquid to distend the uterus for hysteroscopy was reported by several surgeons, but all were concerned about the spill of media through the tubes and into the peritoneal cavity. Thus the technique did not advance because the pressure was kept low and illumination was poor. In 1962 Silander[30] developed the balloon hysteroscope, reflecting the continued concern and difficulty with the distention problem. Although the instrument was an advance with its fiberoptic illumination, it did not solve the irrigation/distention problem because of distortion and poor visibility.

The modern antibiotic era, greater safety with abdominal surgery, and a growing pressure to achieve a good technique of hysteroscopy combined with the development of several distention techniques about 1970 such that modern panoramic hysteroscopy had its foundation finally established. The final steps in development of instrumentation were in place by 1970 with the exception of the distention-control system. Liquid hysteroscopy was developed after a report by Edstrom and Fernstrom[10] that the use of 32% dextran 70 was a safe and effective means of uterine distention. Quinones et al.[24] confirmed this but, because of inability to obtain the 32% dextran solution, adapted 5% dextrose in water for hysteroscopic tubal cauterization. Lindemann[14] developed a CO_2 system and equipment that kept the flow of CO_2 below 100 mL/min and the pressure limited to 200 mm Hg or less. These systems all worked, and the last key problem—endometrial distention and irrigation—in the evolution of hysteroscopy as a workable method was solved.

Thereafter techniques and equipment were refined to make hysteroscopy in the office a convenient diagnostic technique. Operative hysteroscopy also has developed rapidly in the past 20 years, initially through use of mechanical instruments that were borrowed from curettage sets and from cystoscopic instrumentation. Intrauterine scar and septa were the first to be repaired hysteroscopically. In 1976 Neuwirth and Amin[19] reported the adaptation of the urologic resectoscope to the resection of submucous leiomyomas. Laser surgery under hysteroscopic control was introduced by Goldrath et al.[12] in 1981. Most significantly, they reported on the successful hysteroscopic laser ablation of the endometrium to manage menorrhagia. Earlier work by Droegemueller et al.,[8] using a cryosurgical blind instrument, had suggested the possibility of control of menorrhagia. Other reports of hysteroscopic electrosurgery included that of DeCherney et al.,[6] who described successful ablation using a resectoscope. In 1988 Van Caillie[31] reported an electrosurgical ablative method using a rollerball electrode. Subsequent reports indicate that laser and electrosurgical ablative methods are effective in large numbers of suitable patients for prolonged periods of time. Further modification of the hysteroscopic technique has included the continuous-flow instrument, which allows the use of large volumes of low-viscosity liquids for distention but sharply reduces the problem of systemic fluid absorption that can lead to cardiac failure in prolonged surgical procedures.

To summarize, hysteroscopy was introduced about the same time as other endoscopic procedures such as cystoscopy and peritoneoscopy (laparoscopy). It bloomed late because of the special problems of performing endoscopy in the endometrial cavity: bleeding, the high pressure needed, ready absorption of the distending media, the potential for infection, and the small, irregular shape of the uterine cavity. Because of the slow start, gynecologic diagnosis and treatment for various conditions of the uterus moved in other directions. Although the technique developed slowly, since 1970 it has experienced rapid growth in use for diagnosis and treatment, with the catalyst of new parallel technologies and the pressure to contain the cost of medical care while increasing precision, accuracy, and convenience.

ENDOSCOPY OF THE ENDOMETRIAL CAVITY

Endoscopy in the endometrial cavity is a special situation defined by the anatomy of the uterus and its cavity, the abnormalities seen, and the therapeutic objectives. The most important factor is the small space of the endometrial cavity, which causes magnification of most images in hysteroscopy because of the short distance between the objective lens of the hysteroscope and the target. This optical factor also creates a narrower field of view. The optical system found in most of the rigid endoscopes is infinity focus; a normal-sized image is seen at 4 cm to the object. Characteristics of the rigid endoscope include the following:

- Focus
- Resolution
- Image contrast
- Magnification
- Field of view
- Depth of field

A normal endometrial cavity is about 4 to 6 cm between the internal os and the top of the fundus, so most images are magnified. Another problem is the source of illumination, a tungsten or halogen lamp, each of which produces different colors and intensity and often may be less than optimal because of the distance between the illumination and the target. The light transmission is by fiberoptic bundles, although a quartz rod can be used. Because the cavity is lined by a delicate mucosa, bleeding is frequently a problem. This causes blood bubbles in a gaseous medium and bloody discoloration and distortion due to dispersion of blood and mucus in a liquid environment.

Anatomy poses several problems: The cervical canal is a narrow, tough but dilatable, structure about 4 cm long. The narrow, long neck to the cavity creates difficulty in the introduction of manipulating instruments except those passed through the cannula of the hysteroscope. This in turn causes limitation in freedom of manipulation in the cavity. Furthermore, the fundal portion of the uterus extends laterally, making the restriction at the cervical entrance particularly bothersome. This has led to design of offset ocular lenses of the rigid endoscopes, as well as flexible and semiflexible fiberoptic endoscopes to integrate illumination, vision, distention, and manipulation. Compounding the problems of anatomy is the fact that two of the more common disorders to be treated are intrauterine scar and submucous leiomyomas, both of which are randomly distributed in the endometrial cavity and impose design features on the endoscopes. All of these factors make hysteroscopy more difficult as a diagnostic procedure than many other endoscopic procedures, and particularly skill dependent for surgical intervention. Specifically, the lesion must be located and identified entirely, and a manipulating instrument must be guided into place to cut, burn, biopsy, or grasp. To perform certain procedures, a combination of direct, endoscopically controlled maneuvers and semiblind maneuvers may be necessary. The cervix may be dilated preoperatively with laminaria or hydrogels or may be cut in order to gain access with a larger instrument when needed.

DISTENTION OF THE ENDOMETRIAL CAVITY

Examination of the endometrial cavity does not require distention. It can be performed by the contact hysteroscope of Barbot et al.,[1] which has a wide-angle contact lens and can give some information about the endometrial cavity by a series of segmented views. The technique is not adaptable to surgical manipulation. The instrumentation is sophisticated but serves mainly to provide some visualization of the endometrial cavity without the need for a distention system or a specifically designed light source, since the instrument uses ambient light for illumination.

The main power of hysteroscopy rests in panoramic examination of the cervical canal, uterine chamber, and uterotubal junctions. To accomplish panoramic endoscopy, a uterine distention system must be used. The minimal conditions that must be met by the distention systems are an intrauterine pressure sufficient to distend the uterine cavity and a flow rate sufficient to clear debris from the objective lens (Table 58-1). The minimal pressure is in the range of 35 to 50 mm Hg. The maximal pressure should be 200 mm Hg in a normal uterus, and maximal flow depends on the medium used. The pressure parameters are easily understood, that is, the pressure should be sufficient to separate the uterine walls but below the level that will rupture the organ. The minimal flow need be sufficient only to keep the visual field clear. The maximal flow rate is limited by the volume that can be absorbed safely by the body during the procedure. For example, carbon dioxide received much attention early in hysteroscopy as a result of accidents from gas embolization. It has been established from animal data[15] that 100 mL of CO_2 per minute at standard temperature and pressure cannot create clinical gas embolism over a period of 5 to 10 minutes even if all the gas is absorbed into the vascular bed of the uterus. The critical limit for liquids varies with the osmolarity of the liquid, as well as its composition. For example, 32% dextran 70 (Hyskon)

Table 58-1. Conditions and limitations of uterine distention in hysteroscopy

Condition	Limitation
Pressure	35–200 mm Hg
Volume	5–80 mL
Flow	CO_2 < 100 mL/min
Hyskon*	< 500 mL absorbed
Electrolyte solutions (e.g., Ringer's lactate)	< 2500 mL absorbed
Nonelectrolyte solutions (sorbitol, glycine)	< 2500 mL absorbed

*Thirty-two percent dextran 70.

can cause congestive heart failure if 400 to 500 mL is absorbed into the blood stream.[27] It is eliminated slowly. A low-viscosity liquid, Ringer's lactate, will produce similar problems at about 3 L and is eliminated more rapidly. The composition of the liquid is important in that hyponatremia can occur with use of nonelectrolyte solutions such as 5% dextrose in water when absorbed in large volumes such as 3 L; azotemia can occur with use of glycine solutions. Because liquids must be excreted from the body via the kidneys, the total volume absorbed during a procedure is the critical factor.

Carbon dioxide

Several carbon dioxide hysteroscopic insufflators are on the market, all of which are limited in maximal flow to 100 mL/min. The medium is ideal for endoscopy because a colorless gas does not create the optical distortion resulting from refraction of light. It is a problem in the uterus if it causes foaming of blood or mucus, which does produce major optical distortions. Because it is a gas, CO_2 readily leaks from the uterine cavity. Contracervical caps are available to reduce the leakage, but they are now rarely used. Rather, most hysteroscopists are careful to dilate the cervix just enough to introduce the endoscope. This limits the escape of gas around the hysteroscope and permits rapid examination quite conveniently in the office setting under local anesthesia or mild analgesia. Carbon dioxide is not very suitable for operative hysteroscopy because of the problem of uterine leakage, bubble formation in blood, and the inferior lens-washing effect of the gas compared with liquids.

Thirty-two percent dextran 70

Thirty-two percent dextran 70 (Hyskon) is a viscous liquid that has superior optical qualities. The index of refraction is less than that of water and therefore it gives a wider field of view. Because of its viscosity the pressure in the endometrial cavity is less likely to fall quickly unless there is a large leak at the cervix; 32% dextran 70 thereby permits more stabilized viewing. In addition, should blood be present in the endometrial cavity, because of viscosity, it will tend to clump in the Hyskon rather than disperse, permitting hazy but continued vision. It is slippery and sticky and can cause a problem if it drips on the floor. To control drips, as well as to measure output, we clamp a glove over the stem of the Sims speculum to collect the outflow. Allergic reactions have been attributed to dextrans, which are produced by microorganisms to which some humans have sensitivity. Anaphylactic reactions are rare; skin reactions are more common. Hyskon in the vascular systems will act as a plasma expander and consequently produce congestive failure if volumes of more than 500 mL are absorbed. Being viscous, the fluid is hard to pump through hysteroscopes with narrow channels. The product is water soluble, and when allowed to dry will produce a solid residue that binds valves, scissor tips, and cannulas. Consequently the instruments must be washed with hot water and a detergent promptly after use. The delivery system for Hyskon is a problem, because the product is packaged in a glass bottle. The options include a 50-mL plastic syringe attached to a short, wide-caliber Luer-Lok catheter for injection into the port on the hysteroscope cannula. An alternative is the DeCherney pump,* which uses high-pressure carbon dioxide to force the fluid through the endoscope and into the uterus to achieve the needed 80 mm Hg intrauterine pressure. The safety of design of the DeCherney pump was questioned because the system must be fail-safe when the Hyskon is exhausted to avoid gas embolism. The product currently is back on the market and readily available.

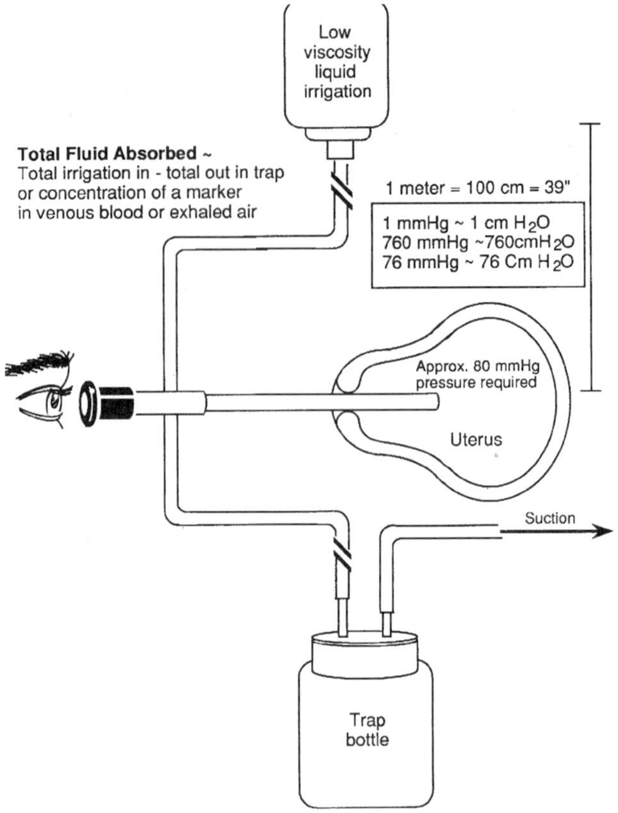

Low-viscosity liquids

The low-viscosity liquids can be categorized as electrolyte solutions such as Ringer's lactate and normal saline, and nonelectrolyte solutions such as glycine, sorbitol, and dextrose solutions. The electrolyte solutions cannot be used with electrosurgery but have the advantage of reducing the risk of plasma electrolyte disturbance secondary to absorption. The nonelectrolyte solutions must be used with electrosurgery, and in large volume can cause problems secondary to electrolyte disturbances or to high levels of glucose or urea from excess absorption of the sugar or glycine. Laser surgery can be conducted in all of these media, including Hyskon. Congestive failure can be precipitated by these media if the volume absorbed in a short interval exceeds the capacity of the circulatory system to accept, redistribute, and excrete the fluid. Low-viscosity fluids can cause heart failure when an excess of 2 L of fluid has been absorbed rapidly.

To control the uterine pressure and volume, as well as the flow of the distension medium, a continuous-flow hysteroscope can be used for the low-viscosity liquids. The container of fluid may be hung above the patient and connected to the hysteroscope or passed through various pumps that are available. Gravity is usually sufficient to

*DeCherney pump, Cabot Medical Devices, Philadelphia, Pa.

Fig. 58-1. Low-viscosity irrigation dynamics.

control the pressure (Fig. 58-1.) The principle of the system is to dam the circulating fluid in the endometrial cavity. This is accomplished by a double-channel hysteroscope (Fig. 58-2). The inner channel is for inflow of the liquid from a bag, which can be raised 50 to 150 cm above the patient. The fluid enters via a valve-controlled port at the cannula base into the inner sheath and flows out the end of the hysteroscope into the endometrial cavity. The outer sheath has multiple fine openings at the tip through which the fluid enters to return via the outer channel to an outflow valve at the base of the cannula. The resistance to liquid outflow into the outer channel of the hysteroscope by the openings at the tip causes a dam effect in the uterine cavity that raises the volume and pressure in the cavity and can be modulated by varying the outflow. The outflow port is controlled by a valve and is connected to a gravity drain or to a suction trap bottle. The surgeon can adjust the outflow valve to vary the outflow orifice and dam or release the fluid pool in the uterine cavity. Thus the outflow valve then can produce a rise or fall in the uterine pressure simply by opening or closing the valve to the vacuum or negative-gravity pressure.

This system readily controls flow, pressure, and volume in the uterus. The continuous-flow method is more complicated to master and the view, although good, is not as clear as that with Hyskon. However, it is a fine technique,

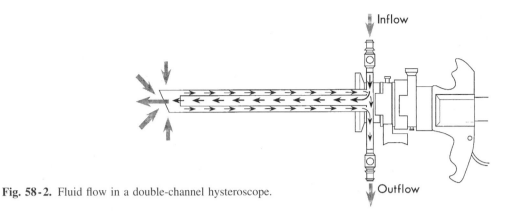

Fig. 58-2. Fluid flow in a double-channel hysteroscope.

particularly for the resectoscope. Because there is high flow with these systems, it is mandatory to monitor the net difference between inflow and outflow to avoid accidental overload and congestive heart failure. Alternatively, a fluid marker such as ethanol may be used[9]; the anesthesiologist then uses a breath analyzer for ethanol to measure the concentration in the exhaled breath, which is proportional to the fluid absorbed. Congestive heart failure may occur because only a small percentage absorption, perhaps 10% to 20% of the flow, can quickly lead to overload if the total volume of liquid used rises to 10 to 15 L. As a means of reducing the risk of fluid overload, carbon dioxide hysteroscopy may often be used to begin an operative procedure, followed by a changeover to a liquid system once the surgery has begun.

All of the liquid systems may create problems of wetness or slippery surfaces if there is no control of leakage. This is important so as not to divert the attention of the surgeon, who must maintain focus on the surgery. The common practice is for a team to become most comfortable with one of the medium and delivery systems.

One of the most important features of all of the distention systems is the appropriate dilatation of the cervix. Clearly the cervix must be open sufficiently to permit entry of the hysteroscope into the uterine chamber. Excessive cervical dilatation is an error because leakage occurs, leading to poor uterine distention. A pursestring suture or a cross-clamp on the cervix may help the problem. In this aspect of the procedure, the technique of hysteroscopy differs significantly from that of dilatation and curettage.

DIAGNOSIS OF ENDOMETRIAL LESIONS

The accurate appraisal of the endometrial cavity is essential for the gynecologist and reproductive surgeon. The techniques available include diagnostic curettage, hysterography, hysteroscopy, ultrasonography, computed tomography (CT), and magnetic resonance imaging (MRI). The purpose of this section is to consider briefly these alternatives for their optimal utilization.

The diagnostic curettage is the oldest of these procedures, dating to the mid-nineteenth century. Essentially it is a means of tactile appraisal of the uterine cavity, as well as

a method for sampling the endometrial wall surrounding the endometrial cavity. The technique rarely misses malignant mucosal lesions unless they are focal or pedunculated. It also generally will identify a submucosal leiomyoma unless it is on a stalk or in one of the horns of the uterine cavity inaccessible to the curette. The technique can miss foreign bodies such as intrauterine devices (IUDs) or ossified remnants of pregnancy, as well as complete septate or subseptate uterus, and produce a false interpretation of a normal cavity. The technique may give false-positive information, such as the impression of a septate uterus or submucous leiomyoma derived from an arcuate configuration of the endometrial cavity. To do a thorough curettage to appraise the endometrial cavity, anesthesia or significant analgesia and sedation are needed.

Hysterography is the time honored diagnostic procedure, having developed after the introduction of radiographic dyes into radiology about 1920.[29] The technique requires little or no analgesia. It outlines the endometrial cavity well but can give false-positive information due to shadows produced by local spasm and bubbles. It gives minimal information about the mucosa, but it does give data about tubal patency unless spasm or debris causes functional blockage of the uterotubal junction. It rarely gives a falsely normal picture unless the cavity is overfilled with the radiopaque dye so as to obscure a filling defect created by a polyp or submucous leiomyoma. The angle of the X-ray camera is also important in this regard, since axial views of the uterus can also miss intrauterine lesions that normally would produce a visible filling defect. The radiation exposure is low but is a consideration with this technique. Posthysterographic pelvic inflammation can occur. (See Chapter 27.)

The hysteroscopic technique dates back to the mid-1970s. It is convenient, accurate but skill dependent, and almost risk free. Perforation should not occur if the examiner does nothing blindly. Local infection has not been seen in our experience since 1975. The method offers not only diagnosis but preoperative appraisal; that is, the abnormality, such as a submucous leiomyoma, can be examined for the feasibility of transcervical removal. Minimal or no analgesia is needed once skill is developed for the office

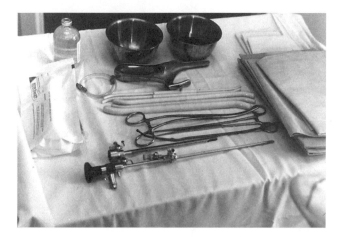

Fig. 58-3. Equipment for office hysteroscopy, including backup bottle of 32% dextran 70 (Hyskon).

examination, because the discomfort comes from cervical dilatation and the gentle pressure needed to distend the endometrial cavity.

Ultrasonography has been more useful for endometrial appraisal since the development of the transvaginal probe. Although ultrasonography is slightly less accurate than hysteroscopy, it is less invasive and can give information about uterine size and the adenexa. A diagnosis of submucous leiomyoma may often be made, but it is not as useful for preoperative appraisal of lesions of the cavity, including differentiation of a polyp from a submucous leiomyoma.

The CT scan and MRI have become useful adjuncts to intrauterine diagnosis in the past 10 years. Leiomyosarcoma may be suggested by MRI. The location of intramural leiomyomas may help in prediction of the success of a submucous myomectomy to correct menorrhagia. At present, however, these two techniques are of occasional help in evaluation and management of disorders of the endometrial cavity. In summary, a variety of techniques are now options to evaluate the uterus and endometrial cavity. Hysteroscopy is a leading method because of the accuracy of diagnosis, convenience of performance, and potential for therapy.

DIAGNOSTIC HYSTEROSCOPY

Techniques

The uterus is a conical potential chamber surrounded by a thick muscular coat with a narrow entrance made of tough but dilatable collagen tissue. To succeed with the technique, the telescope must enter the illuminated chamber after appropriate cervical dilatation as it expands with the distention fluid. The basic prerequisites for hysteroscopy are the endoscopic instrumentation and lighting, the appropriate facility for the procedure, options for pain relief, and the uterine distention system. For office hysteroscopy (Fig. 58-3), the instruments include a 4-mm wide-angle hysteroscope, a one-arm speculum, tenaculum, uterine sound, and

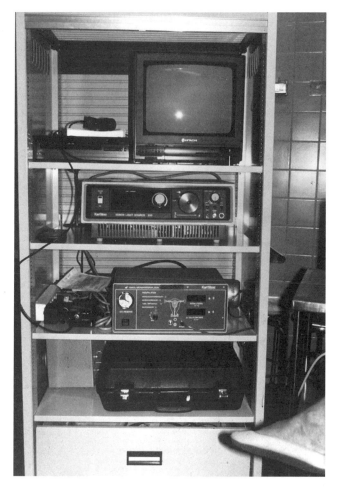

Fig. 58-4. Carbon dioxide system, xenon light source, and television camera and monitor for office or operating room.

cervical dilators up to 8 mm in diameter. In the office the distention system is usually a carbon dioxide insufflation system with pressure limited to 150 mm Hg and flow not to exceed 100 mL/min (Fig. 58-4). Alternatively, Hyskon in a 50-mL syringe with wide-bore tubing leading to the hysteroscopic cannula or a low-viscosity liquid with a continuous-flow system can be used, particularly in the operating room. A local infiltration set for an intracervical block for the office, or general anesthesia may be needed in the surgical suite. Sterile drapes are used in the operating room. For office examination, we use only a preparative solution of povidone-iodine (Betadine) without sterile draping. Sterile gloves are used in the office (Fig. 58-5).

The procedure may be performed on a standard office examination table with the patient in stirrups. The perineum and vagina are prepared with the povidone-iodine. A bimanual examination is performed to note the size and location of the uterus. The presence of tenderness should preclude the examination. The speculum is inserted and the cervix grasped on the anterior lip with the tenaculum. If the cervical canal is narrow (less than 4 mm), it is advisable to place 10 mL of an intracervical block of 1% lidocaine at the

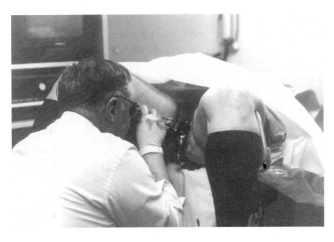

Fig. 58-5. Patient undergoing office hysteroscopy with CO_2 distention.

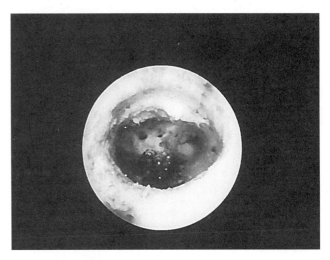

Fig. 58-6. Hysteroscopic view of the internal os, using 12° hysteroscope and Hyskon.

2-, 4-, 8-, and 10-o'clock positions in the cervix before dilatation in the office. Alternatively, local anesthetic can be placed in the cervical canal on a cotton swab. The examination should start by inserting the 4-mm hysteroscope into the canal and advancing it under vision, using CO_2 distention. If the instrument cannot be advanced, the direction of the canal is noted, the uterus should be sounded, and the cervix dilated just to the same caliber as the hysteroscopic sheath. As the field of view is usually a 30° offset, it is important to rotate the hysteroscope to look for the correct path of the canal, which appears as a tunnel, or follow the flow of bubbles as they ascend into the uterus (Fig. 58-6). Once the internal os is passed, the uterine chamber should be inspected systematically, including the cornual regions and tubes, the fundus, side walls, and isthmus. It goes without saying that in the office it is important to keep up a conversation with the patient during the examination to reduce the level of patient anxiety.

Indications

The indications for diagnostic hysteroscopy include all of the indications for diagnostic curettage plus a few others for which the precision, accuracy, and safety of hysteroscopy make it uniquely suitable, such as the search for an IUD when a curettage does not locate it, or the appraisal of a possible uterine perforation. Evaluation of the uterotubal junction is also in this category, as are examination of a known submucous leiomyoma for the possibility of hysteroscopic excision and evaluation of a uterine anomaly. Other indications include evaluation of Asherman's syndrome, evaluation of hysterographic filling defects, and evaluation of irregularities of the endometrial cavity detected at curettage. Clearly the major diagnostic area is evaluation of abnormal bleeding to explore for polyps and leiomyomas in the cavity. Cancer staging has remained controversial, although more groups are now using this technique for appraisal of canal involvement as well as

using the microcolpohysteroscope to aid in determination of the depth of a cone biopsy.

Contraindications

Contraindications are few and include known large perforation of the uterus, presence of a desired pregnancy, upper genital tract infection, and hemorrhage so severe that the procedure cannot be performed satisfactorily because of bleeding. This last contraindication is relative. We have had experience when hysteroscopy in the face of massive bleeding has been successful, as well as clinically important. Specifically, if the source of the hemorrhage is intracervical, hysteroscopy can distinguish this because the endometrial cavity will be free of blood. Cervical bleeding often can be controlled by local paracervical suture. This may then avoid abdominal exploration or hysterectomy to control hemorrhage. Furthermore, heavy bleeding from a submucous leiomyoma sometimes can be controlled by coagulation if specific bleeding points can be identified.

Complications

Complications of diagnostic hysteroscopy are uncommon. In our experience, the frequency of posthysteroscopy infection is very rare. Indeed, in 15 years of office hysteroscopy, we have had no instance of postexamination febrile reaction or other indication of infection. Perforation of the uterus is rare in a diagnostic procedure unless there is a faulty technique or intrauterine synechiae are present. Perforation can occur when blind dilatation with a dilator or the hysteroscope has been performed. These perforations are most frequently at the anterior or posterior isthmus. Fundal perforation can also occur, but mainly during surgery to correct synechiae when the anatomy of the cavity is distorted. Hemorrhage during a diagnostic procedure has been caused by the cervical tenaculum and by trauma to submucous leiomyomas. Complications arising from absorption of distention medium have been reported during diagnostic procedures but are far less frequent than those after surgical procedures. Gas embolisms in diagnostic procedures have not been reported in more than 10 years, and rarely has congestive failure been described. Allergic reactions to 32% dextran 70 continue to be a rare problem in diagnostic procedures and usually involve skin reactions.

HYSTEROSCOPIC SURGERY

Indications

The indications and applications of interventional hysteroscopy have expanded steadily since the establishment of reliable methods in the early 1970s. Initially the major thrust was tubal sterilization. The first efforts were by electrocoagulation of the uterotubal junction.[25] These approaches caused bilateral tubal closure by follow-up hysterography or hysteroscopy in about 80% of cases after one treatment. More important was the finding of a high incidence of cornual ectopic pregnancies after tubal coagulation.[5] Another major problem was the potential to electrocoagulate the full thickness of the uterine wall and cause a burn of adjacent bowel with subsequent necrosis, perforation, or peritonitis. Other approaches were tried,[28] including injection of sclerosing agents and placement of plugs and intratubal devices under hysteroscopic guidance. Although all of these methods worked some of the time, none of the techniques blocked the tubes sufficiently well to replace current techniques of tubal sterilization. Indeed, tubal blockage methods remain one area of important research.

Other indications for surgery that have become established are treatment of intrauterine scar,[13,17] correction of the septate or subseptate uterus,[2,4] repair of obstruction of the uterotubal junction,[3] removal of foreign bodies such as IUDs or fetal bones, removal of polyps and submucous leiomyomas,[7] and ablation of the endometrial cavity. Each of these applications is a separate topic and is covered briefly with the exception of endometrial ablation, which is discussed more extensively.

Contraindications

The contraindications to hysteroscopic surgery are few. They include genital tract infection, a uterine cavity too enlarged to maintain prolonged distention for an operative procedure, precancerous or cancerous lesions of the genital tract, pregnancy, and a relative contraindication of heavy uterine bleeding. Another occasional contraindication is the inability to perform concomitant laparoscopy in selected complicated cases, such as advanced Asherman's syndrome or the presence of large submucous leiomyomas. Simultaneous laparoscopy is at times an important consideration for aggressive hysteroscopic surgery to identify perforation

and avoid visceral injury and may pose a contraindication to the hysteroscopic method.

Complications

Complications of hysteroscopic surgery include infection of the myometrium or adenexa. The frequency of infection is remarkably low, and we have encountered only two of clinical significance in more than 20 years. Uterine perforation is one of the more common complications and can occur because of distorted anatomy, a weakened uterine wall, and surgical error. Cervical bleeding may also occur during manipulation. The use of simultaneous laparoscopy is designed to minimize damage from perforation or penetration, which can include mechanical or thermal injury to surrounding vital organs, usually colon, ileum, or adnexal structures. Hemorrhage may occur from injury to large uterine vessels that cannot be controlled by coagulation or balloon tamponade and necessitates laparotomy. Intravascular overload and pulmonary edema are serious complications and are avoidable by tracking fluid balance. Burn of the intestine without perforation can occur when laser or electrosurgical devices are used. These are related to a thin myometrium, excessive power, or prolongation of thermal contact at one point sufficient to produce a penetrating burn through the uterine serosa and affecting adjacent structures.

Applications

Hysteroscopic treatment of the septate uterus has replaced the abdominal approaches to unification unless a bicornuate uterus exists. Most uterine anomalies are of the septate variety, for which hysteroscopic repair is applicable. Evidence indicates that pregnancy loss is higher in the septate anomaly, and in such a patient septum repair is appropriate. Clearly it is necessary to perform laparoscopy to ascertain that the corpus is fused.

The actual repair is done in the operating room with a laparoscope in place. The septum is transected with scissors, laser, or a resectoscope loop (Fig. 58-7). The dissection proceeds to the level of the intertubal line. As the normal myometrium is reached, typically bleeding can be seen and the dissection is terminated. Some surgeons use an IUD or a balloon as a stent to minimize adhesion formation. The use of postoperative high-dose estrogen, 2.5 mg to 5 mg daily for 3 to 6 weeks, is common. The anatomic results have been excellent (Fig. 58-8). The data indicate that reproductive outcome is also improved. The procedure is brief, the recovery time is short, and the complications are minimal.

Asherman's syndrome is also now treated hysteroscopically. The condition may manifest as a single band or a partial or total obliteration of the cavity that is present (Fig. 58-9). The technical challenge may be very great if the cavity is badly damaged. The etiology is predominantly associated with termination of pregnancy or postpregnancy curettage for retained tissue. The associated factors are

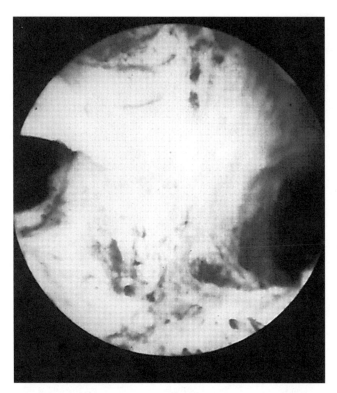

Fig. 58-7. Hysteroscopic view of the septum.

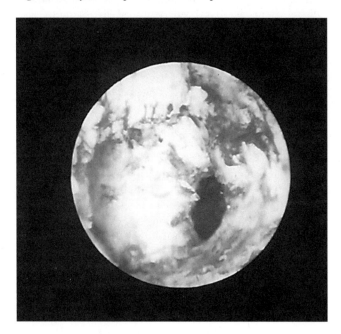

Fig. 58-9. Major adhesion in center of the fundus in a patient with Asherman's syndrome.

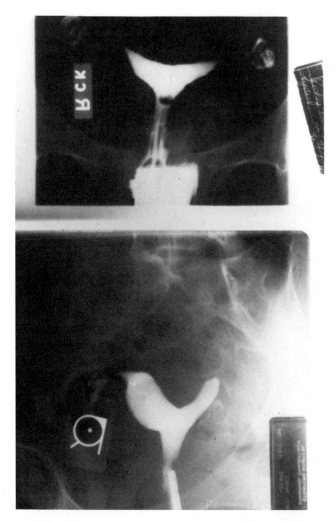

Fig. 58-8. *Lower view,* preoperative hysterogram of a wide septum; *upper view,* postoperative hysterogram 2 months later.

usually clinical or subclinical endometritis. Clearly the normal repair process of the endometrium is impeded by the combination of the curettage, infection, and a hypoestrogenic postpregnancy state that promotes scar formation. Correction of the damage is dependent on restoration of normal anatomy by dissection and the stimulation of the residual normal endometrium to migrate over the denuded areas to reestablish a functioning mucosa (Fig. 58-10). The postoperative hormonal therapy and the techniques of repair, although more complex, are essentially the same as for correction of the septate uterus. The outcome is dependent on the degree of damage present, including any occlusion of the tubes. In our experience about 50% of the women with documented Asherman's syndrome will succeed in having a child after repair.

Removal of foreign bodies, including IUD fragments and bone, are well handled with hysteroscopic control (Fig. 58-11). Removal is dependent first on localization of the foreign body and then retrieval. Typically these patients present with infertility and/or abnormal bleeding. Ultrasonography is more accurate than roentgenography or hysterography for identification of bone or plastic in the uterus. However, specific localization is best done by two-position pelvic X-ray film, with a probe in the uterus,

Fig. 58-10. Preoperative and 2-month follow-up hysterograms in a patient with Asherman's syndrome.

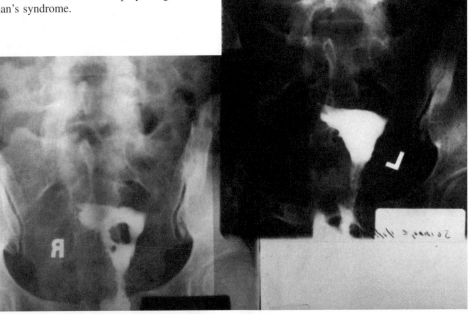

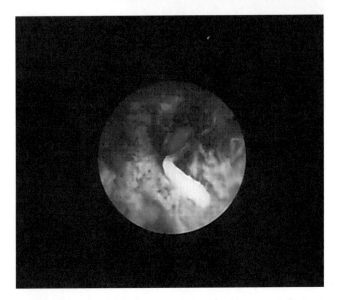

Fig. 58-11. Fractured Dalkon Shield embedded in submucosal myometrium.

or hysteroscopy/laparoscopy. The technique may be very simple or may be complicated by fragmentation of the foreign body as it is removed. Both bone and plastic IUDs may fracture easily if they have been present in the uterus for a long time. This means careful removal of the fragments with forceps. The outcome in terms of relief from abnormal bleeding and restoration of fertility is often dramatic.

Repair of proximal uterotubal blockage is feasible under hysteroscopic control.[21] One advantage of the hysteroscopic technique is that the scar at the uterotubal junction may at times be visualized, so that the possibility of spasm can be eliminated. Other techniques, for example, radio-

graphically controlled balloon systems such as produced by Bard, may also be used but will not distinguish tubal obstruction due to scar from spasm. A blind technique using a cannula introduced into the cornu through which a catheter is passed has been described by Maroulis and Yeko.[18] Tubal patency is determined by injection of fluid into the tube and subsequent ultrasonographic detection of the fluid in the cul-de-sac. These methods are all useful for management of patients who have bilateral obstruction at the cornu on hysterosalpingography.

The advantage of visual control using a hysteroscope and a laparoscope is the precision of diagnosis, as well as control of the repair. The repair may be done with fine clamps and scissors or by special catheters that can be passed through the hysteroscope into the proximal tube (Fig. 58-12). By using a combination of mechanical dissection and fluid pressure by injection through the catheter into a balloon[3] or directly into the tube, obstructions may be opened. We have had successful pregnancies after such recannulation, confirming other reports of success. The procedures can be done on an outpatient basis and clearly have advantages over cornual reimplantation when feasible. Recently a 0.5-mm flexible fiberoptic hysteroscope has become available that will make it possible to visualize the entire interstitial and isthmic tube for diagnosis and control of therapy.

Submucous myomectomy (Figs. 58-13 and 58-14) and polypectomy have been performed hysteroscopically, using a resectoscope and/or various surgical clamps, for more than 20 years. The polypectomy is a straightforward removal semiblindly with ovum forceps or under hysteroscopic control with hysteroscopic forceps and needs no further elaboration here (Fig. 58-15).

The most common indication for hysteroscopic myo-

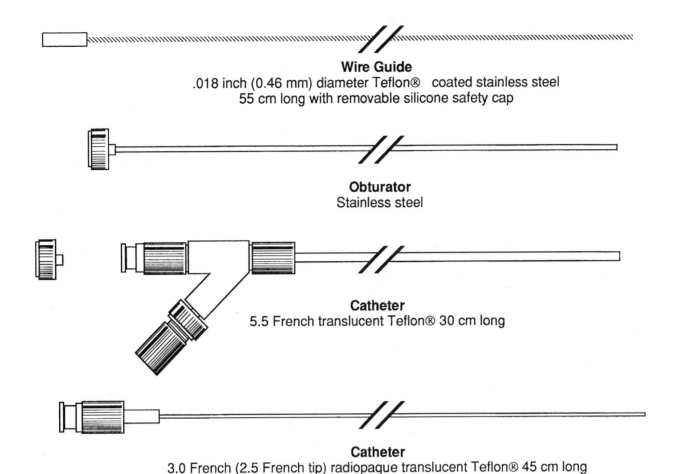

Wire Guide
.018 inch (0.46 mm) diameter Teflon® coated stainless steel
55 cm long with removable silicone safety cap

Obturator
Stainless steel

Catheter
5.5 French translucent Teflon® 30 cm long

Catheter
3.0 French (2.5 French tip) radiopaque translucent Teflon® 45 cm long

Fig. 58-12. Novy cornual cannulation set.

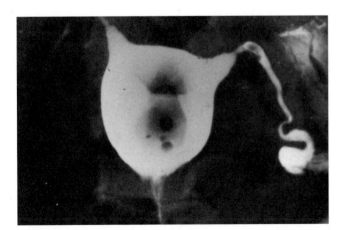

Fig. 58-13. Preoperative hysterogram showing two filling defects in a patient with menorrhagia and infertility.

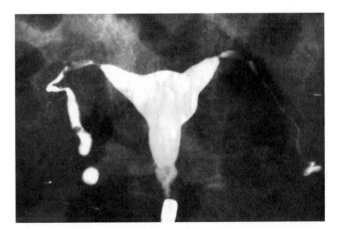

Fig. 58-14. Postoperative hysterogram 2 months later with correction of menorrhagia. The patient subsequently had a term delivery.

mectomy is excessive bleeding. Patients with infertility and recurrent abortion have also been treated. Patients who primarily want control of bleeding to avoid hysterectomy and who have no interest in fertility should have an associated ablation. Such patients in general have done well. Further surgery has been required in about 20% of

patients followed for more than 10 years. Patients desiring fertility have also done well if carefully selected. Many have conceived and about half have had a vaginal delivery. The longer the interval between the myomectomy and menopause the more likely the patient will be forced to be retreated in a pattern similar to the follow-up of abdominal

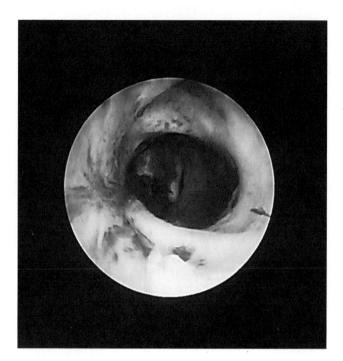

Fig. 58-15. Pedunculated polyp missed at previous curettage.

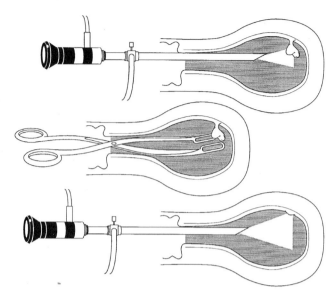

Fig. 58-16. Semiblind hysteroscopic surgery.

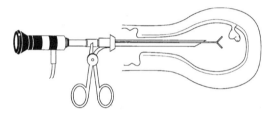

Fig. 58-17. Fixed-distance hysteroscopic surgery. Interventional instrument is attached to the hysteroscope.

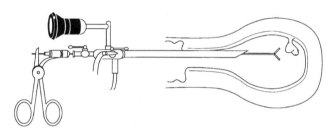

Fig. 58-18. Hysteroscopic surgery with interventional instrument passing through the sheath.

- Mechanical
- Electrosurgical
- Laser

myomectomy. The complications of myomectomy are intraoperative bleeding and perforation. Emergency laparotomy has occurred in about 1% of cases, generally because bleeding was not controlled by cautery or tamponade. The good long-range outcome, speed of surgical recovery, low emergency laparotomy rate, and the shorter operating room time all support the cost effectiveness of the hysteroscopic procedures versus abdominal myomectomy or hysterectomy when they are feasible. (See Chapter 39.) The technique of hysteroscopic myomectomy and the whole topic of ablation are covered in the following sections.

TECHNIQUES OF HYSTEROSCOPIC SURGERY

Successful surgical intervention in the uterus is based on expertise in hysteroscopic surgical techniques:

1. Indirect visual control
2. Instruments fixed to the endoscope
3. Instruments passed through the endoscope
4. Instruments passed adjacent to the endoscope

Visual control is the essence of the surgery. Diagnostic hysteroscopy can be considered a snapshot, whereas hysteroscopic surgery is a motion picture. The methods of the surgery vary. The least complex method consists of surgery guided intermittently with the hysteroscope, which is shown in Fig. 58-16. All other techniques are performed under direct hysteroscopic guidance. The instruments may be attached to the endoscope (Fig. 58-17), passed through the endoscope (Fig. 58-18), or passed around the endoscope (Fig. 58-19). Each method has its own advantages and disadvantages, and the methods often may be switched during the operation. For example, scissors fixed to the end of the endoscope are strong and easily introduced (Fig. 58-20). The problem is that the short, fixed distance from the endoscope to the scissors tip makes the field of view during actual cutting small and therefore restricts the maneuvers with such scissors. Instruments that pass through the endoscope sheath can be moved to and fro but must be slender and flexible, which limits their strength as

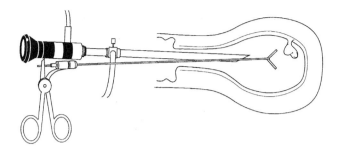

Fig. 58-19. Hysteroscopic surgery with interventional instrument passing adjacent to the sheath.

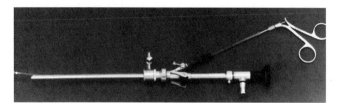

Fig. 58-21. Flexible biopsy forceps in a hysteroscope with an Alberans (deflector) bridge.

well as their lateral maneuverability (Figs. 58-21 to 58-23). Instruments that pass outside the endoscope sheath allow freedom of maneuver but often are difficult to pass into the endometrial cavity with the hysteroscope lying adjacent in the cervical canal. This approach also makes uterine distention difficult because the distending medium can leak out.

Operating instruments

The operating instruments used include catheters, probes, scissors, clamps, biopsy forceps, laser bundles, electrosurgical loops, ball electrodes, and other mechanical, laser, or electrosurgical devices. Each system carries its own special features. For example, electrosurgical devices cannot be used with electrolyte liquids for distention. Laser tips requiring gas cooling, such as a sapphire tip, cannot be used because they deliver high gas flow that may be absorbed and cause gas embolism. Carbon dioxide distention of the uterus is usually not satisfactory for surgery, particularly if laser or electrosurgical devices are used, because of the smoke produced in addition to debris and blood.

Maintenance of visibility

The most critical consideration of hysteroscopic surgery is maintenance of good visibility. Other critical aspects are the surgeon's interpretive skills, uterine distention, and optimal flushing of the endometrial cavity of blood and debris. With the cavity well distended and free of blood, the surgical maneuvers are often not difficult. When procedures using thermal surgery are used (i.e., laser or electrosurgery), the surgeon must also be cognizant of the biophysical

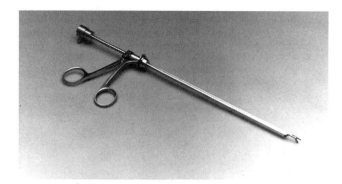

Fig. 58-20. Fixed-scissors instrument without endoscope.

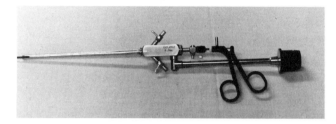

Fig. 58-22. Offset ocular hysteroscopy with rigid electrosurgical scissors passing through the sheath.

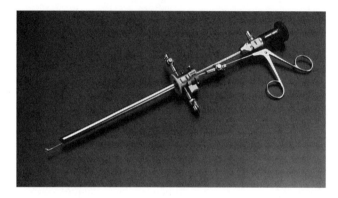

Fig. 58-23. Semirigid scissors passing through a wide-caliber sheath.

variables of the modality. For example, wattage, duration, and degree of contact of an electrosurgical electrode or laser fiber will produce variable impacts and may produce more or fewer surgical and thermal effects than intended. Ultimately, the surgeon's appraisal of the effect determines the course of the surgery.

The distention/irrigation system is the most important part of good visibility. In surgical hysteroscopy, the two systems most widely used involve the noncontinuous direct injection of a viscid medium (Hyskon) into the uterus and the continuous flow of low-viscosity liquids as already described. Hyskon works well because of the viscosity and optical clarity of the material. The major problem is the intermittent pressure/flow delivery imposed by packaging the product in a glass bottle. Hyskon is uniquely advantageous for surgical manipulation with instruments alongside

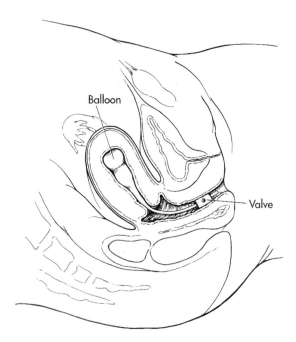

Fig. 58-24. Proper position of Ustasis balloon.

the hysteroscopic cannula. The low-viscosity liquids are best delivered by a continuous-flow system. The field of view is less satisfactory, and debris may cause a problem. But it is a relatively dry method because the outflow goes into the suction bottle and the liquid will not cause the problem with the valves and small channels that occurs when Hyskon congeals.

Blood clots and bubbles are managed by using a small catheter through one of the operating ports of the endoscope to suction the field and keep it clean. The clarity of vision also helps to sustain visual depth of field. As the endoscopes are all infinity focus, the short distance from the distal lens to the target produces magnification and a narrow visual field that may deceive the surgeon as to the true depth of a dissection. With a clear view and this optical limitation in mind, one can compensate for this distortion.

Postoperative care

After surgery, several issues need consideration. Infection, although rare, is probably best avoided by using prophylactic antibiotics. Repair of endometrial surfaces proceeds from areas of normal mucosa. Stenting the endometrial cavity with an IUD or a balloon for several days or a week may be useful if raw surfaces are present. In addition, high-dose estrogen therapy is used to encourage growth and migration of the epithelium. Finally, hemostasis is important, and balloons are useful for postoperative control of bleeding. A Foley catheter is readily available, or a special silastic balloon* can be used (Fig. 58-24). The objective is to distend the balloon with fluid to a pressure

*Ustasis Mentor Corporation, Goleta, Calif.

Table 58-2. Fertility after submucous resection*

	Total patients
Pregnancies	21
Spontaneous abortion	2
Induced abortion	5
Infants	14
Patients with at least one liveborn infant	12

*Fertility reported through 1988 in patients with submucous leiomyomas. Most surgery was done for bleeding, not infertility.

that equals the pressure in the bleeding vessels. Arterial bleeding requires about 80 to 90 mm Hg pressure to form adequate tamponade. In addition, the balloon should be inflated slowly, because excessive volume can raise the intrauterine pressure and rupture the uterus, particularly in the presence of weakened uterine walls after dissection. To avoid rupture, it is important to estimate the probable volume of the cavity and then monitor the pressure in the balloon in order to use no more pressure than needed to achieve hemostasis. The balloon pressure can be released at the bedside and the balloon removed when appropriate. Alternatively, the balloon can be reinflated if hemorrhage recurs after deflation.

Postoperative observation varies from 4 hours to 18 hours, depending on the possibility for hemorrhage. Recovery time from most hysteroscopic surgery is 1 week or less, although the uterine healing may require up to 3 months to complete.

Hysteroscopic myomectomy

Hysteroscopic myomectomy is a special case of hysteroscopic surgery. It is performed generally for two indications, menorrhagia and/or reproductive failure. Diagnostic hysteroscopy is critical for proper diagnosis and preoperative appraisal. If a submucous leiomyoma is present in a patient who is bleeding and future fertility is not an issue, the leiomyoma can be partially or totally excised at the time of endometrial ablation. A residual leiomyoma whose surface has been resected may be incorporated into the postablative endometrial scar, and the outcome will be the same as that after ablation in a patient without a submucous leiomyoma. Resection of the leiomyoma will increase the risk of transfusion and of laparotomy slightly over that for simple endometrial ablation.

If a submucous leiomyoma is found in a patient who has a reproductive problem or desire to maintain fertility, the hysteroscopic myomectomy takes on the character of reconstructive surgery (Table 58-2). Preoperative criteria should include a uterine cavity of 10 cm or less, a leiomyoma that, if sessile, does not occupy more than 3 × 3 cm of surface area of the endometrial wall, and no leiomyoma on the directly opposing wall. If there are "kissing" lesions they should be resected during separate surgi-

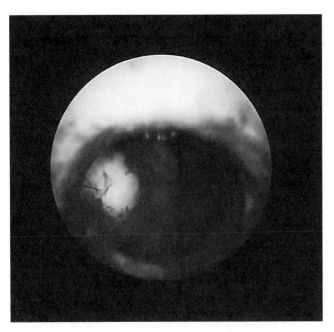

Fig. 58-25. Submucous leiomyoma at the 9-o'clock position.

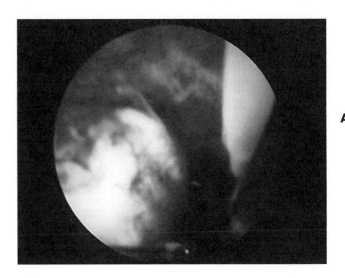

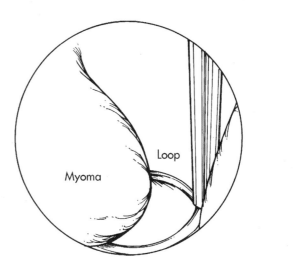

Fig. 58-26. A, Loop extended beyond the leiomyoma to palpate and explore before resection. B, Schematic drawing demonstrates position of loop with respect to the myoma.

cal procedures because of the risk of producing dense bands of scar tissue across the cavity.

Preoperative ovarian suppression with gonadotropin agonists is useful to improve the hematocrit, reduce uterine blood flow, and produce a thin endometrium. Once the surgery is completed, estrogen therapy is started promptly and continued for 14 to 28 days to stimulate endometrial regeneration across the transected base of the myoma.

The technique to remove leiomyomas depends on their size and location. A small pedunculated leiomyoma can be twisted off with polyp forceps and the base reinspected with the hysteroscope. Resection of the leiomyoma is generally carried out with a resectoscope using cutting current at 50 W of power or more, much like a transurethral resection of the prostate. The activated loop should always be drawn toward the surgeon for safety and control. Both the loop and the resectoscope itself can participate in the withdrawal maneuver. A large pedunculated leiomyoma can be partially shaved down on all sides, grasped with an ovum forceps, and twisted out if the cervix is open or transected widely enough at the 6-o'clock position. (See Chapter 39.) This will save time and reduce exposure to distending media. Because these maneuvers are aggressive and blind, laparoscopy is important for safety and control. Laser can also be used for morcellation but is more expensive and cumbersome for this work (Figs. 58-25 to 58-27).

After removal, if hemostasis is needed, an intrauterine balloon can be inserted and inflated to about 80 mm Hg to tamponade bleeding surfaces for several hours.

Clearly hysteroscopic myomectomy is highly skill dependent. Thus results and complications will partially reflect the learning curve. Our transfusion rate has been about

3% and the emergency laparotomy rate about 1% with these procedures over the past 19 years. During those 19 years—as opposed to the numbers in Table 58-2 that only reflect results through 1988—pregnancy has occurred in at least 26 patients, with vaginal delivery in approximately half of those women going to term. The major reason for pregnancy loss has been voluntary termination, because many of the patients chose myomectomy over ablation for menorrhagia control primarily to keep their fertility options open. Eighteen patients have delivered at least one live child.

Endometrial ablation

Ablation is the destruction of a tissue. Endometrial ablation has been studied over the years, using steam, chemicals, freezing, and heat. Droegemueller et al.[8] reported a blind cryoprobe technique to produce endometrial ablation but did not pursue the studies. Goldrath et al.[12]

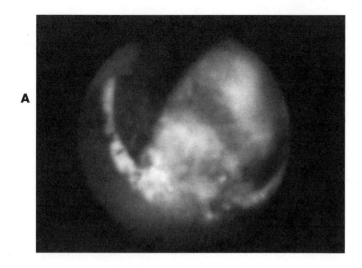

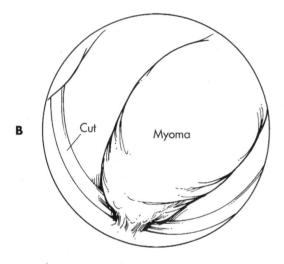

Fig. 58-27. A, Close-up of first cut using pure cutting current in the 50- to 60-W range. B, Schematic drawing demonstrates the location of the cut.

introduced hysteroscopically controlled laser ablation. This report has been followed by many confirming reports and variations of the laser method. A variety of electrosurgical techniques have also been reported. These include loop coagulation, rollerball coagulation, and loop excision techniques. All of these methods use heat to destroy the endometrial mucosa down to the basal layer under the visual control of hysteroscopy. Although laser and electrosurgical energies differ fundamentally as photonic versus electronic power, they are comparable in terms of the wattage applied. The other variables include length of treatment per square centimeter and the efficiency of transmission of the laser or electrosurgical power to the tissue. The tissue interaction with the specific laser or electrosurgical power (i.e., does it penetrate the tissue such as occurs with coagulation current or visible light range lasers?) is also a variable. In the last analysis, all of the factors are controlled by the surgeon's estimate of the damage done, which is usually made through a combination of experience and the appearance of the coagulated or charred tissue as seen through the hysteroscope. Indeed, the principle of thermal ablation is being applied to nonhysteroscopic methods such as a blind radio frequency system recently described[23] in England. Clearly other systems will work and may become a clinical option if they can be made to perform safely and effectively and offer advantages over hysteroscopic methods.

Candidates for ablation are women who would otherwise undergo hysterectomy for menorrhagia in nonmalignant conditions. The indications are medical (i.e., anemia) or pertain to lifestyle (i.e., inability to maintain usual activities because of bleeding). Evaluation of the patient must include a cytologic study and endometrial histology to rule out endometrial cancer or its precursors. The endometrial cavity should not be more than 14 cm in length, because a large endometrial surface will necessitate a long surgical procedure for treatment and increase the absorption of fluid while making endoscopic control of the operative field very difficult.

The patient must be counseled carefully about the risks of the procedure, including possible perforation and/or bleeding. She should also be provided with information about the immediate and long-term results with this method of bleeding control versus results with others such as hysterectomy and hormonal substitution therapy. Combined oral contraceptives may help control menorrhagia, particularly if dysfunctional uterine bleeding is a part of the etiology and there are no contraindications.

Should the patient choose ablation, it is desirable to premedicate her with danazol[11] or a gonadotropin agonist for 1 month before treatment. This should improve the preoperative hemoglobin value, as well as make the endometrium thin and therefore more suitable for controlled thermal destruction of the basalis layer.

The procedure, as done by us, is performed in an operating room under general or regional anesthesia. Consent is obtained for possible laparoscopy and possible laparotomy, as well as for the hysteroscopic ablation. The patient is placed in the dorsal lithotomy position in 20° Trendelenburg. After bimanual examination, the cervix is exposed and grasped with a tenaculum, and the hysteroscope is passed into the uterine cavity for appraisal. If the procedure is to be carried out, usually a rollerball or rollerbar electrode is used with the resectoscope. The bar is extended 3 cm to the midline anterior fundus, and a coagulation current of between 40 and 50 W is used while drawing the tip back toward the distal end to the resectoscope. In this way the electrode, while activated, can be kept under constant view and the effect observed by the surgeon. The necessary speed of movement of the electrode can be determined by the white effect on the endometrium and the fissuring of the adjacent tissue indicating transmission of the heat, which

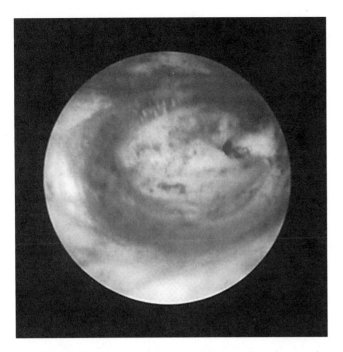

Fig. 58-28. Endometrial cavity under gonadotropin agonist therapy before ablation. Left tube is at the 10-o'clock position.

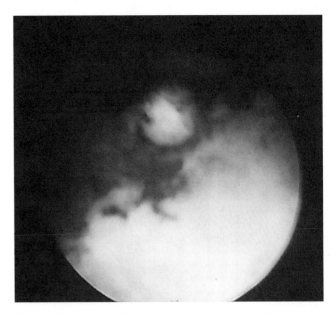

Fig. 58-29. Rollerball during electrocoagulation ablation. The point is coagulation with minimal charring.

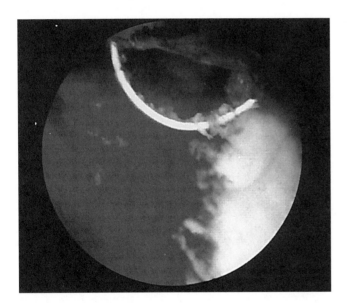

Fig. 58-30. Electrocoagulation with a loop electrode. Wattage may be lower than that for the rollerball unless electroresection is desired.

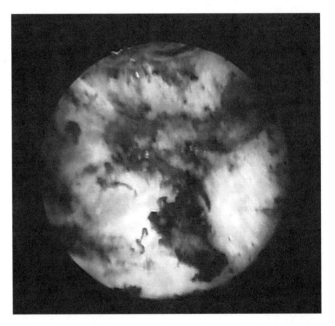

Fig. 58-31. Close-up of endometrium after electrocoagulation burn.

should be to the same distance of penetration as the depth of transmission into the muscle itself underlying the endometrium. The anterior wall is treated first, because bubbles tend to accumulate in this area during the course of the procedure. The top of the uterus and the cornual regions are coagulated and the lateral and posterior walls are done in a concentric fashion. The lower uterine segment may require separate treatment if the resectoscope has not

reached these areas, that is, if the resectoscope has been held fixed and the electrode drawn into the sheath. To reach the lower uterine segment in the same maneuver, which starts at the top of the fundus, the loop can be withdrawn slowly into the tip of the resectoscope while at the same time slowly withdrawing the resectoscope from the top of the fundus. In this way, a burn can be performed in a single maneuver that begins at the fundus and ends at the isthmus. The lower uterine segment should always be checked for

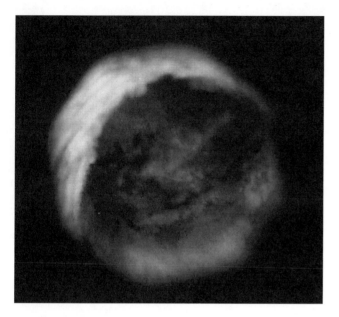

Fig. 58-32. View of the endometrial cavity in same case as in Fig. 58-31. The burn extends only to the isthmus.

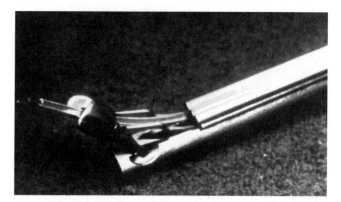

Fig. 58-33. Bare fiberbundle for laser ablation with special deflection bridge.

Table 58-3. Life table analysis of patients who underwent submucous resection

Follow-up (y)	Patients in interval	Cumulative chance of avoiding surgery	Cumulative SE
1	18	0.904	0.030
2	12	0.869	0.039
3	11	0.855	0.043
4	22	0.839	0.047
5	8	0.839	0.048
6	4	0.839	0.048
7	3	0.839	0.048
8	5	0.839	0.048
9	2	0.839	0.048
10	2	0.839	0.331
11	3	0.839	0.331
12	2	0.629	0.329
13	0	0.629	0.439
14	1	0.629	0.439
15	0	0.629	0.439
16	1	0.629	0.439

completeness of the thermal damage whether the uterus has been burned in two segments or burned in a single maneuver as just described (Figs. 58-28 to 58-32).

Laser ablation of the endometrium is carried out in a similar fashion (Fig. 58-33). The differences are that the hysteroscope is inserted into the uterine cavity with the laser fiberbundle, usually with an unpolished tip, and extended to the top of the fundus, which is treated by drawing the bundle slowly across the top. Two techniques are currently in use.[16] In the "touch" technique, the tip of the bundle contacts the endometrium. This will cause a deeper charring burn. In the other technique, the "no touch" technique, the tip of the laser bundle is brought to within a few millimeters of the mucosa and the laser is fired. This will produce a burn of lower temperature and cause less charring and more of a white coagulative effect similar to that seen when the rollerball is used. The wattage that is used for the neodymium:yttrium-aluminum-garnet (Nd:YAG) laser is in the same range as that for the resectoscope, 50 W of power. The laser bundle tip may flare and require cleaning intermittently as a result of touching tissue and developing a coagulum on the tip. This blocks transmission of the laser energy and leads to heat buildup and flaming of the fiberbundle itself, known as a flare. When using the Nd:YAG laser to ablate the endometrium, it is important that goggles be used and/or a protective filter be placed over the ocular lens of the hysteroscope to avoid potential eye injuries to operating room personnel. The laser procedure is carried out in a concentric fashion, similar to the electrosurgical methods. It is technically more difficult to treat the side walls of the uterus with the laser, and dragging techniques of the bundle tip are usually used.

An Alberans bridge can be used on the endoscope to bend the fiberbundle tip so as to angle the beam to a more perpendicular attack on the endometrial surfaces of the lateral walls of the uterus.

Once the endometrial burn is completed, it is our practice to perform a curettage, which provides a mechanical trauma on top of the thermal burn. The endometrial tissue, once coagulated, will lose its cohesion, and superficial endomyometrial tissue may strip off during the course of the curettage. This tissue is sent for pathologic examination. The curettage may also provoke bleeding. If it is important to avoid bleeding, a more profound thermal coagulation may be needed to ensure uniform damage to the true basalis layer of the endometrium. Prophylactic antibiotics are routinely used during the operation.

Once the ablation is completed, the patient is observed for 12 hours for bleeding, infection, and congestive failure, as well as for possible intraperitoneal injury, and then is

Table 58-4. Life table analysis of patients who underwent endometrial ablation

Follow-up (y)	Patients in interval	Cumulative chance of avoiding surgery	Cumulative SE
1	25	1.000	0.000
2	16	1.000	0.000
3	14	0.913	0.059
4	3	0.913	0.064
5	1	0.913	0.064
6	0	0.913	0.064
7	2	0.730	0.186
8	2	0.486	0.313

discharged. Endometrial suppression with a gonadotropin agonist is continued for another 2 or 3 weeks. A pelvic examination and uterine sounding are done 1 or 2 weeks after a procedure performed in the office.

Our experience has been very satisfactory to date. In approximately 300 cases of ablation only, there has been one laparotomy for intraperitoneal bleeding and one laparoscopic injury to the bowel at a time when laparoscopic control was always used during hysteroscopic ablation. We currently do not always use laparoscopic control during ablation. One patient with myometritis requiring 5 days of intravenous antibiotics was encountered. There have not been any cases of congestive failure in this group of hysteroscopic procedures.

The long-term outcome indicates that 82% of patients did not require second procedures for up to 8 years after endometrial ablation (Tables 58-3 and 58-4). These data include a learning curve, and all of the procedures were performed before the introduction of gonadotropin agonists for preoperative preparation. It is important that the immediate results of ablation have produced approximately 90% satisfactory outcome in terms of bleeding control. Only 10% of patients will after 3 months require menstrual protection that is not substantially less than the menstrual protection needed before the surgery. Indeed, about 40% of patients require no menstrual protection. Outcome with regard to pain, in our experience, has been variable. Some patients have noted intermittent pelvic pain, whereas other patients who had preoperative pelvic discomfort report that it disappeared after the ablation. Review of these cases makes it difficult to predict which patients will find relief from pain and which patients will develop discomfort after the procedure.

Since the introduction of gonadotropin agonists administered preoperatively in the last 4 years, results appear to be more satisfactory. A comprehensive comparison has not yet been done. However, the data to date indicate that for suitable candidates the use of ablation to control menorrhagia is a satisfactory approach as an alternative to hysterectomy in the management of benign menopausal bleeding.

It is probable that endometrial ablation will become a routine option to hysterectomy for many of the patients who are now being treated for bleeding by hysterectomy alone.

REFERENCES

1. Barbot J, Parent B, Dubeuesson JB: Contact hysteroscopy: another method of endoscopic examination of the uterine cavity, *Am J Obstet Gynecol* 136:721, 1980.
2. Chervenak FA, Neuwirth RS: Hysteroscopic resection of the uterine septum, *Am J Obstet Gynecol* 141:351, 1981.
3. Confino E, Friberg J, Gleicher N: Transcervical balloon tuboplasty, *Fertil Steril* 46:963, 1986.
4. Daly DC et al: Hysteroscopic metroplasty: surgical technique and obstetrical outcome, *Fertil Steril* 39:623, 1983.
5. Darebi K, Roy K, Richart R: Collaborative study on hysteroscopic sterilization procedures: final report. In Sciarra J, Zatuchni G, Speidel J, editors: *Risk benefits and controversies in fertility control*, Hagerstown, Md, 1978, Harper & Row.
6. DeCherney AH et al: Endometrial ablation for intractable uterine bleeding: hysteroscopic resection, *Obstet Gynecol* 70:668, 1987.
7. Derman S, Rehnstrom J, Neuwirth RS: The long term effectiveness of hysteroscopic treatment of menorrhagia and leiomyomas, *Obstet Gynecol* 77:591, 1991.
8. Droegemueller W, Green B, Mahowski E: Cryosurgery in patients with dysfunctional uterine bleeding, *Obstet Gynecol* 77:425, 1989.
9. Duffy S et al: Ethanol labeling: detection of early fluid absorption in endometrial resection, *Obstet Gynecol* 79:300, 1992.
10. Edstrom K, Fernstrom I: The diagnostic possibilities of a modified hysteroscopic approach, *Acta Obstet Gynecol Scand* 49:327, 1970.
11. Goldrath M: Use of danazol in hysteroscopic surgery for menorrhagia, *J Reprod Med* 35:91, 1990.
12. Goldrath M, Fuller T, Segal S: Laser photovaporization of endometrium for the treatment of menorrhagia, *Am J Obstet Gynecol* 140:14, 1981.
13. Levine R, Neuwirth RS: Simultaneous laparoscopy and hysteroscopy for intrauterine adhesions, *Obstet Gynecol* 42:441, 1973.
14. Lindemann HJ: The use of CO_2 in the uterine cavity for hysteroscopy, *Int J Fertil* 17:221, 1972.
15. Lindemann HJ et al: Der Einfluss von CO_2 Gas wahrend der Hysteroskopie, *Geburtshilfe Frauenheilkd* 36:153, 1976.
16. Lomano J: Laser hysteroscopy. In Baggish M, Barbot J, Valle R, editors: *Diagnostic and operative hysteroscopy*, Chicago, 1989, Year Book.
17. March CM, Israel R, March AD: Hysteroscopic management of intrauterine adhesions, *Am J Obstet Gynecol* 130:653, 1978.
18. Maroulis G, Yeko T: Treatment of cornual obstruction by transvaginal cannulation without hysteroscopy or fluoroscopy, *Fertil Steril* 57:1136, 1992.
19. Neuwirth RS, Amin HK: Excision of submucous fibroids with hysteroscopic control, *Am J Obstet Gynecol* 126:95, 1976.
20. Nitze M: Uber eine neue behandlungs-Methode de hohlen des Menslichen, *Korpers Med Press Wien* 26:851, 1879.
21. Novy MJ et al: Diagnosis of cornual obstruction by transcervical fallopian tube cannulation, *Fertil Steril* 50:434, 1988.
22. Pantaleoni D: On endoscopic examination of the cavity of the womb, *Med Press Cir* 8:26, 1869.
23. Phipps J et al: Treatment of functional menorrhagia by radio frequency-induced thermal endometrial ablation, *Lancet* 335:374, 1990.
24. Guerrero RQ, Durán AA, Ramos RA: Tubal catheterization: applications of a new technique, *Am J Obstet Gynecol* 114:674, 1972.
25. Richard R et al: Female sterilization by electrocoagulation of tubal ostia using hysteroscopy, *Am J Obstet Gynecol* 117:801, 1973.
26. Rubin I: Uterine endoscopy: endometroscopy with the aid of uterine insufflation, *Am J Obstet Gynecol* 10:313, 1925.

27. Schinagl EF: Hyskon, hysteroscopic surgery and pulmonary edema, *Anesth Analg* 70:222, 1990 (letter to the editor).

28. Sciarra JJ: Hysteroscopic approaches for tubal closure. In Zatuchni Z, Labbock M, Sciarra J, editors: *Research frontiers in fertility regulations* Hagerstown, Md, 1980, Harper & Row.

29. Siegler A: *Hysterosalpingography,* New York, 1967, Hoeber Medical Division, Harper & Row.

30. Silander T: Hysteroscopy through a transparent rubber balloon, *Surg Gynecol Obstet* 114:125, 1962.

31. Van Caillie T: Electrocoagulation of the endometrium with the ball end resectoscope, *Obstet Gynecol* 77:425, 1989.

Chapter 59

LASER SURGERY

Dan C. Martin, MD
and Randle S. Corfman, MD, PhD

Lasers have been used in surgery for more than 25 years because of their precise and predictable tissue effects. Additionally, the tissue effects achievable with lasers are diverse, including coagulation, vaporization, and excision. In the performance of any of these procedures, some lateral coagulation occurs, producing hemostasis and tissue distortion. The hemostatic effect offers improvement over use of a scalpel or scissors, which are great incisors but lack inherent hemostatic properties. The tissue distortion induced by high-power-density laser use is less than that induced by bipolar coagulation or mechanical occlusive devices.

Perhaps the most compelling argument for the use of lasers for tubal surgery is the emergence of laparoscopy as the primary access for reproductive surgery. Each of the commonly used lasers can be delivered to the operative site endoscopically, and results equivalent to those achieved by the traditional laparotomy approaches have been reported for many procedures.

LASER BASICS
Power density

Any discussion of laser surgery must be predicated upon a firm understanding of laser physics. In particular, the effects of the lasers are related to specific characteristics of a given wavelength and the general characteristics related to power density. At low-power density, the effects are predominantly those of the wavelength being used. At high-power density, the effects appear to be more related to the speed of vaporization, with lasers of different wavelengths producing similar effects.[25,28]

Detailed descriptions of power density are presented elsewhere,[8] but a common mathematical approximation of this entity is as follows:

$$Pd = W \times 100/sd^2$$

where Pd is the power density in watts per square centimeter, W is the power in watts, and sd is the spot diameter in millimeters. It is easily appreciated that changes in the power density can be obtained with changes in the power settings used, but even more pronounced changes can be obtained by altering the spot diameter. This relationship can be used by the surgeon to control laser-defined variables that affect the surgical result.

The importance of power density has been demonstrated by Taylor et al,[38] who demonstrated that power densities of greater than 5000 W/cm^2 for a continuous waveform and 2500 W/cm^2 for a pulsed waveform resulted in minimal lateral thermal damage to tissue. Falling below these power densities resulted in exponentially increasing later damage. These considerations should be kept in mind when choosing spot diameters and power settings, as well as waveforms, for a laser.

Laser-defined variables include not only the basic type of laser, but also the pulse frequency, the pulse amplitude, and the diameter of the laser beam at the point of impact with the tissue. The laser beam itself is delivered from the laser generator to the target via either a series of mirrors housed within articulating arms or flexible fiberoptic systems. The carbon dioxide (CO_2) laser beam, like other lasers, exits the generator in a specific geometric configuration, transverse electromagnetic mode (TEM$_{00}$), and in a coherent, in-phase form. After bouncing from one mirror to

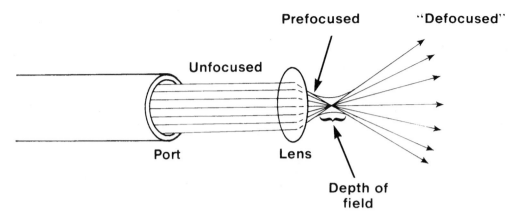

Fig. 59-1. A lens is generally used to focus the CO_2 laser. This can be used with other lasers. (With permission from Martin DC, editor: *Intra-abdominal laser surgery,* 1986, Memphis, Resurge Press.)

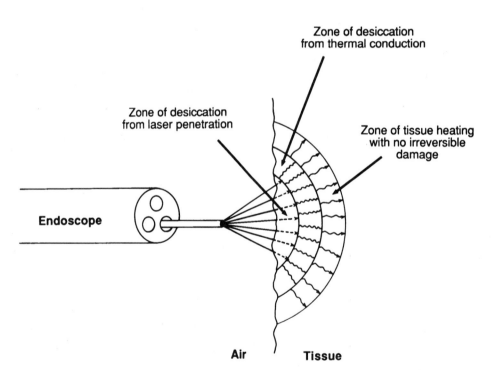

Fig. 59-2. The power density is highest as the laser emerges from the fiber. The power density rapidly decreases until it hits tissue. There is an initial zone of conversion of light energy into thermal energy as the light energy is absorbed by the tissue. Past this zone, there is a thermal conduction zone. With very low heating, reversible thermal damage occurs. Above this level of heat, irreversible thermal damage occurs. Irreversible thermal damage generally occurs in the zone of laser penetration and in the adjacent zone of thermal penetration. Tissue farther away from this has lesser degrees of heating, with reversible thermal damage. (With permission from Martin DC, editor: *Intra-abdominal laser surgery,* ed 2, Memphis, Resurge Press, in preparation.)

Table 59-1. Power densities for CO_2 laser tissue effect

Watts/cm^2	Tissue effect
0–50	Warming
5–200	Superficial desiccation and contraction
400–4000	Slow, wide vaporization and sublimation
> 1200	Rapid, narrow vaporization and sublimation

From Martin DC: Tissue effects of lasers, *Semin Reprod Endocrinol* 9:127, 1991 (with permission).

Table 59-2. The effect of heating tissue

Temperature	Effect
42.5°C	Death of malignant cells
44.0°C	Death of normal cells
60.0°C	Collagen helix uncoils
65.0°C	Coagulation of protein
100.0°C	Vaporization of water
3652.0°C	Sublimation of carbon

From Martin DC: Tissue effects of lasers, *Semin Reprod Endocrinol* 9:127, 1991 (with permission).

Table 59-3. General characteristics of lasers

Type of laser	Color	Wavelength (nm)	Extinction coefficient Water (cm)	Extinction coefficient Tissue (mm)
CO_2	Infrared	10,600	0.001	0.02
Argon	Blue-green	488–515	4,000	0.5
KTP	Green	532	*	*
Nd:YAG	Infrared	1,064	10	1.25

From Martin DC: Tissue effects of lasers, *Semin Reprod Endocrinol* 9:127, 1991 (with permission).
*Approximately equal to argon laser.

the next, the basic configuration is unaltered, permitting a lens system to focus the beam precisely to a large number of spot diameters (Fig. 59-1). In contrast, the laser beam in fiberoptic systems enters the fiber only to bounce along the fiber and exit in a diverging fashion. It is at the exit from the fiber that the laser photons are at their highest-power density (Fig. 59-2).

In an effort to alter this fact of divergence, a variety of lenses have been used with the fiberoptic lasers, including the sapphire and other artificial tips, which attempt to focus the power and increase the power density. Although these systems are inefficient, two effects are noted. First, higher-power densities can be obtained. Second, high temperatures are created at the tip, permitting the tip of the fiber to be used as a heating probe to vaporize tissue.[35] When the initial power density is high enough to exceed the threshold of vaporization, vaporization will be maintained for a short distance from the end of the fiber. Past this, the power density decreases and produces coagulation. As the distance exceeds 1 to 2 cm, the power density is so low that tissue is heated but has no irreversible damage.[19]

The question then arises as to why one would choose a fiber laser over the CO_2 laser. The answer depends on the personal experience of the surgeon. Many surgeons were exposed to the CO_2 laser in the days when articulating arms were more frequently out of alignment than aligned properly, creating unacceptable delays. The fiber lasers were much more flexible, obviating the need for mirror alignment and articulating arms. The new generation of articulating arms, although not perfect, are engineered so as to minimize the possibility of alignment problems.

Tissue effects

The primary effects possible with the lasers include incision, coagulation, and vaporization, each effect arising from a different response of tissue to the laser beam. These responses are, in turn, directly determined by properties of the target tissue. Tissue-defined variables include tissue density, water content, absorptivity, degree of vascularity, and chemical composition. For example, a given exposure to laser energy will produce different effects in ovarian, tubal, and uterine tissues.

As laser energy is absorbed, light energy is converted into thermal energy. The effect of this conversion is depen-

dent on the power and the energy density. At low-power densities, the initial effect is warming or drying (desiccation) of tissue. As the power density increases, the tissue is coagulated or carbonized and there is greater lateral tissue damage. At very-high-power density, water is vaporized, and the solid component—particularly carbon—is sublimated (Table 59-1), producing less lateral tissue damage. As long as the tissue is predominantly water, the temperature at the base of the crater is limited to 100°C. However, dry tissue sublimates at higher temperatures and carbon sublimates at 3652°C.

The potential utility of low-power densities for "welding" of tissues to form a union has been explored, with disappointing results.[21,26] One problem with the use of welding techniques with the laser is that temperatures must be limited to 60°C so that the collagen will unwind but not denature. At this temperature, the collagen will return to its normal state on cooling[15] (Table 59-2).

LASER TYPES

The lasers used in surgery include CO_2, argon, potassium–tantanyl–phosphate (KTP), neodymium:yttrium–aluminum–garnet (Nd:YAG), and helium–neon (HeNe). The HeNe laser is a 2- to 5-mW aiming beam and is not used for gynecologic surgery. The CO_2 laser beam is the most highly absorbed in both water and tissue and is predominantly a surface-effect laser (Table 59-3). On the other hand, the Nd:YAG laser has the least absorption in tissue and is the best-penetrating laser for hemostasis in the case of situations such as gastrointestinal hemorrhage and in surgery of the liver. In gynecology, this has been most useful for endometrial ablation.[22] The argon and KTP lasers have intermediate effects. These have greater penetration in water but are more highly absorbed in tissue than the Nd:YAG laser. This combination is very useful for surgery of the retina.

Although the KTP and argon lasers have significant absorption by hemoglobin, this selectivity is limited to 0.3- to 0.8-mm penetration. Damage to tissue past that point is related to thermal conductivity from the heat produced by the primary absorption.

SAFETY CONSIDERATIONS

Safe use and complications of lasers in surgery are covered extensively in other publications describing the use of lasers.[11,27,33,36] The most important concepts regarding safe use are those that are applicable to medicine and surgery in general. Appropriate indications must exist for the surgery. The approach chosen should be the one most likely to help and least likely to harm the patient. There are situations when the laser may be useful, but it must be recognized that equivalent or improved results can be obtained by using electrocautery or sharp dissection.[8] The skills and limitations of the surgeon need to be recognized realistically; and, even when the surgeon is credentialed, ongoing education is required because of the rapid changes in the field of operative endoscopy. In addition to those concepts, several specific concerns are addressed in the following discussion.

In the dawning of advanced endoscopic surgery it is not uncommon to see a plethora of tubing, wires, light cables, and other paraphernalia on the surgical drapes. Often a foot pedal is present for both the electrocautery unit and the laser. This is a potentially dangerous situation because activation of one may occur when the wrong pedal is depressed. To preclude this event, care must be taken to recognize placement of controlling pedals and to minimize the equipment placed on the operative field. Examples have also been called to the authors' attention whereby the assistant controls the laser or electrocautery pedal for the surgeon. This also is an extremely dangerous practice that has no place in the surgical theater.

Backstops

Backstops are necessary, primarily with the CO_2 laser, so as to obviate damage to unintended structures. Since the CO_2 laser radiation is absorbed by water, solutions are often the easiest to use. These can be introduced into the pelvis or can be injected behind the peritoneum either to dissect the tissue planes or to increase the distance of peritoneal structures from deeper structures.[31,32] An added advantage to use of fluids is that they continually bathe pelvic tissues, providing relief from tissue drying that can occur during both laparotomy and laparoscopy. Although retroperitoneal

placement of these solutions is said in one study to push the peritoneum away from the ureter, the study suggests that this is not the situation in the majority of cases.[13] For adhesiolysis the adhesions themselves often can be used as a backstop simply by impinging the laser beam "end-on." Although these techniques add an extra degree of safety, there is no technique that guarantees safety in all patients.

Concerns regarding the use of backstops are more important for the CO_2 laser than for fiber-propagated lasers. The divergence of the beam of a fiber-propagated laser is generally sufficient to protect distal targets, as discussed earlier in this chapter and demonstrated in Fig. 59-2.

It would be remiss to fail to acknowledge the importance of stepping on the laser pedal only when the HeNe beam or fiber tip is clearly visible. When using the operative channel of the laparoscope it is important to be mindful of the blind spot that exists, which might permit bowel, for example, to sneak into the line of fire, resulting in unintended damage. Any potential damage to vital structures should be thoroughly investigated, even if conversion to a laparotomy is required. Denial, the leading cause of pilot-related fuel mismanagement in aviation (i.e., running out of gas), afflicts surgeons also, with potentially devastating results.

Pulmonary complications

Instructors and participants in laboratory teaching exercises have developed acute bronchitis and pneumonitis when adequate smoke evacuation was not used.[28] Previous studies have shown that laser smoke is particulate. The vaporization of 1 g of tissue produces a mutagenic effect equivalent to three to six cigarettes.[39] Furthermore, this particulate nature increases worries regarding dissemination of other diseases, including human immuno-deficiency virus.[17] Because of this worry, high-flow evacuation systems are used and kept within 1 cm of the surgical site for effective removal of the plume.[28]

Although surgical masks have been designed to filter out the 0.1-to 0.8-μm particles, these masks generally force air around the edges and decrease the effectiveness. Studies have suggested that adequate mask protection will require a fitted face mask with cartridge filters, somewhat close to the masks used to protect from aerosol gases in war.[2]

SURGICAL APPROACH

The extent of surgery to be performed at laparoscopy is controversial.[1,34] Laparotomy is performed when palpation or delicate tissue handling is essential. However, laparoscopy is adequate when techniques are visual and rely more on exposure and visualization than on palpation and delicate control. Lasers themselves are most useful at laparoscopy when the precision and predictability of the cut aid in maintaining delicate control of the surgery. It is acknowledged, however, that the CO_2 laser, in particular, can be utilized with a micromanipulator during laparotomy to gain great precision and control, often with excellent results.

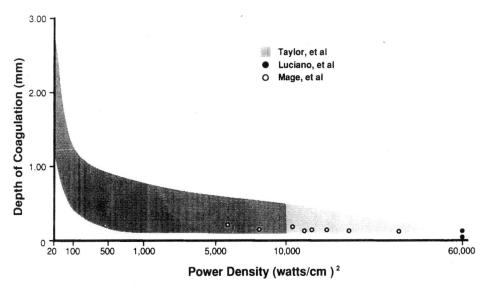

Fig. 59-3. Depth of coagulation of residual tissue, using the CO_2 laser. Coagulation and the remaining tissue after laser vaporization is determined by power density. This is mediated through the speed of the incision. Higher-power densities result in faster incisions and less lateral coagulation. (With permission from Martin DC: Tissue effects of lasers, *Sem Reprod Endocrinol* 9:127, 1991.)

Pelvic adhesions

Pelvic adhesions are one of the most common findings associated with infertility and are found in 15% to 20% of infertile patients.[16] Although uterine immobility, pelvic mass, and tenderness may suggest the diagnosis,[37] these are frequently an unpredictable finding at laparoscopy. Adhesions may interfere with fertility because of mechanical distortion or hormonal abnormalities such as found with luteinized unruptured follicles.[14] In addition, evidence recently has been presented demonstrating nerve fibers in adhesions, supporting a role for adhesions in pelvic/abdominal pain.[20]

Adhesions are lysed by using a multiple-puncture technique. After identification, the adhesions are stretched and excised, with the excision including both margins. When the margins cannot be excised, they are vaporized or coagulated. The bases of all adhesions are excised, because this is a common site for unrecognized endometriosis when it is found in association with adhesions.[30] Without this excision, the diagnosis of endometriosis has been missed by laparoscopic examination only.

When using the CO_2 laser, the superpulse or ultrapulse is used to minimize thermal damage to the remaining tissue. High-power density decreases the time of exposure and the lateral coagulation (Fig. 59-3). A high-flow insufflator with intermittent suction helps keep the smoke cleared. Either irrigation solutions or the adhesions themselves can be used as a backstop.

The argon and KTP lasers can be used with small fibers to create high-power density. The tip of the fiber can be used to touch the tissue directly and thus function as a dissecting instrument.[9] The Nd:YAG laser can be used in a similar fashion with artificial tips.[35] Care should be taken to recognize that the tissue effect of fiber lasers can penetrate further than suspected, increasing the likelihood of intraoperative or postoperative complications.

Although the CO_2 laser is more predictable and precise, studies suggest no difference between this and electrosurgery in the incidence of adhesion re-formation[3,23] or subsequent pregnancy rates.[32] In fact, careless use of the laser, as with any surgical modality, can contribute to adhesion formation and re-formation.

On the other hand, laparoscopy has been shown to decrease the adhesion re-formation rate in a prospective rabbit study[24] and in clinical trials performed by overlapping clinical groups.[10,11] In those studies, new adhesions were identified in 51% of the patients after laparotomy and in only 12% after laparoscopy. In addition, the adhesion re-formation after laparoscopy was of filmy adhesions only, with few dense adhesions found.

Hydrosalpinges

The Bruhat technique[6,29] involves an initial incision into the tube at high-power density, followed by opening of the tube in radial or linear fashion. The tube is then turned back by using a defocused or mode-shifted beam of the CO_2 laser (Fig. 59-4). The defocused beam results in low-power density, resulting in superficial desiccation and contraction,

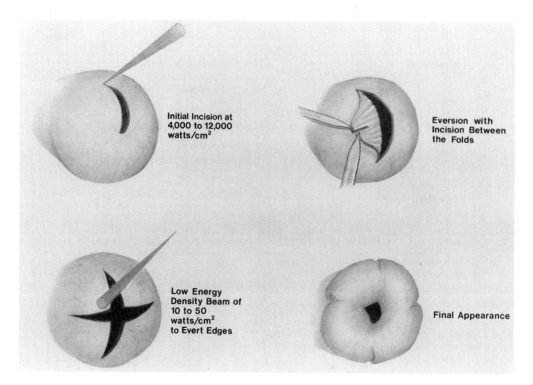

Fig. 59-4. An initial incision in the tube is used to begin the cuff salpingostomy. A series of radial or linear incisions is then made with the endosalpinx under direct vision. The folds are avoided in this incision. A low-power density beam is then applied to the tubal serosa. This everts the edges and turns the endosalpinx outward. (With permission from Martin DC, editor: *Intra-abdominal laser surgery,* Memphis, 1986, Resurge Press.)

which, in turn, induces an eversion effect. Scissor salpingostomy followed by the Bruhat technique is preferred by some surgeons to evert the tubal mucosa and obviate the need for suturing.

Pregnancy rates of 13% to 39% have been reported.[12] Comparative studies by Bruhat and Magee[7] and Tulandi[40] have shown no difference between electromicrosurgery and laser microsurgery. Boer-Meisel et al,[5] using standard microsurgical techniques, reported 77% of patients with stage I disease, 22% with stage II disease, and 3% with stage III disease having intrauterine pregnancies following surgery. Comparison with this specific classification has not been published for lasers. It is anticipated, based on the available data, that the major determinant will be surgical findings and not the equipment or visualization approach.

Tubal anastomosis

Although pregnancy rates of up to 86% have been reported after tubal microsurgery with the CO_2 laser,[18] this has not been the general experience, and a summary of all animal and human studies through 1986 led to the conclusion that lasers should be avoided in tubal anastomosis.[26] This conclusion appears to be related to the observation that at power densities less than 5000 W/cm^2, there is an increasing depth of coagulation in remnant tissue with a subsequent increased chance of tubal stenosis (Fig. 59-5 and 59-6).

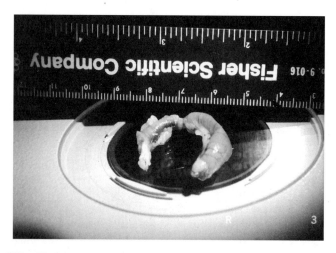

Fig. 59-5. Anastomosis of a rabbit uterine horn resulted in tubal stenosis when power densities of 500 and 1000 W/cm_2 were used. This did not occur at power densities of more than 12,000 W/cm^2.[28] (With permission from Martin DC: Tissue effects of lasers, *Semin Reprod Endocrinol* 9:127, 1991.)

CONCLUSION

The main use of lasers for tubal infertility appears to be at the time of laparoscopy. These are generally used in combination with other laparoscopic equipment, such as bipolar coagulators, thermal coagulators, scissors, grasping forceps, and sutures. The choice of these modalities de-

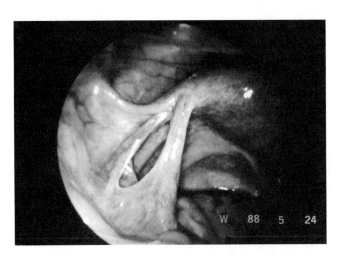

Fig. 59-6. A tubal incision and brushing technique[4] resulted in both stenosis of the anastomotic site and loss of the mesosalpinx. (With permission from Martin DC: Tissue effects of lasers, *Semin Reprod Endocrinol* 9:127, 1991.)

pends on the effect desired, as well as the experience and skill of the operator. Ongoing study is needed to determine which equipment is optimal for a given operative procedure.

REFERENCES

1. Adamson GD: The choice of therapy for the operative treatment of endometriosis is endoscopic laser surgery: pro, *J Gynecol Surg* 7:129, 1991.
2. Akale D, Streifel A, Ahrens R: A method for limiting laser plume during bronchoscopic and other angioscopic surgery. International Laser Safety Conference, Cincinnati, Nov 1990, American Society for Lasers in Medicine and Surgery.
3. Barbot J et al: A clinical study of the CO_2 laser and electrosurgery for adhesiolysis in 172 cases followed by second-look laparoscopy, *Fertile Steril* 48:140, 1987.
4. Bellina JH: Lasers in gynecology, *World J Surg* 7:692, 1983.
5. Boer-Meisel ME et al: Predicting the pregnancy outcome in patients treated for hydrosalpinx: a prospective study, *Fertil Steril* 45:23, 1986.
6. Bruhat MA: Magee G, Jacquetin B et al: Laser CO_2 in tubal surgery. In Bellina JH, editor: *Gynecological laser surgery*, New York, 1981, Plenum Press.
7. Bruhat MA, Magee G: Pregnancy following salpingostomy: comparison between CO_2 laser and electrosurgery procedures, *Fertil Steril* 40:472, 1983.
8. Corfman RS, Diamond MP: Laser, cautery or knife: which is best? In McLaughlin D, editor: *Laser in gynecology*, Philadelphia, 1990, WB Saunders.
9. Diamond MP, DeCherney AH, Polan ML: Laparoscopic use of the argon laser in nonendometriotic reproductive pelvic surgery, *J Reprod Med* 31:1011, 1986.
10. Diamond MP et al: Adhesion reformation and de novo formation after reproductive pelvic surgery, *Fertil Steril* 47:864, 1987.
11. Diamond MP et al: Postoperative adhesion development after operative laparoscopy: evaluation at early second-look procedures, *Fertil Steril* 55:700, 1991.
12. Feste JR: Laser therapy for endometriosis, adhesions, and tubal disease. In McLaughlin DS, editor: *Lasers in gynecology*, Philadelphia, 1991, JB Lippincott.
13. Grainger DA et al: Hydrodissection as a means of protecting the ureter from injury at laparoscopy: evaluation by retroperitoneal exploration. Presented at the American Fertility Society Meeting, Orlando, Fla, Oct 19–24, 1991 (abstract).
14. Hamilton CJCM, Evers JLH, Hoogland HJ: Ovulatory disorders and inflammatory adnexal damage: a neglected cause of failure of fertility microsurgery, *Br J Obstet Gynaecol* 93:282, 1986.
15. Harris DM, Werkhaven JA: Biophysics and applications of medical lasers, *Arch Otolaryngol Head Neck Surg* 3:91, 1989.
16. Hershlag A, Diamond MP, DeCherney AH: Adhesiolysis, *Clin Obstet Gynecol* 34:395, 1991.
17. Jako GJ: CO_2 laser in surgery for prophylaxis of HIV infection, *Lasers Surg Med* 8:139, 1988 (letter to the editor).
18. Kelly RW, Diamond MP: Intra-abdominal use of the carbon dioxide laser for microsurgery. In Dorsey JH, editor: *Obstetrics and gynecology clinics of North America: Lasers in gynecology*, Philadelphia, 1991, WB Saunders.
19. Keye WR, McArthur GR: Laser laparoscopy: argon. In Keye WR, editor: *Laser surgery in gynecology and obstetrics*, ed 2, St Louis, 1990, Mosby–Year Book.
20. Kligman I et al: Immohistochemical demonstration of nerve fibers in pelvic adhesions, *Obstet Gynecol* 82:566, 1993.
21. Klink F et al: Animal in vivo studies and in vitro experiments with human tubes for end-to-end anastomotic operations by CO_2 laser technique, *Fertil Steril* 30:100, 1978.
22. Lomano JM: Laparoscopic ablation of endometriosis with the YAG laser, *Lasers Surg Med* 3:179, 1983 (abstract).
23. Luciano AA et al: A comparison of thermal injury, healing patterns, and postoperative adhesion formation following CO_2 laser and electromicrosurgery, *Fertil Steril* 48:1025, 1987.
24. Luciano AA et al: A comparative study of postoperative adhesions following laser surgery by laparoscopy versus laparotomy in the rabbit model, *Obstet Gynecol* 74:222, 1989.
24a. Magee G, Pouly JL, Bruhat MA: Laser microsurgery of the oviducts. In Baggish MS, editor: *Basic and advanced laser surgery and gynecology*, Norwalk, 1985, Appleton-Century-Crofts.
25. Martin DC: Laser physics and practice. In Hunt RB, editor: *Atlas of female infertility surgery*, Chicago, 1986, Year Book Medical Publishers.
26. Martin DC: Tubal microsurgery. In Martin DC et al, editors: *Intraabdominal laser surgery*, Memphis, 1986, Resurge Press.
27. Martin DC: Laser safety. In Keye WR, editor: *Laser surgery in gynecology and obstetrics*, ed 2, St. Louis, 1990, Mosby–Year Book.
28. Martin DC: Tissue effects of lasers, *Semin Reprod Endocrinol* 9:127, 1991.
29. Martin DC, Diamond MP: Operative laparoscopy: comparison of lasers with other techniques, *Curr Probl Obstet Gynecol Fertil* 9:563, 1986.
30. Martin DC et al: Laparoscopic appearances of peritoneal endometriosis, *Fertil Steril* 51:63, 1989.
31. Nezhat C, Nezhat FR: Safe laser endoscopic excision or vaporization of peritoneal endometriosis, *Fertil Steril* 52:149, 1989.
32. Reich H: Laparoscopic treatment of extensive pelvic adhesions, including hydrosalpinx, *J Reprod Med* 32:736, 1987.
33. Rockwell RJ, editor: *Laser safety in surgery and medicine,* Cincinnati, 1985, Rockwell Associates.
34. Shepard MK: The choice of therapy for the operative treatment of endometriosis is endoscopic laser surgery: con, *J Gynecol Surg* 7:133, 1991.
35. Shirk GJ: Use of the ND:YAG laser with sapphire scalpels. In McLaughlin DS, editor: *Laser in gynecology*, Philadelphia, 1991, JB Lippincott.
36. Sliney D, Wolbarsht M: *Safety with lasers and other optical sources,* New York, 1990, Plenum Press.
37. Stovall TG, Elder RF, Ling FW: Predictors of pelvic adhesions, *J Reprod Med* 34:345, 1989.
38. Taylor MV et al: Effect of power density and carbonization on residual tissue coagulation using the continuous wave carbon dioxide laser, *Colposcopy Gynecol Laser Surg* 2:169, 1986.
39. Tomita Y et al: Mutagenicity of smoke condensates induced by CO_2 laser irradiation and electrocauterization, *Mutat Res* 89:145, 1981.
40. Tulandi T: Salpingo-ovariolysis: a comparison between laser surgery and electrosurgery, *Fertil Steril* 45:489, 1986.

Chapter 60

MICROSURGICAL TUBAL RECONSTRUCTION AND REVERSAL OF STERILIZATION

**Victor Gomel, MD
and Timothy C. Rowe, MD**

Human life ordinarily begins with the bringing together of gametes in the ampulla of the fallopian tubes. When the meeting of the sperm and the oocyte is prevented by distortion or occlusion of the oviducts, conception becomes impossible. Much of the observed increase in the incidence of infertility in the past two decades has been the result of oviductal damage following sexually transmitted infections.

A single episode of pelvic inflammatory disease will leave a residue of tubal damage sufficient to cause infertility in nearly 20% of affected women.[44] Before the development of in vitro fertilization (IVF) and embryo transfer (ET) in women, the only therapeutic option for infertile women with damaged oviducts was an attempt at surgical repair, and the conventional techniques used yielded disappointingly low pregnancy rates.

MICROSURGICAL APPROACHES

Swolin in 1975 described the use of magnification in the surgical correction of distal tubal disease.[38] Magnification, the use of an operating microscope, and microsurgical techniques were subsequently expanded and utilized in the correction of pathologic cornual and midtubal occlusion and in reversal of sterilization.[14,16,27] The ultimate application of microsurgical techniques is, in fact, tubal anastomosis, since magnification enables the precise apposition of tubal segments using very fine suture material. Magnification also allows the recognition of subtle tubal abnormalities even in the presence of tubal patency.

In the treatment of distal tubal occlusion, microsurgical techniques reduced postoperative adhesion formation and improved tubal patency rates; however, the viable pregnancy rates were not significantly better than those obtained by the use of conventional techniques.[21] It has become evident that in distal tubal occlusion the most important factor that predicts outcome is the extent of tubal damage, rather than the surgical technique used. The introduction of microsurgical techniques has allowed the development of tubocornual anastomosis for treatment of proximal tubal occlusion associated with pathologic conditions; it has also allowed tubotubal anastomosis for correction of midtubal occlusion related to pathologic processes, including arrested tubal pregnancy, and for reversal of tubal sterilization. The application of microsurgical techniques has significantly improved the outcome of such procedures.

The assimilation of microsurgical techniques into gynecology has produced benefits beyond improved pregnancy rates. Microsurgery as a *concept* rather than a collection of skills made gynecologists much more conscious of the effects of peritoneal trauma and postoperative adhesions. The conservative and minimally traumatic procedures involved in microsurgery promoted the conservative approaches that are now considered standard care for women undergoing treatment for benign gynecologic disorders. In this chapter are discussed microsurgical principles, the use of magnification, and the instruments involved. Choosing a microsurgical approach in tubal factor infertility may be more controversial in the era of IVF-ET, and the alternatives to microsurgery and their selection are discussed. The general infertility assessment is not considered in detail, but the investigations relevant to tubal and peritoneal factors are reviewed.

INFERTILITY INVESTIGATION

Infertile couples pass through several clearly recognized emotional states in coming to terms with their infertility; these include denial, depression, optimism, frustration, and, finally, acceptance. The identification of a cause of infertility is usually followed by optimism on the part of the couple; but if treatment does not result in pregnancy, despite the elimination of the perceived obstacles, the couple will understandably become frustrated. Such frustration will be especially intense for them if they have not participated fully in the decision-making about treatment. Therefore the significance of any abnormality found as a result of the assessment of the infertile couple must be honestly and accurately discussed with them, and the therapeutic options and their predicted outcomes must be described fully. Although pregnancy is the goal for both the physician and the patient, ultimately the choice of whether or not to undergo a suggested form of treatment lies with the couple.

Even in cases where the history clearly suggests a tubal or peritoneal factor, assessment of other fertility factors is mandatory. At a minimum, a semen analysis and confirmation of ovulation should be undertaken. Other factors should be assessed at the discretion of the investigator. (See Chapter 18.) In the assessment of tubal factors, hysterosalpingography (HSG) is the first step. A properly performed HSG allows the evaluation of the uterine cavity and of intratubal architecture. Proximal tubal occlusion and nonocclusive lesions of the cornu can be identified. HSG also permits assessment of the length, internal patency, and architecture of the proximal segments in the case of a midtubal occlusion or in women seeking reversal of sterilization. With proximal tubal occlusion and nonocclusive cornual lesions, HSG allows assessment of the intramural segment. With terminal tubal occlusion, the presence of ampullary rugal markings is a favorable sign, giving a higher probability of pregnancy after reconstructive surgery; conversely, the presence of intratubal adhesions is an adverse sign. The use of an aqueous contrast medium (diatrizoate meglumine 60% [Hypaque M60]) over oil-soluble media may be preferred, since the former provides a better definition of the tubal mucosa and tubal lesions. Laparoscopy and HSG are complementary procedures in the evaluation of tubal or peritoneal factors. In fertility assessment, laparoscopy is performed *after* HSG, since the hysterosalpingographic information about the status of the uterus and oviducts is important at the time of the subsequent laparoscopy. This is especially valuable when subsequent corrective surgery can be performed laparoscopically. In addition, such information will permit the surgeon to counsel the couple and schedule an adequate length of time for the surgery. Furthermore, if the HSG has shown no abnormality in the uterine cavity, cornua, or tubal lumen, the surgeon who discovers unsuspected adnexal adhesions, tubal phimosis, or distal occlusion can undertake laparoscopic salpingoovariolysis, fimbrioplasty, or salpingostomy with confidence.

SELECTION OF TREATMENT

Surgical skill includes both the technical aptitude for reconstruction and the judgment to decide when surgery is appropriate and when it is not. For the couple in whom there is a tuboperitoneal cause for infertility, or a previously performed sterilization, the only options for achieving a pregnancy are through tubal reconstruction or IVF. Depending on the nature and site of the damage, tubal reconstruction may be effected microsurgically by laparoscopically directed techniques or by tubal cannulation. The choice will be influenced by both nontechnical and purely technical considerations; these are reviewed subsequently. It must be emphasized that the choices are not necessarily mutually exclusive. Undergoing tubal reconstruction does not preclude the possibility of treatment with IVF subsequently and vice versa.

Nontechnical considerations

Irrespective of the potential for surgical therapy, the therapeutic options will be dependent on the local expertise, the respective costs, the age of the woman, and the couple's perceptions of the various procedures.

Costs of treatment. The costs of undergoing one or another treatment for infertility may be considerable, and will be a significant factor when health insurance for these procedures is not available. Another often underestimated potential factor is the economic impact of a multiple pregnancy, which is statistically more likely with IVF. The significance of cost considerations is an individual matter for each couple.

Age of the woman. The age of the woman is a critical factor. There is general agreement, based on a number of data sources, that fecundity begins to decline at about age 31. This trend has been noted both in "normal" couples[42] and in couples with unexplained infertility.[5] In women aged 40 or more who undergo reversal of sterilization, the live birth rate is approximately 45%,[40] a figure significantly less than that in women who are younger. The effect of the age of the woman is even clearer when the results of IVF are considered. There is a rapid decline in "take home baby rate" after the age of 40, falling from a rate of 8.3% per oocyte retrieval between the ages of 40 and 41 to a rate of 2.4% thereafter.[15] This rapid decline in fecundity means that each cycle in which conception is attempted becomes precious. Therefore the physician should be reluctant to offer tubal reconstruction as initial treatment, except for cases of reversal of sterilization, in a woman who is 40 years of age or older. Such couples may well prefer to undergo IVF as initial treatment, since there is likely a higher monthly fecundity rate with IVF and since success or failure is evident within the cycle of treatment. Tubal surgery does, however, offer the possibility of multiple cycles in which conception may occur. If IVF is unsuccessful in a predetermined number of cycles, it may be reasonable to offer tubal surgery subsequently. Interestingly, a number of reports have shown significantly higher pregnancy rates in women over 40 who receive oocytes donated by younger women[29,33]; this topic is beyond the scope of this chapter. (See Chapter 48.)

Perceptions of the couple. The perceptions of the couple regarding assisted reproductive technologies and reproductive surgery will depend on many influences, including the couple's own values and ethical views. Furthermore, partners may not even agree with each other. The physician should aim to provide detailed information for the couple that is as clear and accurate as possible and to abstain from interfering with their decision-making process except to clarify misunderstandings and misinterpretations. The couple's response may be prohibitive (tending to limit gamete manipulation or to restrict interference with "natural" processes or structures) or liberal (favoring performance of any procedure or manipulation that may enhance fertility, regardless of cost, risk, or degree of effectiveness), but most commonly falls between these extremes. The responsible physician will be cautious in dealing with couples desperate to undergo active treatment, since treatment with essentially no chance of success cannot be justified.

Technical considerations

When counseling the couple on therapeutic options for tubal factor infertility it is essential to consider the results achieved in the local center rather than published data available from the literature. This approach provides a factual basis for a decision; in simple terms, this would mean choosing the treatment providing the highest pregnancy rate in the center in which the treatment is carried out. Furthermore, the choice of treatment must be made in the context of the individual couple. Making a choice presupposes that the couple has undergone a full infertility work-up. More than one infertility factor may be present; for example, a couple may have reduced fertility because of tubal disease, as well as oligoovulation or oligospermia.

In certain circumstances, any attempt at tubal repair is contraindicated, making IVF the only option for treatment

(e.g., when both tubes have been removed, when there is a history of tuberculous salpingitis, or when there is severe tubal damage). In other instances, particularly in younger women, tubal reconstruction may be performed first and IVF undertaken subsequently if surgery proves unsuccessful.

In discussing the probability of success after either IVF or tubal surgery, it is important to compare the outcome of each procedure in a standardized manner. It is a common perception among patients that IVF offers a "low" chance of success when compared with the results of tubal surgery; this perception is usually based on the understanding that quoted pregnancy rates after one IVF treatment cycle represent the highest rates of pregnancy that can be achieved. This is clearly not the case, since pregnancy rates remain constant through successive treatment cycles. Data from the Hallam Centre[39] show that after four IVF treatment cycles, an overall cumulative conception rate of 44.6% and a live birth rate of 33.9% can be achieved. Comparative data from a normal United Kingdom population suggest a cumulative probability of pregnancy of 32% after 3 months and 54% after 6 months; therefore IVF can offer pregnancy rates that are comparable to those achieved by a normal population. The outcome of tubal surgery, in comparison, is normally quoted either as a crude pregnancy rate (percentage of patients pregnant after 1, 2, or 3 years) or as a cumulative probability of pregnancy at a fixed point (usually 2 years after surgery) after life table analysis. Although the former rate calculation represents real pregnancies, the latter indicates only a potential.

The risks associated with the various treatment options must be considered and the couple appropriately counseled. IVF, particularly in stimulated cycles, is not without risk. Ovarian hyperstimulation syndrome may result from gonadotropin therapy. Infections of the pelvis or of the gametes may occur, and hemorrhage may follow oocyte retrieval. Multiple pregnancies and their attendant complications represent a real risk of IVF; the twin pregnancy rate is approximately 20%, and triplets or higher-order multiple pregnancies account for 4% of deliveries. The perinatal mortality associated with IVF is just under 10%. Up to 25% of IVF pregnancies may abort, and 6% of clinical pregnancies are ectopic. Regrettably, in the very patients who must choose between tubal surgery and IVF—those with tubal disease—ectopic pregnancy may occur in up to 12% of pregnancies after IVF.[47] Couples making the choice between tubal surgery and IVF should be informed that IVF therapy does not eliminate the possibility of ectopic pregnancy.

The risks of tubal reconstructive surgery, whether carried out by laparoscopy, laparotomy, or tubal cannulation techniques, are small. Tubal cannulation is usually performed with local anesthetic only; laparoscopic surgery and laparotomies carry the risks common to many gynecologic procedures requiring general anesthesia. Concerns regarding general anesthesia may be resolved in some cases by a formal consultation between the patient and the anesthesiologist. It is appropriate to define, for patients with no experience with major surgery, the transient effects on bladder and bowel inherent in undergoing laparotomy. Specific advantages of tubal surgery include the fact that the couple can attempt pregnancy independent of any treatment facility, and can do so over multiple cycles. In addition, the abortion and multiple pregnancy rates in women who conceive after tubal surgery are not different from those of the normal population. The live birth and ectopic pregnancy rates will be governed by the specific nature of the tubal damage, the surgical techniques used, and whether or not the woman has one or both tubes.

RESULTS OF RECONSTRUCTIVE TUBAL SURGERY

Selection of the most appropriate therapeutic approach is a critical part of the surgical management of tubal factor infertility. The results of surgery depend partly on the nature and extent of the tubal damage, but they also depend heavily on the expertise of the surgeon, both in selection of the cases and in technical skills. Selection affects the outcome; if patients with poor prognosis are not operated upon, the overall results will be better. Technical skills are important, since the first surgical attempt is the most likely to be successful. Subsequent surgical procedures must deal with the consequences of the initial surgery, as well as the effects of the disease.

Deciding whether or not surgical treatment is appropriate in an individual case is based on the projected possibility of pregnancy after a particular procedure. Although series of particular procedures can provide an estimate of the probability, the individual case will have features that may alter the prognosis. These features include (1) the nature and extent of the pelvic and periadnexal adhesions, (2) the severity and extent of the disease process affecting the tube, (3) the extent of tubal damage, (4) the final length of the reconstructed oviduct, (5) the presence or absence of additional pelvic disease, and (6) concurrent presence of other factors that might prejudice fertility. An estimate of surgical prognosis must therefore take the preceding factors into account.

Reporting of results must be based on the condition of the "better" adnexa, where the disease process or the damage is less extensive. The following is a review of the reported results from various reconstructive procedures.

Periadnexal adhesive disease and fimbrial phimosis

Laparoscopic management has become the standard approach in treatment for periadnexal disease and/or fimbrial phimosis. Diagnostic laparoscopy not infrequently reveals previously unsuspected periadnexal adhesions. Laparoscopic salpingoovariolysis offers a cumulative live birth rate of 50% to 60% within 12 months, with a 5% ectopic

pregnancy rate. Laparoscopic fimbrioplasty, performed for fimbrial agglutination, phimosis (without occlusion), or prefimbrial phimosis, yields a cumulative live birth rate of 40% to 48%[3,9,10,13,18] within 12 to 18 months.

Distal tubal occlusion

Surgical management of distal tubal occlusion may be performed laparoscopically or by microsurgery via laparotomy. The former technique is becoming the procedure of choice, since the pregnancy rates after laparoscopic surgery appear to approach those yielded by microsurgery.* The outcome in individual cases will depend on a number of variables, including distal tubal diameter, the degree of preservation of the tubal endothelium, and the extent and nature of periadnexal adhesions. A scoring system has been developed based on the preceding parameters.[20] This and other scoring systems allow the surgeon to predict the outcome of surgery and to use this information in counseling patients in the selection of the most appropriate therapeutic approach.

After microsurgical salpingostomy, live birth rates range from 19% to 35% and ectopic pregnancy rates range up to 18% (Table 60-1). Considering that the results that are now being achieved with laparoscopic salpingostomy approach those of microsurgery and that IVF today is a very credible alternative treatment modality, there is a strong argument in favor of performing salpingostomy at the time of the initial laparoscopy.

Proximal tubal occlusion

The diagnosis of proximal tubal occlusion is always tentative when made by HSG or hydrotubation at laparoscopy. A tube may be patent despite failure of dye to pass; such failure can be attributed to cornual spasm, the presence of a mucous plug or synechiae obstructing the intramural or isthmic portion of the tube, or simply poor technique. Selective salpingography and/or fallopian tube cannulation under hysteroscopic, ultrasonographic, or radiographic control will usually allow differentiation of such apparent obstructions from true pathologic occlusions. After tubal cannulation, patency rates have been reported to range from 70% to 90%, and pregnancy rates of 30% to 50% (when at least one tube remains open) have been reported.[36] However, the estimated 70% to 90% patency rate will undoubtedly be partly composed of rates for women whose apparent proximal occlusion was due to faulty hysterosalpingographic technique. We rely heavily on the information yielded by HSG and employ a meticulous technique that is associated with a low false-positive rate for proximal tubal occlusion. This probably accounts for the much lower patency and pregnancy rates obtained after tubal cannulation when compared with those cited in the literature.

The real therapeutic value of tubal cannulation remains

*References 4, 9, 19(pp 230-233), 28.

Table 60-1. Results of microsurgical salpingostomy

Reference	Year	No. of patients	No. of intrauterine pregnancies	No. of viable births (%)[a]	No. of ectopic pregnancies
Swolin[38] [b]	1975	33	9	8 (24)	6
Gomel[15] [c]	1978	41	12	11 (26.8)	5
Gomel[16] [c]	1980	72	22	21 (29.2)	7
Larsson[24] [d]	1982	54	21	17 (31.5)	0
Verhoeven et al.[43]	1983	143[e]	34	28 (19.6)	3
Tulandi and Vilos[41]	1985	67[f]	15	N/S	3
Boer-Meisel et al.[2]	1986	108	31	24 (22.2)	19
Donnez and Casanas-Roux[7]	1986	83	26	N/S	6
Kosasa and Hale[23]	1988	93	37	34 (36.6)	13

[a]N/S, Not stated.
[b]Long-term follow-up.
[c]Follow-up period more than 1 year.
[d]Follow-up period more than 4 years.
[e]Of these, 23 were iterative procedures, among which there were only three (13%) live births.
[f]Of these procedures, 37 were performed using CO_2 laser.

to be proven in a randomized, controlled study comparing cannulation with observation. However, given the minimal risk of morbidity, it is reasonable to attempt tubal cannulation in women whose initial test of tubal patency indicates proximal occlusion. True proximal disease, such as salpingitis isthmica nodosa, extensive fibrosis, or occlusive polyps, will be readily demonstrated in this way. If patency cannot be established, then the choices for therapy are microsurgery and IVF.

Microsurgical tubocornual anastomosis for proximal tubal occlusion associated with pathologic lesions yields live birth rates ranging from 37% to 58%. The ectopic pregnancy rate is of the order of 5% to 7%.[*]

Reversal of sterilization

The primary treatment for reversal of tubal sterilization remains microsurgical anastomosis of the tubal segments. The success of such intervention will depend on the extent of destruction and the length and condition of the residual tubal segments. Provided that the reconstructed tube(s) has a length of at least 4 cm with an ampullary length of at least 1 cm, live birth rates of 60% to 80% can be achieved. The reported ectopic pregnancy rates vary, but average 2% to 5% (Table 60-2).

Kroener sterilization (fimbriectomy = excision of a portion of distal tube) was considered irreversible in the past. However, if at least 50% of the ampulla has been preserved, an ampullary salpingostomy will yield a live birth rate of approximately 30%.[19(p 233)]

In vitro fertilization

Infertility due to tubal damage or occlusion resulting from infection or voluntary sterilization may be managed

either by reconstructive surgery or IVF. The increasing availability of IVF, the simplification of its techniques, and the demystification of gamete manipulation have served to make IVF a more readily acceptable management. IVF-ET is currently the management of choice for significantly damaged fallopian tubes or tubes that have reoccluded after initial surgical reconstruction. The same applies to bipolar tubal disease, since the results of surgical management have been disappointing. Whereas IVF (rather than iterative surgery) is the next therapeutic step after failed salpingostomy, a second surgical procedure may be undertaken after failed tubal anastomosis, especially in cases of reversal of sterilization.

In general, accurate assessment of the condition of the fallopian tubes, along with the other fertility parameters, and a careful and sensitive appraisal of the couple's wishes and limitations will enable the clinician to help the couple reach a decision about the optimal management. It is evident that reconstructive tubal microsurgery remains an important therapeutic approach in appropriately selected cases. The technical aspects relating to such management are discussed below.

SURGICAL TECHNIQUES
General considerations

Equipment and microsurgical instruments. The major equipment includes an appropriate electrosurgical unit and an operating microscope. An electrosurgical unit, which permits both macrosurgical and microsurgical approaches, may be used.

Magnification is best obtained with an operating microscope. In addition to varying levels of magnification, the operating microscope permits precise focusing and provides coaxial illumination and a constant visual field. An objective lens with a focal length of 275 or 300 mm provides a suitable working distance for tubal microsurgery.

[*]References 8, 14, 16, 19, 26, 27

Table 60-2. Results of microsurgical tubotubal anastomosis for reversal of sterilization

References	Year	No. of patients	No. of intrauterine pregnancies	No. of viable births (%)[a]	No. of ectopic pregnancies
Gomel[12]	1974	11		8 (73)	1
Gomel[17]	1980	118		76 (64)	1
Winston[45]	1980	105	63	N/S	3
Gomel[19(pp 237-242) b]	1983	118		93 (79)	2
DeCherney et al.[6 c]	1984	124		72 (58)	8
Schlösser et al.[34]	1983	119		44 (37)	11
Silber and Cohen[35 d]	1984	48		31 (66)	2
Henderson[22]	1984	95		51 (54)	5
Paterson[30]	1985	147		87 (59)	5
Spivak et al.[37 e]	1986	68		34 (51)	6
Boeckx et al.[1]	1986	63	44	N/S	3
Rock et al.[32]	1987	80		49 (61)	10
Xue and Fa[46 f]	1989	117		95 (81)	2
Putnam et al.[31]	1990	86	64	55 (64)	

[a]N/S, Not stated.
[b]Resurvey of 1980 series; follow-up period more than 18 months.
[c]Follow-up period more than 18 months.
[d]Follow-up period more than 4 years.
[e]Follow-up period more than 1 year.
[f]Follow-up period more than 3.5 years.

Automatic foot controls for magnification, focus, and direction of the microscope are preferred, since these changes can then be readily accomplished while the surgeon's hands remain in the operating field. Operating loupes provide lower levels of fixed magnification. They may be used to divide adhesions that extend to the pelvic side wall or cul-de-sac and for dissection of endometriotic lesions located deep in the pelvis.

It is best to perform reconstructive tubal microsurgery while seated. Hence the operating table should be of a configuration that permits the surgeon and assistant to have their knees under the table. For such procedures a stool with a soft bicycle seat may be used.

The basic microsurgery instruments include a microneedle holder, both plain and toothed platform microforceps, and microscissors. The needle holder and the forceps should have rounded rather than pointed tips. A concave-convex configuration on the inner surface of the jaws of the needle holder facilitate positioning and permit a firmer grasp of the needle. Straight iris scissors or a sharp microblade are used for tubal transection, and Teflon-coated rods with rounded tips are used to retract tissue.

A true microelectrode is used to divide adhesions and to coagulate bleeding points. Microbipolar forceps similar to jewelers' forceps may be used for hemostasis involving larger vessels. Although some surgeons have advocated the use of the CO_2 laser for adhesiolysis and tubal transection, there are no current data suggesting that any advantage is derived from the use of this equipment.

In reconstructive tubal microsurgery, generally 8-0 sutures of polyglactin 910 (Vicryl) on a 130-μm shaft with a 4- or 5-mm long, taper-cut needle (Ethicon, Inc. Somerville, N.J.) may be used. This combination avoids the tissue trauma that would result from larger-shaft needles.

Immediate preoperative preparation. It is the surgeon's responsibility to ensure that all necessary equipment is present and in working order before the patient is brought into the operating room. The microsurgical instrument set should be checked to ensure that all pieces are present and functional. The operating microscope should be examined to ensure that it is functioning normally and that all ancillary equipment such as the video camera, monitor, and the electrosurgical unit are working properly.

After induction of anesthesia, the patient is placed in the froglike or lithotomy position. The bladder is catheterized for continuous drainage. A pediatric Foley catheter is passed into the uterine cavity and the balloon inflated. A sterile extension tube attached to this catheter is connected to a syringe filled with dilute dye solution. This allows the syringe to be brought into the sterile field for intraoperative chromopertubation. The patient is then placed in the dorsal position. The abdomen is painted and draped in standard fashion. The scrubbed operating room personnel wash their gloves free of powder and wipe them.

The abdominal incision. A transverse suprapubic incision is the most frequently used incision for reconstructive tubal operations. However, if a midline or paramedian scar is already present, the same route of entry is used to avoid creation of a second scar.

In the last several years, to perform reconstructive tubal microsurgery we have approached the pelvis through a small (minilaparotomy) suprapubic transverse or vertical incision. The length of the incision is dependent on the previous pelvic findings and especially the depth of the patient's subcutaneous adipose layer.

Subcutaneous infiltration of 0.25% bupivacaine hydrochloride (Marcaine) solution precedes placement of the skin incision. Before incising the fascia the rectus muscles are infiltrated with the same solution. When a transverse suprapubic incision is made, it is extended down to the fascia; then the subcutaneous fat is dissected upward and downward over the fascia, which is incised vertically in the midline. The recti are separated in the midline and the peritoneum is incised vertically. At the end of the procedure the subcutaneous tissues are reinfiltrated with the same solution before closure of the skin incision, and a bilateral inguinal nerve block is established. The small incision and the described use of local anesthesia, along with gentle handling of the tissues during the procedure, reduces postoperative discomfort and analgesia requirements. This approach permits prompt mobilization of the patient with discharge from the hospital on the first postoperative day, and has markedly shortened the postoperative recovery period.

Exposure of the surgical field. Once the peritoneal cavity is entered, the surgical personnel thoroughly wash their gloves once again. A wound protector is inserted into the peritoneal cavity, and a small Dennis-Brown retractor is applied. The bowel is displaced into the upper abdomen and kept in place with a Kerlex pad soaked in the heparinized (5,000 U/L), lactated Ringer's irrigation solution. The patient is placed in approximately 10-degree Trendelenburg position. If necessary the table may be tilted slightly toward the surgeon. Although the operating microscope may be draped, this is not necessary, particularly if the microscope is controlled by foot pedals. After elevating the uterus and adnexa by packing the pouch of Douglas loosely with soaked pads, the microscope is brought in over the operating field and focused.

A liter of the irrigation solution in an elevated intravenous (IV) bag is connected via IV tubing to a Gomel microsurgical irrigator. This arrangement permits periodic irrigation of the exposed peritoneal surfaces and ovaries to prevent desiccation during the procedure and to visualize individual bleeders.

Salpingoovariolysis

In contemporary practice it should not be necessary to perform a laparotomy solely for the purpose of salpingoovariolysis. Our primary approach in such cases has been to perform the procedure via laparoscopy, usually at the time of the initial diagnostic laparoscopy.[13,18] Microsurgical salpingoovariolysis is usually performed as part of a reconstructive tubal procedure.

Adhesions involving the fallopian tube or ovary commonly extend to the pelvic side wall, the posterior aspects of the broad ligament, and/or the uterine serosa. It is important to commence by defining the distal margins of the adhesions. These are put on tension and exposed with the use of Teflon rods. They are divided electrosurgically, using the microelectrode, cutting through to the Teflon rod. It is important to divide adhesions one layer at a time. Prominent vessels along the transection line are individually electrocoagulated. Care is taken not to damage or denude adjacent pelvic peritoneum. In the deeper parts of the pelvis, an elongating adaptor may be attached to the handle of the electrosurgical unit to provide easier access. The unit is put in the "blend" setting, which on "cut" mode combines coagulating current with cutting current to provide concurrent hemostasis while dividing adhesions. Pure coagulating current is used (on "coag" mode) to obtain hemostasis of individual bleeders, which are exposed under a jet of irrigation fluid.

Once the adhesions have been divided at their distal attachment the adnexal structures are elevated. This is followed by systematic excision of the adhesions from the tubal serosa and ovarian cortex. Adhesions are frequently composed of two layers (although appearing to be a single layer) and attached to the organ at two levels. It is essential to enter between the two layers of adhesions first. This permits exposure of the demarcation line between the adhesion and the serosa or ovary. Each layer of adhesions is then put on stretch with toothed forceps, the demarcation line identified, and the adhesion transected. Placement of a fine Teflon rod under the incision line enhances exposure. Damage to the serosa or ovarian surface is avoided by keeping the transection line 1 mm away from these surfaces. If tubal serosa or parietal peritoneum is accidentally divided, the denuded area may be reperitonealized by approximating the peritoneal edges using 7-0 or 8-0 sutures, provided this can be accomplished without undue tension. When there is too much tension, the use of peritoneal grafts has been proposed to cover large denuded areas. Such grafts tend to be avascular and may themselves predispose to adhesion formation. In most cases, however, closure of a defect is straightforward with the use of microsutures.

Fimbrioplasty

Partial distal occlusion may result from the agglutination of the fimbria (fimbrial phimosis). In addition, the distal end of the tube may be covered by fibrous tissue that must be incised or excised to gain access to the fimbria. In occasional circumstances the abdominal tubal ostium, located at the apex of the infundibulum, is stenosed (prefimbrial phimosis).

Fimbrial phimosis may be overcome simply by introducing a closed mosquito forceps through the phimotic fimbrial opening, opening the jaws within the tubal lumen, and gently withdrawing the instrument with its jaws open. Deagglutination of the fimbria is achieved by repeating this movement a few times, varying the direction in which the jaws of the forceps are opened. Bleeding is usually negligible provided appropriate gentleness is used.

In cases of prefimbrial phimosis the fimbriated end may have a normal appearance. However, with chromopertubation, the ampulla will distend before any exit of dye solution. A thin Teflon probe is introduced into the lumen of the tube. An incision is placed at the antimesosalpingeal edge of the tube, from the infundibulum, through the stenotic portion, to the distal ampulla. The edges of the resulting two flaps are folded back, and each is secured to the adjacent ampullary serosa with one or two 8-0 Vicryl interrupted sutures.

Any of these variations of fimbrial phimosis may be accompanied by periadnexal adhesions, which must be dealt with first.

Salpingostomy

As with salpingoovariolysis and fimbrioplasty, the primary approach to the management of distal tubal occlusion has been via laparoscopy.

Salpingostomy refers to the creation of a stoma in a tube with a completely occluded distal end (hydrosalpinx). Distal tubal occlusion is usually associated with varying degrees of pelvic and periadnexal adhesive disease, which must be dealt with first. After this is completed, it is necessary to examine the distal end of the tube to ensure that it is free and not adherent to the ovary. If adherent, the tube must be dissected from the ovary until the tuboovarian ligament is exposed. Such dissection will permit the surgeon to fashion the neostomy at the appropriate place.

Salpingostomy may be terminal or ampullary, depending on the anatomic location in which it is performed. In current practice the only place for ampullary salpingostomy is in reversal of previous fimbriectomy (Kroener sterilization). Ampullary salpingostomy was performed in the past when the distal hydrosalpinx was excised because of the presence of significant intratubal adhesions in this segment. Considering the disappointing results yielded by such an approach, its current utilization must be seriously questioned.

The hydrosalpinx is distended by transcervical chromopertubation. The occluded terminal end of the tube is examined under magnification. This allows the recognition of the relatively avascular lines that extend radially from a central

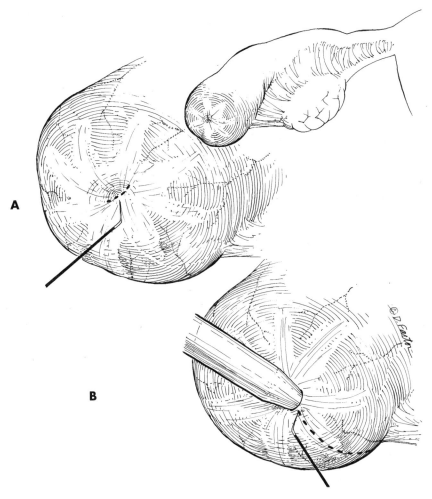

Fig. 60-1. Salpingostomy. **A, B.** (From Gomel V, Rowe TC: Mastering reconstructive tubal microsurgery. In Sanz L, editor: *Gynecologic surgery,* Oradell, NJ, 1988, Medical Economics. Original drawings © David Factor.)

Continued.

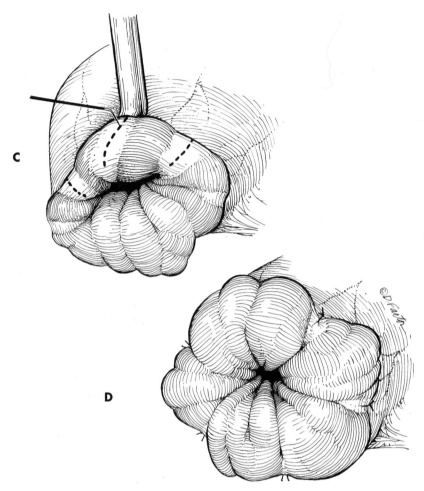

Fig. 60–1, cont'd. C, D. For legend see previous page.

punctum. The tube is entered at this punctum, using the microelectrode, and the incision is extended toward the ovary over an avascular line (Fig. 60-1, **A** and **B**). This fashions a new fimbria ovarica and permits the maintenance of the tuboovarian relationship. At this point it is possible to view the tube from within and to place additional incisions along the circumference of the tube between endothelial folds, over avascular areas (Fig. 60-1, **C**). This approach avoids cutting through the vascular mucosal folds, which will ultimately be shaped as fimbria; bleeding is minimized as a result. Any bleeding points that occur are exposed under a jet of irrigation fluid and coagulated individually with the microelectrode. Once a satisfactory stoma is achieved, the flaps created in the process are everted. They are secured without tension to the ampullary seromuscularis by interrupted 8-0 sutures (Fig. 60-1, **D**).

In the presence of marked thickening or fibrosis of the tubal wall, eversion of the flaps may prove difficult or impossible. Whereas this difficulty may be overcome by incising the serosa transversely at the base of each fold to provide a "hinge" to allow it to evert, such findings

represent a very poor prognosis. The tube will invariably reocclude postoperatively.

In distal tubal occlusion, the prognostic factors are (1) distal ampullary diameter, (2) thickness of the tubal wall, (3) the degree of preservation of mucosal folds, and (4) the extent and nature of pelvic and periadnexal adhesions. Preliminary investigation with HSG and laparoscopy will permit the assessment of these factors. It is also possible to assess the ampullary epithelium by visualizing the ampullary lumen during laparoscopy. By introducing a narrow-caliber telescope (i.e., a hysteroscope) into the ampulla through a small opening made at the distal end of the tube, it is possible to visualize the ampullary portion, which is simultaneously distended with a physiologic solution.

Ampullary salpingostomy for reversal of Kroener sterilization. Tubal sterilization by fimbriectomy results in the removal of varying lengths of distal tube. An ampullary salpingostomy may be considered if more than 50% of the ampulla has been preserved. Otherwise, the postoperative occlusion rate is high and the pregnancy rate is too low.

The technique is similar to terminal salpingostomy. The

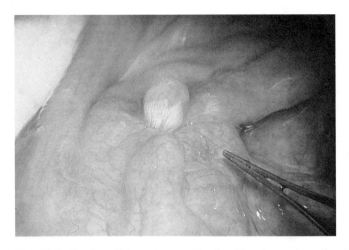

Fig. 60-2. Previous Falope ring sterilization. Note separation of both proximal and distal tubal segments from the Falope ring, which is covered with peritoneum.

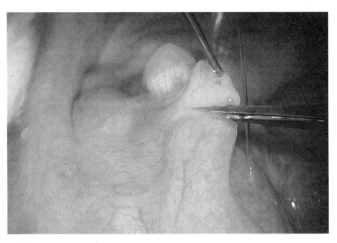

Fig. 60-3. The tube is transected proximal (and distal) to the site of occlusion. It is essential to avoid the vascular arcade in the mesosalpinx, in close proximity to the tube.

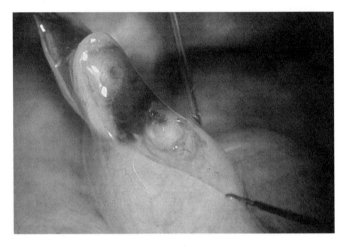

Fig. 60-4. After transection, the dye solution escapes from the lumen of the tube.

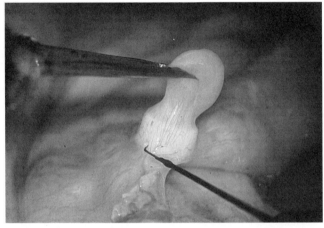

Fig. 60-5. The Falope ring (and the enclosed tubal segment) is excised from the mesosalpinx electrosurgically, using a 100-μm insulated microelectrode with a pointed tip.

oviduct is distended by means of chromopertubation and incised at its most distal point. The initial incision is extended toward the ovary, as in terminal salpingostomy, and further incisions are made along the circumference of the tube, along avascular areas. The resulting flaps are exerted and secured with interrupted 7-0 or 8-0 sutures.

Tubotubal anastomosis

Microsurgery finds its best application in tubotubal anastomosis. The precision afforded by this technique allows total excision of occluded and/or diseased portions, proper alignment, and excellent apposition of each layer of the remaining proximal and distal tubal segments. (See Figs. 60-2 to 60-13.)

Tubotubal anastomosis is performed to reverse a previous tubal sterilization or to remove and reconstruct lesions that are frequently occlusive and affect the tube at sites

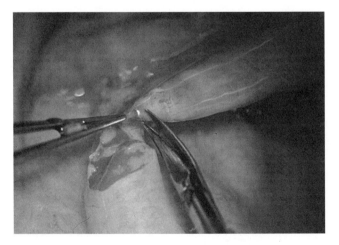

Fig. 60-6. After excision of the serosa from the occluded stump of the ampullary segment, a small opening (corresponding in size to the isthmic lumen) is fashioned in the lumen of the ampulla.

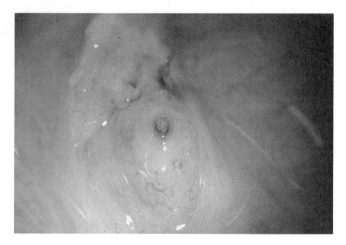

Fig. 60-7. The cut surface of the tube is examined under high magnification.

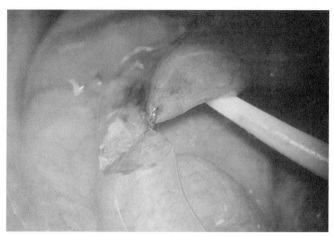

Fig. 60-8. The first suture approximating the muscularis and epithelium is placed at the 6-o'clock position and tied. This apposes the two segments of tube.

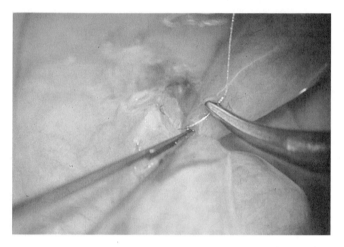

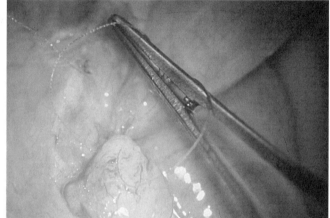

Figs. 60-9 and 60-10. Subsequent sutures designed to approximate the first layer are placed using a single strand of 8-0 Vicryl suture as a continuous series of loops.

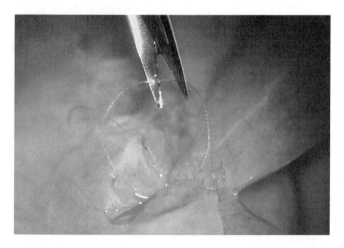

Fig. 60-11. The sutures are tied individually after division of the loop between two successive sutures.

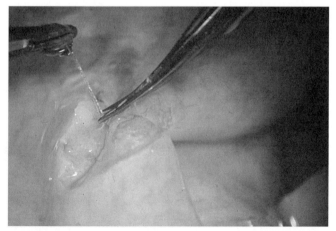

Fig. 60-12. The last suture approximating the epithelium and muscularis has been tied and is being cut.

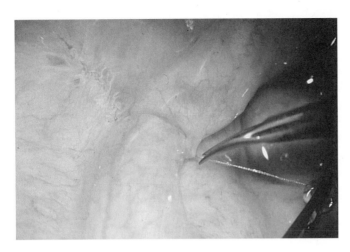

Fig. 60-13. The anastomosis is completed by the approximation of the mesosalpinx (completed) and the serosa of the posterior (completed) and anterior aspects of the tube.

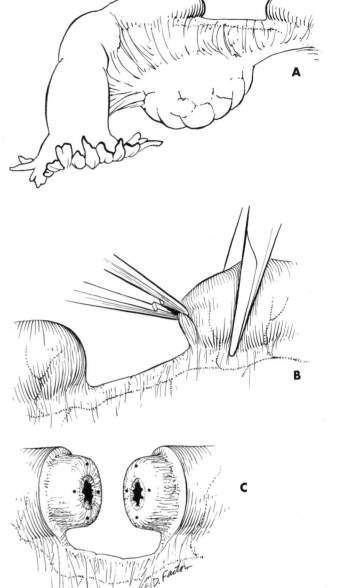

Fig. 60-14. Tubotubal anastomosis. **A,** the occluded segments are elevated on moist pads. **B,** the tip of the occluded segment is grasped with toothed forceps and transected with straight scissors. **C,** the corresponding cardinal points on each segment are identified. The initial suture in the inner layer is placed at the six-o'clock position. (From Gomel V, Rowe TC: Mastering reconstructive tubal microsurgery. In Sanz L, editor: *Gynecologic surgery,* Oradell, NJ, 1988, Medical Economics. Original drawings © David Factor.)

other than the fimbriated end. This section describes the fundamentals of tubotubal anastomosis. The variations necessary to deal with specific types of anastomosis are discussed later in this chapter.

Entry into the abdominal cavity and exposure of the pelvic organs have been described earlier. The pelvis is inspected thoroughly. When present, periadnexal adhesions are divided at their distal margins to mobilize the adnexa. The uterus and adnexa are then elevated toward the abdominal wall by placing them on laparotomy pads that have been soaked in the irrigation solution. The adnexa to be worked on is exposed, and the other one is covered with a wet sponge to prevent desiccation. The microscope is swung into position. The surgeon, assistant, and scrub nurse sit down.

When periadnexal adhesions are present, salpingoovariolysis is first completed as described earlier. Transcervical chromopertubation is carried out to distend the proximal segment of tube. The tube is transected adjacent to the site of occlusion or, in the case of a previous tubal sterilization, near the occluded stump. The tip of the occluded stump is grasped with a strong, toothed forceps (St. Martin-Gomel) to expose the site of transection (Fig. 60-14, **A** and **B**). The tube is transected from the antimesosalpingeal border to the mesosalpinx, using straight iris-type scissors or a sharp microblade. It is essential to halt the incision at the mesosalpinx, in the immediate periphery of the tubal muscularis, to avoid transection of the subtubal vascular arcade. Dye solution will now escape from the lumen of the tube.

The occluded tubal segment is excised from the mesosalpinx, using the microelectrode. The excision line must be kept close to the tube to avoid damage to the vessels cited earlier. The cut surface is examined under high magnification (×20 to ×25) to ensure that the tube is normal. A healthy tube is devoid of scarring, shows normal muscular

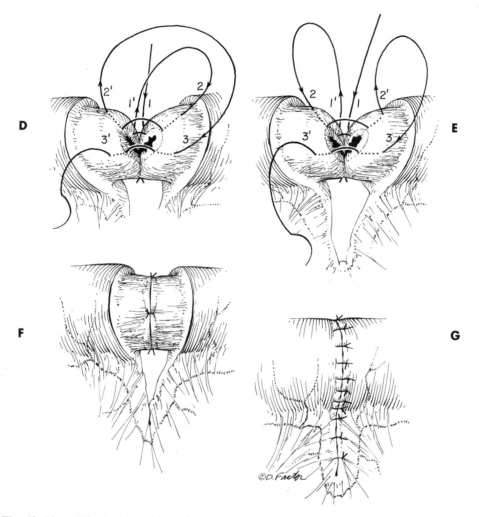

Fig. 60-14 cont'd. D & E, Additional sutures for closure of the inner layer are placed using a single strand of suture in a series of loops. **F,** After closure of the inner layer, chromopertubation should demonstrate tubal patency and a watertight anastomosis. **G,** The defect in the mesosalpinx may be closed in continuous or interrupted fashion.

architecture, and has intact mucosal folds with a pristine vascular pattern. After tubal transection, hemostasis is obtained by precise electrocoagulation of the more significant bleeders. These are located between the serosa and muscularis. They are exposed one at a time under a jet of irrigation fluid, and pinpoint electrocoagulation is achieved by using the insulated microelectrode and coagulating current. Gentle compression of the tube between thumb and forefinger facilitates this process. Electrocoagulation of minor bleeding points is unnecessary because this bleeding stops spontaneously. Electrocoagulation of the tubal epithelium is also unnecessary, and must be avoided for fear of adversely affecting future tubal function. More significant vessels (such as those composing the vascular arcade) may be divided inadvertently or by necessity. These may be electrocoagulated by using bipolar current with appropriate microforceps. Alternatively, the vessel is grasped with a

microsurgical forceps and hemostasis obtained by touching the forceps with a unipolar electrode that is activated. It is essential to avoid overzealous electrocoagulation, to avoid devitalization of the anastomosis site.

In the absence of significant luminal disparity between the two segments, the distal tubal segment is prepared in a similar manner (Figure 60-14, **C**). Patency of the distal segment is tested by descending hydropertubation, injecting a few milliliters of irrigation fluid through the fimbriated end.

Anastomosis of the tubal segments is carried out in two layers. The first of these approximates the epithelium and muscularis and the second the serosa. An 8-0 polyglactin 910 (Vicryl) suture swaged on a 130-μm shaft, 4- or 5-mm long needle is used.

To approximate the inner muscular and epithelial layer the first suture is placed at the mesosalpingeal border (at the 6-o'clock position), in a manner to keep the knot outside the lumen. Except in unusual circumstances, this suture is tied. Accurate placement of this first suture ensures proper alignment of the two segments of tube.

If the distance between the two segments of tube is great or their apposition is difficult because of increased tension, the mesosalpinx adjacent to the cut surface of the two segments of tube may be approximated first, using a single interrupted 7-0 or 8-0 suture. This approximation facilitates the anastomosis by bringing the two segments into close proximity and permits the tying of the anastomotic sutures without tension.

Depending on the site of the anastomosis, three or more additional sutures are required to join the inner layer. These additional sutures are placed by using a single strand of suture as a continuous series of loops, including the muscularis and the epithelium of the two segments (Fig. 60-14, **D** and **E**). The sutures are tied individually, after the division of the loop between two successive sutures. This approach facilitates and speeds up suture placement. The mucosa is not included in the inner suture layer, which is instead placed submucosally. However, evidence suggests this is not of critical importance.[46] Splinting of the lumen is not necessary; it does not facilitate the procedure and may traumatize the endothelium. Staining the mucosa with methylene blue or indigo carmine solution may help the novice because it accentuates visibility of the individual layers.

After approximation of the inner layer, chromopertubation should demonstrate tubal patency and a watertight anastomotic site (Figure 60-14, **F**). The serosa is approximated with two continuous sutures, one run anteriorly and the other posteriorly, starting at the antimesosalpingeal border (at the 12-o'clock position). Finally, the defect in the mesosalpinx is repaired in an interrupted or continuous fashion (Fig. 60-14, **G**).

For reversal of sterilization. The most frequent reason to perform a tubotubal anastomosis is reversal of sterilization. Simply stated, the procedure includes excision of the occluded ends of both the proximal and distal tubal remnants, obtaining hemostasis, and anastomosing the two segments in a way to achieve proper alignment and precise apposition of the lumina.

Depending on the segments that are approximated, tubotubal anastomosis may be

- Intramural-isthmic
- Intramural-ampullary
- Isthmic-isthmic
- Isthmic-ampullary
- Ampullary-ampullary anastomosis
- Ampullary-infundibular

Irrespective of the type, the basic steps of the procedure are the same. These basic steps have been described earlier. The luminal diameter of the tube is not uniform and is significantly greater in the ampullary segment. The techni-

cal variations required are largely dependent on the disparity of the luminal calibers of the two segments to be joined.

Intramural-isthmic anastomosis. In cases of reversal of sterilization, even when the proximal tubal segment appears to be absent, either a minor portion of isthmus or at least the intramural segment will be available. The small isthmic segment that may be present adheres to the uterus, as is frequently the case after tubal electrocoagulation. This is the result of the destruction and retraction of the adjacent mesosalpinx.

It is useful to perform transcervical chromopertubation in order to distend the tiny segment of isthmus, the presence of which should be suspected from earlier HSG. Maintenance of the distention facilitates the dissection of its inferior margin from the uterus. The dissection must be effected carefully to avoid damaging the tube or transecting cornual vessels. This is an important step, because the conservation and appropriate preparation of the segment, even if very small, greatly facilitates the anastomosis.

In the absence of any isthmus, maintenance of uterine distention will indicate the site where the intramural segment should be sought, between the uterine insertion points of the round and ovarian ligaments. The muscularis of the intramural segment is dissected from the surrounding uterine muscle for 1 or 2 mm with microscissors or microelectrode. The tube is then transected with the microscissors, at which point dye solution should stream out of the lumen. The cornual area is very vascular. Dissection in this region will usually cause significant oozing that will hinder visibility. Initial injection of the area with approximately 2 to 3 mL of dilute vasopressin solution (10 U of vasopressin in 60 to 100 mL of normal saline) significantly decreases capillary oozing and facilitates the procedure.

The distal segment is prepared next. Since there is no significant luminal disparity between the intramural and isthmic segments, the latter is simply transected near the occluded end, as described previously.

A two-layer anastomosis is then performed. After the approximation of the endothelium and muscularis, the serosa of the isthmus is approximated to the serosa and superficial muscle of the cornual region. The defect under the tube is repaired by suturing the mesosalpinx to the serosa of the lateral edge of the uterus.

Intramural-ampullary anastomosis. The salient feature of intramural ampullary anastomosis is the considerable luminal disparity that exists between the two segments of tube. The key technical issue lies in the preparation of the occluded ampullary stump. Making a luminal opening that is not significantly larger than that of the intramural tube simplifies the subsequent anastomosis.

The intraluminal segment is prepared as described under intramural isthmic anastomosis. Attention is then turned to the ampullary stump. To identify the tip of the stump, which may be buried between the leaves of the mesosalpinx, a malleable blunt probe may be introduced through the infundibulum and gently threaded toward the stump. Preferably the tube is distended with a few milliliters of dye solution or irrigation solution introduced through the fimbriated end. Using microscissors, the serosa over the tip of the ampullary stump is incised in a circular manner. It is then excised from over the tip of the stump to expose the muscularis. The muscularis over the tip of the ampullary stump is grasped with toothed microforceps and a small incision is made into the ampullary lumen using the microscissors. An opening that corresponds in size to the lumen of the proximal tubal segment is then fashioned at the tip of the stump. Anastomosis is then carried out as described previously.

Isthmic-isthmic anastomosis. Isthmic-isthmic anastomosis is the simplest anastomosis to perform. The lumina are comparable in size. The technique required has been described in the introductory paragraph of the section on tubotubal anastomosis.

Isthmic-ampullary anastomosis. In isthmic-ampullary anastomosis, usually there is also considerable disparity between the lumina of the two segments. The isthmic stump is prepared as described in the basic anastomosis technique. The ampullary stump is prepared as described under intramural-ampullary anastomosis. Once the two segments have been prepared, an anastomosis is completed as described previously.

Occasionally, circumstances will not permit the fashioning of a small opening into the lumen of the ampulla. The proximal end of the ampullary portion may have a fistulous opening that is quite large. A suture or clip might have been applied, which upon removal exposes the ampullary lumen in total. If the opening into the ampullary lumen is inadvertently or by necessity made significantly larger than the lumen of the proximal segment, it is necessary either to enlarge the lumen of the proximal segment or to narrow the ampullary lumen. To enlarge the lumen of the isthmic segment, a 2- to 3-mm slit is made at the antimesosalpingeal border using scissors. The corners thus created are partly excised. This will create an enlarged oval opening. The suture at the 6-o'clock position is then placed and tied. Usually five or more additional sutures will be required to approximate the inner layer. In this variation the suture at the 12-o'clock position approximates the muscularis and epithelium of ampulla to the same tissues at the apex of the slit. The serosa is then approximated and the defect in the mesosalpinx closed as previously described.

Alternatively, to reduce the size of a large ampullary opening, the surrounding muscular layer may be plicated with interrupted sutures and the prolapsing epithelium is invaginated.

Ampullary-ampullary anastomosis. The occluded end of the proximal segment is transected and the occluded stump excised as previously described. An opening is made in the occluded stump of the distal ampullary segment, corresponding in size to the lumen of the proximal segment, as described under isthmic-ampullary anastomosis.

Ampullary-ampullary anastomosis may be complicated by the tendency of the ampullary epithelium to prolapse through the lumen. Although some have advocated excision of the prolapsing mucosal fronds,[45] we prefer not to do this, in order to reduce the likelihood of intratubal adhesions. As the sutures of the inner layer are tied, mucosal fronds are replaced within the lumen by pressure from the irrigating solution, or with the tip of the microforceps or the glass nozzle of a small-bulb syringe. Traction on the ends of the suture as the knot is tightened also usually encourages the fronds to fall into the tubal lumen. It is important not to include these epithelial fronds within the suture or to leave them between tissues that are being approximated. Owing to the larger ampullary circumference (compared with that of the isthmus), a greater number of interrupted sutures will be required to approximate the two segments.

Ampullary-infundibular anastomosis. An ampullary-infundibular anastomosis may be necessary when the prior sterilization has been performed in the distal ampulla close to the infundibulum. The occluded ampullary stump is prepared as described previously. It will then be necessary to fashion an opening into the infundibulum to permit anastomosis of the two segments. A Teflon probe is introduced into the infundibulum from the fimbriated end and an opening is fashioned from the contralateral side using microscissors. The size of the opening that is fashioned should correspond to that of the ampullary segment. A two-layer anastomosis is then performed.

To repair midtubal disease. Midtubal occlusion as a result of pathologic conditions is rare; these conditions usually affect the proximal tubal segment. The causes of midtubal occlusion include endometriosis, tubal moles (the end result of an undiagnosed tubal pregnancy or one treated by observation), and congenital absence of a tubal segment. Another cause, tuberculosis, renders the tube not amenable to surgical repair. A tubal pregnancy treated by linear salpingostomy or by administration of methotrexate may result in tubal occlusion at the gestational site. Surgical treatment of a tubal pregnancy by segmental excision will leave the tube in two segments. Reconstruction of the latter is identical to that of a prior tubal sterilization.

The site of occlusion in an intact tube may be apparent on inspection. Palpation of the tube may identify an indurated segment that is the likely site of occlusion. Transcervical chromopertubation will distend the proximal segment up to the site of occlusion, thus assisting the surgeon in defining the proximal demarcation line. The tube is transected either immediately proximal to the occluded segment or in the occluded segment itself. Successive transection of the tube at 1- to 2-mm intervals will help define the normal segments proximal and distal to the occlusion site. Anastomosis is then carried out as described previously.

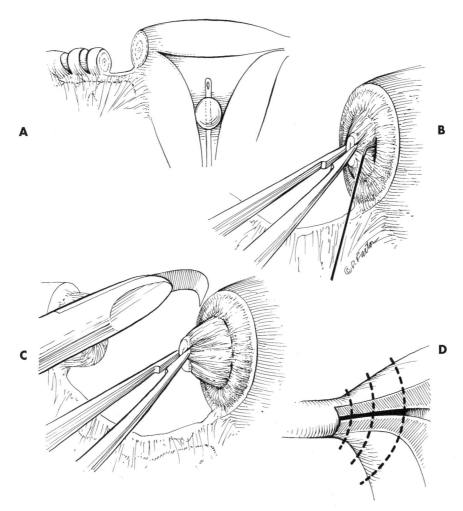

Fig. 60-15. Tubocornual anastomosis. **A, B, C, D.** (From Gomel V, Rowe TC: Mastering reconstructive tubal microsurgery. In Sanz L, editor: *Gynecologic surgery,* Oradell, NJ, Medical Economics. Original drawings © David Factor.) *Continued.*

Tubocornual anastomosis for proximal tubal disease

Various pathologic processes may affect the proximal tube and result in occlusion in the region of the uterotubal junction (UTJ). Histologic studies on such resected segments have identified the causative lesions. In an early series reported by Madlenat et al,[25] the lesions identified from 131 cases of proximal tubal occlusion included the following: salpingitis isthmica nodosa, 45 (34%); endometriosis, 25 (19%); inflammatory sclerosis, 25 (19%); scarring sclerosis, 17 (12.9%); ectopic gestation, 6 (4.6%); and tuberculosis, 5 (3.8%). In 8 (6.1%) no lesions were noted. The percentage of cases without demonstrable lesions varies in different series and may be related to the extent and accuracy of the preoperative investigation.

Traditionally, proximal tubal occlusion arising from pathologic processes was managed by uterotubal implantation. The application of microsurgery to proximal occlusion has made it possible to perform an anastomosis after removal of the affected tubal segment.

Central to the repair of pathologic occlusion in the proximal oviduct is the complete excision of the affected portion of tube, be it intramural or isthmic. In most cases a portion of the intramural segment is spared. This permits the conservation of the segment, rarely of all of it but frequently of part of it.

Initially, the cornual region of the uterus, 1 cm proximal to the UTJ, is injected superficially with a dilute solution of vasopressin (10 U of vasopressin in 60 to 100 mL of normal saline). This is accomplished by using a 30-gauge needle on a 3-mL syringe. Vasoconstriction is recognized by serosal blanching. The tube is then incised at the UTJ (Fig. 60-15, **A**), care being taken not to divide the arteriovenous arcade at the mesosalpingeal margin of the tube. After transection of the tube, patency of the intramural section is assessed by transcervical chromopertubation, and the normalcy of the cut surface is assessed under high magnification (×20 to ×25).

If there is obstruction or abnormal morphology, or both, the intramural segment is dissected from the surrounding

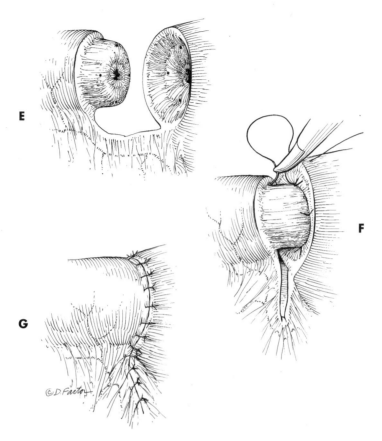

Fig. 60-15, cont'd. E, F, G. For legend see previous page.

uterine musculature 1 to 2 mm at a time toward the uterine cavity. The small portion thus dissected is transected and the cut surface reassessed. It is essential that dissection of the intramural tube from the surrounding uterine muscle be effected at the level of the immediate periphery of the tubal muscularis (Fig 60-15, **B**). The preoperative HSG usually provides information about the length of the normal intramural segment and the extent of excision required. Transection of successive portions of the intramural tube may be achieved either with curved microscissors or a specially designed curved blade (Gomel cornual blade—Spingler-Tritt, Jestetten, West Germany) (Fig. 60-15, **C**). By limiting the excised tissue as described, there is little risk of a large defect developing in the cornu.

Since this dissection must continue until a patent lumen with healthy-appearing mucosa is reached, the anastomosis site may be located in a juxtamural, intramural, or juxtauterine site (Fig. 60-15, **D**).

After the preparation of the cornual end, the occluded and/or abnormal isthmic segment of the tube must be excised. The extent of excision is determined by serial transections of the isthmus 2 to 3 mm apart, commencing at the initial incision site at the UTJ. This is continued until

patent and normal isthmus is identified under high magnification. Patency of the distal segment is confirmed by descending hydropertubation (injecting a few milliliters of irrigation solution through the fimbriated end). After transection, hemostasis is obtained as previously described, by precise electrocoagulation of bleeders that are located between the muscularis and the serosa.

After the preparation of the proximal and distal tubal segments (Fig. 60-15, **E**), these segments are approximated in two layers as follows: The first layer incorporates the muscularis and the mucosa. Usually four interrupted 8-0 Vicryl sutures placed at cardinal points are sufficient. The sutures must be placed in a way to keep the knots external to the lumen (Fig. 60-15, **F**). The initial suture is placed at the 6-o'clock position. If the distance between the two segments of tube is significant or their apposition requires undue tension, approximation of the isthmic mesosalpinx to the uterus with a single 7-0 suture facilitates the procedure.

Once the first anastomotic suture (at the 6-o'clock position) is placed, whether it is tied or not depends on the type of tubocornual anastomosis. If the anastomosis is located deep in the cornu, as in juxtauterine anastomosis, tying the initial suture would render placement of the subsequent sutures difficult if not impossible. In such cases, the suture is held with a clip until the remaining sutures have been placed. The subsequent sutures are placed using a continuous strand of suture, since this facilitates placement and prevents the individual sutures from becoming tangled. If the suture at the 6-o'clock position has not been tied initially, it is tied after the placement of the remainder of the sutures. Thereafter the loop between the succeeding sutures is divided and each is tied in turn. After the first layer (epithelium and muscularis) has been joined, the seromuscularis of the uterus is approximated to the serosa of the tube with 8-0 sutures and the defect in the mesosalpinx is closed by approximating it to the lateral edge of the uterus (Fig. 60-15, **G**).

CONCLUSION

Microsurgery continues to be a mainstay of the management of infertility. However, contemporary options for management also include laparoscopic surgery and IVF. Careful assessment of the potential fertility of the couple must be made before a specific therapeutic approach is selected. The nontechnical considerations that apply to the decision-making process include the age of the woman, the costs of treatment, and the wishes and values of the couple. Technical considerations include the potential risks of each method, complications, and estimated pregnancy rates, and all such considerations should be based on local experience. Incorporation of technical and nontechnical aspects of management will usually allow the couple involved to reach a decision about management that is satisfactory both to them and to the physician involved. Assessment of outcomes demonstrates that tubal microsurgery provides potential both for a satisfactory outcome for the couple and profound technical satisfaction for the surgeon.

REFERENCES

1. Boeckx W et al: Reversibility after female sterilization, *Br J Obstet Gynaecol* 93:839, 1986.
2. Boer-Meisel ME et al: Predicting the pregnancy outcome in patients treated for hydrosalpinx: a prospective study, *Fertil Steril* 45:23, 1986.
3. Bruhat MA et al: Laparoscopy procedures to promote fertility: ovariolysis and salpingolysis: results of 93 selected cases, *Acta Eur Fertil* 14:476, 1983.
4. Bruhat MA et al: La coeliochirurgie. In *Encyclopedie Medicale Chirurgicale Techniques Chirurggie Urologie-Gynecologie,* vol 6, Paris, 1989, Editions Techniques.
5. Collins JA, Rowe TC: Age of the female partner is a prognostic factor in prolonged unexplained infertility: a multicenter study, *Fertil Steril:* 52:15, 1989.
6. DeCherney AH, Mezer HC, Naftolin F: Analysis of failure of microsurgical anastomosis after mid-segment, non-coagulation tubal ligation, *Fertil Steril* 39:618, 1983.
7. Donnez J, Casanas-Roux F: Prognostic factors of fimbrial microsurgery, *Fertil Steril* 46:200, 1986.
8. Donnez J, Casanas-Roux F: Prognostic factors influencing the pregnancy rate after microsurgical cornual anastomosis, *Fertil Steril* 46:1089, 1986.
9. Dubuisson JB et al: Terminal tuboplasties by laparoscopy: 65 consecutive cases, *Fertil Steril* 54:401, 1990.
10. Fayez JA: An assessment of the role of operative laparoscopy in tuboplasty, *Fertil Steril* 39:476, 1983.
11. FIVNAT 1989 et bilan general 1986-1989, *Contracept Fertil Sex* 18:588, 1990.
12. Gomel V: Tubal reconstruction by microsurgery. Presented at the Eight World Congress on Fertility and Sterility, Buenos Aires, Nov 3-9, 1974 (abstract 39).
13. Gomel V: Laparoscopic surgery in tubal infertility, *Obstet Gynecol* 46:47, 1975.
14. Gomel V: Reconstructive surgery of the oviduct, *J Reprod Med* 18:181, 1977.
15. Gomel V: Salpingostomy by microsurgery, *Fertil Steril* 29:389, 1978.
16. Gomel V: Clinical results of microsurgery in female infertility. In Crosignani PG, Rubin BL, editors: *Microsurgery in female infertility,* London, 1980, Academic Press.
17. Gomel V: Microsurgical reversal of sterilization: a reappraisal, *Fertil Steril* 33:587, 1980.
18. Gomel V: Salpingo-ovariolysis by laparoscopy in infertility, *Fertil Steril* 34:607, 1983.
19. Gomel V: *Microsurgery in female infertility,* Boston, 1983, Little, Brown.
20. Gomel V: Distal tubal occlusion, *Fertil Steril* 49:946, 1988.
21. Gomel V, Swolin K: Salpingostomy: microsurgical technique and results, *Clin Obstet Gynecol* 23:1243, 1980.
22. Henderson SR: The reversibility of female sterilization with the use of microsurgery: a report on 102 patients with more than one year of follow-up, *Am J Obstet Gynecol* 149:57, 1984.
23. Kosasa TS, Hale RW: Treatment of hydrosalpinx using a single incision eversion procedure, *Int J Fertil* 33:319, 1988.
24. Larsson B: Late results of salpingostomy combined with salpingolysis and ovariolysis by electromicrosurgery in 54 women, *Fertil Steril* 37:156, 1982.
25. Madlenat P, DeBrux J, Palmer R: L'etiologie des obstructions tubaires proximales et son rôle dans le prognostic des implantations, *Gynecologie* 28:47, 1977.
26. McComb P: Microsurgical tubocornual anastomosis for occlusive cornual disease: reproducible results without the need for tubouterine implantation, *Fertil Steril* 46:571, 1986.
27. McComb P, Gomel V: Cornual occlusion and its microsurgical reconstruction, *Clin Obstet Gynecol* 23:1229, 1980.
28. McComb P, Paleoulogou A: The intussusception salpingostomy technique for the therapy of distal oviductal occlusion at laparoscopy, *Obstet Gynecol* 78:443, 1991.
29. Navot D et al: Poor oocyte quality rather than implantation failure as a cause of age-related decline in female fertility, *Lancet* 337:1375, 1991.
30. Paterson PJ: Factors influencing the success of microsurgical tuboplasty for sterilization, *Clin Reprod Fertil* 3:57, 1985.
31. Putnam JM, Holden AEC, Olive DL: Pregnancy rates following tubal anastomosis: Pomeroy partial salpingectomy versus electrocautery, *J Gynecol Surg* 6:173, 1990.
32. Rock JA et al: Tubal anastomosis: pregnancy success following reversal of Falope ring or monopolar cautery sterilization, *Fertil Steril* 48:13, 1987.
33. Sauer MV, Paulson RJ, Lobo RA: A preliminary report on oocyte donation extending reproductive potential to women over 40, *N Engl J Med* 323:1157, 1990.
34. Schlösser HW et al: Sterilisation Refertilisierung. Erfahrungen und Ergebnisse bei 119 microchirurgisch refertilisierten Frauen, *Geburtshilfe Frauenheilkd* 43:213, 1983.
35. Silber SJ, Cohen R: Microsurgical reversal of tubal sterilization: factors affecting pregnancy rate, with long-term follow-up, *Obstet Gynecol* 64:679, 1984.
36. Simpson CW: Transcervical fallopian tube catheterization, *J Soc Obstet Gynecol Can* 13:37, 1991.
37. Spivak MM, Librach CL, Rosenthal DM: Microsurgical reversal of

sterilization: a six-year study, *Am J Obstet Gynecol* 154:355, 1986.

38. Swolin K: Electro microsurgery and salpingostomy: long-term results, *Am J Obstet Gynecol* 121:418, 1975.

39. Tan SL et al: Cumulative conception and livebirth rates after in-vitro fertilization, *Lancet* 339:1390, 1992.

40. Trimbos-Kemper TCM: Reversal of sterilization of women over 40 years of age: a multicenter survey in the Netherlands, *Fertil Steril* 53:575, 1990.

41. Tulandi T, Vilos GA: A comparison between laser surgery and electrosurgery for bilateral hydrosalpinx: a two year followup, *Fertil Steril* 44:846, 1985.

42. van Noord-Zaadstra BM et al: Delayed childbearing: effect of age on fecundity and outcome of pregnancy, *Br Med J* 302:1361, 1991.

43. Verhoeven HC et al: Surgical treatment for distal tubal occlusion: a review of 167 cases, *J Reprod Med* 28:293, 1983.

44. Westrom L: Incidence, prevalence and trends of pelvic inflammatory disease and its consequences in industrialized countries, *Am J Obstet Gynecol* 138:880, 1980.

45. Winston RML: Reversal of sterilization, *Clin Obstet Gynecol* 23:1261, 1980.

46. Xue P, Fa Y-Y: Microsurgical reversal of female sterilization, *J Reprod Med* 34:451, 1989.

47. Zouves C, Erenus M, Gomel V: Tubal ectopic pregnancy after in-vitro fertilization and embryo transfer: a role for proximal occlusion or salpingectomy after failed distal tubal surgery, *Fertil Steril* 56:691, 1991.

Chapter 61

MÜLLERIAN DUCT ANOMALIES

Howard W. Jones, Jr., MD

Classification
Problems of partial development
    Rokitansky-Küster-Hauser syndrome
    Unicornuate uterus
Problems of lateral fusion
    Obstructive
    Nonobstructive
Problems of vertical fusion
    Obstructive transverse vaginal septum
    Nonobstructive transverse vaginal septum

CLASSIFICATION

Although there are a number of classifications of müllerian anomalies, a very simple one based on defects occurring in the chronology of embryologic development of the müllerian ducts has proven clinically very useful. It is as follows:

- Problems of partial development
- Problems of lateral fusion: obstructive; nonobstructive
- Problems of vertical fusion: obstructive; nonobstructive

Bilateral partial development of the uterus and vagina is often referred to in the literature under the rubric of congenital absence of the vagina. This is misleading in the sense that the vaginal absence is dependent on the absence of the uterus. When the vagina is absent but a uterus is present, the embryologic defect is likely quite different because in the latter circumstance there is essentially never any wolffian duct defect, whereas with the absence of the uterus and the vagina, wolffian and other anomalies are not at all unusual. Unilateral partial development of the müllerian ducts results in a unicornuate uterus.

Problems of lateral fusion of the two müllerian ducts are especially intriguing in that obstructive lesions are almost always associated with ipsilateral wolffian duct anomalies such as congenital absence of the kidney. It is therefore likely that bilateral obstruction of the müllerian ducts would be associated with bilateral kidney agenesis, with lethality early in embryonic development accounting for the clinical absence of such cases. However, there are apparently reported a very few cases that seem to be exceptions to this rule. Invariably, these exceptions have been with extremely low vaginal obstructions with a double uterus and with normal kidneys bilaterally. The lesions described have been so low that one cannot help wondering whether the situations are not those of imperforate hymen with coincidental müllerian duplications rather than obstructions of the müllerian ducts per se.

Attention to obstructive lesions is often necessary soon after the onset of puberty and menses to prevent deterioration of the upper tracks and, of course, to relieve pain when that is a major factor. On the other hand, nonobstructive malformations are seldom encountered until the childbearing age. Correction may be required before reproduction is possible.

The vertical fusion problems, which probably represent a fault in the connection between the down-growing müllerian tubercle and the up-growing urogenital sinus, are especially serious if they are obstructive, and may be clinically manifest in infancy or at the time of puberty when menstruation begins.

PROBLEMS OF PARTIAL DEVELOPMENT
Rokitansky-Küster-Hauser syndrome

Complete agenesis of the müllerian ducts does not seem to have ever been described. In the Rokitansky-Küster-Hauser syndrome there is partial agenesis in that the fallopian tubes, and of course the ovaries, which have a different origin, are quite normal, but the embryologic defect has arrested development just as uterine formation has started. This is precisely at 7 weeks, that is, at 49 days of development. Such patients may have a normally developed lower vagina of a very few centimeters. The usual lesion includes absence of the middle and upper third of the vagina and the uterus, but as just mentioned, the fallopian tubes are generally normally developed.

The diagnosis is seldom made in the newborn, and this may be just as well, because therapy by necessity would need to be delayed to a much later date. Indeed, in some infants it is very difficult to differentiate between congenital absence of the vagina and an imperforate hymen. This differential diagnosis needs to be finalized as puberty approaches, to prevent the accumulation of menstrual blood in those patients who really do have an imperforate hymen. The use of ultrasound or a computed tomographic (CT) scan is useful in differentiation.

Patients with congenital absence of the vagina, that is, with the Rokitansky-Küster-Hauser syndrome, usually seek the advice of a physician at about the time of puberty or later because of failure of menstruation to appear. Otherwise, the growth and development of the patient, including secondary sexual characteristics and the external genitalia, are quite normal.

At age 13 or 14 years, the diagnosis is rather easy to make, but it is necessary to distinguish it from the testicular feminization syndrome, in which situation there may be a shallow vagina with no uterus palpable on rectal examination. It is usually pointed out that patients with the testicular feminization syndrome have little or no pubic hair; although this is sometimes true, it is not always dependable, so that mistakes can be made. Therefore, if there is the slightest doubt, the differential diagnosis can be made easily by a karyotype, because generally there are no karyotypic abnormalities in either the testicular feminization syndrome (46,XY) or the Rokitansky-Küster-Hauser syndrome (46,XX).

Generally speaking it is not necessary for the diagnosis or treatment of these patients to perform a laparotomy, or even a laparoscopy. With a few exceptions, as is noted later, the internal findings are reasonably constant. The tubes and ovaries generally are normal; however, the uterus is represented by a small rudimentary structure suggesting a very immature bicornuate uterus to which the fallopian tube is, of course, connected, and to which a round ligament attaches (Fig. 61-1).

The indications for laparoscopy are for those rare patients with congenital absence of the vagina who, at puberty, do have cyclic abdominal pain of increasing severity. On laparoscopy, these patients are found to have a somewhat enlarged uterine rudiment that needs to be removed, because the menstrual pain is due to a very small patch of functioning endometrium with a cyclic collection of menstrual blood that causes distention and therefore pain (Fig. 61-2). It is to be noted that this amount of endometrium is sometimes very trivial, so that on laparoscopic examination it may be difficult to really be sure that

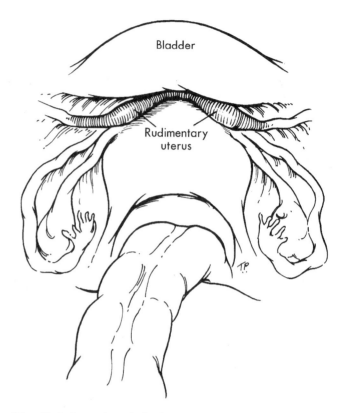

Fig. 61-1. Internal genitalia in Rokitansky-Küster-Hauser syndrome. (Adapted from Jones HW Jr, Rock JA: Reparative and constructive surgery of the female generative tract, Baltimore, MD, 1983, Williams & Wilkins.)

one of the uterine anlagen is abnormal. The incidence of functioning endometrium in one of these uterine rudiments

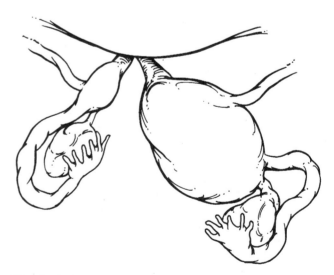

Fig. 61-2. Internal genitalia in Rokitansky-Küster-Hauser syndrome (functional unilateral). (Adapted from Jones HW Jr, Rock JA: Reparative and constructive surgery of the female generative tract, Baltimore, MD, 1983, Williams & Wilkins.)

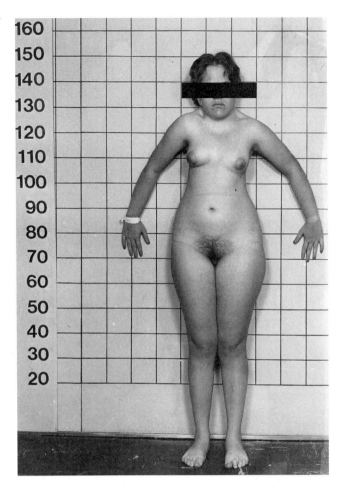

Fig. 61-3. Park-Jones syndrome. (Adapted from Jones HW Jr., Rock JA: Reparative and constructive surgery of the female generative tract, Baltimore, MD, 1983, Williams & Wilkins.)

is in the order of 1%. When it occurs, excision is necessary and the results are dramatic in relieving the patient's cyclic pain.

In the average situation the laterally placed rudimentary structure fades off below, but it almost always fuses with its opposite partner by a thin, fibrous, easily palpable structure about 2 to 3 cm in diameter. This is apparently the undeveloped anlage of the müllerian duct. Actually, this structure can sometimes be felt on rectal examination in a cooperative patient, or under anesthesia. When this can be identified, it tends to confirm the diagnosis of the Rokitansky syndrome, because in the testicular feminization syndrome this structure is not present and therefore not palpable.

Congenital absence of the uterus and vagina with internal pelvic findings exactly as in the average Rokitansky syndrome have been found to be associated in a few cases with shortness of stature, severe bony abnormalities involving the spine (especially of the neck), and sometimes

deafness. This syndrome was originally described by Park et al.,[17] and has been seen by the authors several times since the description of the original case (Fig. 61-3). Interestingly enough, the deafness in this syndrome, when it is present, is associated with bony abnormalities of the small bones of the middle ear (Fig. 61-4). This seems consistent with the disturbance of bony development in the spine, which is mentioned subsequently.

Anomalies of the wolffian duct are associated in a significant number of patients. The percentage of anomalies depends in some measure on the strictness with which one defines the anomalous situation. With major defects such as congenital absence of the kidney on one side or the presence of a pelvic kidney, which sometimes occurs unilaterally, the percentage of anomalies is in the neighborhood of 15%. On the other hand, if more trivial anomalies are included, such as malrotation of the kidney, partial double-collecting system on one side, or malposition of the kidney, the percentage of anomalies can be pushed up to the neighborhood of 40%.

Generally speaking these anomalies are of little clinical significance. However, in rare circumstances, a pelvic kidney will be so located that the normal vaginal position is compromised and the surgical construction of the vagina must be done with great care.

Although it is possible to determine the presence and position of kidneys by ultrasound, for this situation an intravenous pyelogram is required to be certain of the course of the ureters.

Anomalies of bony structures also are not uncommon. It is generally stated that they occur in about 5% of patients. However, this estimation is in large part due to anomalies that are visible in an intravenous pyelogram and are limited to the bones of the lower spine and pelvis. For example, it is not at all unusual in routine intravenous pyelography to observe such anomalies as sacralization of L-5 or the presence of six lumbar vertebrae. However, the cervical vertebrae are sometimes involved and fused, as in the special syndrome of Park and Jones in which fusion of the cervical vertebrae is an inherent part of the syndrome.[17]

Strubbe et al.[20] made a systematic examination for bony abnormalities in 40 patients with the Rokitansky syndrome. They found that, when accurately measured, the hands of almost all patients showed abnormality in that the phalanges were somewhat too short. Although there were serious abnormalities in the hands of only two patients, this study suggests a generalized phenomenon responsible for the bony and müllerian defects. Fortunately, most of the hand defects have little or no clinical significance.

The etiology of this defect has not been elucidated. There have been numerous cytogenetic studies, beginning with the study of Azoury and Jones,[2] but except in very rare and probably coincidental circumstances, such patients are found to have the 46,XX karyotype. Jones and Mermut[11] encountered an example in sisters and were able to find four

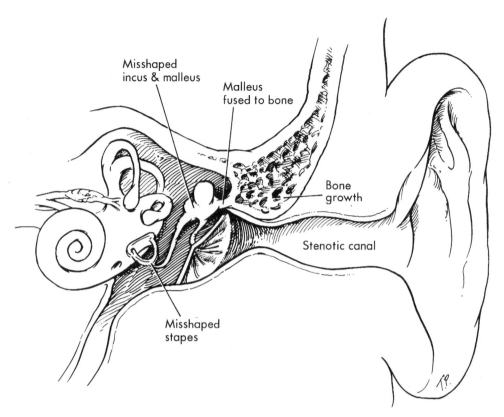

Fig. 61-4. Bones of the middle ear in Park-Jones syndrome. (Adapted from Jones HW Jr., Rock JA: Reparative and constructive surgery of the female generative tract, Baltimore, MD, 1983, Williams & Wilkins.)

other sister siblings with this disorder. Such a finding raises a possibility that the disorder is due to a very rare autosomal recessive problem.

Shokeir[19] reported several sibships in which the disorder seemed to be transmitted in a sex-limited autosomal dominant manner. However, there have been no confirmatory reports.

It is curious and possibly even significant that occasionally a patient exposed to thalidomide during embryogenesis has been found to have the Rokitansky syndrome. This is all the more suggestive as an etiologic agent because thalidomide has a known predilection to affect bony development. Because of the worldwide distribution of cases, thalidomide is certainly not a serious suspect as *the* cause of the Rokitansky syndrome. The experience with the thalidomide children, however, suggests that it is possible that some as-yet unidentified substance or agent that is widely dispersed and easily available may be responsible for this abnormality.

Although the precise cause of the insult is not known, the evidence is rather clear as to exactly when it took place. During embryogenesis, the development of the müllerian ducts at 7 weeks after fertilization, or 9 weeks after the last menstrual period, has reached a state that is very similar to that seen in the müllerian ducts in patients with the

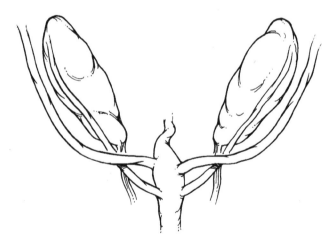

Fig. 61-5. Müllerian duct at 7 weeks of embryogenesis. (Adapted from Jones HW Jr., Rock JA: Reparative and constructive surgery of the female generative tract, Baltimore, MD, 1983, Williams & Wilkins.)

Rokitansky syndrome (Fig. 61-5). This would indicate that development is arrested somewhat uniformly at this period in development.

Suggested treatments have varied from the so-called Frank technique, involving the use of dilators to develop a vagina, to the use of a large variety of materials to line a surgically created vaginal space between the bladder and the rectum.[7] These materials have varied from skin to small and large intestine, to peritoneum, to amnion. Our personal experience of more than 25 years with the use of a split-thickness graft to line a neovaginal cavity has been eminently satisfactory, so that this operative procedure can be highly recommended. This of course does not mean that some effort to dilate the vagina, as in the Frank technique, should not be used.[7] On the contrary, if there is adequate time, a motivated patient, and an anatomic situation that seems favorable (this means a small vaginal path to start with), it is only good sense to make an attempt to create a vagina by manual dilatation. Various dilators can be used. A graduated set of rectal dilators sometimes works well. Plastic centrifuge tubes of increasing size are easily available and make an inexpensive and adequate substitute. Ingram[10] devised a bicycle seat with a special projection that was intended to serve as a vaginal dilator. He found this quite acceptable to most patients and effective among those patients who could use it. Not all patients are amenable to self-dilatation of the vagina, and in that group of patients a surgical alternative needs to be offered immediately.

The question often arises as to the most suitable time to advise surgery. Clearly, the patient should have attained full growth, and this means that the operation should not be undertaken until age 14 or 15 years. It is probably important, however, for patients with this defect to know that an operation can be carried out at any convenient time after that. If the split-thickness graft technique is to be used, it is necessary to use a vaginal mold, and this requires a certain amount of motivation on the part of the patient. This does not seem to develop until at least age 15 or perhaps even 16. Therefore an ideal age to do this is in the summer between school sessions when the patient is about 16 or 17 years of age.

The McIndoe procedure is easier to perform in a patient who has not previously been operated on, but it is possible to use the procedure in patients with previously failed operations. However, by far the most common indication for secondary operations has resulted from a misdiagnosis, when there has been an unwise exploration of the space between the bladder and the rectum in the search for a vagina, and the original diagnosis was an imperforate hymen. In infancy and adolescence, the differential diagnosis among an imperforate hymen, a transverse vaginal septum, and the Rokitansky syndrome may be difficult, as has been mentioned. There is really no reason to hurry the diagnosis, and it is far better to be absolutely certain of the situation than it is to inadvertently open the rectovesical space. In the event this latter does occur, for whatever reason, it is far better to allow the area to heal primarily than to attempt to maintain a cavity by using gauze packs, drains of various kinds, or even a suitable vaginal stent,

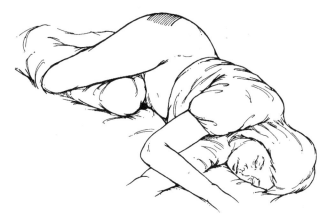

Fig. 61-6. Donor site of split-thickness graft. (Adapted from Jones HW Jr., Rock JA: Reparative and constructive surgery of the female generative tract, Baltimore, MD, 1983, Williams & Wilkins.)

because the mistake is usually made about the time of puberty, and the patient will surely not be cooperative enough to expect to have a functioning vagina.

One of the key steps in the operative procedure is obtaining a suitable satisfactory split-thickness graft. This can be done with any suitable instrument that can secure a graft, which is about 10 cm wide and long enough to be twice the vaginal depth. The Reese electric dermatome serves admirably for this purpose. For the vaginal cavity, a relatively thick graft is desired. A thickness of about 18/1000 of an inch is satisfactory. A thicker graft will sometimes remove so much dermis that healing of the donor site may be delayed.

Any suitable donor site can be used, but it is convenient to remove the split-thickness graft from the buttock so that it can be covered conveniently by swimming gear. With the patient in the Sims position, the uppermost thigh and knee must be secured to the table firmly, the donor site carefully shaved, and the skin prepared with any favorite preoperative technique. The graft should be at least 10 cm wide and 24 to 26 cm long (Fig. 61-6).

The remainder of the operation is carried out with the patient in a lithotomy position. A transverse incision at the site of the vagina is made, with a tendency to make the incision more posterior than anterior so that all available vaginal epithelium can be used to protect the urethra (Fig. 61-7). The development of the vaginal cavity is not difficult in patients who have not previously been operated on. The dissection is most easily developed on one or another side of the median raphe, where the tissue between the bladder and the rectum is often condensed and almost thick enough to call a rectourethralis ligament. However, the spaces are developed by blunt dissection with the fingers, or even with a retractor; the midline condensed band can easily be snipped by scissors and then further dissected bluntly

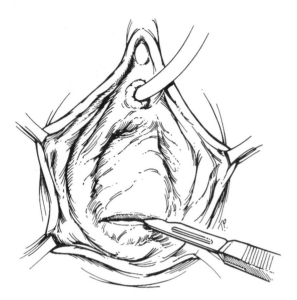

Fig. 61-7. Original incision for the McIndoe procedure. (Adapted from Wheeless.)

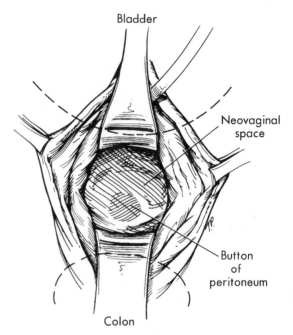

Fig. 61-8. Dissection of the neovaginal space. (Adapted from Jones HW Jr., Rock JA: Reparative and constructive surgery of the female generative tract, Baltimore, MD, 1983, Williams & Wilkins.)

(Fig. 61-8). The dissection should be carried up to the peritoneum, but care must be exercised not to expose too much of the peritoneum lest an enterocele develop at this point after the vaginal cavity has been lined by the graft.

It is necessary to be sure that the cavity is dry so that the graft will not be hampered by underside bleeding; it is interesting that many times no bleeders are encountered that require clamping and tying. Nevertheless, from time to time, there are troublesome bleeding vessels deep in the lateral aspect of the vagina, and these can be caught with a long Kelly clamp and tied with a free ligature (Fig. 61-9).

Several different materials for the prosthesis have been used. We have found that ordinary foam rubber available from any upholstery shop has a very desirable consistency and can be readily sterilized in blocks of about $10 \times 10 \times 20$ cm; these blocks can be whittled down at the time of surgery to a suitable size for a particular patient. The form should be cut so that it is as much as two times the size of the future vagina and compressed by covering it with two rubber sheaths that are ordinary condoms.

The skin graft needs to be sewed to the outer side of the prosthesis, using very fine synthetic absorbable material. A detail is that interrupted vertical mattress sutures should be used so that the exteriorized undersurface of the graft is approximated to the exteriorized undersurface at the suture edges.

After the graft has been inserted into the cavity, the edges of the graft can be sutured to the cut edges of the vaginal epithelium (Fig. 61-10). It is important not to make this suture line too tight, because it is desirable to make a ready opportunity for any serum that might collect under the graft to have an easy route of escape. After trial and error with various types of straps and harnesses for holding the vaginal form in place, it is our experience that none of

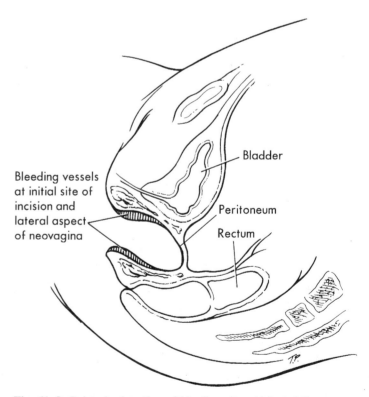

Fig. 61-9. Points in detection of bleeding sites. (Adapted from Jones HW Jr., Rock JA: Reparative and constructive surgery of the female generative tract, Baltimore, MD, 1983, Williams & Wilkins.)

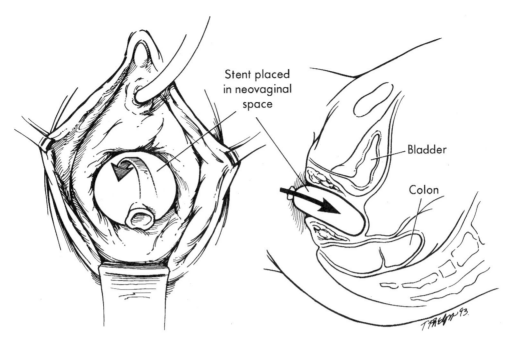

Fig. 61-10. Stent in place. (Adapted from Jones HW Jr., Rock JA: Reparative and constructive surgery of the female generative tract, Baltimore, MD, 1983, Williams & Wilkins.)

these rigs is completely satisfactory. It has been found very satisfactory, however, to use large braided silk sutures through the labia to prevent extrusion of the form. The stitches may be uncomfortable after 1 or 2 days, at which time they can be cut.

A suprapubic catheter is recommended to prevent pressure on the urethra, which would be occasioned by a transurethral catheter that could conceivably result in necrosis of the urethra.

Postoperatively, the patient is kept on a low-residue diet and antibiotics, and generally remains reasonably flat in bed for approximately 1 week; the labial stitches, if they have not been previously cut, then can be severed and the vaginal form removed, the suprapubic catheter withdrawn, and the vaginal cavity irrigated. It is desirable to have available a previously prepared second vaginal form that can be reinserted immediately.

The vaginal form needs to be changed once every 24 hours. This can generally be done by the patient after instruction. As soon as she is able to do this and take a low-pressure, clear water douche, she can be discharged from the hospital.

After about 6 weeks, a Silastic form or one of similar material can be used. This is much easier for the patient to handle, as it can be washed off with tap water. Use of a firm form with Silastic before 6 weeks carries the risk of necrosis of some point of the graft.

Prophylactic antibiotics for the prevention of infection have been a tremendous help in this operation, and since the use of prophylactic antibiotics, one can expect 100%

take of the graft. The vagina should be comfortable and functional in a period of 6 to 10 weeks after the operation.

Unicornuate uterus

The unicornuate uterus occurs when, for whatever reason, there is arrested development on one side. The side with arrested development has the findings common to the Rokitansky syndrome (Fig. 61-11). A unicornuate uterus is essentially asymptomatic and remains undiscovered until the patient either comes in complaining of infertility or has some problem during pregnancy. Most contributions to the literature have consisted of case reports or small series of patients. Reproduction does seem to be compromised by infertility, pregnancy wastage, and premature labor; however, term pregnancies with a viable child from a unicornuate uterus are well known.

Donderwinkel et al.,[5] in the largest series to date, observed 47 pregnancies in 22 patients. Only 20 (44%) of these went to term; 8 (18%) had premature labor, but there was a total of 28 (60%) live babies. There were 10 (22%) first-trimester abortions and 7 (16%) second-trimester abortions. In addition to the 22 patients who were pregnant, Donderwinkel et al.[5] reported 22 additional patients with a unicornuate uterus who complained of primary infertility. In 20 of these patients, it was possible to find another cause for the infertility (mostly endometriosis), leaving only 2 examples of a unicornuate uterus as a possible intrinsic cause of infertility.

These authors presented significant data on wolffian duct anomalies. Among 35 patients who had had an intravenous

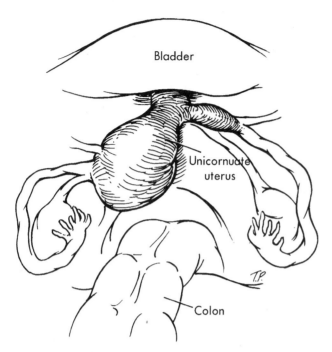

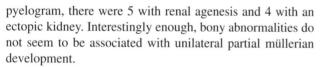

Fig. 61-11. Internal genitalia with a unicornuate uterus. (Adapted from Jones HW Jr., Rock JA: Reparative and constructive surgery of the female generative tract, Baltimore, MD, 1983, Williams & Wilkins.)

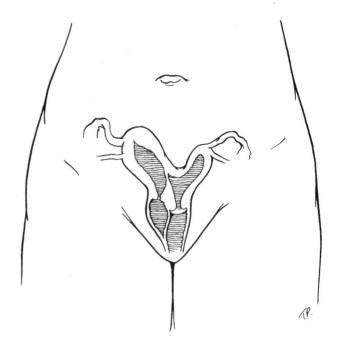

Fig. 61-12. Unilateral vaginal obstruction. (Adapted from Jones HW Jr., Rock JA: Reparative and constructive surgery of the female generative tract, Baltimore, MD, 1983, Williams & Wilkins..)

pyelogram, there were 5 with renal agenesis and 4 with an ectopic kidney. Interestingly enough, bony abnormalities do not seem to be associated with unilateral partial müllerian development.

Thus it is an open question as to whether the unicornuate uterus per se can result in primary infertility. It is unlikely that this is the case. No therapy for this situation is known to exist. On an experimental basis, assisted reproduction might be considered, but there is no extensive experience that would indicate that this is successful. In some instances for patients with repeated spontaneous abortion, the author has removed the contralateral müllerian remnant, which seemed to attach high on the developed side. Term delivery has followed. Andrews and Jones[1] reported the details of reproductive performance in 5 cases.

Cerclage has been recommended and used, presumably with some success in cases of repeated spontaneous abortion and premature labor.

PROBLEMS OF LATERAL FUSION
Obstructive

Unilateral vaginal obstruction. In this section are discussed cases in which there is a unilateral obstruction that may be from low in the vagina upward. The resulting symptoms are very much related to the site of obstruction. In the situation in which development produces what is essentially a uterus didelphys with a double vagina but with

an obstruction very low in the vagina on one side, a large amount of blood may accumulate and the situation may be unrecognized for a number of years after the onset of menstruation (Fig. 61-12). The patient finally becomes aware of cyclic abdominal pain, which fades away several days after it starts. This delayed onset of pain and its characteristics are apparently due to the fact that the distensible vagina can accommodate to the increments of blood resulting from each menstrual period and absorbs enough fluid between periods so that succeeding menstrual flows add to the accumulated blood, but without excruciating pain. This insidious situation is quite unfortunate, because it may result in involvement of the tubes and the development of rather large tuboovarian accumulations of menstrual blood with endometriosis.

It therefore becomes important to diagnose these problems as early as possible and to relieve them by removal of the septum, which is generally an easy procedure. However, sometimes the septum is somewhat thick and contains important arteries that need to be secured.

Patients with this condition, especially those in whom the condition is discovered late (i.e., when they are aged 18 or 19, or even in their early 20s), are always interested in what this obstruction has done to their reproductive potential. This may or may not call for investigation of the tubal status, but in any case, this can certainly be postponed until there have been one or two menstrual cycles after the

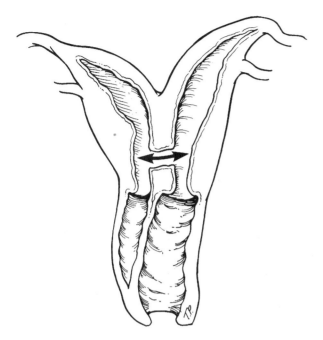

Fig. 61-13. Lateral communicating uterus. (Adapted from Jones HW Jr., Rock JA: Reparative and constructive surgery of the female generative tract, Baltimore, MD, 1983, Williams & Wilkins.)

removal of the septum. If the clinical situation then indicates, one could consider laparoscopy and possibly hysterosalpingography to ascertain the reproductive potential; of course, this evaluation could be postponed until the patient was interested in becoming pregnant.

The epithelium of an obstructed vagina is almost always composed of cuboidal cells, testifying to the müllerian origin of the epithelium. If the obstruction is incomplete, even if the communication with the unobstructed side is extremely small, the cuboidal epithelium seems to have been replaced by squamous vaginal epithelium, presumably by a process of metaplasia that may be the normal embryologic process in the development of the vagina. Thus, when the vaginal septum is removed in obstructed circumstances, the newly opened vagina is lined with adenomatous epithelium. In effect, the patient has vaginal adenosis. This adenomatous epithelium is slowly replaced with metaplasia; but if the area involved is of any size, as when the obstruction is low in the vagina, the metaplastic process will require 2 or 3 years to complete. The patient will experience decreasing vaginal discharge during this metaplastic process. Vaginal creams tending to stabilize the pH of the vagina on the acid side seem to be helpful.

Unilateral vaginal obstruction with a lateral communication. If the obstruction exists as in the foregoing section (i.e., when there is unilateral lower vaginal obstruction) but in addition there is a lateral communication between the two horns of the uterus, a very special situation exists. This communication is usually through the cervix

(Fig. 61-13). When this happens, the obstructive symptoms are even less pressing than when there is a unilateral, low vaginal obstruction, and the patient sometimes complains of a disappearing mass at the vaginal outlet. As one takes the history, one suspects a large Bartholin gland cyst, but on examination such cannot be found. It is interesting and pertinent that the diagnosis is often missed largely because it is not considered. In a series of 11 patients collected by Toaff,[21] the age at which the first symptom occurred was 15.5 years, but the age at which a definitive diagnosis was made and therapy carried out was 23.7 years, indicating the problem in diagnosis.

These patients complain not only of a disappearing vaginal mass, but also of intermenstrual vaginal discharge, sometimes bloody, and particularly occurring immediately after the menstrual period for several days. If attempts are made to make the diagnosis, such as by the use of hysterosalpingography and this is not followed immediately by therapy, a low-grade infection may occur in the obstructed vagina, putting at risk the tubes for future reproduction. Treatment of this particular special situation involves only the removal of the vaginal septum. No treatment needs to be directed at the lateral communication of the uterus, and reproduction is consistent with a duplicated uterus, unless neglect of the original condition has compromised tubal function.

Unilateral uterine obstruction. When the obstruction is in the region of the cervix, the reservoir-like action of the vagina in accommodating the cyclic menstrual blood flow is lost, and symptoms are much more acute and occur far earlier (Fig. 61-14). Such patients seldom have more than three or four menstrual periods before the excruciating pain demands attention. This means that these patients are aged 12, 13, or 14 years. Hysterography through the patent side, ultrasonography, and a CT scan, if necessary, can help to clarify the diagnosis.

The treatment of this condition will clearly vary with the exact point of obstruction. In some instances, it is technically impossible to remove the obstructed side and leave a functioning uterus; therefore, if the cervix is well formed on the unobstructed size, an anastomosis of the obstructed to the unobstructed side is a feasible and useful procedure (Fig. 61-15).

In most instances of this nature, the obstruction involves what amounts to an isolated horn of the uterus with minimal connection to the unobstructed side. When this occurs, early removal is desirable so that retrograde menstruation will not cause endometriosis and then compromise subsequent reproduction. Fortunately, in the rudimentary horn syndrome with obstruction, there is also failure of communication to the cavity of the uterus with a fallopian tube, negating the possibility of spilling menstrual blood. Excisions of these horns give very satisfactory results.

A few examples of pregnancy have been observed in an

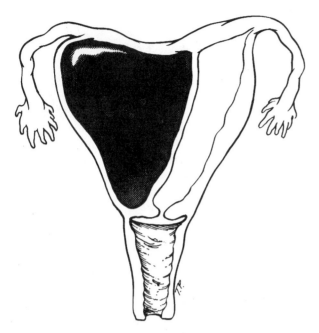

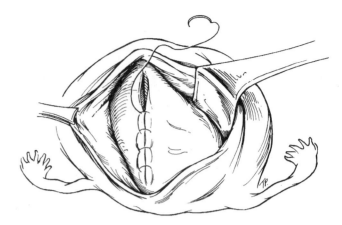

Fig. 61-15. Unilateral cervical obstruction, lateral anastomosis. (Adapted from Jones HW Jr., Rock JA: Reparative and constructive surgery of the female generative tract, Baltimore, MD, 1983, Williams & Wilkins.)

Fig. 61-14. Unilateral cervical obstruction. (Adapted from Jones HW Jr., Rock JA: Reparative and constructive surgery of the female generative tract, Baltimore, MD, 1983, Williams & Wilkins.)

obstructed rudimentary horn. All of these have occurred in very young individuals to whom the exposure to pregnancy occurred soon after puberty, or simultaneously with it, so that there was no opportunity for the trapped menstrual blood to hamper the function of the obstructed horn. In these instances, it is obvious that the fertilizing sperm has ascended through the unobstructed side. Such patients present, as might be expected, with the symptoms of an ectopic pregnancy. In such instances, the ideal treatment is excision of the rudimentary horn. This is sometimes difficult when there is a sharing of a uterine wall with the obstructed side (Fig. 61-16).

With very few exceptions, when there is a failure of lateral fusion of the müllerian ducts with a unilateral obstruction, absence of the ipsilateral kidney is the rule. Therefore determination of the presence or absence of the kidney often may clarify the diagnosis in obscure circumstances.

Nonobstructive

Classification. Under this rubric are considered uterus didelphys, bicornuate uterus, septate uterus, and the T uterus (Fig. 61-17).

Importance of an accurate diagnosis. From a clinical point of view, the importance of an accurate diagnosis in symmetric double uteri without obstruction, identifying the type of uterus, is of extraordinary importance. It is very important to distinguish between a true bicornuate uterus, a septate uterus, and a T uterus for the simple reason that the

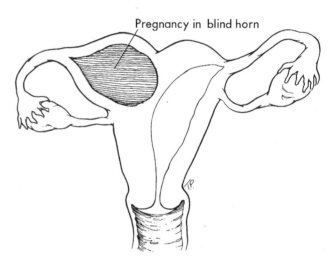

Fig. 61-16. Pregnancy in obstructed horn. (Adapted from Jones HW Jr., Rock JA: Reparative and constructive surgery of the female generative tract, Baltimore, MD, 1983, Williams & Wilkins.)

bicornuate uterus gives only minimal problems with reproduction, whereas the septate uteri or T uteri are almost always the types that are involved in reproductive failure. The practical point is that the distinction between these types cannot be made easily by an examination of a hysterogram. For instance, the images of the cavities of a bicornuate uterus and a septate uterus may be exactly the same. It is the external configuration of the uterus that is key to an accurate diagnosis. In the septate uterus, the external appearance is quite normal and cannot be recognized at laparoscopy or even laparotomy. Sometimes there is a hint of an indentation with a midline raphe, but on pelvic examination the uterus feels normal, except that

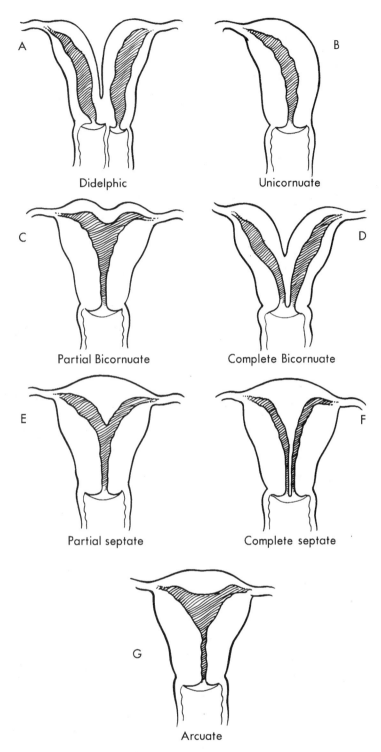

Fig. 61-17. Types of uterine anomalies. **A,** uterus didelphys; **B,** unicornuate uterus; **C,** partial bicornuate uterus; **D,** complete bicornuate uterus; **E,** partial septate uterus; **F,** complete septate uterus; **G,** arcuate uterus. (Adapted from Jones HW Jr., Rock JA: Reparative and constructive surgery of the female generative tract, Baltimore, MD, 1983, Williams & Wilkins.)

sometimes a septate uterus is a little broader than expected. If one can palpate two separate horns on pelvic examination, one can be sure that one is dealing with a bicornuate uterus. The external configuration of the uterus is of such importance that if there is any uncertainty in this regard on simple pelvic examination, an examination under anesthesia or even at laparoscopy may be indicated. Ultrasonography and the more sophisticated CT scan may be helpful and can often make the critical distinction. As already inferred, it is seldom that a bicornuate uterus needs surgical reconstruction. It follows that almost invariably, as has been mentioned, if a double uterus gives reproductive problems requiring surgical attention, it is the septate or T uterus that will be involved.

A special situation pertains to the anomalies associated with and probably caused by exposure in utero to diethylstilbestrol (DES). Kaufman et al.[12] called attention to the varieties of deformities, most of them shaped like a T, in many DES-exposed patients. Haney et al.[8] described the lesion in great detail. Barnes et al.[3] and others have pointed out the unfavorable outcome of pregnancies in DES-exposed women. Treatment for this special situation is difficult, but in selected circumstances surgical reconstruction can be carried out and seems to be helpful, as reported by Muasher et al.[16] and subsequently by Khalifa et al.[13] Although most T-shaped uteri are clearly the result of fetal exposure to DES, T uteri can occur in patients for whom it is certain that there was no history of DES exposure. They represent a rather rare situation but can cause repeated spontaneous abortion, with a history indistinguishable from that associated with a septate uterus.

The diagnosis of a reproductive problem due to a double uterus is essentially made by exclusion. In view of the fact that reproduction in the double uterus, particularly of the bicornuate type, may be essentially normal, it is necessary to determine whether a particular uterus is responsible for the reproductive problem. It follows that there is considerable uncertainty about the relationship of primary infertility to a double uterus. Most often, the reproductive difficulty revolves around repeated spontaneous abortion or premature labor. It is therefore essential in attributing the difficulty to the double uterus that all other causes of reproductive failure be excluded. This would include male factors and such female factors as cervical incompetence; chronic illness; luteal phase defects; and other endocrine disorders, adrenal and thyroid, that may be encountered in the circumstances. Certainly fetal factors would need to be excluded, as would immunologic causes, and particularly karyotypic anomalies in one or another of the potential parents, with a resulting genetically defective zygote. It also would involve such problems as the identification of placental endocrine factors (i.e., failure of progesterone production) that cannot be identified except by a study of placental hormones during a test pregnancy.

A difficult judgmental decision arises when a patient has primary infertility and is found, on investigation, to have a septate uterus as well as a problem that requires an abdominal approach. These include tubal difficulties and/or endometriosis. The question is whether a uterine septum should be treated "prophylactically." Although there is bound to be uncertainty about this point, it is our view that if the abdominal procedure requires surgical therapy, regardless of whether it is laparoscopic surgery or open abdominal surgery, the uterus should be reconstructed at the same time, so that the patient is saved the disappointment of achieving a pregnancy only to have it terminated by a spontaneous abortion. The question of whether this should be done by laparoscopic surgical treatment combined with transcervical resection is a matter of judgment. The fact is that there are no data on the simultaneous approach to this problem by endoscopic techniques. We do know that if the open abdominal approach is used, an 80% term pregnancy rate has been reported by Khalifa et al.[13]

When spontaneous abortion is at issue, the history of the particular miscarriage is critically significant. The characteristic story associated with a septate uterus is of an early midtrimester loss associated with what is in essence a minilabor starting with cramps and followed by bleeding. In primigravidae, the labor may last for only 4 or 5 hours, but results in the delivery of a well-formed but not viable fetus. This is the typical history and one that gives reassurance that the uterus is the cause of the miscarriage. However, there are troublesome exceptions to this history, in that spontaneous abortions do occur earlier and the well-formed fetus rule seems to be violated; but these exceptions are presumably due to the double uterus, since term delivery of normal children follows after the surgical removal of the uterine septum.

Why some septate uteri and those that have a T-shaped cavity, regardless of the etiology of that abnormality, do not behave well reproductively is an unresolved problem. Various mechanisms have been suggested, such as septal endometrial incompetence and septal circulatory inadequacy. Perhaps each or both of these mechanisms play a role. However, clinical experience suggests that regardless of the detail, asymmetric uterine enlargement is undesirable and predisposes to uterine irritability and expulsion of the uterine contents. This observation is confirmed by the occasional occurrence of a pregnancy in both sides of a septate uterus after spontaneous abortions of a pregnancy on one side. It is interesting that these bilateral pregnancies seem to carry to term, suggesting that symmetric bilateral enlargement overcomes the inherent problem.

Surgical treatment is extremely helpful for the bicornuate uterus, the septate uterus, and the T uterus when the work-up has carefully eliminated other correctable endocrine or metabolic causes. The techniques for the repair of each of these conditions are considered later. It therefore goes without much discussion that any correctable endocrine and metabolic causes of reproductive loss should be

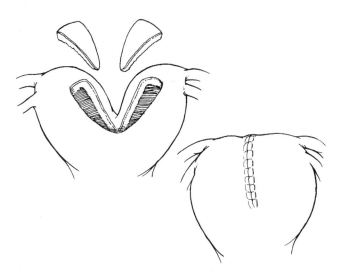

Fig. 61-18. Unification of uterus didelphys.

treated, and only if adequate treatment fails and symptomatology continues should surgical reconstruction be considered.

Uterus didelphys. In the nonobstructed failure of lateral fusion involving both the uterus and vagina (i.e., the uterus didelphys), there are no symptoms related to menstruation. Sometimes dyspareunia may be a problem because of the narrowness of the vagina on one side. The vaginas in this syndrome are by no means always exactly symmetric in size. When dyspareunia occurs, removal of the septum may be required and it is not particularly difficult, although as mentioned in cases in which there is unilateral obstruction, the vagina may be thick and contain blood vessels that yield active bleeding.

Most often, patients with uterus didelphys seek advice when their reproductive function is imminent. There is even more paucity of information in the literature about pregnancy in the uterus didelphys as compared with the unicornuate uterus. Incidentally, the uterus didelphys is but a bilateral unicornuate uterus. A number of examples of simultaneous pregnancies in each side have been reported and is one of the reasons the vaginal septum should not be removed unless dyspareunia is a real problem. These simultaneous pregnancies have generally had a happy outcome for both pregnancies. The literature, particularly the older literature, contains almost miraculous reports of sequential labor with remarkable intervals between the birth of each child. An interval of 24 hours is not unusual, and intervals of several days have been reported. Cesarean delivery would doubtless be used routinely at the present time, and probably accounts for the absence of sequential labor from the current literature. The principal indications for surgical intervention in the didelphic uterus are repeated spontaneous abortion or premature labor, when it is clear that the uterus is responsible for the problem. In this circumstance, the two unicornuate uteri can be united in the midline by unroofing the cavities and suturing them together (Fig. 61-18). If and when this is done, it is important not to unify the cervices, as almost surely a very large incompetent cervix would result. Thus the unification would be confined to the corpus, with a plan to do an elective cesarean section.

Bicornuate uterus. In the bicornuate uterus, as mentioned, the reproductive problem that can be surgically handled is that of premature labor, which gives a very premature baby with all the consequences thereof.

For the bicornuate and T uterus there is no consideration of transcervical operative procedures. It is a matter of an abdominal corrective procedure to make a single functional cavity. In the case of the bicornuate uterus there is a single cervix, so that the unification could result in a single cavity without consideration to the cervix. The operative technique that works well with the bicornuate uterus is the classic Strassman procedure (Fig. 61-19).

Septate uterus. The matter of accurate diagnosis and the clinical setting in which some surgical therapy is to be considered were discussed earlier. The discussion of the septate uterus therefore is confined to its surgical correction. Selection of the most appropriate technique to remove or divide the septum requires the exercise of considerable judgment and experience. It is not a matter of selecting either transcervical resection or abdominal resection alternately for similar lesions, but rather the selection of the procedure most appropriate to the particular situation. If the septum is internal (i.e., occupies space that might be expected to belong to the endometrial cavity so that the hysterosalpingogram reveals a V-shaped image), transcervical resection by operative hysteroscopy seems to yield satisfactory results. This therefore is the procedure of choice if no other intraabdominal procedure is required. However, if there is a hysteroscopic image approaching a T, operative hysteroscopy is inappropriate and dangerous, because often there is only a small intercavitary septum, if any. These uteri are often, but by no means always, the result of exposure to DES, but they can occur spontaneously. T shapes resulting from DES exposure are special and are often quite small; generally they are easily distinguished from spontaneously occurring T uteri. The DES uteri clearly have no resectable intercavitary septum, and therefore are not at all suitable for hysteroscopic treatment.

Thus the transcervical or abdominal approach must be selected according to the particular case. For example, DeCherney et al.[4] found 72 of 103 patients suitable for hysteroscopic resection.

The surgical goal, as stated earlier, in the pathogenesis of the mischief caused by the double uterus is to obtain a cavity that, when it enlarges, will be symmetric.

Technique of transcervical correction. The technique for transcervical transection of a uterine septum is also mentioned in Chapter 58. The septum can be severed by scissors, the cutting current of an endotherm as with a

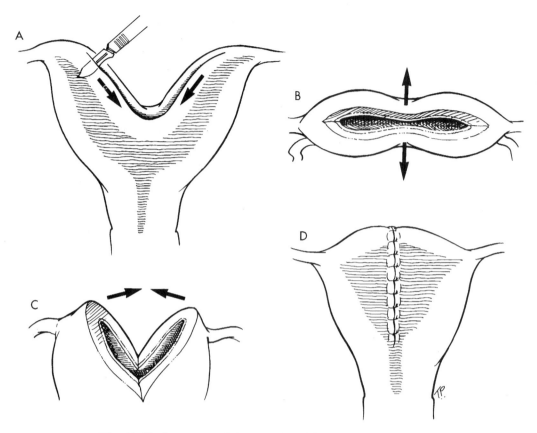

Fig. 61-19. Strassman technique. (Adapted from OB/GYN.)

resectoscope, or the laser. We have found the resectoscope satisfactory and can recommend it. Hyskon is a satisfactory medium for distention. It should be recalled that some patients are sensitive to Hyskon and that absorption from a broad endometrial wound can be considerable. Fatalities have been reported.

With the resectoscope in place and the loop clearly midline, successive cuts can be made until the septum is transected (Fig. 61-20). The most difficult decision is to determine when the septum has been completely transected. This decision is the result of comprehending the extent of the original septum, the evaluation of the configuration of the cavity after successive cuts, and the intensity of the transmitted hysteroscopic light to the laparoscopic observer. The latter presupposes simultaneous laparoscopic observation, which is to be highly recommended, especially for those with little experience.

It does not seem to be necessary to use a balloon or other device to prevent adherence of the adjacent fresh endometrial wounds, although there are limited studies at this point.

A delay of at least 3 months before attempting pregnancy seems reasonable.

Technique of abdominal correction. The classic Strassman procedure is unsuitable for correcting the defect in the septate uterus. As Strassman was working in an era before hysterosalpingography, he operated almost entirely on bi-

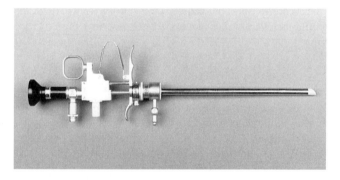

Fig. 61-20. Resectoscope.

cornuate uteri, as his diagnostic techniques were limited almost to a bimanual examination and exploration of the endometrial cavity by curette or other instrument. Tompkins[22] and others have recommended a technique beginning with a midline incision of the uterus until the confluence of the two cavities is reached. After this, the septum is whittled away until the two remaining sides can be united. However, primary excision of the septum by wedge has proven to be an extraordinarily satisfactory procedure and can be recommended. The technique is as follows: The abdomen may be opened by either a transverse or midline incision. The exterior configuration of the uterus, as previously mentioned, may be quite normal, although on occa-

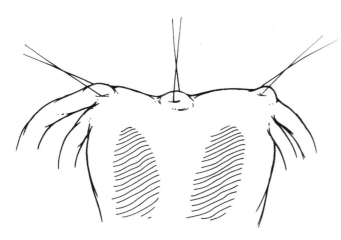

Fig. 61-21. Septate uterus (brilliant green guy sutures). (Adapted from Jones HW Jr., Rock JA: Reparative and constructive surgery of the female generative tract, Baltimore, MD, 1983, Williams & Wilkins.)

sion a small median raphe may be identified. However, on palpation, the presence of the septum can often be confirmed.

It is convenient to outline the incision on the outside of the uterus with brilliant green. The depth of the incision anteriorly and posteriorly will depend on estimation of the size of the septum. The line of brilliant green also ensures that the incision is correct because, after the original cut is made, distortion may occur. Before making an incision, three temporary sutures can be placed—one on each side at the attachment of the round ligaments and one directly in the midline in the area that will be subsequently removed. These sutures are for traction (Fig. 61-21).

To control bleeding, up to 20 U of vasopressin diluted in 20 mL of saline may be injected into the myometrium. This will produce immediate blanching and will diminish the blood loss during the procedure. Many procedures can be carried out with a loss of only 5 mL or so of blood. Because vasopressin may sometimes cause circulatory changes, the anesthesiologist must be alerted when the vasopressin is started. Very satisfactory blanching can sometimes be obtained with only 10 U, so that the possibility of circulatory changes is greatly diminished.

The uterine septum is surgically excised as a wedge. Incisions begin at the fundus and are continued anteriorly and posteriorly. If one incises gently, the endometrial cavity is easy to identify, but care must surely be taken that the cavity is not transected. After the wedge has been removed, very little bleeding will be noted, because of the vasopressin, and the only major vessel that needs to be tied is the ascending uterine artery, which is easily visible at the top of the incision in the region of the tube. It is convenient to clamp and ligate this artery with very fine suture material, even though it may not be bleeding. Generally, it is not necessary to ligate any other vessels (Fig. 61-22).

After removal of the wedge, the uterus may be closed from side to side in three layers with interrupted stitches, using chromic catgut (00) on an atraumatic, tapered needle in preference to synthetic absorbable material, which tends to cut through the myometrium more readily than the catgut. Two sizes of needles are used—a ½-inch half-round needle for the inner and intermediate layers, and a narrow ¾-inch half-round needle for the outer serosal layers. The inner layer must include not only the endometrium but also about one third of the thickness of the myometrium, since the endometrium itself is too delicate to hold a suture and will cut through. The sutures are to be placed through the endometrium-myometrium in such a way that the knot is tied within the endometrial cavity (Fig. 61-23). To facilitate this, an assistant presses together the two lateral halves of the uterus with the fingers and with the guy sutures in order to relieve tension on the suture line and reduce the possibility of cutting through. The stitches can be conveniently placed alternately anteriorly and posteriorly. After the first few stitches are placed and before the final layers are completed, a second myometrium-to-myometrium layer can be started; indeed, as the operation proceeds, the third serosal layer can be inserted. For the serosal layer, a much smaller stitch is appropriate, as for example, 0000 braided Dacron. Theoretically, this should cut down on the opportunity for adhesions to the outside of the uterus.

At the conclusion of the procedure, a single incision is visible, beginning from the back of the uterus from the position dictated by the depth of the septum and continuing anteriorly to a corresponding position in front. Generally speaking, it is not necessary to detach the peritoneal reflection of the bladder, but if there is a particularly deep septum, this may be necessary. If so, the incision in the uterus will in part be covered when the bladder reflection is replaced.

At the conclusion, the uterus appears rather normal in its configuration, but the striking feature will be the proximity of the insertions of the fallopian tubes. It is obviously important in placing the sutures, particularly the ones near the apex, that the interstitial portion of the fallopian tubes not be obstructed by the sutures. At the conclusion of the procedures, the two remaining guy sutures can be removed.

The final size of the uterine cavity seems to be unimportant. Many times a reconstructed cavity is quite small compared with a normal uterus. Of more importance, as has been emphasized before, seems to be the symmetry. A very small, even pencil-like, cavity seems to function normally. Postoperative films often show small dogears, which are left over from the original bifid condition of the uterus. Such dogears do not seem to interfere with function. Although postoperative roentgenograms cannot be considered normal in the sense that it appears like an endometrial cavity, the uterus seems to function satisfactorily (Fig. 61-24).

Blood loss from the procedure if vasopressin is used is minimal. Diminished bleeding from vasopressin lasts ap-

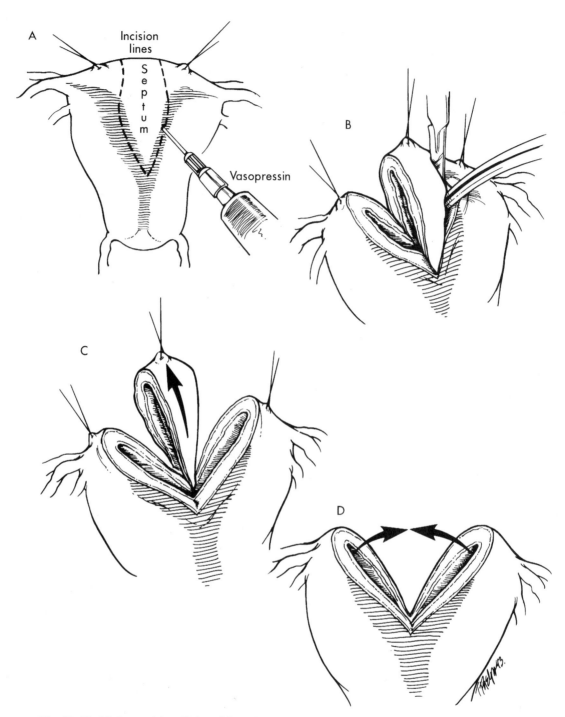

Fig. 61-22. Wedge excision. (Adapted from Jones HW Jr., Rock JA: Reparative and constructive surgery of the female generative tract, Baltimore, MD, 1983, Williams & Wilkins.)

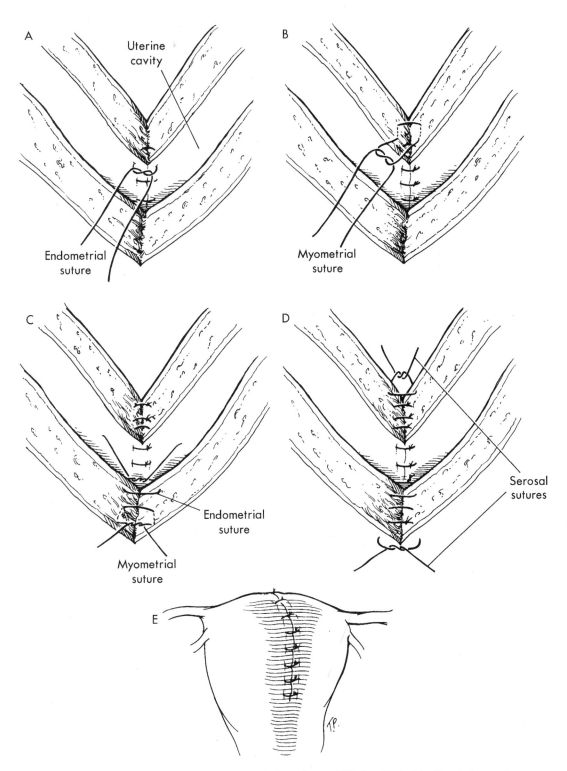

Fig. 61-23. Placement of sutures. (Adapted from Jones HW Jr., Rock JA: Reparative and constructive surgery of the female generative tract, Baltimore, MD, 1983, Williams & Wilkins.)

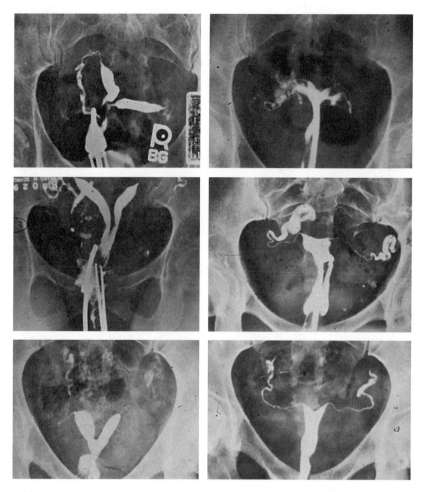

Fig. 61-24. Preoperative and postoperative hysterograms. (Adapted from Jones HW Jr., Rock JA: Reparative and constructive surgery of the female generative tract, Baltimore, MD, 1983, Williams & Wilkins.)

proximately 20 minutes, and the operation normally can be completed well within this time.

If the duplication involves the cervix, it is important not to attempt to unify this for fear of creating incompetence.

Obstetric management. Healing in the nonpregnant uterus is probably not to be compared with healing after a cesarean section. Thus it might be expected that incisions in cesarean-sectioned uteri are less firmly healed than incisions in nonpregnant uteri. Nevertheless, most patients who have had surgical reconstruction of a double uterus have been delivered by cesarean section. This can be recommended as a matter of precaution. Such patients have had a long disappointing reproductive experience. They are often in their late 30s, and in order to minimize the risk of an obstetric catastrophe, an elective cesarean section before the onset of labor seems a conservative approach that avoids all possibility of a uterine rupture.

A delay in becoming pregnant after abdominal surgical reconstruction has generally been advised. This will, of course, have to be modulated by the age of the patient, but a wait of approximately 6 months should be an ideal target.

During this interval, it has been thought not advisable to recommend oral contraceptives because of the deleterious effect of progesterone on healing in the myometrium. Therefore, mechanical contraception with diaphragm or condom has been recommended and has proved to be satisfactory as judged by the ultimate result.

Results. Hassiakos and Zourlas[9] comprehensively reviewed the results from transcervical division of uterine septa from 17 reports from 1974 through 1988. There were 232 patients available, each of whom had had at least one spontaneous abortion. There had been a total of 585 pregnancies, of which 506 (86.5%) were aborted spontaneously. There were but 21 living children from these 586 pregnancies (3.6%). There can therefore be no doubt that this group qualified as being severely handicapped from a reproductive point of view. One hundred and eighty-three patients (i.e., 78.9% of the 232 patients) became pregnant, and 155 (66.8%) carried to term. There was a total of 204 pregnancies, of which 24 (11.7%) were aborted spontaneously. These results, although somewhat lower than those reported for abdominal metroplasty for similar types of patients, are reasonably satisfactory. Of special interest in the review by Hassiakos and Zourlas is the analysis of 36 patients from 8 reports who had primary infertility.[9] Eleven of these 36 (33.3%) became pregnant, but four of these pregnancies were aborted, so that the term pregnancy rate was 7 of 36, or only 19.4%. These data emphasize the point repeatedly made in this chapter, that primary infertility is very unlikely to have a septate uterus as its etiologic agent.

There have been few recent large series of abdominal metroplasty. However, the series of Rock and Jones[18] can be considered representative. Of 47 patients with repeated spontaneous abortions, 45 became pregnant and 38 (81%) had living children. Muasher et al.[16] reported on 22 patients, including 10 who had had early first-trimester spontaneous abortions and therefore abortions somewhat inconsistent with the typical history of spontaneous abortion with a septate uterus; they found that 14 patients (64%) subsequently had a live child. More recently, Khalifa et al.[13] were able to report greater than an 80% term pregnancy rate among 16 patients who had had an abdominal metroplasty, along with an associated other abdominal procedure such as tuboplasty or surgical treatment of abdominal endometriosis. This series included a few patients in whom the uterine septum was repaired "prophylactically" according to the philosophy mentioned previously.

T uterus. Operative correction of the T uterus, whether due to DES exposure or other causes, is quite satisfactory. The goal is to unroof the cross arm of the T and to produce an I. The procedure can be initiated by slicing off the roof or by using a single incision, as in the Strassman, and subsequently removing redundant tissue, if any. The closure is in layers, as described for the septate uterus (Fig. 61-25). Excellent results have been reported in a few patients.[13,16]

PROBLEMS OF VERTICAL FUSION
Obstructive transverse vaginal septum

An obstructed transverse vaginal septum may be symptomatic in infancy, but most often an obstructed septum causes no symptoms until puberty and the onset of menstruation. However, for reasons that are obscure, in some infants a large volume of mucus can collect above the obstruction, and such cases are often described in the literature as examples of hydromucocolpos (Fig. 61-26). Such obstructions need to be relieved promptly, as they present an obvious potential for subsequent reproductive difficulty; however, it is curious that insofar as this author is aware, there is not even a single case report in the literature of reproduction subsequent to the relief of a hydromucocolpos in infancy. As judged by a pedigree study of an inbred Amish community, there is impressive evidence that hydromucocolpos is the result of a rare autosomal gene. McKusick et al.[15] traced five cases of hydromucocolpos in distant cousins. The common ancestors, seven or eight generations before, were the genetically well-known Christian Beiler and Barbara Yoder, eighteenth century migrants to the

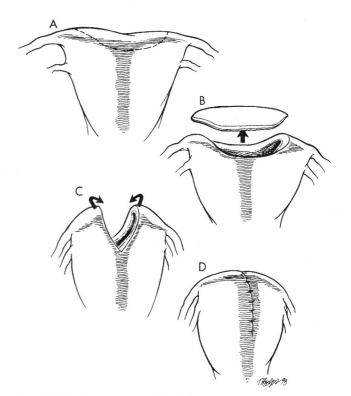

Fig. 61-25. Reconstruction of a T uterus.

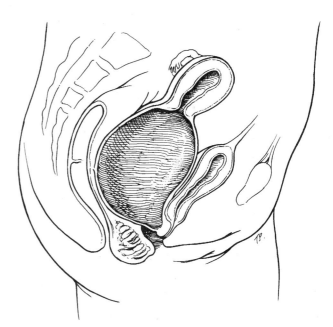

Fig. 61-26. Hydromucopolpos. (Adapted from Jones HW Jr., Rock JA: Reparative and constructive surgery of the female generative tract, Baltimore, MD, 1983, Williams & Wilkins.)

United States. The site of the obstruction may be anywhere along the vaginal canal, but generally it is at the junction between the middle and upper third of the vagina (Fig. 61-27). The diagnosis of this condition in infancy is often missed because the patient presents with an abdominal

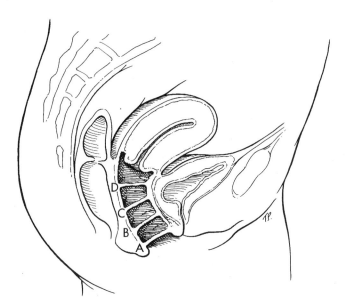

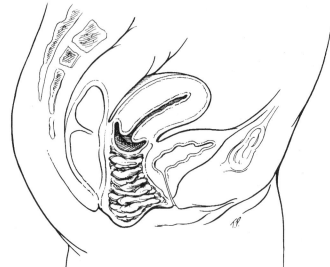

Fig. 61-27. Sites of obstructed transverse septum. (Adapted from Jones HW Jr., Rock JA: Reparative and constructive surgery of the female generative tract, Baltimore, MD, 1983, Williams & Wilkins.)

Fig. 61-28. Long transverse vaginal septum. (Adapted from Jones HW Jr., Rock JA: Reparative and constructive surgery of the female generative tract, Baltimore, MD, 1983, Williams & Wilkins.)

mass and irritability. There is no bulging of the vagina. This mass is the tremendously distended vagina, which in some instances has caused serious urinary tract obstruction. Fatalities from uremia have been reported. The most effective surgical therapy is an operation from below that removes the obstructive membrane. The use of ultrasound-guided needle aspiration has much to recommend it and could be done as a temporary measure with great precautions not to introduce infection. However, permanent relief of the obstruction is urgently necessary, and bilateral Schuchardt incisions may be required to provide access for septum removal. Mandell et al.[14] have especially considered the operative approach to this matter.

Most often, an obstructed transverse vaginal septum does not give symptoms until after menstruation begins. The symptoms are then associated with the outflow of menstrual blood. The character of the obstructing membrane may be quite different in the cases encountered in adults as compared with those encountered in infancy. It is curious and not completely understood why, in some cases, large amounts of mucus collect above the obstructing membrane in infancy, where as in others this does not seem to occur. Whether this is associated with the character of the obstructing membrane is unsure, but in the adult, many times the transverse vaginal septum may be very thick walled, so that its removal is difficult. Indeed, a considerable segment of the vagina can be undeveloped, and if this segment is prolonged to the extent that it involves the whole of the lower portion of the vagina, a situation arises that is described in the literature as congenital absence of the vagina with a uterus present. This situation really is but

an extreme form of transverse vaginal septum (Fig. 61-28). The condition seems to be pathogenetically different from the Rokitansky syndrome because anomalies of the urinary tract and skeleton are unknown with transverse septum, whereas they are quite common in the Rokitansky-Küster-Hauser syndrome. Very rarely, by suitable examination, a uterus is found to be present when the vagina is absent, and in some of these circumstances the endometrial cavity has failed to develop.

An extremely troublesome situation occurs when the defect in development includes the cervix. Thus there may be a functioning corpus that is obstructed and a defect in cervical and vaginal development. In an occasional case of this type, the vagina can be of functional length, but generally speaking it is absent (Fig. 61-29).

When there is accumulation of menstrual blood, symptoms dominated by cyclic pain require therapy usually in the early teenaged years. The duration of the pain in cycles will depend on the size of the obstructed vagina and its ability to act as a reservoir. If the obstructing membrane can be incised by multiple radial incisions with reanastomosis of the upper and lower segments, this is the preferred method.

In some instances the length of the obstructing transverse septum may be such that reanastomosis of the upper and lower segment is impossible. In that circumstance, the connection of the upper and lower segments may be accomplished by developing a space between the rectum and the bladder, as is done in the Rokitansky syndrome. This always presents identification problems at the apex, because it is obviously important to distinguish the blind

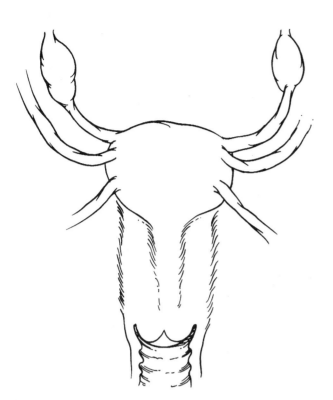

Fig. 61-29. Congenital absence of cervix. (Adapted from Jones HW Jr., Rock JA: Reparative and constructive surgery of the female generative tract, Baltimore, MD, 1983, Williams & Wilkins.)

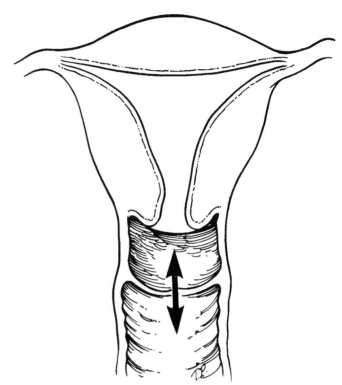

Fig. 61-30. Transverse vaginal septum with opening. (Adapted from Jones HW Jr., Rock JA: Reparative and constructive surgery of the female generative tract, Baltimore, MD, 1983, Williams & Wilkins..)

vagina from the bladder anteriorly and the rectum posteriorly. It is easier to identify the obstructed vagina if there is a considerable amount of accumulated menstrual blood. Because of this, it is a disadvantage to have had the upper vagina drained in any fashion, as has happened in some instances when the accumulated blood in the upper vagina had created a mass of considerable size that was mistaken for some other intraabdominal structure and approached from above. When operating from below, it is often useful to probe with an aspirating needle; when menstrual blood is obtained, identification of the vagina is certain.

After entering the upper vagina, if the upper vagina cannot be anastomosed to the lower vagina, it is necessary to use an indwelling stent. The stent must make provision for menstruation. A very satisfactory one can be made from plexiglass or other suitable material. It is convenient to have a bulbous end that can be placed in the upper vagina, so that as the neovaginal space contracts, the stent will be self-containing. This is a particularly useful point, because these are teenaged patients whose motivation for care of an indwelling stent has proven to be inadequate. The plexiglass stent may be left in place for 4 to 6 months and requires very little care; when it is removed by making a lateral incision, it can be anticipated that the epithelium of the upper and lower vagina will have joined by the proliferation of the edges of the epithelium from above and below.

If the defect in development includes the cervix, as described, one is presented with an extremely difficult therapeutic problem. Preservation of reproductive potential in this situation has been seldom achieved. There seems to be only a scattering of documentation of successful reproduction after agenesis of the vagina, the first one being reported by Zarou et al.[23] Generally, attempts to keep open a fistulous tract between the endometrial cavity and the vagina ultimately are doomed to failure. After repeated dilatations over a number of years, both the surgeon and the patient are happy to solve the problem by the removal of the corpus of the uterus. Nevertheless, efforts to establish a functioning communication between the corpus of the uterus and the vagina have continued. For example, Farber and Marchant[6] reported success in establishing a permanent fistulous opening between the uterine cavity and the cervix in four patients. However, no pregnancies were reported. More recently there are anecdotal reports of pregnancies in this circumstance by the gamete intrafallopian transfer procedure. This is certainly a theoretic possibility.

Nevertheless, all things considered, it seems realistic to recommend hysterectomy as initial primary therapy in these cases, with very, very few exceptions. The status of the fallopian tubes, which are sometimes deformed, would be very key information in arriving at a decision.

Nonobstructive transverse vaginal septum

Most transverse vaginal septa are not complete and therefore do not result in the accumulation of mucus or menstrual blood above them. Under this circumstance, they are likely not to give any symptoms until intercourse is attempted and found to be uncomfortable or even impossible.

Sometimes the opening in the transverse vaginal septum is very small indeed, requiring careful search with a silver probe to find the opening. These openings may be consistent with menstruation, and even pregnancies have occurred (Fig. 61-30). This is very curious, because it indicates that sperm can traverse a gap in the vagina of often a distance of 3 or 4 cm. A number of curious cases have been encountered, as, for example, a patient delivered by cesarian section in whom the lochia became so profuse that it could not be accommodated through the pinpoint opening in the transverse vaginal septum, with the result obstruction and infection, and the necessity for an emergency surgical procedure.

REFERENCES

1. Andrews MC, Jones HW Jr: Impaired reproductive performance of the unicornuate uterus and intrauterine growth retardation: infertility and recurrent abortion in five cases, *Am J Obstet Gynecol* 144:173, 1982.
2. Azoury RS, Jones HW Jr: Cytogenic findings in patients with congenital absence of the vagina, *Am J Obstet Gynecol* 94:178, 1966.
3. Barnes AB et al: Fertility and outcome of pregnancy in women exposed in utero to diethylstilbestrol, *N Engl J Med* 302:609, 1980.
4. DeCherney AH, Russell JB, Graebe RA: Resectoscopic management of müllerian fusion defects, *Fertil Steril* 45:726, 1986.
5. Donderwinkel PFJ, Dörr JRJ, Willemsen WNP: The unicornuate uterus: clinical implications, *Eur J Obstet Gynecol* 47:135, 1992.
6. Farber M, Marchant DJ: Reconstructive surgery for congenital atresia of the uterine cervix, *Fertil Steril* 27:1277, 1976.
7. Frank RT: The formation of an artificial vagina without operation, *Am J Obstet Gynecol* 35:1054, 1955.
8. Haney AF et al: Diethylstilbestrol-induced upper genital tract abnormalities, *Fertil Steril* 31:142, 1979.
9. Hassiakos DK, Zourlas PA: Transcervical division of uterine septa, *Obstet Gynecol Surv* 45:165, 1990.
10. Ingram JM: The bicycle seat stool in the treatment of vaginal agenesis and stenosis: a preliminary report, *Am J Obstet Gynecol* 140:867, 1989.
11. Jones HW Jr, Mermut S: Familial occurrence of congenital absence of the vagina, *Am J Obstet Gynecol* 114:1100, 1972.
12. Kaufman RH et al: Upper genital tract changes associated with exposure in utero to diethylstilbestrol, *Am J Obstet Gynecol* 128:51, 1977.
13. Khalifa E, Toner JP, Jones HW Jr: The role of abdominal metroplasty in the era of operative hysteroscopy, *Surg Gynecol Obstet* 176:208, 1993.
14. Mandell J, Stevens PS, Lucey DT: Diagnosis and management of hydromucocolpos in infancy, *J Urol* 120:262, 1978.
15. McKusick V et al: Hydromucocolpos as a simple inherited malformation, *JAMA* 189:813, 1964.
16. Muasher SJ et al: Wedge metroplasty for the septate uterus: an update, *Fertil Steril* 42:515, 1984.
17. Park IJ et al: A new syndrome in two unrelated females: Klippel-Feil deformity, conductive deafness and absent vagina, *Birth Defects* 8:311, 1971.
18. Rock JA, Jones HW Jr: The clinical management of the double uterus, *Fertil Steril* 28:798, 1977.
19. Shokeir MHK: Aplasia of the müllerian system: evidence for probable sex limited autosomal dominant inheritance, *Birth Defects* 14:219, 1978.
20. Strubbe, EH et al: Evaluation of radiographic abnormalities of the hand in patients with Mayer-Rokitansky-Kuster-Hauser syndrome, *Genetics* 43:167, 1988.
21. Toaff R: A major genital malformation: communicating uteri, *Obstet Gynecol* 43:221, 1974.
22. Tompkins P: Comments on bicornuate uterus and twinning, *Surg Clin North Am* 42:1049, 1962.
23. Zarou GS, Esposito JM, Zarou DM: Pregnancy following the surgical correction of congenital atresia of the cervix, *Int J Gynecol Obstet* 11:143, 1973.

Chapter 62

ASSAYS FOR THE ENDOCRINOLOGIST

Barry D. Albertson, PhD

When Bayliss and Starling proposed the concept of hormones and suggested, at the turn of this century, that they were the instruments of endocrine function, the stage was set for the development of new ways to measure accurately and follow these molecules over time. But the generation of useful endocrine methodologies lagged far behind the demand. Before 1960 it was relatively uncommon for the concentrations of hormones in biologic fluids to be measured. A few steroids could be reckoned with reasonable accuracy, but large volumes of plasma or urine were required and investigators were obliged to withstand exacting procedures and invest large amounts of time to get results. Measurement of other types of hormones was at best a nightmare and at worst a pipedream.[127]

In 1959 and 1960 scientists at two well-known research centers, one at the Veterans Administration Hospital in Bronx, New York, and the other at the Middlesex Hospital Medical School in London, broke through the barriers and published what are now considered the classic papers describing the radioimmunoassay.[51,214] Yalow and Berson[214] had been engaged for several years in investigating the immunologic characteristics and metabolism of insulin in both diabetic and nondiabetic patients. In this effort they characterized a specific insulin antibody and used it as a key reagent in their insulin assay. Oddly enough, the initial attempt to publish their results was met with rejection at the hands of the *Journal of Clinical Investigation*.[213] Ekins,[51] on the other hand, pursued more general microanalytic techniques that were amenable to a wide group of biologic compounds, and in this endeavor relied on a naturally occurring protein, thyroxine-binding globulin, as the specific reagent in his thyroid hormone assay. Interestingly, both of these investigative efforts were hampered by the lack of appropriate radioactive markers possessing adequate specific activity. So it is no surprise that the birthplace of these immunoassays was at "specialized radioisotope centers."[52]

The radioimmunoassay (RIA) defined endocrinology as it is today. It changed forever the way endocrinology was taught and applied, and alone elevated it to a new height among the other medical and research disciplines. But for this single technique to capture the attention of scientists worldwide, other events needed to have fallen into place. One of these was the development of a novel protein radioiodination technique, using the oxidant chloramine-T and relatively small amounts of ^{131}I. This one refinement by Greenwood et al.[71] in 1963 enabled virtually any reputable laboratory to radiolabel polypeptide hormones with high specific activity. ^{14}C-Radiolabeling of steroids came earlier, 20 years or so, but readily available ^{3}H- and ^{14}C-labeled steroid hormones possessing high specific activities for RIA use were developed coincidentally with that of the peptide hormones.[126]

Fractions of cell membranes[103] and cell receptors[20,95] were also used as "reagents" in these new assays with the hope of imparting a greater degree of specificity. Instead of these, it was unique antibody production that played a second crucial role in the development of RIAs. Reagent-class antibodies opened the door to the generation of assays for a vast number of peptide, polypeptide, and glycoprotein hormones. Nonprotein hormones (and a few other compounds or haptens) fell short in terms of their "intrinsic antigenicity," for example, the steroids, thyroid hormones, cyclic nucleotides, and prostaglandins.[52] Antibodies for these delinquent hormones soon were available as a result of some sophisticated chemical manipulations that disguised these hormones so that highly specific and sensitive antibodies could be obtained.

Finally, but certainly not the least important development, was the isolation and purification of protein, peptide, steroid, and other hormones from tissue, blood, and plant sources so that radioligands, antibodies, and assay standards could be generated. The women and men who gave hour upon hour of laboratory tedium for this end have never been given adequate credit.

Thus, with all the pieces available to put the puzzle together, curiosity and necessity stoked the fire that led to what today is a triumph of scientific ingenuity. Thousands of endocrine and non–endocrine researchers daily use these techniques and reagents, described later, the enterprise being fueled by a billion-dollar endocrine diagnostic, research, and development industry that produces state-of-the-art reagents and newer and better assays and assay reagents. The overview presented here is a compilation of the published work and words of many pioneering investigators in the field.

COLORIMETRIC ASSAYS

During the years that sophisticated bioassays and RIAs were being developed, clinical chemists and biochemists, using advances in chemical manipulation, provided the expertise and technology to measure a wide variety of compounds in blood and biologic fluids that were important to both clinicians and researchers. An excellent review of many of these assays was published by Gold[67] in 1975.

Although these assays began as laborious manual methods, they have remained in the armamentaria of hospital laboratories, evolving to what are now automated (autoanalyzer) analysis systems. Current analysis systems measure a wide variety of compounds in very short amounts of time. They include random-access and "stat" sample interventional access. They are relatively expensive, often in the $100,000 range, and take up a significant amount of laboratory floor space. Unfortunately, they represent the ultimate in "black box" technology; that is, the operator loads the samples and appropriate reagents or assay modules, presses the *Start* button, and walks away.

These tests or assays, although usually considered to be

in the purview of clinical chemistry, measure many of the molecules that hormones affect, such as glucose, urea nitrogen, uric acid, calcium, phosphorus, and many others. Two colorimetric assays frequently needed by endocrinologists involved in clinical nutrition research and patient care that remain in the purview of the bench chemist are total serum cholesterol and triglycerides. The principles of these assays, as with all colorimetric assays, are based on the chemical structure and metabolism of the molecules in question and on the addition of specific reagents, including enzymes, to generate quantitative color changes (usually measured spectrophotometrically) that are specific for that particular compound (Fig. 62-1).

A variety of other molecules, such as glycosylated hemoglobin, can also be measured by using colorimetric end points that provide accurate results with very small coefficients of variation, often less than 2%. However, plasma or serum levels of these molecules required for spectrophotometric analyses must be in the microgram or milligram per deciliter ranges. Thus most hormones presented chemists and biochemists with sensitivity obstacles that required much more elaborate technology.

BIOASSAYS

Bioassays were most certainly some of the first endocrine assays. They usually involved the injection of hormone preparations into live animals, ultimately measuring specific endocrine responses. Both in vitro and in vivo bioassays have been developed over the years, often involving complex biologic phenomena such as enzyme activities, gene products, growth factor production, synthesis of complex macromolecules, and the production or inhibition of other hormones. For example, bioassays for growth hormone have been based on body weight changes, the incorporation of amino acids into proteins, or the addition of smaller chemical groups to larger macromolecules.[3] On the other hand, bioassays for luteinizing hormone (LH) and/or follicle-stimulating hormone (FSH) usually require the production of only a single hormone from a tissue or isolated cell population.[47]

In vitro bioassays

In vitro bioassays have been classified as either proximal or distal[68] depending on whether the response is an intermediary one, such as the stimulation of adenylate cyclase, cyclic adenosine monophosphate (cAMP), or other second messenger; or an end response, such as the product of a steroid or protein hormone via trophic stimulation[1] (Fig. 62-2). Proximal types of bioassays provide investigators with an application that offers a wide variety of endocrine tissues from which to choose. Distal response assays, on the other hand, must be individualized for each hormone.[68] Other classifications include bioassays that elicit mitogenic or cytochemical responses. These encompass some of the most sensitive bioassays currently available and often re-

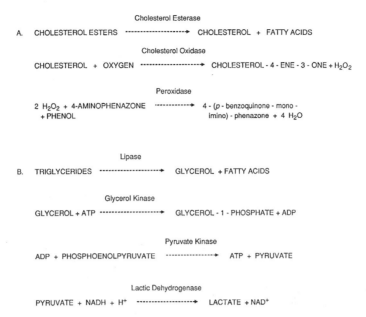

Fig. 62-1. Colorimetric assay methodology for measuring serum cholesterol and triglycerides. **A,** Total serum cholesterol is quantitated by the use of cholesterol esterase, which effectively hydrolyzes cholesterol esters. Then, in the presence of oxygen, all of the free cholesterol in the sample is oxidized by cholesterol oxidase to cholest-4-en-3-one and stoichiometric amounts of hydrogen peroxide (H_2O_2). The H_2O_2 subsequently reacts with phenol and 4-aminophenazone in the presence of peroxidase to form 4-(p-benzoquinone-monoimino)-phenazone, which is pink in color. The intensity of the color formed is proportional to the total cholesterol concentration of the original sample and is measured photometrically at 500 to 600 nm. **B,** Similarly, serum triglycerides can be completely hydrolyzed to free glycerol and free fatty acids by using microbial lipase. The stoichiometrically formed glycerol is subjected to glycerol kinase in the presence of adenosine triphosphate (ATP), forming glycerol-1-phosphate and adenosine diphosphate (ADP). This generated ADP plus phosphoenolpyruvate in the presence of pyruvate kinase produces ATP and pyruvate, which in the presence of the reduced form of nicotinamide-adenine dinucleotide (NADH), H^+, and lactate dehydrogenase (LDH) produce lactate and the oxidized form of NAD (NAD^+). The disappearance of NADH in this final reaction, monitored at between 340 and 380 nm, is a stoichiometric measure of the glycerol formed from the original triglyceride in the sample. (**A** redrawn from Scheme for colorimetric assay for total cholesterol, with permission from Diagnostic Laboratory Systems, Boehringer Mannheim Corporation, Indianapolis, 1988; **B** redrawn from Scheme for colorimetric assay for triglycerides in blood, with permission from Abbott Laboratories, Diagnostics Division, Abbott Park, Chicago; 1984.)

quire that investigators have access to permanent endocrine-responsive cell lines.

In vivo bioassays

In vivo bioassays have been essential for the quantitative standardization of many hormones.[68] These include the murine hypoglycemia test for insulin, the rat tibial growth response for growth hormone, the pigeon crop-sac assay for prolactin, the rat ovarian weight response for gonadotropins, the rat uterine weight response for estrogens, the release of labeled thyroid iodide for thyroid-stimulating hormone (TSH), and the adrenal depletion of ascorbic acid for adrenocorticotropic hormone (ACTH),[169] to mention only a few.

Unfortunately, these in vivo assays may be fraught with insensitivity and nonspecificity, and yield values with broad confidence limits. But, despite these flaws, in vivo bioassays are indispensable for the detection of hormones or regulatory factors unseen by other bioassays or immunoassays. Testimony to this fact has been the description by Manasco et al.[111] of a novel, blood-borne, testis-stimulating factor from boys with gonadotropin-independent precocious puberty, that is, familial male precocious puberty (FMPP), which is undetectable with the most sensitive

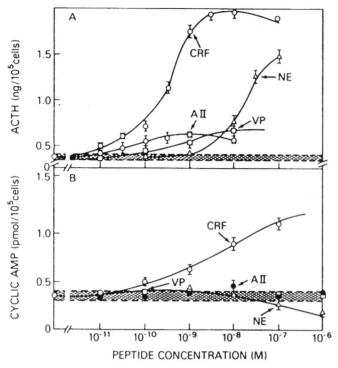

Fig. 62-2. Distal and proximal and bioassays. **A,** Distal hormone response: stimulation of adrenocorticotropic hormone (*ACTH*) release. **B,** Proximal hormone response: cyclic AMP release. Production and release of both cAMP and ACTH are shown in response to stimulation of various doses of corticotropin-releasing factor (*CRF*), vasopressin (*VP*), angiotensin II (*AII*), and norepinephrine (*NE*). Points are the mean of data from duplicate rat pituitary cell incubations. The shaded horizontal bar represents basal response of the ACTH and cAMP of the rat pituitary cell culture system. (From Aguillera G et al: *J Biol Chem* 258:8039, 1983.)

rodent Leydig cell bioassays but can be picked up by using a live intact male monkey bioassay (Fig. 62-3).

The major complication of the bioassay is validation. For example, most endocrine tissue and cells respond to stimulating and inhibitory substances, both of which can be contaminants of the biologic fluids to be tested. Moreover, assay requirements can be quite stringent, requiring enzyme inhibitors, antioxidants, rigorous buffering, and consistency in cell types, tissues, or animal strains. But, despite these drawbacks, bioassays furnish a unique form of hormone quantitation and provide information not available with other assays.[3]

RADIORECEPTOR ASSAYS

Radioreceptor assays are the first cousin of the RIA, measuring the interaction of a ligand hormone not with the use of an antibody, but with specific receptor sites for that hormone on cells or cell membrane preparations that manifest the action of the hormone[34] (Fig. 62-4). Thus the radioreceptor assay shares a kindship with the bioassay; that is, both are functional hormone assays. The first radiorece-

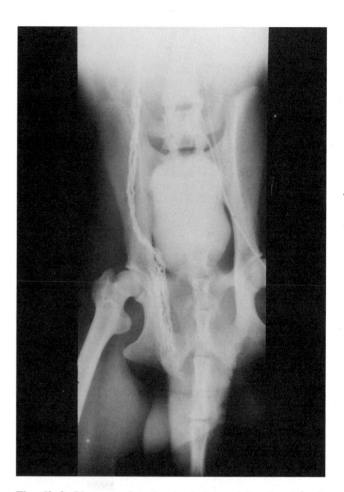

A

Fig. 62-3. Bioassay of testis-stimulating activity. A unique in vivo bioassay using live, intact, male cynomolgus monkeys to detect gonadotropin-like testis-stimulating activity in the blood of boys with familial male precocious puberty (FMPP). Anesthesized monkeys are catheterized via the jugular vein to gain access to the spermatic vein (**A;** note venous plexus) and the femoral artery to gain access the spermatic artery (**B**). Plasma samples from boys with FMPP that have no bioactivity in classic gonadotropin bioassays (rat Leydig cell, etc.) stimulate monkey testis testosterone production after acute injection into the spermatic artery. Vessels are shown by prior injection of radiopaque contrast dye.

ptor assays were developed for ACTH by Lefkowitz and associates.[102,103] The new technology rapidly spread to most other polypeptide and steroid hormones.[28,34,46,189]

The circumstances under which radioreceptor assays distinguish themselves have been described by Gordon and Weintraub[68] (1) as a supplement to RIA data providing (with bioassays) additional indexes of biologic activity, for example, in determining steroid hormone analogue potency for the glucocorticoid receptor; (2) in measuring hormonally active substances for which other assays have not yet been established; and (3) in providing insight into endocrine disorders that involve hormone receptor abnormalities or autoantibodies to hormone receptors.

Hormone target tissues are usually chosen as the source of the receptor preparation, with enzyme-dispersed cells or cell

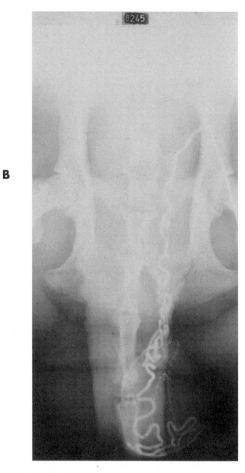

B

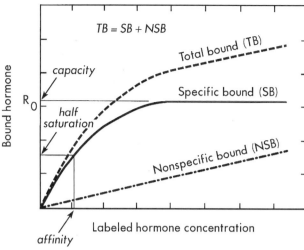

$$TB = SB + NSB$$

Fig. 62-4. Saturation curve of a typical radioreceptor assay showing total binding (*TB*) and nonspecific binding (*NSB*) at different concentrations of labeled hormone (TB − NSB = specific binding [*SB*]). Extrapolation of the asymptotic saturation line to the y axis indicates the total number of receptor sites (R_0) per cell or milligram of receptor protein. The concentration of hormone at half-saturation of receptor sites gives a measure of affinity. (Redrawn with permission from Chrousos GP: Radioreceptor assay of steroids and assay of receptors. In *Hormone assay techniques,* 15th training course syllabus, p 214. © The Endocrine Society, Bethesda, Md, 1989.)

Fig. 62-3, cont'd. For legend see opposite page.

membrane preparations often being employed. The radiolabels ³H and ¹⁴C have been frequently used in these assays; however, the higher specific activity of ¹²⁵I makes this the isotope of choice for labeling both steroid and polypeptide hormones.

Like bioassays, specific conditions must be met when using radioreceptor assays. For example, enzyme inhibitors such as aprotinin (kallikrein/Trasylol) may be needed to inhibit intrinsic protease activities; however, these preparations can actually damage peptide hormone tracers, inhibit binding of the tracer to the receptor, or potentially invalidate the assay in unknown or nonspecific ways. Low incubation temperatures have been used in some receptor assays to minimize assay component degradation, and special buffering systems are often required, since radioreceptor reactions are often pH- and ionic strength-dependent. Radioreceptor assays can be very precise, accurate, and specific, but, like all other assays, they must be rigorously validated before the data are accepted as sound.

Taken together, bioassays and radioreceptor assays provide information to the investigator that other assays do not, that is, an approximation of the true biologic activity of the hormone in question. Moreover, bioassays—along with

radioreceptor assays—measure not only the first step in the biologic cascade but intermediate and final steps, giving an excellent representation of the full biologic effect of these hormones from receptor binding to cell response. Because no other assays have this power, bioassays and radioreceptor assays will continue to be used as essential tools in the investigator's arsenal. However, they come at a high cost in terms of time, money, and assay complexity.[3]

RADIOIMMUNOASSAYS

The principles of RIAs and techniques involved in their development have not changed for 25 years. Detailed treatises of all aspects of the RIA can be found in a variety of publications, textbooks, and assay manuals.*

Because of their specificity, sensitivity, and ease of performance, RIAs have been the benchmark of most, if not all, hormone assays and continue to be the gold standard of hormone measurement for basic and clinical endocrine diagnosis and research. However, when performed in a casual or cavalier manner, results from the RIA can be not only inaccurate but misleading. Oddly enough, the basic tenets of RIAs have not changed from their inception, as evidenced by the fact that many renowned research laboratories continue to use the RIA techniques they established and validated 20 or more years ago. What has changed is the production of better reagents,

*References 4, 8, 13, 33, 53, 67, 80, 84, 102, 129, 195, 212.

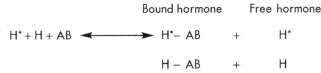

Bound hormone   Free hormone

$$H^* + H + AB \longleftrightarrow H^* - AB + H^*$$

$$H - AB + H$$

Fig. 62-5. Generalized scheme of an RIA. Radiolabeled hormone (H^*) and antibody (AB) are combined such that the percentage binding is between 25% and 35%, usually established during assay setup experiments. The addition of unlabeled hormone (H) in the form of standards or in an unknown sample perturbs (decreases) the H^*-AB binding equilibrium dynamics, depending on the unlabeled hormone concentration. The final step, separation of bound hormone from free hormone, gives ultimate hormone quantitation (measured as radioactivity in bound [pellet] or free fraction [supernatant] after centrifugation or another physical separation procedure). In practice all the components (H, H*, and AB) are added together until equilibrium is established. However, the late addition of tracer (H^*) can improve assay sensitivity. (Redrawn from Albertson BD: Hormone assay methodology: present and future prospects. In Adashi EY, editor: Reproductive endocrinology update, *Clin Obstet Gynecol* 33:591, 1990.)

that is, antibodies with greater specificity (both polyclonal and monoclonal); tracers with higher specific activities, giving greater precision and sensitivity (e.g., multilabeled ^{3}H and ^{125}I isotopic incorporation into steroids, as well as proteins); and the availability of RIA kits, produced by both large and small manufacturers, that include virtually everything an investigator needs to get results.

The basic principle of the RIA is the competitive inhibition of the binding of a labeled hormone to a "specific" antibody by the same unlabeled hormone that is contained in prepared standards or unknown samples[3] (Fig. 62-5). A typical RIA is performed by the simultaneous addition of standards or unknown samples into assay tubes. To these tubes is added a fixed amount of radiolabeled antigen, and then antibody. After an appropriate reaction or incubation time, antibody-bound and unbound labeled antigen are separated by a variety of physical or chemical techniques, a final step that can well determine the ultimate success or failure of the assay.[212]

RIAs have been modified by the incorporation of solid phase–linked reagents and novel radiolabeling procedures that have improved the stability and ease of performing these assays. For example, immunoradiometric assays (IRMAs) have become proverbial. These differ from classic RIAs in that the antibody, usually an immunoglobulin G (IgG), is labeled instead of the hormone. The advantage of this perturbation is that iodinated immunoglobulins can be more stable than iodinated hormones. But IRMAs can produce standard curves that have an upper-level "hook effect"[195]; that is, when high concentrations of the hormone are present in the reaction mixture, a hook in the standard curve and in the unknown samples reverses the slope of the data curve caused by a decrease in bound counts with

labeled antibody at the higher hormone concentrations. Thus biologic samples suspected of being elevated should be measured at more than one dilution to be certain that the hormone concentrations are within the linear portion of the standard dose-response range of the assay.[53,195]

The major drawbacks of RIA and IRMA technology are linked to (1) limitations of the radioactive tracer component, including short and fragile reagent life; (2) the cost of equipment for measuring gamma or beta particles; (3) radiation exposure to users; (4) radioisotope licensing; and (5) serious long-range, environmental problems derived from isotope disposal.

On the other hand, RIAs and IRMAs have provided researchers and clinicians with the tools to measure a host of hormones to concentrations of picograms or even femtograms per milliliter of plasma, serum, or culture media. Thus it is no surprise that these assays are some of the most popular and enjoy widespread use.

Sensitive RIAs have been successfully developed and commercialized for the accurate measuring of low circulating levels of hormones, requiring relatively small volumes of biologic fluids. These assays incorporate (1) purified radiolabeled hormones with high specific activities, so that only trace amounts of hormone need be added; (2) labeled hormones or antibodies that do not affect the specificity or immunoreactivity of the reagents; (3) antibodies (polyclonal and monoclonal) with high affinities and specificities to measure low levels of the desired hormone; and (4) appropriate reference preparations against which the concentration of unknown sample may be dose-interpolated. Features of the key components of RIAs are elaborated in the following sections.

Antibodies

The power of the RIA (or other immunoassays) is married to the quality and specificity of the antibodies used. The more specific the antibody, the better able one is to measure accurately the hormone of interest. Antibodies most commonly used for RIAs have been selected from the immunoglobulin class called gamma globulin, or IgG[72] (Fig. 62-6). IgGs are made up of two heavy polypeptide chains (approximately 450 to 700 amino acids) and two light polypeptide chains (approximately 214 amino acids) symmetrically arranged and covalently linked to each other by disulfide bridges. Because these IgGs possess antibody reaction sites along with antigen determination sites, the IgGs themselves serve as antigens when injected into an animal of another species, an important characteristic used in the production of second antibodies for RIAs.

Although the concentration or titer of a desired antibody is important, the principal determinants of a great antibody are its affinity and specificity for the desired hormone. The antibody-antigen interaction is derived by the combination of events involved in the intricate "locking" of the antigen in a complementary way to the combining site of the

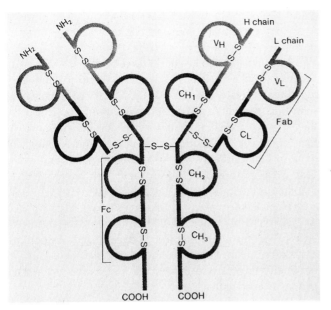

Fig. 62-6. Immunoglobulin model. Immunoglobulin molecules (IgG) are composed of two heavy chain (*H*) and two light chain (*L*) polypeptides. Each IgG has two antigen-binding sites (*Fab*) and a complement-fixing site (*Fc*). Variable regions of the heavy and light chains are shown by solid and gray loops. Folded loops of the protein chains and the chains themselves are joined by disulfide bonds (*S-S*). (From Guttmann RD, editor: *Immunology: a Scope publication*, Kalamazoo, Mich, 1981, The Upjohn Company.)

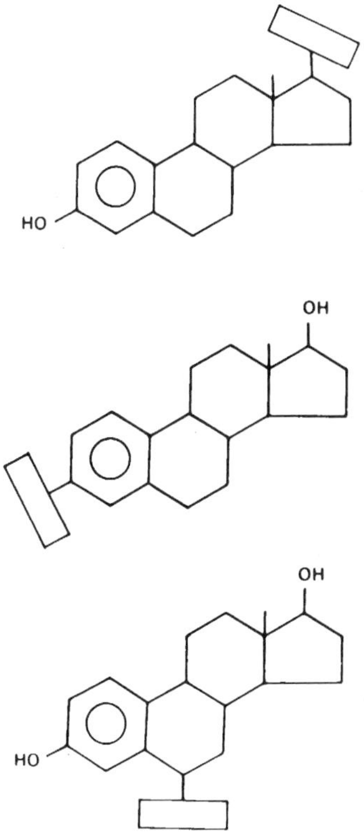

antibody through electrostatic, hydrogen-bonding, and Van der Waals interactions.[42,53,146,195]

The synthesis of specific antihormone IgGs is accomplished by injecting highly purified hormone preparations into laboratory animals. Protein or polypeptide immunogens are usually injected into guinea pigs, rabbits, sheep, goats, chickens, or other animals that are sufficiently foreign to the parent animal species' hormone molecules. If the immunogen has a molecular weight of less than 1000 d, it probably will not intrinsically stimulate antibody production (often termed a hapten). This necessitates linking or chemically conjugating it to a carrier molecule to establish immunogenicity in the animal of choice. A number of carrier molecules, usually ones with intrinsic immunogenicity, have been successfully used for this task and include bovine serum albumin, thyroglobulin, and hemocyanin. Steroids, thyroid hormones, and vitamin D and its precursors must be conjugated to immunogenic carrier molecules for adequate antibody production. For example, steroids differ from each other by small changes in their structure, usually in hydroxyl and/or ketone radicals. An intimate understanding of the chemistry of these reactive sites enabled coupling reactions to be devised.[106] The best known are the mixed-anhydride reaction and the carbodiimide reaction. And, as mentioned earlier, the choice of the exact molecular site of conjugation is essential, that is, through the reactive moiety of the molecule that is least

Fig. 62-7. Molecular sites of conjugation to estradiol. Conjugation on carbon atom 17 (*top panel*) generating antisera capable of detecting all of the major estrogens; on carbon atom 3 (*middle panel*) for estradiol and perhaps estriol; and carbon atom 6 (*lower panel*) that might produce very specific estradiol antibodies.

likely to alter its characteristic stereospecificity[53,195] (Fig. 62-7).

The most widely used method of inducing antibody formation has been to inject the antigen or antigen-conjugate in Freund's adjuvant,[53,63,64] a mixture of mineral oil (included to delay resorption), waxes, and killed bacilli (to sensitize the animal). The technique involves injecting the meringuelike adjuvant-hormone emulsion intradermally or subcutaneously on the back along the paraaortic lymphatic chain (Fig. 62-8). Initially large amounts of antigen were thought to be essential for good antibody production, but the studies by Vaitukaitis et al.[196] demonstrated that very small doses of antigens can be used. Moreover, low doses of immunogen often produce antibodies with the highest affinity; conversely, higher doses of immunogens produce antibodies with lower affinities. High-dose immunization can also induce "tolerance" in the immunized animal, resulting in very low or no measurable antibody titer.[33,53,195]

Primary immunizations are usually begun with complete Freund's adjuvant (with mycobacteria added) or a similar adjuvant and usually takes about 8 weeks for significant levels of antibodies to be detected. Titers and affinities usually peak within 3 to 4 months.[48,53] Blood samples from the animals are obtained by cardiac puncture, by retroor-

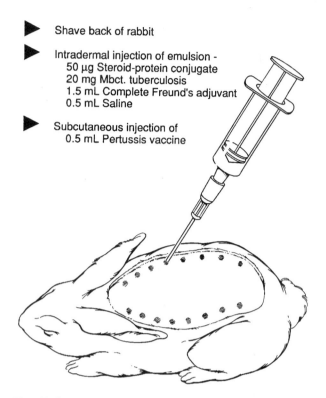

► Shave back of rabbit

► Intradermal injection of emulsion -
   50 µg Steroid-protein conjugate
   20 mg Mbct. tuberculosis
   1.5 mL Complete Freund's adjuvant
   0.5 mL Saline

► Subcutaneous injection of
   0.5 mL Pertussis vaccine

Fig. 62-8. Immunization of a rabbit for production of steroid antibodies for RIA. A similar approach could be used for protein and polypeptide hormones.

bital sinus puncture, or by "nicking" tail veins or the marginal ear veins of rabbits with a sterile scalpel blade. The serum is screened for antibody titer, specificity, and affinity by using an appropriate radiolabeled ligand.

Several alternative non–Freund's adjuvants have been used recently and are selected on the basis of type of cellular response desired. These include alum compounds (especially aluminum hydroxide [Alhydrogel]; water-in-oil emulsions employing microparticulate, stabilized emulsions containing nontoxic, metabolizable oils such as squalene [Hunter's TiterMax; Cytrx Corporation, Norcross, Ga]; oil-in-water–based adjuvants [RIBI adjuvant system; Immunochem Research, Inc, Hamilton Minn]; bentonite; trehalose dimycolate; vinyl acetate copolymers; muramyl dipeptide; liposomes; and pristane [2,6,10,11-tetramethyl-pentadecane]).

The antiserum produced in animals is actually a heterogeneous population of immunoglobulins with different affinities and specificities. Thus each individual animal that is immunized with antigen may produce totally different antibody populations with different titers, affinities, and specificities. This often means that a single rabbit, for example, may be the sole source of a "great antibody" and could elevate that particular animal to an invaluable status. The loss of such an animal could be devastating. This fact, among other particulars, has led to the replacement of polyclonal antibodies with monoclonal antibodies that rep-

resent a single immunoglobulin with a unique affinity and specificity for a single antigenic site of a hormone or other hapten[2,188] (Fig. 62-9).

Monoclonal antibodies have, in general, improved RIAs because (1) they can be produced in large quantity with high titers; (2) they are consistently similar or identical over long time periods of hybridoma clone production; and (3) they are (or can be) quite specific for the hormone of interest, almost to a fault. For example, in the development of a specific antibody for ACTH, monoclonal antibodies have been produced that are so specific for pituitary ACTH that they sometimes do not cross-react with other bioactive ACTH molecules, such as fragments of ACTH or "big" ACTH found in ectopic ACTH syndrome.[150] There are a host of companies currently producing and distributing antibodies in either kit or bulk form that provide users with the ability to pick and choose the best antibody for their particular application.[3]

Radiolabels

The most commonly used isotopes in RIAs are shown in Table 62-1 with some of their physical characteristics. Of these, ^{3}H and ^{125}I have been most routinely used.[166] Historically, tritium has been the tracer of choice for steroid and vitamin D RIAs because the specific activities available are reasonably high, the labeling procedures are carried out by reputable commercial companies that provide assurance of activity and purity, and the costs are sufficiently low to keep budgets intact. ^{14}C-Labeled steroids have been used in RIAs, but the long isotope half-life and thus the low specific activity of these nuclides made them unsatisfactory in terms of yielding good assay sensitivities. Six- and eight-labeled tritiated steroids are available and greatly improve assay sensitivities, often into the low-picogram or high-femtogram range. Recently steroids have been introduced into the market that are iodinated, providing even higher specific activities and higher sensitivities for assay applications.

The most commonly used tracers for polypeptide and thyroid hormones have been isotopes of iodine, beginning with the use of ^{131}I. However, this tracer's 8-day half-life and rather low specific activity quickly led to its substitution with ^{125}I, which has a 60-day half-life.[22,115,166,191] As with tritium, iodination of protein and thyroid hormones is carried out commercially by several reputable companies that ship reagents to laboratories on a frequent basis. However, some investigators continue to iodinate their own hormone preparations in an effort to minimize tracer costs or when only precious amounts of a highly purified hormone are available. Dedicated iodination areas (usually modified chemical fume hoods) are required for these preparations, along with gamma particle–monitoring devices and labeled antigen purification systems, including powdered cellulose absorbent, gel filtration, dialysis, ion-exchange chromatography, cross-linked dextrans (Sepha-

Fig. 62-9. Production of monoclonal antibodies. Preparation of hybrid cells or hybridomas, which secrete homogeneous monoclonal antibodies against a particular hormone or antigen (*X*). Animals (usually rats or mice) are injected with an antigen or antigen-conjugate. Once serum levels of "polyclonal antibodies" are detected, that animal's spleen is harvested surgically and the spleen cells are fused with a non–immunoglobulin-secreting mouse myeloma cell line. Selective growth medium contains an inhibitor (aminopterin) that blocks the normal biosynthetic pathways by which nucleotides are made. The cells must therefore use a bypass pathway to synthesize their nucleic acids, and this pathway is defective in the mutant cell line to which the normal B lymphocytes are fused. Because neither cell type used for the initial fusion can grow on its own, only the cell hybrids survive. Clones are selected from the hybridoma on the basis of antigen specificity and affinity and can be grown ad infinitum for assay application. Although monoclonal antibodies have been widely used and applied to polypeptide and protein hormone assays, their unique specificity can make them problematic for the measurement of altered forms of circulating hormones. (From Alberts B et al, editors: *The molecular biology of the cell*, ed 2, New York, 1989, Garland Publishing, Inc.)

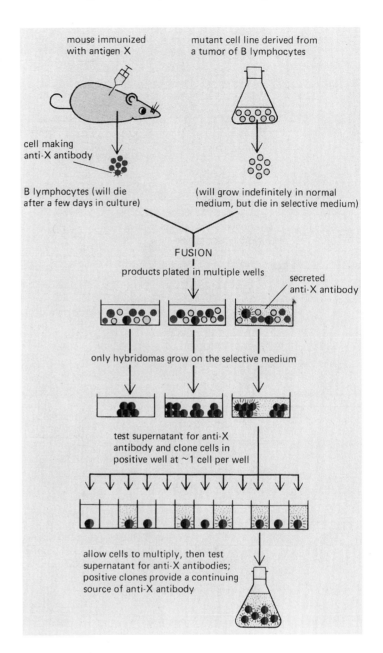

Table 62-1. Isotopes used in RIAs

Isotope	$T_{1/2}$	Decay particle	Detection efficiency	Specific activity
^{14}C	5568 y	β	80%	10-50 mCi/mmol
^{3}H	12.35 y	β	55%	50-200 Ci/mmol
^{75}Se	121 d	g + x	90%	100-300 Ci/mmol
^{125}I	60 d	g + x	90%	2000 Ci/mmol
^{131}I	8 d	g	45%	2000 Ci/mmol

dex), or anion-exchange resins. Purification of the newly labeled hormones by chromatographic methods may be required to reduce "nonspecific" assay binding. Prewashing Sephadex columns with albumin has been used to help saturate absorption sites, and the addition of 2-mercaptoethanol has been used to stabilize a variety of labeled protein hormones during purification and storage.[179,183] In cases when the original antigenic preparation is not pure or when significant antigenic degradation occurs during radiolabeling, additional purification (such as starch gel and polyacrylamide gel electrophoresis, or high-performance liquid chromatography [HPLC]) may be necessary.*

Routinely used iodination procedures include the following: (1) use of the potent oxidizing agent, chloramine-T (originally marketed as a disinfectant), by Greenwood et al.,[71] which converts ^{125}I-labeled NaI to free iodine (a simple mixing of the peptide, sodium iodide, and chloramine-T is required, with the reaction being terminated by the addition of the reducing agent, frequently sodium metabisulfite); (2) the lactoperoxidase method of Marchalonis,[112] in which this enzyme in the presence of a trace of H_2O_2 transfers ^{125}I-labeled NaI to free iodine with

*References 14, 62, 66, 118, 120, 136, 179, 183.

selective incorporation into tyrosyl or histidyl residues (the addition of glucose oxidase to this cocktail, which generates H_2O_2 from glucose in situ, minimizes the potential for protein or peptide damage. A reducing agent is not required to stop the reaction, since sample dilution is sufficient[122]); (3) the method of Bolton and Hunter,[17] or the conjugation labeling technique (Fig. 62-10), in which an intermediate derivative, 3-(*p*-hydroxyphenyl)propionic acid–*N*-hydroxysuccinimide ester, is iodinated by the chloramine-T reaction and then subsequently condensed with amino groups on the polypeptide hormone; (4) the iodogen method of Fraker and Speck,[61] in which a relatively insoluble soluble oxidizing agent (1,3,4,6-tetrachloro-3α,6α-diphenyl glycoluril) is evaporated onto the walls of a reaction vessel from a

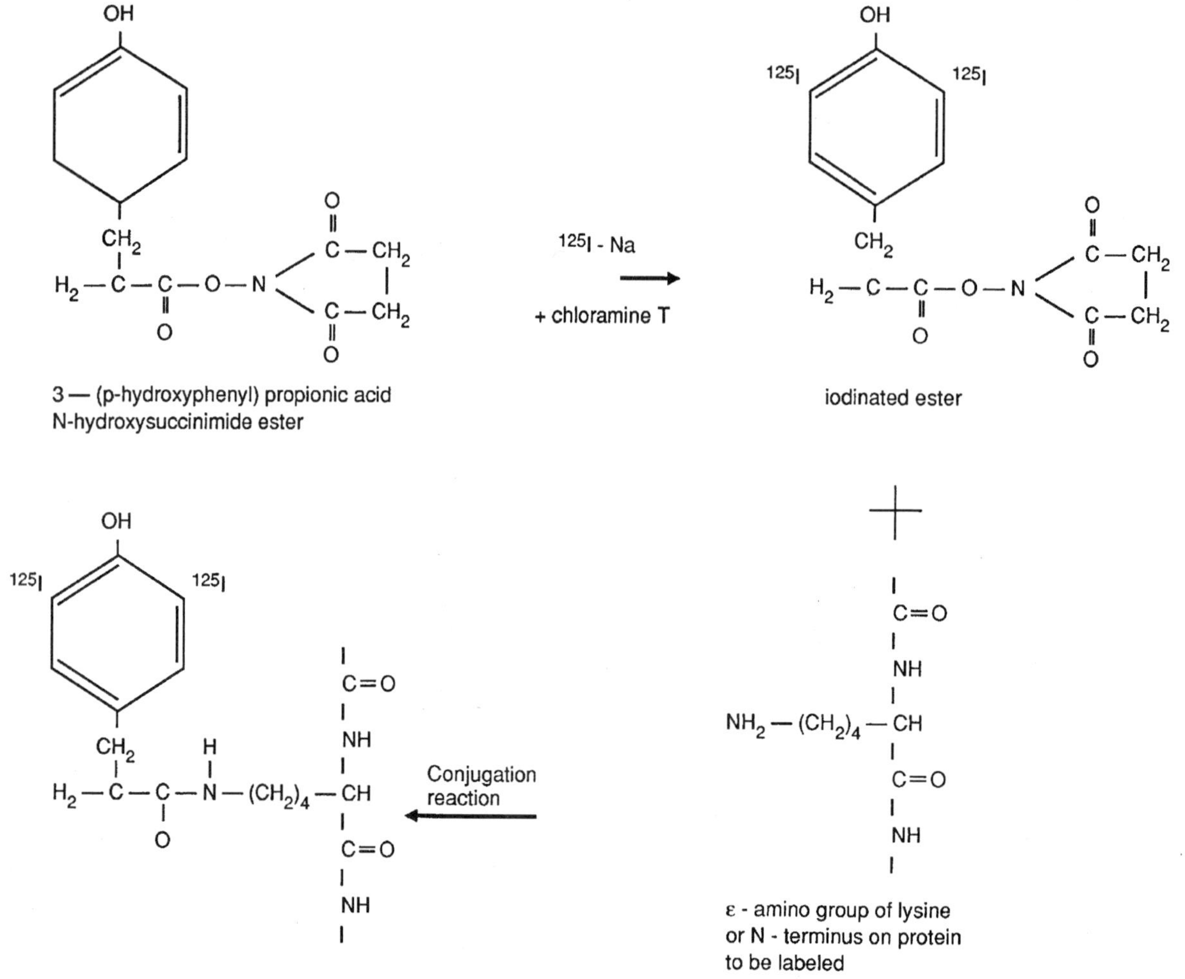

Fig. 62-10. Bolton-Hunter iodination scheme. Schematic representation of the iodination scheme of Bolton and Hunter,[17] using chloramine-T. (Redrawn from Chard T: *An introduction to radioimmunoassay and related techniques.* In Work TS, Work E, editors: *Laboratory techniques in biochemistry and molecular biology,* Amsterdam, 1982, Elsevier Science Publishers, Academic Publishing Division.)

solution in chloroform or methylene chloride, (the polypeptide and ^{125}I are added, and the reaction is terminated when the mixture is removed from the vessel, without requiring the addition of a reducing agent[33]); (5) chlorine/sodium hypochlorite oxidation[151]; (6) iodine monochloride[61]; (7) iodine vaporization[61]; and (8) electrolysis.[134,165] Each of these techniques has the potential of chemically damaging the hormone to be iodinated if vigorous reaction conditions are used. Thus gentle iodination procedures have been adopted; for example, hormone damage can be minimized when labeling with the lactoperoxidase method if the H_2O_2 is added in two or three small aliquots, since this is such a harsh oxidizing reagent.

Small polypeptide molecules that do not contain histidyl or tyrosyl residues may be modified by substituting a tyrosyl group within the polypeptide or at the nonfunctional end of the molecule. Similar approaches have been used with steroids, but in this case iodination is located at a site distant from unique hydroxyl or ketone groups. This position must be carefully chosen so as not to affect the molecule's native conformation. These new tyrosyl analogues can be iodinated by several of the eight techniques just described.

The final specific activity of the newly labeled antigen can be estimated by determining the disintegrations per minute (dpm) of radioactivity found in the molecules at various stages during radiolabeling. By comparing the dpm of the isotopes before labeling with the total dpm of the various labeled fractions (e.g., labeled antigen and free isotope), one can determine the percentage recovery. By knowing this recovery, and the amount of antigen and label initially present, one can estimate the specific activity of the newly formed tracer.[183] One may also wish to check for immunoreactive changes of the labeled antigen, using a quick RIA screen, by assaying the radiolabeled antigen alone and then diluted with unlabeled antigen. A decrease in the immunoreactivity of the tagged hormone would indicate that the molecule had suffered some insult during the labeling procedure.[183]

Separation of bound from free fractions

Once the primary hormone-antibody reaction reaches equilibrium it is necessary to determine the distribution of the hormone between the free and bound forms. This usually requires that the bound fraction be physically separated from the free fraction so that the radioactivity of either the bound or free phase can be measured accurately.[206] Essential in this is the premise that the separation techniques used do not disturb the initial equilibrium attained between hormone and antibody (or receptor). All of the techniques devised to perform this final all-important step of the RIA exploit the physical-chemical differences between the hormone in its free and bound forms. A perfect separation system would completely divide the two components of the assay. In practice, this is never achieved because (1) the free hormone almost always can behave as if it is bound, that is, constituting what is commonly referred to as "nonspecific binding," and (2) there is invariably incomplete separation of the bound-hormone complex.[33] Classic immunologic methods for separation of bound from free hormone fractions have been based on spontaneous precipitation of antigen-antibody complexes, since molar concentrations of these complexes permitted simplistic approaches.[212] RIAs, because of their much higher assay sensitivities, utilize very low molar concentrations of reagents and thus demand specific assay steps that will effect the separation of antibody-bound and free antigens.[211] In considering the best approach to the separation of bound from free antigens several factors should be weighed: the speed of the procedure, simplicity, applicability, effectiveness, and cost.

The earliest methods used for separation of bound and free fractions in RIAs were electrophoretic, including paper chromatoelectrophoresis, starch gel electrophoresis, cellulose acetate electrophoresis, and polyacrylamide gel electrophoresis. The extremely cumbersome nature of these approaches led to techniques that involved nonspecific fractional precipitation of the hormone-antibody complex itself, using salts or organic solvents. Reagents used included ethanol, acetone, dioxane, sodium sulfite, ammonium sulfate[33] (Fig. 62-11), trichloroacetic acid (TCA), and polyethylene glycol (PEG).[183] Although these procedures were immediate and needed no second incubation step, fractional precipitation techniques may have a tendency to bring down other proteins or assay components, causing an incomplete separation of the two fractions.

Solid-phase bonding of either the hormone or antibody components of the RIA was attempted in the early days of RIAs. The solid-phase antibody technique made use of antibodies covalently bonded or fixed to insoluble polymers covalently cross-linked to one another or physically ad-

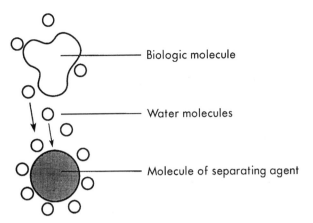

Fig. 62-11. Fractional precipitation of bound and free fractions with ammonium sulfate. The ammonium sulfate molecule takes up water molecules, depriving the protein of its protective hydration shell. (Redrawn from Chard T: An introduction to radioimmunoassay and related techniques. In Work TS, Work E, editors: *Laboratory techniques in biochemistry and molecular biology,* Amsterdam, 1982, Elsevier Science Publishers, Academic Publishing Division.)

sorbed to plastic. These immunosorbents included bentonite particles,[24] bromoacetyl cellulose,[24] Sephadex,[207] Sepharose,[125] Enzacryl AA,[125] and polyacrylamide gels. Although this approach has the advantage that all the components of the assay (antibody, hormone tracer, and the means of separating bound from free fractions simply by decanting or low-speed centrifugation) are within one unit, it necessitated the user to have available large or nearly unlimited amounts of antisera. The use of a solid-phase separation technique such as antibody attachment to polystyrene macrobeads or microbeads or captured in a mesh of polyacrylamide gel has provided the simplest and most user-foolproof approaches to separation of bound and free fractions. But these concoctions are wasteful of antibody and very difficult to produce, especially in relation to batch-to-batch consistency. If unlimited amounts of antibody are available, these approaches can offer true simplicity of this final assay step to the point of being almost instantaneous and automatic.

Physical adsorption of antibodies to polypropylene or polystyrene discs, plastic tubes, or microbeads has been developed, particularly for protein hormones, and has yielded reproducible and highly sensitive assays in which the adsorbed antibodies have a very long shelf life. Separation by solid-phase antigen precipitation has also been successful, being simple, economical, quick, and reproducible.

Adsorption of free antigens has been and probably remains the gold standard for steroid and steroid metabolite RIAs. Free hormone is bound to specific adsorbents, which are then precipitated by centrifugation. Powdered talc and Florisil (magnesium silicates), kaolin, fuller's earth, Lloyd's reagent (aluminum silicates), and cellulose were

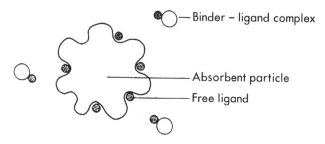

Fig. 62-12. Adsorption separation using powdered charcoal. Free hormone enters "crevices" on the charcoal particle and is firmly adsorbed. Antibody-bound hormone cannot enter the crevices and thus remains in the liquid phase. (From Chard T: An introduction to radioimmunoassay and related techniques. In Work TS, Work E, editors: *Laboratory techniques in biochemistry and molecular biology,* Amsterdam, 1982, Elsevier Science Publishers, Academic Publishing Division.)

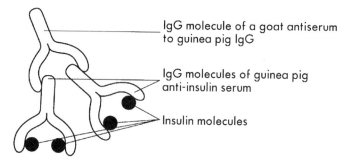

Fig. 62-13. Second antibody separation of bound and free fractions in an insulin RIA. Primary IgG antibodies are raised in guinea pigs against human insulin. Each primary antibody binds two insulin molecules. A secondary antibody produced in a goat is an anti–guinea pig IgG, and binds two primary antibodies. (Redrawn from Chard T: An introduction to radioimmunoassy and related techniques. In Work TS, Work E, editors: *Laboratory techniques in biochemistry and molecular biology,* Amsterdam, 1982, Elsevier Science Publishers, Academic Publishing Division.)

some of the earliest of these adsorbents, many of which were originally used by chemists as decolorizing agents. But one, dextran-coated charcoal, has remained as one of the most used for RIAs[33] (Fig. 62-12). Used primarily in steroid, vitamin D, and small-peptide RIAs, charcoal combines all of the best features of the earlier methods, but more importantly has endured the test of time in its use by many established research and clinical laboratories. There are, however, some requirements for charcoal separation steps to perform well: (1) The preparation of the charcoal (usually Norit A, Norit SG, or Norit G-60) must be rigorous, with multiple washings in distilled water or assay buffer to segregate the fine particles from the usable heavier granules. Dextran T-70 or dextran T-80 is often used to produce dextran-coated charcoal, although this procedure has been found to be unnecessary for good charcoal separation. (2) Conditions (e.g., incubation times and temperature) must be determined under which the separation is complete with minimal stripping of the hormone from its antibody. (3) Optimal centrifugation conditions must be established so that decanting the supernatant into counting vials from the assay tubes does not result in contamination with the pelleted charcoal.

Generally polypeptide hormone assays use the addition of a second antibody for separating the bound from free fractions[33] (Fig. 62-13). Because the initial binding step in polypeptide hormone RIAs produces a soluble hormone-antibody complex, simple centrifugation may not be adequate for separating bound from free fractions. A second antibody, generated against the IgG of the animal species in which the first antibody was generated, is added after equilibrium has been reached in the first antibody-hormone reaction. This second antibody–primary antibody–hormone complex is an insoluble species, and the bound hormone can be separated by centrifugation. For protein or polypeptide hormones, the use of double antibodies (that is, a primary antibody generated against the hormone to be

measured and a secondary antibody generated against the primary antibody) is usually the method of choice. Second antibodies are routinely harvested in large domestic animals such as sheep or goats, since relatively large amounts of antibody (i.e., blood plasma or serum) are often required, especially when hundreds or thousands of samples are anticipated. Goat or sheep antirabbit or antirat IgGs are the most common type of second antibody used (although IgA and IgM fractions have found application) and give excellent separation of the original rabbit, rat, or other IgG species of primary antiserum–antigen complex from free hormone.

The ability to generate large amounts of monoclonal antibodies has further enhanced and simplified the bound from free separation step. These uniform populations of antibodies can be bound to the walls of plastic assay tubes, microtiter plates, or microbeads, making a simple decanting step the method of separating bound from free fractions.

Magnetic field separation of bound hormones has also been developed. In this application ferric oxide is conjugated to the first or primary antibody, and a magnetic field—usually in the form of a strong permanent magnet—is imbedded in the base or sides (and near the bottom) of an assay tube rack or holder. After the initial incubation of reagents of the RIA is completed and the reactants have reached equilibrium, the assay tubes are placed into the magnetic field and allowed to remain there for several minutes. The assay tubes can be singly or simultaneously decanted, blotted, and then counted, thus effectively separating the free from bound fractions en masse. Both steroid and polypeptide hormones can be assayed by using magnetic separation techniques, providing simplicity and quick turnaround time for laboratories performing large numbers of assays.[3]

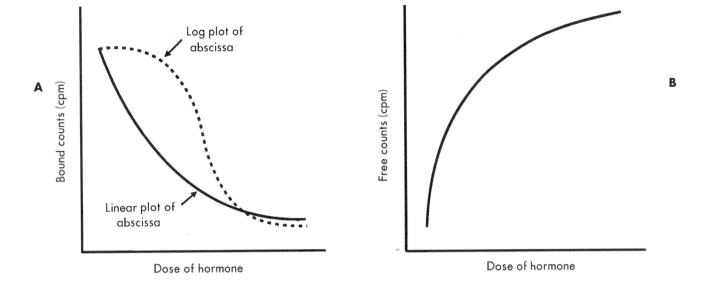

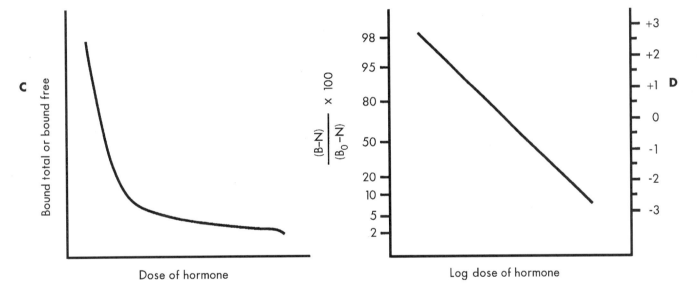

Fig. 62-14. RIA standard curve presentations. A variety of techniques have been used to graph data for RIAs. The simplest of these is shown in **A** and **B**, where either bound or free counts per minute (cpm) or radioactive disintegrations per minute (dpm) are plotted against the dose of nonlabeled hormone (standard curve). **C,** Standard hormone plotted against either the bound over free hormone or the bound over total hormone calculation. All of these plots enable the investigator to determine unknown-sample hormone samples based on the standard curve generated, but all of these generate curvilinear plots, making actual hormone levels difficult, especially when the slope of the plot is flat. Several approaches have been used to linearize these plots, making the determination of unknown samples at the extremes of the standard curve more valid. The most popular of these is the log-logit plot **(D).** This plot employs the number of counts bound to antibody normalized to the maximal number of bound counts (B_0), when only antibody and labeled hormone (i.e., no unlabeled hormone) are incubated together. Nonspecific counts, which reflect physically trapping hormone in the assay tube, are subtracted from both total and bound counts. The resulting log-logit plot is usually a straight line and simplifies visual dose interpolation of unknown samples. (Redrawn from Chard T: An introduction to radioimmunoassay and related techniques. In Work TS, Work E, editors: *Laboratory techniques in biochemistry and molecular biology,* Amsterdam, 1982, Elsevier Science Publishers, Academic Publishing Division.)

1127

The variety of hormones and their unique chemical properties has led to the diversity of techniques for this crucial step in the RIA. Thus it is not surprising that individual laboratories use their own special techniques for this separation step.

Data display and antibody/receptor binding characteristics

There are a variety of methods for handling the data derived from RIAs.[53,60,155-162,164,195] Standard curves are routinely generated and can be displayed graphically as either hyperbolic functions or straight lines, depending on the mathematical manipulation of the data. The simplest of these are depicted in Fig. 62-14.[33,195]

Mathematical derivations of these curves have been summarized by Vaitukaitis[195] and are described below. The basic dose-response or standard curve is constructed by placing the bound over free activity (B/F) or any other partition index between bound and free on the ordinate and the unlabeled antigen or ligand concentration on the abscissa. A log scale of the abscissa yields a sigmoid curve. One of the most-used curve fitting response variables is the logit transformation:

$$\text{Logit } B/B_0 = \text{Log e } (B/B_0)/(1 - B/B_0)$$

where B = antibody-bound radioactivity of each sample and B_0 = antibody-bound radioactivity at the zero dose. On the abscissa is plotted the log scale of the unlabeled hormone and on the ordinate the logit (log base e) of B/B_0 (Fig. 62-14, **D**).[195]

Hormone-receptor or antibody-binding interactions have also been mathematically analyzed by a variety of approaches.[195] In general, when hormone [H] interacts with a specific receptor or antibody [R], a reversible reaction at equilibrium can be defined as

$$[H] + [R] \overset{k_a}{\underset{k_d}{\leftrightarrow}} HR$$

where HR is the hormone-antibody (receptor) complex.

The affinity of the hormone for its antibody or receptor can also be expressed using a rearrangement of the above reaction:

$$Ka = k_a/k_d = [HR]/[H] [R] = 1/Kd$$

where

Ka = Equilibrium association constant in liters per mole
ka = Association constant rate
kd = Dissociation rate
Kd = Equilibrium dissociation constant in liters per mole

When the number of occupied receptors or antibody sites is related to the total number of antibodies or receptors, the following relationship is:

$$[R_0] = [HR] + [R]$$

$$\text{or} \quad [R] = [R_0] - [HR]$$

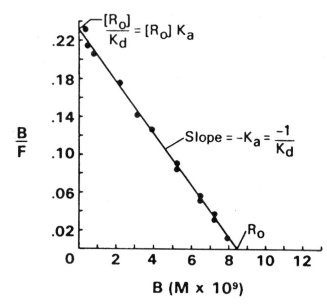

Fig. 62-15. Scatchard analysis of hormone binding data. Bound counts divided by free counts are plotted against the dose of the bound counts. The X intercept of the line drawn through the data points indicates the total binding capacity of cells, antibodies, or membrane or intracellular receptors (*R0*). The Y intercept of the plot indicates the binding equilibrium association constant ([*R0*]*K_a*). The slope of the line gives the binding affinity (−*K_a*). (From Vaitukaitis JL: Hormone assays. In Felig P et al, editors: *Endocrinology and metabolism,* New York, © 1987, McGraw-Hill, Inc. Reproduced with permission by McGraw-Hill, Inc.)

where

R_0 = Total number of antibodies/receptors
HR = Bound receptors or antibodies
R = Free receptors or antibodies

By rearranging the above equations, one can generate a final equation that, when plotted, results in a straight-line relationship of the hormone bound to its receptor or antibody, that is:

$$HR/H = -1/Kd [HR] + [R_0]/[Kd]$$
$$\text{or} \quad = -Ka [HR] = [Ka] [R_0]$$

This represents the Scatchard plot, regarded as the most frequently used transformation of receptor or antibody-hormone binding data[53,170,171] (Fig. 62-15).

From hormone receptor or antibody binding data, one can generate several important binding parameters including the following: R_0, or the total binding sites per cell or protein preparation, i.e., the binding capacity, found from the lines intercept of the abscissa or x axis; the Ka, or equilibrium association constant, for the hormone and its receptor or antibody obtained from the lines intercept of the ordinate or y axis and from the slope of the generated line; and the Kd, or equilibrium dissociation constant, also obtained from the slope of the line.

Scatchard plots are theoretically linear, but when actual binding data are graphed, many are not (Fig. 62-16).[8,33] Nonlinearity can be the result of allosterism between the

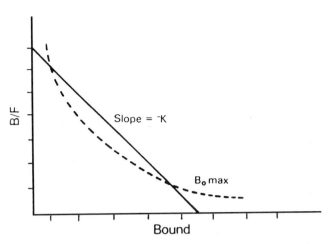

Fig. 62-16. Theoretic and actual Scatchard analysis of data. The straight line shows the theoretic straight-line relationship; the broken line indicates the often observed actual Scatchard data. (Reprinted with permission from Ashkar FS: *Radiobioassays,* vol 1, Copyright CRC Press, 1983, Boca Raton, Fla.)

receptor after initial hormone binding (positive cooperativity) or the converse (negative cooperativity), multiple binding sites per cell or antibody moiety, artifacts of nonequilibrium conditions, inaccurate estimates of assay measurements (e.g., nonspecific binding), and bound and free measurements and different affinities of labeled and nonlabeled hormone.[8,34,40,119,155]

Assay quality control and validation

Optimal utilization and interpretation of RIA data require knowledge of the precision and reproducibility of the methodology. Early RIA data often measured and quantitated very large changes in hormone levels in response to various stimuli, and assay validation and quality control were often ignored. It was no surprise that some laboratories produced results from a single blood sample that showed a tenfold difference from each other.[30] Thus the incorporation of proper and adequate quality control became habitual. Several quality control techniques can be used, involving values derived from assay results, pool sample results, standard curve results, and commercially supplied "plasma or serum" standards. The most commonly utilized quality control parameters for RIAs (and that can be applied to all assays) are (1) specific activity of the tracer (hormone or antibody); (2) amount of tracer; (3) total counts per minute; (4) nonspecific background counts; (5) slope of the standard curve; (6) intercept of the standard curve; (7) the percentage of bound counts in the absence of unlabelled hormone, that is, bound over total counts $(B/T)_0$; (8) within-assay variance; and (9) between-assay variance.[163] The first three parameters relate to the labeling procedure and to the amount of tracer present, both of which are known to influence assay sensitivity. $(B/T)_0$ is affected by the binding capacity or titer of the antibody, the binding affinity of the antisera, the immunoreactivity of the tracer (an index of "damage"), and the assay

incubation conditions.[30] The slope of the standard curve line can be calculated by linear regression analysis or determined graphically. Intercept gives a measure of assay sensitivity. Confidence limits for potency estimates of unknowns are derived from within-assay variance calculations. These parameters and the mathematics involved in determining them are discussed in much more detail elsewhere.[30,155-157,162]

Because RIAs are dependent on the precise interaction of chemicals in accordance with the laws of mass action, the principles of RIA appear quite simple. But a host of nonspecific factors and cross-reacting molecules constantly threatens to interfere with these reactions, jeopardizing the validity of the results.[206] This necessitates that the user validate each assay. Several criteria must be met to assume assay validity.

Specificity. The assay should be specific, that is, measure only the hormone of interest. Assay specificity can be defined as the degree of freedom from interfering substances. Specificity of the antibody for the antigen is influenced by heterogeneity or the absence of purely specific antibodies, cross-reaction with other antigens or metabolic fragments that retain immunoreactive sites, and possible influences of the antigen-antibody reaction owing to the presence of low-molecular-weight substances that may alter the environment of the reaction.[52] Cross-reactivity measurements are an index of assay specificity, that is, evaluation of the uniqueness of the antibody for a specific antigen. Antibody cross-reactivity can occur between antigenic determinants on similar hormones or between multiple hormones and their precursors, fragments, or metabolites, and between different types of steroid molecules. Cross-reactivity may also exist to varying degrees between the same hormones in two different animal species. Cross-reactivity problems with antibodies are minimized by using chromatographic separation procedures to "purify" the sample containing the antigen or hormone.

Sensitivity. The assay should be sensitive enough to measure levels of a hormone under conditions when concentrations are known to be low, but meaningful. Sensitivity can be defined as the the smallest amount of unlabeled antigen that can be distinguished from "no" antigen. This also can be defined by the slope of the dose-response curve with the formula:

$$S = \frac{B/F \times \text{slope } B/F}{1.1}$$

or sensitivity (S) equals the mean difference between duplicate estimates (B/F) divided by 1.1 times the slope of the dose-response curve at B/F.

Accuracy. The assay should be accurate. Accuracy is the ability of an assay to measure exactly in a quantitative way the amount of hormone in a biologic fluid or tissue, when that amount is known. However, until the precise chemical structure and properties of the antigen are known, one can only approximate this "true" value by evaluating a "relative" accuracy. Accuracy is routinely determined by the ability of the assay to measure correctly the amount of hormone "spiked" into a blank sample.

Precision. The assay must be precise. Precision is defined as the ability to have an assay perform consistently in reference to hormone antibody-binding characteristics, separation of bound from free fractions, etc., over long periods of time, assay after assay. As stated by Midgley and associates,[119] "Assay precision is the extent to which a given set of measurements of the same sample agrees with the mean of that set, i.e., the amount of variation in the estimation of unlabelled antigen."

Reproducibility. The assay should be reproducible. The main factor influencing reproducibility, that is, the duplication of the values within or between assays, is the difference in individual techniques in carrying out the same operation.

Proper validation of the assay also requires that the apparent hormone content of an unknown sample be independent of the dilution at which it is assayed, establishing in a sense that all the components of the assay are performing optimally and as expected. Simply stated, the concentration of the unknown must decrease linearly with dilution or, alternatively, a dilution curve of the unknown must be superimposable on a dilution curve of the standard over a wide (100-fold or more) concentration range. Lack of exact superimposability can be due to experimental errors. Superimposability does not prove immunochemical identity of the unknown and standards, but strongly suggests that this is so. A lack of superimposability can be caused by a variety of specific and nonspecific factors and implies that the assay lacks quantitative validity, although it still may be useful clinically.[212]

The actual performance of the RIA and the nuances of each step, from preparing assay reagents to data reduction, are too numerous to elucidate in a single volume. In fact, the subtle distinctions of RIA procedures are usually omitted in written texts and syllabuses. True understanding and expertise come from months or years of training and frequently only in discussions with those who helped father and establish each essential step. These must be mastered at some point if the user expects valid quantitation of extremely small amounts of hormones, regardless of whether assays are set up from scratch in the laboratory or generated from a commercially prepared kit.[41]

NON–RADIOMETRIC ASSAYS

Many informative books and journal review articles on non–radiometric assays have been published over the course of the last decade covering a wide range of methodologies for enzyme immunoassays, electrochemical sensors, bioluminescence assays, fluoroimmunoassays, and chemiluminescent assays.* Of these assays, the enzyme immunoassay (EIA) or enzyme-linked immunosorbent as-

say (ELISA) best typifies the evolution of endocrine assays from a radiometric to a non–radiometric approach.

Evolution of EIA and ELISA

Several factors led to the change from isotopic to non–isotopic assay methodologies in routine work: (1) the critical separation of bound from free step in RIAs was and continues to be an obstacle to RIA automation; (2) the cost of reagents, including radioisotopes and equipment; and (3) the fact that RIAs require radioactive tracers. Researchers and clinical chemists realized the need to protect laboratory personnel and come to grips with the problems of generating large volumes of radioactive waste. The result has been a search for alternative approaches to hormone assay technology.

The principle of the enzyme immunoassay depends on the ability to assay the concentration of a hormone or other analyte by measuring the activity of an associated "enzyme" that is conjugated to either a primary or a secondary antibody.[13] The detection systems required for ELISAs and EIAs range from visual to photometric, quantifying colored, fluorescent, or luminescent products. Reviews of these assays have been published by Voller et al.,[198] Albertson and Haseltine,[4] and others.[†]

The ELISA, first described by Engvall and Perlman[54] in 1971, has been subject to many modifications and refinements. In the ELISA, the basic tenets of immunoassays are conserved, those being the interaction between an antibody and a corresponding antigen. The novelty is that an enzyme that can be easily quantitated acts as the tracer. This enzyme is covalently linked to either the hormone or one of the antibodies in the reaction. After an appropriate incubation period with either standard hormone or sample and a step separating the bound from free fraction (which under certain circumstances may not be necessary), the enzyme activity is measured through the addition of a specific enzyme substrate or chromogen that turns color in the presence of the enzyme in a dose-response relationship, that is, the more enzyme, the darker the color. Assay quantitation can often be made with the naked eye; however, spectrophotometric analysis provides more precise readings and significantly quickens result turnaround time. There are several obvious advantages in the use of enzyme labels. Particular enzymes can be purchased with no licensing regulations, they are available in very pure form, they are quite inexpensive, and they have long shelf lives. There are a variety of enzymes that can be used, providing sensitive assays because of the amplification effect of these enzymes. Some ELISAs and EIAs have been automated, and enzymes (as well as the chromogens used) are nontoxic and safe, posing no disposal problems.

Because the antibody moiety carries the label in the EIA or ELISA, polypeptide or proteins were the first hormones

---

*References 3, 9, 15, 23, 31, 35, 36, 44, 54, 69, 70, 77, 80, 82, 88, 96, 100, 109, 110, 123, 130, 132, 135, 137, 138, 140, 141, 145, 149, 172, 173, 175, 177, 184, 192, 198-202, 208, 209.

†References 15, 123, 137, 175, 199, 208.

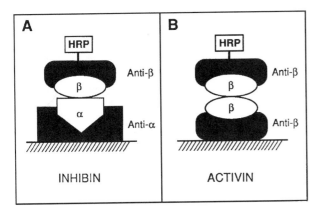

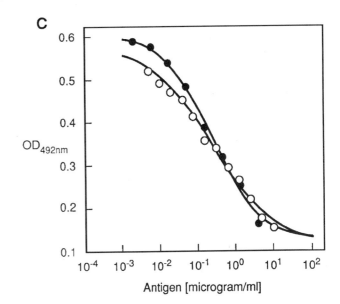

Fig. 62-17. Application of ELISA technology for the measurement of inhibin and activin. For this and other EIAs, 96-well or ELISA plates are frequently used with one of the two antibodies coated to the wells. Because inhibin is a heterodimer, a second antibody, generated against a separate unique binding site, can be conjugated to an enzyme (in this case, horseradish peroxidase, *HRP*) and added as a unique reagent. The amount of enzyme/second antibody bound in this system is directly proportional to the amount of hormone in the sample. After the ELISA plate is washed, the enzyme activity is quantitated with the addition of *o*-phenlyenediamine, the reaction is stopped with sulfuric acid, and the absorbance is measured at 492 nm in an ELISA plate reader. **A** and **B,** Orientation of the assay and its components to measure inhibin or activin by changing the solid-phase–linked anti-alpha (*Anti-α*) or antibody against a beta chain (*Anti-β*). **C,** Competition ELISA of porcine follicular inhibin (•) or pure porcine inhibin (○) when the multiwell ELISA plate was coated with pure porcine inhibin. (Redrawn with permission of John Wiley & Sons, Inc, from Schwall R et al: Approaches to non–radiometric assays for inhibin and activin. In Albertson BD, Haseltine F, editors: *Non–radiometric assays: technology and application in polypeptide and steroid hormone detection,* New York, Copyright © 1988, John Wiley & Sons, Inc.)

routinely measured by these techniques. This was based on the fact that sandwich or double-antibody assays could be developed that utilized antibodies directed toward different antigenic epitopes of the hormone. New assays based on different antigenic sites of subunits of a hormone have also exploited enzyme assay technology. For example, Schwall and his colleagues[176] have devised an EIA scheme that detects two related gonadal peptides, inhibin and activin (Fig. 62-17).

In the basic EIA or ELISA procedure the hormone is sandwiched between two specific and different antibodies: the primary or capture antibody is usually linked to a solid-phase matrix, sometimes a polystyrene tube, microfilm plate well, or sphere; a separate secondary antibody is conjugated to the enzyme tracer. This approach is most frequently applied to molecules that have an appropriate topographic distribution of antigenic determinants and are large enough to bind to two different antibodies without affecting either the binding reaction or affinity. By using 96-well microtiter plates, 8-well microtiter plate strips, and a plate or ELISA reader, one can get results in about 60

seconds (even shorter for the newer, state-of-the-art ELISA plate readers).

The ultimate challenge for enzyme assays was to be able to measure all of the polypeptide and steroid hormones and achieve the same or better assay sensitivity, specificity, accuracy, and precision as that achieved by RIAs. This was not an insurmountable task, and has been achieved in many circumstances.

If the particular protein hormone exists as a monomer and if highly purified preparations of the protein are available, a competitive type of EIA or ELISA can be used. For example, purified antigen is coated to the ELISA plate wells in an overnight incubation step. Limited amounts of the specific hormone antibody and either pure hormone standards or sample are added. Nonspecific binding can be minimized with the addition of blocking agents such as phosphate-buffered saline-Tween 80 (polysorbate 80). After an overnight incubation the plate is washed, and the antibody-antigen mixture is added to antigen-coated 96-well plates and incubated for 1 hour. During this final incubation any antibody that did not bind to the hormone is washed from the wells, and the bound component of the assay is quantitated. One drawback of microtiter plates is the limited surface area available through which to bind hydrophobic compounds. To solve this limitation a variety of macro- and microbeads have been used, including latex or polystyrene, polycarbonate, polyacrylamide, and copolymer beads.[135] The beads can be linked to antibodies and then incubated with the hormone; excess reagent is removed by washing.

The preparation of enzyme-protein conjugates is critical. The functional residues and stabilities of both the enzyme used and the molecule to be coupled will determine the precise chemical cross-linking approach used. Since enzymes themselves are proteins, conjugation methods are as

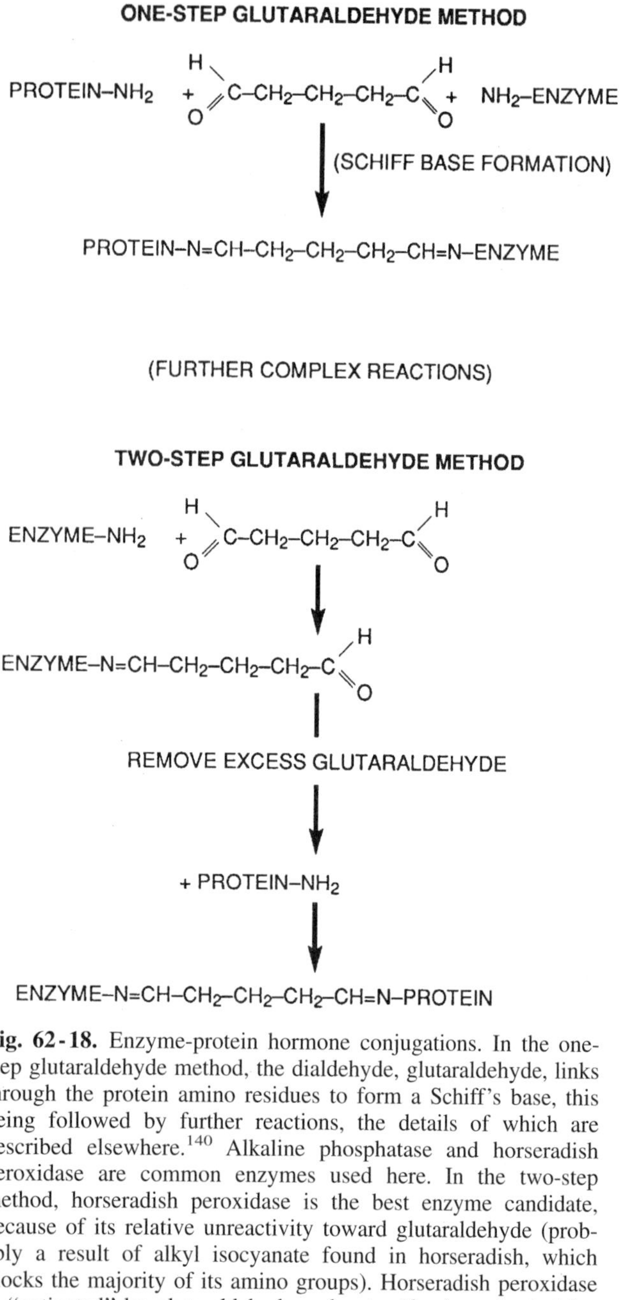

ONE-STEP GLUTARALDEHYDE METHOD

PROTEIN–NH$_2$ + O=C–CH$_2$–CH$_2$–CH$_2$–C=O + NH$_2$–ENZYME

(SCHIFF BASE FORMATION)

PROTEIN–N=CH–CH$_2$–CH$_2$–CH$_2$–CH=N–ENZYME

(FURTHER COMPLEX REACTIONS)

TWO-STEP GLUTARALDEHYDE METHOD

ENZYME–NH$_2$ + O=C–CH$_2$–CH$_2$–CH$_2$–C=O

ENZYME–N=CH–CH$_2$–CH$_2$–CH$_2$–C=O

REMOVE EXCESS GLUTARALDEHYDE

+ PROTEIN–NH$_2$

ENZYME–N=CH–CH$_2$–CH$_2$–CH$_2$–CH=N–PROTEIN

Fig. 62-18. Enzyme-protein hormone conjugations. In the one-step glutaraldehyde method, the dialdehyde, glutaraldehyde, links through the protein amino residues to form a Schiff's base, this being followed by further reactions, the details of which are described elsewhere.[140] Alkaline phosphatase and horseradish peroxidase are common enzymes used here. In the two-step method, horseradish peroxidase is the best enzyme candidate, because of its relative unreactivity toward glutaraldehyde (probably a result of alkyl isocyanate found in horseradish, which blocks the majority of its amino groups). Horseradish peroxidase is "activated" by glutaraldehyde and not self-polymerized. After removing excess glutaraldehyde, the active enzyme is allowed to react further with antigens or antibodies containing amino residues. (Redrawn with permission from O'Sullivan MJ, Bridges JW, Marks V: Enzyme immunoassay: a review, *Ann Clin Biochem* 16:221, 1979.)

likely to produce enzyme-to-enzyme complexes or protein-to-protein complexes as the desired enzyme-to-protein conjugate. Several approaches have been described by O'Sullivan et al.[140] and include the one-step glutaraldehyde method, two-step glutaraldehyde method (Fig. 62-18), periodate method, and the use of *N,N'-o*-phenylene-dimaleimide or *m*-maleimidobenzoyl-*N*-hydroxysuccinimide

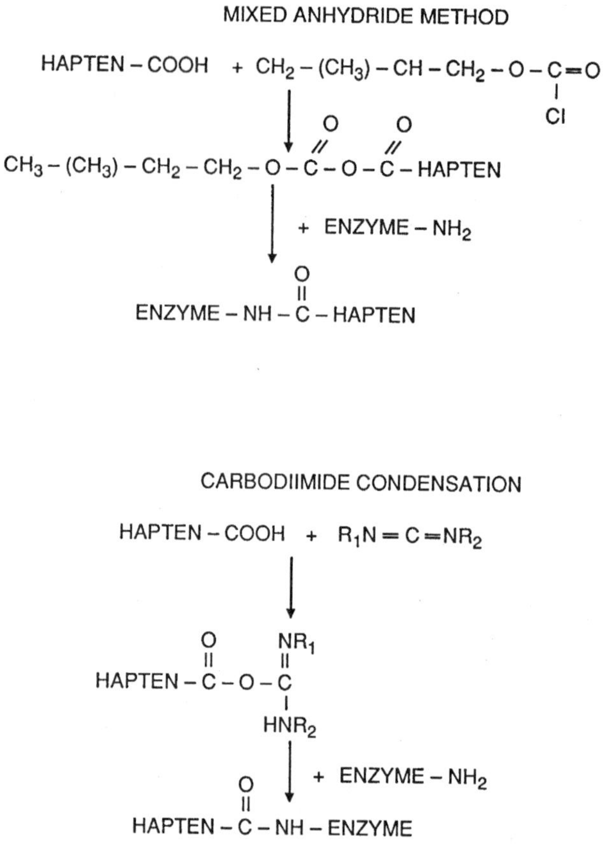

MIXED ANHYDRIDE METHOD

HAPTEN – COOH + CH$_2$ – (CH$_3$) – CH – CH$_2$ – O – C=O
                                                        Cl

CH$_3$ – (CH$_3$) – CH$_2$ – CH$_2$ – O – C – O – C – HAPTEN

+ ENZYME – NH$_2$

ENZYME – NH – C – HAPTEN

CARBODIIMIDE CONDENSATION

HAPTEN – COOH + R$_1$N = C = NR$_2$

HAPTEN – C – O – C
                  HNR$_2$

+ ENZYME – NH$_2$

HAPTEN – C – NH – ENZYME

Fig. 62-19. Enzyme-steroid conjugation methods. These reactions have been successfully used for steroids, for example, estradiol by using the mixed anhydride method and testosterone and cortisol with carbodiimide condensation. (Redrawn with permission from O'Sullivan MJ, Bridges JW, Marks V: Enzyme immunoassay: a review, *Ann Clin Biochem* 16:221, 1979).

(MBS).[140] Hapten-enzyme conjugate coupling reactions are often similar to those used for protein-enzyme cross-linking. Experts caution against linking enzyme molecules to hapten (e.g., steroid) antigenic sites and recommend the use of a different site and cross-linking methods when preparing the enzyme label from that used to prepare the immunogen. The more common methods use mixed anhydrides, carbodiimide, and bifunctional imidates such as MBS (Fig. 62-19).[140]

Basic ELISA formats

Enzyme or other non–radiometric assays can be subdivided into two groups: (1) heterogeneous assays, in which assay formats require a bound from free separation step and in which the enzyme activity is not influenced by the hormone-antibody reaction; and (2) homogeneous assays, in which the enzyme activity of the conjugate is influenced by the hormone-antibody reaction and in which a distinct step for separation of bound from free is not required.

Heterogeneous assays. The basic design of several simple heterogeneous enzyme assays are shown in Fig.

62-20.[138] The competitive enzyme assay (Fig. 62-20, **A**) is analogous to classic RIAs. Enzyme-labeled hormone and unlabeled (sample) hormones (*H*) compete for the binding sites of a limited number of solid-phase bound antigen-specific antibodies (*AB*). Antibody saturation occurs simultaneously, provided that all reactants are incubated together.[138] Sequential saturation may be preferred if the hormone to be measured is in very low concentrations in the fluid to be tested[215]; however, this often reduces the specificity of the assay.[131] The amount of enzyme-labeled antigen bound by the antibody is inversely proportional to the concentration of unlabeled antigen present in the sample.[199]

The reverse of the competitive EIA is the inhibition EIA in which the antigen-antibody interaction between a solid-phase–linked hormone (*H_L*) is inhibited by free sample hormone (*H_S*). This modification is called the immunoenzymatic assay (Fig. 62-20, **B**). Here, enzyme-labeled antibody is allowed to react with antigen, and excess solid-phase antigen is then added. Sample hormone (*H_S*) is added and binds to the enzyme-antibody complex. The remaining free enzyme-labeled antibody is subsequently separated by binding to a solid-phase–coupled antigen, also added in excess. The enzyme activity detected on the solid-phase matrix after separation of bound and free is inversely proportional to the amount of antigen in the sample.

Sandwich assays have also been developed (Fig. 62-20, **C**). Large protein or polypeptide hormones with several dissimilar epitopes or antibody-binding sites are particularly suitable for sandwich antigen assays. Obviously, for this approach, the two assay antibodies should not react with each other but only with their unique epitopes on the hormone. In addition to these formats there are several modifications, that is, assay designs that employ multiple ligand hormones and antibodies that ultimately give either a direct or indirect measure of the particular hormone in question.[54,131,215]

The overall quality of the ELISA depends on the specific characteristics of the enzyme label chosen. For example, in heterogeneous assays, the enzyme activity is usually measured on the washed, bound phase. Therefore, interfering serum or plasma sample factors are usually removed by the washing procedure, making the pretreatment of samples unnecessary. In general, highly purified enzyme preparations produce the most sensitive assays. The most commonly used enzymes meeting this criterion are alkaline phosphatase, horseradish peroxidase, β-D-galactosidase, glucose oxidase, carbonic anhydrase, acetylcholinesterase, catalase, and glucoamylase.[54,140] Although the actual detection of this assay end point, that is, measuring enzyme activity, is usually performed by photometry, chemical luminescence- and fluorescence-producing substrates and have also been used (see later sections).

Enzymes are coupled to the assay antibodies or antigens by a variety of chemical techniques, two of which have just

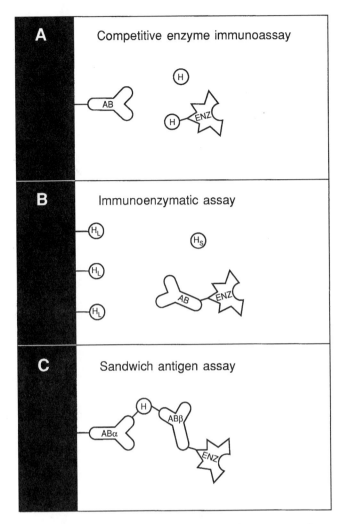

Fig. 62-20. Typical heterogeneous enzyme immunoassay formats. **A,** Competitive enzyme immunoassay. **B,** Immunoenzymatic assay. **C,** The sandwich antigen assay format. *H,* Hormone moiety (*H_S*, hormone in sample; *H_L*, solid-phase–linked hormone); *ENZ,* enzyme, which can be coupled to hormone or antibody (*AB*). The left side of each panel represents a solid-phase support material. (Redrawn with permission from Oellerich M: Enzyme immunoassay: a review, *J Clin Chem Clin Biochem* 22:895, 1984.)

been described. The goal is to incorporate as much enzyme as possible onto the hormone or antibody without compromising its activity or the properties of the coupled complex. The acid test of this step comes in generating a standard curve after the enzyme conjugation is completed.[140]

Systems used in heterogeneous assays to separate bound from free assay fractions usually incorporate a solid-phase matrix, such as polystyrene beads (bound to one of the antibodies), cellulose, and magnetic polyacrylamide agarose or chromium dioxide particles.[54,138] Precipitation can also be used, for example with second antibodies or polyethylene glycol (PEG).

Homogeneous assays. The principal design of the simplest homogeneous enzyme assays has been described by Oellerich[138] and others.[54] Because homogeneous assays do

A

B

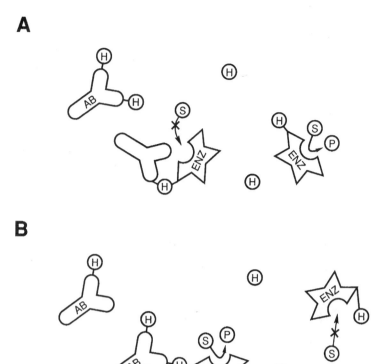

Fig. 62-21. Typical homogeneous enzyme immunoassay formats (EMITs). **A,** Enhanced enzyme multiplied immunoassay. **B,** Inhibited multiplied immunoassay. All the reactants are present in a single reaction medium. *H,* hormone; *ENZ,* enzyme linked to a hormone or an antibody (*AB*). Substrate (*S*) of the enzyme can be converted to product (*P*) if the enzyme is available for this conversion step. *S→P* indicates the completion of the conversion by the enzyme; *S—×→P* indicates inability of the enzyme to catalyze the conversion. (Redrawn with permission from Oellerich M: Enzyme immunoassay: a review, *J Clin Chem Clin Biochem* 22:895, 1984.)

not require a separation step, they are more susceptible to plasma or serum interferences, making the selection of enzyme labels critical. The rule is to choose an enzyme that is absent from and unaffected by such biologic sample factors. Those routinely used are lysozyme, malate dehydrogenase, glucose-6-phosphate dehydrogenase, and β-D-galactosidase. The most common homogeneous assay format is the enzyme-multiplied immunoassay technique, abbreviated *EMIT* (Fig. 62-21).[138] Two very basic approaches can be used, one in which the activity of the enzyme label is enhanced by antigen in the sample (Fig. 62-21, **A**) and one in which it is inhibited (Fig. 62-21, **B**), because the sample hormone (*H*) increases if the conjugate is bound to the antibody.[131,167] In EMIT assays, an enzyme-labeled antigen is required and the ability of the enzyme to catalyze a substrate to a product, which is the final factor to be quantitated, is compromised by the hormone-enzyme conjugation binding to the antibody. Conjugation of the enzyme to the hormone does not destroy the enzymatic

activity; however, binding of the hormone-specific antibody to the enzyme inhibits the enzyme activity. Free hormone in the sample relieves this inhibition by competing for antibody. Therefore, in the presence of antibody, enzyme activity is proportional to the concentration of free hormone.[140] The reverse of this mechanism is found in an EMIT for thyroxine that uses thyroxine-malate dehydrogenase. Here the thyroxine-malate dehydrogenase conjugate is enzymatically inactive basally, but is activated when bound by thyroxine antibodies.[21,140] There are many variations of these basic principles, eloquently described by Oellerich.[138]

A variety of enzyme labels have been used in homogeneous EIAs. EMIT assays invariably use a nicotinamide-adenine dinucleotide (NAD)–dependent glucose-6-phosphate dehydrogenase or other dehydrogenases. They are available in very pure form, are inexpensive, and have activities that can be easily quantitated photometrically. Reviews of EMIT assays have been published by O'Sullivan et al.,[140] Scharpe et al.,[173] and others.[21,54,133]

The final reagent in the EIA or ELISA format is the chromogen, that is, the enzyme substrate or substrate-associated molecule that actually effects the color change. In an assay where β-amylase might be used as the enzyme, starch could be the final indicator, producing a clear end product from a dark black to violet starting point. Other more commonly used chromogens are 2-nitrophenol (with β-D-galactosidase), 4-nitrophenol phosphate or phenolphthalein (with alkaline phosphatase), and o-phenylenediamine (with peroxidase).

EIAs have been used in virtually all previous RIA applications. Assays for the detection of plasma and serum proteins, tumor antigens, drugs, hormones and other haptens, antigens, and antibodies have been developed.[54,138,140,175] Likewise, EIA and ELISA accuracy is affected by the same factors that influence RIAs, plus potentially others. When directly comparing EIAs with RIAs, one finds that they are comparable in terms of both assay accuracy and precision. Coefficients of variation for interassay and intraassay variability are between 2% and 10% when mid–standard curve range values are evaluated.[54,137]

Assay performance, however, can be perturbed because of inherent interference of the enzyme or immunologic reactions in these assay formats. Endogenous enzymes in biologic fluids to be tested may interfere with "assay reagent" enzyme activities and other plasma or serum factors (e.g., proteins), probably far more so in these settings than with RIAs. Thus pretreatment of some serum or plasma samples may be necessary to avoid problematic assay interferences.

EIA and ELISA cross-reactivity (as with the RIA) is primarily dependent on the specificity of the antibodies used and, as in all assays, must be rigorously validated. The sensitivity of EIAs has also been shown to rival classic RIAs.[54,137,139] For endocrine assays, EIA and ELISA hormone values ranging from 0.2 to 50 fmol per tube is not uncommon. Some

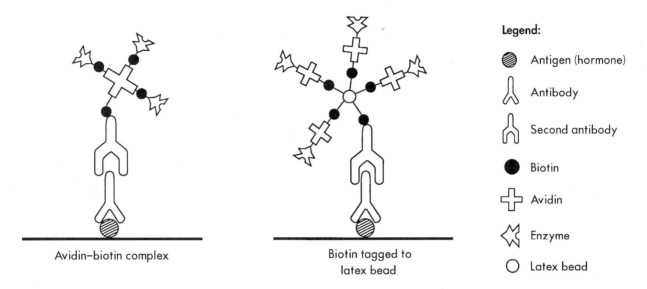

Fig. 62-22. Avidin-biotin enhancement. With the incorporation of avidin and biotin as reagent multipliers, signals can be increased by threefold or fourfold, depending on the specific application. (Redrawn with permission from Nilsson B: assays, *Curr Opin Immunol* 2:898, 1990, Copyright Current Science.)

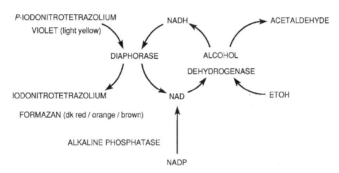

Fig. 62-23. Substrate amplification by enzyme cycling. By substituting NADP as a substrate for alkaline phosphatase in place of *p*-nitrophenyl phosphate and incorporating an enzymatic regenerating system, the color end point of the EIA can be magnified with the production of increased iodonitrotetrazolium formazan by cycling reduced nicotinamide-adenine dinucleotide (NADH/ NAD). (Redrawn with permission from Nilsson B: Enzyme linked immunosorbent assays, *Curr Opin Immunol* 2:898, 1990, Copyright Current Science.)

heterogeneous EIAs can detect analytes in the attomole (10^{-18} mol) per tube range, for example, ornithine-δ-amino-transferase or mouse myeloma IgG.[81,83,178]

In general, to increase the sensitivity of an assay further, the number of substrate conversions per unit of time must be increased by introducing a suitable multiplier in the assay "sandwich" structure.[135] Streptavidin (and the homologous protein avidin) are remarkable for their ability to bind up to four molecules of biotin with exceptionally high binding affinity. By incorporating a biotin label on a second antibody it is theoretically possible to increase the number of labels per sandwich by a factor of three. Further manipulation using more monoclonal antibodies can increase this to four[27,135] (Fig. 62-22).

One other approach to improve assay sensitivity is through substrate amplification by enzymatic cycling. For example, by replacing the alkaline phosphatase substrate *p*-nitrophenyl phosphate with NADP and adding an enzyme cycling system, a significant increase in signal intensity can be obtained[135] (Fig. 62-23). Even better sensitivities have been reported when fluorescent substrates are used to detect end points of enzyme activity.[27] (See Fluorescence Assays; Enzyme-Linked Fluorescence Assays.) It appears, however, that the sensitivity of heterogeneous enzyme assays for hormones is linked to the procedures used to separate bound from free fractions. Solid-phase systems using Sepharose-coupled antisera often lack good sensitivities. Although microcrystalline cellulose-coupled antibodies combined with second-antibody separation steps have sensitivities similar to or better than those with RIAs, generally ELISA or EIA sensitivities for protein hormones are better than analogous RIAs. Steroid EIAs possess sensitivities and reproducibilities related to the steroid conjugates used and antisera employed. Combinations in which the same steroid derivative is used for the preparation of immunogen as label (homologous systems) are more specific, but often less sensitive. But comparable specificities, sensitivities, and reproducibilities to RIAs are obtainable with enzyme assays when the optimal combination of antisera, conjugates, and enzyme labels is chosen.[140] Homogeneous assays can perform even better under optimal circumstances. Wide detection limits using EMIT assays for thyroxine and a number of drugs have been reported to be between 0.1 to 10,000 pmol/mL.

The real advantages of the enzyme-linked substrate immunoassay is the elimination of the issues of using radioactivity, including costs (both in direct and disposal costs), contamination concerns in the laboratory, and exposure of laboratory personnel. With state-of-the-art automation procedures, turnaround time for large-scale enzyme assays have improved dramatically, enabling 400 to 500 (or even more) patient samples to be assayed daily for any particular hormone (antigen/ligand/hapten). References to 1000 samples per day (for example, antibody detection for *Trichinella spiralis*) have been made in the literature.[168]

The future of EIAs and ELISAs is dependent on improvement of critical areas of the assay: production of better enzyme labels, employment of better cross-linking chemistry, development of a better understanding of interfering substances in biologic samples, implementation of monoclonal antibodies in the assay formats, improved chromogen reagents (e.g., chromogen-liposome complexes that give clear-cut and distinctive results), and improvement of the automated setup and detection systems. Currently there are complete EIA systems available that read, wash, dispose, incubate, and process samples and that perform sophisticated, customized data reduction.

FLUORESCENCE ASSAYS

Concurrent with the development of EIAs and ELISAs was the emergence of a variety of other non–radiometric assays applicable to the endocrinologist. Fluorimetric methods and fluorescent probes have gained increasing interest and use over the past several years, since they too can be incorporated into rapid and sensitive assays that offer inexpensive, stable, and safe reagents. Their attractiveness is associated with the fact that, like enzyme immunoassays, a single label can produce many detectable "events" per label molecule, depending on turnover (for enzymes), or in the case of fluorescence, one molecule can cycle many times through the excited and ground state during a short measurement period.[44,128]

Fluoroimmunoassays (FIAs) and immunofluorometric assays (IFMAs) are based on labeling of the immunoreac-

tants with fluorescent probes. The techniques of labeling proteins or antibodies with fluorescent probes is certainly not new. As early as 1941 Coons et al.[38] were describing the immunologic properties of antibodies containing fluorescent groups. The high sensitivity of the fluorescence measurement, combined with the ability of the fluorescent probe to change, depending on its environment, offered the possibility for developing heterogeneous assays in which the concentration of an analyte or hormone could be monitored directly in the reaction mixture,[77] not to mention homogeneous assay formats in which the concentration of an analyte can be measured directly in the reaction mixture without the step of separating bound from free fractions.

The problems with fluorescence immunoassay methods historically centered around their inferior assay sensitivities, usually a result of high background in the fluorimetric measurement. The recent development of solid-phase separation systems, new fluorescent probes, and automated instrumentation has improved the sensitivities of these assays, making them equal to or better than those found in RIAs or enzyme-linked immunoassays.

The basic principle of fluorescence is shown by the simplified Jablonski diagram in Fig. 62-24.[77] Luminescent molecules capable of absorbing energy can transfer that energy within its molecular structure, releasing it as a photon. The absorbed energy excites the electronic field of the molecule from its ground state singlet (S_0) to a higher electronic state (S_1, S_2, S_3, etc.). The excited state then releases or unloads this energy in various forms, and often as fluorescence. After energy unloading, the molecule returns directly back to the ground state (S_0) (Fig. 62-24, **A**). The small loss of energy in luminescence, that is, the difference between excitation and emission energies, or wavelengths, is determined as the Stokes shift. This shift is about 30 to 50 nm for fluorescent organic molecules, but longer for other fluorescent molecules such as the lanthanide chelates (Fig. 62-24, **B**). The ratio between absorbed energy and emitted energy is called the quantum yield. This parameter and others such as the fluorescence molecules absorption spectra, emission spectra, and fluorescence lifetime (that is, the decay rate of the excited state) are quite variable; they are dependent on a host of physical and chemical factors (e.g., temperature, polarity, pH, quenching, and so forth), and are key in the selection of an appropriate fluorescent marker.[77]

However, as in all assay formats, fluorescence analysis is not without unique problems. When organic fluorescent probes with narrow Stokes shifts are used, very high background fluorescence can be observed because of light scattering of the excitation beam, for both soluble molecules (Rayleigh and Raman scattering) and insoluble molecules (Tyndall scattering). The very nature of biologic fluids having high concentrations of protein make them difficult candidates for use in fluorimetric assays. These interfering fluorescence wavelength emissions are usually between 320 and 350 nm and can be as high as 430 to 470

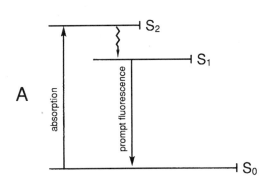
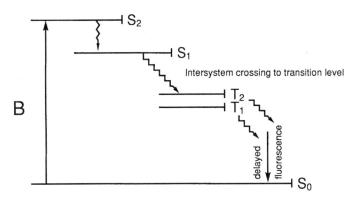

Fig. 62-24. Energy levels and transitions in a typical fluorescent organic molecule (**A**) and in a fluorescent rare-earth chelate (**B**). S_0, ground state; S_1, S_2, excited singlets; T_1, T_2, triplets. Straight arrows indicate radiative energy transfer; wavy arrows indicate nonradiative energy transfer. (Redrawn with permission from Hemmila I: Fluoroimmunoassays and immunofluorometric assays, *Clin Chem* 31:359, 1985.)

nm. Thus the specific emission of usable fluorescent probes should be greater than 500 nm. Pretreatment of plasma and serum samples with proteolytic enzymes and oxidizing or denaturing agents can help eliminate this background contamination. Solid-phase support structures such as microbeads with intrinsically low fluorescence backgrounds can also eliminate nonspecific serum background.[77]

Biologic fluids also contain a host of factors that can quench the fluorescence yields. The pH, the polarity of the probes, and the oxidation state of nearby molecules or heavy ions can also alter fluorescence yields. Some molecules carrying the fluorescence probes can even be self-quenching.

Despite these potential problems a variety of fluorescent probes have proved satisfactory. These probes have a high fluorescence intensity; that is, their fluorescence signal is easily distinguished from background, and their unique chemical characteristics enable them to be bound to antigens (hormones) or antibodies without adversely affecting their properties.

Fluorescence intensity depends on both the absorption of excitation and quantum yield. The molar absorptivity of the probe must be high (greater than 10,000) with as high a quantum yield as possible. Moreover, the emission energy of the probe must be easily and clearly distinguished from background. Thus probes with emissions of greater than 500 nm and large Stokes shifts (greater than 50 nm) are essential.

Coupling of fluorescence probes to other molecules is not unlike other coupling requirements. Immunoreactants must have functional groups such as carboxylic acid, aromatic, hydroxyl, sulfonic acid, or aliphatic amine groups available. Reactive intermediates such as esters, isocyanates, acid anhydrides, isothiocyanates, or *N*-hydroxyl succinimides have been successfully used.[77] Fluorescein or rhodamine derivative probes (having very high fluorescence intensities) are widely used, with isothiocyanate fluorescein derivatives being the most popular.[74,190] Umbelliferone, a 7-hydroxycoumarin compound, has also been applied to fluorescence assays. Although its fluorescence intensity is not as good as that of fluorescein, it has a larger Stokes shift, enabling it to be used to label polymers such as polylysine to increase the yield of steroid tracers.[18,185] These and other fluorescent labels that have endocrine applications are shown in Fig. 62-25. Each of these compounds has its own strong and weak points in specific applications; some have excellent quantum yields, high Stokes shifts, and good photostabilities, but some can also be sensitive to scattering of light, sensitive to background interferences, and self-quenching. Fluorescamine and *N*-pyrene maleimide have been used in fluorescence assays because of their excellent fluorescence enhancement and long fluorescence lifetimes (hundreds of nanoseconds).[18,74,104] Naturally occurring fluorescent phycobiliproteins from algae, along with porphyrins and chlorophylls, have unique fluorescent properties that make them excellent candidates for fluorescent assay applications.*

Because of intrinsic detection limitations, fluorescein- and rhodamine-labeled tracers are applicable only for assaying analytes and hormones that are found in the nanomolar range. For hormones requiring sensitivities in the picomolar range, new approaches were needed. Recently metal chelates, in particular the fluorescent rare earth ions, have been exploited for application in fluorescence assays because of their excellent fluorescent properties and high detection sensitivity (10^{-13} to 10^{-14} mol/L). Most notable of these are the lanthanides, europium (Eu-III) and terbium (Tb-III). When these lanthanides are chelated with organic ligands like 4,

*References 16, 18, 19, 29, 49, 58, 75, 77, 79, 98, 116.

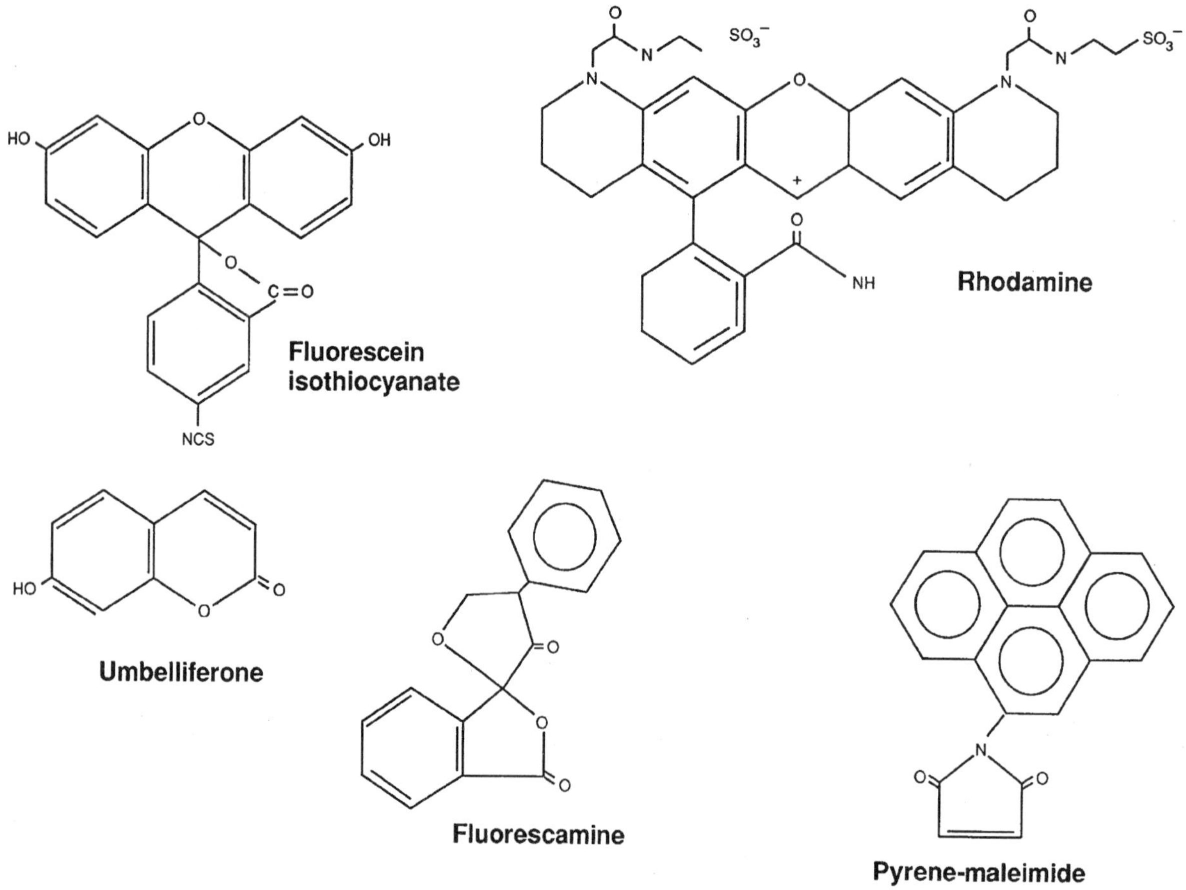

Fig. 62-25. Typical fluorescent compounds (probes) used in fluorescence immunoassays.

7-bis(chlorosulfophenyl)-1, 10-phenanthroline-2, 9-dicarboxylic acid (BCPDA), the resulting compound fluorescence is often characterized by broad excitation in the absorption region of the ligand (250 to 360 nm), reduced fluorescence quenching, decreased serum autofluorescence, large Stokes shifts (greater than 250 nm; fluorescein is about 30 nm), and long fluorescence lifetimes (100 to 1000 microseconds).[44,57,77]

Application with this chelating compound has been made in the Cyberfluor System (Cyberfluor Inc, Toronto). It can be labeled to streptavidin without loss of biologic activity and quantitated in microtiter plate wells, with final fluorescence measured on a solid-phase system using specially designed equipment.[32,45,89,152]

By delaying the measurement of fluorescence after a flash excitation of the sample, background short-lived fluorescence due to serum, solvents, cuvettes, and reagents is essentially eliminated. However, these lanthanides do not form particularly stable (that is, chemically inert) chelates, especially in aqueous biologic fluids. Moreover, they also have a tendency to dissociate and be quenched by water.[77] These flaws or shortcomings have been partially corrected by the development of aqueous, stabilized, chelation systems by polymerization of the chelate to latex particles that

are covalently bound to antibodies or antigens.[77] Polyamino-polycarboxylate chelates of lanthanides have been used more than any other type of complex in producing usable fluorescent assays. Terbium and europium chelated to IgGs using diazophenyl ethylenediaminetetraacetic acid (EDTA), to thyroxine using EDTA and sulfosalicylic acid, or to specific antibodies using EDTA and β-diketones represented the first steps in producing usable and efficient fluorescent labels for routine laboratory use.[77,121]

The use of separate steps for lanthanide dissociation and simultaneous development after the specific immunoreaction has been perfected by LKB-Wallac (Turku, Finland) in its Delfia (dissociation-enhanced lanthanide fluorescence immunoassay) time-resolved system, making it possible to use non–fluorescence bifunctional complexes such as the derivatives of aminophenyl-EDTA or aminobenzyl-diethylenetriaminetetraacetic acid for europium labeling.*

The Arcus time-resolved fluorometer (LKB-Wallac) is essentially identical to other conventional instruments, except that it has added a system for time-gated measurements of only a portion of the total fluorescence emission cycle. During a critical portion of the emission cycle the

*References 56, 77, 78, 87, 107, 108, 117, 144, 180, 187, 193, 197.

photomultiplier is inactive; thus unwanted events go undetected. An example of the sequence might be the following: excitation light flash (1 microsecond), time delay during which short-lived or unwanted fluorescence is decayed (400 microseconds), actual measuring time with active photomultiplier (400 microseconds), and recovery time before the next cycle (200 microseconds). This makes about 1000 flashes (or a 1-millisecond full cycle) for the 1-second well measuring time.[44] Newer gated fluorometers using lasers (often nitrogen lasers) as the excitation source enable these instruments to measure fluorescence from a solid-phase matrix rather than being limited to measurements from solutions.

Fluorescence assay principles are identical with those of the RIA and enzyme-linked assays in respect to reaction conditions, for example, separation of bound from free fractions and assay validation. Fluorescence assays are also classified in a manner similar to RIAs and enzyme assays, that is, those with labeled antigen versus labeled antibodies, those featuring competition between antigens (tracer and free) for a limited amount of antibody versus noncompetitive or excess reagent assays, or as heterogeneous (requiring a separation of bound from free fraction) or homogeneous (not requiring a separation step) assays.[77] Competitive assays using limited amounts of antibodies are similar to most standard RIAs.

Solid-phase–based sandwich assays using labeled antibodies are most common, are termed immunofluorimetric assays, and are analogous to IRMAs. These provide the user with simple procedures and low-background fluorescence. Polyacrylamide beads, polysaccharide microbeads, and magnetized cellulose particle compounds have seen application in these assay formats.[50,77,91,148] Like the IRMA, immunofluorimetric assays use fluorescent probe–labeled antibodies in excess (that is, an excess reagent assay). In these assays the fluorescent signal is directly proportional to the analyte or hormone concentration. The use of excess reagents can shorten the incubation time, provide greater sensitivity, and widen the measurement range of the assay.[77,194]

As in EIAs and RIAs, fluorescence assays can be used to measure protein or polypeptide hormones having two or more distinct epitopic antibody-binding sites, like TSH or hCG.[6,7,85,101,142] The primary or capture antibody is immobilized on a solid matrix, such as polyacrylamide beads or cellulose nitrate or acetate discs. This can then, in turn, be quantitated by a second antibody. Common separation techniques used in RIAs (double antibody, PEG, ammonium sulfate precipitation, etc.) are rarely used in heterogeneous fluorescence assays because of their intrinsic background fluorescence properties. Thus solid-phase separations are most often used. Obviously, all of the solid-phase materials employed in the separation step of these formats must provide ease of handling (that is, be easily washed) throughout the assay procedure, as well as provide intrinsic low fluorescence, scatter, and quench properties.[77]

Microbeads, composed of polysaccharides,[50] polyacrylamides,[39,86,91] or magnetizable cellulose particles[39,148] have received the widest application. The use of polyacrylamide and polystyrene beads and magnetizable particles can eliminate the centrifugation steps during washing sequences, and polyacrylamide and polystyrene beads can be applied to homogeneous assay formats because of their low fluorescence and scattering properties. Dipstick or surface technology can be applied to fluorescence assays by employing cellulose acetate-nitrate substrate or polymethylmethacrylate. Special fluorimeters are available to measure the fluorescence from these solid-state applications.[77]

Homogeneous fluorescence assay formats do not require a "bound from free" separation step to enable final fluorescent measurement, because of the reaction mixtures' direct effect on the fluorescence properties of the labeled antibody or antigen. These assays are simple and rapid, like their RIA and enzyme assay counterparts, but they fall short in terms of assay sensitivities seen using heterogeneous assays because of interference from serum samples and by the chemical nature of the actual assay immunoreaction. Thus homogeneous fluorescence assays are usually found in applications where analytes or hormones are known to be in relatively large concentrations, for example, in drugs and hormones such as cortisol and estriol. Most of these homogeneous fluorescence assays are of the competitive type in which antibody binding induces some change in the labeled antigen fluorescence properties, usually in fluorescence wavelength. Detailed descriptions and useful modifications of both homogeneous and heterogeneous fluorescence assays are provided by numerous investigators.[7,18,44,49,77]

Currently, fluorescence assays with sensitivities equal to or greater than those of RIAs, EIAs, or ELISAs have been developed. This has been fueled by the development of better reagents (antibodies, fluorescent probes, cleaner separation techniques, etc.) and more sophisticated and automated instrumentation. The use of polyfluorescein, rhodamine, and chelated rare-earth lanthanides used in time-resolved measurement fluorometers has enabled fluorescent assays to achieve sensitivities similar to or better than those of the best RIAs and EIAs. Background fluorescence can be decreased with acidic or enzymatic pretreatment of the biologic sample.

Instrumentation has also improved dramatically over the past several years, which has increased the signal-to-noise ratios using improved fluorescence optics, better fluorescence detectors and signal-processing hardware, and special fluorescence filters. The formats of these systems range from carrying out assays in flow cells[105,181] to using disposable cuvettes,[99] microtiter plates or microtiter strips, or plastic strip surfaces (e.g., dipstick formats).[77] The replacement of continuous light with pulsed excitation and lasers has greatly improved the versatility and sensitivity of these assays. Time-resolved fluorescence assays have also

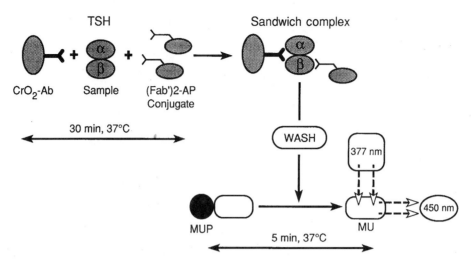

Fig. 62-26. Scheme of sandwich enzyme-linked fluorescent assay (ELFA). The assay format for an ELFA for human TSH (hTSH) employs two monoclonal antibodies specific for hTSH. The capture antibody, which is specific to the intact hTSH molecule, is coupled to chromium dioxide paramagnetic particles (for the separation of bound from free fractions). The detection antibody, which is specific to the beta subunit of hTSH, is conjugated to alkaline phosphatase (*Fab'2-AP*). Sample is dispensed by an automated, robotics type, mechanized system; the particles and alkaline phosphatase conjugate are then added and incubated. After the incubation, the particles are washed, and the fluorogenic substrate, 4-methylumbelliferyl phosphate (*MUP*), is then added for signal generation, using an excitation wavelength of 377 nm and an emission wavelength of 450 nm. (Redrawn with permission of Dr. Thomas Li, Vista Immunoassay System, San Jose, Calif, 1992, Syva Company.)

been established using terbium (TB^{3+}) and samarium (Sm^{3+}), as well as europium (Eu^{3+}).[10,43,99] For conventional fluorescence immunoassays, assay sensitivity is not limited by instrumentation but by the signal-to-noise ratio of the sample. Appropriate filtering must be used to decrease background fluorescence in addition to implementing unique measuring systems, depending on the fluorescence assay system manufacturer.

ENZYME-LINKED FLUORESCENCE ASSAYS

Hybridization of EIA and fluorescence technology has resulted in new sandwich enzyme-linked fluorescent assay (ELFA) formats (Fig. 62-26). Moreover, these systems have been integrated into automated, self-contained assay reagent module formats (Fig. 62-27), enabling the user to measure a wide variety of hormones on a single ELFA monitoring system (e.g., SYVA Co, San Jose, Calif and PB Diagnostics, Westwood, Mass). These approaches, and others, provide state-of-the-art, classic, wet chemistry format assays for polypeptide and glycoprotein hormones, as well as dry chemistry multilayered immunoassay systems for drugs and other antigens. However, it comes as no surprise that virtually all manufacturers or suppliers of these systems have their own unique reagents, dry or wet chemistry modules, and robotic assay systems employing polarization, surface, kinetic, or time-resolved measurements.*

*References 32, 45, 50, 57, 77, 89, 91, 101, 108, 117, 142, 144, 147, 148, 152, 193, 194.

CHEMILUMINESCENCE ASSAYS

Another more recent modification of the original immunoassay scheme employs the utilization of chemiluminescent end points as opposed to colorimetric and fluorimetric end-point determinations. Research using chemiluminescent molecules as immunoassay reagents has been ongoing for over a decade, but the implementation of these assay techniques in routine endocrine measurements is relatively new.*

Chemiluminescence differs from fluorescence in that it involves excited-state formation as the product of an exoergic chemical reaction.[201] The excited-state product molecule relaxes to a ground state and in so doing emits photons. Chemiluminescence incorporates a population of excited states of specific molecules as a consequence of the thermodynamics of the oxidative chemical reaction involved. The photoefficiency of this reaction or the number of photons emitted per molecule of reactant is called the chemiluminescence quantum yield.[202] The kinetics of these reactions can be varied by modifying the chemical reactions involved so that the photon emission can occur immediately (within 1 or 2 seconds) or be slightly delayed (within several seconds to minutes). The actual kinetics of the reactions varies according to the concentration of initiating reagents, but it usually is characterized by a very rapid rise in emission intensity (measured in fractions of a second)

*References 11, 25, 94, 97, 174, 177, 201, 202, 210.

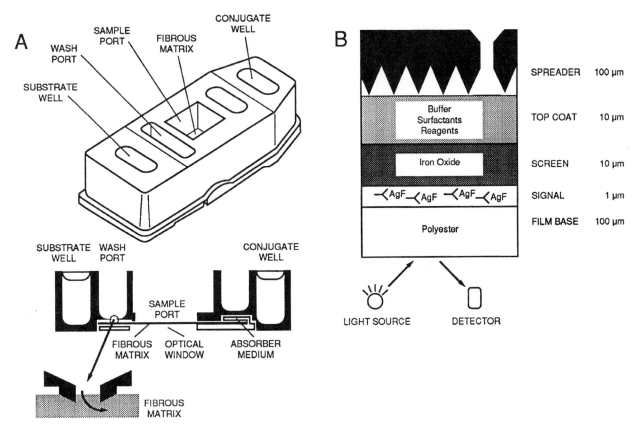

Fig. 62-27. New self-contained immunoassay test modules and dry chemistry multilayer technology. **A,** Top and cutaway views of self-contained test module for automated sandwich enzyme-linked fluorescent immunoassay (ELFA) for glycoprotein hormones. The patient sample is delivered into the sample port, a glass fiber strip (*fibrous matrix*) that serves as the solid phase, which is conveniently sealed in a plastic test module housing. The test module carries appropriate amounts of all necessary reagents, that is, alkaline phosphatase antibody conjugate and wash/substrate (4-methylumbelliferyl phosphate) solutions inside sealed wells within the plastic housing. Fluorescence is measured directly through the sample port optical window. Test modules for a specific hormone are loaded into an automated analyzer that completes all of the pipetting, incubation, measuring, and data-reduction steps. Results are available in less than 30 minutes. **B,** Automated system technology using dry chemistry multilayered immunoassay for total thyroxine. This competitive immunoassay utilizes three polysaccharide layers coated onto a polyester base. The bottom layer, or signal layer, contains an immobilized, high-affinity monoclonal antibody that is in complex with a fluorescent (rhodamine)-labeled thyroxine conjugate (*AgF*). The thickness of the layer is very thin relative to the rest of the element. The next layer, or screen layer, contains the pigment iron oxide that acts as a screen, in order to make possible an optical separation of free from bound conjugate. The top layer contains all necessary buffers, reagents, and surfactants. Ten microliters of serum or plasma are automatically diluted by the analyzer and pipetted into the test module (similar to that in **A**), where a molded plastic grid spreads it evenly across the surface of the multilayer. Thyroxine in the sample diffuses into the multilayer, where it then competes with conjugate for the limited binding sites of the antibody. After several minutes the fluorescence of bound conjugate is measured and the concentration of thyroxine in the sample is interpolated from a standard curve, which is stored in the memory of the instrument. (Redrawn with permission from PB Diagnostics, Westwood, Mass.)

followed by a gradual decay (measured over a few seconds) as the excited states become depolarized.

Good chemiluminescence quantitative techniques have only recently become a reality. The search for efficient luminometry has centered around improving nonspecific luminescence and interferences from the assay system itself. Light detection is achieved by using high-efficiency photomultiplier tubes, but still remains in the 20% to 30% efficiency range. Events are treated in either a digital or an analogue manner, depending on the type of instrument being used. Digital systems operate on a one photon–one event–one pulse basis, with the number of pulses per time

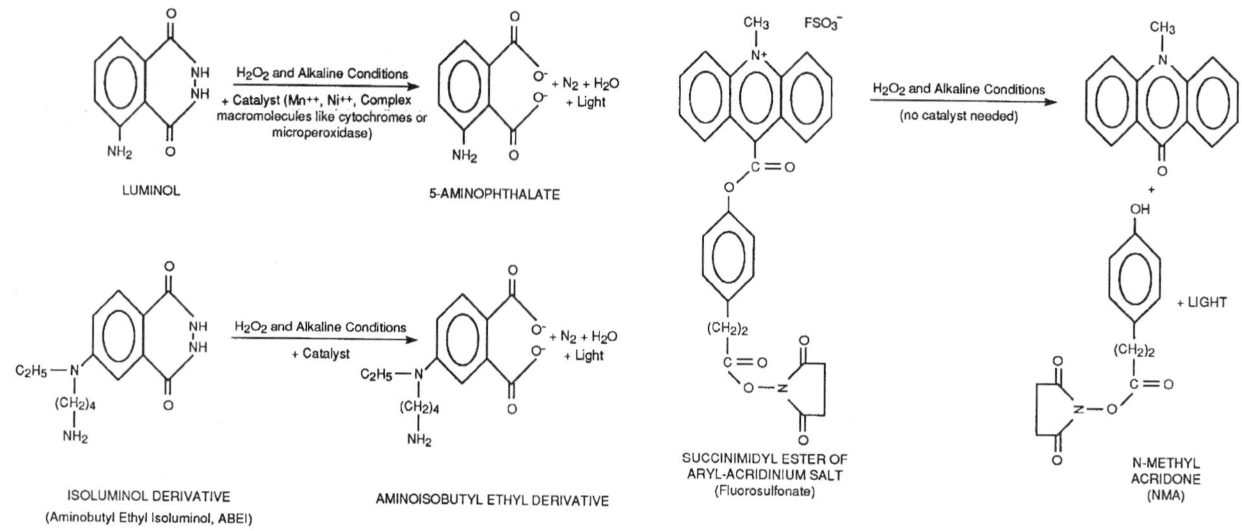

Fig. 62-28. Chemiluminescent molecules (luminol, isoluminol, and an arylacridinium derivative) and their reactions to produce light: simplified chemical reactions of common "labels" in chemiluminescence assays. Luminol and isoluminol require catalysts such as Mn^{++} or Ni^{++}, or complex macromolecules such as cytochromes, horseradish peroxidase, or microperoxidase. Acridinium derivatives offer certain advantages, since the reaction does not require catalysts, making it less susceptible to background and interference effects, and the *n*-methylacridone (NMA) produced in this reaction has a higher chemiluminescence quantum yield because the yield is independent of the chemical modifications required to conjugate the acridinium salt to assay components. (Redrawn with permission from Weeks I, Woodhead J: Chemiluminescence immunoassay, *J Clin Immunoassay* 7:82, 1984.)

being a function of light intensity. Analogue systems involve treating the photomultiplier output as a photocurrent, the magnitude of which is proportional to light emission intensity.[202] New automated luminometric systems must incorporate a sample transportation system, an elevator mechanism that translocates each sample to a light-free chamber near the photomultiplier tube, and an automatic injection system to dispense initiating reagents, all of which are integrated with software programs for operation and data reduction.

Although instrumentation and electronic signal interpretation are important, the success of chemiluminometric assays depends on the ability to produce stable conjugates among the antigen, the antibody, and the label. The first assay prototypes employing chemiluminescent probes encountered assay interferences from a variety of factors that influenced assay catalytic reagent requirements and microenvironmental quenching.

Most of the early published studies of chemiluminometric assays have involved small molecules, principally steroids, because of the well-established procedures for producing externally labeled steroid molecules. Conjugation chemistries (succinate or glucuronide bridging) have also been developed. The derivatives of luminol (e.g., isoluminol) (Fig. 62-28)[202] make conjugation with minimal loss of quantum yield a reality.[174]

Chemiluminescent molecules are covalently linked to either the assay antigen (hormone) or the antibody, and like other assays these reagents can be adapted to either a homogeneous system or a heterogeneous format. Although the homogeneous assays provide simplicity, heterogeneous formats provide higher assay sensitivity.

Endocrine assays have been developed by Kohen and her colleagues for several steroid hormones and their urinary metabolites, including progesterone,[92,93,143] estradiol,[90] estrone-glucuronide,[205] estriol glucuronide,[12] and pregnanediol glucuronide,[55] reaching and/or surpassing assay performance and sensitivities of the best EIA/ELISA and RIAs.[37] These assays have adapted solid-phase methodologies, making the removal of interfering serum factors or other quenchers a part of the assay dynamics. The conjugation of aminobutylethylisoluminol (ABEI) to antibodies has posed some significant problems in terms of quenching and loss of quantum yield. Most investigators have overcome this by adding a dissociation step just prior to luminometry. This usually involves high temperatures and the addition (incubation) of strong alkali. The use of acridinium esters may eliminate this quench, and thus the extra assay step.

Polypeptide assays can be flawed (as just stated) when labels are linked to these proteins producing greatly reduced quantum yields. Other isoluminol derivatives (e.g.,

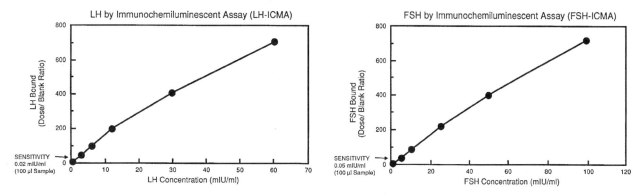

Fig. 62-29. Typical standard curves of chemiluminescence assay of LH and FSH. Sensitivities for comparable RIAs are as follows: LH, 4.0 mIU/mL using a 100-μL sample; FSH, 0.5 mIU/mL using a 100-μL sample. (Redrawn with permission from Dr. Darrel Mayes, Endocrine Sciences, Calabassas Hills, Calif, 1992.)

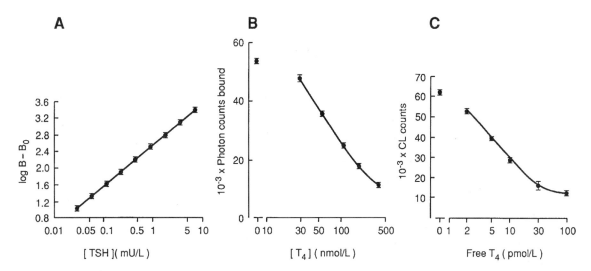

Fig. 62-30. Chemiluminescent assay standard curve for the measurement of thyroid-stimulating hormone (TSH), thyroxine (T_4), and free T_4. **A,** Dose-response curve of a two-site immunochemoluminometric assay for human TSH using a high-affinity monoclonal antibody labeled with 3 mol of acridinium ester per mole of antibody. The assay format comprises (1) mixing sample with labeled antibody (2 hours), (2) adding solid-phase polyclonal antibody (1 hour), and (3) a final wash step with mild detergent to help reduce nonspecific binding (background) to less than 0.1% of added activity. Luminescence of the acridinium component is evaluated with the addition of alkaline hydrogen peroxide. Light intensity is quantitated over a 1- to 2-second period, being directly proportional to the sample's TSH concentration. The ordinate is expressed as the log of specific antibody-bound light emission. Similar assays for total T_4 and serum free T_4 (**B** and **C**) use an acridinium-labeled T_4 antibody incubated with a solid-phase conjugated T_4 moiety, and the unknown sample or standard. After centrifugation to separate the solid-phase immune complexes, chemiluminescence is measured, with the concentration of T_4 in the sample or standard being inversely proportional to the emission of light intensity.[201] Free T_4 assays are technically difficult but can be simplified, as shown here, by the introduction of labeled hormone analogues that bind to the antibody but not to serum proteins. (Redrawn with permission from Weeks I, Sturgess ML, Woodhead JS: Chemiluminescence immunoassay: an overview, *Clin Sci* 70:403, 1986.)

aminohexylethylisoluminol, AHEI) have partially overcome this obstacle.[97,202] The incorporation of acridinium derivatives and other labels has been attempted with encouraging results.[203] Examples of this are gonadotropin assays (Fig. 62-29) that incorporate paired monoclonal antibodies linked to an acridinium ester, providing highly

sensitive and specific procedures when directly compared with analogous IRMA formats. Similarly, assays for TSH, thyroxine (T_4), and free T_4 have been developed that also employ monoclonal antibodies and an acridinium chemiluminescence label (Fig. 62-30).[201-204]

Photons or light intensity can be measured accurately

and precisely by using commercially available luminometers. The earliest models were crude in design, in essence being small, shoebox–sized darkrooms requiring the manual dispensing of catalysts and other luminescent reagents by the operator, and measuring only one assay sample at a time. Current state-of-the-art luminometers are now more accurately classified as chemiluminometric systems that utilize assay-specific reagent modules for chemistry containment. These systems can automatically dispense reagents, incubate reactants, and measure light intensity (either as a flash or a glow) at a variety of postreaction time intervals, integrate this intensity, and report results through computerized data-processing systems.

OTHER ASSAY TECHNIQUES

There are several other assay approaches available to the endocrinologist for the measurement of important molecules. Electrochemical immunoassays combine the sensitivity of bioselective electrode detection with the specificity of the antigen-antibody interaction. Electrochemical methods are not plagued by problems of sample turbidity, quenching, or interferences from the many absorbing or fluorescing compounds found in biologic samples that interfere with other spectroscopic techniques. Both potentiometric (that is, assays based on charge separation across the sample electrode surface, with slow recovery and slow response times) and amperometric (that is, assays based on oxidation-reduction reactions at the electrode surface, resulting in fast response times) assay approaches can be used to monitor immunoassays to provide both rapid and specific analyte analysis.[124] Although these methods adapt to flow-through procedures, sensor fouling remains a common problem and represents a serious limitation to these techniques. Potentiometric immunoassays have proven themselves over the years, but amperometric devices appear to be more promising. Amperometric electrodes have better long-term stability, show little if any interference, and can produce linear responses in an analyte's physiologic range. For example, electrochemical detection can be linked to an enzyme label, that is, an enzyme that is available in very pure form and inexpensive. The product of the enzyme reaction should be nontoxic and easily detected at low levels.[76] One example is alkaline phosphatase, used to catalyze the conversion of an electroinactive substance (phenylphosphate) to phenol (Fig. 62-31). Phenol is separated by chromatography (usually HPLC) and is detected by oxidation in a thin-layer electrochemical cell with a carbon-paste working electrode.[76] This gives an extremely sensitive method of quantitating alkaline phosphatase activity, and thus an application for EIA or ELISA techniques using this or other enzymes. These assays can be formatted as either competitive or sandwich types, and can attain sensitivities using amperometric detections equal to those of other immunoassay techniques (e.g., low picogram per

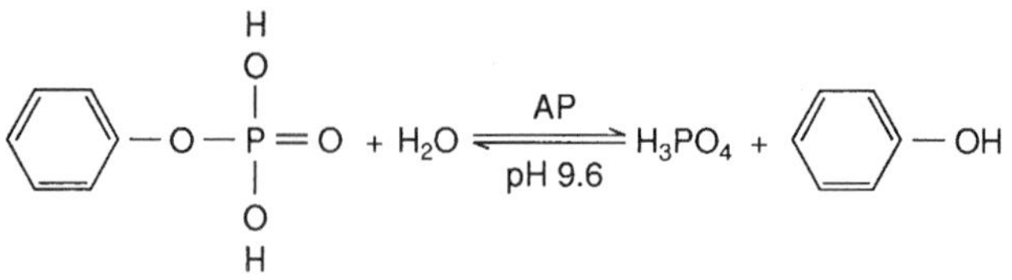

Fig. 62-31. Conversion of phenylphosphate (electroinactive) to phenol (electroactive) for immunoassays with electrochemical detection. *AP*, Alkaline phosphatase. (Redrawn with permission of John Wiley & Sons, Inc, from Heineman WR et al: Immunoassay with electrical detection, *Methods Biochem Anal* 32:345, 1987. New York, Copyright © 1987, John Wiley & Sons, Inc.)

milliliter range on a 20-μL sample volume). Automation of these approaches is currently a high priority for most reagent suppliers and manufacturers.

Other biosensors based on optical (light scattering) or piezoelectric (mass to frequency transducers, i.e., mechanical vibrations translated to electrical signals) techniques have been recently developed.[3,73,145] Capacitative affinity sensors can measure changes in dielectric properties in response to the presence of a particular analyte encompassed on a silicon chip.[3] Pocket-sized blood glucose biosensors utilize a ferocene-mediated response to glucose oxidase. Field-effect transistors have been produced that work by loading or unloading charges to an insulating gate in the transistor. This change in charge alters the net current of the transistor and can ultimately reflect the level of an analyte or chemical in solution. Light-addressable potentiometric sensors[3,73] use an alternating photocurrent through an electrolyte-insulated semiconductor interface to provide a means of measuring small potential changes. A closed circuit is made with a variable voltage source, an electrode, an ammeter, and a biosensor consisting of a silicon wafer covered with an insulating layer that is stable in the presence of biologic solutions. Specific enzymes on the biosensor's surface can produce detectable shifts in the surface potential in the presence of specific molecules of interest.[3] Solid-state or dipstick assays are also currently being designed and improved, as evidenced by the semi-quantitative colorimetric products currently available for monitoring urinary LH and hCG.[3,5,73]

Nephelometry, or the measurement of scattered light, provides a convenient means of quantifying immunoprecipitation reactions. Light scattering occurs as a result of elastic collisions of particles of all sizes with light quanta. The amount and nature of the scatter depend on the size and shape of the particles, the wavelength of light, and the refractive index of the medium.[186] The time course of the nephelometry signal is depicted in Fig. 62-32. Reaction conditions can be selected to cause a maximum of the steepest portion of the curve, that is, the rate curve, to occur within seconds of the injection of the triggering reagent. The use of the rate of change of light scattering is called "rate nephelometry."[186] Rate nephelometry has proven

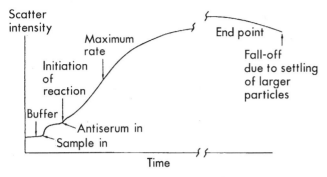

Fig. 62-32. Time course of an immunoprecipitation reaction: variation of intensity of scattered light versus time. (From Sternberg JC: Rate nephelometry. In Rose NR, Freidman H, Fahey JL, editors: *Manual of clinical laboratory immunology,* ed 3, Washington, DC, 1986, American Society of Microbiology.)

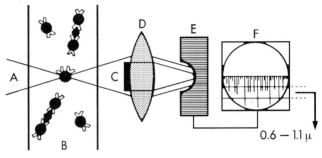

● Latex ⌒ Antibody ◆ Antigen

Fig. 62-33. Quantitation of antigens using particle counting. A collimated beam of white light (*A*) focused to a diameter of 7.5 μm passes through a flow cell (*B*) and impinges on a black spot (*C*). When a particle passes through this beam, light is diffracted past the black spot, collected by the lens (*D*), and focused onto the photomultiplier (*E*). The impulse from *E,* shown on the oscilloscope (*F*), is proportional to the size of the particle. Only agglutinated particles are electronically counted, thus separating bound from free fractions. No physical separation is necessary, making this particular format a homogeneous assay system. (From Masson PL, Holy HW: Immunoassay by particle counting. In Rose NR, Freidman H, Fahey JL, editors: *Manual of clinical laboratory technology,* ed 3, Washington, DC, 1986, American Society for Microbiology.)

itself to be precise and accurate, measuring immunoglobulin; complements C3 and C4; and prealbumin, albumin, and microalbumin.[186] Nephelometric measurements of small, nonantigenic hormones (or haptens) require a variant approach called nephelometric inhibition.[153,186] Although drugs are the most commonly measured haptens using nephelometric inhibition, investigators are pursuing the measurement of hormones by this technique.[186] Currently fixed-time nephelometry is advertised as a third-generation improvement over rate nephelometry, based on the observation that extended assay ranges (on the order of three logs) can be obtained. This ensures that more of the actual measurement signals lie in the linear or near the linear portion of the analyte standard curve, that is, a functional widening of the dose-response curve. This approach always operates in an antibody-excess configuration, and can be used with both homogeneous and heterogeneous formats.

Particle-enhanced immunoassays, employing erythrocytes, clay, or polymer latex as an inert solid-support reagent to increase sensitivities, are based on the measurement of the agglutination of an antigen and its corresponding antibody as a function of the concentration of one of these components.[65] As the immune complex of the antigens and antibodies grows in size, its light-scattering properties change. This change is monitored by visual, spectrophotometric, or nephelometric approaches. Singer and Plotz[182] were the first to describe this approach in detail, in following rheumatoid factor in patients. Currently, commercially available kits and automated instrumentation systems are available but are usually only qualitative or semiquantitative, for example, assays for β-hCG.

Analogous to these are particle-counting immunoassays[113,114] that have been used to measure pregnancy-specific β_1-glycoprotein, TSH, thyroglobulin, thyroid-binding globulin, placental lactogen, somatotropin, T_4, triiodothyronine, and others.[59,113,114] Briefly stated, antigens are quantitated by mixing a biologic sample with antibody-coated latex particles (0.8-μm diameter) suspended in a suitable buffer. Antigen in the sample agglutinates some of the latex particles, so that the number of remaining, dispersed particles decreases. Sample antigen concentration is thus inversely proportional to the unagglutinated particle content (Fig. 62-33).[113]

CONCLUSION

Assays available to the endocrinologist currently incorporate state-of-the-art schemes for the measurement of hormones and endocrine-related molecules for research and clinical uses. They have evolved from simple bench manipulations to assays encompassing complex and sophisticated techniques. Frequent improvements in these assays stimulate and propagate newer and even more elegant improvements; these are usually related to speed of analysis, precision of analysis, and sensitivity of the assay. The result of this effort sometimes appears to be the commercial production of newer kits and/or "perfect" instrumentation systems that are fast, precise, fully automated, versatile, and foolproof.[154] Few, however, are inexpensive. Unfortunately, conjuring up eye-catching marketing strategies to upstage the competition are usually woven into these efforts. Actually, most, if not all, assay "systems" within a particular subgroup are quite similar once the veneer is removed; yet there are quite clever and sophisticated chemistries that certain manufacturing research and development groups have mustered. Unfortunately, the result of these efforts appears to be the demise of true bench chemistry and biochemistry, and the emergence of the "analysis system," often referred to as the "black box." The evolution of assay technology seems to be from laboratory chemist to laboratory instrument custodian.[154] This movement has virtually eliminated the user's true understanding of the nuances of assay technology, and minimizes his or her ability to manipulate reagents or techniques. Trouble-shooting will be left to highly trained laboratory technologists or certified field technicians working for the manufacturers.

One can argue for or against these improvements as being either advantageous or disadvantageous. Simplification and miniaturization of these assays will be a great advantage to some of these efforts, along with development of user-safe and sink-disposable reagents.

Regardless of the changes and improvements, the linchpin of every good assay is inherent in its validation. Greatly improved sensitivities, possibly exceeding clinical or research need, will most certainly be realized, but hopefully not at the cost of diminishing assay specificities. Many more advances in the assays for the endocrinologist will appear by the turn of the century, probably well before. Only time will tell whether the new system methodologies will encompass true improvements over classic or current schemes. As long as the founding principles of immunoassays or other assays remain as central components of the formula, endocrine investigations and discoveries can only advance.

ACKNOWLEDGMENT

The author thanks Michael J. DiMattina, MD, for his review of the manuscript.

REFERENCES

1. Aguillera G et al: Mechanism of action of CRF and other regulators of corticotropin release in rat pituitary cells, *J Biol Chem* 258:8039, 1983.
2. Alberts B, Bozay D, Lewis J et al, editors: *The molecular biology of the cell,* ed 2, New York, 1989, Garland Publishing.
3. Albertson BD: Hormone assay methodology: present and future prospects. In Adashi EY, editor: Reproductive endocrinology update, *Clin Obstet Gynecol* 33:591, 1990.
4. Albertson BD, Haseltine FP: *Non-radiometric assays: technology and application in polypeptide and steroid hormone detection,* New York, 1988, John Wiley & Sons.
5. Albertson BD, Zinaman MJ: Review article: the prediction of ovulation and monitoring of the fertile period, *Adv Contracept* 3:263, 1987.
6. Alfthan H: Comparison of immunoradiometric and immunofluorometric assay for serum hCG, *J Immunol Methods* 88:239, 1986.
7. Arends J, Norgaard-Pedersen B: Immunofluorometry of thyrotropin, for whole-blood spots on filter paper to screen for congenital hypothyroidism, *Clin Chem* 32:1854, 1986.
8. Ashkar FS: *Radiobioassays,* vol 1, Boca Raton, Fla, 1985, CRC Press.
9. Avrameas SP et al: *Immunoenzymatic techniques,* Amsterdam, 1983, Elsevier.
10. Bador R et al: Europium and samarium as labels in time-resolved immunofluorometric assay of follitropin, *Clin Chem* 33:48, 1987.
11. Barnard GJR, Kim JB, Williams JL: Chemiluminescence immunoassays and immunochemiluminometric assays. In Collins WP, editor: *Alternative immunoassays,* New York, 1985, John Wiley & Sons.
12. Barnard GJ et al: The measurement of urinary estriol-16 alpha-glucuronide by a solid phase chemiluminescence immunoassay, *J Steroid Biochem* 14:941, 1981.
13. Behrman HR: A history of hormone assays. In Albertson BD, Haseltine FP, editors: *Non-radiometric assays: technology and application in polypeptide and steroid hormone detection,* New York, 1988, John Wiley & Sons.
14. Berson SA et al: Insulin ^{131}I metabolism in human subjects: demonstration of insulin binding globulin in the circulation of insulin treated subjects, *J Clin Invest* 35:170, 1956.
15. Blake C, Gould BJ: Use of enzymes in immunoassay techniques: a review, *Analyst* 109:533, 1984.
16. Blakeslee D, Baines M: Immunofluorescence using dichlorotriazing-amino fluorescein (DTAF): preparation and fractionation of labelled IgG, *J Immunol Methods* 13:305, 1976.
17. Bolton AE, Hunter WM: The labelling of protein to high specific activity radio-activity by conjugation to a ^{125}I-containing acylating agent, *Biochem J* 133:529, 1973.
18. Brandtzarg P: Conjugates of immunoglobulin G with different fluorochromes: I and II, *Scand J Immunol* 2:273, 333, 1973.
19. Brandtzarg P: Rhodamine conjugates: specific and non-specific binding properties in immunochemistry, *Ann N Y Acad Sci* 254:35, 1975.
20. Brown BL, Ekins RP, Tampion W: The assay of adenosine 3'-5'-cyclic monophosphate by saturation analysis, *Biochem J* 120:8p, 1970.
21. Burd JF et al: Homogeneous reactant-labelled fluorescent immunoassay for therapeutic drugs exemplified by gentamicin determination in human serum, *Clin Chem* 23:1402, 1977.
22. Butt WR: The iodination of follicle stimulating and other hormones for radioimmunoassay, *J Endocrinol* 55:453, 1972.
23. Butt WR, editor: *Practical immunoassay: the state of the art,* New York, 1984, Marcel Decker.
24. Butt WR, Lynch SS: Some observations on the radioimmunoassay of follicle stimulating hormone. In Margoules M, editor: *Proceedings of the international peptide symposium on protein and polypeptide hormones,* Amsterdam, 1969, Excerpta Medica.
25. Campbell AK, Roberts A, Patel A: Chemiluminescence energy transfer: a technique for homogeneous immunoassay. In Collins WP, editor: *Alternative immunoassays,* New York, 1985, John Wiley & Sons.
26. Campbell KL: Solid state assays: reagents and film technology for dip-stick assays. In Albertson BD, Haseltine FP, editors: *Non-radiometric assays: technology and application in polypeptide and steroid hormone detection,* New York, 1988, John Wiley & Sons.
27. Cassano WF: Murine monoclonal anti-avidin antibodies enhance the sensitivity of avidin-biotin immunoassays and immunohistologic staining, *J Immunol Methods* 117:169, 1989.
28. Catt KJ: Radioassays of angiotensins I and II. In *Hormone assay techniques,* 15th training course syllabus, Bethesda, Md, 1989, The Endocrine Society.
29. Chadwick CS, McEntegard MG, Mairin RC: A trial of new fluorochromes and the development of an alternative to fluorescein, *Immunology* 1:315, 1958.
30. Challand GS, Chard T: Quality control in a radioimmunoassay: observations on the operation of a semiautomated assay for human placental lactogen, *Clin Chim Acta* 46:133, 1973.
31. Chan DW, Perlstein MT, editors: *Immunoassay: a practical guide,* New York, 1987, Academic Press.
32. Chan MA, Bellem AC, Diamandis EP: Time resolved immunofluorometric assay of alpha-fetoprotein in serum and amniotic fluid with a novel detection system, *Clin Chem* 33:2000, 1988.
33. Chard T: An Introduction to radioimmunoassay and related techniques. In Work TS, Work E, editors: *Laboratory techniques in biochemistry and molecular biology,* Amsterdam, 1982, Elsevier.

34. Chrousos GP: Radioreceptor assay of steroids and assay of receptors. In *Hormone assay techniques,* 15th training course syllabus, Bethesda, Md, 1989, The Endocrine Society.

35. Collins WP, editor: *Alternative immunoassays,* New York, 1985, John Wiley & Sons.

36. Collins WP, editor: *Complementary immunoassays,* Chichester, UK, 1988, John Wiley & Sons.

37. Collins WP et al: Chemiluminescence immunoassays for plasma steroids and urinary steroid metabolites. In Hunter WM, Corrie JET, editors: *Immunoassays for clinical chemistry* ed 2, London, 1983, Churchill Livingstone.

38. Coons AH, Creech HJ, Jones RN: Immunological properties of an antibody containing a fluorescent group, *Proc Soc Exp Biol Med* 47:200, 1941.

39. Curry RE et al: A systems approach to fluorescence immunoassay: general principles and representative applications, *Clin Chem* 25:1591, 1979.

40. Cutler GB Jr: General features of steroid receptor assays. In *Hormone assay techniques,* 15th training course syllabus, Bethesda, Md, 1989, The Endocrine Society.

41. Dauphinais RM: Solving and preventing problems in ligand assays. In Rose NR, Freidman H, Fahey JP, editors: *Manual of clinical laboratory techniques,* ed 3, Washington, DC, 1986, American Society of Microbiology.

42. Davies DR, Padlan EA, Segal DM: Three dimensional structure of immunoglobulins, *Annu Rev Biochem* 44:639, 1975.

43. Dechaud H et al: Laser excited immunofluorometric assay of prolactin, with the use of antibodies coupled to lanthanide-labelled diethylenetriiminepentaacetic acid, *Clin Chem* 32:1323, 1986.

44. Diamandis EP: Immunoassays with time-resolved fluorescence spectroscopy: principles and applications, *Clin Biochem* 21:139, 1988.

45. Diamandis EP et al: Time resolved fluoroimmunoassay of cortisol in serum with a europium chelate as label, *Clin Biochem* 21:291, 1988.

46. Dufau ML: Radioassays and bioassays of gonadotropins. In *Hormone assay techniques,* 15th training course syllabus, Bethesda, Md, 1989, The Endocrine Society.

47. Dufau ML, Mendelson CR, Catt KJ: A highly sensitive in vitro bioassay for LH and CGs: testosterone production by dispersed Leydig cells, *J Clin Endocrinol Metab* 39:610, 1974.

48. Eisen HN, Siskind GW: Variation in affinities of antibodies during the immune response, *Biochemistry* 3:996, 1964.

49. Ekeke GI, Exley D: The assay of steroids by fluoroimmunoassay. In Pal SB, editor: *Enzyme labelled immunoassay of hormones and drugs,* Berlin, 1978, Walter de Gruyter.

50. Ekeke GI, Exley D, Abuknesha R: Immunofluorometric assay of oestradiol-17β, *J Steroid Biochem* 11:1597, 1979.

51. Ekins RP: The estimation of thyroxine in human plasma by an electrophoretic technique, *Clin Chim Acta* 5:453, 1960.

52. Ekins RP: Basic principles and theory. In Sonksen PH, editor: *Radioimmunoassay and saturation analysis, Br Med Bull* 30:3, 1974.

53. Endocrine Society: *Hormone assay techniques,* 15th training course syllabus, Bethesda, Md, 1989, The Society.

54. Engvall E, Perlman P: Enzyme-linked immunosorbent assay (ELISA) of immunoglobulin G, *Immunochemistry* 8:871, 1971.

55. Esshar Z et al: Use of monoclonal antibodies to pregnanediol-3α-glucuronide to the development of a solid phase chemiluminescence immunoassay, *Steroids* 38:89, 1981.

56. Eskola JU, Nevalainen TJ, Lovgren NC: Time resolved fluoroimmunoassay of human pancreatic phospholipase A$_2$, *Clin Chem* 29:1777, 1983.

57. Evangelista RA et al: A new europium chelate for protein labelling and time-resolved fluorometric applications, *Clin Biochem* 21:173, 1988.

58. Exley D, Ekeke GI: Fluoroimmunoassay of 5α-dihydrotestosterone, *J Steroid Biochem* 14:1297, 1981.

59. Fagnart OC et al: Particle counting immunoassay (PACIA) of

60. Feldman H, Rodbard D, Levine D: Mathematical theory of crossreactive radioimmunoassay and ligand binding systems at equilibrium, *Anal Biochem* 45:530, 1972.

61. Fraker PJ, Speck JC Jr: Protein and cell membrane iodination with a sparingly soluble chloroamide 1,3,4,6-tetrachloro-3α, 6α-diphenylglycoluril, *Biochem Biophys Res Commun* 80:849, 1978.

62. Franchimont P: Dosage radio-immunologique des hormones luteinisantes chorionique et hypophysaire, *Ann Endocrinol* 27:273, 1966.

63. Freund J: Some aspects of active immunization, *Annu Rev Microbiol* 1:291, 1947.

64. Freund J: The effect of paraffin oil and mycobacteria on antibody formation and sensitization, *Am J Clin Pathol* 21:645, 1951.

65. Galvin JP: Particle enhanced immunoassay. In Rose NR, Freidman H, Fahey JL, editors: *Manual of clinical laboratory immunology,* ed 3, Washington, DC, 1986, American Society of Microbiology.

66. Glick SM, Kagan A: Combined immunoassay of insulin and human growth hormone, *J Clin Endocrinol Metab* 27:133, 1967.

67. Gold JJ: Endocrine laboratory procedures and available tests. In Gold JJ, editor: *Gynecologic endocrinology,* ed 2, Hagerstown, Md, 1975, Harper & Row.

68. Gordon P, Weintraub BD: Radioreceptor and other functional hormone assays. In Wilson JD, Foster DW, editors: *Williams' textbook of endocrinology,* ed 7, Philadelphia, 1985, WB Saunders.

69. Gosling JP: A decade of development in immunoassay methodology, *Clin Chem* 36:1408, 1990.

70. Green MJ: Electrochemical immunoassays *Philos Trans R Soc Lond [Biol]* 316:135, 1987.

71. Greenwood FC, Hunter WM, Glover JS: The preparation of ^{131}I-labelled human growth hormone of high specific radioactivity, *Biochem J* 89:114, 1963.

72. Guttmann RD, editor: *Immunology: a scope publication,* Kalamazoo, Mich, 1981, The Upjohn Co.

73. Hafeman DG, Parce JW, McConnell HM: Light addressable potentiometric sensor for biochemical systems, *Science* 240:1182, 1985.

74. Handley G, Miller JN, Bridges JW: Development of fluorescence immunoassay methods of drug analysis, *Proc Anal Div Chem Soc* 16:26, 1979.

75. Hassan M, Landon J, Smith DS: Multifluorescein-substituted polymers as potential labels in fluoroimmunoassays, *FEBS Lett* 103:339, 1979.

76. Heineman WR et al: Immunoassay with electrochemical detection, *Methods Biochem Anal,* 32:345, 1987.

77. Hemmila I: Fluoroimmunoassays and immunofluorometric assays, *Clin Chem* 31:359, 1985.

78. Hemmila I et al: Europium as a label in time resolved immunofluorometric assay, *Anal Biochem* 137:335, 1984.

79. Hendrix JL: Porphyrins and chlorophylls as probes for fluoroimmunoassay, *Clin Chem* 29:103, 1983 (letter).

80. International Atomic Energy Agency: *Radioimmunoassay and related procedures in medicine—1977:* proceedings of a symposium (Berlin, 1977), vol 1, Vienna, Austria, 1978, The Agency.

81. Ishikawa E: Enzyme immunoassay, *Nippon Rinsho* 00 (suppl): 2202, 1978.

82. Ishikawa E, Kawai T, Miyai K, editors: *Enzyme immunoassay,* Tokyo, 1981, Igaku Shoin.

83. Ishikawa E et al: Enzyme labelling with maleimides and its application to the immunoassay of peptide hormones. In Pal SB, editor: *Enzyme labeled immunoassay of hormones and drugs,* Berlin, 1978, Walter de Gruyter.

84. Jaffe BM, Behrman HR: *Methods of hormone radioimmunoassay,* ed 2, New York, 1979, Academic Press.

85. John R, Woodhead JS: An automated immunoradiometric assay of TSH in dried blood filter paper spots, *Clin Chim Acta* 125:329, 1982.

86. Kaplan LA et al: Evaluation and comparison of fluorescence and

enzyme-linked immunoassays with radioimmunoassay for serum thyroxine, *Clin Biochem Anal* 14:182, 1981.

87. Karp MT et al: Time resolved europium fluorescence in enzyme activity measurements: a sensitive protease assay, *J Appl Biochem* 5:399, 1983.

88. Kemeny DM, Challcombe SJ, editors: *ELISA and other solid phase immunoassays,* Chichester, UK, 1988, John Wiley & Sons.

89. Khosravi MJ, Diamandis EP: Immunofluorometry of hCG by time-resolved fluorescence spectroscopy with a new europium chelate as label, *Clin Chem* 33:1994, 1988.

90. Kim JB et al: The measurement of plasma estradiol-17 beta by a solid phase chemiluminescence immunoassay, *Clin Chem* 28:1120, 1982.

91. Kobayashi Y et al: A solid phase fluoroimmunoassay of serum cortisol, *J Steroid Biochem* 16:521, 1982.

92. Kohen F et al: An assay procedure for plasma progesterone based on antibody enhanced chemiluminescence, *FEBS Lett* 104:201, 1979.

93. Kohen F et al: Development of a solid phase chemiluminescence immunoassay for plasma progesterone, *Steroids* 38:73, 1981.

94. Kohen F et al: Chemiluminescence and bioluminescence immunoassays. In Collins WP, editor: *Alternative immunoassays,* New York, 1985, John Wiley & Sons.

95. Korenman SG: Radio-ligand binding assay of specific estrogens using a soluble uterine macromolecule, *J Clin Endocrinol Metab* 28:127, 1968.

96. Kricka LJ, Thorpe GHG: Luminescent immunoassays, *Ligand Rev* 3:17, 1981.

97. Krika LJ et al, editors: *Analytical applications of bioluminescence and chemiluminescence,* London, 1984, Academic Press.

98. Kronick MN, Grossman PD: Immunoassay techniques with fluorescent phycobiliprotein conjugates, *Clin Chem* 29:1582, 1983.

99. Kuo JE et al: Direct measurement of antigens in serum by time-resolved fluoroimmunoassay, *Clin Chem* 30:50, 1985.

100. Langone JJ, Van Vunakis H, editors: Immunochemical techniques, part E: monoclonal antibodies and general immunoassay methods, *Methods Enzymol* 92:1, 1983.

101. Lawson N, Wilson NMR, Pandov H: Assessment of a time-resolved fluoroimmunoassay for thyrotropin in routine clinical practice, *Clin Chem* 32:684, 1986.

102. Lefkowitz RJ, Roth J, Pastan I: Effects of Ca⁺⁺ on ACTH stimulation of the adrenals: Separation of hormone binding from adenyl cyclase activation, *Nature* 228:864, 1970.

103. Lefkowitz RJ, Roth J, Pastan I. Radioreceptor assay of adrenocorticotropic hormone: new approaches to assay of polypeptide hormones in plasma, *Science* 170:633, 1970.

104. Liburdy RP: Antibody induced fluorescence enhancement of an N-(3-pyrene) maleimide conjugate of rabbit antihuman immunoglobulin G, *J Immunol Methods* 28:233, 1979.

105. Lisi PJ et al: A fluorescence immunoassay for soluble antigens employing flow cytometric determinations, *Clin Chim Acta* 120:171, 1982.

106. Loriaux DL: Steroid radioimmunoassay. In *Hormone assay techniques,* 15th training course syllabus, Bethesda, Md, 1989, The Endocrine Society.

107. Lovgren T et al: Determination of hormones by time-resolved fluoroimmunoassay, *Talanta* 31:909, 1984.

108. Lovgren T et al: Time-resolved fluorimetry in immunoassay. In Collins WP, editor: *Alternative immunoassays,* New York, 1985, John Wiley & Sons.

109. Maggio ET, editor: *Enzyme-immunoassay,* Boca Raton, Fla, 1980, CRC Press.

110. Malvanop R, editor: *Immunoenzymatic assay techniques,* The Hague, 1980, Martinus Nijhoff.

111. Manasco P et al: A novel testis-stimulating factor in familial male precocious puberty, *N Engl J Med* 324:227, 1991.

112. Marchalonis JJ: An enzymatic method for the trace iodination of immunoglobulins and other proteins, *Biochem J* 113:299, 1969.

113. Masson PL, Holy HW: Immunoassay by particle counting. In Rose NR, Freidman H, Fahey JL, editors: *Manual of clinical laboratory technology,* ed 3, Washington, DC, 1986, American Society of Microbiology.

114. Masson PL et al: Particle-counting immunoassay (PACIA), *Methods Enzymol* 74:106, 1981.

115. McFarlane AS: Efficient trace labelling of proteins with iodine, *Nature* 182:53, 1958.

116. McKinney RM, Spellane JT: An approach to quantitation in rhodamine isothiocyanate labelling, *Ann N Y Acad Sci* 254:55, 1975.

117. Meurman OH et al: Time resolved fluoroimmunoassay: a new test for rubella antibodies, *J Clin Immunol* 15:920, 1982.

118. Midgley AR Jr: Radioimmunoassay for human follicle stimulating hormone, *J Clin Endocrinol Metab* 27:295, 1967.

119. Midgley AR Jr, Niswender GD, Rebar RW: Principles for the assessment of the reliability of radioimmunoassay methods (precision, accuracy, sensitivity, specificity), *Acta Endocrinol* 63(suppl 142):163, 1969.

120. Midgley AR Jr et al: Use of antibodies for characterization of gonadotropins and steroids, *Recent Prog Horm Res* 27:235, 1971.

121. Milby KH, Zare RN: Antibodies, lasers, and chromatography, *Int Clin Products Rev* 3:10, 1984.

122. Miyachi Y et al: Enzymatic iodination of gonadotropins, *J Clin Endocrinol Metab* 34:23, 1972.

123. Monroe D: Enzyme immunoassay, *Anal Chem* 56:920A, 1984.

124. Monroe D: Amperometric immunoassay, *Crit Rev Clin Lab Sci* 28:1, 1990.

125. Moore PH Jr, Axelrod LR: A solid phase radioimmunoassay for estrogen by estradiol-17β antibody covalently bound to a water insoluble synthetic polymer (Enzacryl AA), *Steroids* 20:199, 1972.

126. Murphy BEP: Some studies of the protein-binding of steroids and their applications to routine micro and ultramicro measurement of various steroids in body fluids by competitive-protein binding, *J Clin Endocrinol Metab* 27:973, 1967.

127. Nabarro JDN: Radioimmunoassay and saturation analysis, *Br Med Bull* 30:1, 1974.

128. Neurath AR, Strick F: Enzyme linked fluorescence immunoassays using β-galactosidase and antibodies covalently bound to polystyrene plates, *J Virol Methods* 3:155, 1981.

129. Newton WT, Donati RM: *Radioassay in clinical medicine,* Springfield, Ill, 1974, Charles C Thomas.

130. Ngo TT, editor: *Electrochemical sensors in immunological analysis,* New York, 1987, Plenum Press.

131. Ngo TT, Lenhoff HM: New approach to heterogeneous enzyme immunoassay using tagged enzyme-ligand conjugates, *Biochem Biophys Res Commun* 99:496, 1981.

132. Ngo TT, Lenhoff HM, editors: *Enzyme-mediated immunoassay,* New York, 1985, Plenum Press.

133. Ngo TT et al: Homogeneous substrate-labelled fluorescent immunoassay for IgG in human serum, *J Immunol Methods* 42:93, 1981.

134. Nielsen ST et al: The electrolytic preparation of bioactive radioiodinated parathyroid hormone of high specific activity, *Anal Biochem* 92:67, 1979.

135. Nilsson B: Enzyme linked immunosorbent assays, *Curr Opin Immunol* 2:898, 1990.

136. Odell WD et al: Radioimmunoassay for human gastrin as an antigen, *J Clin Endocrinol Metab* 78:1840-1842, 1968.

137. Oellerich M: Enzyme immunoassays in clinical chemistry: present status and trends, *J Clin Chem Clin Biochem* 18:197, 1980.

138. Oellerich M: Enzyme immunoassay: a review, *J Clin Chem Clin Biochem* 22:895, 1984.

139. Oellerich M, Haindl H, Haeckel R: Evaluation of enzyme immunoassays (EMIT and ENZYMUN) for detection of thyroxine and of